THE
MERCK
VETERINARY
MANUAL

THE MERCK VETERINARY MANUAL is dedicated to
the Doctor of Veterinary Medicine and
to his colleagues and associates
in the animal sciences.

THE
MERCK
VETERINARY
MANUAL

A HANDBOOK OF DIAGNOSIS
AND THERAPY FOR THE VETERINARIAN

FOURTH EDITION

EDITORIAL BOARD
O. H. Siegmund, *Editor*
C. M. Fraser, *Associate Editor*

J. Archibald
D. C. Blood
J. A. Henderson
D. G. Howell
R. L. Kitchell

Assistant to the Editors
L. Soffer

Published by
MERCK & CO., INC.
RAHWAY, N.J., U.S.A.
1973

MERCK & CO., INC.
Rahway, New Jersey, U.S.A.

MERCK SHARP & DOHME
West Point, Pa.

MERCK SHARP & DOHME INTERNATIONAL
Rahway, N.J.

MERCK CHEMICAL DIVISION
Rahway, N.J.

MERCK SHARP & DOHME RESEARCH LABORATORIES
Rahway, N.J./West Point, Pa.

BALTIMORE AIRCOIL COMPANY, INC.
Baltimore, Md.

CALGON CORPORATION
Pittsburgh, Pa.

CALGON CONSUMER PRODUCTS COMPANY, INC.
Pittsburgh, Pa.

KELCO COMPANY
San Diego, Calif.

HUBBARD FARMS, INC.
Walpole, N.H.

Library of Congress
Catalog Card Number
61–12679

First Printing—June 1973
Second Printing—December 1973
Third Printing—October 1974

SBN 911910–51–4
US ISSN 0076–6542

FOREWORD

The Third Edition of The Merck Veterinary Manual, now out of print, may be the most widely distributed single professional title among veterinary publications in English. Such acceptance brings with it not only great satisfaction, but even greater responsibilities. The editors are keenly aware of this and believe that they can make no better response than to continue to follow closely the objectives set down 20 years ago, when the philosophic basis for the first edition of The Merck Veterinary Manual was formulated: ". . . to provide the veterinarian with concise, authoritative, and readily available information on diagnosis and treatment of the diseases of animals kept by man for use or pleasure".

In this edition we have again used the general organizational scheme of the earlier editions. Important additions to several sections of the book have been made to reflect recent advances. Scarcely a page of the book has not been reworked to some extent; much of the text has been entirely rewritten. Our gratitude, as always, belongs to the nearly 300 authors and reviewers, who unselfishly gave of their skill, erudition and effort. Thanks are also due the many others who helped with the production of The Merck Veterinary Manual, most especially to Mrs. Gertrude Friese for contribution of a large extra measure of effort.

The Fourth Edition of The Merck Veterinary Manual comprises eight Parts. Part I, which is subdivided into 15 sections, deals with diseases of the common domestic animals, large and small. Conditions occurring in North America are emphasized —but because the risk of spread to once-distant places is greater than ever, and because the Manual is now read widely outside the North American continent, increased attention is given to diseases occurring elsewhere.

Part II, Toxicology, is a consideration of the commoner poisons. The current popular and regulatory concern with residues is reflected in the extensive revision of the chapters on pesticides and herbicides. The discussion of poisonous plants has been consolidated into one table, pertaining to the whole of temperate North America. An addition is the table of toxic fungi.

Part III, devoted to the diseases of poultry, has been extensively rewritten to reflect the improved knowledge of these diseases.

Part IV, dealing with management and diseases of fur, laboratory and zoo animals, has been almost completely rewritten. Special attention has been given to diseases of laboratory animals, as well as those of fish and caged birds.

Part V, entitled Nutrition, includes summary descriptions of accepted management and feeding practices as well as considerations of nutrition *per se* and of the important nutritional diseases.

The contents of the Addendum, Part VI, reflect the increasing importance to the veterinarian of such things as laboratory diagnosis and the study of animal behavior. The discussion of body temperature has been included with tabular lists of several other of the more commonly measured physiologic values.

Part VII contains the prescriptions used throughout the Manual. An attempt has been made to bring this list up to date. Whenever possible, generic names are used; when a proprietary name is given, information as to the nature and composition of the product is included. The prescriptions are numbered serially, and arranged, insofar as is possible, into groups having similar pharmacologic activity and clinical indications. Recommendations as to drug usage, either singly or in particular combinations, are those of the various authors. The mention of a specific remedy does not, of course, imply editorial endorsement of such preparations over others of similar or identical composition. In most cases, doses are given in metric measures; conversion tables are included in the four pages preceding the prescription section.

Part VIII is the index. Liberal cross-references provide several routes of access to important subjects. Completeness of coverage and convenience for the reader were the sole objectives in preparing this part.

Efforts have been made to assure accuracy of the scientific names used. In most cases the Seventh Edition of Bergey's Manual of Determinative Bacteriology has been used as the authority for microbial names. In a few instances our authors have recommended newer nomenclature. Organisms likely to be known better by older names (or by other names in other parts of the world) are identified by these in parentheses after the newer ones.

A Guide for Readers is presented on the next page to help the user of this book consult it more effectively.

O. H. Siegmund, Editor
Merck Sharp & Dohme Research Laboratories
Rahway, New Jersey

GUIDE FOR READERS

1. The Table of Contents on p. xiii shows the title of each section of the Manual, and corresponding Thumb Index abbreviation.

2. A list of chapter titles, with subtitles where necessary, is given at the beginning of each section.

3. In most instances, the first statement following a chapter title is a brief definition of the condition to be discussed. In some sections there are no definitions, e.g., Nutrition.

4. Prescriptions are grouped in a separate section (Part VII) which follows the text of the book. Although grouped by action or indication, they are numbered serially and correspond with the numbers of the ℞ symbols in the text. Doses are given in metric quantities. Wherever possible, doses are stated in units per pound of body weight. Where this is not convenient, appropriate doses are given for each species.

5. A number of abbreviations and symbols are used routinely throughout the text. These are listed on p. viii.

6. In the text, the names of proprietary drugs are capitalized; those in the prescription section are shown within quotation marks.

7. Each page heading indicates the last chapter title to be discussed on that page.

8. A large number of tables appear throughout the book, summarizing important data in readily assimilable form. A list of these tables, titled by subject matter, appears on pp. ix to xii.

9. A useful miscellany of information is presented in Part VI, especially arranged for quick reference. This includes the Ready Reference Guides—Weights, Measures, Equivalents and Conversion Tables—on p. 1453.

ABBREVIATIONS AND SYMBOLS

āā	equal parts	mEq	milliequivalent(s)
b.i.d.	twice a day	mg	milligram(s)
BUN	blood urea nitrogen	mo	month(s)
C	centigrade (Celcius)	min	minute(s)
ca.	about	ml	milliliter(s)
cal	calorie(s)	mm	millimeter(s)
cm	centimeter(s)	N.B.	note well
CNS	central nervous system	NF	National Formulary
		NRC	National Research Council
cu	cubic		
DNA	deoxyribonucleic acid	oz	ounce(s)
		p./pp.	page/pages
ECG	electrocardiograph	ppm	part(s) per million
e.g.	for example	pt	pint(s)
EPG	eggs per gram	q.i.d.	four times daily
et seq.	and the following one(s)	q.s. ad	quantity sufficient to make
ex. pulv.	dried	qt	quart(s)
F	Fahrenheit	q.v.	which see
fl	fluid	r	roentgen
ft	foot, feet	RNA	ribonucleic acid
gal.	gallon(s)	rpm	revolutions per minute
gm	gram(s)		
Hgb	hemoglobin	sec	second(s)
i.e.	that is	Sm. An.	small animal(s)
IM	intramuscular(ly)	sp.	species (sing.)
in.	inch(es)	spp.	species (pl.)
IP	intraperitoneal(ly)	sq	square
IU	international unit(s)	subcut.	subcutaneous(ly)
ICU	international chick unit(s)	tbsp	tablespoon(s)
		TDN	total digestible nutrients
IV	intravenous(ly)		
Kcal	kilocalorie(s)	t.i.d.	three times a day
kg	kilogram(s)	tsp	teaspoon(s)
kVp	kilovolt peak	u	unit(s)
L	liter(s)	USP	United States Pharmacopeia
lb	pound(s)		
Lg. An.	large animals	viz.	namely
m	meter(s)	wk	week(s)
M	molar	wt	weight
mA/s	milliampere(s) per second	yr	year(s)
		°	degree(s)
mcg	microgram(s)	μ	micron(s)
ME	metabolizable energy	%	percent
		℞	take

TABLES

Title	*Page*

CONTENTS

PART I

PART I
ALLERGY

ALLERGY AND AUTOIMMUNITY

The Allergic Animal: The allergic animal is one that has become sensitized to a substance and which upon re-exposure to that substance produces an over-reaction to it with effects that are essentially detrimental to the animal's health. Clinical allergies have been most extensively reported in dogs, and also occur in cats, cattle, horses and other domestic animals. Reports of allergic reactions in sheep and pigs are rare but probably occur. Certain breeds of animals seem to have a greater predisposition to these conditions than others, e.g., terrier breeds, Dalmatians, Poodles and Channel Island breeds of cattle. Some families and certain individual animals are highly prone. Animals may exhibit allergic reactivity to a number of allergens, a fact important in diagnosis and prognosis.

The Immunologic Basis of Allergy and Autoimmunity: The terms allergy and **hypersensitivity** are currently used synonymously to denote a state of increased reactivity of an animal to a foreign substance that is harmless to other members of the species. Autoimmunity or autoallergy is the state in which the animal produces an immune response against components of its own tissues. Both allergy and autoimmunity have an immunologic basis and therefore are subject to most of the principles that govern the mammalian immune response. Thus when animals are first exposed to an allergenic substance, certain individuals produce antibodies or specialized lymphocytes that on later exposure to the allergen will interact with it and produce the allergic episode. When antibodies are involved in an allergic disease the reaction occurs soon after challenge with the allergen and in many instances is due to the release of substances such as histamine, serotonin and bradykinin that in turn produce edema, muscle contraction, etc. Such reactions are classified as immediate hypersensitivities. Delayed hypersensitivities are due to the interaction, in tissue, of specialized lymphocytes with the allergen and since the migration of these cells takes some time, hours and even days may elapse after allergen exposure, before signs of allergy appear. In veterinary medicine most of the clinical allergies described seem to be of the immediate type, e.g., respiratory and food allergies; mixed reactions are probably common, e.g., drug allergies; and a few instances of delayed allergies, e.g., contact dermatitis, have been reported.

The autoimmune or autoallergic diseases in animals are likewise due to the production of antibodies or specialized lymphocytes that react with the body's own tissues. It has been suggested that sequestration of certain tissues such as testes, eyes, thyroid and brain or the altered or cross-antigenicity of certain tissues may explain why the body reacts to its own components.

Allergens: Many agents have been implicated in allergic diseases of domestic animals. They are usually biologic in origin and are frequently proteins, e.g., pollens, plant proteins, meats, sera and biologic therapeutic agents. The animal's normal environment and management are important factors in determining the allergens to which it will be commonly exposed and to which it is likely to be allergic. Essentially, an antigenic substance has the potential of producing an allergic response in certain individuals, as have certain low molecular weight compounds such as nickel. Some of the agents commonly associated with allergies in the various body systems are noted below.

Generalized Allergic Reactions and Anaphylaxis: In an allergic animal the state of hypersensitivity is generalized throughout the body. Should the offending allergen reach the circulation, then a reaction will follow throughout the body tissues, predominating in certain "shock" organs, skin, respiratory and gastrointestinal tracts. Large doses of an allergen may be given parenterally and produce a state of profound shock. This happens experimentally in the traditional demonstration of anaphylaxis produced by injection of foreign serum; quite frequently after the parenteral administration of drugs (even in subtherapeutic doses); and infrequently due to the sting of insects. A general allergic reaction also occurs on those occasions when relatively large quantities of an allergen are absorbed rapidly from the gut, the skin, the respiratory tract, or other local site. The manifestations of an acute generalized allergic reaction in an animal depend to a great extent on the species of animal, the amount of the shocking allergen and the route of its administration. Generalized shock, complete collapse, apnea and rapid death are seen in a few very severe cases while in less severe instances the animal may show varying degrees of respiratory distress, cardiovascular irregularities, hypersalivation and lacrimation and skin involvement (pruritus and angioedematous plaques). In addition to these signs, the dog frequently vomits and scours; in the horse, colic is reported; and in cattle, piloerection and edema of the eyelids are commonly seen in a generalized allergic reaction. Mild signs of a generalized allergic reaction may pass unnoticed or the allergen may not be absorbed and produce only localized signs at the site of contact with the various body systems or individual organs as noted below.

Allergies of the Respiratory Tract and Conjunctiva: These allergies are seen frequently in dogs and cats and are described as hay fever or allergic rhinitis. Affected animals rub and scratch their eyes and nostrils and have seasonal attacks of sneezing, lacrimation, and conjunctival infection upon exposure to airborne allergens. Many of these allergies have a marked seasonal incidence due to the shedding of pollen while others are caused by allergens in the bedding or feed and are seen the year-round. Rhinitis and respiratory distress in horses and cattle have also been attributed to respiratory tract allergies. In these instances it is suspected that the animals are sensitive to pollens or allergens from the bedding and feedstuffs. In the horse and cow a single episode may be acute and severe, the animal exhibiting signs of acute respiratory distress, or these episodes may recur and the disease become chronic, e.g., heaves in horses.

Allergy of the Digestive Tract: Recently it has been shown that dogs and cats may be allergic to foods such as milk, animal meats, fish, poultry and various cereals. Shortly after ingestion these animals may vomit and show evidence of abdominal discomfort. Several hours later they void fluid or bloody feces. The absorption of small quantities of the food may cause the appearance of respiratory or cutaneous signs of allergy after a brief lag period. In both horses and cattle copious diarrhea, and in cattle rumen atony and laminitis, may follow the ingestion of an allergenic feed. In large animals the feedstuffs implicated have usually been cereal grains, and skin manifestations such as pruritus, urticaria and angioedema may be seen later in the episode.

Allergy of the Skin: Pruritus, sweating, piloerection, urticaria (hives), angioedema (edematous plaques) and even hemorrhage of the skin may be produced in animals after absorption of an allergen following inhalation, ingestion or absorption by any of the routes described above. Allergic dermatitis can also be produced in the skin at the site of local allergen administrations, e.g., insect bites. In addition to these, contact hypersensitivity has been described in dogs, cats and horses, usually due to prolonged contact with allergens that produce dermatitis at the site of contact. In dogs, pollens and other plant materials may produce allergic dermatitis on the feet or lower extremities, and dyes, mordants and materials used in the processing of carpets may also produce regional dermatitis. In horses, contact dermatitis has been reported in areas of the skin that come in contact with harness to which soaps or preservatives have been applied.

Allergy to Insects: The bites of many insects may produce an allergic response in addition to other damage. In dogs and cats, flea bites have produced acute and chronic allergic dermatitis. In these species the lesions caused by lice and mite infestation may, in part, be allergic in nature; fatal generalized allergic shock following bee sting has been reported.

In Australia, "Queensland itch," an allergic dermatitis, is caused by the bites of the sandfly *Culicoides robertsi*. Similar conditions are due to biting and sucking flies described in America and other parts of the world. In cattle, allergic dermatitis has been attributed to the bites of *Simulium* (black flies) and in both horses and cattle the rupture of *Hypoderma* larvae may produce a local reaction or the generalized manifestations of shock.

Allergy to Therapeutic Agents: Many therapeutic agents have been implicated in allergies in many species of animals. Vaccines, toxoids and antisera, antibiotics, corticosteroids, hormones, and insecticides as well as other drugs have been reported to cause allergies in domestic animals. These reactions are produced in some instances by the drug itself (and sometimes by very small doses); in others, by breakdown products; and in others by stabilizing agents such as carboxymethyl cellulose, which is widely used in the drug and food industries. These agents are administered by various routes and have produced local reactions at the site of injection; for example, in the eye from an ophthalmic ointment or in the lungs following aerosol exposure to an allergenic drug. Once absorbed they may produce a general allergic reaction or a response at a site distant from the point of administration.

Autoimmunity: In recent years autoimmune or autoallergic conditions have been described in animals where certain individuals produce an immune response to components of their own body tissues. In autoimmune hemolytic anemia of dogs (q.v., p. 21) antibodies are produced against erythrocytes resulting in their destruction and the concomitant signs of systemic disease, icterus and anemia. Systemic lupus erythematosus (SLE) has been described in dogs which produce a variety of autoantibodies including antinuclear antibodies. Hemolytic anemia is also associated with this disease and the presenting signs include epistaxis, anorexia, weakness, lameness and vomiting. In cattle, an autoallergic condition known as **milk allergy** is associated with undue distension of the udder with milk. Under these circumstances certain cows absorb **casein** and exhibit signs of urticaria and respiratory distress.

Diagnosis of Allergic Conditions: Since most of these reactions occur soon after challenge with the inciting agent, it is extremely important to obtain an accurate history of the events immediately preceding an allergic episode in an attempt to arrive at a diagnosis of allergy and to incriminate a specific allergen. Changes in season, normal routine or environment, or the administration of new food or a drug should be carefully investigated. A skin test using 0.1 ml of a dilute solution of the suspect allergen intradermally will produce a marked reaction in the skin of an allergic animal within 30 minutes and no reactivity in the normal animal. This method of diagnosis has only recently been used in animals, and it should be borne in mind that many animals have multiple allergies and appropriate controls should be included in testing. Provocative exposure to the allergen after a period of withdrawal, for example, food or a suspect environment may also prove useful in establishing a diagnosis. A limited number of laboratories are available for the investigation of serum for the presence of the autoantibodies of autoimmune conditions.

Therapy of Allergies and Hypersensitivities: Whenever possible it is advisable to remove the animal from any further exposure to the offending allergen. If the allergen is not known, it is desirable to place the animal in an area free of potential allergens, a clean cardboard box for a dog or a clean, loose-box-stall for a large animal. While definitive studies on the drugs used to treat allergies in animals are lacking, the indiscriminate use of therapeutic agents should be avoided lest one produce further allergies in the patient. In acute generalized allergic reactions, epinephrine may be given by injection (R 511). If the situation is life-threatening it may be given carefully by the IV route. A variety of antihistiminic preparations are the most frequent therapeutic agents used in allergies of animals (R 535, 536, 537, 538, 539). Their efficacy in these reactions, particularly in large animals, has still to be fully authenticated. Conservative symptomatic therapy may be initiated at the discretion of the attending veterinarian. In more chronic forms of allergy, including autoimmune disease, the administration of corticosteroids is indicated (R 145, 152, 154, 158). The allergic state may persist in an animal for a long time, even for its entire lifetime. The best way to prevent further episodes is to remove the animal, wherever possible, from further exposure to the allergen. In recent years successful hyposensitization of allergic dogs and cats has been claimed using various regimens of parenteral allergens.

PHOTOSENSITIZATION

A condition in which an animal is rendered hypersensitive to light by the presence of a photodynamic agent. It should be differentiated from sunburn in which the white or lightly pigmented skin of a normal animal becomes inflamed following overexposure to ultraviolet rays. In photosensitization, the active rays are those absorbed by the photosensitizing agent. They often extend into the visual spectrum and usually are quite harmless to the unsensitized animal. In sunburn, the development of lesions is delayed, while in photosensitization, lesions develop very rapidly. The condition is best known in sheep and cattle, but may occur in any animal. It is world-wide in distribution.

Etiology: Photosensitizing substances may be introduced into the body by ingestion or by injection, or become operative through faulty liver function or aberrant pigment metabolism.

Primary photosensitivity: This is caused by the ingestion of photosensitizing agents not normally present in the diet. The best known sources of such compounds are plants of the genus *Hypericum* (St. John's wort or Klamath weed) or *Fagopyrum esculentum* (buckwheat). A large number of other plants have been reported to cause photosensitization, and in the absence of evidence of liver dysfunction it is reasonable to postulate the presence of photosensitizing agents, even though the photoactive principles have not been isolated.

Species of *Trifolium, Medicago* (clovers and alfalfa), *Erodium* and *Brassica* have also been incriminated in serious outbreaks of photosensitization, e.g., "trefoil dermatitis" and "rape scald". Some of these plants are dangerous only at certain stages of growth, e.g., rape and other *Brassica* spp. usually cause trouble only when immature. The keratitis due to phenothiazine sulfoxide is another example of primary photosensitivity.

Hepatogenous photosensivity: This constitutes the most important group. In ruminants, liver dysfunction is by far the most frequent cause of photosensitization. The photosensitizing agent is normally absorbed from the alimentary tract and either detoxified by the liver or excreted in the bile. Anything which interferes with these processes results in the agent reaching the peripheral circulation and photosensitization occurs.

Phylloerythrin is one such substance. It is a porphyrin derived from chlorophyll in the alimentary tract of ruminants and some other animals. It has been incriminated as the photosensitizing agent in the following conditions: occlusion of the common bile duct, facial eczema (q.v., p. 9), a syndrome associated with hepatic pigmentation in Corriedale sheep, congenital photosensitivity of Southdown sheep, and poisoning by *Tribulus terrestris* (devil's thorn or puncture vine), *Lippia reh-*

manni, Lantana camara, Panicum miliaceum (broom corn millet), *Narthrecium ossifragum* (bog asphodel, believed to cause conditions known as "yellowses" and "alveld" in sheep), *Myoporum laetum* and copper.

Photosensitization has also been reported when liver damage or icterus have been caused by blockage of the common bile duct by hydatid cysts or liver fluke, in leptospiral infections and Rift Valley fever, in lupine mycotoxicosis, in poisoning by *Nolina texana* (bunchgrass), *Agave lecheguilla* (lechuguilla), *Holocalyx glaziovii, Kochia scoparia, Tetradymia* (horsebrush or rabbit-brush) species, the algae *Microcystis aeruginosa* (*toxica*), *M. flos-aquae* and *Anabaena flos-aquae,* phosphorus, aniline, carbon tetrachloride and phenanthridinium. It is likely that phylloerythrin is the photosensitizing agent in at least some of these.

Many of the plants which cause hepatogenous photosensitization are toxic only under certain conditions of growth or climate; e.g., "geeldikkop" in South Africa occurs in sheep which graze *Tribulus terrestris* after it has wilted. Prior to wilting the plant is regarded as good sheep fodder.

Aberrant pigment metabolism: In this type, e.g., congenital porphyria, the photosensitizing agents are pigments that are normally absent or present only in minute amounts in the body.

Clinical Findings: The lesions and signs of photosensitivity are the same regardless of its cause. Photosensitized animals show photophobia immediately when they are exposed to sunlight. They seek shade or, if this is not available, turn their backs to the sun. Lesions are confined to white, or lightly pigmented, exposed areas of skin. Erythema develops very rapidly and is followed by edema. If exposure to light is terminated at this stage, recovery occurs promptly. If exposure to light is continued, skin necrosis follows, and the severity of the lesions may be accentuated by trauma from rubbing and by infection. In sheep, the most commonly affected parts are the face and ears, which frequently become thickened and pendulous ("big head"). In cattle, any unpigmented areas may be affected including the tongue, but the teats and udder appear to be especially sensitive.

In St. John's wort poisoning, hypersensitivity to contact with cold water has been reported. Affected sheep may develop convulsions and drown in dips or rivers.

Phenothiazine frequently causes keratitis in cattle and occasionally this occurs also in sheep, pigs and birds. The condition is due to the presence of phenothiazine sulfoxide in the anterior chamber of the eye.

Depending on the cause of the particular condition, there may be lesions and signs other than those associated with the photosensitivity. Some of these are described under facial eczema and congenital porphyria.

Prophylaxis and Treatment: Control of photosensitization can be achieved by preventing access to the offending plants. This is true for both primary and hepatogenous photosensitization, but can prove very difficult in practice, especially when plants are toxic only during certain periods depending on climatic factors. Methods which have proved effective are grazing on plants known to be safe or confining stock to small areas and feeding them hay. The former procedure may involve the growing of special crops for grazing during dangerous periods. In facial eczema, fungicides have proved effective in controlling the saprophytic fungi, and management practices designed to reduce litter may prove of value. Keratitis following the administration of phenothiazine should be prevented by treating the animals in the afternoon and keeping them in the shade during the following day.

In all except primary photosensitivities, the treatment of skin lesions is symptomatic. Attempts should be made to determine the site and cause of primary lesions; however, the stress imposed by photosensitization contributes to the cause of death and symptomatic therapy is helpful.

While photosensitivity remains, animals should be housed or given adequate shade. The topical application of "sun screens" may be useful to prevent further photosensitization (℞ 487, 503). Corticosteroids, given parenterally, may prove valuable. If the skin becomes infected, sulfanilamide powder in oil may be applied to the areas. In the case of sheep, fly-strike should be prevented.

When photosensitivity has ceased, the skin heals remarkably well, even after extensive necrosis. Yet the prognosis and the eventual usefulness of an animal will be governed by the site and severity of the primary lesions. After most toxic liver injuries, adequate regeneration takes place and normal function is restored.

FACIAL ECZEMA
(Pithomycotoxicosis)

A photosensitization of sheep and cattle arising from liver damage caused by the ingestion of toxic spores of the saprophytic mold *Pithomyces chartarum,* which grows on dead litter in pastures. It is, therefore, a mycotoxic disease and its common name is an unfortunate misnomer.

The disease occurs in New Zealand, Australia, South Africa and probably in North America. Weather conditions which result in warm ground temperatures and high humidity are required for prolific growth of this mold. Outbreaks of the disease are confined to hot periods of summer and early autumn. There may be several toxic periods in one season, separated by intervals when the pastures are safe. By following weather conditions and by estimation of spore numbers on pastures, toxic periods can be predicted and farmers warned.

A highly toxic compound, sporidesmin, has been isolated from cultures of the mold and from spores collected from toxic pastures. When sporidesmin is given orally to sheep or cattle at the rate of 0.5 to 1.0 mg/kg of body wt, it produces typical liver lesions and photosensitization. Rabbits, guinea pigs, rats, mice and chickens are also susceptible to the toxicosis.

Clinical Findings: The primary lesions in sheep and cattle are confined to the liver, gallbladder, bile ducts and the urinary bladder. At an early stage, there is inflammation, edema and necrosis of epithelium. Later, fibroblastic repair results in partial or complete obliteration of bile ducts by scar tissue, and 10 to 14 days after the toxic period, both obstructive jaundice and the secondary lesions of photosensitization occur. Livers become firm and fibrous with increased bile duct proliferation around the portal tracts.

Many photosensitized animals die of liver injury and stress 3 to 4 weeks after the toxic period. Others recover slowly, the skin lesions heal and there is nodular regeneration of the liver, which remains misshapen. Some animals that recover may lose condition or die if exposed to stresses such as pregnancy and lactation.

Animals with milder cases often exhibit no icterus or photosensitization, but they have patchy, pale, fibrosed areas in the liver, particularly in the left lobe. (For treatment *see* p. 9.)

Prevention: The application of benzimidazole fungicides to pastures considerably restricts the buildup of *P. chartarum* spores and so reduces pasture toxicity. Control recommendations specify the spraying of pastures in mid-summer with a suspension of thiabendazole (B 359). An area calculated at 1 acre per 15 cows or 100 sheep should be sprayed and animals admitted and maintained on the sprayed areas only when predicted danger periods of fungal activity are current. The fungicide is effective within 4 days after spraying provided that no more than 1 in. of rain falls within 24 hours during the 4-day period. After this time heavy rainfall does little to reduce the effectiveness of spraying since the thiabendazole becomes incorporated within the plants. Pastures will then remain safe for about 6 weeks. After this period spraying should be repeated to ensure protection over the whole of the dangerous season.

CONGENITAL PHOTOSENSITIZATION IN SOUTHDOWN SHEEP

A heritable defect in the hepatic uptake of certain organic anions leading to photosensitization from the accumulation of excessive quantities of phylloerythrin in the peripheral circulation. It appears to be inherited as a simple recessive. Affected lambs become photosensitive as soon as they commence to graze green plants, and the progressive skin injury usually leads to death within a few weeks because pain and stress interfere with eating. If chlorophyll is excluded from the diet or if affected lambs are not exposed to sunlight, they grow normally, and several generations have been bred by allowing affected sheep to graze only at night and protecting them from the light during the day. Icterus is rarely seen, but bilirubinemia can usually be detected. No histologic lesions can be seen in the liver, but hepatic function tests indicate delays in plasma clearance of bilirubin, sodium cholate and injected test dyes. Elimination of carriers of the heritable factor, therefore, is the only control feasible.

CONGENITAL PORPHYRIA ERYTHROPOIETICA
(Porphyrinuria, Pink tooth)

A rare hereditary disease of cattle, swine, cats and man in which defective hemoglobin metabolism results in the production of excessive quantities of Type I porphyrins in the nuclei of developing normoblasts.

The defect in cattle is inherited as a simple recessive factor and usually confined to herds where inbreeding or close line breeding is practiced. The disease has been recognized in the U.S.A., Canada, Denmark, Jamaica, England, South Africa and Argentina.

The heterozygous animal appears as a normal individual, but the homozygous recessive animal is affected at birth and shows reddish-brown discoloration of the teeth, bones and urine. The urine contains excessive quantities of coproporphyrin I and uroporphyrin I, while the discoloration of teeth and bones is due primarily to uroporphyrin I. Bones, urine and teeth (especially the deciduous teeth) exhibit a marked red fluorescence when irradiated with near-ultraviolet light. Prolonged exposure to sunlight causes typical lesions of photosensitization with superficial necrosis of unpigmented portions of the skin. A hemolytic anemia develops that is characterized by normochromicity with macrocytes and microcytes and marked basophilic stippling. Splenomegaly eventually develops and the bones show increased fragility due to a diminished cortex. The animal becomes progressively unthrifty and may die unless protected from the sunlight.

The defect in swine and cats is extremely rare and differs in some respects from that in cattle. Photosensitization is not a feature and the disease is transmitted as an autosomal dominant trait. The disease in swine has been reported only from Denmark and New Zealand; in cats it has been recognized only in the U.S.A.

Diagnosis should be based on the excretion of abnormal uroporphyrins and on the brown discoloration of the teeth which display red-orange fluorescence when irradiated with near-ultraviolet light. Affected animals and their heterozygous sires and dams should be excluded from the breeding program.

BLOOD, LYMPHATIC AND CARDIOVASCULAR SYSTEMS

ANEMIA

A condition of the blood characterized clinically by a reduction in circulating erythrocytes or hemoglobin or both. The anemic condition reflects either (1) a decreased production of red cells or hemoglobin, or (2) an increased destruction of red cells. The **reticulocyte count** is the single most informative laboratory test to determine which of the 2 errors is primarily responsible: a marked, sustained reticulocytosis that is not accompanied by a rise either in hemoglobin and packed cell volume (PCV) is indicative of increased red cell destruction; alternatively, absence of reticulocytes indicates an inadequate red cell production. The following classification of the anemias provides a basis for diagnosis and treatment of this condition.

I. Anemias of Bone Marrow Hypofunction
   A. Anemias due to reduction in red cell production
      1. Nutritional anemia; Deficiency of vitamin B_{12}, folic acid and protein
      2. Injury to marrow stem cells, Hypoplastic and aplastic anemia
      3. Marrow displacement by abnormal cells, Myelophthisic anemia
   B. Anemias Due to Reduction in Hemoglobin Synthesis
      1. Deficient heme synthesis, Deficient iron, vitamin E or B_6
      2. Deficient globin synthesis
II. Anemias of Increased Red Cell Loss—Possible Causes
   A. Hemolytic anemia due to genetically defective red cells
   B. Red cells with abnormal shapes
   C. Red cells with abnormal hemoglobins
      (*These 3 types (above) apparently are unimportant in the common domestic animals, and are not discussed in the Manual.*)
   D. Red cells with abnormal enzyme content
      1. Heinz body anemia (G6PD deficiency)
      2. Pyruvate kinase deficiency in Basenji dogs
   E. Hemolytic anemia due to acquired defects of red cells
      1. Globulin sensitization of red cells (Coomb's positive anemia) due to adsorption of drugs or virus to the red cells
      2. Isoimmune hemolytic anemia
      3. Idiopathic autoimmune hemolytic anemia
   F. Hemolytic anemia due to mechanical damage to red cells
      1. Vasculitis, disseminated intravascular coagulation with microangiopathic hemolytic anemia

III. Anemias Due to Loss or Hemolysis of Normal Red Cells
  A. Hemolysis of normal red cells
    1. Due to increased reticuloendothelial removal, splenomegaly
    2. Due to red cell parasitism
    3. Due to action of bacterial, plant, chemical or physical agents
  B. Loss of normal red cells
    1. External hemorrhage or external parasitism
    2. Internal hemorrhage or internal parasitism

The degree of anemia is determined by the levels of hemoglobin (Hgb), packed cell volume (PCV) and red cell count (RBC). The characterization of the anemia is aided by the calculated red cell indices, mean corpuscular volume (MCV), mean corpuscular hemoglobin (MCH) and mean corpuscular hemoglobin concentration (MCHC). The clinician will seldom use all of these parameters, but their determination may be very useful both in diagnosis and assessment of therapy. As the rubricytes mature in the marrow their mean volume decreases and their mean hemoglobin content increases. A highly responsive marrow will release macroreticulocytes or large polychromatic red cells which have bypassed one or more divisions and thus have a higher than normal cell volume. Thus in an anemia in remission, there is usually an upward shift in the MCV as these large cells accumulate in the peripheral blood. They mature to normal color or lose their polychromatophilic (RNA) staining after 2½ days in the peripheral blood. Reticulocytes or polychromatophilic red cells produced under normal circumstances become normochromic after one day in circulation. These large reticulocytes are an index of erythropoietin stimulation and their detection is an important observation. They are 1½ to 2 times the normal red cell diameter and are called "shift red cells". A polychromatic red cell is one with basophilic staining by Wright's or similar stain. A reticulocyte is a red cell with an RNA reticulum demonstrated with a wet-mount preparation stained with new methylene blue or similar stain. Thus polychromatic red cell and reticulocyte are usually synonymous, but because the wet-mount preparation is more sensitive there are usually more reticulocytes than polychromatic cells in the same blood sample.

A very useful measurement of the marrow response in anemia can be determined from a **corrected reticulocyte count** or **index**. There are in most species, under normal conditions, about 1% of reticulocytes in the peripheral blood. Thus, if the PCV should drop to one-third of normal value, the same production of reticulocytes would be 3% of the peripheral red cells due to their reduced dilution with normal red cells. In addition, if this 3% is made up of shift red cells with a ½-day maturation time then the reticulocyte percentage must be divided by 2½ to account for their longer peripheral blood maturation time. Thus, what might at casual observation appear to be a mild reticulocytosis when fully corrected may indicate a hypofunctional marrow. A reticulocyte index of 3 or more times normal indicates a hyperplastic productive marrow and usually a hemolytic process which is releasing iron available for reutilization. A reticulocyte index of less than 2 times normal, with severe anemia, indicates an impaired marrow response, e.g.,

Reticulocyte Index =

$$\frac{\text{patient PCV, in \%}}{\text{normal PCV for species, in \%}} \times \frac{\text{reticulocyte count, in \%}}{\text{shift red cells, number present}}$$

Example calculations:

(a) $\frac{12}{36} \times \frac{25}{2.5} \simeq 3$ (indicates *hyperplastic* marrow)

(b) $\frac{12}{36} \times \frac{6}{2.0} = 1$ (indicates *hypoplastic* marrow)

Anemia may be masked by dehydration, which can be detected by determining the concentration of plasma proteins (PPC). The level of plasma proteins can be simply and rapidly determined from the refractive index. There is usually enough plasma above the packed cells in the microhematocrit tube for this test providing the plasma is clear. The normal ranges of red cell values for some domestic species are given below:

Animal	PCV %	Hgb gm/100 ml	RBC × 10⁶/cu mm	MCV ml × 10⁻¹²	MCHC %	PPC gm/100 ml
Horse (Light breeds)	30-50	11-19	7-12	34-58	31-37	6-8
Horse (Heavy breeds)	25-45	8-14	6-9	37-52	32-38	6-8
Ox	25-45	8-15	5-10	40-60	26-36	6-8
Sheep	25-50	9-16	8-16	25-50	30-38	6-7.5
Goat	20-37	8-14	8-18	18-34	30-40	6-7.5
Pig	32-50	10-16	5-8	50-68	30-35	6-8.5
Dog	37-55	12-18	5-9	60-77	30-35	6-7.5
Cat	27-45	8-15	5-10	40-55	30-35	6-7.5
Rabbit	35-45	9-15	5-7	60-68	31-35	5-7
Chicken	30-40	9-13	3	127	29	3-5
Turkey	39	11	2	203	29	3-5

Clinical Findings in Anemia: Certain signs are characteristic of anemia regardless of the cause or species. Generally, there is pallor of the mucous membranes, weakness, lethargy, loss of appetite, increased heart and respiratory rates and there may be a systolic murmur due to reduced blood viscosity. If the anemia is acute or hemorrhagic, or both, there may be hypotension and shock. Care should be exercised in the handling and examination of the anemic animal as excitement may cause collapse.

ANEMIAS OF BONE MARROW HYPOFUNCTION

DECREASED RED CELL PRODUCTION

NUTRITIONAL ANEMIA

This category includes those factors whose deficiency leads to a reduction in red cell production as distinguished from a reduction in hemoglobin synthesis. Vitamin B_{12} and folic acid are required for DNA synthesis and in the deficient animal there is a reduction in mitoses in the erythroid precursors and hence a reduction in red cell numbers. The disease in man is classically macrocytic and normochromic and is characterized by ineffective erythropoiesis or the production of abnormal cells that either are not released into the circulation or have a shortened peripheral lifespan, or both. No clear counterpart exists in animals; however, a general deficiency of cobalt and thus of B_{12} occurs with a mild reduction in blood volume but not a marked drop in hemoglobin. Naturally occurring folic acid deficiency anemia in animals has not been recognized, but altered hemopoiesis may result from low levels of folic acid, especially in animals with rapidly growing tumors. Anemia due to carbohydrate starvation is mild, while protein deficiency causes a more severe anemia with accompanying drop in blood volume. The effects appear to be nonspecific and due to general debility and reduced activity. Recovery is slow and plasma proteins appear to be replaced prior to increased erythrogenesis. Thus, there may be an increase in plasma volume and a worsening of the anemia for a time even after improved diets are given.

Decreased red cell production is the prime cause of the anemia of chronic disease although some increase in hemolysis is usually present. The reasons for this type of anemia are numerous and include toxemia of abscessation or uremia and inadequate nutrition. In chronic diffuse liver disease, there is inadequate detoxification of normal metabolites and altered amino acid supply. These changes often result in the appearance of "target" red cells in the peripheral blood.

INJURY TO MARROW STEM CELLS
(Hypoplastic and aplastic anemia)

In hypoplastic and aplastic anemias, the shortage of red cells is not as critical as the lack of platelets and neutrophils.

Death is usually rapid, occurring in 10 to 14 days if there is aplasia due to hemorrhage and sepsis. Rarely there is a pure red cell aplasia in which granulocytes and platelets are maintained; in these cases, the animals survive longer and benefit from blood transfusions (q.v., p. 31).

Damage to marrow stem cells is usually an individual idiosyncrasy and related to drug or toxic exposure. Chloramphenicol and cyclic hydrocarbons will rarely cause marrow aplasia while body irradiation in the 200- to 500-r range will regularly cause aplasia. Bracken fern poisoning (q.v., p. 977), in cattle especially, will cause a herd outbreak of marrow aplasia. The virus of panleukopenia (q.v., p. 320) causes aplasia and pancytopenia in Felidae, but again, death is due to agranulocytosis and thrombocytopenia. Most cases of aplastic anemia are idiopathic. The disease should be confirmed by bone marrow aspiration biopsy and treatment given. This consists of a corticosteroid, such as prednisolone (Ŗ 152), methyltestosterone (Ŗ 177), and antibiotics.

MARROW DISPLACEMENT BY ABNORMAL CELLS
(Myelophthisic anemia)

Rarely an animal with chronic infection will develop myelofibrosis in which the specialized cells of the marrow are displaced by connective tissue. Much more common is the invasion of marrow by lymphoid tumors and less often by other types of tumors, either myelogenous in origin or metastatic sarcomas and carcinomas. In any case, the appearance of nucleated red cells in the peripheral blood, especially if the anemia is mild or absent, should alert the clinician that these cells may be displaced by tumor growth in the marrow cavity. A further search should then be made for tumor cells either in peripheral blood or bone marrow biopsy.

ANEMIAS OF DECREASED HEMOGLOBIN PRODUCTION
(Bone marrow hypofunction)

DEFICIENT HEME SYNTHESIS
(Deficiency of iron, vitamin E or vitamin B_6)

These are deficiency-induced reductions in heme and therefore of hemoglobin synthesis as distinguished from the macrocytic anemias of reduced cellular multiplication. The result is a microcytic hypochromic anemia. The most important cause is iron deficiency.

Copper deficiency may be absolute or molybdenum-conditioned (q.v., p. 1322). Copper is required to recharge the ferroxidase enzyme system and deficiency thus blocks iron utilization and results in an iron deficiency anemia which is again hypochromic and microcytic. In absolute iron deficiency there will be no hemosiderin in bone marrow. In copper deficiency anemias there will be adequate or abundant marrow hemosiderin but a low serum iron. Cobalt and copper are usually added to feeds via a salt block or supplement. All suckling animals are iron-deficient for a time, but only in swine is this deficiency regularly critical. Baby pigs should be given iron either parenterally (R 501) or orally (R 502) during the first week of life. Care should be exercised before iron is administered by either route to insure that the pigs are not vitamin E-deficient; any history of such deficiency (q.v., p. 581) in the herd, or previous evidence of iron toxicity is reason to delay iron administration until at least 24 hours after the administration of vitamin E. A persistent anemia in young pigs that has not responded to previous iron administration should invoke the same precaution. Vitamin E is required for the synthesis of heme and normally there is a large pool of heme present which scavenges any free iron which may result from oral or parenteral administration. Low levels of vitamin E, and therefore heme, allow free iron to circulate, which results in peroxidation of cellular membranes and necrosis, particularly in the heart, liver and skeletal muscle.

Vitamin B_6 or pyridoxine deficiency causes anemia but the condition is not recognized clinically and is presumed to be rare.

DEFICIENT GLOBIN SYNTHESIS

The synthesis of the alpha and beta chains of globin which combine with heme to form hemoglobin are under genetic control. In animals, a globin deficiency has not been recognized, but anemia in the sheep causes a "switching" to alternate globin chains that form hemoglobin "C". This hemoglobin C releases oxygen more readily to the tissues than the normal hemoglobin, A or B; in this respect it is similar to fetal hemoglobin. This "switching" thus appears to be a protective mechanism which permits more efficient oxygen transport at low hemoglobin levels.

ANEMIAS OF INCREASED RED CELL LOSS

RED CELLS WITH ABNORMAL ENZYME CONTENT

Glucose 6-phosphate dehydrogenase (G6PD) deficiency: This enzyme is part of an intererythrocytic metabolic chain that protects hemoglobin from oxidative denaturation. In the deficient cells, oxidants cause globin precipitation resulting in the formation of "Heinz bodies" and rapid cell lysis. Old red cells with a lower G6PD level are more susceptible to oxidation denaturation than are young red cells. Thus exposure to an oxidant drug such as phenothiazine, phenylhydrazine or primaquine causes selective hemolysis of the more senescent red cells. In man low G6PD levels are genetically transmitted deficiencies, while in animals the susceptibility to oxidant drugs occurs mainly in debilitated animals. Usually no treatment is required as the young population of red cells is spared. Blood transfusions should be considered if the PCV drops below 25%. The marrow is usually functional and spontaneous recovery rapid. A similar condition has been observed when test dogs were fed large quantities of onions, and the anemias associated with feeding rape, kale or turnips to herbivores also have a Heinz body pathogenesis. G6PD or Heinz-body anemia can be diagnosed by incubating 0.1 ml of heparinized blood in 100 mg% of acetylphenylhydrazine in 2 ml of buffer for 2 hours at 37°C. Test and control red cells are then stained with new methylene blue and examined microscopically for Heinz-body formation. Normal red cells should contain few Heinz bodies and G6PD-deficient red cells many.

Pyruvate kinase deficiency in Basenji dogs is a genetically transmitted deficiency of the red cells similar to that reported in man.

Hemolytic Anemia Due to Acquired Defects of Red Cells

GLOBULIN SENSITIZATION OF RED CELLS
(Coombs' positive anemia)

Red cells may become the target of antibodies which coat their surfaces and cause them to be removed from circulation by the reticuloendothelial (RE) system. This condition can be diagnosed with reagent antisera specific to the globulin of the species tested. Globulin-coated red cells are precipitated rapidly from suspension by specific combination of the reagent antiglobulin with the globulin on their cell membranes thus constituting a positive Coombs' or antiglobulin test.

The adsorption of drugs, particularly penicillin, to red cells will rarely induce an immune hemolysis in man, but is not known to occur in animals. The adsorption of virus to the red cells may cause a hemolytic crisis during recovery from an otherwise relatively mild disease.

Isoimmune hemolytic anemia (q.v., p. 36 et seq.) occurs naturally in the horse and possibly in the dog and the pig.

Idiopathic autoimmune anemia or autoimmune hemolytic anemia (AIHA) occurs in the dog and is qualitatively similar to the disease in man. The disease is called idiopathic until an inciting antigen, likely adsorbed to the red cells, can be identified. AIHA occurs in the dog as part of the uncommon syndrome of canine systemic lupus erythematosus along with thrombocytopenia and rheumatoid arthritis. The latter disease is believed to be virus-induced. The usual form of AIHA, i.e., unassociated with lupus, is not rare and is characterized by hemolytic crises with a very low PCV (<10%), a marked reticulocytosis, and spherocytosis, frequently with a positive direct Coombs' test.

In chronic cases, icterus will be marked due to ischemic hepatic damage. If blood transfusions are to be given at all, they should be given only with great caution and after matching. Prednisone in high doses of 50 to 100 mg daily for 2 to 3 days will usually result in a marked rise in the PCV and improved color and condition in the dog. The dosage of steroid should be decreased to half, or less, of the initial dose in 2 to 3 days and then to a maintenance dose of 5 to 10 mg daily which should be maintained for 6 weeks. Steroids may be required at high levels for 3 weeks to induce a rise in PCV. Splenectomy is rarely required if steroid therapy is properly administered.

Most therapeutic failures result from steroid therapy being discontinued too soon after remission begins. Should a hemolytic crisis occur after a steroid-induced remission, even higher levels of steroid may be required to again bring the hemolysis under control. Dogs may develop signs resembling those of Cushing's disease during treatment of AIHA but return to normal as the treatment is decreased. Hematinics are usually not required, and iron should not be given.

The adsorption of the agent of equine infectious anemia (q.v., p. 254) to the horse red cell has been shown to result in a similar pathogenesis in this anemia. Idiopathic AIHA probably occurs in species other than the dog. The common association of anemia with lymphoid tumors in many species is now believed to have an autoimmune basis.

HEMOLYTIC ANEMIA DUE TO MECHANICAL DAMAGE TO RED CELLS

Diseases which cause vasculitis necessarily activate the clotting mechanism and cause disseminated intravascular coagulation (DIC) of some degree. The passage of red cells at high velocity through damaged arterioles results in fragmentation of red cells as they impinge on intraluminal strands of fibrin.

The damaged cells are then removed by the RE system. This pathogenesis is referred to as a microangiopathic hemolytic anemia (MHA). It is characterized clinically by anemia with very marked poikilocytosis and reticulocytosis. MHA occurs in young calves with hemolytic uremic syndrome (HUS) where there is severe anemia, poikilocytosis, uremia, hemoglobinuria and collapse. The disease results from thrombotic lesions in the renal cortices and normally follows a rather mild upper respiratory or enteric infection by about a week. Treatment of HUS consists of IV heparin (0.5 mg/kg of body wt every 3 hours until hemoglobinuria clears), and blood transfusions. MHA to a mild or severe degree occurs as a part of the pathogenesis of many other anemias where there is vasculitis, e.g., EIA, malignant catarrhal fever, chronic hog cholera, and in thrombotic purpuras. Anemia with marked poikilocytosis may occur in some parasitic diseases, especially where there is extensive somatic migration as in *Strongyloides* infection. This may have a MHA-type pathogenesis. MHA occurs in cases of malignancy, especially if there are cavernous and necrotic areas of tumor as in hemangiosarcomas.

ANEMIA DUE TO LOSS OR HEMOLYSIS OF NORMAL RED CELLS

HEMOLYSIS OF NORMAL RED CELLS

Hemolysis Due to Increased Reticuloendothelial Removal, Splenomegaly and Hypersplenism: Any condition which causes an enlargement of the spleen will result in an increased erythrophagocytic activity in that organ. An enlarged spleen (splenomegaly) may occur as the result of an immunoproliferative reaction in the organ due to chronic infection, autoimmune disease, or splenic neoplasia. Diseases of the liver resulting in cirrhosis and portal hypertension will cause congestive splenomegaly. The stretching of the splenic reticulum in the enlarged spleen is a specific stimulus to increased phagocytic function. In addition, the enlarged spleen pools blood, and in these areas, low glucose, low cholesterol and high pH results in a premature aging or "conditioning" of the red cells, which causes them to become spherocytic and subject to phagocytic removal from circulation. Splenomegaly then, for hemodynamic reasons alone, progresses to hypersplenism (which is defined as an enlarged spleen of any cause with concurrent reduction in one or more of the cellular elements of the blood), marrow hyperplasia, and hopefully, to timely correction of the cytopenia by splenectomy. The clinical disease resulting from hypersplenism may therefore be a thrombocytopenic purpura or hemolytic anemia or neutropenia or any combination of these. If immune factors are added to the congestive pathogenesis, then the disease is more severe. There is some danger of thrombotic disease in the immediate postoperative period (1 to 2 days) due to loss of splenic control on thrombocytosis. This complication is reflected clinically by cold extremities, particularly of the tips of the ears and tail in dogs. If these signs are marked, heparin should be administered IV at 1 to 2 mg/kg body wt, repeated t.i.d. for 1 to 2 days or until signs of thrombosis subside.

Hemolytic Anemia Due to Red Cell Parasitism: Red cell parasitism may result in IV hemolysis of red cells with hemoglobinemia and hemoglobinuria as in babesiasis (q.v., p. 442). Alternatively, the parasites may be removed from the red cells by the spleen and the cells returned to the circulation, or the erythrocytes may be removed entirely and destroyed by the cells of the RE system. The latter pathogenesis occurs in hemobartonellosis of dogs and cats (*see* p. 324), anaplasmosis in cattle (p. 279) and sheep (p. 279), eperythrozoonsis (p. 310) and malarial merozoites in mammals and birds. Ehrlichiosis (q.v., p. 316) in horses, dogs and probably cattle causes anemia with hemorrhagic manifestations due to platelet and leukocyte infection with the causative organisms, and in thrombocytopenic purpura.

Trypanosomes are common in cow blood in North America but are generally nonpathogenic. Rarely, a dog that has returned from South America will develop an acute hemolytic anemia with marked reticulocytosis and the presence of trypanosomes in the blood. Dogs which have been in the Mediterranean area may become infected with *Leishmania* spp. by arthropod vectors. There is epistaxis, but only mild anemia, and biopsy of bone marrow, lymph node or spleen will demonstrate the *Leishmania* organisms in RE cells.

In general, the marrow is hyperplastic in anemias due to red cell parasitism and there is a marked peripheral blood reticulocytosis. If there is hemoglobinuria with iron and protein loss, then recovery will be slower. The marrow in ehrlichiosis is terminally hypoplastic. Diagnosis of the red cell parasitism is based on demonstrating the organism in the red cells; a wet mount and new methylene blue stain (q.v., p. 1382) is more efficient than examination of a dried-stained blood smear. Treatment and prevention must vary with the disease. The demonstration of *Hemobartonella* in an anemic cat without a marked reticulocytosis is cause to look for an RE neoplasm which has lowered normal immunity. A positive Coombs' test has been demonstrated in some of the anemias of red cell parasitism.

Lysis of Normal Red Cells Due to the Action of Bacterial, Plant, Chemical or Physical Agents: Bacteral hemolysins: (see LEPTOSPIROSIS, p. 347, and BACILLARY HEMOGLOBINURIA, p. 335).

Bartonella bacilliformis causes a generally fatal hemolytic anemia in man, dogs and rodents. The disease is most likely to occur in splenectomized dogs. The disease (Oroya fever) can be diagnosed by demonstration of the intraerythrocytic organisms on stained blood smears. Chloramphenicol given IV at 5 to 10 mg/lb daily for 3 to 5 days is the treatment of choice.

Plant hemolysins: Most of the plants that cause hemolytic anemia such as rape, kale, turnips and onions, do so because of depletion of the red cell enzyme glucose-6-phosphate dehydrogenase with Heinz-body production, and these are discussed above (p. 19) under RED CELLS WITH ABNORMAL ENZYME CONTENT. Direct lysis of the red cell membrane can be caused by saponin from the waxy cuticle of plants, or by ricin from castor beans. Hemolysins are the toxic principles in some spider and snake venoms.

Chemical hemolysins: A wide range of chemical compounds may produce hemolysis and, in addition, an aplastic anemia. The agents most commonly involved with this latter form of anemia are the cyclic hydrocarbons such as benzene, toluene, acetanilide and phenacetin. Heavy metals such as lead and silver inhibit hemoglobin synthesis and arsenicals can cause hemolysis. Phenylhydrazine produces Heinz bodies and hemolysis and is described above (p. 20). Anemias of these causes should be treated symptomatically pending specific toxicologic diagnosis. Lead poisoning produces only a mild anemia and the nervous signs are usually more prominent. The disease causes basophilic stippling of red cells, showers of peripheral blood rubricytes (especially in dogs), the urinary excretion of increased amounts of delta aminolevulinic acid and increased blood levels of lead.

Considerable quantities of copper may be accumulated gradually without apparent harm, but "chronic copper poisoning" results when any one of several "stresses" leads to a sudden release of stored copper which causes acute hemolytic anemia in sheep, pigs and cattle. In sheep, the source of the copper is usually phytogenous, leading to high copper levels in the liver which may then be released by hepatic injury of any cause, such as mild pyrrolizodine alkaloid poisoning (see SENECIO POISONING, p. 1003 on forced exercise. In pigs, copper may be included in rations as a growth stimulant. In marginally vitamin E-deficient pigs which develop hepatosis diaetetica (q.v., p. 581) sufficient hepatic necrosis and release of stored copper may occur to cause a hemolytic crisis and icterus.

Excess molybdenum, usually phytogenous in origin, will inhibit the intermediary metabolism of copper and cause lameness, depigmentation of skin, diarrhea and hypoplastic anemia which is microcytic and hypochromic and molybdenosis (q.v., p. 943). Removal of molybdenum or increased dietary copper is indicated.

Physical agents causing hemolysis: Intravascular hemolysis will follow full thickness skin burns and can be expected if more than 20% of skin is affected. The excessive ingestion of cold water, especially in calves, may cause vascular hemolysis, likely of osmotic origin, with anemia, dyspnea and hemoglobinuria.

LOSS OF NORMAL RED CELLS

Loss Due to External Hemorrhage or External Parasitism: External hemorrhage may occur from wounds, uterine prolapse and lacerations or surgical trauma, especially dehorning and castration. In acute hemorrhage there is hypovolemia and hypotension with a normal PCV. In chronic hemorrhage there will be a low PCV usually with marked reticulocytosis. In acute bleeding, blood transfusions are indicated (*see* p. 32) to replace blood volume and clotting factors. The marrow is usually responsive, and parenteral iron at 3.4 mg/gm of Hgb (estimated loss) and hematinics should be given. In anemias of chronic hemorrhage, transfusions are less likely to be required, especially if the animal is on its feet and bleeding has been stopped for 2 hours. Iron and hematinics should be given as above. Care should be taken in handling the anemic animal as stress may be fatal.

External parasitism may cause anemia, particularly in young animals. In general, bloodsucking insects such as Tabanidae, black flies and mosquitoes cause more irritation than blood loss. Calves occasionally become heavily infested with lice and become thin, weak and mildly to severely anemic. Kittens and puppies can become severely anemic due to a heavy louse infestation, and in endemic areas, bloodsucking ticks infect a wide variety of hosts. These anemias are primarily of blood loss and should be treated with hematinics (℞ 502) and application of insecticides (*see* TICK INFESTATION, p. 714). Cattle especially suffer marrow depression with heavy louse infestation, and recovery is slow.

Loss of Normal Red Cells Due to Internal Hemorrhage or Internal Parasitism: Internal hemorrhage may be acute or chronic and result from surgery, wounds, tumors or abscesses and enteric or urinary tract ulceration. Diagnosis is usually aided by aspiration of the chest, abdomen or subcutis. If generalized bleeding is present, blood should be drawn into a glass vial and the clotting time determined. Thrombocytopenia will cause purpura and poor clot retraction. If platelets are present in adequate numbers, as determined on a stained smear or by platelet count, then the prothrombin time should be determined. Prothrombin levels are low in warfarin or sweet clover poisoning (q.v., p. 990) and hepatic failure. Clotting agents that act to raise blood calcium are generally not efficient and calcium gluconate can be given as easily. If the bleeding has been mild but very prolonged, iron deficiency should be suspected and treated as described above.

Internal Parasitism: (q.v., p. 649 et seq.): Profound anemia may be caused in young dogs and cats by hookworm infection. In severe cases with collapse, blood transfusions should precede anthelmintic treatment. Iron loss in enteric parasitism is not reabsorbed and in chronic cases there may be better response to parenteral iron (℞ 501) than to an anthelmintic. The marrow is usually productive if iron stores are not exhausted, and there will be a marked peripheral blood reticulocytosis, occasionally with severe poikilocytosis. In sheep, acute haemonchosis may cause death due to anemia without debilitation. It should be noted that diarrhea will occur with most enteric parasitisms of the sheep except *Haemonchus*. In calves and yearling cattle, chronic *Ostertagia* infection will cause cachexia, an anemia with poor reticulocyte response and occasionally marked poikilocytosis. Iron may be given parenterally (℞ 501) if there is severe anemia or if serum iron is low.

POLYCYTHEMIA

An excess in the number of circulating erythrocytes per unit volume of blood.

Relative Polycythemia: This results from loss of the fluid parts of the blood. The condition is also called hemoconcentration or apparent erythrocytosis. It is a transient state produced by shock or dehydration following excessive sweating, continual vomiting, persistent diarrhea, or insufficient fluid intake. Insufficient water intake in weakened anemic animals and hemoconcentration (relative polycythemia) superimposed upon the anemia, may mask the true state of affairs with apparently normal erythrocyte, PCV and hemoglobin values.

Secondary Polycythemia: This is a compensatory increase of erythrocytes in conditions of inefficient oxygenation. Newborn mammals show this type of polycythemia temporarily. It is also observed in animals raised at high altitudes or trained for racing and in animals suffering from heart disease. Chemicals such as coal tar derivatives and carbon monoxide may cause temporary transient polycythemia, apparently by contraction of the spleen and release of stored erythrocytes.

Polycythemia Vera: This condition, also known as erythremia or true erythrocytosis, is marked by persistent polycythemia due to excessive formation of erythroblasts in the bone marrow and is accompanied by an increased blood volume and viscosity, an enlarged spleen and cyanosis. Although rare, the condition has been reported in dog and cow. Treatment in the various polycythemias can only be directed toward correction of the causative mechanisms. Phlebotomy is warranted only in polycythemia vera, to provide temporary relief.

CANINE THROMBOCYTOPENIC PURPURA (CTP)

Hemorrhagic disorders in dogs associated with severely reduced numbers of circulating platelets. Since platelets (thrombocytes) are essential to formation of the initial barrier in damaged vessel walls, widely dispersed petechiae and ecchymoses in the skin and mucous membranes are observed clinically.

Etiology: The symptomatic form of CTP occurs when iatrogenic or other known causes are involved. Certain cytotoxic chemicals, such as nitrogen mustard, busulfan, 6-mercaptopurine and cyclophosphamide will destroy platelet-producing megakaryocytes. Hypersensitivity of an individual dog to almost any drug or chemical agent can make it an antigen and result in CTP. Leukemia and aplastic anemia may also produce the disease. Infiltration of the bone marrow by leukemic cells may crowd out normal bone marrow elements, including megakaryocytes, and produce thrombocytopenia. In aplastic anemia, loss of normal marrow constituents often is not followed by replacement. Splenic enlargement due to a variety of causes, including granulomatous inflammation, neoplasia, infarction and generalized splenomegaly of uncertain cause, may be associated with CTP.

The idiopathic form of CTP can accompany certain autoimmune disorders, such as auto-immune hemolytic anemia and systemic lupus erythematosus. In these diseases dogs may develop auto-antibodies against several of their own tissues, including thrombocytes.

Clinical Findings: Petechiae and ecchymoses appear suddenly on visible skin and mucous surfaces. These may be accompanied by epistaxis, melena, hematuria, toenails that continue to bleed after clipping, and extensive bruising following routine clinical palpation. Pallor, weakness, rapid pulse and edema may occur in cases where there is severe anemia accompanying the thrombocytopenia.

Diagnosis: Direct platelet counts on fresh blood collected with EDTA can help assess the role of platelets in this hemorrhagic problem. Counts less than 100,000/cu mm are suggestive and less than 30,000 strongly suggestive of CTP. Other tests, including prolonged bleeding, whole-blood clotting, clot-retraction times and normal Lee-White coagulation and prothrombin times can be helpful in pinpointing this disorder. Positive direct Coombs' tests associated with auto-immune hemolytic anemia and positive LE preparations with systemic lupus erythematosus also support a diagnosis of idiopathic CTP.

Treatment: In dogs developing CTP after prolonged drug therapy or after short-term exposure to a new drug, an iatrogenic cause is a strong possibility; the suspected agent should be discontinued and the patient immediately given corticosteroids (e.g., prednisone, 0.5 to 1.0 mg/lb of body wt daily). Treatment of CTP that is associated with leukemia or aplastic anemia is most difficult, since control of the underlying cause is usually impossible. Remissions of idiopathic CTP can usually be achieved with corticosteroid therapy, but relapses often occur after variable periods. Prednisone is started at 1.0 mg/lb of body wt/day. If no improvement is seen within 24 hours, the dose is increased to the 1.5-mg level. If still no improvement is seen by the third day, the dose of prednisone can be halved and a splenectomy performed, provided the dog is not too anemic. Maintenance doses of prednisone (2.5 to 5 mg/dog daily) are established and given for 4 weeks following splenectomy. Whole-blood transfusions are reserved for emergency use to correct severe anemia secondary to blood loss. To replenish thrombocytes with transfusions, absolutely fresh blood is needed.

HEMOPHILIA AND OTHER HEMOSTATIC DISORDERS IN DOMESTIC ANIMALS

Defects in hemostasis may be inherited or acquired. Normal hemostasis requires normal vessel walls, proper levels of blood coagulation factors and adequate numbers of functioning platelets. Two hemophilias, A and B, are inherited as sex-linked traits and commonly carried by females and manifested clinically only in males, except when hemophiliac males are mated to carrier females. Other inherited conditions are carried as autosomal traits.

Several of the inherited defects in hemostasis which have been described in animals are: (1) Factor VII deficiency in Beagle hounds (stable factor, or proconvertin deficiency); (2) classical hemophilia or hemophilia A due to a deficiency of Factor VIII (antihemophiliac factors, AHF, AHG) in practically all breeds of dogs and in Standardbred and Thoroughbred horses; (3) Von Willebrand's disease in swine (similar to hemophilia A, but inherited autosomally and thought to be a defective control mechanism for Factor VIII production); (4) hemophilia B or Christmas disease, due to a deficiency of Factor IX (plasma thromboplastin component, PTC, Christmas factor) in Cairn Terriers and Black and Tan Coonhounds. Increased activity of the fibrinolytic system has also been recognized in dogs as a cause of excessive bleeding postoperatively or after trauma. Postoperative bleeding and poor wound healing may be related to a lack of fibrin-stabilizing factor (FSF, Factor XIII) but has not been described in animals.

Acquired disorders may result from a number of diverse causes which affect specific components in the hemostatic mechanism. Vessel wall damage with accompanying petechiation occurs in such conditions as equine purpura haemorrhagica (q.v., p. 39) or in vessel wall anoxias due to poor circulation or anemia. Certain coagulation factors in circulating blood may be depressed by agents in the feed, by drugs, or by various diseases, particularly those causing severe hepatic damage. Warfarin or dicoumarin (see SWEET CLOVER POISONING, p. 990) depresses production of prothrombin and Factors VII and X. Anaphylactic shock, incompatible transfusions, or bacterial endotoxins may cause adhesiveness and margination of platelets onto vessel walls and initiate IV clotting and thromboembolism. Amniotic fluid contains thromboplastin and possibly can be introduced into the maternal circulation during dystocias; this also can initiate generalized IV clotting. Since levels of circulating prothrombin and fibrinogen are normally marginal, they are further depleted by IV clotting and a bleeding tendency ensues.

Reduced platelets in the circulation (thrombocytopenia) can result from a number of causes (see CANINE THROMBOCYTOPENIC PURPURA, p. 27).

Thrombocytopathia and thrombasthenia are conditions in which platelet numbers may be normal but their function abnormal. Thrombocytopathia may be either congenital or acquired (hepatic cirrhosis, leukemia, uremia). The platelet phospholipid (Platelet Factor 3), essential for blood coagulation, is abnormal or is not released from the platelet. Thrombasthenia (Glanzmann's disease) has been reported in an intensively bred strain of Otter Hounds. It is manifested by hemorrhagic occurrences due to platelets that react poorly or not at all to normal stimuli of collagen ADP and thrombin. The defect occurs in both sexes and appears to be autosomal.

Diagnosis: Vessel wall: Defects in the vessel wall are diagnosed by prolonged bleeding times in the absence of other defects in the hemostatic mechanism, or obvious evidence of a ruptured aneurysm.

Platelet abnormality: A platelet count should be done on fresh whole blood collected with EDTA and not based on the observation of platelets in a stained smear. Whole-blood clotting time, clot reaction and other clotting tests are abnormally long when the platelet count drops below 10,000 per cu mm. Where platelets may be normal in number but abnormal in function, certain laboratory tests such as the response of platelets to adenosine diphosphate (ADP), thrombin and collagen are required. These and other tests mentioned in this chapter are not usually conducted by the practitioner but can be done in clinical laboratories.

Coagulation abnormalities: Prothrombin deficiencies (warfarin, dicoumarin poisoning) produce a prolonged one-stage prothrombin time (OSPT) and Russell Viper Venom Time (RVVT).

Factor VII deficiency produces a prolonged OSPT. Factor VIII and Factor IX deficiencies can be shown by the results of assay tests such as long whole-blood clotting time in glass and silicone, abnormal thromboplastin generation time (TGT) or partial thromboplastin test (PTT).

Acquired combined deficiencies of blood coagulation may be diagnosed by carrying out specific assays for coagulation factors. Such deficiencies are often associated with disseminated generalized IV coagulation occurring in some hypersensitivities, or resulting from scurvy or hepatic disease. Considerable liver damage must occur before coagulation tests are abnormal.

Since birds do not possess Factor XII (Hagerman factor) their clotting times of whole blood in glass and silicone tubes should be the same.

Treatment: In external bleeding one should use pressure bandages or applications of hemostatic sponge, topical thrombin or epinephrine. Transfusions of cross-matched blood should be used in marked blood loss and when signs of anemia occur. In thrombocytopenia or thrombocytopathy, platelet-rich plasma should be transfused. Such plasma is obtained from blood which has been slowly spun (600 to 800 rpm for 8 to 10 min.). In other coagulation disorders, platelet-poor plasma (blood spun at 3,000 rpm for 20 to 30 min.) may be used. Fresh plasma (not more than a week old) must be used in Factor VIII deficiency. Stored plasma or serum may be used but fresh plasma is preferable in Factor IX deficiency (hemophilia B) or Factor VII deficiency.

Vitamin K (R 554) is indicated in avitaminosis K, prothrombin-time abnormalities, Factor VII deficiency and hepatic disease, and is of limited value in Factor IX deficiency. Natural vitamin K should be used when the prothrombin lack is due to dicoumarin (warfarin). Ascorbic acid (vitamin C) should be used in purpuras or liver disease. ACTH (R 137) and steroids (R 148, 149, 154) are recommended in coagulation disorders, in thrombocytopenia and in areas where increased fibrinolysis is present. These products appear to assist in a nonspecific manner in capillary resistance and may increase the efficacy of transfused plasma given in acute bleedings of unexplained origin. Stilbestrol (R 163) may possibly increase capillary resistance but it may have a paradoxical effect in certain species such as dogs where bleeding has increased because the drug has produced a thrombocytopenia. Tolonium chloride (R 553) or protamine (R 551) can be used to neutralize heparin. Epsilon aminocaproic acid appears to influence excessive fibrinolysis and may be useful in coagulation defects caused by lack of stability of the platelet plug or excessive fibrinolytic activity.

BLOOD GROUPS AND BLOOD TRANSFUSION

"Blood groups" as used here refers to genetically transmitted antigenic components of red cell walls. Some of these groups are complex with many subgroups called factors, and the groups themselves are then referred to as blood-group systems. Each red cell antigen is controlled by a pair of allelic genes, one of which is derived from each parent. Since the progeny of any mating can thus bear only those blood factors that were in either or both of the parents, this forms the basis of parentage testing based on red cell antigens. An individual will not have (iso)antibodies against any of the factors present on its own red cells but may have or be capable of developing antibodies against factors present on red cells of other individuals of the same or different species. In some species (man, sheep, cow, cat, pig and horse), so-called "naturally occurring" isoantibodies may be present in variable but occasionally significant titers. Such isoantibodies are usually absent in the cat and dog or present in very low titers in the cow, and in these species an initial unmatched blood transfusion can be administered without serious risk. Only 20% of cats have naturally occurring isoagglutinins, and most isohemolysins in the dog are due to prior blood transfusions. With random blood transfusion in the dog, there is a 30% chance of isosensitization, and less than 10% of randomly chosen dogs have naturally occurring isoantibodies. In the horse, possibly in mink and very rarely in swine, transplacental immunization of the female may occur. Females of various species may inadvertently be isoimmunized by vaccination, e.g., viral enteritis antigen given to mink and anaplasmosis vaccine to cattle. The isoantibodies are globulins, usually of a gamma-G and -M type. They vary in their mode of action between species and against different factors within the same species, e.g., most blood antibodies (to red cell antigens) are agglutinins, but some are powerful hemolysins which fix complement (dog anti-A).

Blood-Typing Tests: The sera used to identify blood groups are called typing reagents. These reagents may be isoimmune if produced in other species. Most blood-typing tests are carried out as saline hemagglutination systems but in some species such as cattle where the red cells do not readily agglutinate, hemolysins are involved and complement is needed in the system. Other antibodies will act only in serum or are enhanced by the addition of serum to the test system. Additional techniques such as treatment of red cells with papain, ficin, trypsin or dextran may be required to demonstrate specific red cell antigens or serum antibodies. In these cases, the antibodies are termed "incomplete" as they will not cause red cell clumping in the usual saline hemagglutinating test. To detect an antibody on the red cell that does not cause its agglutination, a second antiserum is prepared (usually in rabbits) against the globulin of the species to be tested. This antiglobulin will then detect red cells that have an antibody bound to them. The procedure is called the Coombs' test and is the basis for the diagnosis of autoimmune hemolytic anemia.

The Blood-Group Systems of Some Domestic Species: The table summarizes present knowledge on blood groups in a number of species. In each case, the first character, a capital letter, is the name of the blood-group system. The figure immediately following, in parentheses, is the number of factors identified within each system. The genotypic alternatives exceed the number of factors because if only one factor is present per system, its presence or absence gives 2 alternatives.

SPECIES	SYSTEMS	FACTORS
Cow	13	A(6), B(37), C(11), F-V(4), J(2), L(1), M(2), N(1), N'(1), S(6), R-S(2), T'(1), Z(2).
	reagents are isohemolysins	
Sheep	7	A(1), B(11), C(2), D(1), M(3), RO(2), XZ(2).
	reagents are isoagglutinins and lysins	
Horse	8	A(6), C(1), D(2), F$_{r4}$(1), F$_{r5}$(1), F$_{r1}$(2), J(4), K(1).
	reagents are isoagglutinins and lysins	
Pig	16	A(2), B(2), C(1), D(1), E(8), F(2), G(2), H(3), I(2), J(1), K(5), L(11), M(4), N(3), O(2), S(1).
	reagents are iso- and heteroagglutinins	
Dog	7	A(2), B(1), C(1), D(1), E(1), F(1), G(1).
	reagents are isoagglutinins and lysins	
Cat	2	A(1), B(1).
	reagents are isoagglutinins	
Mink	5	A(3), C(1), D(1), E(1), G(1).
	reagents are isoagglutinins	

SPECIES	SYSTEMS	FACTORS
Rhesus Monkey	6	A(1), B(1), C(1), D(1), E(1), Rh.
	reagents are isoagglutinins and lysins	
Rat (Lewis & Wistar)	4	A(1), B(2), C-D(2), G(1).
	reagents are isoagglutinins	
Mouse (C57)	4	$H_1(1)$, $H_2(20)$, $H_3(1)$, $H_4(1)$.
	reagents are isoagglutinins	
Chicken (DeKalb)	12	A(7), B(21), C(1), D(1), E(9), H(2), I(2), J(2), K(2), L(2), N(1), P(2).

Applications of Blood-Group Typing: Blood-typing of bulls used in artificial breeding units is widely practiced throughout the world. This procedure protects the pedigree of registered stock by allowing a "Parentage Exclusion" test. Since the dam is usually known, all blood factors in the calf which differ from hers must have been derived from the bull in question. Similarly, twin calves frequently have placental fusion that results in a mixing of blood types. If the calves are of opposite sex, the hormonal as well as blood stem cell mixing usually results in a sterile or freemartin heifer and may, as well, cause sterility or reduced fertility in the male. An identical blood type indicates a 97% chance of placental fusion and sterility. The 3% discrepancy is the probability that calves of opposite sex would have inherited the same blood type. In a number of species, especially cattle and chickens, attempts to demonstrate that heritable traits in blood groups and serum proteins can be correlated with growth and production have been inconclusive.

Blood Transfusions: In general, in veterinary therapeutics, the indications for blood transfusion are acute and repeated transfusions are not often necessary. Consequently, an initial unmatched transfusion can be given without serious risk to most species except the horse. Serious reactions to repeated transfusions are likely to occur in cattle and to a lesser extent in dogs. Due to the diversity of blood groups in cattle, only an identical twin is a matched donor. For this reason, if blood is to be administered, an adequate volume should be given initially so that repeated transfusions are less likely to be required.

The amount of blood to be given should at least be roughly calculated and this is most accurately arrived at by considering the degree of anemia and normal blood volume based on body weight. For practical purposes, the young calf and Thoroughbred horse have 45 to 50 ml of blood per pound of body weight, dogs have 35 to 40 ml/lb, cows have 30 to 35 ml/lb, sheep, goats and heavy horses have 28 to 30 ml/lb and mature swine have 25 ml/lb. The "tilt test" in man is a useful rule of thumb to estimate blood loss, and extrapolation to animals suggests that if inducing the animal to stand causes a sustained increase in pulse rate of 30 per minute, there has been a 20 to 25% loss of blood volume or about 8 to 10 ml loss of blood per pound of body weight. In acute hemorrhage, there will be loss of blood volume and likely hypotension but no drop in packed cell volume (PCV) for several hours, until circulating cells are diluted by vascularization of interstitial fluid. In these cases, dextran infusion may be sufficient to prevent shock. Acute loss of ⅓ of the blood volume will cause shock, while a loss of ⅛ to ⅔ of the blood volume may be tolerated over a 24-hour period. If the bleeding has been a prolonged oozing of the latter type, such as may occur following dehorning or castration, then dextran will only further dilute a low PCV, and whole blood should be given. Species with a muscular contractile spleen, such as the horse and dog, will tend to mask the degree of blood loss in acute hemorrhage for 12 to 18 hours. Great care should be exercised in restraining the severely anemic animal as forced exertion may be fatal.

In chronic anemias, the decision to give blood should be based on the marrow response and on the PCV. An animal with a PCV of 15 and a hemoglobin of 5 gm need not be transfused if the drop in PCV was gradual and is arrested and if there is a strong peripheral reticulocytosis. Reticulocytes are not seen in the horse and evidence of increased marrow production should be based on an upward shift in the mean red cell volume, i.e., presence of significant numbers of larger young cells.

Blood for transfusion should be collected into a 2.5% solution of sodium citrate at the rate of 1 part anticoagulant to 4 to 9 parts of blood. The practitioner can easily make up collection bottles using 500-ml rubber-stoppered bottles containing 50 to 60 ml of anticoagulant solution. The bottles are autoclaved and the tops put on while the bottles are hot, which forms a vacuum on cooling. Commercial collection bottles containing anticoagulant solution should be used if the blood is not to be used immediately. There is a progressive loss of red cell enzyme in stored blood which reduces the ability of these cells to carry oxygen. Therefore, fresh blood is most desirable for general use. A transfusion of 7.5 ml of blood per pound of body weight will raise the red cell count by about 1 million red cells per cubic millimeter and the hemoglobin by nearly 3 gm%. All transfusions should be started very slowly for the first 50 to 100 ml to check for signs of reaction (which usually become apparent by respiratory distress). Epinephrine should be available should reaction occur.

Cross-matching of blood should always be carried out prior to blood transfusion in horses and in dogs where autoimmune hemolytic anemia is suspected. In the latter case, transfused cells likely will have a very shortened life-span and transfusion should only be considered if there is impending circulatory collapse. If typing is possible, canine blood for transfusions should always be collected from A-negative donors.

Technique of Cross-Matching: Tube test: 1. Collect anticoagulated blood and serum from donor and recipient. 2. Wash the red cells 3 times in 0.91% saline and prepare a 5 to 10% red cell suspension. 3. Place equal volumes (2 drops) of recipient's serum and donor's cells in a test tube and mix. Place donor's serum and recipient's cells in a second tube. Mix donor's serum and cells and recipient's serum and cells and place in separate tubes for controls. 4. Leave tubes 30 minutes at room temperature, then spin down cells for 1 minute at 500 to 1,000 rpm. 5. Examine tubes for hemolysis (slight hemolysis in dog cells is not specific). Shake tubes against finger to re-suspend cells, check for persistent red cell clumping or agglutination. Transfer a drop of blood to a slide and check microscopically for agglutination. Significant hemolysis or agglutination indicates incompatibility.

Slide test: The above procedure can be simplified by adding a drop of a 50% suspension of washed, donor red cells to a drop of recipient serum on a glass slide, mixing with a rocking motion and examination for agglutination.

These methods are adequate for detecting saline agglutinins but the antiglobulin test is required to detect incomplete antibodies.

HEMOLYTIC DISEASE OF NEWBORN FOALS
(Isoimmune hemolytic anemia, Equine neonatal isoerythrolysis)

Etiology: An acute anemia in which erythrocytes of newborn foals are agglutinated or hemolyzed by specific isoantibodies produced in their dams. Although such foals are normal at birth they can absorb dangerous levels of isoantibodies through their alimentary tract for up to 48 hours later if they obtain colostrum from their dams. Clinically recognizable neonatal isoerythrolysis rarely occurs in foals of primiparous mares and generally is not seen until a mare has had her third or fourth foal. Mares are isoimmunized naturally by focal placental breakdown allowing fetal-placental hemorrhage of incompatible foal blood into the maternal circulation. A fairly large fetal-placental hemorrhage may be required to initially isoimmunize a mare to a significant degree. Restimulation of the mare in subsequent pregnancies requires much less incompatible foal blood of the same type. Also, therapeutic agents such as blood transfusions and incompatible tissue vaccines may contribute to the problem. Neonatal isoerythrolysis can occur only when a foal and its sire possess a blood factor absent in the mare (often factor Q or A'). Certain stallions mated to such mares will always sire susceptible foals because they are genetically homozygous for the offending blood factor. Other stallions (heterozygotes) will sire such foals only part of the time. Although neonatal erythrolysis may occur in foals of any breed it is more frequently seen in Thoroughbreds and mules.

Clinical Findings: The severity of anemia varies considerably depending upon the amount and type of isoantibodies consumed. Hemolytic isoantibodies are the most damaging, and the highest titers exist in the first colostral milk, hence vigorous foals that nurse heartily soon after birth may be the most severely affected.

Signs of the disease may be manifested as early as 8 to as late as 96 hours post partum. They include lethargy, jaundice and hemoglobinuria. The foals show general weakness and dullness, tachycardia and accelerated respiration, but are afebrile. They prefer to spend much of their time lying down; indeed, those severely affected often cannot stand. They seldom have the desire to nurse and do so only for short periods. The conjunctiva, sclera and mucous membranes become progressively icteric in seriously affected foals. Erythrocyte counts range from about 2,000,000 to 4,000,000/cu mm, and the erythrocytes tend to agglutinate in their own plasma. Foals with erythrocyte counts of this level during the first 24 hours require treatment.

Diagnosis: This may be made on clinical grounds. The demonstration of isoantibodies in the mare's serum or colostrum would be a positive indication, but Coombs' test of the anemic foal's erythrocytes provides a definitive answer when the diagnosis is in question. Except for anemia, icterus and sometimes bloody urine, few lesions are regularly seen. Splenomegaly and generalized icterus are often seen in foals dying 24 to 48 hours post partum. Sections may reveal ruptured alveoli, necrosis of hepatic cells and engorgement of the spleen with erythrocytes.

Prophylaxis: If the mare's serum shows a definite antibody titer ($>$1:2) near the end of gestation, or if a test of the mare's colostrum with the foal's cells at birth shows an antibody titer of $>$1:8, the disease may be avoided by taking the foal from its mother immediately at birth for 24 to 48 hours. The foal may be nursed by a normal foster mother or may be bottle-fed on colostrum from nonimmunized mares. Such colostrum can be frozen for this purpose. The mother of the foal should be milked in order to remove most of the colostrum. The foal then may be safely returned to its mother. The disease can usually be prevented by mating mares that have already produced one or more afflicted foals to stallions whose red blood cells are not agglutinated or hemolyzed by isoantibodies present in the mare's serum. However, in such cases, serum antibody levels should be measured during late gestation to detect the possible appearance of new isoantibodies.

Treatment: For those foals that are not seriously affected, ordinary nursing care together with antibiotics (R 11, 44, 54) and restriction of exercise for the first week usually will result in recovery. Exsanguination transfusion is the only known method of saving a severely afflicted foal. In this way, damaged erythrocytes and excess antibodies are removed and replaced by the transfused blood. The blood of either the dam or the sire should not be used in transfusions (but the saline-washed erythrocytes of the mare have been used successfully in treating the foal). A horse should be selected whose red blood cells are not agglutinated or hemolyzed by the serum or colostrum of the mare or the serum of the foal, and whose serum contains no demonstrable isoagglutinins or isohemolysins for the sire of the foal if the sire is available. The erythrocyte count of the foals should be maintained at 7,000,000 to 8,000,000/cu mm until recovery. Usually, removal of 3 to 7 liters of the severely afflicted foal's blood, replaced by 4 to 6 liters of the donor's blood, either by direct transfusion or the use of whole, citrated blood will correct the anemia and relieve the signs. Additional transfusions may be necessary and supportive therapy is essential. Albumin given IV to adsorb bilirubin prior to its removal via exsanguination transfusion may be helpful adjunct therapy in severely icteric foals.

HEMOLYTIC DISEASE OF NEWBORN PIGS

Early postnatal deaths from hemolytic anemia due to iso-immune antibodies have been recorded in pigs from the U.S.A. and several other countries. Although transplacental isoimmunization is possible, the disease probably occurs most often as a consequence of vaccinating sows with hog cholera vaccines produced from swine blood or swine tissues.

The disease can be experimentally produced when parents selected according to their blood types are mated and the gestating sow is inoculated with erythrocytes from the male. The resulting blood group antibodies can be detected in both the sow's serum and colostrum.

Hemolytic disease in pigs resembles that in horses since the transfer of antibodies to the newborn occurs via the colostrum. Pigs born healthy and vigorous may succumb within 24 hours of birth. Various degrees of hemoglobinemia, hemoglobinuria and jaundice may develop, depending on the amount and avidity of the antibodies consumed.

Diagnosis and treatment are similar to those for the corresponding disease in horses (q.v., p. 38).

EQUINE PURPURA HAEMORRHAGICA

An acute, frequently fatal, noncontagious, apparently allergenic disease which is a clinical entity in the horse. The purpura is nonthrombocytopenic and as such, it differs from the idiopathic purpura of the dog and cow and from the isoimmune purpura of neonatal swine, but is similar to Henoch-Schönlein disease of man.

Etiology and Pathogenesis: The disease is a clinical syndrome which may have more than one cause. Characteristically it occurs as a sequela to upper respiratory *Streptococcus equi* ("Strangles") infection, following 1 to 3 weeks after the initial illness. Viruses are not felt to cause the disease directly but other pyogenic infections or bacterin injections (especially *S. equi*) may do so. The disease is likely a type of Arthus reaction and similar to "serum sickness". The pathogenesis is based upon antigen, presumably streptococcal protein, in continuous circulation. In recovery from the acute infection, antibody is produced which combines with the circulating antigen. Because initially the antigen is in excess, the immune aggregates formed are very small and therefore soluble, which allows them to continue in circulation. Complement is taken up by the antigen-antibody reaction and these soluble complexes cause vascular endothelial injury throughout the body with the resulting edema and purpura. Normally, antibody is in excess and the immune aggregates formed are large, insoluble and rapidly cleared from the circulation by the reticuloendothelial system without vascular injury.

Clinical Findings: Subcut. edema and petechiation of the visible mucous membranes of sudden onset are the characteristic signs. Urticarial wheals are often observed. The edema is most prominent around the head, eyes and lips. Dependent edema of the belly (1 to 3 in. thick) and legs is present. Edema is prominent in the viscera and is evidenced by pulmonary edema and occasionally diarrhea or colic due to hemorrhage and edema in the gut. There are petechial and larger hemorrhages on all mucous membranes. The skin over the edematous areas may crack and slough, with oozing and crusting of serum on the surface. In mild cases, the temperature is usually normal or slightly elevated and the heart rate may be increased to 90 to 100/min. There is neutrophilic leukocytosis with nearly normal platelet counts. Anemia occurs in severe cases, or hemoconcentration may occur if loss of plasma has exceeded loss of red cells. The blood clots normally and fibrinogen would be expected to remain at normal levels and complement levels should drop. Urine may be scanty and proteinuria has not been reported but should be expected. The disease lasts 1 to 2 weeks followed by recovery in about 50% of cases. Relapses are common as are secondary bacterial infections. Death may be rapid due to asphyxia, or due to anemia and toxemia of secondary infection in protracted cases.

Lesions: Marked edema is the most characteristic change while hemorrhages may be sparse or extensive. The edematous extravasations are present subcut. and in the IM fascia. There may be edematous blockage of the airways of the head and patchy congestion and edema of both the respiratory and enteric canals. There is usually blood-tinged edema beneath the hepatic and renal capsules with some degree of ascites. There are commonly widely distributed focal lesions in skeletal muscles due to ischemia (pale) or hemorrhage (dark). Deep abscesses or pyogenic cellulitis due to the primary disease, often yielding *S. equi,* are frequently found.

Diagnosis: A history of recent pyogenic infection or immunization and the sudden appearance of angioneurotic edema and urticarial wheals that progress to extensive sharply demarcated dependent edema and edema of the head suggest the diagnosis. The purpura is usually more extensive than the petechiae of EIA (q.v., p. 254). In some cases, there may be no satisfactory history of precipitating disease.

Treatment: Since the disease is likely related to circulating bacterial protein, antibacterial therapy to clear the exciting antigen from the blood is indicated. Penicillin (B 44) with streptomycin (B 56), tetracycline (B 58), oxytetracycline (B 33) or triple sulfa (B 78) may be given. The antibiotics, but not the sulfas, may be given in dosage rates up to twice those indicated. Corticosteroids (B 145) may be indicated in those cases due to bacterin injections but must be accompanied by high levels of antibiotics. Tracheotomy may be necessary if asphyxia is imminent. Blood transfusion is indicated if the anemia is severe (hemoglobin <5 gm and dropping). Bandaging of limbs is helpful and good nursing is indicated.

LYMPHANGITIS OF HORSES

An inflammation of the lymph vessels and nodes, secondary to pyogenic cellulitis and usually affecting the pelvic limbs.

Etiology: This form of lymphangitis develops after infection by streptococci, less frequently by staphylococci or other pathogenic pyogens. Lack of regular exercise may be a contributing factor and the disease is observed more frequently in horses in good condition.

Clinical Findings: Signs develop one to several days after the infection becomes established. Commonly systemic disturbance is observed with fever, anorexia, increased rate of pulse and respiration, leukocytosis, neutrophilia, increased sedimentation rate and slight icterus. Signs in the affected limb are those of a hot, spreading, painful edematous swelling that may involve the entire limb. Severe lameness accompanies the swelling. Lymph ducts are visibly swollen, as are the regional lymph nodes. Exudation of serous fluid may occur at various areas, particularly at the hock and along the medial aspect of the thigh. Small vesicles or abscesses may develop in the skin, rupture and exude a serous or purulent fluid.

The course is acute or peracute. The swelling reaches maximal size in 2 to 4 days. If treatment is successful, the swelling gradually recedes over a period of days or weeks. Severe or untreated cases often become chronic with fibrosis and induration of the leg occurring. Recurrent attacks are not uncommon. Other conditions resembling this disease are ulcerative lymphangitis, North American blastomycosis, sporotrichosis, equine cryptococcosis, the early stages of purpura haemorrhagica and localized cellulitis of the area.

Treatment: Sulfonamides (R 75, 82) and antibiotics (R 11, 25, 44, 58) are indicated and are most effective when used early in the course of the disease. Corticosteroids (R 145, 148, 154) may be useful but some danger attends their use unless the infection has been suppressed. Phenylbutazone (R 150) is indicated to suppress inflammation and pain. Diuretics, particularly furosemide (R 520), are of benefit in stimulating resorption of edematous fluids. Application of warm packs or warm water baths, especially in conjunction with the use of a turbalator will stimulate lymphatic and venous drainage and hasten the reduction of edema. Moderate exercise is indicated. Any vesicles or ulcers should be treated locally with antibiotic or antiseptic powders or ointments.

HEART DISEASE

Although heart disease is infrequently treated in domestic animals, except the dog and cat, cardiac conditions often present diagnostic problems. Those aspects of cardiac disease which are of primary interest to clinicians are outlined under the appropriate headings in this chapter. Recommendations for therapy are limited to those conditions and species in which there has been substantial experience with treatment.

Examination and Diagnosis: A systemic examination is necessary in evaluating the state of the heart. The examination should include palpation of the cardiac region to detect thrills and cardiac displacement, prolonged careful auscultation in the standard areas of auscultation, percussion of the area of cardiac dullness, and palpation of the arterial pulse. Roentgenologic examination of the cardiac silhouette for distortion and enlargement is an important diagnostic procedure in small animals. An electrocardiogram (ECG) should be obtained whenever feasible. In areas where heartworms may be encountered in the dog, the blood should be examined for microfilaria.

The first object of the examination should be to classify the animal with respect to the condition of its heart. Heart disease should be considered present only when a dependable sign is found. It is important to avoid placing subjects in this category on the basis of suggestive signs, since many conditions simulate true cardiac involvement.

In the dog, a diagnosis of heart disease should not be made unless at least one of the following dependable signs can be detected: (1) a Grade IV or greater systolic murmur (q.v., p. 44); (2) a Grade III systolic murmur in the absence of anemia; (3) a diastolic murmur; (4) a palpable precordial thrill; (5) generalized venous engorgement; (6) atrial fibrillation or flutter; (7) paroxysmal ventricular tachycardia; (8) atrial or ventricular extrasystoles consistently present and of frequent occurrence; (9) complete atrioventricular block; (10) left bundle branch block; (11) electrocardiographic right ventricular enlargement (see COR PULMONALE, p. 54) pattern; (12) roentgenologic evidence of gross heart enlargement, enlargement of one or more chambers, or pericardial effusion; (13) pronounced splitting of the second heart sound. Atrial fibrillation or flutter, complete atrioventricular block, pericardial friction rub, precordial thrills and generalized venous engorgement are reliable signs of cardiac disease in horses. The same signs are dependable evidence of heart disease in most domestic species including the ox. Signs which are of controversial significance or questionable specificity include: infrequent ventricular extrasystoles, all arrhythmias and conduction disturbances appearing after exercise, RS-T segment shifts, wandering pacemaker, diastolic murmur (a reliable sign in the dog) and enlargement of the area of cardiac dullness. Diastolic and systolic murmurs are common in normal horses and in the absence of other signs cannot be considered reliable evidence of organic cardiac disease.

Since severe chronic or posthemorrhagic anemia can affect the heart unfavorably, one may consider this a sign of heart disease when the hemoglobin level is below 50% of normal.

The most common and obvious signs in animals with cardiac disease are (1) systolic murmur, (2) dyspnea, (3) coughing, (4) pulmonary edema and ascites and (5) ease of fatigability or weakness, and, while highly suggestive of heart disease, a positive diagnosis should be made only after one or more of the dependable signs have been elicited, or other possibilities thoroughly eliminated. Rarely, in certain degenerative diseases of the myocardium, congestive heart failure may be present without abnormal heart sounds or diagnostic electrocardiographic changes.

HEART SOUNDS AND MURMURS

Normal heart sounds and variants: Four heart sounds are frequently audible in horses. The first (S_1) sound is associated with closure of the atrioventricular valves, the second (S_2) sound with closure of the semilunar valves and ventricular relaxation. The third (S_3) sound occurs in early diastole at the end of the period of rapid ventricular filling. The fourth (S_4) or atrial sound is related to atrial systole. While all these sounds may be heard, often only S_1 and S_2; S_1, S_2 and S_3; or S_4, S_1 and S_2 can be detected.

In cattle only S_1 and S_2 are ordinarily audible. Either S_3 or S_4 are sometimes heard, but less often than in horses. During the IV administration of calcium solutions in cattle with hypocalcemia, either S_4 or S_3 or both may be accentuated and become audible.

In the dog, only S_1 and S_2 are ordinarily heard. Inspiratory splitting of S_2 occurs, but the interval between the 2 components is usually too slight to be audible. Less commonly the first sound may be split.

The characteristics of heart sounds in other domestic mammals (e.g., goats, sheep, swine, cats) have received less study. In general only S_1 and S_2 are audible in these species.

Murmurs and other abnormal sounds: The following arbitrary classification of heart murmurs with respect to intensity is useful: Grade I—the murmur of lowest intensity which can be heard; Grade II—a faint murmur still audible after a few seconds auscultation; Grade III—a murmur which is immediately audible when auscultation begins; Grade IV—loudest murmur which is still inaudible when the stethoscope chest piece is just removed from the chest; Grade V—extremely loud murmur that can still be heard with the stethoscope just removed from the chest wall.

There are 2 general types of *systolic murmurs,* ejection and regurgitant. Ejection systolic murmurs are crescendo-decrescendo in intensity, with the greatest intensity during mid-systole. They are sometimes produced by stenosis of the semilunar valves, infundibular stenosis, dilation of the aorta or pulmonary artery or increased rate of flow through a semilunar valve orifice. Regurgitant systolic murmurs are pansystolic and frequently of constant intensity. They can be caused by mitral or tricuspid regurgitation, or by an interventricular septal defect. These abnormalities do not invariably produce murmurs which can be recognized as either ejection or regurgitant in type.

Diastolic murmurs fall in 3 general categories: (1) the arterial diastolic murmur of aortic and pulmonic insufficiency; (2) the passive atrioventricular diastolic murmur accompanying actual or relative atrioventricular valve stenosis; and (3) the atriosystolic or presystolic murmur associated with mitral or tricuspid stenosis.

Continuous or *machinery murmurs* may be present over arteriovenous fistulas as with patent ductus arteriosus (q.v., p. 61) which is present in animals at birth and is audible in foals, disappearing shortly after birth. This continuous murmur waxes and wanes in intensity with systole and diastole, being of greatest intensity during the second heart sound.

In horses, presystolic, early systolic and early diastolic murmurs are frequently audible in the absence of cardiovascular disease or anemia. The early systolic murmurs are most common and generally heard over the base of the heart (aortic and pulmonic auscultatory areas). A short, high-pitched, squeaking early diastolic murmur, greatest in intensity near the cardiac apex (mitral area), is not infrequently heard in healthy young horses.

Diastolic gallop rhythms: Triple, 3-beat or gallop rhythms resemble the cadence of a galloping horse. The "extra" sound is classified as early diastolic (ventricular), presystolic (atrial) or summation gallop. These sounds represent abnormal accentuations of S_3 and S_4 in animals in which these sounds are normally inaudible. The early diastolic (ventricular) gallop sound (exaggerated S_3) is associated, in the dog, with advanced myocardial disease and congestive heart failure. The presystolic (atrial) gallop sound (exaggerated S_4) becomes audible when the interval between atrial and ventricular systolic (PR interval in the ECG) is prolonged. Summation gallop results from fusion of atrial and ventricular gallop sounds and may occur in congestive heart failure with tachycardia. All 3 of these gallop rhythms may be heard in normal horses and, rarely, in cattle. However, as in the smaller domestic species, they may have pathologic significance since accentuation of S_3 and S_4 in all species is favored by dilation of the heart.

Systolic click: Short, sharp, often transient sounds during systole are known to occur uncommonly in the dog and probably in other domestic species. They usually are single, but may be multiple; and may disappear completely in some beats. Their clinical significance is uncertain, but they have been attributed to such extracardiac causes as tensing of the walls of a dilated aorta or pulmonary artery and pleuropericardial adhesions.

Splitting of the heart sounds: Audible splitting of either S₁ or S₂ may occur in the absence of other cardiac abnormality. S_1 may be markedly split when the contraction of the 2 ventricles is asynchronous, as in bundle branch block and certain ectopic ventricular beats.

S_2 may be split during inspiration in dogs and during either inspiration or expiration in horses. Abnormal splitting of S_2 is associated with pulmonary hypertension as in pulmonary emphysema of horses and heartworm infection of dogs. Other causes in dogs (and possibly in other species) include atrial septal defect, pulmonic stenosis, right bundle branch block, certain ventricular ectopic beats, aortic stenosis and left bundle branch block.

Triple rhythms: The various sounds, outlined in the foregoing, that may produce triple rhythms may be summarized as follows: (a) Physiologic: third heart sound in horses and cattle, fourth heart sound in horses and cattle, and summation gallop in horses during tachycardia; (b) Abnormal: systolic click; (c) Pathologic: diastolic ventricular gallop, diastolic atrial gallop, and diastolic summation gallop.

Splitting of S_1 or S_2 must be distinguished from triple rhythms in which 2 of the sounds are close together as in certain systolic clicks in dogs and when S_4 closely precedes S_1 in horses.

ARRHYTHMIAS IN NORMAL ANIMALS

The rhythm of the dog heart usually is irregular when the animal is at rest, and becomes more regular as the rate accelerates during exercise or excitement or following administration of atropine. This normal variation in rhythm is known as sinus arrhythmia. The heart rate is regularly accelerated and then retarded. This is caused by a waxing and waning of vagal activity usually related to the respiratory cycle, although this is not always the case. The irregularity may be so pronounced that the heart seems to "skip" a beat at intervals. In the dog, this arrhythmia usually is associated with a healthy heart and is likely to disappear in cardiac disease (owing to tachycardia) or to be replaced by another arrhythmia.

In horses, incomplete atrioventricular block with dropped beats and sino-atrial block may be observed in 16 to 20% of animals examined and are commonly believed to be normal variants. In these arrhythmias, ventricular contraction fails at intervals. This, when accompanied by a single auricular sound, is diagnostic of incomplete atrioventricular block and disappears when the horse is exercised sufficiently, excited or given atropine.

ABNORMAL ARRHYTHMIAS

Sinus pause (sinus arrest or sino-auricular standstill): This condition denotes a total arrest of cardiac activity resulting from failure of the pacemaker. It usually is attributed to increased vagal activity. The heart may stop for several beats and then resume its activity or only one contraction may be missed. Certain reflex effects, such as passing a stomach tube in aged subjects, firm pressure on the eyeballs (oculocardiac reflex), firmly grasping the muzzle so as to occlude respiration, and carotid sinus pressure, may produce transient cardiac standstill in dogs. These last 2 maneuvers are useful in determining clinically whether or not vagal cardiac control is present in dogs.

Premature contractions: Premature beats are contractions which occur earlier than expected, i.e., the interval between the preceding contraction and the premature contraction is considerably shorter than the average diastolic pause. The premature contraction may be discovered through palpation and auscultation of the heart and by a shortened diastolic interval, usually followed by a prolonged or compensatory diastolic pause. Since less time has been available for cardiac filling, the pulse and heart sounds are usually weaker than in the regular beats. If the contraction occurs very early, little blood may have entered the heart so that the systole does not open the aortic and pulmonary valves. Then only the first heart sound is heard and no pulse can be palpated. If a long compensatory pause follows, the ensuing heart sounds and arterial pulse are exaggerated. Premature beats may alternate with regular beats producing groups of 2 (bigeminy) or 3 (trigeminy). In this case, a strong beat is paired with 1 or 2 weak beats. This arrhythmia is one of the more common irregularities observed in the presence of heart disease. In the dog, atrial and ventricular extrasystoles occurring frequently and persistently, in the absence of the action of certain drugs, toxins or electrolyte disturbances, have been found associated with myocardial disease in all cases reported. In dogs, therefore, these arrhythmias are considered evidence of myocardial disease. In other species studied, however, although premature beats are common in diseased hearts, they sometimes are observed in animals showing no other signs of heart disease.

Atrial fibrillation: A relatively common arrhythmia found in dogs with serious heart disease. It also has been reported in horses and cattle and probably occurs in all species. In this condition, numerous impulses arise in the atria producing localized contractions of the atrial myocardium at an extreme rate of frequency (several hundred per minute). The ventricular rate is variable and the rhythm and force of contractions are irregular (delirium cordis, total irregularity of the heart, perpetual arrhythmia). In the dog, the ventricular rate is rapid (usually between 190 and 250/min) in untreated cases. In horses, the ventricular rate may be rapid (55 to 105/min) or slow (as low as 16/min) or normal. In the ox, the ventricular rate usually is accelerated (90 to 150/min). When the ventricular rate is increased, some of the diastolic pauses may be too short to permit adequate filling of the ventricles so that little blood is forced into the peripheral arteries. When this occurs, a pulse is not produced in the peripheral arteries and consequently the pulse rate is less than the heart rate (pulse deficit). In the dog, this pulse deficit may be considerable, e.g., heart rate 204 and pulse rate 98/min. The heart sounds are extremely variable in time and intensity. This arrhythmia is an extremely grave prognostic sign in dogs; its inception usually marks the final stages of serious heart disease and, while death may not be imminent, it ordinarily is not delayed more than a few months. In the horse, cases have been reported which were paroxysmal in nature and followed by complete recovery. Although some horses may continue to work despite the presence of auricular fibrillation, strenuous exercise cannot be tolerated and syncope or sudden death may occur.

When this arrhythmia occurs, 2 types of therapy may be used. If marked congestive heart failure is present, it usually is necessary to digitalize the animal (Ŗ 507). If the subject is not in congestive heart failure or following successful digitalization, attempts may be made to abolish the arrhythmia with quinidine sulfate (Ŗ 515, 516). This therapy has been notably successful in the horse but rarely of value in dogs since in this species atrial fibrillation seldom occurs except in the presence of severe underlying heart disease. The prognosis and response to quinidine therapy appear to be better in dogs of giant breeds. If the arrhythmia is not of long standing, the possibility that it may be paroxysmal in nature and disappear spontaneously should be kept in mind, especially when dealing with horses and cattle.

Atrial flutter: This is a form of rapid heart action in which the atria beat regularly, but at an extremely rapid rate (300 to 400/min). It is much less common than atrial fibrillation, but has been observed in the dog. Usually, there is a fixed atrioventricular block of a 2:1 or 3:1 ratio and the ventricles beat regularly at a rate of one-half or one-third the atrial rate. Under most clinical conditions, recognition of this arrhythmia with certainty requires an ECG.

Clinical experience with atrial flutter in dogs is so meager that recommendations for therapy cannot be made with confidence. It is probable that when atrioventricular block is not marked and consequently the ventricular rate excessively rapid, digitalis preparations should be prescribed.

Heart block: A delay or interruption in conduction of the cardiac impulse somewhere in its course from the sino-atrial node to the ventricles. There are 3 types: sino-atrial (SA) block, atrioventricular (AV) block and bundle branch block (BBB). In **sino-atrial block,** both the atria and the ventricles fail to contract occasionally. During the interval of the missed beat, no sound is heard on auscultation. In **atrioventricular block,** conduction between the atria and ventricles is impaired. In incomplete AV block, the conduction time (PR interval in the ECG) is merely increased. In incomplete AV block with dropped beats, the conduction is stopped at intervals so that the ventricles fail to contract periodically. In the resting horse, the atrioventricular conduction time (PR interval) is frequently variable, and incomplete AV block with dropped beats or SA block may occur. With exercise, excitement, or atropine, these variations in AV conduction or SA node impulse formation disappear in the normal horse. In complete atrioventricular block, none of the impulses arising in the auricle is conducted to the ventricles. The auricles and ventricles then beat independently, the latter in response to an ectopic pacemaker in the nodal or ventricular tissue and the pulse rate usually is abnormally slow. Incomplete AV block can only be diagnosed with certainty by means of an ECG. In the horse, when the atrioventricular conduction time is long, S_4 may be heard just prior to S_1. In incomplete AV block with dropped beats, the ventricles fail to contract periodically. If, during the pause, an atrial sound is heard, the presence of incomplete AV block with dropped beats is demonstrated. In the absence of this finding, an ECG is required for diagnosis. In animals other than the horse, incomplete atrioventricular block with dropped beats usually is associated with heart disease. Occasionally, dogs are observed with this degree of atrioventricular block in the absence of other signs of heart disease. Rarely, it may occur as a transient manifestation during the course of infectious disease. Toxic doses of digitalis also may produce this as well as other arrhythmias.

heavy abdominal musculature, it is not clinically detectable unless abdominal paracentesis is carried out. The ascitic fluid in dogs usually is serosanguineous despite the postmortem absence of any gross hemorrhage.

Treatment: A primary aim of therapy in congestive heart failure is to eliminate the edema fluid. This may be done by decreasing the work of the heart (rest and restriction of exercise), reducing the sodium intake, increasing the sodium (and water) elimination through diuretics (℞ 517, 519) and by bringing about cardiac compensation by means of digitalis glycosides (℞ 507).

In dogs, the diet may be regulated to decrease sodium intake. Suitable low-sodium diets are available commercially for dogs with congestive heart failure. In general, foods of animal origin contain much sodium and foods of vegetable origin contain little. Foods low in salt include fresh or frozen vegetables without salt, wheat-based cereals, polished and coated rice, dialized milk and soybean oil meal. Meat, fish and poultry must be limited as should milk and milk-containing foods, although these foods often are tolerated as long as no salt is used in their preparation. Public water supplies usually do not contain much sodium, but well waters may, and softened water nearly always is high in sodium. Distilled water is recommended if the sodium content of the water is unknown.

The use of diuretics to increase sodium (and water) elimination is important. In dogs, the most effective drugs are furosemide (℞ 520) and the chlorothiazide derivatives (℞ 519). Withdrawal of ascitic fluid by abdominocentesis is indicated only when the volume markedly interferes with breathing, and then only to the extent necessary for comfort. Removal of ascitic fluid results in loss of protein and the abdominal fluid will soon be replaced if cardiac compensation and diuresis are not brought about by appropriate medical therapy.

Digitalis glycosides slow the heart and increase the strength of myocardial contraction. While rest, sodium restriction and diuretics are useful adjuncts to the medical therapy of congestive heart failure, digitalis is always the primary therapeutic agent since it acts directly on the failing heart. Digitalization is seldom undertaken in animals other than the dog and cat, and dosage recommendations will be limited to these species. Presumably, general principles for the use of digitalis in the dog and cat apply to farm animals as well. A number of digitalis glycosides are in current use, but evidence regarding their absorption, fate, and efficacy in various species is meager. The most complete studies have been made of the glycoside digoxin in the dog, and a desirable rate of absorption and excretion have been demonstrated. It is supplied in both oral and parenteral dosage forms (℞ 507).

Digitalization has been accomplished only when sufficient drug has been given to produce full therapeutic action. In general, the drug should be given until therapeutic levels are reached, as indicated by amelioration of the clinical signs of congestive heart failure, or until toxic signs become evident. The dosage calculated on a weight basis is effective in most animals, but the amount required to produce optimal effects in a given case is not always predictable and the dosage must be governed by clinical results. Since most forms of heart disease in animals are chronic and progressive, digitalis therapy, once indicated, is usually continued indefinitely. Three methods of digitalization are employed, depending upon the urgency of therapy. They may be termed slow, rapid, and intensive digitalization.

Slow Digitalization is used when signs of heart failure (right or left heart failure) develop gradually and are not severe. The animal is placed immediately on the oral maintenance dose without a prior loading dose. The incidence of toxic signs is low, and digitalization can usually be accomplished within 1 to 2 weeks. If no improvement is noted within 10 days, the dosage should be gradually increased.

Rapid Digitalization is used when signs of congestive heart failure are more severe, and where close observation of the animal is possible during the process of digitalization. Using the oral form, total digitalizing (loading) dose is calculated on the basis of body weight (℞ 507) and divided into 6 equal doses which are given at 8-hour intervals over a 48-hour period. The animal is then placed on a daily maintenance dose.

Intensive Digitalization is used in extreme emergencies such as the acute pulmonary edema of severe left heart failure. The loading dose is administered by the parenteral route (℞ 507). One-half of the calculated dose is given immediately by slow IV injection, followed by one-fourth of the dose in 6 hours and the final one-fourth dose 6 hours later. If a therapeutic effect is obtained, the animal may then be placed on the oral maintenance dose beginning 12 hours later. If a therapeutic effect does not occur, one-eighth of the calculated digitalizing dose is repeated at 6-hour intervals until a therapeutic effect is seen or evidence of toxicity occurs.

Since individual tolerance to digitalis glycosides varies widely, the patient should be observed carefully for signs of digitalis toxicity, particularly in the initial period of digitalization. Mild diarrhea is a common early sign of toxicity but does not necessitate discontinuation of the drug. Vomiting, depression, or the onset of cardiac arrhythmias, however, signal a need to discontinue digitalis therapy immediately. Twenty-four to 48 hours should be given for excretion of the drug and the regression of toxic signs, following which therapy can be reinstituted at a lower dosage level. A therapeutic effect is indicated by slowing of the heart rate and amelioration of the signs of congestive heart failure (decrease in coughing and dyspnea in left heart failure, loss of ascitic fluid due to diuresis in right heart failure).

Heart disease secondary to disordered pulmonary circulation (cor pulmonale) results in right ventricular dilatation and hypertrophy. In severe cases, congestive heart failure may supervene. Pulmonary heart disease, as defined here, is seen in dogs usually secondary to heartworm (*Dirofilaria immitis*) infection (q.v., p. 686). In cattle grazing at high altitudes, pulmonary hypertension occurs in some individuals with consequent right heart failure (*see* HIGH-MOUNTAIN DISEASE, p. 512). In both species, digitalization is helpful in the acute stages. In the dog, surgical removal of the adult filaria may be carried out in heavy infections. However, this surgical technique is not uniformly successful. Cattle stricken with brisket disease are improved when returned to lower altitudes.

THE PERICARDIUM AND ITS CONTENTS

The pericardium may be congenitally absent or only partially formed. Such abnormalities are usually of no clinical significance. Hydropericardium may occur in congestive heart failure and hydremia, e.g., in parasitism with associated anemia. Pericarditis with massive sanguineous effusion is a clinical entity which may occur in dogs. The clinical signs usually first noted by the owner are dyspnea, ease of fatigability and ascites. The diagnostic signs include muffled heart sounds, low electrocardiographic potentials and, on fluoroscopy, the cardiac silhouette is circular, greatly enlarged and cardiac pulsations cannot be easily discerned, or are absent. When the fluid is removed, it is found to resemble blood closely, but does not clot. It is bacteriologically sterile and its removal (in amounts up to 700 ml) results in dramatic alleviation of the clinical signs. The condition may recur, but it usually does not. Similar effusions are sometimes present owing to neoplasms within the pericardial sac (e.g., heart base tumors). In these cases removal of the fluid is merely palliative. (*See also* TRAUMATIC RETICULOPERITONITIS, p. 134.)

THE MYOCARDIUM

Degenerative changes of the myocardium occur in many diseases. Cloudy swelling is seen in febrile infectious diseases and metallic poisoning. Fatty degeneration occurs in severe anemia, infectious diseases and poisoning by such agents as phosphorus, heavy metals, chloroform and ether. Hyaline degeneration sometimes is found in the myocardium of horses that have died of paralytic myoglobinuria and in lambs, calves and foals affected with white muscle disease (q.v., p. 578). Specific degenerative diseases of the myocardium have not been well characterized in domestic animals.

Myocarditis often develops in the course of infectious diseases, such as foot-and-mouth disease, hemorrhagic septicemia, equine infectious anemia, pullorum disease and blackleg. Myocarditis may accompany septicemic diseases in dogs.

Myocardial infarction is rare in domestic animals, although occasionally observed on postmortem examination. In the dog, small foci of myocardial necrosis in various stages of resorption and scar formation are found in association with sclerotic narrowing of small intramyocardial arteries.

Many myocardial lesions, if extensive enough, will produce typical electrocardiographic changes, such as depression or elevation of the ST segment, depression of the T wave, increased duration of QRS, low voltage, abnormal notching of the QRS complex, and certain arrhythmias, such as atrial fibrillation, ventricular extrasystoles, paroxysmal ventricular tachycardia and atrioventricular block. Clinical diagnosis of myocarditis frequently is difficult or impossible in mild cases. The most frequent diagnostic signs of myocardial inflammation or degeneration are electrocardiographic changes listed above, tachycardia out of proportion to the increased temperature, arrhythmias and cardiac enlargement. In severe cases, murmurs of mitral and tricuspid incompetence may appear and signs of congestive heart failure develop.

THE ENDOCARDIUM

Acute endocarditis, usually of bacterial origin, may be found associated with infectious processes elsewhere in the body, e.g., pyemia, septicemia, wound infection, omphalitis, strangles, or swine erysipelas. Acute mural endocarditis of the atria occasionally is seen in dogs and other species on postmortem examination. Bacterial endocarditis is most likely to occur in the presence of pre-existing cardiac lesions, such as congenital defects or chronic valvular endocarditis. Clinical diagnosis is difficult. The affected subject exhibits signs of a severe systemic infection, septic embolism, cardiac disease or possibly only a murmur, and a positive blood culture (bacteremia). In pigs, erysipelas endocarditis is found in animals from 3 months to a year of age. The mitral valve most commonly is involved, the tricuspid and aortic valves more rarely. The lesions consist of cauliflower-like masses on the surface of the valve. Acute valvular endocarditis is not rare in cattle, horses and dogs, but is less common in other species. Treatment of bacterial endocarditis consists of massive doses of bactericidal antibiotics and supportive therapy. In the absence of knowledge of antibiotic sensitivity, penicillin is the antibiotic of choice.

Chronic valvular disease most often is seen in dogs, occasionally appears in horses and cattle, and is rare in sheep, goats and cats. Valvular lesions, characterized by fibrosis with edema and mucinous degeneration, are common in adult dogs. The mitral valve is by far the most commonly affected; next in frequency is the tricuspid valve, then the aortic, and last, the pulmonary valve. In the dog, the most common result of these lesions is insufficiency of the mitral valve.

The signs of clinically significant mitral insufficiency in the dog include cough, dyspnea, rales and restlessness at night. A grade III or louder pansystolic murmur is audible at the mitral area. There are no typical electrocardiographic changes. Atrial arrhythmias are often present in advanced cases, including atrial premature beats, atrial tachycardia, atrial flutter and atrial fibrillation. Left atrial and ventricular enlargement and pulmonary venous engorgement may be observed in thoracic roentgenograms. The cause of the lesion is not known. Possibly, it results from a previous acute valvulitis with subsequent healing, scarring and deformity.

Valvular blood cysts or hematomas are seen in up to 75% of young calves under 3 weeks of age. The atrioventricular valves are most commonly affected. These lesions are also seen in the young of other species and their significance is unknown.

Subendocardial hemorrhages are seen in septicemia and toxemia and are commonly observed in animals bled to death (e.g., slaughter by Jewish ritual).

CONGENITAL ANOMALIES OF THE CARDIOVASCULAR SYSTEM

In recent years, improved clinical methods and greater interest in heart disease have resulted in an increase in the number of cases of congenital heart disease recognized especially in dogs. Certain of these can be corrected surgically. Many types of cardiovascular malformations which occur in man have been observed in animals. Those discussed below have been selected on the basis of their possible clinical significance in veterinary medicine and do not constitute a complete list.

I. Septal defects
  1. Interatrial septal defects
  2. Interventricular septal defects
II. Anomalies of the derivatives of the aortic arches
  1. Persistent ductus arteriosus
  2. Persistent right aortic arch
III. Pulmonic stenosis
IV. Aortic stenosis
V. Tetralogy of Fallot

Recent studies indicate that in dogs brought to a large veterinary clinic about 0.7% have detectable signs of congenital heart disease. The types of lesions seen, in approximate order of their frequency, are: patent ductus arteriosus, pulmonic stenosis, aortic stenosis, persistent right aortic arch, interventricular septal defect and tetralogy of Fallot. Cardiovascular malformations occur predominantly in purebred dogs, and certain specific anomalies are seen more often in certain breeds. This evidence, in addition to familial aggregations of affected dogs, indicates that genetic factors are of etiologic importance in that species. Genetic studies indicate that inheritance is complex (non-Mendelian). Prevalence rates are not known in other domestic animals. From studies made in swine, a prevalence rate similar to that in dogs seems likely.

The basic clinical diagnostic methods used are physical examination, ECG, X-ray and fluoroscopy. Cardiac catheterization and angiocardiography are also useful diagnostic methods.

In mild conditions, such as small interatrial and interventricular septal defects and patent ductus arteriosus, the animals may reach an advanced age without outward signs of heart disease. When the condition is more serious, the newborn animal may show weakness, dyspnea, cyanosis and retarded growth. The most severely affected animals die in the early postnatal period. If the condition is not obvious soon after birth, signs of congestive heart failure may ensue at a later time, usually before maturity, but occasionally as late as at 5 to 7 years of age. The appearance of signs of congestive heart failure in a young or middle-aged animal should alert the clinician to the possibility of an underlying congenital heart defect.

In some instances the early recognition of congenital heart

disease may enable the pet owner to reclaim his investment, or the livestock producer to avoid attempting to raise an animal which is destined to die at an early age. Essentially complete surgical correction of certain defects, notably patent ductus arteriosus, pulmonic stenosis and persistent right aortic arch, is possible without extensive special equipment. Where equipment for extracorporeal circulation or hypothermia is available, correction of other malformations may be attempted.

Signs of congestive heart failure (systemic venous congestion, hepatomegaly, ascites, pulmonary congestion and edema) may occur when the underlying congenital malformation severely impairs cardiac function. Animals with such signs may show dramatic improvement when treated with rest, low-sodium diets, cardiac glycosides and diuretics. Unless the underlying defect is surgically corrected, the response is usually temporary and death eventually results from irreversible congestive heart failure.

In the dog, clinical criteria for the common malformations discussed here are well enough developed that a definitive diagnosis can often be made on the basis of physical, roentgenographic and electrocardiographic signs. When surgical correction is contemplated, or when more complex anomalies are encountered, it is often desirable to perform additional confirmatory studies such as angiocardiography and cardiac catheterization. The clinical features of specific congenital malformations in species other than the dog are not well known, and in them, an accurate diagnosis more often depends on such special studies.

SEPTAL DEFECTS

ATRIAL SEPTAL DEFECTS

The foramen ovale is an oblique opening in the interatrial septum normally allowing flow from the right atrium to the left atrium during intrauterine life. At birth, this opening is forced closed by the increase in left atrial pressure which occurs at the onset of breathing. Anatomic closure of the foramen ovale occurs due to fibrosis during the postnatal period, and the foramen cannot reopen. Anatomic closure of the foramen ovale is complete within a week after birth in the dog, but may not be complete for some months in horses and cattle. Failure of the normal fibrotic reaction to occur results in a probe-patent foramen ovale. Although this may be considered to be an anatomic defect, it causes no functional abnormalities as long as left atrial pressure exceeds right atrial pressure. This "one way valve" may be reopened and allow right to left shunting of blood if right atrial pressure becomes abnormally elevated.

True atrial septal defects are consistently present openings in the interatrial septum. Defects of the septum secundum type are most common and occur in the thin portion of the interatrial septum occupied by the foramen ovale. Septum primum atrial septal defects are situated low in the interatrial septum and usually involve the atrioventricular valves as well.

Functional Pathology: In the presence of a large atrial septal defect, blood passes from the left to the right atrium through the septal defect. This additional blood must be pumped as an extra load by the right side of the heart and in time causes a dilatation and hypertrophy of this portion of the heart. As a result of the greatly increased blood flow through the pulmonary system, pulmonary hypertension may ensue, followed by congestive heart failure. Usually, there is no shunting of unoxygenated blood into the sytemic circulation. However, a slight cyanosis may appear indicating a reversed flow of blood from right to left atrium, particularly where pulmonary hypertension and congestive heart failure are present, or when coexisting lesions (e.g., pulmonic stenosis) cause an increase in right atrial pressure.

Clinical Findings: A small patent foramen ovale may be present without producing detectable clinical signs. In large septal defects, dyspnea, palpitation and cyanosis may be observed. Usually, a harsh systolic murmur is noticed over the base of the heart. The second heart sound is increased in amplitude and may be split. The right ventricle and pulmonary outflow tract are enlarged. Increased pulmonary vascular markings may be evident in thoracic radiographs.

Treatment: The atrial-well technique may be used for surgical correction in dogs. Repair under direct vision is facilitated by heart-lung bypass.

INTERVENTRICULAR SEPTAL DEFECTS

Interventricular septal defects range in size from small openings of little functional importance to almost complete absence of the interventricular septum. The majority of these defects occur in the upper membranous part of the interventricular septum. They may be combined with other congenital anomalies, such as patent ductus arteriosus, interatrial septal defects, pulmonic and aortic stenosis.

Functional Pathology: In small, uncomplicated, interventricular septal defects, the blood is transmitted from the left to right ventricle with considerable force. The amount of blood passing through this opening is small and such a defect has little or no effect upon the general circulation.

In the presence of a large defect without pulmonic stenosis, direction of the shunt depends upon the relative resistance to flow through the intrapulmonary vascular bed as compared with that of the systemic vascular bed. In young animals, the resistance in the intrapulmonary vascular bed is lower than the resistance in the systemic circulation and the shunt is entirely from left to right. As a consequence, the load of the right ventricle is increased and leads to hypertrophy and dilatation of the right ventricle and pulmonary artery. Subsequently, the resistance to pulmonary blood flow may rise due to obliterative changes in the pulmonary vascular bed. In the earlier stages, when the pulmonary resistance reaches the level of the systemic resistance, there may be some shunting in each direction, right to left or left to right, but later, when the pulmonary resistance has risen above the systemic level, the right-to-left shunt predominates and cyanosis usually appears.

Clinical Findings: An uncomplicated small septal defect often does not result in outward signs of heart disease. The physical signs, however, are usually distinctive and appear in the form of a holocystic, rather harsh murmur, frequently accompanied by a distinct thrill. The murmur and thrill are usually most pronounced in the right second to fourth intercostal space near the sternal margin. While the lesion itself may have little functional effect, there is the potential hazard of subacute bacterial endocarditis which may develop along the margins of the septal defect. This complication has been reported most commonly in cattle. Radiographic evidence of right ventricular enlargement and increased pulmonary blood flow is present in defects of moderate to large size. Animals with a large septal defect and extensive occlusive lesions in the intrapulmonary vascular bed have pulmonary hypertension and a right-to-left shunt. They are cyanotic and show all the associated features of cyanotic congenital heart disease, such as fatigability, anorexia, weakness and dyspnea.

Treatment: The surgical correction of interventricular septal defect requires extracorporeal circulation or deep hypothermia. The defect is usually patched with a nonreactive plastic material. Small defects in which functional changes are minimal may not appreciably shorten life if left untreated, but there is some increased risk of bacterial endocarditis.

ANOMALIES OF THE DERIVATIVES OF THE AORTIC ARCHES

Among the embryonic aortic arches which persist in the normal mammal are the right and left third, the left fourth, and portions of the right and left sixth arches. The third pair of arches give rise to the carotid arteries. The left fourth remains as the definitive arch of aorta, while the sixth arches give rise to the pulmonary artery, its branches, and the ductus arteriosus.

PERSISTENT DUCTUS ARTERIOSUS

During fetal life, an important communication exists between the aorta and the pulmonary artery. This connection is formed by the left sixth aortic arch and is known as the ductus arteriosus. Failure of the ductus arteriosus to close shortly after birth leads to an anomaly which is known as a persistent or patent ductus arteriosus. It is one of the most common clinically recognized congenital cardiovascular anomalies of the dog. It may be combined with other cardiac anomalies. It is inherited as a polygenic defect in miniature and toy Poodles.

Functional Pathology: Due to the existence of higher pressure in the aorta than in the pulmonary artery, a part of the arterial blood is pumped during the systole through the patent duct into the pulmonary system (left-to-right shunt). If pulmonary resistance remains low, there is increased flow through the lungs, left heart and ascending aorta, which constitute the path of the shunt. These structures dilate in response to the increased volume of blood they receive. If pulmonary vascular resistance is high, right ventricular hypertrophy and pulmonary hypertension are present, and a right-to-left shunt may occur through the ductus, sending venous blood to the descending aorta.

Clinical Findings: The so-called "machinery" murmur (see p. 45) is present during systole and diastole in the left-to-right shunt. The pulse usually is typical, quickly and strongly distending the artery (water hammer pulse). Electrocardiographic evidence of left ventricular hypertrophy may be present and thoracic radiographs show left atrial and ventricular enlargement, increased pulmonary vascular markings and dilatation of the ascending aorta.

When pulmonary hypertension with a right-to-left shunt is present, the machinery murmur is usually absent, there is accentuation and splitting of the second heart sound, and electrocardiographic and radiographic evidence of right ventricular hypertrophy. Secondary polycythemia is usually present.

Treatment: Ligation or complete surgical division of the persistent ductus arteriosus is recommended.

PERSISTENT RIGHT AORTIC ARCH

A right aortic arch represents a common vascular anomaly in dogs, in which the right fourth embryonic aortic arch persists, displacing the esophagus and trachea to the left. The trachea and esophagus are incarcerated in a vascular ring formed by the arch of the aorta on the right side, the pulmonary artery below, the base of the heart ventrally and the ligamentum arteriosum (or ductus arteriosus) dorsally and to the left.

Persistent right aortic arch is hereditary in the German Shepherd Dog. This anomaly has also been reported in cattle, horses and cats. Other anomalies of the aortic arch system may also result in vascular rings that partially or completely encircle the esophagus and trachea.

Functional Pathology: The pathology of this anomaly arises only from the fact that the vascular ring which encircles the esophagus and trachea may compress these organs with resultant dysphagia and regurgitation. A part of the esophagus cranial to the constriction is usually considerably dilated.

Clinical Findings: The clinical signs include dysphagia, regurgitation of food, and a reducible swelling in the caudoventral cervical region, owing to the dilated esophagus. The typical sign of regurgitation of solid food usually appears when puppies are 3 to 9 weeks old, although it may begin shortly after birth. Occasionally, the condition is discovered incidentally on postmortem examination. A barium swallow reveals dilatation of the esophagus cranial to the heart base.

Treatment: Relief of the constriction of the esophagus and trachea is obtained by surgical division of the ligamentum arteriosum (or ductus arteriosus). Some degree of dilatation of the precardiac esophagus usually remains after section of the vascular ring.

PULMONIC STENOSIS

In the dog, both valvular and subvalvular pulmonic stenosis have been described. In the former, the stenosis involves the valves only, while in the latter, the narrowing is in the outflow tract of the right ventricle below the pulmonic valve. Valvular pulmonic stenosis has been shown to be hereditary in Beagle dogs.

Functional Pathology: The primary functional disturbance is interference with emptying of the right ventricle. Right ventricular systolic pressure is elevated and there is right ventricular hypertrophy. The pulmonary arterial pressure is low or normal. Poststenotic dilatation of the pulmonary artery may occur, producing in advanced cases a rounded enlargement of the vessel resembling an aneurysm (poststenotic dilatation).

Clinical Findings: A harsh, crescendo-decrescendo systolic murmur, frequently accompanied by a thrill, is usually present with its point of maximal intensity located at the third or fourth left intercostal space, slightly below a horizontal line drawn through the point of the shoulder (pulmonic area). The cardiac silhouette shows enlargement of the right ventricular and atrial borders and poststenotic dilatation of the pulmonary artery may be visible. Electrocardiographically, there is usually marked deviation of the mean electrical axis to the right producing an ECG typical of right ventricular enlargement. It is impossible to differentiate between high subvalvular and valvular stenosis without the aid of angiocardiography.

Treatment: Pulmonary valvotomy is recommended for valvular stenosis. In the subvalvular type the infundibular ring is resected.

AORTIC STENOSIS

In the dog and pig, stenosis of the outflow tract of the left ventricle is a fairly common congenital cardiac lesion. It has been reported chiefly in Boxers and German Shepherd Dogs, and has been shown to occur in familial aggregations in these 2 breeds, and in Newfoundlands. Little is known regarding its prevalence in other species. In most instances, the valves are not primarily involved, the narrowing occurring below them in the form of a fibrous ring (fibrous subaortic stenosis).

Functional Pathology: The chief disturbance is obstruction to emptying of the left ventricle with resultant left ventricular hypertrophy. There is often poststenotic dilatation of the ascending aorta.

Clinical Findings: In the dog, the systolic murmur of aortic stenosis is ordinarily located in the third or fourth left intercostal space and right second to third intercostal space. It may be well transmitted to the neck. Fainting and sudden death are not uncommon with this defect. Electrocardiographic evidence of left ventricular hypertrophy may be present, and arrhythmias and conduction disturbances are frequent. Radiographically, left ventricular enlargement and poststenotic dilatation of the aorta are prominent signs. Treatment, when and if practical, is surgical.

TETRALOGY OF FALLOT

This complex malformation consists of pulmonic stenosis, usually of the subvalvular type, and ventricular septal defect with overriding aorta. Right ventricular hypertrophy is present. Tetralogy of Fallot has been reported a number of times in dogs, cattle, horses and cats. It is inherited in the Keeshond breed.

Functional Pathology: The combination of pulmonic stenosis and ventricular septal defect is functionally similar to that of a large interventricular septal defect and pulmonary hypertension. Owing to the obstruction to outflow from the right ventricle, ventricular systolic pressure is elevated, resulting in a right-to-left shunt through the ventricular septal defect. The aorta, which partially overrides the septal defect, receives blood from both ventricles, while pulmonary blood flow is diminished. Mixing of arterial and venous blood results in cyanosis.

Clinical Findings: Cyanosis is usually present from birth, and is worsened by exercise, precipitating dyspnea, and often collapse. Polycythemia may be present, owing to chronic hypoxemia. Despite the marked disability which accompanies this defect, dogs have been known to live for a number of years before dying from congestive heart failure or embolic phenomena.

A loud, harsh systolic murmur is usually heard best in the pulmonic area and right second to third intercostal space, near the sternal margin. A thrill may be palpated in these areas. Right ventricular hypertrophy is indicated by marked right axis deviation in the ECG, accompanied by large S waves in the left precordial leads. Thoracic radiographs reveal right heart enlargement with normal diminished pulmonary vascular markings. The ascending aorta is usually dilated.

Treatment: The creation of an artificial ductus arteriosus (Blalock-Taussig shunt) may increase pulmonary blood flow and alleviate the cyanosis to some degree. Complete correction by relief of the pulmonary stenosis and closure of the ventricular septal defect is preferable, but requires open heart surgery.

THROMBOSIS, EMBOLISM, ANEURYSM

A thrombus is a blood clot still at its site of origin and accordingly may be classified as venous, arterial or cardiac (valvular or mural). Venous thrombosis is uncommon in animals and secondary pulmonary embolism (except for heartworm emboli in dogs) is rare. Cardiac thrombi are usually associated with endocarditis. All or part of a thrombus may break off and be carried downstream as an embolus that lodges distally at a point of narrowing. An aneurysm is a saccular or cylindric dilatation due to weakness of a blood vessel wall. Aneurysms may form at the site of degenerative or inflammatory changes or because of partial rupture of the vessel wall. These changes may disrupt the endothelium as well, and cause overlying thrombus formation with subsequent formation of emboli. Although aneurysm, thrombosis and formation of emboli may be recognized simultaneously, distinct clinical syndromes involving mainly one or the other of these aspects are recognized in certain species.

The most common type of aneurysm occurs in the anterior mesenteric artery of horses as a result of arteritis caused by *Strongylus vulgaris* larval migration. Similar changes in the aorta and iliac arteries cause iliac thrombosis in some horses. Aneurysm of the thoracic aorta occurs in some dogs with esophageal granulomas caused by *Spirocera lupi*. Nonparasitic aneurysms are seen occasionally in all species. Rupture of dissecting aortic aneurysms (q.v., p. 1082) may cause significant losses in rapidly growing young turkeys.

Clinical Findings and Diagnosis: Aneurysms ordinarily do not cause clinical signs unless hemorrhage occurs or an associated thrombus develops. Except for aortic rupture in turkeys (with sudden death), spontaneous aneurysmal hemorrhage is rare and clinical signs usually are related to thrombosis. The signs vary according to the size and location of the thrombus and whether formation of emboli occurs. In some horses with verminous aneurysm and thrombosis, emboli become detached and partially or completely occlude terminal branches of the mesenteric arteries. Affected intestinal segments show changes ranging from passive congestion to hemorrhagic infarction. Clinical manifestations are those of colic, constipation or diarrhea. The colic is usually recurrent and attacks may be severe and prolonged.

Aneurysms of the abdominal aorta and its branches may be felt by rectal examination as hard or elastic pulsating swellings. In the case of excessive thrombus formation, the pulse distally may be delayed and have a slow rate of rise in pressure or may be absent.

Verminous thrombosis with or without aneurysm of the terminal aorta and proximal iliac arteries produces a characteristic syndrome in horses. Although they are normal at rest, graded exercise brings about an increasing severity of weakness of the hindlegs with unilateral or bilateral lameness, muscle tremor and sweating. Severely affected animals cannot endure exercise, they become lame and then fall or lie down. Following a short rest period, the signs disappear and the animal seems normal. Subnormal temperature of the affected limbs may be detectable along with decreased or absent arterial pulsations.

A different syndrome occurs in cats as a result of aortic embolism. In most instances a primary cardiac disorder is present such as endocarditis or myocarditis with associated thrombus formation. When all or part of the thrombus breaks off, it lodges distally in the arterial system. Most often this occurs at the terminal aorta and typically there is sudden onset of posterior paralysis, severe pain and muscle spasm at rest. The hind limbs are cool, rectal temperature is subnormal and femoral pulses are absent. Apparently, vasospasm or other factors must play a significant role since ligation of the caudal aorta does not reproduce the syndrome.

In unclear cases or those in which surgery is contemplated, angiocardiography is helpful in confirming the diagnosis of aneurysm, thrombosis or embolism, and in providing an assessment of collateral circulation.

Treatment: Surgical repair of certain types of aneurysm in a major vessel is technically feasible, but special experience is required. If the aneurysm is more distally located and there is adequate collateral circulation, the affected segment can be reached following appropriate ligations.

In horses an aneurysm rarely ruptures and the chief concern is with thrombosis and formation of emboli. The arteries commonly involved are not readily approachable from a surgical standpoint. Occasionally, there is a spontaneous recovery. The most rational approach in the horse is the prevention and control of strongylosis (q.v., p. 675).

Aortic emboli in cats may be removed surgically; however, recurrent formation of emboli is common. Thrombolytic and anticoagulant drugs have not been sufficiently evaluated in cats or horses to justify therapeutic recommendations.

SHOCK

A term used to describe a state of collapse characterized by an acute and progressive failure of the peripheral circulation.

Etiology: The specific etiology of shock is unknown, but it occurs following many forms of serious stress, including severe trauma, cardiac failure, massive hemorrhage, burns, anesthesia, overwhelming infections, internal obstruction, anemia, dehydration, anaphylaxis and intoxication.

In the less severe forms of shock, the body compensates adequately by accelerating the heart and constricting peripheral vessels (both reflexly), thus preserving the "peripheral resistance". When the shock is more severe, this compensation begins to fail and a vicious cycle appears. The poor circulation deprives the heart, the vasoconstrictor center and the vasoconstrictor smooth muscles of the necessary blood, hence the heart weakens, the peripheral vessels dilate, the blood flow is diminished, cardiac output is lowered still further and the body's ability to maintain its normal pH is reduced. As this sequence proceeds, a point is reached where, if treatment is delayed, the shock becomes irreversible and death soon follows. A number of explanations, on both nervous or humoral grounds, have been advanced for this syndrome; inapparent or underlying infection is doubtless important.

Clinical Findings: While the signs are variable depending on the cause, they include: apathy, prostration, rapid thready pulse, rapid respiration, thirst, low temperature and blood pressure, oliguria and hemoconcentration (except in hemorrhage).

Treatment: The prime goal in treatment is to restore blood volume and pressure. This can best be accomplished by infusions with colloids and buffered multiple electrolyte solutions (e.g., ℞ 565). In severe hemorrhage, the colloid should be in the form of blood; in other types of shock, plasma can be used. Plasma substitutes (e.g., gelatin, dextrans) may be used when neither blood nor plasma is available, but not as effectively, and some undesirable reactions have been seen.

It is generally recommended in the treatment of shock that buffered multiple electrolyte solution should form the bulk of the infused fluid—at least 3 parts electrolyte solution to one part blood. Ten milliliters of total fluid per pound of body weight will approximate one-fourth of the normal volume and is a good rule-of-thumb dose, to be given in an hour. In severe hemorrhage, up to 50 ml/lb should be given in 1 to 2 hours. The following additional measures should be taken: (1) Hemorrhage, if present, should be controlled. (2) Pain should be relieved, not only for the relief of the patient, but because it may aggravate the shock. Morphine (℞ 592) or meperidine (℞ 590) given IV are the most useful drugs for this purpose. (3) Antibiotics are of value in all cases of shock and should be given at once. Full doses of penicillin-streptomycin combinations, or one of the tetracycline series should be given. (4) The corticosteroids (hydrocortisone, prednisone, dexamethasone) and ACTH are often helpful since they have the ability to combat stress (q.v., p. 587). In acute shock states, corticosteroids can be given early, in large doses, IV. (5) Oxygen therapy is useful, but it must be appreciated that the body can withstand the effects of a good circulation of "poor" blood much better than it can deal with a poor circulation of "good" blood. (6) Vasoconstrictor drugs, epinephrine (℞ 511), levarterenol (℞ 513), or pentylenetetrazole (℞ 640) should be given only when shock is characterized by vasodilation (as from spinal anesthesia). In other forms of shock, vessels are, in any case, constricted reflexly, and they then become weakened from anoxia; therefore, these drugs are contraindicated. (7) The body temperature should be maintained but not raised. "Keeping the patient warm" can be overdone to a point where it encourages vasodilation and thus operates to accentuate the shock syndrome.

Animals that require treatment for shock should be observed carefully for some time following apparent recovery, since serious relapses may occur.

CYCLIC NEUTROPENIA IN GRAY COLLIE DOGS

(Gray Collie syndrome, Silver Collie
syndrome, Periodic myelodysplasia)

A rare and apparently heritable hematologic disease, characterized by cyclical recurrence of severe neutropenia, often associated with increased susceptibility to infection. Its heritability appears to be linked to coat color as it has been reported only in the gray Collie, but whether all the lethal effects associated with this coat color can be attributed to the one disease is still to be determined.

Affected dogs are usually noted from 6 weeks to 6 months of age, and unless they are raised under close medical supervision, few live a full year. Both sexes are affected. Such dogs are smaller than their litter mates and commonly suffer repeated infections. During the 1- or 2-day neutropenic phases, which occur at about 10-day intervals, there is fever, anorexia, depression, weakness, arthralgia and sometimes gingivitis with shallow ulcers near the base of the teeth. During an episode the total white blood cell count may range from 5,000 to 7,000 cells/cu mm; no band neutrophils are seen and the total neutrophils may range from 38 to 500 cells/cu mm. Other signs include severe bilateral conjunctivitis and keratitis, vomiting and diarrhea, and commonly a terminal suppurative bronchopneumonia and pleuritis. Bone marrow biopsies indicate that there is a maturation defect early in the neutrophilic series.

Symptomatic and supportive therapy may extend the lives of such dogs, but obviously they should not be used for breeding purposes.

DIGESTIVE SYSTEM

APPETITE

Food intake: Appetite is determined by complex reflex mechanisms and is variable depending essentially on the caloric requirements of the individual and the quality, digestibility, energy content and palatability of the ration. The increased requirements of late pregnancy, lactation and repetitive muscular work result in increased food consumption. The food intake and productivity of grazing animals will vary according to the pasture species, its stage of growth and quality. The composition and the physical form of prepared rations have a marked influence on food intake (*see* nutrition section). There is considerable individual variation with respect to food intake. Many animals, fed to appetite, will consume nutrients in excess of their requirements and tend to obesity. This tendency is marked in certain individuals that are voracious or greedy. Other individuals, although apparently healthy, are poor feeders and just maintain body condition under similar circumstances.

For economic reasons certain classes of farm livestock are kept under conditions of restricted food intake. When such animals are fed in groups, individual variations in appetite and in speed of food consumption coupled with the effect of dominance can result in marked variations in food consumption between members of the group. This variation can lead to problems associated either with excessive food intake, such as fermentative diarrhea in individual calves suckling "cafeteria" style, or to problems associated with severe food restriction, such as reproductive failure in individual sows groupfed on restricted rations during pregnancy.

Palatability: Palatability has a recognized, although ill-defined, effect on appetite. Certain feed constituents are more palatable than others and rations consequently vary in palatability. Substances such as molasses in livestock feeds and sucrose in piglet creep feeds are incorporated in an attempt to increase palatability. Moldy feeds generally cause a temporary reduction in appetite in all species, and the provision of frequent small amounts of fresh creep feed to piglets induces greater consumption in areas where hot and humid conditions may lead to rapid feed deterioration. There is undoubtedly a difference in palatability between various pastures and this may be sufficient to severely reduce food intake. This is one cause of the weaner "ill-thrift" syndrome that occurs in lambs grazing certain pasture species in the autumn months in the Southern Hemisphere.

Overindulgent pet owners sometimes encourage selective appetite in dogs and cats by catering to or developing their taste for certain foods. Frequently this can lead to gross nutritional imbalance and to deficiency disease such as osteodystrophia fibrosa in animals fed solely on lean meat and heart, and to osteodystrophies associated with excess vitamin A in adult cats fed solely on liver. If a conventional diet is offered, these animals may exhibit psychic anorexia. This usually can be overcome by withholding food for a day or 2 until true hunger develops.

Decrease or loss of appetite (inappetence; anorexia): A temporary decrease in appetite may result from fear, excitement, violent exercise or even scarcely apparent changes in the character of the diet. More prolonged inappetence can result from emotional disturbance such as that caused by the housing or yarding of pastured sheep—especially hill-breeds of sheep. Cats may refuse to eat for long periods when confined away from their home environment.

Voluntary restriction of food intake occurs during lactation in sows that were fed to appetite during pregnancy and considerable weight loss will result. A voluntary restriction in food intake of fat ewes occurs in the terminal part of pregnancy and this may initiate pregnancy toxemia.

Impairment of food intake may occur without loss of appetite. Local inflammatory lesions or wounds of the lips or oral structures, pharynx or esophagus may result in a lowered food intake because of pain during eating. Similarly, diseases which impair food intake either through their effect on nervous control (botulism, tetanus) or through their effect on muscles controlling these functions (white muscle disease) will produce a similar syndrome.

A degree of inappetence varying to frank anorexia is present with most disease states and consequently its occurrence is of little diagnostic value; however, the degree to which it is manifest, the speed of its onset and the selectivity of its loss are of some value in differential diagnosis. Inappetence may occur in such diverse conditions as specific amino acid or B-vitamin deficiencies and chronic infectious disease. A severe degree of inappetence is usually present with hepatic or renal disease and with any condition in which there is alimentary-tract stasis, severe pain, high fever, toxemia or septicemia, and dementia or stupor.

Increased appetite (polyphagia): Increased appetite and thirst are seen in pancreatic fibrosis and diabetes mellitus in the dog although emaciation gradually develops. An increased appetite is sometimes seen in chronic malabsorptive states and may accompany certain pituitary tumors and hypothalamic dysfunctions. Helminth infections are said to be accompanied by increased food intake, however inappetence is generally present in animals showing frank clinical signs of parasitism. An increase in appetite occurs following recovery from any disease in which inappetence has been manifest although this may be transient in remittent conditions such as equine infectious anemia. An increase in food intake above the normal occurs following periods of starvation or severe food restriction. Animals gaining access to palatable feeds, especially animals on restricted food intake, will grossly overfeed, and this may be followed by severe digestive disturbances such as rumen overload in the cow and acute gastric impaction in the horse.

Perverted or depraved appetite (pica): A depraved appetite is shown by craving for substances not ordinarily considered as food. The several species vary in their predilection for foreign material. Cattle ingest cloth, leather, pieces of metal, wood, stones and carcass material such as bone and hide. They may also lick larger objects and the sides of buildings. Horses may ingest dirt or sand or chew bones. The tendency for them to chew wooden objects is often merely a vice. Sheep may ingest dirt, bones and frequently wool; puppies frequently swallow sticks, bones, feces and grass, and adult dogs may acquire the vice of ingesting foreign objects. Such activities predispose to traumatic lesions within the mouth, alimentary-tract obstruction and sand colics, botulism and poisoning with substances such as lead.

Pica most commonly is due to nutritional deficiency. It is classically associated with phosphorus deficiency, however, in all species it may occur with deficiency of protein, fiber, minerals and vitamins or salt. Boredom, especially in stabled animals, may lead to excessive licking and chewing, and on occasion apparent simple curiosity may result in the ingestion of foreign material. Pica may also accompany such conditions as gastritis, pancreatic disease, rabies and gingivitis associated with teething. Psychic disturbances in pigs, dogs and cats may result in the savaging and even the ingestion of the newborn by the dam. Animals may show addiction to certain poisonous plants such as Darling pea and locoweed.

Treatment: A careful clinical examination and survey of the diet history is necessary to determine the cause of the altered appetite and to distinguish between the temporary alterations due to the nature of the food, environment, or the physiologic and psychic state of the animal, and those changes due to disease. It is essential that the cause of the altered appetite be determined as in most cases the appetite will not return to normal until this is corrected.

If the loss of appetite is complete, IV feeding with dextrose and protein hydrolysates or oral force feeding or both may be necessary. Liquids or semi-liquids can be pumped through a stomach tube in dogs, horses, cattle, sheep and swine. Cats may be intubated with a No. 8 or 10 soft rubber catheter. Care must be taken to avoid aspiration pneumonia, especially in recumbent animals.

During the convalescent period the return of appetite can often be hastened by the provision of highly palatable feeds. The administration of B-vitamins parenterally, or orally in the form of brewers' yeast, is occasionally beneficial in stimulating the appetite (Ŗ 598). Corticosteroids effectively increase the appetite in some cases and anabolic steroids are used by some for this purpose in dogs and in horses. Various rumenatorics and tonics containing substances such as strychnine, organic arsenicals and vitamins have traditionally been used to stimulate appetite, however their efficacy is open to some doubt. Rumen inoculation (q.v., p. 1417) may be useful in cattle where rumen atony is a factor in anorexia or where the administration of oral antibiotics has resulted in disturbances of the rumen flora.

In cases of pica the nutritional deficiency must be identified and corrected.

DENTAL DEVELOPMENT

One of the many criteria that should be considered in the estimation of age is the appearance of the teeth, but tooth development is subject to variation and dogmatic statements on the age of any individual animal should be avoided. The ages given in the tables of tooth eruption and wear are averages, which will be accurate for most animals, but may be quite erroneous for any individual. The most valuable criterion is eruption, when the tooth breaks through the gum. To make use of this sign, one must know the deciduous and permanent dental formulas, the table of eruption and the difference in appearance between deciduous and permanent teeth.

DENTAL FORMULAS

	Deciduous	Permanent
Horse	$2\left(\text{Di}\frac{3}{3}\text{Dc}\frac{0}{0}\text{Dp}\frac{3}{3}\right) = 24$	$2\left(\text{I}\frac{3}{3}\text{C}\frac{1}{1}\text{P}\frac{3\text{-}4}{3}\text{M}\frac{3}{3}\right) = 40\text{-}42$
Ox Sheep Goat	$2\left(\text{Di}\frac{0}{3}\text{Dc}\frac{0}{1}\text{Dp}\frac{3}{3}\right) = 20$	$2\left(\text{I}\frac{0}{3}\text{C}\frac{0}{1}\text{P}\frac{3}{3}\text{M}\frac{3}{3}\right) = 32$
Swine	$2\left(\text{Di}\frac{3}{3}\text{Dc}\frac{1}{1}\text{Dp}\frac{3}{3}\right) = 28$	$2\left(\text{I}\frac{3}{3}\text{C}\frac{1}{1}\text{P}\frac{4}{4}\text{M}\frac{3}{3}\right) = 44$
Dog	$2\left(\text{Di}\frac{3}{3}\text{Dc}\frac{1}{1}\text{Dp}\frac{3}{3}\right) = 28$	$2\left(\text{I}\frac{3}{3}\text{C}\frac{1}{1}\text{P}\frac{4}{4}\text{M}\frac{2}{3}\right) = 42$
Cat	$2\left(\text{Di}\frac{3}{3}\text{Dc}\frac{1}{1}\text{Dp}\frac{3}{2}\right) = 26$	$2\left(\text{I}\frac{3}{3}\text{C}\frac{1}{1}\text{P}\frac{3}{2}\text{M}\frac{1}{1}\right) = 30$

Deciduous incisor teeth of domestic swine, ruminants and carnivores are distinctly smaller than those of the permanent set. In the horse, the deciduous incisor teeth approach the permanent teeth in size. However, the deciduous teeth have a distinct neck and lack the prominent medial groove of the labial surface of the permanent incisor dentition.

ESTIMATION OF AGE BY THE WEAR OF THE TEETH

Horse: After eruption, it takes about 6 months for the tooth to grow out far enough to be in wear. When the entire occlusal (table) surface is in wear, the outer and inner enamel rings are completely separated by yellow dentin and the tooth is said to be level. Evidence derived from the eruption and leveling of the teeth should be given more weight than the signs given below.

The disappearance of the black cavity or cup in the infundibulum is much used in the estimation of age. It is not wholly reliable because it depends on the depth of the enamel infundibulum and the amount of cementum in the bottom, both of which are variable. The cups are supposed to disappear from lower I 1, I 2, and I 3 at 6, 7 and 8 years, but this sign should be evaluated with the leveling of the teeth. For example, if the cup is gone from I 1, but I 3 is not yet in wear, the age probably is less than 5 years. The cups in the upper incisors are of little use in age estimation.

After the cup has disappeared, the bottom of the infundibulum remains, first as a long oval containing cementum, then as a small round spot of enamel near the lingual side of the tooth. The enamel spot remains in the majority of horses through the 16th year.

The dental star is the darker dentin that fills the pulp cavity as the tooth wears. It appears first at 8 years as a dark-yellow transverse line in the dentin on the labial side of infundibulum of I 1. As the enamel spot recedes toward the lingual side, the dental star becomes oval and moves to the middle of the occlusal surface. It reaches this position in all the lower incisors at 13. At 15, the dental stars are round. The star should not be confused with the enamel spot, which wears more slowly than the dentin and, therefore, remains elevated.

The shape of the occlusal surface changes as the tooth is worn down. At first, it is a long oval with the long diameter transverse. Then the lingual side becomes much more strongly curved, the 2 diameters become equal and the tooth is said to be round. At a later stage, the tooth is triangular with the apex toward the tongue. Finally, the tooth appears compressed from side to side with the long diameter sagittal. This final stage has been called biangular. The transitional forms

ERUPTION OF THE TEETH

	Horse	Ox	Sheep, Goat	Swine	Dog	Cat
Di 1	Birth to 1 week	Before birth	Birth to 1 week	2-4 weeks	4-5 weeks	2-3 weeks
Di 2	4-6 weeks	Before birth	1-2 weeks	6-12 weeks	4-5 weeks	3-4 weeks
Di 3	6-9 months	Birth to 1 week		Before birth	5-6 weeks	3-4 weeks
I 1	2½ years	1½-2 years	1-1½ years	1 year	2-5 months	3½-4 months
I 2	3½ years	2-2½ years	1½-2 years	16-20 months	2-5 months	3½-4 months
I 3	4½ years	3 years	2½-3 years	8-10 months	4-5 months	4-4½ months
Dc	Does not erupt	*Birth to 2 weeks	*3-4 weeks	Before birth	3-4 weeks	3-4 weeks
Dp 2	Birth to 2 weeks	Birth to 3 weeks	Birth to 4 weeks	6-10 months	5-6 weeks	5 months
C	4½-5 years	*3¼-4 years	*3-4 years	5-7 weeks	4-6 months	Upper: 2 months; Lower: none
Dp 3	Birth to 2 weeks	Birth to 3 weeks	Birth to 4 weeks	1-4 weeks	4-6 weeks	4-5 weeks
Dp 4	Birth to 2 weeks	Birth to 3 weeks	Birth to 4 weeks	1-4 weeks	6-8 weeks	4-6 weeks
P 1 (wolf tooth)	5-6 months	None	None	5 months	4-5 months	None
P 2	2½ years	2-2½ years	1½-2 years	12-15 months	5-6 months	Upper: 4½-5 mo.; Lower: none
P 3	3 years	1½-2½ years	1¼-2 years	12-15 months	5-6 months	5-6 months
P 4	4 years	2½-3 years	1½-2 years		5-6 months	5-6 months
M 1	9-12 months	5-6 months	3-5 months	8-12 months	4-5 months	4-5 months
M 2	2 years	1-1½ years	9-12 months		6-7 months	None
M 3	3½-4 years	2-2½ years	1½-2 years	18-20 months	6-7 months	None

* The canine tooth of domestic ruminants has commonly been accounted a fourth incisor.

are hard to classify and I 3 does not follow the pattern very closely. Consequently, the times of change given in the literature vary with the investigator. It is agreed that I 1 and I 2 become round at 9 and 10, and all incisors triangular by 16 and 17.

The so-called 7-year hook is the result of the failure of the lower I 3 to wear all of the occlusal surface of the upper I 3. An overhang is left at the back of the upper tooth. This hook is supposed to appear at 7, wear off at 9 and appear again at 11.

Galvayne's groove is a longitudinal groove in the labial surface of upper I 3. It is located midway in the length of the tooth so that at first it is concealed in the alveolus, then gradually emerges from under the gum as the tooth grows out, and finally disappears as the ungrooved proximal part of the tooth comes into view. The cementum in the groove remains as a dark line, while that on the rest of the tooth is worn off to expose the white enamel. According to Galvayne, the groove appears at the gum line at 10, extends halfway down the tooth at 15, reaches the occlusal surface at 20 and disappears by 30. The groove is of little value as a single indicator of age. If it is present, the horse probably is over 10. The length of the groove or the absence of it can only be used in conjunction with other signs.

There are 3 other general indications of age. The angle formed by the upper and lower incisors, when the teeth are viewed in profile, becomes more acute with age. When the teeth are viewed from the front, they are seen to diverge from the median plane in a young horse and to converge in an old one. The arcade of the incisors, when seen from the occlusal surface, is a half-circle in the young horse and a straight line in the old.

The more useful signs are arranged chronologically in the following list:

5 YEARS: I 1 and I 2 level, labial border of I 3 in wear.
6 YEARS: Cup gone from I 1.
7 YEARS: All lower incisors level. Cup gone from I 2. Hook in upper I 3. Cementum has worn off, changing the color from yellow to bluish white.
8 YEARS: Dental star appears in I 1. Cup gone from I 3.
9 YEARS: I 1 round.
10 YEARS: I 2 round. The distal end of Galvayne's groove emerges from the gum on upper I 3.
13 YEARS: The central enamel spot is small and round in the lower incisors. The dental stars are in the middle of the table surfaces.
15 YEARS: Dental stars round, dark and distinct. Galvayne's groove halfway down.

16 YEARS: I 1 and I 2 triangular.
17 YEARS: I 3 triangular. Enamel spots gone from lower incisors.

Ox: As in the horse, the signs of wear are much less reliable than eruption for the estimation of age.

5 YEARS: All incisors are in wear. The occlusal surface of I 1 is beginning to become level; that is, the ridges on the lingual surface of the tooth are wearing out and the corresponding border of the occlusal surface is becoming a smooth curve instead of a zigzag line.
6 YEARS: I 1 is leveled and the neck has emerged from the gum.
7 YEARS: I 2 is leveled and the neck is visible.
8 YEARS: I 3 is leveled and the neck is visible. I 4 may be level.
9 YEARS: I 4 is leveled and the neck is visible.

Dog: The data given below were found reliable in about 90% of large dogs. Small dogs and dogs with undershot or overshot jaws give misleading results.

1½ YEARS: Cusps worn off lower I 1.
2½ YEARS: Cusps worn off lower I 2.
3½ YEARS: Cusps worn off upper I 1.
4½ YEARS: Cusps worn off upper I 2.
5 YEARS: Cusps of lower I 3 slightly worn. Occlusal surface of lower I 1 and I 2 rectangular. Slight wear of canines.
6 YEARS: Cusps worn off lower I 3. Canines worn blunt. Lower canine shows impression of upper I 3.
7 YEARS: Lower I 1 worn down to root so that occlusal surface is elliptical with the long axis sagittal.
8 YEARS: Occlusal surface of lower I 1 is inclined forward.
10 YEARS: Lower I 2 and I 1 have elliptical occlusal surfaces.
12 YEARS: Incisors begin to fall out.

LARGE-ANIMAL DENTISTRY

Signs of Dental Disease: Of large domestic animals, the horse is most affected by dental irregularities and disease. This section, therefore, is devoted mainly to a consideration of equine dentistry, although in many cases the remarks also apply to cattle.

Foreign bodies may occasionally become wedged between the dental arcades or lodged in the soft tissues of the mouth cavity, causing irritation, discomfort and excessive salivation. Examination of the oral cavity reveals their presence and dictates the method of removal. The possible presence of rabies should be kept in mind.

Dental troubles affect the rate of mastication. During the chewing process, the horse may stop for a few moments, then start again. Sometimes the head is held to one side as if the animal were in pain. Occasionally "quidding", in which the horse picks up its food, forms it into a bolus and then lets it fall from the mouth after partially chewing it, is seen. Occasionally the semi-chewed mass, instead of being dropped, becomes packed between the teeth and cheeks.

In some instances, to avoid using a painful tooth, a horse may bolt its food, with indigestion and colic as a frequent result. Unmasticated grain may be noticed in the feces. However, this sign may indicate nothing more than a greedy feeder.

Other signs include: excessive salivation; blood-tinged mucus from the mouth, usually caused by sharp teeth lacerating the buccal mucosa; fetid breath; swelling of the face or jaw; lack of desire to eat any hard grain; loss of condition; and loss of coat luster.

CONGENITAL IRREGULARITIES OR ABNORMALITIES IN DEVELOPMENT

Abnormal number of teeth: It is rare to encounter a reduction in the number of teeth in the horse. Supernumerary teeth occasionally are encountered in the incisor or molar regions. Their extraction is not recommended unless they cause mechanical interference with mastication or are irritated by the presence of the bit, in which case surgical removal is indicated. For the same reason the removal of wolf teeth is recommended. They may require periodic rasping or trimming to prevent damage to neighboring soft tissues.

Irregularities of development or shedding of the teeth: The eruption of temporary teeth may cause trouble that is transitory. Sometimes the temporary teeth are shed prematurely leaving a depression of the gum surrounded by an inflamed margin. This may cause a temporary loss of condition resulting from the discomfort of eating. The root of the temporary tooth may be absorbed, but the crown persist as a covering or "cap" to the erupting permanent tooth; these retained caps are readily removed with forceps.

Abnormalities in position and direction of individual teeth: This condition may be encountered in the incisor region. Some of these teeth may be rotated on the long axis, or may overlap adjacent teeth. Most abnormal positions of incisors are caused by injuries.

Imperfect apposition of the teeth: (a) **Parrot mouth (overshot jaw),** where the upper jaw overhangs the lower jaw, results in imperfect apposition of the teeth of the upper and lower incisors. (b) **Sow mouth (undershot jaw, prominent chin, bulldog jaw)** is the opposite of parrot mouth, but is less common in horses. If a foal is badly affected, sucking is an impossibility. Treatment, where feasible, in both parrot and sow mouth consists of rasping or shearing the offending points and projections. Braces have been used with some success in parrot mouth in foals. It should be noted that it is possible for the molar arcades to have anterior and posterior projections without parrot or sow mouth.

Ectopic teeth: The best example of this is the dentigerous cyst or so-called temporal odontoma, which most commonly is located in the mastoid process of the petrous portion of the temporal bone and is recognized by the presence of a discharging sinus near the base of the ear. The only treatment is surgical removal of the teratomatous mass of dental tissue and the associated secretory membrane.

IRREGULARITIES OF WEAR

Irregularities are very common in the teeth of the molar region of mature or old horses.

Sharp teeth: This is the commonest dental "disease" in the horse and is characterized by the presence of sharp edges or points on the cheek teeth. The outer or buccal margin of the upper arcade and the inner or lingual margin of the lower arcade are affected. In severe cases, lacerations are seen on the buccal and lingual mucosa. Treatment consists of rasping or cutting the long projections. The aim is to remove the offending edges only.

Shear mouth: This can be considered an extreme form of sharp teeth usually due to arthritis of the tempero-mandibular articulation. There is an exaggerated obliquity of the molar tables. It usually is seen in old horses and may involve 2 or more opposing teeth and may be encountered in all arcades. The signs are identical with those of sharp teeth, except that the buccal edges of the upper teeth may wound the gum of the lower jaw and the lingual border of the lower arcade may injure the hard palate. Treatment is not very satisfactoy, but rasping or shearing is necessary in an attempt to restore as near normal alignment as possible. Hard feed may postpone the necessity for repeated treatment.

Wave mouth: Due to uneven wear of the teeth, a wave-like condition occurs on the molar arcades. The base of the biggest wave and opposing concavity usually occurs at the fourth cheek teeth. In some cases, the teeth are worn to gum level, permitting the opposing teeth to cut into the gum and give rise to alveolar periostitis. Treatment is not very successful despite the removal of the offending wave. Severe cases require attention to the secondary alveolar periostitis.

Step mouth (step-formed tables): In this condition, there is a sudden variation in the height of adjacent molars. It may be caused by the loss or extraction of a tooth from the opposite arcade, or a fracture through the mandible. Clinical signs are the same as those caused by dental trouble in general. Cutters are necessary to remove the elongations. The float should be used after shearing affected teeth. Removal of any affected or loose teeth should be carried out.

Smooth mouth: In this condition, the tables become smooth either through the crown being worn down to the root or through a defect in the tooth substance. This defect is presumed to be due to an equal rate of wear of the dentin and enamel. Clinical signs are not of pain or inability to masticate, but the results of improper mastication, e.g., colic attacks and general unthriftiness. It is most commonly seen in the older horse, but may occur in young animals. Smooth surfaces will be noted on manual examination of the tables. Treatment is unsatisfactory. Feeding mashes or chopped feed will allow time for the different dental tissues to become uneven in wear. Even so, the condition probably will recur.

ALTERATIONS IN THE SUBSTANCE OF THE TEETH

Fractures or fissures of the teeth: The incisors sometimes are affected as a result of trauma sustained in accidents. In the case of the cheek teeth, fracture usually is caused by the horse closing the jaws on some unexpected hard substance, such as a stone or piece of metal. Cows rarely fracture a molar tooth in this way since the object is swallowed immediately after being picked up. The fourth cheek tooth, which bears the brunt of the chewing process, is most commonly affected. If the fracture extends to the root, alveolar periostitis will result.

Treatment consists of removing any obvious spicules and smoothing the remaining roughened edge. If the fracture involves the root, the tooth must be extracted.

Dental caries: There is some doubt that herbivorous animals are affected with caries, the belief being that when this condition does occur, it is secondary to alveolar periostitis. The abnormality may be termed "pseudocaries" or, more expressively, "decayed tooth". The term applies to a destruction of the cement and dentin, the enamel being left comparatively intact since it is much more resistant to decay. In large animals, damage to the tooth and the formation of a small cavity on the table permit food particles to undergo decomposition within the cavity. Bacterial activity aids in the process of destruction until eventually the pulp cavity is invaded and alveolar periostitis results. An early case is seldom brought in for attention, but in such a case, careful examination reveals a small black spot on the table. Other signs usually are those of alveolar periostitis.

ALVEOLAR PERIOSTITIS
(Periodontal disease, Pyorrhoea alveolaris)

Chronic ossifying alveolar periostitis (odontoma, pseudo-odontoma): This is characterized by the formation of an exostosis at the root of the affected tooth. The swelling is slow to develop and greatly hinders the extraction of the affected tooth. The cause is believed to be a low-grade infection of the alveolar periosteum leading to a periostitis and osteitis with subsequent new bone formation over the root of the involved tooth. Removal of the affected tooth is indicated.

Purulent or acute suppurative alveolar periostitis: In this condition, the periosteum usually is thickened and extremely vascular. Erosion of the tooth follows and, if any of the last 3 or 4 upper molars are involved, maxilary sinusitis usually results. In the lower jaw, osteomyelitis and a dental fistula may follow.

Anything which leads to exposure of the alveolus may give rise to the disease, e.g., separation of the gum from the crown, lodgement of food between the teeth, caries, fissures or fractures of the teeth, also where the teeth have become worn down to the level of the gum as sometimes occurs in old horses. The condition affects the cheek teeth and only rarely the incisor teeth, in which case it usually is secondary to compound fracture involving the alveolus or injury to the interalveolar space. The most commonly involved teeth are the fourth and third molars in that order. In cattle, actinomycosis of the jaws predisposes to the condition; it should be considered whenever loose cheek teeth are encountered in cattle.

Very often, the first sign is a purulent, unilateral nasal discharge if the affected tooth has its roots in the maxillary sinus. The pus is fetid and characteristic of the smell of necrotic bone. Other signs, as mentioned under signs of dental trouble, are evident. In the lower jaw there usually is an enlargement of the mandible over the root of the affected tooth. The gum around the tooth is inflamed and recedes from the crown of the affected tooth. Pus also may be evident in and around the socket. There may be displacement of the affected tooth by virtue of the compression of the jaws. In the upper jaw, the tooth is displaced laterally, while in the lower jaw, it is displaced medially. Sometimes, the formation of a dental fistula occurs. When alveolar periostitis is suspected, every tooth and also the entire gum region should be examined with meticulous care. Radiographs are often necessary for an accurate diagnosis. The affected tooth should be removed.

DENTAL FISTULA

A fistula connecting the root of a tooth and the exterior, the maxillary sinus, or the nasal cavity. Causes are alveolar periostitis or external injury with secondary infection. In the former case, the disease spreads from the tooth outwards, while in the latter, the condition originates at the site of trauma and by a process of osteomyelitis extends to the tooth root. Removal of the affected tooth is indicated.

DISEASES AND CONDITIONS OF THE MOUTH (LG. AN.)

CONTUSIONS AND WOUNDS OF THE LIPS AND CHEEKS

In large animals, wounds of the lips and cheeks are most commonly encountered in the horse as a result of falls, kicks, inhumane bits, bites, or tears from projecting objects. The vascularity of the region means rapid healing as a rule, except when a penetrating wound gives rise to a fistula. Treatment is routine. When a laceration involves the border of the lip, suturing should commence at that border to obtain the best cosmetic effect. If penetrating wounds are encountered, deep sutures must be placed in addition to those approximating the skin edges.

LAMPAS
(Palatitis)

A hardening and swelling of the mucous membrane of the hard palate just behind the upper incisor arcade in horses. In young horses, it is largely associated with the change from temporary to permanent dentition. In older horses, it is more in the nature of a passive congestion of the region. Examination of the mouth shows that the most anterior rugae of the hard palate extend below the level of the adjacent incisor teeth, causing pain when the horse attempts to eat. The affected region is hard and swollen.

The animal should be placed on a laxative diet of soft feed. Feeding of roots, such as turnips, is advocated by some. The old horse with this condition should be fed from a manger or rack rather than from the ground. Recovery is generally spontaneous and uneventful.

CLEFT PALATE

This condition is occasionally found in newborn animals of all species. The sole cause was long thought to be hereditary but recent evidence indicates that ingestion of toxic agents by the pregnant female and viral infections during pregnancy are also causes. The initial sign is milk dripping from the nostrils when the newborn animal attempts to nurse. Respiratory infections due to inhalation of food commonly occur. Visual inspection of the mouth readily reveals the cleft palate. Attempts to surgically correct the condition are open to question because of ethical considerations and poor results.

STOMATITIS

A nonspecific inflammation of the mucosa of the oral cavity. Stomatitis may be caused by trauma or chemical irritants. The most common causes of traumatic injury are awns of barley, fox-tail, porcupine grass and spear grass. Chemical stomatitis arises most commonly from oral contact with irritant drugs such as leg blisters. Consumption of plants of the crowfoot family, especially those containing anemenol (buttercups, crocus, pasque flower, cowslips) and prolonged medication with mercurials, arsenicals and iodides also result in stomatitis.

Examination of the oral cavity and tongue reveals local or generalized areas of acute inflammation. In chemically induced stomatitis the buccal mucosa may be edematous and coated with a catarrhal exudate. The regional lymph nodes may be enlarged.

The first clinical sign of disease is excessive frothy salivation, or in the case of plant awns, a reluctance to permit manual examination of the mouth cavity. Animals often exhibit evidence of irritation of the mouth, i.e., stand with their mouths open, loll their tongues or chew with their heads turned sideways. They soon develop difficulty in eating. Usually, the breath has a putrid or sweetish odor. Actinobacillosis (wooden tongue) must be considered in a differential diagnosis in cattle.

Most animals make rapid and uneventful recoveries when the cause is removed. Treatment is necessary only in severe cases. If there is marked inflammation, treatment with a broad-spectrum antibiotic is advisable. Mild antiseptics such as a solution of 0.5% hydrogen peroxide, 5% sodium bicarbonate and 1 to 3% potassium chlorate used as a mouthwash may hasten recovery.

INFECTIOUS BOVINE ULCERATIVE STOMATITIS

A nonfatal, moderately contagious, viral infection of cattle which usually involves most of the animals in a herd. All ages are susceptible.

The most prominent clinical findings are erosions and ulcers in and around the mouth, anorexia and marked loss of weight. The irregularly shaped superficial erosions measure up to 1 cm in diameter and 2 mm in depth. They occur on the tongue, lips, buccal mucosa, palate, muzzle, nostrils, the anterior part of the turbinates and the skin surrounding the mouth. Affected animals usually try to eat, but ordinary rations irritate the lesions. The animals exhibit oral sensitivity and bleeding from the erosions may occur. Diarrhea is absent, which distinguishes it from bovine virus diarrhea, and temperature is normal. The course is 2 to 3 weeks for an individual and 6 to 8 weeks for a herd.

Diagnosis is made on the basis of clinical and pathologic manifestations. There is no confirmatory laboratory test except isolation and characterization of the causative virus.

The most effective therapy is to remove animals from coarse rations and offer them soft feeds, such as chopped green fodder or silage. In particularly severe cases, local treatment with mild antiseptics may be helpful. Development and final resolution of the lesions runs a definite course, regardless of medication. Herd-to-herd transmission can be prevented by sanitary measures.

MYCOTIC STOMATITIS

A distinctive stomatitis of cattle that commonly occurs in the late summer and early fall in the Southern and Western five-eighths of the U.S.A. It does not often appear north of a line drawn from Baltimore to Salt Lake City and extended to Vancouver, Canada.

Etiology: The cause is unknown. Many believe it to be an allergic reaction to fungi that infect pasture grasses in late summer and fall while others believe it is caused by the virus that produces bluetongue in sheep.

Clinical Findings: The chief clinical signs are inflammation of the mucous membranes of the mouth, superficial erosions of the epidermis, and lameness. Stomatitis and epidermal exfoliation generally are more marked in older animals and lameness less marked, while in younger animals, lameness is most pronounced and stomatitis less severe. The first sign is frothy salivation. Shortly, small erosions or ulcers can be detected on the mucosa of the lips, dental pad and anterior margins of the tongue. Within a few days, these lesions become covered with accumulations of necrotic tissue. Usually in about a week, extensive necrosis of the mucosa of the anterior part of the oral cavity and tongue has occurred. In most cases, only the anterior portion of the oral cavity is affected, but in severe cases necrosis of the entire oral cavity, tongue and muzzle occurs. The breath is fetid.

Lameness, apparently caused by laminitis, occurs early in the course of the disease. Affected animals lie most of the time and are extremely reluctant to rise. Severely lame animals generally walk on their heels, with a stiff gait; a few walk on their toes with a stilted gait. In many herds, lameness is the only sign of disease in young animals. Marked edema above the hoof occurs in many young animals. A bluish sensitive line above the coronary band, similar to that described in cases of bluetongue in sheep, occurs in some cases. Some degree of lameness usually persists for 2 to 3 weeks. Many older animals with marked oral involvement exhibit little or no lameness during the entire clinical course.

Exfoliation of the epidermis of the teats, udder and perineal region sometimes occurs. Some animals have nasal discharges. Severely affected animals have profuse diarrhea with much mucus and blood in the feces.

The course varies greatly, but, in extreme cases, recovery usually takes place in 1 to 3 weeks. The herd morbidity rate usually is low (5 to 20%) and the few fatalities observed result from secondary bacterial infection.

Lesions: The only striking pathologic changes, other than the necrotic stomatitis and epidermal exfoliation, are hyperemia, hemorrhage and necrosis of the alimentary canal extending from the omasum to the rectum.

Treatment: No specific treatment is available. Antihistamine drugs may give temporary relief. The use of very mild oral antiseptics helps to remove the necrotic debris and hasten healing. Strong mouthwashes should be avoided. Antiseptic ointments may be used to hasten healing of the teat lesions which cause much discomfort to milking cows. Affected animals should be removed from pasture and fed a soft diet made into a slop or gruel.

PHLEGMONOUS STOMATITIS AND CELLULITIS

An acute, deep-seated, diffuse, rapidly spreading inflammation of the oral mucosa, pharynx and surrounding structures, including the subcut. tissue. It occurs sporadically in cattle of all types and enzootically in some of the intensive dairying areas of the Midwestern U.S.A. The cause is not completely understood, but hemolytic streptococci or coliform organisms usually can be isolated early in the disease.

The onset of clinical signs is sudden. An animal may progress from normal to near death in 24 hours. The first sign is excessive, watery salivation, usually associated with excessive lacrimation. These changes are accompanied by a febrile reaction, with a temperature of 105° to 107°F and an increase in pulse and respiratory rates. The animal usually refuses to eat or drink. There is marked swelling of the tissues of the face, around the mouth and nostrils and in the intermandibular space. The affected tissues are painful and edematous. Breath is foul and large sheets of superficial oral epithelium peel off. A severe toxemia with weakness is characteristic. Large pockets of fluid may form in the mandibular region and along the trachea.

Some of the milder cases recover spontaneously, but the more severely affected animals usually die unless treated.

Treatment: Sulfonamides (R 75, 82) administered IV during the acute phases of the disease, may be effective in controlling the infection. Oral therapy may be employed when the patient is again able to swallow. Penicillin (R 44) is also effective. Injection of part of the dose of penicillin into the diseased tissue is recommended.

Massive submandibular edema, all abscesses, and accumulations of fluid that develop following recovery should be drained surgically.

PROLIFERATIVE STOMATITIS OF CATTLE

A common and relatively innocuous viral disease of calves usually occurring before 6 months of age. A hyperkeratotic diet may be required to initiate the lesion in cattle over a month of age. Up to 5% of the calves which pass through some of the large public stockyards in the upper Midwest (U.S.A.) develop the condition. Cattle over 2 years old are rarely affected. The only clinical signs are wart-like proliferations usually measuring 0.5 to 1 cm in diameter on the tongue, lips, palate and buccal mucosa. Seldom are cases serious enough to warrant treatment. Animals usually recover spontaneously in 1 to 3 months and are immune.

PAPULAR STOMATITIS OF CATTLE

This mild disease of cattle from 1 month to 2 years of age is caused by a virus and up to 100% of a susceptible herd may become affected. Lesions occur on the muzzle, inside the nostrils and on the buccal mucosa, and consist of reddish raised papules measuring 0.5 to 1 cm in diameter which appear active for about a week and then regress. Evidence of the healed lesion may be present for several weeks. There is no systemic disturbance; the disease is important chiefly because of the confusion it may cause in the clinical diagnosis of the several forms of stomatitis of cattle.

ULCEROMEMBRANOUS GINGIVITIS OF SHEEP

This condition has been recorded in sheep in New Zealand and is believed to be identical with trench mouth in humans. *Sphaerophorus necrophorus* has been mentioned as the cause. The condition is encountered in animals from 2 years of age onward. Ulceration of the gums is followed by involvement of the dental alveoli and loosening of the teeth. In the early stages, the IM administration of one-half million units of penicillin daily for 5 days has given good results; even previously loose teeth become firm.

SMALL-ANIMAL DENTISTRY AND DENTAL EMERGENCIES

CONGENITAL ABNORMALITIES OF THE MOUTH

CLEFTS

Clefts are the most common congenital abnormality involving the lips of small animals.

Cheiloschisis, commonly called harelip, is due to failure of the processes making up the jaws and face during embryonic development. The malformation is probably hereditary, although the mode of transmission is not clear. Nutritional deficiencies in the dam as well as certain stresses imposed during pregnancy are also suspected as at least contributory factors. Cleft of the lower lip is rare and usually occurs in the median line. Clefts of the upper lip are generally found at the junction of the premaxilla and maxilla. These may be unilateral or bilateral, incomplete or complete and are frequently associated with clefts of the alveolar process and palate. **Palate cleft** (palatoschisis) may involve the palate only or it may extend from the lip through the alveolar part of the upper jaw into the palate. The anomaly is due to aberrant development of various embryonic processes of the upper jaw. Heredity is again thought to play a definite role in its etiology, although faulty nutrition of the mother and mechanical interference to the fetus are known to cause these defects. Palatal clefts are frequently associated with other abnormalities. They are not readily apparent at birth. Frequently, the first indication of their presence is regurgitation of milk through the nose in small, undernourished puppies. If left untreated, the animals usually die from starvation or secondary infection of the nasopharynx or middle ear.

Treatment: Since clefts are often associated with other more serious congenital defects, the patient should be carefully examined before surgical correction is initiated. Such treatment is effective only if the defect is not too large. Furthermore, if surgical correction is decided upon, it should be carried out during the first few days or weeks of life, before the patient's general health is influenced by the defect. Lip clefts cause marked difficulty in nursing and the animal must be hand-fed until the correction is completed. Correction of palate clefts is much more difficult and usually not as satisfactory. Euthanasia is advisable in animals with gross defects, and those treated successfully should not be used for breeding purposes.

ABNORMALITIES IN THE DEVELOPMENT OF TEETH

Occasionally, imperfect development of the deciduous teeth has been reported, consisting usually of deviation from the normal in number and placement. Such anomalies occur seldom in dolichocephalic breeds, occasionally in the mesocephalic and very commonly in the brachycephalic breeds. Supernumerary teeth are usually unilateral and occur in the upper jaw more frequently than the lower. The number of teeth is seldom reduced except in the brachycephalic breeds. The greatest reduction involves the cheek teeth of the lower jaw.

Deviation in placement usually results from crowding in the dental arch. The upper third premolar is the first tooth to rotate as the muzzle is shortened by selective breeding. Later, all upper premolars may rotate. The molar teeth are seldom affected. Anomalous placements of teeth are more common in the upper than the lower dental arch. Occasionally, teeth are abnormally placed owing to an aberrant development of the tooth germ. Such deviations occur in all breeds.

The above abnormalities require no special treatment unless they cause malocclusion, in which case extraction or repositioning of the offending tooth is necessary.

DENTAL CARIES

Dental decay is not common in small animals, possibly because of the comparative absence of readily fermentable carbohydrates in their diets. In dogs, decay is usually seen on the table surfaces or in the region of the neck of the molar teeth. In the cat, erosion of the enamel is sometimes seen on the buccal surface of the molars and premolars, just below the gingival margin. On superficial examination, the teeth appear normal. Affected cats hesitate to chew their food; they stand over the dish of food and salivate, but do not eat. Seriously affected teeth should be filled or extracted.

DENTO-ALVEOLAR ABSCESS

An acute or chronic inflammation and infection of the apex of a tooth, the periodontal membrane and the periapical alveolar bone, usually originating in the dental pulp.

Etiology: Dento-alveolar abscesses may be caused by injury to the tooth or by infection from the root canal resulting from pulpitis or suppurative pericementitis.

Clinical Findings: Acute alveolar abscesses are seldom diagnosed in small animals but, when they are seen, the animal is usually presented with a history of reluctance to eat. A local swelling, frequently fluctuating, may be seen, but the tooth itself appears sound. A parulis, or gum boil, may be present near the involved tooth; at other times the infection may extend into the surrounding bone with continued pain but without visible evidence of abscessation.

In chronic abscesses, local inflammation of the gums appears near the affected tooth and is accompanied by soreness due to destruction of cortical bone over the apex of the tooth. Most commonly, the upper fourth premolar tooth in the dog is affected. An abscess developing at the root of this tooth may discharge through a fistula into the mouth (alveolar fistula), or it may extend by way of the sinus and rupture superficially on the face, forming a fistula usually below the eye (maxillary fistula). The discharge of pus through such a fistula is almost invariably intermittent in character. After the abscess ruptures, the pressure within the sinus is reduced, the skin lesion heals and the signs subside temporarily. Gradually, the swelling reappears below the eye, becomes larger as the internal pressure increases, until rupture and drainage recur. The complaint of the owner seldom refers to the tooth but to this draining fistula.

Diagnosis: Differentiation of chronic dento-alveolar abscess and chronic suppurative pericementitis may be difficult. In the latter, there ultimately is a pus pocket alongside the root of the tooth, followed by a detachment of the periodontal membrane from the cement. Radiographs of the suspected tooth are valuable in arriving at a diagnosis. Fetid, purulent saliva may be present if a dento-alveolar abscess drains into the mouth. A history of the animal hesitating to chew its food, coupled with an examination revealing reddening of the gingiva around a slightly painful tooth, should suggest a chronic dento-alveolar abscess, although the tooth may appear sound and no discharge is evident. Evidence of an intermittently draining fistula under the eye on the affected side is pathognomonic.

Treatment: If a fluctuant swelling is present near the affected tooth, ventral drainage coupled with parenteral penicillin (℞ 44) is sometimes successful in the treatment of an acute dento-alveolar abscess.

General anesthesia is necessary and endotracheal intubation is to be recommended to prevent aspiration of foreign materials during surgery and to maintain a patent airway. If a maxillary fistula is present, continuity should be established between the fistulous tract and the alveolus of the extracted tooth. Granulation tissue and necrotic bone should be removed by curettage. The tract is flushed daily with benzalkonium chloride solution (℞ 399) until the infection is controlled. Penicillin (℞ 44) or other systemic antibiotics (℞ 11, 29) should be administered for several days to combat local and possible systemic infection. The mouth should be flushed several times daily with salt solution (℞ 431), sodium bicarbonate solution (℞ 433) or benzalkonium chloride solution (℞ 399). A soft diet is recommended.

PERIODONTAL DISEASE
(Periodontitis, Pyorrhoea alveolaris)

An acute or chronic inflammation of the periodontal membrane characterized, in severe cases, by resorption of the alveolar bone, loosening of the teeth and often atrophy of the gums. It may be local, involving only one tooth, but is usually generalized.

Etiology: Mechanical irritation from calculus with subsequent infection probably is the most common cause. In some breeds of dogs, irregularities in form and position of the teeth resulting in food impactions and faulty occlusion (e.g., brachycephalic breeds) may be predisposing factors.

Functional insufficiency of the jaws due to lack of exercise in mastication may cause periodontal disturbance and subsequent disease. Atrophy of the supporting tissues of a tooth due to disuse after loss of its antagonist may lead to food impaction and periodontal disease. Improper feeding and systemic conditions such as diabetes mellitus, low-calcium intake, hyperparathyroidism, and chronic nephritis also may result in periodontal disease.

Clinical Findings: The signs usually noted are excess salivation, occasionally in appetence, but more frequently hesitation to masticate anything but soft foods. The teeth involved are usually painful when tapped or probed with a tartar scraper. Pain seems to be more severe early in the course of the disease, but subsides as the tooth becomes loosened in its alveolus. As the condition progresses, slight pressure on the tooth or gum causes small amounts of pus to exude from pockets around the tooth. Foul-smelling breath is a constant sign.

Lesions: The teeth are usually encrusted with calculus which when first deposited is soft, but soon becomes quite hard. As it accumulates, the calculus extends downward toward the gum, causing a progressive irritation. The gums become congested and swollen and bleed readily; the margin of the gum is pushed away from the neck of the tooth and becomes inflamed. If the calculus is not removed, food material becomes lodged between the edge of the calculus and the gum, and undergoes putrefaction, causing secondary infection around the neck of the tooth. A foul-smelling pus is formed and the tooth becomes loose in its socket. This leads to loss of a part or all of the tissue of the alveolar process, periodontal membrane and surrounding gum.

Patients with chronic systemic conditions, particularly chronic nephritis, have a slow-forming dental deposit which leads to a foul-smelling, low-grade inflammation of the gums which favors periodontal disease. Periodontal disease of the incisor teeth is of common occurrence in toy breeds with low-calcium or improper calcium-phosphorus intake.

Treatment: For the proper restraint of the patient, general anesthesia is to be recommended for the successful treatment of periodontal disease in small animals. All tartar, including that which is below the gum line, should be removed from the affected teeth as the initial phase of treatment. Seriously loosened or diseased teeth should be extracted.

Following removal of large calculus accumulations, involved teeth are usually somewhat loose. Many will regain their normal attachment with treatment.

After scaling and necessary extractions, the gums should be flushed with saline solution and painted with tincture of iodine (℞ 413) or zinc chloride solution (℞ 441). If the gums are hypertrophied, the excess tissue should be removed by electrocautery. Post-surgical administration of broad-spectrum antibiotics (℞ 29, 41) is indicated. Liquid or soft diets should be provided for several days until the gums have had adequate time to heal. Supportive therapy, including high dosages of injectable vitamin B-complex, seems helpful in hastening recovery and preventing recurrence. Daily irrigation of the gum margins (℞ 399, 431) is helpful in preventing food and debris accumulation until the gums are healed. To prevent recurrence, the teeth and gums should be observed closely and early tartar accumulations removed periodically. Owners are encouraged to feed solid foods and to provide large bones or hard rubber toys for gum and tooth exercise.

GINGIVITIS

An acute or chronic inflammation of the gums, characterized by congestion and swelling.

Etiology: Gingivitis may be caused by local irritation, by spread of infection from the other areas of the mouth, or may be secondary to a systemic disease. The most common local cause is dental calculus. Others are physical trauma, foreign bodies, dental caries and irritation from broken teeth. Most diseases of the mouth cause some degree of gingivitis by direct extension of the infection. Among the most prominent general conditions that cause gingivitis are: hypovitaminosis B, uremia and leptospirosis. Cats develop severe gingivitis secondary to most chronic debilitating diseases.

Clinical Findings and Diagnosis: Simple inflammatory gingivitis produces a narrow band of bright-red, inflamed gingival tissue surrounding the neck of a tooth. There may be edema with swelling of the intestinal papillae. The gums are friable and bleed easily. If untreated, the gums become more swollen, ulcerated and finally hypertrophied. Usually, the patient shows little discomfort.

Because gingivitis is frequently secondary to more serious systemic conditions, a thorough physical examination should be carried out in order to diagnose the primary disease.

Atrophic gingivitis is usually encountered in older patients or in animals with chronic gingivitis.

Treatment: Local causes, such as calculus deposits or dental caries, are dealt with by elimination. In systemic diseases supportive therapy must be employed. Hypertrophied gums may be excised if the lesions are not too extensive. Oral hygiene in the form of mouthwashes with benzalkonium chloride (℞ 399) or salt solution should be employed, regardless of the cause.

EPULIS
(Fibromatosis gingivae, Fibromatous epulis,
Ossifying fibroma, Gingival hyperplasia)

A benign, irregular fibrous neoplasm of the gums, usually originating in the region of the alveoli and involving much of the gum margin. It is a relatively insensitive, vascular, tough, fibrous connective tissue structure, with an irregular surface covered with epithelium. The growths usually have a broad base of attachment, are the color of the normal gum and may grow large enough to completely cover the buccal and labial surfaces of the teeth. Some predisposition to these growths seems to exist among certain brachycephalic breeds in which the condition is termed gingival hyperplasia or familial gingival hypertrophy.

The term epulis is also used by some when referring to giant-cell epulis or tumor of the gum of the dog. This tumor is usually single and characterized histologically by bizarre forms and giant cells. Malignant tumors of the gums (e.g., squamous-cell carcinoma or malignant melanoma) may also be called epulis, but should be differentiated and called by their proper names. Histopathologic examination is to be encouraged to assure proper diagnosis and hence treatment and prognosis.

Clinical Findings: Epulis is most common in older dogs. Animals with this condition are usually asymptomatic, although hair, food and debris may collect between the growth and the dental arcade causing irritation and halitosis.

Treatment: Treatment is unnecessary unless growths are large enough to interfere with mastication. If removal is necessary, electrosurgical techniques are most satisfactory. The mouth should be rinsed with benzalkonium chloride solution (℞ 399) for several days following surgery.

HEMORRHAGE FROM THE MOUTH

Etiology: Oral bleeding may be due to acute trauma, may follow extraction of diseased teeth or occur as secondary hemorrhage from a previous disease involving the oral mucosa, gingiva or periodontium. The hemorrhage may be spontaneous and prolonged when associated with hemophilia, diabetes mellitus, blood dyscrasias or infection. Wounds resulting from traumatic injuries are the most common causes of bleeding from the mouth in small animals. Accidental biting of the tongue or lips is not common, but does occur during convulsions. More common is the biting of a tumor in the mouth with subsequent bleeding. Bleeding may occur from ulcers in severe stomatitis or glossitis. Slight hemorrhage is occasionally encountered when the deciduous teeth are shed.

Clinical Findings: Hemorrhage ranging from blood-stained saliva to profuse venous or arterial bleeding is the obvious sign. In the case of foreign bodies or injuries to the mouth, the animal usually shows obvious signs of discomfort and annoyance by pawing and rubbing its muzzle. Larger foreign objects are evident on examination, as are larger wounds. Smaller foreign bodies and wounds may be difficult to locate because of the bleeding and an uncooperative patient. Anesthesia is sometimes needed. Very small wounds may cause profuse bleeding, especially if they are in a very vascular area such as the tongue, hard palate or gums. The constant movement of the tongue over the wound often prevents normal clotting and causes the bleeding to persist.

Treatment: If the wound is small and bleeding not severe, application of a cold pack held in place for a few minutes will usually control the hemorrhage.

Care must be taken to remove all foreign bodies, especially if small (e.g., porcupine quills), as they are easily overlooked if the mouth is not carefully examined. If bleeding is profuse, the damaged vessels must be isolated and ligated. Large lacerations of the mucosa should be sutured, while smaller wounds heal rapidly without repair. The rapid healing of most mouth wounds is probably due to the great vascularity of the tissue rather than to antiseptic properties of the saliva. Gelfoam (℞ 547) or gauze soaked in 1:1,000 epinephrine should be used as packs to place over areas of persistent oozing hemorrhage. Systemic aids to coagulation (℞ 546) may be used, but are not always successful.

In cases of gross laceration or fracture, broad-spectrum antibiotics such as tetracyclines (℞ 29) should be given prophylactically.

Injection of vitamin K (℞ 550) is effective in cases where bleeding is due to liver disease, bishydroxycoumarin poisoning or specific vitamin K deficiency. In rare cases, blood transfusions may be required to promote clotting and replace the blood loss.

POSTEXTRACTION PAIN AND SWELLING

The pain and swelling which occasionally follow extraction are usually due to operative trauma or to infection in the alveolus. This is noted only when several large, well-rooted or infected teeth are removed. It is rare for pain and swelling due to operative trauma to last more than 2 or 3 days following surgery. Infection can appear from one to several days following extraction and is characterized by hesitancy to eat, resistance to examination of the mouth, depression and fever. Examination of the mouth reveals swelling and sometimes suppuration.

Flushing the mouth with benzalkonium chloride solution (℞ 399) or with warm saline solution will keep the mouth relatively clean and prevent accumulation of foreign material in the alveolus. Liquid or soft diets should be given until the gums are healed. If infection is a problem, a systemic antibiotic (℞ 11, 29, 44) or sulfonamides (℞ 68) should be given. Sedatives are seldom needed.

TOOTH LUXATION AND FRACTURE

Since animals employ their teeth for apprehending food, gnawing, tearing, biting, fighting and carrying objects, their teeth are constantly subject to injuries.

Luxation of the teeth ranges from little more than loosening of the alveolus to complete avulsion. Luxation usually occurs as the result of fighting, automobile accidents, or accidental catching of the teeth in fences and cage doors. The teeth are occasionally driven into the nasal cavity, lip, cheek or tongue. If completely avulsed, they may be swallowed.

Luxation usually establishes a compound wound. Soft tissue is lacerated, bone is fractured (alveolus) and hemorrhage is usually present. The complete wound must be considered in treatment.

Totally or partially dislocated teeth are removed. Detached bone or soft tissue should also be removed and the area treated as for typical extraction. If a dislocated tooth is of special importance to the animal, it may be replaced in the alveolus and held in place by wire fixation to an adjacent tooth. These teeth usually become reattached to the alveolus and remain functional, but should be watched carefully and removed if diseased. A systemic antibiotic (℞ 29, 44) or a sulfonamide (℞ 66) should be given.

Fractured teeth are not uncommon in dogs and cats and are usually the direct result of fights or automobile accidents. Puppies may chew on hard objects and fracture their teeth. Evidence of a fractured tooth may be shown by the animal acting hungry, but hesitating to eat. Some animals are unable to retain saliva. Teeth with a part of the crown missing are often discovered during a routine examination of the mouth for other purposes. If the dog shows no sensitivity, the fractured tooth may remain indefinitely without causing trouble, provided the pulp is not exposed. Frequently, the lateral surface of a molar becomes split away, allowing tartar to accumulate and eventually resulting in periodontal disease.

If the pulp cavity is exposed, or if the fractured tooth is sensitive to pressure, heat or cold, either a root-canal procedure or extraction should be considered. In questionable cases, the owner should be advised of the presence of the fractured tooth and instructed to return the patient if the discomfort continues.

Mandibular fractures may result from difficulty at the time of extraction of the canine teeth or larger molars. This is a particular danger in older dogs when the mandible itself is fragile and the alveolar attachments have become ossified, making the tooth difficult to extract. Such fractures are repaired by wiring, pinning or other forms of immobilization.

DISEASES AND CONDITIONS OF THE MOUTH (SM. AN.)

CHEILITIS

An acute or chronic inflammation of the lips or lip folds.

Etiology: Wounds of varying severity comprise the most common lip lesions seen in small animals. Dogs occasionally chew such sharp objects as recently emptied tin cans, which may inflict slight or severe lip wounds. Fight wounds are common, and thorns, awns, burrs and fishhooks may imbed themselves in the lips and cause marked irritation or severe wounds.

Infections of the lips may be secondary to such wounds or

foreign bodies, but are more commonly associated with infections elsewhere on the body or in the mouth. Severe dental disease or stomatitis can produce cheilitis by direct extension. Licking areas of bacterial dermatitis or infected wounds may spread the infection to the lips and lip folds. Severe external otitis, especially in long-eared dogs, may extend to the commissures of the lips. Local or generalized bacterial skin infections in small pups often cause infection of the lips and other parts of the face.

Other causes are hypovitaminosis B, allergic reactions, demodectic and occasionally sarcoptic mange, eczema and other skin disorders and paralysis of the lips due to facial nerve damage. The heavy folds present at the mucocutaneous border of such breeds as Spaniels or St. Bernards may predispose to infections of these areas.

Clinical Findings and Diagnosis: Animals with cheilitis usually scratch or rub at their lips, have a foul breath, and occasionally salivate excessively or have anorexia. With chronic infection of the lip margins or folds, the hair in these areas is discolored, moist and matted with a thick, yellowish or brown, foul-smelling discharge. Removal of this discharge usually reveals hyperemia and sometimes ulceration of the underlying skin. Acute allergic reactions cause the lips to become edematous. Dogs that have been poisoned with bishydroxycoumarin or for other reasons have a clotting defect may show diffuse swelling of both the upper and lower lips due to hemorrhage. Since this swelling may resemble that seen with allergic reactions, a careful search for petechiae and ecchymoses in the skin and visible mucous membranes of other parts should be made. Hypovitaminosis B can cause slightly reddened, dry, crusty lesions with visible cracks in the skin at the commissure of the lips and ulceration and necrosis of the tongue and gums. The cause of cheilitis due to extension of infection from the mouth or from other areas of the body is usually easily detected because of the primary lesion.

Treatment: Wounds to the lips should be thoroughly cleaned, sutured if they are large enough to warrant it, and treated as if infected. A systemic antibiotic (℞ 44) should be administered for several days.

Infectious cheilitis which has spread from a lesion elsewhere usually improves with treatment of the primary lesion, but local treatment may also be necessary. When the infection is severe, hair should be completely clipped from the lesion and the area gently cleaned with a germicidal detergent (℞ 423), dried well and an antibiotic ointment (℞ 406) applied several times daily. Before each ointment application, the lesions may be rinsed with aqueous benzalkonium chloride solution (℞ 399).

Ulcerations and infections involving the skin folds at the mucocutaneous border of the lips are best handled by surgical extirpation. Mild cauterization using 5 to 10% silver nitrate solution is an acceptable alternative method but recurrence is common.

EOSINOPHILIC GRANULOMA OF CATS
(Rodent ulcer)

An inflammatory lesion of unknown origin on the lips of cats, characterized microscopically by ulceration of the surface epithelium, an underlying zone of necrosis and leukocytic infiltration, and a deeper layer containing large numbers of eosinophils. It usually involves the anterior portion of the upper lip, but additional lesions may also be seen on the lower lip, tongue, soft palate, wall of the pharynx and other areas of the oral mucosa.

Clinical Findings: The early lesion is a small plaque on the lip margin. It increases in size gradually and may involve the lip as far up as the nose. As the lesion enlarges, it assumes a typical brown, dry appearance and its edges roll over, giving the lip a characteristic scooped-out appearance. The lesions may be spread, apparently by licking, to other locations, such as the skin on the inner surface of the thigh, popliteal region or ventral abdomen. The cat constantly licks the affected parts, but otherwise they seem to have little adverse effect. Ulcers elsewhere in the mouth may cause some difficulty in mastication and deglutition. There is frequently an associated peripheral eosinophilia.

Treatment: No treatment is entirely satisfactory. Some cats respond dramatically to parenteral or topical corticosteroid therapy (℞ 152, 156). Removal of the lesion by electrosurgical techniques or surgical excision, repeated chemical cautery and radiation therapy have all been used with varying degrees of success. The latter methods usually leave a deformed lip.

STOMATITIS

An inflammation of the mouth which may be a primary disease of the oral cavity or secondary to systemic disease. The inflammation may be localized or diffuse, and the nature and severity of the lesions vary greatly. Glossitis (q.v., p. 106) and gingivitis (q.v., p. 96) are localized forms of stomatitis.

Etiology: Inflammatory lesions of the mouth may arise from infectious diseases, deficiency diseases, trauma or burns. Fusospirochetosis or Vincent's disease (q.v., p. 104) is perhaps the most common infectious stomatitis in the dog. Feline rhinotracheitis is frequently accompanied by ulcerative stomatitis, as is leptospirosis in the dog. Inflammation and secondary infection of the mouth are frequently seen with such systemic conditions as malnutrition, avitaminosis B, anemia and uremia. Local factors which may cause trauma include dental calculus, foreign bodies and burns of thermal, chemical or electrical origin.

Clinical Findings: Clinical manifestations vary greatly with the type and extent of inflammation. In most cases, especially in cats, there is complete or partial anorexia. Excessive salivation, especially when attempting to eat, is common. The oral mucosa is reddened and hyperemic. The epithelium desquamates easily. The animal may paw at its mouth, usually shows evidence of pain, and resents any attempt to examine its mouth. There is often an offensive odor to the breath and in the more serious infections, a thick, brown, foul-smelling discharge from the mouth, which is sometimes accompanied by bleeding. The animal frequently shows increased thirst. Regional lymph nodes may be swollen and tender.

Treatment: The first consideration is to determine the cause and, if possible, eliminate it. Thus, broken or diseased teeth should be extracted, tartar scaled from the remaining teeth and any foreign bodies removed. Oral discharges should be cultured, direct smears made and sensitivity tests performed. Systemic infections, and other disease conditions—e.g., vitamin deficiencies or anemia—should be appropriately treated in conjunction with symptomatic treatment of the stomatitis. Fusospirochetal disease requires vigorous local treatment and administration of penicillin (℞ 44) or penicillin and streptomycin (℞ 41) and injectable vitamin-B complex should be initiated promptly and continued for at least a week. Antimicrobial agents as polymyxin B, chloramphenicol and neomycin and glutamycin sulfate are utilized depending on the infectious agent present. Debridement of necrotic tissue promotes more rapid healing when followed by thorough irrigation of the mouth with mouthwashes, such as potassium permanganate solution (℞ 425), salt solution (℞ 431) or benzalkonium chloride solution (℞ 399). Small, painful ulcers may be cauterized with 5% silver nitrate (℞ 618). In gangrenous stomatitis, debridement or surgical excision of the lesions should be employed if the animal can safely be anesthetized. High dosages of vitamin C and the C-complex vitamins seem to hasten recovery in most types of stomatitis. Animals that are unable or refuse to eat should be given lactated Ringer's solution (℞ 565) or saline-dextrose parenterally (℞ 567) to prevent dehydration. Frequent offerings of a liquid diet and later semisolid foods will encourage eating.

ULCEROMEMBRANOUS STOMATITIS
(Fusospirochetosis, Vincent's infection,
Vincent's angina, Trench mouth)

This disease is caused by fusiform bacilli and spirochetes, which are normal inhabitants of the mouth, after some predisposing factor decreases the resistance of the oral mucosa. It frequently accompanies, or follows other infections or deficiency diseases. In cats it is seen most commonly in animals on a restricted diet and in conjunction with chronic debilitating diseases. The infection appears first as a gingivitis with redness and swelling of the gingival margins which are painful and bleed easily, and progresses to a necrotic gingivitis with ulceration and necrosis of the gingivo-alveolar tissues and the formation of pseudomembranes. Extension to other areas of the oral mucosa is common. There is a characteristic offensive odor, usually accompanied by escape of brown, purulent, slimy, fetid saliva which stains the muzzle and front legs. The infection may spread to the lower portions of the respiratory tract causing pneumonia. Spirochetal sinusitis, secondary to mouth infection, has been seen in cats. The diagnosis is confirmed by demonstrating the organisms in large numbers in stained smears of the exudate from the mouth.

Treatment: *See* p. 103.

GANGRENOUS STOMATITIS

Gangrenous stomatitis is characterized by rapid and massive destruction of tissue and most frequently occurs in avitaminosis B or as a sequela to Vincent's disease. It is also seen in advanced cases of uremia, especially those associated with subacute leptospirosis. The tip and free borders of the tongue are most commonly affected; the gum margin adjacent to the molars and premolars may also be involved and sometimes the condition extends throughout the mouth. It is usually accompanied by marked prostration and toxemia.

Treatment: *See* p. 103.

ULCERATIVE STOMATITIS

Ulcerative stomatitis, in both cats and dogs, is usually associated with systemic disease and is frequently pseudomembranous as well as ulcerative. The superficial destructive changes in the oral mucosa are very marked. In cats with rhinotracheitis, extensive lesions occur in the form of numerous, rapidly developing, shallow ulcers on the tongue and palate, and occasionally on the gums and buccal mucosa. Ulcerative stomatitis may also occur in cats as a primary entity. In these conditions, ulceration usually starts at the tip of the tongue, with reddening and loss of papillae. As the ulcer progresses, the mucosa is lost and a pseudomembrane may form. There is an accompanying increase in the flow of saliva which is clear early in the course, but may become discolored, blood-stained and fetid as the condition progresses. In dogs, ulcerative stomatitis is seen during the course of any severe systemic disease, or as a complication of catarrhal stomatitis. Debilitated or cachectic animals frequently exhibit oral ulceration and it may also accompany long-standing chronic disease, such as nephritis with uremia, or occur as a manifestation of avitaminosis B. In these conditions it usually precedes gangrenous or ulceromembranous stomatitis.

Traumatic ulcers of the mouth occur from irregular, fractured or diseased teeth. Erosions of the buccal mucosa may result from constant abrasion caused by excessive accumulations of tartar. These lesions are usually superficial with only circumscribed loss of epithelium, but they may develop into ulcers with loss of deeper tissues.

Treatment: *See* p. 103.

CATARRHAL AND FOLLICULAR STOMATITIS

In catarrhal stomatitis, the mucosa, particularly that of the soft palate and pharynx, is edematous and slightly reddened in irregular streaks or patches. Grayish-white or brownish-gray adhesive exudate appears on the tongue and in the recesses of the mouth and pharynx. This may be the first lesion of avitaminosis B or of anemia. Systemic causes should be sought, such as catarrhal gastritis or some specific infectious disease.

The more severe and prolonged form of catarrhal stomatitis,

with more marked local tissue changes and more prominent constitutional disturbances, is termed follicular stomatitis. It may be associated with a severe generalized disease, such as distemper, or with malnutrition or unsanitary conditions of environment. The mucous membrane shows vesicles which ulcerate and have shallow, well-defined, grayish-yellow, denuded surfaces. Cats may develop a marked lesion on the mucous membrane at the angles of the upper and lower jaw which sometimes progresses to severe stomatitis and scarring.

Treatment: *See* p. 103.

MYCOTIC STOMATITIS

A specific type of ulcerative stomatitis, caused by *Candida albicans,* of dogs and cats, characterized by the appearance of soft, white to gray, slightly elevated patches on the oral mucosa. The periphery of these small lesions is usually reddened and the surface covered with a whitish tenacious membrane. The lesions may coalesce as the disease progresses. The infection is most likely to occur in young animals following prolonged treatment with a broad-spectrum antibiotic. Similar lesions are usually noted simultaneously in the pharynx and on the anal mucosa. Tentative diagnosis may be confirmed by culture of the material from the lesion.

Treatment: Local treatment with an aqueous solution of gentian violet (℞ 411) or with nystatin ointment (℞ 356) is effective if only a few lesions are present. When the lesions are widespread, the oral administration of nystatin (℞ 355) along with topical application of nystatin solutions is advised.

GLOSSITIS

An acute or chronic inflammation of the tongue. The inflammation may be due to a primary disease of the tongue or may be secondary to a disease process elsewhere. Local causes include irritation from excessive tartar on the lingual surfaces of the molar teeth, penetrating foreign bodies, bite wounds, rubber bands, thread or string looped about or under the tongue, burns and insect stings. A number of other, more generalized processes, including both infectious and metabolic diseases, may also cause tongue lesions.

Clinical Findings: Excessive salivation and a reluctance to eat are common signs, but the cause may go undiscovered for long periods if a close examination of the mouth is not made. Irritation originating in the dental arcade causes reddening, swelling and occasionally ulceration of the edge of the tongue. When a thread, string, or rubber band is looped under the tongue, the dorsum of the tongue may show no evidence of inflammation. The frenum, however, is painful, shows acute or chronic irritation and is frequently cut through by the foreign body. Porcupine quills and plant awns may become imbedded so deeply that they are not palpable. Insect stings cause an acute, massive, edematous swelling of the tongue.

In long-standing cases, in which an ulcerative or gangrenous glossitis exists, there is a thick, brown, foul-smelling discharge and occasionally bleeding. The animal usually resists any attempt to examine the mouth.

Treatment: Foreign bodies, broken or diseased teeth should be removed, under anesthesia if necessary. Infectious glossitis (usually ulcerative or gangrenous) should be treated with a systemic antibiotic such as penicillin (℞ 44) or penicillin with streptomycin (℞ 41), in conjunction with high dosages of injectable B-complex vitamins. Mouthwashes, such as benzalkonium chloride solution (℞ 399) and other antiseptics (℞ 425, 441) should be used to flush the mouth several times daily. A bland diet and parenterally administered fluids (℞ 561, 567) may be necessary. Acute glossitis due to insect stings may require emergency treatment including tracheal intubation or tracheotomy if the respiratory distress is severe. Injections of epinephrine (℞ 511) or antihistamines will aid in reducing the tissue swelling.

If the glossitis is secondary to another condition, the primary disease should be treated. The tissues of the tongue heal rapidly once irritation and infection are eliminated.

MOUTH BURNS

Burns of the mouth are not uncommon and may involve any or all of the structures of the mouth. They may range in severity from mild injury with only temporary discomfort to destructive lesions with loss of tissue, scar formation and contraction of the scar with subsequent deformity. The causes are general and not always due to prehension (see BURNS, p. 755 and ELECTRIC SHOCK, p. 754).

The owner may have observed the incident and be able to provide a history. Although the patient may appear to be hungry, it hesitates to eat or drink, salivates excessively and resents handling of the mouth or face. In untreated cases with marked tissue destruction, there is danger of a secondary ulcerative or gangrenous stomatitis.

If the oral mucosa is reddened but exhibits no tissue defects, no specific treatment is required. These animals should be given a soft or liquid diet until the area has healed. If the burn causes loss of tissue, the area should be cleaned and debrided under anesthesia. The danger of secondary infection should be avoided by giving an antibiotic (R 11, 29, 44) for several days. Local treatment is of little value. If the tissue damage is extensive, frequent flushing with isotonic saline solution will keep the burned areas free of necrotic debris and food particles and hasten healing.

ORAL PAPILLOMATOSIS

A benign neoplastic disease of dogs characterized by the occurrence of single or, more frequently, multiple papillomas on the mucous membranes of the mouth. It is caused by a virus which infects only the dog, produces lesions in or around the mouth and is most common in younger animals (*see* PAPILLOMATOSIS, p. 243). The disease is asymptomatic except in those cases where the warts interfere with eating. Occasionally, if the warts are very numerous, the dog may bite them when chewing and they may then become infected. The papillomas may regress spontaneously within a few weeks. If removal is necessary, it is best accomplished using electrosurgical techniques. The use of commercial or autogenous wart vaccines sometimes effects a cure.

PARALYSIS OF THE TONGUE
(Glossoplegia)

A partial or complete loss of function of the tongue which may be peripheral or central in origin. In the former, rough manipulation and excessive pulling on the tongue during dental examination may be the cause. Glossoplegia of central origin may accompany or follow such conditions as strangles, upper respiratory infection, meningitis, or cerebral abscess.

In the unilateral case, the tongue is deviated toward the nonaffected side. In the bilateral case, the tongue is limp and often protrudes through the relaxed jaws. In mild cases of either central or peripheral origin, a weakness in the muscle power of the tongue is often evident.

Careful nursing, with particular attention to feeding, will aid those cases where spontaneous recovery is likely. Where the condition persists beyond 6 weeks, likelihood of return to normal function is slight.

TONSILLITIS

Etiology: Tonsillitis is a common clinical problem in the dog and rare in the cat. In the dog, it may occur either as a primary disease or secondary to infections in the mouth, pharynx or nasal passages. Chronic tonsillitis may occur in brachycephalic dogs, such as the Boxer, English Bulldog and Boston Terrier, in association with the elongation and hypertrophy of the soft palate and chronic pharyngitis so often found in these breeds.

Hemolytic streptococci and staphylococci are the pathogenic bacteria most often cultured from diseased tonsils. Plant fibers or other foreign bodies which lodge in the tonsillar fossa may produce a localized unilateral inflammation or a peritonsillar abscess. Other physical and chemical agents listed under pharyngitis (q.v., p. 110) may also affect the tonsils.
One should not confuse tonsillar enlargement due to neoplasia, such as malignant lymphoma or squamous cell carcinoma, with tonsillitis.

Clinical Findings and Diagnosis: The earliest signs are fever, listlessness, salivation, inappetence and dysphagia. The mandibular lymph nodes may be enlarged. Frequently there is a short, soft cough which is followed by retching and the expulsion of small amounts of mucus. Swallowing movements, chewing grass or pawing at the base of ears are signs which may appear as the throat becomes sore. Tonsillar enlargement will range from almost inapparent to a size sufficient to cause mechanical difficulty in swallowing. A mucoid exudate containing leukocytes, epithelial cells and bacteria may surround the tonsil. The tonsillar tissue may be edematous and bright red with small necrotic foci or plaques, and will protrude from the crypt in severe cases.

Repeated attacks may lead to chronicity. When this condition exists, the affected dog will be subject to occasional exacerbations of acute signs, generally poor health and lowered resistance to disease. Nephritis with lumbar tenderness may occur subsequent to tonsillitis.

Chronic inflammation will result in a "muddy" tonsil with only slight enlargement. Inflammation of the palatine tonsil may be accompanied by a similar inflammation of the pharyngeal tonsil. Since inflammation of the tonsils may be a sign of generalized or regional infection, the diagnosis of primary tonsillitis should be made only after the existence of any underlying disease has been eliminated by a thorough physical examination.

Treatment: Prompt administration of antibiotics systemically is the key to successful treatment of bacterial tonsillitis. The most effective and economical antibiotic, in most cases, is penicillin (Ŗ 44). It should be given for 10 days. Sulfonamide (Ŗ 75, 82), or tetracycline (Ŗ 58) therapy is effective. Swabbing the tonsils and tonsillar crypts with 2% aqueous iodine solution is beneficial. A soft, palatable diet is recommended for a few days until the dysphagia disappears. The parenteral administration of fluids is required for those animals which are unable to take food by mouth.

Surgical removal of the tonsils during a remission of the disease is recommended for animals with recurrent attacks.

PHARYNGITIS

Inflammation of the pharyngeal mucosa.

Etiology: Pharyngitis usually is infectious and frequently associated with inflammation of adjacent tissues. Retropharyngeal and subparotid lymph nodes may be inflamed or abscessed. Pharyngitis often accompanies systemic infectious diseases, especially respiratory infections, or is the result of extension from adjacent infections such as rhinitis. Trauma to the pharynx may result from foreign bodies or unskilled use of instruments, e.g., balling guns. Irritating chemicals administered in capsule form can cause pharyngitis if the capsule is broken in the mouth or remains lodged in the pharynx. Inhalation or ingestion of chemicals may cause intense irritation. Thermal irritation of the pharynx occurs in the dog as a result of ingesting hot food or liquids. Elongation of the soft palate or eversion of the lateral ventricles in brachycephalic dogs can cause respiratory distress and nasal regurgitation, with resulting pharyngitis and tonsillitis.

Clinical Findings and Diagnosis: Slow, deliberate ingestion of food or anorexia may be the first sign. If pain is great, the animal also may refuse to drink. Palpation of the pharynx shows increased sensitivity. There may be swelling of the submaxillary, retropharyngeal and pharyngeal lymph nodes and the tonsils often are enlarged and inflamed. If there is an accompanying laryngitis, a suppressed cough can be elicited by pressure on the pharynx. If pain causes resistance to opening of the mouth, examination can be facilitated with general anesthesia. Inability to swallow may cause drooling; retching and coughing are common.

Infection in the pharynx is characterized by fever, bilateral purulent nasal discharge and stiffness of the neck. *Pharyngeal paralysis (see below) may be a sign of rabies.*

Prognosis: The course of primary pharyngitis usually is favorable, although the condition occasionally is fatal, due to edema of the pharynx and subsequent asphyxia. The prognosis is less favorable if the process results in formation of diphtheritic membranes and ulcers.

Treatment: Treatment is similar to that of tonsillitis (q.v., p. 109). If the condition has been caused by mechanical trauma (foreign bodies), local application of Mandl's solution (℞ 615), after removal of the offending object, is usually effective. The affected animal should receive soft or liquid foods which can be swallowed easily. Supplementary IV feeding may be necessary during the acute stage.

Large animals should be given sulfonamides (℞ 75, 82) or antibiotics (℞ 44, 54) parenterally. Local treatment of pharyngeal lesions is unwise. In the horse, where swelling and exudates may cause distressing dyspnea, steam vapors with cresol (℞ 394) are helpful and may avoid the need for tracheotomy; abscessed lymph nodes are common and should be given appropriate surgical treatment. The cough may be relieved by applying syrupy expectorants on the tongue (℞ 392). It is unwise to attempt restraint and oral medication because of the danger of causing fatal asphyxiation.

Small animals with systemic signs should be given sulfonamides (℞ 75, 82) or preferably antibiotics (℞ 11, 25, 29, 44, 54). Local treatment with astringent and antiseptic solutions containing iodine (℞ 414), tannic acid and glycerin (℞ 619) or silver nitrate (℞ 617) is helpful in overcoming the inflammation. In chronic pharyngitis, local application of Lugol's solution is helpful. Diphtheritic membranes may be carefully removed and the underlying tissues treated locally. Elongated soft palate or everted lateral ventricles can be corrected surgically.

PHARYNGEAL PARALYSIS

A disorder of central or peripheral origin but that most frequently occurs as a sign of encephalitis and is of special clinical significance in rabies in cattle and dogs. It is also an important sign in encephalomyelitis. It is seen in many intoxications (e.g., botulism), probably some fungus poisoning, as well as with the general paralysis of parturient paresis. Peripheral paralysis is infrequent and may result from injury to the glossopharyngeal nerve, pressure from tumors or abscesses, or injury from fracture of the floor of the cranium. Pharyngeal paralysis also may be idiopathic in the horse.

Clinical Findings: The animal suddenly loses its ability to swallow, food particles and saliva drop from the mouth and nose, and gurgling sounds emanate from the pharynx. If the interior of the pharynx is palpated, no muscular contractions are produced. Such animals die from aspiration pneumonia or exhaustion. The signs of pharyngeal paralysis of central origin are partially or completely masked by others of the fundamental disease. A ready diagnosis of the fundamental disease often results in the pharyngeal paralysis being ignored.

Diagnosis: Probing with the stomach tube suffices to differentiate between peripheral paralysis and esophageal obstruction. Foreign bodies in the mouth of the horse may lead to error in diagnosis. Corn cobs and sticks may become wedged between the upper arcades of the cheek teeth. Of greatest significance is the frequency with which signs of pharyngeal paralysis dominate the clinical picture in rabies in dogs and cattle. Of first importance in diagnosis is to determine whether the paralysis be of central or peripheral origin.

The prognosis is always guarded. When of central origin, it depends upon the fundamental process; when peripheral, upon the possibility of removing the cause. There is always the danger of aspiration pneumonia.

Treatment: There is no treatment for the local paralysis other than efforts to remove the cause of peripheral paralysis and none should be attempted before making a complete examination. In peripheral paralysis, or that present in equine encephalomyelitis, the patient should be fed and watered through a stomach tube. Limiting the process of dehydration may be lifesaving.

INFECTION OF THE GUTTURAL POUCHES

A condition in solipeds usually resulting as an extension of a pharyngitis.

Etiology: Bacteria (commonly *Streptococcus* or rarely *Pasteurella*) or fungi (*Aspergillus*) are the usual organisms associated with the disease, although herpesvirus or myxovirus infections have not been eliminated as inciting causes. The condition usually results from an extension of a pharyngitis into the eustachian tube.

Clinical Findings: The condition may be acute or chronic. Intermittent mucopurulent nasal discharge, especially when the animal lowers its head, is the most common clinical finding. Swelling or displacement of the parotid gland often is present. Pyrexia, epistaxis, dysphagia, abnormal head posture, respiratory abnormalities, ocular changes and facial paralysis have all been associated with the condition, although no feature has been constant.

Diagnosis is made by the clinical signs, and confirmed by examination of the pharynx with an endoscope, or by radiographs showing the fluid line in the guttural pouch.

Treatment: Catheterization and irrigation of the pouches with antibiotics (R. 49) combined with parenteral antibiotic therapy has been effective in many cases. Iodides given orally are frequently effective. Chronic or unresponsive cases may require drainage via Viborg's triangle.

The animal with guttural pouch mycosis, particularly when associated with epistaxis or evidence of cranial nerve damage, indicates a very poor prognosis. Prompt control of pharyngitis will reduce the incidence of guttural pouch infection.

SALIVARY DISORDERS (SM. AN.)

PTYALISM

Hypersecretion of saliva characterized by a profuse driveling from the mouth.

Etiology: The causes of ptyalism are many and varied, the commonest being: (1) drugs or poisons, such as bismuth, mercury, organophosphates, arsenic, and contact with toads; (2) local irritation or inflammation as from stomatitis, glossitis (especially in cats), pyorrhea, teething, foreign bodies in the buccal cavity, neoplasms, injuries and other mucosal defects; (3) infectious diseases, such as rabies and the nervous form of distemper, or other convulsive disorders; (4) disturbances of the nervous system, such as motion sickness or hysteria; (5) reflex stimulation from irritation of the esophagus or stomach, as in gastritis; (6) sublingual salivary cyst; (7) abscesses and other inflammatory conditions of the salivary glands; (8) tonsillitis; (9) administration of medicine in some species (particularly cats); (10) conditioned or natural reflex response to fear, to fondling (in some cats) or in anticipation of food.

Pseudoptyalism is the dribbling of saliva due to difficulty in swallowing. It usually results from paresis of the lips, tongue or pharynx, dislocation or fracture of the jaw, or from an inability to swallow or open and close the mouth, regardless of cause.

Clinical Findings: Driveling is the only conspicuous sign of excessive secretion of saliva. Care should be exercised to eliminate the possibility of rabies before examination is carried out. In the case of certain poisons (e.g., mercury), the salivary gland may become enlarged and painful and the saliva may be irritating.

In pseudoptyalism, there frequently is a drooping of the lower jaw, or sometimes tongue-lolling or drooping of the lips, depending on the location and extent of paralysis or degree of mechanical interference.

Treatment: The underlying cause, local or systemic, should be determined and treated if possible. In cases of poisoning (mercury or arsenic), emetics, cathartics and a gastric lavage should be given if the poison has been recently ingested. BAL (℞ 601) is effective if used soon enough, or sodium thiosulfate (℞ 610) if the former is not available. Atropine (℞ 489) and pralidoxime chloride (PAM, ℞ 608) are indicated for organophosphate poisoning. The possibility of further access to the poisonous substance should be eliminated.

Where inflammation or irritation is the cause, the mouth should be cleansed and foreign bodies, dental calculus or diseased teeth removed.

In nervous and reflex disturbances, sedatives, antimotion-sickness drugs or tranquilizers are helpful. If it is necessary to check the condition until the cause is determined, atropine sulfate (℞ 489) may be used.

Pseudoptyalism related to acute eosinophilic myositis (q.v., p. 582) can usually be corrected by the administration of systemic corticosteroids. Opening of the jaw under general anesthesia is usually required with chronic fibrosing myositis.

APTYALISM

Diminished or arrested secretion of saliva.

Etiology: Aptyalism may result from the use of certain drugs (atropine or belladonna), from extreme dehydration or pyrexia,

just caudal to the eye. Involvement of the zygomatic gland results in divergent strabismus of the affected eye, and exophthalmus with swelling of the membrana nictitans, the temporal area, and in the oral tissues immediately posterior to the last molar tooth.

Abscesses of the zygomatic and parotid glands are particularly painful. The affected animal holds its head rigidly and resents examination of the swelling or opening of the mouth.

Treatment: Mild infections with moderate swelling may respond to systemic antibiotics or chemotherapy ($\mathbb{R}$ 11, 29, 44, 60, 68). More advanced infections which have not localized may benefit from the application of hot packs to the inflamed region several times daily.

If an abscess is present, drainage through the overlying skin or, in the case of the zygomatic gland, drainage posterior and lateral to the last cheek tooth within the oral cavity is indicated. Injection of antibiotics into the nonlocalized lesion is occasionally successful in the early case. Well-developed abscesses should be incised and drained.

If the abscess cavity is large, cautery of the inner lining with tincture of ferric chloride or silver nitrate ($\mathbb{R}$ 618) will hasten healing. A drain may be placed in the abscess cavity for 48 hours, or it should be flushed with saline daily until healing is completed. Penicillin ($\mathbb{R}$ 44), sulfonamides ($\mathbb{R}$ 68), or a broad-spectrum antibiotic ($\mathbb{R}$ 11, 29, 60) should be given for 4 or 5 days following drainage. Recurrence should suggest surgical removal of the affected gland.

SALIVARY FISTULA

A fistulous tract discharging saliva into the mouth, or into the skin in the anteroventral region of the neck or over the parotid gland. Most cases are caused by wounds which penetrate the gland or by the spontaneous rupture of gland abscesses. Healing is prevented by the constant flow of saliva and a fistula develops.

Diagnosis and Treatment: Diagnosis can usually be made by the location of the fistula, the nature of the discharge and the history of previous injury in the area of a salivary gland. Care must be taken to differentiate a salivary fistula from a draining sinus in the neck region due to a penetrating foreign body or from sinuses arising from congenital defects.

Complete surgical removal of the gland and fistulous tract is the only satisfactory method of treatment.

CYSTS AND SINUSES OF THE NECK
DUE TO DEVELOPMENTAL ANOMALIES

Cysts and sinuses of the neck region which are due to imperfect fetal development are of importance mainly because of the desirability of differentiating them from salivary gland infection, salivary cysts and salivary fistulas.

Thyroglossal-duct cyst develops when the early embryonic thyroglossal duct persists after birth. This cyst is quite rare, always single, and found in the midline of the neck, usually at the level of the hyoid bone and larynx. These cysts are smoothly rounded, have a well-defined border and are anchored to the hyoid bone and deep tissues. They are seldom attached to the skin unless there is superimposed infection and, as a rule, they are not tender. They contain clear fluid.

Branchial cyst or **lateral cervical cyst** develops from congenital malformation of parts of the branchial apparatus, usually the second branchial cleft. Branchial cysts may be unilateral or bilateral, have a lateral position in the upper portion of the neck and are usually only very slightly mobile. These cysts vary considerably in size and an individual cyst may vary in size from time to time due to escape of contents through a small opening into the throat or through a small cutaneous fistula termed a **branchial fistula** or **lateral cervical fistula.**

Treatment consists of surgical removal of the cyst.

DISEASES OF THE ESOPHAGUS (SM. AN.)
ESOPHAGITIS

Primary esophagitis is rare in small animals; however, secondary esophagitis may be encountered as a sequela to foreign bodies in the esophagus, wounds, as a consequence of prolonged vomiting, or in association with severe gastritis. It is commonly associated with achalasia, megaesophagus and cardiospasm. It may also develop as a post-surgical complication of cardioplasty. Irritation due to instruments or drugs, the ingestion of caustic materials, neoplasms and the parasite *Spirocerca lupi* (q.v., p. 689) are also causes of this condition.

Difficulty in swallowing, excessive salivation and hematemesis are the primary signs. Extensive necrotic lesions, such as those produced by caustic or corrosive agents, cause violent retching and vomiting. Food is usually refused or regurgitated soon after swallowing.

The lesions vary with the cause and may be catarrhal, ulcerative, or necrotic. Foreign bodies may produce lacerations or punctures of the esophageal wall. Stenosis occasionally follows the healing of extensive lesions. Contrast radiography with fluoroscopy are essential diagnostic aids in many esophageal conditions.

Esophagoscopy allows direct observation of the esophageal wall and an accurate appraisal of the type and extent of the lesions. Stricture following healing can be demonstrated by contrast radiography.

Meperidine (℞ 590), to control pain, is indicated during the acute stages. A soft, bland diet should be offered frequently and in small quantities. Antibiotics (℞ 41) are administered both therapeutically and prophylactically. Steroid therapy (℞ 145, 148, 154), with due regard for possible presence of infection, may be beneficial in counteracting the inflammatory changes.

FOREIGN BODIES IN THE ESOPHAGUS

Foreign bodies, e.g., bones, needles and fishhooks, usually lodge between the thoracic inlet and the base of the heart or between the base of the heart and the esophageal hiatus of the diaphragm.

Clinical findings: Salivation, retching and extension of the neck are constant signs of cervical foreign bodies. When a complete obstruction exists, immediate vomiting follows the intake of food or water. Partial obstruction permits the passage of fluids but not solids, so that liquids are retained, but solid food is regurgitated. The signs produced by a foreign body depend upon its location, its composition, the degree to which it obstructs the esophagus, and the duration of the condition. If the obstruction has existed for some time, anorexia and loss of weight may be the predominant signs.

Dysphagia resulting from esophagitis is often the outstanding sign of small, sharp, nonobstructive objects. Perforation of the cervical esophagus can cause local abscessation or, in the thoracic portion, extensive pleuritis and empyema.

Many foreign bodies can be demonstrated by radiography. The presence of a nonradiopaque object may necessitate the use of a barium suspension. Esophagoscopy is an important diagnostic procedure, since it permits direct examination of both the foreign body and the esophageal wall. Occasionally, large masses in the cervical portion of the esophagus can be localized by external palpation.

Treatment: If the object is in the upper portion of the esophagus, it sometimes is possible to grasp and remove it with forceps. For those in the posterior half of the esophagus, the use of gastric forceps may be useful. An esophagoscope may be passed down to the obstruction and a pair of long alligator forceps used to grasp the foreign body, withdraw it into the esophagoscope and so remove it. All manipulations should be carried out with extreme care to avoid puncture or extensive laceration of the esophageal wall. Foreign bodies, particularly those with sharp edges, should never be pushed down the esophagus.

Surgery may be the preferred approach. The choice of an esophagotomy or a gastrotomy will depend on the location and size of the foreign body. The esophagotomy incision may be presternal or intrathoracic following a thoracotomy. Where the gastrotomy route is followed, it may be necessary to introduce forceps through the cardia to grasp the foreign object and to draw it into the stomach, thence to the outside.

DILATATION OF THE ESOPHAGUS

An increase in the caliber of the lumen of the esophagus which may be generalized or regional.

Etiology: Constrictive bands originating from a persistent right aortic arch or from the ligamentum arteriosum in association with the aorta, pulmonary artery and base of the heart may cause retention of food in the esophagus and lead to esophageal dilatation. Congenital paralysis in which there is an absence of peristalsis in the thoracic esophagus may lead to accumulation of food in the esophagus and eventual dilatation. A similar paralysis has been observed in older dogs and thought to be due to neuromuscular dysfunction resulting from exogenous or metabolic toxins. **Achalasia,** a condition in which the terminal esophagus fails to dilate as foodstuff approaches the cardia, is thought to be due to degenerative changes involving the neural plexus, or to cardiospasm, and may result in retention of food and secondary dilatation. Dilatation of the thoracic esophagus is usually followed by secondary dilatation of the cervical esophagus unless the basic cause is removed.

Clinical Findings: Dysphagia, regurgitation and progressive loss of condition are the cardinal signs. At the onset, regurgitation occurs immediately after swallowing. However, as the condition progresses and the esophagus becomes enlarged, regurgitation is delayed. The puppy with congenital dilatation characteristically appears normal while nursing, but begins to vomit when the diet is changed to solid food. In advanced cases, pulmonary disease develops as the result of aspiration of fluids from the esophagus. This is particularly apt to happen when the animal is confined and spends a great deal of time lying down. Pressure applied to the abdomen may result in ballooning at the thoracic inlet. Roentgenologic examination of the esophagus may reveal extreme dilatation and elongation of the entire organ, dilatation of that portion anterior to the base of the heart, or dilatation of the thoracic esophagus with a cone-shaped obstruction at the cardia.

Treatment: Mechanical dilatation by means of bougies placed in the cardia may alter the contractile power of the sphincter and allow the esophagus to empty in those cases considered to be due to cardiospasm. Surgical correction by means of an extramucosal esophagocardiomyotomy appears to offer the greatest chance for the successful treatment of the condition in the dog. In cases of congenital or acquired paralysis a semiliquid diet must be given in small frequent portions. It is sometimes helpful to feed the dog from a dish placed higher than his head so he must eat while standing on his hind legs. Gravity thus helps food pass into the stomach. Supportive therapy with vitamin B-complex should be routine.

ESOPHAGEAL STENOSIS

A narrowing of the lumen due to pathologic changes in the wall of the esophagus.

Etiology and Clinical Findings: Stenosis of the esophagus of small animals occurs following trauma, surgery which produces scarring, or as a result of tumors of the esophageal wall. In general, the signs are similar to those described under foreign bodies of the esophagus, with dysphagia, regurgitation and loss of condition being the cardinal signs. Radiography, using contrast media, may show a stricture of the esophagus with dilatation or a diverticulum of the portion anterior to the stenotic area. It is important to give small portions of contrast material immediately prior to taking the radiograph in order to demonstrate stenosis of the cervical esophagus.

Esophageal tumors are rare causes of stenosis, but since the incidence of sarcoma of the esophagus is high in animals with *Spirocerca lupi* (q.v., p. 689), this diagnosis should be considered in areas where this parasite is prevalent.

Treatment: Animals for which the surgical approach is not desirable may be maintained on a liquid or semiliquid diet given frequently and in small amounts. Periodic use of mechanical devices to dilate the affected area may be attempted.

DISEASES OF THE ESOPHAGUS (LG. AN.)

CHOKE

An obstruction of the esophagus by food masses or foreign bodies.

Etiology: Horses choke most frequently on greedily eaten dry grains, and less often on ears of corn, potatoes or a bolus of hay, and occasionally on medicinal boluses. Choke in horses often occurs secondarily to stenosis or diverticulum, as well as from inflammation of the esophagus.

Ruminants usually choke on solid objects, such as apples, pears, beets, plums, potatoes, turnips or ears of corn. On rare occasions cattle choke on foreign objects obtained in the feed.

Obstruction in large animals occurs most frequently in the cervical and less often in the thoracic portion of the esophagus.

Clinical Findings: Horse: The affected horse becomes anxious, arches its neck and retching occurs. Salivation is profuse and food and saliva are regurgitated through the nostrils. Coughing is pronounced and the animal may paw at the ground, get up and down and show other signs of distress. Milk runs from the nostrils of nursing foals attempting to swallow. After an hour or so, the forced or spasmodic efforts at swallowing become less frequent and the animal may become quiet.

Cattle: Bloat (q.v., p. 141) and salivation are characteristic signs. The degree of tympany varies with the completeness of esophageal closure and the length of time that it has existed. Chewing movements, protrusion of the tongue, extension of the head and neck, dyspnea, grunting and coughing are also seen.

Diagnosis: The diagnosis is made from the history and the prominent signs. An object causing obstruction in the cervical esophagus may be located by external palpation and passage of a stomach tube. Diagnosis of thoracic obstructions may be confirmed by the careful passage of a stomach tube.

Treatment: Horses: Obstructions from grain and hay tend to resolve spontaneously as the bolus is softened by saliva. The course may be a few hours to several days, however, and there is a risk of pressure necrosis or esophagitis resulting ultimately in a stenosis with dilatation or diverticulum. Inhalation pneumonia may occur.

In the horse, hasty procedures are to be avoided. Controlling the pain with sedatives, confining the animal and allowing it access to water, but not to food, may result in spontaneous recovery. Passage of a stomach tube up to the obstruction and repeated pumping and siphoning may relieve grain choke. Atropine (℞ 489), methylatropine nitrate (℞ 493), or methampyrone (℞ 591) to control the pain and the spasms, is the primary medication required. Tranquilization is often helpful (℞ 361, 369). In some cases, solid thoracic obstructions may be gently pushed into the stomach with a large stomach tube or probang, if the patient is tractable, or anesthetized.

Cattle: Relief of tympany is the first consideration and trocarization of the rumen should be done promptly when indicated.

Solid objects in the cervical portion of the esophagus may be massaged upward and removed through a mouth speculum, or a No. 9 steel wire may be made into a loop, passed through the mouth speculum until beyond the object and then slowly withdrawn. When other methods fail, a probang may be used. Stiff stomach tubes of large caliber work well for this purpose. The disadvantage of this method is the risk of tissue damage and subsequent esophagitis. In a choke near the diaphragm, a rumenotomy may be performed to remove the object. Esophagotomy may be elected in cervical choke in either species but should be resorted to only when usual methods of treatment fail; often it is followed by an esophageal fistula.

ESOPHAGEAL STENOSIS

Etiology: Stenosis may be caused by cicatricial tissue or by compression. Cicatricial tissue in the horse may follow esophageal obstruction which damages the wall, or irritation to the wall from rough handling in attempts to remove the obstruction. On rare occasions, caustic chemicals may cause esophagitis and subsequent scarring. Compression of the esophagus occurs occasionally in cattle with lymphosarcoma and from adhesions and traumatic reticulitis near the esophageal hiatus. Compression of the esophagus by a persistent right aortic arch has also been reported. In sheep, compression from caseous lymphadenitis involving the mediastinal lymph nodes is a rare cause.

Clinical Findings: Stenosis in horses results in repeated choke. Repeated obstruction leads to weakened walls and eventual dilatation or diverticulum. The clinical signs described in the section on choke occur intermittently. Water is swallowed with no difficulty. Animals chronically affected tend to remain thin.

Cattle with this condition tend to be chronic bloaters and may show a tendency to choke.

Diagnosis: Habitual choke in large animals suggests stenosis and esophageal diverticulum. The passage of a fairly large stomach tube will reveal the narrowing. It is sometimes advisable to use tubes of gradually increasing diameter to determine the degree of stenosis. Barium may be used in cervical choke to ascertain the area involved by radiographs.

Treatment: There is no satisfactory treatment. Feeding on sloppy mashes and fine-cut hay will help to prevent obstruction, but this procedure is only palliative and so tedious that the patient is usually sacrificed.

ESOPHAGEAL DIVERTICULUM (DILATATION)

This condition assumes its greatest importance in the horse. It most often occurs secondarily to stenosis and thus may be indirectly associated with esophagitis or chronic choke. Most diverticula are found in the low cervical and thoracic portions of the esophagus. The important signs are usually seen after feeding and are similar to those of choke.

The diagnosis is based on the history and clinical signs. Some cases of cervical dilatation may be palpated and even observed by visual examination. Radiography following the administration of barium has been used in diagnosis. There is no effective treatment.

ESOPHAGITIS

Esophagitis is rarely diagnosed as a clinical entity in large animals. It may occur occasionally in horses where it is due most often to trauma from foreign bodies or the injudicious use of stomach tubes. Irritating chemicals may infrequently be involved. The condition may be secondary to infectious diseases such as virus diarrhea, infectious bovine rhinotracheitis or malignant catarrhal fever.

In severe cases, dysphagia, salivation, spasms of the esophageal and cervical musculature, vomiting and extension of the head and neck may be seen.

Withholding feed and water for 2 days often relieves the condition. Electrolytes, methampyrone (℞ 591), atropine (℞ 489) and corticosteroids should be administered as supportive therapy and to control spasms. Water is then given and if this is tolerated, moistened mashes may be tried. Sulfonamides or antibiotics should be used to control infection.

SPASM OF THE ESOPHAGUS
(Esophagism)

A condition occurring in horses, most commonly in the young. Although the exact etiology is unknown, the condition has been observed in nursing foals when they begin to take solid food; in young animals convalescing from debilitating acute infections; in horses with acute esophagitis, such as that induced by the breaking of a capsule containing some irritant drug; following the use of a stomach tube during which injury to the mucosa may have occurred; and following the injection of large doses of morphine. Esophagism may also occur during routine stomach tube passage and in tetanus.

Clinical signs resemble those of esophageal obstruction, but do not necessarily have any relation to the intake of food. Sometimes, they are brought on by drinking cold water.

There is contraction of the muscles of the neck, pulling the chin down and backward. Some animals make convulsive efforts to vomit, placing the feet under the body and extending the head. Frothy saliva is discharged from the mouth and nostrils and coughing is frequent. Periods of spasm may occur several times a day, or only at intervals of several days. Sometimes there is interference with the passage of a stomach tube. The spasms are symptomatic and cease once the primary cause is removed.

If possible, the primary cause should be treated. Otherwise, treatment is largely symptomatic. Atropine (R 489) seems to control the spasms. Severe spasm may be relieved by morphine (R 592), or by use of spasmolytic agents such as dipyrone (R 492). Tranquilizers (R 361, 369) may control signs in nervous individuals.

GASTRITIS
(Gastric catarrh)

Acute or chronic inflammation of the gastric mucous membrane, often associated with enteritis. The term gastroenteritis is used to describe the condition of inflammation of both stomach and intestinal mucosa. The condition is common in all species of domestic animals. For purposes of this discussion gastritis is taken to include rumenitis. (*See* p. 134 et seq.)

GASTRITIS IN LARGE ANIMALS

Etiology: Gastritis without involvement of other areas of the alimentary tract is rare. Primary gastritis may be caused by the ingestion of caustic or irritating chemicals in all species, but it is usually accompanied by some degree of stomatitis and enteritis. Gastric disturbance with varying degrees of gastritis may follow over-eating, sudden changes in diet or ingestion of feeds that are too hot, frozen, moldy or spoiled, the ingestion of sand or foreign bodies and crib-biting with wind-sucking in horses. Chemical rumenitis may occur with grain overload in cattle (q.v., p. 140) and is frequently followed by a fungal or bacterial rumenitis. Calves incorrectly fed may develop rumenitis when milk spills into the rumen and putrefies. Abomasal ulceration and abomasitis are common in young calves and often appear associated with the ingestion of straw or other poorly digestible roughage and with hair balls. In all species gastrointestinal parasitic infections are a common cause of gastritis.

Abomasal ulcers occur in braxy and in pasteurellosis in sheep, and gastric venous infarction is common in acute septicemic and toxemic disease in swine. Gastritis is common in the erosive and vesicular virus diseases of ruminants and occurs in conjunction with many enteric infections in all species.

Clinical Findings: The clinical syndrome is indistinct and varies with the cause. In the horse, chronic gastritis and milder forms of gastritis are manifest by unthriftiness and periodic bouts of subacute abdominal pain. Laminitis may accompany or follow gastric disturbance. The feces may be dark and tarry if gastric hemorrhage has occurred. The temperature and pulse rate are usually within the normal range. *Habronema* ulceration may be clinically inapparent. More acute attacks and those following overeating are generally the result of gastric dilatation and pyloric spasm. The temperature is usually elevated and the pulse is fast and weak. Severe pain is usually manifest; the horse sweats profusely and violent episodes of severe colic may occur. Retching movements are common and the horse may vomit. Gastric rupture is a possible sequela. Between these episodes, subacute abdominal pain is manifest and the horse may assume a sitting-dog position.

In pigs, vomiting is the cardinal sign of gastritis, with depression, inappetence and evidence of abdominal pain.

In ruminants, abomasitis is manifest by depression, inappetence and a fall in production. The temperature and pulse rate are usually mildly elevated and rumination is depressed. Occasionally a pain response may be elicited by percussion over the abomasum. Acute rumen overload produces a characteristic syndrome (q.v., p. 140). Abomasal ulceration in calves may produce a syndrome of unthriftiness but is usually clinically inapparent unless perforation sufficient to produce local peritonitis occurs. Putrefactive rumenitis in calves is manifest by depression, toxemia and diarrhea. The passage of a stomach tube allows the escape of foul-smelling gas. Passage of a stomach tube and examination of material aspirated may facilitate diagnosis in all species.

Most parasitic infestations of the stomach produce a protein-losing gastropathy with unthriftiness and diarrhea without evidence of abdominal pain. However, haemonchosis may be manifest purely as a severe anemia without diarrhea, and hyostrongylosis in adult pigs may simply produce a syndrome of chronic wasting.

Treatment: First and most important is to remove the cause. The animal should be placed on a restricted diet of easily digested food, such as bran gruels or mashes, and green feed or fine hay. If the condition is due to spoiled or irritating feeds, evacuation of the gastrointestinal tract with a mild laxative, such as mineral oil (℞ 484) is indicated. Antihistamines (℞ 537, 538) should be given to prevent laminitis. If infection is suspected, enteric sulfonamides (℞ 63, 73) or antibiotics (℞ 11, 54) should be administered. To provide protection to the irritated gastric mucosa, protective agents, such as kaolin (℞ 472) or bismuth subnitrate (℞ 468) may be given. In acute gastritis in horses, meperidine (℞ 528) and spasmolytics (℞ 493) are indicated. The passage of a stomach tube may allow relief of gas or of fluid distension. Gastric lavage with isotonic saline should be attempted in cases of chemical gastritis and where impaction has occurred. Intravenous fluid therapy and other measures to combat shock should be initiated. With severe impactions or overload in horses and ruminants, gastrotomy with removal of the food mass is indicated. Following cessation of the signs, the animal should be returned slowly to normal diet. In cattle, gastritis often results in disturbance of the normal rumen flora. Rumen inoculation (q.v., p. 1417) with fresh rumen contents is of considerable aid in hastening recovery in such cases. The administration of a tonic (℞ 499) will speed recovery. With putrefactive rumenitis in calves gastric lavage is indicated. Penicillin is given by mouth and the calf is taken off milk for a 24-hour period. An equal volume of electrolyte solution (℞ 555) is fed during this period and the calf is put back on full milk intake gradually over a further period of 48 hours by increasing the milk and decreasing the electrolyte proportions in the fluid fed.

(For treatment of parasitic gastritis *see* parasitology section.)

GASTRITIS IN SMALL ANIMALS

A low-grade inflammation with shallow erosions of the gastric mucosa caused by overeating, ingestion of spoiled food, ingestion of indigestible material particularly in the growing animal (bones, hair, paper, toys) or the administration of irritant drugs (aspirin). Gastritis is also associated with infectious diseases, such as distemper, viral hepatitis, leptospirosis, acute pancreatitis, pyelonephritis, chronic renal failure and gastrointestinal parasites. Ingestion of caustics, arsenic, mercury, lead, thallium and phenol may produce acute corrosive gastritis.

Clinical Findings: Vomiting, depression and abdominal pain are the cardinal signs. Animals may exhibit excessive thirst but vomiting occurs with the ingestion of water or at any time if there is extensive damage to the mucosa. If corrosive agents have caused the gastritis, the vomitus may contain blood and shreds of gastric mucosa. Food may be refused or animals may exhibit a depraved appetite (licking concrete, chewing dirt). Pain may be manifested by restlessness and objection to palpation of the anterior abdomen. Animals may assume a crouched position or stretch out on a cool surface. When the gastritis is severe there is often an accompanying enteritis. Subacute gastritis is manifested by continued vomiting and signs of weight loss, dehydration and electrolyte imbalance.

Diagnosis: The diagnosis is based on a history of the dietary habits of the animal, the ingestion of foreign or caustic materials and the clinical signs. Gastric radiography may reveal the presence of opaque foreign bodies while the use of a moderate amount of contrast medium in the stomach may facilitate the visualization of ulcers, neoplasms, nonopaque foreign bodies and abnormalities in position or contour of the stomach. Hypertrophy of the gastric rugae is not a constant radiographic finding.

Treatment: In acute gastritis all food and water should be withheld for at least 24 hours. Water intake may be controlled by giving the animal ice cubes to lick. If the vomiting is persistent or if enteritis is present, parenteral fluid therapy must be instituted to offset dehydration and electrolyte imbalance. Ringer's solution (B 566) is indicated in diseases of the upper digestive tract. Other parenteral fluids such as isotonic saline, 5% dextrose in saline, and amino acid solutions may be used.

Phenobarbital (B 531) is given as a sedative and to reduce gastrointestinal hypermotility and secretions. Meperidine (B 590) may be used in cases of corrosive gastritis where there is evidence of pain. Chlorpromazine (B 363), or atropine sulfate (B 489) may be administered to inhibit vomiting. In cases where ingestion of a poison has been established, an emetic, such as apomorphine (B 460), is administered soon after ingestion unless the substance swallowed is corrosive in nature. In cases of poisoning the antidote should be administered immediately or gastric lavage or gastrointestinal lavage with a 2% solution of sodium bicarbonate may be employed to remove the irritant foreign material from the stomach. Gastric sedatives, such as bismuth subnitrate with kaolin (B 468), kaolin and pectin (B 472), or dihydrostreptomycin, kaolin and pectin (B 50) should be given in small frequent doses. After the first 24 hours, broth, soup or boiled milk may be given. The following day a bland diet consisting of Pablum and milk, oatmeal, soft-boiled eggs, cooked rice and milk puddings can be instituted. This diet should be fed in small amounts 3 or 4 times daily and gradually modified until the animal returns to a normal diet. Polyvitamin therapy is a useful adjunct in the treatment of gastritis.

Subacute gastritis occurs when acute gastritis has been improperly treated or when chronic ingestion of irritant materials continues. Chronic vomiting may also be present in gastric neoplasia, or in eosinophilic gastritis. Palliative treatment may be required for gastritis secondary to a systemic disease (B 466) until specific therapy for the underlying condition becomes effective.

GASTRIC DILATATION (SM. AN.)
(Gastric torsion)

A distension of the stomach caused by the accumulation of gastric secretions, food or gases, or gastric torsion.

Etiology: Gastric dilatation in dogs occurs in 2 general forms with vastly different clinical pictures. In the first, there is a compensatory enlargement of the stomach over a long period because of an increased food intake. Etiologic factors in this category include parasitism, inadequate diet and pancreatic insufficiency. With defective pancreatic secretion, digestion is incomplete and the patient tries to compensate by eating larger quantities.

The second form appears as a sudden stormy episode in which there is an acute distension of the stomach with gastric secretions, food and gas. Acute gastric dilatation is seen most often in the larger breeds, but occasionally it occurs in the smaller ones. The exact cause is unknown, but the intake of a quantity of dry food, followed by vigorous exercise and the consumption of a large volume of water, is believed to be a precipitating factor. Torsion of the stomach, which causes occlusion of both orifices and also the gastrosplenic vessels, will produce signs of acute gastric dilatation. It is seen more commonly in deep, narrow-chested dogs, such as those of the Greyhound family.

Clinical Findings: The gastric dilatation which is secondary to malnutrition or pancreatitis usually produces no signs referable to the stomach. Puppies which have overeaten have a noticeably enlarged abdomen and show signs of colic. Pain is evinced on abdominal palpation. There may be attempts to vomit and occasionally the condition is so severe as to cause the animal to collapse. Acute gastric dilatation, with or without torsion, produces a characteristic clinical picture in which the animal initially shows signs of abdominal pain and then rapidly develops abdominal distension, excessive salivation, retching, dyspnea and peripheral circulatory collapse.

Lesions: In the chronic cases, a marked increase in abdominal size is the only abnormality. In acute gastric dilatation, the stomach wall is distended, hyperemic and very thin. When torsion of the stomach occurs, the organ rotates upon the attachments to its lesser curvature.

Diagnosis: When the condition is due to parasitism, pancreatic dysfunction or inadequate diet, the diagnosis will be adequately supported by history and the physical signs.

Gastric torsion and acute gastric dilatation produce identical clinical pictures, and cannot be differentiated with certainty. If a tube can be passed into the stomach, it is safe to assume that no torsion exists. However, it is sometimes impossible to pass a stomach tube in an uncomplicated case of acute dilatation. Laparotomy may be required for a positive diagnosis.

Treatment: The treatment of secondary gastric dilatation consists of treating the primary condition. Simple overloading of the stomach is treated by inducing emesis with apomorphine (℞ 460).

Treatment of acute gastric dilatation must be regarded as an emergency. Initial efforts should be directed toward relieving the tympany. It may be possible to do this by passing a stomach tube, but failing this, the gas must be released through a large-gauge hypodermic needle which is inserted through the abdominal wall into the distended stomach. Meperidine (℞ 590) may be administered to combat pain. If release of the gas does not bring about immediate and marked improvement, a laparotomy should be performed promptly so that the stomach can be completely evacuated and at the same time be examined carefully for possible rotation. Gastropexy may be necessary. General anesthetics are usually contraindicated in the acute case. Anesthesia is obtained by infiltration of a local anesthetic.

Animals which show signs of shock should be given IV corticosteroids (℞ 160), low molecular weight dextran and sodium lactate immediately. Antibiotics and oxygen are highly beneficial. Dogs which survive the acute attack should be starved for 24 hours, placed on a liquid diet for at least 3 days and then placed on a schedule of at least 3 meals a day at which they are given bland foods similar to those described under the treatment of acute gastritis (q.v., p. 129). Since the condition has a tendency to recur, the owners should be advised to take preventive measures against it, such as multiple daily feedings, withholding water for an hour after eating, and prohibiting feed and excess water after vigorous exercise until the dog has relaxed.

GASTRIC FOREIGN BODIES (SM. AN.)

Etiology: Young dogs and cats may swallow any of a variety of foreign objects such as rubber balls, stones, bones, silk stockings, fishhooks and needles. Because of their licking habit, cats often swallow large amounts of hair which may form a mass in the stomach or intestines. A depraved appetite, such as that associated with rabies, pancreatic disease, avitaminosis, or mineral deficiency, frequently causes animals to ingest foreign substances. Some dogs develop a vice of swallowing stones, but, as a rule, these animals show few clinical signs of ill-health.

Clinical Findings: The signs produced by gastric foreign bodies are extremely variable. Many ingested objects do not produce clinical signs of disease and may remain undetected in the stomach for long periods. In such cases there may be a history of intermittent vomiting after the ingestion of solid food. Affected animals often show a gradual loss of condition.

Large, rough foreign bodies produce a more violent reaction and affected animals show signs of gastritis (q.v., p. 129). Sharp and irritating objects may lacerate the mucous membrane and cause hematemesis, or rarely perforation. A characteristic and suggestive sign is vomiting.

Hair balls in the stomach of cats can cause occasional episodes of retching, vomiting and inappetence, and loss of condition. Their presence is sometimes indicated by a change in behavior in which the cat cries frequently for food, eats ravenously when it is offered, but loses interest after a few mouthfuls.

Diagnosis: A tentative diagnosis of gastric foreign body can usually be made on the basis of the history and physical examination. Roentgenography is frequently helpful in arriving at a positive diagnosis. The recommended procedure is to make first a survey film to check for the presence of radiopaque objects in the stomach. If this is negative, further roentgenographs may be necessary following the administration of a radiopaque mixture.

Treatment: Apomorphine (℞ 460) may be given to cause the expulsion of small, smooth objects. However, vomiting should not be induced if the foreign body is of such size or shape that it could injure the esophagus. Small objects can sometimes be removed with forceps through a gastroscope. Small sharp objects, such as needles, pins or tacks, often can be made to pass safely through the intestinal tract by feeding small balls of absorbent cotton which have been mixed with meat or bread soaked in milk, or packed into gelatin capsules. Methylcellulose (℞ 487) or agar compounds are useful in providing bulk. Hair balls in cats are usually passed with the feces after the administration of one or more doses of petrolatum. Many gastric foreign bodies can be removed only by a gastrotomy.

GASTROINTESTINAL ULCERS

In the dog, gastric ulceration is most commonly associated with either tumors of the stomach or hemorrhagic gastritis due to severe uremia.

Gastric ulcers assume major importance in swine and abomasal ulcers in mature cattle and young calves appear to be increasing in importance and to be associated with feeding practices, the stress of high production and confinement rearing. (*See* ULCERATION OF THE ABOMASUM, p. 148) Gastric ulcers are a cause of sudden death in foals. Duodenal ulcers occur rarely, perhaps less rarely in swine than in other species.

ESOPHAGOGASTRIC ULCERS IN SWINE

The incidence of gastric ulcers in swine has increased in the past decade. This ulcer is remarkably similar to the chronic peptic ulcer in man except for location. Peptic ulcers in man occur in the glandular fundic portion of the stomach but in swine are found in the squamous epithelial area of the cardiac portion of the stomach.

Etiology: The cause is unknown. Infectious agents, nutritional deficiencies, feed consistency, feeding methods and toxic substances have all been investigated but none will consistently produce the disease. A combination of confinement rearing, stress due to transportation, deprivation of food, crowding and mixing with unfamiliar pigs results in a significant increase in gastric ulcers in rapidly growing pigs. Mixing pigs and starvation for 18 to 26 hours at the abattoir before slaughter results in a marked increase in gastric ulcers. The disease may be inapparent in a group of rapidly growing feeder pigs or young breeding gilts and some anxiety, tension or physical stress may precipitate the acute illness.

Clinical Findings: Gastric ulcers occur in swine of all ages but are most common in rapidly growing feeder pigs. In the acute form, hemorrhage results in anorexia, weakness, anemia, black tarry feces and death in a few hours or days. In the chronic form, unthriftiness, black tarry feces and anemia are characteristic but the pig may survive for several weeks. In the subclinical form, anemia and black tarry feces are not characteristic but affected pigs do not reach maturity at the expected time and in these the ulcer has usually healed and a scar remains. In some herds up to 90% of the feeder pigs may be affected while in other herds it occurs only sporadically.

Lesions: The typical terminal lesion is found in the wall of the stomach near the esophageal opening in an area which normally is a white, glistening, nonglandular, rectangular patch of squamous epithelium. It is common to find a crater 1 or 2 in. or more in diameter encompassing the esophagus. The crater appears as a punched-out area, cream or gray in color, and may contain blood clots or debris. In acute hemorrhage the stomach and upper small intestine will contain dark blood. Earlier the ulcers are characterized by hyperkeratosis and parakeratosis of the squamous epithelium about the esophageal opening into the stomach. Later, the proliferative lesion erodes to form the ulcer. The healed ulcer appears as a stellate scar.

Diagnosis and Treatment: The appearance of 1 or 2 listless, anemic pigs in a pen, showing anorexia, loss of weight, reluctance to move, the passage of dark feces and sometimes labored breathing, or the sudden death of an apparently healthy pig is suggestive of gastric ulceration. There is no known effective treatment. Access to green pasture has produced some recoveries. Stress conditions such as overcrowding should be avoided. Growing pigs should not be moved from one pen to another but rather raised in the same pen until marketing.

TRAUMATIC RETICULOPERITONITIS
(Traumatic gastritis, "Hardware disease")

A disease of cattle resulting from perforation of the reticulum, and sometimes the rumen, by a sharp object. The condition is under almost constant consideration in the differential diagnosis of diseases of the digestive system in cattle because of the similarity of its signs to those of other such diseases. It is most common in mature dairy cattle and in beef cattle less than 3 years of age. Occasionally, cases have been reported in other species of ruminants.

Foreign objects are common in the stomach of cattle because they lack discrimination against hard materials in the feed and incompletely masticate food at the time of ingestion. The disease is common where silage and hay are made from fields containing old rusting fences and baling wire, or from areas where buildings have recently been constructed, burned or torn down.

Etiology: Swallowed metallic objects, such as nails or pieces of wire fall directly into the reticulum or fall into the rumen and are subsequently carried over the rumino-reticular fold into the lower anterior part of the reticulum. As the exit of this organ, the reticulo-omasal orifice, is elevated above the floor, retention of heavy objects in the reticulum is favored. The honeycomb-like reticular mucosa acts as a trap for sharp objects. Contractions of the reticulum promote penetration of the wall by the metallic object. The volume of the gravid uterus in late pregnancy and straining during parturition or mating are additional factors that may initiate this process.

The foreign object may pierce the wall of the reticulum and its overlying peritoneum resulting in contamination of the peritoneal cavity. A localized peritonitis follows, frequently resulting in adhesions, or a more severe and widespread peritonitis may occur. The object may penetrate the diaphragm and enter the thoracic cavity (causing pleuritis and sometimes pneumonitis) and the pericardial sac (causing pericarditis, sometimes followed by myocarditis, endocarditis and septicemia). Occasionally, other organs, e.g., liver, spleen, may be pierced and infected because the object takes a different course.

Clinical Findings: The initial attack is characterized by sudden onset, with anorexia and a sharp fall in production in lactating cows. The animal may exhibit an arched back, an anxious expression, a reluctance to move and an uneasy, careful gait. Forced sudden movements and the acts of defecation, urination and lying down may be accompanied by groaning. A "grunt" may be elicited by percussing in the area of the xiphoid, or by elevating this area firmly and then releasing rapidly, or by pinching the back. The "grunt" may be detected by placing the detector of the stethoscope over the trachea. Tremor of the triceps and abduction of the elbow may be observed. The pulse rate may be slightly elevated and respiratory movements tend to be shallow and accelerated and are sometimes accompanied by an expiratory grunt. Rectal temperature is often elevated by 1° or 2°F. A pulse rate of over 90 and a temperature over 104°F usually indicate serious complications such as pleuritis, pericarditis or diffuse peritonitis. In these complications toxemia and depression are much more severe. Pleuritis may be unilateral or bilateral and is manifest by fast shallow respiration, muffling of lung sounds and the variable presence of pleuritic friction rubs. Thoracocentesis may allow the drainage of several liters of fluid. Traumatic pericarditis is usually manifest by muffling of the heart sounds with a variable presence of a pericardial friction rub and occasionally the presence of gas and fluid sounds on auscultation. A pronounced atrial jugular pulse is present early in the course and congestive heart failure (q.v., p. 51) is a frequent sequela. In the presence of these complications the prognosis is grave.

Diagnosis: In early cases traumatic gastritis is not always readily distinguishable from peritonitis or indigestion arising from other causes. White blood cell counts usually indicate leukocytosis due to neutrophilia with a variable shift to the left. A history of sudden onset, fever and evidence of pain are not characteristic of ketosis or indigestion due to most other causes. The rapid labored breathing accompanied by rales that are characteristic of pneumonia are not present. Abomasal displacement may be differentiated by history and on auscultation in many cases; it usually occurs after parturition, has a slower clinical onset, is afebrile and accompanied by ketonuria, and percussion in the xiphoid area is unlikely to cause "grunting".

Other syndromes that can be differentiated are abomasal torsion and dilatation, omasal impaction, lymphosarcoma involving the gastrointestinal tract and pyelonephritis. More difficulty may be expected with peritonitis arising from other causes, e.g., trauma, abomasal ulcer, intestinal obstruction. Careful evaluation of the history may help rule these out. Electronic metal detectors are used as diagnostic aids but many healthy cattle carry metal objects in their reticulum.

Cattle that come to notice late in the course of the disease and have not recovered spontaneously may be classified into one of 2 general types, acute and chronic. The acute cases usually present signs of acute peritonitis, pericarditis or septicemia. Chronic cases are recurrent and present a real challenge to the diagnostician and may involve vagus indigestion or diaphragmatic hernia (q.v., pp. 139 and 574).

Prophylaxis and Treatment: Avoiding the use of baling wire, magnetizing the bins used to prepare and store feed, and keeping the animals away from sites of new construction or removal of old buildings or fences are examples of steps that can be taken. As an additional precautionary measure bar magnets may be administered orally, preferably after fasting for 18 to 24 hours. Permanent magnets 2½ to 3 in. long and ½ to 1 in. in diameter, either cylindrical or with a grooved surface, are commonly used. Such a magnet usually remains in the reticulum and holds any ferromagnetic objects on its surface.

Treatment of the typical case seen early in its course may be surgical or medical. Either approach seems to improve the chances of recovery from about 60% in untreated cases to 80 to 90%. The surgical approach involves rumenotomy with manual removal of the object or objects if they can be reached. Medical treatment involves antibacterial therapy to control the peritonitis combined with administration of a magnet to prevent recurrence. Penicillin plus dihydrostreptomycin (℞ 41) or sulfonamides (℞ 82) are in general used for 3 days. It is recommended that affected animals be kept immobilized for 1 to 2 weeks and placed on an inclined plane to help limit further anterior progress for the foreign object. Feed intake should be reduced and, if a laxative seems to be indicated, a mild one such as magnesium hydroxide (℞ 483) is preferred. Use of metal detectors to aid diagnosis and flexible magnetic metal retrievers introduced orally or through an incision in the flank to aid in removal of the objects or magnets is practiced by some.

More advanced cases, those with obvious secondary complications or that do not respond to initial therapeutic measures should be evaluated from an economic viewpoint.

DIGESTIVE DISORDERS OF THE RUMEN

RUMINAL PARAKERATOSIS

A noninfectious, noncontagious disease of sheep and cattle, characterized grossly by hardening and enlargement of papillae and, microscopically, by the accumulation of excessive layers of keratinized squamous epithelial cells on the papillae of the rumen. The disease is caused by fattening on finely ground or pelleted feed and occurs commonly in feed-lot cattle and lambs, in which it is observed at the time of slaughter. The incidence may be high in fattened animals.

Many of the papillae are enlarged and hardened and several may adhere together to form bundles. The papillae of the anterior ventral sac are commonly affected. In cattle, the roof of the dorsal sac may show multiple foci of parakeratosis, each focus being 2 to 3 sq cm in area. In sheep, abnormal papillae may be visible and palpable through the wall of the intact rumen. Microscopically, affected papillae contain excessive layers of keratinized epithelial cells, particles of food and bacteria. The rumens of affected cattle are difficult to clean in the preparation of tripe. The abnormal epithelium, by interfering with absorption, may reduce efficiency of feed utilization and rate of gain.

Ruminal parakeratosis may be prevented by fattening animals on rations which contain unground ingredients in the proportion of one part of roughage to 3 parts of concentrate. At present the necessity and economics of prevention are unknown.

"SIMPLE" INDIGESTION
(Mild dietary indigestion)

A minor disturbance in gastrointestinal function usually associated with a change of feed or overfeeding.

Etiology: Almost any factor which can cause a minor alteration in the environment of the rumen may cause simple indigestion. It is common in dairy cattle that suddenly eat excessive quantities of a highly palatable feed such as corn or grass silage, or root crops and their tops. A sudden change in feed, the use of spoiled or frozen feeds, the introduction of urea to a ration, turning cattle onto a lush cereal grain pasture, and parturient cows eating their placentas can all result in simple indigestion. A degree of simple indigestion is common in feed-lot cattle being introduced to a high-level grain ration.

Clinical Findings: The clinical signs depend upon the type of animal affected and the cause of the disorder. Dairy cattle with simple indigestion due to silage overfeeding are anorectic and milk production drops moderately. The rumen is usually full, firm and doughy; the primary contractions are absent but secondary contractions may be present. Temperature, pulse and respiration are normal. The feces are normal to firm in consistency but reduced in amount. Spontaneous recovery usually occurs in 24 to 48 hours.

Simple indigestion due to excessive feeding of grain results in anorexia and rumen stasis; the rumen is not necessarily full and may contain excessive quantities of fluid. The feces are usually soft and foul smelling. The affected animal is bright and alert and usually begins to eat within 24 hours. The result of a more severe upset from the same cause is described under grain overload (q.v., p. 140).

Diagnosis: This is based largely on the elimination of other possibilities and a history of a change in the nature or amount of the diet. The systemic reaction and painful responses to percussion seen in traumatic gastritis are not observed. The absence of ketonuria, and the history, help eliminate ketosis from consideration. Displaced abomasum can usually be eliminated by auscultation. Vagus indigestion and abomasal torsions become more readily detectable as they progress because they have a longer course, but initial differentiation may be difficult. Rumen overload is soon distinguishable by its greater severity and the pronounced fall in the pH of the rumen contents.

Treatment: Treatment should be aimed at correcting the suspected dietary factors. Spontaneous recovery is usual. Administration of 5 to 10 gal. of warm water or saline via a stomach tube, followed by vigorous kneading of the rumen, may aid in restoring rumen function. Magnesium hydroxide (R 483) given orally, seems to be useful when excessive amounts of feeds having a high-energy content have been ingested. If too much feed containing urea or large amounts of protein has been ingested, acetic acid or vinegar may be administered orally. If the activity of the ruminal microbes is reduced, administration of ingesta from a healthy cow or a commercially available dried concentrate may restore the microflora.

VAGUS INDIGESTION

A group of related clinical syndromes of cattle caused by vagal nerve injury as a result of the lesions of traumatic reticuloperitonitis and other less common suppurative lesions. In some cases vagal nerve injury cannot be demonstrated. It is most common in late pregnancy but can occur in nonpregnant cattle. It is characterized by inappetence and eventually anorexia, progressive distension of the abdomen, varying degrees of dehydration, scant feces and progressive loss of weight. Onset is insidious and most cattle have been ill for several days or weeks when first seen by the veterinarian. The temperature is usually normal, the heart rate may be slower than normal in the early stages but later ranges from 84 to 110 per minute. The rumen is usually distended with fluid and may be atonic or hypermotile. The abomasum may be impacted and palpable externally through the abdominal wall behind the right costal arch or by rectal examination as a large firm doughy mass lying on the right side of the ventral floor of the abdomen. It is not easily palpable in advanced pregnancy but commonly the gravid uterus is displaced dorsally and posteriorly into the pelvic cavity thus giving a false impression of terminal pregnancy. The rectum is usually empty except for sticky mucus. Most affected cattle die from secondary starvation, dehydration, acid-base and electrolyte imbalances.

Treatment: Response to treatment is unsatisfactory. Rumenotomy provides only temporary relief and the use of cathartics, stomach and intestinal stimulants and lubricating substances has been disappointing. If parturition is pending, fluid therapy (℞ 558) and rumen lavage with a large-bore stomach tube are indicated. Parturition may be induced in pregnancies over 8 months using a glucocorticoid hormone (℞ 145); (parturition will occur in 48 hours, the placenta may be retained, the calf is usually born alive and the reduction in the intra-abdominal volume may allow partial return of the motility of the forestomachs and abomasum so that recovery may occur).

GRAIN OVERLOAD
(D-Lactic acidosis, Carbohydrate engorgement, Rumen impaction)

An acute disease of ruminants characterized by indigestion, rumen stasis, dehydration, acidosis, toxemia, incoordination, collapse and, frequently, death.

Etiology: The cause is excessive ingestion of feeds rich in starch or sugars, e.g., cereal grains, corn, fruits, root crops or high-energy prepared feeds. These favor the proliferation of gram-positive bacteria in the rumen whose end-production of fermentation is L- and D-lactic acid. The rumen pH falls to 4.0 to 4.5, destroying the protozoa, cellulolytic organisms and lactate-utilizing organisms as well as impairing rumen motility. Superimposition of lactic acid and its salt, lactate, on the existing solutes in the rumen liquid causes a substantial rise in osmotic pressure which draws fluid into the rumen causing dehydration. Mammals metabolize L-lactic acid more rapidly than D-lactic acid, the absorption of which leads to a more severe and protracted acidosis than an equivalent absorption of L-lactic acid. Progressive acidosis and dehydration may lead to the death of the animal in 1 to 3 days. In protracted cases hypochloremic alkalosis may follow the acidotic phase.

Clinical Findings: About 8 to 12 hours after feeding, the animals may show anorexia, signs of indigestion and irritability progressing to dullness. The rumen may be distended and show reduced motility. Progressive signs include atony of the rumen with increasingly fluid contents, increased pulse and respiration rates, variable rectal temperature, sunken eyes, loss of dermal elasticity, incoordination, collapse and coma. The feces are usually soft and malodorous; they may have a grayish color and small volume in severe cases; other animals develop a profuse diarrhea. Death may ensue within one to several days. Some animals show lameness that may be attributable to laminitis. Animals that survive the acute phase but develop fungal rumenitis remain anorectic, become cachectic and die within 2 weeks.

Diagnosis: Testing a sample of rumen contents discloses low pH (4.0 to 4.8 would be considered diagnostic of the disease). The hematocrit may be greatly elevated (40 to 50), blood pH and bicarbonate values are extremely low and blood lactate is very high. History of deliberate or accidental exposure to an excess of a high-energy feed relatively low in protein or a sudden change in conditions in a feed lot help establish the correct diagnosis.

Treatment: Mortality is high in severely affected animals unless vigorous therapeutic procedures are initiated early. Emergency slaughter should be considered when many cattle are severely affected (recumbent and in shock). Treatment of the severe form necessitates rumenotomy with removal of all ingesta, washing out the rumen and replacing the contents with ingesta taken from healthy cattle.

Alternatively the rumen can be emptied using a large stomach tube (1 in. diameter, 10 ft. long) and irrigating the rumen 15 to 20 times. The rumen is filled using water from an ordinary water hose connected to the stomach tube and then allowed to empty by gravity flow. Fluid therapy using balanced electrolytes (R 558) is necessary to correct the acid-base imbalance and dehydration, and to restore renal function. If balanced electrolytes are unavailable, a saline-bicarbonate mixture (R 568) may be used. Less severely affected animals may be treated with oral antacids to control rumen pH (R 469, 483) and supportive IV fluid therapy (R 558, 568). Ancillary treatment includes: antibiotics to suppress lactic acid formation in the rumen (penicillin, R 41, 43), antihistamines (R 537), glucocorticoids (dexamethasone, R 143) and calcium borogluconate (R 583). However, none of these treatments alone or combined is as effective as the combination of emptying the rumen either by rumenotomy or by lavage and the administration of large quantities of fluids. During the convalescent period, which may last 2 to 4 days, cattle should be given good-quality hay with no grain.

BLOAT IN RUMINANTS
(Tympanites, Tympany, Hoven, Meteorism)

An excessive accumulation of gas in the first 2 compartments (rumen and reticulum) of the ruminant stomach. Mild dis-

tension is of little consequence, but severe bloat causes great
discomfort and is frequently fatal.

Bloat occurs in all domestic ruminants, but is most common
in cattle and in this species may cause heavy losses. It is
particularly important in cattle in Australia and New Zealand
and in other countries where year-round grazing is practiced.
In the U.S.A. and Great Britain, it occurs most commonly on
newly developed, highly productive pastures and is an important deterrent to the development and utilization of such
pastures. It rarely occurs in sheep throughout these countries,
but is of economic importance in this species in restricted
areas in the Western U.S.A.

Although pasture bloat may occur at any time, the incidence
is higher in wet summers on clover-dominant pastures that are
growing rapidly. Bloat occurs less often in animals fed in feed
lots and barns.

Etiology: Bloat may be classified as primary or secondary.
Solid objects, such as corn cobs, turnips, apples, potatoes and
peaches, commonly lodge in the esophagus and, by preventing
eructation, cause secondary bloat. External pressure on the
esophagus by enlarged mediastinal lymph nodes; interference
with cardial innervation, as in vagus indigestion and diaphragmatic hernia; and sporadic cases of bloat in young calves are
further examples of causes of secondary bloat. Primary bloat
is by far the more important.

Primary bloat in animals at pasture or on dry feed is caused
by the interaction of a number of sometimes rather obscure
factors which combine to reduce the ratio of gas eliminated by
eructation to gas produced by fermentation. Overproduction of
gas *per se* is not the important factor, and neither excessive
consumption of dangerous material nor lack of rumen motility
are responsible; most authorities agree that bloat is caused by
a failure of the eructation mechanism.

Lush pastures, particularly those dominated by rapidly
growing leguminous plants, are most commonly the cause of
serious bloating, but such pastures do not always induce bloat,
nor are other types always safe. The primary cause of pasture
bloat appears to be a change in the composition of certain
pasture plants, the change being one that facilitates the development of a stable foam that in turn prevents eructation.
Some animal factors, including individual susceptibility, the
volume and composition of saliva, and possibly habituation,
may influence the hazard of bloat on a given pasture, but if
serious losses due to bloat are to be prevented, it is necessary
to control these changes in plant composition. Alternatively,

or as an interim measure, it is necessary to prevent the development of frothing by chemical or physical means.

Clinical Findings: The first sign is a distension of the left side which may become so severe that the area of the left paralumbar fossa protrudes above the normal top line. Distension on the right side is lateral in direction. Breathing may become labored and, in some cases, there is profuse salivation. Grazing usually ceases when intraruminal pressure becomes moderately high, i.e., between 10 and 30 mm of Hg or when the left side feels firm during the relaxed phase of the rumen motility cycle. Rumen motility can usually be detected until the condition of the animal is critical, although its effectiveness in clearing the cardia is obviously reduced. Eructation usually continues, but with decreased frequency and the amount of gas expelled is apparently reduced as the intraruminal pressure increases. When tympany becomes severe, eructation may eventually cease. At this point, the visible mucous membranes become cyanotic and the gait staggering; the animal may vomit, respiration is labored and eventually collapse occurs. Death usually ensues within a few minutes after the animal falls to the ground. Bloating and death may occur within 36 minutes after the cow has entered the pasture. Usually, however, several hours pass between the beginning of pasture grazing and fatal termination. The clinical signs in secondary (obstructive) bloat do not differ materially from those of the primary (nonobstructive) forms, but eructation may be entirely absent in cases of choke. The causes of death in bloat are not known, although interference with respiration and gross visceral distension are probably important factors.

Diagnosis: The presence of the clinical signs are sufficient for diagnosis in the animal. The mere finding of ruminal tympany at necropsy is not diagnostic of ante-mortem bloat. The most significant findings are congestion and hemorrhage of the tissues of the cranial parts of the body with pallor and ischemia of the caudal parts. These changes are the result of occlusion of the caudal vena cava which causes blood to be shunted to the cranial parts of the body.

Prophylaxis: The prevention of bloat may be attempted by carefully controlled management practices, but these are subject to many inexplicable failures and only guarded recommendations can be made: (1) maintaining pastures that do not exceed 50% legumes; (2) practicing strip-grazing that compels close or whole-plant grazing; (3) feeding at least 10 lb/head of dry, scabrous hay before permitting the grazing of legume-rich pastures, or overnight-feeding of Sudan hay; (4) administering antibiotics, such as procaine penicillin, either orally or in the feed at the rate of 100 to 200 mg every 24 to 48 hours, or in salt (50,000 u/oz) to which the cattle have free access. (Rumen microorganisms may become resistant to antibiotics, hence, the last method is not generally acceptable.) Silicones and household detergents have been suggested as useful anti-foaming agents, but are most unreliable and are not recommended.

The prophylactic administration of either non-ionic surfactants such as poloxalene or nontoxic oils or fats has been found to be generally effective, provided they are given regularly and in sufficient quantity. The oil or fat, usually emulsi-fied with water, may be sprayed on strip-grazed pasture at the rate of 2 to 4 oz per cow per day. If grazing is uncontrolled, the material may be dosed orally, painted on the flanks where the cow can lick it, or mixed with the drinking water to make a 2% emulsion, although the latter method is open to error unless an adequate intake is ensured. The selection of oil or fat to be used depends largely on cost, although freedom from milk-tainting substances and depression of fat-soluble vitamin availability should be considered. In general, peanut oil and tallow are most favored. Poloxalene is administered in feed or mineral licks or blocks at the rate of 10 to 20 gm daily. The ruminal implantation of a slow-release device containing anti-frothing agents is undergoing extensive field trials in Australia. Enzymic activity in the rumen can be reduced by the feeding of an enzyme inhibitor (alkyl arylsulfonate) applied to a floating matrix (vermiculite) and coated (cellulose) for slow release in the rumen. When fed with grain, this built-up compound is capable of greatly reducing legume bloat. Although none of the above methods are highly effective against feed-lot bloat, they are used and, particularly the administration of oil, recommended for trial.

Treatment: When individual animals are to be treated, intra-ruminal pressure should be reduced as quickly as possible. This may be done by passing a large stomach tube which is then manipulated in order to encounter gas pockets. In foamy bloat, the stomach tube method is usually disappointing, but it may have diagnostic value in determining the foaming characteristics of the ingesta. Sometimes, trocarization of the rumen through the left paralumbar fossa is justified. The cannula should be left in place until the danger is past. If the animal is in critical condition or has collapsed, rumenotomy should be performed at once.

Defoaming agents should be given immediately. The more useful compounds are vegetable oils, such as peanut oil, corn oil and soybean oil. Doses of 4 to 8 oz are probably sufficient, but in practice it is usual to administer at least 1 pint. Cream is quite effective in an emergency. Certain household detergents have been recommended by some as being effective in reducing foam. Cresol (30 ml), turpentine (30 to 60 ml), formaldehyde solution (15 to 30 ml) and other so-called antiferments have little effect on gas formation. They are probably no more effective than the vegetable oils and may have undesirable side effects, such as the production of off-flavors in milk. The silicones, for some unknown reason, have proved to be of little or no value in actual practice. The drug or defoaming agent may be given by drench, but, because of the danger of aspiration, administration by stomach tube or, in extreme cases, through a cannula entering the rumen through the paralumbar fossa is preferred. Because bloat can be rapidly fatal, farmers should be advised to dose their animals with oil at once rather than resort to folk medicine procedures.

ABOMASAL DISORDERS

DISPLACEMENT OF THE ABOMASUM

A disease of mature, high-producing, heavily fed dairy cattle, usually near parturition, in which the abomasum is displaced to the left of the rumen. It also occurs in steers, calves, bulls and sheep. Less commonly the abomasum moves anteriorly between the reticulum and the diaphragm.

Etiology: The basic cause of the condition is believed to be a reduction in abomasal tone. This could result from a variety of factors most of which are operative particularly at or about the time of parturition. These include heavy feeding of grain, ketosis, hypocalcemia, toxemias due to metritis, mastitis, etc. and any debilitating illness. It has been suggested that diminution in the size of the rumen due to a low-roughage diet creates a potential space beneath the ventral ruminal sac, and it is by this route that the atonic abomasum moves passively to the left side of the abdomen. Then, due to the absence of peristaltic movements, gas accumulates in the abomasum, causing it to move upwards on the left of the rumen. Mechanical factors associated with the act of parturition are no longer considered important.

Clinical Findings and Diagnosis: The severity of clinical signs varies greatly from case to case. Typically there is intermittent anorexia with marked preference for hay or grass rather than grain. There is loss of weight and diminished milk yield. Feces are usually scant, pasty and mucus-covered, but diarrhea may occur. Rumen movements are present but decreased and may not be noted if the rumen is pushed too far medially. A fullness in the left flank may be noted. A constant sign is a mildly positive urine-ketone reaction, probably secondary to the reduced food intake.

A diagnosis can usually be made by auscultation over the last 3 ribs about halfway down the cow's left side, where occasional resonant splashing or gurgling sounds may be heard. In cases in which these sounds are particularly infrequent they can be elicited by vigorous ballottement low in the left flank. Alternatively, percussion and simultaneous auscultation over the last 2 or 3 ribs on the left gives rise to a clear, resonant "pinging" sound.

Treatment: The simplest method of handling a displaced abomasum consists of rolling the cow on her back and massaging the anterior part of the abdomen from left to right for a few minutes. When the cow is let up she will often start eating at once. However, few cows respond permanently to this technique and in most cases surgery is required. Following surgery, the administration of glucose and propylene glycol (R 643) together with appropriate antibiotic therapy is indicated.

DISTENSION AND TORSION
OF THE ABOMASUM

A condition in which the abomasum becomes progressively distended and eventually undergoes torsion while occupying a position to the right of the midline. Insofar as the basic cause is abomasal atony, it shares a common etiology with left displacement. That the organ does not displace to the left in this condition is thought to be due to local anatomic factors such as the size of the rumen, the tightness of omental attachments, etc.

A history of recent parturition is commonly encountered. During the phase of distension, the appetite is depressed, the milk yield lowered and feces reduced in quantity. The pulse rate progressively increases. Distension of the right flank develops and high-pitched resonant sounds can be heard on auscultation and ballottement of the right flank.

Torsion of the abomasum causes signs of acute abdominal pain, increased pulse rate (90 to 160), subnormal temperature and depression. The feces are usually scanty; there may be diarrhea. Progressive dehydration is a prominent feature. Death usually occurs within 1 or 2 days. Traumatic gastritis, ketosis, displaced abomasum, abomasal ulcers, abomasal impaction, torsion of the cecum and vagus indigestion are all considered in differential diagnosis.

To treat, an incision through the right paralumbar fossa is made and the abomasum drained. The torsion, if present, is corrected manually after releasing gas and removing contents. If the abomasum contracts promptly, it is considered a good prognostic sign, but in most cases this does not happen and mortality is high.

IMPACTION OF THE ABOMASUM

This gastric upset occurs in calves and lambs that ingest indigestible fibrous material such as hair, wool or rags. The impacted mass often contains putrefying casein curds. Ewes fed on grain stubble containing morning glory, and adult cattle and sheep fed poor-quality fibrous feed, may develop fiber balls in the abomasum. Pregnant animals wintered on chopped feed without supplement are most commonly affected. Affected calves and lambs become unthrifty and may develop distended abdomens with excessive fluid detectable in the rumen or abomasum. The feces tend to be soft and discolored and may contain traces of fibrous material. Such animals frequently respond to abomasotomy with removal of the obstructing mass and supportive therapy.

Adult ruminants impacted with fibrous feed show anorexia, very scanty, tenacious, malodorous feces and right-flank distension, initially without systemic involvement. They become weak, dehydrated and recumbent. In advanced pregnancy the uterus may force the impacted abomasum anteriorly making it less accessible to palpation. Many cases of vagus indigestion are complicated by impaction of the abomasum. This is probably due to damage to the long pyloric nerve which results in functional stenosis of the pylorus. Such nerve damage is often a sequela to traumatic gastritis. The prognosis is unfavorable and no treatment can be recommended as being likely to succeed.

ULCERATION OF THE ABOMASUM

Abomasal ulceration occurs in such diseases as bovine virus diarrhea and malignant catarrhal fever; commonly in association with displacement or other causes of abomasal atony; apparently as a result of the stress of heavy milk production; in nursing beef calves, often with marked licking of the haircoat; commonly in calves at weaning time; and rarely with lymphomatosis.

Many affected animals are asymptomatic and heal spontaneously. Others show vague signs of anorexia and loss of condition, sometimes with blood in the feces, sometimes with evidence of sensitivity under the right costal arch. Displacement, atony or both may be present. Occasionally a major vessel is eroded and acute, even rapidly fatal hemorrhage into the lumen of the abomasum follows. In other cases, complete perforation of the abomasal wall leads to rapidly fatal peritonitis. In chronic cases, signs may be limited to unthriftiness, sometimes with evident distension and dehydration.

Definite ante mortem diagnosis is difficult without a laparotomy. The multiple nature of the ulcers makes surgical excision difficult but removal of hair balls in calves may be helpful. Treatment is frequently unrewarding but the use for several days of electrolyte solutions IV (℞ 558) and kaolin and pectin (℞ 472) orally is indicated for valuable individuals. A source of energy, e.g., 5% dextrose, should be supplied with the electrolyte solution.

EDEMA DISEASE OF SWINE
(Colibacillary enterotoxemia, Stomach edema,
Gut edema, Bowel edema)

An acute disease of 4- to 14-week-old pigs, usually associated with weaning or some management change, and characterized clinically by paresis and subcut. edema.

Etiology: Edema disease results from the rapid proliferation of specific serotypes of hemolytic *Escherichia coli* in the upper small intestine with elaboration of toxin. Sudden changes of diet predispose to such proliferations. The disease occurs commonly 1 to 2 weeks after weaning. Following absorption, the toxin causes increased vascular permeability and neurologic disturbances. The etiology of edema disease is similar to that of acute hemorrhagic post-weaning enteritis (q.v., p. 149), and the 2 syndromes sometimes occur together.

Clinical Findings: Unexpected death, usually of the largest pig in the group, may be the first event noticed. In live pigs, eyelid edema, pitting edema of the forehead and ataxia constitute the first clinical signs. The amount of edema is quite variable. The ataxia progresses until pigs become recumbent, and flaccid paralysis develops terminally. Pupillary dilatation and voice changes also occur. The disease is sporadic. The morbidity may be high in affected groups but the herd incidence is usually low. Most affected pigs die.

Lesions: Edema in variable amounts and generalized degenerative arteriopathy are characteristic. Common sites of clear gelatinous fluid accumulation include the subcut. tissues of the forehead, the eyelids, the submucosa of the cecum and cardial gland region of the stomach and the mesentery of the spiral colon.

Differential Diagnosis: The sudden onset of typical neurologic signs and edema in pigs of 4 to 14 weeks of age following several days after a management change indicates edema disease. The isolation and serologic identification of almost pure hemolytic *E. coli* from the intestine immediately following death, helps to confirm the diagnosis. Diseases that may be confused with edema disease include: mulberry-heart disease; salt poisoning; perirenal edema and nephropathy associated with pigweed (*Amaranthus*), lamb's quarters (*Chenopodium*) or fungal toxins in moldy feeds; acute ulceration of the esophageal cardia; Teschen disease; pseudorabies and arsenic poisoning.

Prophylaxis and Treatment: Treatment is largely impracticable. Prophylaxis is aimed at reducing factors believed to predispose to the proliferation of *E. coli*, and at avoiding sudden changes in management. Feeding antibiotics during the critical period may help to reduce the incidence of the disease.

COLIBACILLOSIS OF WEANED PIGS
(Enteritis in feeder pigs)

A disease associated with almost pure infections of hemolytic *Escherichia coli* and characterized by a range of syndromes. The prevalent serotypes of *E. coli* are identical with those of edema disease (q.v., p. 148) and rarely cases of both diseases occur together in the same outbreak. Most outbreaks are in recently weaned pigs but older, and less commonly younger, pigs may be affected.

Most often the disease is manifest in fast-growing pigs by depression, anorexia, fever (105°F), diarrhea and sometimes by bluish discoloration of the skin, especially of the extremities and venter. Occasionally deaths occur with little or no warning and occasionally diarrhea persists for several days with no deaths in the affected group. Frequently morbidity is high in the age group at risk. At one extreme the disease closely resembles salmonellosis (q.v., p. 377) and at the other, swine dysentery (q.v., p. 411). The history of the outbreak may suggest edema disease but the signs usually permit differentiation. Dehydration is usual, as is a stomach filled with feed. There is a severe catarrhal enteritis of the small intestine; the large bowel may exhibit a milder reaction.

Affected pigs should be treated promptly both parenterally (streptomycin, ℞ 54, is a good first choice—time does not permit a prior sensitivity test) and orally (streptomycin, ℞ 51, or nitrofurazone, ℞ 100, in the drinking water). All pigs in the age group should be treated by medication of the drinking water. Clinical experience suggests that feed be restricted for several days.

ENTERITIS (SM. AN.)

An acute or chronic inflammation of the mucous membrane of the small intestine. Enteritis can exist as an isolated disease involving only the small intestine, or more commonly as part of a more generalized process involving the stomach or the colon. It is common to use "enteritis" as a general term which includes both gastroenteritis and enterocolitis, however, the 3 conditions should be clinically differentiated to insure proper therapy.

Etiology: The causes of enteritis are essentially the same as those listed for gastritis. This condition is an outstanding feature of certain infectious diseases, such as distemper, panleukopenia, leptospirosis, "salmon poisoning" and toxoplasmosis, and is manifested to a lesser degree in many other systemic diseases. It is frequently seen in animals harboring helminths or coccidia. Other protozoan parasites, such as *Giardia, Trichomonas, Entamoeba* and *Balantidium* play a somewhat less sharply defined role in enteritis. The ingestion of decaying or contaminated food, sprays or poison baits, irritating medications and foreign bodies are all causes of acute gastroenteritis. An allergic response to a specific food may produce edema of the intestinal wall and signs of inflammation. Certain heavy metal poisonings produce enteritis.

The role of bacteria in the production of enteritis of dogs and cats is not clear. Although *Proteus* sp. are often suggested as the cause of enteric disease, *Salmonella* spp. are the only organisms that are generally accepted as enteric pathogens. *Escherichia coli* and *Vibrio* sp. are perhaps responsible for acute enteritis. The role of virus infection in enteritis has not been fully elucidated.

Clinical Findings: Diarrhea is the outstanding sign of enteritis. This is accompanied by vomiting when the condition involves the anterior portion of the duodenum and the stomach, and by tenesmus when it extends for any distance into the colon. Severe, localized lesions of any part of the small intestine sometimes cause vomiting. The feces are liquid and foul-smelling, and may be dark green or black as a result of bleeding high in the small intestine, or blood-streaked from hemorrhage originating in the lower portions. The temperature may be elevated if the cause is infectious.

The abdomen is tense in acute cases and the animal evinces pain when it is palpated. The dog may lie with its legs outstretched and its abdomen pressed against the cool floor, or may assume a "praying attitude" with the elbows and sternum on the floor and the hindquarters elevated.

Initially, intestinal motility is increased and abdominal auscultation reveals borborygmi. Subsequently, some animals develop a reflex atony which enhances the accumulation of gas. Dehydration, electrolyte depletion and acidosis are the most dangerous complications of prolonged cases. Chronic cases may develop in which the lesions are so slight that they produce no signs other than recurrent diarrhea and slight loss of condition.

Lesions: The lesions seen in enteritis range from a mild hyperemia and edema to extensive necrotic changes.

Diagnosis: The diagnosis of enteritis is readily made from the signs and history, but establishment of the cause may require extensive laboratory work. Radiographic studies utilizing both plain films and barium contrast techniques are valuable in determining the type and extent of the lesions. The feces should be examined grossly and microscopically for the presence of parasites and protozoa. They also may be cultured to check for the presence of pathogenic bacteria. Urinalysis and hematologic studies sometimes yield pertinent information which, when combined with results of the other tests and the physical findings, aids in the establishment of a specific diagnosis.

Treatment: All food should be withheld for the first 24 hours. Thirst is minimized by offering 1 or 2 ice cubes to lick. Vomiting can be controlled by a suitable gastric sedative, such as benzocaine and cerium oxalate (R 470), or by central inhibition of the vomiting reflex with chlorpromazine (R 363). An attempt should be made to offset dehydration and electrolyte imbalance by the parenteral administration of fluids. The choice of the solution to be used depends upon how much vomiting has accompanied the diarrhea. Lactated Ringer's solution (R 565), or isotonic saline (0.9%), alone or with 5% dextrose and amino acids, is frequently used.

Meperidine (R 590) is given to relieve pain. Simple diarrhea is controlled by preparations such as bismuth subcarbonate (R 468), belladonna (R 491), kaolin and pectin mixtures (R 472), tannic acid (R 476), charcoal (R 471), and aluminum hydroxide gel (R 478).

If bacterial pathogens are incriminated, a suitable antibacterial agent should be administered, e.g., phthalylsulfathiazole (R 63), dihydrostreptomycin (R 50), chlortetracycline (R 11) or neomycin (R 24). These agents may be given separately or in combination with the antidiarrheic agents.

After the first 24 hours have elapsed, a bland diet consisting of soups, broths, Pablum, rice, boiled milk, soft-boiled eggs and small portions of lean meat should be instituted. This diet is gradually adjusted until regular feeding is achieved once again.

Hemorrhage as a result of *Ancylostoma caninum* is handled by using a suitable vermifuge and treating the concurrent anemia. Blood transfusions are given to animals with low levels of hemoglobin. Less advanced cases are treated with hematinics.

Enteritis which accompanies infectious diseases or uremia is handled by treating the primary disease and using the foregoing methods for control of the enteritis.

The outcome of poisoning with heavy metals may be favorable if an early diagnosis has been made and treatment with a specific antidote is instituted. Parenteral fluid therapy (R 565) and antidiarrheic agents should be used.

INTESTINAL OBSTRUCTION (SM. AN.)

Etiology: The small bowel is the usual site of acute intestinal obstruction. The common causes are mechanical: foreign objects such as bones, fruit pits and rubber or plastic toys, large numbers of roundworms or tapeworms, adhesions or constriction by fibrous tissue formed following surgery, neoplasms, abscesses or granulomas, or impaction of indigestible material such as hair, bones or bedding materials (*see* IMPACTION, p. 154).

Volvulus, intussusception and hernia cause strangulation of the small bowel when in addition to obstruction of the intestinal lumen, occlusion of the vascular supply occurs. Volvulus may occur during vigorous exercise or following abdominal surgery, but is rare in small animals. Obstruction caused by intussusception of the bowel is more frequent. In the young animal it is usually associated with severe enteritis or intestinal parasitism. A common site of the intussusception is in the jejunum and proximal ileum but a significant number occur at the ileocecal junction. Compression of a loop of intestine by a hernial ring may cause obstruction; the herniated loop becomes firm and filled with gas and fluid, the sequela of any form of intestinal obstruction. Ileus may also be caused by local or generalized peritonitis, gastroenteritis, prostatitis, pancreatitis, torsion of the spleen or postoperatively following routine laparotomy.

Clinical Findings: The higher the site of intestinal obstruction, the more acute are the clinical signs and the more rapid is the course. The outstanding signs are persistent vomiting, severe dehydration, weakness and depression, and rapid loss of condition. Initially, pain is manifested by abdominal rigidity. The animal objects to palpation of the abdomen. Vomiting is an early sign when the obstruction occurs in the anterior intestine. Initially the vomitus consists of ingested food and mucus; later it contains bile. Complete anorexia is common and if vomiting continues, collapse, shock, and death occur because of electrolyte (sodium, chloride and potassium) and water loss, alkalosis and terminally, uremia.

"Chronic" small bowel obstruction may be exhibited by gradual weight loss, and dark-colored loose feces, occasionally blood-streaked. Such animals generally have a long history of unresponsive treatment for diarrhea.

Diagnosis: The history and clinical signs are sufficient to suggest a diagnosis of intestinal obstruction. Palpation of the obstruction or the dilated gas and fluid-filled bowel anterior to the obstruction is usually possible. If abdominal guarding prevents palpation, sufficient relaxation may be achieved by the administration of meperidine (℞ 590) or chlorpromazine

(℞ 363). On auscultation of the abdomen no peristaltic sounds are heard and percussion produces "tinkling" gas and fluid sounds. The peripheral pulse is rapid, hard and bounding. In intussusception a sausage-shaped mass in the mid-abdominal region can be palpated.

Radiopaque foreign bodies in the intestinal tract can be seen on abdominal radiographs, but nonopaque bodies must be outlined by a contrast medium. In either case, the gastrointestinal tract is empty, and gas-capped fluid levels can be seen in the dilated loops of bowel anterior to the obstruction when the abdomen is radiographed in a standing lateral position. If intussusception is present, it may be possible to see the increased radiodensity of the sausage-shaped mass or, more commonly, outlining of the layers of the intussusception by thin layers of gas. A barium enema may be utilized to outline the intussusception.

Treatment: Acute intestinal obstruction is always a surgical emergency. General treatment includes meperidine (℞ 590) to relieve pain and IV electrolyte and fluid therapy. Ringer's solution (℞ 566), isotonic saline or 5% dextrose in saline should be used prior to and during surgery. Animals with severe circulatory dysfunction may need a transfusion of whole blood or plasma. Postoperative care includes IV fluid therapy and broad-spectrum antibiotics for 3 to 7 days. Return to a regular diet can begin in 5 to 7 days.

INTESTINAL IMPACTION—CONSTIPATION

The formation of enteroliths or coproliths in the colon signifies inadequate propulsion of feces. This may result from mechanical obstruction such as: perineal hernia; rectal diverticulum or tumor of the colon; distortion of osseous pelvic structures following fractures; compression of the colon by an enlarged prostate gland or a neoplasm within the abdominal or pelvic cavity; excessive fiber and relatively indigestible material such as hair and bone; infected anal sacs, anal fissures and occlusion of the anus with matted hair and feces.

Failure of the distal colon to relax, as in megacolon, is characterized by a history of chronic constipation, often accompanied by intermittent diarrhea. Affected animals seldom show any signs of discomfort. In many instances constipation results from failure of the defecation reflex. Paralyzed dogs or cats may be unable to defecate due to nerve dysfunction or those kenneled for long periods may suppress the act of defecation.

Clinical Findings: Constipation is exhibited by tenesmus and frequent attempts at defecation, often accompanied by cries of pain. Digital examination reveals a hypersensitive anus and dry impacted feces in the rectum. Blood-streaked feces may be caused by spicules of bone which have lacerated the colon. Paradoxical diarrhea may occur in obstruction of the colon as watery brown stools are passed around the hardened fecal mass.

Diagnosis: A history of difficult defecation and palpation of the large, dilated colon filled with impacted feces is sufficient for a diagnosis of constipation. Abdominal radiographs clearly outline the greatly distended large bowel containing dense fecal masses, or opaque bone spicules.

Treatment and Control: For simple constipation an enema of warm tap water, or 2% sodium bicarbonate is effective. Fecal impactions should be digitally broken, softened by a retention enema of dioctyl sodium sulfosuccinate (℞ 480) and evacuated with enemas. Occasionally general anesthesia may be needed for effective breaking of fecal masses with forceps. In extreme cases, surgery may be necessary.

When constipation has been relieved, dietary regulation and management is important. The feeding of bones should be avoided, adequate exercise ensured and frequent grooming performed. Glycerine suppositories, mucilose flakes orally (℞ 485), surfactant laxatives (℞ 488), or lubricants such as mineral oil or petrolatum-vitamin combinations are helpful in preventing chronic constipation in hospitalized dogs and cats.

ACUTE INTESTINAL OBSTRUCTIONS (LG. AN.)

INTUSSUSCEPTION

The invagination or "telescoping" of a portion of the intestine into an adjacent portion.

Etiology and Occurrence: The mechanical causes of intussusception are irregular or excessive peristaltic movements. Enteritis, intestinal parasites, errors in diet, and tumors of the bowel are possible exciting causes. Intussusception occurs most frequently in cattle and is not infrequent in sheep. It is rare in swine and horses. The most common site is the ileocecal junction with the ileum invaginated into the colon.

Agonal invaginations of the intestine are not uncommon in all species.

Clinical Findings: The signs in horses resemble those of volvulus, and differentiation of these conditions may only be accomplished by rectal examination or exploratory laparotomy. In the horse, the evacuation of dark, blood-tinged feces is less common than in other species.

In cattle the signs are rapid in onset and are those of abdominal pain (kicking at the abdomen, treading and stretching). Anorexia is complete. Bowel evacuations are scanty, contain dark, tarry bloody and may consist of mucus masses mixed with dark blood.

Lesions: The invaginating portion forms a thickened ring enclosing the invaginated part and its mesentery. Compression of the veins results and a bluish-red or purple color soon develops. In true intussusception, the opposed serous surfaces separate with difficulty, if at all, which helps to differentiate it from agonal invaginations.

Diagnosis: A definite diagnosis can be established by locating the intussusception on rectal palpation in the horse and cow. Distension of the small intestine with gas and fluid always occurs. In advanced stages, abdominal peritoneal tap behind the sternum will yield abnormal peritoneal fluid. Early laparotomy is indicated in suspected cases.

Treatment: Laparotomy is performed and the intussusception may be reduced by extrusion or "pushing out" of the intussuscepted part. It is inadvisable to pull at an intussusception. If manual reduction is impossible or if necrosis of the bowel has occurred, the affected portion should be resected and the normal ends anastomosed. In the horse, ileocecal intussusception is difficult to reduce and end-to-side anastamosis into an accessible portion of the cecum is the most successful treatment.

INTESTINAL TORSION AND VOLVULUS

Volvulus is an intestinal obstruction due to a twisting of the bowel on its mesenteric axis; torsion is a twisting of the bowel on its own or long axis. Volvulus may also be due to a loop of intestine strangulating another section of intestine. Volvulus is most common in the small intestine, and torsion is most common in the large intestine and cecum.

Etiology: Volvulus and torsion are most likely to occur following events such as strenuous exercise, rolling, jumping and sudden bodily movements. Although reported in all species, these conditions occur most frequently in the horse. Torsions of the abomasum and cecum occur occasionally in ruminants.

Clinical Findings: In volvulus of horses the onset is sudden with signs of acute abdominal pain. The animal may kick at the abdomen, paw, stretch, sink almost to the ground and show other typical signs of colic. Conjunctival congestion becomes marked and diffuse. The pulse gradually increases in rate and becomes weak or thready. A pulse rate greater than 90 per minute indicates a critical condition. Initially, the temperature may be elevated (103° to 104°F), but it falls to subnormal in the terminal stages. Anorexia is complete; bowel evacuations are suppressed or scanty. Tenesmus is frequent. Peristalsis is slight or absent. Tympany may be noted in the small intestine, and twisting of the mesentery can often be determined by rectal examination. The course is short—a few hours to 48 hours. Terminally, the colic attacks give way to severe depression, the pulse becomes extremely fast and weak, and death ensues.

Signs of cecal torsion in cattle are similar to those of torsion of the abomasum (q.v., p. 146) except that they are slower developing and diagnosis is almost always possible by rectal palpation. The markedly distended cecum can be palpated at the pelvic inlet or even in the pelvis. It is also possible to percuss the distended organ through the right paralumbar fossa.

In torsion in horses, the clinical signs are usually less acute than in volvulus. This is because the rotation of the colon is usually less than 360°, and the obstruction of the blood supply is usually incomplete. The actual torsion may not be within reach, but one can usually determine that there is a displacement by rectal palpation. Pathogenesis of torsion is similar to volvulus but takes longer to develop.

Lesions: Following displacement of a part of the gut, the outflow of venous blood is obstructed, while the thicker walled arteries continue to supply some blood. The affected portion thus becomes dark red, the wall is thickened and the mucous membrane is red, swollen and may be necrotic. Gas accumulates, distending the lumen of the occluded bowel. Serohemorrhagic fluid is present in the abdominal cavity; focal or generalized peritonitis is present; rupture of the intestine may occur.

Diagnosis: A definite diagnosis can be made only by rectal palpation or, if this is impossible, by exploratory laparotomy.

Tapping caudally to the xiphoid cartilage will yield an abnormal peritoneal fluid.

Treatment: Surgical correction with manual reduction undertaken early in the course of the disease is more likely to be successful than rolling and attempts at manual reduction per rectum. It is the preferred treatment in all species. General anesthesia with halothane gas and oxygen is the safest anesthetic in the horse. A standing operation with local anesthesia is preferred in the cow. The right paralumbar fossa is the preferred surgical site in the cow while the ventral paramedian site is preferred in the horse. After accumlated gas is released, the involved viscus can usually be rotated to its normal position. In some cases, completely emptying the distended cecum greatly facilitates repositioning. An abdominal support bandage and post-surgical treatment with IV fluids (lactated Ringer's and Na_2CO_3) and antibiotic therapy are recommended. Prognosis in cases of volvulus is uniformly poor, regardless of treatment, and recoveries are uncommon.

IMPACTION OF THE LARGE INTESTINE IN HORSES

Impaction usually occurs in the small colon and the transverse colon. It also may occur in the large colon, especially in the area of the pelvic flexure. Feed containing a large amount of fiber (e.g., straw, cornstalks, alfalfa hay, mesquite beans) is the usual cause. A contributing factor is the lack of water intake in cold weather.

Clinical Findings: The onset of signs occurs after obstruction is complete. Distension of the large colon with gas causes acute abdominal pain. The usual signs described for colic are seen along with progressive congestion of the conjunctival mucous membranes (indicating toxicity). The pulse gradually increases in rate; above 90 per minute, the condition is critical. The temperature may be elevated in some cases. Rupture of the large colon may occur in the violent stages of colic, in which case there is sudden change in signs, to trembling and cold sweat. Rupture of the bowel terminates in death in a few hours.

Diagnosis: The diagnosis usually hinges on the lack of passage of fecal material, a dry sticky rectum, and the palpation of the impaction by rectal examination. Acute gas distension of the colon will be present cephalad from the impacted mass.

If rupture has occurred, it may be possible to feel fecal contents on the surface of the bowel.

Treatment: Medical treatment will meet with variable success. Mineral oil and magnesium sulfate are popular laxatives. Surface tension agents are also used to penetrate the impacted mass. Antiferments and oral antibiotics such as neomycin are helpful to prevent gas formation. When it is obvious that medical relief is not to be obtained, or if the horse is acutely ill, left-flank laparotomy under local infiltration anesthesia is indicated. This approach is adequate for impactions in the transverse colon, pelvic flexure and small colon. The impacted mass is carefully massaged until it is broken down.

INTESTINAL FOREIGN BODY
(Enterolith)

In the horse, the most common location for an enterolith is at the narrowing of the lumen in the transverse colon. These foreign bodies usually develop in the right or left dorsal or ventral colons and are mineralized masses that start with a nucleus such as a piece of metal. Concentric layers of mineral are built up around the foreign body, and eventually, through peristaltic action, the object may be pushed to the transverse colon and be too large to pass. Signs are then those of acute abdominal obstruction from impaction. The foreign body may be confused with an impaction, but the treatments are identical. In most cases enterotomy will be necessary to remove the foreign body.

Penetrating foreign bodies in the horse: Rarely a horse will have a penetration of the small intestine or stomach by a sharp foreign body, causing signs of acute peritonitis. The metal may puncture adjacent organs and signs vary from case to case. In general, the signs are those of acute abdominal pain, high temperature, and rise in white blood cell count. Peritoneal tap will reveal an abnormal fluid containing a large number of segmented neutrophils. These penetrations usually result in death.

Foreign body penetration in cattle (see p. 1341)

INTESTINAL INCARCERATION

An occlusion of the intestinal lumen by pressure from the serosal surface.

Etiology: A loop of intestine may pass through a rent in the mesentery, an opening in the peritoneum (hernia), or it may be strangulated by the stem of a pedunculated tumor or other fibrous cords or bands, such as adhesions. Scrotal hernia of bulls is one of the most common causes of incarceration in cattle. Adhesions causing partial or complete incarceration may occur following laparotomy incisions in all species. They are, however, more common following midline laparotomy incisions, especially in horses. The changes that occur in a strangulated portion of the bowel are similar to those of volvulus and torsion.

Clinical Findings: The general signs in the horse are similar to those of torsion. In cattle, they resemble those of intussusception, although the abdominal pain may be more marked and there may be complete retention of feces.

Diagnosis and Treatment: Diagnosis is confirmed by rectal examination or exploratory laparotomy. Laparotomy is almost always necessary for reduction since manipulation per rectum is rarely successful.

MUSCULAR HYPERTROPHY WITH STENOSIS OF THE ILEUM

A chronic hyperplastic disease of the ileum of unknown etiology has been reported in pigs, horses, cats and children. It occurs most frequently in pigs in which it has been described as the muscular type of regional or terminal ileitis (Crohn's disease).

The disease appears to be a congenital neurogenic imbalance resulting in hyperplasia of the muscularis with an increased thickness of the wall. It may be familial in Yorkshire pigs and in man, where several siblings may be affected. No anatomic abnormalities have been demonstrated in the ileocecal opening that could have resulted in stenosis with secondary work hypertrophy of the wall. Affected animals may exhibit signs of bowel stenosis, but often nothing is noted until the terminal stage of perforation and peritonitis. Pigs with hypertrophic ileal stenosis appear healthy and thrive normally as long as they are on a predominantly liquid diet. When dry-feed consumption increases, which usually happens at approximately 2 months of age, masses of dry, partly digested food lodge in the diseased ileum. The stasis results in necrosis of the intestinal wall with subsequent perforation, peritonitis and death.

The primary histologic lesion is a diffuse hyperplasia and hypertrophy of both circular and longitudinal layers of the muscularis affecting the terminal 1 to 3 feet of the small intestines. Due to the increase in size of the muscularis, the lumen is reduced in size, and the affected intestine becomes thick and inelastic, resembling a rubber hose. The mucosa and submucosa of the affected section are essentially normal, showing only changes attributable to stasis.

COLITIS (SM. AN.)

A chronic inflammatory disease of the colon.

Etiology: The condition has been ascribed to bacterial infection, allergy and psychogenic disorders. It has been reported in dogs to be associated with diets containing horse meat and has been produced experimentally with anticolon serum. It is now suggested that it is the result of an autoimmune mechanism.

Clinical Findings: The mucosa of the colon is inflamed, edematous, granular, and appears red and shiny with tiny hemorrhagic areas. Ulcers 3 to 4 cm in diameter are present. These tend to coalesce and increase in size. In advanced cases only islands of normal mucosa remain in the thickened granular mucosa of the colon.

Young adult animals are most frequently affected. Colitis is reported more commonly in Boxers than in other breeds. The onset is insidious. There may be no signs of abnormality other than constipation for several months, then a sudden onset of diarrhea occurs which is quickly resolved. As the condition progresses, diarrhea becomes more frequent until periods of remission fail to occur. Rectal stenosis may develop where lesions remain localized. The diarrhea is persistent and does not respond to medication. Tenesmus with the passage of flatus develops. The feces are watery, foul-smelling and contain blood, pus and mucus. The dog loses condition despite a normal appetite and temperature.

Diagnosis: The appearance of the colonic mucosa as seen with an endoscope is characteristic. Such examination may result in hemorrhage. Occasionally, ulcers may be demonstrated radiographically following a barium enema. The history of persistent diarrhea containing mucus, blood and pus, and the failure of the condition to respond to the usual therapeutic measures are diagnostic. Prognosis for a full recovery is poor.

Treatment: The diet should be of low residue, e.g., sugar, eggs, lean meat, gelatin and cooked cereal. Three or 4 small meals should be fed daily. Polyvitamin therapy should be instituted. Whole-blood transfusions may be indicated where anemia is present. Antispasmodics (℞ 489, 493, 492) are indicated, and antidiarrheic preparations such as kaolin and pectin mixtures (℞ 472), bismuth subnitrate (℞ 468) or a mixture of dihydrostreptomycin, kaolin and pectin (℞ 50) provide temporary relief.

The disease in some cases may be controlled by the use of sulfonamides, antibiotics or corticosteroids (℞ 140, 148). Soluble sulfonamides (℞ 64) probably control inflammation more effectively than the enteric sulfonamides. Penicillin and streptomycin (℞ 41), or the broad-spectrum antibiotics (℞ 7, 11, 29) may help control the condition. Systemic corticosteroid therapy (℞ 145) or topical steroids in the form of an enema may prove beneficial.

COLIC IN HORSES

A syndrome caused by diseases of the alimentary tract and characterized by subacute or acute pain. It may be confused with pain in other organs, e.g., hepatitis and urethral obstruction, and with other diseases such as laminitis, lactation and transit tetany, tetanus and peritonitis.

Etiology: Acute colic with severe pain may be caused by engorgement with grain resulting in acute gastric dilation; impaction of the ileocecal valve due usually to feeding of finely-chopped indigestible roughage; intestinal accidents including torsion, strangulation, intussusception and diaphragmatic hernia; enteritis, especially that caused by the ingestion of sand; hemorrhage into the intestinal wall as occurs in purpura haemorrhagica and anthrax; and the accumulation of gas due to the ingestion of lush green feed.

Subacute colic includes the 2 common forms of the disease, impaction of the cecum or colon with undigested fiber, and spasmodic colic due to increased gut motility usually following periods of excitement, unusual activity and long cold drinks. Colic may also be **recurrent or chronic.** This may be due to a deficiency of blood supply caused by a verminous aneurysm; adhesions (due also to migration of *Strongylus vulgaris* larvae), or impaction caused by poor teeth; indigestible roughage in the diet; phytobezoars and enteroliths;

overfeeding; old age and debility; and feeding too large amounts too infrequently.

Clinical Findings: The clinical signs in colic are much the same irrespective of the cause, varying only in their severity. Restlessness is manifested by pawing, kicking at the belly, getting up and lying down and rolling. Looking at the flank is a common sign and affected horses lie down carefully and get up slowly, often adopting a dog-sitting posture. Other abnormal postures, including the adoption of a sawhorse attitude and lying on the back, may also occur. Geldings frequently protrude the penis without urinating.

The pain observed is usually intermittent, especially in the early stages, with longer intervals between bouts in subacute cases and being almost continuous in acute cases. In the most severe cases there is profuse, patchy sweating, "sobbing" respiration, signs of shock including a rapid pulse (100/minute) of small amplitude and a clammy skin. The horse's movements are so violent that it may do itself much physical injury within a short time.

Auscultation of the abdomen is helpful in diagnosis. In flatulent colic, apart from the distended abdomen, there are high-pitched "gassy pings"; in spasmodic colic there are loud gut sounds or borborygmi; and in impaction the normal sounds are decreased or absent. A rectal examination is essential in diagnosis. Distension of intestinal loops is characteristic of flatulent colic; in cases of verminous aneurysm the enlarged, obstructed vessel may be palpable and slack, distended loops of intestine can be found, and in spasmodic colic no abnormalities are detectable. A cylindrical mass in the terminal part of the ileum high up in the right flank is diagnostic of impaction of the ileocecal valve.

Passage of nasal tube may result in the expulsion of large quantities of evil-smelling, green-stained fluid. This usually results from an obstruction of the intestine at any level from the pylorus to the ileocecal valve. Projectile vomiting of similar material may occur and is usually a terminal event causing rupture of the distended stomach.

Treatment: Acute and chronic intestinal obstruction may need to be relieved by surgical means. A verminous aneurysm does not respond to any known treatment but colic due to intestinal disease produced by the aneurysm or thrombus may respond temporarily to therapy. Acutely ill horses suffering shock and dehydration require supportive therapy with alkaline IV infusions in large quantities. The relief of pain is of paramount importance to avoid self-injury. Meperidine (1 to 2 mg/lb body wt by subcut. injection) or chloral hydrate (15 to 30 gm by stomach tube) are best. Tranquilizers may be helpful in mild colic attacks (e.g., ℞ 370). For impaction, mineral oil (℞ 484) is best, and in sand colic, magnesium sulfate (℞ 496) is recommended. In both diseases these treatments may be followed 12 to 24 hours later by an injection of carbachol (℞ 479). The latter treatments may be contraindicated in old or debilitated horses. In cases of spasmodic colic, atropine sulfate, ¼ to ½ grain (15 to 30 mg) is effective quickly when injected subcut. "Myspasmol", 10 to 30 ml of 3% solution, or methampyrone (℞ 492) are recommended for the same purpose. These drugs are antispasmodics and tend to reduce peristalsis.

In all cases, some attention should be given to preventing a recurrence of the disease by providing dental attention, advice on feeding and exercise, and effective parasite control.

COLITIS IN HORSES
(Colitis-X)

A peracute, noninfectious, often fatal enteritis of horses which occurs sporadically or in groups of horses.

Etiology: The cause is unknown; many affected horses have recently been exposed to some form of stress or upper respiratory tract disease but many others have not. Affected horses rapidly become dehydrated, and death appears to be caused by peripheral vascular failure or shock, possibly due to endotoxins from gram-negative organisms.

Clinical Findings: Horses of all ages, other than foals, may be affected, and in a group up to 20% may show clinical signs. The onset is sudden and marked by depression, rapid (100/minute) heart rate and mild-to-moderate abdominal pain. The temperature may rise briefly in the early stages, but in almost all cases it is subnormal when the horse is examined. Death may occur in as short a time as 3 hours without the appearance of additional signs. In less acute cases, life may be prolonged to 24 or even 48 hours and profuse diarrhea and dehydration are prominent signs.

  Lesions: Apart from the general signs of dehydration and peripheral circulatory failure, the only significant lesions are in the large intestine. The cecum or colon or both are distended with very fluid, odoriferous contents, and the mucosal lesions vary from severe hyperemia to an extensive, green-black, hemorrhagic necrosis.

Differential Diagnosis: The disease may be confused with salmonellosis, arsenic poisoning, acute intestinal obstruction or acute arterial occlusion caused by *Strongylus vulgaris* larvae. Colitis-X is much more common than the other diseases mentioned and is the preferred diagnosis pending observation of pathognomonic lesions at postmortem examination or isolation of a specific etiologic agent.

Prognosis and Treatment: The prognosis is very poor indeed. If the patient is seen early and the disorder is not peracute, the frequently repeated IV administration of adrenal corticosteroids and very large volumes of alkaline IV fluids to combat the severe acidosis and dehydration is recommended. Broad-spectrum antibiotics are usually administered in large doses but their value has not been unequivocally ascertained.

EQUINE GRASS SICKNESS

A disease of unknown etiology, attributable to disorder of the autonomic nervous system and usually fatal. Horses, ponies and occasionally also donkeys are affected. The disease has been reported from the United Kingdom, Scandinavia, the Low Countries and Brittany. The Japanese literature contains reports of possibly related conditions, and one suspected outbreak has been seen in the U.S.A. Grass sickness has a peak incidence in 3- to 8-year-old animals and a peak occurrence in spring. However, it may occur at any age, and has been seen occasionally in housed stock without access to grass.

Clinical Findings: Acute, subacute and chronic forms are recognized. Acute cases live for only 4 to 48 hours and subacute cases for about 6 days. Chronic cases continue for several weeks and may occasionally survive.

The disease is afebrile, characterized by profound depression, restlessness, patchy sweating and fine muscular tremors over the shoulders and flanks. There is stasis of the alimentary tract, difficulty in swallowing leads to drooling, and stomach contents may be discharged via the nares. There is passive resistance to passage of the stomach tube. The pulse is soft and very rapid. In acute and subacute cases the rectum contains dark, hard, dry feces often coated with blood-flecked mucus. Chronic cases become progressively dehydrated.

At necropsy of acute and subacute cases the stomach is distended with evil-smelling green fluid, the colon is impacted and the spleen enlarged. In chronic cases the entire gastrointestinal tract is often contracted and virtually empty. Histologically there is degeneration of neurones in the alimentary mural plexuses, the vertebral and prevertebral ganglia and the autonomic centers of the CNS.

Treatment: Prognosis is poor. Evacuation of the stomach and rectum, parenteral replacement of fluid, and administration of massive doses of multivitamins may afford symptomatic relief. In the suspected outbreak in the U.S.A., subcut. administration of 10 ml of a 1:1000 neostigmine solution, given three times daily, was reported to produce dramatic improvement and several complete recoveries.

DIARRHEA OF NEWBORN ANIMALS
(Scours, Colibacillosis)

Neonatal diarrhea occurs in newborn calves, piglets, lambs and foals. Under intensified husbandry the disease accounts for large economic losses.

NEONATAL DIARRHEA OF CALVES

Diarrhea occurs commonly in calves under 10 days of age and is characterized by varying degrees of diarrheic acidosis, dehydration, depression and death losses.

Etiology and Pathogenesis are not well understood. Many infectious agents singly or in combination are thought to contribute to the disease. These include: the enteropathogenic serotypes of *E. coli,* salmonellae, chlamydiae, the virus of IBR and the "Nebraska virus" of enteritis of calves. Susceptibility to the disease may be increased by a combination of factors which include: physiologic immaturity in calves born from dams fed inadequately during gestation, failure of the calf to obtain sufficient colostrum soon after birth and thus a failure to absorb sufficient immune globulins, birth of calves into heavily contaminated environments, overfeeding and the use of inferior-quality milk replacers. These, if they contain indigestible substances such as nonmilk carbohydrates and proteins or heat-denatured skim milk powder, will provide a substrate for normally harmless intestinal bacteria to proliferate and cause the disease.

Regardless of cause the result is a net loss of electrolytes and fluids into the intestinal lumen, resulting in diarrhea. The loss of bicarbonate ion and fluids results in acidosis and dehydration and, if severe enough, shock and renal failure leading to hyperkalemia, which has a toxic effect on the myocardium. Colostrum-deprived calves commonly die of coliform septicemia with or without diarrhea. Colostrum-fed calves more commonly develop diarrhea and if they die, they usually do so as a result of acidosis, dehydration, hyperkalemia and renal failure. Survivors of these acute effects frequently die in several days from physiologic starvation.

Clinical Findings: Colibacillosis in calves is usually characterized by diarrhea and progressive dehydration, but septicemia, toxemia or both may produce peracute illness and death in a few hours without evidence of diarrhea. The feces are usually increased in amount, watery to pasty in consistency, yellowish to greenish or light brown and may contain streaks of blood and excessive mucus. They are frequently very foul-smelling. The intestines may be filled with fluid, thus distending the abdomen in the early stages, but the calf appears gaunt in a few days. The course varies from 2 to 4 days or longer; in the terminal stages the skin is inelastic, the eyes are sunken, the calf feels cold to the touch and the perineum is soiled with feces. At this stage the prognosis is guarded. Arthritis, meningitis and navel ill may be present.

    Lesions: Except in cases too acute for diarrhea to occur, dehydration and absence of body fat are marked; the small intestines are usually fluid filled and the large intestine contains fluid-to-pasty, yellowish feces. In the alimentary-tract form of IBR the lesions consist of asbestos-like accumulations of milk curd and inflammatory debris in the rumen and abomasum and often mucosal hemorrhages are present in the abomasum. Systemic infection commonly results in polyarthritis, meningitis and ophthalmitis.

Diagnosis: It is difficult to make a definite etiologic diagnosis of diarrhea in calves; it is dependent on an accurate history, signs, culture of internal organs for bacteria and virus isolation, and identification of faulty feeding and management practices. A thorough examination of all possibilities is necessary in order to design useful control measures, even though treatment, to be effective, must begin at once.

Treatment: Most important are correction of the acid-base imbalance and dehydration, and treatment of the intestinal and systemic infections, if they exist. In early cases, before dehydration and acidosis occur, affected calves should be starved for 18 to 24 hours and given an antibacterial agent (℞ 473) and an electrolyte solution orally (℞ 477). Severely dehydrated calves urgently require blood or other fluid therapy (℞ 558, 568) over a period of 24 hours or longer. Systemic infection can be treated with antibiotics (℞ 10, 25) or sulfonamides (℞ 75, 82).

The response to therapy will vary considerably between calves, seasons and farms. Reasons for failure include: (1) failure to correct the acidosis and dehydration, (2) failure to restore renal function and the development of a hyperkalemia (severely affected calves should begin to urinate within an hour after the onset of IV fluid therapy), (3) drug-resistant strains of *E. coli* and salmonellae, (4) enteric colonization of *Pseudomonas, Proteus,* yeasts and fungi which may occur in prolonged diarrhea or following prolonged administration of oral antibacterial agents, (5) the alimentary-tract form of IBR and the Nebraska viral disease will not respond to the usual therapy for diarrhea, (6) the starvation syndrome caused by the use of milk replacers containing ingredients which are indigestible by calves under 3 weeks of age, (7) the development of meningitis, polyarthritis and endophthalmitis.

Control and Prevention: The control and prevention of neonatal diarrhea are based on at least 3 assumptions: (1) since newborn calves must be physiologically mature at birth the dam must be adequately fed during pregnancy, (2) most cases of neonatal diarrhea in calves are infectious in origin or at least infection plays an important role in pathogenesis and (3) ingestion and absorption of sufficient colostral immunoglobulins by the calf soon after birth provides protection against coliform septicemia; additionally, the immunoglobulins provide a measure of protection against the effects of diarrhea. Thus effective control and prevention begins with the nutrition (especially vitamin A) of pregnant cows. Calves should be born into a clean dry environment: dairy cattle should calve in a well-bedded clean box stall and beef cattle in small groups away from contaminated buildings or wet overcrowded corrals. All calves should receive at least 2 kg of colostrum that should be ingested within the first few hours after birth even if it requires forced feeding. The navel should be swabbed with tincture of iodine. Early isolation and treatment of scouring calves will help prevent new cases. Dairy calves should be reared in individual stalls until weaned from milk or milk replacer, and fed with separate pails. Whole milk should be fed for at least 10 days before switching to a milk replacer.

Calf barns should be depopulated as frequently as possible to reduce the environmental population of microorganisms. The use of prophylactic levels of antibacterial agents beginning immediately after birth has been tried in problem herds, but its efficacy has been difficult to evaluate. Vaccination of the dams with an autogenous vaccine before parturition has not been successful. Newly purchased calves should be isolated for 3 weeks and the various age groups should be segregated.

NEONATAL DIARRHEA OF FOALS

This is most common in foals up to 10 days of age that are nursing mares with an abundance of milk, but excessive milk intake is not a necessary predisposing factor. Several infectious agents including *Actinobacillus* (*Shigella*) *equuli, Salmonella, E. coli, Corynebacterium equi* and streptococci have been incriminated. (*See also* NEONATAL SEPTICEMIAS, p. 394.)

Clinical Findings: Diarrhea, lethargy, failure to suck and dehydration are common, and colic and flatulence occasional signs. The feces are watery to pasty and foul-smelling. The foal will commonly strain after defecation and the perineal area becomes soiled and irritated. Dehydration is sometimes severe and concurrent pneumonia may occur.

With accompanying septicemia there is fever in the early stages, the foal is acutely ill, and arthritis and tenosynovitis occur commonly while meningitis occurs less often. Affected foals usually remain recumbent for long periods; they may die in 2 days, but some survive a week or longer and become severely dehydrated and emaciated.

Treatment: Foals with diarrhea should be partially or totally starved for up to 24 hours or until beginning recovery from the disease is apparent. The foal should then be muzzled for 2 to 3 days and allowed to suckle for only a few minutes 3 times a day or the mare should be hand milked twice daily so that the foal is able to get only one-third of its normal intake. Oral administration of preparations containing antibiotics or chemotherapeutics with or without protectants such as koalin-pectin, and electrolytes are indicated (R 29, 82, 477). Foals with severe dehydration require fluid therapy (R 558) and those with septicemia need parenteral antibiotics (R 3, 10, 25).

Prevention: Foals should be born in a clean, dry and disinfected stall or on pasture. The umbilical-cord stump should be immersed in tincture of iodine immediately after birth or as soon as it is broken.

Foals should receive colostrum as soon after birth as possible. The perineal area and udder of the mare should be washed after foaling. Mares with excessive quantities of milk should be milked by hand to avoid excessive engorgement by the foal.

NEONATAL DIARRHEA OF LAMBS

An enteric disease of lambs similar in all respects to calf scours and marked by diarrhea and depression. Sporadic cases are caused by dietetic errors, chilling or an unsanitary environment, with the occasional explosive outbreak due to infection. Outbreaks are caused by enteropathogenic strains of *E. coli*. Occasional outbreaks of lamb dysentery caused by *Clostridium perfringens* Types B and C have been recorded (q.v., pp. 338 and 339).

As in calves, signs usually occur during the first few days of life. They include liquid feces, weakness, depression and, occasionally, colic and bloating. Mortality is high in untreated cases, death often occurring within 24 hours.

Treatment must be instituted early with antibiotics or chemotherapeutics given orally (℞ 467, 473) and antibiotics (℞ 10) parenterally. Passive immunity against *Cl. perfringens* Types B and C can be induced by a specific antiserum or by active immunization of the ewes during the gestation period with formalized bacterin. Bismuth (℞ 468) also can be used for diarrhea in lambs.

The ingestion of colostrum within 2 hours after birth is of paramount importance in the control of colibacillosis in newborn lambs. Lambing grounds must be kept dry and overcrowding must be avoided.

NEONATAL DIARRHEA OF PIGLETS

Common in pigs a few days of age under intensified rearing systems, this is one of the most important causes of mortality and economic losses. Explosive outbreaks are especially common in new piggeries where large numbers of gilts are being farrowed; the disease may occur in every litter of piglets and persist for more than a year or 2 and then decline as the breeding stock becomes older and develops a herd immunity and the management improves with experience.

Etiology: There is evidence that colibacillosis in piglets is caused by an overmultiplication of enteropathogenic serotypes of *E. coli*. Septicemia occurs in some piglets, and the mortality rate is much higher than from the diarrheic form of the disease. A similar syndrome may be caused by clostridial infection (q.v., p. 339).

Clinical Findings: Peracute coliform septicemia causes rapid death within several hours with or without diarrhea. Affected piglets are weak, cold and appear blue; there may be distension of the abdomen and dehydration is common.

Enteric colibacillosis is characterized by bright-yellow-colored pasty to watery feces; the tails of the piglets are wet and straight, the creep area contains puddles of feces and the piglets fail to nurse. They are dehydrated and gaunt and many die within 24 hours if adequate treatment is not started immediately. In the early stages a fever may be present but after the onset of diarrhea the body temperature is commonly subnormal.

The entire litter may be affected and die within a few days but some piglets survive and remain unthrifty. Udder engorgement followed by agalactia occurs commonly in a few days if the piglets do not nurse.

Lesions: Piglets with colibacillosis are dehydrated, some are emaciated and the intestinal tract from the duodenum to the rectum contains a yellowish fluid. The mesenteric lymph nodes may be enlarged. The stomach may contain some milk curds.

Diagnosis: Dead piglets should be submitted to a laboratory for a pathologic diagnosis, culture and determination of drug sensitivity and serotype of the *E. coli.*

Treatment: Antibacterial agents are given orally (℞ 96) and parenterally (℞ 10). An isotonic saline-dextrose solution may be given orally or subcut. (℞ 569) for dehydration and to minimize the effects of starvation. The entire litter is usually treated with the oral preparation because the disease will usually affect all the piglets. If treatment is delayed even a few hours after the onset of signs, the rapid progressive dehydration and acidosis results in a high mortality.

Prevention: *E. coli* infection in piglets cannot be eradicated but the incidence of neonatal diarrhea can be reduced to a low level by (1) controlling the bacterial population in the farrowing house with management techniques and good sanitation and (2) by ensuring that piglets are thrifty at birth and receive adequate quantities of colostrum within the first hour after birth. Many trials of vaccines have been disappointing but more recent ones show promise. Early treatment is an important part of control.

As the occupation time of a farrowing house increases, the infection rate increases in almost geometric fashion. Modern farrow-finish swine operations now practice group breeding and group farrowing so that dams will farrow within a short interval. Following lactation the piglets can be weaned from groups of gilts and sows and the farrowing facilities can be cleaned out, washed and disinfected and left vacant for up to a week before the next series of farrowings. The dam should be washed before she enters the farrowing house and again just prior to farrowing. As each piglet is born it should be dried off and the litter collected in a clean warm box until the last piglet is born. When farrowing is complete the udder should be washed and the entire litter allowed to suckle (this allows each piglet to obtain approximately the same concentration of immunoglobulin). If agalactia is present every effort must be made to correct it so that piglets obtain colostrum within hours after birth. If the agalactia is complete, cows' colostrum is an adequate substitute.

DISEASES OF THE RECTUM AND ANUS

RECTAL DEVIATION

A condition of male dogs over 6 years of age usually seen in association with perineal hernia and concurrent relaxation of the structures of the pelvic diaphragm. The rectum is characteristically deviated laterally and feces become impacted within the flexure.

The outstanding sign is tenesmus. The perineum may bulge when the animal attempts to defecate. Digital examination will reveal pouching and lateral deviation of the rectum. Radiographs taken following a barium meal also will demonstrate the deviation.

Treatment consists of castration, which is usually followed by a return of normal tone to the pelvic diaphragm and a reduction in the extent of the rectal deviation. A low-residue, slightly laxative diet should be fed and daily enemas may be necessary. If the condition does not improve, more extensive surgery will be required.

RECTAL PROLAPSE

A complete eversion of the posterior portion of the rectum through the anus, usually characterized by the protrusion of a large cylindrical mass covered with a congested, inflamed and often hemorrhagic mucosa. The anterior part of the rectum or the posterior part of the colon may prolapse into the rectum and extend beyond the anus. This can be differentiated from true prolapse since it is possible to pass a probe some distance between the prolapsed mass and the anal sphincter. **Anal prolapse** is a partial prolapse in which the mucous membrane has moved posteriorly on the muscular coat to form a circular protrusion outside the anus.

Rectal prolapse is encountered most frequently in young, heavily parasitized animals which are depleted in protein, vitamins and fluids, and which have been consuming high-fiber rations. The resultant enteritis, diarrhea and tenesmus bring about the prolapse. It may occur in association with constipation, neoplasms, foreign bodies and lacerations in the rectum, and has been encountered in protracted dystocia and in old dogs suffering from prostatitis. The exciting cause is straining, such as occurs in cases of enteritis or during parturition, particularly where there is vaginal prolapse in ewe and cow.

Rectal prolapse may occur in young animals that have a congenital weakness of the anal sphincter muscles. It appears to develop in Boston Terrier puppies more often than in other breeds. Skunks are susceptible following surgical removal of the scent glands. It is common in young pigs, particularly those fed on large quantities of whey, and in young rams of certain breeds. Straining and prolapse of the rectum may be observed in bovine rabies.

Clinical Findings: Where the rectal mucosa alone is involved in the prolapse, the congested mucosa protrudes from the anus. This may occur only during defecation or when the animal is straining.

Where true prolapse occurs, the eversion of the rectum is complete and a cylindrical mass protrudes from the anus. Immediately after prolapse, the rectal mucosa is red and glistening. As the prolapse persists, the color deepens to dark red and may become almost black. Congestion of the prolapsed portion may proceed to ulceration and necrosis. Small amounts of liquid feces may be passed. Manipulation of the prolapse apparently causes little or no pain.

Treatment: Small animals: In cases of mucosal prolapse, reduction is effected by manipulation or with the aid of a bougie or soft paper cone. Application to the mucosa of cool astringent solutions such as 5% alum (B 612), 1% phenylephrine, or the instillation of a saturated sugar solution into the rectum will prevent recurrence in some cases. If the mucosal prolapse is persistent, it is best corrected by surgery such as pursestring suturing of the anus or colopexy.

Any underlying cause must be corrected and careful attention must be given to the diet and feeding schedule to prevent recurrence. Fluid therapy may have to be instituted to correct dehydration. For the first 24 to 48 hours, a liquid, low-residue diet should be fed. Milk should be avoided as it may precipitate further straining. Therapeutic diets, which are available commercially, may be indicated. Enemas of warmed olive or mineral oil at the rate of 60 to 90 ml morning and night, will produce soft evacuations. Applications of topical anesthetic agents, such as a dibucaine ointment (℞ 589), to the anal and rectal regions may prevent straining. In some cases, it will be advisable to administer a sedative, such as phenobarbital (℞ 531).

Large animals: Reduction and retention are indicated before marked necrosis of the bowel has occurred. Retention is accomplished with purse-string suturing. In the presence of marked necrosis, amputation or submucous resection of the prolapsed rectum should be performed.

ATRESIA

Uncomplicated **anal atresia,** in which the cloacal membrane persists, is a common defect wherein the closure is limited to the region of the anal outlet, and the anal depression and sphincter are normally developed. Not uncommonly, atresia ani in females is accompanied by a persistent communication between the rectum and vagina, producing a type of **recto-vaginal fistula** (vulvovaginal anus).

Anal and rectal atresia involves the anus, and also a variable portion of the rectum, in which an area filled by connective tissue exists between the anal membrane and the blind end of the rectum. In calves and foals the patent gut may terminate in the region of the colon with no evidence of abnormality in the rectum or anus.

If unable to defecate, young animals show marked signs of distress manifested by tenesmus with grunting or whining depending on the species. Examination reveals the absence of the anal orifice in atresia ani and usually some degree of protrusion of the anal region caused by the collection of feces. Tenesmus, absence of feces, and distension of the abdomen are the most obvious signs observed in atresia coli. The anus and rectum appear normal, and the condition must be differentiated from meconium impaction. In atresia coli, even though the anus and rectum are normal, abdominal distension and the absence of feces are obvious. Radiographs, by showing the presence of gas in the rectum or the dilated blind end in the region of the colon, permit an estimation to be made of the distance between the end of the rectum and the anus.

The only treatment is surgical. Colostomy or cecostomy may be considered in calves after insuring that other congenital or hereditary defects are not present.

PERIANAL FISTULA AND SINUS

Although the formation of infected tracts around the anus most commonly accompanies infection of the anal sacs, it may also be the result of minute fecaliths lodging in the pouches between the mucosal columns of the anal canal. The tracts run beneath the skin and into the perianal and pararectal tissue. Constipation, as evidenced by straining, may be a prominent sign before the fistula becomes obvious. Defecation is painful.

Topical and systemic administration of antibacterial agents as determined by the results of sensitivity testing may resolve the condition, but permanent relief is seldom achieved by this treatment. Complete healing is unlikely unless the infected tracts are completely excised.

ANAL FISSURE

A split in the mucosa of the anus, which may extend into the submucosa. Any laceration of the anal region may result in a fissure. The most common cause in dogs is the passage of pieces of bone or other hard or sharp objects in the feces. It may result from the passage of hard feces. In horses and cattle, mucosal lacerations may be inflicted during rectal examination. Care must be exercised to avoid perforation of the rectum during such examinations. Constipation is a prominent sign. The animal is reluctant to defecate because of pain. The feces usually are hard and small, and may have spots of blood on their surface. There may be tenesmus and the animal will resent examination of the anus. Diagnosis is made from the signs and inspection of the anal region.

Oral administration of mineral oil (℞ 484) or olive oil helps maintain soft feces. Topical treatment of the fissure may be attempted by the use of silver nitrate (℞ 618). If the fissure is deep, surgical repair is necessary.

IMPACTION, SUPPURATION AND ABSCESSES OF THE ANAL SACS

Etiology: The 2 anal sacs open on either side of the anus near the junction of the mucous membrane and skin. Their glandular lining produces a gray or brown, sebaceous secretion having an unpleasant odor. The sac ducts sometimes become occluded and the secretion accumulates. This leads to irritation that the dog attempts to relieve by rubbing its anus along the ground, an act known as "scooting". The sacs may subsequently become infected and abscessed.

Clinical Findings and Diagnosis: The first signs are "scooting" and frequent attempts to bite at the anal region. With infection, the characteristic gray-brown secretion is altered in color and consistency, usually becoming thin, yellow, foul-smelling and mixed with pus.

On examination, the anal region appears inflamed and swollen. If the ducts have been occluded for some time, a bulging of the skin is noted over the sacs. If the sacs are infected, abscessation may occur. Unless the owner of the animal is observant, these abscesses may rupture spontaneously, heal and again rupture with the ultimate formation of fistulous tracts leading from the anal sacs to the skin. This condition results in painful defecation and ultimately in constipation.

Treatment: In uncomplicated occlusion of the ducts, simple pressure on the sacs is sufficient to dislodge the contents. This is best accomplished by introducing a gloved finger into the anal orifice and expressing the contents of the sac by pressing on the outside with the thumb.

Where infection has occurred, the sacs should be emptied and flushed with isotonic salt solution. Following this, a mixture of penicillin and streptomycin (℞ 38) or other suitable antibiotics, as determined by sensitivity tests, should be injected into the sacs. Mastitis preparations serve this purpose well. Treatment is repeated weekly until improvement is noted. For refractory or chronic cases in which fistulas have developed, surgical extirpation of the sacs is indicated.

RECTAL STRICTURE

The rectum may be injured by foreign objects (bone, needles, fishhooks) as they pass through the intestinal lumen, or by external factors (accidents, fights, maliciousness). Injured tissue adjacent to the intestinal wall may, in the process of healing, cause constriction of the lumen. An enlarged prostate gland may also result in a diminution of the size of the rectal lumen. Neoplasm is a rare cause. However, narrowing of the lumen of the bovine rectum may occur in abdominal **fat necrosis**. This is due to encircling fat depots undergoing necrosis and hardening. Since lesions are widespread, surgical intervention is not advised. Functional stricture, in the absence of any demonstrable organic lesion, has been described. Digital examination reveals only the presence of muscle spasm producing an annular constriction within the rectum.

If caused by cicatricial tissue, the stricture may be occasionally relieved by frequently passing bougies of increasing size. More usually, extensive surgical resection is necessary.

PERITONITIS

A local or general, acute or chronic inflammation of the peritoneum caused by microbial or chemical agents. Bacterial peritonitis may result, following contamination, from perforation of the stomach, rumen, or intestine, or following perforation of the abdominal wall. It is sometimes caused by the rupture of abscesses within the abdominal cavity, or faulty surgical technique. A variety of oganisms may be found, but the commonest are *Escherichia coli,* staphylococci and streptococci. A specific form of infectious peritonitis is seen in cats (q.v., p. 323).

The introduction of sterile, irritating substances into the peritoneal cavity will initiate a nonbacterial peritonitis. Such substances as talc from surgical gloves, sulfonamide crystals, calcium solutions, blood, and all antiseptic solutions behave in this manner. Special types of chemical peritonitis are caused in some instances in association with pancreatitis or the escape of bile into the peritoneal cavity. While all species are susceptible, clinical observation indicates that peritonitis in horses is a somewhat more serious condition.

Clinical Findings: Abdominal pain is severe. The abdominal wall is tense and tucked-up, and the patient resents palpation. The temperature is elevated. Anorexia is a constant sign and, in small animals, vomiting occurs. In horses there is evidence of severe colic, restlessness, groaning and intermittent episodes of lying down. In cattle rumination ceases and milk production drops. When the animal walks, the gait is stilted. Respiration and pulse rates are accelerated. There is increased reliance on thoracic respiration to minimize the abdominal pain. As the condition progresses, emaciation and dehydration are evident; anemia may be present.

Exudation into the peritoneal cavity leads to reduced peristalsis (paralytic ileus), with subsequent distension of the bowel. The abdomen may become distended due to the accumulation of fluid. The exudation results in hemoconcentration, hypoproteinemia and a reduction in blood volume. Toxemia and bacteremia may lead to anemia. Death results from circulatory collapse (shock).

If "**bile peritonitis**" remains localized, the most serious result is that of visceral adhesions. All the signs associated with other forms of peritonitis are present including emesis, shock and abdominal rigidity. However, an outstanding additional sign is that of icterus.

Lesions: The peritoneal surface becomes covered with a fibrinous exudate. Adhesions occur between abdominal organs. This is particularly true in cattle. In acute cases, a collection of thin slightly colored fluid together with hyperemia and petechiae of the viscera may be the only changes noted. Depending upon the cause, the peritoneal fluid may contain ingesta, urine or bile. The greater omentum frequently adheres to the injured site and may successfully localize the peritonitis. Abscess formation may result. If localization fails, generalized peritonitis ensues. In time, the exudate becomes bloody, purulent, or both.

Diagnosis: The diagnosis is based upon the signs and a history of abdominal injury or surgery. The leukocyte count is elevated and shows a neutrophilia. Paracentesis with subsequent cytologic studies of the peritoneal fluid is useful. In small animals radiography may be used to confirm the presence of fluid in the abdomen and distension of the large intestine. Exploratory laparotomy may be necessary to determine the nature and extent of the injury and for its treatment, if the gallbladder or bile ducts are ruptured.

Treatment: The initiating cause should be removed, e.g., by intestinal resection, repair of a ruptured organ, etc. Antibacterial therapy should be instituted immediately. Paracentesis and culture of the exudate will reveal the nature of the offending organisms and the antibiotics to which they are sensitive. Until such a report is available, the broad-spectrum antibiotics (Ŗ 11, 25) or penicillin and streptomycin combinations (Ŗ 41) should be administered. Antibiotics and sulfonamides given orally are likely to be ineffective if vomiting is present. Intraperitoneal instillation of a soluble nonirritating antibiotic, e.g., streptomycin, may be lifesaving in acute diffuse peritonitis. In addition, surgical drainage of the peritoneal cavity may be indicated. This may be carried out as for peritoneal dialysis, using a solution of a suitable chemotherapeutic as a lavaging agent.

Pain is controlled with meperidine (Ŗ 590) or morphine

(R 592). In large animals, chloral hydrate or tranquilizers are useful. The fluid and electrolyte balance should be maintained with isotonic saline or electrolyte solution. The dog can absorb fluid to the equivalent of its own blood-volume in a 24-hour period. Blood transfusions are indicated if anemia is severe.

Food should be withheld during the first 48 hours of treatment. Parenteral nutrients may be given in the form of amino acids (R 595) and glucose. High dosage of vitamins should be administered daily by the parenteral route. As the condition of the patient improves, food may be given by mouth in the form of liquids and the normal diet achieved gradually.

PANCREATIC DISEASE IN THE DOG

Disease of the pancreas is relatively rare in the dog. The main syndromes are the result of acute pancreatitis, chronic relapsing pancreatitis, and its sequela, fibrosis. In addition, a syndrome characterized by malabsorption is recognized in young dogs but some argument exists as to whether the pathologic lesion is hypoplasia or atrophy. Carcinoma of the acinar pancreas is uncommon, but insidious and devastating in its manifestations. Functional islet cell adenocarcinomas are very rare and cause a syndrome characterized by convulsions due to hypoglycemia.

PANCREATITIS

Etiology: The cause of pancreatitis, whether chronic or acute, is unknown. The underlying lesion is one of necrosis, and many factors including trauma, nutritional deficiencies due to excess fat in the diet, infection, duct occlusion, reflux of bile or intestinal fluid into the gland and distension of the stomach with food have been associated with the disease. The common mechanism is probably ischemia leading to necrosis and release of activated proteolytic and lipolytic enzymes that digest the pancreas and surrounding tissue. Chronic replacing pancreatitis is a continuance or a periodic recurrence of the necrosis. A proportion of chronic cases terminate in diabetes mellitus as a result of fibrosis of the gland.

Clinical Findings: Dogs that suffer from spontaneous pancreatitis tend to be middle-aged, inactive, obese house dogs that often eat fat, either from their master's plates or from garbage containers. Working or athletic dogs are almost never affected, except on the rare occasions when pancreatic necrosis is a complication of abdominal surgery or trauma. The acute disease causes much vomiting and marked abdominal pain, followed in some cases by shock. Hypoglycemia due to sudden release of insulin and hypocalcemia due to calcium combining with fat in the peritoneal cavity are possible complications. The feces usually contain some blood. Jaundice is an unusual complication that occurs when the common bile duct is occluded by the inflammatory reaction or digested by the enzymes released during the attack.

The chronic relapsing form of pancreatitis is characterized by repeated mild attacks of vomiting and abdominal pain of only a few days' duration. Discovery of the true cause of such attacks may come months or years later when a particularly severe attack warrants sufficient investigation to identify the disease. More commonly the problem is recognized after voluminous orange- or clay-colored, rancid-smelling, frequent stools containing undigested food are present. The appetite may be ravenous owing to the malabsorption and, in some cases, the concurrent diabetes mellitus. The pancreas is reduced to a fibrotic cord. Chronic pancreatitis also occurs in the domestic cat.

Diagnosis: The clinical diagnosis of acute pancreatitis may be confirmed by finding an elevated amylase or lipase concentration in the serum. Leukocytosis, hemoconcentration, elevated BUN and the presence of protein and casts in the urine may also occur. The disease may be confused with acute renal failure or intestinal obstruction but the acute pain tends to rule out the former and radiography will rule out the latter. Chronic pancreatitis is confirmed by an absence of trypsin and the presence of fat and undigested meat fibers in the feces (see PANCREATIC FUNCTION TESTS, p. 1385). Amylase and lipase concentrations are not elevated in the serum of animals with fibrosis of the pancreas.

Treatment: The most important aspect of the treatment of acute pancreatitis is initiation of vigorous therapy aimed at combating pain and shock with analgesics such as meperidine (℞ 590), and electrolyte solutions to restore to normal the decreased blood volume, blood pressure and renal function. Propantheline bromide (℞ 494) or atropine sulfate (℞ 489), which have an inhibitory effect on pancreatic secretion, may limit the extension of inflammation in milder cases. Penicillin (℞ 45) and streptomycin (℞ 52) or one of the tetracyclines are given to combat secondary infection of necrotic tissue. Parenteral feeding and good nursing care are essential. Oral feeding should be avoided to minimize pancreatic secretions.

In chronic pancreatitis, replacement therapy must be given for the duration of the animal's life. Three daily feedings of a high-protein, high-carbohydrate, low-fat diet are recommended. Pancreatin granules (℞ 497) are mixed with each meal in a dosage level sufficient to keep the feces normal. This may require as much as 15 gm per day. Absorption of fat is enhanced by the administration of an emulsifying agent, sorethytan mono-oleate (℞ 498), with the meals. Choline (℞ 599) may be added to the diet for its lipotrophic effect, but generally these latter 2 agents are unnecessary for long-term replacement therapy. Tablets of pancreatin should not be used as they are generally passed through the dog's digestive tract intact. The prognosis is good and management is not difficult as long as diabetes is absent. When the endocrine function is also lost, insulin therapy must be used. The prognosis for such cases is poor.

PANCREATIC HYPOPLASIA

This disease is also called juvenile atrophy of the pancreas and it is seen in young dogs, usually before 2 years of age. The pancreas is small, thin and lace-like in form. Affected dogs lose weight in spite of having a ravenous appetite. They do not vomit or suffer abdominal pain. The stools become soft, unformed and voluminous, may take on a putty-like consistency and are passed frequently. Undigested food may be seen in the feces and the hair of the tail and perineal region may become oily because of the excess fat in the feces. Diabetes mellitus is very rare in conjunction with this disease.

The diagnosis is confirmed by the absence of trypsin in the feces and the presence of fat and undigested meat fibers. It must not be confused with intestinal malabsorption where trypsin will be present in the feces. Laparotomy may be necessary to make a positive diagnosis. Treatment is as for chronic pancreatitis without diabetes mellitus.

Pancreatic Neoplasms: (*see* NEOPLASMS OF SMALL ANIMALS, p. 596).

DISEASES OF THE LIVER AND BILIARY TRACT

Most liver disorders are associated with more generalized diseases, e.g., toxicoses, congestive heart failure, parasitism,

and as such are discussed under those specific headings.
Lipidosis (excess storage of fat in liver cells) may be the result
of hepatoxins, a deficiency of lipotropic factors, disturbances
of hepatic-cell metabolism, or simply the result of heavy feeding. Poisoning by bacterial toxins, chloroform, carbon tetrachloride, plant alkaloids, arsenic and phosphorus, among
others; and such metabolic disturbances as diabetes mellitus in
dog, baby pig anemia or ovine pregnancy toxemia all may
result in the condition, but other signs are likely to be much
more marked than those of liver dysfunction.

Fibrosis is usually the result of toxic or parasite damage but
may be obscure in origin. **Primary amyloid disease** of the liver
is rare in animals and the secondary condition scarcely more
common, being seen in chronic pyogenic processes, chronic
tuberculosis, and in horses used for antibody production.
Chronic passive congestion of the liver may result from any
of several thoracic disorders. Relief must be obtained by
treatment of congestive heart failure (q.v., p. 51). **Telangiectasis** (blood-filled, abnormally distended sinusoids) is of unknown
cause, and of significance only because it leads to condemnation for human consumption of about 2% of all cattle livers.
"Sawdust livers", found in fat young beef cattle, contain many
small yellowish necrotic foci, 1 to 2 mm in diameter. These are
foci of hepatic epithelial cells undergoing coagulation necrosis,
and it is suspected that these may be the forerunners of
abscesses or telangiectasis. The condition results in condemnation of about 1% of livers.

Acute infectious hepatitis may be caused by all known infectious agents. More common causes are canine infectious
hepatitis, leptospirosis and clostridial infections. **Abscessation**
is common in cattle, usually, it is believed, as a sequela to a
degree of rumen acidosis occurring with heavy grain feeding.
Most biliary disorders are the result of parasitism or the
spread of infection from the gut.

ENDOCRINE SYSTEM

THE PITUITARY GLAND
(Hypophysis)

Pituitary and hypothalamic disease may result from tumors, encephalitis, abscesses, local hemorrhage or injury. Pituitary tumors may be asymptomatic or produce increased or decreased function. Hormones secreted by the adenohypophysis are somatotropin (STH or growth hormone), thyrotropin (TSH), adrenocorticotropin (ACTH), gonadotropin (which consists of the follicle-stimulating, FSH, and luteinizing, LH, fractions) and prolactin (lactogen). The hypothalamus produces humoral agents called releasing and inhibiting factors which regulate the synthesis and release of the adenohypophyseal hormones which are proteins. All hypophyseal hormones are available in crude or partially purified form and some are now synthesized.

The neurohypophysis stores vasopressin or antidiuretic hormone (ADH) which controls blood pressure and diminishes the loss of urine, and oxytocin which causes uterine contractions and the ejection of milk. Neither the anterior- nor posterior-pituitary hormones are effective when given by mouth and must be injected.

ANTERIOR-LOBE DISORDERS

Because pituitary hormones regulate rates of function of their target organs, malfunction of the pituitary results in an abnormal slowing down or speeding up of the rates at which the thyroid, adrenal cortex or gonads function.

Overproduction of STH leading to gigantism or acromegaly is infrequent and without practical therapy. Genetic selection for rapid growth and large body size results in selection of animals with additional STH output. Underproduction of STH likely produces pituitary dwarfs in animals but such newborn animals seldom survive and therapy with STH is impractical.

Abnormal production of prolactin has not been identified in domestic animals.

Canine Cushing's disease is a complex of signs occurring in many breeds but the incidence is greater in the small breeds. The inciting cause is usually a functional tumor of the anterior lobe of the pituitary, in which overproduction of ACTH stimulates the adrenal cortex to bilateral hyperplasia and increased output of adrenocortical hormone, which produces the majority of changes. In some instances, the primary cause is a tumor of the adrenal cortex (usually unilateral) leading directly to increased activity of the gland. The principal signs are bilateral symmetrical alopecia, dry, hyperkeratotic skin, relaxation of the skeletal muscles, increased abdominal obesity, pot-bellied appearance, and frequently polydipsia and polyuria. Of diagnostic value is the marked lymphopenia and eosinopenia which accompany the disease.

ACTH (℞ 139) administration increases the urinary 17-ketosteroid level several-fold in bilateral hyperplasia, with less elevation in neoplasia.

Surgical removal of the adrenal glands relieves the signs but careful pre- and post-surgical therapy must be given including a mineralocorticoid (deoxycorticosterone acetate, DOCA), a glucocorticoid (cortisone acetate, ℞ 140) and salt. DOCA dosage (℞ 141) must be based on blood sodium and potassium levels for several weeks until DOCA pellet implants can maintain a balance. A good prognosis should not be expected in more than 50% of the cases.

The adiposogenital syndrome is characterized by extreme obesity together with hypoplasia of the gonads. The appetite is voracious, and other signs are lethargy, hypersomnia, hypothermia and often polydipsia and polyuria. It is caused by tumor or destructive lesions also affecting the hypothalamus and usually the posterior lobe. Other pituitary tumors occur, but have little clinical importance.

Pituitary cachexia or **Simmonds' disease** sometimes is seen in dogs and consists of cachexia not explainable by other causes. It usually is caused by a pituitary tumor. There is no cure, but the condition may possibly be alleviated temporarily by the use of anterior-pituitary extracts.

POSTERIOR-LOBE DISORDERS

Posterior pituitary hormone (oxytocin) is occasionally used in hastening normal parturition in small animals if the cervix is dilated (R 173). Manual delivery or cesarean section are preferred in large animals since oxytocin can induce uterine rupture.

Oxytocin regulates the contractility of the myoepithelial "basket cells" around the alveoli of the udder. Nursing produces a neural impulse which travels via the hypothalamus to the posterior lobe of the pituitary gland which instantly responds by releasing oxytocin. This hormone is carried by the bloodstream to the udder where it causes milk let-down. Injection of oxytocin produces the same effect and can also make available the "residual" milk which cannot normally be obtained by milking. Similarly, manipulation of genitalia causes release of oxytocin resulting in uterine contractions (aid in sperm transport) as well as the effect noted on the udder. Because of the participation of the nervous system in this process, lactating females are very sensitive to disturbances or environmental stresses which may as easily prevent release of oxytocin as proper stimuli enhance it. Oxytocin (R 172) can be used to correct agalactia in some postparturient sows, and milk let-down in cows can be augmented.

DIABETES INSIPIDUS

A disorder of the neurohypophysis with chronic manifestations, characterized by the excretion of excessive quantities of very dilute but otherwise normal urine and associated with a severe polydipsia.

Etiology: Diabetes insipidus results from a deficient secretion or release of the antidiuretic hormone by the neurohypophysis. Secretion of this hormone, which controls the rate of water resorption in the distal convoluted tubules of the kidney, is dependent on the integrity of the neurohypophyseal system which includes the supraoptic and paraventricular nuclei and their axon tracts which extend into the posterior lobe. Injury to any part of this system may result in diabetes insipidus. It is occasionally seen in horses and cats, but most often in dogs.

Cases may be separated into 2 main groups. In the idiopathic group, no pathologic organic changes are demonstrable and the cause is unknown. The so-called symptomatic group comprises a number of pathologic conditions. The most common lesion in dogs is a tumor of the neurohypophysis or of the adjacent intracranial structures. However, any intracranial space-occupying lesion that compresses or invades these structures can cause diabetes insipidus. Other causes are metastasis of a tumor to the pituitary or hypothalamus, abscess formation in this region, fracture of the base of the skull and basilar meningitis.

Clinical Findings: The condition is seen more often in older dogs and affects both sexes. The onset usually is insidious, with progressively increasing polydipsia and polyuria if it is due to a tumor; it may be more sudden when due to trauma or meningitis. Enormous quantities of fluid are ingested and excreted: up to 20 liters a day in the dog and 100 liters in the horse. The urine is water-clear and of low specific gravity (1.002 to 1.006 in dogs) and contains no albumin. Housebroken dogs, if confined, are in constant distress as they seek access to the outdoors.

Diagnosis: Diagnosis depends on proof of chronic polydipsia and polyuria, with the production of urine of a constant or slightly fluctuating low specific gravity. Incontinence and increased frequency should, therefore, be distinguished from increased urinary volume. Since tumors of the neurohypophysis may frequently involve the adjacent adenohypophysis and the hypothalamus, diabetes insipidus, obesity and gonadal atrophy frequently coexist. In horses, in which diabetes insipidus is usually due to tumor of the pars intermedia, there is concurrent somnolence and muscle weakness.

Diabetes mellitus is distinguished by glycosuria, by the high specific gravity of the urine (from 1.035 to 1.060 in dogs) and by a darker color: yellow, orange or amber. In diabetes insipidus, the urine is very pale yellow. In compensated chronic nephritis, polyuria also may be present, but will be lesser in extent and the specific gravity will be higher (1.010 to 1.012 in dogs). In addition, albumin and casts often are present; these are absent in diabetes insipidus.

A diagnosis may be confirmed by the parenteral injection of vasopressin tannate in oil (℞ 175). The antidiuretic hormone causes temporary disappearance of the polyuria and polydipsia for 6 to 24 hours, if these are due to diabetes insipidus.

Treatment: The control of diabetes insipidus requires the parenteral use of antidiuretic hormones, usually as vasopressin tannate in oil (℞ 175), the dose being adjusted to the individual case. The effects are only palliative and temporary after each injection. Dietary restriction of urinary solutes, salt and protein, may help reduce urine output.

THE THYROID GLAND

Like other endocrine glands, the thyroid affects or coordinates many body functions. In domestic animals, the most important of these functions are tissue oxidation (metabolism), growth, reproduction, and egg and milk production. The stored thyroid hormone probably is the large protein molecule, iodothyroglobulin, which is present in the colloid within the thyroid follicles. For practical therapeutic purposes, the amino acid L-thyroxine is considered to be the active thyroid hormone. In some species, triiodothyronine has been isolated from the thyroid and blood and may have several times as much physiologic effect as L-thyroxine.

In domestic animals, most of the disorders of the thyroid are characterized by the underproduction of thyroxine. The 2 common causes of hypothyroidism are iodine deficiency and inherited low production of thyrotropic hormone. Hyperthyroidism is occasionally also observed in domestic animals, but it is not commonly diagnosed. The parafollicular cells of the mammalian thyroid secrete the hormone calcitonin in response to high plasma calcium levels. In submammalian species these cells, which are derived from ultimobranchial tissue, form a separate gland. Calcitonin functions to lower excessively high levels of blood calcium.

HYPOTHYROIDISM

Hypothyroidism, which includes goiter, cretinism and myxedema may be the result of inadequate iodine intake. In the so-called goiter belt, the natural feedstuffs and water are deficient in iodine and a reliable supplementary source of iodine, such as stabilized salt, must be fed. Hypothyroidism may result from the presence of goitrogenic substances in feeds or the administration of synthetic goitrogens. Their effect is to interfere with or to prevent the secretion of thyroxine. Raw soybeans, cabbage, rape, turnips, many other natural foods and some drugs have been shown to contain goitrogens. Hypothyroidism may also be the result of inborn errors of metabolism due to a simple autosomal recessive gene. Cases of congenital goiter have been reported in sheep and suspected in cattle.

SIMPLE GOITER
(Colloid goiter, Endemic goiter)

A diffuse, symmetrical enlargement of the thyroid gland with clinical or subclinical hypothyroidism. In the U.S.A., the Great Lakes Basin, the Northern Great Plains States and upper Mississippi Valley, the Rocky Mountains States and the Pacific Coast States should be regarded as wholly or partially deficient in iodine. In other parts of the world, mountainous and inland areas distant from the sea should be regarded as potentially iodine-deficient.

Clinical Findings: Simple goiter due to iodine deficiency is most common in newborn pigs and lambs. It is less common in foals and calves, but may occur in any mammal. The glands usually are at least twice the normal size, frequently larger, soft and dark-red in color. Severely deficient, goitrous pigs and lambs may be dead or weak at birth. The neck is usually grossly enlarged and the skin and other tissues may be thick, flabby and edematous. Pigs, calves and lambs may be partially hairless or woolless, but extreme goiter may exist in the presence of the normal amount of hair or wool. Iodine deficiency in the pregnant mare may result in the birth of goitrous foals. Many foals from severely iodine-deficient dams are weak at birth, unable to suckle and may die. Goiter was common in dogs in iodine-deficient areas prior to the widespread use of iodized salt in human diets and the inclusion of trace minerals in prepared pet foods. Goiter has been reported in cats, but is regarded as rare.

The iodine requirements of the pregnant female appear to be higher than those of other animals and iodine deficiency usually manifests itself in the newborn. Microscopic examination of the thyroid may be necessary to detect subclinical goiter. Gross thyroid enlargement of any animal in the so-called goiter belt, in conjunction with a lack of dietary iodine supplementation, is strong evidence of simple goiter.

Prophylaxis and Treatment: Prophylaxis is more effective than treatment. The use of stabilized iodized salt (containing at least 0.007% iodine) is recommended in all areas known or suspected to be iodine-deficient. In extreme cases, pigs and lambs may be born dead or die within a few days after birth. Among the latter group, treatment does not seem to improve the chance of survival. The use of iodized salt in goitrous animals which do not die usually will result in restoration of normal thyroid function. Specific iodine therapy may be employed (℞ 578, 582).

GOITROGEN-INDUCED HYPOTHYROIDISM

The feeding of raw soybeans, especially in the absence of adequate iodine intake, may produce simple goiter. Present methods of processing, which include heating the meal, destroy the natural goitrogen which soybeans contain. Although goiter has been produced in laboratory animals with natural plant goitrogens, it is not likely to occur in animals receiving adequate iodine. The compounds in plants responsible for goitrogenic activity are thiocyanates, thioglycosides and perchlorates. The *Brassica* spp. (q.v., p. 7) contain a substance named goitrin which is the active goitrogen.

The production of controlled hypothyroidism with goitrogens, such as thiouracil, in attempts to induce fattening in meat animals has had limited experimental application in chickens, swine and sheep. In general, goitrogens may improve fattening and feed efficiency when fed for short periods, but variability in response has limited their use to experimental feeding trials thus far.

CRETINISM

Extreme hypothyroidism in the newborn or young animal resulting from complete absence of the thyroid hormone due to iodine deficiency. The immature animal fails to grow, has irreversible CNS dysfunction, mental dullness, dry brittle coat, thick skin, scaliness, dermatitis, lethargy and obesity. Thyroid preparations (℞ 182) may be tried in animals diagnosed as cretinous, but usually euthanasia is advisable. Iodine is of no value since the thyroid cells are exhausted.

MYXEDEMA

A reaction to a lack of thyroid hormone in the adult, characterized by lethargy, accompanied by cutaneous thickening and edema, especially of the head and limbs. It must be considered, however, that different species of animals vary in relative thyroid activity, some being excessively active (hyperthyroid type) and others much less active (hypothyroid type). Within species, there are breed and individual differences that may be explained as differences in thyroid function.

In farm animals, signs are not likely to occur in the absence of goitrogen administration. Although conclusive evidence is lacking it appears that excessive fattening and lack of sex drive in both sexes may occur. In cows, reduced milk production and silent heat can be a result of hypothyroidism due to high environmental temperatures.

An unequivocal diagnosis of hypothyroidism would require objective measurement of thyroid function, such as lowered basal metabolic rate or reduced radioactive iodine uptake. In older dogs, obesity, lethargy, dryness of the skin and loss of hair are sometimes attributed to hypothyroidism. The administration of desiccated thyroid (℞ 182) or other forms of thyroxine may alleviate these signs.

HYPERTHYROIDISM

Excessive secretion of the thyroid hormone, increased metabolic rate, and hypertrophy and hyperplasia of the thyroid epithelium as a consequence of overstimulation by the thyrotropic hormone of the anterior pituitary gland.

Clinical Findings: The first sign of hyperthyroidism, whether it is spontaneous or induced, is weight loss accompanied by increased appetite. The animal is restless and nervous; heart and respiratory rates are increased and the metabolic rate is elevated. Blood cholesterol is reduced and glycosuria and creatinuria may occur. There is hypertrophy and hyperplasia of thyroid tissue in simple goiter and hyperthyroidism. In simple goiter, the increased cellular activity is the result of an attempt to compensate for inadequate iodine intake. In hyperthyroidism, the increased cellular activity results in excessive thyroxine secretion.

Except possibly in the dog, hyperthyroidism does not often appear spontaneously in animals. The condition is sometimes reported as a cause of poor fattening in steers.

The discovery that thyroxine or thyroactive substances, such as desiccated thyroid and thyroprotein, influence milk production, growth rate, reproduction and, in chickens, egg production and feathering, has led to considerable experimental use of these materials. Thyroid administration during the decline phase of milk production in cattle has been shown to increase both milk and butterfat production. Since the metabolic rate is increased by thyroid therapy, feed intake must be increased if body weight and a high level of lactation are to be maintained. The requirements of certain vitamins, particularly vitamin A and the B-vitamins, are increased. Excessive weight loss which cannot be corrected by feeding, extreme nervousness and excessive cardiac and respiratory rates are indications for the discontinuance of thyroid therapy or reduction of dosage.

Treatment: Spontaneous hyperthyroidism can be dealt with by both surgical and medical means. Complete thyroidectomy, in the absence of accessory thyroid tissue, is followed by hypothyroidism which in turn must be corrected by thyroid administration. Partial thyroidectomy may correct hyperthyroidism, but the thyroid remnants may undergo further hypertrophy and thus re-establish hyperthyroidism.

Thiouracil and its derivatives depress thyroid activity. In dogs, 0.1 to 0.2 gm of thiouracil daily will usually reduce thyroxine secretion. Blood hemoglobin and red and white cell counts should be made before and during therapy since goitrogens may produce anemia, agranulocytosis, fever and skin reactions. Dosage must be determined by giving to effect.

THE PARATHYROID GLANDS

Much of what is known about the function of the parathyroid glands has been learned by studying the parathyroidectomized dog. Complete removal of the glands is followed by a rapid drop in blood calcium and an elevation of inorganic blood phosphorus. There is hyperexcitability of the peripheral nerves, muscular tremors and finally violent convulsions and death.

Primary hyperparathyroidism has been recognized as a clinical entity in the dog. It may·be due to an adenoma of the parathyroid which leads to hyperplasia and overproduction of parathyroid hormone (PTH). The excessive PTH release may lead to demineralization of bones even leading to fractures and bone deformities. Treatment is limited to surgical attempts to remove sufficient hyperactive tissue to reduce the level of hormone production to normal limits.

Secondary hyperparathyroidism is secondary to (1) chronic renal disease or (2) chronic imbalance in the nutritional calcium-phosphorus intake (*see* NUTRITIONAL HYPERPARATHYROIDISM, p. 562 and INTERSTITIAL NEPHRITIS, pp. 854 and 855).

Secondary hyperparathyroidism (renal) of dogs is due to

chronic renal dysfunction which leads to phosphate retention and then calcium depletion (reason unknown). During progressive development of renal lesions the kidney becomes less and less able to excrete phosphate. The resulting elevations in plasma phosphate and altered calcium: phosphate ratio (low calcium) cause hyperactivity of the parathyroid. This causes demineralization of bone, resulting in further increases in plasma phosphate. Since the damaged kidney is unable to excrete phosphate adequately, plasma levels continue to rise. Hypocalcemia then stimulates excessive PTH production and finally parathyroid hypertrophy (see pp. 567 and 855).

The spontaneous occurrence of parturient paresis in dairy cattle and postparturient eclampsia in the bitch is supposedly due to hypocalcemia. There is a physiologic basis for the theory that the sudden demand for calcium cannot always be met by the parathyroid glands and that temporary hypoparathyroidism follows. Until more is known of the specific parathyroid mechanisms involved, the present therapy of calcium salts should be employed. Therapy with PTH is less effective than calcium injection, much slower in effect and generally not recommended.

PTH causes resorption of bone and increased plasma calcium concentration. It decreases phosphate reabsorption in the kidney and promotes, in the presence of vitamin D, the absorption of calcium from the intestine. Calcitonin inhibits bone resorption but does not affect PTH action in the kidney or intestine. Secretion of these 2 hormones is regulated solely by the level of blood calcium.

THE THYMUS

In the late fetus and in the newborn mammal the thymus represents about 1% of body weight. With increasing age the thymus gradually decreases in size and in the adult it is an insignificant, atrophied structure. In the young it regresses following hypophysectomy or as a result of stresses such as severe injury, infection, or injection of cortisone. Its main function lies in its prodigious ability to produce and liberate lymphocytes which migrate to the lymph nodes and the spleen. These lymphocytes give rise to cells which are responsible for most or all immunologic reactions of the body. The activation of antigenic response has also been shown to occur without the migration of whole cells from the thymus. It is probable that the rates of immune reactions are influenced by steroidal hormones.

The thymus, along with other lymphoid tissue, can be involved in the pathology of bovine lymphosarcoma.

DIABETES MELLITUS

A chronic disorder of carbohydrate metabolism due to insulin insufficiency. Although diabetes is seen in the dog, the disease is rarely diagnosed in other domestic animals.

Etiology: No specific cause has yet been found for this condition. In most cases, the insulin-producing cells of the islet tissue of the pancreas have been damaged. In the dog, this damage frequently is associated with disease of the pancreatic parenchyma, such as chronic pancreatitis or pancreatic atrophy or fibrosis. Previous infection may play a part in the onset of this condition. Most cases of diabetes mellitus occur in dogs over 5 years of age. It is more frequent in obese animals.

Clinical Findings: Usually, the disease is fairly well advanced when first seen by the veterinarian, and the patient is emaciated. The onset is insidious, but the owner may have noticed increased thirst or urination or sudden loss of weight in obese animals. The main signs are polyuria, polydipsia, polyphagia, weakness and emaciation. In advanced cases, an acetone odor may be detected on the breath. Acidosis with persistent vomiting occurs in severe cases, especially in dogs. The terminal episode is diabetic coma. Secondary signs are sometimes present in the form of corneal opacity or ulcer and cataract. If the pancreatic parenchyma has been damaged, digestive disorders paralleling those of pancreatitis may be present. Available information indicates that the disease is nearly 3 times as common in female dogs as in males.

Diagnosis: Diabetes mellitus may be diagnosed by finding sugar in the urine of patients showing typical clinical signs. A more certain diagnosis can be made if an elevation of blood sugar can be shown. The normal values for blood sugar in the dog are from 75 to 100 mg/100 ml. In fasting animals, blood sugar levels above 150 mg/100 ml are diagnostic of diabetes mellitus. Values have been reported as high as 500 mg/100 ml. The specific gravity of the urine is usually increased (1.040 to 1.060). The disease can be differentiated from diabetes insipidus, which is rare, by the hyperglycemia and glycosuria, and the high specific gravity of the urine. Chronic nephritis with polyuria can be ruled out in the same way and also by the presence of albumin in the urine and an elevated urea-nitrogen content of the blood.

Treatment is seldom successful on a long-term basis in the dog, but may be attempted where subtotal disease is present and when deficiency of acinar tissues is not a complication. Mild disease may be controlled by change to a semidiabetic diet consisting of meat and milk. The dog should be offered a diet low in carbohydrates and the total amount of carbohydrates equally divided between 3 daily meals. If the diet does not control the disease, injections of insulin should be commenced, using the protamine-zinc form of insulin (R 171), varying the dose until the disease is brought under control and the urine contains only a trace of sugar. Doses usually range from 5 to 50 u/day, depending on the severity of the disease and the size of the animals. The insulin should be given prior to feeding; the feed should be given in frequent small portions and if excessive insulin results in hypoglycemia, 5 to 20 gm glucose should be given orally or parenterally and the daily insulin dose reduced. In mild cases of diabetes, one of the oral hypoglycemic sulfonylureas may be used (R 161). Oral dosing greatly simplifies treatment and encourages owners to carry out home treatment. The sulfonylureas stimulate release of insulin, hence, functional tissue must be present.

In diabetic acidosis, the use of regular insulin (rather than protamine-zinc) along with IV injections of glucose and electrolytes is indicated. These cases must be treated as medical emergencies. The primary objectives are to reduce the ketonemia and to replace electrolytes lost through vomiting. Regular insulin may be given in an initial dose of 10 to 50 u and repeated at 6- to 8-hour intervals depending upon the dog's response.

When insulin therapy has been instituted, it is helpful to check the urine sugar and blood sugar levels at frequent intervals until such time as an adequate maintenance dose is determined.

In diabetes, as in pancreatitis, there is a tendency for fat deposition to occur in the liver. This can be prevented by the addition of choline (R 599) to the diet. Pancreatin and bile salts may also be employed.

THE ADRENAL GLANDS

The adrenal glands consist of 2 parts, the medulla and the cortex. The medulla secretes epinephrine and norepinephrine.

Medullary release of these hormones is under the direct control of the sympathetic nervous system and constitutes the initial response of the animal to stresses such as disease, trauma, extreme temperatures and hemorrhage. Although sympathetic stimulation causes the release of both hormones, norepinephrine-release increases during periods of hypotension, whereas epinephrine release increases when metabolic adjustments such as increased blood glucose levels are needed to meet emergencies. Both cause ACTH release by the pituitary via stimulation of the hypothalamus.

Although the adrenal cortex is known to synthesize some 50 steroids, only a few are of significance. The adrenal sex steroids —androgens, estrogens and progesterone—are of little imporance except during hyperplasia of the adrenal cortex. The glucocorticoids, cortisol (hydrocortisone) and corticosterone, are concerned with intermediary metabolism of carbohydrates, proteins and fats. They, like the medullary hormones, are released during periods of stress and constitute a secondary response to meet emergencies. Their release is under the control of ACTH. The glucocorticoids elevate blood-glucose levels by stimulating liver gluconeogenesis from body protein. They mobilize body fats and proteins and inhibit peripheral utilization of glucose. The glucocorticoids also exert a profound anti-inflammatory effect by suppressing the activity of fibroblasts and depressing vascularization and formation of granulation tissue.

The mineralocorticoids, aldosterone and desoxycorticosterone, aid in the maintenance of normal sodium and water levels in extracellular fluid and are essential for life. They cause increased sodium retention and potassium loss by the kidney tubules. The mineralocorticoids are released in response to low-sodium serum levels and hypotension. Excessive administration of mineralocorticoids can cause death due to potassium depletion. In cases of adrenal hyperplasia where surgical removal of both adrenals is required, the animal must be maintained on mineralocorticoid therapy, usually subcut. desoxycorticosterone pellets, and must receive additional dietary sodium.

Many synthetic steroids possessing enhanced glucocorticoid activity but lessened mineralocorticoid activity are now widely used in veterinary medicine. Most of these represent alteration of the cortisol molecule by unsaturation, fluorination, or methylation. Perhaps the greatest use of glucocorticoids in veterinary medicine is for their anti-inflammatory effects in chronic conditions such as conjunctivitis, arthritis, tendonitis, dermatitis and bursitis. Local application to the inflamed area is preferred whenever possible, although they can be administered parenterally. Dairy cattle with ketosis usually respond to the blood-glucose-elevating properties of the glucocorticoids, and their use is especially indicated when ketotic cows fail to respond or relapse after IV glucose. Massive doses of glucocorticoids are used to alleviate the signs of shock although their exact mechanism of action in this condition is unknown. Because of their anti-inflammatory properties, glucocorticoids should not be administered parenterally for infectious diseases unless accompanied by an appropriate antibiotic. Glucocorticoids are known to cause abortion and retained placenta, so they should not be administered to pregnant animals, especially during the last third of pregnancy. Glucocorticoid administration to sheep partially inhibits wool growth and causes tenderness of the fleece. Similar signs are seen during periods of stress in sheep, presumably due to hyperactivity of the adrenal cortex.

Absence of adrenocortical function leads to **Addison's disease.** This condition is rare in animals although it has been reported in dogs. Hyperfunction of the adrenal gland causes Cushing's disease (q.v., p. 184) and this also has been reported in dogs. Cushing's disease may be caused by a tumor of the adrenal cortex or it may be secondary to a diseased anterior pituitary.

THE GONADS

OVARIAN MALFUNCTION

Hyperestrinism: The excessive production of estrogen by abnormal ovaries, possibly with persistent follicles, follicular cysts, or a granulosa tumor (*see also* p. 606). The usual signs are a disturbed estrous cycle, sterility, excessive or prolonged uterine bleeding and sometimes nymphomania. It is often accompanied by squamous vulvar hyperplasia. The changes in the uterus consist of reddening and thickening of the endometrium, with a roughened surface and glandular hyperplasia. Alopecia (q.v., p. 915) and hyperpigmentation of the skin are also believed to be signs of hyperestrinism. This condition is rather frequently seen in bitches of middle age or older. Spaying is the recommended treatment. However, alopecia is also seen in hypoestrinism.

Certain forms of hyperestrinism are associated with cystic follicles. This condition, which is an important cause of sterility, is seen in swine and cattle. In cows, these lesions are often associated with more or less constant heat and the gradual assumption of external features and behavior characteristic of the male (*see* CYSTIC OVARIAN DISEASE, p. 794). In cattle, the fluid within the cystic follicles rarely contains measurable amounts of estrogens and the clinical signs are difficult to reconcile with this fact. The lack of myometrial tone does not suggest direct estrogen stimulation. Possibly the CNS is abnormally sensitive to estrogens in some of these cases.

Hypoestrinism: A lack of estrogens, or possibly a lack of response by the CNS to estrogens in the entire animal, is fairly common. Silent heat, or ovulation without psychic heat, is often encountered in cattle. In sheep, the same may be observed at the beginning or at the end of the breeding season. The result of a single stimulation by gonadotropin out of the normal season is also an ovulation without heat. In these conditions, the appearance of the accessory organs of the ewe suggest lack of estrogen stimulation.

Hypoestrinism develops as a normal consequence in the spayed animal. One effect of estrogens upon growth is to cause the long bones to ossify so that they cause an early cessation of skeletal growth. Early spaying prolongs the growth period so that the spayed female usually has a larger frame than the unspayed female. The prevention of periodic stimulation and restlessness enables the spayed female to fatten more readily and the carcass quality is generally improved.

In spayed bitches, urinary incontinence may occur, but this usually responds well to the administration of diethylstilbestrol (℞ 163). Spaying may cause some bitches to become fatter than normal.

Hypoprogesteronism is not a common nor easily recognized clinical entity. Most animals get the required progesterone from the corpus luteum; in some species the uterus takes over progesterone production during the latter part of pregnancy. The times when hypoprogesteronism might be clinically evident are (1) when improper corpus luteum formation occurs resulting in short cycles, and (2) at the time when the transfer from ovarian to uterine progesterone should occur—resulting in interruption of pregnancy. This latter time varies with the species. The cow uterus may never take over, the mare uterus may take over in 90 days.

Hyperprogesteronism: Such a condition may exist as a result of persistent corpora lutea, such as seen in cystic glandular hyperplasia of the endometrium (*see* PYOMETRA, p. 841) in the bitch. The same syndrome is seen with the excessive use of exogenous progesterones, or it may follow pseudocyesis (q.v., p. 845). Such a condition may exist as a result of persistent corpora lutea which is really a result of the absence of a luteolytic factor such as prostaglandin from the uterus. This lack of luteolytic factor from the uterus occurs during pregnancy, endometritis and with the presence of a foreign body such as a mummified fetus.

Relation of sex hormones to infection of the genitalia: There is a definite relationship between the susceptibility to infection of the uterine endometrium and the reproductive stage in cows. Cows during the follicular phase are much more resistant to infections than they are during the luteal phase. Pyometritis is more frequently observed in cows with a corpus luteum in the ovaries than in those with follicles. Cows are thought to be more resistant to infections while under the influence of exogenous estrogens or stilbesterol (R 163). Conversely, the injection of progesterone increases the susceptibility of cows to infections of the reproductive tract.

CONTROL OF OVULATION

Follicle-stimulating hormone (FSH) produced by the anterior pituitary causes ovarian follicular development. These follicles produce estrogens which feed back to the pituitary, inhibiting FSH and stimulating luteinizing hormone (LH) release. LH then acts on the follicles causing them to ripen, ovulate and luteinize, changing the hormone production from the ovary to progesterone, which in turn feeds back to the pituitary and inhibits the LH release. This allows the FSH to again proceed toward the development of more follicles and the next cycle. The life of the corpus luteum is set by the species and is ended abruptly by a luteolytic factor a few days before the onset of estrus. Any control of the estrous cycle therefore must come into play in one of 3 ways: (1) induction of ovulation, (2) inhibition of ovulation, (3) induction of corpus luteum regression.

Undernutrition and climate (in seasonal breeders) influence reproduction largely by their effects upon release of gonadotropins from the pituitary. Nervous factors appear to have most influence upon LH secretion and thus upon ovulation. These factors act through the hypothalamus which is a link in the chain influencing the release of gonadotropins. The rabbit, cat, ferret and mink are animals in which a nervous stimulus given by coitus is required for LH release and consequent ovulation. The same effect may be brought about by injecting hypothalamic extracts or stimulants, e.g., picrotoxin.

Superovulation may be induced by injecting a follicle-stimulating preparation. Pregnant-mare serum (PMS) may be used in cattle. It is most effective if it is injected while a declining corpus luteum is present in the ovary. An injection of 2,000 IU of PMS on day 17 of the cycle has been recommended for twin production in cattle. Multiple births are undesirable in dairy cattle, but there may be some advantage in beef cattle production. In sheep, a single injection of 500 IU of PMS (R 168) on day 13 of the cycle may increase the ovulation rate and hence the lambing percentage to a significant degree. In the anestrous season, ovulations and pregnancies have resulted from breeding after a dose of 750 IU of PMS has been given, followed by another 16 days later.

EXTRINSIC SOURCES OF ESTROGENS AND THEIR EFFECTS

In Australia, sheep fed upon pure stands of subterranean clover sometimes develop a form of hyperestrinism exhibited in the female by infertility, uterine prolapse and dystocia arising from aberrant parturition, and in the castrate male, by metaplasia of the accessory sex glands. Cattle have not been similarly affected. Growing vegetation, especially legumes, contain a variety of substances, of which genistin is one, that are mild estrogens. They do not constitute a serious problem in the U.S.A. at the present time. In fact, the beneficial effects of spring grass upon milk yield and fertility have been ascribed to these substances, though without conclusive evidence. However, the estrogen content of pelleted diets for laboratory animals, especially mice, should be carefully watched as an excess has caused breeding problems and misinterpretation of research findings as a consequence. Stilbestrol residues in meat scraps have also caused trouble in mink.

Estrogens and growth: In most mammals, estrogens cause premature ossification of the epiphyses of the long bones. Thus, they generally limit growth, but this effect has not been noted in ruminants. Oral administration of diethylstilbestrol in the feed during the later phases of fattening increases the efficiency of feed utilization by as much as 10% and the rate of growth is correspondingly accelerated. The carcass quality may sometimes be decreased slightly if this method of fattening is used in cattle. In wethers, stilbestrol feeding may cause the development of urinary calculi.

TESTICULAR MALFUNCTION

In general, male hypogonadism, which is not uncommon in domestic animals, has not been helped by endocrine therapy. So-called slow-breeding males may be induced to mate by the injection of the male sex hormone testosterone (R 178). The mere fact that they mate, however, does not ensure fertility and it is essential to check the quality of the semen. (*See* SEMEN QUALITY AND MALE FERTILITY, p. 775.)

EYE AND EAR

VETERINARY OPHTHALMOLOGY

PHYSICAL EXAMINATION OF THE ANIMAL EYE

Examination of the conscious animal's eye and its adnexa may be conveniently accomplished in a dark room or stall. In a quiet environment, ocular movement is minimal and little restraint is needed. The equipment required consists of a binocular magnifying loupe, a small light source (pencil flashlight) and an ophthalmoscope. Using a loupe and the flashlight, all the anterior structures may be inspected. The ophthalmoscope permits closer examination of these and, in addition, a minute examination of the lens, vitreous and fundus.

A staining solution (2% fluorescein), an irrigating solution (isotonic saline), a mydriatic (2% homatropine methylbromide) and a local anesthetic (0.5% tetracaine) are important aids.

EYELIDS

ENTROPION

An inversion of the margin of the eyelids. The lower lids are most commonly involved unilaterally or bilaterally. It may be an inherited defect in young sheep and dogs (especially such breeds as Chows, Bulldogs and Setters). It also occurs following laceration and faulty healing of the eyelid and as a sequela to prolonged blepharospasm associated with conjunctivitis or keratoconjunctivitis. The inversion of the lid margin allows the eyelashes to irritate the cornea. The resultant pain, epiphora and photophobia may be complicated by superimposed infection. Permanent improvement of the defect is afforded by surgical correction of the lid position.

ECTROPION

Eversion of the margin of the lower eyelid. It is common in dogs and most often seen in Spaniels, St. Bernards and Bloodhounds. It may be hereditary or secondary to injury to the eyelid, or seventh cranial nerve. Ectropion results in varying degrees of conjunctival inflammation and epiphora, with accumulation of exudate in the conjunctival folds, and may be followed by pigmentary keratitis. The appearance of the lower eyelid usually is esthetically objectionable.

This defect may be corrected by appropriate surgical procedures.

BLEPHARITIS

An inflammation of the eyelids which may occur as a primary pathologic condition or as an extension of conjunctival or corneal disease. Bacterial or mite invasion of meibomian glands and hair follicles at the lid margin are the common causes. Also, during the course of allergic reactions, these structures frequently are inflamed in the dog.

The lids are swollen, red and partially denuded; pruritus and epiphora are often seen. Crusts of dried purulent material accumulate at the lid margins. The conjunctiva generally is congested.

A 3% rotenone ointment is effective when demodectic mites are identified as the cause of blepharitis, but 10% sulfur ointment is recommended when sarcoptic mites are identified (*see* MANGE, p. 909). An antibiotic-corticoid ophthalmic preparation (℞ 386) provides effective control of the common bacterial invasion of eyelash follicles and reduces the inflammatory changes of the eyelids. Frequent daily cleansing of the lid margins with 3% sodium bicarbonate solution or a similar collyrium is required. The application of ophthalmic preparations containing a local anesthetic (℞ 373, 594) or antibiotics (℞ 374, 375, 381) will relieve pruritus and mitigate infection. The use of topical anesthetics should be closely monitored.

TRICHIASIS, DISTICHIASIS

Cilia at the lid margins occasionally turn and grow inward or are misplaced on the inner margin of the lid. This results in irritation of the bulbar conjunctiva and cornea. The condition may be recognized after 5 weeks of age. Good restraint, proper lighting and magnification are required to see the misdirected lashes.

Plucking the offending cilia affords temporary relief. It may be necessary to repeat this procedure bimonthly. The lash follicles can be destroyed with the epilation needle or surgically removed.

LACRIMAL APPARATUS

The lacrimal sac is occasionally inflamed. In such cases, pressure over the lacrimal sac causes pus to appear at the lacrimal puncta. If ducts are stenosed the sac swells and may rupture. The only clinical signs may be chronic epiphora, mild conjunctivitis and slight fullness over the lacrimal sac. Saline irrigation of the nasolacrimal apparatus will dilate the stenosed ducts, resulting in normal drainage, and ophthalmic antibiotic drops may be used topically for several days to resolve the infection. Imperforate puncta must be surgically opened. Nasolacrimal atresia is rare. Destruction of the lacrimal and accessory lacrimal tissue causes keratitis sicca (q.v., p. 207).

CONJUNCTIVA

SUBCONJUNCTIVAL HEMORRHAGE

Acute hemorrhage of conjunctival vessels frequently fills the subconjunctival space. Short-necked, brachycephalic nervous breeds are most frequently affected. The hemorrhage may occur spontaneously when the animal is being restrained, or as a result of trauma. The animal shows little discomfort. Resorption of the blood usually requires 1 to 2 weeks.

Topical anesthetic ointments, such as 2% butacaine sulfate (℞ 373) or protective collars may be applied if the animal attempts to scratch or rub the eye. Early frequent application of ice packs may lessen the amount of hemorrhage. The intraocular structure should be carefully evaluated, since trauma may produce uveitis. If uveitis is present, it should be treated as the primary condition.

CHEMOSIS

Edema of the palpebral and bulbar conjunctiva characterized by protrusion of the membranes beyond the palpebral fissure. It is usually an allergic reaction, but may be an extension of catarrhal conjunctivitis. Cold compresses and steroids (℞ 380, 384) applied topically afford relief. Chemosis commonly accompanies the viral conjunctivitis in cats.

CONJUNCTIVITIS

Inflammation affecting the mucosa (bulbar and palpebral) of the conjunctival sac. Several types may be recognized clinically: (1) acute catarrhal, (2) acute purulent, (3) follicular or chronic, varying in appearance according to the cause. The characteristic signs include mucoid to purulent discharge, hyperemia, swelling and local pain manifested as blepharospasm. The condition may be unilateral, bilateral, local or associated with systemic disease, depending upon the cause.

Infectious agents, bacterial and viral, may cause primary conjunctivitis (see INFECTIOUS KERATOCONJUNCTIVITIS, p. 213). Redness, swelling, serous to mucopurulent discharge and regional lymphadenopathy are associated with bacterial causes, and marked epiphora and scant mucoid discharge with viral causes. These latter may demonstrate intracellular inclusion bodies in cell scrapings. Allergic conjunctivitis is most often manifest as chemosis. Foreign material of any type or size initiates acute local reaction. In unilateral cases, the inner surface of the membrana nictitans should be carefully examined for embedded material or tissue hyperplasia.

Chemical agents (soaps, tick dips, etc.) are many times the cause of severe, acute, painful conjunctivitis that is often bilateral.

The nematode *Thelazia californiensis* may be found in the eyes of dogs, sheep, cats and deer. The resulting conjunctivitis in affected animals is aggravated by rubbing the eyelids with the forelegs. The threadlike worms are 25 to 400 mm long and may be found singly or in clumps in the conjunctival sac.

Treatment of conjunctivitis should be directed toward frequent and careful cleansing of the sac and lids with an appropriate solution. Infections are best treated topically with chloramphenicol or a combination of neomycin, polymyxin and bacitracin. Either of these ophthalmic preparations should be applied every 2 to 3 hours during the day. Foreign bodies should be removed at once. Chemical agents need to be washed out immediately with large volumes of tap water or saline solution followed by an appropriate neutralizer. Allergic reactions require cold packs and topical instillation of corticosteroid ophthalmic ointments. Chronic follicular conjunctivitis often responds to the use of stimulant astringents (zinc sulfate 0.25%; or yellow oxide of mercury), or to antibiotic and corticosteroid combinations.

Conjunctivitis in cats is manifest chiefly by edematous swelling. Erythema is not a conspicuous sign of conjunctivitis in this species. Prominence of the membrana nictitans is frequently noticed.

Animals with conjunctivitis should be confined in a darkened room or stall. Sedation and restraint may be needed to prevent self-injury to the affected eyes. In small animals, dew-claws should be taped. Antihistamines (R 535, 537) either orally or by injection are sometimes used to help control the pruritus associated with conjunctivitis.

HYPERTROPHY OF THE GLANDS OF THE MEMBRANA NICTITANS

This common ocular lesion of dogs is often improperly referred to as harderian gland enlargement. It is most often seen in young, growing dogs. The unilateral occurrence of this lesion is commonly followed several weeks later by involvement of the second eye.

The sudden appearance of a red mound of lymphoid-appearing tissue is seen at the medial canthus of the eye. The swelling may vary in size with or without treatment. Little discomfort is noticed. A serous or mucous discharge is observed staining the lower lid. Surgical excision of the swollen gland affords prompt relief.

CORNEA

DEGENERATIVE PANNUS

Invasion of vascularized connective tissue in the superficial stroma of the cornea. Hyperplasia of the nictitating membrane is a frequent complication. The condition is most common in the German Shepherd Dog and may affect both eyes, beginning at the temporal limbus, extending centrally as a pink, fleshy peninsula which becomes pigmented. Epiphora and blepharospasm may associate with the disease.

Treatment combines subconjunctival injection of prednisolone at the arc of origin at the limbus, followed by topical instillation of steroid (R 377), which must be used regularly for the life of the patient. Surgical removal by superficial keratectomy and irradiation with strontium 90 (beta-ray applicator) are also temporarily effective.

KERATITIS

An inflammation of the cornea, which may be superficial, interstitial or ulcerative. Keratitis is a common disease of animals. Canine breeds with large, prominent eyes are most susceptible to superficial corneal injury.

Superficial keratitis is caused by external influences which irritate or abrade the corneal surface. Subsequent invasion of the deeper corneal tissue by infectious agents produces clinical keratitis. Failure of the eyelids to cover the cornea properly will result in corneal drying and erosion. Vitamin A deficiencies produce a similar effect.

Keratitis sicca, a destructive drying of the cornea due to lack of adequate tear secretion, may be caused by primary disease of the lacrimal gland or by denervation of the gland. Tears must be replaced by topical administration of 1% methylcellulose solutions ("artificial tears") or by surgical transposition of the parotid duct. Interstitial keratitis is often associated with systemic infections, e.g., canine distemper, infectious canine hepatitis, and with uveitis. It occurs most frequently in younger animals and is most often bilateral. Infectious keratoconjunctivitis (q.v., p. 213) is a specific disease of cattle and sheep characterized by intense lacrimation, photophobia, opacity of the cornea and sometimes ulceration.

Interstitial keratitis is recognized by the dense, sudden clouding of one cornea and, after several days, the other. This inflammation usually follows or is coincident with the occurrence of systemic illness. Variable degrees of pain, photophobia and serous discharge are manifest. Deep vascularization of the cornea occurs, but is not easily identified at first since the fine, brush-like vessels are located within the corneal tissue. The bulbar conjunctiva becomes congested.

Ulceration of the cornea produces a characteristic cloudiness of this tissue, with loss of surface continuity. The conjunctiva is congested. Photophobia and a serous discharge characterize the early signs of corneal ulceration and the exudate frequently becomes purulent. Gross examination of the cornea will generally reveal the site of the erosion. Small ulcers may become visible only after staining with fluorescein solution. Within 3 to 5 days following deep corneal erosion, newly formed blood vessels invade the tissue to surround the zone of devitalized cells. Healing of corneal ulcerations requires from 4 to 8 weeks. Small, dense, white scars often remain at the site of healed ulcers.

Prolapse of the third and fourth layers of the cornea (**keratocele**) may occur if the ulcerative process is not arrested. A keratocele may heal, as does a more superficial corneal ulceration, but usually requires surgical containment. Aqueous humor may escape through the tissues that form the keratocele. If a portion of the iris is drawn into the hernia when a keratocele develops, iridocorneal adhesion (adherent leukoma) follows.

A dense, brownish pigmentation of the cornea is a sequela to keratitis in some animals. This pigmentary keratitis follows a subacute or chronic keratoconjunctivitis and is associated with vascularization of the cornea. There are always inflammatory cells in the epithelial layers. Once the cornea becomes pigmented, the tissue retains the dense, black or brown discoloration.

Treatment of keratitis is most effective when the patients are confined in darkened rooms or stalls. Topical treatment of corneal ulceration includes application of warm compresses following cauterization of the ulcer with iodine tincture or phenol. Purulent exudate should be removed from the corneal or conjunctival surfaces several times daily, using isotonic saline, 3% sodium bicarbonate or 1:5,000 benzalkonium solution. A 1% ointment or solution of atropine sulfate should be applied to relieve ciliary spasm and avoid synechia. Antibiotic preparations (Ŗ 372, 374, 375, 381) should be applied topically. Solutions of nitrofurazone (Ŗ 382) and sodium sulfacetamide (Ŗ 388) may be effective in special cases. Chloramphenicol, 1% topical ointment (Ŗ 374), is usually the drug of choice. Acquired resistance to antibiotics is observed sometimes in the treatment of corneal lesions.

Systemic medications that may be of value in the treatment of corneal ulcerations include the injection of foreign proteins (Ŗ 642, 647). Adequate intake of vitamins A, C, D and B-complex should be assured. Sedation is recommended for nervous animals that mutilate themselves.

In cases of chronic keratitis, radiation therapy, e.g., strontium 90 (see VETERINARY RADIOLOGY, p. 1398), has been employed to destroy blood vessels that are no longer functional in corneal repair. This therapy is effective in arresting neovascular and pigmentary changes in the cornea.

It may be necessary to bandage the ulcerated eye. A deep ulcer or keratocele should be treated surgically by providing a conjunctival flap to cover the affected cornea.

The prognosis of interstitial keratitis is good to excellent and treatment usually is successful. The dense corneal cloudiness which characterizes this disease often clears spontaneously as the systemic infection subsides. Corticosteroids in suspension or ointment form are sometimes combined with topical antibiotics (Ŗ 387) for treating interstitial keratitis without ulceration or bacterial complication.

DERMOID

This benign corneal neoplasm is occasionally seen in all species. The lesion, usually detected in young, growing animals, is a small, flat, skin-like elevation close to the limbus. Hair is frequently found growing from the surface of the neoplasm. Its presence initiates local discomfort, serous discharge, and rarely corneal ulceration. Surgical removal of the dermoid from the globe is recommended at an early age (4 to 6 weeks) to avoid complications.

ANTERIOR CHAMBER

FILARIAL OPHTHALMITIS

On rare occasions, filariid worms of the genera *Setaria* and *Dirofilaria* become lodged in the anterior chamber of the eye; the former is seen in horses, the latter in dogs. Although presence of the worm often causes surprisingly little disturbance to the animal, occasionally severe uveitis occurs. Removal can be accomplished surgically through a small puncture incision through clear cornea close to the limbus.

UVEA

IRITIS

It is unusual for the iris to be inflamed without some evidence of cyclitis and occasionally choroiditis. Inflammation of parts or all of the uveal tract is diagnosed in dogs and cats as well as horses (*see* PERIODIC OPHTHALMIA, p. 214). Iritis or iridocyclitis may be caused by penetrating foreign bodies or may follow severe laceration or contusion of the eyeball. The iris and ciliary body may also become inflamed during the course of certain systemic infections, such as leptospirosis, infectious canine hepatitis, canine distemper, sepsis and autoimmune reactions.

Iritis is characterized clinically by acute onset, photophobia, blepharospasm, epiphora and pain. Affected animals are quiet and depressed. Congestion of the bulbar conjunctiva, haziness of the cornea and swelling of the iris may be detected. The pupil constricts and becomes pin-point. Clumps of leukocytes appear as white precipitates in the aqueous humor. During iridocyclitis the eye is usually hypotonic. However, adhesion of the iris to the lens is a common complication of iritis and may precipitate secondary glaucoma. Vitreal opacities appear when the ciliary body and choroid are inflamed.

Both topical and systemic antibiotic medications are employed when treating iridocyclitis. Corticosteroids may be combined with the topical antibiotic therapy. Steroids are very useful and effective when administered systemically (℞ 154) and subconjunctivally (℞ 385). Mydriatics are used as needed to maintain pupillary dilatation whenever the iris is inflamed. Parenteral injections of foreign-protein solutions (℞ 642) have been given. The use of analgesics, such as meperidine (℞ 590) or corticosteroid-aspirin combinations (℞ 146) are recommended for relief of pain.

EYEBALL

GLAUCOMA

Increased intraocular pressure incompatible with continued health and function of the eye. In dogs, the wire-haired terriers and cockers are chiefly affected. Glaucoma may be classified as primary, secondary and absolute. This classification is based on the distinction that a recognizable, antecedent pathologic condition within the eyeball precedes the occurrence of secondary glaucoma.

Regardless of cause, the glaucomatous eye is grossly abnormal in the later stages. The eyeball is enlarged and bulges. The cornea is hazy and will be opaque if the intraocular tension is very high. The vessels of the bulbar conjunctiva and sclera are congested. The pupil, when visible, is widely dilated and responds poorly, if at all, to light. The eyeballs feel hard. The affected animal is quiet, depressed and irritable. Glaucomatous cupping of the optic disk can be seen in dogs in the early stages, before the cornea has become opaque.

Primary glaucoma must be treated promptly with miotic solutions. Instillation of a 0.1% solution of diisopropyl fluorophosphate (℞ 379), 3% pilocarpine or demecarium bromide (℞ 376) has proved effective when augmented by an oral carbonic-anhydrase inhibitor (℞ 378, 518, 519). Scleral trephining or iridencleisis is generally advisable as soon as the acutely glaucomatous eyeball has become less congested and swollen. Preservation of sight often may be achieved if surgery is successful. Even if vision cannot be saved, the maintenance of a healthy, though nonfunctioning, eyeball is desirable for cosmetic reasons. Secondary glaucoma is associated with antecedent eye disease developing as a complication of uveitis, subluxation or luxation of the lens, complicated hypermature cataracts and accidental or surgical wounds. Treatment must be surgical. Absolute glaucoma is the terminal state of primary or secondary glaucoma and requires enucleation or retrobulbar injection of absolute alcohol for the relief of pain.

LENS

CATARACT

Any opacity of the lens. Almost every dog over 8 years of age will have some degree of lens change (nuclear sclerosis). Congenital and traumatic cataracts are also seen.

The inflammation may subside spontaneously if infection does not develop. Confinement of the affected animal to darkened quarters is important. Analgesics (℞ 590) are useful to relieve pain, and in severe cases, additional sedation may be necessary. The frequent application of warm compresses is recommended. Penicillin or other appropriate antibiotics should be administered parenterally until the inflammation subsides. The formation of orbital abscesses should be carefully watched and surgical drainage provided when necessary. The eye should be covered with a bandage whenever the lids cannot cover the protruded cornea. Every precaution should be taken to prevent desiccation of the cornea by frequent irrigation of the corneal surface with sterile 1% solution of methylcellulose.

INFECTIOUS KERATOCONJUNCTIVITIS
(Pink-eye, Infectious ophthalmia)

An infectious disease of cattle, sheep and goats which is characterized by photophobia, lacrimation, conjunctivitis and varying degrees of corneal opacity and ulceration.

Etiology: In cattle, *Moraxella bovis* is the most common cause although infectious bovine rhinotracheitis virus and other viral agents have been associated with pink-eye; it appears probable that all may cause clinical disease singly as well as concurrently. Ovine infectious keratitis is thought to be caused by *Mycoplasma* or *Rickettsia*. Little effort has been expended to study the disease in goats but a *Rickettsia* is suspected as the cause. Agents causing the disease in cattle, sheep and goats appear to be species-specific.

Clinical Findings: The disease occurs suddenly in the initially affected animals and tends to spread rapidly. Dry, dusty environmental conditions, bright sunlight, feeding in tall grass, or the presence of large numbers of flies tend to propagate the disease. More younger animals than older ones are affected, but all ages may be involved. The initial signs are photophobia and excessive lacrimation, later there is a mucopurulent discharge from the eye. Conjunctivitis and varying degrees of keratitis are present and the animals seek shade. Some animals develop a mild fever with a slightly depressed appetite and decreased milk production. The clinical course varies from a few days to several weeks.

Lesions: The lesions vary in severity from a mild conjunctivitis and keratitis to a severe conjunctivitis and ulcerative keratitis with resultant penetration of the anterior chamber. The conjunctival vessels become hyperemic and prominent. A small ulcer or ulcers occur near the center of the cornea or less often close to the limbus without initial notable corneal discoloration. After a short time the ulcers are surrounded by an opaque ring of varying size due to corneal edema and leukocytic infiltration; the opacity may involve the entire cornea. Regression may occur in the early stages or the lesions may continue to progress. Continued active ulceration may cause rupture of the cornea.

In chronic or recovering cases, the corneal lesions either regress over a long period or the cornea is permanently scarred. Either unilateral or bilateral infection may be present.

Diagnosis: The characteristic lesions serve to differentiate the condition from vitamin A deficiency and ocular inflammation due to factors such as foreign bodies, parasites and allergies.

Prophylaxis and Treatment: Recovered animals often become carriers. Immunity under field conditions is variable but older animals are less frequently affected and some immunity is suspected. Vaccines prepared against agents known to infect the eye have not proven reliable for the control of pink-eye. A number of antibiotics are effective against *Moraxella bovis* (penicillin, chloramphenicol, nitrofurazone and tetracycline) and are beneficial if treatment is initiated early. Rapid response to treatment after severe corneal ulceration cannot be expected. Viral agents in cattle will not be affected by antibiotic therapy but such treatment will help to alleviate secondary bacterial infection. Antibiotics may be administered either topically as solutions or powders, or by subconjunctival injection; repeated ocular applications are necessary and affected animals should be placed in a shaded area. Ophthalmic preparations containing dyes, ocular or subconjunctival injection of prednisolone and injection of vitamin A have been used with variable success. An agent causing the sheep disease is susceptible to penicillin, streptomycin and chlortetracycline.

PERIODIC OPHTHALMIA
(Recurrent iridocyclitis, Moon blindness)

An inflammatory disease of the eyes of horses and mules characterized by sudden onset of acute clinical signs which subside, but recur following quiescent periods of varying length.

The iris and ciliary body are primarily affected, but after repeated occurrences, the lens, retina and vitreous body are involved and vision is impaired.

Etiology: The cause of periodic ophthalmia has not been clearly defined. The disease is neither heritable nor congenital. Nutrition studies indicate that there is an inverse relationship between incidence and the level of riboflavin in the diet. There is evidence that the disease is more frequent where the standard of management is poor.

Positive titers for *Leptospira bovis* and *L. pomona* have been associated with periodic ophthalmia. Infection by *Onchocerca cervicalis* microfilariae which die in the eye also produces ocular disease indistinguishable from periodic ophthalmia. There is evidence that the ocular inflammation may be a localized hypersensitivity or allergic reaction following secondary infection or toxemia.

Incidence: Equine periodic ophthalmia probably occurs throughout the world. In the U.S.A., the disease is more frequent on the eastern seaboard and, to a lesser extent, in the Mississippi and Ohio River Valleys. It is rare in the Rocky Mountains, west coast and southwest regions. Ordinarily, the incidence is low; occasionally, outbreaks involve a rather high percentage of a group. The disease is recognized more frequently in mature horses and mules, probably because the lesions are more pronounced and diagnosis is less difficult. However, the disease has been observed in animals as young as 3½ months of age.

Clinical Findings and Diagnosis: The acute signs appear suddenly, then gradually abate in a few days to a week or more to be followed by a quiescent period which may last for only a few days or, in extreme cases, for several years. Repeated acute exacerbations often occur.

In the **acute stage,** there is sudden onset of photophobia and lacrimation involving one or both eyes. This may be associated with slight depression and a moderate elevation of temperature (1° to 1.5°F). Attention is drawn to the affected eye by its extreme sensitivity to light, the closed eyelid and the excessive lacrimation. Careful examination reveals a severe catarrhal conjunctivitis, with or without some opacity of the cornea. A cellular exudate which may produce a simple diffuse cloudiness of the aqueous humor or a yellowish, flocculent exudate which settles to the lower half of the anterior chamber is present.

Contraction of the pupil is characteristic and the pupil responds very slowly to mydriatics. It is difficult or impossible to see the deeper structures of the eye. Intraocular tension is decreased; severe decrease is a bad prognostic sign. Pericorneal vascular infiltration is observed on the ventral border of the cornea about the third or fourth day. Gradually these vessels extend and, in severe cases in which repeated attacks have occurred, may reach the center of the cornea. The acute signs gradually abate and the eye appears to return to normal.

During the **quiescent stage**, most cases can be detected only by careful ophthalmoscopic examination under favorable light conditions. The most common lesions in the mildly affected quiescent case are opacities in the vitreous body. The presence of such opacities may be detected by a study of the optic disk and retina, using the −3 lens of the ophthalmoscope. If opacities are present, it is difficult to get a sharp image of the retinal vessels and the retina. By using the +8 lens, tiny, pepper-like opacities and strands of fibrillar material may be seen in various parts of the vitreous body. It may be possible to see opacities of varying size, shape and density in the lens. In some cases, there is a persistent adhesion of the iris to the anterior lens capsule which may result in a bit of the iris being torn loose or it may prevent dilatation of the pupil. In such cases, dilatation of the pupil with mydriatics (or even prolonged darkness) results in stretching and tearing of the iris, leaving the pupil irregular and distorted in outline. Occasionally, small yellowish foci or diffuse yellowish discoloration of the iris may be detected. It is rare that corneal vascularization can be detected clinically during this stage.

Of particular diagnostic assistance in the quiescent stage is the **fluorescein test**. Fluorescein dye (℞ 560) injected IV escapes from vessels in affected eyes and appears in the ocular fluid. In severely affected eyes, the dye will appear within less than a minute, whereas in less severely involved eyes, several minutes are required. In sunlight, the dye appears green, while under ultraviolet light, it fluoresces and gives a yellow color. In horses with one eye affected, the contrast between the 2 eyes is striking. The dye stains all mucosae and other vascular structures for a short time and is eliminated unchanged in the urine. Since this dye may produce temporary photosensitization, particularly in gray horses, the animal should not be exposed to sunlight for at least 24 hours after the test.

In the **advanced stage**, blindness of varying degree is present. The eyeball is atrophied, the lens may be opaque, the cornea is reduced in size and increased in convexity. There is definite pericorneal vascularization, posterior synechiae may be seen, the pupil may be fixed in a closed position and the animal may be obviously blind.

An accurate history of recurrent acute attacks aids in the diagnosis, since history of iridocyclitis is typical of periodic ophthalmia. Iridocyclitis may occur in the course of diseases such as equine viral arteritis, and is difficult to separate from periodic ophthalmia, but such occurrences are not common. Injuries to the eye usually can be detected without difficulty because the iris and ciliary body are not affected unless there is perforation of the cornea or sclera.

Prophylaxis and Treatment: Although, under certain circumstances, the addition of rather large quantities of riboflavin (40 mg daily) to the ration has been followed by a significant decrease in incidence, this procedure is of no apparent value in the treatment of the clinical disease. Where there is evidence of infection by *Leptospira,* streptomycin (R 56) for 5 days is recommended. A dark stall contributes to the animal's comfort during the period of photophobia. The instillation of ophthalmic suspensions or ointments containing prednisone or prednisolone with or without antibiotics has given control of the acute signs. Subconjunctival injection of 10 mg of prednisolone at 48-hour intervals will prove more effective than topical preparations and is the preferred method of administration. Atropine (R 371) should be used promptly and often enough to keep the pupil dilated and prevent synechia. In older cases, where adhesions have already become established, atropine may free them, but generally they are too firmly fixed.

DISEASES OF THE EXTERNAL EAR

OTITIS EXTERNA

Otitis externa occurs in most species of animals, but the incidence is greatest in the dog. The domestic cat is less troubled with otitis, and when present in that species it is usually secondary to ear mites or the presence of an adenoma of the ceruminous glands that line the ear canal. Rabbits also suffer from otitis secondary to ear mites. The condition is uncommon in the larger domestic species.

Etiology: The etiology of otitis externa in the dog remains poorly defined. Certain factors are thought responsible for initiating inflammation and predisposing the ear canal to infection with bacteria or fungi or both. These include trauma (sometimes as a result of faulty cleaning), the presence of excessive amounts of dirt, wax, hair and moisture, the presence of foreign objects such as plant seeds, anatomic abnormalities and the presence of new growths in the ear canal. Ear mites (*Otodectes cynotis*) are important. Hot humid weather is also associated with an increased incidence of the disease. Breeds with long hair and pendulous ears are frequently affected, but erect-eared breeds are by no means immune. Otitis can be secondary to generalized seborrhea.

The bacteria infecting the external ear are species of *Proteus, Pseudomonas, Staphylococcus, Streptococcus, Clostridium,* coliforms and diphtheroids, but of these only the *Proteus* and *Pseudomonas* organisms are not found in normal ears. It is thought possible that fecal contamination of the ear canal may result in otitis due to *Proteus* and *Pseudomonas.*

Aspergillus, Penicillium and *Rhizopus* species of molds are found in both diseased and healthy ears. Yeasts are found more frequently (*Pityrosporum* and *Monilia*), both in diseased and healthy ears, but the *Pityrosporum* species are frequently found in diseased ears and may be a primary infection. Allergy may be responsible in some instances as many dogs with otitis also have allergic dermatitis.

Clinical Findings: Animals with otitis externa hold the affected ear low (if one ear is involved), shake their heads violently or rub the ear along surfaces or scratch the ear. This self-mutilation may cause abrasions and bleeding. Excessive head shaking frequently results in hematoma formation in the pinna of the ear. Kittens with ear mites may be so agitated as to appear to be convulsing.

The external ear canal is inflamed, painful and may be ulcerated; the hair will be wet or sticky with the discharge and it will have an abnormal odor. With persistent or untreated otitis externa, the epithelium of the ear canal undergoes hypertrophy and becomes fibroplastic. In extreme cases the ear canal is completely blocked by hypertrophied tissue and hearing is impaired. The nature of the cerumen and the discharge is to some extent characteristic of the microorganisms present. A brownish-black cerumen, resembling shoe polish in consistency, is often associated with *Staphylococcus* and *Pityrosporum,* a crumbly yellow-brown cerumen with staphylococci or yeasts and *Proteus.* A pale-yellow, watery, suppurative and odorous discharge is associated with the presence of *Proteus* or *Pseudomonas* organisms, which are commonly present in chronically infected ears.

Diagnosis: The general diagnosis is obvious in most cases. The specific cause, i.e., the presence of foreign objects or ear mites, will be identified only if the ear is carefully examined with an otoscope both before and after cleaning.

Treatment: Not all cases of otitis externa respond well to treatment. In general, a high percentage of failures and re-treatments can be anticipated. Persistence is essential if the disease is to be cured or the chronic form of the disease prevented.

ACUTE OTITIS EXTERNA

Because of the pain, anesthesia or tranquilization may be necessary prior to inspection and treatment. The ear must be thoroughly examined with an otoscope and foreign objects removed with a small wire loop, an ear spoon or an alligator forceps small enough to pass through the speculum. Swabs of the exudate should be collected for culture and sensitivity testing. The presence of ulcers or ear mites should be noted as well as the condition of the ear drum. If the epithelium is intensely inflamed, probing and swabbing should be avoided. The ear should be cleaned by flushing away the debris and exudate using warm saline or water with a germicidal detergent, and the canal dried as gently as possible. An antibiotic-corticosteroid lotion or ointment should be applied to the ear canal (℞ 443, 459). If the epithelium is raw and acutely inflamed, a thin layer of protective astringent lotion or ointment (℞ 452, 453) can be applied. Antibiotics (℞ 6, 11, 41) should be administered systemically for 4 to 5 days if the ear drum is acutely inflamed or if the animal has a fever. Analgesics or tranquilizers may be necessary. The antibiotic-steroid local treatment should be continued for a week. If antibiotic sensitivity testing is done, then the appropriate antibiotic must be used for the local and systemic treatment. The animal should be examined after 48 hours to ensure that treatment has been effective and again at weekly intervals until the inflammation has subsided. During this time small ulcers in the ear canal should be painted with an astringent solution (℞ 442). Taping the ears over the head may be of value in pendant-eared dogs.

CHRONIC OTITIS EXTERNA

The discharge from the ears should be cultured and a sensitivity test done. The ears should be thoroughly cleaned by gently flushing with a germicidal-detergent solution. If the discharge is particularly waxy, a cerumenolytic agent (℞ 447) may be more useful. Excessive hair should be clipped from the ears. If indicated it may be an advantage to use a solution of antibiotic rather than an ointment for the first 48 hours of treatment. Such preparations must be used frequently (every 2 hours) in order to maintain a high concentration of antibiotic within the ear canal. Subsequently, an ointment containing the antibiotic can be used.

As with acute otitis, astringent solutions (℞ 470) or ointments (℞ 460) should be painted sparingly on locally ulcerated or irritated areas of epithelium. Antibiotic-steroid combinations (℞ 451, 459) may be useful to reduce pain and swelling as well as to control infection.

Surgical treatment may become necessary if therapy has failed or the disease has been neglected.

MYCOTIC OTITIS EXTERNA
(Otomycosis)

Otitis externa in which mycotic organisms have invaded the skin of the ear canal causing the formation of dry, scaly accumulations of epithelium, cerumen and dirt which adhere closely to the underlying skin. The irritation produced may cause the animals to rub and scratch the affected ear, superimposing traumatic damage. Removal of the scaly deposits often causes bleeding. The condition may extend to and involve the tympanum. Although mycotic infections are common in the ears of animals, they are usually associated with bacterial infection and purulent otitis externa. This type of otitis is most common in heavy-eared breeds and those dogs that spend much time in the water or swamps. Culture of the organism on Sabouraud's medium is necessary for positive diagnosis.

Treatment is based first on elimination of moisture from the ear canal. Adequate ventilation is mandatory and can best be accomplished in pendant-eared dogs by taping the ears over the top of the head. The ear canal should be thoroughly cleaned of all superficial scaly deposits with a wire loop or cotton swabs saturated with alcoholic phenylmercuric nitrate solution (℞ 399). Fungicidal ointments (℞ 356, 446, 449, 457, 459) or thymol preparations (℞ 458) should be applied until the scaliness has disappeared.

PARASITIC OTITIS EXTERNA
(Otodectic mange, Ear mange, Otoacariasis)

Otitis externa caused by the ear mite *Otodectes cynotis*. The dog, cat, fox, rabbit and ferret are affected. The mites live on the surface of the skin of the ear and ear canal, and feed by piercing the skin and sucking lymph, with resultant irritation, inflammation, exudation and crust formation.

Clinical Findings and Diagnosis: Ear mites cause the animals to shake their heads and to scratch or rub the affected ears. There is a waxy, dark-brown, sometimes flaky exudate in the ear canal. Examination of the ear canal with an otoscope will reveal the small, white or flesh-colored mites moving on the dark exudate. Mites can also be demonstrated by examining the exudate with a hand lens or under a low-power microscope.

Treatment: Instillation of a bland oil, such as mineral oil, or a cerumenolytic agent (R 447) into the ear canal, followed by gentle massage aids in the cleaning process and kills many of the mites. The use of a wire loop will avoid packing the heavy exudate against the tympanic membrane in the cleaning process. After cleaning, an acaricide such as rotenone (R 444) or dimethyl phthalate (R 457) or a protective-type solution in an oil base (R 452) should be applied and the treatment repeated every third day for 4 applications. This extended treatment will prevent reinfestation by destroying newly hatched parasites. In severe cases, the entire body of the animal should be treated weekly with a parasiticidal powder or dip to kill those mites not in the ear canal. If chronic inflammatory changes are present, a protective ointment (R 453) or antibiotic-corticosteroid preparation (R 387, 443, 448, 459) should be used until the inflammation subsides. Antibiotic ointments are useful for concurrent bacterial infections.

TUMORS OF THE EXTERNAL EAR

Any tumor of the skin or cartilage may be encountered in the external ear. Adenomas of ceruminous glands are probably the most frequent tumors in the ear canal of dogs and cats. Tumor-like polyps of hypertrophied tissue are common in the ear canal of dogs and cats with long-standing irritation or infection.

Treatment: Surgical removal is the only satisfactory method of treatment. Lateral resection of the conchal cartilage is often necessary for removal. Concurrent otitis should be treated.

HEMATOMA OF THE EAR

A subcut. hemorrhage resulting in a soft, fluctuating swelling, usually on the inner surface of the pinna, but occasionally on the outer surface. It occurs commonly in dogs, cats and pigs, and is a particular problem of dogs with pendant ears. It is rare in other species. The hematoma may be small or involve the entire pinna. The cause is trauma, either due to bite wounds or to violent shaking of the head caused by otitis externa. Dicoumarol poisoning may predispose swine to hematoma formation.

Treatment: Small hematomas may be treated by aspirating the blood with a syringe and a fine hypodermic needle and firmly bandaging the ear to the top of the head or to a roll of bandage for 7 to 10 days. Large hematomas require surgical evacuation of the blood clot. The loose skin is then apposed to the cartilage with many sutures placed through all layers of the ear, and the ear is firmly bandaged. Any co-existing otitis must be treated or the hematoma may recur or be produced in the other ear. Wounds in the pinna should be treated at the time of surgery. The animal may require sedation postoperatively to prevent head shaking or scratching of the ear. The bandage and most of the sutures should remain in place for 10 to 14 days.

OTITIS MEDIA AND INTERNA

Otitis media is an inflammation of the tympanic cavity arising because of infection extending from the ear canal or from the eustachian tube. Hematogenous infection is also possible. Otitis media due to extension of infection from the ear canal or due to the penetration of the ear drum by foreign objects is possible in all species, but is most common in the dog, cat and rabbit. Infection from the eustachian tube is common in the dog, cat and pig, the cat being particularly susceptible.

Otitis media can quickly lead to otitis interna and result in deafness and disequilibrium.

Clinical Findings: The signs of otitis media and otitis externa are similar. Head shaking, rotation of the head to the affected side, pain, the presence of a discharge in the ear canal and changes in the ear canal are present. If otitis interna is superimposed, head rotation will be pronounced, the animal will circle to the affected side and fall to the same side, often being unable to rise. Nystagmus and incoordination may be present and the disease can terminate with death of the animal due to meningitis or an abscess in the cerebellum.

Diagnosis: Otitis media should be suspected in cases of severe purulent otitis externa or whenever penetrating plant awns are found in the ear canal. Diagnosis can be confirmed by inspecting the tympanum with an otoscope in the anesthetized animal. If the tympanic membrane is ruptured, one should assume that otitis media is present.

Otitis interna should be strongly suspected if the previously mentioned signs are present. In the case of infection by way of the eustachian tube, otoscopic examination will reveal a discolored and raised tympanic membrane.

In otitis media and interna of long duration, radiographs will often disclose the presence of fluid in the tympanic cavity or sclerotic changes in the bone of the tympanic bulla.

Treatment: Because of the possibility of damage to hearing and the vestibular apparatus, systemic antibiotic therapy should be instituted as soon as the diagnosis is made. Tetracyclines (e.g., ℞ 25) or chloramphenicol (℞ 7) should be used until the results of bacterial sensitivity tests are known. If the ear drum is ruptured, the tympanic cavity should be carefully cleaned under otoscopic examination using long alligator forceps and by flushing the cavity with detergent solutions and rinsing with saline. Solutions containing neomycin and polymyxin B should be placed in the ear canal and the tympanic cavity, in addition to the systemic therapy. The ear drum will heal in time.

In the case of otitis media and interna with a clean, normal external ear, but an abnormal tympanum, incising the tympanum may be advantageous in that it permits culture of the fluid, relieves the pressure and thus the pain and removes the inflammatory exudate that could cause a permanent hearing deficiency. Systemic therapy using the antibiotic selected by sensitivity testing should be continued for at least 10 days and possibly for up to 6 weeks or longer in cases of otitis interna. Any associated otitis externa should be carefully treated. In chronic otitis media with sclerosis and osteomyelitis of the tympanic bulla, a bulla osteotomy may be necessary.

Prognosis: Otitis media with an intact tympanum responds well to systemic antibiotic therapy, but when chronic otitis and a ruptured tympanum are present, the chances of successful treatment are reduced. Otitis interna carries a guarded prognosis. Some neurologic signs (such as the head tilt) may persist for the remainder of the animal's life or the signs may abate after many months. Animals recovering from otitis interna should be given adequate time to adapt to the neurologic deficiencies inflicted by the disease.

DEAFNESS

Deafness in animals can be acquired or congenital. Acquired deafness occurs because of bilateral occlusion of the external ear canals as in chronic otitis externa or because of destruction of the middle ear as in acute or chronic otitis media. Other causes of acquired deafness are trauma to the petrous temporal bone, loud noises, canine distemper, drugs (hygromycin, streptomycin, kanamycin, neomycin, salicylates), neoplasms of the ear or brain and old age. Obviously unilateral deafness or partial loss of hearing is possible in some of the above instances.

Congenital deafness can occur in any species or breed. A syndrome in cats causing white fur, blue eyes and deafness results from an autosomal gene that is fully dominant with complete expression in the production of white fur, with incomplete expression for deafness and with incomplete dominance in the production of the blue iris. Deafness is due to the total or partial agenesis of the organ of Corti, spiral ganglion and cochlear nuclei. White coat color also is associated with congenital deafness in other animals. In the dog, the breeds commonly affected at the present time include the Dalmatian, Bull Terrier, Scotch Terrier, Border Collie and Fox Terrier. This list changes with time due to breed popularity and the elimination of the defect as it becomes a problem. Cocker Spaniels were known, for example, to have a hereditary deafness but it is no longer common in that breed.

Diagnosis: Diagnosis of deafness is very difficult in the young or in animals kept in groups; it is only when the animal is observed as an individual at an age when responses to stimuli can be predicted that deafness becomes obvious. The main sign is failure of response to auditory stimulus. An example of this is failure of noise that excites other dogs to awaken a sleeping dog. Less obvious signs are unusual behavior such as excessive barking, a voice change, confusion when given vocal commands and lack of movement of the pinnae. Electrophysiologic methods of conducting auditory testing have been used on cats, but the technique is not in general use. In the case of acquired deafness, otoscopic examination of the external ear, radiographic examination of the tympanic bullae and a neurologic examination may determine the cause. In congenital deafness, these procedures will reveal normal structure and function (apart from absence of hearing). A careful history and shrewd observation of the animal are necessary in the diagnosis of deafness.

Treatment: Successful removal of an occlusion of the external ear canal will eliminate deafness from this cause. Deafness due to bacterial infections of the middle and internal ear may respond to early antibiotic treatment. Relief from deafness due to loud noise, trauma, or viral infections is dependent on time. Hereditary deafness may be eliminated from a species by test breeding to determine the nature of the inheritance so that the responsible carriers can be eliminated from the breeding program.

INFECTIOUS DISEASES

RABIES

An acute encephalomyelitis caused by a virus. It is a natural disease of dogs, cats, bats and wild carnivores. However, all warm-blooded animals are susceptible. The disease is world-wide except for Australia, New Zealand, New Guinea and Oceania. Sweden, Norway and Great Britain were among the first countries to eradicate rabies. More recently, Japan, Taiwan, Hong Kong and Malaya have eliminated the disease. It is enzootic, and at times epizootic throughout the Western Hemisphere in bats, dogs, foxes and skunks.

Mode of Transmission: The virus may be recovered from the CNS and also from the salivary glands, lacrimal glands, pancreas, kidney and adrenal tissues of infected animals. In nature, it is transmitted from animal to animal by means of a bite introducing the virus-bearing saliva. Rarely, rabies may be transmitted by virus contamination of fresh, already existing wounds. Virus may be present in the saliva and be transmitted by an infected animal several days prior to the onset of clinical signs

Incubation Period: The incubation period is variable, but generally is within 15 to 50 days. In rare cases, it may be much longer, even several months.

Pathogenesis: Infection takes place by the deposition of infected saliva in or near a nerve. The virus is carried to the CNS via the nerve trunks. Experimentally, it has been shown to reach the spinal cord within 24 hours and can be demonstrated in the cord tissue within 4 to 5 days. The virus travels upward in the cord and finally reaches the brain after a variable time, which requires most of the incubation period. The virus usually travels centrifugally from the CNS and reaches the salivary glands via their nerve supply. Although considered invariably fatal, there is evidence to indicate rare instances of recovery.

Clinical Findings: Rabid animals of all species exhibit certain clinical signs which are typical of rabies with minor variations peculiar to carnivora, ruminants, bats and man. The clinical course of the disease, particularly in dogs, can be divided into 3 phases, the prodromal, the excitative and the paralytic. The term "furious rabies" refers to animals in which the excitative phase is predominant, and "dumb or paralytic rabies" to dogs in which the excitative phase is extremely short or absent and the disease progresses quickly to the paralytic phase. In any animal, the first sign is a change in behavior, which may be indistinguishable from a digestive disorder, injury, foreign body in the mouth, poisoning or an early infectious disease. Temperature is not significant and inability to retain saliva may or may not be noted. Animals usually stop eating and drinking and may seek solitude. There is frequently irritation or stimulation to the urogenital tract as evidenced by frequent urination, erection in the male and sexual desire. After the prodromal period of 1 to 3 days, animals either show signs of paralysis or become vicious. Carnivora, swine and, occasionally, horses and mules bite other animals or people at the slightest provocation. Cattle will butt any moving object. The disease progresses rapidly after the onset of paralysis.

Paralytic Form: This form of rabies is characterized by early paralysis of the throat and masseter muscles, usually with profuse salivation and the inability to swallow. Dropping of the lower jaw is a common sign in dogs. Owners frequently examine the mouth of dogs and cattle, searching for a foreign body, or administer medication with the bare hands. These animals are not vicious and rarely attempt or are able to bite. The paralysis progresses rapidly to all parts of the body with coma and death in a few hours.

Furious Form: Furious rabies represents the classical "mad-dog syndrome" in which the animal becomes irrational and viciously aggressive. The facial expression is one of alertness and anxiety, with pupils dilated. Noise invites attack, and it is instinctive in all species to attack. Such animals lose all caution and fear of natural enemies. There is no evidence of paralysis during the excitatory stage; dogs rarely live beyond 10 days after the onset of signs. Dogs with this form of rabies frequently roam streets and highways, biting other animals, people and any moving object. They commonly swallow foreign objects, feces, straw, sticks and stones. Rabid dogs will chew the wire and frame of their cage, breaking their teeth, and will follow a hand moved in front of the cage, attempting to bite. Young pups apparently seek human companionship and are overly playful, but bite even when petted, usually becoming vicious in a few hours. As the disease progresses, muscular incoordination and convulsive seizures become common.

Death from rabies is the result of progressive paralysis. The lesions are found in the bulbar region of the CNS.

Rabid domestic **cats** and **bobcats** attack suddenly, biting and scratching viciously. **Foxes** frequently invade yards or even houses, attacking dogs and people. Rabid foxes and **skunks** are responsible for most pasture cattle losses, and skunks have attacked dairy cattle in barns.

Rabies in **cattle** follows the same general pattern, and those with the furious form are dangerous, attacking and pursuing other animals and man. Lactation ceases abruptly in dairy cattle. Instead of the usual placid expresson, there is one of alertness. The eyes and ears follow sounds and movement. A most typical clinical sign in cattle is bellowing of a character which can hardly be mistaken once encountered. This may continue intermittently until approaching death.

Horses and **mules** show extreme agitation evidenced by rolling as with indigestion. As with other species, they may bite or strike viciously and, because of size and strength, become unmanageable in a few hours. Such animals frequently suffer self-inflicted wounds.

The **vampire bat** is confined at present to South America, Trinidad, Central America and Mexico. These animals fight among themselves but rarely attack other animals except to feed. Their sole food is fresh blood. Although preferring cattle, they may feed on any animal, including man, by biting and lapping blood from the bite wound. Vampire bats sometimes carry living virus in the saliva for an undetermined period as an asymptomatic salivary gland infection. Cattle losses are severe in infected areas. Rabies contracted from vampire bats is almost exclusively of the paralytic form.

In North America there are immense numbers of **insectivorous bats**, both as solitary individuals and in large colonies, which may become infected and transmit rabies. Rabid bats have been found widely distributed throughout the continent. Most of these isolations have been made during surveys, but many have been from bats captured while attacking humans or animals. Several human deaths due to rabies have been attributed to infections from bats.

Differential Diagnosis: Clinical diagnosis is usually possible but may be difficult; in the prodromal stage, rabies may easily be confused with other diseases. Inability to swallow saliva in all species of animals is suggestive of an obstruction in the throat, a foreign body lodged between the teeth, or ingestion of irritating substances. Furthermore, many animals will fight when injured, when provoked, or for possession of food or a mate. Normal cats and squirrels, particularly males, at times make sudden unprovoked attacks on other animals or man. All of these behavior patterns may be present in rabies, but can also be unrelated.

If there is human exposure, the animal should be confined for observation for 10 days. If possible, the suspect animal should not be killed, but be allowed to die. Rabies progresses rapidly and usually typical signs will be evident in a day or two.

Wildlife acting in an abnormal manner should be considered rabid until proved otherwise. The same is true of bats which may be observed flying in the daytime, resting on the ground, attacking people or animals, or fighting. Insectivorous bats, though small, can inflict a wound with their teeth and should never be caught or handled with bare hands.

A complete history and observation period are important in diagnosis. If the suspected animal dies, the brain should be examined in a laboratory. In the past this examination was for the presence of Negri bodies. Most virus diseases, particularly distemper and infectious hepatitis in dogs and panleukopenia in cats, produce inclusion bodies which may be confused with Negri bodies. However, if the brain examination is negative or unsatisfactory, inoculation of mice will provide a definite diagnosis.

The **fluorescent-antibody staining technique** combines the speed of histologic techniques with the greater sensitivity of biologic examination. The test is based on direct visual observation of a specific antigen-antibody reaction. When properly used, it can establish a highly specific diagnosis within a few hours, and it has become the test of choice in most laboratories.

Control Methods: Rabies control programs work best on a countrywide basis and should include the following: 1) Mass vaccination of dogs—this is the single most effective measure. An outbreak can be controlled when 70% of the dog popula-

tion is vaccinated within not more than 2 to 3 weeks. 2) Elimination of stray dogs—strays should be collected and held by a
local pound or humane shelter for several days and, if un-
claimed, destroyed humanely. 3) Reduction of excess numbers
of wildlife vectors—outbreaks of rabies in wild carnivores occur generally when the population of the species becomes
particularly dense in an area. Under official auspices trapping
and poisoning programs are the most effective means of reducing overpopulation to a safe level.

Immunoprophylaxis: Three types of inactivated-virus vaccines
and 6 types of modified live-virus vaccines are available for
dogs. The oldest inactivated type, sometimes called Semple-
type vaccine (℞ 133), is a heat-inactivated, phenol-treated,
fixed virus (20% CNS emulsion) of caprine or ovine origin. Sensitivity to this vaccine has on rare occasions led to
paralysis. There are 2 new inactivated-virus tissue culture
types of vaccines available for dogs (℞ 129, 132). Of
these 3 vaccines, two (℞ 132, 133) are known to protect dogs
for a year; there are no comparable data on duration of
immunity for ℞ 129 (without adjuvant).

Of the 6 modified living-virus vaccines, the oldest and most
widely used in dogs is the low egg passage (LEP) Flury strain
of chicken embryo origin (℞ 127). The high egg passage
(HEP) Flury vaccine (℞ 126) is recommended primarily for
cattle and cats. The remaining modified live-virus vaccines
for dogs are newer cell culture products (℞ 125, 128, 130, 134).
All of the live-virus vaccines are lyophilized, require refrigeration, and should be used within 45 minutes after reconstitution.
They have been shown to protect dogs for at least 3 years.

There are important species differences in response to rabies
vaccines, e.g., the LEP types are for use in dogs only, and
may prove pathogenic in other species. The various vaccine
types and recommendations for dosage and use in the various
species are listed in the prescription section.

Management of Dogs and Cats Bitten by Rabid Animals: Un-
vaccinated dogs, cats and other pets bitten by a known rabid
animal should be destroyed immediately. If the owner is unwilling to do so, the animal should be vaccinated and placed
in strict isolation in a kennel for 4 months or longer. If the
animal exposed has been vaccinated previously within 3 years
with a modified live-virus canine vaccine, or within one year
with an inactivated-virus vaccine, it should be revaccinated
and restrained (leashing, yard or house confinement) for 30
days.

PSEUDORABIES
(Aujeszky's disease, Mad itch, Infectious bulbar paralysis)

A virus infection of swine which occasionally infects non-porcine species in which it causes a fatal encephalomyelitis manifested by severe pruritus and self-mutilation.

Etiology and Epidemiology: Sometimes called *Herpesvirus suis*, the etiologic agent produces cytopathology in numerous tissue cultures and fatal encephalomyelitis upon inoculation of most laboratory animals. Swine are the natural host and principal reservoir. Rats, once suspected as reservoirs, are now considered unimportant in transmission, which in endemic areas (Midwestern U.S.A. and parts of Europe) occurs easily between swine via oral and nasal secretions. Porcine infections are usually inapparent except in suckling piglets which develop a usually fatal encephalomyelitis and in pregnant sows which may abort or produce stillborn or mummified fetuses. Fatal pseudorabies occurs sporadically in nonporcine species contacting swine. These species (*see* clinical signs) are "dead-end hosts" usually uninvolved in further transmission but serving to indicate infection in swine populations. As with other herpesviruses, latent infections may occur.

Clinical Findings: Swine frequently experience inapparent infection. Susceptible suckling piglets, however, develop acute pyrexia, paralysis, coma and death within 24 hours of onset. Occasionally older pigs abort or develop encephalitis with depression and sometimes blindness or convulsions.

Cattle and sheep infected by swine manifest "mad itch", licking, frantically biting, and rubbing themselves against solid objects until the affected areas (back, sides, frequently the vulva) become lacerated, swollen and raw with serosanguinous exudate. The animal becomes recumbent; coma and death follow.

Dogs and cats exhibit intense pruritus and succumb.

Lesions: Gross lesions are those of self-mutilation. Histopathologically, an acute encephalomyelitis with neuronal degeneration, microgliosis, perivascular cuffing and herpetiform inclusions are found. The distribution of skin lesions is frequently explainable by the locale of inflammation in the cord and brain stem.

Diagnosis: Pseudorabies in piglets must be differentiated from transmissible gastroenteritis (q.v., p. 302). In older pigs it could be confused with the viral polioencephalomyelitides and various toxicoses, and in aborting sows it must be distinguished from numerous syndromes.

In sheep, cattle, dogs and cats the clinical picture is unique but could be confused with rabies. Where any question exists specimens should be submitted for rabies examination. Histopathology aids diagnosis. The virus can be identified in tissue cultures or by producing the classic disease by subcut. inoculations of rabbits with brain or spinal cord tissue of suspect animals.

Control: Outbreaks are halted by separating cattle or sheep from swine. Cats and dogs should not have access to dead piglets, placentae, aborted fetuses, or clinically ill animals.

Public Health Importance: Nonfatal human infections have resulted from laboratory accident.

POX DISEASES

Acute viral diseases in man and mammals, characterized by typical vesicular eruptions of the skin and mucous membranes. The individual lesions tend to progress from macules through papular, vesicular and sometimes pustular stages before encrusting and healing. In the fully developed disease, the center of individual lesions tends to be depressed giving typical umbilication. In affected areas of skin and mucous membrane, the epithelium frequently contains typical cytoplasmic inclusions which essentially are intracellular virus colonies. The diseases affect man (smallpox or variola and alastrim); various mammals (cow pox, swine pox, goat pox, sheep pox, horse pox, rabbit pox, q.v., p. 1127, mouse pox, q.v., p. 1140 and monkey pox, q.v., p. 1155); and birds (fowl pox, q.v., p. 1021, canary pox, pigeon pox and turkey pox).

In some of these diseases, infection acquired by inhalation becomes generalized and there tends to be epizootic spread as in smallpox, sheep pox and rabbit pox. In other instances, infection occurs through the skin by contact as in horse pox, fowl pox and mouse pox. In cow pox, infection is also transferred by direct contact to the skin, but the disease remains localized on the udder and teats. The strains of vaccinia virus used in the preparation of vaccine for immunization against smallpox in man have long been propagated in laboratory animals. Many of these strains probably have been derived from the disease in cows. The viruses of smallpox, alastrim, vaccinia, cow pox, rabbit pox, mouse pox and monkey pox, and perhaps horse pox, are immunologically closely related and differ considerably from the pox viruses of sheep and goats and of birds. Swine are affected by 2 viruses, one apparently vaccinia and another which affects swine only.

COW POX
(Variolovaccinia, Vaccinia)

A mild eruptive disease of milk cows usually restricted to the skin of the udder and teats, with little constitutional disturbance. It spreads by contact.

Etiology: While less common than formerly, cow pox still appears sporadically. Practically all the cows in a herd become affected. It seems to spread during the process of milking even when this is done mechanically. Occasional outbreaks, clinically undistinguishable from natural cow pox, have been caused by vaccinia virus introduced by persons recently vaccinated against smallpox. Many outbreaks are not recognized early enough for the source to be traced. The viruses of natural cow pox and of vaccinia can be isolated and distinguished by laboratory methods. Both viruses are resistant to drying and may survive for weeks in scabs or dust.

Clinical Findings: After an incubation period of 3 to 7 days, small congested papules appear on the teats or adjacent areas of the udder. The papules increase in size and are hot and firm to the touch. After a few days, vesicles appear, but tend to rupture early. The fully developed lesions are umbilicated with a raised firm edge and depressed center. The scabs become dark brown in color, and drop off in about 2 weeks. Secondary infection commonly occurs and staphylococcal mastitis may be a complication. Attention may first be directed to the disease in cows by the occurrence of lesions on the hand, arm, or face of milkers. In man, the disease is likely to be more severe, and attended by lymphadenitis and fever, in those who have not previously been vaccinated against smallpox.

After recovery, animals are immune to further cow pox infection for several years.

Diagnosis: Cow pox may be difficult to distinguish from other affections of the teats. The character of the individual pocks with dark-red, firm, raised edges and depressed center and the rapid spread through the herd may be helpful features. Diagnosis can be established by isolation of the virus from the lesions and by serologic tests for its identification.

Control: Animals can be actively immunized by vaccination with commercial smallpox vaccine, but the disease is not sufficiently prevalent or serious to justify widespread use of this practice. When an infected animal is discovered, it should be isolated at once. However, before the disease is recognized on a farm, other animals usually are already infected so that control on that farm by isolation of infected animals may be impossible. There is no specific treatment.

PSEUDO-COW POX
(Milkers' nodes, Paravaccinia)

A poxlike disease on the udders of cows. It may spread to the milkers and cause red papular lesions on their hands. There is no cross-immunity with cow pox. A virus has been isolated in bovine tissue culture, which may be related to the bovine papular stomatitis virus.

SWINE POX

An acute infectious disease characterized mainly by skin lesions that resemble those of pox in other warm-blooded animals. It affects only swine. The disease is prevalent in the U.S.A., particularly the Midwest, where 1 to 5% of all herds may be affected at any single time in areas of dense swine population. It is found throughout the entire year, but is perhaps most common in the warm months.

In some parts of the world, infection of swine with vaccinia is the common type of pox in swine. In such areas, this may be known as swine pox and the type found largely in the U.S.A. may be known as pseudo-swine pox or poxlike disease.

The disease described here is the pox which affects swine only, not vaccinia infection.

Etiology: The causative virus is distinct from other pox viruses. It grows in porcine tissue culture, but growth has not been reported in other cell cultures. It has been found to persist in the tissues of infected swine for 18 to 30 days after initial exposure. It is abundant in the diseased skin, less so in the lymph nodes draining infected areas and is rarely found in the blood stream. The virus is readily transferred from pig to pig by rubbing it into the scarified skin, by lice (*Haematopinus suis*), less often by other insects and by simple contact. Hog lice, once infected, may carry the virus for weeks or months. Other insects apparently act as mechanical carriers.

Hogs may be infected with vaccinia either naturally or

artificially. The virus of vaccinia may produce an abortive type of pox or any grade up to a severe type. Swine immune to vaccinia are fully susceptible to swine pox and vice versa, though a minor antigenic relation between the 2 has been described.

Clinical Findings: Within 5 to 7 days—rarely as long as 12 days —following exposure by skin scarification or infected lice, erythematous, irregularly rounded areas (papules), averaging 4 to 5 mm in diameter, develop on the skin. When louse-borne, the skin involvement is usually confined to the under portions of the body, but may extend up the sides or even affect all parts. Rarely, a few proliferative lesions may appear along the back in lice-free hogs. Flying insects are suspected as carriers in these instances. In 2 or 3 days, the reddened areas along the belly change to "pustules" without much gross evidence of vesicles ever forming. In the pustules the central area is somewhat dried and scablike, surrounded by a narrow raised inflammatory zone so that the entire lesion is usually umbilicated. True scabs are formed within 8 to 11 days after the appearance of the papules. These are shed without scarring 2 to 3 weeks later. All skin lesions do not necessarily arise at the same time—secondary pox lesions may develop after the first ones are well started. Constitutional effects are usually mild during the first 7 to 10 days of the disease and consist of some degree of inactivity, some loss of appetite and failure to grow as rapidly as healthy pigs. Very few pigs die of swine pox. No common secondary infections have been recognized. Other diseases, however, may coexist with pox. In such cases, the impact of the 2 diseases is greater than the sum expected for them. For this reason, swine are not vaccinated for other diseases while in the active stages of pox. An attack of the disease renders animals immune. This may account for the fact that swine pox is rather rarely seen in aged animals.

Lice-free hogs are usually not seriously affected with swine pox. Susceptible hogs should not be exposed to those affected with pox. There is no treatment.

SHEEP POX AND GOAT POX

Sheep pox is a highly infectious and frequently fatal exanthematous disease which at one time had a wide distribution, but is now confined to parts of Southeastern Europe, North Africa and Asia. It is the most severe pox disease of domesticated animals. Goat pox has a distribution similar to that of sheep pox, but the condition is, on the whole, less severe.

Etiology: The viruses causing these 2 diseases are closely related to each other and to the virus of lumpy-skin disease (q.v., p. 275). They grow in various tissue cultures. These agents are highly resistant to desiccation. Infection is readily transmitted by contact or by the inoculation of the contents of the skin lesions.

Clinical Findings: The incubation period in **sheep pox** is from 4 to 7 days. The disease usually causes a severe systemic disturbance with widespread lesions. The eruptions are most prevalent on the cheeks, nostrils, lips and wool-free skin. The vesicular stage may be hemorrhagic: it is followed by the development of pustules and there is a marked tendency to generalization of the lesions. The lungs contain multiple spherical nodules commonest near the pleural surface. Lesions also may occur in the trachea and the alimentary tract. A gelatinous edema of the subcut. and IM tissue is not uncommon. The mortality varies from 5 to 50%.

The incubation period of **goat pox** is from 5 to 10 days. The disease tends to attack male kids and females in milk. In the initial stages, there may be a slight pyrexia, but in most outbreaks, constitutional disturbances are not marked. The lesions are not so widespread as in sheep pox, being confined to the hairless regions of the body, such as the axilla, thigh, nose and mouth. In the female, the udder also may be involved. The lesions are typical pox lesions, but usually are much smaller than those of sheep pox; moreover, the hemorrhagic complication of sheep pox lesions is absent. Some outbreaks of goat pox probably have been confused with contagious ecthyma (q.v., p. 290).

Immunity: Natural attacks of both diseases induce a solid and durable immunity. In countries where sheep pox is enzootic, susceptible animals are immunized by the inoculation of lymph from experimental lesions into the tail region or by the injection of sensitized virus, i.e., virulent vesicular fluid treated with a suitable amount of antiserum. More recently, formalized vaccines, prepared either from natural virus or from cell cultures, have produced immunity. The addition of aluminum hydroxide extends the protection. Similar methods may be used for goat pox. Vaccinia produces no immunity to sheep pox or goat pox.

PAPILLOMATOSIS
(Warts)

Warts of the skin or oral mucosa are self-limiting benign tumors occurring at multiple sites, chiefly in the young, of many species. (They have not been clearly shown to occur in cats or sheep.) They may be cauliflower-like, as usually seen in cattle, or small, scattered horny elevations. Isolated, individual small pedunculated growths that are not true warts can also develop on the skin. These do not change in size and generally do not create a problem.

Etiology and Transmission: Wart viruses are host-specific under natural conditions. The virus appears to infect the basal cells of the epithelium causing some cells to degenerate, while others are stimulated to excessive growth and wart formation. New virus particles form in the degenerating cells and completely replace the nuclear material when the cell reaches the surface; thus, there is much infective virus at the surface of the wart. The virus is quite resistant and may contaminate fences, stanchions or other objects. Skin wounds from such objects frequently lead to infection of susceptible animals. Tattoo instruments or hypodermic needles will transmit the infection in cattle.

Clinical Findings: Cattle: Warts commonly occur on the head, neck and shoulders, and occasionally on the back and abdomen. The extent and duration on an animal depends upon the area infected and dosage of virus, as well as the degree of susceptibility. They may last for a year or longer. Papillomatosis becomes a herd problem when the infection occurs in a large group of young susceptible cattle. Immunity to re-exposure usually develops 3 to 4 weeks after initial infection with the virus, although warts may not be seen until about 2 months after infection. They have been known to recur, probably from loss of immunity.

The bovine wart contains a fibromatous element. This is particularly prominent in the venereal form of the disease in young cattle. Fibropapillomas may be a serious problem on the penis of young bulls and can cause dystocia when affecting the vaginal mucosa of heifers.

There is a form of persistent cutaneous papillomatosis in herds of older cattle in which the warts are small and occur in succession. Although a papilloma-like virus can be seen in such warts, it has not been experimentally transmitted to test animals. Similar persistent warts can occur on the teats and udder of dairy cows. Wart virus has been found in tumors of the urinary bladder of cattle, possibly as a secondary infection of the tumor which probably developed from a carcinogen in bracken fern eaten by the animal. Wart-like lesions in the mouth, esophagus, rumen and reticulum are the result of proliferative (papular) stomatitis virus infection (q.v., p. 90) and not bovine papilloma virus.

Horses: Warts are common when young horses are kept together. The small, scattered warts usually appear on the nose and lips, presumably at the sites of abrasions when colts "nuzzle" each other. They cause no inconvenience and regress in a few months. The fibrosarcoma-like skin tumors produced in the horse by inoculation with bovine papilloma virus and naturally occurring equine sarcoid have no relation to equine cutaneous papillomatosis.

Dogs: Oral papillomatosis is often seen in young dogs and is caused by a virus that does not produce warts on the skin. The oral warts may be quite extensive at times. When skin warts occur, they are scattered, few in number and usually seen in older dogs. They contain a virus but no transmission trials have been reported. Oral papillomatosis has also been observed in coyotes, but its relation to the disease in dogs is unknown.

Rabbits: Both cutaneous and oral warts occur in rabbits. Rabbits immune to one kind are susceptible to the other. The cutaneous papillomas are found as keratinized horny growths in cottontail rabbits in some sections of Midwestern U.S.A. These contain a virus (Shope papilloma virus) that will produce skin papillomas of the domestic rabbit. The skin lesions do not contain infective virus but some become malignant carcinomas.

Oral papillomatosis may occur in colonies of domestic rabbits and can be transmitted to wild rabbits. The small, white, nodular or cauliflower-like warts are multiple. They are caused by a virus different from that of cutaneous papillomatosis.

Goats: Warts have been described in goats affecting various skin areas, and some of those on the teats and udder became carcinomas.

Monkeys: A transmissible cutaneous papillomatosis has been reported in monkeys, but the species specificity was not established.

Deer: A cutaneous fibromatosis occurs in white-tailed deer and is caused by a papilloma-like virus found only in the epithelium covering the tumors. Deer are not susceptible to the bovine papilloma virus.

Diagnosis: Warts can be readily recognized. Whether they can be regarded as infectious in an individual animal depends upon such circumstances as age of the animal and lesion, previous contacts, and presence of warts on other animals of the herd.

Treatment and Control: Infectious papillomatosis is a self-limiting disease, although the duration of warts on individual animals may vary considerably. A variety of chemicals have been advocated for treatment without agreement on their value. Surgical removal is recommended if the warts are sufficiently objectionable. Surgical intervention in the early growing stage of a wart may lead to recurrence and stimulation of growth; therefore, warts should be removed when near their maximum size or when regressing. Affected animals may be isolated from susceptible animals, although with the long incubation period, many will have been exposed to the infection before a problem is recognized.

Vaccines of wart tissues containing formalin-killed virus have been used for treatment with limited success. One controlled trial on experimentally produced warts in cattle indicated that these vaccines were of no value. Since wart viruses are mostly species specific, there is no merit in using a vaccine of wart tissue derived from one species on another species of animal.

When the disease exists as a herd problem it can be controlled by prophylactic vaccination using a suspension of ground wart tissue in which the virus has been killed with formalin. It may be necessary to begin vaccination as early as 4 to 6 weeks of age in calves with about 0.4 ml vaccine intradermally at 2 sites, and repeating the dose in 4 to 6 weeks and at a year of age. Immunity to infection with the virus will develop in a few weeks, but this immunity is not related to the unknown mechanism involved in regression of the wart. Since exposure to the virus may have occurred prior to vaccination, as with a contaminated tattoo instrument, the vaccine-induced immunity may develop too late to prevent development of warts. A program of prophylactic vaccination must be in effect for about 3 to 6 months before its preventive value will be noted. It should be continued for at least a year after disappearance of the last wart since infective wart virus may still contaminate the premises. Stalls, stanchions and other inert materials can be disinfected with formaldehyde fumigation, but this must be done with high humidity and temperature to be effective.

THE EQUINE RESPIRATORY DISEASE COMPLEX

Of the 10 or more viruses associated with acute equine respiratory disease, only those causing arteritis, influenza and rhinopneumonitis produce clinical syndromes and epizootiologic patterns sufficiently distinctive to suggest an etiologic diagnosis. If available, serologic or virologic confirmation should be sought.

The following viruses have been incriminated as causes of acute equine respiratory diseases but their significance is obscure: equine herpesvirus-2 and -3; equine cytomegalovirus; equine paramyxoviruses (parainfluenza 1, 2, 3); equine rhinoviruses-1 and -2; and equine adenoviruses.

Infection with any of these viruses may be complicated by proliferation of bacteria or mycoplasmas.

EQUINE VIRAL RHINOPNEUMONITIS

Etiology and Epizootiology: Designated equine herpesvirus-1 (EHV-1), the virus of equine viral rhinopneumonitis produces acute respiratory catarrh upon primary infection, resulting in annual outbreaks among foals in areas with dense horse populations and sporadic episodes elsewhere. The age, seasonal and geographic distributions vary and are probably determined by immune status and aggregation of horses. In individuals, the outcome of exposure is determined by immune status, pregnancy status and possibly age. Mares may abort several weeks to several months after clinical disease or asymptomatic infection. The reservoir is the horse; a latent carrier state may exist. Transmission occurs by direct or indirect contact with virus-laden nasal discharge, aborted fetuses or placentas.

Clinical Findings: After an incubation period of 2 to 10 days, fully susceptible horses may develop any of the following signs: fever (102° to 107°F) persisting 1 to 7 days and accompanied by leukopenia (neutropenia and lymphopenia), congestion and serous discharge from nasal mucosa and conjunctiva, malaise, pharyngitis, cough, inappetence, sometimes edematous mandibular lymph nodes, and sometimes constipation followed by diarrhea. Frequently bacterial infections with mucopurulent nasal exudate and coughing follow. The infection is mild (CNS signs) or inapparent in horses preconditioned immunologically.

Pregnant mares may abort fresh (minimally autolyzed) fetuses 3 weeks to 4 months after asymptomatic infection. Abortion is most common in the 8th to 11th months of gestation (sometimes occurring earlier). It is usually sudden without premonitory signs and followed by prompt placental expulsion and unimpaired subsequent breeding performance.

Diagnosis: Abortion due to EHV-1 can be tentatively diagnosed when grossly evident focal hepatic necrosis is present in spontaneously aborted, minimally decomposed fetuses with petechiation throughout. Finding intranuclear inclusions in hepatic cells and bronchiolar or alveolar epithelium confirms the diagnosis as does virus isolation. Serology on aborting mares is diagnostically unproductive.

Immunoprophylaxis: Immunity following natural infection appears partially humoral and partially localized in the respiratory tract where it lasts from 3 to 9 months and can be augmented by mild or subclinical respiratory reinfections with EHV-1. Usually 2 to 3 exposures are needed to provide good resistance.

Immunity against abortion is probably humoral, persists longer, but also needs occasional augmentation and requires further study to explain why protection is sometimes incomplete and why the same mare may abort twice.

Intranasally administered modified live virus vaccine (℞ 124) is used on farms where infection has been a problem. Caution is advised in vaccination or introduction of recently vaccinated animals onto farms free of the disease because of the hazard of shedding vaccine virus and vaccine-induced abortion. A parenterally administered vaccine is used in Germany.

Sanitary Management: On small farms with horses in close contact, little is accomplished by attempted isolation after abortions begin. Isolation and strict sanitary precautions are useful in the event of an abortion by a newly introduced mare, especially on large farms with separated groups of mares or in areas where abortion storms are rare or unknown. Efficient quarantine measures should be imposed on unknown mares arriving on a stud farm.

Treatment: Medication is seldom indicated. Confinement with careful observation during the febrile period and several days thereafter is necessary so that serious secondary infections may be handled promptly. There are no treatments for fetal infection. Some prenatally infected newborn foals may survive with diligent care and antibiotics (℞ 11, 25, 41, 58) until 48 to 72 hours after the temperature has returned to normal and the pulmonary congestion and edema are resolved. Appropriate nursing, supportive care and oxygen assist in recovery. *See also* p. 251.

Infections by other herpesviruses: EHV-2 isolated from the pharynx of a horse with respiratory disease may cause respiratory disease. The equine coital exanthema virus does not seem to be pathogenic for the respiratory tract.

EQUINE VIRAL ARTERITIS
(Epizootic cellulitis, "Pink-eye")

An acute contagious viral disease characterized by fever, catarrh, edema and abortion.

Etiology and Epizootiology: Presently unclassified, the arteritis virus is distinct from other equine viruses. Spread is by contact with respiratory secretions. The disease is not commonly diagnosed. It occurs in sporadic outbreaks which are usually attributable to movements of horses. Mortality is low. Clinical signs are most severe in very young or very old horses and those in poor physical condition. Up to 80% of pregnant mares may abort.

Clinical Findings: After an incubation period of 1 to 8 days, fever and leukopenia may be accompanied by lacrimation, conjunctivitis, nasal congestion and discharge, weakness, depression, anorexia and weight loss. Less consistent findings are CNS disturbance, photophobia, colic, diarrhea, icterus and edema of the eyelids, conjunctiva, legs, ventral body wall and sometimes the sheath, scrotum and mammae. Abortion occurs during the febrile period or shortly thereafter.

Lesions: In addition to lesions observable in the animals, the occasional fatal case may have pulmonary emphysema, pulmonary and mediastinal edema, excess fluids in the pleural and peritoneal cavities, enteritis, edema of the intestinal submucosa, and splenic hemorrhage and infarcts. Most gross lesions are attributable to vascular lesions consisting of histopathologically evident thrombus formation, endothelial swelling and a characteristic degeneration and necrosis of the media of arteries, particularly smaller ones.

Diagnosis: Clinical diagnosis usually requires a composite of signs and lesions in several horses. Differential diagnosis includes influenza, equine viral rhinopneumonitis (EVR), influenza, and sometimes African horse sickness, equine infectious anemia and purpura haemorrhagica.

The occurrence of abortion during or just following illness is a valuable diagnostic feature because abortion rarely accompanies influenza and the mare is usually healthy at the time of EVR abortion. Fetuses aborted due to EVR (q.v., p. 246) usually have characteristic lesions while those aborted due to arteritis have neither lesions nor inclusion bodies.

Since few laboratories work with this virus, it is advisable to get instructions from the laboratory prior to collecting specimens for serologic or virologic diagnosis.

Prophylaxis and Treatment: There is no specific treatment; antibacterial drugs and symptomatic therapy are indicated, and good nursing and absolute rest with very gradual return to activity are essential. Since experimentally developed vaccines are not commercially available, prevention is contingent on good hygiene and isolation.

EQUINE INFLUENZA

An acute, highly contagious febrile respiratory disease.

Etiology and Epizootiology: Presently, 2 immunologically distinct influenza viruses are enzootic among horses throughout the world. Myxovirus A-equi-1 has probably been present for decades. Myxovirus A-equi-2 was first recognized in 1963 as a cause of widespread epizootics which subsided leaving the virus established enzootically. The enzootic state is maintained throughout the year by sporadic clinical cases, and by mild or inapparent infection of susceptible horses which constantly join the population by birth, immigration or waning immunity. It is not known if a carrier state exists. Consequences of exposure are largely determined by previous immunologic conditioning, and in susceptible animals vary from mild inapparent infection to a severe disease which is rarely fatal except in very young, very old or otherwise debilitated patients. Epizootics are propagated by contact with respiratory secretions and result when one or more actively infected horses join an aggregation of susceptible horses assembled for show, sales, training or racing.

Clinical Findings: The incubation period is usually 1 to 3 days with a range of 18 hours to 5 and rarely 7 days. The onset is abrupt, with temperature up to 107.5°F, usually lasting less than 3 days unless bacterial infection follows. Coughing is observed early and may persist for several weeks. Nasal discharge is scant. Expiratory dyspnea, anorexia, weakness and stiffness are sometimes present. Mildly affected horses recover spontaneously within 2 to 3 weeks, but those severely affected may convalesce for 6 months. Recovery from the incapacitating signs and cough are hastened by completely restricting strenuous activities.

Complications such as bacterial infections, chronic bronchitis, asthmoid conditions and pulmonary emphysema are best prevented by restricting exercise, controlling dust, providing superior ventilation and practicing good stable hygiene.

Lesions: Usually no lesions are observed in live patients. At necropsy, interstitial pneumonia, bronchitis, peribronchitis and perivasculitis may be seen.

Diagnosis: In individual cases, laboratory assistance may be needed to differentiate influenza from equine viral rhinopneumonitis, equine viral arteritis and miscellaneous equine respiratory viral infections (q.v., p. 246). Equine influenza is usually diagnosed on observation of fast-spreading disease with rapid onset, high fever, weakness and cough; virologic or serologic study require instructions from a consenting laboratory.

Prophylaxis: Where available, bivalent inactivated vaccines should be administered annually. Probability of exposure can be reduced by isolation of additions to stables and by minimizing contact with other horses.

Treatment: Horses without complications require only rest and nursing, but antibiotics (R 11, 25, 41, 58) are indicated when fever persists beyond 3 to 4 days or when purulent nasal discharges or pulmonary involvement are evident. Restricted exercise is mandatory (*see* Clinical Findings).

COMPLICATIONS OF EQUINE VIRAL RESPIRATORY DISEASES

Bacterial infections may appear during or following viral infections and produce a mucopurulent nasal exudate, persistent fever, lymphadenitis, persistent cough, leukocytosis, laryngitis, bronchitis or pneumonia.

Upper respiratory inflammation may extend into the sinuses, eustachian tubes or guttural pouches. Toxicosis or pleuritis may accompany pneumonia. These complications are more frequent and more severe at collection points and racing and training grounds than on farms. *Streptococcus zooepidemicus,* a common secondary invader, is isolated frequently from the upper respiratory tract and sometimes from lungs or pleural exudate. *Actinobaccillus equuli* and *Escherichia coli* are isolated less frequently. *Pseudomonas aeruginosa* may be involved in persistent coughing and other upper respiratory complications. Isolation of *Str. equi* indicates primary or secondary strangles (q.v., p. 391).   Mycoplasmas of unknown significance are sometimes isolated.

PROPHYLAXIS AND TREATMENT OF RESPIRATORY DISEASES AND THEIR COMPLICATIONS

Prophylaxis: Vaccines of variable effectiveness are available for equine influenza, viral rhinopneumonitis and strangles. The cost and hazards of each vaccination must be weighed against the probability of exposure and potential losses in economic and sentimental value. The strength of arguments supporting vaccination increase with probability of exposure.

Treatment: Most acute equine respiratory disease is clinically diagnosed tentatively as rhinopneumonitis, arteritis, influenza, or influenza-like conditions lacking distinctive signs and possibly due to numerous viruses (q.v., p. 246). Rarely is a definite laboratory diagnosis available when therapy is instituted.

Regardless of etiology, restricted exercise, careful observation and confinement in comfortable, draft-free quarters with palatable feed and fresh water are fundamental.

Confinement should begin at onset of fever and continue at least 10 to 14 days and longer if complications appear. Failure to restrict exercise contributes to severity and duration of illness and development of serious sequelae.

Antipyretics and corticosteroids may obscure signs and mask the need for antibacterial therapy, which should be instituted when fever persists beyond 3 to 5 days or when mucopurulent nasal or pharyngeal exudate appears. Penicillin (R 44) and streptomycin (R 54), or both, are common initial choices with supplementation with sulfonamides (R 75, 82, 85) and addition of broad-spectrum antibiotics (R 11, 18, 25, 58) to the regimen in unresponsive cases.

Persistent coughs, unresponsive to antibiotic therapy require rest and may respond to therapy with iodides (R 573, 579, 581) or nitrofuran (R 98) or pharyngeal applications of corticosteroid-antibacterial combinations.

EQUINE ENCEPHALOMYELITIS
(Equine Encephalitis)

The equine encephalitides constitute a group of diseases of Equidae characterized by similar clinical nervous disturbances and generally high mortality. The causal arboviruses infect a variety of other vertebrate hosts including man. These diseases are serious although sporadic public health problems.

Etiology and Epizootiology: Horses may be infected by either group A or B arboviruses. The group A viruses include eastern and western, and group B viruses include Venezuelan and Japanese encephalomyelitis. Eastern equine encephalomyelitis occurs principally in Eastern Canada and the east coastal and gulf states of the U.S.A., but has been identified in the southwestern states, Mexico, South and Central America and some Caribbean islands. Western equine encephalomyelitis occurs principally in Western Canada, Western and Central U.S.A. and Mexico. Both eastern encephalomyelitis and western encephalomyelitis have been found to cause clinical disease in horses in the states of Florida, Louisiana and Texas. The Venezuelan virus is widely distributed in South and Central America, Mexico and now (1971) in southern Texas and Florida. Japanese encephalitis is an east Asian disease.

An unrelated virus causes **Borna disease** in Europe, where it has occurred for years and usually appears during the spring and early summer. Until recently it was not thought to be arthropod-borne but it is now recognized to be transmitted by ticks as well as by ingestion. Clinically, the disease resembles the North American encephalitides. The incubation period is 4 weeks or longer, the course 1 to 3 weeks, the mortality usually high and a characteristic inclusion (Joest body) develops in ganglion cells of the brain.

The Japanese B virus is widely distributed in the Far East causing encephalitis of man and horses, although mortality in horses is low (less than 5%). It causes abortion in swine but provides no other signs in this species. This virus has an arthropod vector-bird-mammalian cycle similar to that of the North American viruses. The Japanese encephalitis virus has not been identified in the Western Hemisphere.

The 3 American viruses, eastern, western and Venezuelan, are maintained in nature by an arthropod-bird or -rodent reservoir from which infection is transmitted to mammalian hosts by biting insects, principally mosquitoes of the genera *Aedes, Anopheles, Culex* and *Culiseta.* Mosquitoes act as biological vectors, i.e., the viruses multiply in the body and persist in the salivary gland. Transmission by arthropods other than mosquitoes is probably unimportant. Wild birds serve as a principal reservoir for eastern and western encephalomyelitis virus. Forest rodents are the most probable reservoirs of Venezuelan virus. Reservoir hosts tend to develop viremia with blood titers adequate to infect mosquitoes, therefore actively contribute to the cycle of virus survival. The horse may be regarded as a dead-end host with the western virus. Horses infected with eastern virus may develop a viremia adequate for infecting mosquitoes, but do not contribute significantly to transmission or persistence of the virus in nature. The Venezuelan virus produces a viremia adequate for infecting mosquitoes, and unlike the other 2 viruses, may also spread between horses and to man by contact or aerosol.

These diseases are more frequent in pastured than in stabled horses and are concentrated in areas having the appropriate combination of reservoir hosts and mosquitoes.

Clinical Findings: Signs include fever, impaired vision, irregular gait, wandering, reduced reflexes, circling, incoordination, yawning, grinding of teeth, drowsiness, pendulous lower lip, inability to swallow, inability to rise when down, paralysis and death.

Those with mild cases may slowly recover in a few weeks, but mortality in horses is about 20 to 50% from the western type of virus, over 90% from the eastern type, and up to 75% from the Venezuelan type.

Lesions: No characteristic gross lesions are observed. Microscopically, hemorrhage, degeneration of nerve cells in the cerebral cortex, thalamus, hypothalamus and other parts of the CNS can usually be demonstrated. Perivascular cuffing with polymorphonuclear and mononuclear cells may be present. Inclusion bodies are present only in Borna disease.

Diagnosis: A presumptive diagnosis may be based on clinical signs, history and seasonal occurrence and is aided by knowledge of enzootic areas or known epizootic activity of a virus type. Demonstration of typical histopathologic lesions of a viral encephalitis strengthens the diagnosis. Further support and improved specificity result from positive virus neutralization or hemagglutination inhibition tests on acute-phase and convalescent serums. Because of the high mortality and rapid death of horses affected with eastern equine virus, it is difficult to obtain paired sera in this disease. However, horses with eastern virus encephalitis often have developed antibody 2 or 3 days after signs appear. Specific diagnosis is dependent on recovery of the virus from brain tissue and subsequent serotyping.

In the differential diagnosis, botulism, rabies, encephalomyelitis, tetanus, listeriosis, fungal toxicosis, chemical poisoning, plant poisoning and X-disease-serum hepatitis must be considered.

Prophylaxis and Treatment: No specific antiviral agent is available. Supportive treatment and good nursing will aid in the recovery of mild cases. Since the disease is primarily spread by mosquitoes, control measures should be directed against these arthropods.

Vaccines (R 118) are prepared from the eastern type and the western type. Since there is little cross-immunity between the 2 types, a bivalent vaccine (R 118) prepared from both types is also available. Intradermal injection of the vaccine—given in 2 doses, 7 to 10 days apart—results in immunity after about 2 weeks which will protect animals throughout the current season. Annual spring vaccination is recommended in endemic areas. In 1971 a vaccine against the Venezuelan-type virus became available, but pregnant mares and very young foals should not be vaccinated.

EQUINE INFECTIOUS ANEMIA
(Swamp fever)

An acute or chronic disease of Equidae, characterized by intermittent fever, depression, progressive weakness, loss of weight, edema and progressive or transitory anemia. It is found wherever there are horses.

Etiology: The virus has been found in all tissues and discharges, and persists in the blood for the life of the horse. It is transmitted by any mechanism that will transfer blood from an infected to another horse. Insect transmission appears to be entirely mechanical and without a biologic phase in the insect. Insertion and withdrawal of a hypodermic needle may provide adequate contamination for transmission.

The virus shows considerable resistance to chemical disinfectants, heating, freezing and drying. If protected from sunlight, infected dried blood retains its virulence for several months.

Ordinarily, the disease spreads slowly and sporadically, but it may occur in epizootic form when circumstances are favorable for its transmission, such as abundance of bloodsucking flies and the promiscuous use of unsterilized hypodermic needles and other surgical instruments.

Clinical Findings: The incubation period usually ranges from 1 to 3 weeks, though periods of 4 days to 3 months have been reported in artificially induced infections. Horses experiencing active disease will have decreased packed cell volume; decreased red cell half-life; and Coomb's positive red cells, using anticomplement (C3) antisera. Haptoglobin values decrease and indirect bilirubin and plasma hemoglobin are transiently increased. The total white blood cell count varies, but usually will be slightly decreased with a relative lymphopenia. Leukocytes contain stainable iron, and are called sideroleukocytes. Hypergammaglobulinemia occurs in horses infected for several months.

Lesions: In acute cases, hemorrhages are occasionally found on the serous surfaces and mucous membranes. The spleen will be enlarged and the abdominal, hepatic and splenic lymph nodes swollen. In subacute and chronic cases, necropsy reveals emaciation, pale mucous membranes, subcut. edema, especially along the ventral abdominal walls and limbs, accentuated hepatic lobular architecture, splenomegaly and enlarged abdominal lymph nodes. The yellow marrow of the long bones may be replaced by red marrow. Intravascular clotting with emboli is frequently observed in advanced or terminal cases.

Microscopically, there is reticuloendotheloid cell proliferation in many organs and periportal and perisinusoidal collections of round cells in the liver with accumulations of hemosiderin in the Kupffer's cells. There may be loss of hepatocytes due to anoxia. Perivascular lymphoid infiltrations may occur in the other organs also. Proliferative glomerulitis is present in some horses and there is glomerular deposition of immunoglobulins (IgG) and complement (C3).

Diagnosis: The development of clinical EIA in a susceptible horse inoculated with blood from a suspect case will establish the diagnosis. Recently, several serologic procedures have been described for detecting antibodies: these include complement-fixation, complement-fixation inhibition, serum neutralization, and immuno-diffusion techniques. The latter, the "Coggins test," is the easiest to run, has proved to be highly satisfactory and has replaced all others for most purposes.

EIA should be suspected when an animal is presented with a history of weight loss, accompanied by periodic fever. In addition, several horses in a group may develop similar signs following the introduction of new animals into a herd. Occasionally, horses on pasture may die without signs of illness having been noticed.

Treatment and Control: No specific treatment or vaccine is available. General supportive therapy may help in an individual case, but an infected animal may serve as a source of infection for other horses. Whenever a diagnosis is established, the infected horse should be promptly isolated from other horses and maintained in isolation, if it is not to be killed. Apparently, the primary vector is the horse fly, and stabling during the fly season provides excellent control.

Control of stable flies, mosquitoes or other blood-sucking parasites might also be desirable by repeated spraying or by screening. Equipment that may cause skin abrasions or absorb secretions or excretions should be avoided or disinfected between horses. Surgical instruments, e.g., hypodermic needles, tattoo instruments, should be sterilized between horses. Infected horses should not be used as brood mares as their foals frequently become infected *in utero* or postnatally.

AFRICAN HORSE SICKNESS

An insect-borne disease of Equidae in which the mortality rate is high. Since the early 1700's, the disease has increased to become a major enzootic plague throughout southern and equatorial Africa. In 1960 it spread throughout the Middle East, in 1966 to North Africa and 1967 to Spain.

Etiology: African horse sickness is caused by a diplornavirus of which there are 9 immunologically distinct serotypes. Natural transmission occurs seasonally via insect vectors and not by contact. Gnats (*Culicoides* spp.) are the principal vectors but the disease has also been transmitted experimentally by mosquitoes. The disease disappears between insect seasons, and recovered animals have not been found to be carriers of the virus. Dogs have been infected by eating infected horse meat, but the role of dogs in the spread of the disease is not significant. Cattle and sheep are refractory.

Clinical Findings: The incubation period is less than 10 days. The disease may take either an acute pulmonary or a more chronic cardiac form although at necropsy the lesions generally indicate some degree of mixing of the forms. Infection of partially immune horses results in a mild, transient fever.

Horses with the **pulmonary form** rarely recover. They develop a high (105°F +) temperature but continue to eat and appear quite normal until the last 24 to 36 hours when pulmonary edema causes increasingly difficult respiration. Terminally there is severe, labored respiration with coughing as the bronchi and upper respiratory passages fill with fluid. The horse dies of anoxia.

Horses with the **cardiac form** are also febrile. The animals continue to eat, but they soon develop localized areas of edema subcut. on the head and neck. The occurrence of edema in the supraorbital and frontal region is characteristic. It may also involve the lips, intramandibular and cervical areas. Stocking or dependent edemas which appear terminally are secondary to cardiac insufficiency. Conjunctivitis, often hemorrhagic and edematous, is common as are petechiae on the ventral surface of the tongue.

Lesions: The dominant gross lesions in the **pulmonary form** are interstitial and alveolar edema, with effusion of fluid filling the bronchi terminally. In the **cardiac form**, in addition to the changes apparent in the live animal, there is hydropericardium, edema and hemorrhage of the coronary fat, myocarditis with varying degrees of hemorrhage and necrosis which is often more striking histologically than grossly. Hemorrhagic gastritis is common. Lymphoid tissue is grossly swollen and histologically reactive. There may be hepatic congestion.

Diagnosis: The clinical and pathologic changes are usually adequate for a diagnosis in enzootic areas. Virus isolation from equine blood at the height of fever may be accomplished in day-old mice or tissue culture and identified by neutralization with known sera. A rise in antibody titer is also diagnostic of recent infection.

Immunity and Control: Seven attenuated, neurotropic strains of African horse sickness virus have been used in a polyvalent mouse-brain vaccine for the past 30 years. Since 1960 all 9 serotypes have been adapted to propagation in tissue culture. The resultant attenuated polyvalent tissue-culture vaccine produces a satisfactory immunity and is safer and easier to produce. Vaccine containing all of the serotypes present in the region of use should be administered annually.

Control is also facilitated by the destruction of insect vectors. Countries free of African horse sickness must prevent the entry of either infected equine animals or vectors. Horses from infected countries should be quarantined for 30 days in insect-free isolation and tested for virus. In view of the multiplicity of strains, antibody is not an index of either the current presence or absence of virus, so should not be a factor in judging safety for importation.

VESICULAR STOMATITIS

The disease caused by the vesicular stomatitis viruses, like foot-and-mouth disease, is characterized by a febrile response accompanied by vesicles on the mucous membranes of the mouth, epithelium of the tongue, the soles of the feet, the coronary band, and occasionally in other areas of the body. Cattle, horses and swine are naturally susceptible. However, the agents have a wide host range, which includes deer, bobcat, raccoon and monkeys and experimentally many rodents and cold-blooded animals. Human infections have been recognized in enzootic areas and in laboratory workers. The disease has been confirmed only in North and South America.

The rod-shaped virus belongs to the group "rhabdoviruses". Such viruses parasitize not only mammals but fish, insects and plants, a diversity of hosts unknown for any other morphologic group of viruses.

Etiology and Epizootiology: In a herd 50 to 75% of the animals show clinical evidence of the disease, but nearly all will develop antibodies. The disease is not as contagious as foot-and-mouth disease.

The virus, found in abundance in the clear vesicular fluid and the vesicular coverings, is most infective at the time the vesicles rupture or shortly thereafter. Five or 6 days later, however, the lesions may be innocuous, indicating that the virus is short-lived. There are 2 serologically distinct viruses, the New Jersey and Indiana viruses. Although only one serologic type of the New Jersey virus is known, there are 3 subtypes of the Indiana virus. There is no cross-immunity between the 2 viruses nor between the viruses of vesicular stomatitis, foot-and-mouth disease and vesicular exanthema.

Vesicular stomatitis usually occurs epizootically in temperate regions and as an enzootic disease in warmer regions. The disease occurs during the warm season of the year, which coincides with the season of activity of mosquitoes and biting flies. At this time, spread can be very rapid, thousands of animals becoming affected within a few weeks. An insect is believed to be the vector. The reservoir for the virus is not known. Sandflies (*Lutzomyia* spp.) may fill both roles.

Clinical Findings: The incubation period is 2 to 5 days. Frequently, excessive salivation is the first sign. Examination of the mouth may reveal blanched, raised vesicles. The lesions vary in size; some are no larger than a pea, while others may involve a portion or the entire surface of the tongue. In the horse, the lesions are principally confined to the upper surface of the tongue, but may involve the inner surface of the lips, angles of the mouth and the gums. In cattle, the lesions may occur also on the hard palate, lips and gums, sometimes extending to the muzzle and around the nostrils. Secondary lesions involving the feet of horses and cattle are not exceptional. In natural infections in swine, foot lesions are frequent and lameness is often the first sign observed. Immediately before or simultaneously with the appearance of the vesicles, there may be a rise in temperature. Ordinarily, there are no complications and the disease is usually self-limiting with recovery in about 2 weeks. In dairy herds, the loss of milk production may be serious and, in some instances, mastitis is a sequela. Animals recovering from a natural infection are immune for less than a year.

Diagnosis: Vesicular stomatitis, while economically important, is of particular significance because of its similarity to foot-and-mouth disease, vesicular exanthema and an enterovirus infection in pigs which was recently found in Europe. Therefore, outbreaks must be accurately identified. When vesicular stomatitis affects horses under natural conditions, there is no serious diagnostic problem because horses are not susceptible to foot-and-mouth disease. The diagnosis is made upon the distribution and character of the lesions and the disease may be differentiated from horse pox by the absence of papules and pustules. When the disease occurs in cattle or swine, a diagnosis is made by recovering the virus from the vesicular coverings or fluid in embryonating chicken eggs or in cell cultures and identifying the agent by the complement-fixation or virus-neutralization tests. Antibodies in serums of recovered animals can also be detected by the same tests. Diagnosis of this disease by animal inoculation tests can be made as described under foot-and-mouth disease (*see* p. 261).

Suspected cases should be immediately brought to the attention of state or federal authorities.

Prophylaxis and Treatment: There is no specific treatment for vesicular stomatitis and no vaccines or hyperimmune serums are commercially available. Secondary infection of the abraded tissue and other sequelae should be treated symptomatically.

FOOT-AND-MOUTH DISEASE
(Aphthous fever, Aftosa, Epizootic aphthae)

An acute, highly communicable disease chiefly confined to cloven-footed animals. Cattle, swine, sheep, goats, buffalo, bison, camel, deer, reindeer, moose, llama, chamois, alpaca, vicuna, giraffe, antelope and hedgehog are generally considered the natural domestic and wild hosts. The dog, cat, rabbit, mouse, muskrat, rat, chicken and other fowl, turtle, snail, monkey and snake can be infected artificially but are not believed to have important roles in spread of the disease. Man, despite his frequent and sometimes intensive exposure, becomes infected only rarely.

Etiology and Epizootiology: There are 7 distinct types of the causal virus; namely, A, O, C, South African Type (S.A.T.) 1, S.A.T. 2, S.A.T. 3, and Asian Type 1, all immunologically distinct. In addition, there are subtypes (currently 56) which are important from epizootiologic and immunologic standpoints. The disease is enzootic in certain parts of Europe, Asia, Africa, and South and Central America. In other regions, such as North America, Great Britain, Australia and New Zealand, where strict measures of prevention and eradication have been implemented, the disease has not become established.

The disease is spread by contact with infected animals or contaminated fomites. The virus is found in the fluid and coverings of the vesicles, as well as in the blood during the febrile stage; and, at times saliva, milk, feces and urine of live animals, and meat or other parts of slaughtered animals, also are infectious. The severity of the disease varies with the strain of virus and the susceptibility of the animal population. Morbidity within a herd may approach 100%. Young animals in excellent health and high nutritional state appear to be most susceptible. The virus may persist to produce healthy carriers which, however, have never been proved to transmit the infection to susceptible animals.

Clinical Findings: The usual incubation period is 2 to 5 days, but extremes of 1 to 18 days or longer have been reported. Onset may be abrupt. The acute disease is characterized by high fever, which in mild cases may be absent or unnoticed. This is followed by eruption of various sized vesicles in the mouth and on the feet. The mouth lesions are blanched, raised, and filled with a clear, straw-colored fluid. Vesicles may appear on the mucous membranes at the border or on the dorsal surface of the tongue, on the buccal surfaces of the cheeks, on the gums and inner surfaces of the lips, on the margins of the dental pad, or along the margin of the angles of the mandible. Anorexia may be complete. There may be severe salivation, and the animal may open and close its mouth with a characteristic smacking sound. Lameness is common. The feet may become swollen, hot and painful about the coronary bands and interdigital spaces. Eruptions similar to those found in the mouth appear on one or more feet. Vesicles may also occur on the udder, teats, conjunctivae, nasal passages, perineum and other thin-skinned areas. The vesicles usually rupture within 24 hours, leaving a raw, eroded area which heals rapidly in uncomplicated cases.

Mortality rarely exceeds 5% of the affected animals; but mortalities as high as 50% have been reported with the malignant form of the disease in which the virus attacks muscular tissue, particularly that of the heart of young animals. Of greater importance are the losses in general productiveness of the animals and indirect losses due to quarantines, embargos and disruption of normal commerce.

Secondary bacterial invasion of the ruptured vesicles, particularly those of the feet, may occur. Other complications are abortion, mastitis, pneumonia and septicemia.

Diagnosis: The main signs are fever, salivation and lameness. The appearance of vesicles in the oral cavity and nostrils, and on feet and teats, should prevent any serious error in reaching a presumptive diagnosis.

Clinical diagnosis of FMD in cattle is complicated by the fact that the lesions are indistinguishable from those of vesicular stomatitis. In swine, the lesions are similar to those of vesicular stomatitis, vesicular exanthema, and an enterovirus infection recently found in Europe. Identification of the virus is usually made by the complement-fixation test. However, virus neutralization, agar-gel diffusion precipitation, and fluorescent antibody tests may also be used. The type involved is differentiated by complement-fixation or by virus-neutralization tests. Subtypes are identifiable by the complement-fixation or other tests.

Differentiation of FMD, vesicular stomatitis and vesicular exanthema can be made by inoculation, usually on the affected premises, of a number of species of animals with the infectious material, and production of the typical disease in only those species known to be susceptible to the particular virus. Usually cattle, swine and horses are inoculated by scarification of the epithelium of the tongue. When cattle and swine develop typical vesicles preceded by a rise in temperature, a diagnosis of FMD is made. A diagnosis of vesicular stomatitis (q.v., p. 257) is made when typical vesicular disease is reproduced in all 3 species. Vesicular exanthema virus effects only swine (q.v., p. 309). It is sometimes difficult to arrive at a definite conclusion from results of inoculating only one group of animals. Because of the importance of an accurate diagnosis, tests should be made only by authorized personnel properly trained to deal with the vesicular diseases.

In many countries, including the U.S.A., all suspected cases must be reported to the regulatory officials by the most expeditious means.

Control: In countries in which the disease is under governmental control, the following measurers are used: (1) quarantine of premises and rigid inspection of areas involved, (2) slaughter and disposal by burial or burning of all infected and susceptible animals exposed to the disease, (3) thorough cleaning with trisodium phosphate or sodium carbonate and disinfection of the premises and all possibly contaminated materials, and (4) testing of the premises by careful restocking with susceptible livestock to ensure eradication of the virus.

The virus of FMD is destroyed at both extremes of the pH range. For practical disinfection, a 2% commercial lye (sodium hydroxide) solution is used, but because of its corrosive nature, some workers prefer a 4%, or stronger, sodium carbonate solution which is quite effective.

Prophylaxis and Treatment: In countries where the disease is enzootic, drastic measures of eradication are not economically feasible. Control is based on a modified system of vaccination and quarantine, using vaccines specific for the type and subtype of virus involved.

Chemically inactivated vaccines prepared from FMD virus propagated in cattle or in a tissue culture system, and suspended in an adjuvant, have been used with considerable success in some countries. However, the immunity is not long-lived, and wanes after 4 to 6 months, requiring revaccination. Vaccines containing one or more immunotypes of the virus are produced in most countries. Vaccination of swine is less successful than is vaccination of cattle or sheep. Recently, vaccines prepared with attenuated virus have been used on a limited scale in restricted areas. Protection afforded by polyvalent or type-specific sera is short-lived (about 2 weeks), and their use has been discontinued.

In countries where the disease is enzootic and not rigidly controlled, treatment is usually directed toward promoting rapid healing of the lesions and preventing secondary infection.

RINDERPEST
(Cattle plague)

An acute viral disease of artiodactyls, particularly cattle and buffalo, characterized by fever, erosive stomatitis and gastro-enteritis.

Etiology and Epizootiology: The causal agent is an RNA virus antigenically related to the viruses of canine distemper and human measles. Although all strains of the virus are immuno-logically identical, they vary markedly in virulence and infectivity. The virus is heat-labile but it will remain viable for weeks in the cold and for months in frozen animal products.

The disease is enzootic in parts of Asia and equatorial Africa. Morbidity and mortality may exceed 90% except in enzootic areas where the indigenous cattle and buffalo possess a high degree of innate resistance. Native swine of Southeast Asia and wild pigs of Africa suffer severely but European breeds of swine show only a mild transient fever.

Spread requires close contact between sick and healthy animals. The virus is present in all tissues and fluids of infected animals and can be isolated from the blood and nasal secretions 1 or 2 days before the onset of fever. It is excreted in the expired air, nasal and oral secretions, and in the feces. Entry is usually through the mucosa of the upper respiratory tract.

Clinical Findings: A prodromal fever follows an incubation period that varies from 3 to 15 days. Within 1 or 2 days of the onset of fever, nasal and lacrimal discharges appear together with anorexia, thirst and depression. The fever reaches its peak 2 to 3 days later when oral lesions emerge. The nasal discharges become mucopurulent, and the breath is fetid. Diarrhea appears as the fever declines and is followed by dehydration, abdominal pain, labored painful respiration and death. The convalescence of surviving animals is long. Recovery confers a permanent immunity and calves of immune dams are protected passively for several months.

Lesions: Gross changes are most apparent in the digestive tract. In the mucosa of the lips, tongue and buccal cavity, small nectrotic foci lose their debris to become superficial erosions which may coalesce. Congestion and hemorrhage of the mucosal surfaces of the abomasum and intestine are prominent; involvement of the crests of the mucous membrane folds results in streaks of inflammation and hemorrhage. The virus also has an affinity for lymphoid tissues, consequently severe necrotic erosion of Peyer's patches is often evident.

Diagnosis: Experienced veterinarians, in countries where the disease is enzootic, make presumptive diagnoses of rinderpest from clinical signs and necropsy findings. In countries free of rinderpest, a presumptive diagnosis must be confirmed by isolation and serologic identification of the virus or by detection of specific antigens. The current prevalence of the virus diarrhea-mucosal disease complex (*see* below), which produces similar changes, enhances the need for confirmatory diagnosis. The specimens required are blood in anticoagulant, lymph node, tonsil and spleen.

Control: Small areas of infection, in otherwise rinderpest-free countries, are customarily eliminated by strict quarantine and slaughter. When the disease is widespread, control can be achieved through vaccination. Strains attenuated by passage through goats or tissue cultures are used as live-virus vaccines. One inoculation confers an immunity of several years' duration.

BOVINE VIRUS DIARRHEA
(BVD, Mucosal-Disease Complex)

An infectious disease of cattle caused by a myxovirus and characterized by erosions and hemorrhages of the alimentary tract and manifested clinically by diarrhea and dehydration. **Mucosal disease** is a variant of the BVD complex which occurs in older calves and cattle and involves failure of antibody production, destruction of lymphoid tissues and necrotic lesions throughout the alimentary canal.

Originally described as 2 disease entities (mucosal disease and bovine virus diarrhea) with somewhat similar but characteristically different syndromes, it is now clearly established that only one virus is involved and that the diverse features of the 2 syndromes exhibit considerable overlap. Recently the same virus has been associated with congenital defects of the CNS.

Incidence and Occurrence: The disease is worldwide in distribution. Primarily a disease of yearlings and up to 2- and 3-year-olds, it can occur in calves and is occasionally observed in adult cows. Morbidity is high on the basis of serologic evidence but low from a clinical viewpoint: many cattle have subclinical virus diarrhea which leaves them with detectable antibodies and future protection from the disease. Likewise, the mortality is low when based on serologic evidence but high in those animals showing obvious clinical signs, particularly severe diarrhea.

Transmission: The transmission of BVD under natural conditions has not been well established. It is assumed to be by direct contact with clinically sick or carrier animals, or by indirect contact (contaminated feed). The incubation period is from 1 to 3 weeks under natural conditions and 7 days experimentally.

Clinical Findings: Affected animals are dull, depressed and anorectic. There is complete rumen stasis and sometimes mild bloat. Early temperatures vary from 104° to 106°F, but these usually return to normal or below in 1 or 2 days and before the animal starts to scour. The diphasic temperature elevation has not been observed in field cases. Heart and respiratory rates are generally increased. Profuse watery diarrhea is usual and the feces may contain mucus, blood and have a foul odor. Tenesmus may be present but defecation is usually effortless. Severe diarrhea causes rapid dehydration. Oral lesions are present in about 75% of clinical cases when the animals start to scour. Typically there is diffuse reddening of the oral mucosa, then mottling of the mucosa with pinpoint lesions, which generally enlarge to 1 to 2 cm as shallow, epithelial erosions. Sites of erosions include the hard palate, soft palate, dorsum and sides of the tongue, gums and commissures of the mouth. In early cases, the cheek papillae are hyperemic and their tips will slough leaving blunt, shortened papillae as the disease progresses. The tongue is usually difficult to grasp and pull from the mouth because of the greasy, necrotic cells on its surface. Additional signs occur sporadically in individual animals. These include hyperemic, encrusted external nares, erosions of the coronary band and interdigital cleft, corneal opacity and abortions. Laminitis and respiratory signs have been reported but their direct association with BVD is unconfirmed. Leukopenia with relative lymphocytosis is common early in the disease. Leukocytes may occur with secondary bacterial infection. The course of the disease varies from 2 to 3 days up to 3 weeks. Patients with acute cases can die in 48 hours, other cattle can have the disease and be anorectic with oral lesions and mild diarrhea for 2 to 4 days then gradually recover and come back on feed. However, if diarrhea is profuse the prognosis is grave and such animals should be salvaged immediately. Failure to make an early diagnosis will mean the animal will have no salvage value because of dehydration and emaciation. The occasional animal that survives the acute disease is usually so badly debilitated as to be an economic liability and will eventually die from secondary necrobacillosis or mycotic infections.

The BVD virus can cause abortion in pregnant cows and has been associated with congenital defects of the CNS of calves.

Lesions: The basic lesion in BVD is an ulcer which develops in association with edema and vasculitis immediately below epithelial surfaces. This results in erosions of the esophagus, forestomachs, abomasum and intestine. Epithelial necrosis occurs but is more prominent in mucosal disease where necrosis and ulceration is marked also in the oronasal areas. Catarrhal enteritis may be marked in more chronic forms of the disease. Necrosis of lymphoid tissues occurs particularly in those associated with the intestine. In the chronic types of mucosal disease, hemorrhage results in dark-red necrotic foci in the ileum representing affected Peyer's patches.

Treatment: Supportive therapy to combat diarrhea and dehydration may be helpful but cattle with BVD cannot be effectively treated.

Control: A modified live-virus vaccine is available which can provide significant antibody titers and offer immunity for a certain time, the length of which has not been established. The best vaccination program would be to vaccinate calves at 6 months of age. The economic justification for vaccination is not well defined. The incidence of the fatal disease is so low in most herds, and the naturally occurring protective antibody is so prevalent in most cattle populations, that widespread vaccination does not seem warranted. Routine use has also been discouraged by reports that the vaccine can precipitate the clinical disease in certain circumstances. These circumstances have not been accurately defined.

MALIGNANT CATARRHAL FEVER

(Malignant head catarrh, Snotsiekte, Catarrhal fever, Gangrenous coryza)

An infectious, usually fatal disease of cattle caused by a virus and characterized by a catarrhal, mucopurulent inflammation of the upper respiratory and alimentary epithelia, keratoconjunctivitis, encephalitis, rapid dehydration and enlargement of the lymph nodes. It is reported in most countries where cattle are raised.

Etiology and Epizootiology: The causative virus is closely associated with the RBC or WBC and with lymph node tissue. It remains active outside the body only for a short time. The incubation period varies from 2 weeks to 5 months or longer, but most often is 3 to 9 weeks. Sheep and latently infected cattle may serve as clinically normal carriers. Morbidity is usually low, but mortality high, reaching 80 to 90%. A high incidence of the disease is rare but it may be markedly persistent on certain farms.

Clinical Findings: The course of the disease varies from the peracute condition of 1 to 2 days to an extreme of 4 weeks (usual range, 4 to 14 days). Signs most commonly observed are clear copious nasal discharge and lacrimation, followed by mucopurulent, dark, nasal discharge with incrustation of the nostrils. The very earliest stages may consist of temperature elevation and congestion of the oral mucosa only.

Five syndromes have been described: peracute, intestinal, head and eye, benign and chronic. The head-and-eye is the most readily recognized form. The signs are marked by their variability with no 2 cases being exactly alike. Respiratory embarrassment may be obvious in some animals. Stomatitis, rhinitis, pharyngitis, laryngitis, cystitis and vaginitis of a serous to an ulcerative nature may be observed. Other signs that may be noted include a partial cloudiness to complete opacity of the cornea and external swelling of the superficial lymph nodes of the head and neck. A vesicular or papular exanthema about the neck, axillae and perineum may develop.

The intestinal form is accompanied by severe diarrhea, with much tenesmus, and the oral mucosa may become eroded or ulcerated. The nervous form is signaled by excitability, hyperesthesia and muscular tremors. Occasionally, these may progress to epileptiform convulsions or an aggressiveness suggestive of rabies.

Regardless of the syndrome, specific histopathologic lesions of the lymph nodes, adventitia and walls of the small blood vessels of any involved organ are considered by some investigators as pathognomonic. The prognosis is grave, with death usually occurring within 10 days. In recovering animals, the convalescence is very slow; others may linger on for weeks and even then may relapse. Blindness occasionally persists.

Lesions: In addition to the lesions already mentioned, the following may be present: nonsuppurative encephalomyelitis, congestion and edema of the meninges, general lymphoid hyperplasia, abomasitis and enteritis, with varying inflammatory exudates. The retropharyngeal and anterior cervical lymph nodes may be edematous and hemorrhagic.

Treatment and Control: Treatment is of little value, although some animals survive, and administration of antibiotics or sulfonamides for control of secondary bacterial infection, and supportive therapy (fluids) may be worthwhile in valuable individuals. Affected animals should be isolated, and the separation of sheep and cattle may be helpful. The incidence usually is not high enough to justify herd disposal.

INFECTIOUS BOVINE RHINOTRACHEITIS (IBR), INFECTIOUS PUSTULAR VULVOVAGINITIS (IPV) AND ASSOCIATED SYNDROMES

IBR is an acute contagious viral infection characterized by inflammation of the upper respiratory tract. Bronchopneumonia may result when complicated by bacterial infection. The virus may invade the placenta and fetus via the maternal blood stream, causing abortion or stillbirth from 2 to 3 months subsequent to the respiratory infection. It also causes encepalitis in 2- to 3-month-old calves and on experimental inoculation produces severe oral and gastric necrosis in newborn calves. In the field, this enteric form of IBR has been observed to cause high mortality in affected calves under 3 weeks of age.

The virus also causes infectious pustular vulvovaginitis (IPV), an acute contagious disease of cattle characterized in the female by inflammation, necrosis and pustule formation on the mucosa of the vulva and vagina, and occasionally in the male by similar lesions on the skin of the penis and prepuce. Vesicle formation does not occur. Venereal transmission is usual although the infection may be transmitted by equipment brought into contact with the genitalia. With the possible exception of South America, the virus is found worldwide.

Etiology: The virus is present in the nasal and ocular secretions of IBR-infected cattle, in the placental tissues and fluids of those which abort, in the tissues of the aborted fetuses and in the brain of calves affected with encephalitis.

When responsible for IPV, the virus is found in the exudate produced in association with vulvovaginitis. Nuclear inclusions are present in infected tracheal epithelium early in infection. Only cattle are susceptible to infection with this virus. It is a member of the herpesvirus group and produces characteristic necrosis and intranuclear inclusion bodies in cell culture.

Epizootiology: IBR is most prevalent in large concentrations of cattle such as are found in feed lots and large commercial dairy operations, while the genital infection (IPV) is confined mainly to small, reproductively active herds, particularly of dairy cattle.

Since IBR frequently occurs from one to several weeks after the addition of new animals, it is believed that recovered cattle may be carriers. Cattle following clinical recovery from IPV also remain shedders of the virus for variable periods. Infection of some animals does not result in disease and can be recognized only by detection of neutralizing antibodies in the serum.

Clinical Findings: The incubation period of IBR is generally from 10 to 14 days. Initially, the temperature ranges from 104° to 108°F, with a serous nasal discharge which in a few instances contains flecks of blood. The animals are mildly depressed, the respiration rate is accelerated, there is profuse salivation and anorexia is present. The majority of cattle do not show other clinical signs and recover without treatment in 10 to 14 days. In about 10% of cases, more severe clinical signs are noted. The muzzle and external nares become hyperemic and encrusted with a dried exudate. When these encrustations are removed, the underlying tissues appear a brilliant red, hence the lay term "red nose". As the disease progresses, the nasal exudate changes in character from serous to mucopurulent, and an inspiratory dyspnea develops because of the presence of a pseudodiphtheritic membrane in the nasal passages and trachea. When complicated by bronchopneumonia, there is considerable weight loss and recovery is prolonged. The morbidity ranges from 15 to 100%; death losses rarely exceed 5% of the affected animals and are due usually to bronchopneumonia.

Calves may be born with the enteric form of IBR or become infected shortly after birth. Some calves will show the respiratory form of the disease as well as an intractable diarrhea. There are oral erosions in most calves, and calves under 3 weeks of age do not respond to therapy.

IPV may exhibit a wide variation in severity. There may be swelling of the vulva with a small amount of sticky exudate on the vulvar hair. Pain is exhibited by reluctance to allow the tail to rest on the vulva and when the animal urinates or the vulva is manipulated in the course of examination. The mucosa is bright red and exhibits varying numbers of small pustules about 2 mm in diameter. These are soft and moist with raised edges and depressed centers. In some cases, the lesions are so numerous that they coalesce to form a plaque. Varying degrees of epithelial necrosis and exudation may be observed in the vagina. Appetite and production are little affected and abortion does not occur as a sequela. While it is probable that fertility is reduced during the acute phase permanent infertility does not result.

Abortion due to the virus may occur in herds which there is a recent history of IBR, without a history of IBR, or following vaccination of pregnant animals against the disease. Prodromal signs of abortion are not obvious; the abortion is rarely complicated by genital-tract infection, and the breeding efficiency of aborting cattle does not appear to be impaired.

Lesions: Petechial to ecchymotic hemorrhages may be found in the mucous membranes of the nasal cavity and the paranasal sinuses of cattle with IBR. The sinuses are often filled with a serous or muco-serofibrinous exudate. As the disease progresses the pharynx becomes covered with a serofibrinous exudate. The pharyngeal lymph nodes may be acutely swollen and hemorrhagic. In the early stages of IBR the trachea exhibits multiple small hyperemic areas or general hyperemia. Later, large quantities of blood are found in or lining the wall of the trachea. The tracheitis may extend into the bronchi and bronchioles and terminate in bronchopneumonia. The pulmonary lymph nodes are extensively swollen.

The erosions found in the oral cavity with enteric IBR are also present in the rumen, abomasum, cecum and colon.

Diagnosis: Diagnosis of IBR and IPV is based on the characteristic lesions and signs of illness, the demonstration of a rising serum-antibody titer between acute and convalescent stages, the occurrence of intranuclear inclusion bodies in biopsy material and the isolation of the virus in tissue culture.

Prophylaxis and Treatment: A modified live-virus vaccine is available for the prevention of the various syndromes caused by the IBR virus. However, pregnant cows should not be vaccinated since the vaccine virus causes abortion. Exposure to recently vaccinated animals has not been proved to produce disease in susceptible stock. The vaccine can be used in open cows prior to the breeding season, in 6- to 8-month-old heifers, and in beef calves as a part of a preconditioning program. It should not be used until cattle have been in a feed lot 3 to 4 weeks, since the vaccine cannot be recommended in the face of an outbreak or for cattle with shipping fever. It should be kept in mind that IBR commonly occurs in vaccinated cattle. More effective vaccines may be developed, particularly vaccines which can be given locally, to produce local antibodies. The immunity from any form of the natural disease appears to provide protection for at least 3 years.

There is no specific therapy. All breeding operations should be suspended in the herd infected with IPV until the animals return to normal. Most animals recover without treatment in about 2 weeks. Secondary bacterial infection of either IBR or IPV should be treated with appropriate antibiotics.

CHLAMYDIAL ABORTION

EPIZOOTIC BOVINE ABORTION (EBA)

An infectious disease of cattle manifested primarily by abortion that is epizootic in California where it is known as "foothill abortion" because of its high prevalence in cows which are pastured on foothill terrain. The disease has been reported to occur in Western U.S.A. and Europe.

Etiology and Transmission: The causative agent is a strain of *Chlamydia psittaci* that is antigenically and pathogenically similar to, if not identical with, the one causing ovine chlamydial abortion (enzootic abortion of ewes, q.v., p. 273). Strains recovered from aborted fetuses of either cattle or sheep can be used to reproduce abortion in either species. The organisms from bovine tissues can be propagated in yolk sac tissues of chicken embryos, in mice by nasal instillation, and less readily in guinea pigs by IP inoculation. The natural mode of transmission is unknown but recent isolations of chlamydial agents from ticks and rodents suggest the existence of a vector-reservoir cycle in nature, with cattle being an accidental host. The disease apparently is not contracted by venereal means, and thus far has been reproduced experimentally only by parenteral inoculation.

In epizootic areas, only heifers in their initial pregnancy and cattle introduced from areas free of the disease are affected. The abortion rate varies from 25 to 75% in such animals. In susceptible herds, cattle of all ages are affected.

Clinical Findings: Naturally infected cattle show few if any signs of infection other than abortion, which occurs usually between the fifth and seventh months of gestation. Occasionally, calves are born alive but invariably die within several days. Temporary retention of the placenta sometimes occurs but the cow's reproductive capacity is not affected. Experimentally infected pregnant cows develop a transient hyperthermia shortly following inoculation. A diphasic serologic response occurs with circulating chlamydial antibodies appearing after inoculation, receding, and then increasing again prior to abortion.

Lesions: The subcut. tissues of aborted fetuses may be edematous and the abdomen distended by excessive amounts of peritoneal fluid; erythema may be present over the skin of the abdomen. Petechial hemorrhages may be scattered throughout the subcut. tissues, over the ventral surface of the tongue, the mucosa of the trachea and the oral cavity, and in the conjunctiva. The liver lesions are the most characteristic of the disease: the liver may be enlarged, granular and friable, and from pale red to reddish orange. About 50% of the fetuses exhibit one or more of the gross lesions associated with the disease; the remainder show no gross changes. Histopathologic lesions occur principally in the liver and brain and are of a granulomatous nature. They occur regularly and range from a wild focal necrosis to a chronic focal reticular cell hyperplasia.

Diagnosis: Tentative diagnosis can be made clinically when typical lesions are present. In their absence diagnosis is based on herd history, circumstances of the outbreak, and histopathologic findings, but conclusive diagnosis rests upon isolation and identification of the agent. Isolation of the agent from fetal tissues often fails, possibly because the organisms have been eliminated by the time the abortion occurs. Serologic evidence obtained by complement fixation tests is of little differential-diagnosis value. No specific serologic test is available at present.

Prophylaxis and Treatment: Although cattle that undergo natural infection apparently become immune, attempts thus far to induce immunity by artificial means have been unsuccessful. Prophylactic therapy with tetracyclines at the level of 2 gm per cow daily throughout pregnancy has been shown to be effective under experimental conditions, but field application is limited because of cost and the problem of maintaining adequate dosage levels.

ENZOOTIC ABORTION OF EWES (EAE)

An infectious disease of sheep manifested by abortion and to a lesser extent by stillbirth or premature lambing. The disease has been reported in Scotland, Germany, Hungary, Roumania, Bulgaria, South Africa and the U.S.A.

Etiology and Transmission: The causative agent is a strain of *Chlamydia psittaci* that is antigenically and pathogenically similar, if not identical, with the one that causes bovine chlamydial abortion (epizootic bovine abortion, q.v., p. 271). Strains recovered from aborted fetuses of either sheep or cattle can be used to reproduce abortion in either species. The organisms from ovine tissues can be propagated in the yolk sac of chicken embroys, in mice by nasal instillation and in guinea pigs by IP inoculation. The natural mode of transmission of the agent appears to be by ingestion although the disease can be produced experimentally by parenteral inoculation. There is no evidence of venereal or arthropod-mediated transmission.

The epizootiology of the disease is not completely understood. It is believed that lambs in aborting flocks become infected during birth or shortly thereafter through ingestion of infectious materials. Open ewes may also become infected at this time. In either case, the infection remains latent until conception occurs. The agent then invades the placenta and fetus, and abortion ensues. Infected ewes may deliver normal lambs at term; occasionally only one lamb of a set of twins will be infected. Ewes which become infected during late gestation may not abort (or deliver prematurely) until the subsequent gestation.

Clinical Findings: Abortion, stillbirth or premature lambing, occurring usually during the second gestation and frequently accompanied by placental retention, are characteristic of the disease. Placental retention occurs more frequently when the ewe aborts than when delivery is premature, and persists from 2 to 10 days. Ewes may carry dead fetuses *in utero*, which sometimes mummify before being expelled. Such ewes lose condition rapidly and some may die shortly after aborting. Apart from these cases, the disease has little effect on the ewe.

Lesions: Placentitis with necrosis of the cotyledons and edema and thickening of the intercotyledonary spaces are the principal lesions. Fetal membranes of EAE-infected ewes resemble closely those of cattle aborting from brucellosis. The subcut. and muscle tissues or aborted fetuses are edematous and hemorrhagic, and blood-tinged fluids are present in the serous cavities.

Diagnosis: Laboratory assistance is essential in differentiating chlamydial abortion from ovine abortion due to other causes. Placentitis, and the demonstration of intracellular elementary bodies in impression smears from the surface of the cotyledons, provides a tentative diagnosis. Isolation and identification of causative chlamydiae constitutes a conclusive diagnosis. Since many ewes normally harbor chlamydial agents in their intestines (and contamination of the placenta with these agents may occur during abortion), isolation of chlamydiae from internal fetal tissues is of more diagnostic value than when isolated from the placenta. Because chlamydia-positive sera are common among flocks naturally infected with intestinal chlamydiae, serologic findings must be specific to be of significance in diagnosis of chlamydial abortion.

Control: Moderate control of chlamydial abortion by vaccination has been reported from Scotland, but this measure has had limited success in the U.S.A. Tetracycline compounds are effective in controlling the abortion, but the cost and problem of administering the antibiotic is a major disadvantage. Since the infection is transmitted predominantly at lambing time, precautionary measures such as segregation of aborting animals, and the careful disposal of infected placentas and fetuses are probably the most effective means of limiting spread of the disease.

Treatment: Tetracycline therapy is recommended for the treatment of infected newborn lambs and ewes that have carried dead fetuses for some time prior to abortion. However, effective doses have not yet been established. Secondary bacterial infection resulting from placental retention lends itself to antibiotic treatment.

EPHEMERAL FEVER
(Three-day sickness)

A benign, arthropod-transmitted viral disease of cattle occurring in Africa, Australia and Asia and characterized by fever, stiffness and lameness. Spontaneous recovery usually takes place within a few days. Other domestic animals are not susceptible.

Etiology: The causal virus, tentatively classified as a cone-shaped rhabdovirus, is present in the blood during the febrile stage. As little as 0.002 ml of blood is infective. The virus has been isolated in the brains of baby mice and also cultured in a baby hamster kidney (BHK) cell line. The disease can be readily transmitted to susceptible animals by IV inoculation of infected blood, but not by other routes. Transmission by direct contact does not occur. Ceratopogonid gnats have been incriminated as important vectors of the disease.

The incidence and severity of the disease vary from year to year and epizootics occur periodically. The virus does not persist in the recovered animal and it is believed that certain fauna are responsible for the carry-over from season to season.

Clinical Findings: The disease usually appears suddenly in a herd, affecting several animals within a few weeks. It is most prevalent during wet summers when conditions favor the multiplication of biting insects. Common signs are fever, rigors, listlessness, inappetence, watering of the eyes and nose, swelling of the eyelids, hypersalivation, dyspnea, atony of the forestomachs and decrease in milk yield, followed by the characteristic stiffness and lameness involving various groups of muscles. The stiffness may be fleeting, often passing from one limb to another. The animal becomes recumbent and remains so for 3 days or more.

In spite of the alarming signs, the course is generally favorable with early recovery. Pneumonia may develop if the patient is neglected. The morbidity seldom exceeds 5% in cattle at range, but it may be as high as 50% in stabled stock. The mortality is less than 2%. The greatest loss is in milk yield and in condition. Immunity usually follows recovery, however, repeated attacks have been reported.

Treatment and Control: Neither treatment nor prophylactic vaccination is recommended. The patient should be carefully nursed and properly housed and fed. Quarantine measures are of no avail.

LUMPY SKIN DISEASE

An infectious, eruptive, poxlike disease of cattle characterized by the appearance of nodules on the skin and other parts of the body. Secondary infection often aggravates the condition.

Lumpy skin disease occurs in many parts of Africa and in

Madagascar. It is a disease of cattle only and is generally fatal in calves.

Etiology and Epizootiology: The infectious agent is a virus closely related to that of sheep pox. The prototype strain is known as the Neethling poxvirus. It has been adapted to embryonated eggs in which it produces macroscopic pox and hemorrhages on the chorioallantoic membrane without any embryo mortality. It can also be propagated in monolayer cultures of calf or lamb kidney cells.

Lumpy skin disease appears epizootically or sporadically. Frequently new foci of infection appear in areas far removed from the initial outbreak. Its incidence is highest in wet summer weather, but it may also occur in winter. It is most prevalent along water courses and on low ground. It is possible that migratory birds, e.g., egrets, help to spread the disease. Since quarantine restrictions designed to limit the spread of the infection have failed, biting insects have been suspected as vectors, but many outbreaks have occurred under freezing conditions where insects practically could be excluded. Because the disease can be transmitted by means of infected saliva, contact infection must be accepted as a method of spread. Sheep are suspected of being possible carriers in Kenya.

Artificial infection can be produced by the inoculation of cutaneous nodule suspensions or blood taken during the early febrile stage, or by feed or water contaminated with saliva from infected animals.

Clinical Findings: A subcut. injection of infected material produces first a painful swelling and then fever, lacrimation, a nasal discharge and hypersalivation, followed by the characteristic eruptions on the skin and other parts of the body. The incubation period varies from 4 to 14 days.

The nodules are well circumscribed, round, flat and slightly elevated and involve the entire cutis and the mucosa of many internal organs, especially of the gastrointestinal tract. Nodules may occur on the muzzle and within the nasal and buccal mucous membranes. The skin nodules contain a firm, creamy-gray or yellow mass of tissue. The regional lymph nodes are swollen and edema develops in the udder, vulva or scrotum. Secondary infection sometimes occurs, causing extensive suppuration and sloughing of the swollen organ. As a result, the animal may become extremely emaciated and may have to be destroyed.

The nodules either persist or resolve entirely. In mild cases, only hairless patches are left. In others, the dead tissue is cast off, leaving deep suppurating craters.

The morbidity varies from 5 to 50% and the mortality from 1 to 75%. The greatest loss is sustained from the decrease in milk yield, the loss in condition and the rejection or reduced value of the hide.

Diagnosis: Since there are many causes of skin eruptions in cattle, a tentative field diagnosis of lumpy skin disease must be based mainly on the severity and extent of the lesions and the similar involvement of several animals. For laboratory confirmation, biopsies of fresh nodules, adjacent skin scrapings and serum samples should be collected. Cultivation of the virus from nodules or skin in embryonated eggs or tissue cultures, neutralization tests, electronmicroscopy, demonstration of intracytoplasmic inclusions resembling those of sheep pox and inoculation of cattle aid in differential diagnosis. Similar, but less severe skin lesions are produced by the Allerton and bovine mammillitis herpesviruses. The organism *Dermatophilus congolensis,* is often found in bovine skin nodules in the U.S.A.

Prophylaxis and Treatment: Quarantine restrictions are useless. Prophylactic vaccination by means of virus attenuated by egg passage offers the most promising method of control. Goat pox and sheep pox virus passed in tissue culture have also been used.

Good nursing and administration of sulfonamides and antibiotics to control secondary infection are recommended.

SPORADIC BOVINE ENCEPHALOMYELITIS
(Buss disease)

Sporadic bovine encephalomyelitis (SBE) has been observed in 16 states of the U.S.A. and in Japan, Australia, Czechoslovakia, Hungary and South Africa, suggesting a worldwide distribution.

Etiology: SBE is caused by a strain of the psittacosis-lymphogranuloma group, now classified as *Chlamydia psittaci.* While all chlamydial strains contain an identical group-specific antigen, cell walls of SBE strains contain an antigen that is similar to that found in strains causing ovine polyarthritis and that distinguishes these chlamydial strains from those causing abortions or pneumonia. SBE organisms are found in the brain and spinal cord, in serous exudates, blood, lymph nodes and internal organs indicating a systemic infection. They are excreted in the feces and urine.

Clinical Findings: The incubation period varies from 6 to 31 days. Inactivity and depression mark the clinical onset of SBE. The affected cattle become anorectic and develop fever which persists until death or recovery. Excessive salivation, dyspnea and mild diarrhea are additional clinical signs in the early stage. Recovery may follow this stage, but most often affected cattle develop nervous signs and have difficulty in walking. They develop a stiff gait, stagger, circle, and fall over small obstacles. The limbs become weaker and signs of paralysis develop. During the terminal stage, the cattle can hardly rise and may exhibit opisthotonos. The course of the clinical disease lasts from 10 to 14 days, but in some instances affected cattle may not die for a month. Cattle of all ages may be affected, but the disease is seen more often in younger cattle. The disease occurs sporadically with a low morbidity, but the mortality of the stricken cattle is over 50%.

Lesions: Nonpurulent, aseptic meningoencephalomyelitis occurs. Macroscopic lesions in the CNS are due to hyperemia and edema. After an acute course, few pathologic changes will be found although the peritoneal and pleural cavities may contain increased amounts of fluid. More chronic cases have serofibrinous exudates in the body cavities. Fibrinous pericarditis, pleuritis and lobar pneumonia may then also be found. Microscopically, all parts of the brain may have vasculitis with perivascular cuffing and parenchymal foci of inflammation composed predominantly of mononuclear cells.

Diagnosis: A definite diagnosis can only be made by isolating and identifying the causative agent in developing chicken embryos from the brain or by histologic examination of the CNS. When typical clinical signs have been observed, a diagnosis of SBE can often be reasonably well substantiated by the serofibrinous peritonitis. Demonstration by complement fixation of strain-specific chlamydial antibodies in serum of affected cattle may confirm the clinical diagnosis, but the presence of group-specific antibodies is meaningless because subclinical intestinal infection of cattle with chlamydiae is common, and these strains stimulate development of group-specific antibodies.

Treatment and Control: No specific means for prevention and control are known. The causative chlamydial agents are sensitive to tetracyclines or tylosin, but effective dosages have not been established. In any case, treatment should be early before irreversible CNS lesions are induced.

ANAPLASMOSIS
(Gallsickness)

A peracute to chronic infectious disease of ruminants characterized chiefly by anemia, icterus and fever.

Etiology and Epizootiology: The exact nature and classification of the causative agent has presented a continuing taxonomic problem. A body in the red blood cell is associated with the disease complex. These bodies are referred to as anaplasmata, anaplasms and "marginal bodies", and are observed in blood smears stained with Wright's or Giemsa stain as small, rounded, basophilic bodies located in the stroma of the erythrocytes near the margins. Anaplasms range in diameter from about 0.3 to 1.0 μ. Electron microscopy reveals that the larger or mature anaplasm is composed of several so-called initial bodies. The initial body is thought by some to be the infective form, capable of invading the erythrocyte and undergoing a type of fission to form the mature body.

Variants of the classic form or related genera have been seen and are being studied. *Anaplasma marginale* has been considered the distinct pathogen of the group, causing anaplasmosis. The disease in cattle is enzootic in warmer parts of the world, but it has now been reported from most states in the U.S.A.; it is, however, most prevalent in the Gulf States, lower plains states and California, particularly in moist or brushy areas where arthropod vectors are abundant. The infection is limited to cattle and related ruminants. Wild ruminants such as deer and antelope harbor latent *A. marginale* infection, and must be considered important factors in maintaining *Anaplasma* infection at high levels in many parts of the world where the disease is enzootic.

In some parts of the world, notably Africa, the relatively non-virulent *A. centrale* occurs with *A. marginale* and is differentiated from the latter by the more central location of the anaplasm. *A. ovis* is normally relatively nonvirulent, but is capable of producing mild anaplasmosis in sheep and goats under certain conditions.

Transmission: Anaplasmosis has been transmitted from infected to susceptible bovine hosts under experimental conditions by the bites of numerous species of ticks (*Boophilus, Rhipicephalus, Dermacentor, Hyalomma* and *Ixodes*), by horse-flies (*Tabanus*), by stable flies (*Stomoxys*) and by mosquitoes (*Psorophora*). It is concluded, logically, that these bloodfeed-ing arthropods may serve as vectors in nature. With fly and mosquito vectors, the transmission is accomplished mechani-cally by the insect's proboscis, which carries fluid blood from infected to susceptible cattle when feeding is interrupted and, therefore, transfer must be immediate to be effective. Ticks, however, ingest infected blood and transfer the infective agent to a susceptible host animal later when feeding is continued on a new host.

Since the infection is easily transmitted by mechanical trans-fer of infected blood, outbreaks of considerable proportions have been traced to mass operations, such as bleeding, dehorn-ing, castrating, ear-tagging and vaccinating.

Clinical Findings and Course: The severity of the disease varies considerably with age. Calves undergo mild infections, with little or no mortality. In yearling cattle, the disease is more severe, but recovery is the rule. Greatest severity occurs in cattle 2 or 3 years of age or older, with marked anemia developing and mortality varying between 20 and 50%. All breeds and types of cattle are susceptible. Most cases occur during warmer seasons when vectors are abundant.

The disease may be peracute, acute, subacute or chronic. The earliest signs include depression, inappetence, indolence and elevation of body temperature, commonly to 104° or 105°F, but as high as 107°F in the severest cases. Lactating cows show a rapid fall in milk production. As the disease progresses, marked anemia develops, evidenced by pale mucous mem-branes, and the animal becomes dehydrated and constipated. Loss of weight is pronounced and dehydration is noticeable in the acute form. In beef cattle, the disease usually is not recog-nized until the affected animal is extremely anemic and weak. A marked icterus may develop Not uncommonly, affected animals succumb from hypoxia when moved or handled for treatment. If the animal survives the period of erythrocyte destruction, it usually recovers gradually. Hemoglobinuria does not occur.

The course of the clinical disease may be as short as a day or less in the fatal, peracute form, several days to 2 or 3 weeks in the more typical acute and subacute forms, or considerably longer in the occasional chronic form. Some animals never re-cover completely, remaining emaciated and unproductive. So far as is known, all recovered animals remain permanent carriers.

Diagnosis: In enzootic areas, anaplasmosis should be suspected in mature cattle showing anemia without hemoglobinuria. Icterus often is an important sign. The only incontrovertible evidence of the disease, however, is demonstration of the anaplasms or marginal bodies in the erythrocytes in stained blood smears. Up to 50 or 60% of the red blood cells may be parasitized. In cases where blood cell destruction has been extensive and the course of the disease prolonged, there may be so few anaplasms present in the circulating red cells that positive diagnosis by microscopy is impossible. A complement-fixation test was developed but is not in general use. A capillary antigen (CA) test is practical and useful in detecting clinical or carrier infection and can be used by practitioners and smaller laboratories.

Necropsy findings are those associated with red blood cell destruction. The blood is thin and watery and icterus usually is evident. The spleen is enlarged and soft. The liver is turgid and often of a mottled mahogany color. The bile is thick and brownish green, and the gallbladder is distended, this appearance being responsible for the old name of the disease, gall-sickness. If death occurs suddenly without anemia or icterus, there might be confusion with anthrax on the basis of the gross appearance of the spleen, particularly in areas where both diseases occur.

Prophylaxis: Prevention is a problem because of the difficulty of significantly reducing the tick, fly or mosquito populations in areas where the disease is enzootic. However, the incidence of the disease can be reduced to some extent by killing vectors on the host or by repelling them with proper chemical dusts or sprays. For these to be effective, cattle must be dipped, sprayed or dusted at frequent intervals during the vector season. Large biting flies, particularly horse flies, are believed to be the most serious vectors in some areas of the U.S.A., e.g., Louisiana and other Gulf States, while ticks appear to be the most important natural vectors in others, e.g., California and Oregon.

Since animals that have recovered from anaplasmosis remain permanent carriers, they should be conditioned for market and sold for slaughter as soon as possible. If the potential breeding value of the recovered animal warrants retention, it should be kept reasonably isolated from other cattle during the season

of greatest danger of transmission, or treated to destroy the
carrier infection (℞ 11).

Spread of the disease by man can be prevented by proper
precautions during mass procedures, such as dehorning, bleeding, eartagging, castration and vaccination. Care should be
taken to use individual, sterilized needles and properly cleaned
and disinfected instruments for each animal.

The inoculation of blood containing *A. centrale,* which gives
rise to a mild infection that protects against subsequent infection with the virulent *A. marginale,* is used with considerable
success in South Africa and certain other countries. This
method is not permitted in the U.S.A.

In certain countries such as Brazil where premunition is
practiced, cattle may be infected by injection of 5 ml of blood
from a carrier of *A. marginale* and protected from severe clinical disease by administration of chlortetracycline (℞ 11) at the
onset of the clinical reaction. The animals quickly recover and
remain immune carriers. Infection can be prevented in cattle
by feeding the antibiotic (℞ 11) at low levels. The use of this
procedure to protect cattle through short periods of greatest
danger of natural infection has proven useful. In enzootic
areas a large percentage of newly introduced cattle may be
protected by administration of single therapeutic doses of
chlortetracycline at 2- or 3-week intervals during the period
of their exposure to natural infection (℞ 11). The effectiveness
of this procedure depends on the drug being introduced at the
time anaplasms are beginning their increase in the red blood
cells, and are most susceptible to the inhibitory action of the
drug. At the dosage recommended, the drug inhibits multiplication of the parasite without interfering with development of
immune carrier state. Work to develop useful vaccines continues.

Treatment: Although favorable claims have been made for
many drugs in the treatment of anaplasmosis, only chlortetracycline (℞ 11) has been shown to have inhibitory action
against *A. marginale.* The time in the course of the disease
when the antibiotic is effective is limited to the period of
anaplasm multiplication. It is of no value against the parasite
after the peak of infection has been reached.

Carrier infection may be eliminated by prolonged daily administration of relatively large doses of tetracycline (℞ 11).
At present, this procedure is costly and appears to be justified
only for valuable breeding animals. Recently several dithio-
semicarbazones used IV have been shown to suppress develop-

ment of the parasite, lessen anemia and increase survival rates
of infected animals.

Symptomatic and supportive treatment is of paramount importance. Transfusion of 4 to 12 liters of normal bovine blood
is the best single treatment and often is sufficient to start an
extremely anemic animal on the road to recovery. The transfusion may be repeated after 48 hours, if necessary. Water
given in large volumes, by stomach tube, is helpful. Parenteral
administration of dextrose also is helpful as supportive treatment. Mild laxatives, such as mineral oil, may be administered
for the relief of constipation. Saline laxatives are to be avoided
because they contribute further to the badly dehydrated state
of the animal.

Treatment procedures should be accomplished with as little
disturbance to the animal as possible, since even mild exertion
may produce hypoxia and death. Driving or rough handling is
to be avoided. If considerable resistance, excitement or struggling is encountered, treatment should be discontinued. Sick
and convalescing animals respond well to careful management
and good nutrition on pasture, with access to shade and fresh
water. Application of suitable insect repellents adds to the
comfort of the animal.

HEARTWATER

A tick-borne, septicemic, rickettsial disease of sheep, goats
and cattle characterized by hyperthermia and nervous signs.
It is restricted to the subtropical lowland regions of Africa and
Madagascar.

All ruminants, including indigenous antelopes, are apparently
susceptible, but some animals, such as the blesbok and wildebeest, which may be reservoirs of infection, develop only an
inapparent transient reaction. Indigenous breeds and Persian
sheep are more resistant than imported breeds.

Etiology and Transmission: *Cowdria (Rickettsia) ruminantium*,
the causal agent, parasitizes the endothelial cells of the blood
vessels and is readily found in preparations made from the
hippocampus, the cerebral cortex and the intima of large veins.
The presence of the agent in sick animals during the febrile
stage can be demonstrated by IV inoculation of blood into
susceptible animals. The incubation period following inoculation varies from 7 to 14 days. Recipient animals should be

immunized against bluetongue, which otherwise could interfere with interpretation. In nature, the disease is transmitted primarily by the "bont" tick (*Amblyomma hebraeum*), a 3-host tick. The tick becomes infected either during the larval or nymphal stage and transmits the disease during one of the subsequent stages. The progeny of infected female ticks are not infective.

The main ways of propagating the infective agent are by serial passage in susceptible hosts, by feeding the larval and nymphal stages of the tick on sick animals, or by passage in ferrets. At room temperature, infected blood loses its potency within a few hours, but the organisms may be preserved by freezing or inoculation of mice, in which the organisms survive for about 90 days.

Clinical Findings: Hydrothorax, hydropericardium, edema of the lungs, an enlarged spleen and sometimes a hemorrhagic gastroenteritis may be found. In **peracute cases,** the animal suddenly develops a fever, collapses and dies in convulsions, usually discharging froth from its nostrils or mouth. The **acute form** is more common. In spite of the fever, feeding and rumination continue for a time, but soon the animal becomes listless and develops an anxious expression, hyperesthesia and other nervous signs. It walks with a high-stepping, stiff, unsteady gait, turns in circles, blinks its eyes and makes chewing movements. The animal will generally collapse in convulsions and die unless treatment has been instituted early in the course of disease. In the **subacute** and **chronic forms,** the signs are less severe.

Diagnosis: High fever associated with nervous signs in ruminants in areas infested with the "bont" tick is presumptive evidence of heartwater. For a positive diagnosis, the infective agent must be demonstrated.

Prophylaxis and Treatment: Control of tick infestation is the most useful prophylactic measure. Virulent blood is used as a vaccine. Young calves under 3 weeks old are fairly resistant and may recover spontaneously. When a reaction is produced in either calves or adults, antibiotic treatment is advised. Tetracyclines (R 11, 25) are specific and will usually effect a cure if administered early. Sheep require a higher treatment level (3 to 4 mg/lb) than cattle (2 to 3 mg/lb). Tetracyclines in oil (1 to 3 mg/lb body wt) have been useful, as have the sulfonamides.

BLUETONGUE

A noncontagious, insect-borne virus disease of sheep, cattle, goats and wild ruminants. The disease occurs widely on the African continent and to a lesser extent in North America, Asia and Europe.

Etiology and Transmission: Bluetongue virus can be propagated in chicken embryos, a variety of cell cultures, and in suckling mice and hamsters by cerebral inoculation. The principal biologic transmitting vector is a biting midge of the genus *Culicoides,* thus the disease is primarily seasonal. The virus can also be transmitted by inoculation of infectious blood, spleen, liver, and selected lymph nodes. The virus exists in a multiplicity of antigenic types, each serologically distinct. At least 16 serologic types have been identified in Africa and a plurality of types probably exist in other continents or countries, including the U.S.A. where at least 6 types have been identified.

Clinical Findings: The incubation period in sheep is from 1 to 7 days. The usual clinical signs in chronologic sequence include: respiratory distress (panting); hyperemia of muzzle, lips and ears; elevation of body temperature (up to 108°F); depression; inflammation, ulcers, erosions, and necrosis of the epithelial surfaces of the mouth, especially the dental pad. Disease signs that may appear, depending on the severity, include a swollen and cyanotic tongue, lameness due to a coronitis, wryneck or torticollis, vomiting, pneumonia and conjunctivitis. Bluetongue in the U.S.A. is considered milder than in Africa, with mortalities ranging from 5 to 30%. Cattle may be inapparently infected or they may develop clinical signs similar to those in bluetongue-infected sheep, while in white-tailed deer the virus often causes an acute fatal hemorrhagic disease.

Diagnosis: Clinical diagnosis can be confirmed by inoculation of blood from suspect cases into susceptible sheep and intravascularly into embryonating chicken eggs. Virus isolated in sheep and then in eggs or initially in eggs can be adapted to tissue culture systems and identified by serum neutralization or fluorescent antibody tests. Diagnosis can be made also by challenging immunity of an inoculated sheep with a known bluetongue virus challenge inoculation. Serologic antibody tests from recovered sheep, cattle, goats, or wild ruminants include serum neutralization, micro-agar-gel diffusion, or complement fixation.

Bluetongue viremia in sheep, cattle and goats is primarily

associated with red blood cells rather than plasma or white cells. A washed erthrocyte fraction of blood obtained during recovery stages often will yield the virus whereas by usual procedures of virus isolation the suspect sample would be considered virus-free. Cattle and goats may serve as important reservoirs of the virus.

Prevention: Monovalent modified live-virus vaccine of chicken embryo or tissue culture origin is available for sheep in the U.S.A.; a polyvalent vaccine propagated in cell culture is used in South Africa. Vaccination in early gestation frequently results in hydranencephalus in the lamb. The same syndrome is believed to occur in the bovine fetus as a result of natural infection of the dam during early gestation. Under experimental conditions, abortion and congenital arthrogryposis-type anomalies have occurred in calves. Current recommendations are against vaccinating pregnant ewes or using vaccine in nonendemic areas as vaccine virus has been transmitted from vaccinated to nonvaccinated sheep by the bite of *Culicoides variipennis*. Passive immunity in lambs lasts about 6 months and interferes with active immunity if the lambs are vaccinated earlier than 6 months. In the face of an epidemic, the decision whether to vaccinate will depend on the existing circumstances. Procedures reducing the number of biting flies should help to minimize the disease.

NAIROBI SHEEP DISEASE

A tick-borne viral disease of sheep and goats characterized by fever and gastroenteritis. Man is susceptible but cattle are not. The locus of the disease is eastern Africa.

Etiology and Transmission: The causal agent is a heat-labile arbovirus that can be propagated in mice intracerebrally and in goat and hamster kidney cultures. It is transmitted naturally by all stages of the brown tick, *Rhipicephalus appendiculatus,* in which it can survive for about 2½ years. Other ticks may also transmit the disease. The virus is in the urine and feces, but the disease is not spread by contact. Wild rodents develop asymptomatic viremias and may be reservoirs of infection.

Clinical Findings: A prodromal fever of 1 to 3 days duration follows an incubation period that ranges from 4 to 15 days. Sometimes the fever is diphasic. Illness is manifested by depression, anorexia, mucopurulent blood-stained nasal discharge, and fetid dysentery causing painful straining. Pregnant animals frequently abort. In fatal cases, death follows about 2 days after remission of the fever. The mortality in sheep varies from 30 to 90%. Goats generally recover.

Lesions: The most marked lesions are hemorrhagic gastroenteritis, hyperplasia of lymphoid tissues including the spleen, hydropericardium and heart hemorrhages. Extensive subcut. and intracutaneous ecchymoses mark the fetus.

Diagnosis: The clinical signs and postmortem findings are suggestive. Confirmation necessitates isolation and serologic identification of the virus in susceptible sheep, mice or cell cultures. Organs rich in virus are blood, lymphoid tissues, liver and cecum.

Prophylaxis and Treatment: Control of tick infestation and vaccination with mouse brain-adapted virus are the only prophylactic measures. There is no reliable treatment.

RIFT VALLEY FEVER

A mosquito-borne viral disease of sheep, goats, camels and cattle characterized by a short incubation period, fever, hepatitis and death in young animals and by abortion in pregnant animals. Man is susceptible and eye complications are common.

Etiology and Transmission: The causal agent is an ungrouped arbovirus that can be propagated in mice, chick embryos and a variety of tissue cultures. It is transmitted by culicine mosquitoes. Man is usually, and readily, infected through contact with infected animals and their tissues.

Clinical Findings: The incubation period varies from 12 to 96 hours in sheep and cattle and 4 to 6 days in man. Signs manifested are fever, listlessness, anorexia, unsteady gait, mucopurulent nasal discharge, diarrhea and abortion, which often is the only clinical finding in adult animals. The mortality in lambs is very high, but in adults rarely exceeds 30%. In cattle, the death rate is lower. In man, the disease assumes an influenza-like character.

Lesions: The striking lesions are the bright-yellow necrotic liver, widespread subserosal hemorrhages, enlarged spleen and gastroenteritis.

Diagnosis: An epizootic in ruminants, characterized by a short incubation period, a high mortality in newborn animals, abortions, necrosis of the liver and contact infection of man, justifies a tentative diagnosis of Rift Valley fever. For a positive diagnosis, isolation in mice or tissue cultures and serologic identification of the virus is necessary. Histologic examination of the affected liver is an aid to diagnosis.

Prophylaxis and Treatment: Removal of stock from low-lying, moist, mosquito-infested regions to higher altitudes, or stabling, is recommended. Prophylactic vaccination is the only practical and reliable method of control. The vaccine employed is a live virus, attenuated by serial intracerebral passage in mice and produced either from infected mouse brains or lamb kidney tissue cultures. Annual vaccination is advisable, but pregnant animals should not be vaccinated. No specific treatment is available.

WESSELSBRON DISEASE

A mosquito-borne viral disease of sheep characterized by high mortality in newborn lambs and by abortion in ewes. Man is susceptible. Overt disease has been recognized only in Southern Africa but antibody surveys indicate that infection of sheep, cattle and horses occurs throughout Africa. The disease resembles Rift Valley fever (q.v., p. 287) in its epizootiology, clinical signs and postmortem findings, but there is no cross-protection. Pigs, guinea pigs, mice and rabbits may be infected experimentally. Prophylactic vaccination with a live-attenuated virus is recommended. No specific treatment is available.

CONGO VIRUS DISEASE

A transient disease of African cattle and goats characterized by fever, depression and anorexia. The causal agent, an ungrouped arbovirus, is transmitted by hard ticks (*Hyalomma* spp.) and is similar to, and may be identical with, the virus causing Crimean hemorrhagic fever in man. The link between Africa and Eastern Europe and central Asia is postulated as being the ectoparasites of migratory birds. Virus isolations in suckling mice have been made from ticks, cattle, man and African hedgehog. Neither vaccine nor treatment is available.

LOUPING ILL

A viral encephalomyelitis of sheep on the tick-infested rough hill pastures of Great Britain and Ireland. It has also been recognized in cattle, horses, pigs and man.

Etiology and Epizootiology: The causal agent is one of the tick-borne encephalitis viruses of arbovirus group B, and is antigenically related to Russian spring-summer encephalitis and Central European tick-borne encephalitis. The disease occurs in spring and autumn, which coincides with periods of maximum activity of the tick vector, *Ixodes ricinus*. Of susceptible sheep placed on a tick-infested pasture, when ticks are active, as many as 60% may die within a period of 2 months.

Ixodes ricinus also harbors and transmits the infective agent of another and distinct disease, **tick-borne fever**. This febrile disease is caused by a *Rickettsia*-like organism which can be observed in the cytoplasm of the granular leukocytes. Tick-borne fever is not fatal, but aggravates the effects of louping ill.

On farms where the disease is enzootic, the losses are mainly confined to sheep under 2 years old, with an average mortality of 10%; the adults of a closed population are mostly immune as a result of abortive and subclinical infections. When, however, the disease appears for the first time, or after a lapse of several years on a farm, sheep of all ages may be susceptible and losses very high.

Clinical Findings: All susceptible animals bitten by infected ticks have a viremia for some days afterwards. During this incubaton period, although their temperature is high, they appear relatively normal, but after about 6 to 14 days, the virus in some individuals multiplies in the nervous system and signs of brain and spinal cord damage become obvious. These are muscular incoordination, tremors of the lips, ears and head, circling, staggering and standing apart from the flock with a lowered head. Finally, paralysis occurs and the animal may remain down with occasional convulsions for many hours before dying. In some chronic cases, there may be only paralysis of the hind legs, but young lambs die quickly, and most are found dead in the morning. Although about half of the infected animals show no clinical signs they remain immune for life and can pass on maternal immunity to their lambs in the milk. In some cases, however, if animals experience "stress" during the incubation period, the clinical signs are induced.

This is thought to be the cause of a number of cases in store lambs transported from sales by truck and which develop the clinical disease when they arrive on tick-free pastures. There is no danger of such animals spreading disease, however, and any ticks which they carry do not survive for long on low ground.

Lesions: There are no macroscopic lesions. Microscopically, there is encephalomyelitis with infiltration of mononuclear cells into the meninges and perivascular spaces, together with diffuse and focal infiltration into the substance of the nerve tissue, and perivascular cuffing. Necrosis and neuronophagia of the motor cells is a constant feature in the ventral horn and brain stem, but destruction of Purkinje cells is variable.

Diagnosis: The disease occurs only on tick-infested farms. Affected animals should be examined for ticks on the head, neck, ears, axillae and inside of the thighs. If the animal has a febrile reaction with no signs of encephalitis, diagnosis of louping ill can be made by examining a serum sample for the presence of specific hemagglutinin-inhibiting (HI) antibodies; the presence of immunoglobulin M (IgM) antibodies is indicative of infection within 28 days and rising titers to IgG is confirmatory. If there is severe encephalitis, the presence of IgM is sufficient presumptive evidence; in animals found dead or sufficiently ill to warrant destruction the brain can be examined microscopically or used to inoculate mice or tissue culture for the recovery of virus.

Prophylaxis: There is no treatment, but preventive vaccination is effective. The antibodies can be detected for 3 years in most sheep which have not been exposed to challenge. Vaccinated ewes pass on maternal antibodies in the colostrum to their first and second season lambs. The vaccine is best given in the autumn to weaned lambs and sheep about to be bred for the first time the following spring. It may be given in the spring if the ewes are injected 28 days before lambing is due, to ensure that antibodies are transferred in the colostrum.

CONTAGIOUS ECTHYMA

(Contagious pustular dermatitis, Sore-mouth, Orf)

An infectious dermatitis of sheep and goats, affecting primarily the lips of young animals. Encountered in all parts of the world, it occurs most commonly in late summer, fall and winter on pasture and winter in the feed lots. The condition may occur in very young lambs in the early spring and rarely in mature sheep.

Etiology: The disease is caused by a highly epitheliotropic virus that produces characteristic skin lesions. Infection occurs by contact, probably associated with injuries to the skin or mucous membrane. The virus is highly resistant to desiccation, having been recovered from dried crusts after 12 years. It also is resistant to glycerol and to ether.

Clinical Findings: The primary lesion develops on the skin of the lips, with frequent extension to the mucosa of the mouth. Occasionally, lesions are found on the feet, usually in the interdigital region and around the coronet. Ewes nursing infected lambs may develop lesions on the udder. In very young lambs, the initial lesion may develop on the gum below the incisor teeth. The lesions develop as papules and progress through vesicular and pustular stages before encrusting. Coalescence of numerous discrete lesions often leads to the formation of large scabs, and the proliferation of dermal tissue produces a verrucose mass under them. Where the lesion extends to the oral mucosa, secondary necrobacillosis frequently develops.

The course of the disease is from 1 to 4 weeks, within which time the scabs drop off and the tissues heal without scarring. During the active stages of the infection, the more seriously affected lambs fail to eat normally and lose condition. Extensive lesions on the feet lead to lameness.

Diagnosis: The proliferative lesion is characteristic. The disease must be differentiated from ulcerative dermatosis (q.v., p. 292), the virus of which produces a different kind of reaction leading to tissue destruction and the formation of crateriform ulcers. Ecthyma usually affects younger animals than does ulcerative dermatosis, although this criterion can only be used presumptively. A positive differentiation may be obtained by the inoculation of susceptible and ecthyma-immunized sheep.

Immunity and Vaccination: Sheep that have recovered from a natural attack are highly resistant to reinfection. Despite a multiplicity of immunogenic virus strains, with an occasional exception, the presently employed commercial single-strain vaccines have produced satisfactory immunity in all parts of the U.S.A. Sheep immunized against contagious ecthyma are susceptible to the virus of ulcerative dermatosis.

Vaccines can be used on infected premises but should not be used on noninfected premises. Vaccinated animals should be segregated from unprotected stock until the scabs have fallen. The vaccine consists of finely powdered dried ecthyma scab, suspended in a diluent immediately before use. A small amount of the suspension is brushed cver light scarifications on the inside of the thigh or axillary region of the lamb. Older lambs and ewes may be vaccinated in the perianal region. Lambs should be vaccinated at about 1 month of age. For best results, a second vaccination about 2 or 3 months later is suggested. Nonimmunized lambs going into infected feed lots should be vaccinated.

Treatment: Medicinal preparations may help to combat secondary bacterial infection. Where indicated to repel screwworm attack, appropriate repellents and larvicides should be applied to the lesions. The virus is transmissible to man and the lesions, usually confined to the hands and face, are more proliferative in man and occasionally are very distressing. Veterinarians and sheep handlers should exercise reasonable protective precautions. Diagnosis in man is established by transmitting the virus to sheep. A complement-fixation test may be of value in the diagnosis.

ULCERATIVE DERMATOSIS OF SHEEP
(Lip and leg ulceration, Venereal balanoposthitis and vulvitis)

An infectious, ulcerative viral disease of sheep manifesting itself in 2 somewhat distinct forms, one characterized by the formation of ulcers around the mouth and nose or on the legs (lip and leg ulceration) and the other as a venereally transmitted ulceration of the prepuce and penis or the vulva (balanoposthitis and vulvitis).

Clinical Findings: The lesion, regardless of anatomical location, is an ulcer with a raw, easily bleeding crater varying in depth and extent, containing an odorless creamy pus and covered from the beginning with a scab. Face lesions occur on the upper lip, between the border of the lip and the nasal orifice, and on the chin. The ulcerative process may, in very severe cases, perforate the lip. Foot lesions occur anywhere between the coronet and the carpus or tarsus.

Posthitis lesions partially or completely surround the preputial orifice and may become so severe as to produce phimosis. In rare cases, the ulcerative process may extend to the glans penis so that the animal becomes unfit for natural breeding.

In the female venereal form, the edema, ulceration and scabbing of the lips of the vulva have less serious consequences.

There are no noticeable early systemic reactions. Very often, the disease remains unrecognized until the lesions have reached such an advanced stage that signs of lameness or disturbed urination become apparent.

Diagnosis: This depends entirely upon recognition of the characteristic ulcerative lesion. Differentiation between this lesion and that of contagious ecthyma (q.v., p. 290), which is essentially proliferative in character, is fundamental. The question of the similarity of the agents of ulcerative dermatosis and contagious ecthyma is not clearly defined, but inoculation of sheep previously immunized against contagious ecthyma will help in arriving at a diagnosis. However, the 2 virus agents appear to be related. It is also difficult and, in some instances, virtually impossible, without resorting to sheep inoculation, to differentiate between bacterial balanoposthitis (sheath rot) (q.v., p. 827) and ulcerative dermatosis.

Prophylaxis and Treatment: Infected animals should be isolated and those with genital lesions should not be bred. The time taken to recover varies from 2 to 8 weeks and is not greatly influenced by treatment. Treatment, therefore, is usually not attempted unless (1) the animals are to be bred in a short time, (2) lip lesions interfere with eating or (3) foot lesions make the animals so lame that they are losing flesh.

Treatment, when given, consists of removing the scabs and all necrotic tissue from the ulcers and applying any one of the following preparations: silver nitrate (styptic pencil), 30% copper sulfate solution, 4% formaldehyde, 5% cresol (sheep dip) or sulfa-urea powder. Foot and lower leg lesions can be treated conveniently with copper sulfate or formaldehyde solutions in foot bath troughs.

SCRAPIE
(Tremblante du mouton, Rida)

A relentlessly progressive, fatal neuropathy of sheep, and less often of goats, characterized chiefly by intense pruritus, altered gait and debility. It is rarely seen in animals less than 2 years of age.

Etiology: Scrapie is usually transmitted from parents to offspring but occasionally by contact. Experimentally it may be transmitted by inoculation of susceptible animals, by various routes, with suspensions of many tissues, but especially brain, from scrapie-affected animals, with cell-free tissue extracts, or with cell culture cell-free fluids. The disease may also be transmitted by mouth. Other features that would permit characterizing the agent as a virus have not been demonstrated, and it has not been detected by electron microscopy. There is complete resistance of the agent to ultraviolet light in the optimum absorptive range of nucleic acids. The agent is nonantigenic, highly resistant to heat and to a surprising number of chemical agents including 12% formalin.

Goats are 100% susceptible and successful experimental transmission in sheep ranges from about 5 to 60% depending on the breed. The disease has been transmitted to mice, rats and Syrian hamsters and back to sheep. Recently, it has been transmitted to mink, Chinese hamsters, voles and gerbils.

Incidence: The disease has been reported in most European countries and has been known in Britain, France and Germany for 200 years. In these countries, it is enzootic and waxes and wanes in different breeds over periods of many years. Males and females are equally susceptible. The incidence in affected flocks varies greatly, usually ranging from 4 to 20%. Over long periods, however, it may be much less than 4%, while occasionally it may approach 50%.

In recent years, small outbreaks, usually traceable to the introduction of sheep from enzootic areas in Europe, have been recorded in Canada, the U.S.A., the Himalayan region of India, and South Africa. Australia and New Zealand are now free of the disease.

Clinical Findings: The onset is insidious. Affected sheep become more excitable, and fine tremors of the head and neck may be observed. The most characteristic feature is intense pruritus, which often begins over the rump, and may extend to other parts. In some cases the pruritus makes it difficult for the animal to feed and rest normally. Nervous signs may be elicited from a quiet but affected sheep through a sudden noise or movement. The wool is dry, separable and brittle, resulting in loss of fleece over large areas. Other areas may be rubbed raw. Sheep will nibble at their limbs in an effort to relieve the itching. Emaciation, weakness and incoordination of the hind-quarters are passive, and inability to rise occurs in the later stages. Occasionally there are epileptiform convulsions. When made to trot, there is often a peculiar high-stepping action of the forelegs, sometimes with galloping movements of the hind legs. Animals live about 6 weeks to 6 months following onset of signs. Recoveries have been reported, but without an unequivocal means of diagnosis such an interpretation remains subject to question.

Lesions: The only macroscopic abnormalities are abrasion of skin over the rubbed areas, and a small increase in volume of cerebrospinal fluid. The histologic picture is of bilaterally symmetrical spongiform encephalopathy, with hypertrophy of astrocytes, and degeneration, including vacuolation, of neurons. These abnormalities vary in intensity and distribution in the different animal species.

Diagnosis: Signs of CNS disturbance, hind-limb weakness and compulsive rubbing, with an insidious onset and a protracted course strongly suggest scrapie. For diagnosis, histologic examination should be made of the medulla oblongata in sheep and goats, and of whole brain saggital sections in small laboratory animals.

Control: Sheep from families in which scrapie has been recognized should not be introduced into other flocks. The eradication program used in the U.S.A. comprises: confirmation of field diagnosis through histopathologic evaluation, quarantine and slaughter of all sheep and goats in the infected flock, identification and slaughter of all exposed animals moved from the flock and their immediate progeny. Similar programs were effective in Australia and New Zealand and are in force in South Africa and Canada. No prophylactic or palliative measures are known.

HOG CHOLERA
(Swine fever)

An eradication program has markedly reduced the incidence of hog cholera in the U.S.A. As of March, 1972, the pigs in 38 states had had no clinical signs of hog cholera for more than a year and these states were declared free of the infection. The remaining states were in the last phase of the program and were eliminating all sources of hog-cholera infection. Vaccination had been outlawed and suppliers encouraged to destroy vaccines in storage. Any new outbreak of hog cholera will be followed by immediate slaughter of the infected herd, decontamination of the premises, and thorough investigation to locate the source of the infection.

Hog cholera is an acute, highly contagious, viral disease affecting all ages of swine. It is characterized by sudden onset, high morbidity and mortality, and a diversity of clinical signs and lesions when caused by virulent strains of the virus. In the chronic form of hog cholera associated with strains of lower virulence the mortality is low in mature swine and only baby pig losses, abortions and stillbirths are found.

Etiology: The disease is caused by an RNA virus similar in structure and antigenically related to the virus of bovine virus diarrhea. It multiplies in cell cultures derived from the pig but most pure strains produce no observable cytopathic effect. The virus is inactivated readily by sunlight, heat and most disinfectants. It is unlikely to survive longer than 4 days in the environment of pig houses except under very cold conditions, but it may survive several months in pickled pork and bacon and several years in frozen carcasses.

Clinical Findings: The incubation period is normally 2 to 6 days but can be up to a month. In acute outbreaks, the first signs are dullness, partial anorexia, transient constipation, hyperemia and fever, which reaches a peak (106° to 108°F) about 4 to 6 days after the onset of signs. The constipation soon changes to diarrhea. The skin frequently becomes cyanotic, particularly over the abdomen, ears and snout. Nervous signs are common but variable and include ataxia, paralysis and convulsions. The morbidity is high; mortality may vary, being highest in young pigs. Some deaths may occur suddenly early in the disease, but most deaths occur 5 to 15 days after the outbreak starts, and chronic cases may linger for 30 days or more. Recovery often results in stunting.

Congenital infections are common. Infection of sows may result in fetal death, mummification, small litter size, stillbirths, anomalies, weak piglets, or congenital tremor.

Lesions: The virus multiplies in all cells of the body, but damage is most evident in the endothelium of the blood vessels. In peracute cases there may be little to see, but in acute cases, petechial and ecchymotic hemorrhages may occur in a variety of organs. Lymph nodes appear edematous, congested and hemorrhagic. None of the gross lesions are pathognomonic but the presence of hemorrhages in the larynx, kidneys and bladder; infarcts in the spleen and kidney; button ulcers near the ileocecal valve and a widening of the white line at the costochondral junction, are strongly indicative of hog cholera. Histologic lesions associated with blood vessels in the CNS are more specific.

Diagnosis: A fairly firm diagnosis can be based on the signs and gross lesions alone, but many outbreaks do not fit the usual pattern, and are frequently confused by concurrent bacterial infections, notably salmonellosis and pasteurellosis. Leukopenia (i.e., leukocyte count less than 10,000) in pigs over 5 weeks of age, is a fairly reliable indication of hog cholera and characteristic brain lesions support the diagnosis. To confirm the presence of hog cholera infection, specific laboratory techniques may be necessary. The most accurate of these are the fluorescent antibody test on frozen sections of tonsil, or isolation and identification of the virus by fluorescent antibody technique on tissue cultures inoculated with tonsil or spleen. Hog cholera must be differentiated from salmonellosis, erysipelas, mulberry heart disease, transmissible gastroenteritis, viral encephalitis (including Teschen disease) and pseudorabies.

Immunity and Vaccination: There is ony one main serotype of hog cholera virus, although minor variants exist. Recovered animals are strongly immune and immune sows confer protection on their offspring through their colostrum. Short-term passive protection can be provided by the injection of hyperimmune anti-hog cholera serum.

Broadly, 2 types of vaccine are in current use, inactivated and live attenuated. Live attenuated vaccines are usually prepared from virus that has been adapted to rabbits (i.e., lapinized) or tissue cultures, or both. Unfortunately, many of these are not fully attenuated and antiserum has to be injected with them. Inactivated vaccines are usually prepared by mild heat inactivation (37°C) and are preserved with crystal violet. The protection provided by inactivated vaccines is not as solid as that from attenuated vaccines nor is there any virus interference before immunity develops. Best results are obtained if 2 doses are given 30 days apart. Vaccines have been prepared from the virus of bovine virus diarrhea, which is antigenically related to hog-cholera virus, but the protection afforded is weak.

Epidemiology and Control: Hog cholera is enzootic and serious in most South American, African, Asian and European countries, but it is absent from Canada and Australia, and has recently been eradicated from Britain where it had been enzootic until 1962. The infection has been reduced to sporadic outbreaks in the U.S.A. by an intensive eradication program.

The virus is transmitted most readily by direct pig-to-pig contact and by feeding uncooked pork scraps. The prohibition on feeding uncooked garbage is essential in any control program. The virus can also be transmitted from farm to farm indirectly, by contaminated feed, water, equipment or clothing. However, the maintenance of a closed herd and careful precautions against entry will usually serve to exclude it. Experience in Britain has shown that the greatest obstacle to eradication is the diagnosis of chronic forms of the disease caused by virus strains of low virulence. Once a slaughter program is under way in an area, vaccination with live virus should be stopped. When a herd is slaughtered because of hog cholera, the premises should be thoroughly cleaned, disinfected, and left empty for a minimum of 2 weeks.

AFRICAN SWINE FEVER

Etiology and Epizootiology: African swine fever (ASF) is a highly contagious viral disease of porcine animals, confined until recently to the African continent, but now also found in parts of Western Europe and recently in Cuba. Although the signs and lesions are in many respects similar to those of hog cholera, the causative virus is immunologically distinct; swine immune to hog cholera are fully susceptible to African swine fever. In Africa, outbreaks of ASF in domestic swine often follow contact (probably via tick vectors) with wart hogs (*Phacochoerus*), bush pigs (*Potamochoerus*) or forest hogs (*Hylochoerus*), all of which may serve as inapparent carriers of the infection. In Europe most outbreaks follow contact with infected domestic swine or fomites from them usually in the form of uncooked pork scraps. Certain argasid ticks that have fed on infected pigs can maintain the virus for months and transmit it to other pigs.

The causative virus, present in all fluids, tissues and excretions of acutely infected swine and periodically liberated in the discharges of carrier animals, is exceptionally hardy, retaining infectivity after 18 months at room temperature, after 1 hour at 56°C, or in commercially processed and stored hams after 6 months. Smears of infected blood were infectious after 24 hours exposure to 1% NaOH, but not to 2%. The virus is relatively resistant to trypsin and acid but sensitive to ether.

Only swine are naturally susceptible. The virus has been passed experimentally in rabbits, chick embryos and tissue cultures. The attenuated strains so evolved have not provided a protective immunity nor have killed-virus vaccines.

Clinical Findings: In closely observed herds, the first sign of ASF is fever; temperatures of 105° to 108°F occur from 5 to

5 days after natural infection. There is an early leukopenia. After about 4 days of fever or about 24 to 48 hours before death, animals usually stop eating and become listless, incoordinate and cyanotic. The pulse and respiration are accelerated and about one-third cough and have dyspnea. Vomiting, diarrhea and eye discharges are sometimes observed. Death often occurs within 4 to 7 days after the onset of fever. With ASF acquired from wild animals, mortality in domestic swine frequently approaches 100%. However, currently in Portugal and Spain, natural passage through domestic swine has somewhat modified the severity of ASF and resulted in a relatively high percentage of survivors. The survivors are usually carriers for life, although the virus is not continually present in the excretions.

Lesions: The rapidly fatal course of ASF in many animals causes them to die in relatively good flesh. Generalized viral damage to the walls of small blood vessels results in varying degrees of edema, congestion and hemorrhage, with some thrombosis. A frequently severe cyanosis of hairless areas is sharply demarcated and edematous. Cutaneous ecchymoses occur on the skin of the legs and abdomen. Pleural, pericardial and peritoneal fluids are excessive. Petechiae occur in the mucous membrane of the larynx, urinary bladder, in the renal cortex and visceral surfaces of organs. Edema is often prominent in the mesenteric structures of the colon and adjacent to the gallbladder.

Diagnosis: Any suspect hog cholera-like disease should be reported immediately. The lesions of hog cholera and ASF are too similar to be certain of a differential diagnosis by gross pathology; however, there are minor differences that may be somewhat helpful. The "button ulcers" of hog cholera rarely, if ever, occur in ASF. Severe edema of lungs and walls of gallbladder and excessive pericardial, pleural and peritoneal fluids are common in ASF and rare in hog cholera. For laboratory diagnosis, samples of the blood and spleen should be taken preferably 2 to 3 days after onset of fever.

In the laboratory the suspect virus may be replicated in swine bone marrow or buffy coat (leukocyte) cultures. Swine red blood cells will adsorb to the leukocytes that are infected with ASF virus and later the virus causes cytolysis of the leukocytes. These reactions do not occur with hog-cholera virus. Fluorescent antibody tests readily differentiate the 2 viruses. Complement-fixation and agar-gel diffusion tests also may be used. Swine immunized with hog-cholera virus will become infected if challenged with ASF virus as the suspect agent.

Control: The spread of ASF to Europe and the absence of a vaccine intensify the international hazard. Cooperative international efforts to prohibit the movement of infected animals, products or vectors help, but veterinarians everywhere must be alert to the recognition of ASF and have access to a competent diagnostic service. A diagnosis must be followed by strict quarantine and slaughter.

VESICULAR EXANTHEMA

An acute, highly infectious, viral disease of swine which is no longer known to exist naturally. It is characterized by formation of vesicles on the snout, the mucous membranes of the mouth, the feet between the toes, and the soles, coronary band and dew claws. Horses and dogs are irregularly susceptible to artificial inoculation.

Vesicular exanthema of swine (VES) is caused by a small RNA virus which belongs to the picornavirus group. There are 13 known immunologically distinct types of the virus. As the signs and course of the disease are clinically indistinguishable from those of foot-and-mouth disease, it is important that an accurate diagnosis be made.

The disease was discovered in 1932 in California. During the 1950's the disease became widespread in the U.S.A., but a vigorous campaign to eradicate the disease has been successful. In 1959 the country was declared free of vesicular exanthema and has remained so to date. The disease has never been reported as a natural infection in any other part of the world.

Diagnosis is based upon fever and the presence of typical vesicles which break in 24 to 48 hours to form erosions. Clinically, the lesions are indistinguishable from those of foot-and-mouth disease, vesicular stomatitis, and a recently reported vesicular viral disease of swine in Europe. A diagnosis can be confirmed serologically using complement-fixation, immuno-diffusion and neutralization tests. Suspected cases of vesicular exanthema should be immediately brought to the attention of the proper authorities.

TESCHEN DISEASE
(Porcine poliomyelitis, Talfan disease)

A viral disease of pigs, closely analogous to human poliomyelitis, and characterized mainly by spinal paralysis.

Etiology and Epidemiology: The causal enterovirus is resistant to wide variations in pH, to many enzyme actions, and to most bacterial disinfectants. It is inactivated rapidly by formalin and by temperatures over 60°C, but may survive several days at room temperatures and long periods in the frozen state. There is only one main antigenic type.

The Teschen virus infects only the pig, in which it causes a subclinical infection of the alimentary tract, particularly the intestine. Occasionally, it gains access to the CNS causing overt disease. The virus is excreted in the feces for 1 to 3 months, after which a local intestinal immunity develops. In herds in which the virus is endemic, infection of the alimentary tract occurs early in life while the CNS is protected by circulating colostral antibodies. These are superseded by antibodies actively stimulated by the infection itself.

A puzzling epidemiologic feature is that although both virulent and avirluent strains of the virus occur in most areas of the world, including North America, serious outbreaks of the disease have been recorded only in mid-Europe and Madagascar. In other countries the disease is sporadic and mild or unrecognized.

Clinical Findings: In severe outbreaks the morbidity and mortality rates may be high, affecting all age groups. The main sign is an ascending paresis progressing to a flaccid paralysis. Pigs so affected may continue to eat if they can get to food. A few pigs may show other nervous signs. In the milder outbreaks, which occur in most Western countries, the disease appears as a mild posterior paresis affecting small numbers of pigs, usually about 8 to 12 weeks of age.

Lesions: There are no gross lesions. Histologic lesions are confined mainly to the gray matter of the posterior brain and spinal cord. The lesions are typical of viral infections, and include neuronal degeneration, glial cell proliferation, and vascular congestion and cuffing.

Diagnosis: A presumptive diagnosis can be made from the clinical picture and absence of gross lesions. The nature and distribution of the histologic lesions provide supportive evidence, but are not specific to Teschen disease. Further evidence may be obtained by demonstrating a rise of neutralizing or complement-fixing antibodies in paired serum samples from early and late stages of the disease. However, a definitive diagnosis can only be made by demonstrating the presence of the virus in the CNS in early cases. This is usually done by isolating the virus in porcine kidney cell cultures.

The disease must be differeniated from Aujeszky's disease, edema disease, hog cholera, encephalitic forms of vomiting and wasting disease, rabies, arsenic poisoning, and various less common forms of poisoning.

Treatment and Control: There is no treatment. Vaccines are used in mid-Europe but not elsewhere.

TRANSMISSIBLE GASTROENTERITIS (TGE)

A rapidly spreading viral disease of swine, characterized by profuse diarrhea and vomiting. The disease results in severe dehydration and high mortality in pigs infected during the first week or 2 of life. In older swine, morbidity may be high but mortality is low. The great majority of outbreaks occur in winter and early spring.

Etiology: The causal coronavirus can be grown in porcine kidney cell cultures. It proliferates in the epithelial cells of the small intestines and may be found transiently in other organs without causing obvious changes. It does not affect common laboratory animals but may infect dogs and foxes subclinically and may be excreted in their feces for up to 2 weeks. It may also be excreted by starlings for short periods. The virus is readily transmitted through feces and fomites; airborne infection may occur. Pigs may shed virus up to 8 weeks after infection. The virus is very labile to sunlight and heat but may remain infective for years when frozen. An important means by which virus is carried over winters is in infected fattening herds receiving weaners from susceptible sources. Transient diarrhea occurs in each freshly introduced batch of pigs.

Clinical Findings and Diagnosis: The incubation period is 14 hours to 4 days. The most pronounced sign, scouring, is often preceded by vomiting. Vomiting is less frequent after the first day of the disease. In baby pigs, the watery diarrhea is typically bright yellow or green. It may contain curds of undigested milk and often drips from the anus without expulsive efforts. Dehydration is rapid and thirst is evident; even the youngest pigs drink water copiously and they continue to suck the sow as long as they have sufficient strength. As dehydration progresses, the feces tend to become thicker. Diarrhea continues in surviving piglets for 5 to 9 days. Most fatalities occur 2 to 6 days after the onset. Mortality in newborn pigs is 75 to 100%. Deaths are unusual in pigs over 4 to 5 weeks of age. In weaned and older swine the diarrhea is most often manifested by projectile expulsion of brownish or yellowish watery feces which may continue for 1 to 5 days. Vomiting is rare in shoats and older animals, except in sows infected near parturition. Sows infected late in pregnancy sometimes have elevated temperatures, but depressed body temperatures are commonly found in other pigs.

Less virulent strains of virus also exist and these produce a milder more chronic form of the disease. The mortality in young piglets is very low but unfortunately the immunity produced in sows is also low, and outbreaks tend to keep recurring in the same herd.

Lesions: The primary lesion is loss of intestinal epithelial cells resulting in extreme shortening of the intestinal villi. This may be seen best 1 or 2 days after infection and before regeneration starts by placing bits of jejunum under water and comparing them with a hand lens or dissecting microscope with duodenal mucosa taken from near the pylorus. Chyle, easily seen in the mesenteric lymphatics of normal and most pigs with enteric colibacillosis, is absent in pigs with TGE. In early stages of the disease, the stomach is usually filled with coagulated milk and the intestine is distended with clear or brightly colored fluid and gas containing bits of milk curd. In later stages the pig is dehydrated, distension of the intestine is less pronounced, but the stomach remains filled. The stomach wall in the fundic region is often severely congested in the terminal stages of the disease. Inflammatory changes are rare early in the disease but may later occur in any part of the intestine.

Diagnosis: Diagnosis of TGE is strongly suggested by the appearance of rapidly spreading diarrheal disease affecting all ages of pigs and fatal only in piglets. Failure of antibiotic therapy may add support to the diagnosis. A specific diagnosis of TGE requires laboratory procedures, such as the fluorescent antibody technique applied to frozen sections of the jejunum, preferably of pigs killed at the onset of disease, or cell cultures inoculated with intestinal materials.

Prophylaxis and Treatment: During an enzootic, persons, animals or public conveyances of any kind from infected, or possibly infected, areas should not be allowed on TGE-free farms. If new stock must be introduced, they should be isolated from the herd until farrowing is completed.

When an outbreak occurs, it is advisable to separate sows near term as widely as possible in small groups or individual houses even when they apparently have been exposed. This practice may not be entirely effective, depending upon the efficiency of personnel, but it usually delays spread. Each day of age gained by baby pigs before infection occurs decreases the mortality rate. New sows about to farrow should not be added to an infected herd for 2 or 3 months after an outbreak.

Sows recovered from natural infection transmit a type of immunity to their pigs. This protection is unrelated to colostral circulating antibodies. It depends upon the presence of antibody in milk and is effective only as long as such milk is in the gastrointestinal tract of the piglets. Largely because of this mechanism of lactogenic immunity, difficulty has occurred in the development of vaccines. Tests on a modified live virus given to sows during pregnancy indicated it was less effective than planned infection with virulent virus but its efficacy in the field remains to be assessed.

Planned infection of sows early in pregnancy with virulent virus stimulates effective immunity. It should be used, however, only where it is inevitable that sows will be exposed on farrowing and where there is no danger of spreading the disease to neighboring droves. This is best carried out by grinding or chopping intestinal-tract material from infected pigs from the same drove and mixing it with the sow feed after withholding feed for one day. Sows, thus immunized, should be isolated from infected pigs at farrowing to reduce the exposure of their pigs to virus.

The carcasses of pigs dying of TGE should be disposed of in a way that eliminates the possibility of their being carried or eaten by dogs or other animals that move from farm to farm.

There is no specific treatment. Some practitioners have observed benefit from orally or parenterally administered antibiotics or sulfonamides in animals more than 4 or 5 days old at onset. Dehydration may be combatted by supplying fresh water or hypotonic saline to the piglets. In some instances it has appeared useful to wean pigs old enough to eat dry feed. Careful attention to providing a warm, dry environment may increase the survival rate.

VOMITING-AND-WASTING DISEASE

(Ontario encephalitis, Viral encephalomyelitis of piglets)

A viral disease of young piglets characterized by vomiting, constipation, anorexia, and either chronic emaciation or acute encephalomyelitis.

Etiology and Epidemiology: The causal coronavirus, the Hemagglutinating Encephalomyelitis Virus (HEV), grows in pig kidney ... and affects only pigs. Infection appears to be widespread ... North America and Western Europe, but is usually subclinical ... in which it is endemic a herd ... immunity ... although occasionally individual piglets ... clinical signs these are rarely diagnosed. However ... enters a susceptible herd during the farrowing ... litters may be affected simultaneously, and the mortality in these may be high.

... : The virus infects all age groups but usually ... of 5 to about 21 days of age show clinical ... signs are anorexia, depression, constipation and ... amount of vomiting. Intestinal stasis occurs and ... abdomen may become bloated with gas. Some piglets ... pharyngeal paralysis and are unable to drink. After 1 to 3 days the disease progresses in 1 of 2 ways. In some outbreaks pronounced signs of CNS derangement develop and the affected piglets soon die.

In other outbreaks, central nervous signs are minimal but the anorexia and constipation persist and the piglets slowly waste away, dying over periods of 1 to 6 weeks.

Lesions: There are no distinctive gross lesions. Histologically, nonspecific lesions typical of viral encephalitides may be found in the brain stem, cervical cord and paravertebral ganglia. These are constant findings in the encephalitic syndrome and may sometimes be found in the wasting syndrome.

Diagnosis: In large outbreaks a fairly firm diagnosis can be made from the clinical and postmortem findings. Diagnosis can be confirmed by demonstrating a rise of neutralizing antibodies. Isolation of the virus from affected piglets is difficult and unreliable. The disease must be differentiated from bacterial meningitis, hypoglycemia, agalactia, hog cholera, Teschen disease and pseudorabies.

Treatment and Control: There is no treatment, and control is difficult. Herdsmen must be encouraged not to sell out and repopulate in the face of an outbreak since the worst loss is usually over by the time diagnosis is made. Sanitation and isolation are the only protection for a susceptible herd.

ENZOOTIC PNEU...MONIA OF PIGS

(Virus pneumonia...of pigs, VPP)

A chronic, clinically mild, econo...mically import...
respiratory disease of pigs, charact...
to become permanently endemic in a...
persistent, dry cough, sporadic "flare ups"...
distress, and a high incidence of lung lesions in slau...

Etiology: The terms "virus pneumonia" and "enzoot...
monia" are frequently used to describe a characteristic
syndrome of undetermined etiology, but recent studies...
shown that *Mycoplasma hyopneumoniae* (*suipneumonia*...
a primary cause, and it has been suggested that the t...
"enzootic pneumonia" should be reserved for pneumon...
caused primarily by this agent.

M. hyopneumoniae is a fastidious pleomorphic organism,
smaller than most bacteria, and difficult to see clearly under
ordinary light microscopes. It can be cultured in specially
prepared liquid or on solid media, but its isolation from field
cases is difficult and generally unreliable. It is rapidly inactivated in the environment and by disinfectants, but it may
survive longer periods in cold weather. It appears to be host-
specific.

Enzootic pneumonia is frequently complicated by other
mycoplasmas, bacteria and viruses, and there is some evidence
that certain strains of *Mycoplasma hyorhinis* and perhaps some
viruses may themselves act as primary agents or trigger mechanisms to produce an enzootic pneumonia syndrome.

Epidemiology: Enzootic pneumonia is of worldwide distribution. In the U.S.A. and in most other countries where modern
pig farming methods are practiced, the lungs of between 30 and
80% of the swine slaughtered show pneumonic lesions of the
type associated with enzootic pneumonia.

Pigs of all ages are susceptible but within a herd pigs usually
become infected in the first few weeks of life from their dam,
or more often from other young pigs after mixing. The incidence of lung lesions is highest in growing pigs between 2 and
4 months of age. Immunity develops slowly, the lung lesions
regress, and adult pigs may recover completely.

Economic Importance: Even in a mild form, enzootic pneumonia may impair the growth rate and feed conversion of
growing pigs. The effect is enhanced where large numbers of
pigs are closely confined in poorly ventilated buildings under

poor husbandry conditions. The effects of the disease are uneven and unpredictable, placing limits on the efficiency and flexibility of large production units.

Clinical Findings: In herds in which the disease is endemic, the morbidity is high but clinical signs may be minimal and mortality is low. Coughing is the commonest sign and is most obvious when pigs are roused. The disease tends to flare up sporadically in individual pigs or groups of pigs into a clinically severe pneumonia. A common predisposing factor is a change of weather, usually to hot, humid conditions, but other stresses, such as transient viral infections, may also cause flareups. The disease is usually more severe when it first enters a herd, and pigs in all age groups may be affected.

Lesions: The lesions in the lungs are gray or plum colored, and most common in the apical and cardiac lobes. Old lesions become clearly outlined. The associated lymph nodes may be enlarged. Histologically, inflammatory cells are present in the bronchioles, there is perivascular and peribronchiolar cuffing, and extensive lymphoid hyperplasia.

Diagnosis: The nonspecific diagnosis "enzootic pneumonia" based on clinical, pathologic and epidemiologic findings is adequate for most practical purposes. However, in special cases it may be necessary to attempt to determine the specific etiology. *M. hyopneumoniae* can be demonstrated in touch preparations of the cut surface of affected lung, identified by the fluorescent antibody technique, and sometimes isolated and identified in culture. Certain serologic tests, principally the complement-fixation test, may be useful on a herd basis.

Enzootic pneumonia should be differentiated from swine influenza (q.v., p. 308), pasteurellosis (q.v., p. 386) and other pneumonias.

Control: When the disease first enters a herd, mass treatment with macrolide antibiotics such as tylosin or one of the tetracyclines helps to control the severity of signs. When the disease flares up in herds in which it is endemic, treatment of individual pigs with antibiotics usually results in a remission of the overt signs, presumably by controlling secondary bacteria.

Inactivated mycoplasmal cultures have been used as vaccines in Sweden and some other countries in attempts to reduce the effects of the endemic disease, but so far their merit cannot be judged.

The economic effects of the disease can be reduced, sometimes almost eliminated, by improvements in housing and husbandry, paying particular attention to ventilation and overcrowding. Carrying litters through in batches, so that litters from older sows go through together, may also be beneficial.

In most large intensive units, complete control is difficult; it is advisable, where possible, to start such units with foundation stock from breeding herds that are enzootic-pneumonia-free and to adopt precautions against direct and indirect contact with other herds. Most commercial herds that are set up in this way remain free of enzootic pneumonia for long periods, and those that become reinfected may develop only an uncomplicated mild form of the disease.

In the U.S.A. and parts of Europe most of the enzootic-pneumonia-free supply herds were established originally by the specific pathogen-free (SPF) swine repopulation technique. Other methods of eradicating the disease have proved less reliable. However, in Britain conventional purebred breeding herds have been found in which enzootic pneumonia could not be detected and these have been used to supply pneumonia-free stock.

The biggest difficulty with enzootic-pneumonia-free herd programs is in ensuring that the causal agents of the disease are indeed absent from all the herds enrolled.

SWINE INFLUENZA
(Hog flu, Pig flu)

An acute, highly contagious respiratory disease caused primarily by a Type-A influenza virus.

Etiology: Although the virus is the primary cause, outbreaks are frequently complicated by *Haemophilus influenzae suis* (*see also* GLÄSSER'S DISEASE, p. 414) and sometimes by other bacteria. Stress is an important predisposing factor.

The virus can be grown in embryonated hens' eggs and in tissue cultures. It is unlikely to survive outside living cells for more than 14 days except in very cold conditions. It is readily inactivated by disinfectants.

Epidemiology: The disease is most common in the Midwestern U.S.A. during the fall and winter. It occurs occasionally in other states, and some other countries (e.g., Germany, Czechoslovakia and Kenya). In the U.S.A. outbreaks occur simultaneously in autumn on different farms within an area. It is thought that the virus is widely seeded before the outbreaks begin. Outbreaks are provoked by the onset of cold, inclement weather, or other stress factors. The disease then spreads rapidly within a herd mainly by airborne infection.

One mechanism of survival between epidemics involves the swine lungworm as a vector. Lungworm eggs containing the virus are passed in the feces of infected pigs and ingested by earthworms, and the infected earthworms are eaten by pigs. The lungworm larvae then migrate to the lungs. The pigs remain clinically normal and noninfective until the disease is precipitated by stress.

The virus may also survive between outbreaks in a subclinical form in noninfective carrier pigs. It has been isolated from the lungs of recovered pigs 3 months after infection.

Clinical Findings: A typical outbreak is characterized by sudden onset and rapid spread through the entire herd, often within 1 to 3 days. The main signs are depression, fever, anorexia, coughing, dyspnea, muscular weakness, prostration, and a mucous discharge from the eyes and nose.

The mortality is generally about 1 to 4%. The course of the disease usually varies from 3 to 7 days, with recovery of the herd almost as sudden as the onset. However, some pigs may become chronically affected. In herds which are in good condition, the principal economic loss is from stunting and delay in reaching market weight.

Lesions: The lesions are usually confined to the chest cavity. The pneumonic areas are clearly demarcated, collapsed, and purplish red in color. They may be distributed throughout the lungs but tend to be more extensive and confluent ventrally. Nonpneumonic areas are pale and emphysematous. The respiratory airways contain a copious mucopurulent exudate and the bronchial and mediastinal lymph nodes are edematous, but rarely congested. There may be severe pulmonary edema or a serous or serofibrinous pleuritis. Histologically, the lesions are primarily those of an exudative bronchiolitis.

Diagnosis: In typical outbreaks, a fairly firm presumptive diagnosis can be made on clinical and pathologic findings alone but, in atypical outbreaks, it may be necessary to confirm the diagnosis by laboratory tests. Embryonated hens' eggs can be used to isolate the virus from nasal swabs or affected lung tissue in the early acute stage of the disease, or a retrospective diagnosis can be made by taking serum samples during the acute and convalescent stages and demonstrating a rise in specific antibodies using the hemagglutination-inhibition test. The development of immunofluorescent procedures may provide a quicker diagnosis in the future.

Control: Prevention of swine influenza is not practical except in conditions where pigs can be reared free from lungworms. Experimentally, vaccines may confer some protection but it is doubtful whether they are justified economically. There is no specific treatment, but antibiotics, good husbandry and freedom from stress help to reduce losses.

EPERYTHROZOONOSIS

An uncommon sporadic, febrile hemolytic disease of swine, sheep, cattle, cats and other mammals caused by a blood parasite found in the plasma and upon the erythrocytes.

The majority of infections are subclinical and the incidence of overt disease is low. The parasite probably occurs in most countries but the incidence of subclinical infection is not known. Different species of parasite exist in different hosts (e.g., *Eperythrozoon suis, E. ovis*), and each appears to be relatively host-specific. Transmission is by bloodsucking insects.

In clinical cases there are varying degrees of hemolytic anemia, fever, anorexia, weakness and icterus. Most cases are mild, transient and unimportant, and are usually secondary to other conditions. More severe cases have been recorded in young pigs and cats.

Differentiation should be made from nutritional anemias (q.v., p. 17) and from ictero-anemic conditions due to other infectious agents or toxic substances. Laboratory diagnosis of acute eperythrozoonosis may be made upon demonstration of large numbers of the blood parasite in Giemsa-stained film taken early in the disease. Smears should be made from fresh, noncitrated blood to avoid alterations in parasite morphology.

Tetracycline or oxytetracycline given IM at not less than 3 mg/lb of body wt is specific in single doses against *E. suis*. Hematinic drugs, such as sodium cacodylate and iron-dextran are indicated. Chlortetracycline added to the drinking water at the rate of 200 mg/gal. is an effective herd treatment. Close confinement in shade to prevent unnecessary exertion is desirable.

CANINE DISTEMPER

A highly contagious viral disease of dogs characterized by a diphasic temperature elevation, leukopenia, gastrointestinal and respiratory catarrh, and frequently pneumonic and neurologic complications.

Etiology and Epizootiology: Canine distemper virus is universal and unless isolated, most dogs are exposed as puppies. Transmission occurs by the aerosol-droplet route and by contaminated objects. The incubation period is 6 to 9 days but the premonitory signs are subtle, so sickness may not be observed until 2 to 3 weeks after exposure. The disease occurs in the Canidae (dogs, foxes, wolves, etc.), the Mustelidae (mink, ferrets, skunk, etc.), most Procyonidae (raccoon, coati mundi, etc.), and some Viveridae (binturong).

Clinical Findings: Canine distemper begins with an elevated temperature lasting 1 to 3 days. The fever then subsides for several days before a second elevation which lasts a week or more. A leukopenia accompanies the fever and may fluctuate or remain low throughout the illness. Mucopurulent material accumulates in the medial canthus of the eyes, the conjunctivae are reddened, photophobia is evidenced by squinting of the eyes and a mucopurulent nasal discharge is often present. The dog is usually depressed and anorectic and often develops diarrhea. A dog can recover from the above signs and then succumb to nervous complications as: (1) convulsive seizures characterized by inability to stand, jerking movements of the head and jaws, and paddling motions of the legs, or (2) encephalic signs in which the dog wanders aimlessly, unaware of its surroundings. The consequences of infection vary from a mild, inapparent infection to severe disease manifested by most of the above signs. The course of the disease may be as short as 10 days, but more often is prolonged for several weeks or months with intervening periods of abatement followed by a relapse. Sometimes when recovery seems imminent, permanent neurologic residua (chorea, tic, flexor spasm, hyperkinesia) appear, manifested by localized twitching of leg or facial muscles.

Lesions: The virus of canine distemper produces cytoplasmic and intranuclear inclusion bodies in respiratory, urinary and digestive epithelium, and an interstitial giant-cell pneumonia. Other lesions depend upon the severity of the attack and the extent of secondary bacterial infection. These may include inflammation of the mucous membranes of the gastrointestinal tract, hemorrhagic enteritis, splenic enlargement, bronchial pneumonia and a pustular dermatitis of the lower abdomen. Occasional hyperkeratosis of the footpads explains the now defunct term "hardpad disease". Lesions found in the brain of dogs with neurologic complications include Purkinje cell degeneration, gliosis, demyelination, perivascular cuffing, nonsuppurative leptomeningitis and intranuclear inclusion bodies predominately within glial cells.

Diagnosis: Distemper should be considered in any febrile condition in puppies. While the typical clinical case is not difficult to diagnose, sometimes the characteristic signs fail to appear until late in the disease. The clinical picture may be modified by superimposed toxoplasmosis, coccidiosis, ascariasis, infectious canine hepatitis, and numerous viral and bacterial infections. Distemper is sometimes confused with leptospirosis and infectious canine hepatitis. A febrile catarrhal illness with neurologic sequelae justify a diagnosis of distemper. Clinical diagnosis is best confirmed at necropsy by histopathologic lesions or by immunofluorescent assay of virus in tissues. In living patients, conjunctival epithelium can be examined with these procedures. Paired sera may be tested for antibody.

Prophylaxis: Successful immunization of pups with modified live-virus vaccines (℞ 109, 110) or with inactivated-tissue vaccines (℞ 108) depends upon the absence of interfering maternal antibody. The age at which pups can be immunized can be predicted from a nomograph if the serum antibody titer of the mother is known. This service is available in many diagnostic laboratories. When this information is not available, many alternative procedures are used. One is to vaccinate the pup with modified live-virus vaccine when it is first seen (usually about 8 weeks of age), and to repeat the vaccination at 3 to 4 months of age to immunize those dogs which the first dose left unprotected due to interference by maternal antibody. Administration of doses of vaccine at 2-week intervals more nearly approaches the ideal. Immune serum (℞ 107) has been used to passively protect dogs; however, because it may block active immunization, the use of antiserum for short-term protection is discouraged. Active immunization with modified live-virus vaccines is more efficacious. A modified live-virus measles vaccine (℞ 121) is available which can be administered at 3 to 4 weeks of age. The effects of this vaccine are short-lived, but will carry the dog through the early months until later vaccinated with a canine distemper vaccine. Many varieties of inactivated and attenuated distemper vaccine are available and should be used according to manufacturer's directions. Modified live-virus vaccines are generally recommended and annual revaccination is suggested.

Treatment: At the first suspicion of distemper, some clinicians administer repeated large doses of anticanine distemper serum (R 107) or antibody concentrates (R 117); others immediately give modified live-virus vaccine. Both these procedures are of questionable value once clinical signs have developed. Other treatments are directed at limiting secondary bacterial invasion, supporting the fluid balance and the overall well-being of the patient, and controlling nervous manifestations. These include antibiotics, electrolyte solutions, protein hydrolysates, dietary supplements, antipyretics, nasal preparations, analgesics and anticonvulsants (*see* PRESCRIPTION section, p. 1457 et seq.). No one treatment is specific or uniformly successful. Good nursing care with attention to the comfort of the patient is essential, but despite all effort some individuals will fail to make a satisfactory recovery.

Treatment for chorea is usually unavailing, but it may be treated as are other neurologic manifestations of distemper, with antispasmodics and sedatives.

INFECTIOUS CANINE HEPATITIS

A contagious disease of dogs with signs varying from a slight fever and congestion of the mucous membranes to severe depression, marked leukopenia and prolonged bleeding time.

Etiology and Epizootiology: The causal adenovirus produces characteristic intranuclear inclusion bodies in hepatic and endothelial cells. Dogs of all ages are susceptible. Exposure usually occurs by ingestion of virus. Airborne transmission is not considered a problem. Direct transmission can occur during the acute illness, when the virus is present in all secretions and excretions. The virus then localizes in the kidney and is eliminated in urine for months afterwards. Virus-containing urine from recovered dogs can spread the disease. Indirect infection may also occur through fomites. The incubation period is 5 to 9 days. The disease occurs throughout the world, antibodies being detectable in almost 80% of adult dogs.

Clinical Findings: The disease varies from a slight fever to a fatal illness. The first sign is an elevation of temperature above 104°F, lasting from 1 to 6 days. Usually, a "saddle" type temperature curve is seen, with an initial elevation for a day, then a drop to near normal for a day, followed by a secondary rise.

On the day after the initial temperature rise, leukopenia develops, and persists throughout the febrile period. The degree of leukopenia varies, and seems to be correlated with the severity of the illness. If the fever is of short duration, leukopenia may be the only sign, but if the fever lasts more than a day acute illness develops.

Signs are apathy, anorexia, thirst, conjunctivitis and serous discharge from the eyes and nose. Intense hyperemia of the oral mucous membranes may be seen, as well as enlarged tonsils, and occasionally signs of abdominal pain. Vomiting may also be observed. There may be subcut. edema of the head, neck and trunk.

There is direct correlation between the severity of illness and the clotting time. Controlling hemorrhage may be difficult. Interference with blood clotting is manifested by hemorrhage around deciduous teeth and appearance of spontaneous hematomas, and may be demonstrated by nicking the edge of an ear. Respiratory or nervous involvements are not usually seen in dogs. Foxes may show convulsions intermittently during the course of illness, and terminal paralysis involving one or more of the limbs, or the entire body.

Upon recovery, dogs eat well but regain weight slowly. Seven to 10 days after disappearance of acute signs, about 25% of recovered dogs develop "hepatitis blue eye", a transient unilateral or bilateral corneal opacity which disappears spontaneously.

Chronic hepatitis may develop in dogs having low levels of passive antibody when exposed. Simultaneous infection with the viruses of infectious canine hepatitis and distemper is sometimes seen (*see* CANINE DISTEMPER, p. 311).

Lesions: Endothelial damage results in intraocular hemorrhages, bleeding in the mouth, "paint-brush" hemorrhages on the gastric serosa, and hemorrhagic lymph nodes. Hepatic cell necrosis produces varying color changes in the liver, which may be normal in size or swollen. The gallbladder wall may be edematous and thickened; edema or petechial hemorrhages of the thymus may be found.

Diagnosis: Usually, the abrupt onset and prolonged bleeding time suggest infectious hepatitis. Clinical evidence is not always sufficient to differentiate infectious hepatitis from distemper. The diagnosis is confirmed if characteristic intranuclear inclusion bodies are found in the liver.

Prophylaxis: A formalized virus vaccine (℞ 113) can be used alone or in combination with inactivated distemper vaccine (℞ 115). Two inoculations (at least 2 weeks apart) are required. Protection from inactivated vaccine lasts 3 to 6 months and inoculations should be repeated accordingly.

Several attenuated live-virus vaccines are available in combination with distemper vaccines (℞ 115, 116).

A passive protection (which interferes with active immunization) is transferred by immune bitches to puppies. As in distemper, 82% of kenneled puppies became immune to infectious canine hepatitis when vaccinated at 9 weeks of age. Unlike the situation found in distemper, 100% were immune when tested at 1 year of age.

For temporary protection, an antiserum is available. An inoculation of antiserum, 0.25 ml/lb of body wt, will protect a dog against virulent virus. It should be repeated every 10 days.

Treatment: Daily blood transfusions are helpful in seriously ill dogs. In addition, 5% dextrose in isotonic salt solution plus 5% protein hydrolysate in an amount of 250 to 500 ml daily should be given, preferably IV. In patients with prolonged clotting time, subcut. administration of fluids may be dangerous. A broad-spectrum antibiotic (℞ 11, 25, 29) should be administered if the disease is prolonged. It is advisable to give antidistemper and hepatitis serum (℞ 114) or canine immune gamma globulin (℞ 117) to prevent simultaneous infection with distemper.

CANINE HERPES
(Herpesvirus infection of puppies)

A fatal viral infection of infant puppies.

Etiology: The causal virus, presently classed with the herpes group, produces a cytopathic effect in dog kidney cell cultures.

Clinical Findings: Puppies less than one month of age usually die within 24 hours of the onset of illness. Experimentally, the virus causes vaginitis in bitches, and puppies that are infected *in utero* die 1 to 3 weeks after birth.

Lesions: The gross changes consist of focal necrosis and hemorrhages involving the liver and, in particular, the kidneys. The lungs are usually pneumonic as a result of extensive necrosis and there is extensive edema with occasional hemorrhages.

Microscopic examination reveals necrotic lesions in most organs and acidophilic intranuclear inclusion bodies are occasionally seen in cells. The most consistent feature is the occurrence of basophilic globular bodies at the nuclear membrane within the nucleus of the degenerating cells.

Diagnosis: This condition may be confused with infectious canine hepatitis, but it is not accompanied by the thickened, edematous gallbladder often associated with the latter. The focal areas of necrosis and hemorrhage, especially those that occur in the kidneys, distinguish it from hepatitis and toxoplasmosis. Canine herpesvirus causes serious disease only in very young puppies. The rapid death and characteristic lesions distinguish this infection from canine distemper.

Prophylaxis and Treatment: There is no available vaccine. Infected bitches develop antibodies and litters subsequent to the first infected litter will usually not be infected.

Removal of puppies from affected bitches by cesarean section and rearing them in isolation has been successful in preventing deaths under experimental conditions. However, infections have been noted even in cesarean-derived puppies.

Deaths are markedly reduced when infected puppies are reared in incubators at elevated temperatures (95°F, 50% relative humidity). Puppies so reared must be given adequate fluids.

CANINE RICKETTSIAL DISEASES

CANINE EHRLICHIOSIS
(Canine rickettsiosis)

A septicemic disease associated with the presence of rickettsiae in the monocytes and neutrophils. The disease occurs in the Mediterranean basin, almost all parts of Africa, Syria, India, Ceylon, the U.S.A. and Aruba (W. Indies). The disease is infectious for dogs and other closely related Canidae.

Etiology: *Ehrlichia* (*Rickettsia*) *canis*, the causal agent, parasitizes monocytes and neutrophils in which it occurs as colonies of coccoid bodies. *Rhipicephalus sanguineus* is the usual vector. The disease is transmitted through the egg, and the tick is infective in all stages. Infection can be induced by the inoculation of blood or organ emulsions from diseased animals.

Clinical Findings: The incubation period varies from 7 to 21 days. The disease is characterized by recurrent fever, muco-purulent discharge from the nose and eyes, vomiting, fetid breath, emaciation and enlargement of the spleen. Erythemato-pustular eruption of the axilla and groin is sometimes seen. Hyperesthesia, convulsions, hysteria, meningoencephalitis and paralysis may occur. Erosions of the buccal mucosa and skin, edema of the hindquarters, ascites, hydrothorax and gastro-enteritis are the most common signs. The death rate may be high, especially if the disease is complicated by babesiasis, trypanosomiasis or haemobartonellosis. Recovered animals re-tain a latent infection. Upon necropsy, ulcerations in the ali-mentary canal, subendocardial hemorrhages, edema of lungs, mottling of liver and kidneys, and a swollen spleen are usually found.

Diagnosis: Blood films made on approximately the 13th day after infection should be examined for rickettsiae. Impression smears from organs also show the parasites. Characteristic signs with the finding of rickettsial bodies in the monocytes and neutrophils are suggestive. The disease is often compli-cated by concurrent infections with red blood cell parasites transmitted by the same tick vector. Splenectomy unmasks the carrier state.

Prophylaxis and Treatment: Tick infestation should be con-trolled. Sulfamethazine (R 82), chlortetracycline (R 11) and oxytetracycline (R 25) are specific. Good nursing is important in aiding recovery. Treatment of concurrent babesiasis (q.v., p. 442) or trypanosomiasis (q.v., p. 432) is essential.

SALMON POISONING COMPLEX

An acute infectious disease complex (not a toxicosis) of the dog family in which the infective agents are transmitted through the various stages of a fluke with a snail-fish-dog life cycle.

Etiology: The disease complex is the result of 2 etiologic agents: (a) *Neorickettsia helminthoeca* and (b) the Elokomin fluke fever agent. *N. helminthoeca* has not been isolated singly in nature. The transmitting vector is a small fluke, *Nanophy-etus salmincola*. The dog becomes infected by ingesting trout or salmon that contain rickettsia-infected, encysted metacerca-riae of the fluke. These may occur throughout the fish, but are especially numerous in the kidney. In the dog's intestine, the larval flukes are digested free, embed in the duodenal mucosa, and introduce the 2 causal agents. Fluke infection alone produces little or no clinical disease.

The infection is apparently maintained by the elimination of infected fluke ova in the feces of the dog or other host. From these, ova develop larval stages which may successively infect the snail and the fish and culminate in the metacercarial stage in the fish. A second dog, eating such fish, completes the parasite cycle and at the same time becomes infected with *Rickettsia*. Dog-to-dog transmission occurs both by aerosol and per rectum by dirty thermometers.

Age, sex and breed appear to be of no importance. The disease may appear at any time, but is more frequent when fish are most accessible. Infected fish are found in the Pacific Ocean from San Francisco, California, to the 59th parallel (off the coast of Alaska). Salmon poisoning in dogs is most frequently reported from northern California to Puget Sound. It is more prevalent west of the Cascade Mountains but is also seen inland along the rivers of fish migration. Mortality in untreated natural infections ranges from 50 to 90%.

Clinical Findings: Signs usually appear suddenly 5 to 9 days after eating infected fish and usually persist for 7 to 10 days. During the first or second day of signs, the body temperature reaches 104° to 106°F and persists or falls slightly during the next few days and is accompanied by great depression and almost complete anorexia. After a febrile peak the temperature drops to below normal before death ensues. At first, there may be diarrhea or the feces may be scanty, frothy and yellowish, but usually soon become bloody. Sometimes almost pure blood is passed. Vomiting occurs at this time. Dehydration and extreme weight loss are conspicuous in the later stages. Thirst is marked but drinking leads promptly to vomiting. Nasal or conjunctival exudate may be observed.

Diagnosis may be confirmed by finding fluke ova in the feces. The ova are oval, yellowish brown, rough-surfaced, about 50 to 75 μ in size and possess an indistinct operculum. During the first day or two, ova may be too scanty to be found readily in direct smear. All lymph nodes are usually enlarged.

Lesions: The disease complex appears to affect chiefly the lymphoid tissue and intestine. Alimentary tract lymph follicles, lymph nodes, tonsils, thymus and, to some extent, the spleen show enlargement with microscopic necrosis, some hemorrhage and hyperplasia. A variable but often severe hemorrhagic enteritis is seen throughout the intestine. This seems to arise from damaged lymph follicles. Microscopic necrotic foci also appear apart from follicles. Flukes embedded in the duodenum account for little tissue damage.

Prophylaxis and Treatment: No vaccine or other prophylactic is currently available. Immunity in recovered cases is strong and persistent.

Various sulfonamides given orally or parenterally have been successful in treatment. Dosage at therapeutic blood levels should be maintained at least 3 days. Experimentally, good results have been obtained with chlortetracycline, chloramphenicol and oxytetracycline. The best results follow administration of large divided doses. If the animal is dehydrated, IV fluid therapy is essential to avoid nephrotoxic effects. General supportive treatment, aimed at correcting and maintaining fluid and electrolyte balance, providing nutritional requirements and controlling diarrhea, often is essential unless there is a prompt favorable response. Treatment in the late stages may not be beneficial.

ELOKOMIN FLUKE FEVER

A fluke-transmitted disease resembling rickettsial infections, of the canine family, bears, raccoons and ferrets. It is seen alone or as a complicating agent in the salmon poisoning complex. It utilizes *Nanophyetus salmincola* in the same manner as described for the salmon poisoning complex. The Elokomin fluke fever agent (as yet unnamed) resembles *Neorickettsia helminthoeca* but is differentiated from it by animal cross-protection, serum neutralization and its wider host range. This agent produces a mortality of less than 10%.

Clinical Findings: The incubation period is longer than seen in the salmon poisoning complex, 9 to 14 days on primary isolation. The temperature curve is of the plateau type with persistence of fever for 4 to 7 days. The bloody diarrhea is absent as is the severe dehydration. Generalized somatic lymph node enlargement is striking. Although the mortality is low, many dogs will exhibit severe weight loss that persists for long periods. Fluke eggs are seen on fecal examination. The lesions of uncomplicated Elokomin fluke fever resemble those seen in the salmon poisoning complex, in which it plays a part, except that the severe intestinal lesions are lacking. There are no prophylactic measures, while treatment follows that of the salmon poisoning complex (*see* above).

FELINE PANLEUKOPENIA
(Feline infectious enteritis, Feline distemper, Feline agranulocytosis, Feline ataxia)

A highly contagious disease of cats, characterized by sudden onset, fever, anorexia, depression, dehydration, marked leukopenia and high mortality.

Etiology and Epizootiology: The disease is caused by a small DNA virus which attacks all members of the cat family (Felidae) and the raccoon, coati mundi, and kinkajou in the raccoon family (Procyonidae). Panleukopenia virus or the antigenically identical mink enteritis virus causes gastrointestinal disease in mink. All secretions and excretions of affected animals contain virus and the infection spreads through direct contact or by means of material contaminated with virus.

Clinical Findings: The incubation period varies from 4 to 10 days. With the onset of fever, animals stop eating, vomit and become depressed and weak. Diarrhea may occur 2 to 4 days after the initial temperature rise. Extreme dehydration occurs rapidly although affected cats seem to desire water. Shortly before the temperature becomes elevated, there is a decrease in leukocytes, later the leukopenia increases markedly to the point that sometimes few leukocytes can be found. The granulocytes are chiefly affected so that a differential cell count will show the few remaining cells to be of the lymphoid series. If the cat recovers, a compensatory leukocytosis may occur. The course of the disease seldom exceeds 5 to 7 days. Mortality is high, especially in young cats, and losses from 60 to 90% are reported. Infection of kittens *in utero* or within a few days after birth results in the destruction of the external granular layer of the cerebellum (cerebellar hypoplasia) which is manifest clinically by incoordination noted when the kitten begins to walk (feline cerebellar ataxia).

Lesions: Lesions correlate closely with signs of illness. There is marked evidence of dehydration and emaciation except in very acute cases where gross changes may be negligible. The first changes are found in lymph nodes and consist of hyperplasia, edema and necrosis. Later, the red marrow of the long bones may become semifluid and appear fatty. Reddening may be seen in the terminal portion of the ileum and sometimes extends to involve most of the small intestine. Microscopically, the epithelium of the villi of affected portions of the intestine shows degeneration and the intestinal wall may be edematous. The liver, kidneys and spleen may appear slightly swollen.

Degeneration of liver cells and tubular epithelium of the kidney is seen. Intranuclear inclusion bodies are found in the cells of the intestinal epithelium and lymph nodes; however, these can be found consistently only early in the disease and may not be found in cats surviving 3 to 4 days. When recovery occurs, a marked myelogenous cellular response is seen.

Prophylaxis and Treatment: Recovered cats are immune. Homologous antiserum (℞ 123) offers good protection for about 10 days. Active immunity is conferred by inactivated vaccines made from tissues of infected cats (℞ 111), feline tissue culture (℞ 112) and mink enteritis virus with adjuvants (℞ 119). Repeated annual vaccination is recommended. An attenuated live virus vaccine (℞ 131) is also available and appears to give an early and long lasting immunity, although it should not be given to pregnant cats or to kittens less than 4 weeks old.

Since antibodies, passively transmitted to the kittens by an immune dam, may interfere with the establishment of active immunity, it is recommended that kittens be vaccinated after weaning at 8 to 10 weeks of age. To assure that maternally transmitted antibodies are no longer at a possibly interfering level, a second dose at 16 weeks of age is recommended.

Treatment should be aimed at combating dehydration, providing nutrients and electrolytes, and preventing secondary infection. During the first few days of treatment, medication should be given parenterally since most patients with panleukopenia will vomit oral medication. Whole-blood transfusions are of considerable value. Five to 10 ml of blood per pound of body weight should be administered daily or every other day during the acute phase of the disease. Dehydration should be counteracted with fluids given subcut. at a rate of approximately 10 ml/lb of body wt per day. A balanced electrolyte solution, Ringer's or lactated Ringer's (℞ 565, 566), is preferred for this treatment. Broad-spectrum antibiotics, e.g., chlortetracycline (℞ 11), oxytetracycline (℞ 25, 29) or chloramphenicol (℞ 7) may be of value in combating secondary infections. Given at the rate of 2 ml/lb of body wt per day in the very early stages of the disease, antiserum may be of some value.

FELINE RESPIRATORY DISEASES

A group of highly contagious upper respiratory infections characterized by sneezing, lacrimation, conjunctivitis and rhinitis. This group includes pneumonitis as well as feline rhinotracheitis, and infections with other viruses often denoted as coryza, influenza or chronic respiratory disease.

Etiology: Feline rhinotracheitis virus, perhaps the most common cause of upper respiratory infections in cats, belongs to the herpes group. In addition to herpesvirus, picornaviruses and reovirus have been isolated from the respiratory tract of cats showing signs of rhinitis and conjunctivitis. The etiologic agent of feline pneumonitis, *Chlamydia psittaci,* belongs to the psittacosis-lymphogranuloma venereum group of organisms. Natural transmission of these agents occurs by the aerosol-droplet route. The incubation period is generally 2 to 6 days, perhaps up to 10 days in the case of pneumonitis, and as long as 19 days with reovirus.

Clinical Findings: The diseases produced by many of these agents are clinically indistinguishable. The onset is marked by frequent sneezing, conjunctivitis, fever and often by salivation. Excitement or movement may accelerate the sneezing. The fever may initially reach 105°F, but soon subsides, tending to fluctuate from normal to 103°F. Initially, serous nasal and ocular discharges are noted. These soon become mucopurulent and copious. By this time depression and anorexia are evident. Ulcers may appear on the dorsal surface of the tongue. Picornavirus infection may produce a severe pulmonary edema and pneumonia. Reovirus infections exhibit no fever and no nasal discharge, and may be restricted to the eye. The respiratory virus diseases tend to be most severe in young kittens. Signs in adults may be limited to sneezing and a slight serous conjunctivitis and rhinitis. Signs may persist for 5 to 10 days in milder cases, up to 3 to 6 weeks in severe cases. Mortality is generally low and prognosis for eventual recovery is usually good with the possible exception of picornavirus pneumonia and rhinotracheitis in young kittens. In any case, the owner should be cautioned that illness is often prolonged, marked weight loss may occur, and that these diseases are occasionally complicated by bacterial infection resulting in pneumonia, meningitis or intractable frontal sinusitis. The agents apparently persist in the cat for long periods and all signs may recur if the patient is stressed.

Lesions: Lesions are confined to the respiratory tract and conjunctiva. The conjunctiva and nasal mucous membranes are reddened, swollen and covered with a serous to purulent exudate. In severe cases of rhinotracheitis, focal necrosis of the mucosa of the nasal passages and turbinates may occur. The larynx and trachea may be mildly inflamed. The lungs may be congested and show small areas of consolidation; however, the pulmonary lesions are not usually remarkable except in picornavirus pneumonia. Ulcerative glossitis and ulcerative stomatitis may occur. The characteristic histopathologic lesion of rhinotracheitis is the acidophilic intranuclear inclusion body in the epithelial cells of the nasal membranes, tonsils, epiglottis, trachea and nictitating membrane. However, because of their transitory nature the inclusions are not demonstrable in long standing cases. These inclusions have not been demonstrated in other upper respiratory virus infections of cats. In the case of pneumonitis, Giemsa-stained sections will demonstrate elementary bodies in the cytoplasm of mononuclear cells from the alveolar and bronchial exudate.

Diagnosis: A presumptive diagnosis is based on the typical signs of sneezing, fever, conjunctivitis and rhinitis. Cytologic examination of Giemsa-stained conjunctival scrapings is of diagnostic value for the feline pneumonitis agent. Definitive positive diagnosis is based upon isolation and identification of the agent from the nasal and ocular secretions.

Prophylaxis and Treatment: A modified live vaccine of egg origin (℞ 122) is available for the prevention of pneumonitis; however, it has no effect against the respiratory viruses. Many antigenically distinct viruses are involved and a natural infection with one does not produce immunity or protect against others. The avoidance of exposure to sick cats, overcrowding and stress provides the best protection against the upper respiratory diseases.

Treatment is largely symptomatic and supportive but the broad-spectrum antibiotics (e.g., ℞ 7, 11, 25, 29) are useful against secondary invaders as well as directly against *Ch. psittaci.* Nasal and ocular discharges should be removed frequently for the comfort of the patient. Nose drops containing a vasoconstrictor and antibiotics (℞ 445, 454) and a bland ophthalmic ointment containing antibiotics (℞ 372, 375, 383) may be helpful. If dyspnea is severe, the animal may be placed in an oxygen tent. Supportive fluids (℞ 561, 566, 567) may be indicated to correct dehydration and force-feeding may be necessary to prevent the severe weight loss. Antihistamines (℞ 534) may be beneficial early in the course of the disease.

FELINE INFECTIOUS PERITONITIS
AND PLEURITIS

A chronic fatal infectious disease of domestic cats and larger Felidae occurring in all ages but more commonly in 1- to 2-year-old cats, especially males. No etiologic agent has yet been isolated, although a virus is suspected. The disease is characterized by an insidious onset, anorexia, depression, dehydration, wasting, dyspnea and abdominal enlargement. Fever (103° to 105°F) is common, more severely affected cats are moribund with a subnormal temperature. Some cats are anemic and exhibit vomiting or diarrhea.

A diagnosis is based on the history of a persistent antibiotic-resistant fever, chronic debilitation, and the presence of usually abundant fluid exudate in the peritoneal or pleural cavity or both. The fluid is characteristically pale yellow to dark amber, clear or slightly cloudy, and has the consistency of syrup and a high specific gravity (1.018 to 1.047). Few cells are found in the exudate, but the protein content is high. Strands or flocculent particles of fibrin are seen grossly and on stained smears. Hemograms typically reveal moderate to severe anemia, relative neutrophilia, and a mild lymphopenia. A shift in serum-protein A/G ratio and an absolute hypergammaglobulinemia is found in most cases. Radiographically there is a homogenous "ground glass" fluid density in the thorax or abdomen, obscuring visceral detail.

The duration of illness is usually 2 to 6 weeks. Treatment is ineffective.

FELINE INFECTIOUS ANEMIA

An acute or chronic anemia of domestic cats caused by a rickettsial agent which multiplies within the vascular system.

Etiology: Infectious anemia of cats is recognized in many parts of the world. The causative agent is generally agreed to be *Haemobartonella felis*, a small, coccoid, rodlike, or ringlike organism. Dimensions of these structures vary from a diameter of 0.2 to 1.0 μ for the coccoid forms and up to 3.0 μ in length for the rod forms. The organisms are usually found in varying numbers on the surface of erythrocytes, but are occasionally seen free in the plasma. They appear as dark red-violet bodies in thin blood smears stained with Wright's or Giemsa stain. The number of red cells affected varies with the severity of infection and with the stage in the life cycle of the parasite. Blood smears made during certain stages of the disease show no parasites. The disease can be transmitted experimentally by parenteral or oral transfer of small amounts of infected whole blood into susceptible cats.

In experimentally induced cases the incubation period varies from 1 to 5 weeks, and recovery does not induce immunity to reinfection.

Methods of natural transmission have not been established; however, there appears to be a higher incidence among cats, particularly males, 1 to 3 years of age. A significant portion of the cat population may carry the infection in a latent form, which becomes exacerbated in the presence of various debilitating diseases or stresses.

Clinical Findings: Any anemic cat may justly be suspected of having feline infectious anemia. In acute cases, there is usually a fever of 103° to 106°F. Jaundice, anorexia, depression, weakness and splenomegaly are common signs. In chronic or slowly developing cases there may be normal or subnormal temperature, weakness, depression and emaciation, but there is less likely to be jaundice and splenomegaly. Dyspnea in both instances varies with the degree of anemia. Gross necropsy findings are not distinctive. The spleen and mesenteric lymph nodes may be enlarged and a bone marrow hyperplasia may be present.

Diagnosis: Laboratory confirmation depends upon identification of the parasite. A series of smears over a period of several days may be required for an accurate diagnosis, since the erythrocytic bodies show up only periodically. Certain artifacts may be mistaken for blood parasites and must be carefully eliminated. The organisms are readily demonstrated in the affected cells when stained with acridine orange and examined under an ultraviolet microscope.

Blood cell changes typical of a regenerative anemia are present in positive smears. These include diffuse basophilia in the larger cells, nucleated erythrocytes, anisocytosis, Howell-Jolly bodies and an increased number of recticulocytes. Red cell counts may fall as low as 1 million per cubic millimeter. Hemoglobin values of 7 gm or less per 100 ml of blood are seen. Mean corpuscular volumes (average cell size) increase. There is a moderate increase in WBC counts with monocytosis in the acute forms of the disease, normal counts in the chronic forms and leukopenia in the moribund cases of the disease.

Prophylaxis and Treatment: Blood transfusion is the most effective treatment, particularly in acutely anemic cases. From 30 to 80 ml of whole blood should be given and repeated as required, perhaps every second or third day. Oxytetracycline (℞ 29), tetracycline hydrochloride (℞ 58) or chloramphenicol

(℞ 7) should be given in full doses. To prevent relapses, drug treatments should be continued over a period of 10 to 20 days. Thiacetarsamide sodium (Caparsolate), an arsenical compound, given IV is reported to be effective; dosage is 0.5 ml/10 lb on day 1, and repeated on day 3. Toxic reactions may occur, and transfusion should precede dosing if the hematocrit is less than 20%.

In view of limited knowledge about the transmission of this disease, little can be recommended with reference to prophylaxis. Extreme care, however, should be exercised in selecting blood donor cats for general transfusions. Such donors should be checked for evidence of the carrier state by trial transfusion into susceptible experimental kittens.

ROCKY MOUNTAIN SPOTTED FEVER

An acute, infectious, febrile disease of man that varies from a mild to a rapidly fatal infection. It is widely distributed in the Western Hemisphere. Its interest to veterinarians arises in that the etiologic agent, *Rickettsia rickettsii,* is maintained in animals and is transmitted to man solely by certain ticks that feed on animal hosts, including man. It multiplies in the cells of the small peripheral blood vessels resulting in thrombosis and extravasation. The rash starts on the extremities and extends to the body. The disease may be reproduced experimentally in guinea pigs and monkeys. Rabbits, young sheep and young dogs are mildly susceptible.

Epizootiology: The maintenance of the organism in nature depends largely on ticks and the animals upon which they feed—rodents, rabbits and hares. In the U.S.A., 5 species of ticks have been recognized as natural carriers of the organism. They are: *Dermacentor andersoni, D. variabilis, Amblyomma americanum, Haemaphysalis leporispalustris* and *D. parumapertus.* The infected tick passes the organism through the egg to its offspring, and the ticks, in any stage of the life cycle, may transmit the infection during feeding.

Exposure may be occupational or recreational, or infected ticks may be brought into the household by dogs. Infected starving ticks seem to harbor an attenuated form of the organism. However, after the ticks have been warmed and allowed to feed, the rickettsiae become virulent. This transition to the virulent form, called "reactivation", may account for the observation that ticks will not transmit disease unless they have fed for several hours.

Transmission of *R. rickettsii* to man and animals is accomplished in most instances through the bite of a tick. It has also been shown that the crushed tissues and feces of infected ticks may spread the infection to the conjunctiva or abraded surfaces of individuals.

Diagnosis: Isolation of the organism or demonstration of its presence in ticks by immunologic methods is a common procedure; however, isolation from naturally infected animals is rarely accomplished. Therefore, in animals, the Weil-Felix (complement-fixation) test is used alone or together with isolation of the organism from ticks feeding on the animal.

Control: Vaccines diminish the severity of, but do not eliminate the disease in man; none are available for domestic animals. Control of tick populations is difficult. Wide-strip spraying of insecticides (℞ 271, 304) around yards, barns, kennels, corrals, holding pens and along trails will control *D. variabilis* and *A. americanum*. Elimination of the small host mammals has been more effective in *D. andersoni* areas.

Clothing barriers can be created by having each outer clothing layer overlap the one above it, e.g., trouser legs tucked in socks. Tick repellents also help (*see* TICK PARALYSIS, p. 721). Since ticks seldom attach themselves immediately and must feed for several hours to transmit the organism, removal of clothing twice a day and searching for ticks is effective. Ticks should be removed with extreme care. The tick should be grasped with forceps, gloves or a piece of paper to avoid contamination of the fingers. Care should be exercised to avoid breaking off the mouth parts in the skin. The wound then should be treated with tincture of iodine.

Q FEVER

A rickettsial infection of man and animals, usually inapparent, but occasionally causing human outbreaks of influenza-like disease; rarely causing chronic endocarditis in man and abortion in sheep and goats.

Etiology and Epidemiology: The etiologic agent *Coxiella* (*Rickettsia*) *burnetii* has worldwide distribution and reservoirs in ticks, cattle, sheep, goats and bandicoots. It is resistant to many disinfectants and desiccation. In enzootic areas, antibody prevalence approaches 80%. The agent escapes from reservoir-hosts in placental materials and milk and during meat processing or necropsy. Transmission to man may be airborne or by direct contact. Tick-to-animal cycles exist in nature.

Diagnosis: Rarely diagnosed clinically, infection is confirmed serologically by complement-fixation or agglutination tests or by isolation of the agent from human blood, milk or placental materials from animals.

Treatment and Control: Man is treated with tetracyclines. Pasteurization of milk and careful disposal of animal placentas reduce infection. An inactivated vaccine has been used to protect laboratory workers.

ANTHRAX
(Splenic fever, Charbon, Milzbrand)

An acute, febrile disease of virtually all animals and man caused by *Bacillus anthracis*. In its most common form, it is essentially a septicemia characterized principally by a rapidly fatal course.

Anthrax has worldwide distribution. Districts where repeated anthrax outbreaks occur exist in southern Europe, parts of Africa, Australia, Asia and North and South America. In the U.S.A., there are recognized areas of infection in South Dakota, Nebraska, Arkansas, Mississippi, Louisiana, Texas and California. Small areas exist in a number of other states.

Etiology: *Bacillus anthracis* is a gram-positive, nonmotile, spore-forming bacterium of relatively large size (4 to 8 $\mu \times 1$ to 1.5 μ). The bacilli grow in chain formation, but may occur singly or in pairs. They form spores, which are centrally located in the cell, after discharge from an infected animal or an opened carcass. The spores are resistant to heat, low temperature, chemical disinfectants and prolonged drying. They may persist for long periods in dry products as feed, animal by-products, stored contaminated objects or in soil.

Outbreaks of anthrax commonly are associated with neutral or alkaline, calcareous soils which have become "incubator areas" for the organisms. In these areas, the spores apparently revert to the vegetative form and multiply when optimum environmental conditions, as soil, moisture, temperature and nutrition, exist. The organisms then have an increased capability to form more spores as environment and biological competition remain favorable. Cattle, horses, mules, sheep and goats may readily become infected when grazing such areas. Infection may also be caused by consumption of contaminated natural or artificial feedstuffs, as bone meal, oil cake and tankage. Swine, dogs, cats, mink and wild animals in captivity frequently acquire the disease from consumption of contaminated meat.

Man may develop localized lesions (malignant pustule or malignant carbuncle) from contact with infected blood or tissues, or acquire a fatal pneumonia (woolsorter's disease) from spore inhalation when handling animal by-products. Occasionally, he develops acute meningitis from systemic involvement, or intestinal anthrax from consumption of meat.

Clinical Findings: The disease occurs in peracute, acute, chronic and cutaneous foims. The **peracute** form is characterized by its sudden onset and rapidly fatal course. Staggering, difficult breathing, trembling, collapse, a few convulsive movements, and death may occur in cattle, sheep or goats, without showing any previous evidence of illness.

In **acute** anthrax of cattle, horses and sheep, there is first a rise in body temperature and a period of excitement followed by depression, stupor, respiratory or cardiac distress, staggering, convulsion and death. During the course of the disease, the body temperature may reach 107°F, rumination ceases, milk production is materiallly reduced, and pregnant animals may abort. Bloody discharges may occur from the natural body openings. Horses may show fever, chills, severe colic, loss of appetite, extreme depression, muscular weakness, a bloody diarrhea and swellings in the region of the neck, sternum, lower abdomen and external genitalia.

The **chronic** form of anthrax with local lesions confined to the tongue and throat is observed mostly in swine, but occurs occasionally in cattle, horses and dogs.

In swine, some animals in a group may die of acute anthrax without having shown any previous signs of illness. Others may show rapidly progressing swelling about the throat, which, in some cases, causes death by suffocation. Many of the group may develop the disease in a mild chronic form and make a gradual recovery. However, some of these when presented for slaughter as normal animals may show evidence of anthrax infection in the cervical lymph nodes and tonsils.

A **cutaneous** or localized form of anthrax, characterized by swellings in various parts of the body, occurs in cattle and horses when anthrax organisms lodge in wounds or abrasions of the skin.

The carcass of an animal dead of anthrax should not be subjected to necropsy. Rigor mortis is frequently absent or incomplete. There may be dark blood oozing from the nostrils and anus with marked bloating and rapid body decomposition. If the carcass is inadvertently opened, septicemic lesions are observed. The blood is dark, thickened and fails to clot readily. Edematous, red-tinged effusions are present and small hemorrhages are common in the subcutis and are frequently seen in serous and mucous membranes. An enlarged, soft spleen of semifluid consistency and dark-red or black color is common. The liver, kidneys and lymph nodes are usually congested and enlarged.

Diagnosis: A diagnosis based on clinical signs may be difficult, especially when the disease occurs in a new area. Therefore, laboratory examination should be utilized to confirm a tentative clinical diagnosis. Blood should be collected aseptically from a peripheral vessel shortly after death and sent to the laboratory on sterile cotton swabs, gauze or suture tape, or as blood smears. The smears should be dried and kept separated during shipment. Tissue specimens obtained at death should be of small size, placed in clean glass containers and sent to the laboratory in sealed, metal mailing tubes surrounded by dry ice and labeled "suspected anthrax". In the case of swine, cervical lymph nodes packed in borax can be sent to the laboratory, as anthrax organisms rarely occur in the blood stream. Usually, ears and splenic tissue are unsatisfactory for making a laboratory diagnosis.

At the laboratory, the methods commonly used in identifying the disease comprise (1) microscopic examination of blood smears stained with polychrome methylene blue or Giemsa to demonstrate encapsulated bacilli; (2) observance of death of guinea pigs or mice within 48 hours following inoculation of blood or tissue suspension, and organism demonstration from stained smears of the blood and spleen; (3) identification of the organism by its growth and characteristics from culture inoculation of blood or tissue suspension, or both, and (4) the use of bacteriophage identification of anthrax bacilli from nonpathogenic bacilli.

Anthrax must be differentiated from other conditions causing sudden death. In cattle and sheep, the clostridial infections and lightning stroke may be confused with it. Also, acute leptospirosis, bacillary hemoglobinuria, anaplasmosis, and acute poisonings from bracken fern, sweet clover and lead must be considered in cattle. In horses, acute infectious anemia, purpura, the various colics, lead poisoning, lightning stroke and sunstroke may resemble anthrax. In swine, acute hog cholera and pharyngeal malignant edema, and in dogs, acute systemic infections and pharyngeal swellings from other causes must be considered.

Treatment and Control: Since anthrax is a highly fatal herd disease, early treatment and rigid control procedures are essential to control it. When an outbreak occurs it is best to use antibiotics for the sick animals and immunize all apparently well animals in the infected herd and surrounding community. In mature cattle and horses, penicillin (℞ 44) administered at levels up to 6 million units or more daily gives good responses in the early stages of the disease. Oxytetracycline (℞ 33) given IV at a daily dosage of 5 gm in divided doses will maintain adequate blood levels to combat the infection. Other antibiotics, e.g., chloramphenicol (℞ 7), erythromycin (℞ 18) or sulfonamides (℞ 82, 85, 86, 90) can also be utilized, but they are less effective than penicillin or the tetracyclines. Prophylactic use of penicillin for exposed cattle has been successful.

Anthrax of livestock can be largely controlled by annual prophylactic vaccination of all animals in the endemic area and the initiation of good control procedures. The noncapsulated Sterne-strain vaccine has essentially replaced the previously used Pasteur-attenuated-spore vaccines. It can be used with comparative safety on all species of livestock, and it produces a high degree of immunity.

Specific control procedures, besides therapy and immunization, are necessary to contain the disease and prevent its spread. These procedures are: (1) notification of the appropriate regulatory official of the disease outbreak; (2) rigidly enforced quarantine of the infected premises or area; (3) prompt disposal of dead animals by cremation or deep burial; (4) destruction of manure, bedding or other contaminated material by burning; (5) isolation of sick animals and removal of well animals from the incubator areas; (6) disinfection of stables, pens, milking barns and equipment used on livestock; (7) use of insect repellents; (8) control of scavengers feeding on animals dead from the disease; (9) general sanitary procedures for persons who contact diseased animals, for their own safety, and to prevent spread of the disease.

CLOSTRIDIAL INFECTIONS

All members of the genus *Clostridium* are relatively large, anaerobic, spore-forming, rod-shaped organisms. The spores are oval, sometimes spherical, and are subterminal or terminal in position. The vegetative forms of the clostridia in the tissue fluids of infected animals occur singly, in pairs, or, rarely, in chains. Differentiation of the various pathogenic and related species is based on cultural characteristics, spore shape and position, and the serologic specificity of the toxin or the somatic antigens. The natural habitats of the organisms are the soil and intestinal tract of animals and man. Pathogenic strains may be acquired by susceptible animals either by wound contamination or by ingestion. The diseases thus produced are a constant threat to successful livestock production in many parts of the world.

The diseases caused by members of the clostridial group can be divided into 2 categories: (1) those in which the organisms actively invade and reproduce in the tissues of the host with the production of toxins that enhance the spread of infection and are responsible for death; (2) those which are characterized by toxemia resulting from the absorption of toxins produced by the organisms within the digestive system (the enterotoxemias) or in food or carrion outside the body (botulism). If treatment of the first group is to be attempted, large doses of antibiotic are indicated to establish effective levels in the center of necrotic tissue where clostridia are to be found.

MALIGNANT EDEMA

An acute, generally fatal toxemia of cattle, horses, sheep, goats and swine usually caused by *Clostridium septicum* and often accompanied by other organisms. A similar infection has often been seen in man. The disease is worldwide in distribution.

Etiology and Routes of Infection: *Cl. septicum* is found in soil and intestinal contents of animals and man throughout the world. The great majority of strains are potentially virulent, unlike most other pathogens. Infection ordinarily occurs through contamination of wounds containing devitalized tissue, soil or some other tissue-debilitant. Wounds caused by accident, castration, docking, unsanitary vaccination and parturition may become infected.

Clinical Findings and Diagnosis: General signs, such as anorexia, intoxication and higher fever, as well as local signs, develop within a few hours to a few days after predisposing injury. The local lesions are soft swellings that pit on pressure and extend rapidly because of the formation of large quantities of exudate that infiltrate the subcut. and IM connective tissue of the affected areas. The muscle in such areas is dark-brown to black. Accumulations of gas are uncommon. Similarity to blackleg is marked, and differentiation made on necropsy is unreliable; laboratory confirmation is the only certain procedure. Horses and swine are susceptible to malignant edema, but not to blackleg.

Rapid confirmation of a diagnosis can be made on the basis of fluorescent antibody staining of the *Cl. septicum* cells from a tissue smear. This cannot be relied upon, however, if the animal has been dead for 24 hours or more, for *Cl. septicum* is an extremely active postmortem invader from the intestine and, consequently, demonstration of its presence in a specimen taken from such a carcass is not significant.

"Braxy" is a type of gas gangrene of the abomasum of sheep due to the action of *Cl. septicum*. It occurs principally in Iceland, Norway and Scotland. The ingestion of frozen grass or roots is thought to be a contributing factor. The wall of the abomasum is edematous, hemorrhagic and necrotic. Lambs are affected during their first winter on pasture or forage crops, and the course is rapidly fatal. If they survive one winter on an infected pasture, they are immune for life.

Prophylaxis and Treatment: Immunization against *Cl. septicum* infection is attained by the use of bacterins as in blackleg. *Cl. septicum* is usually combined with *Cl. chauvoei* (*feseri*) in a blackleg-malignant-edema vaccine (℞ 105). Two doses, some months apart, the first year of life, generally give protection. Annual vaccination is indicated in highly infective areas. In these areas, revaccination is suggested following the occurrence of severe trauma.

Treatment with high doses of penicillin (℞ 44) or broad-spectrum antibiotics (℞ 7, 11, 33, 58) is indicated early in the disease. The animal may be saved in later cases, but the affected tissues may slough, rendering the animal useless.

BLACKLEG

An acute, febrile disease of cattle and sheep caused by *Clostridium chauvoei* (*feseri*) and characterized by emphysematous swelling, usually in the heavy muscles. The disease is worldwide in distribution.

Etiology and Routes of Infection: *Cl. chauvoei* has as its principal habitat the intestinal tract of animals. It probably can remain viable in the soil for considerable periods, although it does not actively grow there. The organisms are probably ingested, pass through the wall of the digestive tract and, after gaining access to the blood stream, are deposited in muscle and other tissues.

In cattle, blackleg infection is usually endogenous, in contrast to malignant edema. The majority of lesions develop spontaneously, being associated with wounds, bruises, or other injuries. Commonly, the animals that contract blackleg are of the beef breeds, in excellent health, gaining weight and usually the best animals of their group. Most cases occur in the first 2 years of life. Animals under 6 months of age are seldom affected, probably being protected by maternal immunity. In sheep, the disease is not restricted to the young, and most cases follow some form of injury such as shearing cuts, docking, crutching or castration. Endogenous blackleg in sheep is uncommon in the U.S.A.; it is much more common in New Zealand where blackleg is seen more frequently in sheep than in cattle.

Clinical Findings: As with other endogenous infections, there is no definite incubation period. Usually within 1 to 5 days, acute lameness, accompanied by depression and fever, develops. Characteristic edematous and crepitant swellings develop in the hip, shoulder, chest, back, neck or elsewhere. At first, the swelling is small, hot and painful. As the disease rapidly progresses, the swelling enlarges, there is crepitation on palpation, and the skin becomes cold and insensitive as the blood supply to the area diminishes. General signs include prostration and tremors. Death occurs in 12 to 48 hours.

Diagnosis: The occurrence of a rapidly fatal febrile disease in well-nourished young cattle, particularly of the beef breeds, with crepitant swellings of the heavy muscles suggests a diagnosis of blackleg. The affected muscle is dark red to black, dry and spongy, has a sweetish odor and is infiltrated with small bubbles, but with little edema. The lesions may be in any muscle, even in the tongue or diaphragm. In sheep, since the lesions of the spontaneously occurring type are often small and deep, they may be easily overlooked. Occasionally, the tissue changes caused by *Cl. septicum*, *Cl. novyi*, *Cl. sordelli*, and *Cl. perfringens* may resemble those of blackleg, and at times both *Cl. septicum* and *Cl. chauvoei* may be isolated from blackleg lesions. This is particularly the case when the carcass has been examined 24 hours or more after death, giving time for postmortem invasion of the tissues by *Cl. septicum*. Confirmation of a field diagnosis can be made by laboratory examination of tissue specimens. These should be taken as soon after death as possible. The fluorescent antibody test for *Cl. chauvoei* is quickly carried out and is quite reliable.

Control: A bacterin (℞ 105) containing *Cl. chauvoei* and *Cl. septicum* is a safe and reliable immunizing agent for both cattle and sheep. Although a single inoculation will often confer sufficient protection, 2 injections, several weeks apart, are required for protection in many areas.

Vaccination is used not only as a routine measure in enzootic areas but also as a preventive procedure at the beginning of an outbreak to check further losses. Penicillin and broad-spectrum antibiotics are used in the treatment of early black-leg, but it is frequently unsuccessful. Treatment of more advanced cases may save the animal, but usually there is so much loss of muscle that it is not practical.

BACILLARY HEMOGLOBINURIA
(Redwater disease, Infectious hemoglobinuria)

An acute, infectious toxemic disease, primarily of cattle, caused by *Clostridium haemolyticum*. It has been found in sheep, and very rarely in dogs. It occurs in the western part of the U.S.A., along the Gulf of Mexico, in Venezuela, Chile, Great Britain, Turkey and probably in other parts of the world. Usually the infection is associated with liver fluke infection.

Etiology: *Cl. haemolyticum* apparently has its only habitat in the animal body. It may survive for long periods in contaminated soil or in bones from carcasses of animals that have been infected with it. Ingested in the feed or water, it ultimately becomes lodged in the liver as latent spores. The incubation period is extremely variable. The onset of the disease is determined by the occurrence of a locus of anaerobiosis in the liver where dormant spores are lying. Such a nidus for spores is most often caused by fluke infection, much less often by high-nitrate content of the diet, accidental liver puncture, liver biopsy or any other cause of localized necrosis. When favorable conditions of anaerobiosis occur, the spores germinate, the resulting vegetative cells multiply and release lethal quantities of hemolytic toxin.

Clinical Findings: In cattle, the appetite is lost, rumination, lactation and bowel movement suddenly cease, and respiration is shallow and labored. The temperature usually rises to a peak of about 106°F but drops to subnormal a few hours before death. A blood-stained mucoid diarrhea may develop and the urine is dark red, translucent and foamy. There is marked dehydration and a rapidly progressing anemia, the red cell count dropping to 1,500,000 or lower just before death, which results from anoxia. Terminally, 60 to 80% of the red blood cells are hemolyzed, and the hemoglobin is excreted in the urine. The duration of clinical signs varies from about 12 hours in pregnant cows to about 3 to 4 days in steers, bulls and nonpregnant cows. The mortality in untreated animals is about 95%. Some cattle suffer from subclinical attacks of the disease, and thereafter act as immune carriers of the organism.

After death, rigor mortis sets in more rapidly than usual. Dehydration, anemia, and sometimes subcut. edema are present. There is bloody fluid in the visceral and thoracic cavities. The lungs are not grossly affected and the trachea contains bloody froth with hemorrhages in the mucosa. The small intestine, and occasionally the large intestine, are hemorrhagic and their contents often contain free or clotted blood. An anemic infarct in the liver is pathognomonic, being slightly elevated, lighter in color than the surrounding tissue and outlined by a bluish-red zone of congestion. The kidneys are dark, friable and usually studded with petechiae. The bladder contains purplish-red urine.

Diagnosis: The general clinical picture usually permits a diagnosis. The most striking sign is the typical port-wine-colored urine, which foams freely when voided or on agitation. A low hemoglobin reading or packed cell volume with normal red cells is characteristic. The presence of the typical liver infarct is sufficient for a presumptive diagnosis. The normal size and consistency of the spleen serve to exclude anthrax and anaplasmosis. Bracken-fern poisoning and leptospirosis should also be considered. Diagnosis should be confirmed bacteriologically by (1) isolating *Cl. haemolyticum* from the liver infarct where possible, (2) demonstrating *Cl. haemolyticum* in the liver tissue by fluorescent antibody test, or (3) demonstrating the toxin in the fluid in the peritoneal cavity or in a saline extract of the infarct.

Treatment and Prophylaxis: Early treatment with penicillin (℞ 44) or broad-spectrum antibiotics (℞ 7, 11, 33, 58) is essential. Whole blood and fluid therapy are also helpful.

Cl. haemolyticum bacterin prepared from whole cultures confers immunity for about 6 months. In areas where the disease is seasonal, one preseasonal dose is usually adequate; where the disease occurs throughout the year, semiannual immunization is necessary. Cattle that are in contact with animals from areas where this disease is endemic should be immunized, for healthy animals from such areas may be carriers.

INFECTIOUS NECROTIC HEPATITIS
(*Clostridium novyi* (*oedematiens*) infection, Black disease)

An acute infectious disease of sheep and rarely of cattle caused by *Cl. novyi* Type B. The organism multiplies in areas of liver necrosis resulting from the migration of liver flukes, and it produces a powerful necrotizing toxin. The disease is worldwide in distribution, wherever sheep and liver flukes coincide.

Etiology and Pathogenesis: Type B strains of *Cl. novyi* probably have the animal body as their principal habitat and pass from animal to animal by contamination and ingestion of spores. Multiplication in the intestine serves both as a source for cells or spores to infect the liver or to infect other animals through contaminated herbage. Focal necrosis caused by immature liver flukes migrating through the liver creates the anaerobic conditions necessary for initiation of the infection. The lethal and necrotizing toxins damage hepatic parenchyma, and thus aid in enlargement of the infected lesion and the production of a lethal amount of toxin.

Clinical Findings: Death is usually sudden with no well-defined signs. Affected animals tend to lag behind the flock, go down in sternal recumbency and die within a few hours. Most cases occur in the summer and early fall when liver fluke infection is at its height. The disease is most prevalent in 1- to 4-year-old sheep and is limited to animals infected with liver flukes. Differentiation from acute fascioliasis is often difficult, but peracute deaths of animals which show typical lesions on necropsy should arouse suspicion of black disease.

Lesions: The most characteristic lesions are the grayish-yellow necrotic foci in the liver which often follow the migratory tracks of the young flukes. Other common findings are the enlarged pericardial sac filled with straw-colored fluid, and excess fluid in the peritoneal and thoracic cavities. There is usually extensive rupture of the capillaries in the subcut. tissue causing the adjacent skin to turn black, hence the common name.

Control: Some reduction in incidence of this disease may be accomplished by reduction of the numbers of snails, usually *Lymnaea* spp., that act as intermediate hosts for the liver flukes or by reducing the fluke infection of the sheep. However, these procedures are not always practical, and active immunization with *Cl. novyi* toxoid or bacterin may be better. A long-term immunity is produced by one inoculation. Following this, only new introductions to the flock—lambs, and sheep brought in from other areas—need to be vaccinated. This is best done before the late summer.

BIG HEAD

An acute infectious disease, caused by *Clostridium novyi*, *Cl. sordelli*, or rarely, *Cl. chauvoei*, characterized by a nongaseous, nonhemorrhagic, edematous swelling of the head, face and neck of young rams. This infection is initiated in young rams by their continually butting one another. The bruised and battered subcut. tissues offer conditions suitable for growth of pathogenic clostridia, and the breaks in the skin offer an opportunity for the organism's entrance. Treatment is with broad-spectrum antibiotics or penicillin.

THE ENTEROTOXEMIAS
(*Clostridium perfringens* infection)

Cl. perfringens is widely distributed in the soil, and in the alimentary tract of animals, and is characterized by its ability to produce potent exotoxins, some of which are responsible for specific enterotoxemias. Six types (A, B, C, D, E and F) have been identified on the basis of the toxins produced, but of these, only 3 are of significance.

TYPE B ENTEROTOXEMIA
(Lamb dysentery)

A highly fatal intoxication of young lambs, calves and foals caused by *Cl. perfringens* Type B. It occurs in England, France, Germany, and other European countries as well as in South Africa. The organism has rarely been found in the U.S.A. It was once present in Australia, but apparently has been eliminated.

Clinical Findings: Type B enterotoxemia occurs as an acute to subacute disease in animals less than 3 weeks of age. Many die before signs can be observed, but some newborn animals stop nursing, become listless and remain recumbent. A fetid diarrhea, sometimes tinged with blood, develops, and death generally occurs shortly thereafter. Some young animals may live for several days.

Lesions: Gross lesions are variable, but generally consist of severe inflammation of the intestine, with foci of ulceration and necrosis surrounded by red zones of hyperemia. The intestinal contents contain varying amounts of blood.

Diagnosis: Diagnosis is based upon the demonstration of Type B toxin in the intestinal contents. Almost pure cultures of *Cl. perfringens* Type B can usually be obtained from the small intestine.

Control: Lamb dysentery can be prevented by dam immunization with Type B toxoid. Newborn animals from nonimmune dams can be passively protected by injection of Type B antitoxin at birth. This immunity lasts up to 3 weeks, thus carrying the young animals through the critical period.

TYPE C ENTEROTOXEMIA
(Struck, Hemorrhagic enterotoxemia)

Cl. perfringens Type C was originally described as the cause of an acute intoxication ("struck") of mature sheep in the Romney Marsh district in England. Since then, it has appeared in the U.S.A. and probably elsewhere. It is an acute intoxication with hemorrhagic enteritis and peritonitis, occurring with greatest frequency in the winter and spring.

Hemorrhagic enterotoxemia is usually a highly fatal intoxication of vigorous suckling calves, lambs or piglets under 2 weeks of age. It is characterized by sudden onset, hemorrhagic enteritis, diarrhea and early death. Affected young are usually from dams that are heavy milk producers. The disease is apparently worldwide in distribution.

Clinical Findings and Diagnosis: Signs vary with the degree of intoxication. Affected animals become listless, stop nursing and display evidence of acute colic, such as uneasiness, straining or kicking at the abdomen. Hemorrhagic diarrhea may or may not occur. The clinical course of the disease varies from 2 to 24 hours. In many cases, the animal dies without signs being observed. Temperature remains normal to subnormal. Mild cases occur and, on recovery, these animals often fail to make normal gains, but they have good antitoxin titers.

Lesions: The postmortem lesions are hemorrhagic in character. The predominant lesion is a necrotic, hemorrhagic enterocolitis with loss of much of the mucosa of the small intestine, which is filled with blood and tissue debris. Petechiae occur on the thymus, heart, and serosal membranes.

Diagnosis: Demonstration of Type C toxin in the small intestinal contents confirms the diagnosis.

Control: The disease can best be controlled by dam vaccination. Two doses should be administered during the first year, the second dose a month or so before parturition. Booster doses should be given to the adult females annually. Antitoxin is used for therapy or for prophylaxis in newborn animals from nonimmunized dams.

TYPE D ENTEROTOXEMIA
(Pulpy-kidney disease, Overeating disease)

An enterotoxemia of sheep, less frequently of goats, and rarely of cattle, caused by *Cl. perfringens* Type D. This is the classic enterotoxemia of sheep. It is worldwide in distribution and may occur in animals at any age. It is most common in the young, either under 2 weeks of age or in weaned lambs in feed lots on a high-carbohydrate diet or, less often, on lush green pastures.

Etiology: The causative agent is *Cl. perfringens* Type D. However, predisposing factors are also essential; the most common of these is the ingestion of excessive amounts of feed or milk in the very young and grain in feed-lot lambs. In young lambs, the disease is restricted to the single lambs, for seldom does a ewe give enough milk to allow enterotoxemia to develop in twin lambs. In the feed lot, the disease usually occurs in lambs on high-grain diets. As the starch intake increases, it provides a suitable medium for organism multiplication and toxin production. Many sheep carry strains of *Cl. perfringens* Type D as part of the normal microflora of the intestine, and they serve as the source of organisms to infect the newborn. Most such carriers show a demonstrable amount of antitoxin in their sera in the absence of vaccination.

Clinical Findings: Usually, the first indication of enterotoxemia is the occurrence of sudden death in the best conditioned lambs. In some cases, excitement, incoordination and convulsions occur before death. Opisthotonos, circling and pushing the head against fixed objects are common signs of cerebral involvement. Hyperglycemia or glycosuria is frequently, but not always, observed. Diarrhea may or may not develop.

Lesions: Postmortem examination may reveal only a few hyperemic areas on the intestine and a fluid-filled pericardial sac. This is particularly the case in young lambs. In older animals, hemorrhagic areas on the myocardium, and petechial and ecchymotic hemorrhages of the abdominal muscles and serosa of the intestine may be found. Bilateral pulmonary edema and congestion are frequently occurring lesions, but usually not in young lambs. The rumen and abomasum contain an abundance of feed and undigested feed is often found in the ileum. Edema and malacia can be seen microscopically in the basal ganglia and cerebellum of lambs. Rapid postmortem autolysis of the kidneys has given rise to the popular name "pulpy-kidney disease" although pulpy kidneys are by no means always found in young lambs, and are seldom found in goats or cattle.

Diagnosis: A presumptive diagnosis of enterotoxemia is based on the sudden, convulsive death of lambs on good feed. Smears of intestinal contents reveal many gram-positive, short, fat bacilli. Confirmation can be made by the demonstration of Type D toxin in the small intestinal fluid. Fluid, not ingesta, should be collected in a sterile vial within a few hours after death, and sent under refrigeration to a laboratory for toxin identification. Chloroform, added at 1 drop for each 10 ml of intestinal fluid, will stabilize any toxin present.

Control: The method of control depends upon the age of the lambs, the frequency with which the disease appears on a particular property, and the details of husbandry. If the disease occurs consistently in young lambs on one property, ewe immunization is probably the most satisfactory method of control. The breeding females should be given 2 injections of Type D toxoid or bacterin (R 106) their first year and one injection, 4 to 6 weeks before lambing, each year thereafter. If the disease occurs only sporadically, it may be best to wait until 1 or 2 cases have occurred and then to passively immunize the single lambs with antitoxin.

Enterotoxemia in feed lot lambs can be controlled by reducing the amount of grain, and increasing the amount of roughage in the diet. However, this may not be satisfactory from an economic point of view, in which case immunization of all animals with toxoid when they first enter the feed lot will probably reduce losses to an acceptable level. Two injections 2 weeks apart will protect them through the feeding period. When alum-precipitated toxoids or bacterins are used, the injection should be given at such a site on the animal that the cold abscesses, which commonly develop at the site of injection, can easily be removed during normal dressing and thus do not leave blemishes on the carcass. Alternatively, antibiotics may be incorporated in the feed for about 10 days (e.g. chlortetracycline, 10 mg/lb of feed).

CLOSTRIDIUM SORDELLI (BIFERMENTANS) INFECTIONS

These are acute infections mimicking those of the other histotoxic clostridia. They are found in the Western U.S.A., South America and Turkey, but are comparatively rare even in these countries. Outbreaks are sporadic.

Cl. sordelli is probably a member of the soil microflora as well as of the animal intestine. It enters the body through breaks in the skin and, apparently, can occasionally pass through the intestinal wall to be picked up in the liver. Most infections are associated with wounds or with liver fluke infection. The etiology of the cases of *Cl. sordelli* infection in feed lots is not known.

There is little to distinguish *Cl. sordelli* infections from those of *Cl. septicum* or *Cl. novyi*. There is a rapidly progressing lesion at the site of infection, with fever, depression and edema that is almost equal to that produced in *Cl. novyi* infections, but which is more blood-stained. The odor is fetid and characteristic. Death is often sudden, with ill-defined necropsy findings. There has been no detailed study of these infections in feed lot of cattle, but the majority of lesions have been found in the throat region with localized edema and hemorrhage.

Bacterins have been used for the prevention of *Cl. sordelli* infections, however, the infrequent occurrence of the disease makes routine vaccination economically questionable. Because death is sudden, little is known of treatment, but large doses of broad-spectrum antibiotics or penicillin would be indicated in suspected cases.

TETANUS

A toxemia caused by absorption of a specific neurotoxin from tissue infected by *Clostridium tetani*. Almost all mammals are susceptible to this disease, although cats seem much more resistant than any other domestic or laboratory mammal. Birds are quite resistant, 10,000 to 300,000 times as much toxin being required for a lethal dose on a body weight basis for pigeons and chickens as is required for horses. Horses are the most sensitive of all species, with the possible exception of man. Although tetanus is worldwide in distribution, there are some areas, such as the northern Rocky Mountain section of the U.S.A., where the organism is rarely found in the soil and where tetanus in man and horses is almost unknown. In general, the occurrence of *Cl. tetani* in the soil and the incidence of tetanus in men and horses is higher in the warmer parts of the different continents.

Etiology: *Cl. tetani* is an anaerobe with terminal, spherical spores, which is found in soil and intestinal tracts of animals and man. In most cases, it is introduced into the tissues through wounds, particularly deep puncture wounds where anaerobic conditions can prevail. Often in lambs, however, and sometimes in other species, it follows docking or castration. Frequently, it is not possible to find the point of entry in a case of tetanus, for the lesion itself may be minor or has healed.

Pathogenesis: The spores of *Cl. tetani* are unable to grow in normal tissue, or even in wounds where the tissue remains at the oxidation-reduction potential of the circulating blood, as this is too high for anaerobic growth. Suitable conditions for multiplication are brought about where a small amount of soil, or a foreign object, causes tissue necrosis and allows multiplication of the contaminating spores. The bacteria remain localized in the necrotic tissue at the original site of infection as they cease growing, the bacterial cells undergo autolysis and the potent neurotoxin is released. It is usually absorbed by the motor nerves in the area and passes up the nerve tract to the spinal cord where it causes ascending tetanus. The toxin causes spasmodic, tonic contractions of the voluntary muscles by nerve cell irritation. If more toxin is released at the site of the infection than the surrounding nerves can take up, the excess is carried off by the lymph to the blood stream to the CNS, causing descending tetanus. Even minor stimulation of the affected individual may cause the characteristic muscular spasms.

Clinical Findings: The incubation period varies from one to several weeks, but usually averages 10 to 14 days. There is first a localized stiffness, often involving the masseter and neck muscles, the muscles of the hind limbs, and muscles in the region of the infected wound. General stiffness becomes pronounced about a day later, and tonic spasms and hyperesthesia become evident.

The reflexes are increased in intensity and the animal is easily excited into more violent, general spasms by sudden movement or noise. Spasms of head muscles cause difficulty in prehension and mastication of food, hence, the common designation "lockjaw". In the horse, the ears are erect, the tail stiff and extended, the anterior nares dilate, and there is prolapse of the third eyelid. Walking, turning and backing are difficult. Spasms of the neck and back muscles cause extension of the head and neck, while stiffness of the leg muscles cause the animal to assume a "sawhorse stance". Sweating is frequently present. General spasms cause disturbance of circulation and respiration, resulting in increased heart action, rapid breathing and congestion of mucous membranes. Sheep, goats and swine often fall to the ground and have opisthotonos when startled. Consciousness is undisturbed throughout the disease.

Usually, the temperature remains slightly above normal during the disease, but it may rise to 108° to 110°F toward the end of a fatal attack. In mild attacks, the pulse and temperature remain nearly normal. Mortality averages about 80%. In the animals that recover, there is a convalescent period of 2 to 6 weeks; protective immunity does not usually develop following recovery.

Prophylaxis and Treatment: Active immunization of valuable animals can be accomplished with tetanus toxoid. If a dangerous wound occurs after immunization, another injection of toxoid to increase the circulating antibody should be given. If the animal has not been previously immunized with tetanus toxoid, it should be treated with 1,500 to 3,000 IU or more of tetanus antitoxin, which will usually give passive protection up to 2 weeks. Toxoid should then be given simultaneously and repeated in 30 days. Yearly booster injections of toxoid are advisable.

All surgical procedures should be conducted with the best possible operative techniques. When large numbers of animals are docked or castrated, instruments should be sterilized before use and thereafter at frequent intervals. After such surgery, animals should be turned out on clean ground, preferably grass pastures. Only the oxidizing disinfectants as iodine or chlorine can be depended upon to kill the spores.

When administered in the early stages of the disease, curariform agents, tranquilizers, barbiturate sedatives, in conjunction with 100,000 to 200,000 IU of tetanus antitoxin, have been effective in the treatment of horses. Such therapy should be supported by drainage and cleaning of wounds and the administration of penicillin (R 44) or broad-spectrum antibiotics (R 7, 11, 29, 58). Good nursing is invaluable to tide the animal over the acute period of spasms. The patient should be placed in a quiet, darkened boxstall with feeding and watering devices high enough to allow their use without lowering the head.

Slings may be useful in cases where standing or rising is difficult.

BOTULISM
(Lamziekte)

A type of food poisoning marked by progressive paralysis, caused by ingestion of the toxin of *Clostridium botulinum*.

Etiology: Botulism is an intoxication, not an infection, and always results from ingestion of toxin in food. There are 8 types and subtypes of *Cl. botulinum*, differentiated on the serologic specificity of the toxins, A, B, C-alpha, C-beta, D, E, F and G. Types A, B and E are of most importance in human botulism; C-alpha in wild ducks, pheasants and chickens; C-beta in mink, cattle and horses; D in cattle. Only 2 outbreaks, both in man, are known to have been caused by Type F. Type G, which was isolated from soil in Argentina, is not known to have been involved in any outbreak of botulism either in men or animals.

In the U.S.A., during the past 10 years, there has been an average of 16 cases per year in man, ranging from a low of 5 cases in 1967 to 47 cases in 1963. The incidence of botulism in animals is not known with such accuracy, but it is relatively low in cattle and horses, probably more frequent in chickens, and very high in wild waterfowl. There are probably from 10,000 to 50,000 birds lost in most years, with losses reaching one million or more during the great outbreaks in the Western U.S.A. The very great majority of birds involved are ducks, although loons, mergansers, geese, and gulls are also susceptible. Type C-alpha is involved in duck botulism. The same type is usually responsible for botulism in pheasants. Dogs, cats and swine are comparatively resistant to all types of botulinum toxin when it is administered by mouth.

Most botulism in cattle occurs in South Africa, where a combination of extensive agriculture, phosphorus deficiency in soil and *Cl. botulinum* Type D in animals creates a condition ideal for bovine botulism. The phosphorus-deficient cattle chew any bones with accompanying tags of flesh that they find on the range; if these came from an animal that had been carrying Type D strains of *Cl. botulinum*, it is likely that intoxication will result, as a gram or so of dried flesh from such a carcass may contain enough toxin to kill a full-grown cow. Any animal eating such material also ingests spores of *Cl. botulinum* Type D. These spores germinate in the intestine and, after death, cells invade musculature which in turn becomes toxic and infective for other cattle. Type C strains also cause botulism in cattle in a similar fashion. This type of botulism in cattle is rare in the U.S.A. A few cases have been reported from Texas under the name of "loin disease", and a very few cases have been encountered in Montana. Botulism in sheep has been encountered in Australia, not from phosphorus deficiency as in cattle, but from protein and carbohydrate deficiency. This results in the eating of carcasses of rabbits and other small animals that sheep find on the range.

Botulism in mink usually is caused by Type C-beta strains that have produced toxin in chopped raw meat or fish. Types A and E strains have been involved, but comparatively seldom.

Clinical Findings: The signs of botulism are associated with the paralysis of muscles, and include progressive motor paralysis, disturbed vision, difficulty in chewing and swallowing, and generalized progressive weakness. Death is usually due to respiratory or cardiac paralysis. "Limber neck" is not always seen in birds as death may occur without it. The toxin prevents synthesis or release of acetylcholine at motor end plates. Passage of impulses down the motor nerves and contractility of muscles are not greatly hindered; only the passage of impulses from nerves to motor end plates are affected. No characteristic lesions develop, and pathologic changes may be ascribed to the general paralytic action of toxin, particularly in the muscles of the respiratory system, rather than to the specific effect of toxin on any particular organ.

Diagnosis: Diagnosis of botulism can be best made by identification of the specific toxin in the serum, in extracts of liver tissue, in contents of the gastrointestinal tract, or in the food of affected animals. The type of toxin is determined by specific antitoxin neutralization. Isolation of the organism itself is not reliable evidence, for it can be present either in food or in intestinal contents without causing botulism. In any suspected case of botulism, a serum sample should be obtained as quickly as possible.

Control: Canned food which is considered unfit for human consumption should not be fed to animals. Control of botulism in wild ducks is difficult unless the water level of the lakes or ponds involved can be drastically lowered. It is generally not possible to eliminate bone-chewing and the resultant botulism in cattle by feeding mineral supplement or by fertilization of the soil with high-phosphorus fertilizer, because too great an area of land is usually involved. Immunization of cattle with toxoid with Types C and D has proved successful in South Africa and in Australia. Toxoid is also effective in immunizing mink, and it has been used in pheasants.

Botulinum antitoxin has been used for treatment with varying degrees of success, depending upon the type of toxin involved and the species of host. Treatment of ducks with Type C antitoxin is often successful, as is the treatment of mink. In cattle, however, such treatment is rarely used. Treatment with guanidine hydrochloride, 5 mg/lb body wt, has been reported to overcome some of the paralysis caused by the toxin, but the drug has not as yet been used sufficiently to be certain of its value.

LEPTOSPIROSIS

A contagious disease of animals and man due to infection with *Leptospira* spp. These are very slender, helical organisms having a characteristic hook in one or both ends. In dogs, cattle, pigs, sheep, goats and horses, infections are usually asymptomatic, but they may result in a wide variety of disease conditions including fever, icterus, hemoglobinuria, abortion and death. Following acute infection, leptospires frequently localize in the kidneys and are shed in the urine, sometimes in enormous numbers for months or years. They survive well in surface waters, and leptospirosis is essentially a water-borne disease.

The common mode of natural infection is from contact with urine or by intake of urine-contaminated feed or water. Artificial infections are readily established by the conjunctival or vaginal routes and through skin abrasions. If shedder animals are introduced into a herd which has been free of the disease, leptospirosis is rapidly disseminated and abortions may occur among animals in the middle or last third of gestation. Clinical signs may be severe, mild, or absent. Recovery is associated with high levels of circulating antibodies and the disappearance of leptospires from the animal except those localized in the kidneys. Leptospiral abortions are not characterized by retention of the fetal membranes or impaired fertility and subsequent pregnancies are usually normal. Most outbreaks of the disease are therefore self-limiting, but the control of some may require rodent depopulation or fencing the herd from surface waters in addition to immunization and chemotherapy.

Diagnostic Procedures: Serologic methods: Of the more than 100 antigenically distinct leptospires, only 6 or 7 cause disease in domestic animals. There is remarkably little cross-immunity, and dual and even treble infections have been reported. Antibodies first appear in the serum of infected animals by the sixth or seventh day, and titers rise rapidly to a very high level. The titer then declines to a more or less constant level which may persist for years. A single positive serologic result indicates either vaccination, passive immunity from the milk of the dam, or current or past infection. Serologic confirmation of a clinical diagnosis of leptospirosis requires the demonstration of a rising titer in consecutive serum samples, the first taken as early in the disease as possible and the second after an interval of 7 to 10 days. Vaccination with bacterins stimulates only low levels of agglutinins. The carrier or shedder state cannot be diagnosed serologically. The serologic methods commonly used include the "plate" agglutination, microscopic agglutination, and complement-fixation tests.

Primary isolations are made by inoculating 1 ml of blood, collected during the acute stage of infection, into laboratory animals or suitable media. A series of 4 or 5 inoculations should be made to ensure isolation. Similarly, urine may be examined for leptospires 2 weeks or longer after acute infection. Negative results do not rule out infection, however.

Histopathogic examination: A clinical diagnosis of leptospirosis can be confirmed by the demonstration of the organisms in sections of kidney and liver stained by the silver-impregnation method of Levaditi or the Warthin-Starry technique. Leptospires do not stain with the common aniline dyes.

Microscopic examination: Fresh material in the form of tissue scrapings from liver or kidney substance or the centrifuged deposit from freshly collected urine may be examined by means of the dark-field microscope. In some cases, the characteristic motile organisms are readily seen, but this method and the previous one are relatively unreliable and require the interpretation of an expert. A fluorescent antibody technique is being studied.

LEPTOSPIROSIS IN DOGS
(Canine typhus, Stuttgart disease, Infectious jaundice)

Leptospirosis in dogs is usually due to infection with *L. canicola* or *L. icterohaemorrhagiae*. *L. pomona* infections have been reported, but are usually inapparent.

Etiology: Infections with *L. canicola* are much more prevalent than those with *L. icterohaemorrhagiae* and frequently produce epizootics of the so-called hemorrhagic type of leptospirosis. The icteric type of leptospirosis is usually due to *L. icterohaemorrhagiae;* rats are a reservoir of infection.

Clinical Findings: Dogs of all ages may be affected. The incidence is much greater in males. The incubation period is 5 to 15 days. In severe cases, the disease may have a sudden onset, characterized by slight weakness, refusal to eat, vomiting, a temperature of 103° to 105°F and often a mild conjunctivitis. At this stage, clinical diagnosis is difficult. Within 2 days, there is a sharp drop in temperature, depression is more pronounced, breathing is labored and thirst is marked. Icterus may appear as the first manifestation of the illness and vary in intensity from lemon to deep orange color. Muscular stiffness and soreness, particularly of the hind legs, as evinced by unwillingness to rise from a sitting position, and pain are usually detected on palpation of the anterior dorsal abdomen or lumbar area. The oral mucous membranes may at first show irregular hemorrhagic patches resembling abrasions or burns, which later become dry and necrotic and slough in sections. A slimy salivary secretion around the gums is at times tinged with blood. Swallowing is difficult. In some cases, the tongue may show necrotic patches or the entire tip may slough. More advanced cases show intense depression and muscular tremors, with the temperature dropping gradually to subnormal, reaching as low as 97°F. Bloody vomitus and feces may be seen, indicating severe hemorrhagic gastroenteritis. Frequent urination with albumin, pus cells and casts in the urine indicate acute nephritis. The eyes become sunken and the vessels of the conjunctiva are injected. The pulse becomes thready and, in severe cases, uremia develops. Mortality seldom exceeds 10%. In fatal cases, death occurs usually 5 to 10 days after onset. Chronic, progressive nephritis frequently follows acute *L. canicola* infections. In such cases, death may not occur until long after the initial illness has subsided.

The leukocyte count may rise to 35,000; the BUN may also be elevated. Other laboratory findings are variable, depending on the severity and stage of the disease.

Lesions: Hemorrhagic gastroenteritis is often the predominant lesion. The tissues may be uniformly bile-stained. The liver is engorged and the lymph nodes are often hemorrhagic. The myocardium may be diffusely hemorrhagic. The organs may have the typical uremic odor. The kidneys are enlarged in the acute phase and may have gray foci or mottling at their corticomedullary junction as in acute interstitial nephritis. Oral ulcers and tongue sloughs may be present in the uremic animal. Chronic cases have varying degrees of interstitial nephritis.

Diagnosis: Diagnosis is made on the basis of clinical and necropsy findings, histopathologic demonstration of leptospires in the kidneys or liver, demonstration of leptospiruria, and serologic tests.

Prophylaxis: To reduce the chances of exposure, owners are well-advised to keep their dogs leashed. During epizootics of leptospirosis, confinement to the owner's premises may be recommended. Bivalent bacterins are available, but apparently must be administered every 6 to 8 months to maintain a significant antibody level.

Chemoprophylaxis (℞ 54) may be recommended for dogs at high risk (show or stud dogs). If leptospirosis is diagnosed in a kennel dog, treatment of all dogs in the kennel should be considered (℞ 54).

Treatment: Penicillin and streptomycin (℞ 41) are recommended for acute infections; dihydrostreptomycin (℞ 54) is recommended in heavy doses for termination of the carrier-shedder state.

Dehydration and acidosis can be treated by giving M/6 lactate solution, alone or in combination with saline-dextrose solution, and high doses of soluble B-vitamins. If the patient is in the anuric phase of the disease, excessive fluid volume must not be administered. The animal should be weighed daily and the fluid volume adjusted so that a 40-lb dog loses approximately 0.2 lb per day. Although expensive and time-consuming, peritoneal dialysis can be lifesaving when used in selected cases with uremia.

LEPTOSPIROSIS IN CATTLE
(Redwater of calves)

Leptospirosis of cattle in the U.S.A. is due to *L. pomona, L. grippotyphosa* and *L. hardjo.*

Clinical Findings: Hemolytic icterus and hemoglobinuria often exist in 50%, or more, of affected young calves. Mortality ranges from 5 to 15%. The acute clinical syndrome occurs in only 2 to 4% of adults, and deaths are rare. Total morbidity may exceed 75% in older stock and usually approaches 100% in calves.

In calves, the classical case presents fever, prostration, inappetence, dyspnea, icterus, hemoglobinuria and anemia. Body temperature rises suddenly to 105° or 106°F. Hemoglobinuria rarely lasts longer than 48 to 72 hours. As it subsides, the icterus rapidly clears and is succeeded by anemia. The erythrocytes begin to increase in number on the fourth or fifth day and the count returns to normal 7 to 10 days later. Most cases show leukocytosis. Some degree of albuminuria is commonly present during the febrile peak.

In older cattle, signs of leptospirosis vary greatly and the diagnosis is often difficult. The signs are particularly obscure in dairy herds infected with *L. hardjo;* lowered milk and calf production occur with few clinical signs. A hemolytic crisis is seen only occasionally. In dry cattle, the infection is so mild that it is generally overlooked, but in milking stock, a sharp drop in milk production is noted. The milk is thick, yellow and blood-tinged, although there is no evidence of mammary inflammation. Abortion is common and takes place 2 to 5 weeks following initial infection. It is commonest about the seventh month of pregnancy. An abortion storm in a breeding herd is often the first indication that leptospirosis exists, the mild initial signs having passed unnoticed. Calves reared by cows that have been previously infected acquire through the colostrum a passive immunity which lasts 1 to 2 months. The calves generally have a higher antibody titer than their dams.

Lesions: Anemia and icterus are prominent features in the acute hemolytic form of the disease. The urine is a clear-red or port-wine color. The kidneys show the most significant lesions in the form of a reddish brown mottling of the cortex, often sufficiently pronounced to be visible through the intact capsule. The liver may be swollen, with minute areas of focal necrosis. Petechiae in the epicardium and lymph nodes are seen in fulminating cases.

Diagnosis: Serology with "paired" serum samples, direct culture in media, or animal inoculation techniques are usually necessary to confirm clinical and postmortem findings. The absence of mammary inflammation despite the gross physical changes in the milk is suggestive of leptospirosis. Similarly, elimination of brucellosis, vibriosis and trichomoniasis as possible causes of an abortion outbreak would point to leptospirosis.

Prophylaxis: In the absence of state or federal regulations for the control of leptospirosis, cattle owners rely on annual vaccinations with commercial *L. pomona* bacterins. Bacterins containing *L. grippotyphosa* and other serotypes are widely used in the U.S.S.R. and elsewhere, and are being developed for use in the U.S.A. Although bacterins confer protection against abortions and death, their efficacy in preventing persistent renal infections has not been proved. Management methods to prevent leptospirosis include: rat control, fencing cattle from potentially contaminated streams and ponds, separation of cattle from swine, selection of replacement stock from herds which have passed serologic tests for leptospirosis, and chemoprophylaxis of replacement stock (℞ 54).

Treatment: No form of treatment will have much effect on the course of the disease once a hemolytic crisis has developed. In the case of valuable animals, the IV transfusion of washed red cells may prove beneficial if the anemia approaches the critical level. Antibiotic therapy—streptomycin (℞ 54), chlortetracycline (℞ 11) or oxytetracycline (℞ 25)—is often successful if it can be given early. Dihydrostreptomycin (℞ 54) is recommended for termination of the carrier or shedder state.

LEPTOSPIROSIS IN SHEEP

Leptospirosis is less prevalent in sheep than cattle, possibly due to less intensive husbandry methods and less frequent association with pigs. In the U.S.A., *L. pomona* is the most common serotype isolated from sheep. The infection can often be traced to carrier cattle. Clinical features, diagnosis and management of the disease are essentially as already described for mature cattle and calves.

LEPTOSPIROSIS IN SWINE

L. pomona is the organism most commonly encountered in leptospiral infection of swine. Swine act as a reservoir of infection for other animals and man as apparently healthy individuals can excrete large numbers of organisms in their urine. Swine have been incriminated so often that the disease in man is known in Europe as "swine-herd's disease". Swine are also commonly infected with *L. grippotyphosa*.

Acute leptospirosis occurs in young pigs due to *L. icterohaemorrhagiae*. It is characterized by fever, icterus, hemorrhages and death. The source of the infection is usually the urine of rats. Porcine leptospirosis is not a clearly defined entity. In some cases, infection may apparently occur without visible signs, while others show only a febrile reaction lasting 3 to 4 days. More severe clinical signs include poor weight gain, anorexia, intestinal disturbances and occasionally meningitis with rigidity, spasms and circling. *L. pomona* has been isolated from aborted porcine fetuses. Abortions, late in pregnancy, represent the most important single sign of leptospirosis in a herd of swine. Antibiotic therapy has been recommended (℞ 14, 36, 54). The use of *L. pomona* bacterin in exposed herds is warranted.

LEPTOSPIROSIS IN HORSES

During investigations on the etiology of equine periodic ophthalmia (q.v., p. 214), serologic testing revealed that a high percentage of affected horses carried high titers to *L. pomona* and the organism has been isolated from horses. By artificial exposure to *L. pomona*, periodic ophthalmia has been experimentally produced in horses. Equine leptospirosis is characterized by an elevated body temperature of 103° to 105°F for 2 to 3 days, depression or dullness, anorexia, icterus and neutrophilia. Periodic ophthalmia or abortion may occur long after the fever has subsided. The incidence of leptospirosis in horses is not known, but the disease may be more widespread than is realized. Many cases of leptospirosis undoubtedly occur without being recognized because of the mild transient course which leaves only the eye lesions as the visible permanent damage. Measures for control and treatment have not been developed.

BRUCELLOSIS

A specific contagious disease primarily affecting cattle, swine, goats and dogs, caused by bacteria of the *Brucella* group and characterized by abortion in the female, to a lesser extent, orchitis and infection of the accessory sex glands in the male and infertility in both sexes. The disease also affects sheep and is prevalent in the U.S.S.R. and countries of the Mediterranean and Near East. Brucellosis occasionally affects horses where it frequently is associated with fistulous withers and poll evil. The human disease, also called undulant or Malta fever, is usually self-limiting.

BRUCELLOSIS IN CATTLE
(Contagious abortion, Bang's disease)

Etiology: The disease in cattle is caused almost exclusively by *Brucella abortus*, but occasionally *Br. suis* or *Br. melitensis* are isolated. Bovine brucellosis is now much less prevalent in the U.S.A. than formerly because of vaccination and eradication programs; a few states are virtually free of the disease.

Epizootiology: The appearance of the infection in a herd that has been free of brucellosis is characterized by rapid spread and many abortions. In the herd in which the disease is enzootic, the typical infected animal aborts only once after exposure, and subsequent gestations and lactations appear to be normal. Following exposure, most cattle develop a bacteremia and a positive blood serum agglutination reaction; the remainder either resist or recover rapidly from infection. The positive blood reaction usually precedes abortion, but in some animals it may be delayed. The organism is shed in the milk and in uterine discharges and the cow may suffer from temporary sterility. The bacteria are found in the uterus during pregnancy, during the period of uterine involution and, infrequently, for a prolonged time in the nongravid uterus. Many infected cows shed brucellae from the uterus at subsequent normal parturitions following an abortion. Secondary infection contributes to the infertility and, by prolonging the period of involution, also may prolong the presence of *Br. abortus* in the uterus and its discharges. The organism is shed in the milk for a variable length of time, some animals shedding it for life. The extremes of susceptibility are seen in the naturally immune cow which never becomes infected and the very susceptible animal which suffers repeated abortions.

Natural transmission of the disease is through ingestion of the organisms that are present in large numbers in the aborted fetus, membranes and uterine discharge. Cattle may ingest feed or water that is contaminated with brucellae and occasionally lick the contaminated genitals of other animals or recently aborted fetuses. Venereal transmission by infected bulls to susceptible cattle by natural service may occur but is rare. Cows may be infected by means of artificial insemination when the *Brucella*-contaminated semen is deposited in the uterus but not when it is deposited in the mid-cervix. Brucellae may enter the body through mucous surfaces, the conjunctivae, injuries and even through the intact skin.

Mechanical vectors, such as dogs, other animals and man can act as a means of spreading infection. Under certain circumstances, the organism will live for weeks outside the body. Brucellae have been recovered from the fetus, and from manure that has remained in a cool environment for more than 2 months. Exposure to direct sunlight kills the organism in a matter of a few hours.

Clinical Findings: Abortion of the fetus is the most obvious manifestation of the disease. Establishment of the carrier state in a large proportion of animals may lead to a 20% reduction in the milk yield of infected cows, the production of dead calves at term and an increased frequency of retained placenta. In uncomplicated abortions, there usually is no impairment of the general health.

In the bull, the seminal vesicles, the ampullae, the testicles and the epididymides may be infected which results in the organism being shed in the semen. Agglutinins may be demonstrated in the seminal plasma of such bulls. Abscesses of the testicles may occur. The organism has been isolated from arthritic joints.

Diagnosis: Diagnosis must be based on bacteriologic or serologic examination. *Br. abortus* can be recovered from the placenta, but more conveniently in pure culture from the stomach and lungs of the aborted fetus. The organisms may be isolated from the genital tract after abortion or normal calving for periods of up to 10 weeks in 50% of infected animals. Most cows cease shedding from the genital tract when uterine involution is complete. The reservoirs of permanent infection are the reticuloendothelial system and the udder, and it frequently is possible to isolate *Br. abortus* from the milk.

Blood serum agglutination tests are the most practical and reliable methods of diagnosing bovine brucellosis. These tests may also be used to detect antibodies in milk, whey and semen plasma. **Vaginal mucus tests** for *Brucella* agglutinins also may be of some diagnostic value. Agglutination at serum dilutions of 1:100 or above for nonvaccinated animals, 1:200 for calves vaccinated between 3 and 9 months of age, or positive brucellosis card-test results, are considered positive for brucellosis.

The latter test differs from the conventional agglutination tests in that it utilizes an acidified, buffered antigen and only a single test dilution. The advantages are selective detection of antibodies most likely to be associated with *Brucella* infection and the ability to conduct the test of farms within a few minutes after blood collection.

Screening diagnostic procedures: (1) *Milk ring test*—In the official control and eradication of brucellosis on an area basis, the milk ring test has proved to be a highly efficient and accurate diagnostic procedure for locating infected dairy herds. Milk samples are collected from each herd at the milk-processing plant or creamery, or at the farm where the milk is collected in large tanks. The brucellosis status of dairy herds in any area can be determined and the disease eradicated by applying the milk ring test at 3- to 4-month intervals with the necessary follow-up blood tests of the positive herds and slaughter of reactors. The cost of such a program is approximately one-tenth of that required to blood-test the cattle of all herds in the same area, whereas the efficiency of the 2 methods in locating infected herds is comparable.

(2) *Market cattle testing*—Nondairy herds in an area also may be screened for brucellosis by testing the marketed cattle. This program is based upon blood testing of nonproductive or surplus adult cattle destined for slaughter through intermediate and terminal markets or at abattoirs. Reactors are traced to the herd of origin, and the remaining cattle in these herds are tested. The unit cost for detecting a reactor by this method is only a fraction of that incurred by area blood testing of the cattle in all herds.

Brucellosis-free areas can be achieved and maintained, both effectively and economically, by a system which combines utilization of both the milk ring test on all dairy herds and the market cattle testing program on all nondairy herds.

Supplementary tests: Supplementary tests may be employed in herds from which brucellosis has not been eradicated despite the continued conscientious application of standard eradication procedures. Utilization of a battery of these tests improves the possibility of detecting the infected animal or animals which have resided in these herds as undetected reservoirs of infection. Supplementary tests currently used include acidified antigen, complement fixation, rivanol precipitation, and mercaptoethanol agglutination tests. These tests are designed to detect primarily the IgG antibodies that are associated specifically with *Brucella* infection. Another supplementary diagnostic procedure is testing of quarter milk samples with milk or whey agglutination tests. The latter procedure is often an excellent method for detecting chronic infection in the udder of cows that may have equivocal blood serum reactions.

Control: No practical effective treatment is known, and efforts are directed at control and prevention. Eventual eradication of the disease depends upon testing and elimination of reactors. Many individual herds have been freed of the disease by this method. The infected herd is tested at regular intervals until 2 or 3 successive negative tests are obtained. When reactors are found, they are removed and the premises thoroughly cleaned and disinfected.

Clean herds must be protected from reinfection. The greatest danger is from replacement animals. Where possible, new additions should be vaccinated calves or nonpregnant heifers. If pregnant or fresh cows must be used, they should originate from brucellosis-free herds and be negative to the agglutination test. It is advisable to segregate such replacements from the herd for at least 30 days and retest them before permitting them to associate with the main herd.

Vaccination with *Br. abortus* Strain 19 (℞ 103) is widely used in calves and is effective in increasing resistance to infection. Resistance is not complete and will break to some extent, depending upon the severity of exposure. Experimental evidence indicates that the immunity following calfhood vaccination does not decline with the passage of time. A small proportion of these animals become persistent positive or suspicious reactors to the agglutination test, with attendant confusion in diagnosis.

Another vaccine, *Br. abortus* 45/20 bacterin in adjuvant, has gained widespread acceptance in some countries. Most studies indicate that 45/20 vaccine, when used as recommended, induces immunity comparable to that of Strain 19. Current recommendations require 2 initial injections at specific intervals and annual booster injections thereafter. The principal advantage of this vaccine is that agglutination test reactors seldom occur after vaccination, since 45/20 is a nonsmooth strain of *Br. abortus.* Therefore, it can be used in adult cattle without greatly interfering with diagnosis. Disadvantages of 45/20 bacterin are the necessity of giving numerous injections at specific intervals and the attendant economic cost, and occasional objectionable local reactions at the site of injection.

Vaccination as the sole means of control has been effective; the degree of reduction of reactors is directly related to the degree that calfhood vaccination is practiced. However, when it is desired to go beyond control to eradication, test and slaughter are necessary, and continued vaccination poses the problem of interpretation of "positive" test reactions.

BRUCELLOSIS IN GOATS

A disease with signs similar to those of brucellosis in cattle occurs in goats. Caprine brucellosis in man (Malta fever) was the first *Brucella* infection to be recognized and described. The disease in goats is prevalent in Southern Europe and was fairly common in the Southwestern U.S.A. until recent years. At the present time, it occurs rarely in this country.

The causal agent usually is *Brucella melitensis,* but occasionally *Br. abortus* is found. Infection occurs primarily through the ingestion of the organism, but conjunctival, vaginal and subcut. inoculation will produce the disease. Abortion occurs about the fourth month of pregnancy. Rarely, arthritis and orchitis occur, and keratitis and chronic bronchitis may be caused by infection with *Br. melitensis.* The diagnosis is made by bacteriologic examination of the milk or of the aborted fetus, or by the serum agglutination test. In the interpretation of this test, if any animal in the herd shows a titer of 1:100, all goats reacting at 1:50 or 1:25 should also be considered infected. The disease is controlled by the slaughter of reacting animals.

Two *Br. melitensis* vaccines have shown promise of preventing caprine brucellosis in controlled experiments and field trials. One is a killed vaccine suspended in an adjuvant and the other is an attenuated vaccine (Rev. 1 *Br. melitensis* vaccine). Vaccination for the control of caprine brucellosis should be considered only in countries where the incidence of the disease is high.

BRUCELLOSIS IN SWINE

The clinical manifestations of the disease in swine vary considerably, but they are similar in many respects to those of brucellosis in cattle and goats. The disease often is self-limiting within the individual animal to a greater degree than in cattle. Despite this self-limitation, the disease has remained in some herds for years. Brucellosis due to *Brucella suis* also occurs in other domestic animals and man. Epidemics of human brucellosis occur among packing-house workers and the usual source is infected swine.

Etiology: The disease in swine is caused almost exclusively by biotypes of *Br. suis,* but *Br. abortus* is also occasionally found. The disease is spread mainly by direct animal-to-animal contact, usually through the ingestion of infected material. Infected boars may transmit the disease during service, and the organism can be recovered from the semen.

Swine raised for breeding purposes constitute the important source of infection. In such herds, infection is likely to persist, whereas in herds used for pork production only, with no outside replacements other than an occasional boar, the disease will eliminate itself after an acute abortion storm following the introduction of an infected animal. Although of infrequent occurrence, natural transmission from infected weanling pigs has been reported. Some suckling pigs may become infected by contact with infected sows, but the majority reach weaning age without becoming infected. The effects of brucellosis usually are more severe in breeding swine than in young pigs, but both age groups are susceptible.

Clinical Findings: Following exposure to *Br. suis,* swine develop a bacteremia in which the organism may persist in the blood stream for periods varying up to 90 days. During and following the bacteremic stage, it may become localized in a wide variety of tissues. Signs depend considerably on the site or sites of localization. Common manifestations are abortion, temporary or permanent sterility, orchitis, lameness, posterior paralysis, spondylitis and, occasionally, metritis and abscess formation in the extremities or other areas of the body.

There is much variation in the incidence of abortion, from as high as 50 to 80% of the females in some herds, to no observed abortions in others. Abortions also may occur early in gestation and be unobserved. Usually, sows or gilts that abort early come in heat a short time afterward and are rebred.

Sterility in sows, gilts and boars is common and may be the only manifestation of brucellosis. In swine herds where sterility is a problem, it is logical to test for brucellosis before attempting treatment. In sows, the sterility may be permanent, but is more frequently of a temporary nature. Orchitis, usually unilateral, may occur. Fertility appears to be lowered, but complete sterility may or may not ensue.

Diagnosis: The principal means of diagnosis of swine brucellosis are serum-agglutination tests. It is generally accepted that the tests are effective in determining the presence or absence of brucellosis in the herd, but have limitations in detecting brucellosis in individual animals. Thus, entire herds or units of herds, rather than individual animals, must be considered in any control program.

Prophylaxis and Control: In almost any sizable herd of swine, low-titered reactions occur in the absence of infection. These same low-titered reactions occur in herds where infection is present and a few infected swine may have no detectable agglutinin titer. Thus, as a rule of thumb, serum-agglutination reactions below the 1:100 dilution are not considered indicative of brucellosis unless there are definite reactors at the 1:100 dilution or higher in the herd. If blood titers at 1:100 or higher are observed, those animals and all exposed to them should be regarded as infected. The brucellosis card test is usually more accurate than conventional agglutination tests since low-titer agglutinins due to causes other than *Brucella* seldom react with it. Supplementary tests designed for cattle can also be used for swine. Caution should be used in the purchase of individual swine that exhibit a low-titered agglutination response, unless the status of the entire herd of origin is known. Swine should be held in isolation upon their return from fairs or shows before entering the main herd. All replacements should be purchased from herds known to be free of brucellosis, or failing this, should be tested, kept in isolation for 3 months and retested before being added to the herd.

Vaccination is unreliable. Control is based on test, segregation and slaughter of infected breeding stock. The following plans can be used to eliminate brucellosis from a herd:

1. Sales of entire herd for slaughter: This plan is usually the quickest, easiest and most economical. Replacement of the infected breeding herd should be from herds free from infection and may be made after the premises and equipment are cleaned and disinfected. The replacement herd should be placed on clean ground (free of swine for at least 60 days). After 2 consecutive negative tests, 60 to 90 days apart, the replacement herd is eligible for validated brucellosis-free status.

2. Test, segregation and delayed slaughter of infected herds: This plan is recommended for use in purebred herds only where it is desired to retain valuable bloodlines. The procedures to be followed are: (a) Separate and isolate (on clean ground) the weanling pigs at 6 weeks of age or younger. Market the remainder of the herd as soon as practicable. (b) Test the pigs saved about 30 days before breeding and save only gilts that are negative. Breed only to negative boars. (c) Retest the gilts after farrowing. If infection is disclosed, repeat plan 2 or abandon in favor of plan 1. The herd is eligible for validated status following 2 negative tests not less than 90 days apart.

3. Slaughter of reactors only: This is not generally recommended except in herds where only a very few reactors are found, no clinical signs of brucellosis have been noted, and there is doubt that the reactor titers were caused by *Brucella* infection. In this plan, retest the herd at 30-day intervals, removing reactors until the entire herd is negative. Following 2 consecutive negative tests not less than 90 days apart, the herd is eligible for validated brucellosis-free status.

Swine breeders in the U.S.A. should be encouraged to validate their herds. Details of procedures for validating herds and areas are available in USDA-ARS publication 91-79, September 1969.

No practical recommendations can be made for treating infected swine.

BRUCELLOSIS IN DOGS

While dogs occasionally become infected with *Br. abortus,* *Br. suis,* or *Br. melitensis,* these are sporadic occurrences, usually in dogs closely associated with infected herds of domestic livestock. Transmission of *Brucella* spp. from dogs to man and other animals is known. Dogs have been considered to be relatively resistant to *Brucella* infection and in most cases the disease appears to be self-limiting. However, in 1966 it became apparent that enzootics of abortion among kenneled dogs were caused by a newly described organism, *Brucella canis*. The dog appears to be the definitive host of this organism; infection in man has been reported. Infection has occurred mostly in Beagles and nearly always in kennels. In some breeding kennels the disease has caused reduction of the number of pups weaned to one-fourth that of pre-infection levels. The disease is rapidly disseminated among dogs closely kenneled, especially at the time of breeding or when abortions occur. Transmission is congenital or venereal or by ingestion of infective materials. All ages and both sexes appear to be equally susceptible.

The main clinical feature is abortion without premonitory signs during the last trimester of pregnancy. Stillbirths and conception failures are also predominant features of the disease. Prolonged vaginal discharge usually follows abortion and repeated abortions during successive pregnancies are common. Infected dogs also develop generalized lymphadenitis and, in males, epididymitis, periorchitis and prostatitis frequently occur. Bacteremia is a constant finding and it persists for an average of about 18 months after exposure. Pyrexia is not characteristic.

Diagnosis is based on isolation of the causative agent or serologic tests. The organism can usually be readily isolated from vaginal exudate, aborted pups, blood, urine, milk, or semen of infected dogs. The most commonly used serologic test has been the agglutination test. The antigen for use must be prepared from *Br. canis* as this organism shows little cross-reaction with other *Brucella* spp. Nonspecific agglutination reactions sometimes occur with serums from dogs proved not to have been infected.

Attempts at immunization or treatment have not been uniformly successful. The most successful control measures have been based on elimination or isolation of infected dogs identified by positive cultural or serologic results. Management factors are also important as the incidence of infection has been observed to be much lower in kennels where dogs were caged individually.

EPIDIDYMITIS OF RAMS

(*Brucella ovis* infection)

A specific bacterial disease of sheep, characterized in the ram by epididymitis, orchitis and impaired fertility; in the ewe by placentitis and abortion; and in the lamb by perinatal mortality. The disease has been reported in New Zealand, Australia, the U.S.A., South Africa, Romania, Czechoslovakia and South America. It is almost certainly present elsewhere. Epididymitis in rams may also be the result of other infections.

Etiology: Initially, the classification of the infective agent presented a taxonomic problem. Assignment of the organism to the genus *Brucella* has now received general acceptance. *Br. ovis* is not known to cause natural infection in other animal species or in man.

Rams as young as 8 weeks have been infected experimentally by the IV, subcut. and intratesticular routes as well as orally, per rectum and by the application of the agent to mucous surfaces, such as the conjunctiva and prepuce. The disease can be transmitted among rams by direct contact but ram-to-ram transmission is increased during the mating season when clean rams acquire infection by serving ewes previously served by infected rams.

Active infection in ewes is unusual but has developed after mating with naturally infected rams. Contaminated pastures do not appear important in spreading the disease. Active infection is frequently persistent in rams, a high percentage being capable of shedding the causative agent in semen over periods in excess of 4 years.

Clinical Findings: The principal clinical manifestations are lesions of the epididymis, tunica and testis of the ram and placentitis in the ewe, with abortion and perinatal death of lambs. In recently infected rams, the lesions may develop rapidly, the first abnormality detectable being a marked deterioration in semen quality associated with the presence of inflammatory cells and organisms in the semen. An acute systemic reaction is rarely observed in the field. Following regression of the acute phase—which may be so mild as to go unobserved—lesions may be palpated in the epididymis and scrotal tunics. Epididymal enlargement may be unilateral or bilateral, the tail of the epididymis being involved more frequently than the head or body. The most prominent lesion in the epididymis is the development of spermatoceles of ariable size containing partially inspissated spermatic fluid. he tunics frequently become thickened and fibrous, and exnsive adhesions develop between the visceral and parietal yers. The testes may show fibrous atrophy. In most cases, ese lesions are permanent; in a few, palpable lesions are ansient, while in others, organisms may be excreted in de·ctive semen over long periods without clinically detectable sions.

Lesions in the fetal membranes of infected ewes vary from a perficial purulent exudate on an intact chorion to a marked lema of the allantochorionic mesenchyme, usually with ecrosis of the uterine surface of the allantochorion and fetal otyledons.

iagnosis: Since not all infected rams show palpable abnormalities of the scrotal contents (nor are all cases of epididymitis due to this specific infection), the remaining rams must e further examined following palpation. Rams shedding rganisms, but without lesions must be identified by cultural xamination of semen samples. Repeated examinations may e necessary to identify those rams which shed the organism nly intermittently. Microscopic examination of stained semen nears may also be helpful. Fluorescent antibody staining is highly specific diagnostic aid. Serologic tests used for eradica.on and accreditation have included complement fixation and ndirect hemagglutination.

Control and Treatment: The incidence and spread of the disase may be reduced by the regular examination of rams prior o the breeding season and the culling of those with obvious enital abnormalities. Since the incidence of infection in rams ises sharply with age, there are advantages in isolating the ounger, clean rams from older, possibly infected rams and eeping the ram flock young.

Immunization of rams by simultaneous inoculation of *Br. bortus* Strain 19 and a killed *Br. ovis* adjuvant vaccine has een practiced extensively in New Zealand. An alternative rocedure now more generally used is 2 inoculations of the *Br. vis* adjuvant vaccine given between 4 months of age and months before mating. Immunization of weaner rams with llberg's Rev. 1 live vaccine has been recommended in South frica. It is an attenuated *Br. melitensis* vaccine. Since inection in ewes apparently originates almost exclusively from he use of infected rams, lamb losses through infection of ewes re believed to be controlled best by vaccinating rams.

Chlortetracycline and streptomycin used together have been

shown to effect bacteriologic cures. Except in specially valu able rams, such treatment is uneconomic, and even if th infection is eliminated, there is no certainty of a return to un impaired fertility.

TUBERCULOSIS

A chronic disease caused by infection with acid-fast or ganisms belonging to the genus *Mycobacterium*. The diseas affects practically all species of vertebrate animals, and befor control measures were adopted, was one of the major disease of man and domestic animals. The signs and lesions are gen erally similar in the various species.

Etiology: Although the disease in all species is known as tuber culosis, the causative agent in all of them is not identical Three main types of tubercle bacilli are recognized: human bovine and avian. Since tubercle bacilli do not multiply excep in infected animals, the principal reservoirs of these types i nature are the animal species for which they are named. Th 3 types differ not only in distribution, but also in cultura characteristics and pathogenicity. The 2 mammalian type are much more closely related to each other than to the avian type.

All 3 types may produce infection in host species other thar their own. The **human** type is most specific; it rarely produce: progressive disease in the lower animals other than primate: and, occasionally, dogs and parrots. The **avian** type is th only one of consequence in birds, but is also pathogenic fo swine, cattle and sheep, though natural infection in the latte is rare. The **bovine** type is the most cosmopolitan and i capable of causing progressive disease in almost all warm blooded vertebrates.

Pathogenesis: The disease commences with the formation o a primary focus which in man and cattle is in the lung in abou 90% of cases; the primary lesion in poultry is nearly always in the intestinal tract (*see* AVIAN TUBERCULOSIS, p. 1045). Lym phatic drainage from the primary focus in mammals leads to the formation of caseous lesions in the corresponding lymph node and this lesion, together with the primary focus, is known as the "primary complex." This primary complex seldom heal: in animals, but may progress slowly or rapidly.

Wherever the organisms localize, their activity stimulates

he formation of tumor-like masses called tubercles. Because
of the continued growth of the organisms these tubercles enlarge often until they become of great size. Sometimes, large
masses of new tissue develop on the serous membranes of the
body cavities. As the granulomas grow, necrosis of their central portions occurs. Finally, these are reduced to cheesy
masses which have a tendency to undergo calcification. In
mammals, tubercles may become enclosed in dense fibrous
tissue and the disease become arrested. When the bacilli
escape from the primary foci they travel via the lymph and
blood streams, lodge in other organs and tissues to establish
other tubercles. When the blood stream is invaded by numerous tubercle bacilli from a local lesion, many tubercles develop in the major organs. This acute form of generalization,
known as miliary tuberculosis, is usually rapidly fatal. If small
numbers of bacilli enter the circulation from the primary
complex, one or more isolated lesions are formed in other
organs. These generalized lesions may become encapsulated
and remain small for long periods, usually causing no detectable signs.

Clinical Findings: The signs exhibited depend upon the extent
and location of the lesions. Small lesions, located in deep
lymph nodes, may occasion no clinical signs, but enlarged
superficial lymph nodes provide a useful diagnostic sign. If the
disease is progressive, the general signs are weakness, anorexia,
emaciation and low-grade fluctuating fever. In mammals, the
organs of the chest usually are involved. When the lungs are
extensively diseased, there is commonly an intermittent, hack-
ing cough. In birds, lesions are usually found in the intestinal
wall, the liver and spleen rather than in the lungs. The principal sign of tuberculosis in birds and in many mammals is
the chronic wasting or emaciation which occurs despite good
feeding and care.

Diagnosis: Clinical diagnosis is usually possible only after
tuberculosis has reached an advanced stage. Most individuals
have become shedders of bacilli by this time and are a menace
to other animals. Radiology is used only in monkeys and the
small domestic animals. The most certain and practical method
of reaching a specific diagnosis in large domestic animals is to
apply the tuberculin test. This test depends upon the fact
that animals suffering from tuberculosis are allergic to the
proteins contained in tuberculin and give characteristic reactions when exposed to them. If tuberculin is deposited in the

deep layers of the skin (intradermally), a local reaction characterized by inflammation and swelling is induced in infected animals, whereas normal animals fail to give such reactions.

Animals suffering from infection with either human- or bovine-type tubercle bacilli react about equally well to tuberculin made from either type of organism. When testing for avian-type tuberculosis, whether in birds or mammals, the avian-type organism must be used, as such animals react less strongly to tuberculin made from the mammalian types.

The dose used in the intradermal tuberculin test is approximately 0.1 ml of a suitably diluted tuberculin. In the U.S.A., the larger mammals usually are injected in one of the folds at the base of the tail, swine in the skin behind the ear and chickens in the skin of the wattle. The injection sites are examined for the characteristic swellings 72 to 96 hours after injection.

Synthetic-medium tuberculin (OT) is still widely used but in Great Britain and some European countries, purified protein derivative (PPD) tuberculins are being used. PPDs are preferable because they are easier to standardize, more stable and slightly more specific. PPD tuberculins are particularly important in the comparative intradermal tests used to differentiate mammalian tuberculosis from infection by other mycobacteria in man and cattle. In cattle, the test is performed by injecting mammalian and avian tuberculin into separate sites in the skin of the neck. The difference in the size of the 2 resultant responses usually indicates whether tuberculin sensitivity is caused by infection with human or bovine type bacilli rather than by the avian type, the Johne's bacillus, or one of the many "opportunist" mycobacteria. The "opportunist" mycobacteria are common in the environment and some types infect wounds in the skin or intestinal tract. Such infections usually do not progress beyond the regional lymph node; however, temporary sensitivity to tuberculin may result. These and other organisms are responsible for many of the false positive tuberculin reactors which present an important problem in the latter stages of bovine tuberculosis eradication programs. The incidence of such reactors can be reduced by the use of the comparative intradermal test applied by a specialist.

Control: Mammalian tubercle bacilli grow only *in vivo*. The main reservoirs are man and cattle. The prevalence of the disease in such reservoirs determines the disease incidence in other species.

There are 4 principal approaches to the control of tuberculosis: (a) test and slaughter, (b) test and segregation, (c) immunization and (d) chemotherapy. In the past, chemotherapy has been of little value in the control of tuberculosis in farm animals, but recent reports from South Africa indicate that it is economically feasible to treat cattle with isoniazid. Many tuberculous cattle recover and become negative to the tuberculin test. The use of chemotherapy may be of value in heavily infected areas, but cannot be relied upon to eradicate the disease.

The test-and-slaughter method consists of the application of the tuberculin test and the slaughter of reacting animals. This method has been widely used in the U.S.A. and Canada. In the Scandinavian countries and Great Britain, where "test and slaughter" would have been impracticable, varying forms of "test and segregation" have been used, with "test and slaughter" only in the final stages.

While BCG (Bacillus of Calmette and Guerin) vaccine is the most successful immunizing agent in humans and reduces the severity of the initial disease in cattle, it does not completely prevent infection and vaccinated cattle react to the tuberculin test. It has, therefore, played little part in the control of bovine tuberculosis.

TUBERCULOSIS IN CATTLE

This disease used to be very prevalent particularly in dairy cattle but control programs have greatly reduced the incidence in many countries. A number of countries have virtually eradicated bovine tuberculosis from cattle. A few infected herds continue to be discovered in many parts of the U.S.A., which launched the first major control program in 1917. The source of infection is usually other infected cattle although in some European countries pulmonary or genitourinary tuberculosis of man caused by bacilli of the bovine type is the source of infection in up to 60% of reinfected herds.

Tuberculous animals with open lung lesions throw infected droplets into the air by coughing. Such animals also swallow sputum and thus contaminate pasture and cowsheds via the feces. Adult animals are infected by the inhalation of airborne dust particles as well as contaminated feed and water facilities. Young calves may be infected by drinking unpasteurized infected milk.

Early lesions are usually found in the chest and sometimes in the lymph nodes of the head or intestine. In advanced stages of the disease, lesions may be found in many organs and tissues that are seldom affected primarily; thus, infection of the udder, uterus, lymph nodes, kidneys and the meninges occurs with varying frequency. The skeletal muscles are very seldom affected, even in advanced cases. Tuberculosis of the udder is of special significance because of contamination of milk with infective organisms.

TUBERCULOSIS IN SWINE

Swine are subject to infection with all 3 types of tubercle bacilli. Infection is most often contracted by the ingestion of infected materials; hence the primary lesions are in the intestinal tract and associated lymph nodes, particularly the submaxillary. With bovine-type bacilli, generalization is often severe and rapid, but infection with the avian or human type is usually limited to the lymph nodes of the head and to the intestinal tract and associated lymph nodes.

Lesions caused by the avian and human types tend to be fleshy and firm and are not strongly invasive, whereas the bovine bacillus usually causes a rapidly progressive disease with caseation and liquefaction of the lesions. Differentiation has to be confirmed by isolating the organism and typing it. Lesions resembling those of tuberculosis are also produced in pigs by certain of the opportunist mycobacteria.

TUBERCULOSIS IN SHEEP

The disease is rare in sheep, but when it occurs the bovine type causes a condition similar to that in cattle. The avian bacillus may also cause severe progressive lesions.

TUBERCULOSIS IN DOGS

Dogs may be infected by the human or bovine type. Up to 10% of dogs necropsied in some cities, when spittoons were commonly used, were found to be tuberculous. The infection now is much less common in most countries, but dogs may still be infected from a human source and may in turn infect man, especially children. The short-nosed breeds appear to be more susceptible and males are more commonly affected than females.

Tuberculous lesions in the dog usually resemble neoplasms, especially the sarcomas. Often the tubercles are grayish white in color and are circumscribed. The large liver lesions are yellowish with depressed centers and crenated hemorrhagic edges. Some of these lesions have soft almost purulent centers; others appear as ragged bloody cavities or may take the form of small, multiple gray nodules scattered throughout the liver substance.

Lung lesions usually consist of grayish-red bronchopneumonic areas; some break down to form cavities. These may open into the pleural cavity or communicate with a bronchus.

Early spreading lesions vary from areas of acute congestion to hepatization. The pulmonary and pleural lesions are invariably exudative in type and there may be a large quantity of straw-colored liquid in the chest. Such lesions may cause collapse of the lower portions of the lung.

False negative tuberculin tests are common in the dog; radiographs and a history of exposure are helpful aids to diagnosis.

TUBERCULOSIS IN CATS

The cat, unlike the dog, is resistant to infection with human tubercle bacilli. It is considerably more susceptible than the dog to experimental bovine-type infection, and most natural infections arise from the ingestion of infected milk, primary lesions being found in the intestinal tract. However, primary respiratory infection does occur and infected wounds sometimes give rise to tuberculous sinuses. At one time, up to 12% of cats necropsied in parts of Europe were found to be tuberculous but, with the elimination of tubercle bacilli from the milk supply, the disease has become rare.

In general, lesions in cats resemble those in dogs. Few isolated primary foci have been recorded and it appears that infection is followed by rapid generalization. Lesions and discharges are usually rich in bacilli.

The tuberculin test is considered unreliable in the cat and radiographic diagnosis is often difficult. Isolation of the bacilli provides evidence of infection, but negative culture results are of questionable value.

ERYSIPELOTHRIX INFECTION

Erysipelothrix insidiosa (*rhusopathiae*) is a cosmopolitan bacterium capable of living for long periods in water, soil, pasture, decaying organic matter, slime on the bodies of fish, and in carcasses, even after smoking, pickling or salting. It is capable of invading the tissues of animals, birds and man with production of some fairly distinct and other less well-defined diseases. The former include swine erysipelas in its various forms; nonsuppurative arthritis in lambs and, less frequently, in calves; post-dipping lameness in sheep; acute septicemia in turkeys, ducks and occasionally geese and other birds (q.v., p. 1046); and erysipeloid in man.

In acute diseases, *E. insidiosa* usually occurs as a slender, gram-positive, nonmotile, nonsporulating rod, about 1 to 2 μ long. In chronic lesions and old cultures it often appears as a mixture of rods and filaments up to 20 μ in length. It is resistant to certain commonly used antiseptics, such as formaldehyde, phenol, hydrogen peroxide and alcohol, but is readily destroyed by caustic soda and hypochlorites. It is very sensitive to penicillin, less so to the tetracyclines and streptomycin and insensitive to most sulfonamides.

SWINE ERYSIPELAS

An infectious disease, manifested in a variety of forms, affecting mainly growing swine. It is fairly common in many swine-raising areas of the world. Although acute septicemic swine erysipelas causes death, probably the greatest economic loss comes from the mild, chronic nonfatal forms of the disease.

Etiology: *Erysipelothrix insidiosa,* the causal agent, can be isolated readily on blood agar plates from the tissues of acutely sick pigs and also from the tonsils of many apparently normal ones. On farms where the organism is endemic, pigs are exposed naturally to *E. insidiosa* while they are young and have maternal antibodies and thus develop a degree of active immunity without visible disease. The organism is excreted from infected animals and survives for long periods in alkaline soil. Recovered animals and those chronically infected may be carriers of the organism for months. *E. insidiosa* can cause an allergic response in the joints of sensitized pigs and results in chronic sterile lesions similar to those observed in rheumatoid arthritis in man.

Clinical Findings: The disease occurs in several forms; acute septicemia, a skin form, chronic arthritis and vegetative endocarditis. These may occur together, in sequence, or separately.

Swine with acute septicemia may die suddenly without previous manifestation of illness. This occurs most frequently in sucking pigs (rarely before 3 weeks), or in pigs between 100 and 200 lb body wt. Most acutely infected animals have high temperatures of 104° to 108°F. Their joints are sore, as evidenced by walking stiffly on their toes, lying on their sternums and by lying about separately rather than piling in groups. They squeal readily when handled or when submitted to any type of body pressure and shift weight from foot to foot when standing. Skin discoloration may vary from erythema and purplish discoloration of the ears, snout and abdomen, to urticaria (diamond-skin lesions) characterized by square, rhomboidal or diamond-shaped, raised hyperemic or purple-colored lesions over all areas of the body, particularly the lateral and dorsal parts. The lesions may occur as variable-sized pink or light purple areas that become raised and firm to the touch within 2 to 3 days of illness. Later they may disappear or progress to a more chronic type of lesion, such as diamond-skin disease or even necrosis of large areas of skin. These may separate from the body. The tips of the ears and tail may necrose and drop off.

Mortality in the acute septicemic form of the disease may vary from 0 to 100% and death may occur up to 6 days after the first signs of illness. Untreated animals may develop chronic arthritis or vegetative valvular endocarditis; these conditions may also occur in pigs that have shown no previous signs of septicemia, particularly in vaccinated herds. Valvular endocarditis is diagnosed most commonly in mature or nearly mature pigs and is manifested by fatigue, heavy respiration, cyanosis or sudden death, which usually results from embolisms. Chronic arthritis produces intermittent mild lameness, but the affected joints are frequently difficult to detect clinically. They may be only slightly swollen, cool to the touch and not excessively painful when palpated. Mortality in chronic cases is low and is largely restricted to valvular endocarditis.

Lesions: In the acute septicemic infection the lesions are similar to those of many other septicemias. Lymph nodes are usually enlarged and congested, the spleen swollen, pulpy and purplish in color, and the lungs edematous and congested. Petechial hemorrhages in sparse numbers may be found in the kidneys. The skin changes have already been described.

In cases of valvular endocarditis, metastatic embolism and infarctions may occur, particularly in the kidneys, brain or heart. In cases of arthritis, which may involve one or more legs, the joint enlargement is firm due to a thickening of the joint capsule and the capsular ligaments. Granulation tissue forms in the articular cavity. There may be erosion of the articular cartilage, with periostitis and osteitis. Ankylosis may occur.

Diagnosis: The diagnosis of acute erysipelas may be difficult in swine showing only high temperature, poor appetite and listlessness. Since *E. insidiosa* is so sensitive to penicillin, the marked improvement within 24 hours following its use provides support for the diagnosis. If typical diamond-skin lesions develop, these are diagnostic. Chronic forms of arthritis and endocarditis are difficult to diagnose specifically since other agents can cause similar syndromes. At necropsy, demonstration of *E. insidiosa* in stained smears or cultures confirms the diagnosis.

Prophylaxis and Treatment: Either killed bacterins or live culture immunizing strains of *E. insidiosa* of low virulence for swine and man, but of immunogenic potency, are currently extensively used. The formalin-killed, aluminum hydroxide-absorbed bacterin is safe in that it does not infect other species of animals or man, but confers an immunity of relatively short duration. In most instances, this will protect the pig from acute forms of the disease until it reaches market age. An oral vaccine of low virulence is used to some extent. Breeding stock should be revaccinated at least once each year.

Although vaccination raises the level of natural immunity, it does not necessarily provide complete protection. Acute cases may still occur following stress, and little protection is provided against the arthritic or cardiac forms of the disease.

If cases of acute erysipelas suddenly occur in an unvaccinated herd, antiserum may be administered to in-contact pigs as a quick-acting prophylactic measure. Penicillin is the drug of choice in affected pigs. Penicillin treatment is sometimes combined with antiserum to provide a longer action.

NONSUPPURATIVE POLYARTHRITIS IN LAMBS

An acute arthritis of one or more of the diarthrodial joints, usually of the limbs, following entry of *Erysipelothrix insidiosa* through wounds or the unhealed navel. Calves also are sometimes affected.

Etiology: The infective agent, *E. insidiosa,* which apparently is widely distributed in alkaline soil and pasture in many regions, gains entry to the body usually through wounds of young lambs, particularly at docking and castration. After a transient septicemia, the organism becomes localized in one or more joints, without leaving evidence of specific infection of the wound through which it entered. Poor condition of the lambs at the time of the operation and adverse weather afterwards appear to predispose to a high infection rate.

Clinical Findings: The characteristic lesion is an acute nonsuppurative arthritis manifested by heat, pain and only slight swelling of the joint tissues. While any of the joints may be affected, those most commonly involved are the hock, stifle, elbow and knee. In most cases complete recovery occurs in 2 to 3 weeks, but because affected lambs are unwilling to move about freely, growth is often seriously depressed. In about 10 to 15% of cases, the infection persists with the production of a chronic arthritis and permanent enlargement of the joint. The mortality is usually low, a few animals dying from acute septicemia or from complications arising from the enforced decubitus.

In outbreaks following docking and castration, the incubation period is remarkably constant, the first cases appearing 9 to 19 days after the operation, and practically all subsequent cases developing within 5 days. The incidence may reach 50% but in most outbreaks it does not exceed 10%.

Diagnosis: In outbreaks following docking and castration, a presumptive diagnosis can be made from the history and clinical signs. Sporadic cases are not easy to diagnose and recourse may be had to isolation and identification of the organism from affected joints. The disease must be distinguished from polyarthritis due to other bacteria (e.g., streptococcal joint ill), white muscle disease, and other causes of lameness.

Prophylaxis and Treatment: The adoption of strict antiseptic techniques and the maintenance of hygienic conditions for docking and castration are highly desirable, but cannot be relied upon to prevent the disease. The so-called "bloodless" methods of carrying out both operations may reduce the chances of wound contamination, but outbreaks are known to follow all of the methods commonly used. Vaccination should be considered where the disease is a recurring problem.

Penicillin, administered as early as possible in the course of the disease, is the best form of therapy.

POST-DIPPING LAMENESS IN SHEEP

A laminitis arising from an extension of a focal cutaneous infection, caused by the penetration of *Erysipelothrix insidiosa* through small skin abrasions in the region of the hoof. The condition, which normally occurs in outbreaks, has been described in most of the large sheep-raising countries of the world.

Etiology: With time and repeated use, dipping solutions or suspensions of insecticidal agents, which exert little or no bacteriostatic activity, become heavily charged with numerous species of bacteria. *E. insidiosa* is a common pathogenic contaminant and its presence in the vat, sometimes in enormous numbers, leads to the infection of any or all skin wounds made during the dipping operation. Small skin abrasions in the region of the hoof and fetlock joint, made by scraping the legs against the sides of the vat, are particularly common. It is the infection of these wounds with the production of a typical erysipeloid lesion extending to the laminae of the hoof that causes the acute post-dipping lameness.

Clinical Findings: Two to 4 days after dipping, a variable number—up to 90%—of the flock are lame in one or more legs. At this stage, the affected leg appears normal except that the hoof and pastern are hot and painful on pressure. Later there is a variable degree of depilation, sometimes extending as far as the carpus or tarsus.

In many outbreaks, most sheep recover spontaneously in 2 to 4 weeks with nothing more serious than a slight loss of body weight. In others, however, the mortality may rise to 5% and, in young sheep particularly, a higher proportion may develop signs of acute and, later, chronic arthritis.

Prophylaxis and Treatment: The addition of copper sulfate to the dipping wash at the rate of 3 to 5 lb/1,000 gal. is an effective means of control. Other agents with bacteriostatic activity against *E. insidiosa* are also used. Where therapy is indicated, penicillin is the antibiotic of choice.

ERYSIPELOTHRIX INFECTION IN MAN

The most common type of *Erysipelothrix* infection in man, the result of wound infection with *E. insidiosa*, is known as erysipeloid. This sometimes occurs in veterinarians whose hands become infected while carrying out necropsies on swine or turkeys. These infections apparently lead to immunity since reinfection rarely occurs.

After an incubation period of 1 to 5 days, the skin at the point of inoculation becomes swollen, painful and red. If untreated, the process may extend to involve the entire hand. It is accompanied by an itching, burning or prickly sensation. There may be fever as well as swelling and tenderness of nearby joints and the regional lymph nodes. Suppuration is absent. Most cases follow a mild course to recovery within 2 to 4 weeks. Antiserum in doses of 5 to 20 ml usually brings about quick relief and recovery. Large doses of penicillin are indicated in treating the infection.

Two other forms of infection occur in man. One is the diffuse or generalized form consisting either of a slow spread of erysipeloid over most of the body or eruption in areas remote from the site of entry. This is usually accompanied by fever and joint pains. A septicemic form of variable symptomatology and duration has also been observed. There may be joint pains and endocarditis. The skin eruption which accompanies this is of value in suggesting the diagnosis. Blood culture is positive.

TRANSMISSIBLE SEROSITIS
(Chlamydial polyarthritis)

An infectious disease affecting sheep, calves and swine. Dogs are susceptible experimentally. Chlamydial polyarthritis of sheep was first described in Wisconsin, and has since been recognized in the West and Midwest in the U.S.A., and in Australia and New Zealand. The disease was identified in calves from the Western U.S.A., Australia and Austria, and in pigs from Austria, Bulgaria and the Midwestern U.S.A. It is caused by infectious agents of the psittacosis-lymphogranuloma group now classified as *Chlamydia psittaci*. Strains isolated from affected joints of sheep and calves are identical, but strain-specific antigens in their cell walls distinguish them from *Chlamydia* causing abortions or pneumonia in sheep and cattle. The causative agent of chlamydial polyarthritis can be isolated most consistently from synovia of affected joints. It is excreted in feces, urine and conjunctival exudates.

Clinical Findings: Chlamydial polyarthritis is observed in lambs on range, from farms and in feed lots. Morbidity may range from 5 to 75%. Rectal temperatures of affected lambs vary from 102° to 107°F. Varying degrees of stiffness, lameness, anorexia and conjunctivitis may occur. They are depressed, reluctant to move and often hesitate to stand and bear weight on one or more limbs, but they may "warm out" of stiffness and lameness following forced exercise. The highest incidence of the disease among sheep on range occurs between late summer and December.

The disease affects calves from 4 to 30 days of age, which are readily detected because they do not want to move and seek to rest. They may have fever, are moderately alert, and usually nurse if carried to the dam and supported while they are sucking. They usually have diarrhea, which can be severe, and assume a hunched position while standing. The joints and tendons of the limbs are usually swollen, and palpation causes pain. Navel involvement and nervous signs are not observed. Experimentally, very young calves developed severe, watery diarrhea after oral inoculation and died within 4 days without developing fever or signs of polyarthritic involvement.

Chlamydial polyarthritis may be recognized in slaughter pigs as well as in young piglets. The affected piglets become febrile and anorectic, and may develop nasal catarrh, difficulties in breathing and conjunctivitis. This condition has not been clearly differentiated from other infections leading to polyserositis and arthritis in pigs.

Lesions: The most striking tissue changes in chlamydial polyarthritis of lambs and calves are in the joints. Enlargement of the joints of polyarthritic lambs is not often noticed, but in long-standing, advanced cases, slight enlargement of the stifle, hock and elbow may be detected. In affected calves, periarticular subcut. edema and fluid-filled, fluctuating synovial sacs contribute to enlargement of the joints. Most affected joints of lambs or calves contain excessive, grayish-yellow turbid synovial fluid. Fibrin flakes and plaques in the recesses of the affected joints may adhere firmly to the synovial membranes. Joint capsules are thickened. Articular cartilage is smooth, and erosions or evidence of marginal compensatory changes are not present. Tendon sheaths of severely affected lambs and calves are distended and contain creamy, grayish-yellow exudate. Surrounding muscles are hyperemic and edematous, with petechiae in their associated fascial planes.

Diagnosis: The history of the disease and careful examination of the pathologic changes in the joints and other organs can be valuable diagnostically. Cytologic investigations of synovial fluids or tissues may reveal chlamydial elementary bodies or inclusions in affected cells. Isolation and identification of the causative agent in developing chicken embryos from affected joints confirms the diagnosis. Bacteriologic cultures of affected joints are usually negative, but *Escherichia coli* or streptococci may occasionally be cultured. If the joints of young calves are polyarthritic and navel lesions are absent, chlamydial polyarthritis should be considered.

Clinical and pathologic features distinguish chlamydial polyarthritis from other conditions that cause stiffness and lameness in lambs. Lambs with mineral deficiency or osteomalacia usually do not have fever. The abnormal osteogenesis in these 2 conditions and the distinct muscle lesions of white-muscle disease are virtually pathognomonic. In arthritis caused by *Erysipelothrix insidiosa* there are deposits on and pitting of articular surfaces, periarticular fibrosis and osteophyte formation. Laminitis due to blue-tongue virus infection can be differentiated clinically and etiologically. Detailed microbiologic investigations are required to differentiate chlamydial arthritis in animals from mycoplasmal arthritis.

Control and Treatment: If begun early, therapy with long-acting penicillin or tetracyclines or tylosin appear to be beneficial. More advanced lesions do not respond satisfactorily. Daily feeding of 150 to 200 mg of chlortetracycline to affected lambs in feed lots reduces the incidence of chlamydial polyarthritis. One has to keep in mind that intestinal chlamydial infection is probably the first event in the pathogenesis of this disease.

SALMONELLOSIS
(Paratyphoid)

A disease of all animal species caused by many species of salmonellae and manifested clinically by 1 of 4 major syndromes: peracute septicemia, acute enteritis, chronic enteritis and the asymptomatic carrier state. The disease occurs worldwide and incidence appears to be increasing with intensification of livestock production. Young calves, piglets, lambs and foals are all susceptible and usually develop the septicemic form. Adult cattle, sheep and horses commonly develop the acute enteritis, and chronic enteritis may occur in growing pigs and old horses.

Etiology and Transmission: The species of salmonellae which commonly cause disease in mammals are: *Salmonella typhimurium* and *S. dublin* (cattle); *S. choleraesuis* and *S. typhimurium* (swine); *S. typhimurium* (horses). With acute enteritis the organism frequently localizes in the gallbladder, mesenteric lymph nodes, liver, lungs, spleen, joints, meninges and brain. Survivors become chronic carriers and intermittently discharge the organism from the gallbladder into the intestine, and thus out with the feces. Inapparent infection occurs in all species but is most common in cattle, pigs and poultry. The source of infection is the feces of infected animals which can contaminate feed and water, milk, fresh and processed meats from abattoirs, plant and animal products used as fertilizers or feedstuffs, pasture and rangeland and many inert materials. The organisms may survive for months in wet, warm areas such as in feeder-pig barns or in water dugouts. Rodents and wild birds are also important sources of infection.

Clinical Findings: Septicemia: This is the usual syndrome in newborn calves, lambs, foals and piglets, and outbreaks may occur in pigs up to 6 months of age. Illness is acute; depression is marked, fever (105° to 107°F) is usual and death occurs in 24 to 48 hours. In pigs, a dark red-to-purple discoloration of the skin is common, especially over the ears and ventral abdomen. Nervous signs may occur in calves and pigs. Mortality is commonly 100%.

Acute enteritis: This is the common form in adults and it may also occur in calves of 3 to 6 weeks. Initially there is a fever (105° to 107°F) followed by severe, watery diarrhea, sometimes dysentery and often tenesmus. In a herd outbreak, several hours may lapse before the onset of diarrhea, and the fever may disappear with the onset of diarrhea. The feces vary considerably: they may have a putrid smell and contain mucus, fibrinous casts and even shreds of mucous membrane; in some cases large blood clots are passed. Feces may contain large quantities of clear mucus, giving them a greasy appearance. Rectal examination causes severe discomfort, tenesmus and commonly dysentery. Abdominal pain is common and severe in the horse. Dehydration and toxemia are usually severe, and mortality is high.

Subacute enteritis: May occur in adult horses and sheep on farms where the disease is enzootic. The signs include mild fever (103° to 104°F), soft feces, inappetence and some dehydration. There may be a high incidence of abortion in cows and ewes, some deaths in ewes after abortion and a heavy mortality due to enteritis in the lambs under a few weeks of age.

Chronic enteritis: This is a common form in pigs and adult cattle. There is persistent diarrhea, severe emaciation, intermittent fever and poor response to treatment. The feces are scant and may be normal or contain mucus, casts, or blood.

Dogs and cats rarely develop septicemia from salmonellae, although outbreaks in puppies and kittens have been reported. Dogs and cats may act, however, as asymptomatic carriers and many of the types important in other domestic mammals and man have been isolated from them.

A number of *Salmonella* spp. appear in foxes, especially in young kits and produce a peracute enteritis. Mink and other fur-bearing carnivores may also be affected. Several rodents such as guinea pigs, hamsters, rats, mice, and rabbits are susceptible (see pp. 1139 et seq.). Rodents commonly act as a source of infection on farms where the disease is endemic.

Diagnosis of salmonellosis is dependent on the clinical signs and on the laboratory examination of feces, tissues from affected animals, feed (including all mineral supplements used) water supplies, and feces from wild rodents and birds which may inhabit the premises. The clinical syndromes are usually characteristic but must be differentiated from several similar diseases: *In cattle:* enteric colibacillosis; coccidiosis; the alimentary tract form of IBR; bovine virus diarrhea; hemorrhagic enteritis due to *Clostridium perfringens,* types B and C; arsenic poisoning and dietetic diarrhea. *In swine:* enteric colibacillosis of newborn pigs and weanlings, swine dysentery, erysipelas, hog cholera, septicemia due to *Hemophilus* spp. and acute pasteurellosis. *In sheep:* enteric colibacillosis, septicemia due to *Hemophilus* spp., or pasteurellae and coccidiosis. *In horses:* septicemia due to *E. coli, Shigella equuli* and streptococci and colitis-X disease.

The **lesions** are those of a septicemia or a necrotizing fibrinous enteritis. Special cultural techniques are usually necessary to recover the organism. Serum agglutination tests are useful as an indicator of herd infection. Because of the intermittent shedding of the organisms from infected animals it is usually necessary to conduct repeated fecal examinations before the organism is recovered or the animal can be identified as negative.

Treatment: Broad-spectrum antibiotics (℞ 27), and sulfonamides (℞ 82) are used parenterally to treat the septicemia, and nitrofurans (℞ 102) are given orally for enteric infection. Treatment should be continued daily for up to 6 days. Oral medication should be given in drinking water, since affected animals are thirsty due to dehydration and their appetite is generally poor. Fluid therapy to correct acid-base imbalance and dehydration is a necessary part of treatment. Calves, adult cattle and horses need large quantities of fluids to correct electrolyte and fluid losses (℞ 558). The results of treatment are often disappointing. Septicemic salmonellosis in swine usually responds favorably if treated early; however, the enteric form is difficult to treat effectively in all species. Although clinical cure may be achieved, bacteriologic cure is unlikely, particularly in adult animals, because the organisms become embedded in the biliary system and are intermittently shed into the intestinal lumen, which causes chronic relapsing enteritis and contamination of the environment.

Control and Prevention: Control and prevention are difficult because *Salmonella* survive for long periods in the environment, and recovered animals act as reservoirs of infection. The ideal of scrupulous sanitation and elimination of carriers is impractical; however, the rate of infection can be reduced. The incidence of salmonellosis in purchased calves is considerably higher than in home-reared calves. Introduction of such potential carriers into a herd should be avoided if possible. If calves are purchased from a variety of sources, they should be kept in isolation for at least 3 weeks after the date of arrival. Infected animals should be identified with the use of serial fecal examinations and raised in isolation. Newborn animals should be reared in isolation away from older infected animals. A thorough cleanup, disinfection and period of vacancy of animal pens is indicated. Vaccines have given inconsistent results. A killed autogenous vaccine made from the isolate on the affected farm is given to the dam in late pregnancy, and the young are vaccinated several weeks after birth. A vaccine composed of live avirulent strains of *Salmonella* has been used recently in calves and pigs, and the immunity is superior to that produced by bacterin.

Major changes in rations should be avoided. Animals to be transported should be handled carefully and rested at intervals. Medication of the feed and water supplies of susceptible animals which have been exposed to infection has been attempted with some success, e.g., for cattle, furazolidone in the feed or water, to provide 8 mg of the active drug per pound of body weight daily for 7 days; for pigs, 0.41 gm of the active drug per gallon of drinking water for 7 days.

LISTERIOSIS
(Listerellosis, Circling disease)

A sporadic, specific, bacterial infection most commonly manifested by encephalitis or meningoencephalitis in adult ruminants, by septicemia with focal hepatic necrosis in young ruminants and monogastric animals, and by septicemia with myocardial degeneration or focal hepatic necrosis in fowls (*see* AVIAN LISTERIOSIS, p. 1047). The various manifestations of infection occur in all susceptible species. Abortion and perinatal infection may occur in all susceptible mammals, but abortion with encephalitis has not been observed.

Etiology and Epizootiology: Listeriosis is caused by *Listeria monocytogenes,* a small, motile, gram-positive, nonspore-forming, extremely resistant, diphtheroid rod. Although it grows well on most of the commonly employed bacterial media, it is sometimes difficult to isolate from infected tissues and body fluids.

Listeriosis in its various forms is ubiquitous. The organism has been isolated from at least 42 domestic and wild mammals, 22 species of birds, as well as fish, crustaceans, insects, sewage, water, feedstuffs and earth. The natural reservoirs of the parasite have not been determined. Listeriosis of cattle and sheep is most prevalent in cold weather and seldom occurs during the summer or in areas of warm climate. Outbreaks often occur 2 to 4 days after a sudden drop in temperature. Reported exceptions are listeriosis in sheep and goats in Central Asia during the extremely hot, dry summer months.

The encephalitic form is only one manifestation of listeriosis, and it seems possible that each form may have a unique pathogenesis. There is evidence, for example, that infection through the eye or upper respiratory tract leads to encephalitis via the trigeminal or facial nerves, or both, and experimental oral or IV exposure of pregnant sheep or goats consistently leads to abortion without signs of CNS involvement. However, other evidence supports possible hematogenous entry into the brain. Ectoparasites may play a role in transmission. A relation between silage feeding and listeric infection has often been observed, but is not well understood: removal or change of silage in the ration often stops spread of listeriosis in feed lot animals; refeeding the same silage months later may produce new cases. Listeriosis in ruminants has occurred 10 to 14 days following feeding of apparently contaminated silage. The alkaline pH of spoiled silage appears to enhance the multiplication of *L. monocytogenes*. A nonbacterial listeriosis-enhancing agent (LEA) has been demonstrated in the blood of infected sheep and in the lymph nodes and blood of cattle with the diarrhea-mucosal disease complex. Intranasal exposure of sheep with a combination of LEA and *L. monocytogenes* results in listeric encephalitis.

The isolation of *L. monocytogenes* from the viscera of apparently healthy pigs, rodents and chickens, from the nasal mucus of sheep, from the reproductive organs of cows, mares and man, and from feces indicates that many animals are nonclinical carriers.

Clinical Findings: The most readily recognized form of listeriosis in ruminants is **encephalitis.** It may affect animals of all ages and both sexes and may appear as an epizootic in feed lot cattle or sheep. The course in sheep and goats is rapid and death may occur 4 to 48 hours after the appearance of signs; occasionally, the animal may survive for several days. In cattle, the disease is less acute and signs may last 4 to 14 days. Spontaneous recovery is uncommon but may occur. Survivors may exhibit manifestations of permanent CNS injury. Lesions are often localized in the brain stem and the signs indicate dysfunction of the third to seventh cranial nerves.

At the onset of the disease, the infected animal becomes solitary. It crowds into a corner or leans against stationary objects as if unable to stand. When walking, it often moves in a circle. Circling is not a constant sign, but when present it is always in one direction. Marked elevation of temperature (105° to 108°F), anorexia, conjunctivitis and blindness may be present. Marked depression, incoordination and paralysis of the muscles of the jaw, eye and ear as well as stringy salivation and nasal discharge are conspicuous signs. There may be intermittent twitching of the facial muscles, strabismus and drooping of one or both ears, but frank convulsions are rare. The muscles of the head, neck and forelegs usually are more tense than in the posterior part of the body. Terminally, involuntary and aimless running movements are common. Many cows display only a paralysis of the facial and throat muscles which makes eating and drinking impossible.

The disease may occur on the same premises in successive years. The number of animals involved in an outbreak usually is small but may reach 30% in a flock of sheep or goats, and 10% in a herd of cattle. Mortality is high.

L. monocytogenes has been associated with **abortion** and **perinatal death** in many animals in addition to sheep, goats and cows, and may be more common than is generally suspected. Abortion usually occurs in late gestation. Focal necrosis of the fetal liver may be masked by autolytic changes. However, *L. monocytogenes* can often be recovered from the placenta and various fetal organs. In some instances, the bacterium can be isolated from the genital tract of the dam and may be shed in the milk for periods varying from days to months. Usually the dam shows no signs of illness or residual damage from listeric abortion. However, fatal septicemia secondary to metritis has occurred. Encephalitic signs and abortion do not usually occur simultaneously on the same premises.

Lesions: In the **encephalitic form** there are usually no gross lesions. At times, however, the meninges appear slightly inflamed with a few very small gray foci, and the amount of cerebrospinal fluid may be increased. The brain may appear slightly congested and, occasionally, sheep brains may be so hyperemic that the entire brain is bright red.

The **septicemic form** is most common in the monogastric mammals. The principal lesion is focal hepatic necrosis. It has been observed in swine, dogs, cats, domestic and wild rabbits, rats, mice, moles, raccoons, skunks, foxes, chinchillas, mink, lemmings, gerbils and several other small animals. These animals may play an important part in the transmission of the disease. This form also has been found in young lambs and calves before the rumen is functional. In young calves, death occurs before 3 weeks of age and often is preceded by dysentery. At necropsy, in addition to focal hepatic necrosis, there is frequently a marked hemorrhagic gastritis and enteritis involving only the small intestine. At present, there is no satisfactory explanation for the higher incidence of septicemia in monogastric animals and of encephalitis in ruminants. Though rare, septicemia has been reported in all the domestic ruminants and deer.

Diagnosis: At present, there is no satisfactory ante-mortem diagnostic test. Listeriosis can be confirmed only by isolation and identification of the specific etiologic agent. Specimens of choice are the brain from CNS cases, and the placenta and fetus from abortion cases. If primary isolation attempts fail, ground tissue should be held at 4°C for several weeks and recultured. Occasionally, *L. monocytogenes* has been isolated from the spinal fluid, nasal discharge, urine, feces and milk of clinically ill ruminants. For isolation from these sources, the use of embryonated hens' eggs or IP inoculation of mice may be preferable to nonliving media. Serologic tests may be of value in some instances but, in general, have proved to be unsatisfactory because many healthy animals show high titers against the bacterium.

In sheep, it is difficult to distinguish between listeriosis, enterotoxemia and pregnancy toxemia, except at necropsy. The fatty liver found in pregnancy toxemia and the characteristic hemorrhages of enterotoxemia are not seen in listeriosis. In pregnancy toxemia, facial and ear paralysis are less likely to occur, but grinding of the teeth is more common than in listeriosis. Acetone may be present in the urine in both diseases. The torticollis of pregnancy toxemia generally is not as rigid as in listeriosis.

In cattle, listeriosis may be easily confused with thromboembolic encephalitis, rabies or poisoning. The only certain differentiation is by culture, demonstration of Negri bodies or mouse inoculation.

Prophylaxis and Treatment: A satisfactory therapeutic agent has not been found, particularly for sheep and goats. In these species, it appears that irreparable damage is done to the CNS before obvious signs develop. In cattle where the disease is less acute and the CNS alterations are not as advanced when signs appear, therapeutic measures may be of value. Chlortetracycline (R 11) or any of the other tetracycline antibiotics in the highest tolerable dose appear to be the medication of choice, but may be followed by fatal relapse despite additional therapy. It is difficult to maintain therapeutic levels in the brain with these antibiotics. The sulfonamides (R 68, 85), and penicillin (R 44) may be of value if given early, but there appears to be a wide variation of susceptibility to penicillin. Adequate supportive treatment should be given to all animals.

Prophylaxis with autogenous bacterins has been attempted, but the results are inconclusive. In an outbreak, affected animals should be segregated. If silage was being fed, use of that particular ensilage should be discontinued on a trial basis. Spoiled silage should be routinely avoided.

Public Health Importance: Despite the apparently low invasiveness of *L. monocytogenes,* all suspected material should be handled with caution. Aborted fetuses and necropsy of septicemic cases present the greatest hazard. Owners and veterinarians have developed fatal meningitis, septicemia and papular exanthema on the arms after handling aborted material. In encephalitis of animals, the bacterium is usually confined to the brain and presents little danger unless the brain is removed. Pregnant animals, including the human, should be protected from this infection because of danger to the fetus.

L. monocytogenes has been isolated from the milk of cows following abortion and from some cases of mastitis. Such infected milk is a hazard because the organism may survive certain forms of pasteurization and thus expose humans who drink raw or inefficiently pasteurized milk. The concept that animals serve as a reservoir for infection of man may be questioned since the organism has been isolated from the feces of a significant number of apparently normal people as well as animals. Low-grade infections in man may be more common than is generally suspected and, in pregnant women, may lead to death of the fetus. Perinatal infections account for almost 75% of all the cases of listeriosis reported in man during the past few years. Meningitis or meningoencephalitis accounts for most of the remainder. Other manifestations of listeric infection are conjunctivitis, endocarditis and urethritis.

BOVINE RESPIRATORY DISEASE COMPLEX
(Pneumonia)

Bovine respiratory diseases cause serious economic losses and present diagnostic difficulties due to the variety of etiologic agents, predisposing conditions and complicating factors. Differential diagnosis hinges on presence or absence of fever, chest or lung sounds, nature of nasal discharges, condition of visible respiratory mucosa and the nature of dyspnea. Field diagnosis is confusing because these signs are inconsistently manifested by sick cattle and variously interpreted by clinicians. Even when pathologic, serologic and microbiologic findings are available, the etiology is frequently controversial or unknown. The term "shipping fever complex" is being replaced by "bovine respiratory disease complex" which includes pneumonic pasteurellosis and nonpneumonic conditions.

The causes include allergic reactions, parasites, viruses, bacteria and mycoplasmas, and may be multiple or complicated. Several agents which have been isolated from the abnormal lungs are still the subject of controversy and uncertainty. These include adenoviruses, rhinoviruses, syncytial viruses, herpesviruses, picornaviruses, mycoplasmas, chlamydiae and *Haemophilus somnus*.

BOVINE PNEUMONIC PASTEURELLOSIS
(Shipping fever)

Pneumonic pasteurellosis is a distinct entity, usually distinguishable from the rest of the bovine respiratory disease complex by clinical signs and a distinctive fibrinous pneumonia evident at necropsy. The term "shipping fever" is losing favor because it is misleading and the term "hemorrhagic septicemia" is best reserved for the septicemic *Pasteurella* infections seen in cattle, swine and beasts of burden in Southern Asia.

Etiology and Epidemiology: Although the details of pathogenesis remain obscure, *Pasteurella multocida* and *P. haemolytica* are closely associated with the characteristic clinical signs and lesions. These organisms are sometimes cultured from healthy cattle, but the frequency of isolation is greater in shipped cattle and an argument persists about whether their role is as primary pathogens or as opportunists colonizing tissues weakened by stress, bacterial or viral infections (of these, bovine myxovirus parainfluenza-3 is the most common suspect). The disease is rarely diagnosed unless the affected animals have been shipped, or exposed to cattle recently transported. The reservoir is probably cattle and transmission of pasteurellae may occur by aerosol or contact with secretions.

Clinical Findings: Affected cattle exhibit depression, anorexia, serous nasal discharge, cough, fever (105° to 108°F), increased pulse rate and rapid shallow respirations. Lung auscultation reveals increased vesicular sounds, bronchial tones and moist rales. As the disease progresses, absence of lung sounds may indicate areas of consolidation or pleural exudate. Occasionally pleuritic friction or crackling associated with emphysema is heard.

Lesions: The anteroventral portions of the lungs are frequently swollen and firm with red and purple discoloration of lobules separated by serofibrinous material in the intralobular spaces. Pleuritis with serofibrinous adhesions may be present. These lesions are grossly and histologically similar to those of contagious bovine pleuropneumonia although severe hydrothorax is uncommon in pneumonic pasteurellosis.

Treatment: Affected cattle should be isolated. Dihydrostreptomycin in combination with penicillin (℞ 41) is effective in the treatment of early cases. The sulfonamides and particularly sulfamethazine (℞ 82) are quite effective, as are the broad-spectrum antibiotics, e.g., oxytetracycline (℞ 27). Regardless of the initial antibiotic or sulfonamide used, the same drug should be used for 3 to 4 days. Treatment begun more than 1 or 2 days after onset of the disease is much less effective.

Control: Where control by preventing stress or contact with transported animals is impossible, numerous vaccines are enlisted to "aid in the control of bovine *Pasteurella* infections". These vaccines contain various combinations of bovine rhinotracheitis, parainfluenza 3 and virus diarrhea viruses as modified live viruses of tissue culture origin, with or without *Pasteurella* or other bacterins. Their value for this purpose is controversial. The use of antibiotics—injected or in the feed —as a means of preventing this disease has yet to be fully evaluated.

PASTEURELLOSIS OF SHEEP AND SWINE

In contrast to the situation in cattle, pasteurellosis of sheep and swine is usually not associated with changes in management. *Pasteurella haemolytica* can produce a septicemia in lambs without evidence of obvious stress. The condition is manifest by high temperature and sudden death. It must be differentiated from other diseases causing sudden death in this age group, i.e., enterotoxemia due to *Clostridium perfringens* Type D.

Pasteurellosis in swine is usually a secondary complication of enzootic (virus) pneumonia of swine.

Treatment and control measures in sheep are similar to those used in cattle. Early antibiotic treatment of swine is necessary to avoid a high mortality associated with extensive lung damage. Control is based on the prevention or control of enzootic pneumonia (q.v., p. 306).

TULAREMIA

An infectious disease of wild rodents, especially rabbits, transmitted to domestic animals and man directly or by insect vectors. The disease occurs primarily in sheep in the Western U.S.A., but it may affect other animals and birds in the U.S.A. and other countries.

Etiology and Transmission: The causative agent is *Francisella* (*Pasteurella*) *tularensis,* a nonspore-bearing, gram-negative organism which has serologic relationship with brucellae. It is easily killed within 10 minutes at 58°C. Transmission in sheep usually occurs by the bites of massive numbers of wood ticks, *Dermacentor andersoni.* Ticks also transmit the disease to pigs, foals and calves. Outbreaks in sheep appear during the spring months and are frequently associated with deaths in rodents that have been infested with ticks. Man is subject to the disease from handling and cleaning infected rabbits, squirrels or game birds, from eating uncooked, infected meat, drinking contaminated water or from arthropod bites.

Clinical Findings: In sheep, other animals and even man, tularemia may occur as a latent infection for long periods without evidence of clinical signs. Heavy infestations of infected ticks in young lambs, pigs or colts are generally necessary to create clinical manifestations of the disease. Fever (105° to 107°F), general stiffness, fatigue and depression, increased respiration, coughing and diarrhea are common. Weakness, incoordination, and eventual recumbency occur within a few days to 1 to 2 weeks.

The most characteristic lesions found at necropsy are miliary, whitish to yellowish foci (2 to 8 mm) in the lymph nodes, liver and spleen. These lesions also appear in rodents. Enlargement and congestion of the lymph nodes may also be present. Care should be taken by human beings to avoid direct contact with infected tissues and ticks on animals dead of tularemia.

Diagnosis: The occurrence of a heavy tick population in the spring months, the finding of dead rodents and the appearance of a generalized septicemia, especially in young lambs, may suggest tularemia. Agglutination tests of the blood serum can be utilized in living animals. Necrotic foci in the liver, spleen and lymph nodes suggest the disease, and they provide culture material for organism identification. Organisms can sometimes be isolated from ticks taken from dead animals.

Tularemia in sheep should be differentiated from tick anemia and tick paralysis. In the latter, an ascending paralysis, usually not observed in tularemia, is present; rapid recovery occurs when the ticks are removed. Other septicemias, e.g., pneumonia, may develop secondarily to tularemia, or as a primary disease.

Treatment and Control: Individual animals respond to treatment with the tetracycline drugs, particularly oxytetracycline, at levels up to 5 mg/lb of body wt daily. Penicillin and dihydrostreptomycin (℞ 41) are less effective.

Flock control in sheep is accomplished by tick control (q.v., p. 718).

GLANDERS
(Farcy)

A contagious, usually chronic, fatal disease of Equidae, caused by *Actinobacillus* (*Malleomyces*) *mallei* and characterized by serial development of ulcerating nodules which occur most commonly in the upper respiratory tract, lungs and skin. Man, Felidae and other species are susceptible and are usually fatally affected. Glanders is one of the oldest diseases known and, at one time, was prevalent throughout the world. It has now been eradicated or effectively controlled in many countries, including the U.S.A.

Etiology: *A. mallei* is present in nasal and skin ulcerative exudate of infected animals and the disease is commonly contracted by ingesting food and water contaminated by the nasal discharge of carrier animals. The organism is susceptible to heat, light and disinfectants and is unlikely to survive in a contaminated area for more than 6 weeks.

Clinical Findings: Following an incubation period of approximately 2 weeks, affected animals usually exhibit septicemia and high fever (up to 106°F), and subsequently develop a thick mucopurulent nasal discharge and respiratory signs. Death occurs within a few days. The chronic disease is common in horses and occurs as a debilitating condition with nodular or ulcerative cutaneous and nasal involvement. Animals may live for months to years, being responsible for disseminating the disease. The prognosis is generally unfavorable, and recovered animals may not develop immunity.

Although nasal, pulmonary and cutaneous forms of glanders are recognized, more than one form may affect an animal simultaneously. In the **nasal form,** nodules develop in the mucosa of the nasal septum and lower parts of the turbinates. The nodules degenerate into deep, crater-like ulcers with raised irregular borders. With healing of the ulcers, characteristic star-shaped cicatrices remain. In the early stage, the submaxillary lymph nodes are enlarged and edematous, later becoming adherent to the skin or deeper tissues.

In the **pulmonary form,** small tubercle-like nodules, which have caseous or calcified centers, surrounded by inflammatory zones, are found in the lungs. Pulmonary lesions are common in all cases of glanders. If the disease process is extensive, consolidation of the lung tissue and glanders pneumonia may be present. The nodules tend to break down and may discharge their contents into the bronchioles, resulting in extension of the infection to the upper respiratory tract.

In the **cutaneous form** ("farcy") nodules appear along the course of the lymph vessels, particularly of the extremities. These nodules undergo degeneration, and form crater-like ulcers which discharge a highly infectious, thick, sticky, yellowish-gray pus. The liver and spleen may also show typical nodular lesions.

Diagnosis: The typical nodules, ulcers, scar formation and debilitated condition may provide sufficient evidence for a clinical diagnosis of the disease. Since, however, these signs usually do not develop until the disease is well advanced, specific diagnostic tests should be applied as early as possible. In addition to the mallein test, which is the procedure of choice, any of several serologic tests may be used; of these, complement fixation is the most accurate. Bacteriologic examination of exudate from lesions will indicate the presence of the causative organism.

Prophylaxis and Treatment: There are no immunizing agents for the prevention of glanders. Prophylaxis and control depend upon the early detection and elimination, by destruction, of affected animals, as well as complete quarantine and rigorous disinfection of the area involved. Treatment is given only in enzootic areas. Antibiotics are not very effective. Sulfadiazine (Ɓ 66) given daily for 20 days has been effective.

MELIOIDOSIS

A granulomatous disease characterized by the formation of caseous or suppurating lesions in lymph nodes and in viscera. It occurs in sheep, goats, pigs, cattle, horses, dogs, cats, a variety of wild animals and man in tropical countries and rarely elsewhere. Of the laboratory animals, hamsters and guinea pigs are highly susceptible.

The disease is caused by *Pseudomonas pseudomallei* (*Loefflerella pseudomallei, Malleomyces pseudomallei, Bacillus whitmori*), a somewhat oval, gram-negative bipolar-staining bacillus. The organisms are found in discharges, e.g., nasal mucus when the lungs are affected, and urine when the kidneys are involved. Transmission is apparently from animal to animal or from soil and water to animals.

Clinical signs vary with the site of the lesions. In domestic animals it is usually chronic but progressive. In sheep and goats, abscesses in the lungs are common and signs of pneumonia are seen. Nasal discharge is evident if the nasal septum is ulcerated. At times joints are affected and the animal is lame. Signs of encephalitis are evident when microabscesses are present in the CNS.

One or more infected abscesses often have been found in clinically normal sheep, goats and pigs. Death occurs when the abscesses are extensive or when a vital organ is involved.

The lesions show no pathognomonic features and diagnosis is by bacteriologic identification of the bacillus. Some organisms not pathogenic for guinea pigs may have many of the bacteriologic features of *P. pseudomallei*. Complement fixation tests on sera are a useful aid to diagnosis in most species including man. Hemagglutination tests can be used on cattle and pig sera.

There is no effective vaccine. Treatment of clinical cases is generally unsatisfactory. Antibiotics (e.g., chloramphenicol or chlortetracycline) and sulfonamides check the disease while they are being given, but there is a relapse when medication is withdrawn.

STRANGLES

A contagious suppurative regional lymphadenitis of Equidae characterized by the occurrence of abscesses in lymph nodes draining the upper respiratory and buccal mucosae.

Etiology and Epizootiology: The causal agent, *Streptococcus equi*, is a beta hemolytic, antigenically unique streptococcus (Lancefield Group C). It is a pathogen peculiar to Equidae.

In its enzootic form, strangles is a disease of the young but animals of any age without previous infection or in which such experience is temporally remote may contract the disease. The source of infection is the diseased animal or an environment contaminated by pus from strangles abscesses. *Str. equi* is capable of surviving in infectious form for months on fomites or in barns. Whether the asymptomatic carrier state exists is unknown. Concomitant or predisposing viral infections are not requisite but apparently contribute to the rapid spread of strangles.

Clinical Findings: The incubation period for experimental strangles is 3 to 6 days. Usually the first sign noticed is refusal to consume feed and water. A temperature as high as 106°F and catarrhal inflammation of the upper respiratory mucosa and lymphadenitis of the lymphoid nodules of the pharynx develop in the first day or two. Mucopurulent nasal discharge appears when these multiple small abscesses drain. Affected animals are reluctant to swallow and may stand with the neck extended. The infection spreads to the dependent intermandibular and parapharyngeal lymph nodes, which become abscessed. The parapharyngeal nodes are those most commonly involved and the infection may extend from this site to the anterior cervical nodes. The disease is usually contained at the parapharyngeal level and when the abscesses mature and drain, fever lyses and in most cases rapid healing occurs. The course of the disease is approximately 2 weeks for individuals but the course of an outbreak in a herd may extend over several months. If prophylactic measures are not adopted, the disease smolders with the addition of new horses to the herd and with the advent of each crop of foals.

Morbidity in the epizootic form is usually high and mortality low (less than 2%). Death when it occurs is frequently the result of infection of the CNS or formation of abscesses in viscera. Nonsuppurative myocarditis may result; electrocardiography has detected abnormalities in about half of the horses affected. These persist for a few days to as long as several months. Purpura haemorrhagica (q.v., p. 39) may occur as a sequela or even during the course of the more chronic forms of the disease. Empyema of the guttural pouches may occur. However, most horses appear to recover without sequelae.

A more chronic form known as "bastard strangles" may occur. This disease affects individuals only and is not an epizootic. It is characterized by abscess formation in many areas of the body over a period of weeks or months and by rapidly progressing cachexia and intermittent fever. This form of disease is likely conditioned by failure of some individuals to muster a serviceable immune response and to confine disease to the lymph nodes of the upper respiratory tract. Treatment of horses with penicillin at an inopportune moment in the course of events that lead to the primary immune response may contribute to the development of "bastard strangles" because of the modification of streptococcal cell wall antigens by the antibiotic.

Diagnosis: When strangles occurs in epizootic form, its clinical features are difficult to mistake. High fever and the formation of abscesses in the lymph nodes of the head and pharyngeal region are almost pathognomonic. Infection of the upper respiratory mucosa and lymph nodes by *Streptococcus zooepidemicus* secondary to viral disease may mimic strangles but the fever and the characteristic rapid development of abscesses serve to differentiate the diseases clinically. Definitive diagnosis depends on identification of *Str. equi*, preferably from pus obtained upon surgical drainage of mature abscesses. Strangles abscesses which drain naturally are rapidly invaded by *Str. zooepidemicus* the presence of which may confuse bacteriologic diagnosis. Identification of *Str. equi* from an individual (whether or not that individual displays typical signs of strangles) is certain evidence or completely reliable warning of the imminence of this disease in the herd.

Prophylaxis: Horses with mucopurulent nasal discharges or other suggestive signs should be isolated and cultures made before such animals are added to herds free of strangles. If *Str. equi* is identified from these, they should be kept in strict isolation until they are free of the infection.

A killed bacterin may be administered as a 30-ml total dose

IM as three 10-ml injections given a week apart. Some practitioners prefer to use three 5-ml doses in yearlings rather than the recommended 10-ml dose. Vaccinated horses may experience a transient elevation of temperature, and a local reaction at the site of the injection consisting of edema and occasionally induration; the severity varies considerably. Abscess formation at the site of the injection usually is caused by immunization of animals in the incubative stage, or those recently recovered from the disease. A severe local reaction following the first or second injection contraindicates continuing the series. Vaccination failure due to antigenic differences in *Str. equi* strains has not been observed.

Treatment: *Str. equi* is very sensitive to penicillin, and resistance to this antibiotic is rare. Sulfamerazine and sulfamethazine are also effective. Early, prompt and continued treatment (℞ 47, 75, 82) may prevent abscess formation. Once instituted, treatment must be continued until the temperature returns to normal and has remained there for several days. After phlegmon or abscess formation occurs, systemic treatment may only prolong the course of the disease.

Complete rest and nursing should be provided. Abscesses may be hot-packed, and when mature should be incised and drained. Severe dyspnea usually indicates compression of the pharynx or larynx from abscessation of the pharyngeal lymph nodes, and a tracheotomy may become necessary.

CORYNEBACTERIUM EQUI INFECTION

Corynebacterium equi causes a purulent pneumonia in foals and often is found in tuberculosis-like lesions in the cervical lymph nodes of swine. It is doubtful whether the microorganism is of much economic importance in swine. Although not common, the infection sometimes arises in foals when they are about 2 to 4 months old. Usually, the affected foal has suffered no previous illness. The onset of the disease is characterized by dullness, increased temperature, rapid pulse and respiration. The temperature remains above normal and sometimes exceeds 106°F. A cough develops, the eyes water and there is a purulent nasal discharge. Moist rales develop in the lungs. The foal becomes weak and emaciated and dies. The course of the disease is 6 to 14 days and the mortality is high.

In most cases, infection appears to start in the lungs as bronchopneumonia, with multiple abscess formation as the most constant lesion. The abscesses are circumscribed, range from 10 to 100 mm in diameter and are filled with a thick, purulent, yellowish-gray exudate. Usually, they are also found in the pulmonary lymph nodes and rarely are seen in the mesenteric, colic and hepatic lymph nodes. They may occur in the liver.

The microorganism has been found in aborted equine fetuses and in the genital tract of barren mares. However, it does not appear to be a common cause of abortion or sterility in the mare. Possibly, the organism lives in soil and infects animals only when conditions are favorable.

Signs and lesions are not pathognomonic. A definite diagnosis depends upon isolation of the causative organism.

Immunizing procedures are of no avail, and prevention appears to be influenced by good hygienic practices in caring for the mare and foal. Presently known chemotherapeutic agents have no effect.

NEONATAL SEPTICEMIAS AND BACTEREMIAS

(Navel ill, Omphalitis, Omphalophlebitis, Joint ill, Pyemic arthritis, Polyarthritis, Viscosum infection, Sleepy foal disease)

These are infectious processes, arising prenatally or soon after birth, and are caused by a variety of microorganisms. The etiology, pathogenesis and manifestations vary with the species affected, the age when infection is contracted, the species of infecting organisms and the site of infection.

Etiology: Foals: Fatal and crippling infections of newborn foals may be caused by *Streptococcus zooepidemicus (pyogenes* var. *equi), Escherichia coli, Actinobacillus equuli (Shigella equirulis, Bacterium viscosum equi), Salmonella* spp., *Staphylococcus aureus* and *Klebsiella* spp., in approximately that order of incidence. Prenatal infections may be associated with metritis or placentitis. Entry of postnatal infection is by ingestion, inhalation or through the umbilicus. Hypogammaglobulinemia, as a result of deficiency in colostrum or failure of immunoglobulin absorption through the intestinal wall during the first 24 hours after birth, is a predisposing factor. (*See also* DIARRHEA OF NEWBORN ANIMALS, p. 166.)

Calves: Birth-related diseases are less frequent than in foals. The organisms most often involved are *E. coli*, streptococci, corynebacteria, staphylococci, *Sphaerophorus necrophorus* and pasteurellae. Prenatal infections may occur in herds with a history of uterine infection, but most infections are postnatal, entering through the umbilicus or by ingestion. Prematurely born calves are more likely to be affected than calves carried to term. Incidence is highest in calves separated from their dams at birth and stabled in groups.

Pigs: Pathogenesis is similar to that in calves, with streptococci, staphylococci and diphtheroids being the organisms principally involved; "wolf tooth" wounds may serve as a portal of entry.

Lambs: Contamination of the umbilicus at birth, docking and castration wounds, and unsanitary lambing quarters are the important sources of infection. *Erysipelothrix insidiosa* causes serious mortality but other organisms cultured from the lesions such as *Sphaerophorus necrophorus*, streptococci and staphylococci are not of great epidemiologic significance. *Corynebacterium pseudotuberculosis* may infect the navel with subsequent abscessation in the liver and other internal organs.

Clinical Findings: Foals: Signs observed depend on localization of infecting organisms. Lethargy, diminishing strength of the suck reflex and inability to get up and stand unaided or hold the sucking position are characteristics of all infections. Convulsions are associated with meningitis and encephalitis; lameness with arthritis and tenosynovitis; increased respiratory rate and colic with pleurisy, pneumonia, diarrhea and peritonitis. An *A. equuli* infection is characterized by extreme sleepiness, nephritis and uremia.

The course of the condition depends on the affected animal's age at onset and nonspecific factors collectively described as resistance. Death may occur within 12 hours or the course may be prolonged into weeks. Recovery depends on site of infecting organisms and institution of, and response to therapy.

Calves: The course is usually less acute than in foals with a greater tendency toward development of umbilical abscesses. Signs are those of a septic process, and joint involvement is less frequent than in other species. Umbilical hernias are an occasional complication.

Pigs: Neonatal infections may be manifest as acute septicemia, pneumonia, abscesses of internal organs, encephalitis, or arthritis. Signs are those common to generalized septic infection or pyemia accompanied by such specific localizations as abscessation of the navel, pyoarthritis or encephalitis followed by retarded growth or stunting.

Lambs: Infection of the navel and castration or docking wounds, with accompanying pyoarthritis and internal abscesses may reach epizootic proportions. The suppurative type usually appears during the first month. Morbidity is high. Lambs with suppurative infection develop acute lameness and one or more joints become distended with purulent fluid. Nonsuppurative types appear at 1 to 5 months and are accompanied by lameness and stiffness, usually involving all 4 legs, with chronic lameness and retarded development in as many as 20% of a flock. There is little enlargement of joints in the acute stage, but thickening of the capsule may occur in chronic cases.

Lesions: These are typical of septic processes in the umbilical area, joints, liver and other tissues although lesions associated with *A. equuli* are characterized by macroscopic or microscopic abscessation in adrenal and renal cortices. *E. coli* commonly causes pleurisy and peritonitis and the carcass will often have a characteristic odor. Streptococci or staphylococci cause macroscopic abscessation.

Diagnosis: Because of the variety of organisms affecting each species and the frequency of undifferentiated common signs, especially in the very young subject, it is difficult to make an etiologically accurate clinical diagnosis. Specific diagnosis usually must await cultural examination of an accessible abscess or following necropsy. Accordingly, it is desirable to select treatment to cover the infections occurring most frequently or causing the greatest loss. Often, this is dependent on local experience.

Prophylaxis: The prevention of infection depends largely on good management, particularly the provision of a sanitary environment for parturition and upon proper care of the navel immediately after birth. The umbilical cord should not be ligated. The stump may be treated with an antiseptic solution or powder. In foals the cord should be left to rupture naturally when the mare gets to her feet after delivery or by the foal struggling in an attempt to stand for the first time. Tincture of iodine applied to the umbilical cord is indicated in all species.

A small wide-mouth bottle half-filled with tincture of iodine is held against the navel, the newborn and the glass inverted as a unit, held for a moment and then righted. In the fly season, a desiccating healing powder, preferably one with fly-repellent properties, should also be applied. In screwworm areas, the navel of the newborn must be treated promptly with an ointment which kills the larvae and repels the flies. Generally the navel which is properly treated at birth requires little subsequent treatment. The administration of donor colostrum is recommended in cases where the mare leaks milk prior to foaling. If this is not available, an injection of dam's plasma (about 250 ml) may provide a measure of protection; cross-matching foal's cells against donor plasma should always be performed prior to transfusion but this precaution is not necessary in calves.

Treatment: The treatment of advanced or chronic infections of the newborn is difficult and unrewarding; however, in the early acute stages, or prophylactically, antimicrobial drugs are effective.

In the newborn foal, prophylactic and therapeutic use of antimicrobial compounds should be directed principally at *E. coli* and *A. equuli,* then at *S. zooepidemicus.* Injectable penicillin-streptomycin mixtures (℞ 41) or neomycin (℞ 24) may be effective. The initial dose should contain a minimum of 1 gm of streptomycin and an additional 0.5 gm should be given at 3-hour intervals for at least 4 days; ampicillin (℞ 3) or cloxacillin (℞ 17) are useful in staphylococcal and streptococcal infections. Joint infection should be treated by the intra-articular and IM or IV routes. Umbilical abscesses should be drained and the sac flushed with tincture of iodine.

For prophylactic treatment a dose containing 1 to 2 gm of streptomycin should be given every 12 hours for 3 days or longer or neomycin, 0.5 gm, b.i.d. Broad-spectrum antibiotics (℞ 11, 25, 58) may also be used either prophylactically or therapeutically. Salmonellosis, *E. coli* and *Klebsiella* spp. infections may be treated with chloramphenicol (℞ 7), or neomycin (℞ 24) which should be given both orally and parenterally, or nitrofurazone (℞ 102) orally, which should be supplemented by an antibiotic administered parenterally. Chemical cauterization of a patent urachus with silver nitrate sticks has assisted in stopping urine leakage and the resulting bladder and systemic infection.

Treatment of calves should follow the same general principles outlined for foals, but economics may dictate only a one-time treatment. Parenteral treatment with broad-spectrum antibiotics or sulfonamide mixtures (e.g., ℞ 78) is preferred because of a less definite pattern in the incidence of infecting organisms. Surgical drainage and local treatment is especially important in calves. If a hernia is present care should be taken not to incise it. Because of the long hair surrounding the umbilical area and a heavy umbilical cord, the incidence of screwworm and other fly maggot infestation is greater and should be considered in local treatment of early infections.

Although individual professional attention to lambs and pigs often may not be economically feasible in some herds, great dependence must be put on sanitary management; treatment of the umbilical cord at birth is economically feasible and should be practiced. Injection of repository antibiotics may reduce risk of immediate neonatal infection.

ACTINOBACILLOSIS

A disease similar to actinomycosis, but which most often affects soft tissues and lymph nodes. Bony structures may be affected as well. It occurs in cattle and swine, occasionally in sheep, and rarely in man. The causative agent is *Actinobacillus lignieresii.*

In cattle the disease usually affects the tongue ("wooden tongue") and less frequently other tissue, such as skeletal muscle and liver. Small abscesses with a diffuse, extensive connective tissue proliferation are a prominent feature. In sheep, actinobacillosis is a purulent disease of the skin, lymph nodes, and soft tissues of the head and neck. Epididymitis is common in rams. In swine, the soft tissue of the head (especially ears) and the mammary glands may be affected.

Pus from actinobacillosis lesions may contain granules or "rosettes" which are less than 1 mm in diameter, and are smaller than the "sulfur granules" of actinomycosis. Stained smears of the pus will reveal rather short gram-negative bacteria, in contrast to the gram-positive filaments which are demonstrable in actinomycosis.

Circumscribed lesions may be treated by complete excision. The response to iodides is usually dramatic (℞ 574, 579, 581). Systemic or local treatment with antibiotics, e.g., oxytetracycline (℞ 25), streptomycin (℞ 56) and erythromycin (℞ 18), are effective as well.

Actinobacillus equuli (*Shigella equirulis*) is the cause of septicemia in horses (q.v., p. 394).

PARATUBERCULOSIS
(Johne's disease)

A chronic infectious disease of cattle, sheep and goats characterized by thickening of the intestinal wall and recurrent diarrhea that usually persists causing a gradual loss of flesh. With few exceptions, the disease progresses until the animal is killed.

It is a disease of the intestinal tract; however, the bacillus, *Mycobacterium paratuberculosis* (Johne's bacillus), has also been isolated from mesenteric lymph nodes, udder, and reproductive tracts of both sexes. Johne's disease is nearly always brought into a clean herd by the introduction of an infected animal, but it may be months before any animals show clinical signs, especially if management and nutrition are adequate. Infection usually occurs by ingestion of infected feces. The organism can survive in fecal material and contaminated soil for more than a year.

Clinical Findings: Calves are more susceptible than older cattle but because of the long incubation period most cases are seen in 2- to 6-year-old animals. However, a few cattle less than 2 years of age will show signs, especially if nutrition or management is suboptimal. A persistent or recurrent diarrhea is the chief sign, temperature and appetite remaining normal. The animal gradually loses weight and hair-coat color may fade. Remissions may occur, especially during pregnancies, but the course is usually inexorable.

  Lesions: The lower part of the small intestine, the ileocecal valve and the adjacent cecum may be found to be much thickened, and the mucosa thrown up in folds.

  The disease in sheep and goats is similar but scouring is less marked than in the disease in cattle. Pigs can be infected, at least experimentally, and thus are potential shedders.

Diagnosis: Although intradermal allergic tests, complement fixation tests and IV johnin tests are of value in detecting infected herds, they are insufficiently reliable for individual diagnosis. To detect early (subclinical) cases is most difficult. Gram-staining of a small fecal sample from an advanced clinical case will frequently reveal the acid-fast organisms, although negative findings do not rule out the disease. Repeated sampling of the feces or of intestinal mucosa from deep within the rectum is indicated. Culturing of feces is the method of choice for detecting subclinical shedders, but positive results are unavailable for 6 to 8 weeks, and negative results mean little. At necropsy the organism may be found in the intestinal lining or the adjacent lymph nodes, either histologically or by culture.

Prophylaxis and Treatment: No satisfactory treatment is known. In some countries, regulatory bodies provide assistance in handling Johne's disease. However the lack of reliable diagnostic methods for preclinical cases is a major problem.

  Intrauterine infection is rare, and a clean herd can usually be established if young calves are separated—immediately at birth —from older cows and anything contaminated with their feces.

Vaccination, which first proved useful in sheep, is also of value for young calves. However, tuberculin tests of vaccinated cattle are difficult to interpret, and bovine vaccination is not authorized in many countries. Even where vaccination is practiced, it should be used in conjunction with sanitary precautions to minimize exposure. In many areas, rigid sanitation itself will provide satisfactory control.

BOVINE WINTER DYSENTERY
(Winter scours)

An acute infectious, enzootic disease of stabled cattle affecting animals of all ages with calves and yearlings being least susceptible. Winter dysentery is characterized by high morbidity, but very low mortality. It leads to dehydration, loss of weight and condition and, in lactating animals, to a sharp fall in milk production.

Etiology: It is still generally accepted that bovine winter dysentery is caused by *Vibrio jejuni*, but the suddenness with which the disease strikes, together with the rapidity with which it spreads from farm to farm, suggests strongly that other more infectious agents, perhaps one or more viruses, may be involved.

Clinical Findings: The period of incubation is short, varying from 3 to 5 days. The onset is sudden and, in many herds, only one animal shows evidence of diarrhea for the first few days, but the infection quickly spreads to the remainder of the herd. Just prior to the onset of diarrhea the body temperature may be moderately elevated. A profuse watery diarrhea is the main sign. The feces often are dark brown in color and tend to become darker as intestinal hemorrhage occurs. In some instances, they contain large quantities of mucus and blood. Unless complications occur, the temperature shows little or no change. The appetite is depressed and the pulse and respiration rates are only moderately increased.

Severely affected animals show evidence of abdominal pain by switching of the tail, kicking at the abdomen, and lying down and getting up at frequent intervals. Coughing is observed in about 30 to 50% of the outbreaks.

Lesions: The outstanding features at postmortem examination are dehydration, catarrhal inflammation of the jejunum and ileum, and hemorrhage into the lumen of the gut.

Diagnosis: The seasonal incidence of the disease, the age and number of animals affected, together with the suddenness of the onset, are helpful in arriving at a correct diagnosis. Mucosal disease and coccidiosis should be considered the differential diagnosis.

Prophylaxis: Owners are well advised to watch their animals carefully as they go into barns for the winter season. Newly introduced animals should be kept in isolation for a period of 2 weeks. Any animal found to be suffering from an acute attack of dysentery, regardless of cause, should be separated from the main herd until fully recovered. Veterinarians and herdsmen, after handling animals with winter dysentery, should make sure of the cleanliness of their clothing and equipment before working with healthy cattle.

Treatment: Although many agents have been used, none have proven highly effective in reducing the duration of the disease. These agents, which include intestinal astringents such as catechu, zinc phenolsulfonate, ferrous sulfate and copper sulfate, have been used alone and in combination. In severely affected animals supportive fluid therapy with blood transfusions, saline, electrolytes and glucose has been of definite value. There is no immunizing agent for the prevention of winter dysentery.

CONTAGIOUS BOVINE PLEUROPNEUMONIA

A highly contagious pneumonia generally accompanied by pleurisy. The U.S.A. has been free of the disease since 1892. In Australia, a national eradication scheme has almost eliminated the disease. It occurs in Africa and India and probably in Central Asia.

Etiology: The causal microorganism is *Mycoplasma mycoides* (*Borrelomyces peripneumoniae*). Infection spreads by susceptible cattle inhaling droplets coughed out by affected cattle. Urine droplets are a possible additional source. The incubation period of the disease varies from 2 to 17 weeks following contact, with most cases occurring within 5 to 8 weeks. In some localities susceptible herds may show 100% morbidity with high mortality, but lower rates of infection are more common. Some animals may, however, show few outward signs of the disease, the pneumonic area of the lung becoming sealed off by the formation of a fibrous capsule. Such animals become carriers. They are infective but whether in this state or when breakdown due to stress occurs, is not clear; in either case they may actively spread infection and thus constitute a serious problem in control programs.

Clinical Findings: The signs, which are typical of pneumonia and pleurisy, are high temperature (up to 107°F), anorexia, thirst, and painful, difficult breathing. The animal often stands by itself in any available shade, its head lowered and extended, its back slightly arched and the elbows turned out. Respiration is rapid, shallow and abdominal and, if the animal is forced to move quickly, the breathing becomes more distressed and a soft, moist cough is noted. In acute cases, the disease progresses rapidly, animals lose condition, breathing becomes very labored and is accompanied by grunting. The animal becomes recumbent, with death ensuing in a few hours. Less acute cases exhibit signs of varying intensity for 3 to 4 weeks. In these cases, resolution of the lesion often takes place gradually and the animal makes an apparent recovery.

Lesions: The thoracic cavity may contain up to a gallon or more of clear yellow or turbid fluid mixed with fibrin flakes. Varying areas of one or both lungs may be involved, the affected portion being enlarged and the consistency of liver. On section, the typical marbled appearance of pleuropneumonia is evident—due to the thickening of the interlobular and subpleural tissue enclosing gray, yellow or red hepatized portions of the alveolar lung tissue. In chronic or carrier cases, the lesion is sequestered in a thick fibrous tissue capsule and is necrotic.

Diagnosis: Diagnosis is made on clinical and postmortem examination. Confirmatory tests are: the complement-fixation on serum, the precipitin test on lesions (to detect specific antigen) and bacteriologic and histologic examination of lesions. Subclinical disease is detected by use of the complement-fixation test. As soon as an outbreak is suspected, slaughter and detailed postmortem examination of a suspect animal are advisable.

Control: In developed countries, where cattle movement can readily be restricted, the disease can be eradicated by quarantine, blood testing and immunization with live vaccine. Where cattle cannot be confined, the spread of infection can be limited by vaccination. Tracing of the source of infected cattle detected at abbattoirs, blood testing and imposition of strict rules for cattle movement can also contribute to the control of the disease in such areas. The disease is "notifiable", and would be eradicated by slaughter of all infected and exposed animals in many countries.

Treatment is not recommended because necrotic lesions may already be established and these will continue to harbor live organisms.

CONTAGIOUS CAPRINE PLEUROPNEUMONIA

An infectious respiratory disease of goats in which pyrexia, coughing, nasal discharge and signs of respiratory distress may be seen. The incidence is highest in the winter. The incubation period may be from 3 to 28 days. Mortality and morbidity are high and death may ensue rapidly after the onset of signs. Abortions may occur in affected pregnant animals. The disease occurs commonly in many African countries, in Turkey, Iran and India and less commonly in Mediterranean countries of Europe, in Afghanistan, China, Mongolia and Burma. Sporadic outbreaks have occurred in Mexico.

Frequently the pneumonia is confined to one lung. In hyperacute cases, the lung is markedly congested and excess pleural fluid is present. In acute cases, in addition to the excess pleural fluid, the lung has a variegated appearance due to the presence of different stages of hepatization and the distension of the interlobular septa with fluid. Masses of spongy fibrinous exudate overlie affected areas of the lung and adhere to the chest wall. In nonfatal acute cases the lesions rarely sequestrate but slowly resolve and become noninfective.

The disease is usually diagnosed on history, signs and the characteristic lesions. Isolation of the causal *Mycoplasma* is not always successful.

The pleural fluid in acute cases contains abundant branching filamentous forms of *Mycoplasma* visible by dark-field microscopy. Serologic procedures for diagnosis are inadequate at present and indeed it is not certain that the same *Mycoplasma* causes the disease in the different countries.

Vaccines prepared from infected lung and pleural fluid by treatment with formalin are supplied from laboratories in some of the countries where the disease occurs, but their effectiveness is not well documented. Experimentally, live vaccines prepared from attenuated organisms have been more successful. Treatment of the disease with tetracyclines or tylosin has been reported to be effective but would be of limited value unless given in the early stages of the infection.

BOVINE GENITAL VIBRIOSIS

A venereal disease of cattle caused by *Vibrio fetus venerealis* and characterized by infertility and early embryonic death. Abortion occurs in a small percentage of infected cows. The distribution is worldwide.

Etiology: *Vibrio fetus* is a gram-negative pleomorphic rod that has a short, "comma" shape when recently isolated from the tissues. Adaptation to artificial media results in a relatively long, spiral-shaped organism, motile by means of a polar flagellum. *V. fetus* is differentiated from nonpathogenic vibrios in that it produces catalase but not hydrogen sulfide. Exposure to heat, light and drying, quickly destroys the organism, but it may remain viable in manure, hay and soil in a cool, dark environment for up to 3 weeks. Cultures can be stored at room temperature for 2 weeks. Lyophilized cultures remain viable for many months, but frozen material should not be stored for more than 1 or 2 weeks. Fresh specimens are best for diagnosis. If, however, there is a delay before the material can be submitted to the laboratory, it may be frozen. Although *V. fetus* from sheep is morphologically similar to *V. fetus* from cattle, there is no evidence of cross-infectivity.

Transmission: Bovine vibriosis is transmitted either by coitus or artificial insemination. While other possible methods of spread have been suggested, effective control programs can be based on the assumption that the disease is exclusively venereal. Since the disease may be spread by contaminated semen, it is also possible that the infection can be spread by using contaminated instruments for examination and treatment. The infection rate in susceptible females may be almost 100%. Cows develop a resistance to the disease so that in a herd where the condition is enzootic, the disease rate drops, but reinfection often occurs.

The disease may spread from one bull to another in an artificial-insemination stud when a number of bulls are used on the same teaser. Contact of the penis with the rump or escutcheon of the teaser is believed to be the means of transmission. On occasion bulls *may* become infected from contaminated bedding.

Clinical Findings: The primary effect of vibriosis is temporary infertility; abortion is of secondary importance. Irregularity of the estrous cycle is a prominent sign. The long cycles are explained on the basis that conception takes place and is interrupted by infection. The embryo is resorbed and a new cycle begins. If the embryo is expelled, it is often so small that the abortion goes unrecognized. The variable degree of endometritis, and the slight vaginitis and cervicitis sometimes produced may also be overlooked.

Under range conditions the first evidence is a high percentage of the herd returning for service after the bulls have been with the herd 60 days or longer. Calving over a long period and an unusual number of open cows in the fall are 2 suggestive signs; great loss of flesh in the breeding bulls, suggesting overwork due to repeated breedings, is another. Conception rates of 40 to 50% or lower occur in newly infected herds. Various abortion rates have been reported; the majority of abortions occur about the fifth or sixth month of gestation and are accompanied by placental retention. The placental and fetal lesions are not characteristic enough to be diagnostic.

Diagnosis: The history may include evidence of the introduction of animals from herds where vibriosis, or at least infertility, is known to exist. Trichomoniasis and vibriosis are clinically similar, but differ in that pyometra does not occur in vibriosis, and trichomonad abortions occur only prior to the fifth month of pregnancy. Occasionally, the diseases are found concurrently in a herd. Suspected vibriosis may be confirmed by one or more of the following diagnostic procedures:

1. The vaginal mucus agglutination test: A 3 × 3 in. surgical sponge to which an 18-in. piece of string is attached, is placed in the anterior part of the vagina. After 15 minutes, this tampon is recovered and placed in an airtight vial to prevent evaporation. In the laboratory, the mucus is extracted in saline and the agglutination test carried out. While there is no official standard, complete agglutination at 1 to 20 or higher is considered positive. The copious amount of mucus in the vagina during and immediately after estrus dilute the agglutinins so that false negative results may be obtained. Blood, either from injury of the vagina or from postestrous bleeding, may cause a false positive reaction. Highest titers can be expected in mucus collected about the middle of the diestrous period. The vaginal mucus titer becomes positive approximately 60 days after infection. The titer usually persists for at least 4 months, and has been known to last for as long as 2 years. The average is about 7 months. The test is used to make a herd diagnosis and animals should be selected in order to get those that are most likely to react.

2. Isolation of V. fetus from the female genital tract: Vibrios may be isolated from the estrous mucus in the vagina, from the cervical mucus, from an endometrial biopsy or from the uterine fluid discharged during the few days after abortion. They can usually be isolated from the stomach contents and the amnionic fluid of aborted fetuses.

3. Isolation of V. fetus from the bull: The semen from infected bulls may be used for isolation but, because the organisms are frequently masked by contaminants, several samplings may be required. The organisms may be isolated from the preputial membrane by the use of gauze sponges which are placed in special medium following which the medium fluid is filtered to remove contaminants. Culture requires careful technique.

4. Transmission test: This test consists of breeding suspected bulls to virgin heifers and then subjecting the heifers to vaginal mucus culture 4 to 10 days after breeding.

5. Fluorescent antibody diagnostic procedure in bulls: A fluorescent antibody procedure utilizing the fluid recovered from preputial douching may be the most specific procedure in diagnosing infected bulls.

Treatment and Control: If there are no gross uterine changes and reinfection is avoided, 75% of cows will recover in a short time, 24% require from 2 to 12 months and a few cows will carry the infection through a normal pregnancy and harbor the infection in the genital tract after parturition. If no reinfection occurs, a herd may be regarded as free of the disease after 2 years. The best method of bringing the disease under control is to use artificial insemination. Semen for this purpose should either be from known noninfected bulls or should be treated with penicillin and streptomycin. Vibriosis is not transmitted in semen provided it is diluted at least 1:25 and 500 u of penicillin and 0.5 mg of streptomycin are added to each milliliter of the diluted semen and provided also the treated semen is held at 40°F for at least 6 hours before being used.

If natural service must be continued, the infected or exposed cows should be placed in one group and the unexposed (usually only virgin heifers) in a second. Only noninfected bulls are used on the clean animals. The clean herd is gradually increased as the infected herd is reduced. Eventually, only the clean herd remains. The isolation must be strictly maintained if this procedure is to be effective. Although spontaneous recovery in the female is the rule, this may be accelerated by the use of intra-uterine infusions of streptomycin (℞ 55) or streptomycin and penicillin (℞ 40).

In treatment of bulls, no procedure has been uniformly successful. Streptomycin, 25 gm given IM and 5 gm in 10 ml of sterile isotonic saline held in the sheath and massaged around the penis for 5 minutes daily for 3 days, has been successful as based on post-treatment negative preputial fluid examinations (3 consecutive weekly tests). *V. fetus* inhabits the surface of the penis and sheath, and it is probable that any antibiotic effective against the organism, if applied thoroughly to this area will effect a cure. Treated bulls should be tested by breeding them to heifers and subsequently testing the heifers by culture of vaginal mucus for the organisms.

Vaccination is effective in controlling the disease, especially in beef herds kept under range conditions. Usually vaccination is done at least 2 weeks before breeding and is repeated annually. Bulls may be vaccinated but the value is unknown.

OVINE GENITAL VIBRIOSIS

An infectious disease caused by the organism *Vibrio fetus* and characterized by abortion. The most serious economic loss from this disease occurs in sheep in the Rocky Mountain area of the U.S.A., but it has been diagnosed in many other parts and other countries.

Etiology and Transmission: *Vibrio fetus intestinalis* causes epizootics of abortion in sheep. In cattle the *intestinalis* variety causes only sporadic abortion. In both sheep and cattle the route of transmission of *V. fetus intestinalis* is oral. *V. fetus venerealis,* which is transmitted venereally, causes infertility and early abortion in cattle (*see* p. 405). This variety apparently does not infect sheep.

The incubation period of the ovine disease is 10 to 50 days. An outbreak of vibriosis in a flock produces immunity sufficient to prevent the appearance of the disease among exposed ewes for at least 2 years. Repeated outbreaks among susceptible replacement ewes are not uncommon. Nonpregnant ewes may carry the organism in the uterus for long periods. It has also been isolated from other internal organs, including gallbladder and intestine.

Clinical Findings: Abortion during the last 8 weeks of pregnancy or, in some instances, the delivery of weak lambs at term constitutes the typical syndrome. There is usually no indication of the impending abortion. A few animals may show a vaginal discharge. Recovery is prompt and fertility in subsequent breeding seasons is usually good. Occasionally, abortion is complicated by metritis and subsequent death. The ewe mortality varies from 0 to 5%. Usually, the incidence of abortion does not rise above 10 to 20%. In some outbreaks, however, as many as 70% of the ewes have lost their lambs.

Lesions: In some aborted fetuses, the liver shows gray necrotic foci varying from 1 to 3 cm in diameter. This is not a constant finding and is most frequent in near-term fetuses. The fetus is usually edematous and the body cavities contain a reddish fluid. The fetal membranes also are edematous and the cotyledons large and necrotic. There is wide variation in the lesions and it is necessary to have bacteriologic confirmation of the diagnosis.

Diagnosis is confirmed by microscopic demonstration of typical *V. fetus* organisms in the stomach contents of aborted lambs or by isolation of *V. fetus* from stomach contents, liver, lung, or placental fluids. Care must be taken to differentiate vibriosis from ovine chlamydial abortion (q.v., p. 273) as this latter disease produces nearly identical clinical findings and can occur concomitantly.

Treatment and Control: Aborting ewes should be isolated and strict hygienic practices adopted, including removal of aborted fetuses and associated discharges. If possible, unaffected ewes should be moved to a clean area and provided uncontaminated feed and water.

It has been reported that penicillin and streptomycin (R 41) will control an outbreak. A bacterin is effective if ewes are vaccinated shortly before mating, again in 8 weeks and annually thereafter. Feeding oxytetracycline, 80 mg/ewe/day over the last 7 to 8 weeks of pregnancy will reduce the incidence of abortion, and may be economical in some situations. Usually adequate sanitation is effective and more practical.

CORYNEBACTERIUM PSEUDOTUBERCULOSIS INFECTION

(In sheep: Caseous lymphadenitis, Pseudotuberculosis
In horses: Ulcerative lymphangitis)

An infection by *Corynebacterium pseudotuberculosis* (*ovis*), occurring in sheep, horses, cattle, goats, deer and rabbits. The organism has been isolated from the lymph nodes and appendix of man. It causes caseous lymphadenitis in sheep, ulcerative lymphangitis in horses and occasionally skin lesions in cattle. Caseous lymphadenitis occurs in sheep rather generally in the Western U.S.A. and Canada and is reported also from Argentina, Uruguay, Chile, Australia and New Zealand. It is a chronic disease, in which clinical signs and lesions may not be observed until several months after infection. The superficial, particularly the precrural and prescapular, lymph nodes usually are the primary sites of the lesions. Later, the visceral lymph nodes may be involved, particularly the mediastinal, bronchial and sublumbar. In generalized cases, the lesions may be distributed throughout the lungs, liver, kidneys and spleen, and the corresponding lymph nodes.

The affected lymph nodes become enlarged by abscesses containing a caseous, greenish-yellow, odorless pus. In lesions of long standing, this pus becomes a rather dry, firm mass, usually arranged in concentric "onion ring" layers within a thick fibrous capsule. The capillaries surrounding the abscesses may be filled with masses of organisms.

Some affected animals in the early stages of an extensive involvement of the lymph nodes are found in excellent condition at the time of slaughter, but if allowed to live, gradual emaciation develops, followed by general weakness and death.

Sheep of 2 to 4 years of age contain the highest percentage of infected animals. Twenty percent of all animals found infected on postmortem inspection are condemned. *C. pseudotuberculosis* is believed to enter the body largely through skin abrasions, principally at the time of shearing. A few animals are infected through the unhealed navel and through docking and castration wounds.

Ulcerative lymphangitis in **horses** resembles the cutaneous form of glanders. It is characterized by nodules, ulcers and inflammation of the lymph vessels, especially in the region of the fetlock, but occasionally extending up the leg. The nodules may enlarge to 1 in. in diameter. They are tough and rather insensitive at first, but later become soft and painful, and finally rupture, exuding a greenish-white pus. The onset is slow and usually manifests itself by pain. The marked involvement of the lymph nodes, so characteristic of the disease in sheep, is absent in the horse. Infection by inhalation of contaminated dust may also occur, the primary lesions then developing in the lungs.

Chronic single or multiple abscesses, known as **false distemper,** is another manifestation in horses. The disease is characterized by abscess formation, most frequently in the pectoral region, but in some animals extending to involve the mammary gland. These abscesses may reach a size of 5 to 20 cm; there is extensive peripheral edema. The abscesses may be a manifestation of systemic infection and develop slowly over several weeks. Systemic disturbance seems confined to leukocytosis and neutrophilia. Abscesses most often rupture externally, discharge viscid creamy pus and heal spontaneously. Generalized involvement occurs occasionally, in the form of abdominal abscesses, often perirenal. External abscesses may be found concomitantly. Vague clinical signs, such as depression, anorexia and loss of weight are recorded. Pathogenesis and transmission are unknown. Distribution corresponds to that of sheep in western states.

In **cattle,** there have been a few reports of this infection. It has been found in a case of bronchopneumonia in a cow and also in calves and in the so-called "skin lesions" of tuberculosis of cattle in Utah, California and Idaho. In areas where skin lesions are commonly found, *C. pseudotuberculosis* has been isolated from some of the lesions taken by biopsy or at postmortem examination of lesion-free tuberculin-reactor animals.

Diagnosis: Serologic tests alone are not diagnostic. Diagnosis of caseous lymphadenitis in sheep can be made by careful palpation of external lymph nodes or by the appearance of the characteristic lesions at necropsy. The organism can be easily isolated from the lesions in both sheep and horses. In ulcerative lymphangitis and in all other forms of lymphangitis in horses (q.v., p. 41), a positive diagnosis must be established in order to rule out the possibility of glanders (q.v., p. 388).

Prophylaxis and Treatment: Prevention of the disease in sheep is directed toward reducing the opportunities for infection of wounds sustained during shearing and around feed bunks and watering troughs. Where the disease is prevalent, the younger sheep should be shorn first. The older animals should be sorted by palpating the superficial lymph nodes and all suspected animals shorn last. Shears and other equipment should be thoroughly disinfected whenever an abscess is accidentally incised. As the animals are shorn, they should immediately be turned onto pasture or open range. This reduces the exposure of sheep with shearing wounds to infected animals with ruptured or incised abscesses and to the dust of contaminated yards and holding paddocks. Vaccines have been unsuccessful. The infection can be reduced if young sheep are carefully examined for skin lacerations immediately after shearing. All wounds must be cleaned and the skin sutured if necessary. Penicillin-streptomycin topical ointment or other appropriate antibacterial therapy (℞ 41) should be begun at once.

In horses, the disease seems to be less prevalent where the animals are kept under conditions of good husbandry and stable management.

The great majority of cases of ovine caseous lymphadenitis go untreated because the disease is usually diagnosed for the first time in animals of good condition at the time of slaughter. When the lesions are so extensive that general signs are apparent, the patient is usually beyond successful treatment. Encapsulated abscesses rarely regress in response to therapy; surgical intervention may be advisable in valuable animals.

In horses with the lymphangitis form without abscesses, administration of oxytetracycline, 2 mg/lb of body wt IV, daily for 5 days or longer is useful. Bandaging and continued local antibiotic treatment of infected areas should be repeated as indicated.

When chronic abscesses are present, antibacterial therapy prolongs the disease by delaying their maturation. This may be hastened by use of ointments or heat. Irrigation of the drained abscess cavity with suitable antiseptics and systemic administration of oxytetracycline may hasten healing. Prognosis is poor if internal abscesses develop.

SWINE DYSENTERY

(Bloody scours, Vibrionic dysentery,
Hemorrhagic dysentery)

A common important mucohemorrhagic dysentery which occurs in most of the swine-producing countries of the world and is characterized by inflammation of the large colon, cecum and rectum.

Etiology: The bacterium *Vibrio coli* has received the most attention as the cause of this disease; however, its role, if any, has not been established. The syndrome has been reproduced experimentally by feeding pure cultures containing the spirochete *Treponema hyodysenteriae*, but whether this is the only agent involved is not yet known. Infection is spread mainly or solely through ingestion of infected feces.

Epidemiology: A subclinical carrier state is common. Recovered animals, whether treated or untreated, and in-contact pigs which never developed overt signs of infection, may remain carriers for long periods.

New outbreaks in herds from which the disease was previously absent usually follow the introduction of new stock. No other method of transmitting the disease between herds is known. The highest incidence of the disease is in feeder units, particularly those which repeatedly introduce weaners from other herds. Once the disease has entered a herd, it usually remains permanently endemic.

Any age of pig is susceptible but the incidence is highest between 8 to 14 weeks of age. The incubation period is usually 6 to 14 days, but it may be much longer. In untreated outbreaks the death losses may range from 5 to 15% and the morbidity from 5 to 95%.

Clinical Findings: The first evidence of disease is usually a partial loss of appetite and the appearance of soft mucoid feces. Diarrhea then becomes more pronounced, staining the perineal region, sometimes with increasing amounts of blood. Dehydration and loss of weight follow rapidly and sometimes occur when diarrhea is mild or absent. The body temperature may rise early in the disease and fall below normal terminally, but in most affected pigs it is in the normal range. In the later stages of the disease, the feces may contain desquamated tissue and coagulated exudate.

The course of swine dysentery may vary from 2 days to 4 weeks or longer. Remissions and exacerbations are common. Surviving animals may be stunted or unthrifty.

Lesions: These are confined almost entirely to the large intestine, cecum and rectum and end abruptly at the ileocecal valve. Catarrhal inflammation occurs in early cases and swelling of the wall, mucus exudation and patchy hyperemia may be seen. Necrotic inflammation may be observed in advanced cases and is characterized by focal necrosis and yellow or gray diphtheritic accumulation on the mucosal surface. The mucosal surface is usually reddened and hemorrhagic. Hemorrhagic inflammation, although striking when present, is not a constant lesion.

Portions of the sloughed membranes may be seen in the contents of the cecum and colon, giving them the appearance of "rice water".

Diagnosis: Diagnosis is based on the history; clinical signs; characteristic gross lesions; and epidemiology, particularly the persistent endemic nature of the disease and the occurrence of relapses. Demonstration of large numbers of spirochetes in the feces or on the mucosal surface of the colon, lends support to the diagnosis but is not specific, since nonpathogenic spirochetes which are morphologically similar to the pathogenic spirochetes, occur in healthy swine.

Swine dysentery may be mistaken for salmonellosis, post-weaning coliform diarrhea, terminal ileitis, hog cholera, hemorrhagic bowel syndrome, TGE and gastric ulcers. It may also be confused with other conditions of unknown etiology which initially appear similar to swine dysentery, but which differ from it in that they resolve spontaneously and rarely recur.

Prophylaxis: For the prevention and control of swine dysentery, maximum use should be made of hygiene, quarantine and isolation. Because the disease usually is brought into a healthy herd by hogs from an infected herd it is important to be careful when purchasing replacements. Disease history of the herd of origin should be determined, and new arrivals should be quarantined for 2 or 3 weeks; any suspected of carrying dysentery should get high levels of antibacterials (see below) in the water during the quarantine. However, this does not entirely eliminate the danger of asymptomatic carriers. When outbreaks occur, pens and yards should be thoroughly cleaned and disinfected between treatment and at frequent intervals after treatment is discontinued. Sometimes complete disposal of the herd, disinfection and restocking may be advisable.

Several chemotherapeutic agents are useful in controlling the disease in herds in which the condition is endemic. Most commonly used are organic arsenicals (℞ 326) and tylosin (℞ 61). More recently the nitroimidazoles have come into use in Europe. All these drugs are included in the rations at prophylactic levels. However, it should be noted that the causal agents slowly become resistant to repeated drug usage, and therefore only one drug should be used at a time and the others held in reserve.

Treatment: The same agents may be used at higher levels for treatment. Treatment is most effective when the drug is administered to affected pens of pigs in the drinking water for repeated periods of 3 to 7 days. The partial loss of appetite which occurs in affected pigs reduces the effectiveness of feed medication. Recurrences requiring further treatment are not unusual, particularly if hygiene is neglected.

GLÄSSER'S DISEASE

A fibrinous polyserositis of swine. The classical syndrome is caused by encapsulated strains of *Haemophilus suis* or *H. parasuis* (synonym: *H. influenzae suis*). Stress factors, such as weaning or transport, predispose to the disease. Similar syndromes may be caused by *Mycoplasma* spp., notably *M. hyorhinis*. (*M. granularum* commonly causes arthritis, but not polyserositis.)

The disease may be acute or chronic. After an incubation period of 1 to 5 days, septicemia occurs with fever (106° to 107°F), anorexia and depression. Some pigs become lame with warm swollen joints. Occasionally, mild signs of nervous derangement may be observed. Some pigs may die early in the disease, but in others the fever may subside after several days. They may remain lame and debilitated for variable periods but most eventually recover.

The classic lesion is a pronounced serofibrinous or fibrinopurulent exudate, associated with pleuritis, pericarditis, peritonitis, polyarthritis and meningoencephalitis, which is usually subclinical. The diagnosis "Glässer's disease" is based on the typical signs and lesions but the precise cause may be difficult to determine. Neither *Haemophilus* nor *Mycoplasma* are easily demonstrated in smears but they may be isolated in cultures.

Haemophilus infections usually respond well to penicillin and streptomycin (R 41), and to sodium sulfathiazole (R 90). *Mycoplasma* infections may respond to tylosin, lincomycin or erythromycin, but fixed doses have not been established.

STREPTOCOCCAL LYMPHADENITIS
OF SWINE
(Jowl or cervical abscesses, SLS)

A benign, infectious, and contagious disease characterized by the development of one or more heavily encapsulated abscesses in the soft tissues of the ventral or lateral or both aspects of the neck. Pork industry losses in the U.S.A. are estimated to exceed $8 million annually, largely as a result of product devaluation.

Epidemiology and Etiology: In herds where it is endemic, streptococcal lymphadenitis occurs in each new generation of pigs and in healthy adult swine introduced for breeding purposes. The etiologic agent is a *Streptococcus*. It first colonizes in the palantine tonsils, from which large numbers reach the regional lymph nodes via the lymphatics. Recovered swine continue to carry the *Streptococcus* in their palatine tonsils. It has been shown experimentally that carrier pigs may infect contact pigs for at least 21 months after initial infection. The agent has been isolated from deep nasal swabs of sows on premises where the disease was endemic.

Clinical Findings: Experimentally, initial high fever for 5 or more days, neutrophilia, elevated total leukocyte counts, depression, reduced feed intake, and constipation occur. These signs no doubt occur in field cases, but may be overlooked, and the principal observation is cervical abscessation. Except for the persistent neutrophilia and elevated total leukocyte counts, affected swine appear to be clinically normal after the initial period until developing abscesses become visible approximately 21 days after the initial infection. As a rule, affected swine appear thrifty and make satisfactory weight gains.

Pathogenesis: Scattered miliary abscesses develop in the swollen, affected lymph nodes within 7 days after infection. By about 21 days the internal structure of an affected lymph node is completely destroyed, and its distended capsule proliferates to form the thick, fibrous capsule of a large, single-cavity abscess containing greenish exudate. Abscesses measuring 5 to 8 cm in diameter are common. Incidence commonly exceeds 50% in a given lot of market hogs and may approach 100%. Developing abscesses reach the skin, rupture, and drain in 7 to 10 weeks. No tendency for deep-seated abscesses to drain into the pharynx has been reported. The drained lesions heal by granulation leaving a dense fibrous subcut. tract which is absorbed after several weeks.

Diagnosis: A tentative diagnosis, made on finding abscesses in several pigs, may be confirmed by identifying the agent. Swine that have only deep-seated abscesses may escape detection until they reach the packing plant. If swine have more than one very superficial abscess (which may be removed), the inspector will likely condemn the entire head.

Prophylaxis and Treatment: The introduction of carrier swine must be avoided. Agglutinin titers are detectable for some weeks after recovery and may permit reliable detection of carriers. A modified live vaccine is available (R 135). The *Streptococcus* is quite sensitive to a broad range of antibiotics, including penicillin and the tetracyclines, and has shown little tendency to develop resistant strains. Once pigs have visible lesions, antibiotic therapy is of doubtful economic value. If diagnosis can be established early, antibiotics mixed in feed (P. 14, 36) will prevent the development of additional abscesses. Continuous feeding of low levels of antibiotics (25 to 50 gm/ton of feed) can be used as a prophylactic measure.

SYSTEMIC FUNGUS INFECTIONS

The concept that the soil is the original source of the infectious pathogenic fungi is now widely accepted. In this habitat, the fungi exist as saprophytes on specialized substrates such as decaying keratinized animal tissue and dung. While a few mycoses are highly contagious and are passed from animal to animal without resort to a soil-inhabiting phase, most systemic mycoses are noncontagious, each animal becoming infected from the soil reservoir. Lesions produced by systemic fungus infections are characterized by granulomatous inflammation, necrosis, calcification, abscessation, ulceration, formation of fistulous tracts, fibrosis and nodule formation, and can occur in any organ of the body. The widespread use of antibacterial agents, both therapeutically and prophylactically in foods, may predispose animals to systemic fungal infection.

The following methods are useful means of confirmation when a systemic fungal disease is suspected:

1. Direct microscopic study frequently permits identification of the causative fungus. When exudate (pus, sputum, fetal stomach contents) can be obtained, a drop of it is placed on a glass slide together with a drop of 20 to 40% potassium hydroxide solution. A coverslip is added and the slide gently heated (do not boil). After a few minutes, the slide is placed between 2 sheets of blotting paper and by gently pushing down on the coverslip, excess KOH is removed. This squash preparation is examined microscopically under low and higher power using subdued light. Yeast-like cells, thread-like hyphae, and spherules with endospores may be distinguished by this method.

2. From a small portion of a lesion, such as a large lymph node, the margin of an ulcer or thickened cotyledon, a fragment may be cleared in KOH as described, and examined microscopically for fungi.

3. Spinal fluid may be centrifuged and the sediment examined as described for pus. If budding cells are seen, a por-

tion of the sediment should be placed in a drop of India ink to demonstrate the presence of capsules characteristic of *Cryptococcus neoformans*.

4. Intradermal tests may be employed for the detection of histoplasmosis and coccidioidomycosis in dogs.

5. Five milliliters of clear serum should be submitted to a mycology laboratory for a serologic test when histoplasmosis, blastomycosis or coccidioidomycosis is suspected.

6. Specimens from all suspected cases of fungus infections should be submitted to a mycology laboratory for culture. Antibiotic-supplemented (chloramphenicol, 0.05 mg/ml) brain-heart infusion and Sabouraud's dextrose agar serve for routine isolation. Incubation should be at both 25° and 37°C. For mailing purposes, specimens are best inoculated onto suitable media before shipment rather than being sent in a sterile container. Mold-like growths are examined using cellotape and yeast-like growth using Gram's stain.

7. A portion of a specimen should be fixed in 10% neutral formalin for submission to a pathology laboratory. Special histologic stains for fungi and fluorescent antibody techniques have proved to be the most reliable methods to differentiate various systemic mycotic infections.

HISTOPLASMOSIS

A disease caused by *Histoplasma capsulatum* and characterized by coughing, dysentery, pulmonary nodules demonstrable by X-rays, emaciation, ulceration of mucous membranes and lymphadenopathy. In the Central U.S.A., histoplasmosis is the most frequent systemic fungus disease encountered in dogs and man. Cats, cattle, horses, sheep, pigs and wild animals also become infected, but histoplasmosis is not a serious problem in these species. *H. capsulatum* grows in soil. The disease is not contagious. Infection is acquired by inhalation of the fungus, or rarely by the oral route.

Clinical Findings: Dogs are presented with a chronic intractable cough or diarrhea or both. Enlarged bronchial lymph nodes and pulmonary nodules cause a deep, nonproductive cough. Ulceration of gastrointestinal mucosa is responsible for the diarrhea. Other signs include anorexia, irregular fever, emaciation, vomiting, dermatitis and enlarged visceral lymph nodes. Careful palpation through the abdominal wall frequently reveals enlarged mesenteric lymph nodes. Ulceration of the buccal mucosa and enlarged tonsils sometimes occur. Acute histoplasmosis is nearly always fatal after a course of

2 to 5 weeks. Eight percent of the affected animals slowly develop a cough or diarrhea of 3 months' to 2 years' duration and are classified as having chronic progressive histoplasmosis.

Diagnosis: Histoplasmosis should be suspected in dogs having a therapeutically unresponsive chronic cough or diarrhea. In such cases, the intradermal test should be performed using histoplasmin prepared specifically for dogs. A dose of 0.1 ml is injected intradermally at the lower edge of the flank skin fold. The presence of at least 5 mm of edema or induration at the test site when examined 48 hours later characterizes a positive reaction. Such a reaction indicates present or past infection with *H. capsulatum*. There is some cross-reaction with blastomycosis and coccidioidomycosis which must be ruled out by signs, lesions or microscopic examination of exudate from a lesion. Rarely, in the terminal stages of acute disseminated histoplasmosis, the animal is anergic and therefore insensitive to histoplasmin.

Chest radiographs reveal enlarged bronchial lymph nodes and nodules in the lung. The pulmonary nodules vary from granulomatous foci, 2 to 5 mm in diameter, to miliary calcifications. Since tubercles in canine tuberculosis do not calcify, the observation of calcified pulmonary lesions on radiographs aids differential diagnosis. In addition, blastomycosis, nocardiosis and coccidioidomycosis must be considered.

Assistance in diagnosis is provided by serology. Five milliliters of clear serum is submitted to a qualified laboratory for complement fixation (CF), latex agglutination, immunodiffusion, and immunofluorescence (FA inhibition) tests. In combination, the last 2 tests can be helpful when sera are anticomplementary. Advantage should also be taken of the opportunity to prove diagnosis by culture, animal inoculation and histologic demonstration of the small organism (1 to 5 μ).

Prognosis and Treatment: Acute disseminated histoplasmosis usually is fatal; however, over half of the animals with the chronic condition will eventually recover with symptomatic therapy. Since *H. capsulatum* is disseminated through the sputum, feces, vomitus and urine, infected dogs should be handled carefully to avoid unnecessary contamination of the premises. Amphotericin B (R 351) may be useful but is toxic, and effectiveness depends on the dog's ability to tolerate the drug.

COCCIDIOIDOMYCOSIS

A highly infectious but noncontagious disease of man, cattle, sheep, dogs, wild rodents, cats, horses, pigs, buffaloes and several other mammals, characterized primarily by single or multiple pulmonary and thoracic lymph node granulomas and a tendency to disseminate to other tissues. *Coccidioides immitis,* the causal fungus, is present in the soil of the low-elevation deserts of the Southwestern U.S.A. and similar areas in Mexico, Central and South America. The infection is contracted by inhalation of airborne arthrospores. Of the domestic animals, cattle and dogs are the most important hosts.

Clinical Findings: The onset of coccidioidomycosis in dogs is insidious and the course variable, usually 2 to 5 months, with termination of progressive cases most frequently made at the wish of the owner. Although the dissemination rate in dogs is several times that for man, the majority of infections are subclinical with uneventful recovery. Coughing, dyspnea and other respiratory distress and fever are the most frequent signs. The cough is probably referable to the extensive swelling of bronchial or mediastinal lymph nodes and the granulomas or abscesses in the lungs. Variable appetite, weight loss, listlessness and diarrhea are commonly noted. Pleural, pericardial and peritoneal effusion, as well as cardiac insufficiency, icterus and uremia occur along with granulomas in the pleura, pericardium, heart, liver, spleen or kidney. Lameness and muscular atrophy follow invasion of bones and joints; fluctuating abscesses and ulcers indicate cutaneous dissemination; postural abnormalities or circling point to brain or meningeal infection, and glaucomatous swelling with corneal opacity to involvement of the eye.

Cattle infections are benign and asymptomatic; lesions are limited to lungs and thoracic lymph nodes, and carcass quality is not affected.

Diagnosis: Coccidioidomycosis should be suspected in all cases of intractable illness in animals that have lived in endemic areas. Pulmonary nodules, which rarely calcify, or enlarged lymph nodes may be noticed in chest radiographs of infected dogs. For CF, precipitin, or FA inhibition tests, 5 ml of clear serum, preserved by adding 1 part of 1:1,000 aqueous thimerosal to 9 parts of serum, should be submitted to a qualified laboratory. The coccidioidin sensitivity test will indicate the possibility of exposure. Strict intradermal injection of 0.1 ml of undiluted coccidioidin is made at the lower edge of the flank skin fold. A positive reaction is characterized by a focus of at least 5 mm of edema or induration at the test site 48 hours after injection. Occasionally, a severely infected dog will be anergic, giving negative serologic and coccidioidin tests.

Coccidioidin-sensitive animals may cross-react to histoplasmin, but the reaction to the specific antigen is larger. In tissues or smears, the fungus occurs as round, nonbudding, thick-walled bodies, 20 to 200 μ in diameter, known as spherules. Demonstration of endosporulating spherules in exudate or sections of biopsy material is adequate confirmation. The fungus is easily cultured as a cottony white growth on Sabouraud's agar, but cultures are dangerously infective and should be handled only by persons acquainted with the necessary safeguards.

Coccidioidomycosis in animals must be differentiated from tuberculosis, actinomycosis, actinobacillosis, nocardiosis, histoplasmosis and blastomycosis.

Treatment: Amphotericin B has been used with variable results in treating human coccidioidal infection. It has a similar record of use in the dog (R 351), in which treatment must be accompanied by strictest precaution to avoid kidney damage.

BLASTOMYCOSIS
(North American blastomycosis)

A chronic disease of dogs, horses, cats and man caused by *Blastomyces dermatitidis* and characterized by granulomas, abscesses and ulcers in the lungs, skin and other organs.

Clinical Findings: In dogs, the systemic type of disease is encountered more frequently than the cutaneous form. Depression, fever, anorexia and weight loss are followed by chronic nonproductive dry coughs. Numerous nodules and abscesses are distributed throughout all lobes of the lungs giving them a grayish-white and pink-mottled appearance. Focal or diffuse consolidation of entire lobes may occur. Central necrosis without calcification occurs in the granulomatous nodes. Extension of infection from the lungs results in enlargement and abscessation of the bronchial and mediastinal lymph nodes and pleuritis. Dissemination from the primary pulmonary site results in destructive lesions in bones, peripheral lymph nodes and meninges. Less frequently, blastomycosis is manifested by solitary or multiple skin granulomas which eventually undergo central liquefaction, necrosis and ulceration.

Diagnosis: Blastomycosis should be suspected in dogs with nodules or abscesses in the skin, and respiratory distress. Chest radiographs reveal noncalcified nodules or consolidation of the lungs and enlarged bronchial and mediastinal lymph nodes. For confirmation of the diagnosis, a biopsy of skin nodules should be performed or pus aspirated from abscesses or sputum collected. *B. dermatitidis* appears microscopically as single or budding spherical cells 8 to 16 μ in diameter with a thick refractile wall. In coverglass preparations, the wall gives a "double contoured" appearance. For a complement-fixation test, 5 ml of clear serum should be collected.

Prognosis and Treatment: Blastomycosis is usually fatal once infection is disseminated. Cutaneous lesions may persist for months. Surgical excision of cutaneous nodules is indicated since the infection responds poorly to drug therapy. Amphotericin B (B 351) is the treatment of choice for canine blastomycosis. Early diagnosis improves the chance of therapeutic success. Caution should be exercised in handling blastomycosis cases, even though contagion has not been established with certainty.

CRYPTOCOCCOSIS

A subacute or chronic disease of dogs, cats, cattle, horses, sheep and goats as well as numerous wild and captive animals and man; caused by the yeast *Cryptococcus neoformans.*

Clinical Findings: Dogs: Cryptococcosis in dogs usually involves the brain, meninges and paranasal sinuses, resulting in incoordination, circling, rotation of the head, changes in behavior, lameness, hyperesthesia and nasal discharge. Mucopurulent inflammation of the paranasal sinuses, ethmoturbinates and nasal cavity as well as small cystic centers in the brain and meninges are found at necropsy. Subcut. granulomas are seen around the ears, face and feet.

Cats: Crytococcosis should be suspected in cats, particularly older cats, having chronic nasal and ocular discharge, blindness, incoordination, fever, cough and swelling in the nasal cavity and pharynx. *Cryptococcus* invades the nasal cavity and pharynx causing the formation of expanding masses resembling neoplasms. Posterior extension of the infection from the nasal cavity results in penetration of the cranial cavity and the optic nerves, leading to blindness. Some cats manifest only an intractable chronic respiratory infection; in others, the disease is limited to subcut. tumor-like masses which are granulomas of gelatinous appearance.

Although there is no evidence that this disease is contagious, contact with infected cats should be kept to a minimum.

Cattle: Decreased milk flow, anorexia, severe swelling and firmness of the udder and enlarged lymph nodes are the first signs of infection. After several weeks, the milk becomes viscid, gray-white and mucoid; sometimes the secretion consists of watery serum with flakes. Contaminated udder infusion equipment and drugs are a source of infection. The organism has been isolated from pigeon feces and soil, as well as from milk from apparently healthy cows. A high percentage of cows in a herd may be infected. Rarely, metastatic lesions appear in the lungs following accidental inoculation of the fungus into the udder via the teat canal. Prevention of this type of infection depends on the use of aseptic udder infusion technique and sterile infusion media.

Horses: Respiratory signs and nasal discharge result from nasal granulomas. Granulomatous foci and necrosis occur in the lungs or may be generalized in the viscera. (*See also* EPIZOOTIC LYMPHANGITIS, below.)

Diagnosis: Cryptococcosis should be suspected in dogs or cats with unexplained respiratory and central nervous disease, and in cows with a viscid, gray, mucoid mammary secretion. An indirect FA technique and a tube agglutination test both for *C. neoformans* antibodies, and a latex agglutination test for crytococcal antigens have been developed. For maximal diagnostic coverage, all 3 serologic tests should be used concurrently. Exudative secretions, tissue from a lesion or spinal fluid in coverglass preparations should be examined microscopically. Other specimens can be mounted in undiluted Giemsa stain or India ink under a coverglass as an aid to demonstration of the mucoid capsule of the organism. *C. neoformans* in tissues appears as a round, single-budding, thick-walled, yeast-like organism, 5 to 20 μ in diameter. The entire organism is surrounded by a refractile gelatinous capsule that stains red with the mucicarmine stain. Biopsy material may be examined histologically or cultured for confirmation of the diagnosis.

Prognosis and Treatment: Pulmonary, cerebral, meningeal, or paranasal cavity involvement is fatal. Amphotericin B therapy has been evaluated favorably in human infections and in experimental animal cryptococcosis. Its use in the spontaneous disease of animals is probably justified (℞ 351). Spontaneous recoveries occur in accidental cryptococcal bovine mastitis.

EPIZOOTIC LYMPHANGITIS

A chronic, nodular and suppurative disease of the skin, superficial lymph vessels, lymph nodes and mucous membranes of horses in Europe, Africa and Asia. Infections have also occurred in the mule, donkey and Asian camel. Authenticated human cases are rare. The etiologic agent has been named *Histoplasma farciminosum* (*Cryptococcus farciminosus, Blastomyces farciminosis*) although there is yet no acceptable morphologic or serologic basis for including the organism in the genus *Histoplasma*. In lesions, the fungus appears as round or oval cells that reproduce by budding. The organism is 2.5 to 4 μ in diameter, has a thick wall and is gram-positive.

Cutaneous nodules appear on the skin of the hind legs in the region of the hock after an incubation period of 1 to 2 months. Similar nodules occur on the skin of the forelegs, neck, lips, saddle and harness areas. Infection spreads to adjacent superficial lymph vessels which appear as tortuous cords. Regional lymph nodes become swollen and eventually ulcerate. Skin nodules develop into multiple furuncles and skin ulcers coalesce to form large granulations. Nodules and ulcers sometimes appear in the nasal mucous membranes.

Ulceration of skin nodules, with lymphadenitis and lymphangitis, leads to a presumptive diagnosis of epizootic lymphangitis. Microscopic demonstration of the thin-walled, budding cells characteristic of *H. farciminosum*, or culture of the fungus provides a confirmatory diagnosis. Efforts should be made to differentiate the disease from sporotrichosis, glanders, strangles and *Corynebacterium* infection.

Some animals with mild cases recover spontaneously in a month. In most animals, the disease becomes extensive and incurable. Surgical excision of localized nodules or ulcers is the treatment of choice. Emphasis should be placed upon control by slaughter of infected animals, followed by disinfection of the stable and grooming equipment.

SPOROTRICHOSIS

A disease of horses, mules, dogs, cats, rats and man caused by *Sporothrix* (*Sporotrichum*) *schenckii* characterized by subcut. and lymphatic nodules which sooner or later ulcerate and discharge pus. Internal organs may be involved especially in the dog. *S. schenckii* is a saprophyte which grows in the environment of animals and man, causing disease when accidentally inoculated into the tissues of a susceptible host. After an incubation period of 3 to 12 weeks, an elastic nodule forms at the site of a skin wound; the hair over the nodule falls out leaving a moist exudate which eventually dries to form a crust. Multiple nodules appear and many then ulcerate.

Skin nodules of obscure etiology in horses and less frequently in other animals should be examined for *S. schenckii*. Aspirated material from a fluctuant unopened lesion should be submitted to a laboratory for mycologic examination. Since the small, gram-positive, cigar-shaped yeasts are difficult to demonstrate by direct examination of pus, it is best to confirm the diagnosis by culture of the organism. Biopsies of lesions, even when sections are stained by selective fungal stains, usually reveal few fungus cells.

Potassium iodide (R 579) should be given orally or sodium iodide (R 580) IV to the point of producing signs of iodism. The medication is continued for several weeks after apparent recovery to prevent recurrence. Tincture of iodine should be applied to the skin ulcers. If iodine therapy is instituted before dissemination of the infection, the prognosis is favorable.

CANDIDIASIS
(Candidamycosis, Moniliasis, Candidosis, "Thrush")

Candidiasis is a general term covering diseases caused by mycelial yeasts of the genus *Candida*, especially by *Candida albicans*. Infections are usually restricted to the alimentary canal where the yeasts normally exist as harmless commensals. Dissemination to the skin, placenta, lungs, kidneys and heart may occur. *Candida* species have also been implicated in bovine mastitis. Among animals, candidiasis of poultry and other birds is of particular importance, while infections of piglets and calves seem to be increasing. Other domestic animals found affected include horses, dogs and cats. Immature and debilitated animals are most susceptible. Infections are occasionally associated with antibiotic-supplemented diets or prolonged antibacterial therapy.

Lesions occur most frequently in the mouth and esophagus and consist of large single or small multiple, elevated plaques of soft, whitish yellow pseudomembranous exudate on the mucous membranes. When removed, they leave a hyperemic base which bleeds easily.

Since *C. albicans* or related yeasts may be present on mucous membranes as normal commensals or in other specimens as contaminants from the gastrointestinal tract, it is necessary to demonstrate the fungus in lesions associated with a host reaction. Appropriately stained histologic sections are therefore required. Microscopic examination of scrapings from mucosal or cutaneous lesions usually reveal both yeast cells (2 to 4 μ in diameter) and a tangled mass of hyphae. In such cases, the presence of hyphal filaments provides a tentative diagnosis of candidiasis. Diagnostically useful immunodiffusion and indirect FA techniques have been developed for the detection of serum antibodies to *C. albicans*. Yeasts of the genus *Candida* grow readily on Sabouraud's dextrose agar.

Many treatments for avian candidiasis have been attempted

or postulated: 1% gentian violet, 1% Lugol's iodine, nystatin either alone (up to 300,000 u/kg body wt, b.i.d. for 10 days, 100 mg/kg of food) or in combination with copper sulfate (up to 1 gm/L) in drinking water. Oral amphotericin B has been shown experimentally to be 4 to 5 times as effective as nystatin. Hygienic conditions and concurrent feeding of a high-vitamin-content diet are also important measures. Addition of 20 ml of 15% formic acid per 100 gm food for 15 days has been demonstrated to reduce the severity of avian candidiasis. Mucosal or cutaneous lesions in other animals can be treated with oral (℞ 355) or topical (℞ 356) nystatin.

THE PHYCOMYCOSES

The phycomycoses are not a uniform group but have in common the presence of broad hyphae which have few septa and which usually stain well with hematoxylin.

MUCORMYCOSIS

An opportunistic fungal infection which usually occurs in the presence of lowered or altered host resistance and which may affect any organ of the body. Causal fungi belong to the general *Mortierella, Absidia, Mucor,* and *Rhizopus*. Infection follows ingestion, or occasionally inhalation of fungal elements from moldy feed. Animal hosts include the cow, pig, horse, mule, goat, sheep, dog and cat as well as many wild and captive animals and birds. The organs chiefly attacked are the lymph nodes of the alimentary canal and the gastric and intestinal mucosa. Dissemination to the pregnant uterus, lungs, brain, kidneys and liver may occur. Subcut. nodules and cutaneous ulcers have been described in horses (hyphomycosis destruens). Clinical signs observed include diarrhea, convulsions, respiratory distress, abortion and failure to respond to antibiotic therapy.

Cultures may be misleading as the causal fungi are common saprophytes in animal environments, and the chief difficulty lies in deciding whether an isolate is of causal significance or simply a contaminant. Microscopic examination of KOH preparations from lesions may be a useful aid in diagnosis. Hyphal elements are often associated with blood vessels and may be missed unless the material is thoroughly examined. A useful staining method is to make supplementary mounts in a solution of equal parts of Parker blueblack "Quink" ink and 40% KOH. Mucoraceous hyphae generally stain rapidly in this preparation. However, in all cases, histologic techniques are essential to demonstrate the characteristic, coarse, branching, rarely septate hyphae and associated host response. Immunodiffusion tests have proved of value in confirming mycotic abortion in cattle due to *Mortierella wolfii*.

Mucormycosis in animals must be distinguished from tuberculosis, actinobacillosis, necrobacillosis, coccidioidomycosis, aspergillosis, candidiasis and malignancy.

Amphotericin B has been used with variable results in treating human mucormycosis.

ENTOMOPHTHOROMYCOSIS

Primarily a disease of the subcut. tissues and nasal mucosa of otherwise healthy animals—horse, mule, man—by *Basidiobolus haptosporus* (*meristosporus*) and *Entomophthora coronata*. These fungi are ubiquitous and occur in decaying vegetation, soil, and with *Basidiobolus* species, the gastrointestinal tract of reptiles. *B. haptosporus* has been found associated with skin lesions and probably gains access to the tissues following minor trauma and insect bites. The mode of infection of *E. coronata* is probably by inhalation of spores which then invade the nasal mucosa. Lesions are limited to nasal polyps and granulomas.

Specimens are collected by biopsy or after surgical removal of the lesions. Direct examination and isolation procedures are similar to those already described for mucormycosis (*see* p. 425). Histologic techniques reveal the characteristic picture of a granuloma in which coarse, irregular, rarely septate hyphae surrounded by a collar of eosinophilic granular material, are readily visible. Nasal polyps in entomophthoromycosis must be distinguished from those of rhinosporidiosis (q.v., p. 427).

Surgical removal of lesions has been found satisfactory.

ASPERGILLOSIS

A primary respiratory and occasionally generalized infection caused by species of *Aspergillus,* especially *Aspergillus fumigatus*. It is worldwide in distribution and has been recorded in almost all domestic animals and birds as well as many wild species. The disease is characterized by the formation of yellowish caseous nodules or plaques and has been known to affect almost every organ of the body. The most common forms of aspergillosis are respiratory infections in poultry (q.v., p. 1064) and abortion in cattle.

Present knowledge on mycotic abortion is limited to the fetus and membranes, for no signs have been noted in the dams prior to abortion. The cotyledons frequently retain much of their maternal caruncle portion, and are greatly thickened, especially at the margins. Central necrosis is also common. The maternal surface of the intercotyledonary areas of he chorion sometimes has a leather-like consistency with disrete-to-confluent thickenings. Skin lesions may be present on he fetus.

Diagnosis is by the demonstration (KOH, histologic) of characteristic regular, septate hyphae in lesions and by isolaion of the etiologic *Aspergillus* on Sabouraud's dextrose agar. Diagnostically valuable immunodiffusion precipitin tests are available for respiratory infections in man. Similar tests should be applicable to animals. Aspergillosis in animals must be differentiated from tuberculosis and other granulomatous diseases. As the many causal fungi of mycotic abortion induce similar changes, abortion due to aspergilli should be distinguished by histologic and culture techniques from that caused by phycomycetes and *Candida*.

Amphotericin B therapy has been evaluated favorably in human infections. Its use in the spontaneous disease of animals is probably justified.

MISCELLANEOUS MYCOTIC INFECTIONS

Rhinosporidiosis: A chronic, nonfatal, granulomatous disease of cattle, horses, mules and man found in warmer countries, especially India. It is characterized by the production of nasal polyps in animals although in man other sites may be infected as well. The etiologic agent, *Rhinosporidium seeberi*, has never been cultured. It is not contagious and the frequent history of prior extended exposure to water of pools and rivers suggest that *R. seeberi* has a natural habitat in water.

Unilateral tumor-like nasal polyps are 2 to 3 cm in diameter, may either be pedunculated or sessile, are lobulated, soft, pink in color, bleed readily, and are dotted with small white specks (the sporangia). The diagnosis is made by finding sporangia in KOH mounts and in stained tissue sections of polyp biopsies. Spores may be present in the nasal discharge. The large size of the sporangia allows them to be distinguished from the much smaller spherules of *Coccidioides immitis,* and their thin walls from those of *Emmonsia crescens* and *E. parva*. Rhinosporidiosis must be differentiated from entomophthoromycosis, aspergillosis and cryptococcosis of the nasal cavity; from "nasal granuloma" caused by *Helminthosporium* and from nasal schistosomiasis.

The standard treatment is surgical excision of the infected growths.

Adiaspiromycosis (Haplomycosis): A chronic respiratory disease of wild animals, especially burrowing mammals, caused by *Emmonsia crescens* and *E. parva*. Skin sensitization has

been reported in cattle and man. Presumably, infection occurs following the inhalation of spores from the soil. Adiaspiro
mycosis is characterized by the formation of large, thick-walled
yellowish spherules in the lungs of otherwise normal animals.
Reaction of the lung tissue is often minimal. Diagnosis is
based on the finding (KOH, histologic) of characteristic lung
spherules, and on isolation of the causal fungi.

Eumycotic Mycetomas (Eumycetomas): A supposedly rare
fungal disease of dogs, horses, cats and man, that induces
chronic inflammatory reactions and the development of granulomatous nodular masses on various parts of the body. Available culture findings indicate that only 3 fungi, *Curvularia
geniculata, Allescheria boydii* and *Helminthosporium spici-
ferum,* are agents of eumycotic mycetomas in animals. These
fungi are basically saprophytes with the inherent capacity to
parasitize both plants and animals. Blackish, or in the case
of *A. boydii,* whitish, granules are present in the lesions. They
are composed of dematiaceous mycelium and chlamydospores.
Complete surgical excision is the only effective treatment.

Geotrichosis: An opportunistic oral, intestinal, bronchial or
pulmonary infection of dogs, man and birds in captivity
caused by *Geotrichum candidum.* The fungus is frequently
isolated from fruits, soil and dairy products. Intracellular yeast
elements of *G. candidum* closely resemble those of *Histoplasma
capsulatum.*

PATHOGENIC ACTINOMYCETES

Although it has been the custom in the past to include actinomycete diseases under mycotic diseases, there is now no
justification for this; actinomycetes are bacteria, the diseases
they cause respond to antibacterial therapy, and techniques of
isolation and identification are typically bacterial. (*See* ACTINO-
MYCOSIS, below.)

ACTINOMYCOSIS

A local or systemic chronic suppurative and granulomatous
disease chiefly of cattle, horses, swine, sheep, pigs, dogs and
cats (rarely of wild animals) caused by *Actinomyces bovis.*
Human infections are caused by *A. israelii, A. eriksonii* and
A. naeslundi. Another species, *A. odontolyticus,* has been regularly isolated from deep carious dentine, while a filamentous
microorganism first isolated from gingival plaques of hamsters
with periodontal disease, has been named *A. viscosus.*

ACTINOMYCOSIS IN CATTLE
(Lumpy jaw)

Bovine actinomycosis usually is a chronic disease of the mandible, maxilla, or other bony tissues of the head; seldom does it involve soft tissue. Actinomycosis of the mandible and maxilla is characterized by swelling, abscessation, fistulous tracts, extensive fibrosis, osteitis and granuloma. The teeth loosen and eating is difficult; swelling of the nasal cavity causes dyspnea and there is gradual emaciation. Incision of the lesion reveals coalescense of abscesses containing a viscid, mucoid, yellow pus and "sulfur granules" 2 to 5 mm in diameter. Fistulous tracts extend through the skin, discharge pus for a period, then indurate leaving indented fibrotic scars in the skin.

Diagnosis: A history of a slow-developing swelling on the maxilla or mandible with fluctuating abscesses or fistulous tracts suggests actinomycosis. For confirmation, pus should be collected in a tube and shaken with saline to dissolve mucus. The contents then are poured into a Petri dish, "sulfur granules" picked out, crushed on a glass slide and stained by Gram's method. Under the oil-immersion objective, *A. bovis* appears as gram-positive filaments, rods, cocci, branching or club-shaped forms. Finding these structures differentiates it from actinobacillosis (q.v., p. 398) and staphylococcosis which also produce pus containing yellow granules.

On brain-heart infusion agar with 0.2% dextrose under anaerobic conditions (the presence of 5% CO_2 in the anaerobic environment is advantageous), *A. bovis* produces soft, convex colonies that are smooth and dull white. Stained smears show gram-positive diphtheroid forms. Branching is rarely observed.

Treatment: Actinomycotic lesions always take a chronic course of many months' duration. Infection of the maxilla or mandible seldom can be completely stopped, except when diagnosed and vigorously treated at its onset. When the lesions are small and circumscribed, surgery is the treatment of choice. This is followed by packing the wound with gauze tampons soaked in streptomycin solution or tincture of iodine. If the lesion is not circumscribed or if abscessation is advanced, the fistulas and abscesses should be curetted and packed with tampons soaked in tincture of iodine.

Injection of streptomycin around actinomycotic lesions aids persistent cases. The dosage may be 5 gm daily for 3 days or 2 to 6 gm every other day for 5 treatments. Sulfanilamide, sulfapyridine and sulfathiazole have also been used successfully in cattle. One gram per 15 lb of body wt daily for 4 to 5 days is recommended. Also, isoniazid (3 to 5 mg/lb of body wt, orally or IM) for 2 to 3 weeks has been used.

Once rarefying osteitis becomes extensive, treatment prolongs the life of the animal, but complete recovery should not be expected. X-ray therapy at the rate of 500 r every other day for 5 doses will temporarily reduce the size of the maxillary or mandibular lesions. However, irradiation does not destroy the infection and must be repeated.

ACTINOMYCOSIS IN OTHER SPECIES

Swine: *Actinomyces bovis* causes primary chronic granulomatous and suppurative mastitis in sows, which destroys the affected gland. Small abscesses in the udder contain cohesive, viscid, yellow pus surrounded by a wide zone of dense connective tissue. As in cattle, yellow mineralized granules are scattered throughout the pus. Some of the deep-seated abscesses rupture and discharge exudate through fistulas. Large, irregular, granulating skin ulcerations can be seen at the opening of the fistulas. Granulomatous nodules or abscesses also are seen under the skin of the abdomen. Occasionally, *A. bovis* causes generalized infection with purulogranulomatous nodules throughout the lungs, spleen, kidneys, and other viscera.

The prognosis is poor since one or more mammae are destroyed and the infection does not respond favorably to chemotherapy. It is often necessary to resort to surgical excision of the infected mammary gland to save the life of the sow and make her acceptable for slaughter.

Horses: *Actinomyces bovis* or an anaerobic diphtheroid, synergistic with *Brucella abortus* or *Br. suis,* causes the common diseases of horses known as fistulous withers and poll evil (q.v., p. 551). *A. bovis* alone causes abscesses with fistulous tracts in the submaxillary, pharyngeal and cervical region. The lymph nodes of the region contain nodules, abscesses and discharging fistulas.

Surgical drainage of the infected bursa, if performed prior to its rupture, gives most satisfactory results. It is recommended that 1 gm streptomycin be given initially followed by 0.5 gm every 3 hours on the day preceding surgery and to continue for 3 days afterwards. At the time of surgery, 1 gm of streptomycin is injected into the bursa. Once fistulas have developed, neither surgical nor medical treatment is satisfactory.

Dogs: *Actinomyces* sometimes are found to cause chronic granulomatous pleuritis. Frequently, subcut. lesions (abscesses, fistulous tracts) are present as well. The prognosis is poor since the infection usually is noticed too late.

NOCARDIOSIS

Nocardiosis of animals is a chronic infection resulting from soil-borne organisms of the genus *Nocardia*. Etiologic agents are *Nocardia asteroides*, *N. farcinica* (which does appear to be a distinct species), *N. brasiliensis*, *N. caviae* and *N. dassonvillei* (which is probably indistinguishable from *Streptomyces griseus*). Cattle appear to be the most frequent animal host. Other animals affected include dogs, horses, cats, sheep, goats and poultry, as well as a wide variety of wild and captive animals. The disease is characterized by generalized purulo-granulomatous nodular lesions.

Clinical Findings: Cattle: Nocardial mastitis has been the predominant infection reported in cattle. Systemic illness—prolonged high temperature, anorexia, loss of condition, increased lacrimation and salivation—may or may not be evident. Affected mammary glands may become enlarged and firm. The whitish, viscid exudate contains discrete blood clots and small (1 mm diameter) whitish clumps (microcolonies) of bacteria. Small draining sinuses are often formed, while in severe cases the gland may rupture. Metastasis to lungs and supramammary lymph nodes may occur. Bovine farcy, abortion, pulmonary and generalized infections have also been recorded.

Dogs: The clinical signs of canine nocardiosis include fever, soreness, lameness, dyspnea, empyema, enlarged abdomen, lymphadenitis, and fluctuating subcut. or salivary gland abscesses. Granulomatous swellings resembling actinomycotic lesions are seen—frequently on the extremities of dogs. Superficial abscesses rupture and discharge pus-containing flakes of necrotic tissue. The lungs and bronchial lymph nodes nearly always contain suppurative and granulomatous lesions. Well defined microcolonies are seen in pleural exudates.

Diagnosis: Nocardiosis should be suspected in dogs with unexplained pulmonary disease, with subcut. and salivary gland nodules or abscesses. Chest radiographs have revealed diffuse, noncalcified, soft nodules in several lobes of the lungs.

For diagnostic purposes, pus, sputum, or a biopsy specimen from a lesion is collected, smears are prepared, dried, stained with gram stain and examined under oil immersion. The organisms appear as beaded, gram-positive, weakly or irregularly acid-fast, branching filaments 1 μ or less in diameter. *Nocardia* are easily cultured on plain Sabouraud's dextrose agar, which should be incubated at both 25° and 37°C.

Specific diagnosis of mastitis in cattle depends upon culture of clumps in the milk from the affected quarter. Complement-fixing antibodies and precipitins have been demonstrated in the sera of infected cattle. Cutaneous hypersensitivity reactions have proved of diagnostic value.

Prognosis and Treatment: Nocardiosis frequently terminates fatally despite vigorous chemotherapy. Nevertheless, the canine disease has been arrested by daily treatment with oxytetracycline (R 25, 29) for up to 3 weeks, with 1 to 2 gm of sulfadiazine (R 66) by mouth daily for 6 to 12 weeks and with novobiocin, 25 mg/lb by mouth daily. Cutaneous or subcut. abscesses or nodules should be surgically excised, followed by local application of iodine.

Bovine mastitis caused by *Nocardia* has been successfully treated with udder infusion of 500 mg of novobiocin combined with 25 to 40 ml of 0.2% nitrofurazone, b.i.d. for 3 to 5 days.

THE TRYPANOSOMIASES

A group of allied protozoan diseases of animals and man caused by some species of the genus *Trypanosoma*. Members of this genus infecting mammals are divided into 2 sections, principally on grounds of life cycle and pathogenicity. Those in the section Stercoraria normally follow a cycle of development in an insect vector with the forms infective to the mammalian host being transmitted "contaminatively" in the vector feces. None cause disease excepting *T. cruzi*. Most members of the section Salivaria follow a cycle of development in tsetse flies (genus *Glossina*) and are transmitted to the mammalian hosts by the bites of the flies during feeding. Exceptions are, first, *T. equiperdum* which is a venereal infection, and second, *T. evansi* and *T. equinum* which are assumed to be transmitted "directly" (i.e., without a cycle of development) from a parasitemic to a susceptible mammal in the mouth parts of blood-sucking flies when their feeding is interrupted. All salivarian species are considered capable of causing disease and concurrent infection with 2 or more species can occur.

Many synonyms are extant both for species names of trypanosomes and for the diseases they may cause. In the simplest terms the name "nagana" can collectively describe the tsetse-transmitted animal infections (*T. vivax*, *T. uniforme*, *T. congolense*, *T. simiae*, *T. suis* and *T. brucei*); "sleeping sickness" can describe the tsetse-transmitted human infections (*T. gambiense* and *T. rhodesiense*); "surra" the animal infections with either *T. evansi* or *T. equinum*; "dourine" the equine infections with *T. equiperdum*; and "Chagas" disease the infection of man and animals with *T. cruzi*.

The pathogenicity of salivarian trypanosomes in the field may vary with the species of mammal infected, with breeds within a domestic species, with exposure to stress, including intercurrent disease, with the strain of the trypanosome and with the size and frequency of the infective dose or doses. TABLE 1 therefore only describes a commonly accepted pathogenicity of trypanosome species to domestic animals.

TABLE 1. THE COMMONLY ACCEPTED PATHOGENICITY OF SOME MEMBERS OF THE GENUS *TRYPANOSOMA* TO DOMESTIC ANIMALS

Trypanosoma	Dogs	Horses	Pigs	Camels	Cattle	Sheep/Goats
Stercoraria (selected species only):						
T. theileri	R	R	R	R	—	R
T. melophagium	R	R	R	R	R	—
T. cruzi	—	0	—	0	0	—
Salivaria:						
T. vivax	R	**	R	**	**	**
T. uniforme	R	**	R	**	**	0
T. congolense	*	**	*	**	***	**
T. simiae	0	0	***	***	0	0
T. suis	0	0	*	0	0	0
T. brucei	***	***	*	***	*	**
T. gambiense	—	0	—	0	—	—
T. rhodesiense	0	0	0	0	—	—
T. evansi	**	***	—	***	*	**
T. equinum	**	***	0	0	0	0
T. equiperdum	0	**	0	0	0	0

*	**	***	degrees of pathogenicity
			symptomless infections
	R		refractory to infection
	0		insufficient known

NAGANA
(Tsetse-transmitted animal trypanosomiasis)

Distribution: The nagana trypanosomes in Africa are related to the distribution of tsetse flies (*Glossina* spp.) which are found between latitudes 14°N and 29°S. A trypanosome indistinguishable from *T. vivax* on grounds of morphology and host susceptibility has also been recovered from 2 islands in the West Indies, from South American countries bordering the Caribbean, and from Mauritius in the Indian Ocean, but is directly transmitted in these localities.

Epidemiology: The natural transmission cycles of nagana trypanosomes involve tsetse flies and wild animals, principally Bovidae, which usually have symptomless infections. The trypanosomes become important when domestic animals become available as alternative hosts for the tsetse flies.

There are 22 known *Glossina* species which can be broadly classified into forest, riverine or savanna species according to their preferred habitat. The most important economic situations relate to the transmission of *T. congolense* and *T. vivax* by savanna species whose presence denies the use of thousands of square miles of land to cattle and other livestock. Cattle populations may sometimes persist in relation to low densities of forest or riverine species.

The importance of noncyclical methods of transmission in Africa is probably small, at least in those parts of Africa where nagana seems to be eradicated with the tsetse. This, however, raises the question of how *T. vivax* persists in countries outside Africa and in some parts, e.g., the Sudd, of Africa.

Diagnosis: The field veterinarian most often has to rely on clinical appearance together with the demonstration of trypanosomes using thick and thin blood smears, wet blood smears, or lymph node—of which the first is the most effective method. Since bovine nagana is usually seen as a chronic wasting disease associated with a degree of anemia and intermittent fever, and trypanosomes may be easily demonstrated in tissue smears from such cases, diagnosis in cattle is best made on a herd or an area basis. Horses and dogs may, in addition, show corneal opacity, and horses can show edema of the limbs and ventral surface of the abdomen. Trypanosomes in all susceptible animals are most easily seen in the initial stage of the infection or in acute cases. *T. simiae* infections in pigs are always hyperacute with death intervening even a few hours after the onset of signs.

Injection of laboratory rodents with blood from suspected animals will reveal most *T. brucei* infections and some *T. congolense* infections, but *T. vivax* will at best only rarely produce a transient parasitemia. A similar result is obtained using blood agar cultures at room temperature. None grow on mammalian tissue cultures. Recently developed laboratory methods which may assist the field veterinarian are the use of the hematocrit centrifuge to concentrate trypanosomes in the blood, the anion exchange column, and an indirect fluorescent-antibody test. The antigenic lability of trypanosomes within a species makes difficult the development of other serologic methods of diagnosis.

Treatment and Control: It appears that nagana can be eliminated, at least from much of Africa, by eradicating the tsetse vectors but this is not always practical. Drugs are used extensively in the control of nagana but their use can only be palliative as reservoir infections in wild animal hosts are not being attacked. A list of drugs commonly used in the treatment of the trypanosomiases in domestic animals is given in TABLE 2 (p. 437). Another drawback to drug prophylaxis is the ease with which trypanosomes become resistant. In order to try to overcome this difficulty some African countries have adopted a procedure whereby a single chemotherapeutic drug is put into common use, reserving diminazene aceturate to control only drug-resistant situations. Diminazene aceturate was chosen for this role as for many years no field strains of trypanosomes were discovered to be resistant to it. In recent years, however, resistant trypanosomes populations have been commonly reported from Nigeria together with isolated cases from other African countries.

Immunization of cattle using vaccines has not been found possible due to the antigenic lability of trypanosomes, but introducing the cattle to a light tsetse challenge and treating with diminazene aceturate when parasitemias are discovered has been successful on an experimental basis.

SLEEPING SICKNESS
(Tsetse-transmitted human trypanosomiasis)

T. gambiense and *T. rhodesiense* are morphologically similar to *T. brucei* and are distinguished from this species principally by their ability to infect man. It has recently been shown that differentiation can be effected by incubating the trypanosomes with human plasma. *T. brucei* loses the ability to infect rats after this treatment, whereas *T. rhodesiense* and *T. gambiense* continue to be infective. Epidemiologic evidence makes it clear that wild animals and, in certain circumstances, cattle are important reservoirs of *T. rhodesiense*. There is at present no evidence that animal reservoirs play a part in the transmission of *T. gambiense*.

SURRA

(Animal infections with *T. evansi* or *T. equinum*)

Distribution: It is probable that these 2 trypanosomes are derived from *T. brucei* which has become adapted to non-cyclical methods of transmission outside the distribution of tsetse flies. Movements of livestock have introduced the trypanosomes into new areas and countries. *T. equinum* is probably not a distinct species but a synonym for *T. evansi*. Exposure to trypanocidal drugs will often cause *T. evansi* to apparently lose its kinetoplast and the organism is then indistinguishable from *T. equinum*. The disease occurs in the Middle East, Asia, the Far East, Central and South America, and in the areas of Africa north of the distribution of tsetse. The distribution of surra overlaps that of nagana but delineation is difficult due to the similarities of morphology and animal host range between *T. evansi* and *T. brucei*.

Epidemiology: All domestic mammals are susceptible to infection but whereas fatal disease can occur in camels, horses and dogs, the infections of buffaloes, cattle and pigs are normally nonpathogenic and these animals often form reservoirs of infection. Reports of infections in wild animals generally relate to fatal episodes, e.g., the capybara of South America and deer of Mauritius.

The principal method of transmission of surra is assumed to be "direct" by the interrupted feeding of blood-sucking flies. Carnivores can be infected from eating meat derived from parasitemic animals, and the vampire bat is a proven vector in South America.

Diagnosis: As with nagana, the field veterinarian most often has to rely on clinical appearance together with the demonstration of trypanosomes using thick and thin blood smears, wet blood smears, or lymph node biopsy smears. Clinical diagnosis is again not easy as the disease is associated with a degree of anemia, edema and intermittent fever. Posterior paralysis is said to occur in camels in the Sudan and horses in South America. The disease in dogs is usually more acute with marked edema, opacity of the cornea and rapid emaciation.

Trypanosomes are best demonstrated in early infections or in acute disease. As well as the examination of tissue smears, suspected parasitemic blood may be inoculated into laboratory rodents. No method is known, however, of culturing *T. evansi*. The demonstration of increased serum immunoglobulins by precipitation with mercuric chloride has allowed efficient and simple diagnosis of surra in camels. Unfortunately the technique does not work in cattle with nagana. The recently developed methods for diagnosing nagana trypanosomes can also be expected to be of use in relation to *T. evansi*.

Control: The control of surra is almost entirely by diagnosis and treatment (TABLE 2). Resistance to suramin is not un-

TABLE 2. DRUGS COMMONLY USED IN THE TREATMENT OF THE TRYPANOSOMIASES IN DOMESTIC ANIMALS

Drug	Synonyms	Animal	*Trypanosoma*	Main Action
Diminazene aceturate, (℞ 328)	Berenil, Babesin (as the dilactate salt), Ganaseg	Cattle Dogs	*vivax, congolense, brucei, evansi,* *congolense, brucei, evansi*	Curative (with the possible exception of *brucei*)
Quinapyramine sulfate, (℞ 340)	Antrycide sulfate	Cattle Horses Camels Pigs Dogs	*vivax, congolense, brucei, evansi,* *brucei, evansi, equinum, equiperdum* *evansi* *simiae* *congolense, brucei*	Curative Curative Curative Curative Curative
Quinapyramine (prophylactic), (℞ 340)	Antrycide prosalt	Cattle Pigs	*vivax, congolense,* *simiae*	Prophylactic
Homidium bromide, (℞ 329)	Ethidium bromide	Cattle Equids	*vivax, congolense, brucei* *vivax*	Curative
Homidium chloride, (℞ 329)	Novidium chloride Babidium chloride Ethidium chloride	As for the bromide salt		
Prothidium (℞ 338)		Cattle	*vivax, congolense*	Curative and Prophylactic
Metamidium		Cattle	*vivax, congolense*	Not marketed commercially
Isometamidium (℞ 333)	Samorin M & B 4180	Cattle	*vivax, congolense*	Curative and Prophylactic
Suramin (℞ 345)	Moranyl, Naganol, Antrypol, Bayer 205, Naphuride, Germanin	Horses Camels Dogs	*brucei, evansi, equinum* *evansi* *brucei, evansi*	Curative

common, but the organisms remain fully susceptible to quinapyramine sulfate.

DOURINE
(Equine infections with *T. equiperdum*)

Distribution: The disease is recognized on the Mediterranean coast of Africa, the Middle East, Southern Africa and South America. The distribution is probably wider than reported due to the often very chronic nature of the disease.

Diagnosis: The classical signs may develop over periods of weeks or months. Early signs include edematous swelling of the external genitalia with mucopurulent discharge from the urethra in the stallion and from the vagina in the mare followed by gross edema of the genitalia. Later, characteristic plaques 2 to 10 cm in diameter appear in the skin and the animal becomes progressively emaciated. The mortality in untreated cases is 50 to 70%.

Demonstration of trypanosomes from the urethral or vaginal discharges, the plaques on the skin, or peripheral blood is not easy unless the material is centrifuged. Infected animals can be detected with a complement-fixation test but only in areas where *T. evansi* or *T. brucei* do not exist as they have common antigens.

Control: In endemic areas horses may be treated (TABLE 2). Where eradication is required, strict control of breeding and elimination of stray horses has been successful. Alternatively, infected animals may be identified using the complement-fixation test and compulsorily destroyed.

CHAGAS' DISEASE
(*T. cruzi* infection of man and animals)

The normal transmission cycle is between opossums, armadillos, rodents and wild carnivores, and bugs of the family Reduviidae. Distribution is in Central and South America and localized areas of Southern U.S.A. Domestic animals may become infected and introduce the trypanosome into human dwellings in situations of low standards of living where the bugs will exist. Man then becomes infected by the contamination of wounds or eyes or food with bug feces containing metacyclic trypanosomes. The trypanosome is pathogenic to man, and possibly to young dogs and cats, but other domestic animals act as reservoir hosts. Chagas' disease is of great importance in South America.

NONPATHOGENIC TRYPANOSOMES OF DOMESTIC ANIMALS

T. theileri or markedly similar trypanosomes have been detected by culture of peripheral blood on biphasic blood agar from cattle in every continent. Infection with similar trypanosomes has also been detected in domestic and wild buffalo and a variety of other wild ungulates. In the few areas studied, transmission is contaminative following a cycle of development in species of tabanid flies. Although the majority of parasitemias are subpatent, the trypanosomes may be accidentally seen by a veterinarian in a blood smear being examined for pathogenic protozoa, in a hemocytometer chamber, or as a contaminant of primary monolayers derived from bovine tissue. Allegations of pathogenicity have never been proven experimentally.

T. melophagium of the sheep also has a worldwide distribution and is transmitted by the sheep ked. *T. theodori,* reported from goats, may be a synonym for the same trypanosome.

BOVINE TRICHOMONIASIS

A contagious, venereal, protozoan disease of cattle, characterized by sterility, pyometra and abortion. The disease exists wherever cattle are found.

Etiology: The causative pyriform protozoan, *Trichomonas foetus,* is 10 to 15 μ in length by 5 to 10 μ in width. There is considerable pleomorphism and those organisms cultivated in artificial media tend to become spherical. At the anterior end of the organism there are 3 flagella which are approximately the same length as the parasite. An undulating membrane extends the length of the organism and is bordered by a marginal filament which continues beyond the membrane as a posterior flagellum. The organism can be held in isotonic saline or Ringer's solution at 4°C for 24 hours without appreciable loss of numbers. Many of them die if the specimen is frozen, although some will survive the freezing procedure used for storing semen. They will not survive drying or high room temperature.

Epizootiology: The organism is found only in the genital tract of the cow and bull. Although it may survive long enough on the rump or escutcheon of a "teaser" animal or on contaminated hands of handlers and instruments to allow transmission between bulls used for artificial breeding, control measures can be based on the assumption that transmission occurs only during coitus. The bull remains permanently infected unless properly treated. The infected cow that undergoes 90 days sexual rest post partum or 3 noncoital estrous cycles will usually make a spontaneous recovery, provided normal involution of the uterus has occurred. Rarely, a cow may remain infected throughout pregnancy and discharge trichomonads from the genital tract following calving.

Over 90% of females become infected when bred by a diseased bull. Transmission by artificial breeding can occur, but normal semen dilution methods markedly reduce the chances of spread by this means.

Trichomoniasis, like vibriosis, is insidious and may be present in a herd for months before its existence is recognized. When it first enters the herd, the infection rate is high. As females develop resistance, however, the fertility may reach such a level that the owner is unaware of the presence of the disease.

Clinical Findings: The most common and important sign is infertility caused by early embryonic mortality, and characterized by repeat breeding and long, irregular estrous cycles. An average as high as 5 services per conception may be reached in infected herds. If the embryo survives longer than 10 days, the interval between heat periods is extended. If pregnancy continues into the third month, then a recognizable abortion may occur. Embryonic or fetal death and the resulting abortion always occur prior to the end of the fifth month. Cows that carry their calves beyond this time usually deliver a live calf.

Trichomoniasis is the only common cause of postcoital pyometra in cattle and, in infected herds, this condition usually occurs in less than 5% of the animals. It results from the death and maceration of the developing fetus. The corpus luteum and, in some instances, the cervical seal persist so that there is no discharge of pus. More frequently, however, the cervix opens and there is a slight nonodorous uterine discharge. As in all pyometras, estrus does not occur and the condition may persist for many months. Vaginitis, cervicitis and balanitis are rare.

Diagnosis: A tentative diagnosis may be based on the history and signs, but confirmation rests upon finding the organism in at least one animal in a herd. The organisms may be found in the placental fluid, in the stomach contents of an aborted fetus, in the uterus for several days after abortion and in the pyometra fluids. In recently infected cows, they can be found in the vagina where they are present in large numbers 12 to 19 days after infection. Subsequently the numbers rise and fall in a regular manner according to the phase of the estrous cycle, being highest 3 to 7 days before each heat period.

In the bull, the organisms are present in the prepuce, frequently in small numbers. By careful attention to detail, diagnosis should be more than 90% accurate. The bull should be withheld from service for a week prior to examination, since coitus reduces the number of organisms present. The application of therapeutic agents to the mucous membranes of the prepuce and penis may reduce the number of organisms below diagnostic level for as long as 2 months. Animals that contaminate the prepuce by masturbating or mounting other bulls should be isolated until collection of a clean sample is possible. While trichomonads may be found in all parts of the sheath and on the penis, they occur in the greatest numbers in the fornix and on the glans penis. Samples should be taken from these areas.

Three sampling techniques can be used. A cotton gauze sponge soaked in isotonic saline is passed to the fornix of the prepuce. This region is swabbed with a back-and-forth motion and then several drops of the fluid are squeezed onto a microscope slide and examined. In the pipette method, preputial fluid is collected from the deep portion of the prepuce by means of a 20-in. plastic pipette equipped with a 4-oz (120 ml) rubber bulb. The material is examined directly. The douche method consists of injecting 250 ml of saline into the prepuce, agitating it by barbotage for a few minutes and then recovering the fluid and centrifuging it for 10 minutes at 2,000 rpm, and the sediment is used for direct examination. If no organisms are found, special culture media, not available in most small laboratories, should be inoculated.

All specimens should be examined using 100X power. A larger volume of fluid may be examined if no cover slip is used. The organisms may not be numerous and careful, systematic examination is often necessary. Identification can be made at low power and is based on the size and shape of the organisms as well as the characteristic, aimless, jerky motion. Only living organisms are used for diagnostic purposes.

Diagnosis in the bull may be made by breeding several virgin heifers and examining the vaginal fluid 12 to 19 days after service.

Treatment and Control: Animals with pyometra or other genital abnormalities should be treated or eliminated from the herd. The remainder of the cows will recover if artificial breeding is used for at least 2 years. If artificial insemination is not possible, the herd must be divided into exposed and unexposed groups. Service in the unexposed group is resumed, using uninfected bulls. In the exposed group, recognizable uterine disease is treated and the entire group is allowed 90 days sexual rest or 3 noncoital estrous cycles. Pregnant cows should be re-examined at 6 months to determine if any abortions have occurred. For breeding, the exposed herd should be divided into as many groups as possible, with one bull for each group. Bulls and cows should be re-examined to determine if reinfection has occurred in any group.

Since this disease is rare in North America, slaughter of bulls is to be recommended over treatment. However, successful treatment is possible: the penis is drawn from the sheath (a pudendal nerve block or tranquilization, or both, is necessary) and the surface cleaned by washing with a nonirritating detergent or soap, and then 20 ml of 1:1,000 solution of acriflavine is injected into the urethra and held there while the penis is being treated. The penis and the entire mucous membrane of the prepuce are massaged for 30 minutes with 250 gm of Bovoflavin ointment, where this is available, or otherwise a 0.5% acriflavine ointment. Treatment is repeated 10 to 14 days later. Concurrent with this local treatment, the animal should be given 5 gm of sodium iodide per 100 lb body wt IV for 5 consecutive doses at 48-hour intervals. Diagnostic tests to confirm the success of treatment should be commenced 2 months after treatment and conducted at regular intervals subsequently.

THE BABESIASES
(Piroplasmosis)

A group of tick-borne diseases of animals caused by species of *Babesia* which develop within the red blood cells of the mammalian host, and within various cells of the tick vectors. Babesiasis is a significant disease problem in domestic and wild animals, especially in the equatorial zone, with foci of infection extending into the temperate zones on either side of the equator. Normally, the parasites are transmitted from affected to susceptible animals by ticks which act as true biologic vectors. In enzootic areas, young animals become infected while they are still carrying the resistance conferred by colostrum; repeated exposure to infected ticks maintains a carrier state so that clinical manifestations occur rarely in these areas. Upsetting this equilibrium by the continued introduction of susceptible animals, or by mixing infected and susceptible hosts on the margin of an enzootic area, often results in an explosive epizootic.

Development in the Vertebrate Host: The development in the mammalian host follows a similar pattern in all the large species of *Babesia*, e.g., *B. bigemina, B. caballi.* Within the red blood cell, an anaplasmoid body, consisting mostly of chromatin, is invested with cytoplasm and becomes a signet-ring trophozoite. During this stage the protozoa exhibit rapid ameboid motility, increase in size, and finally form the typical double pear-shaped bodies, 2 to 4 μ in length and 1.5 to 2.0 μ in width, joined at the pointed ends. The daughter parasites escape from the red blood cells with or without lysis, and invade new red blood cells. The so-called small babesiae, such as *B. equi* and *B. rodhaini,* have a similar developmental cycle except that the number of daughter cells within an erythrocyte is 4. They often are arranged as a "Maltese cross" for a time; this form is diagnostic for infection with these piroplasmata.

Transmission, aside from the tick, can be achieved by mechanical means, i.e., contaminated instruments or needles, or in some cases, by intra-uterine transfer.

Clinical Findings: Babesiasis may be peracute, acute, chronic, or inapparent, depending on the number and virulence of the parasites introduced at the first exposure. Pathogenesis and severity are largely dependent upon 3 factors: (1) agglutination and packing of the enlarged, turgid, infected red blood cells in the capillaries of the organs leading to organic dysfunctions, (2) a rapid increase in number of parasites within the red blood cells causing hemolysis sufficiently severe to produce marked anemia, anoxia and death, (3) a sensitization of the host caused by circulating antigen-antibody complexes after antibody production has been elicited.

If the infection is initiated by a large number of parasites, multiplication can be observed in less than 24 hours. The signs observed are dependent upon the organ or organs in which the greatest sludging occurs. The most common signs are pneumonia, digestive disturbance, kidney dysfunction and encephalitis. The body temperature may go as high as 108°F. The appetite is greatly reduced. Icterus is not present in peracute forms of the disease, but the visible mucous membranes are usually congested. Agglutination of infected red blood cells is more characteristic of infection with the larger piroplasmata, such as *B. bigemina, B. caballi,* or *B. bovis.* In the peracute form of infections with the smaller piroplasmata, such as *B. equi* or *B. microti,* 90% or more of the red blood cells become parasitized and lyse easily, resulting in an acute anemia.

When detectable antibodies appear (5 to 8 days after parasites are seen in the peripheral circulation), the course of infection is markedly altered, and the classical syndrome attributed to infection with blood parasites is seen. The capillaries and small vessels become more permeable resulting in edema along the belly, flanks and legs. The red blood cell count decreases rapidly, and the packed cell volume may fall to 9 or 10%. The leukocytes increase in number and activity. The animal becomes more lethargic, and icterus is usually apparent, indicating liver damage. Petechial and ecchymotic hemorrhages occur on most of the serous membranes.

If the infection is initiated by a very small number of parasites, the incubation period may be from 10 to 30 days. Except for a slight elevation of temperature, the infection is inapparent; in these cases, the parasite is extremely rare and difficult to find in stained blood films, and serology must be employed to confirm the diagnosis.

Diagnosis: In the past, diagnosis was possible only if the protozoa could be demonstrated in blood films stained with Romanowsky-type stains, or if the disease could be transmitted to a susceptible animal by subinoculation of blood. The first method often fails and the second is expensive and requires expert interpretation of results. Serologic procedures, including complement fixation and indirect hemagglutination tests as well as precipitin tests, are now used for diagnosis of the babesiases.

Treatment and Control: Acute babesiasis responds well to chemotherapeutic agents. Trypan blue (Ŗ 346) given IV lowers the parasitemia during the acute stages. Quinuronium derivatives (Ŗ 341) have been effective. Acridine derivatives have been particularly effective against the small babesiae.

Since 1939, a number of aromatic diamidines have been more effective. Berenil produced varying results, and phenamidine (Ŗ 337), while more toxic, proved more effective against many of the babesiae. Diampron (Ŗ 349) was introduced in 1960 and was less toxic than phenamidine, but just as effective, at least in cattle. Imidocarb (Ŗ 332), introduced in 1968, has been an effective and less toxic babesiacide. A number of other drugs, such as quinacrine, quinine, tetracycline and neo-arsphenamine, have been used with varying success.

Tick control programs historically have been the method of choice for reducing the incidence of these diseases, but the emergence of drug-resistant strains of ticks has complicated the picture.

Graded doses of living parasites have been used to premunize cattle against *B. bovis* and *B. argentina* in Australia. Vaccines consisting of killed parasites apparently have little prophylactic effect.

There are 72 recognized species of babesia in domestic and wild animals. The following species are important in domestic animals:

1. *Babesia bigemina*—occurs throughout the tropics and many subtropical countries, including parts of South and Central America, Africa, Australia and Europe, causing one of the most widespread and important diseases of bovine animals. It is one of the larger babesiae measuring 4 to 5 μ in length and 2 to 3 μ in width. The parasite is known to be transmitted by at least 8 species of ticks: *Boophilus annulatus, B. microplus, B. calcaratus, B. decoloratus, Haemaphysalis punctata, Rhipicephalus appendiculatus, R. bursa* and *R. evertsi.*

2. *Babesia bovis*—occurs in cattle mainly in the temperature zones of Europe, Africa, Asia and the East Indies. It is one of the smaller babesiae and usually measures about 2.5 by 1.5 μ. The principal vectors are *Booph. microplus, Ixodes persulcatus* and *I. ricinus. Babesia argentina* and *B. berbera* are morphologically indistinguishable from, and may be synonymous with, *B. bovis.*

3. *Babesia divergens*—occurs in northern Europe and has been confused with *B. bovis.* It is one of the smaller babesiae measuring less than 2 μ in length, and is usually observed on the periphery of the red blood cell as a double piriform body. The tick vectors are primarily *Ixodes ricinus* and *Haemaphysalis punctata.*

4. *Babesia motasi*—occurs in sheep and goats in southern Europe and Asia, northern Africa, Russia and Indochina. It is relatively large, measuring 2.5 to 4 μ in length. It is known to be transmitted by *Rhipicephalus bursa, Dermacentor silvarum* and *Haemaphysalis punctata.*

5. *Babesia ovis*—occurs in sheep and goats in most of the tropical world as well as in parts of southern Europe and Russia. *B. ovis* is smaller than *B. motasi,* ranging from

1 to 2 μ in length. *Rhipicephalus bursa* is the principal vector.

6. *Babesia caballi*—occurs in Equidae throughout most of the tropics, and is common in southern Europe, Asia, Africa, Central and South America; it has been enzootic in southeastern Florida since 1962. It is one of the larger piroplasmata, measuring 2.5 to 4 μ in length. The known vectors are: *Dermacentor nitens, D. marginatus, D. pictus, D. silvarum, Hyalomma anatolicum, H. dromedarii, H. marginatum, H. volgense, Rhipicephalus bursa* and *R. sanguineus.*

7. *Babesia equi*—has even wider distribution in Equidae than does *B. caballi.* It occurs on all continents except Australia. It is one of the smaller babesiae, which develop into tetrads and is less than 2 μ in length. Many workers put this species and others from rodents into a separate genus, *Nuttallia.* Forms arranged in a Maltese cross are diagnostic. The parasites are transmitted mostly from stage to stage by the following ticks: *Dermacentor marginatus, D. pictus, Hyaloma anatolicum, H. dromedarii, H. marginatum, H. uralense, Rhipicephalus bursa, R. evertsi* and *R. sanguineus.*

8. *Babesia trautmanni*—occurs in swine of Europe, Asia, Central and South America and Africa. It is one of the larger babesiae, from 2.5 to 4 μ in length. It is known to be transmitted by *Rhipicephalus sanguineus* and possibly species of *Hyalomma* and *Dermacentor.*

9. *Babesia perroncitoi*—has been reported only in swine in North Africa. It is a small babesia measuring from 1 to 2.8 μ in length. The tick vector is unknown.

10. *Babesia canis*—has occurred in dogs on all continents of the world including Australia. It will infect most canine animals. It is one of the largest babesiae, measuring up to 5 μ in length. The chief transmitter is *Rhipicephalus sanguineus,* although *Dermacentor marginatus, D. pictus, D. andersoni, Haemaphysalis leachi* and *Hyalomma marginatum* are also known to be vectors.

11. *Babesia gibsoni*—occurs primarily in Canidae of India and the Far East, but has been recorded from North America. It is smaller than *B. canis,* and measures 1 to 2.5 μ in length. It is transmitted by *Rhipicephalus sanguineus* and *Haemaphysalis bispinosa.*

12. *Babesia felis*—occurs in Felidae of Africa and Asia. It measures less than 3 μ in length and usually divides into 4 daughter cells.

THE THEILERIASES

A group of diseases caused by protozoan parasites of the genus *Theileria*, which invade but do not destroy the red blood cells, giving rise to acute or chronic febrile infections that rarely cause anemia.

Both *Babesia* and *Theileria* are Haemosporidia. *Theileria* appears in the red blood cells during the acute state of the disease, but unlike *Babesia* it does not multiply after invading the erythrocytes. After inoculation into the blood stream of the susceptible animal, the parasites enter lymphoid cells of the spleen, lymph nodes and liver, where asexual multiplication or schizogony takes place. The schizonts in the lymphocytes are called Koch's blue bodies and are of diagnostic value. They are of 2 types, macroschizonts and microschizonts. The particles of the latter break away from the host cell and invade the erythrocytes. These erythrocytic forms can be ingested by a vector tick and enable the infection to be passed on to the next bovine host. The most important *Theileria* infection is East Coast fever of cattle.

EAST COAST FEVER
(Coastal fever, Theileriasis of cattle, Rhodesian redwater, Rhodesian tick fever)

An acute disease of cattle characterized by high fever, swelling of the lymph nodes, emaciation and high mortality, and caused by *Theileria parva*. The disease is a serious problem in East, Central and South Africa.

Etiology and Transmission: *Theileria parva* appears in the red blood cells as ovoid, pear-shaped, discoid or rod-shaped bodies varying in size from 0.5 to 3.0 μ. One to 4 organisms may be found in each red cell and attached forms never are seen. Schizonts or Koch's blue bodies, 3 to 10 μ in diameter, are found within lymphocytes of the spleen, liver and lymph nodes and occasionally are observed free in the blood stream. Transmission is through ticks of the genus *Rhipicephalus*, especially *Rh. appendiculatus*. There is no transmission through ova, as in *Babesia bigemina*.

Clinical Findings and Diagnosis: The onset is characterized by high fever lasting several days, dyspnea, evacuation of dry or liquid hemorrhagic feces, swelling of the external lymph nodes, emaciation and weakness. Up to 90% of the erythrocytes may be parasitized at the peak of fever. Sometimes, there may be cough, salivation, conjunctivitis and rhinitis. The disease runs an acute course, death usually occurring with 2 weeks. Mortality may reach 90 to 100%. Recovered animals are free from infection and immune; they do not remain carriers as do animals that have recovered from other theileriases.

Diagnosis is presumptive on the basis of acute, febrile onset with swollen external lymph nodes in cattle in areas known to be enzootic for East Coast fever. In the live animal, demonstration of Koch's blue bodies in smears from lymph nodes or spleen is confirmatory. The absence of anemia and icterus aids in differentiating East Coast fever from cattle tick fever. On necropsy, the most characteristic changes are petechial hemorrhages on the serous membranes, swellings of the lymph nodes, a liver showing friability, brownish discoloration and small grayish-white foci, and kidneys showing white nodules and spots. The white foci, nodules or spots on the liver and kidney represent aggregations of lymphocytes. Pulmonary edema is probably the immediate cause of death.

Control: The incidence of East Coast fever can be reduced by measures aimed at tick control. The most effective method of eradicating the disease is slaughter of affected and exposed animals and keeping the land free of cattle for 15 months, during which time the infection dies out in the tick population. During this period, nonsusceptible animals such as sheep, goats and horses may be grazed on the land. Infected ticks that engorge on nonsusceptible animals free themselves of the parasite and take no further part in transmission of the disease. Efforts are being made to develop methods of immunization by causing actual infection in the animal and controlling the severity of the reaction by administration of drugs such as chlortetracycline.

Chemotherapy has proved satisfactory only when animals are treated in the very early stages of the disease but unfortunately diagnosis is usually not made until it is well advanced. Treatment must be commenced before clinical signs develop, preferably at the time of infection. Whereas hitherto experimental infection was effected by the attachment of ticks, now it can be brought about by the injection of infective particles derived from infected ticks and cryogenically preserved. Chlortetracycline (R 11) and oxytetracycline (R 33) will inhibit further development of the schizonts so that no additional red blood cells can be invaded. To be effective in halting clinical signs, the drug must be given very early in the infection. Pamaquine (R 336) causes degeneration of the erythrocytic forms when administered during the incubation period, reducing or destroying the infectivity of the blood for ticks.

OTHER THEILERIASES

Theileria annulata (*dispar*) causes a disease of cattle resembling East Coast fever in Africa, the Mediterranean coastal area and the Middle East. The disease has been called "tropical piroplasmosis", "tropical theileriasis" and "Transcaucasian fever". Transmission is effected by ticks of the genus *Hyalomma*. Signs are generally milder and mortality lower than with East Coast fever.

Theileria mutans is the causative agent of so-called "Tzaneen disease" of cattle in Africa, a usually mild infection with low mortality. This parasite has also been recognized in Europe, Asia, Australia and the U.S.A., and is usually considered nonpathogenic in these areas. The transmitting ticks are species of *Rhipicephalus*.

Theileria lawrencei has been described as the causative agent of "corridor disease" of cattle in South Africa. The disease occurs in cattle moved to areas occupied by buffalo, which harbor the parasite as a silent infection. The signs and postmortem lesions resemble those of East Coast fever.

Theileriasis of sheep and goats is caused by *Th. ovis* and *Th. hirci* (*Th. recondita*). *Th. ovis* causes a disease of sheep and goats in Algeria, Egypt, Yugoslavia, the Middle East and the Caucasus. The chief signs are high fever, anemia, icterus and sometimes hemoglobinuria, and the mortality may be as high as 50%. *Th. hirci* has about the same geographic distribution, but the infection is mild and seldom fatal.

BESNOITIOSIS

A protozoan disease of the skin, subcutis, blood vessels, mucous membranes of the upper respiratory tract and some other tissues, caused by various *Besnoitia* spp.

Etiology: Previously known as *Globidium*, the causal agent of the cutaneous disease in cattle is now named *Besnoitia besnoiti* and that of horses *B. bennetti*. *B. jellisoni* has been described from rodents and opossums, *B. tarandi* from reindeer and *B. darlingi* from lizards. Viscerotropic strains of *B. besnoiti* have been isolated from blue wildebeest and impala and an unidentified *Besnoitia* sp. has been found in goats. These *Toxoplasma*-like organisms invade and multiply by endogeny in macrophages. Eventually, characteristic thick-walled cysts filled with many thousands of organisms are produced.

Transmission: Certain biting flies are capable of transmitting *B. besnoiti* mechanically from chronically infected cattle, which serve as reservoirs of the disease. It is also possible to transmit *B. besnoiti* artificially to cattle, rabbits and some laboratory rodents by inoculation of tissues containing trophozoites or cysts.

Clinical Findings: The incubation period is approximately 2 weeks. In cattle the disease commences with fever followed by anasarca, which is usually more noticeable along the ventral portions of the body, such as the dewlap, brisket, scrotum and limbs. Inappetence, photophobia, rhinitis, swollen lymph glands and signs of orchitis are also seen. Anasarca gives way to sclerodermatitis. The skin becomes hard, thick and wrinkled, and develops cracks allowing secondary bacterial infection and myiasis to develop; movement is painful. There is loss of hair and epidermis causing varying degrees of alopecia. Severely affected animals become very emaciated. Cysts appear in the scleral conjunctiva and nasal mucosa.

Although the mortality is low, convalescence is slow in severe cases. Permanent sterility often occurs in severely affected bulls. The disease may be inapparent, showing no clinical signs except a few cysts in the scleral conjunctiva. Affected animals remain life-long carriers.

In horses, signs are similar to those of cattle.

Prophylaxis and Treatment: Infected animals should be isolated and symptomatic treatment applied.

MAMMALIAN COCCIDIOSIS

Usually an acute infection caused by the invasion and destruction of the intestinal mucosa by *Eimeria* or *Isospora* spp., characterized by diarrhea, intestinal hemorrhage and emaciation. Coccidiosis is a serious disease in cattle, sheep, goats and also in rabbits, in which the liver as well as the intestine may be affected (*q.v.*, p. 1132). It is less serious in swine, dogs and cats, and is unimportant in horses. Under modern husbandry conditions (off-floor housing) it is rarely a problem in mink. Intestinal infections occur in deer, camels, antelope, buffalo and other wild animals, but little is known of their etiology.

Etiology: Infection of the host results from ingestion of infective oocysts. In the intestine, the protozoan excysts, invades the mucosa, multiplies asexually then sexually, forming resistant oocysts which are discharged in the feces. Under favorable conditions of moisture and temperature outside the body, the oocysts sporulate and become infective; sporulation requires several days to a week or more. Sporulation consists of segmentation of the protoplasm into small bodies called sporozoites which lie within secondary cysts or sporocysts within the oocyst. In the genus *Eimeria*, the sporulated oocyst has 4 sporocysts each containing 2 sporozoites, while in *Isospora* there are 2 sporocysts each containing 4 sporozoites.

When the sporulated oocyst is ingested by a susceptible animal, the sporozoites escape from the oocyst, invade the intestinal mucosa or epithelial cells in other locations and develop intracellularly into schizonts. These produce many infective bodies, called merozoites, which enter new cells and repeat the process. After 2 or more asexual generations, microgametocytes and macrogametes develop; each of the former gives rise to many microgametes, which fertilize the macrogametes. A resistant wall is formed around the zygotes, which are then called oocysts; these are discharged in the feces of infected hosts.

Clinical coccidiosis is more likely to occur under conditions of poor sanitation and overcrowding, or after the stresses of weaning, shipping, sudden changes of feed or severe weather. Coccidiosis predominantly affects young animals, but may occur in older animals which have had little previous exposure to coccidia.

Pathogenicity: Some coccidia are more pathogenic than others. Frequently, 2 or more species contribute concurrently to the effects on the host. In *Eimeria zurnii*, and *E. bovis* of cattle and *E. ninakohlyakimovae* of sheep, the crypts of Lieberkühn are affected.

The asexual or the sexual stages of the various species destroy the intestinal epithelium, and frequently the underlying connective tissue of the mucosa. This is usually accompanied by hemorrhage into the lumen of the intestine, catarrhal inflammation, and diarrhea. Signs may include discharge of blood or tissue or both, tenesmus and dehydration. Serum protein and electrolyte levels may be appreciably altered but hemoglobin or packed cell volume changes are seen only in severely affected animals. There is usually no consistent change in the blood cells.

Immunity and Carrier Infection: Most animals acquire coccidial infections of varying degree while young. Older animals may have sporadic inapparent infections but are usually resistant to clinical disease. Such clinically healthy, mature animals, however, may be sources of infection to young susceptible animals.

Diagnosis: Clinical coccidiosis is diagnosed by finding appreciable numbers of coccidial oocysts, of pathogenic species, in diarrheic feces. Usually, diarrhea precedes the heavy output of oocysts by a day or 2 and may continue after the oocyst discharge has returned to low levels. Therefore, it is not always possible to confirm a clinical diagnosis of coccidiosis by finding oocysts in the feces. The numbers of oocysts present in feces are influenced by the number of infective oocysts ingested, stage of the infection, age and condition of the animal, consistency of the fecal sample, and method of examination. Therefore, the results of fecal examinations must be related to clinical signs and intestinal lesions (macroscopic and microscopic).

Prophylaxis of clinical coccidiosis is based on controlling the natural intake of sporulated oocysts by young animals so that the infections become established in immunizing proportions without causing clinical signs of the disease. Good feeding practices, good management and attention to the principles of animal sanitation accomplish this purpose. Young, susceptible animals should be provided with quarters that are clean and dry, and feeding and watering devices should be kept clean and protected from fecal contamination.

Stresses associated with shipping and sudden changes in feed should be minimized; prophylactic treatment as described below may be advisable under conditions conducive to outbreaks of coccidiosis.

Where conditions permit, the outdoor, individual portable-pen system for dairy calves has proved effective for reducing losses from coccidiosis as well as other infectious diseases. Moving the pens once a week effectively prevents a build-up of sporulated oocysts, thus allowing light infections to induce immunity.

Low-level feeding of sulfaguanidine (R 74) during the first month of feed-lot confinement has prophylactic value in lambs. Control of coccidiosis has been effected in sheep and goats by low-level feeding of nitrofurazone (R 101) and in cattle by administration of sulfaquinoxaline (R 89) in the drinking water. It has been reported that low levels of amprolium in feed or drinking water are effective in controlling outbreaks in calves, lambs and kids.

Treatment: Sulfonamides remain the drugs of choice in the treatment of mammalian coccidiosis despite the development of many other promising drugs. Although clinical infections are self-limiting and subside spontaneously within a week or so, prompt medication usually results in shortening the course of infection, reducing the discharge of oocysts, alleviating hemorrhage and diarrhea, and lessening the likelihood of secondary infections and mortality. Enteric sulfonamides, such as sulfaguanidine (℞ 73) or the readily absorbed sulfonamides, such as sulfamerazine (℞ 75), or sulfamethazine (℞ 82), may be used. Sulfaquinoxaline (℞ 89) has given excellent clinical results in beef and dairy calves, sheep, dogs and cats. The soluble sulfonamides may be given orally or parenterally and are more effective than enteric sulfonamides. In severe outbreaks of coccidiosis in calves or lambs in feed lots or on lush pastures, consideration should be given to prophylactic treatment of healthy exposed animals as a safeguard against additional morbidity.

Favorable results have been reported for nitrofurazone (℞ 101) in sheep, goats, pigs and dogs. Amprolium has been reported to be effective against experimental and field outbreaks of coccidiosis in cattle, sheep and goats. Synthetic or natural vitamin K preparations may be used to increase coagulability of the blood in individual animals with severe hemorrhage (℞ 549, 550, 554). If transfusions are given, provision should be made to counteract the anticoagulant added to transfused blood.

Sick animals should be treated individually whenever possible to guarantee therapeutic levels of the drug. Symptomatic treatment for diarrhea may often be helpful. Sick and convalescent animals should be provided with clean, dry bedding, good shelter, fresh water and appetizing food.

COCCIDIOSIS OF CATTLE

Eimeria zurnii and *E. bovis* are the species most often associated with clinical cases; *E. ellipsoidalis* and *E. auburnensis* may be mildly or moderately pathogenic. Coccidiosis is commonly a disease of young cattle from 1 or 2 months to 1 year of age. The disease usually is sporadic during the wet seasons of the year, but may occur at any time in severe epizootics in animals confined to feed lots. Particularly severe losses have been reported in the U.S.A. in certain western states in cattle confined to feed lots during periods of extremely cold weather.

The pathogenic coccidia of cattle may cause damage to the mucosa of the lower small intestine, cecum and colon. The first-generation schizonts of *E. bovis* appear as white macroscopic bodies in the mucosa of the villi of the small intestine. The incubation period for bovine coccidiosis caused by *E. zurnii, E. bovis* or *E. auburnensis* is 15 to 20 days; for *E. ellipsoidalis* it is 8 to 13 days. In light infections the most characteristic sign is watery feces, but little or no blood is apparent, and the animal shows only slight indisposition lasting a few days. Severely affected animals may develop a diarrhea consisting of thin bloody fluid or thin feces containing streaks or clots of blood, shreds of epithelium and mucus. The diarrhea may continue for 3 to 4 days to a week or more; the animal loses its appetite, becomes depressed and dehydrated, loses weight, and the hindquarters and tail become soiled with fecal discharges. Severe straining at defecation is common. Death may occur during the acute period, or later from secondary complications, such as pneumonia. If the animal survives the week or 10 days of the most severe period, it may recover but may have a significant weight loss which is not quickly recovered.

Diagnosis, Prophylaxis, Treatment: *See* pp. 452, 453.

COCCIDIOSIS OF SHEEP AND GOATS

Clinical coccidiosis of sheep and goats is usually caused by *Eimeria ahsata* or *E. ninakohlyakimovae* or both; *E. crandallis, E. faurei, E. arloingi* and *E. parva* may be mildly or moderately pathogenic. The most serious outbreaks are seen in lambs in feed lots, usually within 2 to 4 weeks after confinement. In farm flocks coccidiosis is most likely to occur in lambs 1 to 3 months old. Coccidiosis is a sporadic problem of farm-raised goats.

The localization of infection is predominantly the middle and terminal thirds of the small intestine, and the large intestine. Small whitish or yellowish-white circular lesions are sometimes visible in the mucous membrane, representing groups of developing oocysts of *E. arloingi*. Macroscopic schizonts, similar to those of *E. bovis* in cattle, can be seen with the unaided eye in the mucosa of sheep or goats infected with *E. arloingi, E. parva* or *E. ninakohlyakimovae*. Lambs with mild coccidial infections show only slight indisposition and inappetence, and a transient diarrhea with soiling of the hindquarters. Severe coccidiosis, is characterized by copious diarrhea with straining and discharge of dark, liquid, bloody feces, loss of weight and appetite, and dull appearance. Mortality may be 10% or more in severe outbreaks, with pneumonia and other complications developing frequently. The course for animals that recover is from a few days to 10 days, following which there is an extended return to normal weight and condition. Schizonts and merozoites of an unknown species of *Eimeria* occur in the mucosa of the abomasum in sheep and goats. The schizonts attain a macroscopic size and are visible as white bodies known as globidia; the effect of these on the host is unknown.

Diagnosis, Prophylaxis, Treatment: *See* pp. 452, 453.

COCCIDIOSIS OF SWINE

Coccidiosis is less important in pigs than in cattle and sheep. *Eimeria debliecki, E. scabra, E. spinosa* and *Isospora suis* may be pathogenic under certain circumstances. Inflammation may occur in the small or the large intestine. The incubation period is usually 6 to 10 days. Usually, bloody diarrhea is not associated with coccidiosis in swine. Insufficient experimental infections with single species have been induced to enable valid conclusions as to the effects of these on pigs of various ages. Improper sanitation and crowding increase the likelihood that coccidiosis will occur.

Clinical signs are diarrhea, loss of weight, inappetence and general unthriftiness. The disease usually affects young pigs 1 to 3 months old, and unless microscopic diagnosis of coccidiosis is made, the signs are likely to be attributed to ascariasis or other factors. The course usually is 7 to 10 days, with many pigs remaining unthrifty.

Diagnosis, Prophylaxis, Treatment: *See* pp. 452, 453.

COCCIDIOSIS OF DOGS AND CATS

Isospora bigemina and *I. rivolta* apparently occur in both dogs and cats; *I. canis* apparently occurs only in dogs and *I. felis* only in cats. *I. bigemina* is pathogenic for both dogs and cats and *I. canis* is pathogenic for dogs; *I. felis* and *I. rivolta* are less pathogenic and may cause only a slight catarrhal enteritis. The endogenous stages occur in the small intestine. *I felis* occurs in epitheial cells, *I. rivolta* and *I. canis* predominantly in subepithelial cells, and *I. bigemina* in both types of cells. However, *I. felis* and *I. rivolta* are also known to occur in extraintestinal sites. The prepatent period is 5 to 9 days. The oocysts of *I. bigemina* undergo partial or complete sporulation by the time they are discharged from the host. *Toxoplasma gondii* (q.v., p. 456) is now known to have coccidia-like sexual stages in the small intestine of cats, resulting in discharge of oocysts similar to those of *I. bigemina*.

Coccidiosis is a disease of young dogs and cats. In dogs,

clinical infections vary in severity from those with mild diarrheas to severe infections causing bloody diarrhea, anorexia, weakness and emaciation. The course may vary from a few days to 10 days, but seldom is fatal, unless complicated. Clinical coccidiosis may also occur occasionally in kittens. The results of treatment with the usual therapeutic agents are highly variable, but sulfamethazine (R 82) seems to give consistently favorable results, while amprolium is also reported as effective.

Diagnosis, Prophylaxis, Treatment: *See* pp. 452, 453.

TOXOPLASMOSIS

A protozoan infection caused by *Toxoplasma gondii*, which may be acquired or congenital in all domestic animals, in many wild mammals and birds and in man. The infection has been demonstrated on all continents under all climatic conditions. *Toxoplasma gondii* is now classified as a coccidium. The sexual phase (schizogony and gametogony with formation of oocysts) takes place only in the intestinal epithelium of the cat family. Trophozoites and tissue cysts, developed asexually, are widely dispersed throughout the world, occurring in all homothermic animals so far examined. The proliferative active trophozoite is an obligately intracellular, motile organism, which is capable of invading and multiplying in any nucleated cell. It is found in the acute phase of the infection.

Unstained, the trophozoite is boat-shaped, measuring 4 to 8 μ by 2 to 4 μ. In fixed tissue preparations the organism shrinks and may appear ovoid or spherical. The parasite is gram-negative and Feulgen-positive, and can be stained by the usual staining methods (Giemsa, methylene blue and hematoxolin-eosin). Multiplication takes place by endodyogeny (daughter cell formation within the mother parasite).

The cyst, measuring 30 to 150 μ, is found in the brain, eye, heart and muscle tissue in the chronic infection. It is usually a spherical collection of closely packed, viable toxoplasmas surrounded by a resilient cyst membrane which is argyrophilic and Schiff-positive.

All strains isolated from man or animal seem to be serologically identical.

The trophozoites as well as the tissue cysts are delicate organisms which are killed by conventional disinfectants and by desiccation. Conversely, the oocyst is highly resistant and has been found to remain infectious for up to 17 months in a humid environment. The 3 forms are all killed at temperatures above 50° to 60°C and cyst forms are killed at temperatures of −20°C.

The parasites actively invade the cells where multiplication takes place. The cell eventually bursts, liberating toxoplasmas which can either infect neighboring cells, or after hematogenous spread, infect cells throughout the body. In older infections, when antibodies are present, cysts can be demonstrated.

Clinical Findings: Although most infections seem to run a latent or oligosymptomatic course, acute generalized, often fatal toxoplasmosis has occurred in relatively isolated animals as well as in concentrated populations. Enzootics have occurred in kennels, and in mink, rabbit, fox and pig farms.

Generally, the infection runs the same course in most species and may be present in either latent or clinical forms. The clinical infection is either an acute, generalized disease in the younger animal or a chronic disease with CNS involvement in the older.

Acquired or congenital toxoplasmosis in dogs and cats occurs in all parts of the world, but most cases are subclinical. The clinically apparent infections often occur in dogs whose resistance is decreased because of a simultaneous distemper infection. Young animals are the most frequently and seriously affected. The signs include fever, apathy, anorexia, cough, dyspnea, enteritis, jaundice, emaciation and nervous-system disturbances with tremor, incoordination and paralysis. Premature birth and abortion have been observed. Lesions include ulceration of the gastrointestinal tract, lymphadenitis, myocarditis, pneumonitis, swelling and focal necrosis of the liver, and a characteristic encephalomyelitis which has also been demonstrated in sheep.

Latent toxoplasmosis may occur in 25 to 50% of sows. In acute infections, suckling pigs have shown signs of lung involvement, especially dyspnea, and at necropsy, pneumonia, lymphadenitis, ulcerative enteritis as well as hepatitis, nephritis and splenitis are present. Healthy sows may transmit the infection to their young in utero, or to nursing pigs since *Toxoplasma* may be present in the milk.

Positive serologic reactions are relatively rare (10%) in cattle. In acutely infected calves, the signs are dyspnea, cough, fever and weakness as well as CNS disturbances including depression, ataxia and tremors. In adults, extreme excitability in the early stages is observed more frequently than depression.

Serologic studies have revealed that toxoplasmosis is widespread (up to 50%) as a low-grade infection in sheep. Most cases are subclinical. The chronic form presents the usual signs of CNS and respiratory involvement. It is also an important cause of outbreaks of abortions and stillbirths in sheep. In the fetal membranes, multiple fine white flecks or white foci, 1 to 2 mm in diameter, are evenly distributed in the cotyledons, which are pale and usually quite firm in consistency. In the acute stage, focal necrosis and vascular damage of the CNS are found, and in the more advanced cases, glial nodules, vascular repair and calcification.

Serologic surveys show a relatively low incidence (4 to 6%) of toxoplasmosis in horses, but little is known of clinical manifestations.

Diagnosis: Clinical examination can give only a presumptive diagnosis. Confirmation is accomplished by demonstration of specific antibodies or by isolation studies. The method of choice is isolation of *Toxoplasma* in mice or tissue culture inoculated with tissues, blood, spinal fluid, or exudates from animals suspected of having the infection. Direct microscopy is not definitive because of the morphologic similarity between *Toxoplasma* and numerous other organisms.

The Sabin-Feldman dye test and the complement-fixation (CF) tests are specific, and quantitative serologic tests which should be carried out simultaneously, since the CF test becomes positive later and negative earlier than the dye test. A 5- to 10-fold rise in dye-test titer and a 4-fold rise in CF titer, or maximal positive titers in both tests indicate active infection. The indirect fluorescent antibody and indirect hemagglutination tests seem to give similar information as the dye test. Intracutaneous injection of an extract of *Toxoplasma* induces a reaction of the delayed tuberculin type. It is a qualitative test and requires standardization.

Treatment: For animals other than man, treatment is seldom likely to be warranted. Sulfadiazine (33 mg/lb body wt) has been found to act synergistically with pyrimethamine (0.2 mg/lb) in the treatment of acute severe toxoplasmosis in laboratory animals and man. Since these drugs seem to affect only the free organisms it is important that treatment be instituted as early as possible. This therapy may produce a reversible toxic depression of the bone marrow which may be prevented by B-vitamins and folinic acid.

Transmission and Prophylaxis: Toxoplasmosis is transmitted to the fetus when the dam has an acute infection with parasitemia before antibodies are present, but congenital infection does not seem to occur if the acute infection occurs before pregnancy. Infection may be acquired by ingestion of contaminated or infected raw meat or via the respiratory tract. Meat is rendered noninfectious by freezing, cooking, curing, smoke-curing and drying. Sputum, nasal secretions, feces, urine, milk and eggs may be infectious.

Although available evidence suggests that most infections in man are acquired by eating inadequately cooked, infected meat, the role of the cat should be noted. Cats kept confined and fed no raw meat do not appear to be dangerous. Other cats, allowed to stray, or fed raw meat, may shed oocysts—although the incidence of clinical human toxoplasmosis in relation to the number of people who keep cats suggests that the hazard is slight. Such hazard as does exist may be minimized by good sanitary habits; cat litter should be disposed of daily, and disposable litter boxes may be used. Women who are pregnant and who have no antibodies to the disease may wish to leave the handling of the family cat to others.

Sero-negative veterinarians should exercise caution in handling animals with acute septic toxoplasmosis. In hospitals, sputum, feces, urine and spinal fluids as well as gowns, dressings, instruments and glassware should be considered infected until disinfected by boiling, autoclaving, or soaking in 5% phenol solutions.

Laboratory work with trophozoites and tissue cysts is reasonably safe as long as good hygiene and correct laboratory procedures are observed. Discovery of the resistant oocyst indicates, however, that the hazards involved in laboratory work are greater than was formerly appreciated, and laboratory infections have occurred. Experimental work with oocysts requires specially equipped laboratories where the walls and floors, etc., may be sterilized by boiling water or steam. Staff must be provided with caps, eyeglasses, masks, coats, pull-on-trousers, and rubber boots.

A vaccine is not yet available.

SARCOSPORIDIOSIS

A disease caused by invasion of the skeletal musculature by the protozoan *Sarcocystis*. Different species names are given to members of *Sarcocystis* affecting different hosts: *S. bertrami* (horse), *S. hirsuta* and *S. cruzi* (cattle), *S. miescheriana* (pig), *S. tenella* (sheep), *S. moulei* (goat), *S. muris* (mouse), *S. cuniculi* (*leporum*) (*rabbit*) and *S. rileyi* (duck). Evidence now suggests, however, that the infective agent is a fungus with little, if any, host specificity. Both warm- and cold-blooded vertebrates are affected.

Etiology: The parasites invade muscle fibers and grow to produce elongate, spindle-shaped structures called Miescher's tubes or sacs. Within the Miescher's tubes develop sickle- or crescent-shaped spores known as Rainey's corpuscles. The tissues most commonly affected are the skeletal muscles and the muscles of the tongue, heart, diaphragm and esophagus. In many hosts, the lesions are microscopic, but in sheep, cattle and ducks the cysts are often conspicuous macroscopically, rendering part or all of the carcass unfit for human consumption.

The mode of transmission of the parasite from animal-to-animal is incompletely understood. Experimentally, the infection has been transmitted by feeding infected flesh to animals.

Clinical Findings: In most animals, the disease appears harmless, and usually is discovered only at slaughter. Unless a massive infection is present, infected animals seem to experience little discomfort. Occasionally, heavily infected sheep may die and heavily infected pigs may present signs of muscular weakness and become extremely emaciated.

Diagnosis: At necropsy, grayish macroscopic streaking or strippling of muscles may be seen. In some cases, discrete yellowish elongated cysts may be seen embedded in the muscle tissue. Microscopic examination of the lesions reveals *Sarcocystis*.

Control: Good management, sanitation and hygiene are important. No effective treatment is known.

SULFONAMIDE THERAPY

Pharmacology: Mechanism of action: Sulfonamides inhibit bacterial growth by competitive antagonism of PABA which is essential for the synthesis of folic acid by susceptible bacteria. This action prevents the organism from reproducing and enables the host's defenses to overcome the infection. Sulfonamides are ineffective against organisms which can utilize preformed folic acid.

Spectrum of activity: Sulfonamides as a group possess a rather wide antibacterial spectrum. Susceptible organisms include streptococci, staphylococci, *Pasteurella, Bacillus anthracis, Escherichia coli, Vibrio, Shigella, Haemophilus, Proteus, Acti-*

nomyces, Chlamydia and a number of less important infectious agents. Since the spectra of the individual drugs of this group are alike, if an organism exhibits resistance to one sulfonamide, it is likely that it will be resistant to other members of the group.

Absorption: Certain sulfonamides are relatively well absorbed from the gastrointestinal tract, while others are poorly or slowly absorbed. The sulfonamides which are well absorbed include sulfanilamide, sulfathiazole, sulfadiazine, sulfamerazine, sulfamethazine, sulfapyridine, sulfaquinoxaline, sulfacetamide, sulfisoxazole and sulfabromomethazine. The rate of absorption of these compounds varies among different species, but therapeutic blood levels for systemic infections may be obtained in large and small animals by oral administration. The poorly absorbed sulfonamides include sulfaguanidine, succinylsulfathiazole, phthalylsulfathiazole and phthalylsulfacetamide. These compounds are employed for treating infections of the gastrointestinal tract.

Fate and distribution: After absorption, sulfonamides may occur in the body in 3 main forms: acetylated, protein-bound and in the free form, in varying states of equilibrium depending upon many factors. The percentage of these different forms varies with the species of animal, and more work is needed to establish the practical importance of acetylation and protein-binding. For practical purposes, it is perhaps best to consider both acetylated and protein-bound sulfonamide as being therapeutically inactive. Little attention has been given to the distribution of sulfonamides in various species, but in the dog and other smaller animals it has been shown that these compounds are widely distributed in body tissues and fluids. These include eye fluids, peritoneal and pleural fluids, synovial fluids, cerebrospinal fluids and prostatic and bronchial secretions. Sulfonamides are secreted in the milk following oral or IV administration, but the levels attained in the milk are insufficient to treat mastitis effectively.

Excretion: Sulfonamides are excreted largely in the urine where they are found in greater concentration than in the blood. They are also found in the milk, and close attention should be given to the cautions of the manufacturer regarding withdrawal times and periods following treatment during which the milk should not be used for human consumption.

Blood levels: The blood level attained depends on the rate and completeness of absorption, and rates of elimination and destruction of the drug. There is marked variation in blood levels obtained with a particular sulfonamide in different species of animals and also with different compounds within the

same species. In general, sulfathiazole, sulfadiazine and sulfapyridine produce relatively low levels when compared with
sulfamerazine, sulfamethazine and sulfanilamide. For effective
therapeutic action, it is recommended that sulfonamide blood
levels of 5 mg/100 ml be established and, in severe infections,
levels of 10 or 12 mg/100 ml may be desirable. However, there
is empirical evidence that, in many cases, such levels are never
achieved, yet recovery quickly follows treatment, indicating
that in certain disorders the lower concentrations may be quite
as effective. In recent years, a series of sulfonamide compounds
have been introduced which produce prolonged blood levels.
Examples of these are sulfabromomethazine, sulfadimethoxine
and sulfamethoxypyrazine. These are characterized by a high
degree of protein-binding and a low percentage of acetylation.
Unfortunately, it appears that the prolonged blood levels occur
only in cattle.

Toxicology: The toxic effects of the sulfonamides vary with
different compounds, species and individual animals. Toxic
signs are more likely to occur with prolonged administration.
In animals, the following toxic signs have been observed:
anorexia, diarrhea, constipation, emesis, anemia, leukopenia,
agranulocytopenia, cyanosis, oliguria, hematuria, crystalluria,
skin rash, urticaria, excitement, depression, hyperesthesia, peripheral neuritis and convulsions. In cattle, decreased milk
production has been observed following sulfonamide therapy
and, in chickens, a reduction in egg production has been reported.

There is little information on the relative toxicity of the
different sulfonamides for domestic animals. However, on the
basis of experience in man and experimental animals, sulfamerazine, sulfamethazine and sulfadiazine appear to be less
toxic than sulfanilamide, sulfathiazole and sulfapyridine. The
sulfonamides that are poorly absorbed have a very low
toxicity when administered orally.

The presence of dehydration enhances the possibility of the
sulfonamides crystallizing in the urine with consequent renal
damage. Crystalluria may be avoided by ensuring an adequate
urine flow through the use of fluid therapy and the use of the
more soluble sulfonamides (sulfanilamide, sulfamethazine, sulfisoxazole, sulfacetamide). Another approach in the prevention
of renal damage is the use of combined sulfonamides, since it
has been shown that in a mixture, the therapeutic activity is
equal to the total amount of sulfonamide present, while, on
the other hand, each compound possesses its own individual
solubility.

Therapeutic Uses: Selection of a sulfonamide: The principal considerations in the selection of a sulfonamide relate to their pharmacologic characteristics rather than any major difference in antibacterial spectrum. Sulfathiazole, for example, is the most potent sulfonamide *in vitro*, but it is excreted so rapidly that it is difficult to maintain effective blood levels. It is also more toxic than either sulfamerazine or sulfamethazine. Sulfisoxazole is highly soluble over a wide pH range and is, therefore, less likely to produce renal damage. For this reason, it is probably the sulfonamide of choice with which to treat urinary-tract infections. Solutions of sulfacetamide have a neutral pH and hence are the least irritating for instillation in the conjunctival sac. Sulfadiazine and sulfapyridine attain the highest levels in the cerebrospinal fluid and are probably indicated for the treatment of encephalitis or meningitis caused by sensitive organisms. A mixture of sulfonamides is preferable for the treatment of systemic infections as adequate blood levels can be maintained with little danger of renal toxicity.

The poorly absorbed sulfonamides are most frequently employed in treating enteric infections. These compounds do not penetrate the intestinal wall but remain in high concentrations in the lumen. Some investigators are of the opinion that the well-absorbed sulfonamides are of more value in enteric infections since they may act on infections which lie within the wall of the intestine. Phthalylsulfacetamide is poorly absorbed, but it is stated that it penetrates into all strata of the gut tissue and it, therefore, would appear to be a desirable compound for this type of infection.

Local use of sulfonamides: When applied locally, sulfonamides are likely to produce a foreign-body reaction which delays wound healing. For this reason, the use of sulfonamides in clean surgical wounds is not recommended.

Local therapy with sulfonamides appears to be of value in the treatment of certain contaminated wounds of animals. The more soluble compounds, such as sulfanilamide, sulfacetamide, sodium sulfacetamide and homosulfanilamide are less likely to act as foreign bodies, although the latter compound is more likely to delay wound healing than other sulfonamides. Homosulfanilamide is not inhibited by the high concentrations of PABA found in purulent exudate and necrotic tissue; hence, it is of particular value in the treatment of suppurative lesions. In local therapy, careful consideration should be given to the amount of sulfonamide applied to a wound. In general, wounds which must be sutured should receive a "light frost" (50 mg/sq in.), while open or heavily contaminated wounds require a "heavy frost" (100 mg/sq in.). It should be stressed that

accepted medical and surgical procedures should not be neglected in favor of the use of a sulfonamide. It also is important
that powders employed for local therapy should be sterile since
tetanus spores may be present in nonsterile preparations.

In treating infected wounds, homosulfanilamide possesses the
advantage of being less inhibited by pus and tissue debris;
however, as mentioned above, it may interfere with wound
healing. A mixture consisting of 9 parts sulfanilamide and 1
part homosulfanilamide is reported to possess desirable characteristics for local wound treatment. Sulfanilamide and sulfathiazole may be combined in a ratio of 3 or 4 to 1 for topical
therapy. This mixture provides the advantage of the relatively
high solubility of sulfanilamide and the longer action and wider
bacterial spectrum of sulfathiazole.

Dosage and Administration: Effective therapy with sulfonamides depends upon the establishment and maintenance of
proper blood levels. Sulfonamide dosage is based on the body
weight of the animal and is ordinarily expressed in terms of a
daily dose. The initial dose is usually equal to a total daily
dose and serves to produce a rapid rise in the blood level.
Subsequent fractional doses are given at proper intervals to
maintain an effective blood concentration.

Sulfonamides are most frequently administered orally as
powders, tablets, boluses, capsules, emulsions and soluble sodium salts. In some species, the compounds may be administered in the feed. They can be used to permit chickens salvaged from an epizootic of bacterial disease to reach market
weight.

Under certain conditions, IV or IP therapy may be desirable.
This is true when it is impractical to use oral administration
or when it is deemed necessary to produce effective blood
levels quickly. For parenteral administration, solutions of sodium salts are available in concentrations of 5 to 25%. These
solutions are highly alkaline and, therefore, they should be
given slowly and precautions taken to prevent their leakage
into perivascular tissues where they may cause marked irritation.

In most conditions which respond to sulfonamide therapy,
treatment for a maximum of 6 days is sufficient. In general,
if a condition does not show a favorable response within 3
days, it is probable that no response will be obtained. Prolonged therapy should be avoided since it is conducive to toxic
reactions. On the other hand, treatment should be continued
long enough to avoid the possibility of relapse.

SULFAMERAZINE

Clinical reports indicate that sulfamerazine is of value in treating pneumonia, strangles and other upper respiratory infections of horses. It also has been employed for fistulous withers and poll evil, as well as enteric and septicemic diseases of foals, which are often caused by gram-negative organisms.

In cattle, sulfamerazine is of value in cases of acute mastitis complicated by septicemia. Local and systemic therapy is indicated in these cases and a combination of antibiotic and sulfonamide therapy often is most effective. In calf pneumonia, very favorable results have been obtained with sulfamerazine and it or sulfamethazine appears to be the sulfonamide of choice in these conditions. In foot rot of cattle, sodium sulfamerazine has been employed with good results. Other conditions in cattle which have shown a favorable response to sulfamerazine are calf diphtheria, calf scours and metritis.

Sulfamerazine and sulfamethazine appear to be the sulfonamides of choice in treating *Pasteurella* infections of sheep, such as mastitis and pneumonia. In pneumonia of swine, often caused by *Pasteurella* organisms or *Haemophilus suis*, sulfamerazine alone or in combination with sulfamethazine has been employed with success.

Sulfamerazine is useful in treating bacterial infections secondary to canine distemper. In treating pneumonia of dogs, sulfamerazine alone or in combination with antibiotics gives good clinical results.

Sulfamerazine has been used in the treatment of feline panleukopenia, in which, presumably, a number of mixed bacterial infections are included. Favorable responses have also been obtained in certain nonspecific infections of the upper respiratory tract in cats.

In rabbits, sulfamerazine is of value in the prevention and treatment of hepatic coccidiosis (*Eimeria stiedae*) and in the treatment of intestinal coccidiosis (*E. perforans*).

Sulfamerazine has been found to be effective in reducing the mortality of several poultry diseases including pullorum disease, paratyphoid infections, fowl typhoid and infectious coryza.

Dosage: Sulfamerazine is administered orally to all domestic animals in a daily dose of 60 mg/lb of body wt, divided into 2 fractional doses, given at 12-hour intervals. The sodium salt is given IV in a dose of 30 mg/lb of body wt. For poultry, sulfamerazine may be administered in the feed in a 0.4 to 0.5%

concentration or the sodium salt may be mixed with drinking water in a 0.1 to 0.2% concentration.

SULFAMETHAZINE
(Sulfadimidine)

In horses, sulfamethazine is of value in the treatment of pneumonia and upper respiratory infections, such as strangles. It also has been employed with success in fistulous withers, navel ill (joint ill) of foals and against the gram-negative organisms which frequently are involved in enteric and septicemic diseases of foals.

Chronic catarrhal mastitis of cattle due to streptococci has been treated by udder infusion with a solution of sodium sulfamethazine. Penicillin (100,000 u) often is included in the sulfonamide solution. In acute mastitis complicated by septicemia, sulfamethazine has been employed, either alone or combined with antibiotics, for local and systemic treatment. In calf pneumonia, sulfamethazine or sulfamerazine is the sulfonamide of choice. Calf diphtheria, metritis and calf scours respond to sulfamethazine therapy and, in the latter condition, some workers consider it to be more effective than nonabsorbable sulfonamides. Sodium sulfamethazine is also of value in foot rot of cattle.

In sheep, sulfamethazine or sulfamerazine appears to be superior to other sulfonamides for treating pneumonia or mastitis due to *Pasteurella* organisms.

Sulfamethazine has been found useful in the treatment of infectious enteritis, navel ill, pasteurellosis and pneumonia due to *Haemophilus suis* in swine. It also is useful for treating various bacterial infections secondary to canine distemper. In rabbits, it has been used for the treatment of intestinal coccidiosis and in the prevention and treatment of hepatic coccidiosis.

Sulfamethazine is reported to be effective against coccidiosis in chickens and turkeys, although today there are better drugs for this purpose. It may be useful in reducing the mortality rate in pullorum disease, paratyphoid, typhoid, fowl cholera and infectious coryza of chickens.

Dosage: In the horse, cow, sheep, pig and cat, sulfamethazine is employed in a single daily dose of 45 mg/lb body wt, administered in equal fractional doses at 12-hour intervals. Sodium sulfamethazine is given IV in a dose of 30 mg/lb body wt. For poultry, sulfamethazine may be administered in the feed in a concentration of 0.4 to 0.5%, or sodium sulfamethazine may be added to drinking water in a concentration of 0.1 to 0.2%.

SULFADIAZINE

Sulfadiazine is not frequently used for treatment of animal diseases. In general, it appears to be less toxic than sulfanilamide, sulfathiazole, or sulfapyridine. Sulfadiazine is of value in calf pneumonia, but sulfamerazine and sulfamethazine seem more effective. It is useful in treating postdistemper bacterial infections in dogs and in urinary infections of small animals. For these purposes it is often combined with other sulfonamides. In *Salmonella* infections of chickens (e.g., pullorum disease, paratyphoid infections and fowl typhoid), sulfadiazine is reported to reduce the mortality.

Dosage: Sulfadiazine is given orally in daily doses of 60 mg/lb body wt. In the horse, cow, sheep and cat, this amount is divided into 2 doses given at 12-hour intervals, while in the dog and pig, equally divided doses are administered at 8-hour intervals. In poultry, sulfadiazine may be administered in the feed in a concentration of 0.5%.

SULFANILAMIDE

In the horse, sulfanilamide produces fairly persistent blood levels and is effective against the common organisms involved in pneumonia and in upper respiratory infections, such as pharyngitis, bronchitis and strangles. It also has been employed in a limited number of cases of chronic nasal catarrh and sinusitis. Sulfanilamide may be of some value in fistulous withers and poll evil. Hemolytic streptococci are frequently involved in infected wounds of horses and local or systemic use of sulfanilamide is reported to be effective in these cases.

Oral administration of sulfanilamide in the cow is reported to restore the milk to a normal appearance in many cases of chronic catarrhal mastitis due to *Streptococcus agalactiae*. However, systemic therapy is of little value in bringing about bacteriologic cures in these cases. Sulfanilamide is also of some value in treating pasteurellosis of cattle, although sulfamerazine and sulfamethazine are superior for this purpose.

In sheep, sulfanilamide has been recommended for treatment of joint ill due to streptococci and it is reported to bring about some clinical improvement of infectious enteritis and coccidiosis.

Sulfanilamide is probably now little used in small animals, but is effective in cases of cystitis in dogs due to *Escherichia coli* and streptococci. Bacterial infections secondary to canine distemper may respond to sulfanilamide, but it would appear that other sulfonamides (e.g., sulfamerazine and sulfamethazine) are of more value in these cases.

Dosage: For the horse, cow and pig, sulfanilamide is administered orally in a daily dose of 60 mg/lb body wt. This is divided into 2 fractional doses at 12-hour intervals. For the dog and cat, the daily dose is 90 mg/lb body wt, divided into 2 equal doses at 12-hour intervals.

SULFATHIAZOLE

Sulfathiazole is effective against many common pathogens when tested *in vitro*; however, it is relatively more toxic than sulfamerazine or sulfamethazine and its rapid excretion makes it difficult to maintain effective blood levels.

In cattle, sulfathiazole is of value in treating pasteurellosis, calf pneumonia and calf diphtheria. However, sulfamerazine and sulfamethazine appear to be more effective in these conditions. Since the alkaline urine of herbivores tends to insure solubility of sulfathiazole, it is of value in treating urinary-tract infections. Sodium sulfathiazole has been employed for foot rot in cattle.

Diseases in swine which respond to sulfathiazole therapy are infectious enteritis, pneumonia and pasteurellosis a 3% sulfathiazole ointment has been employed topically in treating seborrheic conditions of the skin in pigs.

In dogs, sulfathiazole is effective in treating urinary-tract infections due to *Staphylococcus aureus, Proteus vulgaris, Escherichia coli* or beta hemolytic streptococci. It is also employed in bacterial infections secondary to canine distemper. In cats, sulfathiazole has sometimes been found useful in treating feline pneumonitis. Topical therapy with sulfathiazole powder has been employed in various skin conditions of this species. Sulfathiazole is reported to reduce the mortality rate in fowl cholera and infectious coryza of chickens.

Dosage: In the horse and cat, sulfathiazole is administered in daily doses of 90 mg/lb body wt. For these animals, 3 equal fractional doses are given every 8 hours. The daily dose for the cow, sheep, pig and dog is 120 to 180 mg/lb body wt and, in these animals, equal fractional doses are administered at 4- to 6-hour intervals.

SULFAPYRIDINE

In cattle, sulfapyridine is of value in vaginitis and calf diphtheria. It is also effective for pasteurellosis, but sulfamerazine and sulfamethazine are probably superior. Sodium sulfapyridine has been employed IV in a dose of 60 to 90 gm for foot rot in cattle. Other conditions which respond to sulfapyridine are secondary bacterial infections in canine distemper, pneumonia in dogs and swine, and pneumonitis in cats. In most of these conditions, sulfamerazine and sulfamethazine appear to be safer and more effective.

Dosage: Sulfapyridine is administered in daily doses of 60 mg/lb body wt. In all animals except the pig, this amount is divided into equal fractional doses administered at 12-hour intervals. In the pig, one dose per day is suffucent to maintain adequate blood levels.

SULFAQUINOXALINE

Sulfaquinoxaline is readily absorbed from the gastrointestinal tract and produces persistent blood levels. The drug is excreted partly in the urine and partly through the intestinal tract in the feces.

In some species (e.g., the dog) sulfaquinoxaline may cause hypoprothrombinemia, which can be prevented by the administration of vitamin K simultaneously.

Sulfaquinoxaline is useful for the treatment of coccidiosis of chickens and for the prevention and treatment of this disease in turkeys. Although sulfaquinoxaline is also used as a prophylactic agent against coccidiosis of chickens, other newer and more effective drugs have largely supplanted it. It has been used in combination with amprolium. The combined drugs used at the rate of 0.0006% of each in feed offer protection against all of the common species of coccidia. When used for prevention of cecal or intestinal coccidiosis in chickens, sulfaquinoxaline may be fed either intermittently or continuously.

Sulfaquinoxaline added to mash is useful in controlling mortality from acute fowl cholera (*Pasteurella multocida*). Losses due to fowl typhoid (*Salmonella gallinarum*) in turkeys can often be reduced by giving sulfaquinoxaline in the drinking water.

Sulfaquinoxaline is also effective in the prevention and control of intestinal coccidiosis of calves, lambs, dogs and cats, as well as hepatic and intestinal coccidiosis of rabbits.

Dosage: Because of the varied forms in which this drug is prepared, and the several treatment schedules recommended, the directions of the manufacturer should be followed. (*See also* COCCIDIOSIS of poultry, p. 1066.) In mammals, the daily dose is 60 mg/lb body wt orally for infectious diseases, but only $\frac{1}{10}$ of this (6 mg/lb body wt) for coccidiosis.

SULFISOXAZOLE

This sulfonamide is relatively soluble and well absorbed after oral administration. In the dog and cow, experimental studies indicate that sulfisoxazole does not produce as prolonged blood levels as sulfamerazine or sulfamethazine. The drug is excreted rapidly in the urine in high concentrations and this, together with its high solubility, recommends it for use in urinary-tract infections. Compared to other sulfonamides, the acute toxicity of sulfisoxazole is relatively low.

In dogs, sulfisoxazole has been used to treat postdistemper bacterial infections and urinary-tract infections. In cattle, the drug is useful for foot rot, pasteurellosis and pneumonia. Locally it is used for mastitis.

Dosage: A daily dose of 60 or 90 mg of sulfisoxazole per pound of body weight probably will be needed in most species in order to maintain adequate blood levels. The daily dose should be divided and administered at 6-hour intervals.

SULFABROMOMETHAZINE
("Sulfabrom")

Bromination of the fifth carbon of the pyrimidine nucleus of the sulfamethazine molecule results in a prolongation of the blood levels attained when this compound is given orally or IP. Sulfabromomethazine retains the excellent antibacterial activity of the parent compound and its unique long-acting effects make it particularly attractive as a sulfonamide for use in large animals. Single doses of this compound in cattle result in therapeutic blood levels that persist for 48 hours and longer. The advantages of this property to the large-animal practitioner are obvious. Unfortunately, prolongation of blood levels does not reliably occur in other species, although the drug is as clinically effective as other sulfonamides. There appears to be little danger of crystalluria occurring, even with repeated doses of sulfabromomethazine.

Dosage: In cattle, sulfabromomethazine is given orally in boluses in doses of 60 to 90 mg/lb of body wt. The solution may also be given orally as a drench, at the same dose. Solutions of buffered powder may be administered IP at 60 to 90 mg/lb. These doses may be repeated after 48 hours, if necessary.

SULFACETAMIDE

This sulfonamide is well absorbed after oral administration and rapidly excreted in the urine in high concentrations. Compared to other sulfonamides, it possesses a relatively high solubility and is reported readily to penetrate the tissues of the renal tract and the eye. These properties recommend it for use in urinary and eye infections.

Sulfacetamide is used topically as a lotion for dermatologic and ophthalmologic infections in small animals. Orally, it is recommended chiefly for urinary-tract infections, especially those due to *Escherichia coli*.

Dosage: Orally, the drug is given in a daily dose of 60 mg/lb body wt.

SULFAGUANIDINE

Sulfaguanidine is employed for treating various intestinal infections in a number of species, but today other sulfonamides, such as succinylsulfathiazole and phthalylsulfathiazole, are considered to be superior for these purposes. It has been replaced by other drugs for the prevention and treatment of coccidiosis in poultry.

Dosage: Sulfaguanidine is given to mammals at an initial dose of 120 mg/lb of body wt, followed by daily maintenance doses of 60 mg/lb. It may be administered to poultry in the feed in a concentration of 1 to 1.5%.

SUCCINYLSULFATHIAZOLE
("Sulfasuxidine")

This sulfonamide is poorly absorbed and is employed for treating infections of the gastrointestinal tract. These include bacillary dysenteries of dogs and cats, calf scours and necrotic enteritis in swine.

Dosage: Succinylsulfathiazole is administered orally in daily doses of 90 to 210 mg/lb body wt. This amount may be divided into 2 or more fractional doses.

PHTHALYLSULFATHIAZOLE
("Sulfathalidine")

Phthalylsulfathiazole, being a poorly absorbed sulfonamide, is used for treating intestinal infections only and is of value in calf scours and in infectious enteritis of swine and dogs. It is considered to be less toxic and more effective than sulfaguanidine.

Dosage: The daily dose range for animals is 60 to 135 mg/lb body wt.

HOMOSULFANILAMIDE HYDROCHLORIDE
("Sulfamylon")

Homosulfanilamide differs from other commonly used sulfonamides in being less active against beta-hemolytic streptococci and staphylococci. It is less inhibited by the presence of pus and necrotic tissue than other sulfonamides, because it is not antagonized by the high concentrations of PABA found in such lesions.

Homosulfanilamide is primarily employed by local application in the treatment of infected wounds and is especially suitable for infections due to gas-forming bacteria. A powder containing 1 part homosulfanilamide and 9 parts sulfanilamide is reported to be of value in these conditions. For metritis in cattle, introduction of a suspension containing both homosulfanilamide and sulfanilamide powder into the uterus is recommended.

PHTHALYLSULFACETAMIDE

Phthalylsulfacetamide does not enter the blood stream after oral administration. However, unlike other poorly absorbed sulfonamides which remain largely in the lumen of the gut, it is reported to penetrate all layers of the intestinal wall.

Commercially, phthalylsulfacetamide is most often found as one of the active ingredients in antidiarrheal preparations. It is recommended for use in treating enteric infections in young animals of all species.

Dosage: The drug is given in a daily oral dose of 40 to 120 mg/lb body wt. This is divided into 3 fractional doses.

SULFADIMETHOXINE

This is a newer sulfonamide which is structurally related to sulfadiazine. In cattle it produces prolonged blood levels. An oral dose of 90 mg/lb of body wt results in peak blood levels in 12 to 24 hours and effective levels persist for 48 hours. The degree of acetylation and protein binding is similar to that of sulfamethazine.

Sulfadimethoxine is reported to be an effective treatment for a variety of bacterial infections in dogs and cats which include tonsillitis, pharyngitis, bronchitis, pneumonia, sinusitis, metritis and dermatitis. Of particular interest is its use in treating salmonellosis in Greyhound dogs. This is a condition which does not respond readily to other sulfonamides or antibiotics. Large oral doses (25 mg/lb of body wt, 3 times daily) of sulfadimethoxine in conjunction with concentrated globulins have been used with good results in canine coccidiosis. Presumably in cattle, sulfadimethoxine should be of value in the same diseases for which other sulfonamides are used.

Dosage: For cattle an initial dose of 50 mg/lb body wt followed by a daily dose of 25 mg/lb will maintain effective blood levels. Doses employed clinically for dogs and cats have been considerably less than this. An initial dose of 7 to 14 mg/lb followed by daily doses of 3 to 7 mg/lb have been used.

OTHER NEWER SULFONAMIDES

Several other new sulfonamides which produce prolonged blood levels in cattle have been studied pharmacologically but have not been used therapeutically to any extent in this country. These include **sulfamethoxypyridazine, sulfapyrazine-methoxyine** and **sulfachloropyridazine.** The latter compound is reported to be of value in treatment of calf scours due to *Escherichia coli* when given orally in a daily dose of 35 mg/lb body wt.

ANTIBIOTIC THERAPY

Antibiotics are primarily effective against bacterial infections in animals; some of the large viruses and several protozoa and fungi are also sensitive to these drugs. Certain antibiotics are effective for salmon poisoning in dogs, due to a *Rickettsia*-like organism. They may be either bacteriostatic or bactericidal in action depending in large part on dosage. They act primarily through interference with bacterial growth, and are most effective in acute infections when bacteria are in a rapid-growth stage.

Antibiotics are somewhat selective in their antibacterial actions. Streptomycin, for example, is mainly effective against gram-negative bacteria, while penicillin is most active against gram-positive organisms. Other antibiotics (e.g., chlortetracycline) have a wider range of activity and are effective against both gram-positive and gram-negative bacteria. These are called broad-spectrum antibiotics to distinguish them from the more selective ones, such as penicillin. Under clinical conditions, it is often not possible to establish the exact nature of the causal organisms. If an infection does not respond to a particular antibiotic within a reasonable time (approximately 48 hours) consideration should be given to changing the therapy to another antibiotic or other antibacterial agent. Whenever possible, a culture should be obtained for purposes of testing the susceptibility of the pathogen to antibiotics. Bacteria sometimes develop resistance to an antibiotic to which they were formerly susceptible, particularly if it is used initially in doses which are too low.

Antibiotics are less inhibited in their action by the presence of organic matter (i.e., pus, blood, tissue debris) than are sulfonamides. However, sulfonamides excel antibiotics in their ability to diffuse into cavities, such as joints, the pleural sacs and the subarachnoid space. Antibiotics are less likely to produce toxic effects than sulfonamides. While the serious allergic reactions to antibiotics sometimes observed in man have not been a major problem in animals, reactions are known to occur, particularly to penicillin.

Antibiotics may be applied locally for treating infections of the skin, ear, eye, udder and other accessible areas. It is known that combinations of some antibiotics with one another can produce synergism, but antagonism can also result. The possibilities of the latter occurring may be greater when a narrow-spectrum and broad-spectrum antibiotic are used in combination. Combinations of penicillin and streptomycin may be synergistic and are widely used. The interaction of antibiotics is conditioned by many factors and requires further evaluation. If the local infection is severe, a combination of local and systemic therapy is usually indicated.

Antibiotics are commonly administered by the intramammary route for the treatment of bovine mastitis, leading to a high concentration in the milk. A problem of major concern is the presence of antibacterial substances in market milk. Much of the attention has been directed toward penicillin, but the presence of any antibacterial agent is an adulteration and such milk should be discarded. In addition, antibiotics may appear in milk following systemic therapy as well as by infusion of the udder. Repository forms of penicillin (e.g., benzathine penicillin) may appear in milk for as long as 8 to 10 days after IM injection and the tetracyclines as long as 48 hours. Close attention should be given to the manufacturer's instructions regarding periods after treatment during which the milk should not be used for human consumption.

Antibiotics may be added to rations for the purpose of promoting growth in animals. Studies have shown that the addition of small amounts of chlortetracycline, penicillin, oxytetracycline, bacitracin or streptomycin to the feed promotes growth in young animals, although the first 3 antibiotics appear to be more consistent in their action. Five to 15 gm/ton of feed is suitable except for streptomycin where larger amounts (probably 20 to 50 gm/ton) must be employed.

Addition of much higher concentrations of antibiotics to feeds (e.g., 25 to 200 gm/ton of feed) or to the drinking water (e.g., 0.5 to 1.0 gm/gal.) has been advocated for the prevention and treatment of diseases of poultry and swine. Such practice is often quite effective where many animals are to be treated. CAUTION: In some countries, laws now restrict or forbid addition of antibiotics to feed or water. It is essential to conform to local requirements.

PENICILLIN

Penicillin is derived from cultures of *Penicillium notatum* or *P. chrysogenom*. Several types are commonly produced; type G is the form in most common use.

The sodium, potassium, procaine and benzathine salts of penicillin are commonly available. In addition, certain biosynthetic forms, such as penicillin-V, are in use. When it is desirable to obtain high blood levels rapidly, aqueous solutions of sodium or potassium salts are employed. Repository forms, such as procaine penicillin or benzathine penicillin, are used for maintaining blood levels over extended periods.

Penicillin is well absorbed following IM injection, which is generally used. Special formulations are available for oral and IV use. Following absorption, penicillin diffuses to most fluids and tissues and is rapidly eliminated from the body by urinary excretion.

The toxicity of penicillin is very low. The severe allergic reactions encountered with penicillin in man are infrequent in animals. An acute anaplylactic reaction has been reported in cattle. Dyspnea, salivation, staggering, collapse and in some cases death within one-half hour have been seen after use of penicillin, streptomycin and the tetracyclines. Mild reactions involving the skin and mucous membranes are sometimes seen in dogs and horses.

Clinical Indications: Penicillin is mainly effective against grampositive bacteria. A new broad-spectrum form of penicillin, ampicillin, is available but has not been extensively used in veterinary medicine. Penicillin is an effective agent for the treatment and control of bovine mastitis due to *Streptococcus agalactiae*. When proper sanitary and husbandry measures are enforced, bacteriologic cures can be obtained in 80 to 90% cases of this type, particularly if treatment is started before extensive changes in udder tissue have occurred.

Many types of vehicles have been used for intramammary

infusion of penicillin. These include sterile water, oils and ointments. Penicillin itself does not appear to be irritating to udder tissue. It also is effective against bovine mastitis caused by *Str. agalactiae*. Penicillin is of value in staphylococcal mastitis, but it is definitely less effective than for the streptococcal forms. Combinations of penicillin and other antibacterial agents are commonly used for the treatment of mastitis.

Penicillin is of some value in the treatment of infectious cystitis and pyelonephritis of cattle due to *Corynebacterium renale*. In certain cases, alleviation of signs and disappearance of organisms from the urine occurs, but in others, little or no response may be obtained. For best results, penicillin should be employed early in the course of the disease.

Clinical evidence indicates that penicillin is of value in a number of bacterial infections in which the exact etiology is unknown. Among these are calf pneumonia and secondary bacterial infections associated with distemper in dogs. Metritis of cattle, often associated with a mixed infection, has been treated successfully by instillation of penicillin suspension directly into the uterus. Penicillin also can be useful in treating anthrax and infections due to *Erysipelothrix*.

Penicillin has been employed in the form of ointments or solutions for treatment of localized infections of the skin, eyes and ears. For infected wounds of the skin and in ear infections, penicillin ointments have been used topically with some success. In severe infections of the eye, skin or ears, it is ordinarily desirable to use both systemic and local treatment. Penicillin given orally has shown some merit in the prevention and control of bloat in cattle. However, like many agents used in this condition, considerable variation in response occurs.

Added to bull semen in the concentration of 1,000 to 2,000 u/ml, penicillin is reported to effectively retard bacterial growth for a period up to 8 days. It is also used for this purpose combined with streptomycin (1,000 u of each antibiotic per milliliter).

Dosage and Administration: The dose varies with the type and severity of infection; in most instances, a dose of 2,000 u/lb body wt IM is considered to be minimal. In severe infections, this is increased to 5,000 to 10,000 u/lb body wt, or more. The frequency at which penicillin is administered varies with the type of preparation. The following is recommended: for aqueous vehicles, every 3 or 4 hours; oil and beeswax, every 12 hours; for repository forms containing procaine penicillin in water or oil, every 24 hours or longer; for benzathine penicillin, every 24 hours or longer. In severe infections, it may be desirable to use a sodium or potassium salt combined with a procaine salt, since the former gives a prompt high blood level, while the latter maintains a concentration for a prolonged period.

Government regulations now restrict the maximal single dose of penicillin for intramammary infusion in bovine mastitis to 100,000 u. This may be administered in the form of a solution in sterile water, a suspension in oil, or incorporated in an ointment base.

Oral therapy with penicillin is not widely used for treating infectious diseases of animals. In general, much larger doses are necessary than by the IM route and absorption is variable. Special forms of penicillin (e.g., penicillin-V) are available for oral use.

Preparations: Amongst these are: penicillin powder for aqueous solution, penicillin in oil and beeswax, procaine penicillin in oil, procaine penicillin in aqueous suspension, benzathine penicillin in aqueous suspension and penicillin tablets for oral use. Ophthalmic ointments containing penicillin appear to be preferable for treating conjunctival infections since they require less frequent application than do solutions. Combinations of penicillin with other antibiotics are commonly available.

STREPTOMYCIN AND DIHYDROSTREPTOMYCIN

Streptomycin is produced by cultures of *Streptomyces griseus*. Dihydrostreptomycin is formed by chemical alteration of streptomycin. Both streptomycin and dihydrostreptomycin are relatively stable in the dry form or in aqueous solution, and possess similar antibacterial activity.

Streptomycin is adequately absorbed from subcut. or IM sites of injection; absorption from the gastrointestinal tract is minimal. Applied topically, streptomycin has poor powers of penetration. After absorption, it is well distributed in body tissues and fluids, including the pleural and cerebrospinal fluids. It is mainly excreted in the urine by glomerular filtration.

In large doses over prolonged periods, streptomycin may be toxic, the most significant effect being vestibular disturbances which are reversible. Occasionally, a permanent loss of hearing may result. For normal short-term therapy using conventional doses, CNS damage or allergic reactions do not constitute a serious problem. Contact dermatitis may develop in persons handling the drug. Dihydrostreptomycin may produce permanent deafness and for this reason its parenteral use should be restricted to those cases in which the infection is not susceptible to other antibacterial therapy.

Clinical Indications: Streptomycin and dihydrostreptomycin are primarily effective against gram-negative bacteria, although a few gram-positive organisms also are susceptible. Bacteria may acquire a resistance to the antibiotic, especially when exposed to continued low concentrations of the agent.

Both antibiotics are useful in the treatment of bovine mastitis due to gram-negative organisms, particularly *Escherichia coli, Aerobacter aerogenes* or *A. cloacae*. Streptomycin has been used combined with penicillin in the form of a solution, ointment or bougie. These preparations offer the advantage of a wider antibacterial spectrum. Streptomycin is of some value in actinomycosis of cattle due to *Actinomyces bovis.* It has been successfully used in treating calf pneumonia; this should be continued for at least 4 to 5 days. Intrauterine and preputial infusions of streptomycin are reported to be of value in overcoming bovine infertility due to vibriosis. It also has been combined with penicillin and infused in the uterus, for treatment of metritis in cattle.

Streptomycin is useful in the treatment of septicemia in newborn foals, although a combination of penicillin and streptomycin often is more advisable as both gram-negative and gram-positive organisms may be involved. In the horse, streptomycin has been used for treating cystitis due to *E. coli.*

In dogs, this antibiotic is useful in the treatment of acute nephritis and given orally is successful in treating infectious dysentery. Local therapy with streptomycin has been used for treatment of otitis externa in dogs. In cats, IM streptomycin injections are reported to be of value for infectious feline panleukopenia when combined with an injection of feline antibacterial serum. In general, single daily doses of 0.20 to 0.25 gm have been employed and treatment continued for 2 to 8 days.

Oral administration of streptomycin or dihydrostreptomycin is often useful against enteric infections. Streptomycin has been used to treat leptospirosis in swine and dogs and has been successful in eliminating organisms from urine. By local injection, streptomycin and dihydrostreptomycin are of value in the treatment of infectious sinusitis in turkeys. Chronic respiratory disease of chickens has also been effectively treated with streptomycin given in the water, feed or by inhalation. The drug is also of some value in control of fowl cholera and fowl typhoid.

Streptomycin in concentrations of 250 to 1,000 mcg/ml of bull semen is effective in inhibiting bacterial growth and does not adversely affect spermatozoa for periods up to 20 days. Combinations of penicillin and streptomycin may also be used for this purpose and have the advantage of being effective against gram-positive and gram-negative organisms.

Dosage and Administration: For small animals, the recommended maximum daily dose of streptomycin or dihydrostreptomycin is 20 mg/lb body wt by IM or subcut. injection. This amount may be divided and administered in 2 to 4 doses per day. In foals, 0.5 gm every 3 to 4 hours are given by IM injection, while in horses, 1 to 2 gm every 3 to 4 hours have been used. Oral medication is indicated for enteric infections and the suggested dose for dogs, calves and swine by this route is 1 gm daily in a single dose or divided into 2 or 3 equal doses. In bovine mastitis due to *E. coli, A. aerogenes,* or *A. cloacae,* the suggested dose is 0.5 gm streptomycin twice daily by intramammary infusion. In acute coliform mastitis, the use of 5 gm by intramammary infusion combined with 5 to 7 gm given IM has been recommended. These doses are repeated twice daily. The usually recommended dose for parenteral administration in poultry is 15 to 50 mg/lb body wt, a quantity much higher, proportionately, than used in mammals. Streptomycin and dihydrostreptomycin may be toxic to turkeys if they are very ill.

Preparations: Streptomycin is supplied in the form of a powder in sterile vials as streptomycin or dihydrostreptomycin sulfate. For oral medication, streptomycin sulfate is available in solutions for administration in drinking water and dihydrostreptomycin in the form of tablets combined with other agents. Topical ointments containing streptomycin or dihydrostreptomycin alone or in combination with other antibiotics may be obtained and combinations of dihydrostreptomycin and other antibiotics for subcut. or IM injection are also available. No reliable depot form of this drug has been developed and parenteral doses must be repeated every 6 to 8 hours.

TETRACYCLINE
("Achromycin")

This antibiotic is formd by chemical alteration of chlortetracycline. It is well absorbed after oral administration. Intramuscular injections may cause pain and swellings at the injection site. Tetracycline may be given IV in a 2.5% solution. Following absorption, it is widely distributed in body fluids. Appreciable concentrations of the active form are excreted in urine and feces and, to some extent, in milk. Tetracycline produces a golden-yellow fluorescence of bone, visible under ultraviolet light. The significance of this in bone metabolism is not yet known, but faulty egg-shell formation, enamel hypoplasia of the teeth and inhibition of long-bone growth have been reported. It does not appear to delay fracture healing.

Tetracycline has a broad antibacterial spectrum, being effective against gram-positive and gram-negative bacteria and against certain rickettsiae and large viruses.

The toxicity of tetracycline is relatively low. However, following oral administration some dogs and cats may show nausea, vomiting and diarrhea. Oral dosage is not recommended for adult ruminants as the antibiotic is likely to affect the normal bacterial flora of the rumen.

Clinical Indications: Tetracycline is used for a wide variety of infections in large and small animals including: endometritis, pneumonia, tonsillitis, strangles in horses, foot rot in cattle, bacterial infections secondary to canine distemper and feline panleukopenia, bronchitis, pharyngitis, nephritis, calf scours, pyelonephritis, otitis externa and infected wounds.

Dosage: Orally, tetracycline is given to large animals at the rate of 5 to 10 mg/lb daily in divided doses. The oral dose in small animals is much larger: 25 to 50 mg/lb daily in divided dose. The dose is much reduced when the drug is given IV or IM, large animals receiving 2 to 5 mg/lb and the small species 5 mg/lb daily in divided doses.

Preparations: Tetracycline is prepared as boluses of 500 mg and capsules of 50, 100 and 250 mg for oral administration. It is also available as a soluble powder of the hydrochloride salt for the preparation of oral solutions, and sterile vials of 100 and 200 mg for making injectable solutions. A phosphate complex of tetracycline, reported to be more completely absorbed from the gastrointestinal tract, is also available.

N.B.: The term "the tetracyclines" has come into common usage to designate all of the tetracycline antibiotics as a group, i.e., chlortetracycline, oxytetracycline and tetracycline. While therapeutically the distinction is probably not important, the veterinarian should not confuse the general term with the name of the specific drug.

CHLORTETRACYCLINE
("Aureomycin")

Chlortetracycline is produced from cultures of *Streptomyces aureofaciens*. It is available in the dry state as chlortetracycline hydrochloride, a yellow crystalline powder which is quite stable. It is well absorbed when administered orally and this route may be employed to obtain therapeutic blood levels, except in adult ruminants where it is likely to disturb the normal ruminal microflora. It may be injected IV, but one should use freshly prepared solutions and prevent leakage into perivascular tissue. Chlortetracycline seems to be well distributed in the body. It crosses the placenta and attains levels in the fetal blood that are 50% those observed in the maternal blood. It is excreted mainly in the urine. Studies in cattle have shown that appreciable amounts are excreted in the milk.

In experimental studies the toxicity of chlortetracycline is low, and there appear to be no clinical reports on serious toxic reactions in animals. In adult ruminants, high oral doses may produce digestive upset as the result of its effect on the bacterial flora in the rumen. Likewise, dogs and cats may show vomiting, diarrhea and anorexia when the antibiotic is given orally, especially when therapy is prolonged. Subcut. injections of the hydrochloride may produce irritation and even necrosis at the injection site.

Clinical Indications: Chlortetracycline has a broad antibacterial spectrum and is active against many gram-positive and gram-negative bacteria as well as some large viruses and rickettsiae. It has been used to treat streptococcal and staphylococcal mastitis in cattle, but there are other antibiotics of equal or greater effectiveness. Other infections in cattle have been successfully treated with chlortetracycline. These include metritis, foot rot, shipping fever, sinusitis, pneumonia, calf scours, and necrotic laryngitis due to *Corynebacterium pyogenes* infections. Intra-uterine treatment has proved clinically successful in "repeat breeder" cows with subclinical metritis. The antibiotic may be of some value in treating listeriosis of cattle. Chlortetracycline causes a 30- to 60-day disappearance of transmissible anaplasmosis from the blood of carrier animals, and experimental infection can be prevented by feeding the antibiotic. Feeding low levels of chlortetracycline (75 mg/day) reduces the incidence of liver abscesses in feeder cattle.

In dogs, chlortetracycline has been used to treat tonsillitis, pharyngitis, pneumonia, urinary-tract infections, coccidiosis and bacterial infections secondary to canine distemper. It may have some beneficial effect against *Leptospira icterohaemor-rhagiae*. In cats, the antibiotic is used to treat bacterial infections secondary to feline panleukopenia, infectious coryza and pneumonitis.

Several infections of horses—strangles, shipping fever, pneumonia and septicemia in newborn foals—respond to chlortetracycline.

Enteric infections in swine may respond to chlortetracycline therapy; these include necrotic enteritis, salmonellosis and swine dysentery. The use of 50 gm of chlortetracycline per ton of feed produced a marked decrease in incidence of cervical abscesses in swine.

In poultry, chlortetracycline is of value in the control of infectious synovitis when given in feed at the rate of 100 to 200 gm/ton. It is also of some benefit in the control of fowl typhoid and bluecomb disease. In pigeons, use of 0.89% of the antibiotic in feed for 30 days is reported to control ornithosis. The use of continuous low levels of chlortetracycline in feed has proved of value as a growth stimulant in several species, especially in swine and poultry (*see* CAUTION, p. 475).

Local application of a 3% chlortetracycline ointment has been employed in treating external infections in dogs and cats, including otitis externa, conjunctivitis, blepharitis, keratitis, dermatitis and infected wounds. However, it would appear that 1% ointments and 0.5% buffered solutions are more satisfactory dispensing forms for ocular application by animal owners. Aqueous solutions of chlortetracycline are irritating if accidentally injected outside a vein or if applied to wounds.

Dosage and Administration: For oral administration, chlortetracycline hydrochloride is employed in an initial dose of 10 to 25 mg/lb followed every 12 hours by 5.0 to 12.5 mg/lb body weight.

The recommended IV dose is 2 to 5 mg/lb body wt followed by one-half of this dose at 12-hour intervals. Injections should be made slowly, using a 2.5% solution.

In the treatment of bovine mastitis, the usual dose by intramammary infusion is 200 to 400 mg every 24 to 48 hours. For this purpose, ointments are ordinarily employed.

Preparations: Chlortetracycline is available as: crystalline chlortetracycline hydrochloride powder buffered in sodium glycinate (for preparing solutions for injection); 100-mg, 500-mg and 2.5-gm vials; chlortetracycline hydrochloride capsules, 50 and 250 mg; chlortetracycline hydrochloride tablets, 50 and 250 mg; ophthalmic ointment, 10 mg/gm of base; and topical ointment, 3%. A calcium salt of chlortetracycline is also available for topical and oral administration.

OXYTETRACYCLINE
("Terramycin")

Oxytetracycline is derived from cultures of an actinomycete, *Streptomyces rimosus*. In the dry form, crystalline oxytetracycline hydrochloride is quite stable at room temperature, but solutions are unstable and should be administered soon after preparation. Solutions intended for IM injection will keep for approximately 5 days at refrigerator temperature. A solution of oxytetracycline in propylene glycol is stable and has a good shelf-life.

Oxytetracycline is well absorbed in the gastrointestinal tract and from IM injections. In dogs, oral doses produce peak blood levels within 1 to 2 hours. Single IM injections in dogs result in peak blood levels within 15 to 30 minutes, with significant blood levels persisting for 8 to 12 hours. After absorption, oxytetracycline is well distributed in body tissues and fluids except cerebrospinal fluid. Relatively large amounts of oxytetracycline are excreted in the urine where it is concentrated and, after oral administration, significant amounts appear in the feces.

High levels of oxytetracycline administered orally to adult ruminants may disturb the normal rumen flora. Acute anaphylactic reactions and some deaths have been reported following parenteral administration in cattle. In dogs and cats, oral doses may cause vomiting and diarrhea, especially when therapy is prolonged.

Clinical Indications: In cattle, oxytetracycline is used by intramammary infusion to treat mastitis. Systemically, it has been used to treat a number of diseases including shipping fever, metritis, foot rot, calf scours, acute mastitis and anthrax. It may be used either IV or IM or by including small amounts in feed. In dogs and cats, the antibiotic is usually given orally; occasionally the IV route is employed. Several conditions in small animals show a favorable response to oxytetracycline therapy. These include bacterial infections secondary to canine distemper and feline panleukopenia, pneumonia, enteritis, endometritis and infections of the urinary tract.

Parenteral injections of oxytetracycline are useful in treating anthrax, strangles and pneumonia in horses. For treatment of fistulous withers, a combination of systemic and local therapy has been used. In sheep, diarrhea and enterotoxemia are reported to respond to oxytetracycline in the feed. It also has been used to treat necrotic enteritis, atrophic rhinitis and leptospirosis of swine. In the latter disease, levels of 500 gm/ton of feed are reported to eradicate shedding of *Leptospira* in urine and to reduce the incidence of abortions. *Eperythrozoon suis* responds to a single IM injection of 3 mg/lb of body wt.

For poultry, oxytetracycline administered in feed is of value in the control of infectious synovitis, erysipelas, bluecomb and chronic respiratory disease. Generally, a level of 200 gm of antibiotic per ton of feed is required. Oxytetracycline, at low levels (5 to 25 gm/ton of feed), has been used as a growth stimulant and as a prophylactic against diseases of the newborn in several species, including pigs, calves, lambs and poultry.

Topically, oxytetracycline hydrochloride is used in combination with corticosteroids and other antibiotics for the treatment of infections of eyes, ears, skin and wounds.

Dosage and Administration: Oxytetracycline may be administered orally to all species of animals with the exception of adult ruminants, where it can exert an unfavorable influence on the ruminal microflora. For oral administration, daily doses are recommended, which range from 5 to 10 mg/lb body wt (livestock), and from 25 to 50 mg/lb body wt (small animals), given in divided doses every 6 hours. For dogs and cats, the IM dose is 3 to 10 mg/lb body wt daily. In large animals and poultry, the parenteral dosage is 2 to 5 mg/lb body wt daily given IV, IM or subcut. and repeated at 24-hour intervals unless oral therapy is instituted.

Preparations: Oxytetracycline hydrochloride is available as: tablets for oral use in 50 mg and 125 mg; capsules for oral use in 125 mg and 250 mg; boluses for oral use in 250 mg; preconstituted parenteral solutions containing 50 mg/ml; soluble powder for oral use containing 25 gm/lb; ophthalmic ointment for topical use containing 5 mg/gm; aerosol spray for topical use containing 300 mg/2 fl oz; intramammary preparation containing 30 mg/gm; preparation for topical and intramammary use containing 200 mg/10 ml.

CHLORAMPHENICOL
("Chloromycetin")

Chloramphenicol is produced by *Streptomyces venezuelae* and is also prepared by chemical synthesis. It is a broadspectrum antibiotic, being effective against gram-positive and gram-negative bacteria and certain rickettsiae and large viruses. It is well absorbed from the gastrointestinal tract and, in dogs, therapeutic blood levels may be obtained by this route. Peak blood levels are obtained in 2 to 4 hours. High levels of the antibiotics are found in the kidney and liver of the dog, progressively lower concentrations in the lung, spleen, heart, muscle and brain. Although only small amounts of the active compound are excreted in the urine, this may still provide a sufficient concentration for antimicrobial activity in the urinary tract.

Daily doses of 200 mg/lb body wt have been administered orally to dogs without causing undesirable effects. Other studies in dogs indicate that oral doses of up to 50 mg/lb body wt given twice daily for periods up to 133 days do not cause significant alterations in hemoglobin levels or red or white blood cell counts.

Clinical Indications: In dogs and cats, chloramphenicol is effective in pneumonia, metritis, cystitis, nephritis and bacterial infections secondary to canine distemper and feline panleukopenia. In dogs, infectious enteritis (*Escherichia coli* or *Proteus* organisms) responds to chloramphenicol either alone or in combination with dihydrostreptomycin. Limited studies indicate that it is effective against infectious bronchitis, or so-called "kennel cough", and in salmon poisoning in dogs. In the conditions described above, chloramphenicol was administered orally or IM.

Few reports have appeared on the use of chloramphenicol in large animals. Intravenous administration is of value in the treatment of hemorrhagic septicemia of cattle. In calves, oral administration has been employed in white scours and in limited experimental trials it was found to be of value for treatment of contagious bovine pleuropneumonia due to *Mycoplasma mycoides*.

Local application of chloramphenicol in the form of ophthalmic ointments or ophthalmic solution has been found to be effective in certain ocular infections. These include corneal ulcers and abrasions, keratitis, conjunctivitis and iritis. Ointments may be applied every 3 hours, while solutions require more frequent application (usually every waking hour for the first day and every 2 to 3 hours thereafter). In some cases, oral medication can also increase concentrations of chloramphenicol in the ocular fluids.

Dosage and Administration: In dogs and cats, oral administration appears to be satisfactory using 25 to 75 mg/lb body wt given daily in 4 divided doses. Intramuscularly, it has been used for these animals in a dose of 10 to 15 mg/lb body wt at

8-hour intervals. For colts and calves, the daily oral dose is 1 to 2 gm, while for lambs 500 mg daily has been employed.

Preparations: Chloramphenicol is supplied in capsules containing 50, 100 or 250 mg. An ophthalmic ointment and powder for preparing solutions as well as a special preparation for IM administration also are available.

NEOMYCIN

Neomycin is produced by cultures of *Streptomyces fradiae*. Clinically, it is used as neomycin sulfate, a white amorphous powder which is relatively stable in the dry form. Neomycin is soluble in water, but insoluble in organic solvents. Since little or no neomycin is absorbed from the gastrointestinal tract when the antibiotic is given orally, this method of administration is limited to treatment of gastrointestinal infections. When initially introduced, neomycin was not recommended for parenteral use because of its tendency to produce renal damage. However, today it is recognized as being clinically safe when given by injection if proper precautions are taken. These include the restriction of therapy to 5 days or less of recommended dosage.

Clinical Indications: Neomycin has a wide range of antibacterial activity and is effective against a number of gram-positive and gram-negative bacteria, including certain strains of *Pseudomonas* and *Proteus* organisms.

Neomycin sulfate is of some value in treating bovine mastitis due to *Pseudomonas* organisms. In reported trials, 29 to 57% of infected quarters were freed of infection. The efficacy of neomycin in the treatment of streptococcal and staphylococcal mastitis is variable. Some reports indicate that it is quite effective, but in other cases, it was found to be inferior to penicillin for these infections. In a few instances, neomycin has been successfully employed for coliform mastitis. It has been used combined with parenteral steroid preparations for treatment of mastitis.

Oral administration of neomycin is used for treatment of bacterial infections of the gastrointestinal tract and for pre-operative sterilization of the bowel. Indications for systemic administration are not well characterized and neomycin is not often used parenterally.

Topical application of neomycin is of value in treating wounds and infections of the skin, ears and eyes. Ointments containing neomycin in combination with other antibiotic substances (e.g., polymyxin, gramicidin) or other agents (e.g., corticoids) are not available.

Dosage and Administration: In bovine mastitis, the recommended dosage for neomycin sulfate is 0.5 gm per infected quarter. This may be administered by intramammary infusion in the form of an aqueous solution, water-in-oil emulsion or as an ointment. For dogs, a daily oral dose of 5 to 10 mg/lb of body wt may be used.

Preparations: Neomycin sulfate is available as a sterile powder for preparing aqueous solutions for topical or oral use. Topical or ophthalmic ointments containing neomycin alone or in combination with other antibiotics are also available.

BACITRACIN

Bacitracin is obtained from cultures of *Bacillus subtilis*. In the dry state, it is stable except at high temperatures. In solution at room temperature, it is relatively unstable, but, if kept refrigerated no significant loss of potency is noted for approximately 3 weeks. In the form of an anhydrous ointment, it is stable for periods of a year or longer.

Bacitracin is very poorly absorbed after oral administration. Apparently, large amounts of bacitracin are destroyed in the gastrointestinal tract, and only a portion of that given orally can be recovered in the feces. Experimental studies showed that bacitracin was likely to produce renal toxic effects when administered parenterally and, therefore, its use by injection is not recommended. In man, it is used for topical application.

Clinical Indications: Bacitracin, like penicillin, is mainly effective against gram-positive organisms. Some organisms which are resistant to penicillin are sensitive to bacitracin and the reverse also is true.

Bacitracin has been employed in a solution by intramammary infusion for treating cases of bovine mastitis due to *Streptococcus agalactiae*. In general, results were as satisfactory as those obtained with penicillin or sulfonamides.

Bacitracin has been found to be useful when applied topically in such conditions as infected wounds, otitis externa and conjunctivitis in dogs. Ointments containing 500 u of bacitracin per gram or solutions containing 500 u/ml have been employed. Abscesses may be injected directly with 0.2 to 5.0 ml of the solution. Infectious keratitis in cattle is reported to respond to treatment with an ointment of the above concentrations.

Preparations: Bacitracin is available as tablets, and as topical and ophthalmic ointments containing 500 u/gm as ointment base. Ointments containing a combination of bacitracin and other antibiotics also may be obtained.

TYROTHRICIN

Tyrothricin is produced by cultures of *Bacillus brevis*. It is composed of a mixture of several substances, of which gramicidin and tyrocidine are present in the greatest quantities. Tyrothricin is relatively insoluble in water, but is soluble in alcohol and propylene glycol. Unlike the majority of antibiotics, it is stable under most conditions.

Clinical Indications: Tyrothricin is effective against gram-positive organisms, but its activity against gram-negative bacteria is low. Little or no absorption of tyrothricin occurs after oral administration and since it is quite toxic when injected parenterally, it is recommended only for topical use.

Tyrothricin is used in the treatment of bovine mastitis due to *Streptocococcus agalactiae,* but generally it is irritant to udder tissue. The average dose of 20 mg per quarter is infused, in an aqueous or oily vehicle, into dry cows only—but other more effective products are available for this purpose.

Tyrothricin in the form of a 0.5% ointment or as a solution has been employed in treating infected wounds and for irrigation of osteomyelitic lesions in bone. Wound exudate and tissue debris do not markedly inhibit its antibacterial action. Endometritis of cattle responds to irrigation of the uterus with aqueous or oily solutions containing 2 mg of the drug per cubic centimeter. Repeated treatment may be necessary. For topical therapy, tyrothricin may be combined with other antibiotics or sulfonamides.

Preparations: Tyrothricin is available in aqueous alcoholic solution, emulsion, ointment and cream.

POLYMYXIN

Polymyxin is produced by cultures of *Bacillus polymyxa* (*asterosporus*). Several polymyxins are identified as A, B, C, D and E. Polymyxin B has the most desirable therapeutic characteristics and is said to be least toxic. Polymyxin B sulfate is the form ordinarily employed. It is readily soluble in water and solutions remain stable for periods of approximately 2 months if kept under refrigeration.

After oral administration, large amounts of polymyxin appear in the feces and there is little absorption from the gastrointestinal tract. Following IM injection, the antibiotic is rapidly absorbed. In horses severe inflammatory reactions may occur at the site of IM injections.

Polymyxin B is effective against a large number of gram-negative bacteria and its action is accompanied by the development of little bacterial resistance. It is notably effective against many strains of *Pseudomonas aeruginosa*.

Clinical Indications: Initially, polymyxin was recommended for topical use only. However, recent studies report its parenteral use in combination with neomycin. Conditions which respond favorably to such treatment include shipping fever and foot rot in cattle, strangles in horses, and tonsillitis and post-distemper bacterial infections in dogs. For large animals, the recommended dose is 100,000 to 200,000 u/100 lb body wt every 12 hours and for dogs a total dose of 50,000 to 100,000 u. Both polymyxin and neomycin may produce nephrotoxic effects and therefore they should be used parenterally with caution.

Topically, polymyxin, either alone or combined with other antibacterial agents, such as bacitracin and neomycin, is used for treatment of infections of the skin, ear and eye.

Preparations: Polymyxin is available in a sterile parenteral solution containing 100,000 u of polymyxin B sulfate and 100 mg neomycin sulfate per milliliter. Various types of ointments, tablets and solutions for local use are also available.

ERYTHROMYCIN
("Ilotycin")

Erythromycin is produced by cultures of *Streptomyces erythraeus*. It is poorly soluble in water, but readily soluble in alcohol and alcoholic solutions may be further diluted with water. Solutions are stable at room temperature for approximately 24 hours.

Experimental studies on dogs and cats have shown that erythromycin is rapidly absorbed after oral administration and the unmetabolized portion is rapidly excreted in the urine. In dogs, the antibiotic crosses the blood-brain barrier and enters the cerebrospinal fluid. Oral doses of 25 mg/lb body wt have been administered to dogs and cats for periods up to 3 months without producing toxic signs or changes in the formed elements of the blood. A dose of 25 mg erythromycin IM during the first 24 hours of life is reported to reduce the incidence of and mortality due to infectious diarrhea in pigs. Doses of 10 mg/lb daily have been used to treat the condition.

Erythromycin base is readily destroyed by the acid of gastric juice. For this reason, enteric-coated tablets are preferred for oral administration. The consequent delay in absorption may be corrected somewhat by the use of one of its salts such as the propionate.

Like penicillin, erythromycin is primarily active against gram-positive organisms. Bacterial resistance (but not cross resistance to penicillin) is developed relatively quickly.

Clinical Indications: Erythromycin has been employed in dogs to treat such conditions as secondary bacterial infections of distemper, pneumonia, pharyngitis, urinary-tract infections, enteritis, tonsillitis and otitis. In these cases, the antibiotic was administered orally in daily doses of 300 to 600 mg. These amounts are ordinarily divided into 3 or 4 fractional doses.

Preparations: Erythromycin, either as the base or in the form of one of several salts, is available as 100- and 250-mg tablets, as an oral suspension (100 mg of antibiotic in each 5 ml) and as a 1% ointment. Combinations of erythromycin and other antibiotics and sulfonamides are also available.

NOVOBIOCIN
("Albamycin", "Cathomycin")

Novobiocin is derived from *Streptomyces spheroides*. It is freely soluble in water, and solutions are stable when refrigerated. The antibiotic is well absorbed when given orally or IM and peak blood levels are obtained in dogs within 2 to 4 hours. High levels are still present 12 hours later. Following absorption, it is well distributed in most body fluids, but does not readily enter cerebrospinal fluid. Novobiocin is excreted primarily in the feces; only low levels appear in the urine.

Novobiocin is effective chiefly against the same gram-positive bacteria that are sensitive to penicillin, although a few gram-negative organisms are also sensitive. It is reported to be especially active against staphylococci even if these are resistant to penicillin.

Clinical Indications: Novobiocin has been used for the treatment of a variety of infections in dogs and cats. These include bronchitis, cystitis, metritis, nephritis, pharyngitis, peritonitis, tonsillitis, staphylococcal skin infections, pneumonia and bacterial infections secondary to canine distemper and feline panleukopenia. In cattle, the antibiotic has been used for treatment of pneumonia, metritis and mastitis. In chickens, it is reported to be of value in treating staphylococcal synovitis. It is also of value when a penicillin-resistant pathogen is encountered.

Dosage: In dogs and cats, novobiocin is given orally in a daily dose of 10 to 15 mg/lb of body wt and IM and IV at the rate of 2 to 7 mg/lb of body wt.

For cattle, the IM and IV dose is 1 to 3 mg/lb of body wt daily. In all instances, the daily dose is given in 2 equal parts.

Preparations: Novobiocin is available in 250-mg capsules, as an oral syrup (25 mg/ml) and as a sterile powder for parenteral use. Combinations with other antibiotics are also available.

CARBOMYCIN
("Magnamycin")

Carbomycin is derived from *Streptomyces halstedii*. It is soluble in water, and refrigerated solutions are stable for about a week. It is absorbed from the gastrointestinal tract and is excreted primarily in bile. Only relatively small amounts appear in the urine. The antibiotic is effective mainly against gram-positive organisms. It is reported to be particularly active against penicillin-resistant staphylococci and enterococci.

Clinical Indications and Dosage: Carbomycin has been used in small animals to treat a variety of infections including bacterial infections secondary to canine distemper, infectious enteritis, tonsillitis, metritis and pneumonia.

For dogs and cats, the oral dose of carbomycin is 15 to 30 mg/lb of body wt daily, given in 3 or more divided doses. Carbomycin is available as 100- and 250-mg tablets.

OLEANDOMYCIN

This antibiotic is produced by *Streptomyces antibioticus* and is primarily effective against gram-positive bacteria. For parenteral administration, it is used as the phosphate salt, and for oral use triacetyl oleandomycin gives best results. After IM or oral administration, peak blood levels are observed within 3 hours and maintained for 4 to 6 hours.

Oleandomycin has been used to treat acne, furunculosis and deep pyodermas in dogs. The phosphate salt may be given in daily IV doses of 250 mg for 7 days, or triacetyl oleandomycin may be used orally in a dose of 250 mg twice daily for 10 to 14 days. In pigs, the antibiotic is reported to increase weight gains and feed efficiency when supplied at the rate of 20 gm/ton of feed.

TYLOSIN

Tylosin is produced by *Streptomycetes fradiae* and is mainly effective against gram-positive organisms, but some gram-negative bacteria, spirochetes, certain vibrios and PPLO (*Mycoplasma*) are also susceptible. It may be given orally or parenterally, usually as the tartrate salt.

In swine dysentery the antibiotic has produced good results when given in a dose of 200 mg IM followed by 40 to 100 gm/ton of feed or when supplied initially in drinking water (1 gm/gal.) for 48 hours and then in feed. Tylosin is effective in treating infectious sinusitis due to *Mycoplasma gallisepticum* in turkeys when injected into sinuses in a dose of 1 to 6 mg or when given parenterally or in drinking water.

NEWER ANTIBIOTICS

Several new antibiotics have been introduced in recent years for human medicine, but their use for animals has been quite restricted. Various penicillin preparations having a broad antibacterial spectrum are now available, e.g., **potassium phenethicillin, sodium methicillin, ampicillin.** Spiromycin, an antibiotic effective mainly against gram-positive organisms, is reported to be quite effective in treating sinusitis (mycoplasmosis) in turkeys and chickens. In turkeys, a dose of 100 mg may be injected directly into infected sinuses. **Kanamycin** is of value in treating staphylococcal infections resistant to other antibiotics and has been used to treat infections due to *Escherichia coli* in calves and in combination with penicillin to treat streptococcal and staphylococcal mastitis, interdigital furuncles and actinobacillosis in cattle. **Virginiamycin (staphylomycin)** is mainly effective against gram-positive micrococci. In combination with polymyxin B it is reported to give good results in the treatment of otitis externa due to streptococci or staphylococci in dogs.

The **cephalosporins,** a group of antibiotics formed by a species of *Cephalosporium,* are bactericidal and have a wide spectrum of activity. They have not been evaluated in veterinary medicine but appear promising for the future.

Several antibiotic agents having a fungistatic action have been found useful. These include **griseofulvin, nystatin** and **amphotericin-B.** Their uses are described in the chapters on fungal diseases in which they have their effect (*see* SYSTEMIC

FUNGUS INFECTIONS: HISTOPLASMOSIS, p. 417; COCCIDIOIDOMY-
COSIS, p. 418; NORTH AMERICAN BLASTOMYCOSIS, p. 420; CRYPTO-
COCCOSIS, p. 421 and CANDIDIASAS, p. 424).

NITROFURAN THERAPY

The nitrofurans are a group of synthetic antimicrobial compounds, chemically based upon the furan ring to which a 5-
nitro group has been added. The nitrofurans are effective
against many gram-positive and gram-negative bacteria; certain nitrofurans are also active against protozoa, fungi and
some large viruses. They are more bactericidal than bacteriostatic, acting as inhibitors of the carbohydrate metabolism of
the bacterial cell. At therapeutic concentrations they do not
interfere with phagocytosis; most are less effective in the
presence of blood, serum, pus and milk.

Nitrofurans have a low tissue toxicity. Their prolonged use
may lead to a few side effects—such as gastrointestinal irritation, depressed weight gain; depressed spermatogenesis has also
been reported. Clinically only negligible resistance to nitrofurans has been recognized, except in coccidiosis.

In employing the nitrofurans as therapeutic agents, it is
important to select the drug most suitable for the infection
being treated.

NITROFURAZONE
("Furacin")

Nitrofurazone possesses *in vitro* activity against a wide range
of organisms including gram-negative (*Aerobacter aerogenes,
Brucella, Escherichia coli,* pasteurellae, salmonellae, vibrios, and
some strains of *Proteus* and *Pseudomonas*) and gram-positive
pathogens (clostridia, corynebacteria, staphylococci, streptococci and diplococci).

In various dosage forms, nitrofurazone as a topical agent is
effective against bacterial infections of surface lesions of the
skin, eye, udder and genital tract. It is useful in infectious
enteritis in large and small animals and in canine and avian
coccidiosis.

The topical preparations of nitrofurazone are applied as a
0.2% ointment directly on the lesion or on gauze, several
times daily, or left beneath an occlusive dressing for at least
24 hours. The drug does not penetrate intact skin in therapeutic amounts. Solutions of the same concentration are given
by intra-uterine infusion in genital infections.

A suspension containing 2% nitrofurazone and procaine penicillin G is used in treating topical bacterial infections of domestic farm animals as well as dogs and cats.

Nitrofurazone is also available in a 4.59% water-soluble powder for use in infectious necrotic enteritis of swine, for the control of outbreaks of cecal and intestinal coccidiosis (due to *Eimeria tenella* and *E. necatrix*) of chickens and in gray diarrhea of mink. The rate of administration in enteritis and coccidiosis is 330 gm of the powder in 36 and 50 gal. of drinking water, respectively. For mink, 330 gm of the powder is added to every 150 lb of feed. It is given for 1 to 3 weeks. Aqueous solutions of this preparation will deteriorate if allowed to remain in continuous contact with metal for over 7 days.

Nitrofurazone is available in a number of other formulations for topical or oral use in skin, eye or ear infections, and in genital or gastrointestinal infections.

NITROFURANTOIN
("Furadantin")

Nitrofurantoin is rapidly and nearly completely absorbed from the gastrointestinal tract. The antibacterial spectrum covers most urinary-tract pathogens, including many strains of *Proteus* and *Aerobacter*. The drug is useful in the treatment of epizootic tracheobronchitis (kennel cough) in dogs. After oral administration, approximately 45% of the dose appears in the urine; it is supposed that its solubility eliminates the danger of crystalluria. Nitrofurantoin is given 3 times a day at the rate of 2 mg/lb body wt for 4 to 7 days or longer. It should be given with caution in the presence of renal impairment. It is available as a suspension and as tablets.

FURAZOLIDONE
("Furoxone")

Furazolidone is an effective antimicrobial agent for a number of poultry disease including: coccidiosis, fowl typhoid, pullorum disease, histomoniasis, hexamitiasis, synovitis and certain susceptible secondary bacterial infections associated with the chronic respiratory disease complex (CRD) and nonspecific enteritis. Furazolidone improves the efficiency of feed utilization in poultry. It is effective in the treatment of bacterial enteritis and infectious hemorrhagic enteritis of swine, and enteritis and *Pasteurella* pneumonia of rabbits. Furazolidone is available as 11% and 22% premixes. It is also prepared as a 25% dust for aerosol administration in treating CRD and as a liquid suspension for treating bacterial enteritis (colibacillosis or white scours) in baby pigs.

Continual treatment in poultry and large animals may give rise to resistant strains of *Salmonella* and coccidia.

NIHYDRAZONE
("Nidrafur")

Nihydrazone is effective against a wide spectrum of gram-negative and gram-positive organisms, and some protozoa. It is used as a prophylactic for broiler and layer-replacement chickens to prevent CRD, pullorum, typhoid, paratyphoid, coccidiosis and histomoniasis. Nihydrazone is available as a 22% premix and is administered as a final feed containing 100 gm of nihydrazone per ton, or 0.011%.

FURALTADONE
("Valsyn")

Furaltadone as an antibacterial agent may be used in treating lactating or dry cows with mastitis caused by staphylococci (hemolytic and nonhemolytic); *Streptococcus agalactiae, Str. dysgalactiae,* or *Str. uberis; Escherichia coli;* and *Corynebacterium bovis.* Furaltadone is available as a peanut-oil suspension containing 500 mg per 15-ml dose; and in combination with procaine penicillin G 100,000 u/15 ml.

NIFURALDEZONE
("Furamazone")

Nifuraldezone is used to treat enteric bacterial infections in calves. It is effective against many gram-negative and gram-positive bacteria, including the virulent strains of *Escherichia coli* often found in calf enteritis.

The drug is available in boluses containing 1 gm nifuraldezone plus bismuth subsalicylate. The dose is 1 bolus for each 150 lb of body wt administered twice daily for 2 or 3 days.

NITROFURFURYL METHYL ETHER
("Furaspor")

Nitrofurfuryl methyl ether may be used to treat dermatomycoses, and their secondary bacterial infections. It is active against such dermatophytes as *Candida* (*Monilia*), *Microsporum* and *Trichophyton*. It is fungicidal to spores as well as to vegetative mycelia and possesses good antibacterial activity.

It is available as a liquid containing 0.4% nitrofurfuryl methyl ether, 15% benzyl benzoate and 0.5% of a quaternary ammonium compound. It is applied topically, once daily, in the treatment of dermatomycoses, and their complicating secondary bacterial infections, seborrheic and pyogenic dermatitis and parasitic dermatoses caused by mites (demodectic mange). If lesions are extensive, half the involved areas may be treated in the morning and the other half at night. Continuous application may lead to sensitization. It is contraindicated for cats.

METABOLIC DISTURBANCES

KETOSIS IN CATTLE
(Acetonemia)

A metabolic disease of lactating cows occurring within a few days to a few weeks after calving. It is characterized by hypoglycemia, ketonemia, ketonuria, inappetence, either lethargy or high excitability, loss of weight, depressed milk production and occasionally incoordination. In most areas, the incidence is highest in high-producing cows during the stall-feeding period.

Etiology: General agreement on the etiology of primary ketosis has not been reached. Some regard the disease as having its origin primarily in a carbohydrate deficiency, usually associated with a defect in metabolism, but sometimes an absolute deficiency, while others believe that it involves a temporary, relative adrenal insufficiency. Secondary ketosis is commonly caused by a depression of appetite resulting from a primary disease such as metritis, mastitis, traumatic reticulitis or abomasal displacement.

The carbohydrate deficiency hypothesis is based on the observation that, of the various forms of carbohydrate ingested by the ruminant, little is absorbed as glucose. The animal's principal sources of energy are the acetic, propionic and butyric acids arising from microbial fermentation; of these 3, propionic acid is generally accepted as the major carbohydrate precursor and the only one having antiketogenic properties. If this is so, the lactating cow receives little or no surplus of carbohydrate beyond that required for the synthesis of the lactose secreted in the milk. An inadequate caloric intake can occur when the food is insufficient or unpalatable or when the balance of ketogenic and antiketogenic substances in the diet is disturbed, e.g., by the feeding of certain silages.

The biochemical events that lead to ketosis have not been precisely defined. Ketosis occurs when the dietary intake of carbohydrate or its precursors is inadequate or when there is a defect in metabolism. As only a minority of lactating cows develop ketosis, there is obviously some deviation in the metabolism of susceptible animals. This metabolic defect remains undiscovered, but since the endocrine glands influence the function of the various biochemical pathways, it might well be due to some endocrine imbalance.

The "temporary adrenal insufficiency" hypothesis is based on evidence of altered liver metabolism, histopathologic change in the pituitary and adrenals, and the response to glucocorticoid therapy. The stress of late pregnancy, at parturition and immediately afterwards results in a stimulation of the pituitary, which releases the adrenocorticotropic hormone (ACTH). This hormone stimulates the adrenal glands to secrete glucocorticoids which help the cow to withstand the stress, in part by increasing the mobilization of glucose and the formation of new glucose from protein. It is postulated that in the cow that develops ketosis, the stress becomes excessive, leading to exhaustion of the adrenal cortex and failure to produce sufficient glucocorticoids.

It remains to be ascertained whether the pituitary-adrenocortical malfunction is primary or secondary. Although glucocorticoids are undoubtedly effective in the treatment of bovine ketosis, this could be due to pharmacologic action rather than replacement therapy. There is little doubt that the endocrine disorder in the ketotic cow is complex and involves hormones other than glucocorticoids.

Clinical Findings: The signs of ketosis usually appear a few days to a few weeks after calving. They include inappetence, constipation, mucous-covered feces, depression, a staring expression, rapid loss of weight, a drop in milk production, incoordination and paresis. While most animals show lethargy, a few become highly excitable. Respiration is shallow and there is an acetone odor on the breath. Hypoglycemia, ketonuria and ketonemia are always present. Hemoconcentration is frequently observed and there may be a rise in the eosinophil count.

Lesions: The lesions show some similarity to those seen in animals experimentally exposed to stress. They include regressive changes of the anterior lobe of the pituitary gland, hypertrophy and patchy degeneration of the adrenal cortex, involution of the thymolymphatic system, acute involution of the pancreas, gastrointestinal inflammation and ulcers, nephrosis and, most obviously, a profound fatty infiltration of the liver. Liver glycogen levels are low.

Diagnosis: While a negative urine or milk test (Rothera's or "Acetest") will rule out ketosis, the mere presence of hypoglycemia, ketonemia and ketonuria is not sufficient for a positive diagnosis of ketosis. Any abnormality, such as metritis, pneumonia, traumatic gastritis, or mastitis, that causes a cow to go off feed, will produce some degree of secondary or fasting ketosis. Such conditions, of course, may accompany the true ketotic syndrome. A modified urine test, which can be used in the field (℞ 632) may be helpful in differentiating primary and secondary ketosis. Sometimes, it is advisable to reserve judgment until the response to treatment has been observed. Failure to get a definite response to glucose or hormone therapy is cause for reconsideration of the signs and possible complications.

Prophylaxis: Animals susceptible to ketosis should be maintained on a relatively high-energy intake before calving, and the level should be increased substantially after parturition. Rations which induce a high production of propionic acid in the rumen may contribute materially to the prevention of ketosis when fed for a few weeks before and after calving. For example, a ration of finely ground and pelleted-alfalfa hay plus a steam-heated cereal (flaked corn, barley, etc.), in which the ratio of hay to steamed cereal may be as great as 8:1, effects a high production of propionic acid. For this ration to be effective, the animal must not have access to long hay, straw, shavings or other unground roughage. When large amounts of silage are being fed, its replacement by hay may be advantageous. Addition of sodium propionate (℞ 646) to the feed will reduce the incidence. In order to limit the degree of stress, precautions should be taken to avoid marked changes in the environment of the animal during the parturient period.

Treatment: The IV injection of glucose (℞ 562) is not sufficiently effective, even when repeated daily for 3 to 4 days, to be recommended as a sole form of treatment. However, it is commonly used as an adjunct to either the injection of glucocorticoids (℞ 140, 148, 154) or the oral administration of propylene glycol (℞ 643). An injection of glucose results in a prompt increase in blood sugar that is followed by a decrease within the next several hours to a value usually below normal, but still greater than the pretreatment level; the blood sugar may not return to normal for several days, even in cows which show a good response.

Following the IM injection of glucocorticoids, blood glucose usually returns to normal within 8 to 10 hours and may rise to a value considerably above normal within 24 hours, especially when the cause is inadequate calorie intake. In such cases a marked improvement in appetite and general behavior usually occurs within 24 hours and a return to normal blood ketone levels by the third to fifth day. Milk production increases rapidly by the second to third day after treatment.

Sodium propionate (℞ 646), propylene glycol (℞ 643), or lactate mixtures (℞ 587) administered by mouth will bring a recovery in many cases. Compared with other treatments, however, the response is slower and treatment must be extended over a longer period. These substances appear to be of greatest value when used as supportive treatment following the use of glucocorticoids or glucose. Sodium acetate given orally is less effective. Chloral hydrate (℞ 525) sometimes is used in conjunction with other treatments and is especially helpful if hyperexcitability is exhibited. When the appetite has recovered following any of the above treatments, good feeding is required to restore the animal to full health and production.

Since it is often difficult to distinguish between primary and secondary ketosis when the patient exhibits signs of other disease conditions, it may be advisable to treat both for ketosis and the complicating condition.

PARTURIENT PARESIS
(Milk fever)

COWS

An afebrile disease, occurring most commonly at or soon after parturition, manifested by circulatory collapse, generalized paresis and depression of consciousness.

Etiology: Although the exact cause of this disease is unknown, it is usually associated with the sudden onset of profuse lactation in mature cows. The most obvious and consistent abnormality displayed is an acute hypocalcemia in which the serum calcium level drops from a normal of about 10 mg% to levels of 3 to 7 mg% with an average of 5 mg%. Signs usually appear when the serum calcium falls to 7 mg% or lower. Serum magnesium levels may be elevated or depressed and influence the clinical picture observed, low levels being accompanied by tetany and high levels by a flaccid paralysis and somnolence. The disease may occur in cows of any age but is most common in dairy cows from 5 to 9 years old. There seems to be higher incidence in the Jersey breed.

Clinical Findings: Parturient paresis usually occurs within 72 hours after parturition, but occasionally before, during, or even some months thereafter. The disease is sometimes the cause of dystocia arising from inadequate expulsive efforts.

Early in the onset, the cow may exhibit some unsteadiness as she walks. More frequently, the cow is found lying on her sternum with her head displaced to one side, causing a kink in the neck, or turned into the flank. The eyes are dull and staring and the pupils dilated. Anorexia is complete, the muzzle tends to be dry and the extremities are cool. The pulse usually is 50 to 85/min, and the temperature normal or subnormal. The digestive tract is atonic with suppressed defecation and a relaxed anus. If treatment is delayed many hours, the dullness gives way to coma, which becomes progressively deeper, leading to death. With approaching coma, the animal assumes lateral recumbency, which predisposes to bloating, regurgitation and aspiration pneumonia. Treatment in the early stages is always more successful and fewer relapses occur. Those cases which occur at or within a few hours of parturition appear to develop more rapidly and be more severe than those which develop at other times. Diseases which may be confused with parturient paresis are metritis, ketosis, mastitis, grass tetany, acute indigestion, traumatic gastritis, coxofemoral luxations, obturator paralysis, lymphosarcoma, spinal compression and fracture of the pelvis. Some of these diseases and, in addition, aspiration pneumonia and degenerative myopathy, may also occur as complications.

Prophylaxis: The feeding of high-phosphorus, low-calcium diets during late pregnancy helps to prevent parturient paresis, but such rations are difficult to devise in a practical form and, if continued for long periods in heavy-milking cows, may result in dangerous depletion of skeletal mineral reserves. Delayed or incomplete milking after calving, by maintaining pressure within the udder, is of doubtful value in reducing the number of attacks and may aggravate a latent infection into acute clinical mastitis. Massive doses of vitamin D (20 to 30 million units daily), given in the feed for 5 to 7 days before parturition, will reduce the incidence, but if administration is stopped more than 4 days before calving, the cow is more susceptible. Dosing for periods longer than those recommended should be avoided because of the danger of toxicity. A single IV or subcut. injection of 10 million units of crystalline vitamin D given 8 days before calving is an effective preventive. Occasionally, animals show a severe reaction after the IV injection.

Treatment: Effort is directed toward returning the serum calcium level to the normal range. Calcium borogluconate is most commonly used (R 583). Preferably it is injected IV but the subcut. and IP routes are also used. Subcut. administration permits slow absorption of the calcium ion and may lessen the danger of cardiac arrest. Strict asepsis and limitation of the volume injected at one site to about 50 ml reduce the chances of local reactions. Animals that relapse or fail to get up after 8 to 12 hours should be re-treated.

In those cases in which there is an accompanying hypomagnesemia, response is better if magnesium (R 584) is added to the injectable calcium preparation. In cases complicated by ketosis 250 to 500 ml of 50% dextrose should be given IV. In the absence of blood analysis it is often impossible to decide which element is low, and in the field it is a common practice to treat nonresponsive cows with one of a variety of commercial preparations containing not only calcium and magnesium but also glucose and phosphorus.

In the few cases in which there is failure to respond to any other treatment, the udder may be inflated. Each quarter is inflated through a sterile teat tube until firm and, if necessary, the teats are gently tied with gauze to prevent escape of the air. The gauze is removed after 3 to 4 hours and the udder is

partially milked out. If necessary, inflation may be repeated
6 to 8 hours later.

EWES

A disturbance of metabolism in pregnant and lactating ewes
characterized by acute hypocalcemia and the rapid development of hyperexcitability, ataxia, paresis, coma and death.

Etiology: The exact cause is unknown, but the conditions under
which field outbreaks take place are fairly well defined. The
disease occurs at any time from 6 weeks before to 10 weeks
after lambing, principally in highly conditioned older ewes at
pasture. The onset is sudden and almost invariably follows—
within 24 hours—an abrupt change of feed, a sudden change in
weather or short periods of fasting imposed by circumstances
such as shearing, crutching or transportation.

Clinical Findings: Characteristically, the disease occurs in outbreaks. The incidence is usually less than 5%, but, in severe
outbreaks, 30% of the flock may be affected at one time. The
earliest signs are slight hyperexcitability, muscle tremors and a
stilted gait. These are soon followed by dullness, sternal
decubitus, often with the hind legs extended backward, mild
ruminal tympany and regurgitation of food through the nostrils, staring eyes, shallow respiration, coma and death within
6 to 36 hours.

Diagnosis: This is based on the history and clinical signs. In
outbreaks occurring before lambing, pregnancy toxemia offers
the main problem in differential diagnosis. A tentative diagnosis of acute hypocalcemia can readily be confirmed by a
dramatic and usually lasting response to calcium therapy.

Prophylaxis and Treatment: Treatment consists of IV or subcut. calcium therapy, preferably with some added magnesium
(R 584). Affected sheep should be handled with care lest sudden deaths occur from heart failure. Prevention is largely a
matter of avoiding the predisposing causes.

LACTATION TETANY OF MARES
(Transit tetany, Eclampsia)

A condition associated with hypocalcemia and sometimes
with alterations in blood magnesium levels, occurring most
often in mares about 10 days after foaling or 1 to 2 days after

weaning or in nursing mares on lush pasture, but occasionally in nonlactating horses, usually following some stress such as prolonged transport. Uncommon since the passing of the draft horse, it is characterized by incoordination, tetany, sweating, muscle tremors, rapid, violent respiration, and a thumping sound from within the chest, considered by many to be a spasmodic contraction of the diaphragm. While handling may exacerbate signs, affected horses are not hypersensitive to sound, and there is no prolapse of the third eyelid as in tetanus. The body temperature remains close to normal, and the appetite appears unimpaired but during an attack the animal is unable to eat, urinate or defecate. Mildly affected animals may recover spontaneously; severely affected ones go down in about 24 hours, develop tetanic convulsions and usually die within the next day.

Response to IV injections of calcium solutions (℞ 583) given very slowly is generally good. If associated with transport, it may be advisable to incorporate magnesium in the solution (℞ 584). Sedation is often indicated for excitable mares.

TRANSPORT TETANY OF RUMINANTS
(Railroad disease, Railroad sickness, Staggers)

A condition affecting well-fed cows and ewes in the advanced stages of pregnancy, during or immediately after long-continued transportation and stress.

The specific cause is unknown, but the condition is believed by some to be a form of acute hypocalcemia brought on by adverse conditions during shipping. Crowded, hot, poorly ventilated rail cars or trucks with no provision for feed or water seem to be contributing factors.

Clinical Findings: Evidence of the condition is more commonly observed at destination, but may develop while in transit. Early signs of restlessness and uncoordinated movements are followed by a partial paralysis of the hind legs and a staggering gait. Later, in a prone position, the animal assumes an attitude similar to that observed in parturient paresis. A pulse rate of 100 to 120 may be noted, while respiration is rapid and labored. The temperature may be elevated slightly and congestion of the mucous membranes commonly occurs. Extreme thirst may develop, while anorexia is regularly observed with a reduction or complete cessation of peristaltic and rumen activity. Abortion may occur as a complication.

Progressive paralysis, gradual loss of consciousness and death result unless suitable treatment is undertaken soon after onset.

Prophylaxis and Treatment: Animals in advanced pregnancy should be given only dry feed for a day or 2 preceding shipment. Loading should be accomplished with a minimum of excitement and overcrowded, poorly ventilated vehicles should be avoided. For transport involving long periods, suitable arrangements should be made to have the animals fed, watered and rested. Promazine hydrochloride or other suitable ataractics given IM ½ hour before loading are effective in alleviating the stress of transportation and may help to prevent the disease. For treatment, IV injections of calcium borogluconate (℞ 583), or calcium borogluconate with magnesium sulfate (℞ 584) given very slowly, preferably with 250 to 500 ml of 50% dextrose solution, followed by stimulants such as amphetamine (℞ 634) are recommended. Sedation is indicated in the presence of hyperexcitability.

ECLAMPSIA
(Puerperal tetany)

A disease of bitches and queens, occurring during late pregnancy, the puerperium or early lactation.

Etiology: The cause is unknown although hypoparathyroidism has been suggested. The signs are generally alleviated by the IV administration of calcium salts. The disease resembles, in some respects, milk fever in ruminants.

Clinical Findings: Early signs include anorexia and a stilted gait. The animal shows restlessness and an increased respiratory rate. It may fall and lie in a position of opisthotonos. Tonic and clonic convulsions occur with increasing violence. Consciousness is retained. The temperature usually is elevated, sometimes reaching 109°F. There is a resemblance to heat prostration, but the patient's sex, recent or impending parturition, and engorged mammae are important diagnostic aids.

Diagnosis: The signs usually occur in nursing animals with large litters, but occasionally are seen during the last 2 weeks of pregnancy. Plasma calcium falls from a normal level of 9 to 12 mg/100 ml to below 7 mg/100. The disease may be confused with tetanus; however, tetanus is gradual in onset, is characterized by tonic convulsions and does not respond to

IV calcium therapy. Strychnine poisoning and rabies may also offer a problem in differential diagnosis. Untreated cases of eclampsia usually die.

Treatment: The signs subside quickly following the IV injection of calcium gluconate (℞ 585). It is advisable to administer the solution IV to relieve the tetanic spasms and then to give an additional half-dose of a buffered solution by IM injection. Narcotics, such as meperidine (℞ 590) or small doses of pentobarbital (℞ 530) may be used to control the convulsions. Relapses requiring further treatment are not uncommon. Corticosteroids (℞ 152) are reported to prevent recurrence. Oral administration of calcium salts and vitamin D during pregnancy may prevent the occurrence of the condition. Adequate nutrition, with emphasis on the calcium content of the diet, should be ensured. Nursing should not be permitted during the acute stage. Weaning of the young should be considered. If this is not feasible then supplemental feeding of the young to reduce the stress on the mother may be combined with the administration of calcium, vitamin D and adequate nutrition to the mother.

GRASS TETANY IN CATTLE AND SHEEP
(Grass staggers)

A metabolic disturbance, characterized by hypomagnesemia, occurring most commonly in adult cows and ewes, especially those which are lactating heavily and are grazing on lush grass pastures. It also occurs in cattle of any age or condition, particularly beef cattle that are grazing on wheat or other cereal crops, or that are undernourished and exposed to changeable, cold weather. It is manifested by irritability, tetany and convulsions.

Etiology: Grass tetany may be considered to occur in 2 stages: first, the development of hypomagnesemia and second, a triggering of the clinical conditions. The rate of onset of hypomagnesemia depends upon the degree of deficiency; it is rapid in lactating cows allowed lush pasture after being housed over the winter and slow in undernourished beef cows. The low levels of magnesium and high levels of potassium and nitrogen in grass and wheat pastures combine to limit magnesium absorption. Excitement, act of milking, adverse weather and concurrent low blood levels of calcium are all possible trigger mechanisms.

Serum magnesium levels below 1.5 mg% should be regarded as suspicious and levels below 1.0 mg% as positive for hypomagnesemic tetany. Serum magnesium levels in affected animals may return to almost normal during the convulsive stage. Serum calcium levels are usually moderately depressed (5.0 to 8.0 mg%).

Clinical Findings: In the most acute form of the disease, affected cows, which may be grazing in an apparently normal manner, suddenly throw up their heads, bellow, gallop in a blind and frenzied manner, fall and undergo severe paddling convulsions. These convulsive episodes may be repeated at short intervals and death usually occurs within a few hours. In many instances, animals at pasture are found dead without illness having been observed. In less severe cases, the cow is obviously ill at ease, walks with a stiff gait, is hypersensitive to touch and sound, urinates frequently and may progress to the acute, convulsive stage after a period of as long as 2 to 3 days. Grass tetany may accompany parturient paresis and the classical signs of the latter disease are obscured by the tetanic convulsions. Similarly, it may accompany ketosis. In all cases of grass tetany, the loudness of the heart sounds and the rapidity of the heart rate are characteristic signs.

The disease in sheep occurs under essentially the same conditions and has the same clinical signs as the disease in cattle.

Prophylaxis: Prevention is largely a combination of increasing the intake of magnesium in danger periods and of management. Daily oral supplements (2 oz to cattle and ⅓ oz to sheep) can be incorporated in the concentrate feed or in licks containing molasses, but not in mineral blocks. Magnesium alloy "bullets" have been developed for cattle and sheep to give a slow release of magnesium in the rumen. Fertilization with magnesium limestone or magnesium oxide to increase herbage magnesium is successful only with certain soil types. Dusting of herbage with powdered magnesium oxide (110 lb/acre) gives good short-term prevention against grass tetany under suitable weather conditions.

Out-wintered stock should be protected from wind and cold and provided with supplementary food; grass-dominant pasture should not be fertilized with nitrogen; sheep and cattle should have access to hay or dry pasture.

Treatment: Affected animals require treatment urgently. Usually treatment includes administration of magnesium and calcium compounds and sometimes sedatives if the convulsions and tetany are severe. An IV injection containing both calcium and magnesium is used (℞ 584), but it must be given slowly and the effect on the heart beat watched carefully. A less risky alternative is to give the calcium IV and magnesium sulfate subcut. (℞ 563). Unless the animal is removed from the tetany-producing pasture, and fed hay and concentrate, the blood-magnesium level is likely to fall again to dangerously low levels 24 to 36 hours after therapy. To prevent this, follow-up treatment with magnesium by mouth should be started, giving 2 oz of magnesium oxide daily for at least a week, and then withdrawn gradually.

HYPOMAGNESEMIC TETANY OF CALVES

Tetany in calves, characterized by hypomagnesemia, and commonly hypocalcemia, is clinicaly identical with grass tetany in adult cattle. Because of its occurrence in 2- to 4-month-old calves on a sole milk diet, or in younger calves on milk replacer or with chronic scours, the disease is considered to be due to inadequate absorption of magnesium from the gut. The inadequacy may be due to a primary deficiency of magnesium in the diet or to rapid passage of the ingesta through the intestines. Affected calves require prompt treatment with a 10% solution of magnesium sulfate (100 ml subcut.) followed by the oral administration of 10 to 15 gm magnesium oxide daily. This level of oral dosing with magnesium oxide is also effective as prophylaxis.

PREGNANCY TOXEMIA IN EWES

(Pregnancy disease, Lambing paralysis,
Twin-lamb disease, Ketosis)

A disease of preparturient ewes, primarily characterized clinically by impaired nervous function.

Etiology: The primary predisposing cause is undernutrition in late pregnancy, with over-fat ewes carrying twins or triplets being more susceptible than ewes in poor condition and those carrying single lambs. Stresses, such as storms, change of environment, transport, short periods of fasting, and excessive heat, also play a role when coupled with undernutrition.

The early clinical signs suggest a hypoglycemic encephalopathy, and the evidence indicates this to be the primary lesion. The hypoglycemia is due to an inability of the fasted or underfed ewe to supply sufficient glucose from products of digestion or catabolized tissues to meet the carbohydrate demands of large multiple fetuses and the ewe. The defect appears to be in maintenance of the blood glucose level since utilization of available glucose is unimpaired. As the disease progresses, severe ketosis and acidosis may develop, together with hepatic, renal and possibly endocrine disorders. The blood sugar may rise without alleviating the signs of encephalopathy. At this stage the ewe is refractory to treatment. Irreversible encephalopathy, probably similar to that in this disease, can be readily produced by insulin hypoglycemia.

Clinical Findings: Early clinical signs may be erratic and difficult to detect. The usual course, lasting 2 to 5 days, comprises listlessness, inappetence, aimless walking, "propping" against any kind of obstruction, twitching of the muscles of the ears, around the eyes and perhaps of other parts, unusual postures, grinding of the teeth, progressive loss of reflexes, blindness, ataxia and finally sternal decubitus, coma and death.

Laboratory tests usually reveal hypoglycemia early, with normoglycemia or hyperglycemia later, and hyperketonemia. Acidosis (low plasma CO_2-combining power) and high blood nonprotein nitrogen are variable concomitants. Necropsy findings include fatty livers, indistinguishable from those found sometimes in apparently healthy ewes underfed near term. The adrenal glands may be swollen, hyperemic or grayish. The pulmonary changes are associated with recumbency.

Differential Diagnosis: Acute hypocalcemia (parturient paresis or milk fever) before lambing offers the main problem in differential diagnosis. In this, the course is shorter (deaths occur within 24 hours), and there is usually a marked, immediate and persistent response to IV calcium therapy.

Prophylaxis: Flock management should aim to prevent obesity in early pregnancy and to provide adequate supplies of good feed during the last 6 weeks of pregnancy. Feed supplementation depends on the condition of the pastures and the weight of the ewes. Where the pastures become very poor, heavy feeding may be necessary to prevent losses. If adequate and suitable feed is not available for the whole flock during late pregnancy, the more susceptible ewes can be identified by gentle driving. They can be separated from the flock and given special care and nourishment. In susceptible flocks, stresses due to adverse environmental conditions changing the environment should, if possible, be avoided.

Treatment: Once the advanced signs have developed, no treatment has been shown to improve the ewe's chances of survival. The mortality rate of untreated cases is about 80%. With early diagnosis, such as may be made by gentle driving of the flock, particularly where the disease has been induced by relatively sudden fasting, the glucogenic materials, glycerol or propylene glycol, given orally (4 oz twice daily) decrease the mortality. Glucose therapy does not reduce the mortality because of the short-lived effect on blood glucose. Insulin is contraindicated. ACTH and glucocorticoids are probably only effective through increasing blood sugar. Removal of the young by cesarean section early in the course of the disease usually leads to recovery and, provided the ewe is near term, the offspring may be saved. Good husbandry procedures, such as protection from excessive heat and cold and the provision of palatable feed and water, should also be observed. Twice daily force-feeding with finely ground dried grass given by stomach tube may be a worthwhile practice with specially valuable animals, treatment being continued until the appetite returns.

ACUTE HYPOGLYCEMIA
IN NEWBORN PIGS

A sudden fall in the level of blood glucose (below 50 mg%) in newborn pigs, occurring commonly under natural conditions. Since gluconeogenesis is not well developed during the first few days of postnatal existence, a dietary source of readily available carbohydrate is essential.

Death losses in pigs are often high during the first few days of life. Since the cause of death, in many instances, remains obscure, these losses are often ascribed to such ill-defined entities as "baby pig disease" or "3-day pig disease". It is certain that acute hypoglycemia accounts for a significant proportion, but not all, of these early losses.

Acute hypoglycemia may be caused by anything that prevents intake or assimilation of suitable food during the first few days of life, including any other disease. The most common causes are agalactia or dysgalactia in the sow. Congenital weakness or too-large litters may be contributing causes; exposure aggravates the condition, hastening its development and shortening its course.

Signs include shivering, pilo-erection, a characteristic squeal, weakness, hypothermia, deviation of the eyeballs, torticollis, running movements and coma. Without treatment, death usually occurs in 24 to 36 hours.

Treatment involves providing a warm environment, supplemental feeding and, if signs are well developed, IP injection of 10 to 15 ml of 5% glucose solution given every 4 to 6 hours. Evaporated milk diluted with one-half volume of water is a generally satisfactory supplement. Treatment is of little value after nervous signs have become prominent.

Preventive measures include the selection of breeding stock of docile temperament as well as high lactational ability and the provision of supplemental heat for pigs farrowed during the cooler seasons.

OBESITY

A condition due to increased intake of food, possibly accompanied by a metabolic disorder in which excess fat is stored in the body. The deposition of fat may be general or local.

Etiology: Obesity results when caloric intake exceeds the energy requirements. It is due primarily to excessive ingestion of food and lack of exercise. It may be further complicated by hypometabolism, or incapacity to mobilize fat stores. Lesions of the hypothalamus may cause a voracious appetite and the resulting obesity is accentuated by a low metabolic rate and reduced activity. Free-choice diet in such cases results in polyphagia. Animals usually gain from 2 to 3 times their normal body weight before equilibrium is reached. If lesions are present in both the pituitary and hypothalamus, the pathologic appetite cannot be controlled.

Hypopituitarism (dystrophia adiposogenitalis) is occasionally seen in dogs. There is an accumulation of subcut. fat and a depression of sexual function in these animals. Endocrine disorders primarily determine the distribution of fat in the body. Obesity may develop either in the presence or absence of secretions from one or more of pituitary, gonads, thyroid, adrenal and islet cells. It is believed that mobilization of fat stores may be inadequate, leading to hypoglycemia, which causes increased appetite. Castrated animals may tend toward obesity; whether it is due to imbalance or because the castrate is phlegmatic, is undetermined.

Inheritance is a factor in fat utilization and storage as exemplified by lard-type and bacon-type hogs and beef-type or dairy-type cattle.

Clinical Findings: The most obvious sign is the increased subcut. fat. There may be dyspnea after exertion and ease of fatigability. Affected animals show intolerance to heat and may manifest digestive disturbances and skin disorders. Heart, liver, kidney, or pancreatic disorders may result and produce secondary signs.

Treatment: Exercise should be increased gradually as the heart may already be taxed beyond capacity. The caloric intake should be reduced to a point below the animal's normal requirement. A high-protein, low-carbohydrate and low-fat diet is generally effective. Animals are best fed 3 times daily. Commercially prepared diets are available for the control of caloric intake while maintaining a balanced diet. Rapid results should not be expected.

Where the condition is associated with hypothyroidism, treatment with thyroid extract (℞ 180) gives gratifying results. Thyroid extract will increase the basal metabolic rate in hypothyroidism. Metabolic stimulants such as amphetamine sulfate (℞ 634) are useful where there is a low metabolic rate. This drug increases the physical activity of the animal without elevating the basal metabolic rate and is an appetite depressant.

Where the condition is due to hypogonadism, as in castrated animals, treatment with the appropriate hormone may be helpful (℞ 163, 179). Pituitary or hypothalamic disorders are not responsive to currently available medicaments.

HIGH-MOUNTAIN DISEASE

(Brisket disease,
Pulmonary hypertensive heart disease)

A noninfectious disease of cattle characterized by the clinical signs and lesions of congestive right heart failure. It affects animals residing in the mountainous altitudes (usually above 7,000 ft) of the Western U.S.A. and South America and has been observed in certain other mountainous areas of the world. The syndrome is specific for cattle. The possibility of it occurring in certain other ruminants (sheep and deer) under extreme stress cannot be excluded. A similar disease is of clinical importance in chickens in the Andes Mountains. The incidence of the disease in any one herd ranges from 0 to 5%, but is usually less than 2%. Occurrence is related to, but not exclusively dependent upon, the resident altitude. Newly introduced cattle reportedly have a greater incidence than native stock in some geographic regions. The disease occurs primarily during the fall, with a reduced incidence in winter and still less in spring months, and affects all age, breed and sex groups—but not necessarily equally. Variations occur geographically, seasonally and with breed, sex and age.

Etiology: The disease is unequivocally related to the chronic hypoxia of a high altitude environment, which causes pulmonary hypertension. The necessity of some other inciting or causative factor or factors is a moot point. Right ventricular hypertrophy and moderate to severe pulmonary hypertension have been shown to develop in cattle kept at high altitude under controlled conditions. Marked variation in individual susceptibility occurs, with a strong indication that this susceptibility is inherited. The pathway by which the pulmonary hypertension proceeds to congestive right heart failure varies. In some animals it appears related to individual susceptibility and permanent pulmonary vascular damage, while in others it is associated with increased circulatory stress—pneumonia, lungworm infection, inclement weather, chronic pulmonary lesions, ruptured diaphragm, etc.—superimposed upon the already partially compromised pulmonary circulation.

Clinical Findings: The disease usually develops slowly. The affected animal is first noted to be depressed and to remain apart from the herd. As the syndrome progresses, subcut. edema develops in the ventral pectoral (brisket) region and may extend anteriorly to the intermandibular space and posteriorly along the ventral abdominal wall. Ascites and marked distension and pulsation of the jugular vein are usually present, and diarrhea may develop. Respiration is labored and the animals may appear cyanotic. They are reluctant to move, may become recumbent and upon forced exertion may collapse and die. Denudation of muzzle epithelium may or may not be observed, depending upon stage of the disease and age of the afflicted animal.

Lesions: Generalized anasarca is usually present, with edema of the subcutis, skeletal musculature, perirenal tissues, mesentery and alimentary tract wall. Ascites, hydrothorax and hydropericardium are present. The liver lesions, due to chronic passive congestion, vary from an early "nutmeg" appearance to severe central lobular fibrosis. The lungs show varying degrees of atelectasis, interstitial emphysema and, in some cases, pneumonia. Marked right ventricular hypertrophy and dilatation of the heart are present. Displacement of the cardiac apex to the left gives the heart an enlarged rounded contour. Occasionally the large pulmonary arteries contain recently formed thrombi. Microscopically, hypertrophy of the media may be observed in the small pulmonary arteries. This disease must be differentiated from other diseases causing congestive right heart failure in cattle, such as traumatic pericarditis, chronic pneumonia, congenital anomalies and primary myocardial lesions.

Treatment: It is essential that affected animals be moved to a lower altitude with minimal restraint, stress and excitement, where some will recover spontaneously. General supportive therapy, including antibiotics to combat pneumonia, should be administered. Digitalis and diuretic (℞ 508, 514, 519, 521) therapy has proven of benefit. Reduction of pulmonary arterial pressure at high altitude can be accomplished by the admininstration of oxygen and may be of value in the treatment of valuable animals. Since the disease may recur, recovered animals should not be returned to high altitudes. Since an inherited susceptibility is suspected, afflicted cattle should not be retained for breeding.

POSTPARTURIENT HEMOGLOBINURIA

Primarily a disease of high-producing dairy cows which occurs 2 to 4 weeks after parturition. It is characterized by intravascular hemolysis, hemoglobinuria and anemia.

Etiology: The cause is unknown. The disease is rare in beef animals or animals under 3 years of age, and is uncommon more than 4 weeks after parturition. The incidence is generally low but up to 50% of affected animals may die. Diets high in cruciferous plants (such as rape or kale) or beet pulp and prolonged feeding on phosphorus-deficient diets are said to be predisposing factors. In North America the disease may occur after prolonged stabling. The hemoglobinuria is believed to be associated with hypophosphatemia since serum phosphorus levels are always subnormal (0.8 to 1.4 mg%) in acutely ill cows.

Clinical Findings: Rapid intravascular hemolysis leads to hemoglobinuria, icterus and profound anemia. Dehydration, weakness and a marked drop in milk yield are prominent signs. The temperature may be elevated to 103°F. Some respiratory distress may be seen. Intravascular hemolysis continues for 3 to 5 days and, in cows which recover, the return to normal is slow.

Treatment: Transfusion of large quantities of whole blood may be the only effective treatment of severely affected animals. In less severe cases, 2 oz of sodium acid phosphate in 300 ml of distilled water may be administered IV followed by subcut. injections at 12-hour intervals or by daily oral doses of the same amount of phosphate. If injected, sodium acid phosphate should be well distributed in the subcutis to avoid tissue necrosis. Bone meal should be added to the ration. Hematinics (℞ 500, 502) may be beneficial.

MUSCULOSKELETAL SYSTEM

LAMENESS IN HORSES

Lameness may be defined as a departure from the normal stance or gait, occasioned by disease or injury. At least 90% of the cases of lameness are due to pain. The remainder comprise those in which anatomic changes produce what is called "mechanical lameness". Lameness must be differentiated from defective gait caused by faulty conformation and stiffness due to age or fatigue; stiffness usually passes off with exercise. Lameness is not a disease, but a sign of disease, pain, impediment, deformity, or weakness.

Terms such as shoulder lameness, hip lameness and hock lameness are often used to describe so-called regional lamenesses. It should be noted, however, that these regional lamenesses do not specifically indicate the structure involved. In shoulder lameness for instance, the term does not indicate whether the causal lesion is in the scapulohumeral joint, tendon of the biceps, the bicipital bursa, or any of the muscles in that region. A horse's action does not denote the precise region involved, although it may give an indication or clue as to the approximate seat of the trouble.

Etiology: The causes of lameness may be classified as (a) predisposing and (b) exciting. Under predisposing causes may be mentioned immaturity or poor condition, faulty conformation, systemic disease, bad shoeing and lack of attention to the feet. Under exciting causes may be listed trauma, either direct or indirect; incoordination of muscle action, as may occur in tired animals; and bacterial infection, especially of tendon sheaths and joints.

Diagnosis: The history may be valuable if it is objective and complete. Lameness may be evident (a) during rest, (b) during progression and (c) on passive movement, manual examination and testing with hoof testers or hammer.

During rest: Pointing of a forelimb may be evident. No significance is attached to the pointing of a hind leg. A horse may "nurse" or favor a leg by holding it off or just in contact with the ground. The attitude or position adopted by the lame leg may give an indication of the cause. In upward fixation (subluxation) of the patella, the affected leg is rigidly extended backward with the wall of the toe resting on the ground. Abnormal mobility of part of a limb, even while standing, may indicate a ruptured tendon or fractured bone. Adduction or abduction of a leg also may be noted.

During progression: Following the visual examination, the horse should be trotted at once and not walked beforehand, since it may "warm out" of a mild lameness. Most lamenesses are best manifested at the slow trot on hard even ground. Splint lameness, however, shows up better at a fast trot. It is important that the handler lead the horse with enough slack to permit head movement. A horse lame in the foreleg raises its head when the lame limb bears weight and nods or drops the head when the sound leg is in support. In a very slight lameness, the raising of the head is not as evident as the nodding or dropping of the head; hence, the latter probably is more important.

Provided the horse is unshod or shod all around, the sound made by each hoof as it strikes the ground may give an indication as to the lame leg.

If a horse is lame in both front legs and the causes are the same (e.g., navicular disease) or of equal severity, head nod is not apparent. Careful examination will reveal, however, that although the horse seems to be "going even" in front, the gait is "pottery" or stilted and the stride of both legs is shorter than normal. If, however, the lameness in both front legs is of unequal severity, the head nod will be present as in unilateral lameness. When such a case is presented, the less lame leg is very likely to be overlooked unless careful attention is paid to its action. In addition, if the leg with obvious lameness is subjected to nerve blocking in order to desensitize the painful area, that leg may appear sound and the head movement indicate that the other leg also is lame. In suspected hind-limb lameness, attention should be directed to the movements of the croup or quarter. The croup on the affected side generally is raised when the lame leg is in support, the degree of elevation of the croup varying with the seat of lameness. When both hind legs are lame, both legs move stiffly and often the owner believes that the trouble is in the lumbar region. In severe cases, the animal may even appear to crouch. Backing in such cases is accomplished with difficulty.

As the horse is moved toward or away from the examiner, it should be noted whether the legs are carried in a straight line or are adducted, abducted or circumducted while in motion. Attention also should be directed to the body axis to determine whether or not the axis is in the same line as the direction of movement. Trotting the horse along the foot of a hill may give an indication as to the lame limb because of its effect on collateral ligaments.

The action of the horse then should be viewed from the side. By this means, variations in the length of stride and diminished flexion of joints are more readily observed.

Some types of lameness in the foot, e.g., fracture of the wing of the os pedis, are best seen when the patient is trotted or turned in a small circle. Finally, the horse should be backed in order to ascertain if any disability is present which might hinder the action of backing.

When the lame leg is evident, attention should be concentrated upon it and the following points noted: degree of flexion of the joints, length of stride, adduction or abduction of the limb, placement of the foot, and the height to which the hocks are carried.

Manual examination is carried out to determine the exact site of lameness and should be done in a systematic manner so that every part of the leg will be scrutinized. This may include removal of the shoe.

Historically, most cases of forelimb lameness involved the foot, while the hock was the most frequently affected region of the hind leg, but in view of the present-day predominance of the light horse, most cases of forelimb lameness are to be found "from the fetlock downward". In Thoroughbreds in training, however, the carpus is frequently involved.

During examination of the lame limb, frequent comparison should be made between it and the unaffected leg. All identifiable structures should be gently but thoroughly palpated, with the foot both on the ground and raised. The presence of heat in a part should be noted.

If the cause of lameness is thought to be in the foot, the shoe should be removed and the hoof thoroughly cleaned and tested for soundness of both wall and sole with a light hammer, and by application of the hoof tester. Excessive wear of the toe or quarter of the shoe may afford a clue as to the cause of the lameness. The foot should always be examined closely when the lameness seems to be below the olecranon or the stifle joint.

Passive movement of a supposedly affected joint is most useful in the forelimb for detecting limitations of flexion in the carpus and fetlock. It should, however, always be interpreted in the light of the normal range of movement of the limb, especially in older horses. This test should also be carried out on the contralateral leg.

With regard to hind-limb lameness, especially when the lameness appears to be in the hip region, a rectal examination should be carried out. Since the stifle and hock joints move at the same time, pain in the stifle may give rise to limitation of hock movement and vice versa.

The additional weight of a rider on the horse's back often accentuates lameness, but this advantage often is lost to the examiner on account of the pull of the bit on the horse's mouth interfering with the movements of the head.

If, after the above examination procedure has been carried out, a diagnosis has not been made, the horse should be ridden, lunged, or driven for an hour or so, rested for approximately half an hour and reexamined.

Blocking of the nerves to a suspected area is another aid to diagnosis. If, after anesthetizing the nerve supply to the area in question, the horse goes sound, then it may be concluded that the seat of lameness is supplied by the anesthetized nerve. A volar nerve block offers the best confirmatory evidence of foot lameness. Too much reliance should not be placed on the posterior digital nerve block, either unilateral or bilateral, since anastomotic branches of the nerves concerned may create a false interpretation of the results.

Very often, radiography permits the only reliable method of confirming or denying the physical findings, and offers a more realistic prognosis than is possible by clinical examination alone.

CURB

A thickening or "bowing" of the plantar tarsal ligament due to strain.

Etiology: Inflammation and thickening may occur after falling, slipping, jumping or pulling. Poor conformation of the hock is a likely predisposing factor in bilateral cases.

Clinical Findings: There is an enlargement over the posterior surface of the fibular tarsal bone which is easily seen when observing the animal from the side. A curb which has recently and suddenly formed is characterized by acute inflammation and lameness. The horse stands with the leg at rest and the heel elevated.

Treatment: If the condition is due to acute inflammation, cold packs and rest are indicated. When cooled out, the area over the enlarged ligament may be point-fired. Rest is essential.

OSSLETS
(Osselets)

An inflammation of the periosteum on the lower anterior epiphyseal surface of the large metacarpal bone and the associated capsule of the fetlock joint. The proximal end of the first phalanx is involved later. Hence, this condition constitutes a form of arthritis which may progress from the serous to the ankylosing type.

Etiology: The exciting cause is the strain and repeated trauma of hard training in young animals.

Clinical Findings and Diagnosis: The affected horse moves with a short, choppy gait. Palpation and flexion of the fetlock joint produces pain, and examination reveals a soft, warm, sensitive swelling over the front and sometimes the side of the fetlock joint. Radiography in the initial stages may show no evidence of new bone formation in which case the condition is called "green osslets". Later, demineralization of the bone in the area of the distal epiphysis of the large metacarpal bone and the attachment of the fetlock joint capsule to the first phalanx may be seen. This is succeeded by progressive new bone formation or "calcium proliferation" some of which may break off and appear as "joint mice".

Treatment: Rest is very important. The inflammation may be relieved by the application of cold packs over a period of several days. Systemic, anti-inflammatory agents such as phenylbutazone may also be employed. After the acute inflammation has subsided, many Thoroughbred trainers still request the area be point-fired or blistered or both, after which the animal should be rested for 6 months. Some prefer the intra-articular injection of a corticosteroid, however, this and other forms of anti-inflammatory medication, if used along with continued training or racing lead inevitably to destruction of the joint surfaces.

SORE SHINS
(Bucked shins)

A periostitis of the anterior surface of the large metacarpal or metatarsal bone. The condition is most often seen in the fore-legs of young Thoroughbreds in training and racing.

Etiology: This condition is generally brought about by con-cussion (driving, training and racing) in young Thoroughbreds. Recently, radiographic evidence has shown that in some cases there is cortical infraction of the cannon bone, constituting a stress fracture ("saucer fracture"). In milder cases, the con-dition is associated only with stretching or tearing of the overlying periosteum. Trauma of the periosteum from other causes may be involved.

Clinical Findings and Diagnosis: There is a warm, painful swelling on the anterior surface of the large metacarpal or, less frequently, the metatarsal bone. The horse is lame, the stride is short, and the severity of the lameness increases with exercise.

Treatment: The affected horse must be removed from training. The acute inflammation may be relieved by application of cold packs. Rest is necessary until all soreness and inflamma-tion have disappeared. It is common practice with race horses to apply counterirritants or point-fire the area, which enforces several months' rest. If the condition is one of cortical infrac-tion, counterirritation is contraindicated.

CARPITIS
(Sore knee, Popped knee)

An acute or chronic inflammation of the joint capsule and associated structures of the carpus. Exostoses may be present in old cases. The acute form is common in Thoroughbreds in training.

Etiology: The acute form of the disease usually is attributed to concussion from hard training, especially in horses still some-what "soft". Injury to the knee, especially in hunters and jumpers, is a common cause. Some exostoses may be the re-

sult of undetected slab or avulsion fractures of the small
carpal bones (see below). The inflammation occasionally
appears, however, without any obvious signs or history of a
causative agent. Poor conformation may play a part.

Clinical Findings and Diagnosis: Lameness usually is evident
at once. Swelling is always present in acute cases and may
consist of distension of the joint capsule and related synovial
structures or be a true soft-tissue swelling. The chronic case
may show well-developed exostoses. The diagnosis usually is
simple; however, it is necessary to keep in mind the possibility
of fracture of the carpal bones. This, as well as the presence
of exostoses, can best be determined by radiologic examination.

Treatment: Rest is the best treatment and, when sufficient
rest can be given, the prognosis for acute cases is good. Pain
may be relieved by aspiration of excess fluid from the joint
and the intra-articular injection of a corticosteroid, but adequate rest is still mandatory. This procedure may be repeated
after 4 or 5 days if necessary. Blisters (℞ 625) often are used
and occasionally chronic cases are fired. The chief benefits from
these latter procedures probably are gained in the subsequent
compulsory rest given the horse. The presence of degenerative
bony changes in the carpus immediately predicates an unfavorable prognosis. Temporary relief may be obtained in some instances by the use of a corticosteroid or phenylbutazone (℞
150), but knees so affected never are wholly sound again. Anti-
inflammatory treatment combined with continued training and
racing will accelerate the degenerative process within the knee.

ARTICULAR FRACTURES OF THE CARPAL
BONES, PROXIMAL SESAMOIDS
AND FIRST PHALANX

Until radiographic examination became common, "popped
knees", sesamoiditis, and involvement of the proximal end of
the first phalanx were often incompletely or incorrectly diagnosed. These productive exostotic lesions frequently begin
as fractures of an avulsion, shear, or chip type.

Most fractures of the carpal bones are caused by "shear"
stresses; they usually occur towards the end of a race when the
possibility of the joint going into maximum overextension is
greatest. Most occur in the anterior aspect of the carpal joint,
especially involving the radial and third carpal bones. Only
the latter is commonly affected with the shear fracture re-

ferred to as a slab fracture. Chip fractures of the proximal end of the first phalanx are quite common, and must be differentiated from other injuries of the fetlock joint.

Fractures of the proximal sesamoid bones also follow fatigue with coexistent overextension. The lateral proximal sesamoid in the hind leg in the Standardbred may be fractured as a result of torque forces induced by shoeing with a trailer-type shoe. The fractures may be apical, basal, multiple, and may involve one or both of the sesamoids.

Clinical Findings and Diagnosis: Articular fractures often occur towards the end of a race. Chip fractures may produce no signs until the animal is cooling out, when swelling of the fetlock or carpus with accompanying lameness may be noticed. Slab or compression fractures of the carpal bones and severe fractures involving the proximal sesamoids usually result in immediate swelling and severe supporting lameness. It may be difficult to clinically differentiate between a fracture of the proximal sesamoids and rupture or severe strain of the flexor tendons or the suspensory ligament.

If the fracture is incomplete or if the fragment is small, the animal may be walking relatively soundly in 7 to 10 days following simple anti-inflammatory measures such as rest and cold applications to the part. Intra-articular injection of steroids and administration of phenylbutazone also relieve the inflammatory signs. However, lameness will recur with any strenuous work.

A diagnostic set of radiographs entails the exposure of 5 plates in the case of the carpus, and 4 for the fetlock. Anteroposterior, mediolateral, obliques of both the medial and lateral aspects, and mediolateral flexon views are necessary to insure that the fracture line is not missed. The flexion view may be omitted for the fetlock.

Treatment: The combination of intra-articular or systemic anti-inflammatory treatment and continued work usually leads to degenerative changes within the joint. Surgery often is the treatment of choice. The 3 contraindications applying to all surgical interventions into joints are: 1) the chip is very small and does not involve the articular surfaces, 2) there is radiographic evidence of coexistence of degenerative osteoarthropathy, 3) a corticosteroid has been injected into the joint within 8 weeks prior to the date of surgery.

Fractures of the proximal sesamoids may be treated conservatively by allowing stall rest for an extended period (6 to 12 months) to permit fibrous union. In some instances, severing the branch of the suspensory ligament proximal to the sesamoid followed by an extended period of rest is indicated.

BOG SPAVIN
(Articular thoroughpin, Tarsal hydrarthrosis)

A chronic synovitis of the tibiotarsal joint characterized by distension of the joint capsule.

Etiology: Faulty conformation may lead to hock joint weakness and increase production of synovia, especially in the bilateral case. The unilateral case is more likely to be a sequela to a more acute cause such as a sprain.

Clinical Findings and Diagnosis: The affected horse usually is not lame unless the condition is complicated by bone involvement. Distension of the joint capsule occurs in 3 places. The largest swelling is on the anterior medial surface of the hock, while a smaller swelling occurs on each side of the proximal posterior aspect. Bog spavin, unless complicated by bony changes, rarely interferes with the usefulness of the animal, but does constitute an unsightly blemish. Spontaneous appearance and disappearance may occur in weanlings and yearlings.

Treatment: The excess fluid within the joint capsule may be aspirated and replaced with 5 ml of one of the corticosteroids developed for intraarticular injection, and the procedure repeated at weekly intervals for 3 weeks. Other treatments such as blistering sometimes meet with success. The condition has a tendency to recur, especially if poor conformation is a contributary cause.

BONE SPAVIN

Spavin is usually described as a periostitis or rarefying osteitis involving the bones of the hock joint, usually the distal row of tarsal bones on the medial side, and subsequently resulting in exostosis and terminal ankylosis. However, some refer to the condition as a chronic, local periarthritis, medial to the gliding articulation of the hock.

Etiology: Among the theories advanced to explain the condition are faulty hock conformation, excessive concussion and mineral imbalance.

Clinical Findings and Diagnosis: The horse tends to drag the toe. The forward flight of the toe is shortened and hock action is decreased. The heel becomes high. The exostosis often is visible on the lower medial aspect of the hock. When standing, the horse may rest the toe on the ground with the heel slightly raised. The lameness quite often disappears with exercise and returns after the horse has been rested. In so-called occult spavin, there is no visible exostosis and the lameness sometimes is continuous as the bone lesion is within the articular surface. The spavin test may be a useful aid to diagnosis: the leg is picked up and held with the hock, but not the fetlock, acutely flexed for a few minutes; the lameness will be accentuated for the first few steps immediately after release of the leg. This test, less dependable in older horses, should also be carried out on the other leg. Lameness from a gonitis also is accentuated by the "spavin test".

Treatment: The horse should be rested. Point-firing may be performed to hasten ankylosis of the affected bones, but this result is not always achieved. More recently, arthrodesis has been achieved by using a surgical drill and bit. Corrective shoeing consists of raising the heel and rolling the toes. If the exostosis lies under the cunean tendon, tenotomy of this structure may give relief. Wamberg's peripheral neurectomy has also been employed.

SPLINTS

This condition involves primarily the interosseous ligament between the large and small metacarpal (less frequently the metatarsal bones). This reaction is a periostitis with production of new bone (exostoses) along the involved splint bone.

Etiology: Trauma from concussion or injury, bone disease associated with mineral imbalance, strain from excessive training, especially in the immature horse, faulty conformation, or improper shoeing may contribute to the development of this condition.

Clinical Findings and Diagnosis: Splints most commonly involve the medial rudimentary metacarpal and, occasionally, the small metatarsal bones. Lameness is observed only when splints are forming and seen most frequently in young horses. Lameness is more pronounced after the animal has been worked. In the early stages, there is no visible enlargement, but deep palpation may reveal local painful subperiosteal swelling. In the later stages, a calcified growth appears. Following ossification, lameness disappears, except in occasional cases where the growth encroaches on the suspensory ligament, flexor tendons or carpal articulation.

Radiography is warranted in many cases to differentiate splints from fractured splint bones.

Treatment: Complete rest is indicated. In Thoroughbred practice, it is traditional to point-fire a splint, the aim being to accelerate the ossification of the interosseous ligament. However, should radiographic examination disclose a fracture, irritant treatments are contraindicated. Surgical removal of the distal segment is then the treatment of choice. In the case of impingement exostosis against the suspensory ligament, removal of the encroaching exostosis is sometimes carried out. The local use of steroids will delay the consolidation process and is therefore contraindicated.

FRACTURES OF THE SMALL METACARPAL AND METATARSAL (SPLINT) BONES

Fractures of the second and fourth metacarpal and metatarsal (splint) bones are not uncommon. The cause may be from direct trauma as from interference by the contralateral leg, but more often follows prior suspensory desmitis with its resulting fibrous-tissue build-up and encapsulation of the distal, free end of the bone. The usual site of the fracture is through the distal end approximately 2 in. from the tip. Immediately after the fracture occurs, signs of acute inflammation are present at the site. The suspensory ligament usually is involved in the inflammatory process. A supporting lameness is noted; this may recede after several days rest and recur only after working.

Chronic, long-standing fractures cause a supporting lameness at speed, particularly at the trot. Thickening of the suspensory ligament at and above the site results. The fracture usually shows little tendency to heal, instead a false joint forms, often with a considerable build-up of callus at each end of the fracture.

Diagnosis is confirmed by means of an oblique radiograph setting out the bone involved. Surgical removal of the fractured tip and of the callus is the treatment of choice.

TROCHANTERIC BURSITIS

("Whirlbone" lameness)

An inflammation of the tendon of the middle gluteal muscle, of the bursa between this tendon and the trochanter major, or of the cartilage of the trochanter major.

Etiology: This condition is encountered most commonly in Standardbreds and, in some cases, is concurrent with a pre-existing spavin.

Clinical Findings and Diagnosis: The weight is placed on the inside of the foot so that the inside wall of the foot is worn more than the outside wall. The stride of the affected leg is shorter and the leg is rotated inward. The horse tends to carry the hindquarters toward the sound side. In long-standing cases, the muscles between the external and internal angles of the ilium are atrophied, giving a flat appearance to the croup. Pressure over the greater trochanter gives evidence of pain.

Treatment: If the inflammation is acute, the animal should be rested and hot packs applied over the affected area. Injection of an intra-articular corticosteroid into the bursa will relieve the inflammation. In chronic cases, the injection of Lugol's solution (℞ 576) into or around the bursa gives good results.

BICIPITAL BURSITIS

An inflammation of the intertubal or bicipital bursa between the tendon of the biceps and the bicipital groove of the humerus. The usual cause is trauma to the point of the shoulder. Pyosepticemia ("navel ill") or other systemic bacterial infections may occasionally result in a chronic involvement of the bursa.

Essentially the condition produces a swinging-leg lameness, the forward phase of flight being shortened. The animal may stumble due to the toe not being lifted sufficiently to clear the ground. In severe cases, a supporting leg lamness may also be present. Forced extension of the leg usually causes a pain reaction, particularly if the tendon is also involved. Deep digital pressure over the bursa and the tendon of the biceps may elicit a pain response. Radiographs may be of aid if the bursa can be outlined.

Rest is indicated, particularly in acute cases. Intrabursal injection of a steroid (℞ 155, 159) at weekly intervals for 3 or 4 injections may be successful. Phenylbutazone (℞ 150) and administration of oral steroids (℞ 144) are useful. Injection of a counterirritant (℞ 575) around the bursa is often used in chronic cases.

ARTHRITIS OF THE SHOULDER JOINT

An inflammation of the structures of the joint itself. These may consist of changes in the joint capsule, or more frequently, bony changes of the articular surfaces of the humerus or scapula. Occasionally, fractures involving the articular surfaces are present.

Trauma to the point of the shoulder is the usual cause. Bacterial infection of the joint from puncture wounds or of hematogenous origin (pyosepticemia) may be the cause of a purulent arthritis.

A swinging- and supporting-leg lameness is present in severe cases. In milder cases, only the swinging-leg lameness may be noted. The forward phase of flight is shortened. The toe may be worn. The leg often is circumducted to avoid flexion of the joint. Forced extension of the leg, pulling the shoulder forward, often causes pain. Crepitation may be noted if fractures of the humerus or scapula are present. Radiographs of the shoulder joint may demonstrate the arthritic changes.

Treatment often is ineffective due to severe arthritic changes. Intra-articular injections of steroid (℞ 155, 159) at weekly intervals may be of some benefit. Systemic steroids (℞ 144) and phenylbutazone (℞ 150) may relieve signs of pain in some animals. Injection of a counterirritant (℞ 575) is often used, but rarely is beneficial.

COXITIS

Inflammation of the coxofemoral articulation. Most cases are traumatic in origin, occurring secondarily to tearing the rim of the acetabulum, fractures through the acetabulum, or injury to the articular surfaces. Localization of a systemic infection, particularly pyosepticemia in young animals, is not an uncommon cause.

Both a supporting- and swinging-leg lameness is noted. In severe cases the leg may be carried. In less severe cases the gait is rolling, the affected quarter being elevated as weight is born on the leg. The leg is advanced in a semicircular manner with the forward phase of the stride shortened. The toe may be worn from dragging. The animal often stands with the leg partially flexed, the stifle turned out, and the point of the hock turned inwardly. Atrophy of the heavy muscles of the quarter occurs in cases of long duration. Rectal palpation often reveals an enlargement over the acetabulum, particularly if a fracture through it has occurred. Radiographs of the joint may confirm the diagnosis.

The prognosis is generally poor. Rest is indicated in acute cases. Elevating the heel may be of some benefit. Intra-articular injections of a steroid (℞ 155, 159) may relieve the lameness temporarily in milder cases. Phenylbutazone (℞

593) or systemic use of steroids (R 144, 145, 154) is often useful.

GONITIS

An inflammation of the stifle joint. The joint is complex, and the condition may be precipitated by multiple causes: persistent upward fixation of the patella, injuries to the medial or lateral collateral ligaments of the joint, injuries to the cruciate ligaments of the menisci, erosions of the articular cartilage, and bacterial infection of the joint from puncture wounds or of hematogenous origin (pyosepticemia).

The severity of signs is remarkably variable, depending upon the cause and the extent of the pathologic changes. Usually the joint capsule is distended, pouching out between the distal patellar ligaments. Occasionally, the femoropatellar capsule is distended, the enlargement then being noted just below the patella.

A swinging-leg lameness is noted in all cases, the forward phase of flight being shortened. At rest the leg often is turned out from the stifle downward and the fetlock flexed with only the toe touching the ground. In moderately severe cases both a supporting and swinging-leg lameness is noted. In very severe cases, the leg may be carried in a flexed position. Crepitation may be noted if the menisci, cruciate ligaments, or the collateral ligaments of the joint have been ruptured. Radiographs of the joint may be of considerable value in confirming the diagnosis.

The prognosis is poor if the condition is of long duration or if severe injuries to the articular surface ligaments or the menisci have occurred. Rest is indicated. Medial patellar desmotomy is indicated in upward fixation of the patella. Intra-articular injections of steroids (R 155, 159) at weekly intervals may be useful. Phenylbutazone (R 150) and systemic steroids (R 144) may relieve the lameness in less severe cases. Those cases due to rupture of ligaments or damage to the menisci rarely respond satisfactorily.

STRINGHALT
(Springhalt)

A myoclonic affection of one or both hind legs manifested by spasmodic overflexion of the joints during progression. (Cases of foreleg involvement are extremely rare.) The etiology is unknown. Degeneration of the sciatic or peroneal nerve and affections of the spinal cord have been suggested as possible causes. Horses of any breed may be affected.

Clinical Findings: All degrees of flexion are seen, from the mild, spasmodic lifting and grounding of the foot, to the extreme case where the foot is drawn sharply up till it touches the belly and then struck violently on the ground. Stringhalt may be intermittent in character and thus may pass unnoticed at the time of examination. The ailment is most obvious when the horse is sharply turned or backed. In some cases, the condition is seen only on the first few steps after moving the horse out of its stall. The signs are often less intense or even absent during warmer weather.

Although it is regarded as a gross unsoundness, stringhalt does not materially hinder the horse's capacity for work, except in severe cases when the constant concussion gives rise to secondary complications. A severe case may also make the horse unsuitable for equestrian sports.

Diagnosis: Diagnosis is based on clinical signs. If in doubt, the animal should be observed as it is backed out of the stall after hard work for a day or two. False stringhalt sometimes appears as a result of some temporary irritation to the lower pastern area.

Treatment: Best results have been obtained by performing peroneal tenectomy using the standard or radical method. In the latter operation, a portion of the muscle is also removed. Prognosis following surgery should be guarded.

SWEENEY
(Swinney, Shoulder atrophy, Slipped shoulder)

An atrophy of the supraspinatus and infraspinatus muscles of the horse. This atrophy is of 2 types, disuse and neurotrophic.

Disuse atrophy, sometimes involving the triceps also, follows any lesion of the leg or foot which leads to prolonged diminished use of the limb.

Neurotrophic atrophy is due to damage to the suprascapular nerve, which supplies the supraspinatus and infraspinatus muscles. The resulting syndrome is termed suprascapular paralysis or slipped shoulder. The triceps is not involved in this type of atrophy.

In most cases, the condition is due to damage to the nerve, either through bruising with effusion or occasionally the nerve may be severed as a result of injury.

Clinical Findings and Diagnosis: If there is no evident trauma, pain may be absent and lameness may be difficult to detect until atrophy occurs. If injury is evident, there is usually some difficulty in extending the shoulder.

As atrophy proceeds, there is a noticeable hollowing on each side of the spine of the scapula, especially in the infraspinous area, resulting in prominence of the spine. Since the tendons of insertion of the 2 affected muscles act as lateral collateral ligaments to the humeroscapular joint, atrophy of the muscles leads to a looseness in the shoulder joint. Abduction of the shoulder follows and, in severe cases, is sometimes erroneously diagnosed as a dislocation. The affected limb, when advanced, takes a semicircular course and, as weight is borne by the leg, the shoulder joint moves laterally (shoulder slip). At rest, along with abduction of the shoulder, there is an apparent abduction of the lower part of the limb.

Prognosis: The prognosis of disuse atrophy depends on removal of the primary cause. In neurotrophic atrophy, the prognosis is guarded; a mild case should recover in 6 to 8 weeks, but where damage to the nerve has been severe, recovery may take many months if it occurs at all. If the nerve has been severed, recovery is most unlikely.

Treatment: Treatment for disuse atrophy consists of removing the cause of the failure to use the limb. For neurotrophic atrophy, rest at pasture is the best treatment. Massage with stimulating liniments or by an electrical vibrator may be of benefit. So-called inward blisters (℞ 577) have been used.

FOOT AILMENTS OF HORSES

LAMINITIS
(Founder)

An inflammation of the sensitive laminae of the foot. It may be acute or chronic and it may involve 1 or all 4 feet. Most commonly both forefeet are affected.

Etiology: The exciting causes are well known and include: ingestion of cold water by an overheated animal; ingestion of excessive amounts of grain; concussion during hard, fast road work; hard work by an unconditioned animal; toxemias as sequelae to pneumonia or metritis (so-called "parturient laminitis") and superpurgation. Allergic reactions have been incriminated. Grain founder is the commonest type. Ponies, in particular, have been known to founder when at pasture.

Clinical Findings: In acute laminitis, onset is sudden. Both general and local signs may appear. General signs include a rise in temperature up to 106°F with accompanying increase in respiration and pulse rate. In some cases, the pain is so excruciating as to produce clonic spasms and profuse sweating. If the forefeet only are affected, the animal places them forward to relieve them from weight, bringing the hind feet forward under the body for support. If the hind feet are affected, they are placed forward with the forefeet under the body to support the weight. The animal lies down and rises only reluctantly. If standing, the animal resists movement. The first steps are accomplished with intense pain which subsides to a slight extent as the animal "warms up".

Local signs are marked. The affected feet are warm to the touch. The pulse of the digital artery on the affected feet is hard and bounding. Even mild pressure by hoof testers applied across the quarters produces great pain. In mild cases, recovery may occur in about 10 days. In severe cases, the prognosis is poor and the condition is likely to terminate in chronic laminitis. Infiltration of serum takes place in the space between the horny and sensitive laminae with the result that the os pedis is displaced so that the anterior portion of this bone points downward. This displacement is assisted by the pull of the deep flexor tendon. The hoof becomes distorted; the anterior wall becomes concave, the hoof longer, the heels higher, and the hoof wall corrugated. It is important not to confuse so-called "grass rings" with the rings produced by chronic laminitis.

Diagnosis: In acute cases, diagnosis is made by consideration of the case history, the posture of the animal, the increased temperature of the hooves, the hard pulse of the digital artery, the expression of pain and anxiety, and the reluctance to move. Mild cases with no visible hoof deformity may be discovered on X-raying the affected feet.

Treatment: The prognosis is very guarded because of the possibility of hoof deformity and alteration in position of the os pedis. Only if the case is mild and treatment is prompt and adequate, is there much hope of avoiding a dropped sole. In **acute laminitis,** especially in cases of excessive grain consumption and provided superpurgation is not the primary cause, a purgative (℞ 479) is recommended. Oral administration of 1 gal. of mineral oil will act as a laxative and tend to prevent absorption of toxic material from the intestinal tract. Purgation should not be employed in cases following pneumonia or in parturient laminitis of mares. In the latter condition, the uterus usually requires attention. Cold packs or ice packs applied to the affected feet are advocated by some, but newer evidence suggests that hot packs used early in the course of the disease would be more beneficial. Soluble antihistaminics have given favorable results. Corticosteroids may be of value early in acute laminitis but should not be used after the second day of the disease; the use of phenylbutazone is preferable.

Treatment of **chronic laminitis** consists of attempting to restore the normal alignment of the rotated coffin bone by lowering the heels, removing excess toe, and protecting the dropped sole. This may be accomplished by a competent farrier and may require full leather pads or a steel plate shoe in addition to trimming the hoof. Acrylic compounds may be useful in conjunction with proper trimming to build up the toe and to protect the sole. The hoof should be trimmed and the shoe reset at 6- to 8-week intervals.

THRUSH

A degenerative condition of the horn commencing in the central and collateral sulci and eventually involving the entire frog. The predisposing causes are unhygienic conditions that require the animal to stand in mud, urine- or feces-soaked earth or bedding, failure to clean the hoof at regular intervals and atrophy of the frog as found in contracted hoofs. In all probability, there is more than one causal organism, and among them can be listed *Sphaerophorus necrophorus*.

Thrush may be found in any or all of the feet, but is more common in the hind feet. A characteristic foul odor always is present. The affected sulcus is moist and contains a black, thick discharge. When probed, the sulcus is deeper than normal and sensitive in its depth. The characteristic odor and the black, thick discharge in the sulci of the frog are adequate for diagnosis.

The prognosis is good. Treatment should begin by providing dry, clean standings and cleaning the hoof gently to avoid unnecessary injury to the affected part. Any of the recognized astringent lotions will effect a cure, following removal of the diseased tissue. The use of a bar shoe may help in the regeneration of the frog, after the disease process has been arrested. If the cuneate matrix has been damaged, radical surgery should be employed to remove diseased frog tissue.

CANKER

A chronic hypertrophy of the horn-producing tissues of the foot, involving the frog, the sole and, at times, the wall. It is most often found in the hind feet. Canker is seldom encountered today, being primarily a disease of the heavy draft horse. The cause is unknown.

Clinical Findings: The disease is frequently well advanced before detection, attention being directed to it by the fetid odor. The frog may appear to be intact, but has a ragged, oiled appearance. The horn tissue of the frog loosens easily, revealing the swollen, ill-smelling corium covered with a caseous, whitish exudate. The surface of the corium is not smooth, but shows a characteristic vegetative growth. The disease process may extend to the sole and even to the wall, showing no tendency to heal. The tissue bleeds easily if not handled with extreme care.

Diagnosis: The offensive odor, the moist appearance, the soft, swollen, sensitive tissue and the loss of the horny frog established the diagnosis.

Treatment: The prognosis is not good. Treatment must be persistent. All loose horn and affected tissue should be removed. A mild antiseptic and astringent dressing (℞ 616) is applied under pressure and renewed daily at first. The use of caustics (℞ 614) may be indicated. Dressings may be retained by transverse strips of thin metal, springing the ends under the shoe, or by means of a metal sole screwed to the shoe. By this latter method, the horse, if not lame, can be returned to work with less likelihood of the dressings being lost. Maintenance of pressure on the affected part during treatment appears beneficial.

GREASE
(Grease heel, Scratches, Dermatitis verrucosa)

A chronic dermatitis characterized by hypertrophy and exudation on the posterior surface of the fetlock and pastern. The hind legs are more commonly affected. The disease often is associated with poor stable hygiene, but no specific cause is known. Heavy, coarse-legged horses seem most susceptible.

Clinical Findings: Because of the "feather", the disease may progress somewhat before it is noticed. The skin is itchy, sensitive and swollen during the acute stages; later, it becomes thickened and most of the hair is lost. Only the shorter hairs remain and these stand erect. The surface of the skin is soft and the grayish exudate has a fetid odor. The condition tends to become chronic and vegetative granulomatous growths known as "grapes" appear, caused by hypertrophy of the papillae. Lameness may or may not be present. As the condition progresses, there is thickening and hardening of the skin of the affected region, with very rapid hypertrophy of subcut. fibrous tissue. This assumes elephantiasis-like proportions in cases of long duration.

Treatment: The prognosis is guarded, but persistent treatment is usually rewarding. Treatment consists of washing with warm water and castile or green soap, to remove all soft exudate, drying, and applying an astringent dressing (℞ 403, 621). If granulomatous lesions appear, they should be cauterized.

CORNS
(Pododermatitis circumscripta)

Bruising of the sole, in the angle between the wall and the bar, usually in the inner quarter and most commonly in the forefeet. Corns may be classified as dry, moist, or suppurating.

Etiology: Predisposition to corns is usually due to faulty foot conformation, such as straight walls which tend to turn in at the quarters, or contracted feet. More direct causes may be excessive trimming of the sole, thus exposing the sensitive tissue to contusion, or neglect of the feet, to the extent that they become long and irregular. Shoes which have been allowed to remain on until overgrown by the hoof, or shoes which have been fitted too closely at the quarters, may also cause the condition.

Clinical Findings: When the foot is raised and the volar surface freed of dirt and loose horn, a discoloration, either red or reddish yellow, is noted at the site of the corn. A supporting leg lameness is an early sign. Tapping with a light hammer over the area or applying pressure with a hoof tester causes great discomfort. If infection has gained entrance, pain is pronounced when pressure is applied, and if not promptly treated, pus may burrow through to the coronet to produce quittor or a suppurating sinus.

Diagnosis: The lameness, the sensitiveness over a circumscribed area when pressure is applied and the discoloration of the horn usually are adequate for a diagnosis.

Treatment: The prognosis is favorable. In simple, uncomplicated dry corns, relief from pressure on the affected area is the first consideration. This may be achieved by shortening the toe if it is excessively long and by applying a bar shoe to promote frog pressure. A ¾ bar shoe may be of value in relieving pressure.

If the corn is suppurating, it should be drained at once by a surgical opening directly through the sole. It may be advantageous to thin the area around the opening, in order to relieve pressure. Following drainage, the lesions should be irrigated with a mild antiseptic and the foot dressed to prevent drainage from being arrested. Hot foot baths and agents such as Antiphlogistine are helpful. The horse should be kept in a dry, clean box stall. After infection is controlled in suppurating corns, the cavity should be loosely packed with oakum and a metal or leather sole placed between the shoe and the foot. Systemic antibacterial therapy may be indicated in severe septic cases.

BRUISED SOLE

A term applied to bruises on the volar aspect of the foot other than those found at the seat of corn. The cause usually is direct injury from stones, irregular ground or other trauma. Bad shoeing, especially in animals with flat feet or dropped sole, also may cause the condition; in this case, the bruised area is usually around the periphery of the sole.

Signs and treatment are very similar to corns, except that in bruised sole, the infection tends to spread more rapidly under the horn of the sole. Persistent bruised sole not responding to treatment should arouse suspicion of pedal osteitis (q.v., p. 544).

PUNCTURE WOUNDS OF THE FOOT
(Suppurative pododermatitis, Gathered nail, "Nail bind")

The results of such wounds vary from a transient indisposition to an incapacity which eventually necessitates the destruction of the horse. In severe cases, an acutely painful foot is the most obvious sign. Abscess formation quite commonly follows within 10 to 14 days of the infliction of the wound.

The foreign body should be removed and the infected area drained. Tetanus immunization should be carried out in all cases of puncture wounds in the foot. When pain is severe, a volar nerve block provides temporary relief. Systemic antibiotic therapy may be indicated.

QUITTOR

A chronic, purulent inflammation of the lateral cartilage, characterized by necrosis of the cartilage, and one or more sinus tracts extending from the diseased cartilage through the skin in the coronary region. Quittor follows injury to the coronet over the region of the lateral cartilage, by means of which infection is introduced into the deep tissues to form a subcoronary abscess, or it may follow a penetrating wound through the sole.

The first sign is an inflammatory swelling over the region of the lateral cartilage. This is followed by abscessation and sinus formation. During the acute stage, lameness occurs.

The prognosis should be guarded. If extensive damage has been done and the tract has pushed close to the joint capsule anteriorly, the prognosis must be poor. Surgery for the purpose of removing the diseased cartilage is the treatment of choice in most instances.

WOUNDS OF THE CORONET

These are commonly seen following treads from the opposite foot. Varying degrees of damage to the coronary region may be caused. Apart from suppurative coronitis or chronic coronitis, damage to the underlying tissues may result in quittor, necrosis of the extensor pedis tendon, or abnormal enlargement of the hoof wall at the quarter (false quarter).

SAND CRACK

Any break in continuity of the wall of the hoof which begins at the coronet and parallels the horn tubules. Depending upon their location, they are known as toe cracks or quarter cracks and may be classified further as complete, incomplete, deep, or superficial.

Etiology: Sand crack is caused by trauma of the coronet, excessive drying in combination with work on hard streets, excessive thinning and alternate wetting and drying. Cracks are most common in the quarter of a forefoot and in the toe of a hind foot. Extensive injury to the coronet may give rise to the condition commonly known as false quarter.

Clinical Findings and Diagnosis: The presence of a crack in the horn is the most obvious sign. Lameness may be present, although the majority of cases show no lameness. If infection is established, a discharge of pus or blood may follow, accompanied by signs of inflammation.

Treatment: Therapy lies almost entirely in the fields of surgery and corrective shoeing, which change the distribution of the weight borne by the hoof. Growth of new horn may be encouraged by the application of a counterirritant (℞ 624) to the coronet over the crack. If the crack has become infected, an antiseptic pack saturated with 2% cresol solution is indicated. As a protective dressing for the horn, following surgical procedures, a heavy, waxy dressing (R 421) is recommended. A patented patching technique may be successful; unfortunately, it is expensive and not at present widely used. Stripping the horn of the wall completely, being careful not to damage the coronet, is often the treatment of choice in an early and severe quarter crack. The hoof is then bandaged tightly with a pine-oil dressing. The animal is shod with a three-quarter shoe to relieve any pressure over the stripped portion of the wall.

SEEDY TOE
(Hollow wall, Dystrophia ungulae)

A condition affecting the hoof wall in the toe region, characterized by loss of substance and change in character of the horn. It may result from a close-fitting toe clip which produces a chronic inflammation of the laminae. It also may be a sequela to chronic laminitis. Defective development of horn has been considered as the cause or at least as a predisposing cause of seedy toe.

Lameness is infrequent. The outer surface of the wall appears sound, but upon dressing the volar surface of the hoof, the inner surface of the wall is seen to be mealy. There actually may be a cavity due to loss of horn substance. Tapping on the outside of the wall at the toe elicits a hollow sound over the affected portion. The disease may involve only a small area or nearly the entire width of the wall at the toe.

The prognosis is usually good. The diseased portion should be curetted and packed with juniper tar and oakum. If the condition is extensive, it may be necessary to remove the outer wall over the affected area. The shape of the shoe must be modified to protect the thinned anterior wall, if the animal is to be worked.

KERAPHYLLOCELE
(Keratoma)

An inflammatory growth of horn on the inner surface of the wall, usually at the toe. It is not a tumor. It is believed to follow a chronic inflammatory process of the laminar matrix caused by "nail bind", mechanical injury to the wall or coronet, or following hoof-grooving.

The nature of the disease often is not obvious until the growth is well advanced. Examination of the volar surface shows that the growth, commonly of a cylindrical shape, has pushed the white line in toward the center of the sole. The prognosis should be guarded, since pressure atrophy of the pedal bone commonly follows severe cases. Surgical removal of the mass is indicated. In mild cases, corrective shoeing may give some temporary relief.

CONTRACTED HEELS

A condition most commonly seen affecting the quarters and heels of the front feet of light horses. It may be caused by improper shoeing that draws in the quarters and does not allow frog pressure, and is favored by excessive rasping of the foot and trimming of the bars.

The frog is narrow and shrunken. The bars may be almost parallel to each other. The quarters and heels are markedly contracted and drawn in. Lameness is evident when the horse is worked at speed, although it may disappear after exercise. The length of stride is shortened. Excessive heat may be noticed around the heels and quarters and the pulsation in the digital artery may be marked.

The prognosis is guarded as recovery in well-developed cases takes 6 to 12 months. The most important factor in treatment is to restore normal frog pressure. This can be achieved by means of a bar shoe with the addition of shims between the frog and bar to permit direct pressure on the frog. Thinning the wall of the quarters just below the coronary band with a rasp, or grooving the walls parallel to the coronet, ¾ in. below the hairline, from the heel halfway to the toe, will aid in expanding the heels; second and third grooves should be ½ in. apart, and parallel to the first. A hoof dressing should be applied regularly. The operation must be repeated as the quarters grow out until the heels and quarters are normally expanded.

SIDE-BONE

(Ossification of the lateral cartilages)

Ossification of the lateral cartilages of the third phalanx. The disease is commonest in the front feet of heavy horses used at rapid speeds on hard surfaces. It is also frequent in hunters and jumpers, but rare in Thoroughbreds.

Etiology: Repeated concussion to the quarters of the feet may be the essential cause. The condition is believed to be promoted by improper shoeing which inhibits normal physiologic movement of the quarters. Some cases arise from direct trauma.

Clinical Findings: Loss of flexibility of either one or both of the lateral cartilages is indicative of side-bone. Since the rigidity of the cartilages is accompanied by ossification, the cartilages may, in some cases, protrude prominently above the coronet. Lameness may or may not be a sign depending upon the stage of ossification, the amount of concussion sustained by the feet and the character of the terrain. Lameness is most likely when side-bone is associated with a narrow or contracted foot. Mules often have prominent side-bones, yet reveal no lameness. Walking the horse at right angles to an inclined slope may exaggerate the soreness. The gait may show a shortened stride.

Diagnosis: Normally, side-bone can be diagnosed by palpation or by observation. In some cases when side-bone is suspected but cannot be palpated, radiologic examination may be useful.

Treatment: When lameness is present, corrective shoeing to promote expansion of the quarters and to protect the foot from concussion often is of value. Grooving the hooves, along with a blister to the coronary region to promote hoof growth, also may promote expansion of the wall.

RING-BONE
(Phalangeal exostosis)

A periostitis or osteo-arthritis leading to exostosis involving the first or second phalanx of the horse.

Etiology: The condition may result from faulty conformation, improper shoeing and repeated concussion through working on hard ground. It may follow trauma and infection, especially wire-cut wounds. In light horses, the straining of ligaments and tendinous insertions of muscles in the pastern region are most frequent causal factors.

Clinical Findings: Lameness due to the inflammation of the periosteum may appear in the early stages before enlargements occur. After these are well developed, lameness may or may not be present, provided the articular surfaces are not affected. However, lameness is constant if such surfaces are involved and, in some cases, the articulation becomes ankylosed.

Diagnosis: A positive diagnosis of ring-bone cannot be made prior to the development of enlargements, since it is based on the presence of enlargements on either of the phalanges. In some cases, the enlargements may be difficult to detect unless the area suspected is compared with its opposite. When small, symmetrical enlargements, about equal in size, appear, the diagnosis is difficult or even impossible to make. Radiography offers the only dependable means of diagnosis in the early stages.

Treatment: Complete rest is the first and most important requirement. In the early stages with no involvement of the articulation, treatment consists of cold and astringent applications. When the acute stage has subsided, but lameness is still present, counterirritation in the form of a blister (R 627) may be used, but only in the early stages before dense bony accumulations have formed. Deep point firing may also be used for this purpose, and may be of value as a means of creating ankylosis when the pastern joint is involved. The action of an animal with an ankylosed joint may be improved by fitting a rocker shoe to assist an easier break-over.

NAVICULAR DISEASE

The fact that navicular disease has been described as a chronic osteitis of the navicular bone, associated with navicular bursitis and inflammation of the plantar aponeurosis suggests that this is a syndrome rather than a specific disease entity. It is primarily a disease of the forefeet, but on rare occasions it may appear in the hind feet.

Etiology: The cause is unknown. It has usually been considered a disease of the more mature riding horse, and it is doubtful whether the condition referred to as navicular disease in some 3-year-olds is really anything more than a simple bruising of the heel region. The foot becomes abnormal in conformation, being upright and narrow and having a small frog. It should be noted, however, that navicular disease is rare in the donkey and mule. Defective shoeing which inhibits the physiologic action of the frog and the quarters should be considered.

Clinical Findings: Navicular disease is insidious in onset and rarely appears suddenly. Attention is first directed to the affected foot or feet by the attitude of the animal when at rest. The horse relieves the pressure of the deep flexor tendon on the painful area by "pointing", that is, by advancing the affected foot. If both forefeet are affected, they are pointed alternately. Lameness is manifested early in the course of the disease. The stride is shortened and there is a tendency to stumble. The animal stands more comfortably with the heels high.

Diagnosis: Clinical diagnosis is not easy until the condition is well advanced. It is arrived at by the history of pointing, followed by the appearance of lameness. Radiography is of assistance in diagnosis and confirmation of clinical suspicions. It will also help to differentiate navicular disease from fracture of the navicular bone. Posterior digital nerve blocks may be employed as an aid in diagnosis. Application of pressure over the navicular bone with a hoof tester assists in locating the sensitive area.

Treatment: The prognosis is poor. Rest is indicated. In the early acute stage, cold packs to the feet may give relief. Thinning the quarters with a rasp may tend to relieve if the foot is contracted. Toes should be shortened to facilitate the "break-over" when the foot is carried forward. A shoe with branches which thicken toward the heel should be used to relieve tension on the deep flexor tendon. Double digital neurectomy may render relief from pain and prolong the usefulness of the animal. Volar and especially median neurectomy should not be done in light horses that work at speed, and no neurectomy should be considered curative. Intrabursal injection of corticosteroid is likewise palliative rather than curative.

PEDAL OSTEITIS

A rarefying osteitis of the pedal bone. Osteo-arthritic factors have been cited as causes, although repeated concussion, laminitis, persistent corns and chronic bruised sole also may be incriminated. The signs are those of discomfort referable to the hoof region. There is often tenderness of the sole on percussion and pressure. Before the use of X-rays in diagnosis, the condition often was confused with navicular disease, especially if the inflammatory lesion was in the posterior part of the foot. Rest and shoeing with protection to the sole may give relief in mild cases.

PYRAMIDAL DISEASE
(Extensor process disease, Buttress foot)

This condition is usually due to a traumatically induced periostitis and osteitis or avulsion fracture of the extensor process of the third phalanx caused by excessive pull of the tendons inserted on it.

Because of the close association of the extensor process with the distal phalangeal joint, arthritis is very likely to supervene and lameness is seen in most cases. In the early case, heat and pain on pressure may be manifest. An enlargement of the foot just above the coronet is usually present.

FRACTURE OF THE OS PEDIS

This condition may arise as a result of a penetrating wound of the foot, as a result of concussion—the horse that "pounds" is susceptible to this type of fracture—or as a sequela to neurectomy or to a pathologic process in the bone.

Clinical Findings: The degree of pain manifested is variable, many cases showing moderate lameness which is greatly increased when the horse is turned or made to pivot on the affected leg. Hoof testers usually yield positive results in a recent case.

Diagnosis: The signs may suggest the condition, but the only conclusive means of diagnosis is by radiography. More than 2 different views are often required before the fracture line is evident, especially if X-rays are taken immediately after the fracture occurs and if it is of a hairline nature.

Prognosis: When puncture wounds are the cause, the prognosis depends on the presence or absence of infection. Where concussion is the cause, the prognosis is guarded. Fracture following a pathologic process merits an unfavorable outlook. A guarded to favorable prognosis will, however, depend on the fact that the articular surface is not involved and that adequate rest and immobilization of the part are enforced. Disappointment sometimes follows cases in which a small splinter of bone forms a sequestrum, with prolonged and persistent lameness as a sequela.

Treatment: Insofar as possible, the foot is immobilized by the fitting of a plain bar shoe with a clip placed well back on each quarter to limit expansion and contraction of the heels. Rest from work for a year is advised, lesser periods not giving as good results. Where infection or sequestration is present, surgery must be performed. A posterior digital neurectomy may be of value if a pedal osteitis follows the healing process.

ARTHRITIS AND RELATED DISORDERS (LG. AN.)

(Articular rheumatism, Polyarthritis)

Inflammation of the tissues associated with a joint. While frequent in all large animals, arthritis is best known in horses because of the importance of interference with locomotion in this species. (*See also* LAMENESS IN HORSES, p. 518.)

Specific Types of Arthritis: Acute serous arthritis usually is due to trauma and involves only one joint. The joint capsule becomes distended with clear, watery fluid, and is evident upon palpation and movement of the joint. The synovial membrane becomes hyperemic and the tissues surrounding the joint edematous and hot.

Purulent arthritis is commonly associated with navel ill of foals, calves and lambs, or follows trauma. It is characterized by distension of the joint with an accumulation of pus and is extremely painful. The pyogenic organisms enter the joint through wounds or by hematogenous extension. The articular cartilage and subchondral bone are likely to be eroded. The condition may be polyarticular. Early cases appear as acute serofibrinous arthritis.

Chronic arthritis (chronic osteoarthritis) is the type of arthritis most commonly seen in the horse. Ringbone and spavin are common examples. Faulty conformation, chronic trauma and undue stress are factors in producing the disease. Most cases lead to periarticular periosteal exostoses which may become large and extensive. The condition is commonly observed in the stifle joints of older bulls and cows.

Infectious Swine Arthritis is a common term for a group of bacterial and mycoplasmal arthritic infections in younger pigs. In newborn pigs infectious arthritis is usually due to intrauterine or navel infection with *E. coli, Corynebacterium, Streptococcus,* or *Staphylococcus,* and treatment is best directed towards reducing the possibility of infection from the environment. Older pigs will sometimes develop arthritis as a sequela to infection with *Haemophilus, Erysipelothrix,* or *Mycoplasma,* and although diagnosis in the early stages of the condition is not difficult, the more chronic stages can be confused with articular lesions produced by dietary hypervitaminosis A. The infectious arthritides are discussed under the headings of the specific diseases.

Clinical Findings: Arthritis produces pain and altered function of the joint. If the process is active or recent, the joint capsule is usually distended and the surrounding tissues swollen and hot. Manipulation of the joint causes pain. In long-standing chronic cases, normal movement is greatly reduced and crepitation may be felt when the parts are moved. Careful palpation of the joint for pain and swelling is important in diagnosis. In many cases, X-ray examination is necessary for positive diagnosis.

Treatment: Treatment of **acute serous arthritis** requires absolute rest until the joint has returned to normal. Application of cold water or ice to the part helps to relieve pain. If the joint capsule is distended, aspiration of the fluid with a sterile needle and syringe gives added relief. Provided the joint cavity is sterile, the injection of corticosteroids (℞ 155, 159) usually exerts a prompt anti-inflammatory action and aids in preventing a recurrence of excessive fluid within the joint. **Purulent arthritis** demands prompt treatment before irreparable damage is done. In these cases, systemic therapy with antibiotics (℞ 44, 54) may be usefully combined with local therapy. Daily aspiration of the joint contents and replacement with antibiotics (℞ 48, 55) provide a high concentration of the drugs at the site of infection. Phenylbutazone (℞ 150) relieves pain and allows movement so that fibrous restriction of the affected joint is reduced.

Chronic arthritis and **periostitis** may be treated satisfactorily only if diagnosed early and treated promptly before the lesion becomes extensive or ankylosis occurs. Where early diagnosis is established, X-ray therapy may be of value. Other treatments include the use of counterirritants, such as blisters (℞ 628), ultrasonic therapy and point-firing and surgical fusion. After any type of treatment, the patient must be rested for at least 6 months. Treatment usually is unsuccessful in the **chronic deforming and adhesive arthritis** of old bulls and cows. However, restricted exercise, good feeding, housing and management may prolong the life of the patient, and this may be worthwhile in the case of valuable breeding animals. In bulls that are unable to mount, semen for artificial breeding purposes may be collected with an electro-ejaculator. The intra-articular injection of corticosteroids (℞ 155, 159) may relieve the discomfort.

BURSITIS

Acute or chronic inflammation of a bursa may occur in all species, but is more common and important in the horse.

Etiology and Clinical Findings: The most commonly involved bursae are those that are superficial and located over bony prominences or between tendons. Common locations are the bursae overlying the tuber ischii (car bruise), the olecranon process (capped elbow, shoe boil), the tuber calcis (capped hock), the trochanter major (trochanteric bursitis), the bicipital groove (intertubercular bursitis) and the navicular bone (navicular bursitis).

Acute serous bursitis is usually due to severe trauma and is characterized by rapid swelling, local heat and pain. Infection of bursae may be hematogenous or follow penetrating wounds or nonsterile surgical treatment of a serous bursitis. As the bursitis becomes chronic, the local swelling and heat subside, but the area may show evidence of pain on palpation or movement. Atrophy of muscles may occur if the bursitis causes reduced function of a limb.

Treatment: The pain in acute serous bursitis may be relieved by application of cold packs, aspiration of the contents and injection of 2% procaine solution. Prednisolone (℞ 155) or its derivatives have proved beneficial when injected into bursae. Phenylbutazone (℞ 150) will give relief from pain. The bursa should not be incised. If the condition becomes chronic, aspiration followed by repeated injection of half-strength tincture of iodine (℞ 622) or Lugol's solution (℞ 576) may cause the swelling gradually to subside. X-ray therapy (*see* p. 1398) is often beneficial. The application of counterirritants (℞ 623, 628) over the distended area may also help to reduce the swelling. Infected bursae require drainage and systemic treatment with antibiotics. Recovery is slow.

TENOSYNOVITIS

Acute or chronic inflammation of the synovial sheath of a tendon. It is more common and important in the horse.

Etiology: Synovitis often occurs in conjunction with tendinitis. Most cases arise from excessive strain on the tendons from overwork. Others are caused by bruising of the tissues by bumping against hard objects. Infection of the synovial sheath may come about by penetrating foreign bodies, or by metastasis in certain infectious diseases of horses.

Clinical Findings: If primary, the condition usually affects only one synovial sheath. If secondary or metastatic, usually it is seen in several sheaths. Acute synovitis shows the classical signs of acute inflammation together with accumulation of excessive amounts of synovia. If it becomes chronic, pain and heat disappear, but the excess fluid remains. In synovitis due to foreign-body penetration, there is usually exudation of pus and synovial fluid. In horses, chronic synovitis is common in locations such as the synovial sheath of the deep flexor tendon at the hock (thoroughpin) and the sheath of the deep flexor tendon over the distal-third of the metacarpus and metatarsus (tendon sheath gall). Thoroughpin should be differentiated from bog spavin (*see* p. 526) end tendon sheath gall from chronic distension of the capsule of the fetlock joint.

Treatment: In the acute stage, the use of cold packs or cold-water showers, the injection of steroids (℞ 155) into the affected sheath, repeated after 3 or 4 days, and absolute rest are advisable. If infection is present, or if the condition is secondary to another disease, systemic administration of antibiotics (℞ 44, 54) is indicated. For chronic synovitis, application of counterirritants (℞ 628) followed by massage and bandaging results in temporary reduction of the distension. Injection of corticosteroids (℞ 155, 159) into the synovial space may be followed by prompt and more lasting reduction of the swelling, reinjection is dependent on whether the swelling recurs.

TENDINITIS
("Bowed tendon")

Acute or chronic inflammation of a tendon. Tendinitis is seen most commonly in horses used at fast work, particularly race horses. The flexor tendons, the suspensory ligament and the check ligament are more frequently involved than the extensor tendons, and those of the foreleg more commonly than those of the hind. Of these, the superficial flexor is most frequently involved in the common "bowed tendon" of race horses. The primary lesion is a rupture of the tendon fibers with associated hemorrhage and edema. In Thoroughbreds, the "leading" or "inside" foreleg (which depends on whether they race in a clockwise or counterclockwise direction) is more frequently affected than the other.

Etiology: Tendinitis usually appears during forced exercise. The commonest causes include overexertion without proper training, continuance of training after first signs of tendon soreness have appeared, fatigue and fast work on muddy, rough or hard track surfaces. Improper shoeing, by placing extra strain on the flexor tendons, also predisposes to tendinitis. Poor conformation and training at too early an age also may result in tendon breakdown.

Clinical Findings: The horse is severely lame and stands with the heel elevated to ease the tension on the tendons. The structures involved are hot, painful and swollen. Chronic straining of the flexor tendons and associated ligaments in the cannon region ultimately leads to fibrosis, with thickening and shortening of the tendons. In chronic tendinitis, the patient may go sound while walking or trotting, but the tendon rarely holds up under hard work.

Treatment: Tendinitis is best treated in the early, acute stage. The horse should be given absolute rest by confinement. The swelling and inflammation should be reduced by applying cold packs and the leg may be immobilized in a plaster cast for 6 to 8 weeks, but many clinicians prefer not to use casts. Good results have also been obtained by injecting the inflamed area of the tendon with prednisolone or its derivatives followed by the application of a plaster cast. The injection is made by inserting a 20-gauge needle through the tendon and depositing 0.5 to 1.0 ml of prednisolone as the needle is withdrawn. The injections are spaced at half-inch intervals over the entire area of the swelling. Rapid reduction of inflammation usually follows. X-ray therapy, in conjunction with immobilization, may also be used for acute tendinitis.

After removal of the cast, the patient should be given additional rest and the leg supported with bandages for another 4 weeks. Exercise should be mild and gradually increased. Ideally, training should not be resumed until at least a year of rest has been given.

Chronic tendinitis usually is treated by deep point-firing directly into the affected tendon, although the results of firing are questionable in many of these cases. A counterirritant (℞ 628) is applied immediately after firing. Starting about a week after firing, the leg is treated daily with leg paint (℞ 626) for 2 to 3 weeks. A year's rest should be prescribed. The latter is doubtless the chief element in recovery. An alternative is the injection of the tendon at half-inch intervals of a sclerosing agent (℞ 645) after which the horse is rested for 6 to 8 months. For the first 4 weeks after injection, the horses' heels, which are elevated about 1 in. with a special shoe, are gradually lowered to normal position and the animal is given light exercise.

CAPPED ELBOW AND HOCK

Inflammatory swelling of the subcut. bursa located over the olecranon process and tuber calcis, respectively. Trauma from lying on poorly bedded hard floors, kicks, falls, riding the tail gate of trailers, iron shoes projecting beyond the heels and chronic lameness enforcing long periods of recumbency are frequent causes.

Circumscribed edematous swelling occurs over and around the affected bursa. Lameness is rare in either case. The affected bursa may be fluctuating and soft at first, but in a short time, a firm, fibrous capsule forms, especially if there is a recurrence of an old injury. Initial bursal swellings vary in size from hardly noticeable enlargements to those of sizable proportions. Chronic cases may progress to abscessation.

Acute early cases may respond well to cold-water applications, followed in a few days by aseptic aspiration and injection of a corticosteroid (℞ 155, 159). Older encapsulated bursae are more difficult to aspirate and are more refractory to treatment. Aspiration may be followed by repeated injections of iodine (℞ 576, 622). The bursa may also be reduced in size by the application of a counterirritant paint (℞ 623, 628) or radiation therapy. Surgical removal is recommended only for capped elbows, either of the advanced encapsulated type, or those that have abscessed. A shoeboil roll should be used to prevent recurrence of a capped elbow in those animals in which the condition has been caused by the heel or by the shoe.

FISTULOUS WITHERS—POLL EVIL

Two inflammatory disorders of horses which differ from one another essentially only in their location in the respective supraspinous and supra-atlantal bursae. The following account deals with fistulous withers but, except for anatomic details, the remarks apply in general also to poll evil.

In the early stage of the disease a fistula is not present. When the bursal sac ruptures or when it is opened for surgical drainage, and secondary infection with pyogenic bacteria occurs, it usually assumes a true fistulous character. The term bursitis is, therefore, the more appropriate designation for the initial clinical entity.

Etiology: Various theories have been advanced regarding the cause of this disease. Mechanical injury has received some support. Experimental evidence suggests that the condition is primarily infectious in origin. A high proportion of positive reactions to the agglutination test for brucellosis has been observed in horses with bursitis and a low incidence in horses not so affected. Further, *Brucella abortus* and occasionally *Br. suis* can be isolated from the fluid aspirated from the distended but unopened bursa. That the connective-tissue wall of the bursal sac is regularly infected with *Actinomyces bovis* is further evidence for the infectious theory.

While the injection of cultures of *Brucella* or *Actinomyces* failed to produce a typical bursitis, the simultaneous injection of both into the supraspinous bursa produced the characteristic lesion. Furthermore, at times, the 2 infections in cattle occur simultaneously with the appearance on the premises of bursitis in horses. Outbreaks of brucellosis in cattle have followed contact with horses with open bursitis. This suggests that fistulous withers and poll evil result from a dual infection with both organisms.

Clinical Findings: The inflammation leads to considerable thickening of the wall of the bursa. The bursal sacs increase in size by distension and dilatation. Rupture may occur where the sac has little covering support. In older, advanced cases the ligament and the dorsal vertebral spines are affected, and occasionally necrosis is observed in these structures.

The bursitis in the early stage consists of a distension of the supraspinous bursa with a clear, straw-colored, viscid exudate. The distended bursa gives rise to a rounded, puffy swelling of the withers. The bursa may pouch out from under the ligamentum nuchae and under the trapezius muscle or upward between the lateral portions of the ligament. The swelling, therefore, may be dorsal, unilateral, or bilateral, depending on the arrangement of the bursal sacs and the direction which they follow between the tissue layers. Some of the pockets are not attached to the ligamentum nuchae. It is an exudative process from the beginning, with considerable amounts of coagulated fibrin accumulating as it proceeds, but no true suppuration or secondary infection occurs until the bursa ruptures or is opened.

Prophylaxis: It is reasonable to keep horses separate from *Brucella*-infected cattle, and horses with discharging fistulous withers from cattle.

Treatment: The earlier treatment is instituted, the better the prognosis. In some of the early cases, the bursa can be enucleated with fair chances of success. The protracted treatment required in long-standing cases often exceeds the value of the animal. *Brucella* vaccines have not proved helpful.

Treatment is essentially one of the surgical drainage, which may be facilitated by the use of streptokinase-like preparations. The number and extent of the openings will depend on the ramifications of the bursal sacs. Radical surgery is undesirable, but the removal of necrotic bone and ligament is usually necessary. The administration of full doses of streptomycin (℞ 54) for several days before and after surgery is regarded as useful. The standard operating procedure for atlantal bursitis is more universally successful than for complicated cases of supraspinous bursitis.

Oxytetracycline may be given IV, IM (℞ 25) and orally (℞ 29). It may also be applied locally. In some cases, iodine therapy appears to be of considerable benefit, possibly due to its action against *A. bovis*.

ARTHRITIS AND RELATED DISORDERS (SM. AN.)

Inflammatory disorders of the joints are common in dogs, but rare in cats. Several distinct types of arthritis are described in human medicine, but their counterparts in animals are not nearly as well defined. Rheumatoid arthritis, as seen in man, does not occur in small animals. Traumatic arthritis occurs as a sequela of direct injury to a joint. The exudate is serous or, if bacteria are present, fibrinous or purulent. Septic arthritis may cause erosion of the articular surfaces and extreme pain on movement of the joint. One of the most common arthritides in the dog is that associated with congenital dysplasia of the hip. Osteoarthritis, or degenerative arthritis, is commonly observed in dogs and is usually associated with advancing age.

OSTEOARTHRITIS

Osteoarthritis is frequently seen in dogs and is characterized by proliferative and degenerative changes in the affected joint.

Etiology: The cause of osteoarthritis is not completely understood, but the normal aging processes are thought to be contributory. It frequently follows trauma. Osteoarthritis of the hip joint may result from luxation, congenital subluxation or an unstable joint. Osteoarthritis of the knee joint may result from previous ligament injuries. Vascular disturbances, metabolic disorders and hormonal imbalances have been suspected. Obesity may be a predisposing factor.

Clinical Findings: Destruction of the articular cartilage occurs in degenerative osteoarthritis. It may be eroded or pitted and may even disappear. Osseous deposition occurs within the joint and as bone proliferation (lipping) at the edges of the joint.

The hip and knee joints are most frequently affected. Slowly developing lameness is the outstanding sign. Pain of varying degrees is always present. Stiffness on arising is common, but this usually lessens with movement. Crepitus may be present and atrophy of associated muscles may occur.

Diagnosis: The onset is insidious, the course progressive. Although frequently associated with advancing age, osteoarthritis is common in certain of the larger breeds (Boxers, Collies, Great Danes) which often show premature senility. It may occur in young dogs following trauma or in dogs with congenital abnormalities of the joints. Radiography is the most valuable diagnostic aid. Radiographs of affected joints reveal varying degrees of proliferative and degenerative changes. There may be a disproportion between X-ray findings and the signs of the disease.

Treatment: Acetylsalicylic acid (℞ 588) is the drug of choice for symptomatic relief of pain. Corticosteroids (℞ 154) have proved useful, but should not be used indiscriminately. Phenylbutazone (℞ 150) has also been recommended. Intra-articular injections of certain corticosteroids (℞ 159) may be beneficial in selected cases. Weight reduction should be attempted if obesity is present. Warm, dry quarters should be provided. Other forms of treatment include the use of heat pads or heat lamps, gentle massage of the affected joints and ultrasonic therapy.

SUPPURATIVE ARTHRITIS
(Septic arthritis)

This condition is usually caused by the introduction of infection into a joint by trauma. The affected joint is swollen, hot and painful, and the body temperature is elevated. Marked lameness is present. Examination may disclose a wound leading into the joint. A discharge composed of pus and synovial fluid may be present. Pus in the joint cavity may have a lytic effect on the articular cartilage.

Aspiration of pus may be attempted and if unsuccessful, surgical drainage of the joint may be necessary. The pus may be cultured and antibiotic sensitivity tests performed. Appropriate antibiotics should be used locally as well as systemically. Intrasynovial injection of corticosteroids (℞ 159) together with antibiotics often aids in shortening the acute inflammatory phase.

BURSITIS

Trauma to the area of a bursa is the usual cause of this condition. The most common site in dogs is over the elbow prominence. Serous bursitis occurs more frequently in the very large breeds, particularly Great Danes, Irish Wolfhounds and Saint Bernards. The weight of these dogs, coupled with the manner in which they customarily lie down, may be contributory. It is seen occasionally in other breeds, such as German Shepherd Dogs and Bloodhounds.

Clinical Findings: A soft to firm swelling occurs at the level of the olecranon process. Palpation reveals very little pain except in those instances where the bursa has become infected. The bursal effusion is usually serous. If continued trauma can be eliminated, recovery may occur spontaneously.

The condition usually recurs in the larger breeds and eventually becomes chronic. In chronic bursitis, the endothelial lining of the bursa degenerates and the bursal wall becomes thickened and fibrous. In cases of long standing, the skin over the center of the bursal swelling occasionally becomes eroded and develops into a typical indolent decubital ulcer.

Treatment: The fluid should be aspirated and, if infection is suspected, a cultural examination of the effusion should be made. If infection is present, an antibiotic (℞ 38) should be injected directly into the bursa. In the absence of infection, aspiration of the bursa and injection of corticosteroids (℞ 159, 176) may be beneficial.

In all cases of bursitis, prevention of further trauma to the affected site is essential. Protective, padded bandages may be applied. Mattresses or suitable bedding should be provided.

Surgical removal of the bursal sac may be indicated if it is large, unsightly and chronically affected. Superficial bursae are not essential and may be safely excised. However, deep bursae are important to function and, moreover, may communicate with a joint.

SPONDYLITIS

Spondylitis denotes inflammation of the vertebral body characterized by destructive changes. Cats are less commonly affected, however it has been reported in patients with hypervitaminosis A. Although trauma and infection must be considered as contributing factors, the etiology is unknown. Spondylitis occurs in all regions of the vertebral column. The destructive changes may involve the end plate the intervertebral disk as well as the vertebral body. Bone proliferation will be provided by layers of the bone cortex.

Clinical Findings: Pain is the most common sign. The onset may be sudden. It may be difficult to localize the sensitive area accurately. Affected animals are reluctant to move, and they resent being handled or picked up. The gait usually is stilted and lameness suggestive of a nerve deficit may develop in the hind legs. Pressure on the spinous process of the affected vertebrae will cause the animal to wince. In those with acute pain, the back is arched and constipation may be a complicating factor as well as rapid weight loss. As the disease progresses, resulting in increased spinal ankylosis, the signs often subside.

Diagnosis and Treatment: Radiography is the most useful diagnostic aid. The predominant lesion is a lytic focus in the vertebral body. Involvement of the disk will result in narrowing of the disk space. Bone proliferation irregularly occurs. Soft tissue swelling is sometimes noted.

Acetylsalicylic acid (℞ 588), corticosteroids (℞ 154) and phenylbutazone (℞ 150) may be used to alleviate discomfort. Warm, dry quarters should be provided and constipation should be prevented. Ascorbic acid (℞ 597), anabolic steroids (℞ 157) and calcium gluconate (℞ 586) are occasionally beneficial. Antibiotic or sulfonamide therapy is useful in many cases.

SPONDYLOSIS DEFORMANS

A degenerative condition involving the vertebrae characterized by the development of osteophytes at the ends and near the ventral border of the vertebra. Degenerative arthropathy may occur at the articular processes. The disease usually occurs as a chronic progressive disease of older dogs. It may occur in all breeds, but is particularly noted in the larger breeds of working or sporting dogs. Ventral protrusion of the nucleus pulposus associated with changes in the annulus fibrosus is one of the known causes of spondylosis.

The majority of dogs with spondylosis deformans reveal no clinical signs. Signs will develop in association with injury or trauma to the ankylosing new bone. Pain becomes evident and affected dogs are reluctant to move with characteristic freedom.

Radiographically the osteophytes have sloping smooth ventral or lateral surfaces which blend with the cortex of the vertebral body. The disk spaces are of normal width. One or several pairs of vertebral bodies may be involved. Treatment is indicated only in the event of pain. Acetylsalicylic acid alone (℞ 588) or in conjunction with cortisone is beneficial. Anabolic steroids and calcium may hasten the repair of fractures involving the osteophytes.

PATELLAR LUXATION

A partial or complete dislocation of the patella, most commonly seen in dogs and horses and occasionally in cattle. Small breeds of dogs are more frequently affected than the larger breeds. Dorsal and lateral luxations of the patella are also encountered in horses, the dorsal displacement being most common. It is particularly prevalent in ponies, where it often occurs as a bilateral affliction in the first few months of life. In other breeds of horses, it appears most often as a unilateral condition during the first 2 or 3 years of life. It is often congenital because of malalignment of the limb but may be acquired due to ligamentous strain or muscular weakness.

In the dog, intermittent or recurrent luxations are characterized by the animal appearing normal one minute and carrying a hind limb the next. No pain is evidenced and palpation is not resented. Lameness is marked if attempts are made to use the leg. The luxation is usually medial, the stifle being adducted and the hock rotated outward. The affected limb has a "pigeon toed" appearance. The patella can usually be replaced with little difficulty by applying gentle pressure when the stifle joint is fully extended. Persistent luxations cause continuous lameness or abnormal gaits. Rotation of the tibia on the longitudinal axis and bowing of the distal end of the femur and proximal end of the tibia are commonly noticed on radiographs of dogs affected with congenital patellar ectopia. Lateral luxation is infrequent and usually the result of severe trauma. Bilateral luxation is rare and is evidenced by difficulty in standing, and walking with a hopping movement.

Dorsal luxations in the horse may be momentary, recurrent or complete. The stifle and hock joints are fully extended and the fetlock is flexed. The anterior wall of the hoof rests on the ground, so that the entire plantar surface of the hoof is visible from the rear. If forced to walk, the animal will drag the hoof along the ground. The first few times luxation occurs, the horse usually exhibits signs of varying degrees of pain, particularly in cases of complete luxation. Backing is extremely difficult or impossible. In cattle the gait disturbance is not as well defined as in the horse.

In all cases the treatment is surgical.

RUPTURE OF THE CRUCIATE LIGAMENTS

In dogs, this is a common serious derangement of the stifle joint. The anterior (cranial) cruciate ligament is more commonly ruptured than is the caudal (posterior) ligament. Rupture of one or both of these may be accompanied by rupture of the medial collateral ligament, and commonly also by medial meniscal damage.

Osteoarthritis may predispose to or follow rupture of the cranial cruciate ligament. Patellar luxation may contribute to the development of the osteoarthritis.

Chronic lameness involving the stifle joint with distension of the joint capsule is characteristic. Instability of the joint can be demonstrated by exerting pressure on the head of the fibula with the limb held in semiflexion. Inward rotation of the tibia should be prevented while general forward pressure is applied. Cranial displacement of the tibia by thumb pressures indicates rupture of the cranial cruciate ligament.

Surgical treatment, replacing the anterior cruciate ligament with skin or fascia, is the method of choice. The damaged medial meniscus is usually removed. The prognosis is good providing osteoarthritis is not severe.

In large animals, the cranial (anterior) cruciate ligament is ruptured more commonly than the caudal (posterior) cruciate ligament. In many cases, the medial collateral ligament of the femoro-tibial joint is also ruptured or damaged. Bulls are more commonly affected than other large animals. The injury commonly occurs when the bull is hit by another bull on the lateral side of one stifle joint while breeding a cow. Severe mechanical stresses in horses may also rupture these ligaments. Occasionally the same effect results from fracture of the tibial spine instead of ligamentous rupture. Severe lameness is evident, often accompanied by sound of crepitation when the animal walks. Distension of the femoro-patellar pouch is present between the patellar ligaments.

Motion between the femur and tibia can usually be produced by a quick pull on the top of the tibia and then release. When the tibia is released it will often slide forward to produce a typical "drawer" movement. These movements are diagnostic. Rupture of the medial collateral ligament is checked by applying pressure from the outside of the stifle joint and pulling outward on the foot. If opening of the joint can be produced on the medial side, one can assume that the medial collateral ligament is ruptured. The injury must be differentiated from fractures of the femur and tibia.

Replacement of the anterior cruciate ligament with a piece of skin has been done successfully in cattle but not in horses. Success in treatment has also been obtained in bulls by immobilization of the affected limb in a modified Thomas splint for a 6-week period. Prognosis is unfavorable because usually there is damage to the medial meniscus in addition to the ligamentous tearing. Arthritic changes are often irreversible.

CANINE HIP DYSPLASIA

A disease of the hip joints which occurs in young dogs of the large breeds. The abnormality may vary from slightly poor conformation to complete dislocation of the femoral head and acetabulum. Since the condition is not detectable at birth, there is objection to the use of the term congenital. Some of the predisposing factors may be present at birth but as yet these have not been identified. The disease is considered to be polygenic and the occurrence can be lowered by selective mating of dogs with normal hips, and breeding of affected animals is to be discouraged. Environment influences manifestation of the defect.

At birth the hip joints appear normal, both physically and radiographically. The maintenance of sound hip joints, both in shape and form, depends upon full congruous contact between the femoral head and the acetabulum. Dysplasia begins to develop shortly after birth if the femoral head fails to maintain full contact in the acetabulum. At this time, the femoral head and most of the acetabulum are still cartilaginous and the shapes of these 2 parts are easily changed if stresses are increased. Joint looseness is caused by an inherited lack of strength and the related supporting tissues (muscles, tendons, ligaments, and joint capsule). When varying degrees of displacement occur between the femoral head and acetabulum, it is known as subluxation if there is a partial separation, or luxation if the femoral head is dislocated entirely out of the acetabulum. Degenerative joint disease (remodelling change in cartilage and bone) occurs later as a secondary complication of the dysplasia.

Incidence is highest in heavy and rapidly growing pups of the large breeds. At least 50% of most large breeds are affected, but the condition seldom occurs in dogs maturing at less than 25 lb. It has not been reported in Greyhounds, which have from one-half to twice as much pelvic muscle mass, comparatively, as other dogs. The quantity and strength of the supporting pelvic muscle mass is thought to be the key to preventing the disease. There is no sex difference in occurrence. Hip dysplasia also occurs in chickens, cats, pigs, horses and cattle, as well as in man and the dog.

Clinical Findings: Dogs which develop hip dysplasia give evidence of pain in the hip joints starting at 5 to 6 months. This is due to remodelling changes associated with microfractures and tearing of the attachment of the ligaments, tendons and capsule of the hip joint. By 9 to 11 months the joints stabilize and the gait of most dogs is sound if work and exercise are limited. The disease is best diagnosed radiographically and can be detected by 5½ to 6 months of age or even earlier in well-defined cases. Proper positioning for radiographs is extremely important. In most instances, the lesion is bilateral and consists of a shallow acetabulum with a loosely fitting, flattened femoral head. If the changes are mild, the dog may be past a year of age before the disease is recognizable radiographically.

Treatment: Pain relieving drugs (℞ 588) or corticosteroids (e.g., ℞ 154) are useful during the period of joint remodelling. Femoral head resection brings relief if pain persists after the dog is mature. Surgery is usually not needed if exercise and work are restricted.

RUPTURE OF THE ACHILLES TENDON

A partial or complete disruption in the continuity of the gastrocnemius and superficial flexor tendons. It may be the result of trauma from automobile accidents, laceration from mowing machinery or wire, extreme stress during a race or hunt, or occasionally, a severe local infection. Lacerations may occur anywhere along the course of the tendon; however, ruptures are usually at the point of insertions on the calcaneus, in connection with an avulsive fracture of the tuber calcis, or at the juncture of the muscle and tendon.

Rupture of the gastrocnemius muscle (q.v., p. 584) produces a gait identical to that of rupture of the Achilles tendon. Careful examination, both radiographic and by palpation, should be carried out to determine the exact nature of the lesion and the possibility of bone involvement.

There is a characteristic alteration of the stance and gait. The animal is no longer able to stand or walk on the toes of the affected limb. The degree of flexion of the hock is increased without concurrent flexion of the stifle. The plantar surface of the metatarsus may touch the ground. On palpation, the tendon is flaccid and sometimes swollen. Pain is not an outstanding sign.

The treatment is surgical. Ruptures with sharp division of the tendon are easier to repair than indistinct lacerations. After surgical repair, the leg should be immobilized in a slightly flexed position for at least 3 weeks.

DYSTROPHIES ASSOCIATED WITH CALCIUM, PHOSPHORUS AND VITAMIN D

The principal causes of osteodystrophies are deficiencies or imbalances of dietary calcium, phosphorus and vitamin D. Their interrelationships are not easily defined and there may be absolute or relative (i.e., conditioned or secondary) deficiencies of any of the three. Deficiencies must be assessed in relation to availability and growth rate.

An absolute or relative deficiency of calcium causes hyperparathyroidism in all species with the development of osteoporosis (lack of bone) or osteodystrophia fibrosa or both. Calcium deficiency does not cause rickets or osteomalacia in mammals. Absolute deficiency is less common than deficiency conditioned by excess phosphorus.

Phosphorus deficiency causes rickets in growing animals and osteomalacia in adults. There may also be osteoporosis. Phosphorus deficiency occurs mainly in grazing ruminants, being rare in animals consuming grain or meat. Poor appetite and growth rate, pica and abnormalities of gait occur. Decreased milk yield, infertility and, occasionally, anemia (*see* POST-PARTURIENT HEMOGLOBINURIA, p. 514) are seen in cows.

Vitamin D deficiency is the classic cause of rickets (growing animals) and osteomalacia (adults). It usually results from insufficient exposure of animals or their feed to sunshine. It is influenced by deficiencies or imbalances of calcium and phosphorus; high levels of carotene in green feed may also produce signs of vitamin-D deficiency.

More than one disease due to deficiencies and imbalances of calcium, phosphorus and vitamin D may coincide in an animal or group of animals, and descriptions of such cases as pure deficiencies have confused the interpretation of naturally occurring osteodystrophies. At present the diagnosis of these osteodystrophies is based on histologic criteria. Bone ash and serum analyses will generally not allow separation of the various diseases.

There are 2 major hindrances to the logical understanding of the pathogenesis of these osteodystrophies. First, since vitamin D acts to facilitate intestinal absorption of calcium, and in deficiency rickets or osteomalacia occur, it is reasoned that calcium deficiency should mimic vitamin D deficiency. Second, since phosphorus deficiency causes rickets and osteomalacia, conditions characterized by failure of mineralization, then calcium deficiency should cause defects in calcification. In answer to the first point it is suggested that vitamin D is necessary for maturation and mineralizability of bone matrix as well as for transfer of calcium across cell membranes, and that the failure of matrix maturation is important in the development of the diseases. With regard to the second point, the initial step in the mineralization process is concentration of phosphate in the matrix, and calcium, which has a great avidity for phosphate, is then deposited even in the deficiency state. Accordingly, phosphorus deficiency retards mineralization but calcium deficiency does not because calcium is transferred from serum to bone even to the extent of producing tetany.

NUTRITIONAL HYPERPARATHYROIDISM
(Osteodystrophia fibrosa)

A condition affecting all species caused by an absolute or conditioned deficiency of calcium. The lesions and signs are related to excess parathyroid hormone secreted in response to declining serum ionized calcium. In general, growing animals are most severely affected because their requirement for calcium is high, and fast growth rates increase the likelihood of development of disease. This is the most important osteodystrophy of domesticated animals. A large proportion of the osteodystrophies diagnosed as rickets and osteomalacia and osteogenesis imperfecta of kittens and puppies are manifestations of nutritional hyperparathyroidism.

Etiology: Diets consisting solely of grain or grain products (for horses, pigs, cattle and sheep), meat or liver (for dogs and cats) or fruit (for monkeys) cause the condition.

Clinical Findings and Diagnosis: The combination of lameness, bone deformities and osteoporosis in young animals should suggest the diagnosis. In kittens and puppies lethargy, obscure lameness, progressing to posterior weakness and hyperextension, and deviation of carpal-metacarpal and tarsal-metatarsal joints may occur within 6 weeks of weaning onto meat diet. Kyphosis, scoliosis, pelvic deformities and fractures, both macroscopic and microscopic, can also occur within this period if no source of calcium is added to the meat. The onset of signs may be delayed, but not prevented, in kittens fed milk. Milk supplies calcium but also phosphorus, and insufficient milk is consumed to balance these minerals.

Radiographs show generalized demineralization. Growth plates are normal unless rickets is superimposed. Bones are soft, may be deformed and often brown due to subperiosteal hemorrhage. Parathyroid hyperplasia is sometimes recognizable grossly; usually microscopic examination is required. Serum calcium is often normal in response to the parathyroid hormone, therefore analyses may be uninformative. Fibrous tissue proliferation in the marrow with irregular trabeculae showing microfractures and osteoclasia are characteristic of the condition. All bones are affected; fast-growing bones most severely. Treated and adult animals may have deformed bones with normal strength and ash. Pelvic deformities in such animals can cause obstipation or dystocia.

In pigs, lameness and bone deformities occur. Fractures of subchondral bone lead to collapse of articular cartilage. In severe cases bones of the head, including the mandibles, are enlarged. Fractures of long bones may occur and some cases of slipped upper femoral epiphyses and femoral neck fractures in sows may be manifestations of nutritional hyperparathyroidism.

The overt effect of nutritional hyperparathyroidism is well-known in horses as *bran disease, millers' disease* and *big-head*. Many of the obscure lamenesses of horses have been attributed to nutritional hyperparathyroidism and such cases probably constitute a more important effect of the disease. The pathologic changes are similar to those in other species with the provisos that the bones of the head are particularly affected in severe cases and that gross or microscopic fractures of sub-chondral bone, with consequent degeneration of articular cartilage and tearing of ligaments from periosteal attachments, are a dominant influence on the clinical signs.

Nutritional hyperparathyroidism is rarely reported in cattle and sheep. The disease may occur under feed-lot systems. Marrow fibroplasia is not a feature of the condition in these species. Osteoporosis is the dominant lesion.

Treatment: Calcium given orally, and rest are required. Vitamin D without calcium is contraindicated because it stimulates bone resorption. Phosphorus, along with calcium, as in bonemeal, or milk, is contraindicated because it hinders the establishment of optimum Ca:P ratios. Injectable solutions containing calcium should be reserved for immediate treatment of severe cases in small animals. Parenteral treatment is not an efficient means of supplying calcium in bulk.

A cheap and efficient treatment is calcium carbonate, which contains 40% calcium by weight. Half a gram of $CaCO_3$/100 gm of meat corrects the Ca:P ratio and provides sufficient calcium for kittens and puppies. Meat may also be deficient in vitamins A and D and in iodine.

Generalizations regarding requirements for calcium are less meaningful in horses and pigs than in small animals. Factors as growth rate and activity should be considered. Recommendations for 1.2% calcium and 1% phosphorus in the ration have been made recently. These levels are nearly twice "normal levels" and will be influenced by the type and therefore the quantity of feed consumed. Zinc at 100 ppm is required with the high calcium.

Horses require a Ca:P ration of around 1.4:1 and the ratio is apparently quite critical. Calcium should constitute about 0.4 to 0.6% of the ration.

RICKETS

A disease of growing animals characterized by interference with mineralization, and consequently with normal resorption, of growth-plate cartilage and interference with mineralization of bone matrix. Rapidly growing plates in rapidly growing bones are most severely affected.

Etiology: Deficient intake or absorption or both of vitamin D or phosphorus or both are most often causative. In housed animals vitamin D deficiency is important; pastured animals are more likely to be phosphorus-deficient. Increased requirements for vitamin D as occurs, for example, in uremia or inherited biochemical defects, should be considered in rachitic animals on apparently normal diets. Failure to absorb vitamin D may be caused by steatorrhea.

Clinical Findings and Diagnosis: In severe cases there is lameness associated with enlargement of the ends of fast-growing bones, and deformities of the weight-bearing long bones. Lameness and enlargement of the joints is more commonly due to chronic polyarthritis. Radiographs of rachitic bones show wide growth plates and demineralization. Demineralization in nutritional hyperparathyroidism is accompanied by normal growth plates.

Widening of the growth plate due to failure to resorb cartilage is not pathognomonic of rickets. Any factor which interferes with normal metaphyseal vascularization or sinusoidal invasion of cartilage or both may cause widening of the plate. This point should be considered when interpreting radiographs of single joints. Rachitic animals usually have a Ca:P (mg%) product of less than 30. This is a useful aid to diagnosis if serum is collected before any therapy or dietary change has been instituted. Confirmation of the diagnosis in mild cases requires histologic examination including study of active growth plates and of bone matrix in normal tissue. Since rachitic animals may be hypocalcemic, histologic changes of hyperparathyroidism may be present.

Treatment: Accurate diagnosis is imperative as vitamin D without calcium exacerbates those conditions associated with nutritional hyperparathyroidism. Rickets caused by simple deficiencies of vitamin D or phosphorus should be treated according to standard nutritional recommendations after detailed consideration and, if possible, analysis, of the existing diet. Secondary deficiencies require correction of the underlying cause.

OSTEOMALACIA
(Adult rickets)

A failure of mineralization of bone matrix resulting in softening of bone. Osteomalacia occurs in adult animals after bone growth has ceased. Osteomalacia has become a general term applied to soft bones without regard to the reason for the softness. The term is used correctly to describe an osteodystrophy of particular histologic appearance and is not synonymous with soft bones *per se.* According to this usage, osteomalacia is common only in areas of endemic phosphorus deficiency—most of the osteodystrophies diagnosed as osteomalacia are cases of osteodystrophia fibrosa.

Etiology: The same general comments made for rickets apply to osteomalacia.

Clinical Findings and Diagnosis: There is a herd history of low fertility, poor growth, pica, spontaneous fractures and maybe anemia. Serum phosphate is low. Radiographs may show a reduction of bone density but even fractured bones sometimes show no evidence of abnormal density and microscopic examination of mineralized bone is required for confirmation of the diagnosis. Affected bones show an increase in the number and width of layers of unmineralized matrix on bone surfaces.

Treatment: Phosphorus supplements should be added to the diet. Specific procedures used will depend on economic and management factors and the magnitude of the problem.

DEGENERATIVE ARTHROPATHY OF CATTLE
(Degenerative joint disease, Osteoarthritis)

A nonspecific condition affecting mainly the hip and stifle joints. The condition is characterized by degeneration of articular cartilage and eburnation of subchondral bone, distension and fibrosis with ossification of the joint capsule, excess synovial fluid and osteophytes.

Etiology: A variety of causes and predisposing factors probably influence the development, age of onset and severity of the condition. Inherited disposition to degenerative arthropathy occurs. Certain conformations, for example straight hocks in beef bulls, are incriminated. Nutritional factors involved in some cases are high-phosphorus, low-calcium rations, which probably influence the strength of subchondral bone. Copper deficiency may also act in a similar way. Theoretically, anything causing degeneration of articular cartilage, which is irreversible, can initiate the sequence leading to degenerative joint disease. The role of infection is unclear. Infectious arthritis in calves usually produces severe changes in the hock but degenerative arthropathy rarely involves this joint.

Clinical Findings and Diagnosis: Young bulls fed for show on high-grain diets may become lame as early as 6 to 12 months but most cases are first noticed at 1 to 2 years. Lameness is of gradual onset usually affecting both hip joints. Stifle involvement in young bulls is rare. Signs progress concomitantly with degeneration of cartilage and development of osteophytes. Lameness to the point of incapacitation, with crepitation of degenerate joints may develop in a few months; however, correlation between pathologic changes and clinical signs is poor. The earliest changes occur on the dorsomedial surface of the femoral head with complementary lesions of the acetabulum. In cows, the stifle joint is mostly affected and the medial condyle of the femur shows the earliest changes. Onset of signs is later than in bulls, usually occurring in adult animals. Since degenerative arthropathy may result from any of several initiating factors no specific diagnostic tests are available. Diagnosis is based on clinical signs and history.

Treatment: Most animals have irreversible changes in the joints by the time the diagnosis is made. Palliative treatment in valuable breeding animals should be influenced by the knowledge that the condition may be inherited. Specific recommendations regarding prevention are impossible. In general the diet should be carefully inspected, analyzed and if necessary corrected. This is especially important in fast-growing animals. Adequate exercise is indicated and overfattening should be avoided.

RENAL RICKETS
(Renal secondary hyperparathyroidism, Osteodystrophia fibrosa, Rubber jaw)

A disease characterized by decalcification of the bones, particularly of the jaws and the head, and associated with chronic renal insufficiency. It is usually seen in older animals with impaired kidney function due to chronic renal insufficiency. The renal lesions cause retention of phosphates which elevates the serum phosphorus with consequent reduction of the serum calcium. The hypocalcemia induces parathyroid hyperplasia and hyperfunction which leads to a mobilization of calcium from the bones.

In advanced cases the bones of the jaw are soft and pliable. Fractures may occur during routine examination. The teeth are usually loose. The blood urea nitrogen level is elevated. There is usually acidosis, polydipsia and polyuria, and anemia is not uncommon. The appetite is poor and gastrointestinal signs, particularly vomiting, may be prominent.

Chronic nephritis is usually present. The kidneys are small and firm. The surface is rough and the parenchyma is largely replaced with fibrous tissue. The parathyroid glands are enlarged and hyperplastic. This secondary hyperparathyroidism leads to resorption of bone and its replacement by fibrous connective tissue. These changes are particularly striking in the bones of the jaws and head.

There is no satisfactory treatment. The use of fluids, alkalizing agents, calcium preparations and attention to the diet may delay the inevitable end—death from renal failure (*see* CHRONIC RENAL FAILURE, p. 855).

HYPERTROPHIC PULMONARY OSTEOARTHROPATHY
(Marie's disease)

A condition in which osseous changes are associated with intrathoracic lesions. It has occurred in conjunction with tuberculosis, bronchopneumonia and pulmonary abscesses. More commonly it is associated with primary or metastatic pulmonary neoplasms. It has occurred in association with granulomatous processes in the thoracic cavity and esophageal tumors related to *Spirocerca lupi* infection (q.v., p. 689). The disease has been reported in the horse, ox, sheep, deer, lion, dog, cat, fowl and mink.

Etiology: The cause is unknown. One theory holds that the osseous lesions result from deficient oxygenation of the tissues. Another suggestion is that an increased peripheral blood flow is responsible, possibly resulting from vagal nerve reflexes.

Clinical Findings: Affected animals usually are presented with the history that their legs have become progressively thicker during the past few months. The thickening may or may not cause lameness. There is sometimes a history of chronic cough with some dyspnea, especially after mild exercise, together with the obvious leg abnormalities. The appetite and eliminations usually are normal. In advanced cases, there may be a stilted gait or even an inability to stand. There may be pain on movement or palpation of the affected bones. The thickened limbs are warm and the pulse often is easily palpable in the affected areas.

Lesions: The long bones of the limbs (radius, ulna, tibia, fibula, metacarpals, metatarsals and phalanges) are most frequently involved. The affected bones are either partially or completely covered with uneven and irregular periosteal new bone deposits that are external to the cortex. They are in the form of smooth, irregular, diffuse deposits overlying the shafts of the bones, or they may have a verrucose appearance. The joint surfaces are not involved, but there may be a swelling of the soft tissue around the joints and a thickening of the joint capsules. The osseous deposits do not form, or are very slight, in areas where tendons move in close proximity to the bone.

Diagnosis: This is based on physical examination and characteristic radiographic findings. Radiographs reveal extensive proliferation of new bone along the shafts of the long bones and outside the normal cortex. These deformities are almost always bilateral. This bilateral distribution of new bone, together with the absence of cortical erosion, helps to distinguish the condition from bone neoplasia. Radiographs of the chest may disclose a lesion in the lung, mediastinum, pleura or thoracic esophagus.

Treatment: There is no specific treatment for the condition, although treatment of the intrathoracic lesion by surgery or chemotherapy may lead to a regression of the bone changes.

OSTEOCHONDROSIS
(Osteochondritis)

Osteochondrosis is a noninfectious disease characterized by aseptic bone necrosis (osteosis) and attempted regeneration occurring at several sites in the developing skeleton.

The use of the term "osteochondritis", originally employed, is a misnomer, because inflammation is not seen. Bone growth centers, especially those vulnerable to traction or compression, are subject to the disease, especially in rapidly growing animals.

The following forms of osteochondrosis may be distinguished:

1. **Osteochondrosis** or **avulsion of the tibial tuberosity** (the human counterpart of which is Osgood-Schlatter disease) is seen in young dogs, particularly in the large breeds.
2. **Osteochondrosis of the proximal femoral epiphysis** (the human counterpart of which is Legg-Perthes disease) occurs principally in small and medium-sized breeds of dogs. This condition sometimes is mistaken for hip dysplasia. A true fracture of the growth plate is rare in the dog, but common in rapidly growing young swine.

3. **Osteochondrosis of the head of the humerus** (unilateral) occurs in dogs at the age of 2 to 3 weeks.
4. **Osteochondritis dissecans** involves a small area of cartilage, the subchondral plate, and small fragments of underlying bone that separate from the articular surface of either proximal surface of the humerus or the femoral condyle. The piece of articular cartilage may lie loosely in the joint space ("joint mouse"). This lesion is fairly common in the giant breeds of dogs and in pigs.

Etiology: In most instances, the cause of separation or disruption of the tissue is not well established. Obstruction of the circulation and trauma from either excessive traction or compression are thought to be the immediate causes. The tissues, however, may already be weakened by such conditions as lack of minerals, lowered oxygen tension, hormonal imbalance, vitamin deficiency and metabolic disease.

Clinical Findings: Lameness is the outstanding sign. Evidence of pain is usually elicited when the affected area (usually unilateral) is manipulated or palpated. If the damage is severe, atrophy of the muscles in the affected area occurs. There may or may not be a history of trauma.

Osteochondrosis is principally a disease of young animals. In the dog it appears from 3 to 10 months of age, and in the horse between 1 and 2 years of age. The onset is relatively slow, and considerable time may elapse between the appearance of the first signs and the presentation of the animal by the owner for examination. Many mild cases probably pass unnoticed.

Diagnosis: History, age and signs are useful, but good radiographic films are essential for a diagnosis. The characteristic lesion is an area of radiolucency, adjacent to a joint or a growth plate. Osteochondrosis may be confused with small fractures, a solitary cyst, or a focal abscess.

Treatment: For the most part, treatment consists of rest and prevention of weight bearing on the affected limb. The disease is self-limiting and lesions usually heal satisfactorily. The prognosis for complete functional recovery should be guarded, but most animals regain satisfactory use of the limb by the time they reach maturity.

In cases of osteochondritis dissecans, the loose fragment (joint mouse) should be removed surgically.

OSTEOMYELITIS

Inflammation of bone, usually caused by pyogenic bacteria.

Etiology: Infection may result from contaminated compound fractures. Orthopedic surgical procedures may result in osteomyelitis if strict asepsis is not observed. Bite wounds are also a common cause. Usual sites are the face and the legs. In the cat, it is frequently seen in the sacral and coccygeal regions as a result of bites. Severe dental disease may also lead to osteomyelitis of the jaw. Hematogenous focus of infection elsewhere in the body is also encountered.

Clinical Findings and Diagnosis: Pain and swelling characterize the early lesion and, if a limb is involved, the adjacent joint may also be swollen. The patient is reluctant to move the affected limb and usually carries it. If the condition is of long standing, discharging sinuses may be present. Fluctuating swellings should be aspirated and their contents cultured bacteriologically. Fever, leukocytosis and increased blood sedimentation rates are common general findings.

Radiographs of typical osteomyelitis reveal a "moth-eaten" appearance of the affected bone, together with sequestration. Certain cases may be difficult to differentiate from bone tumors.

Lesions: Following its introduction into the bone, the infection spreads in the bone marrow and may erupt through the cortex and spread along the bone surface. Necrosis of bone often follows and there may be sequestrum and involucrum formation and the development of sinuses draining pus to the skin surface.

Treatment: This should begin without delay, even before the causative organism has been identified by culture and its antibiotic sensitivity determined. It is customary to start with full therapeutic doses of penicillin (℞ 44, 46) and sufadiazine (℞ 66). Sensitivity tests may indicate the desirability of treatment with broad-spectrum antibiotics (℞ 7, 11, 29). In cases of mycotic infections, amphotericin B has been used with varying success. Chemotherapy should be continued for at least a week after clinical signs have disappeared. Since many antibiotic agents are hindered in their action by tissue debris and pus, enzymatic debriding agents (℞ 571, 572) may be used for local instillation into sinuses leading from the affected bone.

Immobilization may be advisable if the affected part is a leg. Surgical intervention is often required to curette and remove necrotic bone or sequestra. In severe, chronic cases, amputation of the affected part may be necessary.

Hypoproteinemia and dehydration may occur as complications of osteomyelitis. Protein supplements and fluids should then be administered. Suitable supplements of B-complex vitamins should be given to avoid deficiency during long periods of antibiotic therapy.

ABDOMINAL HERNIA

A protrusion of abdominal contents into the subcutis through a natural or abnormal opening in the body wall. Protrusion through the diaphragm is termed diaphragmatic hernia or rupture (q.v., p. 574). Herniation as a result of a severe blow leading to tearing of the abdominal aponeurosis is frequently called a rupture and not a hernia. The best examples of a nontraumatic hernia are the umbilical and inguinal or scrotal hernias, the latter being merely an extension of an inguinal hernia. The term "delayed hernia" is employed to indicate the type of inguinal/scrotal hernia that occurs in mature stallions or bulls.

In cattle, insufficient attention appears to have been paid to the hereditary nature of umbilical hernia. No matter the breed or species, the surgical correction of this transmissible and undesirable characteristic is questionable. However, not all cases of umbilical hernia are caused by a hereditary mechanism. Improper care of the newborn in the form of excessive traction of the oversized fetus and cutting the umbilical cord too close to the abdominal wall are other possible causes.

In the case of scrotal or inguinal hernias in all species (apart from the delayed variety) surgical correction almost invariably involves simultaneous castration. Perineal hernia is encountered mainly in mature dogs and differs from the other types of abdominal hernias in that the peritoneal lining of the hernial sac is either absent or thin and degenerate. Although many factors have been cited, the actual cause of perineal hernia is unknown.

Femoral (crural) hernia is relatively rare in domestic animals, especially in the larger species.

Clinical Findings and Diagnosis: Two types of hernia are recognized: reducible and irreducible. The **reducible type** is characterized by a noninflammatory, painless, soft, elastic, compressible swelling. It may vary in size from time to time. The swelling can be made to disappear by manipulation or by placing the patient in a suitable position. The diagnosis of perineal hernia in the dog is made from the presence of a swelling at the side of the anus or vulva, between the tail base and sciatic tuber. The hernia can usually be reduced more easily if the hind quarters of the animal are elevated.

Irreducible hernias have the same characteristics as reducible ones, except that the contents cannot be returned to the abdominal cavity. This is due either to adhesions between parts of the hernial contents, to narrowing of the ring, or to distension of a loop of intestine. The contents may be incarcerated or strangulated.

Umbilical abscess may be confused with hernia and both are frequently found together, especially in pigs and cattle. Exploratory puncture is sometimes necessary for differentiation. Hematomas may also be confused with hernias. If the area can be reached by rectal palpation, the diagnosis of an inguinal/scrotal hernia can be definitely determined by locating the ring and the contained bowel.

Inguinal hernia in the male pig is common and the process usually extends to the scrotum. In these cases, palpation of the scrotum reveals the characteristic elastic swelling. In the female pig, this defect is invariably accompanied by arrested genital development; such animals are sterile and surgery is indicated only when the size of the process is a threat to the growth of the pig to market weight.

Inguinal hernia in the male foal often resolves spontaneously during the first year of life. For this reason, corrective surgery is not indicated unless the hernia is of such a magnitude that it interferes with the gait of the animal or is strangulated. Strangulated inguinal hernia in stallions is fairly frequent and is characterized by signs of constant and severe abdominal pain. It is readily recognized by rectal palpation. When diagnosed early, the condition often may be relieved by rectal manipulation of the incarcerated intestine with the animal under general anesthesia. If this fails, immediate radical surgery is necessary.

Inguinal hernia is rare in cattle, however, it is sometimes encountered in the male. Surgical correction when carried out to conserve the breeding potential of the bull is not always successful.

Perineal hernia, which may be either unilateral or bilateral, can be surgically corrected. Whether prostatectomy in the mature male dog is indicated at the same time is a matter of debate, although the consensus appears to favor the simultaneous removal of that gland.

Treatment: Umbilical hernias with very small rings may sometimes be corrected by blistering over the site, or injection of saline into the hernial ring, but hernias are usually treated by surgical repair. Advisability and need for treatment vary with the type of hernia and the purpose for which the animal is kept.

DIAPHRAGMATIC HERNIA

A break in the continuity of the diaphragm with a resultant protrusion of abdominal viscera into the thorax.

Etiology: External violence, such as automobile injuries, kicks or falls, is the usual cause. In younger animals it may be congenital and involve the pericardial sac (peritoneopericardial hernia). The tear in the diaphragm may be large or small. It may be in the central tendinous part, the peripheral muscular portion or along the costal attachment. In cattle, the diaphragm adjacent to the reticulum may be weakened by penetrating foreign bodies permitting partial herniation of the reticulum. Abdominal organs which may herniate into the thorax include one or more lobes of the liver, the omentum, intestine, stomach or spleen. A considerable volume of abdominal viscera may gradually herniate through a relatively small tear because of the negative pressure in the thoracic cavity. Adhesions between the abdominal and thoracic viscera are common in long-standing cases. A collection of serous exudate is usually present.

Clinical Findings: Dyspnea with or without cyanosis is the main finding. Incarceration of stomach or intestine may cause signs of obstruction, while cardiac compression may cause signs of heart failure (peritoneopericardial hernia). Lung or heart sounds may be inaudible on auscultation of the chest.

Radiographically, the heart shadow is enlarged and globe-shaped with widening of the shadow at the diaphragmatic pericardial junction (peritoneopericardial hernia). With traumatic hernia the diaphragmatic line is disrupted. Liver, gas-filled loops of intestine, spleen and stomach may be seen in the thoracic cavity. Radiocontrast materials aid in visualizing viscera penetrating the diaphragm. Fluid may obscure radiographic shadows.

Diagnosis and Treatment: Diagnosis is based on history (trauma), clinical signs and radiographic evidence. Other diseases which cause dyspnea must be considered in the differential diagnosis—pneumothorax, hemothorax, hydrothorax, chylothorax, intrathoracic inflammation and neoplasia. Surgical repair is the only treatment.

MYOPATHIES AND RELATED CONDITIONS IN DOMESTIC ANIMALS

The rather limited response of muscle tissue to injury has led to some confusion in the identification and differentiation of myopathies on the basis of their histopathology. Furthermore, the possibility that concurrent and sometimes widely differing lesions in other tissues might have a common etiology has often been overlooked. Recent research has made it possible to study many of the myopathies from the point of view of etiology, not only as separate entities, but as part of much wider syndromes in which, to a greater or lesser degree, changes in other tissues participate.

Myopathies of various kinds have been described in most of the domestic and laboratory animals, under a variety of names, including paralytic myoglobinuria (azoturia), myositis ("tying or cording up") eosinophilic myositis, polymyositis, muscular dystrophy, white muscle disease (WMD), nutritional myopathy (NM), stiff lamb disease, white flesh, fish flesh and waxy degeneration. (It has been suggested that the expression "muscular dystrophy" be reserved for the classic types of purely degenerative heritable myopathies of unknown etiology. Such types are now recognized in certain strains of sheep, chickens, turkeys and mice as well as man. With the exception of the dystrophies occurring in man, these are at present purely of academic interest.)

Associated with some of the myopathies, degenerative changes in other tissues often occur, notably liver necrosis, subcut. and pulmonary edema with exudation into the large serous sacs, and steatitis and other changes in the fat tissues. Disease entities of similar etiology exist in which some of these latter changes predominate or constitute, apparently, the sole pathology, as, for example, in exudative diathesis (q.v., p. 1349) and encephalomalacia (q.v., p., 1353) in the chick, steatitis in the cat and mink (q.v., pp. 580 and 1115), multiple necrotic degeneration (heart, liver, muscle and kidney) in the mouse, dietary liver necrosis in the rat and, perhaps, massive liver necrosis in the sheep.

In addition to structural changes in the various myopathies, chemical changes may be detected in the muscle tissue and in the blood and urine. Lowered levels of muscle creatine are generally observed, with increased sodium and decreased potassium. Blood serum from myopathic animals has been shown to contain decreased levels of alkaline phosphatase and increased levels of lactic dehydrogenase, serum glutamic oxalacetic transaminase, serum creatine phosphokinase and, in some cases, myoglobin. The urine frequently has an increased creatine:creatinine ratio, as a result of increased creatine excretion, and may contain myoglobin.

Many of the myopathies and some of the related conditions listed have been attributed to a deficiency of vitamin E, sometimes induced by the presence of unsaturated fatty acids and other similar-acting substances in the diet. More recent evidence has implicated other dietary constituents, particularly selenium, which is a required element in animal nutrition. When the selenium content of feeds approaches the critical required level, substances that enhance or interfere with selenium metabolism become important. Good examples of these are vitamin E and sulfur.

The interrelations between selenium and vitamin E in metabolism remain obscure. Some myopathies and related conditions respond only to selenium, some only to vitamin E, others to either selenium or vitamin E. While vitamin E cannot satisfy the need for all selenium, it can reduce the amount required to protect against exudative diathesis. The converse is also true. A vitamin-E deficiency in chicks apparently leads to the development of encephalomalacia and muscular dystrophy even in the presence of selenium sufficient to protect against exudative diathesis (on a low-methionine, low-cystine diet). Similarly, selenium cannot replace vitamin E to prevent the sterility and myopathy in some experimental animals (rabbits) nor encephalomalacia in chicks produced by vitamin E-deficient diets. Conversely, a naturally occurring infertility in ewes, sometimes associated with a high incidence of WMD in lambs in the presence of adequate vitamin E responds remarkably to minute supplements of selenium, as does alopecia in rats and primates. The necrotic liver degeneration observed in rats and swine appears to respond to either nutrient.

In general, the disorders covered in this chapter are nutritional, metabolic or congenital derangements. For convenience the myopathies and certain conditions apparently related etiologically have been brought together in this chapter.

AZOTURIA AND TYING-UP IN HORSES
(Cording-up, Myositis)

Tying-up or cording-up is thought to be a mild form of azoturia and therefore to have a similar etiology. The former occurs mainly in light horses, the latter in heavier breeds; both are associated with skeletal myopathy.

Etiology: The cause of these entities is unknown, but as some cases of tying-up apparently respond to selenium-alpha tocopherol therapy it is possible that these substances may be involved. Both conditions are directly associated with forced exercise after a period of rest during which feed has not been restricted.

Clinical Findings: In both tying-up and azoturia the first signs are profuse sweating and rapid pulse followed by stiffness of gait, particularly of the hindquarters, disinclination to move and, in severe cases, myoglobinuria. In azoturia the disease quickly progresses to recumbency, often with nervous signs. Elevated serum glutamic oxalacetic transaminase (SGOT) and creatine phosphokinase (CPK) are useful indications of the extent of muscle damage. The prognosis depends on the extent of the muscle damage and is good for those that remain standing. It is also fairly good for those animals that go down, because of loss of use of their hindquarters, providing that they remain quiet and contented and the pulse returns to normal within 24 hours. However, survivors sometimes suffer from lameness and prolonged or occasionally permanent muscle atrophy.

The prognosis is bad for nervous, restless, recumbent animals that are not quieted by sedatives or tranquilizers and for those that are forced to continue moving after the signs become apparent. It is also bad if after 24 hours the patient shows progressive inability to roll up on its sternum and retain that position. A weak or irregular pulse is a most unfavorable sign.

Treatment: Good management is of first importance. The patient should be kept as quiet as possible from the time that signs are first recognized, and attempts should be made to keep the animal standing. Close attention should be given to the horse's comfort and precautions taken against the development of decubital ulcers. Nervous, restless individuals, or those showing evidence of pain, should be given sedatives such as chloral hydrate (℞ 526) or tranquilizers (℞ 363, 364, 367, 369). If conditions indicate a period of recumbency an oily laxative should be given. Quick-acting purgatives, such as arecoline and physostigmine, should not be used.

When signs are slight, there is no previous history of occurrence and serum enzyme levels are not significantly elevated, moderate tranquilization may be sufficient. More severely affected horses should not be moved but should be provided with on-the-spot shelter. They should be rubbed dry and blanketed according to the weather. Selenium-vitamin E appears to give favorable results in many cases and may be given every 4 to 6 months prophylactically.

WHITE MUSCLE DISEASE
(WMD, Stiff lamb disease, Nutritional myopathy)

A myodegeneration most frequent in calves and lambs whose dams have been fed during gestation or longer on feeds, especially legumes, grown in certain areas. The disease has been recorded in various parts of the U.S.A. and in many other countries. It has been produced experimentally in several species of animals on low-selenium intake. A similar myopathy occurs naturally in goats, deer, foals and dogs but proof of the etiology is lacking.

Etiology: The cause of WMD is not fully understood. It is undoubtedly associated with low levels of selenium in animal tissues, but interfering or lack of enhancing substances, one of which is vitamin E, and another possibly sulfur, are necessary requirements to precipitate the clinical disease.

Clinical Findings: The congenital type may result in heavy mortalities at or within 2 or 3 days of birth, usually with involvement of the myocardium. The delayed type of WMD is associated with cardiac or skeletal muscle involvement, or both, and may be precipitated by vigorous exercise. Affected animals may move stiffly with an arched back and frequently become recumbent. If the condition is severe enough to prevent nursing, death results from starvation. Sometimes there is profuse diarrhea. In chronic cases there may be relaxation of the shoulder girdle and splaying of the toes. With severe cardiac damage death may be sudden. In progressive cardiac failure, dyspnea results. In some areas unthriftiness may be the only sign associated with selenium deficiency.

Lesions: Skeletal muscle lesions are invariably bilaterally symmetrical and may effect isolated or many muscle groups. Grossly, the affected muscle is paler than normal and may show distinct longitudinal striations or a pronounced chalky whiteness. Cardiac lesions occur as well-defined subendocardial plaques, which are often more pronounced in the right ventricle. With heart involvement, pleural, pericardial and peritoneal effusions, together with pulmonary congestion and edema, are not uncommon.

Diagnosis: In lambs, outbreaks of infectious nonsuppurative arthritis produce a clinical picture similar to that of WMD, and sudden deaths from heart failure might be confused with enterotoxemia. The history and necropsy findings, however, are usually quite characteristic. In mild cases and in very young lambs, laboratory studies such as histopathologic examination, estimation of SGOT and CPK levels and urinary creatine:creatinine ratios may be necessary.

Prevention: For the prevention of congenital WMD or WMD occurring within 4 weeks after birth give selenium (ewes 5 mg, cows 15 mg), orally or subcut. 4 weeks before expected parturition.

For the prevention of delayed WMD give lambs 0.5 mg Se and calves 5 mg Se at 2 to 4 weeks of age and repeat twice at monthly intervals. A selenium-vitamin E mixture is advocated in some areas.

Treatment: Lambs and calves may be given sodium selenite-vitamin E in aqueous solution, subcut. at the rate of 0.25 mg selenium per pound of body weight. This may be repeated after 2 weeks, but not to exceed 4 doses. Larger doses are sometimes advocated but approach the toxic level.

MYOPATHIES IN HERBIVORA DUE TO VITAMIN E DEFICIENCY

Evidence has accumulated indicating the occurrence of myopathies in various herbivores, including rabbits, guinea pigs, calves and lambs, when the diet is low in vitamin E. More commonly these myopathies result from interference with the biologic activity of dietary vitamin E by lipid peroxides formed from unsaturated fats or other similar-acting substances. Routine administration of cod-liver oil to pail-fed calves, for example, has caused a high incidence of this type of myopathy. Experimentally, acceleration of avitaminosis E has been induced by the presence in the diet of organic antagonists, such as tri-o-cresyl phosphate, pyridine, o-cresyl succinate, carbon tetrachloride and sodium bisulfite, and by ferric chloride.

Clinical Findings: Signs are frequently lacking and sudden death from heart failure following slight exertion is not uncommon. When degeneration of the skeletal musculature occurs, it may result in weakness of stance, an awkward gait and an inability to rise or walk unaided if the large muscles of the limbs are affected. Acute cases following severe exercise may show a myoglobinuria.

Lesions: Pathologic pictures vary considerably, depending on the intensity and duration of the vitamin E deficiency. Creatinuria and myoglobinuria, as general indicators of muscle damage, are usually present. Mild cases show slight swelling of the muscle fibers and some degree of hyaline degeneration and proliferation of sarcolemmic nuclei. In some severe cases extensive myonecrosis occurs.

Changes also occur in the chemical composition of muscle; usually the potassium content falls and the sodium content rises. These changes are not specific for vitamin E deficiency; they also occur in other myopathies, including those caused by a disturbance of selenium metabolism.

Diagnosis: To differentiate vitamin E deficiency from other myopathies, diagnosis should include evaluation of the vitamin E status of the diet in relation to both sources of the vitamin and the presence of factors—especially cod-liver oil and other unsaturated fats—likely to interfere with its metabolism. Presence of natural or synthetic antioxidants in the diet will reduce the influence of such factors.

Treatment: Where simple vitamin E deficiency is apparent, dietary supplementation with alpha tocopherol or substances rich in this vitamin should be instituted. Minimum dosages have not been established; however, cures have been reported following daily doses of 5 mg alpha tocopherol to rabbits; 500 mg alpha tocopherol, initially, followed by 100 mg on alternate days to lambs; and 600 mg alpha tocopherol acetate initially, followed by daily doses of 200 mg, to calves. When the causative diet contains substances antagonistic to vitamin E, these must be removed. Dry concentrates of vitamins A and D may substitute for cod-liver oil, thus removing a potential source of oxidative damage.

STEATITIS IN CATS
("Yellow-fat" disease)

A disease characterized by a marked inflammation of adipose tissue and the deposition of "ceroid" pigment in the interstices of the adipose cells.

Etiology: It is believed that an overabundance of unsaturated fatty acids in the ration, together with a deficiency of vitamin

E, results in the disposition of "ceroid" pigment in the adipose tissue. Most naturally occurring and experimentally produced cases have had fish, or fish by-products, as all or part of the diet. A more recent report incriminates fish oil as the primary agent.

Clinical Findings and Diagnosis: Affected animals are frequently plump and well fed, usually young, and may be of either sex. They show loss of agility and general unwillingness to move. Resentment is exhibited on palpation of the back or abdomen. In advanced cases, even a light touch will cause pain. Fever is a constant finding and anorexia may be present.

The typical laboratory finding is an elevated leukocyte count, with neutrophilia and sometimes eosinophilia. A biopsy of the subcut. fat shows it to be yellowish brown in color, with a nodular or granular appearance. Microscopic examination reveals severe inflammatory changes and associated ceroid pigment.

Treatment: Elimination of the offending food from the diet is imperative. The administration of vitamin E, in the form of alpha tocopherol, at least 30 mg daily, is necessary. Antibiotics are of doubtful value, in spite of the fever and leukocytosis. Parenteral use of fluids is not advisable unless dehydration exists. Patients should be handled as little as possible.

CARDIAC AND SKELETAL MYOPATHIES AND HEPATOSIS DIAETETICA IN SWINE

There are several specific entities of swine in which muscle degeneration may be very extensive, including **mulberry heart disease** (MHD) and **enzootische herztod** (EH), and others where the degeneration is frequently less conspicuous, including **hepatosis diaetetica** (HD).

Etiology: The causes of MHD and EH are not fully understood but it is widely thought that they are nutritional in origin. HD is definitely associated with diets low in selenium and vitamin E.

Clinical Findings: All 3 conditions have certain characteristics in common; losses tend to occur sporadically, affecting rapidly growing pigs between 6 and 16 weeks of age, and death almost invariably occurs suddenly.

Lesions: In MHD the characteristic lesion is a grossly distended pericardial sac containing straw-colored fluid and fibrin flakes, together with extensive hemorrhage throughout the myocardium. Microscopically, in addition to interstitial hemorrhage, there is usually extensive myocardial necrosis together with fibrinoid thrombi in capillaries. If animals survive for a few days, nervous signs are seen, resulting from focal encephalomalacia.

In EH, which seems to be confined to Europe, there is less pericardial effusion and myocardial hemorrhage than in MHD. Additional lesions are gross pallor of skeletal musculature and degenerative changes in adrenal and thyroid glands.

In HD there is often subcut. edema together with varying amounts of transudate in serous cavities. Fibrin strands adhere to the liver, which has a characteristic mottled appearance caused by irregular foci of parenchymal necrosis and hemorrhage. Focal lesions of myocardial necrosis and, less frequently, skeletal myonecrosis may be apparent.

Prophylaxis and Treatment: As the cause of MHD and EH is not understood a change of diet is suggested. In HD, dietary errors should be corrected and selenium or vitamin E therapy, or both, introduced.

EOSINOPHILIC MYOSITIS IN DOGS

An acute relapsing inflammation of the muscles in dogs. The disease is common in German Shepherd Dogs and affects most frequently the muscles of mastication. The cause is unknown.

Clinical Findings: The onset of the disease is usually abrupt. During an attack, the muscles of mastication swell symmetrically and interfere with drainage from the retrobulbar tissues, producing edema of the conjunctiva, prolapse of the membrana nictitans and exophthalmos. The mouth is held partially open and the animal eats with difficulty. The attacks last from 1 to 3 weeks and are accompanied by a marked eosinophilia. After each attack, the affected muscles become more atrophied. The periods between attacks vary from 3 weeks to 6 months. With each succeeding attack, the severity decreases and the interval between attacks tends to lessen. In the last stages of the disease, involvement of the esophagus produces difficulty in swallowing.

Lesions: During acute attacks, the affected muscles are enlarged and doughy in consistency, dark in color and hemorrhagic with focal pale areas. The regional nodes are enlarged and firm. During early attacks, the lesions are confined to the muscles of mastication; as the attacks continue, additional muscles may become involved. The histologic lesion is an acute inflammatory myositis in which the primary infiltrating cell is the eosinophil. Although the eosinophilic infiltration is usually quite diffuse, the actual muscle involvement is patchy. Frequently, necrotic muscle fibers appear to be the focus of the reaction.

Diagnosis: The periodic nature of the disease and its unusual selectivity for site and breed usually makes diagnosis obvious. Eosinophilia associated with the syndrome can normally be considered diagnostic. If any doubt remains, histologic examination of a muscle biopsy can be used to confirm the diagnosis.

Treatment: The disease is progressive and no therapy has yet been able to alter its recurrent nature and course. The use of the corticosteroids (℞ 140, 154), and ACTH (℞ 139), however, has a marked effect in minimizing the discomfort and muscle swelling during an attack.

EOSINOPHILIC MYOSITIS IN CATTLE

A focal myonecrosis associated with large numbers of eosinophilic granulocytes. The cause is unknown in most instances but the presence of degenerate *Sarcocystis* in the center of some of the necrotic lesions suggests that they may be implicated. This condition is seen at slaughter as focal greenish-gray discolorations in skeletal and occasionally in cardiac musculature.

MISCELLANEOUS MYOPATHIES

Maxillary Myositis of the Horse: A disease of horses resembling azoturia both clinically and pathologically, except that it is inclined to be more enzootic, more chronic in its course and involves more frequently the muscles of mastication and deglutition. Myocarditis is common. The cause is unknown.

Myopathy of Potassium Deficiency: A degeneration of both cardiac and skeletal muscle occurring in rats, rabbits and possibly other species, kept on a potassium-deficient ration. Dosing with sodium salts accelerates the process. The lesions present a picture of diffuse degenerative changes, including hyaline degeneration, accompanied by loss of striation and eventual loss of sarcoplasm. Interstitial edema is evident in the early stages. The addition of potassium to the diet arrests the degenerative changes.

Reversible Metastatic Calcification (Nutritional Calcification): A deposition of calcium salts in the soft tissues, especially in the muscles of the limbs, resulting from an excessive intake of milk. (The condition is similar to "milk drinker's syndrome" in man.) It may occur when show calves are kept for an unusually long time on nurse cows. It is seen also in dogs and other experimental animals kept on high-milk diets, especially when there is some additional calcium intake. The considerable inorganic salt deposits in the muscles cause pain and limit movement. A history of high-calcium (milk) intake will have a bearing on the diagnosis. Withdrawal of the offending diets results in spontaneous reabsorption, although this may take some time.

Congenital Myodysplasia in Calves: An inherited myopathy, the result of a recessive factor, marked by the absence of normal skeletal muscle development and associated with hydrocephalus. Grossly, the large skeletal muscles are undeveloped and light in color, having a yellowish tinge. The cranium shows the characteristic enlargement of hydrocephalus. Microscopically, there is a disarrangement of the normal muscle structure resulting in a tangle of undeveloped muscle fibers and connective tissue. Usually the animals are unable to stand and soon die.

Myopathies from Plant Intoxication: Degeneration of skeletal and cardiac muscles results when cattle and some other animals feed on certain plants. *Karwinskia humboldtiana* (*coyotillo*) and *Cassia* spp. have been incriminated, but other species may also cause damage. There is pallor of severely degenerated muscles. Microscopic lesions consist of hyaline necrosis and granular degeneration. Some blood enzymes are elevated and myoglobinuria may occur. Treatment consists of removal of animals from offending range and supplemental feeding.

Rupture of the Gastrocnemius Muscle in Cattle: An acute myopathy of unknown etiology except that it appears to result from undue stress on the muscle. It sometimes is a sequela to parturient paresis. There is no satisfactory treatment.

Muscle Hyperplasia in Calves and Lambs (Doppellendigkeit, "Double muscle"): A congenital anomaly occasionally occurring in calves and rarely in lambs. The larger muscles are enlarged due to excessive fibers and their outlines show prominently under the skin. The heritable characteristics are not well understood, but evidence suggests that a recessive factor is responsible.

Brown Atrophy of Bovine Muscle (Xanthosis): A brown pigmentation of the skeletal and heart muscles, of unknown etiology, occurring occasionally in debilitated or aged dairy cows. Grossly, the muscles and heart are brown. Microscopically, very minute brown or yellowish granules are visible in these tissues.

Albino Muscle in Cattle: An apparently physiologic anomaly in which all muscles, except the cardiac, diaphragmàtic and coccygeal, appear lighter in color than normal. There is no apparent histologic or functional alteration.

Myocardial Lipidosis: A lesion sometimes encountered upon necropsy of animals which have suffered from debilitating diseases, especially those associated with anemia. The myocardium loses its normal tone, and seen through the endocardium, has a freckled appearance. With appropriate staining, minute and more or less regularly spaced globules of lipid can be demonstrated within the myocardial fibers.

Fatty Infiltration of the Muscle: A hyperplasia of adipose tissue within the skeletal musculature. It may arise following myodegeneration, but usually occurs for no adequately explained reason. In its severest form a whole muscle may be replaced by fatty tissue. A mild form is normally observed in fattened animals. It is only diagnosed at slaughter.

Nonspecific Muscular Degeneration in Dogs may be responsive to vitamin E-selenium therapy. Ascorbic acid orally at 4 mg/lb of body wt daily seems to ameliorate idiopathic muscular soreness.

MYOCLONIA CONGENITA
(Trembles, Shivers, Dancing pigs)

A congenital disease of pigs, cause unknown, manifest at birth or after several days of apparent normalcy by muscle tremor of varying intensity and persistence. Frequently a disease of litters rather than herds, it commonly affects about 40% of a litter. Severe trembling may lead to difficulty in sucking and death. Survivors improve gradually over a period of days or weeks. The signs are most prominent when attempts are made to stand, and may disappear during rest.

While it has been associated with hog-cholera vaccination of pregnant sows this obviously does not explain all cases. Inheritance, viral infection and improper nutrition have all been suggested causes. Probably there is not a single cause.

Diagnosis may be made on the basis of the typical signs in a number of baby pigs in a litter. There is not yet general agreement as to lesions, but vasculitis, spinal hypomyelinogenesis and cerebellar hypoplasia are among those reported. In some instances no lesions were detected.

No treatments are available. Occasionally a sow will give birth to more than one affected litter. There is some reason to believe that particular boars are responsible for spread of an etiogenic agent.

SPLAYLEGS IN PIGLETS
(Spraddled legs)

A condition of newborn pigs in which the rear legs are spread apart or extended forward. The front legs may also be spread. Affected piglets usually learn to stand within a few days. The incidence within and between litters varies widely and tends to be higher in Landrace than other breeds. The immediate cause of spreading is weakness of the adductor muscles relative to the abductors. Affected pigs are susceptible to overlaying, starvation and chilling because of poor mobility.

Etiology: It has been shown experimentally that the incidence of splaylegs can be increased or decreased by selective breeding. However, hereditary factors are not the only ones involved. The general nutrition of the sow, and particularly the choline and vitamin E levels, may influence the incidence. In addition, a predisposition to splaylegs is exacerbated by slippery floors and cold conditions.

Diagnosis: The clinical signs are distinctive. In differential diagnosis, infections involving the nervous system such as Ontario encephalitis or bacterial meningitis should be considered.

Prophylaxis and Treatment: The herdsman should provide bedding to prevent slipping, protect the pigs from injury by the sow and ensure adequate sucking. If the affected pigs cannot stand, even on bedding, it is advisable to tape the rear legs together above the hocks with a loose figure 8 of tape for 2 to 4 days. Genetic factors and nutritional deficiencies should be considered in prevention, but the immediate step is to avoid the birth of pigs onto slippery floors.

ADRENOCORTICAL AND RELATED THERAPY

The quantitatively and physiologically important steroid hormones secreted by vertebrate adrenal cortices are (1) the glucocorticoids—cortisol (hydrocortisone), corticosterone and cortisone, (2) the mineralocorticoids—aldosterone and desoxycorticosterone (DOC) and (3) steroids with androgenic activity. In addition to cortisol, cortisone and desoxycorticosterone, a large number of steroids are produced commercially whose biologic activities mimic the effects of the endogenously secreted steroids.

Pharmacology of the adrenal cortical steroids: 1. The androgenic steroids are of rare clinical importance only when enzymatic deficiencies of the adrenal cortex diminish cortisol secretion. Under these circumstances a secondary increase in pituitary corticotropin secretion formulates the production of abnormally large quantities of adrenal androgens resulting in the **adrenogenital syndrome.**

2. The secretion of mineralocorticoids permits the body to maintain normal renal secretion or retention of sodium and potassium. Excessive doses stimulate sodium retention by the kidney and excretion of potassium into urine. With continued administration of the mineralocorticoids, the animal with normal cardiovascular function "escapes" from the sodium-retaining effects, but potassium excretion continues at a high level. Aldosterone is the primary mineralocorticoid secreted by the adrenal cortex, but is expensive to produce. The commercially available mineralocorticoids are the acetate ester of desoxycorticosterone, DOCA (desoxycorticosterone acetate) and the 9 alpha-fluoro derivative of cortison, fludrocortisone.

3. Glucocorticoids have profound effects on the metabolism of carbohydrate and proteins and also influence lipid metabolism. Pharmacologically their primary effects are characterized by (1) gluconeogenesis, a shift in the amino-acid pool of the skeletal muscle mass and of the stomach and intestine from protein synthesis into the production of carbohydrate, (2) a significant reduction in lymphoid tissue and lymphocyte formation and (3) inhibition or diminution of all aspects of both the acute and chronic phases of inflammation.

The structural and functional integrity of the adrenal cortex is maintained by the secretion of pituitary corticotropin (ACTH). Increasing concentrations of glucocorticoids in plasma tend to suppress the secretion of ACTH by a direct inhibitory action on the pituitary gland as well as by inhibition of the hypothalamic neurohormone (corticotropin-releasing hormone) which stimulates ACTH production. Long-term administration of glucocorticoids thereby depress the hypothalamo-pituitary system and leads to functional and in some species morphologic atrophy of the adrenal cortex.

Corticosteroids produce other less tangible effects such as stimulation of appetite, increased activity and a sense of "well-being". The last term is borrowed from human medicine, but seems applicable to animals, because of their improvement in behavior and interest in surroundings. Finally, the endogenously produced glucocorticoids, such as cortisol, possess a significant degree of mineralocorticoid activity.

Chemistry and pharmacology of derivatives of cortisol and cortisone: The primary goals in the production of new steroids have been first, to formulate drugs with more potent anti-inflammatory effects, which second, may minimize the sodium-retaining effects of the glucocorticoids and third, may also diminish the toxic side-effects inherent in the glucocorticoid or anti-inflammatory responses. The first and second goals have been achieved but the third remains elusive. The first major modification was the formation of the Δ-1 steroids by inserting a double bond between carbons 1 and 2 of the steroid A ring to produce prednisolone from cortisol and prednisone from cortisone. For a comparable degree of sodium-retaining effects, the anti-inflammatory responses of the Δ-1 steroids are 3- to 5-fold greater than for the parent compounds. A second modification was halogenation of the endogenous steroid. When a fluorine atom is placed on carbon 9 in the alpha position, both glucocorticoid and mineralocorticoid activity, but particularly the latter, are markedly enhanced. This compound, fludrocortisone is used for its anti-inflammatory activity only in topical preparations.

Halogenation in the 9-alpha position of prednisolone and additionally inserting an hydroxyl or methyl group on carbon 16 produces the most marked pharmacologic changes. For example, 16-alpha-methyl-9-alpha-fluoroprednisolone, dexamethasone, has anti-inflammatory activity which is 15- to 25-fold greater than that of cortisol and additionally is virtually devoid of mineralocorticoid activity. Other halogenated steroids with this pattern of activity include triamcinolone and betamethasone.

The enhanced glucocorticoid and anti-inflammatory activity of these derivatives results from a more avid binding of cytoplasmic receptor protein molecules. Additionally, the 9 alpha-fluoro compounds undergo a much slower metabolic transformation. The esterification of the hormones with fatty acids, for example, triamcinolone acetonide or betamethasone valerate, alters the distribution of the steroids permitting them a longer sojourn in the body and hence longer lasting biologic effects.

Clinical Application: Although they do not produce primary cures, corticosteroids are used for the treatment of a wide variety of diseases. The hormones usually control signs or check pathologic changes and, in certain instances, gain enough time to permit other drugs to be used to cure the disease. They should be used in the early stages, before irreversible changes have taken place. When steroids are used in the presence of frank or suspected infection, vigorous anti-infective therapy must be included as part of the therapeutic regimen. In view of the breadth of action of these hormones, their clinical application should be restricted to defined routes of administration in the various diseases. Their use should be safeguarded by carefully established diagnoses, since unwanted side effects may complicate indiscriminate use. The 2 principal uses of corticosteroids are (1) for their anti-inflammatory and anti-allergic actions in a wide range of disorders, (2) for treatment of several metabolic conditions, including stress disease, in which they may possibly act as replacement therapy.

Route of Administration: Because corticosteroids can produce powerful hormonal effects, it is preferable, whenever possible, to use them locally rather than systemically. The routes of administration include (1) external application for treatment of ear, skin and eye diseases; (2) local injection, such as subconjunctival, intra-articular, periarticular and infiltration of tissue; (3) the oral route and (4) parenteral administration, via the IV or IM route.

External uses: For treatment of ear, skin, or superficial eye lesions, hydrocortisone, prednisolone, betamethasone or dexamethasone, combined with antibiotics, may be used as ointments or lotions. All phases of inflammation, including hyperemia, cellular exudation, swelling and pain, are markedly and often rapidly reduced. The anti-inflammatory action is at the cell level and systemic absorption of corticosteroids has not been reported except where a compound of higher potency has been used. Skin diseases which respond to corticosteroid treatment include dermatitis, alopecia, and certain forms of eczema. Corticosteroids may be combined with antibiotics for the treatment of pustular dermatitis. Miliary eczema in cats, acanthosis nigricans in dogs and nonspecific skin diseases reportedly respond to corticosteroid treatment. However, relapses sometimes occur, particularly if treatment is stopped suddenly. When extensive lesions are present, systemic use of steroids may be required.

Many eye conditions respond to topical use of these substances, e.g., conjunctivitis, keratitis, panophthalmia, periodic ophthalmia and certain post surgical conditions. The use of corticosteroids for the treatment of superficial corneal ulcers should be initiated only when the lesion no longer stains with fluorescein. Concurrent antibiotic therapy is essential whenever infection is present or impending. The subconjunctival injection of corticosteroids is sometimes used.

Intra- or periarticular use: Several corticosteroids, preferably with antibiotics, are used for cases in which single accessible joints or tendons are affected. Tendon and muscle injuries have been treated with corticosteroids, with variable results. Conditions which have been treated successfully with corticosteroids include arthritis, bursitis, periostitis, synovitis, tendonitis, tenosynovitis and navicular disease in horses. The most spectacular effect of intra-articular injection occurs when it is used in early stages of serous arthritis when changes are not yet irreversible. Corticosteroids and an appropriate antibiotic are also used in suppurative arthritis such as "joint ill" in foals. Where possible, identification of the causal organism from synovial fluid is advised. The parenteral use of an antibiotic is also recommended. Certain forms of stifle lameness in dogs may respond to intra-articular corticosteroid treatment. Periarticular infiltration of shoulder and hip joints in dogs has produced good results.

Subconjunctival use: The subconjunctival route of administration is of special value where the deeper structures of the eye are involved. Hydrocortisone, prednisolone, dexamethasone or betamethasone in combination with appropriate antibiotics may be used. The volume of injection is approximately 0.5 ml. More than one injection may be necessary.

Systemic use: Systemic administration has proved valuable in the treatment of bovine ketosis, general arthritic conditions and dermatitis. Clinicians frequently use corticosteroids as supplementary therapy in conditions such as infection, shock, acute mastitis, pneumonia, selected cases of colitis in dogs, eosinophilic myositis, burns, feline enteritis, rodent ulcers (cats), laminitis and following surgery. In most cases, it is essential (a) to use antimicrobial or chemotherapeutic substances or specific sera for treating the primary cause, (b) to discontinue the steroid therapy gradually and (c) to maintain use of the specific antimicrobial therapy for at least 24 hours after the corticosteroid drug administration has been discontinued.

The IV injection of corticosteroids is primarily reserved for emergencies, such as postoperative or traumatic shock, or other severe and acute stress syndromes. Only the IV forms of corticosteroid preparations should be used by this route.

Clinical Evaluation of Steroid Therapy: Most corticosteroids have a wide scope of action and versatility. Because of this versatility and such factors as differences in stages of disease in different animals, it is difficult to devise controlled studies for clinical evaluation of these substances. The glucogenic response can be assessed by changes in the blood sugar and liver glycogen levels. This enables the clinician to determine which preparation has the most powerful glyconeogenic property. However, for other effects the appreciation of these drugs rests largely on individual assessment and experience of clinicians. In general, clinical observation would indicate that steroids are useful in the treatment of:

1. **Inflammatory conditions** of many types affecting the skin, ears, joints, tendons, muscles and sometimes the eyes. In small animals, 80 to 90% of nonspecific skin conditions appear to improve with steroid treatment. While relapses do occur, the risk of their occurrence may be reduced by gradual withdrawal of the corticoid used.

2. **Mastitis:** Although some intramammary preparations contain corticosteroids, controlled trials have shown that there is little, if any, advantage in the inclusion of these substances in such formulations. The parenteral use of corticosteroids in certain acute cases of mastitis as adjunctive treatment to appropriate antibiotic therapy can be advantageous.

3. **Bovine ketosis:** The rationale for using corticosteroids in ketosis is based on their ability to stimulate gluconeogenesis and to promote other nonspecific effects such as stimulating the appetite. On parenteral administration, the steroids produce a rise in blood glucose within a few hours. The acetone content of the urine declines and milk production rises to normal, usually within 48 hours depending on the duration of the disease and the milk yield. Several corticosteroids including betamethasone, dexamethasone, prednisolone, prednisone and trimethyl prednisolone have been used. Blood sugar levels are increased to a varying degree after injection of one of the

preparations. Most glucose levels are back to preinjection levels within 38 to 72 hours, except where betamethasone is used as the alcohol suspension, after which increased blood glucose levels have been maintained for 3 to 4 days. Because of the complex nature of ketosis, however, corticosteroids may not always afford specific treatment. In treating any condition with these substances, the nutritional status of the animal should also be considered and full use should be made of supportive treatment with other agents as indicated.

4. **Miscellaneous conditions** embracing a wide variety of otherwise unrelated diseases, usually those assumed to be caused or exacerbated by "stress", have been treated with corticosteroids either alone or in combination with other drugs. Clinical impressions of such treatment are generally favorable, but further critical evaluation is required. In infections, corticosteroids should only be used in conjunction with antibiotics or other chemotherapeutic agents. The latter should be continued for a few days after discontinuing corticosteroid administration.

Contraindications: In veterinary medicine, corticosteroids are used chiefly to treat acute conditions for a limited period; consequently side effects, although known, are infrequent and easily reversed by withdrawing the drug. However, contraindications do exist. The most important contraindications include: (1) acute infections, unless full doses of antimicrobial drugs are included; (2) degenerative eye diseases; (3) dendritic ulcers of the cornea; (4) diabetes mellitus; (5) pregnancy toxemia in sheep; (6) chronic diseases in which tissue changes are irreversible; (7) corneal opacity due to infectious canine hepatitis and (8) cardiac and terminal stages of nephritis.

Dosage: There is no fixed dosage, but usually 1 to 5 mg of cortisone per pound of body weight is recommended for small animals (*see* TABLE for relative potencies). Following remission of the signs of disease the dose is gradually reduced until the drug is either discontinued or a satisfactory maintenance dose is found. This particularly applies to the treatment of chronic skin conditions and to certain forms of lameness. Some dogs and cats have been kept free of signs for long periods on small doses given only once a week.

For the current information on indications, methods of administration, duration of treatment and the precautions to be observed, the reader is advised to follow the recommendations supplied by the manufacturers of the various steroid products available.

RELATIVE BIOLOGIC POTENCIES IN MILLIGRAM
EQUIVALENTS OF COMMONLY USED CORTICOSTEROIDS*

Corticosteroid	Potency	
	Anti-inflammatory	Mineralocorticoid (Na-Retaining)
Hydrocortisone*.................	1	1
Cortisone.................	0.8	0.8
Desoxycorticosterone.................	None	30-50
Fludrocortisone.................	10	125
Prednisone.................	4-5	0.8
Prednisolone.................	4-5	0.8
Methylprednisolone.................	5-6	0.5
Triamcinolone.................	4-5	None or Na-excreting
Dexamethasone.................	30	None or Na-excreting
Betamethasone.................	30	None or Na-excreting

* Hydrocortisone expressed as unity.

Adrenocorticotropic Hormone (ACTH): This hormone is obtained from the anterior lobe of the pituitary gland. It acts by stimulating the adrenal cortex to produce corticosteroids. Its effects are, therefore, similar to, although slower, than those of cortisone acetate. Its use has been superseded by the corticosteroids. Small doses of ACTH are sometimes used following sudden cessation of corticosteroid therapy to prevent withdrawal signs.

NEOPLASMS

NEOPLASMS

Excessive, autonomous new growths of tissue, persisting with or without their original stimuli. The term neoplasm does not apply to compensatory hyperplasias, proliferative infectious diseases, cysts, malformations or inflammatory and reparative masses. Viruses are being incriminated as causal agents in an increasing number of animal neoplasms. Circumstantial and experimental evidence indicates, however, that the origin of some are related to parasites, chemical carcinogens, irradiation, trauma and mechanical transplantation of cells.

Diagnosis: For each domestic species, patterns and types of neoplasms most frequently encountered are well known. Some tumors are consistently malignant. When doubt exists as to the malignancy of a neoplasm, a clue can sometimes be obtained on clinical grounds since those that are large, deeply ulcerated, fixed to the skin over a wide zone and those that are multiple, tend to be malignant. A reliable decision as to whether the mass is truly neoplastic and, if so, whether it is malignant can be obtained on histologic examination. A pathologist can often suggest a likely prognosis should the tumor have been surgically removed. Ideally, punch or wedge biopsies of neoplasms should be histologically examined so that the surgeon's procedures can be guided by knowledge of the tumor type; practically, it is seldom possible to acquire this information fast enough and in veterinary practice it is usual for the surgeon to remove all of the tumor on the primary exposure.

Exfoliative cytology of body cavity fluids or solid tumor masses is occasionally useful in establishing a diagnosis and cytological examination of the blood may identify reticuloendothelial tumors.

Treatment: Many tumors in animals, including most of those arising from visceral organs, are beyond the range of present therapeutic methods by the time a diagnosis of neoplasia can be made. Skin tumors lend themselves to therapy because they are likely to be recognized early and because they are accessible. Many of them do not become malignant and even malignant ones tend to metastasize late in the disease process.

Surgery is the preferred therapy for all tumors, although it should be recognized that bovine cutaneous papillomas and genital fibropapillomas, canine oral papillomas and genital fibropapillomas, canine oral papillomas and venereal tumors, and feline cutaneous fibromas will spontaneously regress in 30 to 90 days. X-ray therapy is useful in selected cases and is used most often in flat infiltrating skin tumors of epithelial origin under circumstances which would not allow adequate skin coverage following surgical removal. It can be used most successfully on basal cell tumors, perianal adenomas, hemangiomas, some papillomas and transmissible venereal tumors. X-ray therapy is not likely to be effective in the treatment of malignant sarcomas and melanotic or deep-seated tumors.

Hormonal chemotherapy in dogs will achieve temporary reduction in the size of perianal gland tumors (estrogen) and mammary tumors (androgen), but may cause blood dyscrasias on prolonged or high use levels. Several of the chemical therapeutic agents used in man have been found to have similar, and at least temporary, beneficial effects on cancerous lesions of domestic animals.

Although medicinal therapy may effect a complete cure in the animal with neoplasia, the usual response will be remission with recurrence in 6 months to 2 years.

NEOPLASMS OF SMALL ANIMALS

The highest incidence of neoplasia in dogs and cats appears after the animals are 5 years old. Boxers have a higher incidence of neoplasia than the general dog population. Benign tumors usually grow slowly, appear as round or ovoid masses, are well encapsulated and exert their harmful effect on the host by occupying space or mechanically interfering with other tissues in the body. Malignant tumors are seen in all sizes and shapes, invade and destroy normal tissue and are usually disseminated through the blood stream or lymphatics (metastasis). Carcinomas, tumors of epithelial origin, usually spread first by means of the lymphatics and later enter the blood stream and become widely disseminated throughout the body. Sarcomas, tumors derived from mesenchymal tissue, usually spread directly via the blood stream. Variations from these generalities will be pointed out in the following text, which will deal only with the more common neoplasms found in each organ system. (*See also* DERMOID, p. 208.)

TUMORS OF THE SKIN

Histiocytomas are single or multiple nodules found in the skin of dogs under 2 years of age. They most frequently are found on the legs and the feet. Grossly they are 1 to 2 cm in diameter and are often ulcerated. The cut surface is pale gray with minute red stippling. Microscopically, histiocytomas are composed of dense accumulations of round cells with ovoid or indented nuclei that have indistinct cytoplasmic borders and many mitotic features. These tumors do not metastasize, but the ulcerated nodules may become infected in which case surgical excision is the treatment of choice. Spontaneous regression may occur 3 to 4 weeks after the tumors develop if they are not excised.

Mast-cell tumors are most commonly found as single or multiple nodules on the posterior half of the body, particularly on the scrotum and the limbs. Grossly, they are usually small nodules located within the dermis. Frequently the overlying skin is ulcerated. The cut surface is gray with no visible capsule. Impression smears of the tumor, stained with Wright's stain, will show typical mast cells with dark-blue cytoplasmic granules and a round nucleus. Microscopically it is composed of cords and sheets of mast cells with varying numbers of eosinophils scattered throughout the lesion. The tumors infiltrate locally with occasional metastasis to the draining lymph node. There is a strong tendency for these tumors to recur locally, making wide excision a necessity in surgical removal. It is reported that the use of corticosteroids will help control mast cell tumors when they are widespread.

Occasionally, mast-cell tumors become systemic in both dogs and cats. The liver, spleen and lymph nodes are packed with mast cells and circulating mast cells may be visible on a peripheral blood smear. It is not known whether systemic mast cell tumors represent metastases from primary skin tumors or are of multicentric origin within the reticuloendothelial system. There is no known treatment for this systemic form.

Papillomas are very common skin tumors in aging dogs and occur as single and multiple projecting nodules, most commonly found around the head, feet and mouth (see ORAL PAPILLOMATOSIS, p. 108 and PAPILLOMATOSIS, p. 243).

Squamous-cell carcinomas may arise from the skin but are most frequently located near body orifices. Grossly, they have a broad base with an ulcerated surface which extends downward into the underlying tissue. The cut surface is pink or pink-gray in color. Microscopically, they are composed of large polygonal cells resembling squamous epithelium. The cells form sheets and cords as they infiltrate the dermis and subcutis. Frequently these cells form clusters which contain keratin in their center. These structures are recognized as "epithelial pearls". Squamous-cell carcinomas are highly invasive and destructive. They metastasize readily to the regional lymph nodes and there is no effective treatment. The prognosis is poor.

A peculiar form of this tumor occurs on the ear tips of cats. It is generally considered to result from the solar radiation. The tumor develops slowly on the tip of the ear but has all the biologic properties and the histologic appearance of other squamous-cell carcinomas. Early amputation of the pinna of the ear is required to prevent the spread of this tumor.

Basal-cell carcinomas occur as small nodular growths in the skin, usually on the anterior half of the body. This tumor arises from the undifferentiated basal layer of cells in the epidermis. Grossly, these small spherical nodules may or may not be pedunculated and they frequently ulcerate. The cut surface is firm, gray and lobulated. Microscopically, basal-cell carcinoma in dogs is composed of undifferentiated basal cells which occur in a ribbon pattern or have a stellate appearance within the dermis. In cats, the neoplastic cells are usually arranged in solid sheets or small nests of cells. Basal-cell carcinomas do not metastasize but infiltrate locally. Wide excision is necessary to prevent recurrence.

Tumors of the perianal gland arise from the modified sebaceous glands normally present around the circumference of the anus, at the base of the tail and in the preputial skin. Male dogs are more commonly affected than females and the tumor usually occurs in the older age groups. Grossly, the tumors appear as smooth, spherical masses in the subcutis; often they ulcerate and bleed. The cut surface is tan in color, has a definite capsule and a firm rubbery lobulated surface. Microscopically, polyhedral eosinophilic cells densely clustered in an expanding mass are observed. The tumor is usually benign and grows slowly. A rare malignant form of this tumor is a nonprojecting mass most easily detected by rectal palpation. Adenocarcinomas of the perianal gland metastasize readily to the iliac and sublumbar lymph nodes which may obstruct the colon as it enters the pelvic canal. Partial control of the benign form of the tumor can be achieved by the use of stilbestrol. Hormone treatment is particularly useful in controlling the bleeding which accompanies ulceration of these tumors. Definitive treatment requires surgical excision of the tumor.

Melanomas are common tumors found in the skin, oral cavity and scrotum. Grossly, they appear as solitary, small raised nodules which may or may not be ulcerated. The cut surface is often visibly black. Microscopically, melanomas are composed of immature elongate cells which usually contain melanin granules in their cytoplasm. The cells form whorls, sheets and small packets. The tumors may metastasize early via the lymphatics and they should always be considered potentially malignant, regardless of the size of the primary nodule. Early wide excision of the primary nodule is essential.

Smooth, firm, ovoid cysts are commonly found in the skin and subcutis of dogs. Often a small communication exists between the lumen of the cyst and the skin surface through which drainage of the cyst contents occurs. Grossly, the cysts contain either pale-yellow, curdy exudate or dry, crumbly, brown material. Microscopically, this material is composed of keratin, necrotic debris and inflammatory cells if the cyst wall has been ruptured. The cysts are **hair matrix tumors** (benign), **keratoacanthomas** (benign), or **epidermal inclusion cysts** (nonneoplastic), depending on the kind of epithelial cells forming the cyst wall. Since cells are continually shed into the cyst lumen, expression of the cyst contents only provides temporary relief. Frequently, the wall of the cyst is ruptured while trying to express its contents, allowing the contents to escape. This produces an intense inflammatory reaction resulting in persistent purulent drainage from the area. Consequently, regardless of the type of cyst, surgical excision of the entire cyst is the treatment of choice.

TUMORS OF THE VASCULAR SYSTEM

Hemangiomas usually are seen as a single mass in the subcutis, often on the limbs or in the spleen. Grossly, the tumor in the subcutis is a soft, spongy, encapsulated mass which has a dark-red cut surface that oozes blood. In the spleen this tumor is circumscribed, dark red-black and when cut, oozes red-black fluid. Microscopically, the tumor is composed of a spongy mass of thin-walled vascular spaces lined with low-lying flat endothelium. Hemangiomas are slow-growing tumors. They do not metastasize and surgical excision is curative.

Hemangioendothelioma, the malignant counterpart of the hemangioma, may also occur in the skin but is usually found in the spleen or liver. Grossly, in the spleen this tumor may reach a size of 15 to 20 cm in diameter and contains large areas of clotted blood due to infarction. Microscopically (excluding areas of infarction and necrosis), the tumor is composed of large immature endothelial cells which form ill-defined vascular channels. This tumor grows rapidly and metastasizes early. If splenectomy can be performed before metastasis has occurred, it may be curative. Thorough examination of the abdominal viscera and a chest X-ray should be performed in conjunction with splenectomy.

TUMORS OF THE RESPIRATORY TRACT

Adenocarcinomas of the nasal cavity arise from nasal epithelium in both dogs and cats. These tumors are destructive and invasive. Radiographically they are seen as a dense mass filling the nasal cavity on the affected site. Grossly, the tumor appears as a reddened, rough, ulcerated, bleeding mass occupying the nasal cavity, frequently causing purulent discharge from the nares. Microscopically, it is composed of invading cords of columnar epithelium, some of which may form mucus-secreting glands. The tumor grows primarily by local invasion and is destructive to the normal structures of the nasal cavity. There is no satisfactory treatment.

Adenocarcinomas of the lung may arise from the alveolar cells lining the alveoli or from the epithelial cells lining bronchi and bronchioles. Consequently this tumor is often known as a **bronchioalveolar cell carcinoma**. If squamous metaplasia occurs within the tumor, it is then identified as a **bronchogenic carcinoma**. Regardless of the type of tumor, adenocarcinomas in the lung are yellow-gray in color and may be seen as multiple small nodules or as a single large mass within the lung. The cut surface of the nodules is yellow and may contain mucus-filled cysts. The animal is usually in extremis before extensive metastases occur. Microscopically, depending on the origin of the cells, the tumor nodules are composed of sheets of cells or poorly formed acini. Adenocarcinomas of the lung grow rapidly and secondary metastases may shower the lungs with numerous smaller nodules. Metastasis to the bronchial lymph nodes is frequent. This tumor usually spreads before the diagnosis is made; consequently, there is no known effective treatment and the prognosis is poor.

TUMORS OF THE GASTROINTESTINAL TRACT
(*See also* TUMORS OF MUSCLE, p. 602.)

Adenocarcinomas may occur anywhere in the digestive tract from the stomach to the rectum. They arise from the mucosa and infiltrate the muscularis. Grossly, they are invariably recognized by a large mucosal ulcer that has a raised, thickened, umbilicate margin. The cut surface of the nonulcerated portion of the tumor, which has a firm, gray appearance, can be seen occupying the zone between the serosa and the mucosa. Adenocarcinomas that involve the large and small intestine grow in an annular fashion and produce constriction of the gut, with subsequent partial obstruction. Microscopically, the tumor is composed of irregular, poorly formed glands with extensive fibrous stroma surrounding them. These tumors are locally invasive and metastasize to the draining lymph node. Occasionally, the tumor may become implanted on the peritoneal surface of the abdominal cavity and will appear as numerous tiny nodules. Early resection of the tumor can be curative.

Adenocarcinoma of pancreatic acinar cells occurs infrequently and may arise in any portion of the pancreas. Grossly, it is usually seen as a small, firm, white nodule in the parenchyma of the gland. Microscopically, it is composed of large polyhedral cells arranged in irregular acinar formation. This tumor metastasizes very early, first to the liver, then to other organs, frequently as numerous small, gray nodules throughout the abdominal cavity on the mesentery, omentum and peritoneum. The widespread metastases are often conspicuous and the primary nodule in the pancreas overlooked. If the tumor is detected prior to metastasis, partial pancreatectomy can be curative.

Tumors of the islet cells of the pancreas are usually functional. Due to their insulin production, clinical signs of hypoglycemia (ataxia, weakness, convulsions, fainting) aid in their diagnosis. Grossly, the tumor appears as single or multiple, firm white nodules in the pancreas. Microscopically, groups of islet cells form a slowly expanding mass within the gland. This tumor is almost always benign and, if partial pancreatectomy is performed, it can be expected to be curative. The rare adenocarcinoma of islet cells metastasizes via the lymphatics to the regional lymph nodes and the liver. Extreme care should be taken when performing partial pancreatectomy not to damage pancreatic ducts leading to the duodenum. A thorough visual and tactile search for additional small nodules in the pancreas should be made at the time of surgery.

TUMORS OF CONNECTIVE TISSUE

Fibromas may occur anywhere but are most commonly found in the subcutis and the wall of the vagina. Grossly, they are usually circumscribed, firm spherical nodules with a rubbery pearl-gray surface. Microscopically, fibromas are composed of broad bundles of mature fibroblasts which produce appreciable amounts of collagen. Surgical removal is the treatment of choice.

Fibrosarcomas most commonly arise in the mammary glands, on the limbs and around the head. Grossly, they are irregularly shaped, poorly encapsulated, lobulated, white fleshy masses. The cut surface is usually gray and may have blotchy zones of red and yellow, representing hemorrhage and necrosis, respectively. Microscopically, the tumor is composed of spindle-shaped cells arranged in irregular whorls with little evidence of collagen production. These tumors expand rapidly by infiltrative growth. They are late to metastasize, but when metastasis occurs, it is widespread. Early complete surgical excision is the only means of treatment. This is often difficult due to the infiltrative nature of the tumor.

Lipomas are common in old dogs and occur as single or multiple nodules in the subcutis of the back, sternum and abdomen. Grossly, they are usually well-defined spherical or lobulated masses which look like normal fat on the cut surface. Microscopically, the tumor cells are indistinguishable from normal fat cells. These tumors grow slowly and need only be removed when they mechanically interfere with normal structures.

Liposarcomas are very rare in dogs and cats. These tumors are poorly defined masses that grow by infiltration rather than by metastasis. Their biologic behavior is similar to that of a fibrosarcoma.

Hemangiopericytomas occur in the skin and subcutis and are found almost exclusively in dogs. They are most often found in the subcutis of the trunk and on the extremities near joints. Grossly, they are poorly encapsulated, often infiltrating between the fascial planes and muscle bundles of the limbs. The tumor is mottled gray and has a firm consistency. The microscopic pattern is variable but is usually a collection of elongate cells arranged in short interlacing bundles or in a whorled pattern around small vascular spaces. Hemangiopericytomas spread primarily by infiltration and have a strong tendency to recur following surgical removal. Because of this tendency to recur, it is recommended that, when the tumor occurs on a limb, amputation rather than local excision be performed. Hemangiopericytomas are similar in many respects to the much less common neurofibroma.

TUMORS OF MUSCLE

Leiomyomas are benign and arise from smooth muscle cells. They are most frequently found in the gastrointestinal tract, uterus and vagina. These tumors usually form a single, large, spherical mass that has a smooth, translucent gray surface. Although these tumors may reach considerable size, the cut surface appears avascular. Microscopically, the tumor mass is composed of spindle-shaped cells with elongate blunt-ended nuclei arranged in irregular broad fasciculi. Leiomyomas grow slowly by expansion and exhibit little tendency to infiltrate locally. The malignant form of the tumor, **leiomyosarcoma,** appears in the same locations as the benign counterpart, but metastasizes readily to the regional lymph nodes. Complete surgical excision is usually curative.

Rhabdomyomas are very rare in dogs and cats. They arise from striated muscle and should all be considered potentially malignant. Histologically, the cells are similar to those of a fibrosarcoma except that cross-striations can be visualized in the cytoplasm thereby identifying the cells as arising from striated muscle.

TUMORS OF CARTILAGE

Tumors derived from cartilage are most often found as part of a mixed mammary tumor in dogs. A relatively frequent tumor in cats, it usually involves the ribs, pelvis and sternebrae. Grossly, chondromas appear as single masses of varying size. The cut surface is translucent blue-gray and frequently contains red-brown areas of necrosis. Microscopically, the cells in the benign tumor closely resemble mature hyaline cartilage, with peripheral collections of immature chondrocytes. Chondromas and the malignant counterpart, chondrosarcomas, grow primarily by expansion. All tumors arising from cartilage should be considered potentially malignant regardless of their histologic appearance. Consequently, radical excision is the treatment of choice.

Osteosarcomas, frequent in dogs, particularly the giant breeds, usually form a large mass projecting from the cortex of the affected bone. The ribs, limbs and lungs are the most common site. On the limbs, this neoplasm is usually located in the metaphysis of long bones. These tumors are firm and may contain spicules of mature bone or cartilage. They destroy normal bone and stimulate periosteal proliferation by their presence, thus producing the characteristic radiographic "sunburst" effect. Microscopically, the tumor cells are quite pleomorphic in appearance and may produce mature bone spicules, immature bone spicules, cartilage and fibrous connective tissue. Osteosarcomas are very invasive locally and they metastasize readily, particularly to the lungs. Early amputation is necessary when the tumor is located on a limb. This tumor always carries a poor prognosis.

TUMORS OF THE LIVER

Hepatomas are infrequent in dogs and are most often recognized at necropsy. Grossly, these tumors are large, ill-defined, spherical masses that are separated from normal liver tissue by a thin, distinct capsule. They are soft and usually protrude above the surface of the liver. The cut surface is usually yellow-gray and often has irregular zones of dark-red hemorrhage. Microscopically, the tumor cells appear very similar to normal liver cells, but they form solid sheets of cells without the orderly cord arrangement of normal liver. Central veins, portal triads and bile ducts are absent. The tumors grow by local expansion. Secondary metastases may occur within the liver, causing numerous, smaller, ill-defined spherical masses. Extrahepatic metastases are rare. Surgical removal of a single liver lobe, when feasible, may be curative.

Bile duct **carcinomas** arise from the epithelial cells lining the bile duct and usually form a single large mass frequently with secondary extrahepatic metastases. Grossly, they usually form a spherical, nonlobulated, poorly encapsulated mass. The cut surface is gray-white and firm. Microscopically, the tumor cells form incomplete and poorly defined bile ducts which may contain mucin. Besides being locally infiltrative, they metastasize readily to the regional lymph nodes and abdominal viscera. There is no effective treatment.

TUMORS OF THE KIDNEY

Adenocarcinomas of the kidney are usually seen as a unilateral mass arising from the renal tubular epithelium. Grossly, the mass is spherical, white and yellow with deep-red striae visible on the cut surface. It is well demarcated from normal kidney parenchyma although a visible capsule may not be present. Microscopically, the tumor cells form incomplete tubules amidst varying amounts of fibrous connective tissue. Adenocarcinomas metastasize early and one-third of the time there will be tumor in the opposite kidney by the time the diagnosis is made. The primary lesion grows by expansion in the affected kidney and may metastasize to the regional lymph nodes. Early diagnosis of the tumor in a single kidney and the removal of that kidney may be curative.

Embryonal nephroma arises from the metanephros and is composed of multipotent, undifferentiated, vestigial renal tissue. It is unilateral, rare in dogs and cats, and is detected in young animals usually under a year of age. Grossly, the tumor is large, encapsulated and may fill most of the abdomen. The cut surface is divided into many lobules by connective tissue stroma and is soft, fleshy and white-gray in color. Fluid-filled cysts of varying size may be visible on the cut surface. A small zone resembling kidney tissue can usually be found compressed along one border of the tumor. Microscopically, the tumor cells may form tubules, incomplete glomeruli, connective tissue, cartilage and bone, illustrating the primitive tissue from which this tumor arises. Surgical removal in the absence of metastases is curative even when the tumor has reached immense size.

Transitional cell carcinomas arise from the transitional epithelium in the urinary tract. They are found in the renal pelvis, ureter, bladder or urethra. Grossly, they appear as broad-based pedunculated masses which are ulcerated and friable on the luminal surface. The cut surface is gray to yellow, firm and often blotched with red. Microscopically, the tumor cells may form acini or they may undergo patchy areas of squamous metaplasia. Transitional cell carcinomas metastasize early to the regional lymph nodes and are locally invasive. Surgical removal is generally impossible.

TUMORS OF THE TESTICLE

Sertoli-cell tumors arise in the seminiferous tubules and are often found in retained testicles, but may be present in either or both scrotal testicles. The opposite unaffected testicle is invariably atrophic. About 50% of Sertoli-cell tumors produce signs of feminization in the dog (atrophy of the uninvolved testicle, bilaterally symmetrical alopecia, nipple enlargement, attraction for other males). Grossly, the tumor appears as a lobulated, grayish-yellow, greasy mass within the contours of the testicle and may enlarge the overall size of the testicle. The cut surface is finely lobulated and contains soft red areas. Microscopically, the tumor is composed of numerous tubules filled with Sertoli cells. It grows primarily by expansion and rarely metastasizes. Castration is curative.

Seminomas are usually seen as a solitary nodule arising from the spermatogenic epithelium of the seminiferous tubules. Grossly, they are small, firm, whitish-gray spherical nodules within the parenchyma. Microscopically, the tumor cells form solid masses of large, round, germinal epithelial cells with prominent nucleoli. The tumor cells can be seen to have broken out of tubules and invaded the interstitium of the testicle. Although seminomas are potentially malignant, they grow primarily by expansion within the gland. Metastasis is rare in dogs. Castration is curative.

Interstitial-cell tumors are very common in aging dogs. They often appear as solitary nodules under 1 cm in diameter. They exert no known hormonal effect on the dog and rarely distort the size or shape of the testis. Grossly, the tumor appears as a light-brown, spherical mass with zones of deep reddish-brown hemorrhage scattered throughout the cut surface. Microscopically, the tumor cells form sheets which are interrupted by zones of hemorrhage. The tumors grow slowly by expansion and are the least likely testicular tumors to metastasize. Castration is curative.

Adenocarcinomas of the prostate gland are seen as focal or diffuse tumors arising from prostatic epithelium. The gland may or may not be enlarged. An interesting side effect occurs when the tumor cells invade the neck of the bladder in the area of the trigone and block one or both ureters, causing secondary hydronephrosis. By rectal palpation the prostate gland containing an adenocarcinoma usually can be felt to be adherent to the floor of the pelvis due to fibrous adhesions developed between the neoplastic gland and the normal intra-pelvic tissue. Grossly, an affected gland may be larger or smaller than normal and it is usually somewhat asymmetric. The cut surface of the tumor is gray, firm and often distinct from the normal glandular tissue. Adhesions to the pelvic wall and the neck of the bladder are common. Microscopically, the tumor cells may form solid cords or ill-defined acini. Inflam-matory cyst formation and fibrosis often accompany the tumor. The tumors metastasize early and widely. Invasion of the neck of the bladder is common. There is no known effective treatment, since complete surgical removal of the neoplastic tissue is generally impossible. (*See also* PROSTATIC NEOPLASMS, p. 849.)

TUMORS OF THE OVARY AND UTERUS

Granulosa cell tumors arise from the granulosa cells of ovarian follicles. They have the potential to secrete estrogen or androgen. However, just what hormone, if any, is secreted in dogs and cats has not been established. Grossly, the tumor is usually seen as a large unilateral multilobulated grayish-yellow mass. The cut surface frequently contains numerous cysts. Microscopically, the neoplastic cells generally produce follicle-like structures. The tumors grow by expansion and metastasis is rare. If the tumor ruptures, implantation of tumor cells may occur on the peritoneum, forming numerous small botryoid masses. Ovariohysterectomy is curative in the absence of metastasis.

Dysgerminomas are rare ovarian tumors in dogs which may appear in one or both ovaries. They have a smooth, glistening surface and the cut surface is grayish pink. Microscopically, they have the histologic features of a seminoma. There is no known hormonal effect on the host. Dysgerminomas should be considered potentially malignant. Ovariohysterectomy is cura-tive.

Adenocarcinoma of the uterus is a rare tumor in dogs and cats which arises from the glandular epithelium of the uterine mucosa. It is usually found close to the cervix, hence both intact and spayed female dogs may have this tumor. It usually occurs in dogs over 10 years of age. Clinically, a persistent sanguinous discharge from the vagina in an old female is suggestive of adenocarcinoma of the uterus. Grossly, the tumor is broad-based and seldom projects into the lumen but rather penetrates through the mucosa into the muscular layers of the uterus. The luminal surface is frequently ulcerated and the tumor grows in annular fashion around the organ. The cut surface is pink-tan and firm. Microscopically, the tumor cells form irregular ill-defined acini amidst abundant fibrous stroma. These tumors are locally invasive and only rarely metastasize to the iliac or sublumbar lymph nodes. Consequently, surgical removal of the uterus or uterine stump including the cervix may be curative.

MAMMARY TUMORS

Mammary tumors are among the most frequent tumors in dogs. They represent 25% of neoplasms in female dogs. They occur most frequently in intact bitches and are extremely rare in male dogs, thus indicating the possible role of estrogen in their pathogenesis. The caudal 2 mammary glands are more often involved than the anterior 3 glands. Grossly, mammary tumors appear as single nodules in one or more glands on the same side of the abdomen, ranging in size from 1 to 25 cm. The cut surface is usually lobulated, gray-tan and firm, often with small and large fluid-filled cysts. Mixed mammary tumors, those which contain both neoplastic epithelial tissue as well as neoplastic mesenchymal tissue, are usually benign and often have grossly recognizable bone or cartilage present on the cut surface. Microscopically, mammary tumors may be divided into 4 categories: (a) **Adenomas**—rare benign growths of glandular epithelium. (b) **Adenocarcinomas**—frequently fast-growing tumors composed of glandular epithelium which often metastasizes to the lungs. (c) **Benign mixed mammary tumor** —the most frequent tumor, which contains neoplastic epithelial and mesenchymal tissue. These tumors grow slowly, may obtain considerable size and may undergo malignant transformation after a certain time. (d) **Malignant mixed mammary tumor**—grossly resembles its benign counterpart and has a tendency to rapidly increase in size. Histologically, either the epithelial or mesenchymal component may have the characteristics of malignant growth, as seen by invasion of lymphatic and blood vessels, anaplasia and metastasis.

From a practical standpoint mammary tumors should be regarded as potentially malignant regardless of the size or the number of mammary glands involved. Treatment requires mastectomy, ovariohysterectomy and removal of the appropriate draining lymph nodes. The caudal 3 glands on each side have a common lymphatic system and drain into the inguinal lymph node. The anterior 2 glands also have a common lymphatic system and drain into the axillary lymph node. Since the malignant mammary tumors metastasize readily to the lungs, radiography should always be performed prior to surgical removal of affected glands in order to rule out previous metastasis.

TUMORS OF THE ADRENAL GLANDS

Adenomas of the adrenal cortex are frequently seen in old dogs. They have no known hormonal effect. Grossly, they appear as discrete small to large tan-yellow nodules within the cortex that may encroach upon the medulla or may project irregularly from the surface of the gland. Microscopically the tumor cells are large polygonal cells with foamy cytoplasm, that form solid nodules. These benign tumors grow slowly by expansion and are usually recognized only at necropsy. Therapy is not considered necessary.

Carcinoma of the adrenal cortex is exceedingly rare in dogs. Histologically, it may be confused with another rare tumor of the adrenal gland, **pheochromocytoma**.

TUMORS OF THE PITUITARY GLAND

Pituitary gland tumors may be adenomas or adenocarcinomas. They are rare and have been reported to be responsible for producing canine Cushing's disease and canine adipose genital syndrome. Grossly, the pituitary gland is enlarged asymmetrically and may expand dorsally via the infundibulum into the hypothalamus. The cut surface of the tumor is gray, firm and frequently contains irregular zones of hemorrhage. Microscopically, the tumor cells may be recognized as chromophobe cells, pituitary basophils or pituitary eosinophils. Tumors of the pituitary gland grow by dorsal expansion and invasion of the hypothalamus since the gland normally lies in a closely confined osseous crater at the base of the skull. These tumors are usually recognized at necropsy.

TUMORS OF THE THYROID GLAND

Tumors of the thyroid gland are most frequently carcinomas. At the time of diagnosis approximately 25% of these tumors are present in both glands. Grossly, they may appear as an enlarged firm thyroid gland of normal shape or, more commonly, they may appear as a thick-walled cyst 1 to 3 cm in diameter filled with necrotic blood and fluid. Microscopically, the tumor cells are cuboidal epithelial cells which may form ill-defined acini or grow in broad solid sheets. Invasion of blood vessels by the tumor cells is common and subsequent thrombosis and infarction may contribute to the gross cystic appearance. Approximately 35% of thyroid carcinomas metastasize to the opposite gland directly via the lymphatic communication at the hilus of the 2 glands. Metastasis also occurs to the lungs, cervical lymph nodes and viscera. Bilateral thyroidectomy is always advised regardless of the gross absence of nodules in the opposite gland. Care should be taken to leave the unattached anterior parathyroid glands in place. Daily administration of thyroid hormone is essential for the remainder of the dog's life following surgery.

AORTIC-BODY TUMORS

Aortic-body tumors arise from the chemoreceptor cells in the aortic body and are usually found in the *sinus transversus pericardii,* the space between the aorta and the pulmonary artery at the base of the heart (heart-base tumor). There is no known hormonal function of these tumors. Brachycephalic breeds such as Boxers and Boston Terriers have a higher incidence of this tumor than other dogs. Grossly, the tumor is a firm, fleshy, nodular, spherical mass that infrequently obstructs the pulmonary artery or the aorta, although it is closely applied to each of these major vessels. The cut surface is lobulated, pink and firm. Microscopically, the tumor is composed of small, round cells with pale eosinophilic or vacuolated cytoplasm. Usually, these tumors do not directly invade the atria, aorta or pulmonary artery, but may be seen in small blood vessels or lymphatics. Aortic-body tumors grow principally by expansion. Metastasis is uncommon. There is no known effective treatment.

Carotid-body tumors have a similar appearance and biologic activity, but are located at the junction of the carotid arteries near the angle of the mandible.

TUMORS OF THE CENTRAL NERVOUS SYSTEM

Astrocytomas arise from the glial astrocytes and are usually found in the cerebrum or cerebellum. Compression of the third or fourth ventricle, or sylvan aqueduct may produce secondary hydrocephalus. Grossly, these tumors appear as an ill-defined mass within the nervous tissue that may be soft and gelatinous. The cut surface is gray and may contain small zones of hemorrhage. Formalin fixation of the brain frequently more clearly differentiates the neoplastic tissue from normal brain. Microscopically, the tumor appears in various patterns ranging from sheets of fibrous stellate cells to large nests of undifferentiated elongate, spindle-shaped cells. These tumors grow by local infiltration and rarely metastasize. There is no known treatment.

Oligodendrogliomas are also derived from glial cells and are seen most commonly in the cerebrum and cerebellum. Grossly they are firmer than normal brain tissue. Microscopically, the tumor is composed of cells closely arranged with scant cytoplasm and uniform, dark, round or oval nuclei. This tumor grows by local invasion and expansion. There is no known treatment.

Meningiomas are more common in cats than dogs. The tumor arises from the dura mater and usually encroaches upon the cerebellum or cerebrum. Grossly, it is seen as a well-lobulated, spherical, firm, white mass that compresses adjacent areas of normal brain tissue. Microscopically, the tumor cells are usually spindle-shaped and arranged in well-defined whorls. Meningiomas grow by expansion, causing compression atrophy of the underlying brain. Invasion of the CNS by these tumors is rare. There is no known treatment. However, if this tumor were diagnosed early enough, it could be surgically removed, since it rarely invades nervous tissues. The signs produced are caused by compression atrophy of the adjacent nervous tissue.

NEOPLASMS (LG. AN.)

Cattle: While accurate reporting and documentation of the occurrence of neoplasia in cattle have never been accomplished, over 100 types have been recorded. The most common tumor of cattle is papilloma (q.v., p. 243); however, since this is benign, most cases are not reported. Of the malignant tumors, the most common is squamous cell carcinoma of the eye and orbit (q.v., p. 612). Lymphoid tumors (q.v., p. 615) are probably the second most common malignancy of cattle. Studies of bovine malignant lymphoma indicate rates as high as 40 per 100,000 cattle in the U.S.A. and even higher rates in some European countries.

At a lower level of incidence are hemangiomas of the heart and liver, fibromas of the heart, lipomas of the peritoneal cavity, and carcinomas of the uterus, ovary and gallbladder. Cartilaginous tumors are the most frequent of the skeletal neoplasms but are not common. Multiple neurofibromas have been reported but are rare in cattle.

Horses: The commonest tumor in horses is the cutaneous "sarcoid" which usually appears around the head but can be transferred to other sites. Sarcoids and papillomas (warts) in young horses are probably virus-induced; however, sarcoids do not ordinarily regress spontaneously and must be removed surgically. Recurrences at the surgical site are frequent.

In gray or white horses, melanomas are the commonest tumors, and these can metastasize widely from the usual primary perineal site giving rise to signs of colic and general loss of condition. The second most prevalent tumor in stallions and geldings is squamous cell carcinoma of the glans penis. These cauliflower-like or smooth tumors are slow to metastasize and are often good subjects for surgical removal. Squamous cell carcinomas of the vulva of mares occur at a slightly lower incidence. The second most prevalent tumor, occurring in both sexes, is squamous cell carcinoma of the eye which tends to be slow-growing but nonetheless malignant.

Tumors found in the mouth, nasal cavity and throat regions are squamous cell carcinomas, fibrosarcomas, and carcinomas from the nasal sinuses and squamous tumors of the salivary glands. Signs of swallowing difficulty may be present but often the tumor is discovered as a visible and palpable mass in the ventral neck region. Older horses show a moderately high incidence of cholesteatomas of the brain, and are rather prone to thyroid and pituitary adenomas, the latter often associated with a long hair coat.

Visceral tumors are rare in the horse and renal carcinoma has by far the highest incidence of these. Hemangiosarcomas of the liver and spleen are the most common neoplasms of these organs, although hepatic carcinomas and lymphoid tumors do occur. Reticuloendothelial tumors are more likely to be myeloid than lymphoid. Lipomas of the peritoneal cavity and skin are moderately prevalent. Any of these visceral tumors can give rise to signs of colic and chronic inanition. Gastric squamous cell carcinomas in older horses may be accompanied by a persistent anemia as well as emaciation.

In the mare, granulosa cell tumors and teratomas occur rarely in the ovary, while in the stallion, seminoma is the most common (but still infrequent) testicular tumor. Mammary carcinoma has been reported in the mare.

Sheep: Lymphoid tumors are the most commonly encountered neoplasm of sheep. Hepatic tumors are less often seen and in some areas of the world, squamous tumors of the skin are quite frequently encountered. Tumors of the skeleton (mostly cartilaginous) are more common in sheep than in other large animals, while a moderately high incidence of ovarian tumors parallels the situation in cattle. Neoplasms of the nasal passages and sinuses are not infrequent. Renal tumors, respiratory carcinoma and carcinoma of the eye may be encountered with moderate frequency. A high regional incidence of intestinal carcinoma is found in New Zealand and Australian sheep. Very few other tumors have been recovered from sheep.

Pigs: The incidence of tumors in pigs is very low and about two-thirds of those occurring are either lymphoid (and related) tumors or embryonal nephromas of the kidney. Melanomas and hemangiomas of the skin account for most of the remainder, while hepatomas occur but are rare. About 20 other types of tumor have been recorded.

OCULAR CARCINOMA IN CATTLE
(Cancer eye)

A term used clinically to designate any apparently malignant neoplastic growth involving the eye and orbital region. This is almost invariably a squamous cell carcinoma originating on the bulbar conjunctiva, eyelids, or membrana nictitans.

Incidence and Etiology: Ocular carcinoma is one of the commonest neoplasms of cattle. Significant economic loss, second only to that due to lymphosarcoma, results not only from condemnation or reduction in salvage value of carcasses but from a shortened productive life-span. Usually, the disease is infrequent before 6 years of age but increases in frequency thereafter. An hereditary basis has been demonstrated and is apparently related more to ocular pigmentation than to the neoplastic process itself; pigment in the lid epithelium or limbus has a significant inhibitory effect on tumor development. High levels of sunlight and nutrition both have an important influence on enhancing the disease. Involvement of a virus has been suggested but not proved.

Clinical Findings, Diagnosis and Treatment: On the bulbar conjunctiva, the pathogenesis proceeds from a hyperplastic plaque, sometimes with an intervening papillomatous stage, to a carcinoma. On the lids, the sequence proceeds from keratosis or focal ulceration. Carcinomas originate more frequently from the lids, membrana nictitans, and lacrimal caruncle; bulbar tumors are less prone to infiltrate and metastasize than those at other sites. Metastasis is usually to regional nodes.

Treatment is generally surgical, the extent being determined by the type and location of the tumor. Small, superficial tumors, usually on the limbus or lids, may be surgically excised, followed by silver nitrate cautery. Broad-based and deep tumors are best controlled by enucleation. Any tumor on the membrana nictitans has a high malignant potential and excision of the entire structure is recommended. Close follow-up of a treated animal is required to control recurrences and the development of new tumors in the same or opposite eye. Lesions originating in the lacrimal lake are especially difficult to control. Irradiation and chemotherapy in various forms, as the primary or as an ancillary mode of treatment, have been used with some success. Therapy is not generally undertaken in cases with metastases unless the procedure will enhance the slaughter value of the animal or permit it to calve or wean a calf.

Since pigmentation is highly heritable, a long-range control program is possible by selecting for breeding only animals with increased amounts of pigmentation in and around the eyes.

CANINE MALIGNANT LYMPHOMA
(Lymphoblastoma, Lymphosarcoma, Lymphocytoma, Lymphatic leukemia, Pseudoleukemia)

A progressive, fatal disease of dogs characterized by neoplastic proliferation of lymphoid tissue, lymphadenopathy and various signs depending on organs involved.

Incidence: Malignant lymphoma with multiple lymph node involvement is the form most commonly seen. It occurs in approximately 5 of every 1,000 dogs that are hospitalized, and in natural dog populations rates as high as 24/100,000 dogs per year have been reported. All breeds are affected and no sex prevalence has been found. The age incidence is from 2 to 12 years.

Solitary or regional lymph node involvement is not common, but may occur in the superficial or internal nodes.

Clinical Findings: The outstanding early clinical sign is a painless enlargement of the superficial lymph nodes. Subsequently, there is a gradual development of weakness, inactivity, occasional vomiting, partial anorexia, diarrhea or constipation, sometimes thirst and polyuria, and often coughing and dyspnea. In the terminal stages, the patient is cachectic and exhibits purulent nasal and ocular discharges and pale mucous membranes. Unilateral or bilateral exophthalmos, jaundice, ascites and ptosis of the third eyelid may be observed. The duration of the disease, from its inception to death, varies from about 6 weeks to 6 months.

Lesions: In typical cases there is bilateral, symmetrical enlargement of all superficial and internal lymph nodes. The latter are gray-tan in color and may be discrete or fused, firm or soft. Usually the spleen is greatly enlarged, with rounded edges and a tense capsule. The liver frequently is enlarged and the portal markings are made more prominent by innumerable, minute, grayish nodules or by a fine, gray reticular surface pattern. Other gross lesions that may be present are hydrothorax, hydropericardium, thickening of the walls of the gallbladder and enlarged tonsils. Microscopically, not only the lymph nodes, spleen and liver, but also most other organs may contain nodular or diffuse infiltrations of neoplastic lymphocytes.

With multiple lymph node involvement, anemia and a tendency to thrombocytopenia are usually present. In most animals a nonspecific neutrophilia occurs. Occasionally, there is a true leukemia, with numerous lymphoblasts present in blood smear. Aspiration of bone marrow often reveals the presence of abnormal numbers of lymphocytes in addition to hyperplasia of myeloid tissue.

Malignant lymphoma involving solitary lymph nodes or regional groups has histopathologic characteristics similar to those of the multiple lymph node type. There are no specific blood or bone marrow changes in cases with solitary or regional lymph node involvement, except for terminal anemia.

Diagnosis: Positive diagnosis is made by microscopic examination of a section from an enlarged node. Aspiration of bone marrow (most easily accomplished from the iliac crest) often reveals the presence of lymphomatous cells. Examination of the blood usually is inconclusive. In arriving at a diagnosis, one has always to consider that mycotic or bacterial agents can produce marked enlargement of lymph nodes.

Treatment: Although there is no known cure, the useful life of some dogs may be prolonged by the serial use of chemotherapeutic agents; the corticosteroid hormones (e.g., prednisone), alkylating agents (cyclophosphamide, chlorambucil) and folic acid antagonists (e.g., methotrexate) are relatively effective in relieving the signs of malignant lymphoma. Eventually, each of these drugs loses its effect, thereby necessitating a change in therapy. Periodic clinical and laboratory examinations are imperative during the course of treatment since the drugs employed are cytotoxic. Overdosage results in leukopenia, thrombocytopenia and anemia. Clinically, the signs of toxicity are susceptibility to infection, purpura and lassitude. If toxic signs develop, the offending drug should be withdrawn for 10 to 14 days, or until normal hematologic values are regained.

As treatment is an attempt to balance the effects of the drug on the neoplastic cells against the development of toxicity, no rigid treatment schedule exists. The following regimen is suggested: Prednisone, 1.0 mg/lb/day, is given until the lymph nodes have regressed to approximately normal size. The dose is then halved and cyclophosphamide (Cytoxan) is added at 1.0 mg/lb/day. Chlorambucil (Leukeran) is employed next, 0.1 mg/lb/day. Finally, methotrexate is given IV every 10 to 14 days, 1.0 mg/lb. The duration of a drug-induced remission varies with each dog and cannot be reliably predicted.

BOVINE LEUKOSIS

(Bovine leukemia, Lymphosarcoma, Reticulum cell sarcoma, Malignant lymphoma)

A malignant neoplasm of lymphoreticular cells with variable clinicopathologic manifestations. In some countries, usually in areas where dairy cattle are a principal industry, it is endemic; there is usually a lower frequency in beef cattle. Bovine leukosis is now reportable in some areas of the world, and attempts are being made in some countries of Northern Europe to eradicate it by a slaughter program. Total lymphocyte counts persisting above normal are used for detection of the pretumorous form of disease; this is the basis for the official test used in countries with control programs.

Clinicopathologic variations occur by age, being uniquely different in calves (birth to 6 months), adolescents (6 to 18 months), and adults (older than 2 years). A fourth form, skin leukosis, occurs usually in adults. Sporadic leukosis usually occurs in calves, adolescents and in adults with skin leukosis, while epizootics usually are restricted to adult cattle. A virus has been hypothesized by several investigators as the causal factor; however, proof is still lacking. A few research workers have been apparently successful in transmitting the disease with whole cells. The mode of natural transmission is suggested to be vertical by way of the placenta, milk or by semen at time of conception. A genetic predisposition in some cow families has been implicated by some investigators.

Clinical Findings: A pretumorous form of leukosis usually is described in adult cattle in areas where the tumor phase is enzootic. The only sign is persistent lymphocytosis which may be present months or years before tumors are detected.

Signs of the tumorous form of the disease may appear quite suddenly followed by death after a relatively short clinical course. Remissions are relatively frequent in the pretumorous form but rare after tumors occur, except with skin leukosis. Once tumors develop, the prognosis is invariably bad. Apart from loss of weight and milk production, the animal may show signs related to involvement of any organ.

Lesions: Calves almost always show generalized lymph node enlargement and bone marrow infiltration. Nodular or diffuse lesions of the spleen, liver, kidney and bones are seen less frequently. Anemia and presence of lymphoblasts and atypical lymphocytes in peripheral blood are common findings. Adolescent animals may show involvement of only regional groups of nodes and the thymus. Anemia and bone marrow involvement are less common than in the young calf. Lymphoblasts and atypical lymphocytic cells may be found in peripheral blood. Animals with skin leukosis have nodular lesions in the dermis which frequently regress spontaneously, only to recur later with generalized lymphadenopathy and organ involvement similar to the adult form. Lesions in adult cattle usually include involvement of lymph nodes, abomasum and heart. Less frequently, the uterus, kidneys, liver, spleen, peripheral spinal nerves, and retrobulbar tissue are infiltrated. Any tissue may be involved.

The neoplastic tissue appears grayish white or yellowish gray. Tumors are moderately soft, edematous or friable; however, some may be firm and relatively hard. Necrosis is a prominent feature of the larger lymph nodes and tumor masses.

Diagnosis: Massive enlargements of multiple lymph nodes is indicative of leukosis. Histologic sections of biopsied enlarged nodes or lesions in involved organs will generally confirm the diagnosis. Visceral involvement without peripheral node enlargement is less rapidly diagnosed except by rectal palpation and exploratory laparotomy. Smears made from aspirations of masses and bone marrow infiltrations are confirmatory, while blood examination in the presence of detectable lesions will often be helpful; but many affected animals, particularly adults, have normal leukocytic counts. Total lymphocytic counts are frequently elevated, but caution should be exercised in using such counts in the absence of lesions as the only basis for making a diagnosis of the tumorous form of leukosis. Bone marrow aspirations are extremely helpful in confirming a diagnosis of the calf form, but less useful in the adolescent form and of little value in the adult form.

A differential diagnosis is more difficult in the adult form and must include a variety of diseases that have similar signs, including other malignancies and fat necrosis. Few diseases other than leukosis, however, have accompanying generalized lymphadenopathy or a massively enlarged thymus gland.

Treatment and Control: Anticancer drugs used to treat leukemias of other animals are useful in prolonging the life of cattle, but are generally impractical. No cure or prevention is known.

FELINE VISCERAL LYMPHOMA
(Lymphosarcoma)

A malignant lymphoid tumor occurring primarily in thoracic and abdominal viscera and lymph nodes. Lymphoid malignancy in the cat differs in distribution of lesions from that seen in dogs and cattle where superficial node involvement is extremely common. Visceral lymphoma is the most common feline malignancy. It occurs most frequently in cats over the age of 2 years but has been seen as early as 6 months of age. There is no significant breed or sex predisposition.

Clinical Findings: Frequently, the affected cat shows a chronic, nonspecific wasting disease with anemia, lethargy and anorexia. In the thoracic form, dyspnea, difficult swallowing and a gagging cough may prevail. Clinical examination should be supplemented by roentgenographs of the cat in standing position, before and after aspiration of thoracic fluid. Stained smears of the aspirated fluid should be examined for malignant lymphoid cells. Differential diagnostic problems include diaphragmatic hernia, chylothorax, pyothorax and hydrothorax. The signs in the abdominal form are often those of an obstruction. If both kidneys are involved, signs of uremia will be present, and in liver involvement, jaundice and anemia. Frequent differential diagnostic problems in the abdominal form are hair balls or infectious feline peritonitis (q.v., p. 323). Radiographic examination of the abdomen, including a barium series and pyelography, is of great diagnostic value. Treatment usually is hopeless.

Lesions: There are 2 main categories of lymphoid tumors based on location, a thoracic and an abdominal form. In the former, the neoplasms originate most frequently in the precardiac mediastinum, either from the mediastinal nodes or from the thymus. At necropsy, the anterior ventral thoracic cavity is filled with white, lobulated lymphosarcoma, which embeds the heart and displaces the lungs dorsally and posteriorly. The lungs are atelectatic due to compression by the tumor and its accompanying hydrothorax. In the abdominal form, the organs affected are, in decreasing order of frequency, intestine (ileum), kidneys, liver, mesenteric nodes and spleen. Leukemia is present in less than 20% of cases. Experimental studies have shown that feline lymphoma can be transmitted from cat to cat with cell-free material. In addition, C-type RNA virus similar to that of avian and murine lymphomas can be demonstrated in affected cats.

NERVOUS SYSTEM

CLINICAL EXAMINATION OF THE NERVOUS SYSTEM

An examination of the nervous system should be part of a general physical examination because the activity of the nervous system may reflect generalized disorders as well as neurologic disease. Interpretation of the results of a neurologic examination requires a general understanding of factors that affect the excitability of neural tissue. The excitability of neural structures is in general controlled by a balance of excitatory and inhibitory influences within the CNS, thus neural responses may be hyperactive or hypoactive depending upon the relationship of these influences. Organic lesions within the CNS may result in increased excitability of other portions of the nervous system through the removal of inhibitory or the enhancement of excitatory influences, or may result in a decrease in excitability through the removal of excitatory or the enhancement of inhibitory influences. Because of the complex interrelationships of CNS structures, some neural activities may be abolished by lesions of the nervous system while others are simultaneously enhanced.

It is important for the diagnostician to realize that the examination of a patient may in itself alter neurologic responses; an excited or frightened animal may often reflect seemingly gross neurologic deficiencies, whereas the same animal in a relaxed state is normal.

CRANIAL NERVES

I. Olfactory: Subjective observation of the animal by an informed owner is usually the best indicator of loss of function. Tests commonly described for testing olfaction utilize smoke or acrid odors but these produce trigeminal (V) mediated avoidance responses rather than olfactory responses.

II. Optic: Total or functional blindness is usually detected by the presence of dilated pupils and a history of bumping into objects. Loss of portions of the visual fields may be estimated by utilizing visual placing reflexes which measure the ability of an animal to detect a supporting object in the lateral visual field and place its feet upon it for postural support. Neurologic blindness may be due to lesions of the retina, optic nerve, optic tract or lateral geniculate nuclei of the thalamus. Neurologic blindness may result from compression of the optic nerves at the optic chiasm from hypophyseal tumors. Deficiencies of the visual cortex do not produce total blindness of domestic animals, but markedly diminish visual acuity. Such deficiencies may occur following severe anoxia. The animal can usually detect the difference between light and dark and can locate an open door due to differences in light intensity, but may bump into objects within a room. The pupillary light reflexes may be utilized to examine the integrity of the retina, optic nerve, optic tracts, pretectal area of the midbrain, oculomotor nucleus, oculomotor nerve, ciliary ganglion and sphincter muscle of the iris. The neural pathway for these reflexes exhibits bilateral distribution at the optic chiasm and in the pretectal area; thus stimulation of one retina will normally invoke pupillary constriction in both eyes. The pupillary light reflexes are carried out by closing both eyes for a few seconds, then one eye is opened and pupillary constriction is noted (simple or direct pupillary light reflex). The opposite eye is then opened and a further constriction of the pupil first examined is observed (indirect or consensual pupillary light reflex). The procedure is then repeated with the opposite eye being opened first. Evaluating pupillary accommodation for far and near vision also tests the neural structures involved in the pupillary light reflexes, but additionally it depends upon the integrity of the visual cortex and is therefore a test for the visual capability of the animal. If the animal is observed focusing upon objects within the environment, the pupil will constrict when focusing on near objects and dilate when focusing on far objects.

The visual blink reflex, in another test for visual capability, is checked by passing an object near or toward the eye (with care taken not to stimulate the eyelids or cornea with air currents) to elicit a blink. This response depends upon the ability of the animal to see the object, intact rostral colliculi, and an intact innervation of the orbicularis oculi muscle by the facial nerve. If the orbicularis oculi muscle is paralyzed, the animal will withdraw from an approaching finger thrust. The visual blink reflex thus provides a test of the visual cortex and visual pathways of the brain, as well as the integrity of the midbrain, pons and facial nerve.

III, IV, VI. Oculomotor, Trochlear, Abducens: These nerves innervate the extrinsic muscles of the eye and therefore control ocular movements. The oculomotor nerve also provides parasympathetic innervation to the ciliary body and muscles of the iris, and innervates the levator of the upper eyelid. Damage to one or more of these nerves or their nuclei may result in an abnormal rotation of the eye (strabismus) or an inability to rotate the eye in various directions. Damage to the abducens nerve results in a medial strabismus and an inability to rotate the eye laterally. Damage to the trochlear nerve is difficult to detect unless the animal has an oval pupil (as in cats) where a rotation of the eyeball around its longitudinal axis in a lateral direction is observed. If a strabismus is observed, the lateral aspect of the eyeball is rotated to a ventrolateral position. Damage to the oculomotor nerve results in a lateral strabismus, inability to rotate the eye in a medial, dorsal or ventral direction, ptosis, a loss of both simple and consensual pupillary light reflexes on the affected side, and a persistent dilation of the pupil.

V. Trigeminal: This nerve is responsible for general sensation (pain, touch, temperature) of the oral and nasal cavities and the skin of the face and head. Caudal, wedge-shaped areas of skin between the ears dorsally and in the mandibular space ventrally are excepted. The nerve innervates the muscles of mastication. Its functional integrity may be tested through the utilization of corneal blink, lacrimation and salivation from stimulation of the oral mucosa; avoidance responses and skin twitch reflexes in response to pin pricks to the skin of the head; and examination of the masticatory muscles for altered tone or atrophy. In unilateral paralysis, the lower jaw drops on the affected side and chewing movements are altered. The efferents for these reflexes involve the facial (VII) or the glossopharyngeal (IX) nerves. Trigeminal reflexes, however, may be utilized to examine the integrity of the hypoglossal (XII), vagus (X) and glossopharyngeal (IX) nerves through the lick and swallow reflexes. These reflexes may be elicited by opening the mouth for a few seconds and allowing the oral mucosa to dry. Upon release of the animal, licking of the lips and swallowing will be initiated. Licking allows an examination of the hypoglossal nerve and swallowing depends upon the integrity of the vagus and glossopharyngeal nerves. Damage to the motor component of the trigeminal nerve may result in paralysis of the muscles of mastication.

VII. Facial: This nerve innervates the lacrimal gland, the salivary glands, the glands of the nasal cavity and the muscles of the face, ear and eyelid. Its integrity may be tested with the blink, lacrimation, and cutaneous twitch reflexes. Flaring of the nostrils during respiration, particularly in large animals, and the normal attitude of the ears are dependent upon the integrity of the facial nerve. With loss of facial nerve function, the animal may reveal a drooping of the lips and ear, dry cornea (paralysis of orbicularis oculi), and accumulation of food in the vestibule of the mouth (paralysis of buccinator). Due to the close proximity of the facial nerve fibers and the nucleus of the abducens nerve, CNS lesions often result in a loss of function in both nerves. Such a set of clinical signs is indicative of an organic lesion in the caudal pons and rostral medulla.

VIII. Vestibulocochlear: This nerve is involved in both auditory and vestibular functions. Deafness is produced if this nerve is destroyed bilaterally, but is rarely produced by lesions. Examination for deafness is difficult to interpret as animals are often cued by the activities of the clinician. Absence of an alerting response in the animal to unexpected noises or to the animal's name are indications of deafness. Electroencephalographic arousal in a lightly anesthetized animal in response to sound is a helpful means of examining an animal for deafness where such apparatus is available. Deafness is most often congenital, but may be acquired due to bilateral inner ear infections.

The vestibular component of this nerve is responsible for the maintenance of normal posture and eye reflexes that are initiated by movements of the head. Damage to the vestibular system may result in the production of nystagmus, which usually is inapparent grossly within a few hours, but can be detected for 1 to 2 days in an ophthalmoscopic examination. Usually a turning of the head toward the affected side, with a torticollis (twisting of the neck around its longitudinal axis) is exhibited and requires 2 to 3 weeks for near complete accommodation. In acute involvement, circling or rolling activity may be elicited. Due to the turning of the head and the torticollis, varying degrees of incoordination will be exhibited.

The integrity of the vestibular system and its CNS connections can be determined in dogs and cats by the head-righting response and the vestibular placing reflex. In examination of the head-righting response, the animal is held by the trunk in a head-up position and slowly rotated to a head-down position; the normal animal will maintain the head in a nearly normal position relative to the field of gravity until tilted to a position in which this is impossible, and will then turn the head to one side or the other. The vestibular placing reflex is elicited by elevating the animal from a supporting surface and accelerating it in for a few inches toward the supporting surface. The animal will reach out toward the support with the forelimbs due to visual placing reflexes and will flare the toes of the forelimb due to activity of the vestibular system.

IX, X. Glossopharyngeal and Vagus: These nerves are examined as indicated above with the lick and swallow reflexes. An additional test is the gag reflex, in which the vagus and glossopharyngeal nerves serve as the afferent and efferent limbs of the reflex arc.

XI. Spinal Accessory: This nerve is generally not tested in a neurologic examination, as malfunctions are difficult to detect clinically. In large animals, atrophy of the sternocephalicus muscle may be noted.

XII. Hypoglossal: This nerve innervates muscles of the tongue and is examined with the lick and swallow reflexes as outlined above. In unilateral paralysis, the tongue protrudes and is inclined toward the affected side.

CEREBRUM

Neurologic disorders involving the cerebrum may manifest themselves in a variety of behavioral patterns, such as circling, general depression or excitement, convulsions, continual pacing, unconsciousness and alterations in temperament. Unilateral lesions of the cerebral cortex generally result in abnormalities of the contralateral side of the animal. There are no specific reflex tests for the involvement of the cerebrum in neurologic disorders other than those described for cranial and spinal nerves which depend upon the cerebral cortex for their elicitation. Electroencephalographic studies are often quite helpful in detecting abnormalities of the cerebral cortex and brain stem.

CEREBELLUM

The cerebellum functions in the control of the range and direction of somatic motor activities. Abnormalities of the cerebellum therefore result in hypermetria or hypometria, and locomotor muscular incoordination. Opisthotonus and tremor may be present. Signs which resemble abnormalities of the vestibular system, such as torticollis and nystagmus, may result from lesions of the cerebellum. Unilateral lesions of the cerebellum generally result in motor abnormalities of the ipsilateral side of the animal.

SPINAL NERVES

Reflexes may be used to test the integrity of the spinal nerves (both afferent and efferent fibers) as well as the CNS components of the reflex arcs. The activity of reflex arcs, however, is dependent upon influences which are imposed upon the spinal cord by the brain. Examination of spinal nerve reflexes therefore also provides an insight into the integrity of the brain. Abnormalities of the brain or its descending fiber systems which pass in the spinal cord may result in the production of hyperreflexia or hyporeflexia. The clinician must be aware of the intensity of reflex activity which should be elicited in the intact normal animal.

Myotatic reflexes: These reflexes are normally functional in the maintenance of muscle tone. The examination of muscle tone by palpation provides some insight into the integrity of the nerves innervating the muscle. To elicit the myotatic reflexes in a clinical examination, a quick stretch is applied to the tendon. In small animals, including calves, foals and young swine, the stretch is applied by striking the tendon with the finger tip or reflex hammer, while supporting the limb with the free hand. The reflexes are difficult to apply in the larger animals. The straight patellar (patellar reflex), triceps (triceps reflex), biceps and brachialis (biceps-brachialis reflex) tendons and the tendons of the ulnaris lateralis and flexor carpi ulnaris tendons (carpal reflex) are well suited for examination of myotatic reflexes. To elicit these reflexes, with the exception of the patellar reflex, it is necessary to utilize the forefinger of the right hand to tense the tendon and apply a stretch to the tendon by tapping the right forefinger with the left forefinger or by using the reflex hammer. In the normal animal only the patellar reflex is brisk, the remainder being ba____ detectable. In conditions which involve transection of des____ ing pathways from the brain, however, all myotatic ____ are more readily obtained.

Hopping and tactile placing reflex: These reflexes ___ to test the integrity of proprioceptive innervation o___ limb muscles, but also depend upon ascending and ___ pathways of the cerebral cortex and brain stem ___ sponse. They are useful, therefore, as survey refle___ ination of a large portion of the CNS. The h___ are elicited in small animals by supporting the ___ with the exception of one limb, which bears ___ mal's weight. The animal is then moved in a ___ tion, and the weight-bearing limb will hop to ___ postural support. Hypermetria or hypometr___ be indications of cerebellar malfunction. ___ flexes are examined by supporting the b___ body and moving him horizontally towar___ face. Upon touching the dorsal surface of ___ supporting surface, the animal should step ___ support its body weight.

In large animals, the tactile placing reflexes can be examined by blindfolding the animal and walking it over level ground without obstacles. Normal placing of the limbs indicates that the proprioceptive reflex pathways are intact. A common sign of loss of proprioceptive sense is crossing of the limbs in an animal with an otherwise normal standing attitude.

Withdrawal (flexor) reflexes: The application of a noxious stimulus to a limb will result in the withdrawal of the limb from the stimulus. This protective reflex may be present in an animal with a spinal cord transection which precludes perception of pain. If the reflex is accompanied by pain perception, however, observation of blinking of the eyes, licking of the lips, or looking around at the stimulated limb provides evidence of the integrity of the CNS. In animals with a transection of descending fiber systems from the brain, the withdrawal reflex is accompanied by an extension of the contralateral limb (crossed extensor reflex).

Pin pricks applied to the skin of the thorax and abdomen result in a twitch of the cutaneous trunci muscle (panniculus reflex). This reflex arc utilizes the lumbar or thoracic nerves as afferent pathways and the caudal pectoral nerve which arises from the brachial plexus. The panniculus reflex, therefore, is useful in localizing spinal cord lesions between these 2 levels. A similar reflex can be elicited in the cervical region, where the afferent limb of the arc is the cervical nerves and the efferent limb is the facial nerve which supplies cervical us muscles.

neck reflexes are best observed in the unrestrained s the animal raises its head, the forelimbs tend to the rear limbs flex; with lowering of the head, the observed. As the head is turned to one side, the that side will extend and that of the opposite side ese reflexes depend upon the integrity of the and of fiber systems within the spinal cord the segments which innervate the musculature

reflex is elicited by stimulation of the anal le stimulus and is expressed by a contraction al sphincter and depression of the tail. It of the perineal nerves and the sacral seg- cord.

REBROSPINAL FLUID

e pressure and composition of cerebro- assistance in determination of the eti- . Examination can be carried out by puncture of the cisterna magna in small animals, or the subarachnoid space at the lumbosacral junction in large animals. Elevations of pressure above about 170 mm water indicate the presence of space-occupying lesions or a defect in drainage of cerebrospinal fluid into the venous system. Elevation of protein is an indication of either encephalitis or meningoencephalitis. Elevation of cellular content is usually a reflection of infection of the CNS. The presence of neutrophils is indicative of bacterial infections, subarachnoid hemorrhage (erythrocytes are also present) or brain abscess. The presence of increased numbers of lymphocytes in indicative of viral infections or toxoplasmosis. Cultures of cerebrospinal fluid will often demonstrate the causative agent in microbial encephalitis.

INHERITED DISEASES AND CONGENITAL MALFORMATIONS OF THE CNS

Congenital defects of the CNS are common and may be either structural or functional defects. Some are known to be inherited, while others are caused by environmental factors (toxic plants, nutritional deficiencies, viral infections), but for many the cause is still unknown. In animals born with a well-developed nervous system (foals, calves, lambs and pigs), inherited neurologic disorders may be recognized at birth. In kittens and puppies, born less well developed, neurologic disorders may not be noticeable until they would normally walk. All grades of disorders occur, ranging from defective skeletal coverings to absence of the brain.

Anencephaly, agenesis of the brain, is regularly combined with defects of the cranial skeleton. **Cyclopia** and **cebocephalia** are severe defects involving cranial as well as facial skeleton. The cause in lambs is ingestion of the range plant *Veratrum californicum* by ewes at day 14 of gestation. **Cranioschisis,** a cleft in the cranial skeleton, is usually associated with herniation of the meninges and parts of the brain. Such hernias are termed **meningoceles** or **encephaloceles,** depending on the herniated parts. These defects are rare; they are inherited in piglets and have no established cause in other species.

Hydrocephalus may be internal or external, and may be associated with other structural defects. Obstruction of the ventricular system may produce internal hydrocephalus, which is moderately common in all domestic animals and may be inherited or occur spontaneously. It may be secondary to a primary inflammatory process or anomaly of the ventricular system, which impedes circulation of cerebrospinal fluid.

Achondroplastic calves are usually affected with internal hydro-cephalus (*see* BOVINE DWARFISM, p. 793).

Arthrogryposis in calves is characterized by fixation of joints in either flexion or extension due to regressive changes in skeletal muscles together with loss of the motor cells in the ventral horn of the spinal cord. A similar syndrome is seen in foals, lambs, pigs and puppies but is related to anomalous closure of the neural tube. **Dysrhaphism** of the brain or, more commonly, the cord leads to arrest in muscle development and subsequently to fixation of joints and distortion of limbs. Less severe defects of the cord may lead only to muscle weakness. One form of this syndrome is "**syringomyelia**" of Weimaraner dogs.

Hereditary neuraxial edema (autosomal recessive transmission) in Hereford calves is characterized clinically by extensor spasms and inability to stand. Histologic examination reveals edema of the terminal portions of myelinated bundles.

Lipid dystrophy or the deposition of abnormal lipid substances in the nerve cells has been described in dogs in Europe and North America. Neurologic signs include progressive ataxia and blindness simulating other encephalitides. A **non-lipid leukodystrophy** has also been observed in several breeds of dogs. A disease in calves referred to as **pseudolipidosis** occurs in Australia and New Zealand. The disease is relatively common in Aberdeen-Angus cattle and is caused by an inborn error of metabolism due to an absolute deficiency of alpha mannosidase. Some calves are affected when about 4 weeks old and others up to 15 months. The disease is progressive or static and abnormalities of gait become progressively pronounced until ataxia is conspicuous. There is widespread deposition of oligosaccharides in tissues.

CEREBELLAR DISORDERS

Congenital cerebellar lesions have been described in many species of domestic animals. These include **agenesis** and **aplasia** (absence or imperfect development), and **hypoplasia.** In the light of recent findings that prenatal infection (kittens with feline panleukopenia virus and calves with bovine virus diarrhea virus) causes cerebellar hypoplasia, the pathogenesis and causes of congenital cerebellar diseases have to be reevaluated. The main signs consist of ataxia at birth or shortly after, lack of equilibrium, violent muscular movements, coarse tremors and opisthotonos. The pathologic features include atrophy of all, or parts of, the layers of the cerebellar cortex but particularly loss of the Purkinje cell layer. Cerebellar hypoplasia, in puppies and kittens, is often accompanied by hypoplasia of the pons, the inferior olivae and sometimes the optic tracts. Clinical signs consist of tumbling, circling and ataxia; a head tremor is often present.

A further type of cerebellar disorder has been seen in calves of the Jersey and other breeds of cattle in North America. The lesions differ from the above in that the cerebellar white matter is predominantly affected. Lesions also occur in other parts of the brain and these are most obviously a lack of myelin formation. In Britain, a condition of **hypomyelinogenesis congenita** somewhat similar to these lesions in calves has been described in newborn paralytic lambs. Throughout the entire nervous system, axis cylinders develop but myelination is deficient. Myoclonia congenita in pigs (q.v., p. 585) may represent a variation of hypomyelinogenesis congenita.

EYE AND OPTIC NERVE

Hereditary (recessive) retinal disease has been described in several breeds of dogs, notably Gordon Setters, Irish Setters and Swiss Spaniels. The dogs are not affected at birth and the disease is a degenerative phenomenon of the normal retina. Congenital optic nerve hypoplasia has been described in blue merle Collies. Congenital aplasia of the optic nerves has also been described in mice and cats. Congenital microphthalmia and congenital retinal detachment have been observed in calves. Hypoplasia of optic nerves in calves and pigs may be due to congenital vitamin A deficiency. Microphthalmia combined with macrophthalmia occurs as a congenital lesion in pigs.

DISEASES IN WHICH LESIONS HAVE NOT BEEN DEMONSTRATED

A **spastic syndrome** is observed in cattle over 6 years of age and is characterized by sudden spastic muscular contractions of one or both hind legs. Early signs occur when the animal arises from a sternal position. The hind legs are stretched and rigid and the muscles of the neck and back exhibit coarse tremors. Initially, attacks may last only a few seconds but progressively they lengthen to as long as several minutes. At first, the attacks are separated by long intervals which become progressively shorter as the disease advances. No treatment is known to effect a permanent cure. Temporary relief may be obtained by the administration of mephenesin (R 529).

Epilepsy is a functional disease of the brain characterized by recurrent periodic tonoclonic convulsions, usually of short duration. It appears to be similar to epilepsy in man. "Idiopathic" epilepsy has been described in many species of animals but probably is seen most often in the dog. The typical history is that of recurrent convulsive seizures with few or no other physical signs. Convulsions may begin in the first year of life, but more frequently begin in the second year.

A high incidence has been noticed in Cocker Spaniels. The typical seizure lasts for 1 or 2 minutes consisting occasionally of a staring appearance, falling on the side and then typical running movements of the extremities. Evacuation of the bladder and bowel is common during epileptic seizures. After the convulsion, the animal may quickly regain its normal state or act dazed and uncoordinated for a few minutes. Convulsions in dogs have also been associated with deficiencies of vitamins A and B, hypocalcemia, intestinal parasitisms, intestinal obstructions and hyperthermia. Convulsions may precede the paralysis of tick paralysis.

Since the cause of the epilepsy is unknown, treatment must be based on the clinical signs. The most effective drug in controlling canine epileptic seizures is primidone (℞ 532). Other drugs commonly used are phenobarbital (℞ 531) and diphenylhydantoin (℞ 527). These may be given singly or in combination.

DISEASES OF THE SPINAL CORD

It is important to conduct a detailed systematic evaluation of spinal-cord dysfunction in the differential diagnoses of paresis, paralysis and paraplegia in animals. Following are some of the more common pathologic conditions in the various species.

DISEASES OF THE SPINAL CORD IN DOGS

Infections which may produce signs of spinal involvement are distemper, rabies, Aujeszky's disease, tetanus, toxoplasmosis, systemic mycoses, meningitis, osteomyelitis and epidural abscesses.

Meningitis is not considered contagious in the dog but usually results from an extension or metastasis of other infections. Usual signs are muscular rigidity, fever, hyperexcitability and abnormal spinal fluids. Antibiotics which pass the blood brain barrier, e.g., chloramphenicol, may be helpful.

Osteomyelitis of the spine generally occurs from wounds and may involve the introduction of foreign bodies. Characteristic bone erosion and proliferation occur with or without clinical signs of meningitis or paralysis. A fistulous tract may be present. Surgical debridement of affected bone, decompression of the cord and antibiotic therapy should be used where indicated.

Noninfectious inflammatory disorders and some diseases of questionable etiology include dural ossification, spondylosis, postvaccination rabies paralysis, tick paralysis, botulism, and so-called "coon dog" paralysis.

Dural ossification (pachymeningitis ossificans) occurs in the German Shepherd Dog and in other large breeds after maturity. Bone plaques cause pressure on the cord and nerve roots which results in pain and gradually increasing paresis. The lesions may be visible in radiographs of excellent quality.

Spondylosis is characterized by development of ventral spurs on adjacent vertebrae which may progress dorsolaterally to cause pressure on nerve roots. Pain, paresis and the typical exostosis are characteristic. Symptomatic relief in spondylosis and dural ossification can be obtained in early stages with salicylates (℞ 588), phenylbutazone (℞ 593) and corticosteroids (℞ 148, 154).

Postvaccination rabies paralysis can result from the use of phenolized brain tissue vaccine. Pain, paresis and paralysis are seen 2 to 3 weeks after inoculation. Some affected animals may die.

Tick paralysis is usually due to *Dermacentor* infestations. It is characterized by flaccid paralysis, or paresis. It must be differentiated from botulism or "coon dog" paralysis (*see* below). Prompt recovery is seen when the ticks are removed.

Many other parasites have been the cause of bizarre signs, when they have been located in CNS tissue. Some of these include *Babesia*, tapeworm and roundworm larvae, heartworms and *Cuterebra* larvae.

Botulism. The type A toxin of *Clostridium botulinum* causes a flaccid paralysis in dogs. This toxin may be present in decaying carcasses or discarded home-canned vegetables.

"Coon dog" paralysis is a rapidly progressing flaccid paralysis of field dogs with gradual recovery after 4 to 6 weeks. The etiology is undetermined; however, some think this condition and botulism are the same. Another theory is that the bite or scratch of a raccoon serves as an antigenic stimulus that triggers immunologic disturbance that damages Schwann cells. Nursing care and supportive treatment are important.

Spina bifida and **hemivertebra** are skeletal malformations most frequently observed in brachycephalic breeds such as the

Boston Terrier. These conditions may be clinically silent or, in extreme cases, may contribute to or cause a spinal compression.

Syringomyelia and **spinal dysrhaphism** are among the congenital ageneses and functional deficiencies in the cord which result in slowly progressive clinical signs in the growing puppy. Abnormal posture, bizarre reflex patterns, ataxia, paresis and a hopping gait are observed.

Krabbe's disease has been reported primarily in Cairn Terriers and West Highland White Terriers and is hereditary. CNS signs are seen in young puppies (visual and locomotor deficiencies). There is no known treatment.

Congenital and probably hereditary disorders have been seen as **atlantoaxial luxations** (usually in miniature breeds) or in more caudal **cervical subluxations** (C6-7) seen in young Great Danes. Signs are characteristic of cord compression, such as pain and motor deficiencies. Surgical correction has been effective in the atlantoaxial luxations especially.

Neoplasia may be either vertebral or intraspinal. The various spinal bone tumors are manifested clinically by signs of compression of the cord. Meningiomas cause compression of the cord and produce profound pain, paresis, or paralysis. Medullary spinal-cord tumors may also cause signs characteristic of compression, but their progress is very rapid. Myelography is frequently needed to pinpoint the location.

Compressions of the spinal cord may be due to osteomyelitis, bone cysts, meningitic abscesses, epidural abscesses, dural ossification, spondylosis, spondylolisthesis, vertebral malformations, neoplasia, spinal fractures, spinal luxations and disk protrusions. Characteristic clinical signs of a spinal compression include pain, paresis and incoordination, and paralysis (flaccid or rigid). If the lesion is at the thoracolumbar junction, the knee-jerk reflex is generally exaggerated, while the toe pinch is normal or diminished. The placing reflex is generally absent. If there is no pain response associated with the toe-pinch reflex, the prognosis of recovery is not favorable, regardless of treatment. If extensor rigidity in the front legs is constant and profound, much spinal-cord damage has occurred and the prognosis is unfavorable. Fractures, luxations and disk protrusions should be confirmed by careful radiographic examination. They frequently require surgical decompression. Pain due to mild spinal compressions may be reduced by salicylates (℞ 588), phenylbutazone (℞ 593) and corticosteroids (℞ 144, 154). Infectious conditions, such as abscesses and osteomyelitis require surgical correction and antibiotic therapy.

INTERVERTEBRAL DISK ABNORMALITY

An affection of the intervertebral disk characterized by herniation or by calcification with or without protrusion. Disk abnormalities are most commonly found in dogs, but they have also been reported in cats, rabbits and other species. Lesions usually occur in the terminal thoracic and lumbar segments, but occasionally affect the cervical region. The most susceptible breeds are the so-called chondrodystrophoid group, e.g., Dachshund, Pekingese, Beagle and Cocker Spaniel. Many believe that the multiple disk changes, often seen in dogs of this group, represent a definite systemic degenerative disease. Clinical neuropathy results from pressure on the spinal cord or nerve roots.

Clinical Findings and Diagnosis: Signs vary with the nature, extent and position of the injury. There may be pain, paresis, flaccid or rigid paraplegia, or evidence of acute progressive ascending paralysis resulting from hemorrhagic myelomalacia or hematomyelia.

Pain may be localized over the affected disk or it may be generalized. An arched back, abdominal tenseness and reluctance to move up and down stairs are signs of thoracolumbar-disk protrusion. Extreme pain on moving the head or neck is characteristic of cervical protrusion. Paresis or weakness may accompany the pain. With thoracolumbar-disk protrusion, the hind legs may be affected; with cervical-disk protrusion, front leg weakness may be seen. Thoracolumbar protrusions are usually characterized by rigid or flaccid paraplegia. The paraplegia is accompanied by urinary and fecal retention or incontinence. Disk protrusions that result in an acute progressive ascending paralysis usually cause respiratory paralysis followed by death within 3 to 7 days.

Positive diagnosis and location of the lesions are obtained only by careful neurologic and radiologic examination. Contrast myelography is usually unnecessary.

Treatment: The treatment of the condition depends largely on the extent of the lesion and the severity of clinical signs produced. Acute progressive ascending myelomalacia does not respond to treatment and is usually fatal. Certain paraplegics will recover with conservative treatment. This treatment consists largely of symptomatic care and good nursing. Adequate rest, good nutrition and maintenance of urine and fecal elimination are essential. An analgesic (R 588) and anti-inflammatory drugs (R 593) are indicated if pain is severe and rest is enforced. Physiotherapy in the forms of hot water baths, whirlpool baths, or ultrasound are helpful.

Surgical treatment is indicated when the location of the herniation can be determined and the spinal cord compression is of relatively few days' duration. Sudden and severe compression may require decompression within a few hours to prevent irreversible damage to the spinal cord. Surgical procedures include disk fenestration, hemilaminectomy, dorsal laminectomy, or a combination of the first 2 of these. Disk fenestration involves lateral or ventral curettage of the affected disk to relieve the pressure on the cord. Hemilaminectomy exposes the cord by removal of one side of the bony arch of the spinal canal. The protruding mass can then be completely removed. Dorsal laminectomy generally allows for decompression but no extensive removal of the lesion.

DISEASES OF THE SPINAL CORD IN HORSES

Abnormality of the vertebral column as a result of trauma is the most common cause of paralysis in the horse. It frequently involves the cervical vertebrae, and results from kicks, accidents during halter breaking, injury while tied to a stationary object and falls while running. The degree of paralysis is dependent on the severity of the accompanying spinal lesion and the location.

Equine incoordination or equine ataxia (wobbles) is a characteristic and progressive incoordinate condition of undetermined etiology. Proposed etiologic agents are toxic food materials and congenital abnormalities of the vertebral column, with or without accompanying trauma. Clinical signs are characteristically first seen in the hind limbs of young horses less than 2 years of age, with a higher incidence in males. The condition is progressive regardless of whether the onset is slow or sudden. In some cases the forelegs are also affected with the weaving, drunken gait being accentuated by swaying of the head and neck. Walking the animal in a tight circle, turning abruptly on a lead, or forcing the head and neck into flexion while backing may accentuate the signs. Necropsy of affected animals may or may not disclose pathologic changes in the cord. If present, the spinal lesion is seen as malacia of the gray or white matter, and may be accompanied by osteoarthritis of the affected articulation or a congenital abnormality of the intervertebral processes. Gross lesions are found primarily in the cervical region, and are probably due to compression or stretching of the spinal cord.

Other proposed causes of spinal disorders in the horse are:

equine encephalomyelitis, nutritional deficiencies, primary parasitism or aberrant migration of parasites in nervous tissues, neoplasms of the spinal cord, unidentified substances in certain hybrid pasture grasses, myelitis following rabies vaccination, and neuritis of the cauda equina.

DISEASES OF THE SPINAL CORD IN CATTLE

Practically all inflammations or infections involving the spinal cord affect the meninges. True spinal myelitis is rare, except in Aujesky's disease (q.v., p. 237).

The most frequent pathologic condition is compression causing sudden or progressive paraplegia. Spinal injury and fractures usually are accompanied by sudden motor and sensory paralysis. Tumors and abscesses usually produce progressive motor paralysis. The most common tumor to be involved is bovine lymphosarcoma (affects the cord in about 20% of generalized cases) but osteosarcoma, osteochondrosarcoma, angioma and lipoma may occur. Abscesses of the spinal cord are metastatic, usually from umbilical or castration infection, metritis, mastitis or traumatic peritonitis.

Spondylitis is common in mature cattle, especially bulls. Spinal fractures occasionally occur in newborn calves from mineral deficient dams, however, the most frequent occurrence is in 3- to 4-month-old calves which have been on inadequate diets and with little or no exposure to sunshine. Such fractures occur when the calves are turned out to pasture in the spring.

Tubercular spinal spondylitis is now rare. Rabies may cause an ascending paralysis and anesthesia. Temporary paraplegia may occur in the cow in heat after much "riding" by other cows.

DISEASES OF THE SPINAL CORD IN SWINE

The most common infectious causes of paresis, paralysis, or paraplegia are hog cholera, Teschen disease, brucellosis and pseudorabies. Bacterial toxemias, as seen in edema disease, are also of diagnostic importance. Toxemias due to plant and chemical origin may cause spinal cord damage. Nutritional causes include calcium, phosphorus, vitamin A and various vitamin B deficiencies. Fractures and disk problems have become more numerous in recent years due to the elongation of the bacon-type hog being raised in confinement, and probably to the inadequacy of diets formulated for older types of slower growing pigs.

DISEASES OF THE SPINAL CORD IN SHEEP AND GOATS

Spinal cord irritation and damage in the sheep and goat may be caused by exotoxins of *Clostridium botulinum, Cl. perfringens* and *Cl. tetani*. Maternal copper deficiencies of pregnant ewes and does may result in "enzootic ataxia" (q.v., p. 1323). Maternal vitamin A deficiency, congenital syndromes, e.g., "border disease" (q.v., p. 647) and fetal viral infections such as bluetongue may be incriminated.

Epidural abscesses (usually metastatic), tumors, ingestion of toxic plants (e.g., *Veratrum californicum*) by pregnant ewes, senile atrophy, and focal symmetrical spinal poliomalacia are recorded causes. Spinal cord lesions may follow subacute *Phalaris tuberosa* poisoning. Osteodystrophic diseases, vitamin D and mineral deficiencies may cause maldevelopment and fractures of the vertebral column.

FACIAL PARALYSIS

Facial paralysis in the cat and dog is not uncommon and is frequently related to trauma or inflammation of the inner ear and lesions in the medulla of the brain. A transient idiopathic neuritis, similar to Bell's palsy in man, has been observed in the dog. The horse may suffer from facial paralysis as a result of trauma to the superficial branches of the facial nerve as it crosses the mandible. Trauma to the petrosum of the temporal bone and guttural pouch infections also occasionally damage the nerve. Listeriosis in cattle often affects the facial nucleus or nerve or both.

Clinical Findings: Total unilateral facial paralysis is characterized by the absence of a palpebral reflex, immobility of the ear, and flaccidity of the muscles of facial expression with subsequent deviation of the nose toward the normal side. The palpebral fissure is opened widely and in response to the menace test the animal may retract the globe resulting in flicking of the third eyelid instead of blinking.

Depending upon the site and degree of injury to the nerve, total or partial facial paralysis may be demonstrated. For instance, in the horse, damage to the buccal branches may only result in slight deviation of the nose and flaccidity of the lips. The site of facial paralysis can frequently be localized to the inner ear by the concomitant vestibular disturbance manifested by a head tilt, nystagmus and incoordination in the acute stages. Lesions of the brain stem in the vicinity of the facial nucleus may cause bilateral signs. In addition, the presence of limb weakness and other cranial nerve deficits are helpful in differentiating a central disease from peripheral lesions.

Treatment: Traumatic and idiopathic neuritis of the facial nerve often heals spontaneously within a few weeks. Corticosteroids (R 142) are useful in controlling acute edema and inflammation (most useful for relief of edema of nervous tissue within 24 hours of injury). Infections must be treated vigorously with the appropriate drug. Protective ophthalmic ointments or surgical closure are necessary to prevent keratitis when the eyelids are paralyzed. With impairment of the prehensile lips of horses, providing wet bulky mashes and deep water containers constitute important supportive care.

PARALYSIS OF THE FORELIMB

The innervation of the foreleg is commonly damaged by direct trauma, pressure by improperly restraining heavy animals in lateral recumbency, and occasionally by tumors. Severe traction on the forelimb resulting in excessive abduction of the shoulder can avulse or severely stretch the entire plexus. The radial nerve is most vulnerable to injury at the level of the first rib and at the humerus where it lies in the musculospiral groove. With total destruction of the brachial plexus, the animal is unable to flex or extend the joints, and the limb is desensitized.

Of the 5 major nerves of the plexus (suprascapular, axillary, radial, ulnar and median), injury to the radial nerve proximal to the elbow produces the greatest motor disability because the elbow, carpus and digits cannot be extended to bear weight. A lesion of the nerve distal to the elbow will result in knuckling of the digits and carpus only. Damage to the other 4 nerves produces only a slight motor disability of the forelimb. In chronic cases, severe muscle atrophy will develop in the denervated muscle groups.

An accurate history and a careful neurologic examination of the foreleg are essential and usually adequate to establish the diagnosis. Radiographic evidence of fractures may suggest the site of injury. The prognosis is guarded where sensory loss is complete and 2 to 4 months' convalescence may be necessary if nerve regeneration is to occur.

With acute contusion of the nerves, the object is to relieve edema and pressure. Where severance of a nerve(s) is suspected, surgical exploration and repair is indicated. If the foot is continually dragged and prone to laceration, it may be protected with a leather boot. Amputation of the limb in small animals may be necessary in irreversible cases.

OBTURATOR PARALYSIS

A paralysis of adductor muscles of the hind legs resulting from injury of the obturator nerve. This is most frequently associated with dystocia. Occasionally other pelvic nerves are also affected, and the signs are of posterior paralysis or posterior ataxia. The condition is commonest in the cow, but the mare, ewe and bitch may also be affected. Injury of the nerves occurs when the fetus lies in the pelvic canal for an extended period, or a large fetus is forced through the pelvic canal. There is nearly always some degree of posterior paralysis in cattle when a hip lock exists for more than an hour.

Paralysis or paresis of the muscles of the hind leg result in ataxia or inability to stand. When only the obturator nerve is affected, the animal may lie on its sternum in dorsal recumbency with the hind legs in extreme abduction. Paralyzed animals are bright and alert in contrast to animals with other postparturient diseases such as milk fever. The condition should be differentiated from fractures, muscle trauma, tumors and abscesses involving the pelvic nerves and posterior spinal cord.

Treatment consists of stimulants and good nursing care while the patient is recumbent. Ample dry bedding and easy access to feed and water are essential. Many animals will recover in the recumbent position, but should be turned from one side to the other at least twice daily. Although some prefer to raise the animal in a sling each day, extreme care should be observed in using a hip sling since severe trauma frequently results. Unless recovery occurs in 7 to 10 days, the prognosis is unfavorable. Some animals apparently fail to realize that they have recovered and should be stimulated daily to try to rise. Animals that can stand but are ataxic recover in 1 to 4 days. They should be maintained in an area of good footing so that they do not slip and become discouraged when attempting to rise. If animals are on a slippery surface, tying burlap bags over the rear feet will provide better traction.

DISEASES OF THE CNS CAUSED BY HELMINTH PARASITES AND INSECT LARVAE

Several helminths, particularly their larval stages, occur in the CNS. Whether actual disease is caused by their presence depends upon several factors, especially location, activity and size. There is also the possibility that helminth larvae entering the CNS may transport and facilitate the multiplication of pathogenic microorganisms. In some instances, lodgement in the CNS may possibly have some biologic significance, such as facilitating, by incapacitation, the capture of the intermediate host, e.g., in coenurosis, but in other instances, migration into the CNS occurs when the parasite enters an unusual host and it is in such hosts particularly that signs may be encountered. There may be motor weakness, ataxia, staggering, circling, head deviation, paralysis, blindness and drooping of the ear or eyelid.

In contrast to these erratic invaders, there are several parasites for which the CNS is the usual location for some phase of development. This applies particularly to the nematodes, of which several species are neurotropic. A pathologic feature of these nematode infections is that, whereas they have become adapted to their natural hosts, in which they cause little or no damage, when they gain access to other hosts, even closely related ones, they may cause severe damage.

An example of a neurotropic cestode is the larva of *Multiceps multiceps* which is considered below. This parasite usually occurs in the brain of the sheep. There are no neurotropic trematodes in domestic animals, but the immature forms of *Paragonimus westermani* sometimes lodge in the brain, where it may be found in the cat, dog, or pig.

CESTODES

COENUROSIS

The common names (gid, sturdy, staggers, etc.) betoken prominent clinical signs. The disease is found in sheep, cattle, other herbivores and occasionally man.

The adult *Taenia (Multiceps) multiceps* occurs in the small intestine of dog, fox and jackal. Tapeworm segments are voided onto pasture, so that onchospheres are ingested by herbivorous hosts and migrate to the CNS (the route is not understood) where they become coenuri. The cycle is completed when scolices within the *Coenurus* are eaten by the definitive host. Coenurosis is most common in sheep, less common in cattle.

In infected herbivores, initial invasion can cause acute suppurative meningoencephalitis. In the chronic phase, the mature cyst (which may attain 5 to 6 cm in diameter in 7 months) may cause increased intracranial pressure. Depending on neuroanatomic location, the cyst gives rise to various neurologic signs. These may be general, such as somnolence, inappetence and wasting, or focal, such as turning, circling or other locomotor disturbances.

CYSTICERCOSIS

The definitive host of *Taenia solium* is man; infection occurs from eating pork containing the larval stage (*Cysticercus*). Cysticerci may also occur in man when eggs are swallowed and onchospheres reach the muscles. In man, pigs and dogs, cysticerci may occur in the brain where they often assume an irregular shape (*Cysticercus racemosus*). They may cause epileptiform convulsions, various mental signs and disturbance of locomotion.

ECHINOCOCCOSIS

The definitive host of *Echinococcus granulosus* is the dog; infection occurs from eating viscera of sheep and other ruminants containing hydatid cysts; sometimes they occur in the brain producing signs resembling those of tumors. Cerebral infections occur in man, cattle and horses. The definitive host of *E. multilocularis* is the fox; multilocular hydatids have been reported in the human brain, but not in domestic animals. The usual intermediate hosts are rodents. There may be little surrounding reaction in the brain other than a fibrous gliosis, and lymphocytic and eosinophilic infiltration.

NEMATODES

Setaria (*Artionema*) *digitata* occurs in the peritoneal cavity of cattle and buffalo; microfilariae reach the blood, are ingested by mosquitoes and thereby transmitted to new hosts, sometimes to abnormal hosts, such as sheep, goats and horses. In such hosts, the infective larvae migrate from the skin and may gain access to the nervous system. In their neural migrations, they cause traumatic focal malacic lesions, with neurologic signs of varied kinds, such as paralysis. A disease, characterized by lumbar paralysis and termed "cerebrospinal nematodiasis" has been ascribed to this nematode. It has been reported in Asian countries, especially Ceylon, India, Japan and Korea.

Other filarioid nematodes and their larval stages occur in the brain of domestic animals, but are rarely discovered; they include *Parafilaria multipapillosa, Dirofilaria immitis* and *Onchocerca* spp.

A few strongyloids, such as *Strongylus* spp. and *Stephanurus dentatus* have been observed to cause lesions in the nervous system of horses and pigs, respectively. *Trichinella spiralis* has been found in the brain in fatal human cases. Ascarids, particularly those whose larval stages migrate in the tissues of intermediate hosts, e.g., *Baylisascaris columnaris* and *Toxocara canis*, frequently gain access to the CNS.

Of particular importance, in this regard, are the metastrongyloids or lungworms. Several species in this group undergo a migration through the brain before reaching the lungs or even mature in the CNS, releasing their eggs and larvae via the lungs. It would appear that the effects of this sojourn in the CNS are not ordinarily manifested in the usual host, but when infective larvae are ingested by other hosts, signs of nervous involvement may occur.

Skrjabingylus spp. are known to cause superficial hemorrhage and meningitis in skunks and weasels. *Aelurostrongylus abstrusus* and *Angiostrongylus vasorum* are lungworms that have been found in the nervous system of cats and dogs, respectively. *Angiostrongylus cantonensis* occurs in the brain of rats but not in domestic animals. The metastrongyloid nematodes of ruminant animals are important in northern regions as a cause of neurologic disease. *Pneumostrongylus tenuis* normally occurs in the white-tailed deer (*Odocoileus virginianus*) in North America without causing disease, but where deer and moose occur in the same location severe effects may occur in the latter, as a result of damage by the worms to the dorsal horn region of the spinal cord.

A similar situation exists in Northern Europe and Asia, where several species of the genus *Elaphostrongylus* are found in the CNS of deer and reindeer, in which they may cause neurologic signs, such as paresis and ataxia.

INSECT LARVAE

Larvae of some Diptera find their way into the CNS of animals and cause neurologic signs. Larvae of *Oestrus ovis*, the nasal fly of sheep, normally inhabit the nasal passages and paranasal sinuses. Sometimes the larvae penetrate the ethmoid bone and reach the forebrain, or an associated pyogenic infection of the sinuses spreads to the brain; this results in neurologic manifestations such as headshaking, high-stepping gait, incoordination and paralysis.

Larvae of the "warble fly" of cattle, *Hypoderma bovis,* in the course of their migration to the subcut. position, normally reside for several months in the spinal canal, where their presence causes inflammation, and necrosis of epidural fat. Despite such regular intraspinal migration, associated neurologic disorders have seldom been reported. However, transient neurologic signs, varying from a stiff, unsteady gait to severe ataxia and weakness of the limbs, may occur in calves given systemic insecticides, e.g., organophosphates, when large numbers of larvae are present in the spinal canal. Onset is rapid and recovery usually occurs in 48 to 72 hours after the calves receive the insecticide. Supposedly, the syndrome is made manifest by the pronounced irritation of epidural tissues which accompanies rapid killing of many larvae. Cerebral invasion by larvae of *H. bovis* also has been reported in cattle and sometimes occurs in horses. Perhaps the most practical approach to dealing with parasitic infection of the CNS is the use of appropriate and effective prophylactic measures.

Treatment: Attempts have been made to apply various forms of treatment to parasitic infection of the CNS. Surgical removal hardly seems practicable with animals. Successful chemotherapeutic treatment has been reported with diethylcarbamazine for cerebrospinal nematodiasis in India at a dose of 45 mg/lb. It should, however, be borne in mind that to kill worms may remove the traumatic effect, but may provoke further damage through toxic or suppurative effects.

MENINGITIS

Inflammation of the meninges is most commonly encountered as a sequela to coliform or streptococcal septicemia of neonatal calves, lambs and piglets but rarely in foals. Fibrinopurulent meningitis may occur in feeder pigs due to *Haemophilus* infection with or without evidence of a generalized polyserositis (*see* GLÄSSER'S DISEASE, p. 414). Encephalitic listeriosis in lambs, sheep, goats and cattle often causes a basilar purulent meningitis. Primary or secondary meningitis is comparatively rare in dogs, cats and mature animals. It may occur in cattle following dehorning and sinusitis. In dogs, cats and pigs, it may complicate a middle-ear infection. It may follow bite wounds, infected surgical or traumatic wounds about the head or vertebral column, or primary nasal cryptococcosis in cats. A focal granulomatous meningitis has also been reported in cats with infectious feline peritonitis (q.v., p. 323).

In the acute stage, meningitis is classically characterized by high fever, hyperesthesia, pain on movement of the body, and in extreme cases, opisthotonos. If depression, coma or paralysis develops, the infection has advanced to meningoencephalitis or myelitis or both. Chronic spinal meningitis, especially of the dog, can be misdiagnosed since the classical triad of signs may not be present at the initial examination. A cerebrospinal fluid examination (q.v., p. 626) is specific for the diagnosis of meningitis. The fluid is often opaque and has a high neutrophil and protein content.

An attempt to obtain a culture and sensitivity of the causative organism(s) from the spinal fluid is advisable, to permit administration of the appropriate antibiotic at the maximum safe dosage. If there is no response to the treatment or if the organisms cannot be cultured, an intensive regime of broad-spectrum antibiotics is often effective (℞ 28). The treatment must be continued until there is a permanent remission of signs and the spinal fluid returns to normal. Corticosteroids are contraindicated. Analgesics, high-quality diet and supportive care are beneficial.

THROMBOEMBOLIC MENINGOENCEPHALITIS OF CATTLE (TEME)

An acute infectious disease primarily affecting the CNS, characterized by fever, severe depression, weakness, ataxia, blindness, paralysis, coma and death within one hour to several days. It is most common in feed-lot cattle but may occur in pastured animals.

Etiology and Pathogenesis: The organism which is most consistently isolated from affected animals is a *Haemophilus* sp., tentatively classified as *H. somnus*. It produces a septicemia with diffuse vasculitis and thrombosis in a variety of organs. The most severe lesions are usually evident in the brain. TEME may occur concurrently or follow outbreaks of pasteurellosis (q.v., p. 385), or it may occur as a disease entity of its own.

Clinical Findings: Temperatures in the early stages may be as high as 108°F but fall to normal or subnormal very rapidly.

Other characteristic signs are stiffness, knuckling at the fetlocks, severe depression, ataxia, paralysis and opisthotonos, followed by coma and death within 1 to 48 hours. Most affected animals are blind, and retiral hemorrhages with grayish foci of retinal necrosis may be observed with an ophthalmoscope. Other signs such as hypersensitivity, convulsions, excitement, nystagmus and circling occur inconsistently. Occasionally animals are found dead without showing any signs of illness. Morbidity is usually below 5% but may be as high as 30%; mortality may reach 100%.

Lesions: The most characteristic lesions are evident in the brain and these consist of focal areas of hemorrhagic necrosis 0.5 to 1.0 cm in diameter which are most prominent on the cut surfaces. Similar hemorrhagic areas may be evident in skeletal muscles, myocardium and kidney. Other but less consistent lesions are fibrinous pleuritis, pericarditis, and polyarthritis most commonly in the stifle joints.

Treatment and Prophylaxis: Clinically affected animals should be segregated and treated immediately with penicillin and streptomycin IM (R 41). Oral medication, preferably in the drinking water, with high levels of chlortetracycline (R 11) may be indicated when large numbers of animals are involved. Treatment is most effective in the early stages of the disease; after the animal becomes recumbent the prognosis is very poor. Since early detection and treatment are of utmost importance, animals should be checked at least every 2 hours in feed lots where the disease has been confirmed.

In severe outbreaks the reduction of concentrates and increasing the roughage of the diet may help control the disease. Attempts to immunize animals with a *Haemophilus* vaccine have yielded variable results.

POLIOENCEPHALOMALACIA
(Cerebrocortical necrosis)

A noninfectious neurologic disease of cattle, sheep, goats and deer, characterized clinically by amaurosis, anorexia, incoordination and depression of ruminal movement. Animals which do not recover from these early signs either spontaneously or after treatment progress to a state of recumbency and opisthotonos, and tonic-clonic convulsions. Characteristic lesions are most frequently found in the cerebral cortex as multifocal or diffuse yellow zones of cortical necrosis. Polioencephalomalacia is the term used in the U.S.A., Canada, Australia and

New Zealand while cerebrocortical necrosis is the term used to describe what is apparently the same disease in the United Kingdom, France and Germany.

Etiology: Results from several countries indicate that animals with polioencephalomalacia are in a state of thiamine (vitamin B_1) depletion. Because ruminants with a normal rumen derive adequate thiamine from symbiotic ruminal activity, the inadequacy is thought to be a result of intraruminal thiamine destruction either by the enzymes or toxins of fungi or other microbes. Structural analogs of thiamine formed by complex intraruminal biochemical reactions may be present and interfere with thiamine metabolism. Thiamine functions as a coenzyme in carbohydrate metabolism, and its lack can be expected to cause increases in the blood concentrations of pyruvic, lactic and alpha-ketoglutaric acids, and a decrease in activity of the enzyme transketolase. The dependence of neurons and glial cells of the brain on carbohydrate catabolism accounts for the prominent neurologic signs.

Clinical Findings: The disease occurs more frequently in young cattle on high-energy diets. Sudden depression, disturbances of gait and blindness of cortical origin are the usual presenting signs, but a short period of prodromal anorexia may be observed. The rumen usually is contracting, but the action is weak and infrequent. Hyperesthesia, head-pressing, muscular tremors and twitching of ears, eyelids and muzzle may also occur. Occasionally papilledema and elevated cerebrospinal fluid pressures are noted. Unless convulsions follow, temperature, pulse and respiration rates remain within normal limits. Bradycardia and arrhythmias may occasionally be detected. In untreated recumbent cattle the mortality is close to 100%. The morbidity in feed-lot cattle is usually less than 5% but in 3- to 5-month-old calves the morbidity may be as high as 50%.

Diagnosis: Diagnosis should be based on signs or lesions and, where possible, on detection of increases in blood pyruvate and lactate concentrations (especially the pyruvate:lactate ratio) and a decrease in blood or tissue transketolase activity.

Included in the differential diagnosis should be lead poisoning, chlorinated hydrocarbon toxicity, infectious thromboembolic meningoencephalitis, brain abscesses and Type-D clostridial enterotoxemia of sheep.

Treatment and Control: Thiamine, alone or in a B-complex preparation, administered IV at a dose of 3 to 5 mg/lb of body wt every 6 hours for 24 hours, is the treatment of choice in cases diagnosed early. Recovery may not always be complete, but the animal's place as an economic unit in the herd is often restored. Since others in the herd are probably also at risk, dietary cereal content should be decreased and additional good quality roughage supplied for a period of 5 days prior to a gradual return to higher energy rations. Supplemental dietary thiamine can be added to the diet temporarily. Since carbohydrate metabolism is impaired in the disease, the use of IV dextrose is contraindicated except in the convalescent stages.

Animals severely affected for more than 24 hours cannot be expected to respond well to treatment.

HYDROCEPHALUS

The presence of excessive amounts of cerebrospinal fluid (CSF) within the cranial cavity. It may be external, with the fluid accumulating in the subarachnoid space around the brain, or internal with the fluid being contained within the ventricular system. In communicating hydrocephalus the excess fluid is present in both locations.

Etiology and Pathogenesis: Hydrocephalus usually results from: (1) overproduction of fluid by the choroid plexuses, (2) obstruction of fluid flow at some point in the CSF pathway, or (3) inadequate resorption of fluid into the venous system via the arachnoid villi.

Recent work has shown that in vitamin A deficiency, an increase in CSF fluid pressure and subsequent hydrocephalus may be associated with a decreased absorption of CSF in the arachnoid villi. Other nutritional deficiencies have been cited as possible causes of some forms of congenital hydrocephalus. Other congenital forms are related to mechanical obstruction of the tentorial foramen or cerebral aqueduct, although such obstructions are generally difficult to demonstrate morphologically. Hydrocephalus in small animals occurs most commonly in the small dogs such as the Chihuahua, Boston Terrier, Pekingese and the toy breeds.

Hereditary forms of congenital hydrocephalus have been reported in Holstein-Friesian and Hereford calves. These are probably due to a single autosomal recessive gene. Achondrodysplastic calves frequently also have congenital hydrocephalus and the conditions are usually inherited as a simple recessive character. The condition may be acquired, most often by obstruction of the CSF pathways as by a tumor or meningitis.

In aged horses, cholesteatomas of the choroid plexuses frequently are associated with some degree of internal hydrocephalus.

Clinical Findings: Many cases of congenital hydrocephalus remain subclinical and well-advanced lesions have been observed as incidental findings on postmortem examinations. The most prominent feature of congenital hydrocephalus is an enlarged head. Hydrocephalus may cause open fontanelles and suture lines. The animal may exhibit depression, abnormal reactions to stimuli, incoordination, paralysis, prostration and sometimes convulsions. Loss of vision and papilledema of the optic disk are frequently evident. Occasionally an affected dog will become irritable, resent being handled and whine without apparent cause. Pneumoventriculograms have been successfully used as a diagnostic aid in dogs. Changes in temperament have also been reported in the horse.

The use of vitamin A, multiple B-complex, improved nutrition and diuretics may be beneficial in an occasional case. Aspiration via cerebrospinal tap may be beneficial in the event of overproduction or inadequate resorption. Surgical treatment consisting of various shunting devices has been described. The prognosis, however, is generally unfavorable.

BORDER DISEASE
("Hairy shaker" disease)

Border disease in Britain and "hairy shaker" disease in New Zealand are clinically identical diseases of sheep. As the infectious agents are not yet characterized, for practical purposes they may be considered as one entity. The condition probably occurs in other countries, including Western U.S.A.

Affected flocks will probably first be recognized at lambing time by the presence of a number of undersized lambs with excessively hairy and sometimes excessively pigmented fleeces. Some of these exhibit involuntary muscular tremors of variable severity that may be confined to the head and neck or affect the whole body. The tremors are reduced at rest and exacerbated with movement. These hairy lambs have a poor survival rate and many die before weaning. However, in the few that survive, the nervous signs will gradually disappear within 3 or 4 months. In affected flocks there is an associated infertility problem with up to 8 times the normally expected number of ewes failing to give birth to lambs. Abortions occur at all stages of pregnancy, some of the aborted fetuses being mummified and many of those occurring late in pregnancy having obviously hairy fleeces. There are no characteristic placental lesions but the aborted fetuses are almost always undersized.

Incidence: Up to half of the hairy lambs seen alive may show nervous signs, but usually the proportion is much less than this. The number of lambs affected may be quite small in the first season in which the flock becomes infected, but the incidence may subsequently increase in the following 2 or 3 seasons to as high as 50% of the lamb crop and then decline to a very low incidence.

Diagnosis: The clinical picture in a flock will usually allow a diagnosis. Some normally smooth-coated breeds of sheep have genetically controlled hairiness of the fleece but confusion should not arise because such lambs will not have any associated nervous signs. Histologic evidence of hypomyelinogenesis provides confirmation. The disease agent is present in the tissues of affected lambs and fetuses and experimentally may be transmitted to ewes in the first 2 months of pregnancy parenterally or by the oral or conjunctival routes.

Control: Introduction of sheep from infected flocks should be avoided. Ewes which have given birth to affected lambs acquire a strong immunity to subsequent infection. Susceptible ewes in their last third of pregnancy may be exposed to infection without any ill effects, but it is not yet certain if they thus acquire any worthwhile immunity.

The natural mode of transmission is unknown and the possibility of spread by the venereal route has not been excluded. There are currently no methods available for the artificial stimulation of immunity.

PARASITIC DISEASES

GASTROINTESTINAL PARASITISM
(LG. AN.)

The digestive tract is inhabited by many species of parasites. The development of clinical parasitism depends on the number and activity of these parasites, climatic conditions and management practices, and the resistance, age, plane of nutrition and level of concurrent disease in the host. The economic importance of subclinical parasitism, now well established in ruminants, is determined by the same factors. Animals that show no clinical signs of disease often perform less efficiently, even under feed-lot and dairy conditions. Advances in therapy and our understanding of epidemiology make possible control, and even prevention, of most losses from parasites. This goal is accomplished by coordinating management practices, diagnostics and strategic anthelmintic applications as an integral part of comprehensive herd-health programming.

Since the advent of effective broad-spectrum anthelmintics, most worm infections of ruminants are diagnosed and handled as general parasitoses and not as specific infections. Diagnosis, treatment and control of the gastrointestinal helminthiases of ruminants are therefore dealt with collectively following the separate discussions of parasite species rather than under each species (*see the table of contents*, p. 649).

CATTLE

Haemonchus, Ostertagia AND *Trichostrongylus*
INFECTION

The common stomach worms of cattle are *Haemonchus placei* (large stomach worm, wire worm), *Ostertagia ostertagi* (medium or brown stomach worm) and *Trichostrongylus axei* (small stomach worm, bankrupt worm). In some tropical countries *Mecistocirrus digitatus*, a large worm up to 40 mm long is present and causes severe anemia. Adult males of *Haemonchus* are as long as 18 mm and the females are up to 37 mm. *Ostertagia* adults are 6 to 9 mm in length and those of *Trichostrongylus* are smaller, about 5 mm. The life cycles of the 3 groups are generally similar. Under favorable conditions, larvae hatch from the eggs shortly after they are passed in the feces and are infective within about 5 days. If conditions are unfavorable, embryonated eggs may remain dormant for weeks, with the subsequent emergence of large numbers of larvae when conditions become favorable.

The prepatent period (time from ingestion of larvae until eggs are passed in the feces) is normally 21 to 25 days. About 3 days after their ingestion, *Ostertagia* larvae have migrated into the glandular crypts of the mucosa where they remain during most of the prepatent period. In heavy infections, the larvae apparently return to the lumen over an extended period, possibly for as long as several months.

Under some conditions a high proportion of the developing *Ostertagia* enter the mucosa and become retarded or inhibited (hypobiosis). In this state they are not very vulnerable to anthelmintics. The worms resume development after some weeks or even several months and produce the Type II disease. The factors which cause developing worms to become inhibited, and those which stimulate resumption of development are not precisely known. In certain climatic regions it is chiefly the infective larvae that are ingested in the autumn that become retarded (e.g., in Scotland). Among the causes that stimulate resumption of development are the parturient state, lactation, removal of a concurrent infection with mature worms and perhaps changes in husbandry and nutrition or even simply the lapse of time. The significance of this aspect of the life cycle is that outbreaks of the Type II disease may occur as long as several months after the infection was acquired and that repeated treatment with an anthelmintic at short intervals (2 to 3 weeks) may be required to cure the disease.

Clinical Findings: Young animals are more often affected, but mature animals frequently show signs and succumb to infection. Digestive disturbances are common in infections with all the stomach worms and may develop during the prepatent period through the activity of the larvae. *Ostertagia* and *Trichostrongylus* infections are characterized by profuse watery diarrhea which usually is persistent. In haemonchosis, there may be little or no diarrhea, but possibly intermittent periods of constipation. Anemia of variable degree is a characteristic sign of haemonchosis.

Concurrent with the anemia of heavy *Haemonchus* infection, there is often hydremia and edema, the edema being most easily observed in the tissues of the submandibular region ("bottle-jaw"). Very heavy infections can produce death before clinical signs appear. Other variable signs include progressive loss of weight, weakness, rough hair coat and anorexia.

Lesions: In heavy *Haemonchus* infections, the folds of the abomasum are usually edematous and may show many minute hemorrhages on the surface where the worms have perforated the mucosa to suck blood. The most characteristic lesion of *Ostertagia* infection is the presence of innumerable small nodules 1 to 2 mm in diameter, raised just above the surface of the mucosa. These are the result of the penetration of the larvae into the crypts.

A minute depression can usually be seen in the center of the nodule. In very heavy infections, these nodules are less discrete, but the mucosa will be thicker and have a rough, irregular surface. In many cases, minute, grayish-white necrotic foci may be seen within the mucosa. Some crypts become greatly dilated as a result of larval invasion and form small vesicles which are quite similar to (but less numerous than) the cystic lesions seen in the abomasal mucosa in bovine hyperkeratosis. Lesions are most marked in the fundic portion, but may extend over the entire abomasal mucosa. Minute hemorrhages and variable congestion may be present in heavy infections. There may be extensive edema. In Type II

Ostertagia infection, the mucosa is thickened, there are numerous confluent nodular lesions, and there is a general "cobblestone" or "morocco leather" appearance. Malabsorption of nutrients and elevated plasma pepsinogen and abomasal pH levels interfere significantly with the digestive process and are important factors in the pathogenesis of ostertagiasis.

In *Trichostrongylus* infections, the mucosa of the abomasum shows moderate to severe congestion. Superficial erosions, covered with a slight fibrino-necrotic exudate, are sometimes seen and, in heavy infections, this exudate is extensive.

Diagnosis, Treatment and Control: *See* p. 662 et seq.

Cooperia INFECTION

Several species of *Cooperia*, referred to collectively as cooperids, occur in the small intestine of cattle; *C. punctata*, *C. oncophora* and *C. pectinata* are the commonest species. The adults vary from 5 to 8 mm in length and are thus difficult to observe grossly. Their life cycle is essentially the same as that of *Haemonchus*. These worms apparently do not suck blood. Most of them are found in the first 10 to 20 ft of the small intestine. The prepatent period is 12 to 15 days.

Clinical Findings: In heavy infections with *Cooperia* there is profuse diarrhea, anorexia and emaciation, but no anemia. The eggs of the cooperids can usually be differentiated from those of the other common gastrointestinal nematodes by the fact that the sides are practically parallel.

In heavy infections the upper portion of the small intestine shows marked congestion of the mucosa, with small hemorrhages. The mucosa may show a fine lace-like necrosis superficially. It is usually necessary to make scrapings of the mucosa to demonstrate the worms, which must be differentiated from *Trichostrongylus, Strongyloides papillosus* and immature *Nematodirus*.

Diagnosis, Treatment and Control: *See* p. 662 et seq.

Bunostomum INFECTION

The adult male of *Bunostomum phlebotomum* is about 9 mm and the female up to 18 mm in length. Hookworms have well-developed buccal capsules into which the mucosa is drawn in attaching and feeding. The prepatent period is approximately 2 months. Exposure may be by ingestion or skin penetration.

Clinical Findings: These worms are active bloodsuckers. Anemia and rapid loss of weight are consequently characteristic signs of clinical bunostomiasis. There may be intermittent constipation and diarrhea. Hydremia and edema may be present, but "bottle-jaw" usually is not as marked as in haemonchosis. During the patent period, a diagnosis may be made by demonstrating the characteristic eggs in the feces.

On necropsy, the mucosa appears congested and swollen, and often shows numerous small hemorrhagic points where the worms were attached. Most of the worms, which are large and easily seen, are in the first few feet of the small intestine. As few as 2,000 to 3,000 worms may cause death in calves. Local lesions, edema and scab formation may result from penetration of larvae into the skin of resistant calves. Infected cattle do not utilize copper effectively.

Diagnosis, Treatment and Control: *See* p. 662 et seq.

Strongyloides INFECTION

The intestinal threadworm, *Strongyloides papillosus,* has an unusual life cycle. Only female worms occur in the parasitic phase of the cycle. These are 3.5 to 6 mm long and are embedded in the mucosa of the upper portion of the small intestine. Small embryonated eggs are passed in the feces, hatch rapidly and may develop directly into infective larvae or into free-living adults. The offspring of these free-living adults may also develop into infective larvae or another generation of free-living adults. The host may be infected by penetration of the skin or by ingestion. The prepatent period is approximately 10 days.

Clinical Findings: Signs are rare, but may include intermittent diarrhea, loss of appetite and weight, and sometimes the presence of blood and mucus in the feces. Large numbers of worms in the intestine produce a catarrhal enteritis with petechial and ecchymotic hemorrhages, especially in the duodenum and jejunum. Skin penetration of the larvae may elicit inflammatory reactions, particularly between the claws where it may resemble early stages of foot rot.

Diagnosis, Treatment and Control: *See* p. 662 et seq.

Nematodirus INFECTION

The adult males of *Nematodirus* are about 12 mm and the females 18 to 25 mm in length. The eggs develop slowly, the infective third stage being reached within the shell in 2 to 4 weeks. Even after the infective stage has been reached, the larvae may remain within the shell for several months. Eggs may accumulate in pastures and hatch in large numbers after rain to produce heavy infections over a short period. After ingestion of infective larvae the adult stage is reached in approximately 3 weeks. The worms are most numerous 10 to 20 ft from the pylorus.

Clinical Findings: Clinical signs include diarrhea, anorexia and weakness. The signs usually develop during the third week of infection before the worms are usually sexually mature. This makes diagnosis more difficult. During the patent period, diagnosis is easily made on the basis of the characteristic eggs. Relatively small numbers of eggs are produced by this parasite. Resistance to reinfection develops rapidly and the adults are mostly eliminated within 2 to 3 months. Postmortem findings may only include a thickened, edematous mucosa.

Diagnosis, Treatment and Control: *See* p. 662 et seq.

Oesophagostomum INFECTION

The adults of *Oesophagostomum radiatum* (nodular worm) are 12 to 15 mm long. The eggs are very similar to those of *Haemonchus placei* and often are grouped with them on routine fecal examination. The life cycle is direct and resembles that of *Haemonchus* but within 24 hours after ingestion, the larvae penetrate the intestinal wall where they remain for 5 to 10 days and then return to the lumen as fourth-stage larvae. The prepatent period is approximately 6 weeks, but may be greatly extended if larvae become retarded in the mucosa.

Clinical Findings: The appetite may be affected in 2 to 3 days after infection. Diarrhea develops in 7 to 15 days. Loss of weight, severe emaciation and general weakness are associated with the diarrhea. The general condition usually improves by the time egg production begins. Although it is not common, the presence of large numbers of adults may produce signs that develop several months after the initial infection. Small nodules are produced in the wall of the intestine as the result of the larval damage. At first, these are only slightly raised areas about 1 mm in diameter, but later they increase appreciably in size and often are filled with pus. Nodule production is not as pronounced in cattle as in sheep. Nodular lesions may predispose to intussusception. Immature worms are often found in the feces. On necropsy, the worms and lesions can be demonstrated.

Diagnosis, Treatment and Control: *See* p. 662 et seq.

Chabertia INFECTION

Adults of the large-mouth bowel worm, *Chabertia ovina*, are about 12 mm long and bent ventrally at the anterior end. There is a typical direct life cycle, with the larvae penetrating the mucosa of the colon shortly after ingestion. The prepatent period is at least 7 days.

Clinical Findings: Diarrhea, with blood and mucus, develops about a month after infection and persists for a month or two. The colon is congested with some erosion of the epithelium. Edema and small hemorrhages are present. The larvae suck blood, and as the adult worm digests the teat of mucosa that is pulled into the large buccal cavity, some blood is ingested. Diagnosis may be difficult since most of the signs occur before eggs are being passed. Often, immature worms can be found in the feces during the period of diarrhea.

Diagnosis, Treatment and Control: *See* p. 662 et seq.

TAPEWORM INFECTION

The anoplocephaline tapeworms *Moniezia expansa* and *M. benedeni* are commonly found in cattle. The tapeworms of this group are characterized by the absence of a rostellum and hooks, and the segments usually are wider than long. The eggs are triangular or rectangular and are ingested by free-living oribatid mites which live in the soil and grass. After a period of 6 to 16 weeks, infective cysticercoids are present in the mites. Infection occurs by ingestion of the mites; the prepatent period is approximately 5 weeks.

Moniezia is commonly considered nonpathogenic, but occasionally in young calves the worms apparently cause diarrhea.

Diagnosis, Treatment and Control: *See* p. 662 et seq.

SHEEP AND GOATS

A number of species of nematodes and cestodes are capable of producing parasitic gastritis and enteritis in sheep and goats. The most important of these are *Haemonchus contortus*, *Ostertagia circumcincta*, *Trichostrongylus axei*, intestinal species of *Trichostrongylus*, *Nematodirus* spp., *Bunostomum trigonocephalum* and *Oesophagostomum columbianum*. *Cooperia curticei*, *Strongyloides papillosus*, *Trichuris ovis* and *Chabertia ovina* may also be pathogenic in sheep; these and related species are discussed under helminths of cattle (q.v., p. 652 et seq.).

Haemonchus, Ostertagia AND Trichostrongylus
INFECTION

The principal stomach worms of sheep and goats are *Haemonchus contortus, Ostertagia circumcincta* and *Trichostrongylus axei* and in some tropical regions also *Mecistocirrus digitatus*. Cross-transmission of *Haemonchus* between sheep and cattle can occur, but not as readily as in infections with the homologous species. Sheep are more susceptible to the cattle species than are cattle to the sheep species. For information on the size of these worms and on their life cycles, *see* the discussion under CATTLE, p. 652.

In the U.S.A., as in most parts of the world, all 3 types of stomach worm are widely distributed. *Haemonchus* is most common in areas receiving summer rainfall, while *Ostertagia* and *Trichostrongylus* are found most commonly in areas with predominantly winter rainfall.

Clinical Findings: Sheep infected with *Haemonchus* may die quickly without showing significant signs. In predominantly *Haemonchus* infections, the animals are more likely to show constipation than diarrhea. The latter is characteristic of ostertagiasis and trichostrongylosis. It must be emphasized that mature animals may develop heavy, even fatal, infections when exposed to large numbers of larvae. This is particularly true of lactating ewes. Death may occur during the prepatent period. The principal lesions of haemonchosis are those associated with anemia. The abomasal contents are commonly stained a reddish-brown color. The lesions and signs of *Ostertagia* and *Trichostrongylus* infections appear to be essentially the same as those found in the corresponding infections of cattle.

Ostertagia in sheep shows the same type of retarded development (hypobiosis) as recorded in cattle. A similar phenomenon has been seen with *Haemonchus*.

Diagnosis, Treatment and Control: *See* p. 662 et seq.

INTESTINAL TRICHOSTRONGYLOSIS
(*T. colubriformis, T. vitrinus, T. rugatus*)

The life cycle of intestinal *Trichostrongylus* is essentially the same as that of the nematodes found in the abomasum of cattle. Shortly after infection, the developing larvae burrow superficially into the crypts of the mucosa. The prepatent period is approximately 3 weeks.

Clinical Findings: Common signs are emaciation and persistent diarrhea. Clinical anemia is not a common sign, but trichostrongylosis is often associated with malnutrition and the combined effects may result in anemia. At necropsy, diffuse congestion of the mucosa may be seen, but usually there is only emaciation and diarrhea. Coccidiosis may accompany trichostrongylosis and there may then be an obvious enteritis. *Trichostrongylus* females produce relatively small numbers of eggs. No diagnostic lesions are found on necropsy.

Diagnosis, Treatment and Control: *See* p. 662 et seq.

Bunostomum INFECTION

Adults of *Bunostomum trigonocephalum* (hookworm) are found in the jejunum. The life cycle is essentially the same as that of the cattle hookworm, as are the clinical findings.

Diagnosis, Treatment and Control: *See* p. 662 et seq.

Nematodirus INFECTION

The species of *Nematodirus* occurring in the small intestine of sheep are similar in morphology and life cycle to those in the intestine of cattle. The prepatent period may be as short as 14 days in sheep. Clinical *Nematodirus* infections are of considerable importance in Great Britain, New Zealand and Australia where death losses of 20% of the lambs in the affected flocks have been reported. The parasites are endemic in some parts of the Rocky Mountain area in the U.S.A. where they occasionally cause clinical disease in lambs.

In those areas where clinical infections are common, the disease often has a characteristic seasonal pattern. Many of the eggs passed by affected lambs lie dormant through the remainder of the grazing season and the winter, with large numbers of larvae appearing during the early grazing period of the following year. It is only when susceptible lambs are exposed to a heavy intake of these infective larvae that the disease develops. Most clinical infections occur in lambs 6 to 12 weeks old. In Great Britain and part of Europe, *N. battus* is the chief cause of the severe outbreaks seen in lambs. In other countries this species does not occur but other species are present and cause a similar disease. Due to different climatic and husbandry conditions the epidemiology of the disease is not as precise as that seen with *N. battus*. Outbreaks often follow rain after a period of dry weather when the eggs have accumulated and then hatch in large numbers to produce heavy infections over a short period. *Nematodirus* spp. often occur in low-rainfall regions (e.g., the Karroo in South Africa and inland Australia) where other parasites rarely cause disease.

Clinical Findings: The disease is characterized by sudden onset, "loss of bloom", unthriftiness, profuse diarrhea and marked dehydration, with death occurring as early as 2 to 3 days after the beginning of the outbreak. Nematodirosis is commonly confined to lambs or weaner sheep, but in low-rainfall country where outbreaks are sporadic, older sheep may experience heavy infections. The lesions usually consist of dehydration and a mild catarrhal enteritis, but acute inflammation of the entire small intestinal tract may occur. Counts of at least 10,000 worms, together with characteristic signs and history, are indicative of clinical infections. The affected lambs may pass large numbers of eggs, which can be identified easily; however, since the onset may precede the maturation of the female worms, this is not a constant finding.

Diagnosis, Treatment and Control: *See* p. 662 et seq.

Oesophagostomum INFECTION

The sheep nodular worm *Oesophagostomum columbianum* is similar morphologically and in its life cycle to the nodular worm of cattle (q.v., p. 656).

Clinical Findings: Diarrhea usually develops during the second week of the infection. The feces may contain an excessive amount of mucus as well as streaks of blood. As the diarrhea progresses, the animals become emaciated and weak and have a stilted gait. These signs often subside near the end of the prepatent period, but the presence of large numbers of adult worms may result in a more chronic type of infection in which signs may not develop for several months. The animals become weak, lose weight despite a good appetite and show intermittent periods of diarrhea and constipation.

Nodule formation is usually more pronounced in sheep than in cattle. The nodules are often found in other organs, especially the liver and lungs. Intussusception may be associated with severe nodular worm infection.

The diagnosis is difficult during the prepatent period, at which time it must be based largely on clinical signs, although the nodules can often be palpated by digital examination per rectum.

Diagnosis, Treatment and Control: *See* p. 662 et seq.

Chabertia INFECTION

The adult worms cause severe damage to the mucosa of the colon with resulting congestion, edema and small hemorrhages. Immature worms are bloodsuckers. Infected sheep are unthrifty and the feces are soft and contain much mucus, often streaked with blood.

Diagnosis, Treatment and Control: *See* p. 662 et seq.

Strongyloides INFECTION

Heavy infections with adult worms cause a disease resembling trichostrongylosis. Damage to the skin between the claws, produced by skin-penetrating larvae, resembles the early stages of foot rot. Most infections are transitory and inconsequential.

Diagnosis, Treatment and Control: *See* p. 662 et seq.

Trichuris INFECTION

Heavy infections with whipworms are not common, but may be associated with congestion, edema and a yellowish discoloration of the cecal mucosa, accompanied by diarrhea and unthriftiness.

Diagnosis, Treatment and Control: *See* p. 662 et seq.

TAPEWORM INFECTION

The pathogenicity of *Moniezia expansa* in sheep has long been debated. Many earlier observations which associated this infection with diarrhea, emaciation and loss of weight did not accurately differentiate between tapeworm infections and infection with certain of the small nematodes (e.g., *Trichostrongylus colubriformis*). Tapeworms are relatively nonpathogenic, but heavy infections may result in signs of disease or the animal may be predisposed to enterotoxemia. Diagnosis may be made on the basis of presence of yellowish proglottids in the feces or protruding from the anal opening, or the demonstration of the characteristic eggs on fecal examination. The life cycle involves a tiny mite which lives in the mat of pastures. The prepatent period in sheep is 6 to 7 weeks. Lambs develop resistance quickly and infections are lost from most sheep by about 4 to 5 months.

Thysanosoma actinoides, the "fringed tapeworm" inhabits the small intestine, as well as the bile and pancreatic ducts. They are commonly found in sheep from the Western U.S.A. Their presence has not been associated with clinical disease.

Thysanosoma is of economic importance because livers are condemned when tapeworms are found in the bile duct during meat inspection. The proglottids are pearl-white and bell-shaped.

Diagnosis, Treatment and Control: *See* below.

DIAGNOSIS OF GASTROINTESTINAL PARASITISMS IN RUMINANTS

The clinical signs associated with gastrointestinal parasitisms are shared with many diseases and conditions; however, presumptive diagnosis based on history and signs is often justified and can usually be confirmed by demonstrating eggs on fecal examination. In evaluating clinical importance of fecal examinations, the following points should be remembered: (1) The number of eggs per gram of feces often is not an accurate indication of the number of adult worms present because of a) negative counts despite the presence of large numbers of immature worms, or b) suppression of egg production by immune reaction or previous anthelmintic treatment. (2) The egg-producing capacity of different worms varies greatly (being significantly lower for *Trichostrongylus*, *Ostertagia* and *Nematodirus* than for *Haemonchus*). (3) Specific identification of eggs is often impractical. The ova of *Nematodirus*, *Bunostomum*, *Strongyloides* and *Trichuris* are distinctive but reliable differentiation of the more common species of ruminant nematode ova is difficult for most stockmen and practitioners. Fecal cultures will produce distinctive third-stage larvae if ante-mortem differentiation is important. The advent of safe and effective broad-spectrum anthelmintics has reduced the need for species or generic differentiations of these parasites.

In many management situations experience has shown that significant infections can be taken for granted, particularly after favorable temperatures and rainfall conditions in certain seasons. "Diagnostic drenching" is recommended in cases where eggs are few or absent, yet history and signs suggest infections. A clinical response to a safe, broad-spectrum anthelmintic permits a tentative diagnosis in retrospect.

Postmortem examinations are the most direct method to identify and quantitate gastrointestinal parasitisms. The demise of one or more animals can provide valuable parasitologic data about the status of the rest of the herd or flock. Routine postmortem examinations are invaluable to diagnosis and are recommended.

On postmortem examination, *Haemonchus*, *Bunostomum*,

Oesophagostomum, Trichuris and *Chabertia* adults (or advanced immature worms) can be seen easily. *Ostertagia, Trichostrongylus, Cooperia* and *Nematodirus* are difficult to see except by their movement in fluid ingesta. Clinically important infections are easily overlooked with these genera. Samples of digestive contents and scrapings of the mucosa should be examined microscopically (low-power magnification). These smaller nematodes can be stained (5 minutes) with a strong iodine solution. After the background ingesta and tissue are decolorized with 5% sodium thiosulfate, the small nematodes are easily seen. The type and severity of gross lesions may also be of considerable diagnostic value.

Multifactorial causation should be considered in evaluating clinical, laboratory and necropsy findings. Mixed parasite infections are the rule. Shipping fever, nutrition-related digestive disorders, salmonellosis, Johne's disease, mucosal-disease complex and trace-element deficiencies, etc., should be considered in making a differential diagnosis.

TREATMENT OF GASTROINTESTINAL PARASITISM IN RUMINANTS

Effective worm control cannot be obtained by drugs alone; however, anthelmintics play an important and sometimes critical role in parasite control. Only when the application of drugs is coordinated with the other methods of control can the most satisfactory economic result be realized.

The "ideal anthelmintic" should be safe, highly effective against adults and immature stages of the important worms of the host, it should be rapidly and completely metabolized in a variety of convenient formulations and economical to use (inexpensive, ineffective drugs are not economic). No drug completely satisfies all of these requirements although thiabendazole (℞ 237) and levamisole (℞ 222) come closest. Both are highly effective against the adults of all nematode species (except *Trichuris*) and have good activity against the immature stages of most species. Thiabendazole has a wider range of safety and is the drug of choice in treating heavy mixed infections in debilitated animals. Higher dosages are indicated for *Cooperia*. Levamisole also kills *Dictyocaulus* (the ruminant lungworm). It is more effective against *Cooperia*, but less effective against *Trichostrongylus axei* than thiabendazole.

Coumaphos (℞ 204), Haloxon (℞ 217) and phenothiazine (℞ 226) are other anthelmintics available for use in ruminants. None are as broad spectrum in their activity as the above.

Coumaphos, an organophosphate, is effective against *Haemonchus, Ostertagia, Cooperia, Nematodirus* and *Trichostrongylus; Bunostomum* and the large intestinal nematodes are not removed. The drug is approved (in the U.S.A.) for feed administration to cattle over a period of 6 days. If anthelmintic treatment of lactating dairy animals is indicated, coumaphos would seem to be the drug of choice. Haloxon, another organophosphate, is effective against *Haemonchus, Ostertagia, Trichostrongylus, Cooperia* and *Strongyloides.* Haloxon is approved as a drench for sheep and cattle. Coumaphos and Haloxon alone are safe at recommended dosage; however, concurrent use of other organophosphates (such as insecticides) or phenothiazine may lead to toxic reactions, particularly in debilitated animals. Dichlorvos (℞ 207) is effective against *Trichuris* infection in sheep.

As a therapeutic agent, phenothiazine (℞ 226) is usually effective against adult *Haemonchus* and *Oesophagostomum* but progressively less effective against *Trichostrongylus, Ostertagia* and the small intestinal species. It is relatively ineffective against immature stages.

The continuous administration of phenothiazine at the rate of 2 gm daily, usually in salt or mineral, is effective in reducing larval development in the feces and hence the population of infective larvae on the pasture. If intake can be assured, low-level phenothiazine is helpful in preventing heavy exposure to susceptible animals by reducing contamination. This procedure has often failed to give consistent results because of erratic consumption of the drug.

Toxic reactions following phenothiazine therapy are unusual in ruminants although photosensitization may result. If this is a concern, treatment should be given in the afternoon and the animals kept in the shade for the following day. The metabolized drug is excreted in the urine as a red dye which stains wool. In feed-lot animals a transitory reduction in appetite has been associated with therapeutic dosages.

The development of drug resistance by populations of *Haemonchus contortus* has been demonstrated against phenothiazine, thiabendazole and some of the newer drugs. Increased dosages of thiabendazole can deal with unresponsive strains of *Haemonchus.* It has been shown that finer particle size and increased purity significantly improve the anthelmintic efficiency of phenothiazine. NF-grade phenothiazine, which is approximately 95% pure, may be as much as 25% less efficient than material that is 99% pure.

Lead arsenate (℞ 221) and niclosamide (℞ 224) are effective against tapeworms in cattle and sheep with the exception that only niclosamide shows promise (at doses of 200 to 250 mg/kg) against *Thysanosoma actinoides*. Lead arsenate may be mixed with suspensions of thiabendazole or phenothiazine to make a more general-purpose anthelmintic.

Consideration should be given to the following points when treating clinically affected animals: (a) providing adequate nutrition, (b) minimizing continuous ingestion of large numbers of larvae after treatment, (c) treating all animals in the herd as a preventive measure and to reduce pasture contamination, and (d) the hypobiotic larvae of *Ostertagia* are not satisfactorily killed by any of these anthelmintics. Repeated treatments, at 2- to 3-week intervals, are often necessary because these larval stages have been protected from prior treatments. After the adults are removed, the larvae emerge and continue their development. (e) Alternation of anthelmintics should be encouraged to maximize the best characteristics of different drugs and minimize the possibility of resistance.

Some compounds used chiefly against *Fasciola hepatica* are also effective against *Haemonchus* (rafoxanide, clioxanide, bromosalans and carbon tetrachloride). The older drugs, copper sulfate either alone or combined with arsenicals or nicotine, are effective but much less so than the broad-spectrum drugs and organophosphorus compounds.

Disophenol administered by subcut. injection has prevented reinfection by *Haemonchus* for about 2 months. It would seem particularly useful for breeding ewes where problems of tissue residues do not arise.

GENERAL CONTROL MEASURES FOR GASTROINTESTINAL PARASITISM IN RUMINANTS

The word "control" generally implies the suppression of parasite burdens in the host below that level at which economic loss may occur. To do this effectively requires an intimate knowledge of the epidemiologic and ecologic factors governing pasture larval populations and the role of host resistance to infection.

The goals of control can be summarized as: (1) to prevent heavy exposure in susceptible hosts (recovery from heavy infection is always slow), (2) to reduce overall levels of pasture contamination, (3) to minimize the effects of parasite burdens, and (4) to encourage the development of immunity or resistance.

Strategic use of anthelmintics has a seasonal basis and is designed to reduce worm burdens and thereby the contamination of pastures at periods based on a knowledge of the seasonal changes in infection. Tactical use is based on prompt recognition of conditions likely to favor the development of parasitic disease, e.g., weather, grazing behavior, malnutrition. Strategic and tactical timing of treatment must be based on a knowledge of the regional epidemiology of the various helminthoses.

For example, in Great Britain, where the pattern of disease caused by *Nematodirus* infection in sheep is clearly defined, strategic treatments with 3 doses of anthelmintic at 3-week intervals beginning just before the disease characteristically appears is recommended.

In other countries similar controls may be used if the seasonal pattern of the disease is known, but in most regions a tactical use of anthelmintics may be required, e.g., within 2 or 3 weeks after rain that follows dry weather.

SHEEP—SPECIAL CONSIDERATIONS

A special strategic treatment is required in most regions to counter the post-parturient relaxation of resistance (parturient rise, etc.) seen in ewes. The precise timing of such treatment will vary between regions and for different species of parasites, but in general, treatment within the month before and again within the month after parturition appears desirable. A treatment 2 weeks before breeding, as part of a "flushing" program, is another strategic application of anthelmintics. Supporting management after a treatment includes movement of sheep from contaminated pastures to pastures which have not been grazed by sheep for at least 6 weeks. Most infective larvae die before the pasture is grazed again; hence, re-exposure is reduced. The improvement of nutrition by better pasture utilization also results. Grazing crops or supplementary feeding also reduce exposure to infective larvae.

Sheep are more consistently susceptible to the adverse effects of worms than other livestock. Clinical disease is more common. Resistance is not strong and frequent treatments may be required, particularly during the first year of life.

CATTLE—SPECIAL CONSIDERATIONS

Pasture rotation is a much less effective means of control in cattle than in sheep because the fecal mass may protect infective larvae from adverse environmental factors for 3 or more months. Optimal pasture utilization and nutritional considerations are more important than pasture contamination factors, although a change to cleaner pastures should ideally follow each treatment. Cattle are more likely than sheep to develop relatively firm resistance, hence subclinical infections are more frequent.

Treatment at the time of weaning is probably of greatest strategic value in beef. Creep-feeding is an effective parasite control practice. If indicated, feed-lot animals should ideally be treated before shipment to the finishing lots. Worming as soon after arrival as feasible is the second choice. Replacement dairy heifers often suffer serious effects from worms due to inattention. Worm control and improved nutritional practices combine to prevent many problems.

A strong immunity in the host animal is clearly desirable. Many parasite-control programs accept exposures to calves under conditions that produce immunity without disease. Such "vaccination" has been an unrecognized element in traditional cattle husbandry, and has allowed the industry to survive and grow. But the economics of contemporary livestock production have placed great stress on this once adequate system.

Judicious pasture and animal management should be designed to avoid conditions conducive to an outbreak while encouraging immunity. However, when the relationships between exposure, host resistance and nutrition get out of balance, as they frequently do in intensive livestock farming, anthelmintic drugs are necessary to prevent losses. In some situations, e.g., intensive grazing or feed-lot fattening, parasite control is virtually impossible without medication.

SWINE

Hyostrongylus, Ascarops AND *Physocephalus*
INFECTION

Three types of stomach worms occur in swine; a thin, stomach worm *Hyostrongylus rubidus* (known as the red stomach worm), and 2 thick stomach worms, *Ascarops strongylina* and *Physocephalus sexalatus*. The thin stomach worm is about 6 mm long and very slender, while the thick stomach worms are 12 mm or more in length and much stouter than *Hyostrongylus*. The thin stomach worm requires no intermediate host. Thick stomach worms are acquired when swine eat infected coprophagous beetles.

Clinical Findings: These worms are quite common and generally are not associated with any significant signs or lesions. When present in large numbers or when the host's condition is reduced by poor nutrition or other factors, they may cause a variable appetite, diarrhea, or loss of weight. *Hyostrongylus* characteristically is found under a heavy catarrhal or mucous exudate and may produce erosions of the mucosa, and sometimes fatal hemorrhage. *Hyostrongylus* has a tissue phase when it is present in the mucosa as a retarded (hypobiotic) form, analogous with that of *Ostertagia* in ruminants. In sows the retarded worms resume development about the time of parturition. The sow may suffer severe gastritis and in addition contaminate the environment of the young pigs.

Diagnosis and Treatment: Clinical signs other than unthriftiness are not obvious. Fatal hemorrhages have been reported in hyostrongylosis. Fecal examinations may show the distinctive ova of *Physocephalus* and *Ascarops*—small (35 to 40 μ by 20 μ) thick-shelled eggs containing an active larva. *Hyostrongylus* ova resemble those of other strongyle worms, *Oesophagostomum, Necator, Trichostrongylus* and *Globocephalus,* and fecal cultures are required to obtain infective larvae for differential diagnosis.

At necropsy, adult worms, especially *Physocephalus* and *Ascarops* are readily seen. Mucosal scrapings for microscopic examination are essential for detection of immature *Hyostrongylus*.

Thiabendazole (R 237), levamisole (R 222) and dichlorvos (R 207) are effective against *Hyostrongylus*. Carbon disulfide (R 203), or the complex with piperazine (R 232) which releases carbon disulfide in the stomach, are usually recommended against *Physocephalus* and *Ascarops,* but precise data are lacking.

Ascaris INFECTION

The adults of the large roundworm, *Ascaris lumbricoides* var. *suis,* are found principally in the small intestine, but they may migrate into the stomach or bile passages. They are 30 cm or more in length and quite thick. A female produces large numbers of eggs (as many as 250,000 per day) which develop to the infective stage in 2 to 3 weeks and are very resistant to chemical agents. When the eggs are ingested, the larvae hatch in the intestine, penetrate the intestinal wall and enter the portal circulation. After a period of growth in the liver, they are carried by the circulation to the lungs, where they pass through the capillaries into the alveolar spaces. About 9 or 10 days after ingestion, the larvae leave the lungs by passing up the bronchial tree and return to the digestive system where they mature in the small intestine. The first eggs are passed 2 to 2½ months after infection.

Clinical Findings: Adult worms may significantly reduce the growth rate of young animals; if they are sufficiently numerous, they may cause mechanical obstruction of the intestine (in which case rupture of the intestine may result), or they may migrate into the bile passages and occlude them, producing icterus. The latter is fairly common, especially in hogs having long periods without feed in transit to slaughter.

The larvae are much more pathogenic. During active migration, most of the damage is mechanical, but a toxic principle may be produced which causes tissue degeneration. The most extensive damage is in the liver and lungs with less in the kidneys. There is some degeneration of the parenchymal tissue of the liver with subsequent cirrhosis. The "white-spotted livers" are condemned at meat inspection. Most of the fibrosis of the liver occurs just under the capsule. In the lungs, there is a variable amount of intralobular hemorrhage. Verminous pneumonia may develop. The animals so affected show marked respiratory signs, commonly referred to as "thumps". There is usually a marked increase in the number of eosinophils both in the tissues and in the circulating blood during the larval migration.

In addition to the respiratory signs, the animals show marked unthriftiness and loss of weight. Permanent stunting may result. The greatest harm comes to pigs up to 4 to 5 months.

Diagnosis: During the patent period, the diagnosis may be made easily by demonstrating the typical eggs in the feces. However, many young pigs show signs (especially respiratory involvement) during the prepatent period. A presumptive diagnosis can be made at this time on the basis of history and signs, and this can be confirmed by demonstrating immature worms on necropsy. In acute cases in which no worms are found in the intestine, it may be possible to recover larvae from the affected lung tissue.

Treatment: Supportive treatment and therapy for the secondary bacterial invaders may be necessary during the respiratory phase of the infection. Many drugs have been used to remove adult ascarids. The most popular ones at present are those that can be administered successfully in the feed or water: piperazine (R 228), dichlorvos (R 207), levamisole (R 222), sodium fluoride and cadmium compounds.

The piperazine preparations (R 228) have a low toxicity and are very effective against the immature worms in the intestine as well as the adults. The piperazine salts have been used in food or water. Sodium fluoride and cadmium oxide are less expensive, but more hazardous to use and have a narrow spectrum of activity. Dichlorvos (R 207) is effective and may be administered in the feed. Levamisole (R 222) is also very effective when administered in water or feed.

The antibiotic hygromycin (R 219) is active against the ascarids when administered as a low-level additive to the feed. Many drugs have been tested for efficacy in destruction of the migratory stages. Pyrantel (R 233) shows greatest promise in this regard. The beneficial effects of reduced lung and liver damage deserve close study.

Macracanthorhynchus INFECTION

The adults of *Macracanthorhynchus hirudinaceus* (thorny-headed worm) usually are in the small intestine. They may be 30 cm in length and 3 to 9 mm in width and slightly flattened when alive, sometimes being mistaken for tapeworms (swine have no adult tapeworms). The outer covering is transversely wrinkled and white or bluish white in color. The anterior end bears a spined retractable proboscis or rostellum by means of which it is firmly attached to the intestinal wall. The eggs are ingested by the grubs of various beetles that serve as intermediate hosts.

The signs are not specific. There is an inflammatory reaction at the site of attachment. This may have a necrotic center surrounded by a zone of inflammation. These lesions can usually be seen through the serosa. The rostellum may perforate the intestinal wall with a resulting peritonitis and death.

There is no effective treatment for the removal of these parasites. Ante-mortem diagnosis is difficult, as the ova do not float reliably in salt solutions. Control depends on avoiding the use of contaminated permanent hog lots or pastures.

Strongyloides INFECTION

The life cycle of the intestinal threadworm *Strongyloides ransomi* is apparently very similar to that of *S. papillosus* of cattle (q.v., p. 655), except that transmission of larval *Strongyloides* occurs through the colostrum, explaining the serious nature of the infection in baby pigs. The adult worms (only females in the parasitic cycle) burrow into the wall of the small intestine. In light and moderate infections the animals usually show no signs. In heavy infections, diarrhea, anemia and emaciation may be observed. Death may result.

Demonstration of the characteristic small, thin-shelled

embryonated eggs in the feces or of the adults in scrapings from the intestinal mucosa is diagnostic. *Strongyloides* ova must be differentiated from the larger *Metastrongylus* (swine lungworm) ova, which are also embryonated in fresh feces. At necropsy, immature worms may be recovered from minced tissues placed in a Baermann isolation apparatus.

Thiabendazole (℞ 237) is effective against intestinal infections. Recent studies have shown that some imidazole anthelmintics administered in the feed for several days before and after parturition reduced considerably the colostral infections in piglets.

Oesophagostomum INFECTION

Oesophagostomum dentatum is the most important of the nodular worms in hogs. The adults are found in the lumen of the large intestine; they are 8 to 12 mm in length, slender and white or gray in color. The life cycle is direct, with infection resulting from the ingestion of the larvae. These penetrate the mucosa of the large intestine within a few hours after ingestion and return to the lumen in 6 to 20 days. Infective larvae may be carried by flies. In nodular-worm infections of hogs, adult animals are often as heavily infected as the younger animals. The mucosa of the large intestine from the ileocecal valve to the rectum may be covered by a brownish material composed mostly of coagulated serum. The wall is 2 to 3 times its normal thickness. The serosa shows small nodules, a hypersensitive response as a result of previous infections. Heavily infected animals may show anorexia, emaciation and digestive disturbances.

See *Hyostrongylus* (p. 667) for comment on differential diagnosis when strongyle eggs are found in feces. At necropsy the worms and lesions are readily seen. Scrapings from the mucosa, with microscopic examination, may be required to detect immature worms. Thiabendazole (℞ 237), levamisole (℞ 222), piperazines (℞ 228, 230) and dichlorvos (℞ 207) are effective.

Trichuris INFECTION

Trichuris suis is 5 to 8 cm long and consists of a slender anterior portion and a thickened posterior third. Exposure is by ingestion of embryonated ova. Heavy exposure is associated with poor sanitation. Heavy infections with whipworms may cause inflammatory lesions in the cecum and adjacent large intestine accompanied by diarrhea and unthriftiness. The double operculated eggs are diagnostic. Dichlorvos (℞ 207) is effective.

HORSES

Gasterophilus INFECTION

Horse bots are the larvae of bot flies. The adult flies are not parasitic; they die as soon as the nutrients brought over from the larval stage are used, usually in about 2 weeks. The 3 important species in the U.S.A. can be differentiated in any stage of their development. The eggs of *Gasterophilus intestinalis* (the common bot) are glued to the hairs of almost any part of the body, but especially the forelegs and shoulders. The larvae hatch in about 7 days when properly stimulated, usually by the animals' licking. The eggs of *G. haemorrhoidalis* (the nose or lip bot) are attached to the hairs of the lips. The larvae emerge in 2 or 3 days without stimulation and crawl into the mouth. *G. nasalis* (the throat bot) deposits eggs on the hairs of the submaxillary region. They hatch in about a week without stimulation.

The larvae of all 3 stages apparently stay for about a month around the molar teeth or embedded in the mucosa of the mouth, after which they pass to the stomach where they attach themselves to the cardiac or pyloric portions or, less frequently, to the mucosa of the first part of the small intestine. After a developmental period of about 8 to 10 months, they pass out in the feces and pupate in the soil. The adult emerges after about a month.

Clinical Findings and Diagnosis: The most commonly encountered clinical sign is a nonspecific digestive disturbance. "Bots" produce no signs in most animals, particularly if the host is well nourished. Specific diagnosis of *Gasterophilus* infection can be made by demonstrating larvae as they pass in the feces at the end of the period of larval development. Infection is often assumed in the fall of the year. History of the individual animals, knowledge of the seasonal cycle of the fly in the particular locality and observation of bot eggs on the animal's hairs are all helpful.

Treatment: Most parasite control programs assume horses are infected in the fall. Piperazine-carbon disulfide complex (R 232), dichlorvos (R 207) or trichlorfon (R 241) have largely replaced carbon disulfide (R 203). A single treatment is usually adequate. It should be given approximately a month after the first killing frost has destroyed the flies in the fall. There is no satisfactory method for protecting exposed animals from attack by the flies, which are responsible for much annoyance during the summer months. When applied on a region basis to all horses, bot control programs markedly reduce fly numbers and bot problems.

Habronema INFECTION

GASTRIC HABRONEMIASIS

The adults of the large stomach worms *Habronema muscae*, *H. microstoma* and *Draschia megastoma* vary in size from 6 to 25 mm. *Draschia* occurs in tumor-like swellings in the stomach wall. The other species are free on the mucosa. The eggs or larvae are ingested by the larvae of house or stable flies which serve as intermediate hosts. Horses are infected by ingesting the infected flies or the larvae which emerge from flies feeding on the lips.

Clinical Findings: An inflammatory reaction of the mucosa, contributing to gastric irritability, poor digestion and sometimes colic may result from the presence of as few as 200 to 300 adult worms. *Draschia* produces the most severe lesions, tumor-like enlargements as much as 10 cm in diameter. These may be filled with necrotic tracts and masses of worms. The tumors may rupture and lead to a fatal peritonitis. Larvae of *Habronema* have been found in the lungs of foals associated with *Corynebacterium equi* abscesses.

Diagnosis and Treatment: Diagnosis is usually established during postmortem examination. Ante-mortem diagnosis is difficult since the thin-shelled eggs are destroyed by the common flotation solutions used in fecal examinations. Worms and eggs may be found by gastric lavage. An examination of *Musca* or *Stomoxys* taken near stables will often reveal *Habronema* larvae up to 3 mm long, which is a clear indication that horses are likely to be exposed.

The anthelmintics tested have shown little or no activity against these stomach worms.

CUTANEOUS HABRONEMIASIS

(Summer sores, Jack sores, Bursatti)

A skin disease of Equidae caused at least in part by the larvae of the large stomach worms, especially *D. megastoma*. When the larvae emerge from flies feeding on pre-existing wounds, they migrate into and irritate the sore, resulting in the production of a granulomatous reaction. The lesions become chronic and healing is protracted. The diagnosis of cutaneous habronemiasis may be made by demonstrating the larvae in scrapings of the lesions. Many different treatments have been used for summer sores, most of them with poor results. Organophosphate pesticides, e.g., ronnel, administered orally have given encouraging clinical response. Surgical removal or cauterization of the excessive granulation is usually necessary. The commonly employed screwworm smears containing lindane in pine oil make a good dressing for these lesions. Control of the fly hosts and the regular collection, stacking and treatment of manure will help control *Habronema*.

Trichostrongylus INFECTION

The small stomach worm of horses, *Trichostrongylus axei,* is the same species as found in ruminants. The adults are very small and slender, measuring up to 8 mm in length. The details of the cycle in Equidae have not been carefully studied, but it is known that the larvae penetrate the mucosa.

These worms produce a chronic catarrhal gastritis and may result in rapid loss of condition. The lesions comprise a characteristic thickening of the glandular mucosa with marked congestion and a variable amount of heavy mucous exudate. The lesions may be rather small and circumscribed (in which case they often are irregularly round) or involve most or all the glandular portion of the stomach. Occasionally, the only lesion is a nodular thickening of the mucosa.

Definite diagnosis on the basis of fecal examination is difficult because the eggs are so similar to some of the strongyle eggs. The feces can be cultured and, in about 5 days, the infective larvae identified.

No drug has been shown to have significant activity against *T. axei* in the horse. This may be due in large part to the protection provided the worms by the heavy mucous exudate. Massive doses of thiabendazole may be worth a trial.

Parascaris INFECTION

The adults of the equine ascarid *Parascaris equorum* are stout worms up to 30 cm or more in length, with the 3 lips being very prominent on the anterior end. The life cycle is essentially the same as that of the hog ascarid. The infective eggs may persist for years on contaminated soil. Adult animals usually harbor very few worms and the principal source of infection for the young foals is soil contamination with eggs from foals of the previous year.

In heavy infections, the migrating larvae may produce respiratory signs. Foals show unthriftiness, loss of energy and digestive disturbances. Diagnosis is based on the demonstration of the worms or eggs in the feces. During the prepatent period, diagnosis must be made on the basis of signs and history.

On farms where the infection is common, most foals become infected soon after birth. As a result, most of the worms are maturing when the foals are about 2½ to 3 months of age. Treatment should be started when foals are 8 weeks old and repeated at 8-week intervals until they are yearlings. Piperazine (℞ 228) or piperazine-thiabendazole (℞ 238) are effective against the adult worms and have considerable activity against the immature stages. All of the broad-spectrum equine anthelmintics are effective, therefore, ascarids are readily controlled in a multiple treatment program.

LARGE-STRONGYLE INFECTION

The large strongyles of horses are also known as blood worms, palisade worms, sclerostomes, or red worms. The 3 species and their respective sizes are: *Strongylus vulgaris*, 12 to 25 mm; *S. edentatus*, up to 35 mm; and *S. equinus*, 30 to 50 mm. The adult worms are attached to the mucosa of the cecum and colon. Under favorable conditions, the larvae develop to the infective stage within 7 days after the eggs are passed in the feces. The larvae are resistant to drying and to low temperatures. Infection is by ingestion of infective larvae only. The larvae of all 3 species migrate extensively after entering the intestine before developing to maturity in the large intestine. The prepatent period is from 16 weeks to a year. The larvae of *S. vulgaris* migrate extensively in arteries, being particularly evident in the anterior mesenteric and nearby arteries where they may cause parasitic thrombosis and aneurysms. Larvae of the other 2 species may be found in various parts of the body (under the parietal peritoneum, in the liver, lungs and pancreas). These species do not produce aneurysms in the mesenteric arteries. Mixed infections of these species and small strongyles are the rule.

Clinical Findings: The strongyles are active bloodsuckers and anemia is the most characteristic sign. Weakness, emaciation and diarrhea also are commonly observed. The intestinal mucosa is damaged where the worms attach and suck blood. *S. vulgaris* is especially important because of the damage done to the mesenteric arteries in which thrombi and aneurysms may form. As a result of the interference with the flow of blood to the intestine, any one of several conditions may follow: Colic and gangrenous enteritis are the most common and serious.

Intestinal stasis, torsion or intussusception and possibly rupture may also occur. Emboli may pass into the posterior aorta or femoral vessels and produce lameness.

Diagnosis and Treatment: Diagnosis generally is based on demonstration of the eggs in the feces. Differential diagnosis can be made by identification of infective larvae. Aneurysms may be palpable per rectum.

Parasite control programs often assume that grazing horses are infected; hence, routine treatments are administered to minimize the risks associated with migrating *S. vulgaris* larvae.

Phenothiazine (R 226) has been the traditional treatment, but because of toxicity, drug resistance and development of drugs with broader spectrums of activity, it is no longer recommended except in combination with other drugs. The long-popular low-level treatment programs should only be used in conjunction with periodic treatment with other drugs.

Mixing phenothiazine with piperazines (adipate, citrate, dihydrochloride or carbodithioic acid) in amounts which supply 1.24 gm of phenothiazine and 4.0 gm piperazine base per 100 lb body wt, results in improved efficacy against most large and small strongyles. These drugs are available in combination with carbon disulfide (R 231).

Thiabendazole (R 208) is active against both large and small strongyles and is one of the best drugs for strongyle control because it is highly effective against immature worms and is of very low order of toxicity. Trichlorfon (R 241, 242), dithiazanine iodide (R 211), dichlorvos (R 207) and pyrantel (R 233) in combinations, or alone, are effective against adult worms. Strongyle control, particularly in grazing animals, should be on a routine basis. Treatment generally should be repeated at 6- to 16-week intervals. The frequency necessary for satisfactory control will vary with the value of the animals, their access to pasture, and management practices. Proper programs will reduce pasture contamination and risk due to verminous colic and aneurysm. Fecal egg counts can monitor the adequacy of the program. Treatment against migrating worms is difficult. Large doses of thiabendazole (200 mg/lb) will kill migrating *S. vulgaris* in the early stages of development. Verminous colic due to aneurysms has been successfully treated with this regimen.

Colic may be associated with the use of anthelmintics. Special precautions are necessary when organophosphorus products (trichlorfon and dichlorvos) are used. Concurrent use of other organophosphates and phenothiazine compounds (including tranquilizers) may have untoward effects. Succinylcholine should not be used sooner than 30 days after administration of organophosphates. Label precautions and use instructions should be strictly observed with all anthelmintics, particularly in the horse.

SMALL-STRONGYLE INFECTION

Many species in several genera of the small strongyles are found in the cecum and colon. Most of them are appreciably smaller than the large strongyles, but some may be almost as large as *Strongylus vulgaris*. One species, *Triodontophorus tenuicollis*, produces rather severe ulcers in the wall of the colon. Most of the small strongyles do not appear to be bloodsuckers. There is apparently no extra-intestinal migration of the larvae in the host, the larval development taking place in nodular enlargements of the wall of the large intestine. Although these are much less important than the large strongyles, they play a part in the development of the common clinical parasitism. *See* the discussion of the large strongyles (above) for the recommended treatments.

Oxyuris INFECTION

The adults of the horse pinworm, *Oxyuris equi*, are found mainly in the cecum, colon and rectum. This species is the largest known pinworm, the female being 7.5 to 15 cm in length. Male worms are smaller and fewer in number. The gravid females pass toward the rectum; some are passed in the feces, while others crawl out of the anal opening onto the perineum. When the latter occurs, they usually rupture, leaving around the anus a yellowish, crusty mass composed of fragments of worms and eggs. The eggs, which are flattened on one side, become embryonated in a few hours and are ingested before they hatch.

Pruritus is the most common sign. Rubbing of the tail and anal region, with resulting poor hair growth around the tail and buttocks, is a characteristic sign and should suggest the presence of pinworms. Samples collected around the perineal region often contain dried female worms or eggs. Application of cellophane tape to the skin of the perineum may be used to recover ova for microscopic examination. The worms also may be found in the feces.

Piperazine (℞ 228), piperazine combinations (℞ 231, 232, 238, 242), thiabendazole (℞ 237), dichlorvos (℞ 240), trichlorfon (℞ 241) and pyrantel (℞ 233) as recommended for the strongyles, are effective against the adult pinworm. Dithiazanine iodide with piperazine citrate (℞ 211) is also effective against the adults and somewhat more effective against the immature worms.

Strongyloides INFECTION

Strongyloides westeri is found in the small intestine. Recent work on *Strongyloides* in pigs suggests that colostral infections might be expected. In heavy infections, it may produce digestive disturbances and diarrhea. Details of the life history of the worm in the horse are not known to differ significantly from that of *Strongyloides* in cattle. Thiabendazole (℞ 237) is an effective treatment.

TAPEWORM INFECTION

Three species of tapeworms of the anoplocephaline group are found in horses: *Anoplocephala magna, A. perfoliata* and *Paranoplocephala mamillana*. They vary in length from 8 to 25 cm (the first one usually being the longest and the last the shortest). *A. magna* and *P. mamillana* usually are in the small intestine, but may also be in the stomach. *A. perfoliata* occurs mostly in the cecum, but may occur in the small intestine. The life cycle is like that of *Moniezia* in ruminants. Diagnosis is made by demonstrating the characteristic eggs in the feces. In light infections, no signs of disease are present. In heavy infections, digestive disturbances are common and anemia has been reported. Ulceration of the mucosa occurs quite commonly in the area of attachment of *A. perfoliata*. Specific treatment is seldom attempted but bithionol and dichlorophen have been recommended.

AMEBIASIS

An acute or chronic enteric disease, common in subhuman primates and sometimes observed in the dog but rare in cattle, swine and cats, and characterized by a persistent diarrhea or dysentery.

Several species of ameba occur in the large intestine of domestic herbivores, but the only known pathogen is *Entamoeba histolytica*. Man is the natural host for this species and usually the source of infection for dogs.

Clinical Findings: *E. histolytica* may live in the lumen of the large intestine as a commensal or invade the intestinal mucosa. In dogs, tissue invasion may result in a mild-to-severe hemorrhagic enteritis, with occasionally irregular macroscopic ulcers. Diarrhea may persist for weeks to months in chronic cases with or without mucus or blood in the feces. Rarely, there may be hepatic abscesses or even septicemia. Patients with acute cases either develop fulminating dysentery, which may be fatal, progress to chronicity or show spontaneous recovery. Amebiasis in subhuman primates tends to resemble the human infection.

Diagnosis: Presumptive diagnosis is based on the demonstration of *E. histolytica* in smears of fresh or specially preserved feces, but its presence may be secondary to other etiologic agents. The pathogenic ameboid form is 20 to 40 μ in diameter and distinguished from nonpathogenic species by the morphology of the nucleus or the presence of ingested red blood cells. The cyst stage is rarely found in dogs.

Treatment of Dogs: In limited experimental trials, paromomycin (1.25 to 10 mg/lb body wt orally for 10 days) and fumagillin (0.15 to 0.6 mg/lb b.i.d. for 5 days per week for 2 weeks) were effective against intestinal infections. The chance of toxic manifestations are less with the former compound. The older drugs (Carbarsone, Diodoquin, chiniofon and Vioform) are only effective at therapeutic levels 2 to 4 times those required for humans.

CANINE HOOKWORM DISEASE

Etiology: *Ancylostoma caninum* is the principal hookworm in dogs in the U.S.A. *A. braziliense* occurs in both dogs and cats in the Southeast. *Uncinaria stenocephalus* is more northern in its distribution than either of the above. It is the principal canine hookworm in Europe, the only cause of canine hookworm disease in the British Isles, and occurs in dogs in Canada and Northern U.S.A. where it is primarily a parasite of foxes. Mature females of *A. caninum* are about 15 mm long; the males are about 12 mm. *U. stenocephala* and *A. braziliense* are somewhat smaller.

Most infections are acquired by ingestion, but infective larvae are capable of penetrating the skin. In susceptible dogs, most of the larvae ingested develop to maturity without leaving the intestine. In dogs which have acquired some degree of immunity through repeated infections, many of the larvae are stimulated to migrate through the tissues. It is in these dogs and those acquiring infection through the skin, that infection may be transferred to the unborn offspring. The process of growth and maturation requires 18 to 21 days. In prenatal infections, eggs may be passed by the pups as early as the 12th day after birth. Most of the adult worms are found in the second quarter of the small intestine, but, in heavy infections, they may be present throughout its entire length. The females lay several thousand eggs per day. These are easily identified on microscopic examination of the feces. Under favorable conditions, the eggs hatch within 48 to 72 hours and the larvae develop to the infective state within 5 to 7 days. Shaded earthen runways offer an especially favorable environment for the larvae during warm weather.

Clinical Findings: The presence of a few worms in a mature dog may result in no demonstrable signs, but hookworm disease may be produced in young puppies by relatively small numbers of worms. In areas where the parasite is common, heavy infections in mature dogs are rare unless the acquired immunity is broken as the result of malnutrition or some other disease process. Animals with a moderate to heavy infection appear unthrifty, may be weak and the pale mucous membranes give evidence of anemia. The presence of many hookworm eggs in the feces will confirm the diagnosis. With less severe infections, unthriftiness alone should lead to a suspicion of hookworm infection and the examination of the feces for eggs.

In young puppies exposed to large numbers of larvae, there may be sufficient pulmonary migration to produce evidence of pneumonia followed by a sudden onset of blood-loss anemia with black tarry stools before the worms are old enough to produce eggs. A less severe but equally abrupt onset of anemia may occur in very young pups due to prenatal infection.

Lesions: The pathologic changes are those associated with blood loss. A hypochromic microcytic anemia is characteristic of clinical infections. Small hemorrhages occur at the point of attachment and persist for some time after the worms move. In heavy infections, there is considerable blood in the lumen of the intestine. The liver may be pale and show evidence of some fatty change. Dermatitis has been shown to be a serious problem with *U. stenocephala* in both Ireland and England under conditions of continuing exposure to reinfection, particularly in Greyhounds. It is seen on all parts of the body but is severe in the interdigital spaces. Secondary bacterial infection may lead to deformities. Although dermatitis is not reported as a problem with *A. caninum* in the U.S.A., it has been produced experimentally and hookworm should be considered when such a dermatitis occurs in dogs closely confined under unsanitary conditions.

Prophylaxis: Since the presence of a few worms is of little pathogenic importance in the well-nourished growing or mature dog, the main problem consists of preventing exposure to massive infections, particularly in young puppies. Puppies should be whelped in quarters where strict sanitation has been followed and should be maintained on dry runways, or washed surfaces, such as concrete, which are exposed to sunlight as much as possible. They should never be confined to areas which have recently been occupied by mature dogs unless such premises are first thoroughly disinfected. Sodium borate (10 lb/100 sq ft), applied several times during the spring and summer, will aid in control by preventing development of larvae in the soil. This cannot be used on grass runs since it is a herbicide.

Treatment: Disophenol (R 209) appears to be the drug of choice. It requires no withholding of food or other preparation nor is any post-treatment purging necessary. Tetrachloroethylene (R 235) is also effective in treatment but produces its best results when administered (orally) after 12 hours' starvation and followed after 2 to 3 hours by a saline cathartic (Epsom salt or Glauber's salt). Toluene (R 240) and n-butyl chloride (R 202) or a combination of both are still widely and effectively used, particularly for very young puppies. Bephenium hydroxynaphthoate (R 199) is commonly used for *U. stenocephala* in Europe where this infection is common. Dithiazanine (R 210) is also effective but must be given daily for 10 days. In severe hookworm anemia, iron salts (orally or parenterally—R 500, 503) or transfusion are indicated. Neither, however, will have any long-range value unless the dog is placed on a high-protein and otherwise well-balanced diet.

CANINE STRONGYLOIDOSIS

Etiology: The causative organism is a small, slender nematode, a few millimeters long, which, when fully mature, is buried in the mucosa of the anterior half of the small intestine. The worms are almost transparent and at necropsy, it is all but impossible to see them with the unaided eye. Some evidence suggests that the species found in dogs is identical with that found in humans (*Strongyloides stercoralis*); it may, however, be a distinct species. Since the disease in man can be quite serious and is resistant to treatment, extreme caution should be exercised in handling cases in the dog.

The parasitic worms are all females, an unusual circumstance among nematodes, and the eggs which they deposit in the intestinal mucosa develop parthenogenetically. The eggs embryonate rapidly and hatch before they are evacuated in the feces. Under appropriate conditions of warmth and moisture, extracorporeal development is rapid. The third larval (infective) stage may be achieved in little more than a day. The molted filariform larvae are excellent skin penetrators, but also may infect a host via the oral mucosa. They migrate by way of the circulation and lungs, reaching the intestine usually as fourth-stage organisms which molt and begin their adult life. Progeny may be shed in the feces within 7 to 10 days after infection.

Some of the larvae shed from a patent infection develop into infective larvae; others develop into characteristic free-living male and female worms which mate and produce progeny that are infective for a new host.

Clinical Findings: Strongyloidosis, at the clinically apparent level, is a heavy infection which, under natural conditions, has been building up for some weeks. The disease usually is characterized by a blood-streaked, mucoid diarrhea. Emaciation is prominent and failure to make appropriate growth may be one of the first signs of infection. The appetite usually is good and the animal is normally active in the earlier stages of the disease. In the absence of intercurrent infections, there is little or no elevation of temperature. In advanced stages, the prognosis is grave. Usually, there is shallow, rapid breathing and pyrexia and, at necropsy, evidence of a verminous pneumonia with large areas of consolidation in the lungs. Marked enteritis, with hemorrhage, mucosal exfoliation and much mucus secretion is also seen.

Prophylaxis: Less than excellent sanitation and the association of susceptible dogs and puppies lead to a rapid build-up of the infection in all animals and ultimately to the occurrence of diarrhea in some or all animals in a kennel or pen.

Animals with diarrhea should be promptly isolated from the healthy or apparently healthy and an effort made to achieve strict sanitation. Direct sunlight, elevated soil or surface temperatures and desiccation are deleterious to all free larval stages.

Treatment: Enteric-coated gentian violet (℞ 215) has been reported as useful, but treatment must be prolonged—a week or more—and sometimes must be repeated. Dithiazanine iodide (℞ 210) has been a satisfactory anthelmintic for infection in both man and dogs. Thiabendazole will prevent mature *Strongyloides* infections in dogs when fed continuously at levels between 0.01 and 0.05% of the ration. Diethylcarbamazine (R 208) has also been employed successfully.

Spontaneous cures apparently due to the development of an acquired immunity also occur, thus complicating the problem of evaluating successful treatment.

ASCARIASIS (SM. AN.)

Etiology: The large roundworms (ascaridoid nematodes) of dogs and cats are commonly encountered, especially in puppies and kittens. There are 3 species involved, namely *Toxocara canis, Toxascaris leonina* and *Toxocara cati.* The most important species is *T. canis,* not only because of its public health importance, but because heavy infection may occur in very young pups. It has also been recorded in cats. *T. leonina* occurs most often in adult dogs, more rarely in cats. *T. cati* occurs in young cats and only exceptionally in dogs. Distribution varies throughout the world; in some areas, e.g., Alaska, *T. leonina* is much more common in dogs than *T. canis,* in others, e.g., Australia, *T. canis* is much more common than *T. leonina.*

These species occur also in wild carnivores and probably gain access to the definitive host by the ingestion of other larvae-infected animals. This mode of infection can occur also in both dogs and cats, especially in cats with *T. cati* and *T. leonina.* The usual mode of infection with *T. canis* is by prenatal infection of puppies from larvae in the tissues of the bitch. When embryonated infective eggs of *T. canis* are swallowed by adult dogs, the larvae do not reach the intestine after migration, but are distributed in muscles, connective tissue, kidneys and many other tissues. From there they migrate into the developing fetus and eventually reach the intestine within a week or so after birth; eggs may appear in the feces of puppies within 3 weeks of birth. At this time, eggs may also be passed by the lactating bitch, as, by licking the feces of her pups, she may swallow some of the larvae which fail to maintain a hold in the intestine of the puppy. Infection with *T. leonina* can be direct by swallowing eggs, as occurs mostly in dogs, the larvae developing in the intestinal wall. It can be indirect, as occurs with cats, by ingestion of rodents, in which larvae may be found encapsulated in the gut wall, mesenteries, diaphragm, abdominal wall and adjacent tissues.

Larvae of ascaridoid nematodes may migrate in the tissues of many animals, including man. Migrating larvae, especially those of *T. canis,* are associated with lesions in liver, kidneys, lungs, brain and eye. The larvae cause mechanical damage and are often associated with granuloma formation and eosinophilia.

Clinical Findings: The first indication of infection in young animals is lack of growth and loss of condition. Infected animals have a dull haircoat and are often pot-bellied. Worms may be vomited and are often voided spontaneously in the feces. In the early stages, pulmonary damage due to migrating larvae may occur; this may be complicated by superimposed bacterial pneumonitis, so that respiratory distress of variable severity may supervene. Cortical kidney lesions (granulomata) containing larvae are frequently observed in dogs.

Diagnosis: Infection in dogs and cats is diagnosed by detection of eggs in feces. It is important to distinguish the spherical, pitted-shelled eggs of *Toxocara* spp. from the oval smooth-shelled eggs of *T. leonina,* owing to the public health importance of the former.

Treatment: Piperazine salts (℞ 228) are highly effective against these roundworms. Hexylresorcinol (℞ 218) is also effective, but should not be used for treating cats. n-Butyl chloride (℞ 202) and diethylcarbamazine (℞ 208) are widely employed; the latter, however, may cause emesis. Dithiazanine (℞ 210) has been reported as effective. Dichlorvos (℞ 207) has proved suitable for removal of ascarids and may be given either by capsule or in older dogs with the daily ration of canned food or meat. Fenthion (℞ 213) is used as an injectable and also results in removal of ascarids. Thiabendazole, fed continuously, at levels between 0.01 and 0.05% of the ration, prevents the embryonation of eggs of *T. canis* in feces of dogs.

It is important that puppies be treated before eggs appear in the feces, particularly if there are children in the household. It is recommended that the first treatment be given to pups at 2 weeks after birth, also that bitches nursing the puppies be treated at the same time. Repeat treatments are necessary if eggs appear in the feces.

Control: The eggs of *T. canis* tend to adhere to inanimate objects—walls, etc.—and to become mixed in soil and dust. For this reason it is important to prevent accumulation of dog feces near the house. This applies particularly to lactating bitches, whose feces should be collected and burnt throughout the suckling period. As eggs may be adherent to the paws and hair, children should not handle lactating bitches or young puppies until successful treatment has been established.

CANINE TRICHURIASIS
(Whipworm infection)

Etiology: The adults of *Trichuris vulpis* are 40 to 70 mm in length and consist of a long, slender anterior portion and a thickened posterior third. They inhabit the cecum and colon where the worm is firmly attached to the intestinal wall, its anterior end being deeply embedded in the mucosa.

Thick-shelled eggs with a bipolar plug are passed in the feces and become infective in 2 to 4 weeks in a warm, moist environment. Although eggs may remain viable in a suitable environment for up to 5 years, they are extremely susceptible to desiccation.

The life cycle is direct. Following the ingestion of infective eggs larval development occurs in the jejunum and the adults mature in the large intestine in about 10 weeks, where they may remain for up to 16 months.

Clinical Findings: No signs are seen in light infections, but as the worm burden increases and the inflammatory, and occasionally hemorrhagic, reaction in the large intestine becomes more pronounced, loss of weight and diarrhea become evident. Also, as fresh blood may accompany the feces of heavily infected dogs, anemia occasionally follows.

Prophylaxis: Besides a regular treatment of dogs with an anthelmintic, advantage should be taken of the susceptibility of the eggs to desiccation. By maintaining cleanliness and eliminating moist areas the infection of dogs can be reduced considerably.

Treatment: The treatment of *T. vulpis* has been cumbersome and largely inefficient with the use of drugs such as n-butyl chloride, but there are now at least 3 acceptable treatments. Phthalofyne (℞ 227) has proved quite useful either orally or IV. Dichlorvos (℞ 207) can be administered either by capsule or in feed and glycobiarsol (℞ 216) may be given orally as a tablet or crushed in the feed.

HEARTWORM INFECTION
(Canine filariasis)

A clinical or inapparent infection with the parasite *Dirofilaria immitis,* which occurs frequently in the dog and rarely in the cat. Several filarial species have been reported from dogs in different parts of the world. At the present time, only 2 of these, *Dirofilaria immitis* and *Dipetalonema reconditum,* are known to occur in dogs in the U.S.A. *D. immitis* is of great pathogenic importance, while *D. reconditum* is apparently harmless. The frequent occurrence of the 2 species in dogs in this country requires that discretion be exercised in the diagnosis and treatment of filarial infections.

Etiology: Adult females are about 27 cm long and males about 17 cm. The fertilized eggs develop and hatch within the uterus of the female. The precocious active embryos, known as microfilariae, are about 315 μ long. They are discharged into the blood stream where they remain active for up to a year or more, but are incapable of further development until ingested by the intermediate host—various mosquito species. Within the mosquito, development from the microfilaria to the third stage (infective) larva is completed in about 2 weeks. The infective larvae then migrate to the mouth parts and gain entrance into the dog when the mosquito feeds again.

The immature stages develop and grow in the subcut. tissue, muscle and adipose tissue of the dog and begin arriving in the right ventricle 2 to 4 months after infection. An additional 4 months are required for the worms to reach maturity; thus microfilariae first appear in the peripheral circulation about 8 months after infection. Adults may live and continue to produce microfilariae for several years. The adult worms live in the right ventricle and the adjacent blood vessels from the posterior vena cava, hepatic vein and anterior vena cava to the pulmonary artery.

Geographical Distribution: *Dirofilaria immitis* is most commonly encountered within 100 miles of the seacoast from New Jersey south along the Atlantic and Gulf Coast into Texas. As high as 50% of the hunting dogs and strays may be infected. Nevertheless, heartworm disease may be encountered any place in the U.S.A. and in southern Ontario. It appears to be endemic but with a low rate of infection on the west coast, and is a growing problem in the Midwest, with infection rates from 20 to 40%. High prevalence rates are always associated with high mosquito densities.

Clinical Findings: In classical heartworm disease, the first clinical evidence of infection is either a chronic cough without evidence of upper respiratory infection, which is aggravated by exercise, or tiring on exercise, or both. As the disease advances, chronic coughing, dyspnea, collapse on exercise, and ascites develop; hydrothorax, a hard palpable liver, anasarca and azotemia may be evident. Cor pulmonale is evident in long-standing infections but may appear early. Death is due to general deterioration or collapse on severe exercise.

The acute hepatic syndrome is usually seen in young dogs with the worms preponderantly in the venae cavae. The findings which differentiate these cases from the more common and classical cardiac pulmonary cases described are: (a) absence of any history of chronic coughing, tiring on exercise, or ascites; (b) sudden onset of critical signs in contrast to the gradual onset in the casual heartworm patient; (c) presence of hemoglobinuria, and (d) death very shortly after clinical onset, commonly within 24 to 72 hours. Death appears to be due to hepatic and renal failure.

Occasionally, a dog is seen with the acute hepatic syndrome and the cardiac pulmonary signs of chronic heartworm disease.

Lesions: The most constant lesion is "rugose" or "villose" endarteritis in the pulmonary arteries. As the disease progresses, numerous thromboemboli, both from dead worms and from the rugose lesions, produce a succession of acute inflammatory reactions followed by fibrosis. These lesions combined with the mechanical interference of the blood flow by the worms themselves lead to cor pulmonale and pulmonary hypertension. The classical picture of heartworm disease is undoubtedly the combination of these lesions.

In the acute hepatic syndrome, the physiopathology includes hemoglobinuria, bilirubinuria, and reduced liver function (100% sulfobromophthalein retention for at least 30 minutes). Anemia and icterus are common but not always present. Histopathology reveals enlarged hepatic venules associated with chronic passive congestion. As the disease advances, thickening of the hepatic vein and centrolobular tubules of the kidney with heme casts in the medulla are frequently seen.

Diagnosis: A tentative diagnosis of the clinical infection can be made on the basis of the history and signs. Since at least 2 filariids are known to occur in dogs in the U.S.A., specific diagnosis of *Dirofilaria* infection must be based on the identification of the microfilariae. In general, the microfilariae of *D. immitis* are far more plentiful in the peripheral blood than are those of *Dipetalonema*. Living microfilariae may be seen in whole blood, concentrated in the serum from clotted blood, or concentrated in blood hemolyzed by the addition of a few drops of fresh saponin solution. The microfilariae of *D. immitis* actively thrash about with a series of kinky movements without any appreciable progress. Those of *Dipetalonema* have a smoother more graceful movement; they may coil and uncoil for a short time in one place, then quickly move across and out of the microscopic field with a typical serpentine movement.

The microfilariae may also be readily identified through the use of the modified Knott technique: 1 ml of whole blood is mixed with 9 ml of 2% formalin; the sample is centrifuged for 5 to 8 minutes at 1,000 to 1,500 rpm. The supernatant is discarded and a drop of the sediment mixed with a drop of 1:1,000 aqueous methylene blue. The microfilariae are stained and may be differentiated.

	Dirofilaria immitis	*Dipetalonema reconditum*
Anterior end	Tapering, well-stained	Blunt, lightly stained
Posterior end	Straight, tapering and well-stained	Button hook-shaped, blunt end, lightly stained

Prophylaxis: Chemical prophylaxis may be accomplished 1 of 2 ways. Arsenamide (thiacetarsamide) will destroy most or all of small preadult worms entering the heart. It should be administered IV at the therapeutic dose, 3 to 5 months after the end of the mosquito season in the temperate zones; and twice a year in tropical and neotropical areas where mosquito transmission continues most of the year.

The daily administration of diethylcarbamazine (℞ 208) orally, usually in the food, starting a month before the mosquito season and continuing for 2 months after the end of the mosquito season will destroy the developing stages in the tissues before they reach the heart. In tropical and neotropical areas, this means the continuous feeding of diethylcarbamazine throughout the life of the dog. Preventive medication with diethylcarbamazine should not be initiated in dogs already microfilaria-positive; such dogs should first be treated with arsenamide followed by elimination of microfilariae with another microfilaricide; thereafter they may be started on the preventive medication.

House dogs may be given some measure of protection by being kept within screened houses during the evening and night when mosquitoes feed most actively. Mosquito control may be an important factor in prevention, especially in isolated kennels.

Treatment: Recommended treatment consists initially of the administration of a drug to destroy the adults. It is generally desirable to follow this in approximately 6 to 8 weeks with a microfilaricide.

Arsenamide (℞ 239) is effective in destroying the adults. The improved dosage schedule appears to have eliminated almost all toxic effects of the drug, retained 98 to 100% efficiency and shortened the time of treatment. However, dogs with the acute hepatic syndrome or other evidence of liver or kidney insufficiency are not good therapeutic risks until the basic problem is treated. Of the liver function tests, serum glutamic pyruvic transaminase (SGPT) test is the most useful; normal SGPT values are about 40 and the dog with the value twice that (80) is a poor therapeutic risk. When pulmonary reactions occur, excellent results are obtained with one IM injection of 20 mg of prednisone followed by daily injections of antibiotics. All treated dogs should be closely confined for 3 to 4 weeks and should not be worked hard or allowed unrestricted run for 2 months.

Dithiazanine (℞ 210) is perhaps most commonly used as a microfilaricide. The more recently introduced fenthion appears to be the most effective microfilaricide; a single subcut. injection will eliminate all of the microfilaria in over 60% of the dogs and only a rare dog will require more than a second injection. Fenthion (℞ 214) is an organophosphate and the recommended dose must not be exceeded and no other organophosphate should be used simultaneously.

Stibophen and arsenamide are microfilaricides but now little used for that purpose. Diethylcarbamazine **is not recommended for treatment** because severe reactions and even deaths occur following the destruction of microfilariae with this drug despite the fact that the drug *per se* is not toxic.

SPIROCERCA LUPI IN DOGS

Etiology: Adult *Spirocerca lupi* are bright red worms 30 mm (male) to 80 mm (female) long. They generally are located within nodules in the esophageal wall. Dogs are infected by eating an intermediate host (usually dung beetle) or a transport host (e.g., chicken). The larvae migrate via the wall of the thoracic aorta where they usually remain for about 3 months. Eggs are passed in feces about 5 to 6 months after infection.

Clinical Findings: Most dogs with *S. lupi* infection show no clinical signs. When the esophageal lesion is very large, as it usually is when it has become neoplastic, the dog has difficulty in swallowing and may vomit repeatedly after trying to eat. Such dogs salivate profusely and eventually become emaciated. These clinical signs, especially if accompanied by enlargement of the extremities characteristic of osteoarthropathy, are strongly suggestive of spirocercosis with associated neoplasia, particularly in regions where the parasite is prevalent. Occasionally, a dog will die suddenly as the result of massive hemorrhage into the thoracic cavity following rupture of the aorta damaged by the developing worms.

Lesions: The characteristic lesions are aneurysm of the thoracic aorta, reactive granulomas of variable size around the worms and, often but not always, deformative ossifying spondylitis of the posterior thoracic vertebrae. Esophageal sarcoma, often with metastases, is sometimes associated (apparently causally) with *S. lupi* infection, particularly in hound breeds. Dogs with *Spirocerca*-related sarcoma often develop hypertrophic pulmonary osteoarthropathy.

Diagnosis: A positive diagnosis can be made by demonstration of the characteristic eggs on fecal examination using a flotation method with saturated sodium nitrate or zinc sulfate solution. A gastroscopic examination may occasionally reveal a nodule or an adult worm. Since eggs are sporadically voided in feces and are often missed, a presumptive diagnosis can be made by radiographic examination when it reveals dense masses in the esophagus. Barium will help define the lesion. Spondylitis of the ventral surface of the bodies of posterior thoracic vertebrae is an inconsistent sign of *S. lupi* infection.

Most infections are not diagnosed until necropsy. The granulomas vary greatly in size and location in the esophagus, but are usually so characteristic as to be diagnostic, even if the worms are no longer present. Worms and granulomas may be present in the lung, trachea, mediastinum, wall of stomach, or other abnormal location. Healed aneurysms of the aorta persist for the life of the dog and are diagnostic of previous infection. When sarcomas are associated with the infection, the esophageal lesion is usually larger and often contains cartilage or bone. Metastases of these lesions are frequently present in lung, lymph nodes, heart, liver, or kidney.

Control: Effective control will necessitate prevention of infection or destruction of developing worms by chemotherapy before severe lesions have developed. Neither is practical with information presently available, but in endemic areas dogs should not be fed raw chicken scraps.

Preliminary studies have shown that dithiazanine and disophenol may have some effect on the worms. Surgical removal is usually unsuccessful because of the large areas of the esophagus involved.

STEPHANOFILARIASIS
(Filarial dermatitis of cattle)

Stephanofilaria stilesi is a small filarial parasite responsible for a circumscribed dermatitis along the ventral midline of cattle. The parasite has been reported throughout the U.S.A., but is more common among cattle in the Western and Southwestern regions. The adult worms are 3 to 6 mm long and are usually found in the dermis, just beneath the epidermal layer. Microfilariae are 50 μ long and are enclosed in a spherical, semirigid vitelline membrane. They occur in the dermal papillae. The intermediate host for *St. stilesi* is the female horn fly, *Haematobia irritans* (q.v., p. 738). Horn flies feeding on the lesion ingest microfilariae that develop to the third stage infective larva in 2 to 3 weeks. The infective larva is introduced into the skin as the horn fly feeds.

Clinical Findings and Diagnosis: The dermatitis develops along the ventral midline, usually between the brisket and navel. With repeated exposure to additional parasites the lesion spreads, often involving skin posterior to the navel. Active lesions are covered with blood or serous exudate, while chronic lesions are smooth, dry and devoid of hair. Hyperkeratosis and parakeratosis occur in the epidermis of the parasitized area.

Deep skin scrapings are macerated in isotonic saline and examined microscopically for adults or microfilariae. Microfilariae must be differentiated from *Rhabditis strongyloides* (q.v., p. 898), a small free-living nematode that is occasionally responsible for a moist, superficial dermatitis. The rhabditiform esophagus, so characteristic of the nematode, does not occur in filarial nematodes.

Prophylaxis and Treatment: No treatment is available for stephanofilariasis, but control of horn flies will break the biologic cycle.

ONCHOCERCIASIS

Onchocerca cervicalis is a filarial nematode parasitic in the ligamentum nuchae of horses. Adult females are 250 to 300 mm long, the males 60 to 70 mm. Microfilariae are 200 to 240 μ long, very slender, and have a short, but sharply pointed tail. Microfilariae occur in the dermis or dermal lymph vessels just below the epidermis. They are most numerous in skin overlying sites occupied by the adult females. *Culicoides nubeculosus* is the intermediate host. Microfilariae ingested by these midges develop to infective larvae in about 24 days. Infective larvae are introduced into horses as the midges feed.

Clinical Findings: Adult *O. cervicalis* and their microfilariae are an enigma. They have never been clearly incriminated as etiologic agents for any disease of the horse, nor have they ever been completely exonerated. The adults are frequently associated with fistulous withers and poll evil (q.v., p. 551), but their contribution to these conditions is probably minor.

The microfilariae tend to be found in areas of inflammation. As a result, they are often blamed for dermatitis about the face, neck, shoulders and breast. Dermatitis is caused by a multitude of external irritants, allergens and infectious agents (q.v., p. 895), and microfilariae undoubtedly contribute in some degree.

Microfilariae also accumulate in the eye of horses with equine periodic ophthalmia (q.v., p. 214). Because of their predilection for inflamed areas, microfilariae could easily be in the eye as a result of the disease rather than as the cause. Since the cause has not been clearly defined, however, microfilariae must be considered as possible etiologic agents.

Diagnosis: Biopsy of lesions and demonstration of microfilariae in histologic sections is a satisfactory method, but the most effective method is to excise a piece of skin about 1 or 2 cm in diameter, macerate in isotonic saline, and examine microscopically for the characteristic microfilaria. The microfilaria of *O. cervicalis* must be differentiated from the microfilaria of *Setaria equina*. The latter are sheathed and have an obvious inner body. They must also be differentiated from the larva of *Habronema* spp., the etiologic agent of cutaneous habronemiasis (q.v., p. 673). This larva is in the third stage of development and possesses a spiked knob on the caudal extremity.

Treatment: No treatment is available against the adults or microfilariae of *O. cervicalis*. The treatment recommended for dermatitis (q.v., p. 895) is often of value, even when microfilariae are present in the lesions.

ELAEOPHOROSIS
(Filarial dermatosis; Sorehead; "Clear-eyed" blindness)

Elaeophora schneideri is a normal parasite of deer inhabiting mountains of the Western and Southwestern U.S.A. Adult parasites are 60 to 120 mm long and are usually found in the common carotid or internal maxillary arteries of their host. Microfilariae of *E. schneideri* are about 275 μ long and 15 to 17 μ thick. Microfilariae normally occur in capillaries of skin on the forehead and face. The intermediate hosts are species of horse flies in the genera *Tabanus* and *Hybomitra*. Development in the horse fly requires about 2 weeks. Infective larvae invade the host as the horse fly feeds. Infective larvae go into the leptomeningeal arteries of the host and develop to the fifth (adult) stage in about 3 weeks. These young adults migrate against the blood flow and establish in the common carotid arteries, where they continue to grow. About 6 months later the parasites reach sexual maturity and begin producing microfilariae. The life span of the adults is 3 to 4 years.

Clinical Findings: Clinical disease has not been reported in deer; therefore, they are considered to be the normal definitive hosts. When horse flies transmit the infective larva to elk calves or yearlings, development of the larva in the leptomeningeal arteries causes ischemic necrosis of brain tissue, resulting in blindness, brain damage and sudden death. Blindness in elk is characterized by absence of opacities in the refractive media of the eye, thus the popular name "clear eyed" blindness.

Domestic sheep, especially the lambs and yearlings, may die suddenly 3 to 5 weeks after infection. Death is usually preceded by incoordination and circling. Convulsions and opisthotonos are also common signs. These signs are identical to those of enterotoxemia (q.v., p. 340). Numerous thrombi occur in the cerebral and leptomeningeal arteries. One or more young adult *E. schneideri* accompany each thrombus. If sheep survive the early infection, 6 to 10 months later they develop a raw, bloody dermatitis on the poll, forehead or face, thus the popular name "sorehead". Lesions occasionally occur on the legs, abdomen and feet. These lesions are an allergic dermatitis in response to the microfilariae lodged in capillaries. Lesions persist, with periods of intermittent and incomplete healing, for about 3 years, followed by spontaneous recovery. Hyperplasia and hyperkeratosis occur in the epidermis of the parasitized area.

Diagnosis: Elaeophorosis should not be considered unless sheep are known to have been in enzootic areas of the disease during the summer months. Diagnosis of the disease in lambs, or yearling and calf elk, is usually done at necropsy. Numerous thrombi and parasites will be found in the common carotid, internal maxillary, cerebral and leptomeningeal arteries. Presumptive diagnosis in mature sheep is based upon history, and location and type of lesion. The skin lesion must frequently be differentiated from ulcerative dermatosis (q.v., p. 292). Confirmation is by recovery of microfilariae from the lesion, or postmortem recovery of the adult parasites. A skin biopsy of the lesion is macerated in isotonic saline, and allowed to stand for at least 6 hours at room temperature. The skin is strained off and the fluid examined for the typical microfilariae.

Prophylaxis and Treatment: The dermal form of the disease in sheep is amenable to treatment with stibophen (℞ 234). Piperazine salts are extremely effective at 100 mg/lb body wt orally. Complete recovery will occur in 18 to 20 days. No treatment is available for the cerebral form of the disease.

GIANT KIDNEY-WORM INFECTION IN THE DOG AND MINK

Etiology: The giant kidney worm, *Dioctophyma renale*, occasionally occurs in dogs. The females are the largest nematodes known; adults range from 75 to 100 cm in length and up to 1 cm or more in diameter. Males are smaller, up to 45 cm in length.

The adult worms are bright red in color and as mature adults live in the renal tissues, almost invariably the right kidney. The renal parenchyma is gradually destroyed as the female worm grows and passes eggs in the urine of the host.

The pitted thick-shelled eggs have a bipolar plug and, if ingested by oligochaete annelids, parasitic on crayfish, they hatch and infective larvae develop. By ingesting this host, or fish which have fed on infected annelid worms, the carnivore becomes infected with *D. renale*. Larvae migrate from the stomach or duodenum of the dog to the peritoneal cavity and occasionally the liver before becoming mature adults in the kidney. Eggs are passed in the urine 4 to 6 months after infection. There are less than 200 reported cases in dogs but surveys of incidence in mink range from 2 to 5%.

Clinical Findings and Diagnosis: Signs develop when the parasites approach or reach maturity. The sequence involves a marked loss of weight, as much as one-third to one-half in a few weeks, hematuria, frequent urination, restlessness and evidence of severe abdominal or lumbar pain. The animal may cry, stretch and exhibit a nervous trembling. Anemia may occur secondary to the blood loss. The disease is diagnosed from the signs and the presence of the parasite eggs in the urine. The adult worm may sometimes be detected radiographically.

Prophylaxis and Treatment: Curtailment of the ingestion of raw fish or other aquatic organisms is recommended, especially in areas where the parasite is known to occur in wild animals. Nephrectomy, in the early stages of the infection, leads to rapid recovery.

SWINE KIDNEY-WORM INFECTION

Etiology: The adults of the swine kidney worm, *Stephanurus dentatatus* (25 to 35 mm in length and about 2 mm in diameter) are found in the kidneys, the wall of the ureters and in the perirenal fat. The eggs hatch shortly after being passed in the urine; the larvae reach the infective stage in about 3 to 5 days and are susceptible to cold, desiccation and sunlight. They usually are ingested, but may penetrate the skin through abrasions. They migrate to the liver and, after extensive wandering through the liver tissue and beneath the capsule for 2 to 3 months, most pierce the capsule and enter the abdominal cavity. After some wandering, the larvae settle in the kidney, its adnexa and, occasionally, in other tissues or organs. Patent infections in pigs younger than 5 months of age are acquired prenatally. The kidney worm is found worldwide and, next to *Ascaris,* is the most important parasite of swine, especially in warm climates.

Clinical Findings: Heavy experimental infections of kidney worms have been shown to affect growth adversely. Pleuritis and peritonitis are quite common. The principal economic loss results from the condemnation of affected organs and tissues on meat inspection. Inasmuch as migrating worms may invade and damage a number of organs and tissues, lesions and signs are variable; most commonly observed are lesions of the liver, kidney and surrounding tissues and lungs. The most severe lesions are in the liver, which shows cirrhosis, scar formation, extensive thrombosis of the portal vessels and a variable amount of necrotic tissue.

Diagnosis: When worms are in the kidney or ureter, or have established communication with them, eggs may be recovered in the urine. Otherwise, a definite diagnosis is dependent on demonstration of the worms or lesions at necropsy.

Control: Although feeding a concentration of 0.1% thiabenda-zole in the ration for 14 days has prevented migration of kidney-worm larvae, no satisfactory treatment has yet been developed for the elimination of the adult worm. However, the parasite is eradicated from a pasture in 12 to 18 months after egg contamination is stopped. Only first-litter gilts may be used as breeding stock and these disposed of when their pigs are weaned; this program is effective because the worms may require as long as 10 months to attain significant egg-laying potential. Older boars should also be removed from the infected herd and replaced with young boars from clean herds or the gilts hand-bred.

After the kidney worm has been eradicated, the gilts may then be kept in the breeding herd if it is maintained as a closed herd and care is taken to prevent the introduction of infected animals. A longer period will be required to eradicate the parasite from shaded feed lots than from pastures because the larvae live longer when protected from the sun.

TRICHINOSIS

A parasitic disease of primary importance as a public health problem. Human infections are established through the consumption of infected, insufficiently cooked meat, usually pork or bear. Contrary to common opinion, the prevalence rates are generally higher in dogs and cats than in swine. Among wild animals, natural infections are often reported in carnivores. It has also been reported in such diverse noncarnivores as rats, beavers, opossums, walruses and whales; and probably all mammals are susceptible.

Etiology and Epizootiology: *Trichinella spiralis* is the causative nematode. Infection occurs by ingestion of muscle tissue containing viable trichinae. The cyst wall is digested in the stomach and the liberated larvae partially penetrate the duodenal and jejunal mucosa. Within about 2 days, the larvae develop into sexually mature adults which mate. The females (3 to 4 mm) penetrate deeper into the mucosa and discharge living larvae beginning by the fourth to seventh day. The minute larvae (0.1 mm) migrate to the muscle by 2 routes, either following the lymphatic and portal systems to the peripheral circulation or through connective tissue. Those larvae that reach striated muscle penetrate individual muscle fibers and grow to 1 mm in length. They then coil up and are encysted by host reaction. A myositis is produced. The larvae may remain viable in the cyst for several years. The diaphragm, tongue, masseter and deltoid muscles are among the most heavily involved muscles. The larvae also may invade organs and tissues other than striated muscle but usually are destroyed by local inflammatory reaction. Heart and nervous system damage may occur.

Early in the disease, before maturation, some of the infective larvae may pass through the intestine and be eliminated in the feces. These larvae are infective to other animals. A single adult female generally produces 500 to 1,000 larvae over a 2- to 6-week period, depending on the host. Following reproduction, the adult trichinae die and usually are digested.

Clinical Findings: Light infections generally produce no detectable signs and go undiagnosed. In heavy infections that produce serious illness and occasional deaths, 3 clinical phases are evident:

The **intestinal stage** commencing about 24 hours after ingestion of trichinous meat and continuing through the first week, results in a nonspecific gastroenteritis which may include diarrhea, slight fever, signs of mild abdominal pain, nausea and vomiting.

The **muscle invasion stage,** beginning about a week after infection and usually extending several weeks, is characterized by anorexia, emaciation, muscular pains, dyspnea, edema, low fever and eosinophilia. The invaded muscles are hard, swollen, tense and painful, especially the muscles of respiration, mastication, deglutition and movement. The degree of eosinophilia depends on the host species and may be related to infective dosage. The peak eosinophilia usually occurs 2 to 3 weeks after infection and then declines gradually. Deaths are most common in this stage.

The **convalescent stage** generally begins 5 to 6 weeks after infection. Signs usually recede, although in severe infections muscular stiffness, neurologic disorders, myocardial weakness, nephritis or pulmonary disorders may be seen as a result of previous tissue damage.

Diagnosis: Although ante-mortem diagnoses in animals other than man are rare, swine, dogs and cats with the above signs are prime suspects, especially if there is a history of feeding garbage containing raw or insufficiently cooked pork. Microscopic examination of a muscle biopsy sample will confirm but not necessarily rule out trichinosis. In animals, biopsy usually is not feasible and examination of muscle tissue normally is not made until necropsy. The indirect fluorescent antibody test is probably the most reliable of currently available serologic tests for infections in animals.

Prophylaxis: Although infected wild animal carcasses are also important, most domestic animals are infected by eating garbage containing raw or insufficiently cooked pork. The role of rats is now considered of limited importance.

The general objectives are to prevent the ingestion by animals or humans of viable trichinae present in meat. For swine and other animals this can best be accomplished by (1) elimination of feeding of garbage and wildlife carcasses; or (2) cooking all garbage (212°F) for 30 minutes. Rodent control programs should be carried out as a precautionary measure.

Inspection of meat for viable trichinae at the time of slaughter has proved effective in many countries. Methods of meat inspection and processing in the U.S.A. are currently based on the assumption that all pork may be infected with trichinae; pork products which appear to be "ready to eat" must be processed by adequate heat, freezing or curing to kill trichinae before marketing. Similar pork products lacking the governmental inspection seal or raw pork products should be cooked to at least 170°F before eating.

Treatment: Treatment consists mainly of symptomatic and supportive therapy to alleviate pain until the infection has subsided. ACTH and adrenal corticosteroid hormones are commonly used. Infections in man can be treated successfully with thiabendazole, but this is generally less practicable for animals.

LUNGWORM INFECTION
(Verminous bronchitis, "Husk", "Hoose")

An infection of the respiratory tract by any of several parasitic nematodes. Species of veterinary importance include *Dictyocaulus viviparus,* the lungworm of cattle, *D. filaria, Protostrongylus rufescens, Muellerius capillaris* in sheep and goats, 3 *Metastrongylus* spp. in pigs and *Aelurostrongylus abstrusus* in cats.

The cattle lungworm causes economic loss in young animals in N.W. Europe, particularly the British Isles; North America, in areas with moderate temperatures and high humidity; and in many other areas of the world. The sheep lungworms are important pathogens of sheep in Australia, S.E. Europe and North America, causing losses particularly in lambs maintained with ewes. Lungworms are of less importance in swine but outbreaks of the disease occur sporadically. *A. abstrusus* has been reported to occur in up to 20% of free-ranging cats.

Transmission and Epidemiology: *D. viviparus* and *D. filaria* have direct life cycles. Eggs, laid in the large air passages, are coughed up, swallowed and hatch as they pass through the alimentary tract. Larvae are passed in the feces and reach the infective, third stage, in 3 to 7 days at moderate temperatures (67° to 70°F). Grazing animals ingest the infective larvae which migrate to the lungs via the lymphatic system. The infection becomes patent in 3 weeks. Viability of infective larvae is enhanced by moderate temperatures and high humidity. Lush pasture occurring under these conditions promotes production of semifluid feces which spread larvae more widely on the herbage. Older animals with silent infections act as a source of larvae for young animals. The disease is usually observed in groups of young animals in their first season at pasture. Infective larvae can overwinter at low temperatures if covered by snow.

Eggs of *Metastrongylus* of swine are passed in the feces and are ingested by earthworms in which they develop to the infective stage. *P. rufescens, M. capillaris* and *A. abstrusus* require slugs or snails as intermediate hosts. Ingestion of these intermediate hosts is necessary for infection to occur.

Pathogenesis: Most lungworms are pathogenic due to their location in the trachea and bronchioles. They cause direct irritation, stimulate excess mucus production and predispose to secondary bacterial infection.

Clinical Findings: The most consistent sign in cattle is tachypnea. Rapid shallow breathing is found in both light and heavy infections. A loose husky cough, exacerbated by exercise, is often present. Heavily infected animals stand with their heads stretched forward, mouths open and drool saliva. The animals are often in poor condition. Lung sounds are particularly prominent at the level of the bronchial bifurcation. Infected animals are afebrile unless secondary bacterial infection is present.

The signs in sheep infected with *D. filaria* are similar to those in cattle. Pulmonary signs are not usually associated with *M. capillaris* and *P. rufescens* in sheep, but in heavy infections general unthriftiness may occur. This is also true of *Metastrongylus* infections in swine, although occasionally pulmonary clinical signs are seen. Coughing and dyspnea occur in cats and kittens heavily infected with *A. abstrusus*.

Lesions: *Dictyocaulus* in both cattle and sheep elicit the formation of sunken, plum-colored areas of atelectasis in the postero-dorsal diaphragmatic lobes of the lung. These worms can be most easily found by cutting along the bronchi leading to these areas.

The lesions caused by *M. capillaris* and *P. rufescens* in sheep are also found in the dorsal areas of the diaphragmatic lobes. The lesions may be brownish areas of consolidation up to 2 cm in width or smaller, shot-like, greenish-gray areas of calcification approximately 2 to 3 mm in diameter.

The lesions of *Metastrongylus* are usually plum-colored consolidated areas situated along the posteroventral edges of the diaphragmatic lobes, approximately 2.5 cm in diameter. Worms may be found in the bronchioles leading to these areas.

The lesions of *A. abstrusus* are scattered throughout the diaphragmatic lobes of the lung and are yellowish nodules up to 1 cm in diameter. Eggs, larvae and adult worms may be found on examination of the cut surface of a nodule.

Diagnosis: This is made on the evaluation of 4 criteria; clinical signs, epidemiology, the presence of first-stage larvae in the feces, and necropsy of animals in the same herd or flock. Larvae will not be found in the feces of pneumonic animals in the prepatent stage of the disease.

First-stage lungworm larvae cannot be recovered using most fecal flotation techniques. The most efficient method for recovering larvae is by some modification of the Baermann technique. A 25-gm fecal sample is wrapped in tissue paper or cheese cloth and suspended or placed in water contained in a tumbler. The water at the bottom of the tumbler is examined for larvae after 4 hours; in heavy infections larvae may be present within 30 minutes. In the early stages of an outbreak, larvae may be few in number or absent.

At necropsy, white thread-like worms, up to 8 cm in length are found in the bronchi, often in tangled masses in heavy infections.

Control: Calves should not be pastured with cattle subclinically infected with lungworm, or placed in pastures recently grazed by infected cattle. Infections usually terminate after approximately 3 months and confer a high level of resistance to subsequent infection. In housed dairy calves the disease is usually the result of such poor husbandry practices as feeding hay from the floor of pens.

Vaccination against the disease is practiced widely in Britain and N.W. Europe. The vaccine is comprised of 2 doses of attenuated (X-irradiated) infective larvae. The vaccine is administered by mouth and the second dose is given from 2 to 5 weeks after the initial dose. The animals are housed during the vaccination procedure and for 2 weeks after the second dose to ensure development of adequate resistance before release to pasture.

Those lungworms that require an intermediate host may be controlled by measures designed to eliminate, or to avoid contact with, the intermediate hosts.

Treatment: Since adult lungworms are usually expelled spontaneously, recovery may occur without therapy. Several drugs are useful in cattle: cyanacethydrazide (R 205) is effective against adult but not immature forms; diethylcarbamazine (R 208) is highly effective against immatures but not against adults; methyridine (R 223) and tetramisole (R 236) are effective against all stages of lungworms and also against many of the gastrointestinal helminths which may cause concurrent infections. These drugs are also used in the treatment of *D. filaria* in sheep. Cyanacethydrazide has been reported as effective in the treatment of *Metastrongylus* infections in pigs.

Supportive treatment is of value. The animals are moved to clean pastures or clean, well bedded quarters and their level of nutrition raised.

LIVER FLUKE INFECTIONS
OF RUMINANTS

Fasciola hepatica, the most important trematode of domestic ruminants, is the commonest cause of liver fluke disease in the temperate areas of the world. In extensive areas of Africa, Asia and Hawaii, *Fasciola gigantica* is economically important, and in parts of North America and Europe, *Fascioloides magna* is limited in distribution. In North America, *Dicrocoelium dendriticum* is confined mainly to New York, New Jersey, Massachusetts and the maritime provinces of Canada. It is also found in Europe and Asia.

FASCIOLA HEPATICA
(Common liver fluke)

Etiology: *Fasciola hepatica,* 30 mm long and leaf shaped, has a worldwide distribution and a broad host range. Economically important infections occur in cattle and sheep in 3 forms: **chronic,** which is rarely fatal; **acute,** primarily in sheep and often fatal; and **"black disease",** almost exclusive to sheep and usually fatal.

Eggs passed in the feces develop miracidia in about 10 days and hatch in water. Miracidia infect lymnaeid snails, especially *Lymnaea* spp. in which development and multiplication occur through the stages of sporocysts, rediae, daughter rediae and cercariae. After 1 to 2 months' development, cercariae emerge from snails and encyst on aquatic vegetation. Encysted cercariae (metacercariae) may remain viable for many months unless exposed to desiccation.

After ingestion by the host, usually with herbage, young flukes are released in the duodenum, penetrate the intestinal wall and enter the peritoneal cavity. The young fluke penetrates the liver capsule and wanders in the parenchyma for several weeks, growing and destroying the tissues. It enters a bile duct and matures, beginning to produce eggs about 10 weeks after infection occurred. The minimum egg-to-egg cycle is about 4 months and the adult fluke may live for years. Prenatal infections have been reported in cattle.

Clinical Findings: Fascioliasis in ruminants ranges in severity from a devastating disease in sheep to an asymptomatic infection in cattle. The course usually is determined by the numbers of metacercariae ingested over a short period. In sheep, acute fascioliasis occurs seasonally and is manifest by a distended, painful abdomen, anemia and sudden death. Deaths can occur within 6 weeks after infection. The acute syndrome must be differentiated from infectious necrotic hepatitis (q.v., p. 337). In subacute disease, survival is not unusual even in cases with great damage to livers. Cases of chronic fascioliasis occur in all seasons; signs may include anemia, unthriftiness, submandibular edema and reduced milk secretion, but even heavily infected cattle may not show diagnostic signs.

Sheep do not appear to develop resistance to infection, and chronic liver damage is cumulative over several years. In cattle, there is evidence of reduced susceptibility following calcification of the bile ducts.

Lesions: Immature, wandering flukes destroy liver tissue and there is hemorrhage. Extensive damage leads to acute fascioliasis in which the liver is enlarged and fibrinous deposits form on the capsule. In chronic cases, cirrhosis develops. Mature flukes damage the bile ducts, which become enlarged, even cystic, and have thickened, fibrosed walls. In cattle, cystic ducts are seen and the walls are greatly thickened and often become calcified. Flukes are frequently found in the lungs.

Tissue destruction by wandering flukes may activate the spores of *Clostridium novyi* and the resulting multiplication of this organism leads to necrotic changes and a fatal toxemia (infectious necrotic hepatitis, q.v., p. 337).

Diagnosis: The eggs, oval, operculated, golden, 130 to 150 μ by 65 to 90 μ, must be distinguished from those of paramphistomes (stomach flukes), which are larger and gray. Eggs of *F. hepatica* cannot be demonstrated in feces during acute fascioliasis. In subacute or chronic disease, the number varies from day to day and repeated fecal examinations may be required. The SGOT concentration may serve as an indicator of hepatic damage caused by immature flukes and to indicate the effectiveness of anthelmintics against migrating stages.

At necropsy, the nature of the liver damage is almost diagnostic. Adult flukes are readily seen in the bile ducts, and immature stages may be squeezed or teased from the cut surface.

Control: Control measures for *F. hepatica* infections are designed to reduce the number of flukes in the host animal and to reduce the snail population in the environment. Routine treatments of livestock in autumn and in late winter are advisable; additional treatments are determined by a knowledge of the local epizootic factors. Animals brought into feed lot may require treatment. When drug safety permits, pregnant animals should be treated a few weeks before parturition to ensure that they are not anemic during lactation. Certain products are forbidden in dairy cows.

Older remedies included carbon tetrachloride, hexachlorethane, hexachlorophene, bithionol and Hetol. These compounds had varying degrees of efficacy against adult flukes but treatment was frequently followed by signs of toxicity.

More recently a number of compounds have become available such as Hilomid, clioxanide, oxyclozanide, rafoxanide, nitroxynil and menichlopholan. These compounds have increased efficacy against immature and adult flukes.

The selection of a fasciolicide should be based on the disease situation, host animal and local environmental conditions. Contraindications should be observed and use precautions followed.

The snail intermediate host may be controlled by drainage of land, by suitable management and by use of molluscacides. The ideal compound would kill snails and their eggs when used in low concentration, and be harmless to mammals and fishes. Routine treatment of an area several times a year may be necessary to achieve adequate control. Copper compounds, pentachlorphenates and Frescon are the commonly used molluscacides and are very effective if applied correctly.

Suitable management and fencing may be used to exclude grazing animals from snail habitats. Control is complicated by reservoir infections in wildlife, e.g., deer and rabbits. When sheep and cattle graze together, it is necessary to treat both in a control plan.

FASCIOLA GIGANTICA
(Giant liver fluke)

Fasciola gigantica is similar in shape to *F. hepatica* but is larger (75 mm) with less clearly defined shoulders. It occurs in warmer climates in cattle and buffalo, in which animals it is responsible for chronic fascioliasis, and in sheep, in which the disease is frequently acute and fatal. Control measures should be based on those described for *F. hepatica*.

FASCIOLOIDES MAGNA
(Large liver fluke, Giant liver fluke)

Etiology: *Fascioloides magna*, 75 mm long, thick and oval in outline, is distinguished from *Fasciola* spp. by the lack of an anterior projecting cone. It occurs in ruminants, domestic and wild. Deer are probably the normal hosts. The life cycle resembles that of *Fasciola* spp.

Clinical Findings: The life cycle is not completed in cattle. In this host pathogenicity is low and losses are confined primarily to liver condemnations. In sheep and goats, a few parasites can produce death due to the inability of the host to limit the migration of the flukes in the liver parenchyma.

Lesions: In deer, there is little tissue reaction and the parasites are enclosed in thin fibrous cysts that communicate with bile ducts. In cattle, *F. magna* cause severe tissue reaction resulting in thick-walled encapsulations that do not communicate with bile ducts. In sheep, encapsulations do not develop and the parasites migrate extensively causing tremendous damage. On section, infected livers of cattle and sheep show black tortuous tracts formed by the migrations of young flukes.

Diagnosis: While the eggs of *F. magna* resemble those of *F. hepatica*, this feature is of limited use, as in cattle usually no eggs are passed. Recovery of the parasites at necropsy and differentiation from *F. hepatica* and *F. gigantica* is necessary for definite diagnosis. Where domestic ruminants and deer share the same grazing, the presence of disease due to *F. magna* should be kept in mind.

Control: Little is known of the effects of anthelmintics. It is probable that deer are required for the completion of the life cycle and if they can be excluded from the areas grazed by cattle and sheep, control may be affected. Control of the intermediate host may be possible once it has been identified in a region and the nature of its habitat examined.

DICROCOELIUM DENDRITICUM
(Lancet fluke, Lesser liver fluke)

Etiology: The lancet fluke is slender and 12 mm long. It has a wide distribution in many countries and will infect a wide range of final hosts including domestic ruminants. The first intermediate host is a terrestrial snail (*Cionella lubrica* in the U.S.A.) from which cercariae emerge and are aggregated in a mass of sticky mucus (slimeball). The cercariae are ingested by ants and encyst in this, the second intermediate host. Metacercariae, in the subesophageal ganglion of the ant, cause abnormal behavior which in turn increases the probability of ingestion by the final host. The young flukes migrate to the liver via the bile duct and begin egg laying, about 10 to 12 weeks after infection.

Clinical Findings and Diagnosis: Clinical signs are not obvious, but in massive infections jaundice may be seen. The eggs are distinctive but are very small (40 μ by 25 μ) and not readily seen upon fecal examination.

    Lesions: There does not appear to be any immunity and very heavy infections may accumulate (50,000 flukes in a mature sheep). Cirrhosis occurs and the bile ducts may be thickened and distended. Economic loss is due primarily to condemnation of livers.

Control: The complex life cycle makes an attack on the intermediate hosts difficult unless aggregations of snails and ants can be located and eliminated. Anthelmintics commonly used against *F. hepatica* are not usually effective, but there are reports that Hetolin is very active and that thiabendazole and Hetol may also have efficacy.

PARAMPHISTOMES
(Amphistomes, Stomach flukes, Conical flukes)

Etiology: There are numerous species in ruminants in many countries. Adult parasites are pear-shaped, pink or red, up to 15 mm long, attached to the lining of the rumen and reticulum. Immature forms in the duodenum are 1 to 3 mm long.

The life cycle in the snail host resembles that of *Fasciola hepatica*, but the snails commonly infected are planorbids or bulinids. In the ruminant host, the young flukes remain in the small intestine for 3 to 6 weeks before migrating forward to the rumen and reticulum. Eggs are produced 8 to 14 weeks after infection occurs.

Clinical Findings: Adult flukes do not cause overt disease and large numbers may be encountered. The immature worms attach to the duodenal mucosa by means of a large posterior sucker and cause severe enteritis. Affected animals exhibit anorexia, polydipsia, unthriftiness and severe diarrhea. Extensive mortalities may occur especially in young cattle and sheep. Older animals can develop resistance to reinfection but may continue to harbor numerous adult flukes.

Diagnosis: The large, gray, operculated eggs are readily recognized, but in acute paramphistomiasis there may be no eggs in the feces. Examination of the fluid feces in these cases may reveal immature flukes, many of which are passed. Diagnosis is commonly made at necropsy.

Control: The snail hosts may be attacked as described in the control of fascioliasis. The immature flukes in sheep are susceptible to niclosamide, menichlopholan and rafoxanide, but resorantel is considered to be the anthelmintic of choice as it is effective against both immature and adult stomach flukes in cattle and sheep.

HEPATIC DISTOMATOSIS (SM. AN.)

A slow, inevitably fatal fibrosis of the hepatic duct, due to massive infection with the trematode *Metorchis conjunctus*. The parasite was first recorded in 1934 in dogs in Northern Canada. It has also been reported in South Carolina and the same parasite, or a very similar one, has been found occasionally in cats and raccoons in the Northeastern U.S.A.

The fluke (*M. conjunctus*) is found in an area extending from the Laurentian Mountains into northern Saskatchewan and in the region south of the Hudson Bay. The geographic distribution coincides with that of its 2 intermediate hosts, the snail *Amnicola limosa porata* and the suckerfish *Catostomus commersonii*. Infection of the mammalian host occurs by ingestion of raw fish.

Infected dogs show progressive weakness, ending in complete exhaustion, coma and death. Severe ascites and signs of obstructive jaundice may accompany the infections in cats. The liver is 2 to 3 times normal size. The hepatic duct is distended, thickened and fibrosed, the interlobular connective tissue is hypertrophic. Adult worms may occur in large numbers in the hepatic duct. The diagnosis is made from the presence of the embryonated, operculated eggs in the feces.

All fish fed to dogs in the enzootic area should be sterilized by boiling or the equivalent. No specific treatment has been developed.

CESTODES OF DOGS AND CATS
IN NORTH AMERICA

Because the majority of dogs and cats in North America are highly domesticated, fed largely on prepared foods and rarely have access to their natural prey, cestode parasitism, with few exceptions, is not a serious problem. The more important exceptions are infections of dogs with *Dipylidium caninum*, with its stage in the flea, and infections of cats with *Taenia taeniaeformis*, with its infective larval stage in rodents. Suburban, hunting and farm dogs are in a special category, in that they may occasionally eat rabbits, hares and rodents, as well as raw offal from sheep, cattle, pigs and big game. In the latter case, they may, on rare occasions, become infected with *Echinococcus granulosus* or *E. multilocularis* and present a public health hazard. The importance of some species, e.g., *E. granulosus*, *T.*

CESTODES OF DOGS AND CATS OF NORTH AMERICA
(In order of their importance)

Name*	Definitive Host	Intermediate Host and Organs Invaded**	Diagnostic Features of Adult Worm	Remarks
Dipylidium caninum (Double-pored dog tapeworm)	Dog, cat, coyote, wolf, fox and other animals.	Fleas and more rarely lice; free in body cavity.	Strobila 15 to 70 cm in length and up to 3 mm in maximum width. 30 to 150 rostellar hooks of rosethorn shape in 3 or 4 circles; large hooks 12 to 15 μ, smallest 5 to 6 μ in length. Segments shaped like cucumber seed with pore near middle of each lateral margin.	Probably most common tapeworm of dogs, less common in cats; cosmopolitan. Occasionally infects man, particularly infants.
Taenia taeniaeformis	Cat, dog, lynx, wolf and other animals.	Various rats, mice and other rodents; in large cysts on liver.	Strobila 15 to 60 cm in length, 5 to 6 mm in maximum width. 26 to 52 rostellar hooks in double row; large hooks 380 to 420 μ, small hooks 250 to 270 μ in length. No neck. Sacculate lateral branches of uterus difficult to count.	Common cestode of cats; rare in dogs; cosmopolitan.
Taenia pisiformis	Dog, cat, fox, wolf, coyote, lynx and other animals.	Rabbits and hares, rarely squirrels and other rodents; in pelvic cavity or peritoneal cavity attached to viscera.	Strobila 60 cm to 2 m in length, 5 mm in maximum width. Around 34 to 48 rostellar hooks in double row; large hooks 225 to 290 μ, small hooks 132 to 177 μ in length. 5 to 10 lateral branches on each side of gravid uterus.	Particularly common in suburban, farm and hunting dogs, which eat rabbits and rabbit viscera.
Taenia hydatigena	Dog, wolf, coyote, lynx, rarely cat.	Domestic and wild cloven-footed animals, rarely hares and rodents; in liver and abdominal cavity.	Strobila to 5 m in length and 7 mm in maximum width. Around 26 to 44 rostellar hooks in double row; large hooks 170 to 220 μ, small hooks 110 to 160 μ in length. 5 to 10 lateral branches on each side of gravid uterus.	In farm dogs, more rarely hunting dogs; cosmopolitan.

Diphyllobothrium spp.***	Man; dog, cat and other fish-eating animals.	Encysted in various organs, or free in body cavity of various fish.	Strobila to 10 m in length and 20 mm in maximum width, but usually smaller. Scolex with 2 grooves (bothria) and no hooks. Genital pores ventral on midline of segment.	Canada; Alaska and various other states of the U.S.A.
Echinococcus granulosus (Hydatid tapeworm)	Dog, wolf, coyote, possibly fox and several other wild carnivores.	Sheep, goats, cattle, swine, horses, deer, moose and some rodents; occasionally man and other animals; commonly in liver and lungs, occasionally in other organs and tissues.	Strobila 2 to 6 mm in length with 3 to 5 segments; 28 to 50, usually 30 to 36, rostellar hooks in double row; large hooks 27 to 40 μ, small hooks 21 to 25 μ in length.	Uncommon in North American domestic animals although foci, especially among range sheep, are known; sylvatic moose-wolf cycle where these animals occur; probably cosmopolitan.
Echinococcus multilocularis	Cat, dog, arctic red and gray foxes and coyotes.	Microtine rodents, occasionally in man; in the liver.	Strobila 1.2 to 2.7 mm in length with 2 to 4 segments; along with previous species smallest tapeworm in dogs; 26 to 36 rostellar hooks in double row; large hooks 23 to 29 μ, small hooks 19 to 26 μ.	Alaska and Midwestern U.S.A. and Canada.
Mesocestoides spp.	Many wild canids, felids, mustelids, and other animals including dog and cat.	Complete life history unknown; juvenile tetrathyridia in abdominal cavity and elsewhere of various mammals, birds and reptiles; now known tetrathyridia from body cavity of dogs may enter intestine through intestinal wall.	Strobila 10 cm in length and 2 to 5 mm in width. Scolex with 4 suckers, but no rostellum or hooks. Genital pore ventral in midline of worm. Gravid segments with parauterine organ.	Reported from dog and cat in Midwest and West; in wild animals elsewhere in U.S.A. and Canada.

CESTODES OF DOGS AND CATS OF NORTH AMERICA
(In order of their importance)
(Continued)

Name*	Definitive Host	Intermediate Host and Organs Invaded**	Diagnostic Features of Adult Worm	Remarks
Taenia multiceps multiceps	Dog, wolf, coyote and fox.	Sheep, goats and other domestic or wild ruminants; usually in brain and spinal cord.	Strobila 40 to 100 cm in length and 5 mm in maximum width. Scolex with 4 suckers and 22 to 32 hooks in double row; large hooks 150 to 170 μ, small hooks 90 to 130 μ in length. Vagina with reflexed curve near lateral excretory canal. 9 to 26 lateral branches on gravid uterus.	Rare in domestic carnivores in Western North America; more common in wild animals.
Taenia serialis	Coyote, wolf, dog and fox.	Rabbit, hare, squirrel; in subcut. connective tissue, or retroperitoneal.	Strobila 20 to 72 cm in length and 3 to 5 mm in width. 26 to 32 hooks in double row; large hooks 110 to 175 μ, small hooks 68 to 120 μ in length. Vagina with reflexed curve near lateral excretory canal. 20 to 25 lateral branches on gravid uterus.	Primarily in wild canids. Considered by some authorities as not distinct from *T. multiceps*.
Taenia balaniceps	Bobcat and dog.	Unknown.	Strobila 24 cm in length and 2 to 4 mm in width. Scolex acorn-shaped with 28 to 32 hooks in double row; large hooks ca. 145 μ, small hooks 93 to 98 μ in length. No neck. Uterus with appearance of lobed sac.	Reported from the West (U.S.A.).
Taenia crassiceps	Fox, wolf, coyote, dog (experimentally).	Various rodents and perhaps other animals; subcut. and in body cavities.	Strobila 70 to 170 mm in length and 1 to 2 mm in width. Double row with 30 to 36 hooks in double row; large hooks 126 to 132 μ, small hooks 121 to 140 μ in length. 16 to 21 lateral branches on uterus, sometimes becoming diffuse.	Reported from Canada and Northern U.S.A., including Alaska.

	Definitive host	Intermediate host	Description	Distribution
Taenia krabbei	Wolf, coyote, dog and bobcat.	Moose, deer and reindeer; in striated muscle.	Strobila ca. 20 cm in length and 9 mm in maximum width. Scolex small with 26 to 36 hooks in double row; large hooks 146 to 195 μ, small hooks 85 to 141 μ in length. 18 to 24 straight and narrow lateral branches on gravid uterus.	Reported from Canada and northern U.S.A., including Alaska.
Taenia ovis	Dog, cat (rarely).	Sheep, and goat; in musculature, but rarely elsewhere.	Strobila 45 to 110 cm in length and 4 to 8.5 mm maximum width. Scolex with 32 to 38 hooks in double row; large hooks 160 to 202 μ in length. 20 to 25 lateral branches on gravid uterus. Vagina crosses ovary on poral side of segment.	Occasionally from farm dogs in Western North America; cosmopolitan.

* *Taenia polyacantha* recorded rarely from dogs in Alaska is excluded here.

** In all cases where the life cycle is known, cats and dogs become infected by eating animals, or parts therefrom, which contain the infective larval stage of the tapeworm. These intermediate hosts become infected by ingesting tapeworm eggs (except in the case of *Mesocestoides* spp. and *Diphyllobothrium* spp., which have an extra stage), which are passed in the feces of the definitive host.

*** Several species of *Diphyllobothrium* have been recorded from North American dogs and cats; they require extensive study before they can be identified with certainty.

LARVAL CESTODES
OF PUBLIC HEALTH IMPORTANCE*

	Taenia saginata	Taenia solium	Diphyllobothrium latum	Echinococcus granulosus	Echinococcus multilocularis
Host of adult worm.	Man only.	Man only.	Man; dog, cat and other fish-eating carnivores.	Dog, wolf, fox and several other wild carnivores.	Canidae and the domestic cat.
Name of intermediate larval stage.	Cysticercus bovis. "beef measles".	Cysticercus cellulosae "pork measles".	Plerocercoid.	Hydatid cyst.	Multilocular or alveolar "cyst" or hydatid.
Measurements of larval stage.	9 × 5 mm.	6-10 × 5-10 mm.	About 5-10 mm in diameter.	Diameter sometimes 150 mm.	Variable, penetrates like neoplastic tissue.
Principal intermediate hosts.	Cattle.	Pig, dog (man may be both definitive and intermediate host).	Fish.	Sheep, cattle, swine, moose, deer; rarely, dog, cat, man.	Field mice, voles, lemmings, sometimes domestic mammals and man.
Site of larval stage.	Intermuscular connective tissue.	Intermuscular connective tissue. Occasionally, nervous system.	Mesenteric tissues, testes, ovary, muscles.	Commonly in liver and lungs, occasionally in other organs and tissues.	Various organs and tissues.

* See also CESTODES OF DOGS AND CATS IN NORTH AMERICA, p. 707.

hydatigena and *T. ovis,* depends upon the effects of the meta-cestode on the intermediate host, either as it affects the host itself or the suitability of the carcass or offal meats for human consumption.

In general, cestodes very rarely give rise to well-defined clinical signs in dogs and cats. Pathogenicity varies with the different species, the degree of infection and the age and condition of the host. When signs are observed, they are usually those of general unthriftiness, malaise, irritability, capricious appetite, shaggy coat, colic, mild diarrhea and, occasionally, emaciation and epileptiform fits. Lesions are usually limited to varying degrees of enteritis. Diagnosis of infection is usually based on the presence of eggs or segments in the feces. Data on the range of definitive and intermediate hosts, the diagnostic features of the adult worms and other relevant information are contained in the accompanying table.

Treatment: In the control of tapeworms of dogs and cats, treatment combined with prevention of reinfection is essential for satisfactory results.

The problem of preventing reinfection, however, varies considerably, depending on the nature and range of the intermediate hosts. It is particularly difficult, for example, with *Dipylidium caninum,* where fleas are the intermediate host. Furthermore, some tapeworms are difficult to eliminate by treatment of the definitive host because the neck of the worm is prone to break, leaving the scolex to regenerate a new strobila.

Two related compounds, arecoline hydrobromide (℞ 198) and arecoline acetarsol (℞ 212) cause expulsion of cestodes from the gut by temporary paralysis of the tapeworm scolex and increased peristaltic action in the host. Both compounds may produce undesirable side effects—excessive salivation, superpurgation and temporary collapse. Neither compound has a high efficiency in removal of *Echinococcus.*

Bunamidine hydrochloride (℞ 200) and bunamidine hydroxynaphthoate (℞ 201) are the most effective against *Echinococcus,* but can be toxic in excitable dogs suffering from liver dysfunction.

Dichlorophen (℞ 206), niclosamide (℞ 224) and its piperazine salt (℞ 229) are highly effective against the large tapeworms but of little value against *Echinococcus.*

Feces which may be infected with *Echinococcus* should be handled and disposed of carefully to reduce the risk of infection to man and other animals.

TICK INFESTATION
(Acariasis)

Tick infestation causes local irritation and discomfort, leading to loss of production of meat, milk, wool and eggs. Infectious organisms introduced by contaminated mouth parts of the tick result in abscesses or the transmission of disease. If present in sufficient numbers, ticks remove substantial quantities of blood. Attempts by the animal to rid itself of the ticks may produce bleeding and sores, which in turn may become infested by screwworms or other maggots. Ticks are vectors of several diseases, including Rocky Mountain spotted fever, babesiasis, anaplasmosis, Q fever and tularemia. Each of these diseases is discussed separately in the section on Infectious Diseases (q.v., p. 226). They also may cause tick paralysis. One species causes sweating sickness.

There are 2 families of ticks, the Ixodidae or "hard ticks" and the Argasidae or "soft ticks". The ixodid ticks of major importance as parasites in the U.S.A. are: the Lone Star tick, *Amblyomma americanum*; the gulf coast tick, *Amblyomma maculatum*; the Rocky Mountain wood tick or spotted-fever tick, *Dermacentor venustus (andersoni)*; the American dog tick, *Dermacentor variabilis*; the brown dog tick, *Rhipicephalus sanguineus*; the winter tick, *Dermacentor albipictus*, and the cattle fever ticks, *Boophilus annulatus* and *Boophilus microplus*. *Boophilus annulatus* has now been eradicated in the U.S.A. in so far as resident populations are concerned.

Among the argasid ticks, only 2 cause significant and widespread damage to North American livestock. One, *Argas persicus,* is the fowl tick (q.v., 1095) and the other, *Ornithodoros (Otobius) megnini* is the spinose ear tick.

Hard ticks: When hard ticks are viewed from above, the mouth parts can be seen protruding from the body. The scutum or shield of male ixodids covers much of the dorsal surface, but in the unengorged female, the corresponding structure covers only the front half of the dorsum. As the body of the male is not capable of much distension, it takes relatively little blood. When the female engorges with blood, the posterior portion of its body becomes tremendously distended into a blood-filled sac.

Most hard ticks mate on the host and feeding is then accelerated. After about a week the engorged female drops to the ground and spends about a week digesting the blood. Eggs are then deposited under debris at the surface of the soil.

In warm weather the eggs may hatch in about 2 weeks into

tiny 6-legged larvae or "seed ticks". The larvae crawl up plants to await the passing of a host animal. Seed ticks can live for 8 months or longer without a host to feed on provided the microclimate of their habitat is favorable. When a host animal brushes against a tick-covered plant, the larvae transfer to its body and crawl to a site suitable for attachment. After several days, they become distended with blood and drop to the ground, where they molt and become nymphs which are somewhat larger than the larvae and bear 4 pairs of legs. The nymphs crawl up on vegetation and repeat the process of awaiting a host. They may survive for several months without food.

After transferring to an animal, the nymphs suck blood for about a week before becoming engorged. Once more they drop from the host to molt, become adults and crawl up on vegetation to await a new host.

Ticks that feed as larvae on one animal, as nymphs on another animal and attack a third animal as adults are referred to as 3-host ticks, whether the 3 animals be of the same or 2 or 3 different species. A few species of ticks spend all stages of their development on a single individual and are referred to as one-host ticks. All the important species on small animals are 3-host ticks. Examples of one-host ticks in North America are the cattle-fever tick and the winter tick.

If one is familiar with the species native to a particular region, identification of a specimen is possible with the aid of a hand lens.

(a) The **Lone Star tick** is abundant in the Southern U.S.A., in the region extending from Oklahoma to Virginia and southward. Attacking both wild and domestic animals, this tick prefers to attach on parts not densely covered with hair. It is a 3-host tick and all 3 stages attack domestic animals and man. It is capable of transmitting Rocky Mountain spotted fever of man. The season of activity extends from early spring until late fall. The scutum of the male is marked with a silvery pattern; the scutum of the female has a single silvery-white spot (a "lone star") near the posterior end.

(b) The **gulf coast tick** occurs from Texas to the Atlantic, in a region extending about 200 miles inland from the Gulf of Mexico. The adult stages of this tick attack deer, horses, sheep, hogs and dogs, but the tick is important as a pest of cattle, where it is found principally attached to the inside of the outer ear. The tick is dark brown in color and scutum of both sexes is freely marked with silver lines and spots. Cattle are attacked principally during the later summer and early fall. Summer droughts sometimes delay the seasonal occurrence of this tick. The gulf coast tick is also a 3-host tick, but the larvae and nymphs are primarily parasites of ground-nesting birds, such as meadowlarks.

(c) The **Rocky Mountain wood tick** occurs in the north-western part of the U.S.A. It is a 3-host tick. The larvae and nymphs feed on rodents, while the adults attack domestic and the larger wild animals, attaching chiefly on the head and ears of the host. This tick is reddish brown. The male has the whole scutum beautifully marked with white or silver. The scutum of the female is almost solidly silver-colored and it contrasts strongly with the reddish-brown of the back. This species has an unusually long life cycle, frequently requiring 2 years or longer to develop from larva to adult. The ticks over-winter as nymphs or adults and adults are seen on livestock during the spring and early summer.

(d) The **American dog tick** is abundant in the central and eastern portions of the U.S.A. It occurs in smaller numbers over the entire country, except for the Rocky Mountain area and the Pacific Northwest. In appearance, the tick is quite similar to the spotted-fever tick, but it occurs in a different geographic area. The dog tick is a 3-host tick. The larvae and nymphs feed on small rodents, chiefly meadow mice. The pre-ferred host of the adult is the dog, but it also attacks man, cattle, horses and wild animals, such as foxes and raccoons. The tick is most important as a vector of Rocky Mountain spotted fever in the Eastern States, but it is sometimes an annoying pest of livestock and is a vector of certain livestock diseases.

(e) The **brown dog tick** survives in outdoor areas only in mild climates. The tick is a real problem, however, in heated areas wherever it occurs. In the U.S.A. this tick is primarily a parasite of dogs, only occasionally attaching to man and other animals. The brown dog tick can become a major annoyance in houses and kennels where dogs are kept. It is a carrier of canine babesiasis.

(f) The **winter tick** is distributed from the gulf coast to Canada. It is unique in that it attacks animals in the winter or early spring. It is a one-host tick, parasitic on deer, moose, elk, horses and cattle. It is especially serious as a pest of range horses. The larvae attach over the entire body of the host and spend about a month developing to the adult stage. The en-gorged females drop to the ground through the winter and deposit their eggs during the spring months. The eggs hatch in 3 to 6 weeks, but the larvae remain clustered tightly to-gether throughout the summer and do not attach to hosts until the cool weather of late fall.

(g) The **cattle-fever tick** (*Boophilus annulatus*) was once a grave danger to the cattle industry of the U.S.A., primarily because of its transmission of babesiasis, but also by virtue of its specific effects upon the host. This tick has now been eradicated from the U.S.A., but a closely related species, *B. microplus,* occurs in a small portion of southern Texas and is plentiful in Mexico, Central and South America.

Soft ticks: It is difficult to distinguish the sexes among the argasids. Both sexes take considerable amounts of blood. They resemble bedbugs in their habits, living in cracks and crevices and emerging during the night to take many short blood meals when the host is sleeping. Many argasid ticks infest cave-dwelling or burrowing animals.

(a) The **fowl tick,** *Argas persicus,* is a severe pest of domestic poultry, especially in the Southwestern U.S.A. Blood loss from gross infestations may greatly weaken or even kill fowls. It can carry spirochetosis of fowls.

(b) The **spinose ear tick** differs from the usual argasid life-history pattern. Its larvae crawl into the ears of cattle, horses, dogs, sheep or wild animals and spend 1 to 7 months developing through the nymphal stage. They then drop out of the ears and crawl to fences, barns, feed bunkers, salt troughs and trees to molt to adults, mate and deposit their eggs. Spinose ear ticks are a major pest of livestock in the arid and semi-arid regions of the Southwestern U.S.A. They are more common in animals kept in small enclosures than in range stock.

Clinical Findings: Without exception, ticks are dependent upon blood for their existence. Most animals tolerate a few ticks, but become irritated and restless as the numbers increase, and set about to rid themselves of the pests by rubbing, scratching, licking and biting. These efforts in turn usually aggravate the situation, leading to the development of irritated or raw areas, which may become secondarily infected. Small ticks may become engulfed in the swelling tissue. Tick bites frequently heal slowly.

If present in large numbers, any species will produce anemia. The toxins in the saliva cause irritation at the site of the bite and apparently systemic effects. As a consequence animals lose weight, fail to eat and become lethargic. Some ticks cause paralysis (*see* TICK PARALYSIS, p. 721).

The **gulf coast tick,** tending to concentrate around, on and in the ear, causes cattle great annoyance. It also attacks the hump region of Brahman cattle and sometimes feeds along the top of the neck of all breeds. However, the main damage is to the ear. The ticks feed in clusters and cause marked irritation. As a result, the ear becomes swollen and painful.

The **spinose ear tick** causes pain and irritation and occasionally leads to screwworm or other maggot infestation. Horses are difficult to bridle and cattle and dogs hold their heads in unusual positions. Infested animals also rub their ears, attempting to dislodge the parasites. On examination, larvae and nymphs can be seen deep in the ear, half buried in waxy exudate and debris. The spiny appearance of the bodies of the nymphs is distinctive. The ears frequently are lopped and may discharge a foul-smelling mixture of wax and tick debris.

The **winter tick** causes general depression, lack of appetite, long hair coat without luster and general debilitation. In the more severe cases, an edema develops extending from the jaws to the hind flanks. At this stage, death is imminent and the animal requires skilled nursing if it is to recover.

The **Rocky Mountain wood tick** is a serious parasite of cattle, horses and sheep and is important from a public-health standpoint since it attacks man as well as animals. It is especially notorious as a vector of Rocky Mountain spotted fever.

The first evidence of the presence of ticks on small animals usually is the effort of the animal to dislodge them. Ticks in the ear canal cause great distress, often leading to almost hysterical activities of the animal. Head shaking, crying and inappetence are common in small animals.

Diagnosis: Frequent sites of tick attachment are the ears, neck, flanks and the interdigital spaces, but ticks can be found over the entire body surface. Ticks, particularly soft ticks, frequently are deep in the ear canal and can be located only by the use of an otoscope. Since all 3 stages of the tick may occur on the animal, the size of the tick may vary from that of the tiny larva ("seed tick") to that of the engorged female, 0.5 cm or more in length.

Treatment: When only a few ticks are present on an animal, they may be removed by simply plucking them off, taking care that this is done without breaking off the mouthparts or "head". If this does occur, care must be used to remove the broken parts. Any abscess or ulcerated area that develops should be appropriately treated as such. Most of the irritated areas heal rapidly, with little attention, once the tick is removed properly. Larvae are easily overlooked because of their small size, and treatment of the entire animal best effects their removal.

Ticks on livestock: The control of ticks on livestock is usually a matter of herd or flock treatment, but the same treatment can be applied to individual animals. Ear ticks may be removed from the ear canal manually, but this is usually more difficult and laborious than spraying, dipping or squirt-can treatment.

Although many acaricides have shown usefulness in reducing tick populations, a number of them leave undesirable residues in meat or milk. Because no residues of acaricidal agents in milk are tolerated under the requirements of the United States Food and Drug Administration, and only minimal specified residues are permitted in the fat of meat-producing animals, the earlier recommendation of some materials has been suspended.

In the U.S.A., arsenic (As_2O_3) at 0.175 to 0.19% concentration in solution; pyrethrins plus synergists at 0.1 and 1.0%, respectively, as a wet spray, or 1.0 and 10.0%, respectively, as a mist spray; rotenone, 2 to 4 oz of 5% derris powder per gallon of water; or crotoxyphos at 0.1 to 0.3% in water, have been suggested for tick control on lactating dairy cattle as conforming to the aforementioned restrictions. *Current regulations and label directions should always be consulted since these vary from time to time and from country to country.*

For control of ticks on beef cattle, horses, sheep, goats and hogs, lindane at 0.025 to 0.03%, Delnav at 0.15%, toxaphene or malathion at 0.5%, ronnel at 0.75%, coumaphos at 0.25 to 0.5% concentrations have been suggested for use. Toxaphene, lindane, Delnav and coumaphos are usually recommended as dips. In the dipping of sheep and goats, the concentration of toxaphene and of coumaphos may be reduced to 0.25 to 0.3%. The 0.5% concentration, for safety, must be restricted to adult cattle, horses and hogs.

The recommendations for dairy cattle may also be used for the other species.

Solutions, emulsions or suspensions may be used as dips or sprays, each being effective and of equivalent toxicity. Regardless of the material or method used, it is of prime importance that a uniform dispersion of the acaricide be maintained to avoid erratic dosage and possible poisoning of the animals.

In spraying livestock, freshly mixed dispersions are used and, in a power sprayer, the agitator helps to keep the spray at a uniform concentration. For dips, large quantities of acaricide are used to charge the vat and the dip frequently is re-used over a period of months. It is difficult to stir dipping vats thoroughly and there is the further hazard that the dip may deteriorate on standing, with the result that cattle may be improperly treated. Therefore, although properly dispersed dips are as safe as sprays, there generally is less risk of injuring livestock if spray treatments are employed.

Dips maintained at proper strength are usually more effective than sprays. However, sprays applied thoroughly also give good control. Sprays may be applied at any desired pressure, there being little if any difference in the effectiveness as long as the hair is thoroughly wetted. High-pressure sprays (200 to 400 lb/sq in.) penetrate more uniformly and rapidly and, therefore, are generally preferred.

In addition to dips and sprays, direct application into the ear is often utilized against ear ticks. Low-pressure sprays of toxaphene at 0.5% concentration may be directed into the ears. Squirt-type oil cans or syringes may be used for the same purpose, with any preparation containing 0.5% of lindane or toxaphene. Ronnel, coumaphos or malathion may be used in the same manner. Repetition of these treatments is usually required, according to the degree of infestation.

Ticks on small animals: Dogs may be freed of ticks by treating them with an acaricide. Washes are usually more effective than sprays or dusts as they penetrate the hair better and reach all the ticks. A wash or spray should contain one of the following materials: 0.5% of malathion, or 0.05% of lindane or rotenone. Delnav has shown excellent capacity for tick control on dogs and cats when used at concentrations of 0.15 to 0.25%. If a dip is preferred (immersing the dog except for the head), one-half these concentrations should be used. Concentrates of these agents, which should be mixed with water to give the desired strength, are available. If a dust is preferred, products containing 5% of arylam (Sevin), 1% of lindane, 4 or 5% of malathion, or 3 to 5% of rotenone (derris or cube powder) are available. Lindane should not be used on cats. Dichlorvos in collars and as a topical application is also useful.

Pyrethrins (R 280), with or without synergizing compounds, are effective tick killers, but have practically no residual activity and in general are comparatively expensive.

Always consult and follow label instructions.

Premises: Infestations on premises must be eliminated if reinfestation is to be avoided. This is generally economically impossible for large acreages, but around houses, barns, kennels and the like is highly desirable.

Premises may be cleared of ticks, including the brown dog tick, by application of the following: chlordane as a 2 to 3% spray or 5 to 6% dust, diazinon, dichlorvos, or lindane as 0.5% sprays, malathion as a 2 to 3% spray or 4 to 5% dust. Due consideration must be given to the presence of birds, children, pets and other susceptible species.

Baseboards, door and window casings, edges of carpets, behind pictures and draperies, and all other possible hiding places should be painted, sprayed or dusted.

These materials should be used on limited areas only. Food, water, dishes, or utensils should not be contaminated. Children or pets must not be allowed in treated areas until the acaricide has had time to be effective and the excess chemical has been removed.

Treatment of premises should always be supplemented by treating dogs with a product labeled for such use.

Cautions: The preparations used for tick control may be toxic to man and animals if contacted or ingested in sufficient quantities (*see* Toxicity of Organic Insecticides and Acaricides, p. 962) and should be used with due regard for this fact.

Manufacturers are careful to recommend their products within specified limitations. In all cases, the recommendation of the manufacturer, as stated on the label, together with precautions on the label, should be followed to the letter.

Products must be plainly labeled for animal use. If only plant recommendations appear on the label, then the product must not be used on animals regardless of the circumstances.

Home-devised mixtures of various acaricidal agents and additions of detergents to liquid preparations must not be used.

Most acaricides and insecticides are toxic to fish and quantities of these materials should not be allowed to enter streams.

TICK PARALYSIS

Pyrexia may precede the clinical syndrome of a flaccid, afebrile, ascending motor paralysis produced in domestic and wild animals and man by any of certain species of ticks harboring the causal agent, a neurotoxin. Some but not all strains of these species serve as vectors, and not all infested animals become paralyzed.

Etiology: Although the disease has a worldwide distribution, the vectors have not been identified in all countries. The incidence largely depends upon the seasonal activity of the transmitting ticks. Important vectors are: in Australia (*Ixodes holocyclus*), the U.S.A. (*Dermacentor venustus*, *D. variabilis*, and possibly *Amblyomma maculatum* and *A. americanum*), Canada (*D. venustus*), Bulgaria (*Haemaphysalis inermis*, *H. punctata*), Yugoslavia (*H. punctata*, *Hyalomma scupense*), and South Africa (*Rhipicephalus evertsi*); and the incidence is highest in spring and summer. In European and Asian U.S.S.R. (*Ornithodoros lahorensis*), Yugoslavia and Crete (*I. ricinus*) and South Africa (*I. rubicundus*), the incidence is highest in autumn and winter. Eleven other ixodid species may be responsible for sporadic cases in animals and man. *Argas persicus* causes paralysis in poultry in South Africa, the U.S.A. and Turkey.

Sheep, dogs and humans appear to be particularly susceptible, one tick frequently being capable of causing complete paralysis. Before the application of effective prophylactic measures in 1958, the annual losses were estimated at several thousand sheep in South Africa. During the last 6 decades more than 400 human cases have been recorded, from Canada (250), U.S.A. (123) and Australia (30), and of these 9% died. Prompt removal of vectors undoubtedly saved many lives. Severe outbreaks with considerable losses of cattle have occurred in Montana and British Columbia. The disease has also been produced experimentally in marmots, guinea pigs, hamsters and other animals.

It is generally accepted that tick paralysis is caused by a neurotoxin produced by the female tick during feeding, and usually has its effects over this period. This may be true only for *Ixodes* spp. where males do not feed on the host. Adult males of *D. venustus* (Canada), *Hyalomma truncatum* and *Rhipicephalus simus* (South Africa) have been responsible for tick paralysis in humans.

Clinical Findings: The onset is gradual, paralysis first becoming evident as an incoordination in the hind limbs resulting in an unsteady gait. Reflexes are lost, but sensation may be present. The paralysis ascends over a period of 1 to 2 days from its onset, at the end of which time the victim may be completely immobilized. Further advance results in respiratory failure and death. Immunity is of very short duration. Reinfestation 14 days after recovery may result in another attack.

Lesions: Generally there is only local irritation at the site of the tick bite, with no pathologic changes. However, in South Africa tick paralysis is accompanied by edema of the lungs, hyperemia of the meninges, enlargement of lymph nodes and atrophy of the spleen.

Diagnosis: Tick paralysis in livestock, due to its general appearance, may be mistaken for plant or pesticide poisoning. Full consideration should be given to the fact that the signs do not appear until the tick has been attached and feeding for about 6 days. It also is noteworthy that in livestock, ticks frequently attach themselves in the region of the head. In humans, any covered portion of the body may provide a site for attachment.

Prophylaxis and Treatment: Prevention consists of avoiding tick-infested areas during the tick season, or if tick-infested, spraying with coumaphos at 0.125%, dioxathion at 0.15%, or toxaphene or carbaryl at 0.5%. Treatment may be repeated after 2 to 3 weeks. Prompt treatment or removal of the ticks by hand will check an outbreak. In the U.S.A., if all ticks are removed, signs normally disappear within a few hours with no observable after effects. Tick paralysis in other countries frequently does not disappear after removal of the ticks and, in some cases, paralysis does not develop until after the tick has dropped off on completing its engorgement.

Humans frequenting infested areas should wear close-fitting garments of a smooth, tight texture, with tucked-in trousers and shirts. Clothing and the body should be examined daily for ticks. Excellent protection against ticks can be obtained by spraying clothing with insect repellents, such as diethyltoluamide, dimethyl phthalate or ethylhexanediol.

SWEATING SICKNESS

An acute, febrile, tick-borne toxicosis characterized mainly by a profuse, moist eczema and hyperemia of the visible mucous membranes. It is essentially a disease of young calves, but adults are not entirely immune. Sheep, pigs and goats have been infected experimentally. It occurs in east, central and southern Africa, and probably in Ceylon and southern India.

Etiology: The etiology was in doubt until 1956 when it was shown to be caused by a toxin which is produced by certain strains of *Hyalomma truncatum* (*transiens*). The toxin develops in the tick, not in the vertebrate host. This toxin is retained by ticks for as long as 7 generations. Attempted experimental transmissions between affected and normal animals by contact or inoculations of blood have not been successful.

Graded periods of infestation of a susceptible host by "infected" ticks have different effects on the host. A very short period has no effect, but the animal remains susceptible. A period just long enough to produce a reaction may confer an immunity, but if the infestation is prolonged over 5 days, severe clinical signs and death may result. Recovery confers an immunity which lasts up to 13 months.

Clinical Findings: After an incubation period of 4 to 11 days, signs appear suddenly and include hyperthermia, anorexia, listlessness, watering of the eyes and nose, hyperemia of the visible mucous membranes, salivation, necrosis of the oral mucosa and hyperesthesia (as in heartwater). Later, the eyelids stick together. The skin feels hot and a moist dermatitis soon develops, starting from the base of the ears, the axilla, groin and perineum, and extending over the entire body. The hair becomes matted and beads of moisture may be seen on it.

The skin becomes extremely sensitive and emits a sour odor. Later the hair and epidermis can be readily pulled off, exposing red, raw wounds. The tips of the ears and the tail may slough away. Eventually the skin becomes very hard and cracked, and predisposed to secondary infection or screwworm infestation. The animal is very sensitive to handling, shows pain when moving and seeks shade.

Often the course is rapid and death may occur within a few days. In less acute cases, the course is more protracted and recovery may occur. The mortality in affected calves varies from 30 to 70% under natural conditions. Morbidity in enzootic areas is about 10%. The severity of infection is influenced by the number of ticks as well as the length of time they remain on the host.

Lesions: Emaciation, dehydration, diphtheroid stomatitis, pharyngitis, laryngitis, esophagitis, vaginitis or posthitis, edema and hyperemia of the lungs, congested liver, kidneys and meninges, and atrophy of the spleen are found in addition to the skin lesions described above.

Diagnosis: It is essential to determine the presence of the vector. There is typically a generalized hyperemia with subsequent desquamation of the superficial layers of the mucous membranes of the upper respiratory, alimentary and external genital tracts, and a profuse moist dermatitis followed by a superficial desquamation of the skin.

Prophylaxis and Treatment: Control of tick infestation is the only effective prophylactic measure. Removal of ticks, symptomatic treatment and good nursing are indicated. Antibiotics (℞ 11, 25, 41) or sulfonamides (℞ 75, 82, 90) are useful in combating secondary infection.

PEDICULOSIS
(Louse infestation, Lousiness)

Various species of biting lice (order Mallophaga) and sucking lice (order Anoplura) infest domestic animals. Sucking lice are known to occur only on mammals. Biting lice are found on both mammals and birds (*see* ECTOPARASITISM of poultry, p. 1094).

Etiology: Cattle are most commonly infested with the cattle-biting louse, *Damalinia bovis,* and with 2 species of Anoplura, the short-nosed cattle louse, *Haematopinus eurysternus,* and the long-nosed cattle louse, *Linognathus vituli.* Anoplura less commonly found on cattle include the little blue louse, *Solenopotes capillatus,* the tail louse, *H. quadripertusus* (Florida and gulf coast) and the buffalo louse, *H. tuberculatus* (Old World and tropics).

Horses are commonly infested by 2 species of lice, the common horse-biting louse, *Damalinia equi,* and the horse-sucking louse, *Haematopinus asini.*

Swine are commonly lousy, but only one species is involved, the hog louse, *Haematopinus suis* (Anoplura).

Sheep are most commonly infested with the sheep-biting louse, *Damalinia ovis,* and the sheep-foot louse, *Linognathus pedalis* (Anoplura). Less commonly found on sheep are 2 other species of Anoplura, the face louse, *L. ovillus* and the goat louse, *L. stenopis.*

Goats harbor many louse species, the commonest being the red louse, *Damalinia caprae* (Mallophaga), and the blue louse, *Linognathus stenopis* (Anoplura). Two other Mallophaga, *D. limbata* and *D. crassipes,* are also frequently found.

Dogs and **cats** may be infested with either sucking or biting lice. The parasites involved are *Linognathus setosus* (Anoplura) and *Trichodectes canis* (Mallophaga) in dogs, and *Felicola subrostrata* (Mallophaga) in cats. Other kinds of lice have been found on dogs, e.g., *Heterodoxus spiniger* (Mallophaga).

The Anoplura are bloodsucking lice with mouthparts reduced to stylets which are retracted within the body when not in use. The Mallophaga are provided with obvious ventral chewing mandibles and live on epidermal products as well as blood and exudates when available.

Louse eggs are glued onto hairs or feathers and are pale, translucent and suboval. About 3 to 4 weeks are required to complete one generation, but this varies with species and climatic conditions.

Clinical Findings and Diagnosis: Pediculosis of both types is manifested by pruritus and dermal irritation with resultant scratching, rubbing and biting of infested areas. A general unthrifty appearance, roughened hair coat and lowered production in farm animals are common. In severe infestations, there may be loss of hair and local scarification. Extreme infestation with sucking lice can cause anemia. In sheep and goats, the rubbing and scratching often results in broken fibers giving the fleece a "pulled" appearance. In dogs, the hair coat becomes rough and dry and, if the lice are numerous, the hair may be matted. Sucking lice cause small wounds which may become infected. The constant crawling and either piercing or biting of the skin causes nervousness.

The hair should be parted and an examination, under strong light, made of the skin and proximal portion of the hair coat. The hair of large animals should be parted along the topline, on the neck and dewlap, on and in the ear, on the escutcheon, on the tail base and in the tail switch. The head, legs and feet should not be overlooked, particularly in sheep. On small animals, the ova (nits) attached to the hair are readily seen. Occasionally, where the coat is matted, the lice can be seen when the mass is broken apart. The active biting lice can be seen moving through the hair, while the sucking lice usually are found with the sucking mouthparts embedded in the skin.

In dairy herds, the young stock, dry cows and bulls may escape early diagnosis and suffer more severely. Infestations, particularly of the several sucking louse species, may become so severe as to produce signs suggestive of a grave ailment. Young animals, e.g., calves, may die. Treatment which effectively removes the lice results in prompt improvement.

Pediculosis on farm animals in the Northern U.S.A. is most prevalent during the winter. Shortly after livestock are turned out to pasture in the spring, louse infestations are greatly reduced in severity.

Transmission usually occurs by host contact. Lice dropped or pulled from the host die in less than a week, but disengaged ova may continue to hatch over a period of 2 to 3 weeks in warm weather. Premises recently vacated by infested stock should, therefore, be disinfected before being used for clean stock.

Treatment: Louse control requires direct dermal application of insecticides. Zero or very low tolerances for pesticides in milk limits the highly effective insecticides that may be used on dairy cattle and dairy goats to crotoxyphos (℞ 256), crotoxyphos plus dichlorvos (℞ 255), 0.03% coumaphos (℞ 246) and rotenone (R 294, 296 [but *see* below]). Beef cattle, sheep, goats and swine should be treated with coumaphos (R 246), dioxathion (R 266), lindane (R 271), malathion (R 273), methoxychlor (R 276), carbaryl (R 245), ronnel (R 286), crufomate (R 253, 254) or toxaphene (R 304). Crotoxyphos and crotoxyphos plus dichlorvos may also be used on these meat animals. Rotenone should not be used on swine, but is safe for use on other animals where current regulations permit its use.

Spraying or dipping should be thorough, and usually 2 treatments 14 days apart will eradicate lice. Effective spraying requires soaking the hair to the skin: cattle and sheep require a minimum of 1 gal., but as much as 3 gal. may be required on large long-haired cattle. At least ½ gal. per head should be applied to swine. Dipping is more dependable than spraying, but only rotenone, coumaphos, dioxathion, ronnel, lindane, crufomate or toxaphene should be used in dips. Toxaphene should be used at 0.25%, half the spraying strength, for dipping sheep and goats; 0.03% diazinon (R 261) is an effective spray against lice on sheep. In cold climates, dusting of sheep for louse control is favored over sprays and dips. Large power dusters for large bands of sheep have proved practical. Best results are obtained when treatment follows shearing. Special oil-weighted dust (R 297) should be used in power dusters. Also very effective as dusts are 2% diazinon (R 263), 0.5% coumaphos (R 250) and 3% crotoxyphos (R 259); and for hand application, 50% methoxychlor (R 279).

Cattle lice can be controlled, but not eradicated, by wintertime use of back-rubber devices or dust bags similar to those used against flies in the summer. Effectiveness depends on frequent use by all cattle in the herd (R 251, 252, 257, 258, 259, 260, 267, 274, 277, 289, 305, 306). Use only crotoxyphos, dichlorvos, or coumaphos (R 251, 257, 258, 259, 260) on dairy cattle. Cattle louse populations can also be reduced by handdusting with malathion, toxaphene or methoxychlor (R 275, 278, 305) on beef cattle or rotenone or crotoxyphos (R 259, 296) on dairy or beef cattle.

Dogs can be treated with dips, washes, sprays, or dusts containing rotenone (R 294, 296, 297), methoxychlor (R 276), diazinon (R 261, 263) or malathion (R 275). On cats, only rotenone and pyrethrum preparations should be used.

Lice on swine can be controlled with dips and sprays of lindane (R 271), dioxathion (R 266) and methoxychlor (R 276), and sprays of malathion (R 273), carbaryl (R 245), coumaphos (R 246), toxaphene (R 304), crotoxyphos plus dichlorvos (R 255), crotoxyphos (R 256) and ronnel (R 286).

The United States Food and Drug Administration (USFDA) strictly specifies tissue residue limits of insecticides and carefully regulates their use in livestock products. Similar regulatory agencies exist in most countries. Regulations elsewhere are not identical to those of the USFDA, and such regulations, in the U.S.A. and elsewhere, are subject to change. Users of the MANUAL are cautioned to familiarize themselves with pertinent current local laws and requirements. The treatment of meat and dairy animals must be restricted to uses specified on the labels and all label precautions carefully observed. Tissue residue tolerances and minimum drug withdrawal times between treatment and slaughter are given under TOXICITY OF ORGANIC INSECTICIDES AND ACARICIDES, p. 962). Some states have further restrictions on use of pesticides, e.g., lindane and toxaphene may not be used in New York. Note also the cautions given with the prescriptions.

FLEA INFESTATION

Fleas are small, wingless, laterally compressed, bloodsucking external parasites. All adult fleas feed only on blood and, in feeding, cause intense pruritus and irritation to the hypersensitive host.

Etiology: Several species of fleas infest the dog and cat, 2 of these being the cat flea, *Ctenocephalides felis*, and the less common dog flea, *C. canis*. The flea spends much of its adult life on the body of the host. Eggs are laid either on the ground or on the host from which they fall to the ground. The eggs hatch into larvae which feed on organic matter in the bedding of the host or in cracks and crevices in floors. When mature, the larva spins a loose cocoon attached to bits of debris, and pupates. After about 5 days under optimum conditions, the adult emerges from the cocoon and seeks a host in order to feed and continue its life cycle.

Clinical Findings: Fleas irritate the host by their constant biting and the salivary secretion of toxic and allergenic products. In hypersensitive animals flea bites produce intense pruritus. The animal becomes restless, and bites and scratches to relieve the irritation. By so doing the animal produces an acute, discrete dermatitic patch ("hotspot") or a chronic nonspecific dermatitis. The former lesions are usually subauricular, interscapular or about the rump or thighs. The chronic nonspecific dermatitis usually is restricted to the lower back and perineum. Secondary infection is a common complication in both syndromes. Such self-inflicted trauma often leads to a cycle of constant irritation and pruritus.

Diagnosis: A careful examination of the animal will reveal the fleas or flea debris in the hair. Fleas often can be found in greatest number around the head, the rump and the tail head.

Treatment: To control fleas, both the animal and its environment must be treated. Many of the insecticides will remove fleas from the host's body, but others will return unless they and the immature forms are killed in the bedding or other places.

To kill fleas on pets, commercial preparations of either pyrethrum or rotenone powder may be applied. These materials kill quickly and are safe. Powders or sprays containing lindane or malathion, in concentrations recommended by the manufacturer, are also highly effective, but should not be used on cats. In addition, the organic phosphorus compounds, administered both topically and orally (℞ 285) have been employed successfully to control fleas. "Flea collars" impregnated with organic phosphorus compounds are a convenient means of applying these compounds. As with other insecticides, an appreciation of the toxic or allergic potential of the organic phosphorus compounds is essential. Pendants containing these compounds have been recently introduced and when attached to collars may help avoid the rare allergy or dermatitis and yet permit adequate flea control. Adequate precautions and instructions should be given to the client.

The use of insecticides should relieve much of the animal's discomfort. Treatment of self-inflicted dermatitis should be directed towards controlling secondary infection and relieving the pruritus. The topical application of bacitracin in combination with neomycin, and polymyxin ointment, with or without hydrocortisone, and the oral or parenteral administration of cortisone, prednisolone-hydroxyzine hydrochloride (℞ 153), aspirin, phenobarbital or tranquilizers (℞ 369), achieves these purposes. Care should be taken to clean the dermatitic areas before initiating treatment; hexachlorophene (℞ 423) is ideal for the purpose.

Control of breeding places of fleas is easy when the pet has a sleeping box or basket. The old bedding should be discarded and then the box or basket and surrounding area treated with any of the insecticides mentioned below. Animals should not be allowed to reoccupy the area before surfaces are dry. Other areas where the animal spends considerable time should be treated similarly.

If there is a general flea infestation in a home, 0.5% malathion sprayed along baseboards will control a mild infestation. In truly heavy infestations, it is probably better to call in a professional exterminator.

In addition to malathion (R 273), lindane (R 272), rotenone (R 296), and pyrethrum dusts (R 298) can be used for flea control in buildings. Chlorinated hydrocarbons cannot be used in cats, but dusts containing rotenone and pyrethrins with synergists give excellent results. These powders can be liberally dusted in the hair and also sprinkled around the animal's habitat.

For the hypersensitive patient, a program of hyposensitization with flea antigen (R 120) is worth trying. One can expect approximately 25% success. Hyposensitization, when effective, should be repeated yearly before the flea season.

THE SHEEP KED
(Sheep tick)

The sheep ked (*Melophagus ovinus*) is one of the most widely distributed and important external parasites of sheep. It is a true insect, a wingless fly and not an acarine. The adult is about 7 mm long, of a brown or reddish color and covered with short, bristly hairs.

The female does not lay eggs but gives birth to a single fully developed larva which is cemented to the wool and pupates within 12 hours. A young ked emerges after about 22 days and may live 100 to 120 days if a female and about 80 days if male. During this time about 10 larvae are produced by each female. The entire life is spent on the host. Keds that fall off the host usually survive less than a week and present little danger of infestation to a flock.

To feed, keds pierce the skin with their mouthparts and suck blood. They usually feed on the neck, breast, shoulder, flanks and rump, but not on the back where dust and other debris collect in the wool.

Ked numbers increase during the winter and early spring when they spread rapidly through a flock, particularly when sheep are assembled in close quarters for feeding or shelter.

Clinical Findings: The skin irritation when the keds feed causes sheep to rub and bite, and the fleece becomes thin, ragged and dirty. The excrement of the keds causes permanent discoloration, which is likely to reduce the value of the wool. Infested sheep may lose vitality and be unthrifty, particularly lambs and pregnant ewes. Keds also transmit *Trypanosoma melophagium* which is said to be nonpathogenic for sheep.

Control: Shearing removes many pupae and adults. Thus shearing before lambing and the subsequent treatment of the ewes with insecticides to control the remaining keds can greatly reduce the possibility of lambs becoming heavily infested. Sheep are usually treated after shearing and best results are obtained if an insecticide is used whose residue remains at least 3 to 4 weeks. By this means the keds which emerge from the pupae will also be killed. Modern fly dips, giving freedom from blow fly strike for 6 to 20 weeks, will also eradicate the keds.

Formerly, efficient control of keds was obtained by the use of chlorinated hydrocarbons—DDT, lindane, gamma BHC, dieldrin, aldrin, and toxaphene—but owing to the cumulative effect of toxicity from absorption of these products and their persistence, particularly in animal fats, their use is now prohibited in the U.S.A. and most other sheep-producing countries of the world.

The insecticides that were recommended in the U.S. Department of Agriculture Handbook No. 331 (1968) were: (a) as **dips:** dioxathion 0.15%; malathion 0.5%; ronnel 0.25%; diazinon 0.05%; (b) as **sprays:** dioxathion 0.15%; malathion 0.5%; pyrethrins 0.1% (plus 1% of sulfoxide or piperonyl butoxide, which act as synergists); ronnel 0.25%; diazinon 0.03% (or 0.06% at low pressure); (c) as **dust:** coumaphos 0.5%; malathion 4 to 5%; diazinon 2%. In some countries the organophosphorus compounds chlorfenvinphos, dichlofenthion, fenchlorphos, carbophenothion, pyrimithate, and trichlorfon are in general use, mainly as dips or sprays. Not all have been approved for this purpose in the U.S.A. (*see* TOXICITY OF ORGANIC INSECTICIDES AND ACARICIDES, p. 962).

It is important to note that, while many organophosphorus compounds give effective control of keds, lice and maggot flies (fleeceworms), the only effective compound where control is also required against the sheep scab mite *Psoroptes ovis*, is diazinon now that the use of gamma BHC is no longer permitted.

Dipping: When sheep dipping vats are available, dipping is regarded as the most effective method of treatment. Completely submerging the sheep ensures the destruction of all keds present but in most instances does not kill the pupated larvae, unless a long-acting insecticide is used so that the ked newly emerging from its pupa, is killed by the residue in the fleece of the sheep. Large flocks of range sheep should be treated in a permanently constructed sheep dipping vat. Smaller flocks and farm flocks may be successfully treated in portable galvanized-iron dipping vats or in smaller tanks, tubs or in canvas dipping bags. In areas where the water used in dipping vats is considered hard, it is well to use commercial wetting agents or household detergents.

Spraying as a method of treatment for the control of sheep keds is generally regarded as not being as effective as the dipping method, but is more convenient in some areas. Pressures of 100 to 200 lb/sq in. for short wool and 300 to 350 lb/sq in. for long wool are commonly used. Power spraying may be carried out in portable or permanent pens and there are various types and designs of spray equipment used for applying the insecticide. The purpose is to obtain an even distribution of the insecticide over the whole body, and the concentration of the active ingredient in the spray solution should be twice that used for dipping. A useful type of such equipment is the spray "boom", an endless pipe of rectangular or oval shape, fitted with a series of spray nozzles. The boom is placed in the chute and, as the sheep are driven through, the spray is turned on and they are sprayed from all sides simultaneously. A similar principle is used to apply insecticidal dusts.

Shower dipping is also sometimes used. In this procedure, the sheep are held in a special pen and showered from above and below until the fleece is saturated. The run-off is returned for recirculation and the concentration of insecticide used is the same as for dipping.

Jetting: This technique involves the forceful application of the insecticide by means of a multiple-jet comb drawn through the short fleece. Although a little slower, it is thought advantageous for smaller flocks, as it is economical and does not require a permanent installation.

Dusting: Power dusting is a method which fits well into management practices at shearing time. It is rapid and economical, and avoids wetting the animals. Various types of equipment for dusting are available commercially.

FLIES AND MOSQUITOES

BLACK FLIES AND BUFFALO GNATS

Members of the dipterous family Simuliidae are characterized by a strongly humped thorax, a marked enlargement of the anterior wing veins and the absence of simple eyes. Few species exceed 5 mm in length. Gray, olive and black are their common colors.

The immature stages are aquatic in all known species and most require swiftly flowing water for successful development of larval and pupal stages. An important exception is the southern buffalo gnat which emerges in great swarms from such slow-moving streams as the Arkansas, White River and Red River. The eggs of many species are laid at the water's edge on stones, vegetation or debris so that they are kept moist or occasionally submerged. The southern buffalo gnat drops its eggs into water or crawls below the surface on vegetation to deposit the eggs while submerged. Some of the species in the Adirondack Mountains develop from egg to adult in less than 3 weeks, but others overwinter in the larval stage and so have a larval period of several months.

Only 2 of more than 100 species of black flies in North America have caused severe losses of farm animals. The southern buffalo gnat, *Cnephia pecuarum,* is an annual spring pest in the lower Mississippi Valley, and in outbreak years thousands of mules and cattle have been killed in Louisiana, Arkansas and Mississippi. Flooding of the lower Mississippi and its large southern tributaries appears to increase black fly numbers, and annual spring outbreaks sometimes occur for 2 or 3 years following a major overflow. *Simulium arcticum* killed many cattle in Saskatchewan during the periods of 1913 to 1919 and 1944 to 1946.

It is generally believed that the rapid death of animals following attack by large numbers of black flies is due to toxic substances injected by the insects. The serious effects in animals observed in the Saskatchewan black fly outbreaks appeared to be the result of an increase in the permeability of the capillaries with a consequent loss of fluid from the circulatory system into the tissue spaces and body cavities. Tissues are edematous and reveal internal hemorrhages. This is interpreted as due to a direct toxic action without previous sensitization. The possibility of anaphylaxis has not been completely ruled out since animals that suffer 2 fairly closely spaced attacks sometimes fare worse during the second attack.

Certain species of black flies sometimes cause losses to poultry either by direct attack or through the transmission of *Leucocytozoon* disease (q.v., p. 1077).

Control: Since large-scale control of black flies is difficult and expensive, livestock men usually resort to repellents for the protection of their animals. Dense smudges have saved many southern animals during outbreak years. The animals soon learn to crowd about a smudge for protection. Open flames must be avoided since livestock sometimes crowd so near the source of smoke that they are severely burned. Cold-mixed lubricating-oil emulsion has been widely used for years. Temporary relief may be afforded dogs, horses and valuable cattle by sprays of pyrethrum plus synergist and repellent (℞ 281, 282, 283).

If public funds and trained supervisory personnel are available, large-scale control of black flies is possible by treating breeding streams with methoxychlor. Pesticide treatments involving water surfaces or large land areas are frequently subject to governmental regulation and must be done with due regard for possible deleterious environmental effects and residues in food products.

MOSQUITOES

Mosquitoes of the genera *Aedes* and *Psorophora* sometimes attack livestock in such numbers that deaths or serious production losses occur. Both of these genera lay their eggs on the ground where they are hatched by subsequent rains that submerge them. Both overwinter in the egg stage. The total egg production of millions of adults may be suddenly hatched by a spring rain, or by melting snow, and a vast plague of adults then emerge. Some *Psorophora* spp. have several generations each summer, and a season characterized by alternate dry periods and heavy rains will bring them out in unbelievable numbers. In the rice-growing areas of Arkansas and Louisiana, *Psorophora confinnis* is a severe pest of both animals and man, their abundance being a consequence of the manipulation of irrigation water on large areas of land.

In general, *Psorophora* spp. mosquitoes occur from the latitude of Delaware and Kansas, south through the American tropics, while the *Aedes* spp. are the mosquito pests of livestock, to a greater or lesser degree, all over the U.S.A. and Canada. *Mansonia* spp. are severe on livestock in Florida.

The injury that mosquitoes inflict on livestock consists of outright killing (though this is rare), severe annoyance and blood losses, and the transmission of several diseases. It also is suspected that toxins injected by the insect at the time of biting may cause severe systemic effects. Equine encephalomyelitis can be transmitted by at least 10 species of *Aedes* mosquitoes, but the most important vector is *Culex tarsalis*. The microfilariae of the dog heartworm often are mosquito-transmitted. In Central and South America, *Dermatobia hominis,* the parent of the notorious and destructive torsalo grub, fastens its eggs to a species of *Psorophora* mosquito which then transmits them to the mammalian host where they hatch as the mosquito feeds. Instances of the apparent transmission of fowl pox by mosquitoes have been reported.

Control: It is almost impossible for the individual stockman to protect his animals; residual sprays on the animals do not prevent attack and repellents that will confer adequate protection during heavy outbreaks are unknown.

Valuable animals should be housed in closed or screened buildings and the mosquitoes inside killed with a fog or aerosol of synergized pyrethrum (℞ 282) or dichlorvos (℞ 264). Temporary relief may be afforded by sprays of pyrethrum, synergist and repellent, or crotoxyphos and dichlorvos (℞ 256, 260, 281, 282, 283). The insecticidal residual deposits suggested for stable-fly control (p. 737) will aid in mosquito control outside barns.

Area control of mosquitoes is a specialized procedure that can be carried out successfully only by experienced personnel with proper equipment. Responsibility for execution of control programs should be turned over to official agencies or reliable firms specializing in this type of insect eradication and aware of regulatory conditions.

Insecticides currently in use against mosquito larvae include methoxychlor, malathion, MLO oil, Abates, Dursban, fenthion and aprocarb. Caution is advised with any larvicidal procedure as fish and other beneficial aquatic organisms may be killed.

HORSE FLIES AND DEER FLIES

Horse flies and deer flies belong to the family Tabanidae. They are characterized by 3-jointed antennae with the last segment terminating in a series of rings, the costal vein extending entirely around the wing, large squamae and the almost complete lack of body bristles. Three genera, *Chrysops, Hybomitra* and *Tabanus,* contain most of the important pest species in North America. *Tabanus* and *Hybomitra* (horse flies) are generally larger than *Chrysops* (deer flies) and are more serious pests of animals. Various horse flies and deer flies are important pests more or less locally in different parts of the world.

The larvae of horse flies are largely aquatic or semiaquatic. Egg masses of most species so far studied are deposited on vegetation, rocks or debris projecting from the water or near the water's edge. Eggs usually hatch in 5 to 10 days. The young larvae fall into the water, but most of them soon find their way to the mud near shore where the larval period is spent in search of annelids, insect larvae, small crustaceans and other minute animals that form the larval diet. As time for pupation approaches, larvae travel to drier areas a few feet farther from shore where there is less danger of prolonged submergence during the pupal period. Most of those studied have a single brood each year, and overwintering occurs in the larval stage.

Livestock production losses caused by horse flies are due principally to annoyance and loss of blood. A few individuals of the larger species can prevent a herd from feeding normally and add to the loss by the overactivity they stimulate. Blood loss becomes a significant factor when dozens of flies feed on an animal for several hours each day during the summer. As many as 200 flies have been seen on single isolated animals. Horse flies take from 0.1 to 0.3 ml of blood at a feeding. Moderate infestations may rob an animal of 100 ml of blood daily over long periods.

Horse flies can transmit the causal agents of anthrax, anaplasmosis, tularemia and equine infectious anemia. They are suspected as transmitters of the virus of equine encephalomyelitis. In the Philippines, they carry the trypanosome of surra between animals, while in Africa, they transmit several trypanosomes pathogenic to livestock, including those responsible for nagana. In all of the above instances, transmission is purely mechanical, flies never serving as intermediate hosts for the causative agents.

Control: Horse flies are among the most difficult to control of any of the bloodsucking flies. While the majority of the new organic insecticides will kill horse flies even at low dosages, they will not do so fast enough to prevent biting. Repellents are the only present answer and the synergized pyrethrins have given the best results. Wetting the haircoat heavily (1 to 2 qt/cow) by spraying with an emulsion (℞ 281) is recommended for maximal protection. Protection may last up to 3 days, when treatment must be repeated. Addition of a synthetic repellent may increase effectiveness (℞ 282). Stable flies and horn flies also will be repelled. Allethrin may be substituted for some pyrethrins. Oil-base sprays (℞ 260, 282, 283) afford some protection, but pyrethrin, synergist and repellent concentration must be higher than for less aggressive flies. They are applied from a hand or electric atomizer, using not more than 2 oz per head. Dairy cattle need treatment at each milking. Automatic sprayers are convenient for lactating cows.

STABLE FLIES

While resembling the house fly in size and general appearance this species, *Stomoxys calcitrans,* has a needle-shaped proboscis that at rest protrudes noticeably in front of the fly's face. The larvae develop in manure and in moist, fermenting vegetable matter. Hay or green chop on the ground around outdoor feeding racks is one common habitat for larvae, and refuse from vegetable processing plants is another; others are peanut refuse left in fields to become wet, and bay grasses often washed ashore in windrows along the coastlines of New Jersey and Florida. The cycle from egg to adult can be completed in 3 weeks during the summer, and the females live 4 to 6 weeks.

The bite is more painful to livestock than that of most bloodsucking flies. The wounds bleed freely after the fly has left and are attractive to screwworm flies, house flies and other smaller Diptera. Both sexes are hematophagous. The decreased production caused by stable flies is principally due to annoyance and blood loss. They also may mechanically transmit anthrax and possibly other livestock diseases. It has been estimated that milk production may decrease as much as 50% during heavy infestations and that weight losses of 10 to 15% may occur. Livestock deaths have been reported.

Control: Since individual stable flies visit their hosts frequently and only for short periods, spray applications on the host are not highly effective in reducing populations. Spraying the outside of all livestock quarters on farm premises, as well as fences and other observed resting places, has given some control but is expensive and entirely impractical for range beef herds or even for dairy herds when pastures are well removed from the barnyard. Recommended materials for this purpose are diazinon (R 262), ronnel (R 288), or methyoxychlor (R 276). Livestock barns should be sprayed with dimethoate (R 265), ronnel (R 288), Rabon (R 302), fenthion (R 270), or diazinon (R 262) to thoroughly control stable flies as well as the ubiquitous house fly.

Because of rapid action, synergized pyrethrum or crotoxyphos stock sprays prevent stable flies from feeding and kill most of the flies that come to feed (R 256, 260, 282, 283). Care must be taken to treat well the preferred feeding sites on the legs of animals. Barns should be fogged with synergized pyrethrum (R 282) or dichlorvos (R 264) to kill stable flies.

HORN FLIES

The horn fly, *Haematobia* (*Siphona*) *irritans,* is morphologically very similar to the stable fly, but only half its size. The mouthparts are almost identical in structure and the wound is made in the same manner. The habits and life history are entirely different. The horn fly spends most of its adult life on its host, almost exclusively cattle, using the latter both as a source of food and as a resting place between feedings. It leaves only to deposit eggs on its host's dropped feces. At times, the flies cluster in a thick ring about the base of the cow's horns.

The horn fly's life-cycle, like that of the house fly, is among the shortest known for flies. Eggs sometimes hatch in less than 24 hours, larval stages may be completed in as few as 3 days and the pupal period in 6, making a total cycle of 10 days. Hot, humid weather favors the species.

Since they occur over the entire U.S.A. and can build up enormous populations in short periods, horn flies probably cause greater losses in livestock production in the country than any other bloodsucking fly. As many as 5,000 to 10,000 flies have been reported on a single cow. The blood loss under these conditions is severe. The flies feed at least twice a day and 10,000 flies would extract about a liter of blood a day. Infested animals spend much time fighting the flies and grazing time thereby is reduced. They also crowd together closely for protection and many horn and kick wounds results.

Control: Because of their habit of living almost continuously on the host, horn flies are controlled easily. Methoxychlor (R 276), carbaryl (R 245), malathion (R 273), crufomate (R 253), toxaphene (R 304), coumaphos (R 246) and ronnel (R 286) are all highly effective as sprays but should only be used on beef cattle (except for 0.03% coumaphos). Beef cattle may be treated for horn-fly control in pens or chutes by spraying the backs of the cattle with a high-pressure hydraulic sprayer. There is no need to completely cover the animals with spray; 1 or 2 quarts per head is adequate, not more often than once every 3 weeks. The only sprays permitted on dairy cattle (to avoid residues in milk) are crotoxyphos, dichlorvos (R 256, 260) and 0.03% coumaphos (R 246).

Horn flies also may be controlled by using "back rubbers" available commercially, or lengths of chain or barbed wire heavily wrapped with feed sacks and suspended loosely between 2 posts about 15 feet apart. The sacks are saturated thoroughly with insecticide in number 2 fuel oil or diesel oil.

Effective insecticides include 5% methoxychlor, 1% crotoxyphos, 1.5% dioxathion, 2% malathion, 1% coumaphos, 0.8% crotoxyphos plus 0.2% dichlorvos, 5% toxaphene, or 1% ronnel (℞ 251, 257, 258, 267, 274, 277, 289, 306). Only crotoxyphos, dichlorvos or coumaphos (℞ 251, 257, 258) may be used on lactating dairy cattle.

Daily spraying dairy cattle with a good oil-base stock spray (℞ 260, 264, 282, 283) will give excellent horn fly control. If stock sprays are not used, the dairy farmer may resort to dusts of methyoxychlor every 3 weeks, crotoxyphos not more often than every 2 weeks, or malathion every 10 to 14 days (℞ 259, 275, 279). Labor can be minimized by using dust bags filled with crotoxyphos or coumaphos (℞ 252, 259) in lanes or on pasture. Utmost care must be taken not to allow the dust to contaminate milk or milking utensils, or illegal residues in milk will result.

Dust bags may also be used for horn fly control on beef cattle, using crotoxyphos, coumaphos, methoxychlor or toxaphene (℞ 252, 259, 278, 305).

FACE FLIES

The face fly, *Musca autumnalis,* was introduced into Nova Scotia from Europe sometime during 1950-51. Two years later it was found in the Northeastern U.S.A. and by 1970 had been reported from most of the states. It is morphologically similar to the common house fly, *M. domestica*; members of both species have mouth parts that consist of sponging labellae, both have 4 longitudinal stripes on the thorax. The face fly is slightly larger but this difference is difficult to detect in the field. It is preferable to collect a number of flies and submit them to an entomologist who can differentiate them by the closeness and angles of the interior margins of the eyes and by the distinctive coloration of the face and abdomen.

Face flies breed only in fresh feces and therefore their presence and prevalence will depend on how the animals are maintained. Common house flies will breed in almost any type of manure or decaying organic material. One may be assured face flies are present if large numbers of flies are found on the face and muzzle of livestock.

Face flies are important primarily as a source of irritation, particularly when they feed around the eyes. Only a few flies are sufficient to cause irritation. When large numbers are present the animals will often bunch up in groups with their heads together. Control is difficult. Since the flies do not follow the host into barns they do not come in contact with residual sprays. Control of larvae in the field requires the scattering of all feces within 3 to 5 days of deposit. In treating the face, it is necessary to use safe materials at frequent intervals since secretion of tears by the animals will cover or dilute the spray. Dust bags containing a suitable insecticide have been used in beef cattle herds but results have been variable.

At present, the most effective control is a Ciodrin or dichlorvos emulsified spray applied to the face of the animal. The addition of a small amount of sugar (10 to 15 gm/L) may increase the attractiveness of the spray to the flies. A 1% Ciodrin or dichlorvos oil solution or a combination of Ciodrin plus dichlorvos may be used at 1 to 2 oz per head per day. A list of insecticide formulations appear in the sections on control of horn flies and stable flies (q.v., p. 737 and 738).

SCREWWORMS IN LIVESTOCK

Screwworms were once among the most important pests of livestock in the Southern and Southwestern U.S.A., causing annual losses estimated at 50 to 100 million dollars. They are obligatory parasites, and under optimal environmental conditions the flies oviposit on almost every wound that occurs— even abrasions as small as tick and fly bites.

It is important to distinguish between screwworms and the secondary maggots which frequently infest necrotic tissues. Primary screwworm myiasis should be diagnosed promptly so that livestock owners in the community may be alerted to detect new infestations.

Biology: Screwworms are the larvae of the blow fly, *Cochliomyia hominivorax* (*Callitroga americanum*), a member of the family Calliphoridae. The bluish-green screwworm fly is similar in appearance to the common blow flies, but differs in that its larval development occurs only in the tissues of living warm-blooded animals.

The screwworm fly deposits 200 to 400 eggs on the edge of a wound in rows overlapping like shingles. After about 12 hours incubation larvae covered with dark spines are visible through the translucent shells and the egg mass has a gray appearance. Upon hatching, the larvae crawl into the wound and burrow into the flesh. The maggots feed on the wound fluids and live tissues and complete their growth in about 6 days. The larvae then drop from the wound and burrow into the soil to pupate. The pupal period varies from 8 days to 2 months depending on temperature. Freezing of the soil kills pupae.

The adult insects mate when 3 or 4 days old and gravid females oviposit at 6 days of age. In warm weather, the life cycle may be completed in 21 days.

Grown screwworm larvae are about 12 mm long. The body is tapered with the anterior end being pointed and the posterior blunt, roughly resembling a screw. A pair of tracheae extend from the posterior spiracles forward into the body cavity. For about one-third of their length, these tracheae are deeply pigmented. They may be seen through the skin of the maggot as a pair of parallel lines and are characteristic of the screwworm. When fully grown or nearly so, the larvae are pinkish in color.

Clinical Findings: Screwworms feed as a colony, burrowing deeply into the flesh. The wound exudes a profuse reddish-brown fluid which almost completely covers the larvae and which may stain the hair or wool for several inches as it drains.

An aid in recognizing screwworm infestation in range animals is the change in the animal's behavior. Even a small and relatively inconspicuous wound infested with screwworms attracts not only screwworm flies, but house flies and blow flies which seek the wound primarily to feed on the exudate and are extremely annoying to the infested animal. As the annoyance increases, the infested animal seeks protection by retreating to the densest possible shade of trees or bushes.

Prognosis: If an infestation continues without treatment for as long as 2 weeks, at a time when ovipositing flies are numerous, the host animal will almost certainly be killed. Wounds treated within 4 days after infestation usually heal within a month.

Bacterial infections often complicate screwworm cases. In general, cattle are quite resistant to infection and the wounds usually heal promptly with good treatment, but sheep, goats and horses frequently develop secondary infections.

Control: The most important control measures are prevention of wounds during the season when flies are most active, the prophylactic treatment of unavoidable wounds, regular and frequent inspection of range animals to detect infestations promptly, and treatment of existing wounds to kill larvae and prevent reinfestation.

Breeding should be controlled so that young are not born during the fly season. The navel of the newborn animal is a preferred site for oviposition and should be treated promptly with a recommended screwworm prophylactic if young are born during the fly season. Castration, dehorning, docking and branding should be carried out in cold weather. If surgery is performed during the fly season, the wound should be coated with a screwworm remedy (e.g., EQ 335) and the treatment repeated as necessary until the wound has healed.

Flies and ticks should be controlled by the proper use of insecticides. Each animal on pasture should be seen twice weekly. Animals that are not with the herd, but are solitary and in dense shade or other dark places, should be examined closely.

Eradication Program: In 1958, the United States Department of Agriculture (USDA), in cooperation with livestock authorities of the southeastern states, initiated a program to eradicate screwworms from the Southeast.

Screwworm larvae were reared on artificial media and, 2 days before fly emergence, the pupae were exposed to gamma irradiation at a dosage which caused sexual sterility but no other deleterious effects. Sterile flies were distributed over the entire screwworm-infested region in sufficient quantity to outnumber the native flies, at the average rate of 400 male flies per square mile per week. The female mates only once and, therefore, when mated with a sterile male does not reproduce. There was a decline in the native population each generation until the native males were so outnumbered by sterile males that no fertile matings occurred and the native flies were eliminated. The last case in Florida was found in June 1959 and sterile-fly releases were discontinued in November. The states east of the Mississippi have remained screwworm-free since that time except for brief infestations resulting from import of infested animals from western states.

In 1962 a more extensive program of eradication was undertaken in the southwestern U.S.A. This program has virtually eliminated all the losses caused by screwworms in these states. Native populations of flies were eradicated from all states except Arizona and California in the winter of 1963–1964 and again in the winter of 1964–1965. Unfortunately much of Texas and New Mexico has been periodically reinfested by mated female flies from Mexico. There is evidence that the flies are capable of flying over 200 miles, and no natural barrier exists to block their northward movement during favorable seasons. At present, sterile flies are distributed along both sides of the Mexico-U.S.A. boundary in sufficient numbers to counteract most of the northward migration, but permanent elimination of screwworms from the U.S.A. by the sterile-male technique cannot be hoped for until they are also eradicated from Mexico.

Veterinarians in the U.S.A. can greatly assist the eradication effort by promptly reporting all suspected cases of screwworms to regulatory officials. If myiasis is found, larvae should be preserved in 70% ethanol and forwarded for identification.

Treatment: The USDA has developed 2 remedies, either of which can be used for the protection of wounds from screwworm infestation and for treating infestations. EQ 335 is a mixture containing 3% lindane in a gel base. Smear 62 is an older remedy which utilizes benzene as a killing agent and diphenylamine as a protectant against infestation or reinfestation by newly hatched larvae. A phosphorus insecticide, ronnel, has also been incorporated into a wound dressing similar to EQ 335. All 3 smears are best applied with a 1-in. paint brush. Careful application is necessary in deep wounds to be sure that the smear reaches all the many pockets formed by the burrowing maggots. A thin layer should also be applied to the skin surrounding the wound.

Sprays and dusts may also be used for screwworm control. The topical application of a dust containing 5% coumaphos is an economic and effective means of killing the maggots in a wound. In regions where screwworm flies are very active, it is often advisable to spray livestock with either coumaphos or ronnel as a prophylactic measure. If properly applied, these sprays will kill all larvae and protect animals from infestation for 2 weeks or longer.

WOOL MAGGOTS
(Fly strike, Fleece worms)

Several species of blow flies occasionally deposit their eggs in the wool of sheep. The commonest wool maggots in the U.S.A. and Canada are the black blow flies *Phormia regina* and *Protophormia terraenovae,* and the green bottle fly *Phaenicia sericata. Lucilia illustris, Cochliomyia (Callitroga) macellaria* (secondary screwworm) and other species are sometimes found on "struck" or "blown" sheep, though usually as secondary invaders. *Phaenicia cuprina (pallescens)* is the most important primary blow fly in Australia, *P. sericata* in Great Britain and *P. sericata* and *Calliphora stygia* in New Zealand.

The resulting maggots attack the wool first, but soon begin feeding on the skin and flesh. Some infestations are traceable to soiled wool about the anus, which attracts the flies and encourages them to oviposit. In other cases, entirely clean wool is suddenly blown with maggots. This usually occurs during hot weather following rain. Such a weather sequence often causes a fermentation of the wool near the skin and the resulting odor is highly attractive to blow flies. Once initiated, such infestations progress rapidly, regardless of subsequent changes of weather. The first few maggots release excretory products that are far more attractive to the flies than the original fermenting wool. A single mass placed on a sheep's back will, during a period of less than a week, produce a complete band of infestation around the animal's body. The maggots then progress toward the head and tail until infestation is complete. Since the maggots stay below the surface of the wool, their attack is highly insidious and may remain undetected until a large percentage of a flock is infested and many animals are down. It should be emphasized that wounds are not a necessary prerequisite for wool maggot infestation. When maggot infestation does originate in wounds, screwworm infestation should immediately be suspected.

Since wool maggot infestations can be rapidly fatal, early diagnosis is imperative. The habits of the blow flies make control a complex problem. Blow flies are probably present within striking distance of every flock in the country during the summer. They are strong fliers and their olfactory sense is highly developed.

Control: Blow-fly infestation of the breech region can be effectively controlled for about 6 to 8 weeks by "tagging", whereby the wool is shorn from the area between the hind legs and around the tail. In a similar fashion, complete shearing will control outbreaks involving other parts of the body. To prevent wound infestation, agents such as EQ 335, or 0.5% coumaphos dust (B 250), applied locally at weekly intervals until the wounds have healed, are highly beneficial.

Chemical prophylactic measures consist of wetting the wool and skin of susceptible areas with suitable insecticidal and larvicidal preparations such as ronnel, coumaphos, dioxathion, or diazinon (B 246, 261, 266, 286, 287).

These substances may be applied locally as, for example, around the breech, but more commonly they are used as dips or sprays, the aim being complete saturation of the fleece. Effective protection is usually afforded for a period of at least 6 to 8 weeks and sometimes longer. In some countries, organophosphate insecticides have been applied as "tip-sprays". For this purpose, smaller quantities of more highly concentrated solutions are applied as a fine spray only to the outer surface of the fleece.

Destruction of all carcasses by burning or deep burying

(preferably after poisoning of the carcass) has been recommended for the general reduction of blow fly numbers. While this is a valuable general hygienic measure, it may have little effect on the incidence of primary "strikes", because of the effects of competition between the larvae of primary and secondary flies on the struck sheep.

In small flocks, where individual treatment is carried out, the wool should be completely removed from and around the struck area and the lesions then treated with suitable agents such as EQ 335.

CATTLE GRUBS
(Ox warbles, Cattle maggots)

Cattle in the Northern Hemisphere are commonly infested by myiasis-causing larvae belonging to the genus *Hypoderma*. The adult stages are heel flies or bomb flies. South American cattle may be infested by larvae of the genus *Dermatobia* (*see* FLIES AND MOSQUITOES, p. 735).

Biology: Two species of bot flies (order Diptera, family Oestridae) attack cattle. The smaller species (*Hypoderma lineatum*) develops into the common cattle grub, the other (*H. bovis*) into the northern cattle grub. The adults, hairy flies about the size of honeybees, with a general coloration much like bumblebees, are rapid fliers. Their whitish eggs, about 1 mm long, are fastened to the hairs of the legs and lower portions of the animal's body.

In 2 to 6 days, depending on the temperature, the eggs hatch. The young maggots crawl down the hair to the skin and burrow directly into the tissues. There is a period of several months after the maggots enter the body, during which their movements are not well known. They apparently travel continuously and almost exclusively through connective tissue. They have been found in the connective tissue of the spleen, rumen, intestines, thoracic cavity, muscles, spinal column, heart and esophagus, and rarely, in the CNS. The maggots secrete proteolytic enzymes, which dissolve the tissues, producing readily ingestible food and facilitating their forward movement. The majority of *H. lineatum* congregate for a period of 2 to 4 months in the submucosa of the esophagus, increasing several fold in size and weight. *H. bovis* migrate along the nerves and congregate for a similar period in the epidural fat of the spinal canal. The larvae, now about 15 mm in length and 1 to 2 mm in diameter, begin their final migration, again through connective tissue. Eventually they arrive in the subdermal tissue of the back, where each makes a breathing hole through the skin. Although cysts are formed around them, the breathing pores remain open. Their presence irritates the cyst walls; the serum exuded into the cysts and abundant secondary invading organisms furnish food for the maggots. After a 40- to 60-day period of growth in these cysts, during which 2 molts occur, they emerge through the holes, drop to the ground and pupate. By this time, they have grown to a length of 25 mm and a diameter of 8 mm and have changed in color from creamy white to dark brownish gray. The adult heel flies emerge in 1 to 3 months, depending on weather conditions. They may mate within an hour after emergence and are ready to spend their brief adult life terrorizing their bovine hosts. The adults do not feed and live an average of a week.

Distribution and Seasonal Activity: In much of the Southern U.S.A. *H. lineatum* is common, but *H. bovis* is absent or rare in native cattle. Elsewhere to the north in North America, both species are pests wherever cattle are raised.

Where both are present, the seasonal events for the 2 species are similar, except that those for *H. lineatum* are about 6 to 8 weeks earlier. These events vary considerably from year to year and may be fairly well correlated with local and regional climatic conditions. In Texas, larvae ordinarily make their first appearance about mid-September; progressing northward, this first appearance is gradually later, until in Montana, it is about December 25, and in some of the higher mountain areas, it may be a month or more later. In Texas, the first emergence of the grubs from the back takes place during the last half of February. Where both species are present, grubs may be found in the back for about 5 to 6 months; where only *H. lineatum* is present, for about 4 to 5 months. In Texas, the heel fly season is at its height during January, February and March; in the Northern States, during May, June and July.

Domestic cattle and American bison are the only mammals known to be regularly infested with large numbers of *H. bovis* and *H. lineatum.* Increasing numbers of horses seem to be experiencing light infestations in recent years. On rare occasions, man becomes infested. In these cases, the grub usually is found in the subdermal tissues of the upper extremities. Other species of grubs may be found in the tissues of mammals (*see* CUTEREBRA INFESTATION OF SMALL ANIMALS, p. 750).

Clinical Findings and Diagnosis: Signs of heel fly attack: During periods of sunshine on warm days, cattle run wildly, often blindly, tails high in the air. Careful observation will sometimes permit detection of a pursuing heel fly. Refuge from the flies is found in shade and in water holes. Not all stampeding of this kind is due to heel fly attacks, however, for this activity occasionally is observed in seasons or regions known to be free of heel flies.

Signs of internal infestation: In otherwise normal cattle, the presence of *H. bovis* and their secretions in the epidural fat of the spinal canal is associated with dissolved connective tissue, fat necrosis and inflammation. Sometimes the inflammation extends to the periosteum and bone, producing a localized area of periostitis and osteomyelitis. Occasionally, the epineurium and perineurium may become involved. In rare, severe cases, paralysis or other nervous disorders may occur. Similarly, the presence of *H. lineatum* in the submucosa of the esophagus may cause inflammation and edema in the surrounding tissues sufficiently severe to hinder swallowing.

Signs of external infestation: The penetration of the skin by the newly hatched maggots produces a hypodermal rash. The points of penetration are painful, inflamed and usually exude a yellowish serum. Grubs in the back may occur from the tailhead to the shoulders and from the topline to a point about one-third the distance down the sides. The cysts or warbles are firm and raised considerably above the normal contour of the skin; in each there is the breathing hole, ranging in size from a very small slit to a round hole, 3 to 4 mm in diameter. Secondary infection may result in large suppurating abscesses. The emergence of the grub, its forced expulsion, or its death within the cyst, usually results in healing of the lesion without complications. Carcasses of cattle infested with cattle grubs show marked evidence of the infestation and may be penalized upon inspection.

The number of warbles in an infested animal may range from 1 to 300 or more; infested herds may have animals with no grubs. Infestations are progressively lighter with age.

Treatment: Many of the organophosphorus insecticides, when properly applied, are absorbed by the host and kill the migrating grubs in all parts of the body. Effective grub control can be obtained with these drugs, but important precautions must be taken.

Cattle, especially calves, in areas where grub numbers per animal are known to be high, should be treated as soon as possible after the adult heel fly season is over. They should not be treated later than 8 to 12 weeks before the anticipated first appearance of grubs in the backs, as adverse reactions may develop. Migratory *H. lineatum* larvae congregate in maximum numbers at this time in the submucosal tissues of the esophagus. If rapidly killed by systemic insecticides, a massive, usually transitory, inflammatory edematous reaction may result. The swelling may partially or completely occlude the lumen, swallowing may become difficult or impossible, profuse drooling of saliva may occur, eructation may cease and the calf may become bloated. Recovery is usually rapid and complete (48 to 72 hours after treatment) but in severe cases the calf may die of bloat. Rupture of the esophagus may be caused by attempted passage of a stomach tube.

Migratory *H. bovis* larvae also may appear in maximum numbers during this period in the epidural fat of the spinal canal. If they are rapidly killed by systemic insecticides, a massive, usually transitory irritation of the spinal tissues may result. Mild to severe paraplegia may develop. Again, recovery is usually rapid and complete; rarely, a calf becomes permanently paralyzed.

Five different systemic insecticides, in varied formulations, are available for treatment. Pour-on treatments using coumaphos, famophos, ruelene, or trichlorfon may be used, (℞ 249, 269, 300, 301, 308). A measured amount of the material should be poured evenly along the midline of the animal's back, making sure it runs down the sides of the animal for maximal skin wetting and absorption.

Sprays may be applied using ruelene (℞ 299), coumaphos (℞ 248) or trichlorfon (℞ 307). The spray must be applied carefully so that the entire surface of the skin is thoroughly wet to permit maximum absorption. Coumaphos (℞ 247) also may be used as a dip.

As additives to the diet, famophos (℞ 268) and ronnel (℞ 290, 291, 292) will effectively control grubs only if the treatment regimen ensures adequate intake of the drug. For example, ronnel as an additive to the mineral mix (℞ 290) is generally effective, but in some regions range cattle will not eat enough of the mineral mix to effect a complete grub kill.

No systemic insecticide should be used in conjunction with another since their actions may be synergistic. Their use is prohibited in lactating dairy animals since these drugs are excreted in the milk. Residues are present in all animals for varying periods after treatment.

No systemic insecticide should be used except in strict accord with the manufacturer's recommendations. The TOXICITY

OF ORGANIC INSECTICIDES AND ACARICIDES is discussed elsewhere in this MANUAL (q.v., p. 962).

Where organophosphates cannot be used, and rotenone is approved, grubs can be controlled by external applications of rotenone to the warbles after the grubs have taken up their subdermal positions in the back. Since new grubs continue to appear in the back and since rotenone kills only those it contacts through the breathing holes, it is necessary to repeat treatment every 6 weeks or oftener during the grub season. Washing or dusting by hand with crude rotenone (R 295, 296) gives good results. The wash or dust should be sprinkled over the animals' back and worked into the grub holes with a stiff brush or the tips of the fingers. This treatment, if properly applied, will kill 90 to 100% of the grubs present in the back.

Mechanical extraction: On small groups of tractable animals, instrument extraction or hand expulsion (by squeezing) of the individual grubs is effective. Rarely, when this procedure is carelessly performed, the grub is crushed in its cyst and an anaphylactic reaction may result.

SHEEP NOSE BOTS

The fly, *Oestrus ovis,* is worldwide in distribution and it is one of the most widely distributed of the parasites of sheep in the U.S.A. Goats occasionally are affected and rarely man is attacked, mainly in the eyes. A related species is found in the nasal passages of deer.

Biology: The adult fly is grayish brown and about 12 mm in length. The female deposits larvae in and about the nostrils of sheep without alighting. These larvae are very small, initially under 2 mm in length, and are of a clear white color. They migrate into the nasal cavity, many of them spending at least some time in the paranasal sinuses. As the larvae mature, they acquire a cream color, then darken, finally showing a dark or black band on the dorsal surface of each segment. The larval period, which is usually shortest in young animals, is said to vary from 1 to 10 months in length.

When mature, the larvae leave the nasal passages, drop to the ground, burrow down a few inches and pupate. The pupal period lasts from 3 to 9 weeks, depending upon the environmental conditions. At the end of this time, the fly emerges from the pupal case and pushes its way to the surface. Mating soon occurs and the female begins to deposit larvae.

Clinical Findings: Once the larvae begin to move about in the nasal passages, a profuse discharge occurs, at first clear and mucoid, but later mucopurulent and frequently tinged with fine streaks of blood emanating from minute hemorrhages produced by the hooks and spines of the larvae.

Continuing activity of the larvae, particularly if they are numerous, causes a thickening of the nasal mucous membranes which, together with the mucopurulent discharge, leads to impairment of respiration. Paroxysms of sneezing accompany the migrations of the larger larvae. Larvae present in the sinuses are sometimes unable to escape and die, and gradually become calcified or lead to a septic sinusitis. The purulent inflammation produced in the sinuses may occasionally spread to the brain with fatal results. Occasionally, a mass of larvae blocks the sheep's air supply producing convulsions and, in some instances, death. However, the principal effects of the nose bot are annoyance and debilitation of the sheep. Infestations may consist of 80 or more larvae, but most commonly only 4 to 15 are found.

To avoid the fly's attempts at larval deposition, a sheep may run from place to place, keeping its nose close to the ground, may sneeze and stamp its feet or shake its head. Commonly, especially during the warmer hours of the day when the flies are most active, small groups of sheep gather for mutual defense, all facing to the center of a circle, heads down and close together.

Control: Ruelene given orally as a drench at the rate of 45 mg/lb should afford good control. Do not use within 14 days of slaughter. Observe all warnings on the label of the product. Rafoxanide, given orally as a drench or bolus is effective, but not yet approved for this use in some countries.

CUTEREBRA INFESTATION (SM. AN.)

The presence of the maggot of the rodent bot fly, *Cuterebra* sp., in the subcutis.

Etiology: Adult *Cuterebra* are nonparasitic and seldom observed. Females usually deposit eggs in the burrows of wild mammals during the summer months. Tiny larvae (1 mm in length) hatch from the eggs and wait for contact with an animal in the burrow. Larvae penetrate the skin of the nose and mouth and make their way to various subcut. locations in different hosts. The exact route of migration is unknown. The maggot increases greatly in size, and may reach an inch in length and ⅜ inch in diameter. Black cuticular spines give fully developed maggots a dark color. Larval development takes approximately one month, after which the maggot exits from its subcut. location to pupate in the soil. They mature in about 300 days. Adult flies live approximately 2 weeks and are said to lay up to 2,000 eggs per female.

Clinical Findings: A subcut. abscess of variable size forms around the developing larva. Pus may exude from the breathing hole made through the skin by the parasite. An aberrant larva sometimes invades the brain and causes fatal CNS disturbances.

The usual hosts are burrow-dwelling mammals such as mice, chipmunks, rabbits and squirrels. Dogs and cats sometimes become infested, presumably from investigation of such burrows. Lesions are found most often under the skin of the neck and chest during late summer and early fall.

Treatment: The lesion should not be squeezed since rupture of the parasite may result in anaphylaxis. The breathing hole through the skin should be enlarged surgically to permit careful removal of the maggot. The lesion is then treated as any abscess with flushing and instillation of antibiotic preparations.

PHYSICAL INFLUENCES

ACCIDENTS (SM. AN.)

WOUNDS

Wounds may result in loss of continuity, loss of function, pain and hemorrhage. The lesions produced by trauma are susceptible to infection. The most frequent causes of wounds in small animals are automobile accidents, bites from other animals, broken glass, other sharp objects and unintentional ligatures. The location, nature and extent of the lesions vary from the smallest abrasion to gross lacerations that are badly soiled and accompanied by complicating injuries, such as fractures or ruptured internal organs.

Before proceeding with treatment of the obvious lesions one should consider the possibility of complicating injuries. Therefore, the following routine should be followed: (1) inspection of the body orifices for the presence of blood; (2) palpation of the abdomen for the presence of excess fluid; (3) palpation of the urinary bladder; (4) testing the animal for its ability to stand and to flex all joints without pain; (5) viewing the visible mucous membranes for pallor; and (6) observation of the nature of the animal's pulse and respiration.

Treatment: The following procedures are mandatory in the treatment of any accidental wound: (1) control hemorrhage, (2) relieve pain and control the patient, (3) treat shock, (4) control infection, (5) clean and close the wound and (6) provide after-care.

To control hemorrhage, compression bandages are recommended as a first-aid measure and tourniquets are to be avoided. Later, bleeding vessels are sutured, ligated or coagulated by electrocautery. Pain is controlled with the use of meperidine hydrochloride (℞ 366) together with a tranquilizer (℞ 363, 367, 368), if necessary to quiet the animal. Atropine (℞ 489) is also indicated, especially in those animals that are salivating badly.

Hypovolemic shock may be present as a result of blood or fluid loss to the exterior, into a body cavity or into the tissues. The degree of shock is assessed by an estimate of the blood or fluid lost, by examination of pulse rate and pressure, and by hemoglobin or hematocrit determinations. For handling of shock, see p. 67.

Infection is controlled mainly by adequate wound cleaning and debridement. Antibiotics such as penicillin (℞ 44) or a combination of penicillin and streptomycin (℞ 41) parenterally, and local application of a soluble antibiotic in solution (℞ 2) to the wound before it is closed are used in severely contused and contaminated wounds.

Successful wound management depends upon cleaning, debridement and suturing. To cleanse the wound, it is covered with a sterile dressing while the hair about the wound is clipped, then the skin is scrubbed with a sponge and germicidal soap. The wound dressing is removed, and the wound is cleaned with a mild soap and irrigated with large volumes of sterile saline. In small wounds in tractable animals, this manipulation is made possible by infiltration of the periphery of the wound with local anesthetic solution. In major wounds, general anesthesia is usually required. Debridement is necessary to remove all nonviable tissue and foreign material. Debridement is minimal in incised wounds and in the extremities to retain blood and nerve supply to the foot.

Incised wounds of less than 24 hours duration can usually be closed immediately. Dead space should be eliminated; drains are often necessary, and excess skin tension can be managed by the use of tension sutures. All contaminated wounds should be treated with topical antibiotic solution (℞ 2) before closure. Puncture wounds are always infected; the immediate systemic administration of penicillin (℞ 44) is imperative since overzealous local treatment of puncture wounds often does more harm than good. Washing such wounds with forceful irrigation with nitrofurazone solution is an effective means of both cleansing and introducing antibacterial agents.

The treatment of chronic, obviously infected wounds requires the removal of all foreign material and devitalized tissue by surgical, chemical or enzymatic means. In wounds where phagocytosis and enzymatic action have accomplished self-debridement and healthy granulation tissue is present, nothing but protection of the wound and the avoidance of exuberant granulation is necessary. This process may be assisted by the use of proteolytic enzymes (℞ 408). Most wounds heal by contraction and epithelization, however, in some, skin-grafting or reconstruction is required. The application of a well-padded, firm bandage aids in elimination of dead space, reduces movement in the wound and protects against self-mutilation.

ELECTRIC SHOCK

Electric shock in puppies and kittens is usually a result of their chewing on electric cords. Burn wounds of the mouth, tongue and lips are consistent lesions. The dyspnea and cyanosis of pulmonary edema are common causes of emergency presentation. Stupor, unconsciousness, coma and death also occur. (See LIGHTNING STROKE, p. 760). A striking feature of electric burns is the marked necrosis of large areas of tissue which occurs days or weeks after the burn is inflicted; this is because preferential passage of electricity along vascular channels commonly causes thrombosis.

Treatment of electrical burns is palliative; in time, necrotic tissue is replaced by granulation tissue. Severe manifestations of pulmonary edema may be immediately alleviated by phlebotomy and removal of 10% of the animal's blood volume. Since this procedure may be repeated, blood should be preserved in an appropriate anticoagulant to allow transfusion at later stages of recovery. As there are often signs of shock and inadequate peripheral perfusion, this procedure of phlebotomy is rarely indicated. Instead the animal should be given oxygen therapy (q.v., p. 1402), steroids, (℞ 142, 148, 151) diuretics (℞ 520, 522) and bronchial dilators (℞ 504). Antibiotics (℞ 41) and sedatives (℞ 363) are used as the animal's needs dictate.

DROWNING

Drowning is rare since most pet animals swim instinctively and with considerable efficiency from birth. Occasionally, one hears of an animal (e.g., certain bulldogs) that apparently cannot swim. Treatment consists of establishing an open airway, drainage of the trachea by suspending the patient head down, or by actual mechanical aspiration, and artificial respiration. Heart stimulants or general stimulants are of doubtful value and are usually employed only in cases of complete or impending cardiac arrest. Restoration of body heat also is needed, although excessive heat may be harmful. Of paramount importance, however, is restoration of an adequate oxygen intake by any means available.

BURNS

The destruction of the epithelium or deeper tissues by heat, friction, electricity, or corrosive chemicals.

Etiology: Thermal burns result from scalding with hot liquids, contact with hot objects or exposure to flame or radiant heat. Frictional burns most commonly are caused by rubbing rough ropes against the skin during restraint of large animals. Electrical burns most commonly are caused by lightning stroke in open pastures and less frequently by contact with live electric wires (*see* p. 754). Corrosive chemicals include acids, phenols and strong alkalies.

Clinical Findings: Burns of animals are not strictly comparable to those of man. First-degree burns with reddening of the skin may occur but formation of vesicles and blisters is uncommon. The usual lesion of a moderately severe burn in animals is diffuse edema of the skin and subcut. tissues, with or without formation of small vesicles and sloughs. Charring of tissue occurs in severe burns.

If the burn is severe, the skin may be wholly devitalized and the injury extend into the deeper structures. Sloughing of the skin may follow, leaving large denuded areas from which constant exudation or effusion of serum can lead to considerable loss of protein and fluid. Healing is hastened by feeding a diet high in protein.

Burns of small areas of the body may cause only minor discomfort. Animals with more severe burns are reluctant to move, resent handling and may be indifferent to normal stimuli. Extensive burns with loss of considerable plasma may result in shock. A pressure bandage may prevent swelling, but will not reduce existing swelling. Removal of a pressure bandage after exudate has dried may cause additional tissue damage. Burns characterized by complete destruction of the skin are highly susceptible to contamination and infection. Such burn wounds heal slowly with extensive fibrosis. The prognosis depends on the total area of the burn, the depth of penetration, the location, and the age and condition of the patient.

Treatment: Chemical burns require neutralization of the irritant. Weak acetic acid solution may be applied to alkali burns, alcohol to phenol burns, solutions of sodium bicarbonate to acid burns, and for burns caused by unknown chemicals, saturated solutions of sodium bicarbonate or sodium thiosulfate may be applied. Following the neutralizing bath, the wound should be washed with mild soap (℞ 434) and rinsed with large quantities of isotonic salt solution (ISS). A wet pack should then be applied to the part and kept moist with ISS or sodium thiosulfate solution.

Animals with severe burns over more than 50% of the body should be euthanized. Burns of less than 15% of the body surface can usually be treated on an ambulatory basis. Although pain may be severe initially, it usually will disappear rather quickly. Systemic antibiotic treatment usually is not necessary nor is there need for special modification of fluid or food intake. The use of various dyes, local anesthetics, tannic acid, salves and oils are contraindicated. A hydrophilic ointment containing antibiotics, nitrofurazone or proteolytic enzymes (℞ 398, 408, 418, 419, 437) should be applied and covered with a sterile bandage. Inspection of the wound for the presence of infection should be made every 2 or 3 days and the dressing changed if necessary.

Burns of more than 15% of the body surface require systemic treatment. Examination of the patient should include evaluation of the pulse, respiratory rate, temperature and packed red cell volume and sedimentation rate. The pharynx and larynx should be inspected for edema. Fluid therapy should be started immediately. Oral administration of fluids has proven to be very effective. Saline solution, one teaspoonful of sodium chloride and one-half teaspoonful of sodium bicarbonate per liter of water, may be given orally, at the rate of 10% of body weight the first day and 5% the second day. Such treatment is contraindicated by vomiting or diarrhea. Blood, dextran or plasma (0.5 ml/kg of body wt) and electrolyte solution (1.5 ml) (℞ 565) may be given for each 1% of body surface burned.

Corticosteroids (℞ 145, 152, 158) may be useful during the severe stress. The amount should be gradually reduced as the animal improves. ACTH (℞ 137) may be given if the function of the adrenal cortex seems unduly depressed. Antibiotics (℞ 11, 46) or sulfa drugs (℞ 69, 72) are indicated by the presence of systemic infections. Local therapy may utilize the open method, the closed method, or excision of the burned area. The open method seeks to produce a dry crust over the burned area, by subjecting the wound to a flow of air warm enough to prevent chilling the patient. A crust will begin to form after 1 to 2 days and will remain for about 2 weeks. The crust will slough as the epithelium regenerates. In deep burns the scab will have to be removed by surgery and skin-grafting performed.

In the closed method, a hydrophilic ointment containing antibiotics such as neomycin, polymyxin, bacitracin combinations, nitrofurazone, or proteolytic enzymes (R 398, 408, 418, 419, 437) with or without urea is placed upon the wound and covered with a thick layer of absorbent material. The final covering is either lightly impregnated petrolatum gauze or a nylon fabric commercially prepared for this purpose. The bandage is left in place for 7 to 10 days. This form of therapy is not generally satisfactory in veterinary practice because of the difficulty of keeping the bandage in place and the probability of infection. The animal may be controlled by reasonable use of tranquilizers or other forms of chemical or physical restraint indicated during convalescence. Emphasis should be placed on maintenance of good nutrition.

Small full-thickness burns should be immediately excised and treated as any other surgical wound.

The use of oils, petroleum jelly, or ointments should be avoided in chemical burns. Friction burns are treated with simple protectives such as petroleum jelly (R 422) or antibiotic ointment (R 398) and may be further protected with sterile dressings. Electrical burns may sometimes require local treatment as described for thermal burns.

Suitable restraint to prevent biting, scratching or rubbing of burn wounds must be employed. This may require the use of Elizabethan collars in small animals, proper tying of large animals in stalls, or the ingenious use of dressings. If immobilization of the part can be accomplished, healing will be greatly facilitated. A plaster cast may be employed to effect complete immobilization of the part.

SUNBURN

A superficial inflammation of the skin caused by actinic rays from the sun or ultraviolet lamps.

Etiology: Actinic rays may cause inflammation of skin insufficiently protected by pigments or hair. Although true sunburn is uncommon among animals, it may occur following exposure to bright sunlight after long confinement under cover and in sheep and dogs after shearing. It is a frequent condition in Hereford cattle in the spring when reflection of sunlight from the snow burns the udder and can cause great losses in calving groups if untreated.

Clinical Findings: The effects of overexposure to actinic rays usually are most severe after 12 to 24 hours, varying from mild erythema and discomfort to vesiculation and peeling of the skin. There may be anorexia and increased thirst. Affected animals seek cool or sheltered places. Pigs wallow in available puddles or mudholes. Conjunctivitis and blepharitis are common sequelae. In dairy cattle, the teats are often involved. Peeling and itching of the skin occur during healing. The course is short and the prognosis is favorable, but severely sunburned pigs sometimes develop fever and weakness and may collapse.

Prophylaxis and Treatment: Preventive measures need be taken only with white pigs and recently shorn sheep and dogs. These animals should be introduced to bright sunlight only in short exposures of increasing duration over a few days. In Hereford cattle prevention is accomplished by painting the udder with gentian violet dye just prior to calving. This will help as a form of treatment as well. Treatment consists of removing affected animals to shade and dusting the affected skin areas with soothing powders such as equal parts of zinc oxide and talcum powder or boric acid. Where vesiculation and itching are pronounced, a soothing preparation, such as soft zinc oxide paste ($\mathbb{R}$ 438), may be applied.

SUNSTROKE
(Heat exhaustion, Heat cramps, Heatstroke)

The above terms refer to 3 different manifestations of disturbance of the heat-regulating mechanisms of the body. In general, they all result from high environmental temperature, high humidity and inadequate ventilation. Exposure to direct rays of the sun may be a contributory factor.

Etiology: All domestic animals are susceptible. Dogs confined to close quarters in hot weather, cattle, horses or other stock being driven in large numbers or being transported in hot weather are most commonly affected. Predisposing factors include physical effort, obesity and stagnation of air.

Heat exhaustion: This form of heatstroke occurs in draft horses, cattle and swine. It is unusual in dogs. Prolonged exposure to high environmental temperature causes the peripheral blood vessels to dilate. When dilatation occurs without a compensatory increase in blood volume, circulatory collapse may ensue.

Heat cramps: This form of heat stroke is most common in animals doing hard work in intense heat. Animals with the ability to sweat are most commonly affected, e.g., draft horses. Heat cramps are rare in dogs other than those working or racing in a hot environment, e.g., hounds. Deranged electrolyte balance (acute salt loss) is the factor responsible.

Heatstroke: This serious reaction is most common in dogs, but it also occurs in other animals. The cause is obscure, but it is associated with exposure to high temperature, high humidity and inadequate ventilation.

Clinical Findings: Heat exhaustion: The outstanding signs are weakness, muscular tremors and collapse. There may be hyperpnea and rapid pulse. The body temperature is not necessarily elevated. The onset of heat exhaustion is not as sudden as that of heatstroke.

Heat cramps: The outstanding sign is severe muscle spasm. Working animals are most frequently affected. Sweating stops in horses and working animals other than dogs.

Heatstroke: The outstanding signs are hyperpnea and collapse. There may be a staring expression of the eyes. Vomiting is not uncommon. The rectal temperature is greatly elevated—up to 110°F. The onset of heatstroke is very sudden and it is likely to result in death.

Treatment: Heat exhaustion: Cool water should be applied to the body. The animal should be moved to a cool and shaded place. Cool water with salt (0.5 gm NaCl per pint of water) may be given by mouth. Isotonic saline may be given IV but it must be administered with caution, as the circulation is already impaired and too much fluid given IV could result in pulmonary edema.

Heat cramps: Cool water with salt may be given by stomach tube, unless vomiting is present. It may be more convenient to administer isotonic saline IV.

Heatstroke: Rapid and heroic measures are necessary if death is to be avoided. Dogs respond best to immersion in ice cold water. Cold water should be applied to the body of any animal suffering from heatstroke. Ice packs applied to the cranium and cold water enemas also are useful. High body temperatures should not be lowered too suddenly. The rectal temperature should, therefore, be checked every 5 minutes.

LIGHTNING STROKE AND ELECTROCUTION

Injury or death due to high-voltage electrical currents may be the result of lightning, fallen transmission wires or faulty electrical circuits (*see also* ELECTRIC SHOCK, p. 754). Occasionally puppies and kittens chew through the insulation of an electric cord and receive a severe burn or die from electric shock. Lightning stroke is seasonal, and tends to be geographically restricted.

Certain types of trees, especially those which are tall, spreading, and have well-developed root systems just beneath the ground surface, tend to be struck by lightning more often than others. Electrification of the root system charges a wide surface area, particularly when the ground is already damp; passage of roots beneath a shallow pool of water causes that pool to become electrified. A tile drain may spread an electric charge over an entire field. Fallen transmission wires may also electrify a pool of water. Differences exist in conductivity in soil, varying with geologic composition; loam, sand, clay, marble, and chalk (in that order) are good conductors, while rocky soil is not.

Accidental electrocution of farm animals usually occurs as a result of faulty wiring. Electrification of a water or milk line, metal creep or guard rail can result in widespread distribution of an electric current throughout the stable.

Death from electric shock usually results from cardiac or respiratory arrest; passage of current through the heart usually produces ventricular fibrillation; involvement of the CNS may affect the respiratory or other vital centers.

Clinical Findings: Varying degrees of electrical shock may occur; in most instances of lightning stroke, death is instantaneous, the animal falling down without a struggle. Occasionally the animal becomes unconscious but may recover completely in a few minutes to several hours. Some of these latter animals have residual nervous signs, for example, depression, paraplegia, cutaneous hyperesthesia; these signs may persist for days or weeks. Singe marks on the carcass, damage to the immediate environment or both occurs in about 90% of cases of lightning stroke. Singe marks tend to be linear, and are more commonly found on the medial sides of the legs, although in rare instances much of the body may be affected. Beneath the singe marks, capillary congestion is common; the aboreal pattern characteristic of lightning stroke can be visualized best from the dermal side of the skin by subcut. extravasations of blood. Singe marks are difficult to find on the recovered animal.

Animals periodically receiving electric shocks while tied in stanchions are restless and nervous; they may kick at the stanchion or dividing rails; those which have received intermittent shock eat and drink with care. Smaller animals such as pigs that contact electrified water bowls or creeps may be killed instantly or, from the strength of the shock, be thrown across the pen.

Diagnosis: History of a recent storm may be confusing; finding a dead or injured animal under a tree or near a fence is significant only if one finds evidence of recent burning of bark, splitting of fence posts, welding of wire, etc. *Rigor mortis* develops and passes quickly; postmortem distension of the rumen occurs rapidly and differentiation from antemortem ruminal tympany (q.v., p. 141) must be made. In both conditions, the blood tends to clot slowly or not at all. The mucosae of the upper respiratory tract, including the turbinates and sinuses are congested and hemorrhagic; linear tracheal hemorrhages are common but the lungs are not compressed as in bloat. All other viscera are congested and petechiae and ecchymoses may be found in many organs. Due to postmortem ruminal distension, the poorly clotted blood is passively moved to the periphery of the body, resulting in postmortem extravasation of blood in muscles and superficial lymph nodes of the head, neck and thoracic limbs, and, to a lesser extent, in the hindquarters. Probably the best indication of instantaneous death is the presence of hay or other feed in the animal's mouth; the presence of normal ingesta (especially in the rumen, and lack of frothy ingesta—frothy bloat), absence of a distended gallbladder, and presence of normal feces in the lower tract, and occasionally on the ground beside the animal are supportive evidence.

Treatment: Those animals that survive may require supportive and symptomatic therapy.

FROSTBITE

Destruction of superficial tissues as a result of exposure to cold with secondary structural and functional disturbances of the smaller surface blood vessels. Frostbite is not uncommon in young animals, especially young, poorly nourished cattle and horses exposed to storms and extreme cold. Pigs farrowed in extreme cold may suffer from frosting of exposed parts, especially the ears and tail. Sometimes the combs of chickens are affected.

Clinical Findings: Slight frosting causes the skin to become pale and bloodless. This is soon followed by intense redness, heat, pain and swelling. In such cases, the hair may fall out and the epidermis may peel. Usually, the inflammation subsides, the swelling disappears and only an increased sensitivity to cold remains. There may be irritation and itching for some time.

If freezing is more severe, the affected part becomes swollen and very painful, remains cold and later begins to shrivel. In severe cases, patches of skin are devitalized and a line of demarcation forms between the affected and the normal parts. Finally the destroyed portion drops off, leaving a raw surface.

Treatment: Small, simple lesions caused by freezing may be treated with mild antiseptics and thoroughly covered with healing ointment. Simple frostbites are treated by rapidly warming the affected part by water bath or pack (105° to 108°F) for 15 to 20 minutes, and by applying antiseptic dressing such as 5% carbolized ointment or oil, 1% solution or ointment of silver nitrate or zinc chloride. Gentle daily massage of the area may help to reduce pain and stimulate circulation.

Severe freezing may be treated by conservative means until a line of demarcation appears. The necrotic portion of severely affected tissue should then be removed surgically and the defect treated as an open wound.

RADIATION INJURY

Radiation injury is the result of energy changes in the atomic matter of living tissues, caused by ionizing radiation. Ionizing radiation may be electromagnetic, such as gamma rays and X-rays, or particulate, such as alpha and beta particles. Electromagnetic radiation has no mass and travels at the speed of light. Particulate radiation, because of its mass, has a greater probability of ionization in tissue. Thus alpha particles are absorbed by a few layers of cells, beta particles are absorbed by a few millimeters of soft tissue and X-rays and gamma rays may pass entirely through the body of an animal without interacting. The greater the number of interactions along a given path, the greater the absorbed energy and the greater the radiation injury.

Because electromagnetic radiation, such as X-rays and gamma rays, has the property of penetrating tissue, it can cause damage to organs deep within the body. Alpha and beta particles originate from radionuclides, called internal emitters, which gain entrance to the deep organs of the body through food, water or air, to cause internal damage. Beta radiation may cause superficial skin and eye damage. The extent of injury depends upon the absorbed dose.

Ionization which affects energy bonds within a molecule causes a change in its chemical properties. Injury is subsequent to the alteration of molecules important to normal cell functions. The direct effect of irradiation refers to the condition in which energy is absorbed by or ionization occurs in a critically important molecule. When the injury is due to secondary reaction of free radicals formed in irradiated tissue molecules or water, it is regarded as an indirect effect.

The severity of damage to a living organism depends on the amount of energy absorbed, total of the area of the body exposed, the specific organs within the exposure field and the frequency of exposure. Total body irradiation would be expected to cause more damage than partial body irradiation.

Clinical Findings: The lethal range for total body radiation of animals with gamma or X-rays lies above 200 r. It is difficult to detect clinically any effect of irradiation of animals with doses of less than 25 to 50 r. Very few mammals will survive a whole body dose of 1,000 r. If a low daily dose (less than 50 r) is given over an extended period, high cumulative doses may be tolerated.

While all cellular structures are equally affected by the initial ionization, there are differences in histopathologic sensitivity to radiation. The most rapidly proliferating cells are the most sensitive to radiation. In proliferating cell systems there will be inadequate replacement of the more differentiated forms because of damage to the sensitive precursor cells. Maximum cellular destruction following irradiation occurs earliest in the hemopoietic tissues, and soon thereafter in the intestinal epithelial lining and the germinal layer of the skin. Nerve and muscle cells do not divide in adult mammals and extremely high levels of radiation are required in order to cause histopathologic evidence of damage to these tissues.

The hemopoietic tissues are very sensitive to radiation and generally their sensitivity determines the maximum lethal dose for mammals. Although maximum damage to the hematocytoblasts may be observed in a few hours, maximum depression of circulating blood cells will not be observed for a few days. The differentiating forms of developing blood cells are less sensitive than the hematocytoblasts; and the circulating blood cells, with the exception of the lymphocyte, are relatively radio-resistant. In most mammals the life span of circulating leukocytes is somewhat less than a week, of platelets somewhat greater than a week; and the life span of circulating erythrocytes may be 3 or 4 months. The lymphocyte has apparently a very short life span and is also very sensitive to the direct action of radiation. A lymphopenia may be seen less than a day following whole-body irradiation. Great decreases in the other blood cells follow in order of their circulating life expectancies. Death due to damage to hemopoietic tissues will occur around 2 weeks following irradiation because of the leukopenia with resulting antibody loss. Petechial hemorrhage may occur at about the same time because of the decrease in numbers of platelets. Septicemia develops because of the lack of defenses against bacteria normally present within the body.

Damage to the small intestines can lead to death if the doses are high enough. Although the proliferative rates of cells in the intestinal crypts are slightly less than for the precursor cells in the hemopoietic tissues, severe clinical effects are observed earlier. This is because of the rapid migration of the intestinal epithelial cells to the tips of the villi where they slough into the lumen. Deaths from intestinal damage will occur less than a week following irradiation due to loss of fluids and electrolytes and failure to reabsorb them, particularly in the first part of the small intestine. Sensitivity to radiation decreases distally, with the colon and rectum being only moderately sensitive.

Partial body irradiation may be extensive without serious injury to the whole animal. Localized exposures of 1,000 r or greater, even if distributed over a long period may, however, initiate skin or blood neoplasms.

Acute whole-body irradiation of upwards to 10,000 r may cause damage to the relatively resistant nervous tissue, causing severe CNS disturbances and early death.

The acute dose to the gonads required to cause permanent sterilization of animals is greater than the lethal dose if the whole body is exposed. There will be temporary impairment of fertility with doses less than lethal. It is possible, however, to produce permanent sterilization with doses less than that required to produce severe clinical effects.

Exposure of a fetus to 5 to 25 r during organogenesis may cause developmental defects or initiate leukemia. Genetic effects, even with higher levels of irradiation, are not a serious problem in animals because of the practice of selective breeding.

Treatment and Control: Treatment for whole-body irradiation is symptomatic and aimed toward maintaining homeostasis until the body can repair itself. Blood transfusions and bone marrow implants may be used until the hemopoietic tissues repair. Antibiotics are necessary to combat infections resulting from the leukopenia. Parenteral fluids and electrolytes must be given to balance those lost in the damaged intestine. The beneficial effects of therapy are extremely limited following exposures much greater than the median lethal dose.

Contamination of domestic animals is of concern because of the resulting food products which may enter the human biologic cycle. The radionuclides will be metabolized in the same manner as their stable isotopes. Their removal from the animal's body is dependent both on biologic removal and on the half-life of the particular radionuclide.

In veterinary practice the greatest radiation hazard is the diagnostic X-ray machine. This is a potential hazard for the veterinarian and his co-workers. Practical radiation control should include use of lead gloves and aprons, cones or diaphragms on the X-ray machine and intensifying screens in the cassettes. Personnel should never be in the direct X-ray beam. Because ionizing radiation can be detected only by its eventual biologic effects or by special detecting devices, those working with any type of ionizing radiation should wear dosimeters (film badges or ionization chambers).

MOTION SICKNESS

A systemic condition characterized by excessive salivation, nausea and vomiting brought about by continued motion, as in travel by car, sea or air. Man and many of the domestic animals are susceptible. The principal mechanism involved in motion sickness is concerned with the vestibular apparatus of the ear. Fear of the vehicle is a contributory factor in the case of dogs and cats.

Clinical Findings: The outstanding signs are salivation, nausea and vomiting. The animals may yawn and show definite signs of uneasiness. These signs disappear promptly as soon as vehicular motion ceases.

Control: Motion sickness can be overcome by having the animal become accustomed to travel. With the advent of the ataractic and antinauseant drugs, therapy for the alleviation or prevention of motion sickness is much more effective and specific. A number of these have been used with good results in dogs. Perhaps phenobarbital sodium (℞ 531) alone or with methylatropine nitrate (℞ 464) is the commonest; the latter combination shows effectiveness in controlling salivation. Promethazine HCl (℞ 465) actively inhibits both vomiting and drooling. Perphenazine (℞ 368), promazine HCl (℞ 369) and mepazine (℞ 365) are all useful in control of nausea. Chlorpromazine (℞ 363) and a number of other preparations (℞ 461, 462, 463) with both psychic and antiemetic effects are also used successfully in small animals to control the signs of motion sickness. With the exception of the phenobarbital sodium, all the above drugs are more effective if oral medication is started early, 2 doses usually being given, the first 12 hours and the second, 1 hour before the time of departure.

In cases of habitual motion sickness in small animals, the IV or IM injection of propiopromazine (℞ 370) given 1 hour before the trip will be effective for a minimum of 12 hours.

REPRODUCTIVE AND URINARY SYSTEMS

REPRODUCTIVE PHENOMENA

The data presented in the following tables summarize the temporal and physiological features of the reproductive cycle in the more important domestic and laboratory animals. For detailed information, the reader should refer to standard texts.

GESTATION PERIODS*

DOMESTIC ANIMALS	Days	WILD ANIMALS	Days	Months
Ass	365	Ape, Barbary	210	
Cat	63-65	Bear, black		7
Cattle, Aberdeen-Angus	281	Bison		9
Ayrshire	279	Camel	410	
Brown Swiss	290	Coyote	60-64	
Charolais	289	Deer, Virginia	197-220	
Guernsey	283	Elephant		20-22
Hereford	285	Elk, Wapiti		8½
Holstein-Friesian	279	Giraffe		14-15
Jersey	279	Hare	38	
Red Poll	285	Hippopotamus	225-250	
Shorthorn, beef	282	Kangaroo, red	32-34**	
Shorthorn, milking	282	Leopard	92-95	
Simmental	289	Lion	108	
Dog	58-63	Llama		11
Goat	151	Marmoset	140-150	
Horse, heavy	333-345	Moose	240-250	
light	330-337	Muskrat	28-30	
Pig	112-115	Otter		9-10
Sheep, mutton breeds	144-147	Panther	90-93	
wool breeds	148-151	Porcupine	112	
		Pronghorn	230-240	
LABORATORY AND FUR ANIMALS		Raccoon	63	
		Reindeer		7-8
		Rhinoceros, African	530-550	
Chinchilla	105-128	Seal		11
Ferret	42	Shrew	20	
Fisher	338-358	Skunk	62-65	
Fox	49-55	Squirrel, gray	44	
Marten, European	236-274	Tapir	390-400	
Pine Marten	220-265	Tiger	105-113	
Mink	40-75	Walrus		12
Monkey, macaque	150-180	Whale, sperm		16
Mouse	18-20	Woodchuck	31-32	
Nutria (coypu)	120-134	Wolf	60-63	

* *See also* SOME PHYSIOLOGIC DATA (Laboratory Animals), p. 1160.
** Delayed development as long as a "joey" is in the pouch.

INCUBATION PERIODS

DOMESTIC BIRDS	Days	CAGED AND GAME BIRDS	Days
Chicken	20-22	Budgerigar	17-31
Duck	26-28	Dove	12-19
Muscovy duck	33-35	Finch	11-14
Goose	30-33	Parrot	17-31
Guinea fowl	26-28	Pheasant	21-28
Turkey	26-28	Pigeon	16-18
		Quail	21-28
		Swan	21-35

FEATURES OF THE REPRODUCTIVE CYCLE

Species	Age at Puberty	Cycle Type	Cycle Length	Duration of Heat	Best Breeding Time	First Heat after Parturition	Remarks
Cattle*	4 to 8 months. Usually first bred about 15 months.	Polyestrous, all year.	21 days (18 to 24).	18 hours (10 to 24).	Insemination, from mid-heat until 6 hours after end.	Varies,* best to breed at 60 to 90 days.	Ovulation 10 to 12 hours after end of heat. Uterine bleeding about 24 hours after ovulation in most.
Horse	1 year.	Seasonally polyestrous. Early spring on.	Very variable, about 22 days.	6 days (2 to 11).	Last few days; should be bred at 3-day intervals.	4 to 14 days.	Ovulation 1 to 2 days before end of heat. Twins are usually aborted.
Sheep	7 to 8 months.	Seasonally polyestrous. Early fall to winter. Prolonged seasons in Dorsets and Merinos.	16½ days (14 to 19).	30 to 36 hours.	Little significance.	Next fall.	Ovulation near end of heat.
Swine	5 to 8 months.	Polyestrous, all year.	20 to 22 days.	2 to 3 days.	Little significance.	About 7 days after weaning.	Ovulation usually about 36 hours after beginning of heat.
Goat	7 to 8 months.	Seasonally polyestrous from early fall to late winter.	20 to 22 days.	2 to 3 days.		Next fall.	Many intersexes born in hornless strains.

* Many normal cows ovulate as early as 8 to 12 days after parturition with or without detectable external signs of estrus.

Dog	6 to 8 months or later.	Monestrous. All year, but mostly late winter and summer.		About 1 week.	Several months.	Proestrous bleeding 7 to 10 days. Ovulation usually 1 to 3 days after first acceptance. Ova shed before 1st polar body has been extruded. Pseudopregnancy (pseudocyesis) usually ends between 60 and 70 days.
Cat	6 to 15 months.	Provoked ovulation. Seasonally polyestrous spring and early fall.	15 to 21 days.	9 to 10 days in absence of male. Four days if mated.	4 to 6 weeks.	Ovulation 24 to 56 hours after coitus. Pseudopregnancy lasts 36 days.
Fox	10 months.	Monestrous. December to March, but mostly late January to February.		2 to 4 days.	Next winter.	Ovulation usually on 1st or 2nd day of receptivity. Ova shed before 1st polar body has been extruded. No proestrous bleeding.
Mink	10 months.	Provoked ovulation. Seasonally polyestrous. Mid-February to early April.	Waves of follicles at intervals of a few days.		Next spring.	Ovulation begins 47 hours after coitus which must last ½ hour at least.
Chinchilla	4 months.	Polyestrous, all year.	24 days.	2 days. Mate at night.	12 hours.	
Nutria	5 to 8 months.	Polyestrous, all year.	24 to 29 days.	2 to 4 days.	48 hours.	

continued on next page

FEATURES OF THE REPRODUCTIVE CYCLE (*Continued*)

Species	Age at Puberty	Cycle Type	Cycle Length	Duration of Heat	Best Breeding Time	First Heat after Parturition	Remarks
Rabbit	5 to 9 months.	Provoked ovulation. Breed all year, more or less.		To 1 month.	When vulva is enlarged and hyperemic.	Immediately, but blastocysts die if doe suckles large litter.	In United States do not breed well in summer. Ovulation 10½ hours after coitus. Pseudopregnancy lasts 14 to 16 days.
Rhesus Monkey (*Macaca mulatta*)	3 years.	Polyestrous all year; tendency to anovulatory cycles in summer in United States.	27 to 28 days (23 to 33).	Most matings near ovulation time.	Near ovulation.		Menstruation lasts 4 to 6 days. Ovulation usually about 13 days after onset.
Rat	37 to 67 days.	Polyestrous, all year.	4 to 5 days.	About 14 hours (12 to 18). Usually begins about 7 p.m.	Near ovulation.	Within 24 hours.	Ovulation a little after midnight. Cervical stimulation causes pseudopregnancy lasting 12 to 14 days.
Mouse	35 days (28 to 49).	Polyestrous, all year.	4 or 5 days, usually.	A few hours from 10 p.m. on.		Within 24 hours.	Ovulation soon after midnight. Stimulation of cervix causes pseudopregnancy lasting 10 to 12 hours.
Guinea pig	55 to 70 days.	Polyestrous, all year.	16½ days.	6 to 11 hours. Begins usually in evening.	Mid-heat on.	Usually immediately.	Ovulation about 10 hours after onset of heat.
Hamster	7 to 8 weeks.	Polyestrous, all year. Few pregnancies in winter.	4 days.	At night.		After weaning.	Ovulation about 1 a.m. Pseudopregnancy lasts 7 to 13 days.

ARTIFICIAL INSEMINATION

The technique involves collection, examination, dilution, storage and insertion of semen into the female genital tract.

SEMEN QUALITY AND MALE FERTILITY

Veterinarians are frequently asked to certify the fertility of male breeding stock as well as freedom from diseases which may be transmitted during natural or artificial mating.

The only reliable measure of fertility in the male is a demonstration of his ability successfully to inseminate by natural service the required number of females, in the requisite period, at the appropriate time of the year and under the prevailing conditions of husbandry, or to make available an adequate supply of properly prepared semen which can be used for artificial insemination (AI). Since these requirements obviously vary considerably, both within and between species, fertility is a relative term.

The fertility of any individual animal is subject to change due to environmental influences, seasonal effects, mating frequency and disease. The more important of the environmental influences are sudden changes in feed supply and weather conditions, rapid loss of body weight, shipping from one place to another and intercurrent disease. Seasonal variation is especially important in seasonally breeding species, e.g., in stallions and rams; changes in the ratio of daylight to darkness are reflected in the quantity and quality of the semen. While in temperate zones there is little seasonal effect of temperature, in other regions, high temperatures deleteriously influence the fertility of bulls and rams. In general, high mating frequency depresses semen volume and quality and if extreme, results in lowered fertility. Sexual rest, however, leads to recovery usually within one week; however, it should be noted that it takes 6 weeks for sperm to develop from the basement membranes in the seminiferous tubules to functional maturity. After prolonged inactivity, semen quality and fertility are usually low for the first few services. Any objective assessment of fertility must consider these factors and relate them to the anticipated reproductive demands to be made upon the male.

In the absence of actual proof of fertility from breeding data, it becomes necessary to make an assessment of the probable fertility status by other means. This should be based on the combined information obtained from an examination of the animal itself, its desire and ability to mate, its reproductive organs and representative specimens of its semen. The following discussion deals with semen evaluation. (*See* INFERTILITY

IN LARGE ANIMALS, p. 796, for a brief account of the examination of the male reproductive organs.)

SEMEN EVALUATION

Between males of the common domesticated species, there are wide differences in the nature of the semen produced which are related to differences in the reproductive organs of the corresponding females. For all species, however, the fertilizing capacity of semen appears to be a function primarily of the morphology, number, motility and viability of the spermatozoa and, secondarily, of the volume and physical and biochemical properties of the seminal plasma. For any species, therefore, it is possible to set up average standards to which normal semen should conform under stated conditions of age of donor, frequency of service, time in relation to breeding season, and methods of collection and examination. Obvious deviations from these normal standards can then be recognized and correlated with fertility. However, as the range between what is normal and abnormal narrows, the difficulty of accurate assessment increases and, for any individual animal, the semen findings by themselves, unless blatantly obvious, must be interpreted with caution.

The various methods of collecting semen and average semen volume and density are described under artificial insemination for each species. Since more is known about semen evaluation in bulls than in other species, the following account is based specifically on the standards set for this species. Equivalent standards for other species have not been clearly established and interpretation of the findings must, therefore, be somewhat arbitrary.

Gross Examination: After a representative specimen has been collected, with due care to prevent contamination and temperature shock, the volume is measured, the color noted and preliminary observation is made for evidence of motility, density and absence of foreign material.

Average **volume** is lower with young males, may fall with increasing frequency of service, is higher with adequate prestimulation and usually lower when collection is made by electro-ejaculation than with an artificial vagina. However, it may be difficult, when collecting with the electro-ejaculator, to tell when a complete ejaculate has been obtained.

Normal semen has a creamy or milky opalescent **color.** A yellow color in bull semen is a hereditary character, due to a single autosomal recessive and having no effect upon fertility.

In normal bull semen, sperm **concentration** per cubic millimeter may be roughly estimated from its gross appearance, thus: creamy (1,000,000 to 2,000,000), milk-like (500,000), cloudy (100,000), slight turbidity (less than 50,000) and clear (aspermia). Finally, by gross examination, a rough estimate of motility may be made, in that vigorous activity in a dense specimen gives rise to a characteristic rapidly changing vortex or wave pattern. From these 4 criteria, the experienced observer can obtain a fair estimate of the quality of specimens collected routinely from known individual bulls. Further examination, however, is usually carried out and is essential with unknown animals.

Motility: This should be tested within a few minutes of collection and the tests carried out under controlled temperature conditions. Usually, 4 separate observations are made: (1) gross motility, (2) individual directional motility and the percentage of motile spermatozoa, (3) the duration of motility and (4) the percentage of live spermatozoa (ratio of dead to live cells).

Gross motility is assessed on the type of movement of the spermatozoa and the wave pattern in a drop of undiluted semen placed on a warm slide (85° to 90°F) and observed under the low power ($\times$ 100) of the microscope. It is an estimate of the combined effect of density and motility and, as such, is one of the most reliable tests in the evaluation procedure. Four categories are usually recognized: (1) stationary bunting or weak rotatory movement, (2) oscillatory or rotatory movement with no waves or eddies, (3) progressive movement of spermatozoa with slow-moving waves or eddies, (4) vigorous progression with rapidly forming waves and eddies.

Individual motility: For this observation, the semen is diluted with warm (90°F) isotonic saline to the extent that the activity of individual spermatozoa can be recognized under the high-power ($\times$ 500) magnification. An estimate is then made of the percentage motile spermatozoa (this should correlate closely with the "dead to live" ratio) and the percentage of spermatozoa showing active progressive movement. The specimen is then ranked according to the following classification: (1) motile 0 to 20%, progressing 0%; (2) motile 20 to 40%, progressing 0 to 10%; (3) motile 40 to 60%, progressing 25%; (4) motile 60 to 80%, progressing 75%; (5) motile 80 to 90%, progressing 90%. This is also a convenient time to observe the movement of abnormal forms, e.g., those with bent midpieces, returned tails or no heads, and the number and position of protoplasmic droplets.

Duration of motility: In this test, a portion of the specimen is diluted 1:15 with a suitable diluting fluid (egg yolk-citrate) and incubated at 100°F, the motility being checked at regular intervals until all activity has ceased.

The **percentage of live spermatozoa** (dead to live cell count) is usually determined by making a smear (as a blood smear is made) from one drop of nigrosine-eosin stain to which has been added and mixed on the slide about $\frac{1}{10}$ of a drop of undiluted semen. After drying quickly, a count is made of the dead spermatozoa, which stain pink, in relation to the unstained "live" cells outlined against the dark background of the nigrosine. The percentage live cells should approximate the percentage motile spermatozoa.

By this system of classification of motility in fresh bull semen, critical values indicating some reduction in fertility are usually taken to be less than Grade 3 in the 2 motility scales and less than 12 hours in the duration test. In this respect, it is important to note that in stored semen, particularly that of horses, rams and boars, fertilizing capacity may readily be overestimated from the degree of motility shown. On the other hand, it is possible to underestimate the fertilizing capacity of frozen bull semen from its motility.

Hydrogen Ion Concentration: In the field, the pH is usually measured with a suitable indicator paper or solution and a color scale. The normal pH of bull semen ranges from 6.3 to 6.9. Values above 7.0 are associated with lowered fertility. The test must be done soon after collection, otherwise fructolysis and respiration lead to the accumulation lactic acid and carbon dioxide and a consequent fall in pH; in fact, the rate of change has been used as a measure of density and motility.

Semen Density: The number of spermatozoa per unit volume may be accurately measured by a hemocytometer count, (as for erythrocytes), or more commonly by the faster and less laborious photelometer or absorptiometer techniques. The normal concentration of spermatozoa in bull semen ranges from about 1 to 1.5 million per cubic millimeter and anything less than 500,000/cu mm is usually regarded as substandard, at least for AI purposes. Specimens collected by electro-ejaculation tend to be less dense than those taken with an artificial vagina.

Morphology: Nigrosine-eosin-stained smears may be used for the examination of morphologic abnormalities. Casarett's staining technique also gives excellent results. In this, the smear is fixed in equal parts of alcohol and ether for 3 minutes and then immersed for 5 minutes in the stain consisting of 2 parts of 5% aniline blue, 1 part of 5% aqueous eosin B and 1 part of 1% phenol, warmed to 50°C. Examination is best conducted with oil-immersion microscopy.

Except for specimens showing large numbers of grossly abnormal spermatozoa, reliable evaluation of semen on the basis of the more obscure and subtle types of abnormality can be done only by those with considerable experience. More than 20% of primary abnormalities is indicative of reduced fertility. Final judgment in all cases, however, should not be made until at least 3 specimens have been studied and the reproductive organs carefully examined for evidence of disease.

Evidence of Infection: Semen characterized by excessive thickness may be an indication of genital infection. Pus cells in large numbers will cause a coagulated appearance of the specimen. If there is any reason to suspect inflammation of the genital organs, a smear of the semen should be stained with Wright's stain and a differential white-cell count made. Semen plasma agglutination tests may also be conducted if there is the possibility of genital brucellosis. Suitable culture procedures may be used.

ARTIFICIAL INSEMINATION IN CATTLE

In cattle, AI is utilized primarily as a means towards livestock improvement. Its worldwide adoption for this purpose in dairy cattle breeding has been made possible by the development of milk recording and the use of these data as an objective measure of performance on which to base the selection of superior bulls.

The development of objective measures of quality in beef cattle, such as growth rate, carcass conformation and composition, and feed efficiency, and thus the more accurate selection of sires led to an increase in the number of beef cattle artificially bred. Labor costs and management systems are factors limiting the use of AI in beef cattle.

Collection of Semen: In cattle, semen may be collected by the use of an artificial vagina, an electro-ejaculator or, less preferably, massage of the accessory sex glands.

The **artificial vagina** is used universally in artificial breeding centers. Bulls are induced to serve into this instrument while it is held by an operator alongside the flank of a "teaser" cow, a bull or a phantom teaser. With experience, bulls soon become accustomed to this procedure. Any that are, or with time become, slow breeders can be stimulated by allowing them to watch other bulls serve, or by having the cow or another bull mount the slow bull. Teasing of bulls in these ways also increases the number of spermatozoa per ejaculate.

In preparing the artificial vagina for use, nonspermicidal lubricant is used and the temperature, which is a critical factor in stimulating ejaculation, is maintained between 105° and 118°F according to the individual preference of each bull.

At each collection, up to 3 services may be permitted, yielding a total of about 10 to 20 ml of semen. For the maintenance of normal fertility, collections can be made, on average, only about once every 5 days.

Electrical stimulation of ejaculation is a valuable means of collecting from bulls which are unable to mount. It is now commonly carried out with a rectal "probe" with a series of banded electrodes attached to a variable current and voltage source.

The bull to be ejaculated should be restrained in a chute, because the stimulation results in vigorous contraction of various muscle groups, particularly those of the back. After emptying the rectum, the probe is placed so that it is entirely within the anus. A hand-operated rheostat permits intermittent impulses to be given as the voltage is gradually increased. The response varies considerably, but it is common to use 2- to 4-second impulses repeated at 5- to 7-second intervals. After a variable number of such stimulations, erection and protrusion of the penis occurs, followed by a flow of seminal fluid, the latter part of which is rich in spermatozoa. The semen may be collected by any convenient method; some operators use a modified artificial vagina and others an insulated bottle. In some bulls, ejaculation occurs only after a final series of momentary impulses, at 1- to 2-second intervals, is applied. Older bulls normally require a high voltage. A few bulls ejaculate within the prepuce. Semen collected by electrical stimulation is as fertile as that collected with an artificial vagina.

An alternative method is widely used in South America: The electrodes of the electro-ejaculator terminate in finger rings rather than in a solid rectal probe. A ring is placed on each of the first and third fingers of the gloved hand, the hand is inserted in the rectum, and the techniques of electro-ejaculation and massage are combined.

During collection by **massage** of the accessory sex glands per rectum, erection seldom occurs. The sheath should, therefore, be cleaned by douching with 500 ml of sterile saline containing 1 million units of penicillin and 1 gm of streptomycin. After completely emptying the rectum, the seminal vesicles are massaged with a backward motion until a few milliliters of fluid drop from the sheath. The ampullae are then massaged, an assistant collecting the semen with a glass funnel and vial. This method is not always successful and the quality of the semen is usually lower than that collected by the other 2 procedures. It should only be used as a last resort.

The volume of ejaculate varies from 4 to 8 ml and the concentration from 1 to 1.5 million per cu mm.

Dilution of Semen: After a specimen has been examined and met the required quality standards, it should be diluted or "extended" as soon as possible. Diluting fluids commonly used are the egg yolk-citrate diluter (℞ 629), the egg yolk-phosphate diluter (℞ 631) or a mixture of heat-treated homogenized milk and glycerol (℞ 630). All extenders must be prepared with utmost care. Before mixing, the diluting fluid and semen should be approximately the same temperature, between 80° and 90°F. The dilution ratio varies according to semen quality and may be as high as 1:200. It should be such that each milliliter of diluted semen—the usual inseminating dose—contains not less than 15 million live spermatozoa.

Glass or plastic ware should be used in handling semen, and all equipment must be scrupulously clean. Water used for rinsing glassware or in preparing diluents should be glass-distilled.

Storage of Semen: To store semen effectively for more than a few hours outside the body, the motility and metabolic activity of the spermatozoa must be reduced. This may be done by cooling, by freezing, by special extenders, for example, those containing caproic acid, or by sealing under a high CO_2 or N tension.

In routine artificial breeding the diluted semen is usually stored at 4°C, at which temperature it retains its fertilizing powers without appreciable loss for 3 days. Sometimes it is held for an additional 4 days but decreased conception rates must be expected.

By freezing to —79°C, the temperature of solid CO_2 (dry ice), or to —195.8°C, the temperature of liquid nitrogen, semen may be stored for several years with little loss of fertilizing capacity. (*See* FREEZING OF BULL SEMEN, p. 788.)

By applying a high tension of CO_2 or N in a sealed ampule, spermatozoa may be immobilized without cooling or freezing. Storage under these conditions is effective for up to a week, and the method has the great advantage of avoiding the need for any form of refrigeration during transport. Temperatures that are too high, however, may kill the spermatozoa. Such semen should be kept within the range of 4° to 32°C. Considerable care must be taken to avoid ampule leakage.

Insemination Procedure: The external genitalia are thoroughly cleaned. One hand is then inserted into the rectum and the cervix is grasped through the floor of the rectum. The other hand introduces a pipette, 5 to 6 mm in diameter and 40 cm long, containing 1 ml of diluted semen, through the vagina and deeply into the cervix where the semen is deposited. The hand within the rectum manipulates the cervix in such a way that the passing of the pipette is facilitated. Semen deposited into the anterior half of the cervix results in a conception rate equal to that of semen deposited in the body of the uterus. This form of insemination reduces the danger of causing abortion through accidental insemination of a pregnant cow.

Other things such as management and disease being equal, the conception rate following artificial breeding is equal to that of natural mating. Normally, the best time for insemination is between mid-heat and 6 hours after the end of estrus.

ARTIFICIAL INSEMINATION IN SHEEP

Collection of Semen: Of the 2 methods available for collection of ram semen, the artificial vagina is more commonly used. It is prepared for collection by the introduction of warm water (42° to 45°C) and air between the outer casing and inner sleeve, lubrication with petrolatum or paraffin of the end where intromission of the penis will occur, and attachment of a collecting glass at the opposite end. The rams should have been trained previously to mount a ewe, preferably in estrus, and restrained.

For collection by electro-ejaculator, the ram may be restrained on its side. The moistened bipolar electrode is inserted into the anus. The withdrawn penis may be held with a piece of gauze to facilitate insertion of the glans into a 1.5 to 2 cm graduated collecting tube. Ejaculation occurs after a few short electrical stimulations, and "stripping" of the urethra may be helpful when expulsion of semen is incomplete. In general, electro-ejaculation is less reliable than use of the artificial vagina and the specimens vary in quality and can be contaminated with urine.

The volume of ejaculate collected with the artificial vagina varies from 0.5 to 1.5 ml and the concentration from 2,500 to 6,000 million spermatozoa per milliliter. Semen obtained by the electrical method generally is of larger volume but of lower concentration.

Examination, Dilution and Storage of Semen: Immediately after collection the volume of semen and motility and concentration of spermatozoa are assessed. The ejaculate may be diluted up to 5-fold, depending on the initial concentration. The commonest diluents used are whole, skimmed and reconstituted cow's milk which has been heated for 8 to 10 minutes in a water bath, and egg yolk-glucose-citrate (15% egg yolk; 0.8% glucose, anhydrous; 2.8% sodium citrate, dihydrate; in glass-distilled water). The volume of inseminate can vary from 0.05 to 0.20 ml and should contain 50 to 100 million motile spermatozoa.

The semen may be stored for up to 24 hours by cooling the diluted semen to 2° to 5°C over a 1½- to 2-hour period and by holding at this temperature. Although a proportion of the chilled spermatozoa may remain motile for 1 to 2 weeks, their fertilizing capacity decreases rapidly after 24 hours and generally is quite low by 48 hours.

Freezing and storage of ram semen at the temperature of liquid nitrogen (−196°C) is a more difficult process than is freeze-storage of bull semen. Recently considerable progress has been made and use of thawed ram semen which had been pellet-frozen with raffinose-citrate-yolk-glycerol or lactose-citrate-yolk-glycerol diluents has resulted in a 50% lambing rate.

Insemination Technique: Estrus may be controlled in the ewe by suitable progestogen treatment. Estrus occurs 2 to 4 days after cessation of treatment. Insemination is recommended at the next estrus, 17 to 20 days after cessation. Ewes in estrus are identified by vasectomized rams carrying some suitable "marker" device on the brisket. Ewes should be inseminated while the vaginal mucus is copious, thin and clear to cloudy in appearance.

For insemination, the ewe is restrained to limit movement and to present the hindquarters at a convenient height for easy access to the vagina. After cleaning the vulvar region, the cervix is located with the aid of a speculum and suitable illumination, and the insemination made as deeply as possible into the cervical canal. For this purpose, a graduated 1- to 2-ml syringe, attached to a long, fine inseminating tube is preferred; alternately, a semiautomatic inseminating device can be used. The relatively long, tortuous and firm-walled cervical canal of the ewe usually precludes penetration by the tube for more than one centimeter. In old multiparous ewes, as a consequence of distortion of the tissues, difficulty may be experienced in locating the external os and, in some instances, the semen must be deposited about the posterior folds of the cervix. In maiden ewes in which insertion of the speculum and dilation of the vagina is difficult and can cause injury, the semen should be deposited into the anterior vagina. All these difficulties are minimized by experience.

ARTIFICIAL INSEMINATION IN HORSES

The horse industry has failed to take advantage of the scientific technology that has been applied to other species; to date, few major horse breeds have registry regulations that permit utilization of artificial insemination (AI). Reproductive efficiency is lower in the horse than in any other species of farm animal, and there is at least one stallion for every 7 mares.

A successful AI program requires considerable knowledge of reproductive anatomy and physiology of both mare and stallion, familiarity with semen handling techniques and the proper equipment. However, it offers substantial benefits. It maximizes the opportunity for early recognition, selection and extended use of genetically superior sires; permits disease control; and reduces the possibility of injury to mares or stallions. Stallions with poor breeding habits or injury may be used when natural service is not possible. Semen may be evaluated at each collection, thus permitting immediate observation of minor changes in the least time, thus shortening breeding and foaling seasons. It aids in identification of reproductive problems, prevents overuse of a stallion, particularly early in the breeding season, and permits more effective use of older, more valuable stallions. More mares can be bred to a young stallion providing earlier progeny evaluation, and mares can be bred more often at the most opportune time for maximum conception. Additionally, an AI program favors an accurate record keeping system.

Collection of Semen: Semen for AI should be collected with an artificial vagina designed to separate the gelatinous secretion (gel) from the remainder of the ejaculate. Since the semen must be maintained at body temperature from the moment of collection to insemination, everything that contacts it must be temperature-controlled. Immediately after collection, the gel and filter are discarded and gel-free semen volume measured (in ml). Spermatozoa can be counted electronically or by hemocytometer. If a sperm count cannot be done on each ejaculate, it should be done at least once a week. Motility should be estimated microscopically at body temperature after the semen has been diluted 1:20 in an extender that prevents clumping of the spermatozoa. It is recommended that no less than 4 ml, and no more than 30 ml, of semen containing between 500 million and 1 billion motile spermatozoa be used per insemination dose. Other measurements such as pH, morphology and bacteriologic examination are not routinely essential.

Until the efficacy of semen extenders has been proved, their use for AI of horses is not recommended. Mares should be prepared for insemination prior to semen collection and inseminated as soon after collection as possible, i.e., within an hour.

Insemination of the mare is accomplished with a 20-in. plastic catheter attached to a syringe by a rubber connector. The hand, in a sterile (or disinfected) and lubricated glove and sleeve, is inserted into the vagina and the magnitude of the cervical opening determined. If the cervix is open, the hand is withdrawn to the posterior portion of the vagina. The catheter tip is picked up, carried to the cervix, inserted through the cervix into the body of the uterus where the semen is deposited. The hand is withdrawn in a manner to prevent entry of air.

Insemination should begin on day 2 of standing heat and continue every other day until cessation of heat. If only one day must be selected, day 3 or 4 appears most appropriate. From a practical point of view, semen should be collected from the stallion every other day and all mares in standing heat for 2 days or more inseminated.

ARTIFICIAL INSEMINATION IN SWINE

The possibilities of prevention of spread of disease transmitted via breeding stock, and of greater use of genetically superior boars have made artificial insemination (AI) of swine attractive to producers. With careful, frequent inspection of the sow for heat, semen from fertile boars and application of presently developed techniques, AI of swine is quite feasible. Despite the labor required for accurate detection of heat (in the absence of approved ovulation control procedures), AI of swine will work using the following procedures.

Collection of Semen: Semen may be collected from a boar while he mounts a sow in heat or a dummy sow. Boars can be readily trained to mount a dummy sow, which is the preferred method of collecting semen. Grasping the corkscrew tip of the boar's penis firmly with a surgically gloved hand will provide the stimulus for ejaculation which takes 4 to 6 minutes. The semen can be collected nearly aseptically by directing the tip of the penis into an insulated, sterile, 500-ml collection bottle at 35°C. The liquid, sperm-containing portion of the ejaculate can be decanted or strained through a strainer cap to remove the gelatinous portion. The volume of an ejaculate is 150 to 500 ml containing 30 to 100 billion sperm. Collections should not be made oftener than every 3 days.

Dilution and Storage of Semen: Semen should be handled carefully to avoid bacterial contamination and sudden drops and repeated changes in temperature. Storage of extended semen can be accomplished at 7°C for up to 30 hours in egg yolk-glucose-antibiotic solutions or in heat-treated milk. Boar semen stored at 15°C in sealed glass ampules in a synthetic medium saturated with CO_2 will retain fertilizing ability for at least 4 days. Longer storage periods result in a lower conception rate and reduced litter size. At least 2 billion sperm in 50 to 100 ml of volume are essential for optimum fertility.
Insemination: Ovulation occurs normally about 40 hours after the onset of heat. The optimum time for insemination occurs 12 hours before ovulation and coincides with the time during heat when most gilts and sows will tolerate heavy pressure on the loin area. Inseminations performed at this time will result in a farrowing rate of about 75%, while inseminations at other times will result in 30 to 40% conception rate. Animals should not be restrained during insemination.

At insemination a disposable plastic pipette is inserted into the cervix by keeping the tip of the pipette against the dorsal surface of the vagina. The semen is slowly forced into the uterus from a plastic squeeze bottle or syringe. Careful determination of the optimum time for insemination and patience during insemination are critical for success.

ARTIFICIAL INSEMINATION IN DOGS

In most countries it is necessary to obtain Kennel Club permission to carry out AI if one expects to register the progeny. It is usually also necessary to obtain a license from the Department of Agriculture (or like body) before one may import canine semen from abroad.

Collection of Semen: Semen may be collected by digital manipulation or by means of an artificial vagina, the latter being preferred for both hygienic and esthetic reasons. The presence of a "teaser" bitch greatly facilitates collection.

The ejaculate of 2 to 15 ml is passed in 3 distinct fractions; the first from the urethral glands in the mucosa is a clear watery fluid devoid of spermatozoa, the second from the testicles is rich in spermatozoa, while the third and largest fraction is again devoid of spermatozoa and is prostatic secretion. From a complete ejaculate the sperm concentration should be about 125,000,000/ml.

If an "on the spot" insemination is to be carried out, the entire ejaculate may be immediately injected into the bitch, but if the semen is to be preserved for some time, only the second or sperm-bearing fraction must be used. This second fraction is isolated by changing the collecting tube on the artificial vagina between the passing of the fractions.

Dilution and Storage of Semen: Using the second or sperm-bearing fraction of the ejaculate only, canine semen may be diluted 1:8 with such extenders as heat-treated milk or egg yolk-citrate for preservation, and will keep under such conditions at 4°C for about 6 days. Normal untreated semen will only remain viable for about 18 hours.

Canine semen may also be deep-frozen. The technique is similar to that used on bovine semen (q.v., p. 788) except that the prefreezing glycerolization time must be reduced from 6 hours to 2 hours. Using such semen, conceptions have been obtained after many months of storage.

Insemination: It is important that the bitch be at the correct stage of her estrous cycle for AI. One may test the bitch with a male and observe her reactions or examine vaginal smears microscopically. Ovulation occurs about 48 hours after the commencement of true estrus, at which stage the vaginal smear contains cornified epithelial cells. This phase is usually 10 to 14 days after the proestrual bleeding begins, while blood cells will reappear in the vaginal fluid 24 to 36 hours after ovulation.

When inseminating, the plastic pipette is inserted until the tip is in the region of the cervix. It is almost impossible to inseminate directly through the cervical os. A speculum and suitable illumination may be used to facilitate passing the pipette. The pipette is connected to the glass syringe and the semen slowly injected. It is usual to elevate the bitch's hindquarters while inseminating to avoid semen loss. After the pipette has been removed, and while the bitch is still in the elevated position, a gloved finger is inserted into the bitch's vagina for about 5 minutes. This action simulates the "tie" of natural mating and appears to enhance conception.

ARTIFICIAL INSEMINATION IN CATS

Toms of suitable temperament are readily trained to ejaculate into an artificial vagina (AV) in the presence of a "teaser" queen. A 2 ml rubber bulb-pipet with the bulb end cut off makes a suitable AV. This is fitted over a 3 x 44 mm test-tube, the unit is inserted into a 60 ml polyethylene bottle filled with water at 52°C, and the open end of the rubber tube is stretched over the mouth of the bottle to seal it. The AV opening is lightly lubricated, and slipped onto the penis of the tom as he mounts the teaser. Triweekly collections appear to be desirable.

The average ejaculate volume is about 0.04 ml, and contains 5.7 x 10⁷ sperm. This is diluted with isotonic saline to 1.0 ml and of this, 0.1 ml is used per insemination. Queens in full heat, as determined by behavior and vaginal smear, are induced to ovulate by IM injection of 50 IU of human chorionic gonado-tropin. The diluted semen is deposited in the anterior vagina or posterior cervix with a 9 cm long, 20 gauge needle "bulbed" at the tip. Conception rates are substantially improved if a second insemination and a further 10 IU of gonadotropin are given after 24 hours.

ARTIFICIAL INSEMINATION IN POULTRY

This subject is discussed in the section on Poultry, p. 1081.

FREEZING OF BULL SEMEN

Semen diluted in milk (R 630) can be frozen by the follow-ing steps: The diluted semen is held at 5°C for 6 hours. One milliliter of the diluted semen is then placed in each precooled Pyrex glass ampule and flame-sealed in such a way as to avoid temperature rise of the semen in the bottom of the vial. The sealed vials are placed into isopropanol or ethanol at 5°C and the temperature lowered by adding periodically small amounts of crushed dry ice. With the aid of a thermometer and the circulating alcohol bath, the temperature should be reduced as follows: 1°C per minute from 5° to −15°C, 5°C per minute from −15° to −50°C and 20°C per minute from −50° to −79°C (or below if liquid nitrogen is used). Different opera-tors vary this temperature schedule and use rates as low as 0.25°C per minute from 5° to −15°C followed by 3°C per minute, until the final temperature is reached.

Frozen semen must be stored at a temperature not higher than −79°C (the temperature of dry ice—solid carbon dioxide). If the temperature rises above −70°C, the fertilizing capacity of the semen is reduced.

The egg yolk-citrate diluter is also used for freezing semen. Citrate buffer solution is prepared (R 629) and egg yolk is used to make up 25% of the final mixture. The solution is divided into 2 equal parts and to one part sufficient glycerol added so that the glycerol makes up 14% of the solution, by volume, of this one part. The semen is added to the unglycerolated portion and cooled to 5°C; the glycerolated portion is added in 3 equal parts, at 10-minute intervals. This mixture, which now contains 7% glycerol, is allowed to equilibrate for 6 hours, then frozen as indicated above. Semen may also be frozen using liquid nitrogen as the refrigerant. In this procedure, all steps are the same except that the semen ampules are cooled by passing varying amounts of cold nitrogen and air over the ampules. The final temperature is −195.8°C (the temperature of liquid nitrogen), and the semen ampules are stored by placing them in liquid nitrogen.

HORMONAL ESTRUS CONTROL

When injected into certain animal species, progesterone and progestins are able to cause suppression of estrus for varying periods. In some species feeding of a progestin will suppress estrus as long as the medicated feed is ingested. Estrus and subsequent ovulation generally occur within 3 to 5 days after withdrawal of the medicated feed. The following estrus is also synchronized. In swine, certain orally administered progestins may result in an increased incidence of multiple cystic ovarian follicles.

Experimental work indicates that estrus and ovulation may be effectively controlled by oral progestins used alone or with other hormones. Further studies may determine the economic advisability of using these procedures, particularly in conjunction with artificial insemination. Estrus synchronization and a high-conception rate have been obtained in **sheep** by the insertion of vaginal tampons impregnated with a progestin. The tampon is left *in situ* for 17 days. Estrus in **goats** may be similarly synchronized by treatment during the regular breeding season. Experiments during the anestrus period have been less successful. Research is in progress with cattle.

Estrus synchronization by a nonsteroidal pituitary gonadotropin inhibitor, methallibure, is quite satisfactory in **swine** and perhaps in **poultry** production. In **bitches**, progestins may be used to suppress estrus for indefinite periods although there is a possibility of inducing cystic endometrial hyperplasia. Progestins are not satisfactory for estrus control in the **mare**. Premature involution of the corpus luteum may be produced in **cattle**, thus changing cycle time, by injecting 50 to 150 units of oxytocin daily during the first week of the estrous cycle. Prostaglandins are also luteolytic in **cattle**.

CONGENITAL ANOMALIES OF THE GENITOURINARY TRACT

Congenital anomalies may be hereditary or result from the effect of some toxin or infectious agent on the embryo or fetus. Developmental accidents may also occur.

Anomalies of the urinary system are unusual. Defects of the **kidneys** include occurrence of cysts, horseshoe kidney, ring kidney, hypoplasia and aplasia. They are uncommon in domestic animals. In the dog and cat, they may result in signs indicative of diseases of the urinary system. Diagnosis is by urinalysis and X-ray. The penile **urethra** may open on the ventral surface of the penis (hypospadias) or on its dorsal surface (epispadias).

Cryptorchidism refers to the retention of one or both testicles in the abdominal cavity. It occurs most frequently in swine and horses, and is hereditary in these species. It is suspected to be hereditary in dogs and cats. Bilateral retention results in sterility due to thermal suppression of spermatogenesis. The normal temperature of the scrotum necessary for spermatogenesis is 1° to 8°F below the normal body temperature. Unilateral cryptorchids have normal spermatogenesis in the scrotal testicle, are fertile, and pass the trait on to their offspring. Abdominal testicles produce male hormones, and cryptorchids have normal secondary sex characteristics and mating behavior. Animals with cryptorchid testicles should be castrated. Gonadotropic hormones administered to prepuberal animals may sometimes cause descent of the testicles.

Monorchidism, anorchidism and hypoplasia occur. The hereditary gonadal hypoplasia of Swedish Highland cattle has now largely been eliminated by a control breeding program. A similar gonadal hypoplasia has not been observed in the U.S.A. Idiopathic hypoplasia occurs frequently. Other anomalies of the testis and the epididymis are rare. **Ovarian** agenesis or the presence of supernumerary ovaries is extremely rare and hypoplasia is infrequent.

Prolapse of the prepuce in bulls occurs as a breed characteristic or may result from edema following trauma. Prolapse predisposes to further injury and if untreated results in abscessation, scarring, adhesions and phimosis. Prolapse of the prepuce can be corrected by surgical removal of redundant tissue. Secondary infection following surgery may result in adhesions and stenosis.

Deviations of the penis in the bull may result from injury but in most cases the etiology is obscure; a heritable factor has been suggested. Deviations are lateral, downward or upward, and if severe prevent copulation. Surgical correction by removing 1 or 2 pieces of tunica albuginea on the convex side has been done. Such operations are difficult because of the chance of infection and the difficulty in removing exactly the right amount of tissue.

Corkscrew penis is observed in some bulls. This is a result of extreme erection in which the dorsal and lateral tunica albuginea of the penis stretches more than does the thicker and stronger tunic around the urethral groove. Most bulls eventually overcome this difficulty without treatment. They learn to insert the penis before the corkscrew occurs, or libido may decrease so that there is a less vigorous erection. Corkscrew penis is sometimes seen when using high voltages for electro-ejaculation.

Persistent frenum in young bulls can be cut with scissors. The penis of bulls may be congenitally **short. Diphallus** occurs rarely in the bull.

Hermaphroditism or intersexuality may occur in all species of domestic animals. The true hermaphrodite has both ovarian and testicular tissue. Such a condition is usually bilateral and may result in anomalies of the external genitalia. The most common hermaphrodite is in fact a **pseudohermaphrodite** in which there are present either ovaries or testes, and there is an anomaly of the external genitalia, which resemble, to some degree, those of the opposite sex. Pseudohermaphroditism is most frequently seen in goats and swine.

The most frequent congenital disorder of the **uterus is segmental aplasia** which occurs in inbred cattle. Although often referred to as **white heifer disease** this is a misnomer as it has no connection with coat color. The portion of the uterus without outside opening may fill with fluid causing a distended cyst-like structure. Aplasia may occur at various levels including the cervix so that the description of the condition is quite variable between animals. The vagina may be involved in some cases and this may fill with mucus. These animals are sterile and there is no treatment.

Cattle frequently have a **double cervix.** In most cases this is not a complete double cervix but rather a double external os with 2 cervical canals that join before reaching the internal os. This condition is inherited. It has no effect on fertility and in most cases is found only incidentally in a genital examination. **Cystic Gartner's ducts** on the floor of the vagina are of no clinical importance. Rarely, cows may have an **imperforate hymen** that causes accumulation of fluid in the vagina.

One of the most frequent congenital anomalies of cattle is the **freemartin**, a female born co-twin with a normal male. Over 90% of such females have such extreme hypoplasia of the genital tract that the uterus and ovaries may be observed only histologically. The anterior portion of the vagina is hypoplastic, while the vulva and the posterior portion of the vagina are usually normal. Diagnosis of freemartinism based on vaginal hypoplasia can be determined in most cases by a vaginal examination of the calf with either the finger or a suitably small speculum. The fusion of the placental circulation of the twins allows interchange of embryonic cells and possibly also hormones. The interchange of cells results in a dual genetic pattern in the twins and this can be detected by the combination of 2 different blood types in a single animal. This specific blood-typing test is available through the Purebred Cattle Associations.

PROLONGED GESTATION IN CATTLE

An endocrinologic defect of genetic origin, which renders the fetus incapable of initiating the events leading to parturition. The cow seldom undergoes any preparation for parturition (mammary development, relaxation of the pelvic ligament, softening of the cervix, etc.). Labor, which is invariably very weak, is initiated only on death of the fetus. There are 2 principal forms (Types 1 and 2) of the disease and each appears to be conditioned by a single autosomal recessive gene.

In the U.S.A., the oversized fetus or Type 1 is the most common in Holstein-Friesian cattle: The fetus is beyond term and may weigh 200 lb or more. The skeleton is heavy and the musculature is weak. There is minimal development of the adrenal cortex, and the adenohypophysis, smaller than normal, is characterized by poorly granulated acidophils. In fetuses delivered alive by cesarean section there is an adrenal insufficiency as indicated by a marked and persistent hypoglycemia. To keep such calves alive by therapy (e.g., ACTH) is impractical. In order to save the cow, a Type-1 fetus should be delivered only by cesarean section.

Type-2 calves may appear in a number of breeds, but in the U.S.A. it appears to be most prevalent in Guernseys. Type-2 fetuses are usually premature in appearance and tend to be small, averaging about 50 lb. They are grossly abnormal, often exhibiting hypotrichosis, and some are classifiable as monsters (pseudocyclops). All Type-2 fetuses fail to develop the adenohypophysis and the monsters usually lack the entire gland. Diagnosis of Type-2 fetuses usually can be made at or after normal term by palpating the middle uterine artery where the blood supply indicates a pregnancy of about 7 months and remains constant thereafter. Death of the fetus can take place during normal gestation or up to 200 or more days beyond term. While some cows can expel the dead fetus, most require assistance. To terminate pregnancy, cesarean section is recommended.

BOVINE DWARFISM
(Achondroplasia)

Achondroplasia of genetic origin occurs in most breeds of cattle. The forms range from the so-called Dexter "bulldog" lethal, which is invariably stillborn, to those animals which are so mildly afflicted that diagnosis by visual inspection alone is unreliable.

Of chief concern are the brachycephalic and dolichocephalic dwarfs. The **brachycephalics**, most commonly seen in Herefords, are characterized by short faces, bulging foreheads, prognathism, enlarged abdomens and short legs. They appear to be about half the size of their normal contemporaries. The **dolichocephalics**, most commonly seen in Aberdeen-Angus, have the same general body conformation as the brachycephalics, but lack the bulging forehead, prognathism and short face. Short-faced calves are frequently referred to as "snorter" dwarfs because of their labored, audible breathing, but the dolichocephalic calves also breathe heavily. Both types are low in viability and extremely susceptible to bloat. Since their carcasses are undesirable, they are rarely saved except for experimental purposes.

Various mating experiments indicate that brachycephalic dwarfs, dolichocephalic dwarfs and various types of **"comprest"** animals are all part of the same "genetic complex" which may also include the Dexter lethal. Typically, comprests represent a line of small compact Herefords and are often difficult to distinguish from their nonachondroplastic contemporaries. Analogous comprest types also occur in other breeds. Few of these animals are now being used in breeding. Originally, it was believed that a single, autosomal recessive gene, with complete penetrance, would account for the brachycephalic dwarfs, and this still appears to be the case when matings are confined to comprests. However, when matings are confined to nonachondroplastic "carriers", the ratio of nondwarfs to dwarfs approximates 15:1, thereby implicating recessive genes at 2 loci. At present, however, there is no single genetic hypothesis which will account for all the various achondroplastic types. Considerable progress is being made in the effort to decrease the frequencies of the major dwarf-conditioning genes by eliminating from the breeding population any animal which has produced a dwarf calf.

Genes conditioning achondroplasia are by no means confined to the beef breeds. The Holstein-Friesian Association of America lists the genes for achondroplasia and dwarfism among the undesirable recessives which that organization is attempting to eliminate from the breed.

CYSTIC OVARIAN DISEASE

COWS AND SOWS

One or more forms of cystic ovarian degeneration (cystic Graafian follicle, luteal cyst, cystic corpus luteum, atrophic cysts) which occur commonly in cattle and swine and uncommonly in other animals, characterized by either nymphomania or anestrus.

Etiology: The condition is caused by an aberration of pituitary gonadotropic activity leading to an insufficiency of the luteinizing hormone (LH), which in turn results in a failure of ovulation and the formation of large cystic follicles, luteal cysts and cystic corpora lutea. Most affected animals exhibit signs of increased and persistent estrogenic stimulation, probably from estrogens produced in the cystic follicles.

Incidence is higher in dairy than in beef cattle and high milk production appears to be a predisposing factor. The disease occurs most commonly during the first 8 weeks after parturition during the peak of lactation and more often in parous cows than in heifers. Among heifers, the incidence is higher in those kept many months without breeding or conceiving. In some countries, there is definite evidence of heritable predisposition.

Clinical Findings: The sexual behavior of cattle with cystic ovaries shows considerable variability. Short and irregular intervals between heat periods, the heat periods themselves often being prolonged, progress to marked masculine behavior, the animal pawing, bellowing and making excessive attempts to mount other cows but refusing to be mounted itself. About 25% of cows with cystic ovaries fail to show any sign of estrus. In many cases, the vulva is edematous. There usually is an obvious relaxation of the sacroiliac and sacrosciatic ligaments. In advanced chronic cases, there is thickening of the neck and shoulders and the development of a masculine or "staggy" appearance and an elevated tail head (sterility hump). The condition in swine is characterized by an absence of estrous cycles. The ovaries contain multiple follicular cysts. Physical body changes similar to those seen in cattle are not observed in swine.

Lesions: Follicular (or luteal) cysts, 20 to 60 mm in diameter, are usually present in one or both ovaries. The lining membranes of some of the cysts show patches of a thin layer of yellowish or amber luteal tissue. The stratum granulosum varies from a fairly normal arrangement to almost complete absence of its cells. The theca interna is often edematous and shows cellular degenerative changes. The cyst fluid is thin, clear or yellowish in color.

The uterus is frequently large, flabby and atonic and the cervix relaxed and open. Changes in the endometrium may be marked and are quite variable. Hyperplasia and cystic dilatation of some of the glands are evident on close examination.

Diagnosis: The condition of the ovaries, the history, unusual sexual behavior and the condition of the pelvic ligaments (in some animals) form the chief basis for diagnosis. In cows, the presence of one or more cystic follicles is usually detectable by palpation of the ovaries. There is an absence of normal corpora lutea.

Prophylaxis and Treatment: Careful selection of bulls from families known not to be affected has reduced the occurrence of cystic ovaries in some countries. Avoidance of "forced" milk production, such as occurs from heavy feeding and milking more than 2 times daily, helps in prevention. A few cows may recover from cystic ovaries without treatment, but the calving interval may be unprofitably prolonged. Hormonal therapy has proven highly satisfactory. A single IV treatment of desiccated sheep pituitary gland or a single IM injection of chorionic gonadotropin seems equally effective (℞ 167). A single IV injection of pituitary gonadotropin (℞ 166) with a high content of luteinizing hormone is also effective.

Treatment induces the formation of functional luteal tissue with the re-establishment of an estrous cycle. Breeding may be delayed until the second normal estrus following treatment to reduce the chance of multiple conception; however, breeding at the first estrus often is successful. Repeated treatments may be necessary in some cows. Swine may be treated with the same gonadotropic products as are used for cattle; however, the results are generally not as good. Estrogens should not be used for the treatment of anestrous swine.

MARES

Etiology and Clinical Findings: Abnormal sexual behavior in mares may be 1 of 2 distinct entities: The first is a common, possibly physiologic, condition characterized by prolonged, frequent or nearly continuous estrus of 2 to 16 weeks' duration seen in barren or maiden mares early in the breeding season, even though ovulation may occur. These mares revert to a normal behavior pattern without treatment later in the breeding season. The second is the true pathologic nymphomaniac condition characterized by an extremely psychotic sexual-behavior pattern. Although these mares exhibit signs of constant exaggerated estrus by tail switching, squealing and urine squirting, they refuse to copulate and are also vicious and dangerously aggressive toward man and other horses. Normal cycles and ovulation usually do not occur in these mares and their ovaries are small.

Treatment: For the first condition, small or large doses of luteinizing hormone, progesterone and testosterone have been tried with questionable or erratic results. Many of these mares conceive if bred at the time of true estrus, or near ovulation, as determined by examination of the vagina or rectal examinations of the genital tract and ovaries. In the second condition, although a few mares respond temporarily to tranquilization, ovariectomy is the only treatment that has been shown to be of value and even this may fail when the condition has been of long duration and the mare's vicious habits are well established. Nymphomania associated with cystic ovaries, as observed in cattle, is extremely rare in horses.

INFERTILITY (LG. AN.)

IRREGULARITIES OF ESTRUS AND ANESTRUS IN COWS AND MARES

COWS

Anestrus or irregular estrous cycles in the cow may result from a number of factors, including poor management, diseases or injury, or disturbances in endocrine functions. One of the most important of the management factors is failure to observe estrus. The average duration of estrus is 18 hours; in many cows it is only a few hours. A systematic program for observing cows in heat is important for getting cows bred at the right time. A husbandryman must be familiar with all signs of estrus. Aids in heat detection, such as the use of teaser bulls, or a device attached to the tailhead of the cow which reveals when other cows have been riding, may be valuable adjuncts to the heat-detection program.

Accidental access of bulls to cows and failure to keep proper breeding records often result in pregnancy without service history.

Silent heat refers to normal follicular development and ovulation without the psychic signs of estrus. Frequency decreases as lactation progresses, so that by the fourth postpartum month the incidence of silent heat is low. Some animals presumed to have silent heats have very short cycles and the observation methods mentioned above will help detect these. Those with true silent heats may be detected only through rectal palpation of the ovaries.

The 21-day cyclic changes in the ovary, particularly in the period of 3 to 4 days prior to ovulation, at the time of ovulation, or 3 or 4 days after ovulation, generally can be recognized and the time of the cycle estimated. The corpus luteum regresses approximately 3 days before the mature follicle appears. It becomes smaller in size and changes from the diestrus, liver-like structure to a more fibrous structure. Estrus is determined by the presence of a palpable follicle, an absent or regressed corpus luteum, and firm uterine tone. The vaginal mucosa reveals edema, the cervix is relaxed and hyperemic and clear serous mucus of variable amounts is frequently observed at the vulva, which is puffy and swollen. The immediate postpartum period is characterized by blood in the mucous discharge, and an ovary with a corpus haemorrhagicum, which on palpation is recognized as a soft area in the ovary, usually between 5 and 7 mm in diameter. The new corpus luteum is detectable by the fourth or fifth day as a small and somewhat softer structure than the mature corpus luteum.

During almost half of the cycle the examiner can predict the next estrus with reasonable accuracy. With this information at hand the husbandryman can watch the cow closely for the next anticipated heat. In cows that are approaching ovulation, the appropriate time can be estimated and the cow bred, regardless of whether she shows psychic signs or not. Should the estimate be in error and the cow exhibits psychic signs a few days later, she can be rebred. These cows are normal; they lack only psychic signs of estrus, hence endocrine treatments are not indicated.

When a cow exhibits anestrus, or the interval between heats is irregular and prolonged, it invariably indicates death of the embryo 10 or more days following coitus. The uterine contents frequently terminate in pyometra or mummified fetus, which if left untreated may persist for a year or more. The common practice of removing corpora lutea has little to recommend it; retention of the corpus luteum in the presence of a normal, non-gravid uterus is rare or does not occur.

When circumstances dictate removal of the corpus luteum, it should be done only in those cows in which the structure can easily be delineated and can be enucleated without rupture. The occurrence of hemorrhage and adhesion is greatly increased when the corpus luteum is fragmented during the enucleation procedure. The cow should show psychic estrus 3 to 7 days following enucleation and may be bred. If clinical heat is absent, the cow may be bred on the third or fourth day following removal of the corpus luteum.

Approximately 25% of the cows with cystic ovarian follicles are anestrus. Cystic corpus luteum is not a cause of anestrus.

Under certain circumstances nonfunctioning ovaries will be encountered. They can be recognized as smooth, small bean-shaped structures on a single examination, or reveal no activity or change after several examinations over a period of 3 weeks. The most common cause is low total energy intake during late-winter or during peak production in high-producing cows. This condition tends to correct itself when pasture becomes available, when there is sufficient supplemental feeding, or when production drops to a level commensurate with the food intake. The stress of chronic or severe disease or injury may interrupt ovarian activity and result in anestrus. Congenital defects, such as freemartinism and ovarian hypoplasia, result in estrual failure. Certain ovarian tumors may cause anestrus. The treatment for the inactive ovary is correction of the basic cause. These ovaries usually do not respond to gonadotrophic or steroid hormone treatment. A treatment that may be tried is to inject a combination of pregnant mare serum and chorionic gonadotrophin. (℞ 169).

MARES

The mare is seasonally polyestrus with the normal breeding season extending from February through the summer months in the Northern Hemisphere. Foaling mares usually come in heat on approximately the ninth day post partum and regularly thereafter at 21-day intervals. Breeding is recommended on the 30th day. Barren mares may have irregular estrous cycles characterized by long estrus, frequent short estrus, or long diestrus. The most common abnormality is long estrus during the early spring. As the season progresses, these mares usually revert to normal by April or May. If the mare fails to show estrus or has irregular estrus as indicated by the teaser, the time of ovulation, which in many cases is at the normal 21-day interval, can be detected by rectal and vaginal examination. For many years only the vaginal examination was used and the mares were bred when there was extreme relaxation, hyperemia and edema of the cervix and an accumulation of clear serous mucus in vagina. Recently, rectal examination to determine the presence and maturation of a follicle has supplemented or replaced the vaginal examination. The follicle in the mare is at least 1 in. and sometimes 3 to 4 in. in diameter, prior to ovulation. It is firm up to 24 hours before ovulation, and during the last 24 hours the internal pressure decreases so that ovulation may be anticipated and the mare bred at this time.

Normal estrous cycles may be initiated earlier in the season by placing mares in stalls with controlled lighting. Beginning in December, with lighting time the same as daylight for that time, the amount of light is uniformly increased daily to 19 hours per day on April 1. For the average stall 200 to 300 watts of incandescent light are satisfactory. A substantial number of mares will conceive in February with this system.

The most successful treatment for anestrus and estrual irregularity in mares is proper observations and examination. The use of endocrine products, including pregnant mare serum, is not indicated.

INFERTILITY IN SWINE

Infertility in swine may manifest itself as complete reproductive failure with no production of viable offspring or as a partial failure with reduction in numbers of live piglets born or weaned.

SOWS

Studies have indicated that the average healthy sow ovulates 17 ova, farrows 10 pigs and weans 7.5 pigs. Losses due to non-infectious factors tend to occur during the time from fertilization to implantation or at time of farrowing. Principal causes are believed to be defective ova or spermatozoa, congenital anomalies or aplasia of the tubular genitalia, and inadequate progesterone production by the corpora lutea. Defects such as aplasia of the tract are seen primarily in gilts since they tend to be self-eliminating. Studies on the use of progesterone in these problems have shown no increase in embryonic survival.

Faulty management practices can contribute to infertility and small litter size. Use of immature boars or the overuse of older boars also may be contributing factors (see p. 801). The sow should be mated late on the first day of estrus or early on the second day or both. Since ovulation generally occurs late on the second day of estrus, this should result in optimum fertilization rates. Breeding of the sow twice during the estrous period apparently will increase fertilization but this practice requires the use of additional boars.

Recently, there is an apparent increase in problems of anestrus and poor conception rates, especially in confinement-type operations. At least part of the problem appears to be failure of estrus detection in confined or tethered sows. It may also be related to stress caused by close-confinement housing and a resultant increase in production of sex steroids by the adrenal cortex.

Animals that are overly fat may have farrowing difficulties. Limited feeding of the sow seems to give best results, with some increase in feed allowance during severe cold weather. An average daily intake of 4 lb/day of a corn-soybean diet with vitamin and mineral supplements added appears adequate in most cases. Adverse environmental factors, particularly high temperature and humidity seem to contribute to failure of estrus and early embryonic mortality. Once the pregnancy has been established, high temperatures seem to have little or no effect on gestation.

Sows may show anovular estrus 3 to 4 days after farrowing; normal uterine physiology is reestablished by 20 to 25 days post partum. Sows will usually exhibit estrus 6 to 8 days after weaning at 3 weeks post partum. Ovulation rates may be normal if nutrition has been adequate. Use of exogenous follicle-stimulating hormone preparations such as pregnant-mare serum (℞ 168) at doses of 1000 u at weaning may help insure good follicle development and ovulation rate.

Poor lactation is a significant cause of neonatal mortality in swine (see MMA, p. 823).

Estrogenic material in the diet resulting from mold infestations, usually of the *Fusarium* group and usually found in moldy corn, also cause swine infertility. Production of the toxin in the food is enhanced by cool temperatures following warm, humid conditions. Signs can include anestrus, enlarged vulva, irregular estrous cycles, occasional abortions and failure of lactation. In lactating sows, estrus may occur with almost immediate cessation of lactation.

Infectious diseases including brucellosis, leptospirosis, toxoplasmosis, pseudorabies, and those caused by miscellaneous bacteria and SMEDI viruses may result in frank abortions or early embryonic mortality and mummification of some of the fetuses. In such instances, the pregnancy will continue and the mummified fetuses will be expelled at term with the live pigs. The SMEDI viruses appear to be responsible for a syndrome characterized by stillbirths, mummified fetuses, embryonic deaths and infertility. Serologic or other diagnostic methods are of limited usefulness in the diagnosis of these agents. Serologic tests for brucellosis and leptospirosis, however, are useful for diagnostic purposes.

Diagnosis of causes of infertility in the sow is difficult. Enlargement of the vulva or clitoris may be helpful in diagnosis of hyperestrogenic syndromes. Purulent vaginal discharges must be interpreted with caution, especially in postpartum sows. The discharge may originate from the involuting uterus or from the vagina and cervix with no involvement of the uterus. Uterine involution is usually complete 20 to 25 days after farrowing and normal fertility can be anticipated after that time.

BOARS

Infertility in the male is frequently caused by absence or malformations of the duct system. Boars should not be used until approximately 8 months of age, and should not be expected to produce more than one ejaculate per day as an average, if maximum litter size is to be maintained. Boars that have not been used for more than 4 weeks should be ejaculated once or twice before being put in use in order to remove degenerate spermatozoa present in the tract. One boar for no more than 10 to 12 sows is suggested, especially if hand-mating is not practiced.

Aids to diagnosis of male infertility are careful palpation of the scrotal contents, and collection (with an artificial vagina or by electro-ejaculation) and examination of a semen sample. Testicular biopsy should also be considered.

In testicular hypoplasia the testes will be small and softer than normal but libido may be normal. Acute or chronic orchitis signals the appearance of abnormal sperm production or its complete cessation.

ABORTION (LG. AN.)

Most abortions in large animals result from fetal infection, which usually follows uterine infection by days or weeks. There is no treatment for the animal that is aborting as a consequence of infectious disease. The primary need in such cases is to identify the cause of the abortion so that preventive measures may be taken.

The important infections which may lead to abortion are discussed under their respective headings. For **cattle,** see brucellosis (p. 353), leptospirosis (p. 350), listeriosis (p. 380), IBR-IPV (p. 268), bovine virus diarrhea (p. 264), epizootic bovine abortion (p. 271), vibriosis (p. 404) and trichomoniasis (p. 439). Mycotic abortion is usually caused by either *Aspergillus* or *Mucor.* These agents apparently reach the uterus by a hematogenous route and cause abortion in late gestation. In many of these fetuses the skin is not affected; in others the mold causes ringworm-like lesions. The placenta is frequently severely affected with necrosis of the cotyledons and thickening of the intercotyledonary areas. Diagnosis is based on identification of the mold through culture of the fetal or placental tissues, histologic examination of these tissues, or direct examination of cotyledons after clearing with potassium hydroxide solution. These abortions are almost always sporadic, and the only means of control is reducing exposure of the cows to the molds.

There are presently many cases of bovine abortion for which no diagnosis can be made. Almost certainly other infectious agents will be identified as causes of outbreaks of abortion. In addition to the specific causes of abortion mentioned above, numerous other agents such as parainfluenza-3 virus, *Pasteurella multocida, Pseudomonas aeruginosa, Corynebacterium pyogenes, Streptococcus bovis* and *Staphylococcus aureus* have been isolated from sporadically aborted fetuses.

In **horses,** the most common cause of abortion is the equine herpesvirus 1 (q.v., p. 246). Equine arteritis (q.v., p. 248) is an infrequent cause.

Bacterial infection of the placenta and the fetus probably results from ascension of the agents from the infected vagina through the cervix. The most frequently found agent is *Streptococcus zooepidemicus.* At a much lower frequency, *Escherichia coli,* staphylococci, *Corynebacterium equi* and *Actinobacillus equuli* are found. The prevention of bacterial abortion in the mare is based on hygienic breeding procedures and treatment of genital disease prior to breeding. The same bacterial infections may cause disease of newborn foals, which can be successfully treated with antibiotics. *Salmonella abortivoequina* is currently not a cause of equine abortion in the U.S.A.

In **sheep,** in the U.S.A., the most common cause of abortion is vibriosis (q.v., p. 407). Other agents that have been associated with abortion in sheep, and which are discussed elsewhere in the MANUAL are: *Toxoplasma gondii* (p. 456), bluetongue virus (p. 285), *Brucella ovis* (p. 362), chlamydiae (p. 273), leptospires (p. 352), *L. monocytogenes* (p. 389) and *Salmonella* (p. 377).

Similarly, the important infectious diseases causing abortion in swine are discussed elsewhere: brucellosis (p. 358), leptospirosis (p. 352) and hog cholera (p. 295). Other viruses have also been incriminated.

MISCELLANEOUS CAUSES OF ABORTION

Trauma, fatigue, surgical shock, poisons, certain drugs and chemicals have been incriminated as causes of abortion but specific proof is usually lacking. Nitrate poisoning has frequently been mentioned as a cause of abortion; however, all controlled experiments and observations concerning the effects of nitrate on the fetus have failed to link this chemical with fetal disease or abortion. The above-listed factors may affect pregnancy through stress or direct effect on the fetus. In all probability most chemicals which affect the fetus do so by crossing the placenta and entering the fetus or the placenta or both. Such chemicals may cause fetal or embryonic death, and anomalies of varying severity. The resistance of the fetus to the effects of chemicals increases with the age of the fetus. Thus, a substance that is sufficiently irritating to a fetus to produce resorption, death or abortion early in gestation, may have little or no deleterious effect on the fetus at a later stage of development. Chemicals vary in their effect, depending upon the dosage, the duration of ingestion or exposure to the material, and the specific time of gestation. For example, *Veratrum californicum* produces adenohypophyseal aplasia in fetal lambs when ingested on the 13th day of gestation. Later than this it has no effect.

Most equine twin pregnancies end in abortion. Twisting of the umbilical cord causes abortion in the mare. Introduction of bacterial contaminants in the uterus by artificial insemination pipette, or by other means, may cause abortion or death of the fetus.

The vitamin A deficiency which occurs in range cattle sometimes causes abortion, retained placenta, or weak newborn calves. Many forms of malnutrition, dietary deficiency, or chronic disorders that result in severe cachexia may lead to abortion.

INDUCED ABORTION

Pregnancy may be interrupted with subsequent abortion or resorption of the fetus and its membranes by manually decapitating the fetus. This can be done on fetuses up to approximately 100 days of age. Decapitation is accomplished by grasping the fetal neck between the thumb and forefinger of the hand placed in the rectum. Older fetuses require considerable pressure, and the maximum age at which this procedure can be carried out will depend on the ability of the operator to exert enough pressure on the neck to decapitate the fetus.

Heifers consigned to feed lots can usually be caused to abort by administering a repository form of diethylstilbestrol. The drug should be given IM in doses of 100, 125 and 150 mg during the fifth, sixth and seventh months of pregnancy, respectively. Abortion occurs within 5 to 10 days in 90% of the treated animals.

Removal of the corpus luteum in cattle will cause abortion through the fifth month of pregnancy. It is a particularly useful means of terminating pregnancy when carried out 14 days after breeding. The danger of hemorrhage and adhesions increases as pregnancy advances and the corpus luteum becomes more firmly imbedded in the ovary. Occasionally, fatal hemorrhage results from this procedure.

Douching the uterus with dilute antiseptics, saline or antibiotic solutions will result in abortion in the mare at any stage of pregnancy. About 500 ml of infusion, depending on the stage of pregnancy, is sufficient. During the first few weeks of pregnancy in the cow, the same procedure, using dilute antiseptics, is also satisfactory. In the mare, abortion may be induced by dilating the cervix.

Induction of abortion should be avoided during late pregnancy as it often is complicated by injury to the perineum, vaginal prolapse and uterine infection.

VAGINITIS AND VULVITIS (LG. AN.)

Bruising or laceration of the vagina and vulva frequently result from parturition. Infrequently, traumatic vaginitis may result from malicious injury, service from a large and vigorous bull or prolapse of the vagina. The inflamed vagina is painful, edematous, and often there is a fetid exudate indicating infection with saprophytic organisms. Usually vaginal lacerations are limited to the retroperitoneal area, and cellulitis with accompanying edema, necrosis and fetid discharge are common, often with an accompanying acute metritis. There may be tenesmus and swelling of the vulva. The degree of depression, loss of appetite and fever depends on the severity of the infection. Malignant edema occasionally establishes itself in the injured tissue.

Examination and treatment must be done with a clean, well-lubricated gloved hand in order to minimize pain and straining. If the fetal membranes are retained, they should be removed if this can be done easily and quickly. Since the uterus is usually affected, it should be treated with antibiotics. Antibiotics placed in the uterus will escape through the vagina and assist in treating the infection there (R 13, 34, 40, 99). Oily antibiotic preparations may be placed in the vagina with a catheter (R 42). Animals with severe vaginitis should be treated by parenteral administration of antibiotics or sulfa drugs (R 41, 58, 75, 82). Tenesmus in traumatic vaginitis is usually transitory or caused by examination. It should be controlled by epidural anesthesia. Inflammatory changes usually prevent prolapse in these cases.

Granular veneral disease (Granular vaginitis): This condition is characterized by the presence of spherical nodules, about 1 mm in diameter, on the vulvar mucosa of cattle. Similar hyperplasia may occur in the lymphatic follicles on the bull's penis. This condition should be considered a response of the lymphatic tissue in this area to an irritant or an antigen. It is nonspecific and is not a disease in the classic sense. The agent stimulating the hyperplasia is usually unknown. One disease known to produce this hyperplasia after recovery from the acute infection is IPV (q.v., p. 268). Treatment of females is not indicated and the condition subsides spontaneously in several weeks to several months. Young animals are most frequently affected since these experience the most exposure to new antigens. In the female the condition is not related to fertility, although the predisposing agent may influence fertility.

The condition in bulls tends to be more persistent and affected bulls may refuse to breed. They should be treated by massage of the anesthetized prolapsed penis and sheath with a suitable antibiotic ointment (R 42). This should be repeated sufficiently often to assure elimination of any existing infection. If the nodules persist, they should be cauterized with silver nitrate sticks. Following cautery, the penis should be washed and protected with an antibiotic ointment.

A condition characterized by hyperemia of the vagina and the accumulation of as much as 50 ml of yellow mucoid exudate, occurs as an epizootic in some herds. A virus has been isolated from some of these animals although in many instances no etiologic agent has been isolated. It is postulated that this agent is an enterovirus and gains access to the vagina either by coitus or by extension from a contaminated vulva. The effect on fertility is slight and recovery is spontaneous.

VAGINAL PROLAPSE

Eversion of the vagina through the vulva. In complete prolapse the bladder is frequently contained within the prolapsed vagina. The condition occurs in all species, but is most frequently observed in sheep and cattle.

Etiology: The condition most frequently occurs in mature females in late pregnancy. A number of causes appear responsible, e.g., excessive abdominal pressure, relaxation of pelvic musculature, flaccid, loosely attached structures to the wall and floor of the vagina. The condition may be an inherited weakness in some families and occurs in young animals without regard to pregnancy.

In sheep, the primary etiologic factors are inheritance; distention of the digestive tract, which creates high intra-abdominal pressure; grazing on hill country; and estrogen in the feed. In cattle, a similar etiologic basis may be presumed. The fact that most prolapses occur in pluripara suggests that stretching of the vagina predisposes to eversion. Relaxation of the vulva and the vagina in late pregnancy allows intermittent prolapse when the animal is lying down. This leads to irritation of the mucosa which results in straining and creates a continuous complete prolapse.

Clinical Findings: The signs are obvious. Usually the floor of the vagina prolapses first and repeated prolapsing may result in a diverticulum of one or, less frequently, both sides of the vagina. Complete prolapse results in the cervix appearing at the vagina. Usually pregnancy is not interrupted, although the external os of the cervix may be greatly enlarged and congested. The urethra may be occluded and prevent urination. Failure to treat results in uremia, vascular stasis, necrosis, infection and eventually death.

Prevention and Treatment: Elimination of families predisposed to the condition and those animals that have previously suffered from the condition will reduce the incidence. Feeding practices should be examined and estrogenic sources eliminated, if possible. Sometimes, where pasture is the source of feed, this cannot be done and treatment measures must be continuously applied. Animals should be kept on level ground during late pregnancy. Methods such as rope harnesses and Caslick operations to prevent partial prolapse during recumbency in late pregnancy are useful in cows. For sheep that are pastured on estrogenic feed and chronically affected with prolapse, a commercially available plastic pessary is very useful. The pessary, in the shape of a "T" with the vertical member approximately 6 in. long, and the cross member approximately 8 in. long, is placed with the vertical part in the vagina and the ends of the cross member tied to the wool.

Treatment, to be effective, should follow these steps: (1) wash the organ with soap and water and rinse thoroughly; (2) empty the bladder if necessary; (3) reduce congestion by applying gentle pressure if necessary; (4) replace the vagina and apply antibiotic (℞ 42); and (5) retain the vagina in position. Only the last procedure presents serious difficulty. The irritation of the vaginal mucosa results in extreme tenesmus and retention devices must be strong in order to prevent recurrence. Replacement and retention for a short period can be accomplished with epidural anesthesia. More permanent retention is accomplished through various methods of suturing the vulva. If interrupted sutures are used, they are usually deeply placed about ¾ in. apart and the entire vulva is closed. Another method consists of placing loops on either side of the vulvar lips, which are then laced together. Metal prolapse pins with heavy buttons or similar devices have also been used. Perivaginal sutures, resection and removal of some of the mucosa of the vaginal wall, or cervical or vaginal wall fixation are other methods for providing long-term solutions to chronic prolapse. Fly control may be necessary.

UTERINE PROLAPSE

Prolapse of the uterus may occur in any species; however, it is most common in dairy cows and somewhat less frequent in ewes. Etiology is not clear and occurrence is sporadic. Recumbency with the hind quarters lower than the fore quarters, invagination of the uterus, and excessive traction to relieve dystocia, all have been incriminated as causes. Prolapse of the uterus can occur only within a few hours after parturition when the cervix and the uterus are open and lack tone. Prolapse is always complete, and the mass of uterus usually hangs below the hocks of the affected animal.

Treatment involves removing the placenta, if it is still attached, and thoroughly cleaning the endometrial surface. The uterus is then returned to its normal position by one of several methods. If the cow is in the standing position, epidural anesthesia should be administered in order to replace the uterus. When replacing the uterus of a cow in a standing position, the uterus should be elevated to the level of the vulva on a tray, or by means of a hammock held by 2 assistants. The uterus is then replaced beginning at the cervical portion and gradually working toward the apex. Once the uterus is replaced, the hand should be inserted to be sure that there is no remaining invagination. If the cow is recumbent, she should be placed in a position so that the hind quarters are elevated. This can be done by moving her onto a sloping area, or elevating the hind quarters with some type of lift attached to the hind legs. The uterus is held at the level of the vulva and replaced as indicated above. When the hind quarters are elevated in the recumbent position, epidural anesthesia is usually unnecessary.

Following return of the uterus to its normal position, antibiotic is placed in the uterine cavity and oxytocin administered (R 13, 34, 173, 174). The prognosis depends upon the amount of injury, contamination and infection of the uterus. Prompt replacement of a clean minimally traumatized uterus results in uneventful recovery. There is no tendency for the condition to repeat in subsequent parturitions.

Complications tend to develop when laceration, necrosis and infection occur or when treatment is delayed. Shock is an important factor in prolonged prolapse and requires supportive therapy. In some instances the bladder is in the everted cavity and distended, and the intestines may prolapse into the everted uterus; these require careful replacement before the uterus is returned. The bladder may be drained with a catheter or trocar. Elevation of the hind quarters and pressure on the uterus will aid in replacement of bladder and intestines. It may be necessary to incise the uterus in order to replace these organs.

Amputation of a badly traumatized uterus may be the only means of saving the cow or ewe. This may be accomplished by incising the dorsal side of the uterus, ligating the 2 middle uterine arteries, placing a heavy ligature around the uterus in the region of the cervix and amputating distal to the uterine and vascular ligatures. The stump is replaced in the vagina. Supportive treatment and antibiotic therapy are indicated.

MASTITIS (LG. AN.)

Mastitis is of greatest economic importance in the dairy cow, but the disease may affect any species and is handled in much the same way in all of them. Brief notes on mastitis in sheep, goats and swine are given separately.

Mastitis may be defined as inflammation of the mammary gland due to the effects of infection of the gland by bacterial or mycotic pathogens. Technical factors that predispose to establishment of infection within the gland are poor milking hygiene, milking machine faults, faulty milking management, teat injuries and teat sores.

A diagnosis of mastitis is based on: (1) clinical signs, (2) culture and identification of a mastitis pathogen from a sample of milk collected aseptically and (3) results of tests designed to detect increases in the leukocyte content of milk (in subclinical cases). In clinical cases a provisional diagnosis is usually based on signs and knowledge of the predominant pathogens in the herd but it should be backed up by culture of the secretion and sensitivity tests.

The 4 clinical types of mastitis are: (1) peracute—in which swelling, heat, pain and abnormal secretion in the gland are accompanied by fever, depression, anorexia and often by other signs of toxemia; (2) acute—in which similar changes in the gland occur with only slight to moderate fever and depression; (3) subacute—in which there are no systemic changes and the changes in the gland and secretion are less marked; and (4) subclinical—where the inflammatory reaction within the gland is only detectable by tests, such as the California Mastitis Test (CMT) (q.v., p. 817), the Wisconsin Mastitis Test and the Whiteside test, which are used at intervals to detect a persistently high-leukocyte content in the milk.

Changes in the secretion can vary from a slight wateriness with a few flecks (e.g., subacute staphylococcal mastitis) through wateriness with large yellow clots (e.g., acute and peracute streptococcal and staphylococcal mastitis) to watery, brownish secretion with fine mealy flakes (e.g., coliform mastitis). Peracute and acute cases of mastitis usually have a sudden onset. Without treatment the affected quarter gradually loses its productive capacity and may either atrophy or slowly develop firm nodular granuloma-like masses within the parenchyma.

The bacterial pathogens most commonly responsible for bovine mastitis (in approximate decreasing order of frequency) are: *Staphylococcus aureus, Streptococcus agalactiae,* other streptococci, coliform organisms, *Corynebacterium pyogenes* and *Pseudomonas aeruginosa.* Less commonly, mastitis may be associated with infection of the gland by *Nocardia asteroides, Clostridium perfringens, Mycobacterium* spp., *Mycoplasma* spp. and yeasts.

Treatment of Mastitis: In cases of peracute mastitis systemic treatment with antibiotics, such as penicillin-streptomycin combinations (R 41) or oxytetracycline (R 25) or ampicillin (R 1), is indicated together with a mastitis infusion of the same antibiotic into the affected quarter every 24 hours for 3 to 4 treatments. The affected quarter is infused after the evening milking and repeatedly stripped out during the day. Single or repeated injections of an antihistamine (R 539) or the administration of a corticosteroid (R 147) with IV-administered, isotonic, balanced electrolyte solutions may be of use as supportive therapy in toxemic cases. In acute mastitis, intramammary antibiotic infusions with or without systemic antibiotics initially (depending on the severity) are usually sufficient if the organism is sensitive to the antibiotic in use. Certain antibiotics such as the penicillin ester, penethamate hydriodide (R 39) and erythromycin (R 21) reach much higher levels in the milk than in plasma after systemic administration and are useful in acute cases. Subacute infections are best treated by a 3- to 4-day course of an appropriate intramammary antibiotic infusion. Subclinical infections may preferably be treated by infusing an appropriate long-acting antibiotic preparation into the affected quarter at drying off.

Depending upon which antibiotic and base is infused into the udder and what repository form is injected, the milk collected from the cow for as long as 96 hours following treatment must not be used for human consumption.

SPECIFIC TYPES OF BOVINE MASTITIS

Streptococcal Mastitis: *Streptococcus agalactiae* requires the mammary gland for its perpetuation in nature. All other streptococci, whether saprophytes or potential pathogens, enter the mammary gland by chance and are not dependent upon it for survival. Therefore, *Str. agalactiae* mastitis is a specific infectious disease that can be completely eradicated from dairy herds. The organism enters the gland through the teat opening and resides in the milk and on the surface of the milk channels. It does not penetrate the tissue. Its action on the parenchyma is through an irritant that forms in the milk. For this reason, it is necessary to evacuate the infected glands completely at each milking. Leaving a small amount of milk in the gland leads to an increase in the intensity of the inflammatory reaction which, in turn, produces a deterioration of the functional structures and stimulates the proliferation of the connective tissues.

Streptococcus agalactiae spreads from cow to cow during the milking act and, therefore, shedder-cows should be milked after the non-infected portion of the herd. Calves fed on milk containing the pathogen may transmit it to the immature glands of penmates if they are permitted to suck each other's teats. Therefore, during an eradication program, it is essential that calfhood infections be prevented; otherwise, at some later date, an animal infected as a calf may reintroduce *Str. agalactiae* into the lactating herd during its first lactation.

The other streptococci that may cause mastitis are *Str. dysgalactiae, Str. uberis, Str. zooepidemicus* and Lancefield groups G and L streptococci. Both *Str. dysgalactiae* and *Str. uberis* are common to the environment of dairy farms. *Str. uberis* may contribute significantly to the bacterial count as bacterial numbers per milliliter of milk from infected glands commonly are much greater than is the case with *Str. agalactiae* or staphylococci. *Str. zooepidemicus* is a common pathogen of horses and has been found in purulent conditions of swine. Its occurrence in the mammary gland has been more or less limited to small dairy herds where cows and other farm animals are run together.

Penicillin is specific for *Str. agalactiae,* but some of the other streptococci appear to be more resistant. The antibiotic is infused into the infected gland through the teat canal (℞ 194). Chlortetracycline (℞ 185), oxytetracycline (℞ 193) or sodium cloxacillin (℞ 186) also may be used. Variable results have been reported for neomycin (℞ 192). Benzathine cloxacillin (℞ 187) and penicillin-novobiocin (℞ 196) combinations may be used in dry-cow treatment.

Staphylococcal Mastitis: This is the most important type of mastitis in most dairying areas today because (1) the organism is ubiquitous and can colonize the cow's skin and teat sores, as well as the udder, (2) a high proportion of isolates in many herds are now penicillin resistant, (3) treatment with appropriate antibiotic infusions is less successful than in *Streptococcus agalactiae* infections.

In herds in which staphylococcal mastitis is a problem, 50% or more of the cows may have subclinical infections. *Staphylococcus aureus* may cause peracute mastitis, peracute gangrenous mastitis (in which the skin of the quarter and teat becomes cold and bluish in color and eventually sloughs), as well as the acute, subacute and subclinical types. Infections of a year or more in duration are often refractory to treatment because of the development of a tissue barrier between the antibiotic and the organism.

Treatment of cows with subclinical infections during lactation is not as successful as dry-cow treatment, hence these should be treated at drying off with an appropriate long-acting infusion, e.g., benzathine cloxacillin (℞ 187). A high proportion of staphylococci are sensitive to the penicillinase-resistant drug cloxacillin.

Peracute and acute staphylococcal mastitis may be treated systemically with an appropriate antibiotic, e.g., erythromycin (℞ 21), streptomycin (℞ 53), chlortetracycline (℞ 11). For intramammary therapy, cloxacillin (℞ 186) is recommended but sensitivity tests may reveal that others such as erythromycin (℞ 189), lincomycin (℞ 191), penicillin-streptomycin (℞ 197), chlortetracycline (℞ 185) and neomycin (℞ 192) infusions may be more effective in some instances. Staphylococcal vaccines have been recommended but their value in the control of the disease is debatable.

Coliform Mastitis: The coliform organisms most frequently encountered have been *Escherichia coli* and *Aerobacter aerogenes*. Coliform mastitis is a disease of the normal lactating mammary gland. Coliform bacteria are prevented from multiplying by even low numbers of infiltrating leukocytes, but in cell-free milk, they multiply rapidly, producing a large pool of potential endotoxin. The inflammatory reaction which follows destroys the coliform population, thereby releasing the endotoxin. The resulting toxemia produces the local and systemic signs of peracute mastitis. The temperature ranges from 103° to 108°F, milk secretion ceases even though only one gland usually is the seat of the infective process, and anorexia, depression, dehydration and rapid loss of weight are prominent. The secretion of the affected quarters is usually brownish and watery. Diarrhea also commonly occurs. A unique feature is that, upon recovery, the udder tissue generally returns to normal so that, in a subsequent lactation, no fibrosis is found and the gland is capable of producing to capacity.

Older cows, producing leukocyte-free milk, are especially susceptible to attacks of acute coliform mastitis due to increased patency of the streak canal. Foremilk leukocyte numbers of 50,000/ml should be tolerated in older cows as a protective barrier against spontaneous acute coliform mastitis. Acute coliform mastitis should be treated locally and parenterally with dihydrostreptomycin sulfate (℞ 53) or ampicillin (℞ 1). Chlortetracycline (℞ 185), oxytetracycline (℞ 193) and neomycin (℞ 192) have been used in a similar manner, but with variable results. In the absence of systemic signs, the most specific therapy consists of dihydrostreptomycin sulfate in a water-in-oil vehicle (℞ 188) but other drugs may be used depending on sensitivity tests.

***Pseudomonas aeruginosa* Mastitis:** *Pseudomonas* is occasionally important as a cause of mastitis. Generally, a persistent infection occurs which may be characterized by intermittent acute or subacute exacerbations. *Ps. aeruginosa* is a soil-water organism common to the environment of dairy farms. Herd-wide infections have been reported following extensive exposure to intramammary treatments administered by milkers. The indications are that failure to employ aseptic techniques for udder therapy may lead to the establishment of *Ps. aeruginosa* infections within the mammary glands. Severe peracute mastitis with toxemia and high mortality may follow immediately in some, while subclinical infections may occur in other cows. The pathogen has been observed to persist in a gland for as long as 5 lactations, but on the other hand, spontaneous recovery may be anticipated.

A satisfactory treatment for mastitis caused by *Ps. aeruginosa* has not been developed. The pathogen is often sensitive to streptomycin, neomycin and carbenicillin *in vitro* but variable results have been reported when these drugs have been infused into the udder. Carbenicillin (℞ 184) appears to be the drug of choice.

***Corynebacterium pyogenes* Mastitis:** This pathogen is commonly encountered in suppurative processes of cattle and swine and it produces a characteristic mastitis in dry cows. It is occasionally observed in mastitis in the lactating udder, but may be a secondary invader. The pathogen produces an inflammation typified by the formation of profuse, foul-smelling, purulent exudate. The foul smell is not caused by *C. pyogenes*, but by an anaerobic micrococcus, *Peptococcus asaccharolyticus* (*Micrococcus indolicus*) that commonly is found in association with the former. In the rare instances of *C. pyogenes* mastitis in which *P. asaccharolyticus* is not present, the exudate is odorless.

Corynebacterium pyogenes mastitis may occur in epizootic form among dry cows kept in small enclosures during a protracted wet period. To combat this occurrence, it is important to move the nonaffected animals to dry quarters or to pasture. Surgical removal of the teat, to establish drainage, thus far has proved to be the most satisfactory method for handling well-established clinical cases. Cows or even young heifers with multiple udder abscesses due to *C. pyogenes* or other infections should be slaughtered. Peracute and acute cases should be treated with systemic and intramammary penicillin (R 194). Long-acting penicillin infusions (R 195) at drying off and half-way through the dry period may prevent *C. pyogenes* mastitis in dry cows.

Unusual Forms of Mastitis: *Mycoplasma* mastitis, caused by pleuropneumonia-like organisms (PPLO), is a severe form of mastitis that has been reported in the U.S.A., England, Israel and Australia. The infection may spread rapidly through a herd with serious consequences. Typically, all quarters become involved following a rapid onset. Loss of production is often dramatic, secretion soon being replaced by a serous or purulent exudate. Initially, a fine granular or flaky sediment is characteristic of the material removed from infected glands. Despite the severe local effects on udder tissue, the cow usually does not manifest signs of systemic involvement. The infection will persist through the dry period. Since there is no satisfactory treatment, affected cows should be slaughtered and sanitary measures strictly enforced.

Nocardia asteroides causes a destructive mastitis characterized by an acute onset with high temperature, anorexia, rapid wasting and marked swelling of the udder. Pathology in the udder is typical of a granulomatous inflammation leading to extensive fibrosis and formation of palpable nodules. Herd histories suggest that infection of the udder may be associated with failure to ensure asepsis in intramammary treatment of the common forms of mastitis. Slaughter is recommended for obvious clinical cases, while intramammary infusions of a furaltadone-penicillin preparation (R 190) may be successful in removing latent and subclinical infections.

In recent years, mastitis due to a variety of yeasts has appeared in a number of dairy herds, especially following the use of penicillin in an attempt to eradicate *Str. agalactiae*. Yeasts grow well in the presence of penicillin and if accidentally introduced during treatment they may be able to multiply and cause mastitis. Signs may be severe and accompanied by a high temperature followed by spontaneous recovery in about 2 weeks or by a chronic destructive mastitis.

A chronic indurative mastitis similar to that caused by the tubercle bacillus has been reported to be caused by acid-fast bacilli derived from the soil when such organisms are introduced into the gland along with antibiotics, especially penicillin, in oil or ointment vehicles. The oil is required for the organisms to become invasive for the mammary tissue.

CONTROL OF BOVINE MASTITIS

There are 7 related points to consider: (1) Milking machine function and milking procedures—these should be checked and corrected where necessary. The following factors have been associated with higher incidences of mastitis: (a) Excessive irregular vacuum fluctuation in the teat cup and in the vacuum or milk line. This sometimes occurs due to faulty handling of teat cups (letting excess air into the system) or to inadequate vacuum reserve. (b) Vacuum level—levels of 2 in. of mercury or more above and below the recommended 15 in. are undesirable. (c) Blocked air admission holes in the claw pieces. (d) Narrow-bore milk liners (<1 in. internal diameter) are preferred to wide-bore liners). (e) Gross abnormalities in pulsation rate (normal 40 to 60/min) and ratio (40 to 50 rest:50 to 60 vacuum usual) are undesirable. (f) Clusters should be removed as soon as cow has milked out, i.e., avoid overmilking. (g) Adequate stimulation is essential prior to applying teat clusters.

(2) Milking hygiene should be observed and corrected. A recommended hygiene system is: (a) Initially remove residual milk in teat and discard. (b) Wash teats in clean running water, using antiseptic soap and disposable paper towels. (c) Back-flush clusters with clean water or pasteurize clusters between cows (optional—depending on shed labor). (d) Dip teats of cows at end of milking in a hypochlorite solution yielding 4% available chlorine, a chlorhexidine solution, 0.5%, or an iodophor solution containing 5,000 ppm iodine. (e) Milkers should wear rubber gloves and disinfect their hands when going from cow to cow.

(3) Detect infected cows by repeat CMT's and cultures. Isolate infected cows and milk last. Milk clean heifers first, then clean cows, then recently treated cows and then infected cows.

(4) Treat clinical infections as they occur, but treat subclinical infections preferably at drying off (especially *Staphylococcus aureus* infections). Cows carrying *Streptococcus agalactiae* infections may be treated during lactation with a reasonable degree of success. Preferably treat all quarters at drying off with an appropriate long-acting antibiotic infusion.

(5) Cull any cows that have had 5 or more clinical attacks of mastitis during the lactation or have failed to respond to repeated therapy including dry-cow therapy.

(6) Examine all introductions to herd by udder palpation, culture and CMT of secretion from all quarters.

(7) Maintain client interest and awareness of the mastitis problem by furnishing regular reports or CMT results of cows in his herd.

MASTITIS IN GOATS

The etiology of infectious mastitis in goats and cattle is similar. *Streptococcus agalactiae* produces a subacute mastitis, *Staphylococcus aureus* may cause either subacute or gangrenous mastitis, coliform mastitis has been encountered both sporadically and as a herd-wide infection, and *Corynebacterium pyogenes* produces multiple nodular abscesses.

Programs for diagnosis, control and treatment of mastitis in the goat should be similar to those discussed for the cow.

MASTITIS IN SHEEP

This can be quite an important disease in ewe flocks, with incidences of 2% or more. Apart from deaths from peracute infections, the disease can be a cause of lamb mortality from starvation, or of depressed weaning weights of lambs. Peracute, peracute gangrenous (usually due to *Staphylococcus aureus*), acute, subacute and probably subclinical types occur. The organisms most commonly involved are *S. aureus*, streptococci, *E. coli*, *Pasteurella hemolytica*, and *Corynebacterium pyogenes*.

The principles of diagnosis and treatment used in bovine diagnosis can be applied to the ewe. Little is known about the control of ovine mastitis.

MASTITIS IN SOWS

Mastitis can be important in swine-raising units. Peracute mastitis can affect sows and gilts and is most commonly associated with coliform (*E. coli*, *Aerobacter aerogenes* and *Klebsiella* infections. It most commonly occurs at or just following parturition, and affected sows have a moderate to severe toxemia. The sow's temperature may be elevated to 107°F or may be subnormal. The affected glands are swollen, purple in color and have a watery secretion. Sow mortality is high and the litter will also die unless fostered or fed artificially. Recovered sows may have impaired milk production in the next lactation. The treatment of peracute coliform mastitis in sows is similar to the treatment of this condition in the cow (q.v., p. 810). Ampicillin (℞ 1), dihydrostreptomycin (℞ 53) or oxytetracycline (℞ 25) systemically have been used.

Subacute mastitis may occur in older sows and lead to induration of one or more glands and impair the sow's ability to suckle a large litter adequately. This form of mastitis is more likely to be associated with infection by streptococci or staphylococci. Granulomatous lesions in the mammae of sows have been associated with *Actinobacillus lignieresi, Actinomyces bovis* and *Staphylococcus aureus* infections. *Sphaerophorus necrophorus* and *Corynebacterium pyogenes* have also been incriminated in sow mastitis. A thorough examination of the mammary glands of the sow is important to diagnose any of the above peracute and subacute types of mastitis.

The control of porcine mastitis has not been extensively investigated but isolating sows in adequately disinfected farrowing pens prior to, during and for an adequate period after farrowing should help prevent the severe losses associated with coliform mastitis.

CALIFORNIA MASTITIS TEST (CMT)

A kit consisting of the plastic paddle plus all the necessary reagents is available commercially. Equal quantities of reagents and milk are mixed in the depressions of the plastic paddle by a swirling motion. Negative samples are free from gel formation, positive samples show various degrees of precipitate, which is a reflection of the degree of udder inflammation. There is a high degree of correlation between the CM test and the microscopic examination for leukocytes in milk. The CMT may be used to estimate the leukocyte count of bulk herd milk, bucket milk or quarter milk.

MISCELLANEOUS DISEASES OF THE BOVINE UDDER

UDDER ACNE

A disease of dairy cows characterized by occurrence of pustules on the skin of the udder and teats, often on the udder near the base of the teat. It has a tendency to spread in some herds. Staphylococci can usually be isolated from the pustules. A predisposing factor may be excessive teat cup "crawl" at milking associated with a prolonged interval between cessation of milk flow and teat cup removal. The affected skin should be thoroughly washed with chlorhexidine solution (5,000 ppm) and either chlorhexidine ointment or a neomycin ointment (R 417) applied twice daily after milking. The use of iodophor or chlorhexidine solutions as udder washes and post-milking teat dips will help prevent the spread of the disease.

BOVINE ULCERATIVE MAMMILLITIS

A severe ulcerative condition of the teats of dairy cows which can occur in outbreaks resulting in marked loss of milk production and a high incidence of secondary mastitis in affected herds. Reported from Great Britain, it probably also occurs in other countries. It is caused by a herpesvirus very similar to the Allerton strain of Group II lumpy-skin-disease viruses.

The lesions commence as one or more thickened plaques of varying size on the skin of one or more teats. Vesiculation quickly occurs within these plaques and the surface sloughs leaving a raw ulcerated area which becomes covered with a dark black-brown scab. The scabs tend to crack and bleed especially if milking is attempted. In some cases a large proportion of the teat wall is involved and often the lesion includes the teat orifice, predisposing to mastitis and obstruction of the streak canal. In the early stages of the lesions before vesiculation is marked, intranuclear inclusions may be detected in the cells of the dermis. The disease is more severe in cows that have recently calved, especially those with udder edema. Severe lesions may take several weeks to heal.

Diagnosis is based on the signs and confirmed by histopathology or by virus isolation from early lesions. Serum virus neutralization titers rise quickly and the first sample must be taken very early in the course of the disease.

Affected cows should be isolated and separate milking utensils used. Emollient ointments used before milking may reduce trauma and hemorrhage. Prophylactic infusions for mastitis should be considered if the teat orifice is involved. Iodophor solutions (V/V 1:320) may be useful as teat and udder disinfectants to aid control in infected herds.

TRAUMATIC DISEASES

Superficial wounds to udder and teats are treated as open wounds with antiseptic solutions, powders, or ointments. If such wounds occur in a cow with edema of the udder (q.v., p. 822) serous fluid will escape from the wound for a number of days, but treatment is the same, although healing may be slightly delayed. Superficial wounds of the teats may be bound with adhesive tape or an elastic bandage, which helps control granulation and pain in milking, and hastens healing. Chapped teats usually are treated by application of antiseptic ointments and eliminating moisture and irritants from contact with the teats. Superficial wounds involving the teat orifice should be carefully treated twice daily with an antiseptic solution or ointment and the wound bandaged between milkings to prevent udder infections. Superficial wounds to the udder may cut a large milk vein and severe hemorrhage may result, requiring prompt compression and ligation. Many slight cuts of teats should be sutured, both to favor optimum healing and to prevent development of fistulas.

Deep wounds to the udder and teats are treated similarly to the superficial ones. However, deep wounds of all types, especially teat wounds, should promptly be cleansed carefully and sutured to promote first-intention healing. Adequate local anesthesia in conjunction with chemical and physical restraints greatly assists in the repair of severe teat wounds and fistulas. Aftercare should include the infusion of the affected quarter with antibiotic preparations and the maintenance of high antibiotic blood levels by parenteral therapy, especially with deep udder wounds.

Contusions and hematomas of the udder and teats produce painful swellings and frequently result in bloody milk. Temporary stenosis of the teat canal or orifice may occur. Cold applications of water, ice, or snow, applied for several days, are indicated in the early treatment of this condition to control swelling and pain. Later, warm applications, hot packs, liniments and gentle massage may hasten the resolution of the swelling.

Hematomas of the udder or around the milk veins usually are sequelae of severe contusions and should be treated in the same manner. Rarely, large hematomas may interfere with the circulation of blood in the skin of the udder and necrosis and infection may occur. Hematomas should not be incised or drained unless they become infected, as they will disappear in time.

Abscesses of the udder may be secondary to wounds, advanced mastitis, infected hematomas, or severe contusions. These abscesses should be incised and drained when they are chronic and near the surface of the udder. The wound should be packed for 2 days with gauze containing a counterirritant and washed daily thereafter with an antiseptic solution.

Bloody milk may be due to contusions, wounds, or hematomas of the udder or teats, or lesions of the lining of the teat or gland cistern. It is frequently seen following calving when the udder usually is severely congested and edematous. This latter condition is observed most commonly at the first to third parturitions. Most cows with bloody milk recover without treatment in 4 to 14 days. Wounds, contusions and hematomas resulting in bloody milk are treated as described previously. In these conditions, as well as in the case of lesions of the parenchyma or lining membrane of udder and teats, milking should be done in a gentle manner, preferably by hand. Where large clots form in the lumen of the teat and cistern, great care and often several attempts are necessary to break up and remove the clotted blood.

Teat stenosis is characterized by a marked narrowing of the teat sphincter and orifice or canal and occasionally is observed as a hereditary condition, affecting all teats and making milking very difficult. More often, however, it is the result of a contusion or wound of the teat that produces swelling or formation of a blood clot or scab causing an acute stricture. In these acute cases, conservative treatment as outlined for wounds and contusions is indicated. The use of the milking machine should be temporarily discontinued in favor of hand milking of the affected teats. In rare cases, a teat cannula taped in place may be used, with proper aseptic precautions, for withdrawing the milk. Many acute cases of stenosis progress to the more chronic form, characterized by a fibrous thickening of the canal lining and sphincter muscle, if teat dilators are used routinely or a wound is present in or around the teat orifice, or if the milking machine is applied for excessive periods over the course of several weeks. In these chronic cases, surgical intervention may be necessary to correct the stenosis. All injuries to, or surgical procedures on, the teat should be handled carefully to prevent the introduction of infection. Prophylactic infusions of the quarter are indicated in all surgical procedures or wounds involving the teat or teat orifice. The so-called teat "spider" is a fibrous thickening of the teat or teat sphincter as described above.

Complete teat obstruction is caused by the same factors that cause teat stenosis, or by a congenital membranous obstruction. Treatment is similar to that for stenosis, but the prognosis usually is more guarded. Occasionally, if the injury is severe enough, milking of the quarter should be discontinued for the remainder of that lactation period or permanently.

Occasionally, teat obstructions may be due to corpora amylacea, firm blood clots, small pedunculated tumors of the teat lining or foreign bodies, such as match sticks or teat dilators in the teat cistern, that cause an intermittent obstruction of the teat orifice. These may be removed by massage or by dilation or incision of the teat orifice and grasping and removing the object with a fine pair of forceps.

"Leakers" is a term referring to cows with teats that drip milk continuously or after the stimulus causing milk letdown. These animals usually have sustained a severe teat injury. In general, little can be done to correct this condition satisfactorily. Injecting small amounts of Lugol's solution into the teat sphincter with an intradermal syringe or cauterizing the external teat orifice or teat end as well as surgical correction have been tried with limited success.

Eversions and vegetative growths on the external teat orifice are usually due to the use of a milking machine with too high a vacuum, or to leaving the machine on the cow for an excessive period at each milking. Residual milk at the site of vegetative lesions after milking favors bacterial growth at the external teat orifice, an undesirable condition favoring the development of local infection, ulcers ("black scab") and mastitis.

"Blind" or nonfunctional quarters usually are the result of a severe infection which may occur either in the dry or lactating cow or in the heifer, due to sucking by other heifers or calves. If treated, the infection may be overcome and the quarters milk fairly satisfactorily during the next lactation if fibrosis is not extensive. Blind quarters that still contain a small amount of pus may be dried up permanently by the injection of silver nitrate (R 617). Rarely, blind or nonfunctional quarters may be congenital.

CONGENITAL OR PHYSIOLOGIC DISEASES

Congenital aberrations in the bovine udder include many structural defects, such as fusion of the front and hind teats, large-base or funnel-shaped teats, very small short teats, improperly placed teats, "cut-up" udders, predisposition to pendulous or swinging udders, hypoplasia of front- or hind-quarters of an udder and supernumerary teats. With the exception of the latter condition, there is no treatment. These defects should be eliminated by breeding.

Supernumerary teats may be located on the udder behind the posterior teats, between the front and hind teats, or attached to either the front or hind teats. They are easily removed with a pair of sharp scissors when the animal is from 1 week to 12 months of age. Removal just prior to lactation or during lactation is undesirable as a teat fistula often forms which is difficult to correct. The practice of removing supernumerary teats from dairy heifers is desirable in order to make the udder look better, to eliminate the possibility of mastitis in the gland above the extra teats and to facilitate milking. It is best done at 3 to 8 months of age.

Inversion of the teat orifice is a congenital condition which may be hereditary. It is not desirable, even though usually associated with ease in milking, because the teats frequently spray. This type of teat orifice favors udder infection.

Agalactia is occasionally observed in heifers and probably is a hereditary condition associated with an imbalance of the hormones controlling either udder growth and development, or lactation. No treatment has yet proved of definite value. Occasionally, this condition is due to a severe systemic disease in the recently fresh animal, or it may be associated with advanced chronic mastitis with extensive fibrosis of the mammary gland. Animals affected with the latter condition will never produce a normal supply of milk.

Failure of "letdown" of milk is observed occasionally after parturition in young dairy cattle. This condition may be caused by the pain and discomfort of a large and edematous udder. If usual methods of massage, use of warm compresses, calves sucking and frequent milking fail to result in proper letdown of milk, the administration of posterior pituitary extract (℞ 174) or oxytocin (℞ 173) may be successful. This treatment may have to be repeated for several milkings or even for several days. Development of letdown failure may be prevented by using a milking machine from the very start, i.e., never milking by hand. An exact milking and feeding routine is important in training heifers to develop a proper letdown habit.

Physiologic udder edema and congestion is commonly observed in high-producing dairy cattle prior to and after parturition. This problem cannot be controlled satisfactorily, but several practices may help. Some veterinarians advise milking cows before parturition as a means of reducing the congestion and edema. The level of feeding has been shown to have no influence upon the amount of udder edema, which is apparently determined genetically, and excessive restriction of grain intake, especially after parturition, may result in acetonemia. Frequent milkings may be helpful. Massage and the use of hot compresses and udder ointments and liniments stimulate circulation and promote reduction of the edema in the udder tissues. This massage should be repeated as often as possible. When milk letdown fails, udder edema and congestion will appear to increase. In severely affected cows, the udder will often "break down" and become pendulous. The use of diuretics, such as chlorothiazide (℞ 519), or a similar preparation (℞ 521, 524), have proved highly beneficial in reducing udder edema, especially in young cattle.

Necrotic dermatitis is observed in cows or first-calf heifers with large edematous udders several weeks after calving. In heifers, the area involved is usually the lateral aspect of the udder and medial aspect of the thigh as the udder is pressed tightly against the leg causing chafing, dermatitis and finally necrosis. In cows, it usually is observed at the anterior portion of the udder between the 2 forequarters. Possibly, poor circulation due to the extensive edema is the cause of the necrosis at this site. In heifers, treatment consists of reducing udder congestion as rapidly as possible (℞ 519, 521, 524), limiting movement, daily cleansing of inflamed skin and application of soothing powders, antiseptic oils, or astringents. In cows, the swollen necrotic area at the front of the udder should be washed daily to control the objectionable odor, and astringent and drying powders should be applied along with fly repellents during the summer months. There is no specific treatment to hasten the normal tissue sloughing and repair in this area. Large doses of oral sulfonamides are useful, especially if *Sphaerophorus* infection is present. Sulfur iodide in oil with 10% formalin (℞ 436) is an effective local treatment.

Urticaria or allergic swelling of the udder and teats is observed in association with generalized urticaria (q.v., p. 917), and occasionally, it may be a localized condition where cows are bedded on buckwheat straw or other allergenic plants.

LACTATION FAILURE IN THE SOW
(Metritis-mastitis-agalactia syndrome, MMA)

A prevalent noninfectious syndrome of the gilt or sow that becomes apparent to the producer within 2 or 3 days after parturition. It occurs during all seasons of the year, frequently appearing shortly after such stresses as drastic feed changes, sow confinement in a new or remodeled facility or extremely variant ambient temperatures. It is characterized by a decrease in or absence of mammary gland secretion with resultant starvation of pigs. Neither large litter size nor prolonged parturition are constant features. It is more prevalent in second- or third-litter sows. Death of the affected sow is rare and most will recover in 3 to 5 days without treatment although some remain in a poor state of health.

Etiology: The cause is unknown although various microbial agents have been incriminated. Coliform bacteria are most frequently isolated from affected mammary glands and uteri but will not reproduce the disease. Microbial endotoxins, *Mycoplasma* spp. and poor management practices, as improper housing, bedding, feeding and lack of climatic control, have all been suggested as causes. The disease does occur, however, under ideal management systems and no infectious agent seems uniformly present. Bacterial invasion of mammary gland tissue frequently occurs but appears to be a secondary factor that prolongs the course of the disease. It appears that hormonal imbalance or insufficiency (possibly stress induced) results in mammary gland failure. All hormones associated with lactation have been incriminated but not proved. Adrenocortical-function increase in affected sows has been demonstrated.

Clinical Findings: Listlessness and anorexia several days before farrowing is sometimes seen. Usually the affected sow will reveal signs of disease at the time of parturition or within 2 or 3 days after (the disease has not been recognized later in the lactation period than the first few days). Hunger in piglets is often the first-noticed manifestation. Close observation of the affected sow will reveal several of the following: reluctance to rise or to allow nursing, presence of one or several firm, warm mammary glands, refusal to eat, increased heart and respiratory rates, febrile response, viciousness, comatose condition or normal attitude. Clinical signs are indeed variable; they may appear in one sow only, in many sows, or in a progressive manner suggestive of contagion. The sign most frequently seen is involvement (edema, congestion and frequently small foci of mastitis due to bacterial invasion) of one or several mammary glands, rarely all glands. The milk is more alkaline than normal. Cyanotic splotches in the skin covering the mammary glands are seen on occasion in white sows.

    Lesions: Vaginal discharge is frequently seen in affected sows and may be of a different character than the discharge seen from normal sows, but gross pathologic and histologic examinations of uteri reveals no differences between affected and normal sows. Atretic ovarian follicles and decreased follicular fluid have been found in affected sows.

Treatment: Therapeutic measures vary in effectiveness from farm to farm. Immediate relief from unusual stress factors as extreme heat or cold, poor-quality feed or rough handling is indicated. Clinical trials with various hormones suggest that desirable results can be obtained without multiple drug therapy but conventional treatment includes oxytocin (℞ 172), antibacterial (℞ 41) and corticosteroid (℞ 145) medication repeated at 12- or 24-hour intervals. Oxytocin may be given more frequently if necessary. Vitamin B complex injections appear to stimulate appetite. Intra-uterine infusions appear to create an improvement despite the proved absence of metritis in the majority of cases.

It may be necessary to remove the pigs to other sows for supplemental feeding or to use milk replacer or fresh cow's milk warmed to body temperature and placed in a shallow pan. Corn syrup (1 tablespoon per pint) may make the milk more acceptable. Antibacterials can be added to the milk. Baby pigs should be fed 6 times daily during days 1 and 2; 4 times daily during days 3 and 4; and 3 times daily during day 5 through day 7. Ten-minute feedings are satisfactory. A dry commercial pig starter can be gradually substituted for the milk. If the client is educated to recognize signs in the sow before the pigs are hungry, earlier treatment and additional pig survival are possible.

Prevention: Since this disease syndrome can appear under all forms and types of management systems it is difficult to recommend satisfactory preventive procedures. Stress should be minimized. The recommended rules of feeding during gestation, and sanitation suggestions for swine-farm management should be followed. Phosphorus, calcium, vitamin E and selenium deficiencies have been incriminated and should be guarded against. Autogenous and commercial bacterins have been used extensively and appear to decrease the severity of the syndrome where management practices allow bacterial build-up. Clinical trials indicated that corticotropin (℞ 138) used within one week before farrowing is useful.

CONTAGIOUS AGALACTIA

This disease of goats and sheep occurs in most Mediterranean countries and in Portugal, Switzerland, Iran, the U.S.S.R., Pakistan and India. Mortality is low but morbidity of 25% is common. Lactating animals are affected after parturition when mastitis develops and the milk yield declines. Arthritis usually accompanies the mastitis and the resulting lameness may persist for months. Occasionally keratoconjunctivitis may be present.

Diagnosis made on the history and clinical signs may be confirmed by isolation of the causal organism from infected milk, eyes or joint fluid and its identification as *Mycoplasma agalactiae*. A recently developed complement-fixation test is worthy of more extensive use in diagnosis.

The organism may be shed in milk for months after the onset of the infection, by which time signs may not be evident. The infection may be spread to healthy animals by hand-milking. Control measures should include the removal of infected animals from the flock and attention to hygiene, especially during milking. Treatment with tylosin (2 to 5 mg/lb body wt daily, IM), instituted early, may be beneficial. Prevention by the use of living, attenuated or of killed vaccines has shown promise experimentally and has been used widely in several countries with apparent success.

MASTITIS (SM. AN.)

Acute or chronic inflammatory change in one or more mammary glands, often accompanied by abscessation.

Etiology: Acute mastitis usually occurs from traumatic injury to the mammary gland by nursing young, with acute metritis or following weaning. With the latter, failure of drainage of the glands (galactostasis) may be an underlying cause. Infection, usually with streptococci or staphylococci may occur. Metritis may result in metastatic mammary infection or the presence of bacterial toxins in the milk. Galactostasis may be promoted by malformations of the nipples. Chronic mastitis (cystic hyperplasia, polycystic disease) is more common in older animals and its occurrence is probably hormone-influenced.

Clinical Findings: The initial signs are swelling and inflammation of the involved mammary glands. Discoloration and abscessation may occur. As the infection progresses, pyrexia, lethargy, dehydration and bacteremia follow. Metritis may be present. Young nursing an affected female may die unless weaned and hand-fed. Chronic mastitis is characterized by cyst formation in mammary tissue. These cystic enlargements can be confused with neoplasia and may, in fact, be preneoplastic.

Treatment: The litter should be weaned and hand-fed. Antibiotic therapy should be instituted as early as possible (℞ 11, 22, 29). Abscesses should be lanced and drained. This may be followed by flushing with hydrogen peroxide and instilling local antibacterial medicaments. Estrogen therapy (℞ 163) may be employed to lessen milk flow. Judicious use of corticosteroids should be considered to relieve inflammation. In cases where galactostasis is pronounced, a breast pump may be used 2 to 3 times daily. Hot followed by cold compresses, applied to the glands 2 to 3 times daily, may be helpful. If the animal shows signs of toxemia, supportive fluid therapy, such as 5% dextrose in lactated Ringers' solution (℞ 557) should be employed. In chronic mastitis, excision of the mammary cysts and, in some cases, ovariohysterectomy should be recommended.

BACTERIAL POSTHITIS AND VULVITIS IN SHEEP
(Sheath rot, Pizzle rot)

A spreading ulceration of the epithelium of the prepuce, sometimes involving the penis (balanoposthitis), and also of the vulva in sheep, related to diet, but caused by a bacterium which hydrolyzes urinary urea and initiates ulceration. Variants of this bacterium are found in more severe ulcers. Lesions of similar appearance are produced by the venereal transmission of the virus of ulcerative dermatosis (q.v., p. 292).

Etiology: Bacterial posthitis is common in Australia and New Zealand. In grazing sheep, an increase in the clover and presumably the protein content of pasture and the urea content of the urine are often associated with a higher incidence. The disease shows well-marked seasonal fluctuations, with most new cases developing in the autumn, winter and spring. This disease is most important in older wethers, although young sheep may be affected. Rams are sometimes affected and ewes may show analogous vulval ulceration.

Clinical Findings: The early stage, characterized by external lesions only, is an unimportant clinical condition. In the internal form (sheath rot), however, there is extensive ulceration around the preputial orifice, marked swelling and distension of the sheath with foul-smelling urine, pus and necrotic detritus, and staining of the surrounding wool. Affected sheep, especially in cases where there is difficulty in passing urine, rapidly lose condition. They may be humped and walk stiffly and the hind fetlocks are frequently stained from kicking at the sheath. Fly strike may be an added complication.

Lesions: The disease develops slowly. The first ulcers commence adjacent to the preputial orifice in areas which become wet during urination. From an initial diameter of a few millimeters, the ulcers, covered with scab, may extend or coalesce with others, developing lesions which ultimately surround the preputial orifice. The phagedenic process sometimes extends into the sheath, involving, in advanced cases, the whole of the prepuce, the urethral process and the glans penis. Scabbing and stenosis frequently cause occlusion of the preputial orifice leading to distension of the sheath with urine. The results of such injury, obviously, may be more serious in rams than in wethers. In ewes, ulceration on the vulva may be extensive, but swelling is minimal and extension to the vagina infrequent.

Diagnosis is usually based on the history and clinical signs. The only certain differentiation between bacterial posthitis and the infectious venereal form of ulcerative dermatosis is by transmission experiments in sheep. Material from the former will produce lesions only on the prepuce and vulva, and not on other parts of the body.

Prophylaxis and Treatment: Wethers are treated prophylactically with testosterone (e.g., 60 to 90 mg testosterone propionate) implants with a variable degree of success.

Treatment of early lesions may be aided by moving affected sheep temporarily to the poorest pastures available or by the provision of a restricted diet of oaten or wheat straw with free access to water for up to 10 days. In more advanced cases testosterone implants (e.g., 100 to 150 mg testosterone propionate) can be used in association with local treatment of the sheath using preparations such as 10% copper sulfate ointment, concentrated alcoholic solutions of a quaternary ammonium compound (e.g., 20% cetyl trimethyl ammonium bromide), chlorhexidine digluconate solutions or aluminium paste with silicone. Prior to treatment affected sheep should be isolated, wool clipped from around the prepuce and all pus, urine and debris removed from the sheath.

In severe cases surgical drainage by a longitudinal incision in the ventral aspect of the prepuce is indicated and may be combined with testosterone implantation and the IM injection of procaine penicillin. The results are permanent and enable wethers to be fattened for disposal.

BOVINE CYSTITIS AND PYELONEPHRITIS

A sporadic inflammatory disease of the urinary tract of cattle, and sometimes other species, caused generally by *Corynebacterium renale*.

Etiology: The causative agent in the vast majority of cases of bovine cystitis and pyelonephritis is the diphtheroid bacterium *C. renale*. The organism has a predilection for the urinary tract and rarely produces pathologic changes in other tissues. *Escherichia coli*, *C. pyogenes*, streptococci and unidentified diphtheroid bacilli also have produced urinary-tract infections. These organisms may be the sole agent involved or may be present as a mixed infection with *C. renale*.

Epizootiology: Aberrant *C. renale* infections have been reported in the horse, sheep and dog. The disease is of economic importance in cattle and occasionally in swine. Cows are affected more commonly than are bulls. The short, wide and often traumatized urethra of the female probably offers a predisposition to infection by allowing the entrance of the organism into the bladder.

C. renale has been cultured from the vulva, vagina and penile sheath of apparently normal cattle. The bacteria which have been isolated produced experimental pyelonephritis in laboratory albino mice. The incidence of carrier cows has been found to be significantly higher in herds with clinical cases than in herds with no clinical signs of pyelonephritis before a sporadic case appears. The transmission of bovine pyelonephritis is possibly favored by grooming animals with contaminated brushes, vulvar contact with urine-soiled bedding, tail switching and the use of improperly sterilized obstetric instruments and particularly urinary catheters.

Susceptibility to the disease appears to be increased by the stress of heavy feeding, high production, advanced pregnancy, or cold, uncomfortable weather.

Clinical Findings: A gradual loss in condition occurs over a period of weeks or months. Animals in the advanced stages of infection are emaciated and dehydrated. The appetite is often poor. Generally, the temperature, pulse and respiratory rates are normal.

Restlessness, kicking the abdomen, switching the tail, frequent urination and straining are common signs. The passing of bloody urine containing clots of blood is considered to be almost pathognomonic of pyelonephritis.

The animal's stance may resemble that associated with traumatic pericarditis, gastritis, or indigestion.

Lesions: The urethra of infected cattle is inflamed, edematous and streaked with submucosal ecchymoses. The bladder contains considerable cellular debris, clotted and free blood, and a characteristic "sandy" deposit. The bladder wall is greatly thickened and edematous. Its mucosa is hemorrhagic, may show ulceration, and large vesicle-like swellings usually are present over most of the epithelial surface. The ureters are usually greatly enlarged, from several times their normal diameter up to 2.5 cm. The walls are thickened, edematous and hemorrhages are present. The lumina often are filled with clots of blood, pus and necrotic kidney tissue.

Although the infection may be unilateral, both kidneys are generally involved. The kidneys may be 2 to 3 times their normal size and weight. The external cortical lobulations frequently are ill-defined and the surface may be almost smooth.

The capsule may be adherent. The calyces are filled with a gray, slimy exudate, shreds of necrotic tissue, clotted blood and urine. Calculi and sand-like precipitate are present. A strong odor of ammonia is emitted. Numerous abscesses and hemorrhages occur throughout the medullary and cortical areas. Atrophy of the parenchyma and considerable fibrosis occur in advanced cases. In general, the infection is characterized by an active, extensive and diffuse necrotizing inflammatory process.

Diagnosis: The signs of the disease are most helpful in establishing a diagnosis. Generally, there are only 1 or 2 animals with pyelonephritis in the herd at any one time. Herd history may indicate that sporadic infections have occurred in the past. Pyelonephritis should be differentiated from other diseases such as leptospirosis and bacillary or postparturient hemoglobinuria, in which hematuria or hemoglobinuria are constant findings.

Rectal palpation of the bladder, ureters and kidneys will reveal the characteristic abnormalities which should establish the diagnosis. Palpation of the ureters by the vaginal route in mature cows or mares reveals a cordlike ureter often containing crepitating blood clots. The ureters are most accurately located several inches proximal to their entrance into the neck of the bladder.

The sediment of a centrifuged urine sample from an animal with pyelonephritis will contain numerous *C. renale*. A smear of this sediment stained by the Gram method will show clumps and parallel arrangements of gram-positive, pleomorphic bacterial rods. Urine from suspected cases may be cultured on bacteriologic media for the presence of *C. renale*.

Prognosis depends principally upon amount of functional kidney tissue present, virulence of the microorganism, and its susceptibility to therapy. The increased functional demand on the kidney during pregnancy may mean that cows with a marginal amount of functioning kidney tissue (approximately 30%) will die when the metabolic load is greater than can be handled.

In advanced cases, the outcome is usually unfavorable. If the clinician can detect the enlargement of the ureters before they exceed 10 mm in diameter, the prognosis may be favorable. Relapses are not uncommon, even after the animal appears to have recovered. In general, a guarded prognosis should be given.

Treatment: *C. renale*-infected animals usually respond dramatically to penicillin therapy (℞ 41, 44) for 8 to 15 days, while those infected with *E. coli* do not. The effectiveness of the therapeutic agent may be reduced in the presence of necrotic tissue debris. Therefore, the effects of therapy should be checked by bacteriologic examination of the urine sediment. To prevent relapse, treatment should be repeated if the organism is present in urine sediment a month after cessation of therapy. Other antibiotics may be of value, but critical studies of their efficacy have not been reported. In general, the sulfonamides have not proved as valuable as penicillin products in the treatment of pyelonephritis.

Routine symptomatic and supportive treatment is indicated. Special attention should be paid to keeping the cow eating and to furnishing the necessary nutritional elements to help maintain body weight. Rest from pregnancy and lactation is desirable.

URINARY CALCULI
(Urolithiasis)

Concretions formed within the urinary tract by precipitation of salts normally excreted in the urine. Although the basic causes are not well understood, it is believed that an organic matrix is present in the urinary system around which the crystalline salts are precipitated. Processes which lead to increased concentration of salts in the urine, or which alter urinary colloids believed to prevent precipitation, favor calculus formation. Predisposing factors include: (1) increased concentration of salts in urine due to reduced water intake or heavy dietary mineral consumption; (2) urinary tract infections; (3) the presence of organic debris such as fibrin, mucus, red blood cells, epithelial cells and leukocytes, all of which are favored by urinary infections and urinary stasis; (4) inherited predispositions (sex-linked at least in some instances).

Calculi occur in all species, but are commonest in cattle, sheep and dogs. Their chemical composition varies with the pH of the urine and with the species of animal. Phosphates and carbonates are easily precipitated in alkaline urine, while urates, oxalates and cystine are generally precipitated in neutral or acid urine. Calculi of **cattle** are generally calcium, magnesium and ammonium phosphates; of **sheep,** calcium, magnesium, or ammonium phosphates or silicates; of **horses,** calcium carbonate, calcium phosphate and magnesium carbonate; of **dogs** and **cats,** calcium, magnesium and ammonium phosphate or ammonium urate or calcium oxalate or cystine; of **swine,** ammonium magnesium phosphate, calcium and magnesium carbonate, magnesium phosphate or magnesium oxalate. Varying amounts of organic material may be present in any calculus.

Formation starts commonly in the bladder, less frequently in the kidney and rarely in the prostate. Ureteral and urethral calculi are in passage from the site of formation. The lodging of calculi during passage varies with the species of animal and is determined primarily by anatomical narrowing of the urinary passage. In all cases the result is irritation to the lining of the urinary tract, pain and interference with urine flow varying from partial to complete obstruction.

UROLITHIASIS IN RUMINANTS

Urolithiasis is one of the most important diseases in feeder cattle and sheep and a significant number of cases also occur in mature breeding males. Clinical urolithiasis is seen most frequently during the winter months and particularly in steers and wethers on full feed. Affected animals are usually 5 to 10 months old but it may occur much earlier or later.

Although formation is probably equal in both sexes, the short, large urethra of the female affords little opportunity for obstruction, hence the greater clinical incidence of obstruction is in males. Renal or cystic calculi are usually without noticeable clinical effect in ruminants in the absence of obstruction. Calculi originating in the kidney or bladder lodge at points where the urethra changes direction or is limited in dilatability, commonly the ischial arch and the sigmoid flexure in cattle and sheep and the urethral process in sheep. A single calculus is usually responsible for obstruction in cattle, but sheep are commonly affected with multiple calculi blocking the urethra for several centimeters. Occlusion of the urethra may lead to rupture of the urethra due to pressure necrosis or to rupture of the bladder due to the accumulating urine.

Urethral obstruction: Early urethral blockage in ruminants is expressed by restlessness, twitching of the tail and straining. Partial obstruction results in dribbling blood-stained urine. In complete obstruction, the preputial hairs are dry. Minerals may be precipitated on the preputial hairs. As blockage persists, colic-like signs develop, and the animal kicks at its abdomen, rolls on the ground, and may lie down and rise frequently. The tail is held away from the body and secondary rectal prolapse is common. A pulsating urethra is frequently observed, but is not pathognomonic. Hypersensitivity in the region of the sigmoid flexure of cattle may be evident, and deep palpation may locate the swelling resulting from the obstructing calculus. The urethral process of sheep can be prolapsed and the obstruction visualized. The bladder may be in various stages of distension, with severe distension developing 24 to 36 hours after complete blockage.

Other conditions causing signs of abdominal pain are indigestion, consumption of large quantities of cold water, digestive tract stasis or obstruction, primary enteritis, coccidiosis, rabies and rectal prolapse. Urinary tract infection often causes straining along with frequent attempts to urinate.

In sheep, amputation of the urethral process is simple and allows the immediate passage of urine. Such surgery does not interfere with the ram's breeding capability. Several other techniques for urethrostomy, which by-pass the obstruction via an incision proximal to the occlusion, are successful except that they end breeding capabilities. In breeding animals a urinary calculi retriever may be tried; a urethrostomy can still be performed if results are not successful. Postoperative antibiotics are recommended to prevent infection (℞ 41).

Ruptured urethra: Pressure necrosis and perforation of the urethral wall is common if urethral obstruction is not relieved. Urine then collects subcut. along the sheath and umbilicus to cause the characteristic swelling called **water belly.** This swelling is cold and edematous; aspiration yields a clear fluid, frequently without the smell of urine. Urine may still dribble from the sheath, but signs of abdominal pain and colic are no longer seen, and appetite and bowel function are normal. The BUN concentration begins to rise following rupture of the urethra. While complete skin necrosis is rare, sloughing may be seen due to delayed or incomplete treatment.

Instances of ruptured urethra resemble traumatic injury, subcut. abscesses, and umbilical or ventral hernias. In breeding animals, laceration of the prepuce, with resultant prolapse and infection of the sheath and subcut. tissue, may resemble the urine accumulation following urethral rupture. Hematoma of the penis must also be differentiated.

Treatment of urethral rupture is by urethrostomy and drainage of the subcut. urine. Urethrostomy is performed slightly dorsal to the site employed for relief of urethral obstruction, since hemorrhage and edema are present due to the rupture. The skin over the subcut. urine accumulation is lanced in numerous places to permit drainage for several days. Topical antiseptics (℞ 405) and fly repellents (℞ 264, 283) may be applied to these ventral wounds. Parenteral antibiotics (℞ 41) are administered postoperatively as for uncomplicated obstructions. Electrolyte (℞ 558) or dextrose solutions (℞ 556) are given to correct dehydration and promote urine flow if necessary.

Rupture of the bladder: The most serious sequela to untreated urolithiasis is rupture of the bladder. Sudden relief from the signs of urethral obstruction and pain occur at the time of rupture. The animal may then appear improved for several days before signs of uremia develop. However, dry preputial hairs indicate an absence of recent urination, and the BUN concentration will be greater than 50 mg/100 ml of blood. As urine accumulates in the peritoneal cavity, feed and water consumption decrease and the animal's abdomen becomes progressively swollen. Ballottement allows detection of the fluid, and from behind the animal the abdomen appears pear-shaped. A collapsed bladder and other abdominal organs are felt floating or partially submerged in the urine by rectal examination. Confirmation is obtained by paracentesis through the ventral abdominal wall. Urine is very irritating and will cause peritonitis. The animal is weak and depressed, and the fluid in the peritoneal cavity is red and has a strong odor of urine.

A recently ruptured bladder may be diagnosed by dry preputial hairs, collapsed bladder, a history of abdominal pain and colic-like signs. Once abdominal distension is present, rupture of the bladder must be differentiated from rumen tympany, diffuse peritonitis, tumors of the peritoneal cavity and digestive tract obstructions.

Treatment requires the establishment of ability to urinate, providing for healing of the bladder, and assisting in the correction of uremia. The use of a trocar to drain the urine from the peritoneal cavity will help relieve the uremia. A urethrostomy should be performed to provide free passage of urine. Attempts to repair the ruptured bladder have largely been unsuccessful. Spontaneous healing of the bladder frequently occurs following urethrostomy and removal of the abdominal fluid, although these animals are best salvaged within 3 to 4 months to avoid further complications. Some cases of bladder rupture treated by paracentesis and urethrostomy will fail to pass urine within 48 hours following surgery. Urine will again accumulate in the peritoneal cavity due to lack of bladder healing. Such animals may be treated by performing a cystotomy, suturing a plastic drain into the bladder, and then exteriorizing the other end of the tube through the posterior ventral abdominal wall. Antibiotic (℞ 58) and fluid therapy (℞ 556, 558) may be employed following the procedure since infection and shock are potential complications. These animals should be salvaged within a few months. Occasionally, neglected animals are examined which have a ruptured bladder and severe uremia. Treatment as outlined above may be attempted, but the prognosis is poor.

Prevention: Since the specific cause of urolithiasis is still unclear, no specific prevention is available. Management practices intended to reduce predisposing factors for calculi formation vary widely. In all cases, abundant water should be constantly be available and should be heated in cold weather. It is useful to further increase water consumption by including 5 to 10% sodium chloride in the ration. The addition of a broad-spectrum antibiotic (℞ 11) to the ration has also been useful to control urolithiasis in certain instances. Compounds, such as ammonium chloride (℞ 541), to alter urinary pH are available, but have not been widely successful. Careful observation of susceptible animals by experienced persons several times daily will allow early detection and more successful treatment.

UROLITHIASIS IN DOGS AND CATS

Urolithiasis is relatively uncommon in cats. The debris obstructing the penile urethra of male cats is not organized as are uroliths and the term urolithiasis does not accurately describe the problem. Distinct uroliths do occasionally form in the bladders of cats, occur more frequently in females and are usually phosphate calculi. The treatment and attempts at prevention are the same as they are for dogs.

Renal calculi in dogs are encountered far less frequently than cystic calculi. During the early formation of renoliths, signs are often absent. Discovery of such renoliths is usually through a radiograph taken of the abdomen for another purpose. Pyuria, microscopic hematuria and bacteriuria may be present if urinalysis is performed at this time. Extensive pyelitis or pyelonephritis associated with renoliths may cause depression, anorexia, hematuria and reluctance of the patient to move. There may be pain when the area of the kidneys is palpated. If extensive infection is present there may be fever, palpable enlargement of the affected kidney and a marked leukocytosis with considerable immaturity in the neutrophil series. Signs of uremia are ordinarily absent unless both kidneys are extensively involved, or unless the opposite kidney is absent or otherwise seriously diseased. The treatment is usually surgical removal of the affected kidney. Nephrotomy is indicated if the opposite kidney is absent, also affected, or seriously impaired in function.

Ureteral calculi are uncommon in dogs or cats. When they occur, the signs are depression, fever and pain as determined by abdominal palpation. The dog walks with his back arched and has an anxious expression. Complete obstruction permits no urine to enter the bladder and the urinalysis is normal. In partial obstruction of the ureter, hematuria, pyuria and proteinuria is usually found on urinalysis. Both partial and complete ureteral obstruction will lead to varying degrees of hydronephrosis. The diagnosis is usually confirmed with radiographs. The calculus is best visualized on the lateral radiograph in a well-prepared patient. The use of a contrast agent (R 637) may aid in visualizing a calculus. An excretory urogram has the additional advantage of helping to assess function in the opposite kidney, which is of prime importance since the usual treatment for ureteral calculi is nephrectomy. Efforts to salvage the affected kidney and ureter should be reserved for those instances in which the opposite kidney is absent or seriously diseased. The prognosis, in these circumstances, is less favorable. Postoperative care in cases of nephrectomy for either ureteral or renal calculi should consist of adequate fluid intake, either orally or parenterally, to result in good urine flow. Because infection is such a common finding in urolithiasis in dogs, antibacterial drugs (R 7, 41, 84, 91) should be routinely administered until several days after the urinalysis is normal. Additional urinalyses should be performed at monthly intervals for several months to detect possible recurrence of infection. The specific antibacterial drug should be selected on the basis of results of culture and sensitivity testing.

Cystic calculi: The urinary bladder is the most common location for uroliths in dogs. Signs are usually dysuria, hematuria and frequent attempts to urinate with only small quantities passed at each attempt. Cystoliths can be palpated in most instances either by feeling multiple stones grate against each other or by palpating the hard, unyielding solitary cystolith. Rectal palpation should also be performed to be sure no calculus is in the pelvic urethra. The urinalysis reflects the accompanying cystitis; abnormal findings consist of increased numbers of leukocytes, erythrocytes, proteinuria, often an elevated pH and frequently bacteriuria. Generalized signs, leukocytes and abnormal blood chemistry ordinarily do not occur.

The diagnosis can be confirmed with radiographs. Usually a flat radiograph is adequate, but a pneumocystogram or a positive-contrast radiograph using 2.5 to 5% diatrizoate sodium (R 637) may be helpful in visualizing radiolucent calculi.

The treatment for cystoliths is cystotomy followed by adequate antibiotic therapy (R 41, 91) selected as described for postoperative care for renoliths. Long-term, carefully monitored therapy is helpful in reducing recurrences.

Urethral Calculi occur predominantly in male dogs, with the calculi lodging primarily at the posterior end of the os penis, infrequently at the ischial arch. The condition is a complication of cystitis and cystic calculi associated with the inability of the male dog to pass calculi. The signs of urethral calculi are straining, frequent attempts to urinate resulting in the passage of only small amounts of bloody urine or none at all. The animal is restless, walks in a crouched position and appears uncomfortable. A hard painful bladder can be palpated in the posterior abdomen. If not relieved, the animal becomes progressively more depressed, and shows signs of uremia (vomiting, depression, ammoniacal odor to breath, episcleral injection, dehydration, elevated BUN and creatinine concentrations). Such severe distension of the bladder results in serious loss of bladder tone, and days or weeks may be required before normal tone returns. Eventually, the bladder may rupture. The presence of a ruptured bladder can be confirmed radiographically by injecting air into the bladder, then taking a standing lateral radiograph and finding the air in the dorsal portion of the peritoneal cavity.

An attempt may be made to relieve the obstruction by having an assistant compress the pelvic urethra on the pubis. Sterile saline is then injected through a teat infusion tube while sealing the urethral orifice around the infusion tube with the fingers. The saline dilates the urethra. If the pressure on the urethral orifice is relieved suddenly and the infusion tube withdrawn, in some animals the calculi will be flushed out with the saline. The compression of the pelvic urethra by the assistant prevents the saline from entering the bladder. Sedation of the dog may be necessary.

In some dogs a fiber catheter can be passed into the bladder to relieve the distension. If the dog is severely depressed and uremic, the catheter should be left in place for one or more days. The catheter can be held in place by circling it several times with adhesive tape and then suturing through the tape and the prepuce. An Elizabethan collar may be necessary. When the condition of the animal is improved, the catheter is withdrawn and the calculi are then removed by urethrotomy. If a catheter cannot be passed, an emergency urethrotomy may be performed under local anesthesia to relieve the obstruction. The cystoliths are removed by cystotomy at a later time when the condition of the patient is less critical. Postoperative care consists of antibacterial drugs and careful reevaluation as described for renal calculi.

Prevention of Urolithiasis in Dogs: The approach to preventing recurrence of uroliths varies with the composition of the urolith. For all calculi the following generalities have some use:

1) Following surgery, control infection as described above, selecting the antibacterial drug on the basis of culture and sensitivity testing. Results should be evaluated by observing the patient and by repeated urinalyses until the results are normal. Additional urinalyses should be performed to ensure against relapse. 2) Induce polyuria and polydipsia by adding additional salt to food, water (¼ teaspoon per pint) or by administering as tablets. The dose is 1 to 10 gm daily in 2 or 3 divided doses depending upon the size of the dog. An increased urine flow is helpful in preventing excessive concentration and precipitation of minerals in the urine. For phosphate calculi, a diet restricting intake of minerals, especially calcium and phosphorus has been advocated though the benefits are not clear cut.

D-Penicillamine given in the feed at 7.5 mg/lb body wt, b.i.d., appears to be of specific benefit in preventing recurrence of cystine calculi, which are caused by a renal tubular defect in the reabsorption of cystine resulting in a persistent cystinuria. The disease is considered to be an inherited metabolic defect, and therefore affected dogs should not be used as breeding stock. Acidifiers, especially those containing methionine, should not be given since a low urine pH enhances cystine precipitation and oral methionine may increase cystine excretion. Urinary acidifiers should also be avoided for urate urolithiasis since urates are less soluble in an acid urine.

PREVENTION AND TERMINATION OF PREGNANCY IN THE BITCH

The commonest and most popular method of preventing pregnancy in the bitch is ovariohysterectomy. This is unacceptable in breeding stock and has the disadvantage of subjecting the animal to the risks of surgery, as well as possibly being associated with urinary incontinence in later years. The progestagens will suppress estrus and thus pregnancy, but it is unwise to employ these agents in breeding bitches as the long-term effects are uncertain. Progesterone is useful to suppress estrus temporarily.

Pregnancy may be prevented following undesired mating by administration of estrogens. Diethylstilbestrol (℞ 162) and estradiol (℞ 164) are effective in preventing implantation if given within 5 days after mating, but the signs of estrus frequently persist for 2 to 3 weeks. A more serious complication of estrogen therapy is the development of aplastic anemia or a hemorrhagic syndrome due to thrombocytopenia following excessive doses. The various repellents are of little value in repelling males attracted to a bitch in estrus.

Pregnancy can be terminated safely by ovariohysterectomy until the middle of the term. After this, the risks involved are unwarranted. Other methods of surgical interference are seldom performed in bitches because of the lack of knowledge about their effectiveness, complications and long-term effects.

DISEASES OF THE REPRODUCTIVE TRACT (SM. AN.)

HYPERESTRINISM
(Nymphomania)

A condition arising from the excessive production of estrogenic hormones in which the female is attractive to males, but lacks sexual desire herself. Active ovarian cysts are usually the source of the estrogen. The primary cause, however, may be in pituitary or adrenal dysfunction.

The bitch or queen suffering from hyperestrinism is usually nervous, irritable and sometimes vicious. The bitch will mount and ride males, toys and members of the family, but will rarely permit copulation. The queen shows intense and exaggerated manifestations of estrus and copulates freely. The vulva is usually swollen, reddened and occasionally there may be a bloody discharge. Such animals are commonly sterile.

Prolonged periods of excessive sexual desire, usually without copulation, and without conception if breeding is permitted, together with the swollen appearance of the vulva, indicate nymphomania. Since infection of the vulva, vagina and cervix can produce discharges having an odor which excites males sexually, careful examination of these structures is necessary in arriving at a diagnosis.

Injection of chorionic gonadotropin, 100 to 500 IU to luteinize the cysts and establish a regular estrual cycle, has been tried with variable results. Ovariectomy is the most satisfactory treatment. In valuable breeding animals one may perform a unilateral ovariectomy if the cysts are confined to one ovary. Successful pregnancies have been reported following this procedure. If vulvitis, vaginitis, or cervicitis is the etiologic factor, treatment is as indicated for these diseases (q.v., p. 860). The use of 17-alpha hydroxyprogesterone (1.8 mg/lb body wt, orally, daily) will often suppress the signs but does not effect a cure.

Satyriasis: The comparable problem in the male, exaggerated sexual desire, can occasionally be troublesome in dogs because the frequent attempts to mount other animals, objects or persons are annoying. Administration of an estrogen, obedience training or, ultimately, castration, usually results in alleviation of signs.

METRITIS

An acute or chronic inflammation of the uterus.

Etiology: Metritis usually results from infection acquired at the time of parturition or estrus, or shortly thereafter. Retained fetal membranes, dead fetuses, blood and exudate provide suitable substrates for bacteria which gain entry through the open cervix. Sometimes, infection is introduced by careless use of instruments, and it may also occur at the time of breeding, being introduced either by the stud or attempts to dilate a small vagina. The organisms causing the infection are the common gram-negative bacteria found in the feces, plus streptococci and staphylococci. Hyperplastic endometritis is discussed under the heading PYOMETRA IN DOGS (q.v., p. 841).

Clinical Findings: Acutely ill animals exhibit fever, polydipsia, depression, vomiting and sometimes diarrhea. Occasionally there is a uterine discharge which may be mucopurulent or bloody.

The signs of chronic metritis are not constant. A persistent or intermittent uterine discharge may be apparent. Failure to conceive or the delivery of dead or weak pups, which die soon after birth, is suggestive. Sometimes the condition is asymptomatic.

Diagnosis: A history of abortion, dystocia, or even normal parturition accompanies most cases of acute metritis. Occasionally, a thickened, indurated uterus can be palpated through the abdominal wall. Radiography may reveal a uterus of abnormal size or density. A leukocytosis is usually found, especially in acute metritis. Repeated failure to conceive or the delivery of weak or dead pups suggests chronic metritis. A history of frequent or prolonged estrual bleeding indicates endometrial changes that can be regarded as chronic metritis.

Treatment: Treatment of acute metritis includes supportive therapy, such as parenteral fluids, and a prolonged course of antibiotic therapy. Very small repeated doses of posterior pituitary hormone (℞ 174) may increase uterine tone and help it to discharge the contents. This is, however, contraindicated if the uterus is grossly distended. Introduction of 5 to 15 ml of 0.2% nitrofurazone into the uterus via a sterile metal bitch catheter may be useful. A helpful procedure in acute metritis when hemorrhage is not excessive is to combine an antibiotic with estrogen (R 163): the antibiotic may be penicillin 10,000 u/lb daily IM, chloramphenicol 15 mg/lb daily subcut. divided into 2 or 3 doses, or tetracycline 3 to 5 mg/lb given IV every 12 hours; the estrogen is given until signs of estrus appear. This increases the antibiotic concentration in the uterus and facilitates a more rapid debridement of the endometrium. Intensive antibiotic therapy is most effective when used at the beginning of estrus. The treatment of chronic metritis is the same except that hormone therapy is contraindicated and prolonged treatment with antibiotics is often necessary. Ovariohysterectomy is indicated if resistance to chemotherapy is encountered.

PYOMETRA IN DOGS
(Hyperplastic endometritis)

An accumulation of pus within the uterus accompanied by hyperplastic changes in the uterine mucosa.

Etiology: This condition most frequently is encountered in bitches over 5 years of age. The disease is attributed to ovarian dysfunction with increased progesterone secretion. The contents of the affected uterus may be sterile though in some cases there is gross bacterial contamination. The organisms most commonly found are *Escherichia coli* and *Streptococcus*. *E. coli* is seldom to be found in the purulent material, but can usually be isolated from the hyperplastic endometrium. Most evidence suggests metritis to be most commonly a bacterial infection while pyometra appears to be of endocrine origin. Pyometra is less common in cats and can remain asymptomatic for long periods.

Clinical Findings: Anorexia is usually the first sign followed by depression, polydipsia and polyuria. Vomiting frequently follows drinking and the animal will drink and then vomit as long as water is provided. At this stage, the respiratory rate is increased and the temperature may be elevated, but, as the condition progresses, the temperature falls and finally becomes subnormal. Progressive weakness develops and eventually the animal is unable to stand. The abdomen is distended and pain may be manifested on palpation. Discharges often have a characteristic "sickly-sweet" odor and small quantities may accumulate on the hair around the vulva and on the tail. The vulva is often enlarged and occasionally a persistent diarrhea accompanies the disease. Neglected or untreated animals commonly die.

Diagnosis: There is usually a moderate to severe neutrophilic leukocytosis with immature cells being common. The distended uterine horns are easily detected by palpation. Radiographic confirmation is a simple procedure, the pus-filled cornua being clearly evident. Many animals with pyometra also have renal failure and its associated biochemical changes. These findings, together with a history of nonpregnancy or pseudocyesis and the clinical signs, point to a fairly positive diagnosis. A salient point in the history is the occurrence of signs 2 to 8 weeks after estrus.

Treatment: Ovariohysterectomy should be undertaken as soon as the electrolyte and fluid imbalance is corrected. During the delay occasioned by the replacement of fluids and electrolytes, antibiotics should be administered in heavy dosage. The extent of dehydration should be estimated (mild—5% of body weight, moderate—8 to 10%, severe—12%) and that quantity of replacement fluid (lactated Ringer's solution, ℞ 565) should be administered over a period of several hours. A maintenance dose of 20 ml/lb/day in small dogs to 10 ml/lb/day in large dogs should then be given during the remainder of the time parenteral fluids are needed. If excess fluid losses occur such as in polyuria, vomiting or diarrhea, additional fluids should be given. If the weight is carefully monitored, one can detect fluid accumulation by excessive gain, or inadequate fluid therapy by excessive loss. After surgery all patients should be monitored for signs of renal failure. Antibiotics, such as penicillin and streptomycin combinations (℞ 41) or chlortetracycline (℞ 11), should be given. Medical treatment alone may be attempted on selected patients; satisfactory results, however, are rare. Hormones, such as diethylstilbestrol (℞ 163), followed by posterior pituitary hormone (℞ 174) 3 or 4 days later, may be administered in an attempt to evacuate the uterus.

VAGINAL HYPERPLASIA ASSOCIATED WITH ESTRUS

Enlargement of the mucosa of part of the vaginal floor or wall in bitches during estrus believed to be due to estrogen overstimulation. The condition occurs in bitches of all breeds, but is most commonly seen in brachycephalic types, particularly Boxers.

The excessive hyperplastic reaction usually involves a small portion of the vaginal mucosa, other areas showing only the normal changes of estrus. Difficulty in breeding or in urination often calls attention to the hyperplasia. Frequently, the mass protrudes through the vulvar orifice.

The coexistence or recent history of estrus and the appearance of the swelling are diagnostic. Examination reveals that the mass originates from the vaginal floor or wall, usually between the cervix and urethra. The condition may be confused with tumor or prolapse of the uterus or vagina. In hyperplasia, however, the mass is dome-shaped and often pedunculated, while in prolapse of the vagina or uterus the protruding tissue is more voluminous and broadly based.

The swelling usually subsides soon after estrus. Spaying will hasten involution of the residual hypertrophy and prevent its recurrence. Both spaying and surgical removal of the tissue may be necessary with massive hypertrophy. Surgical removal is always indicated when a large, protruding mass becomes abraded, ulcerated or infected. In the brood bitch, surgical removal is usually practiced, but the owner should be cautioned that the condition may recur at subsequent estrous periods. Such patients may be bred by artificial insemination.

STERILITY IN DOGS

In the study of infertility, the dog has been largely neglected. Consequently, little information is available. Even less appears to be known about the anomalies of reproduction in the cat.

The nature of the estrous cycle in the bitch, gonadal malfunctions and certain more or less well-defined anomalies in sexual behavior in both sexes, are referred to in REPRODUCTIVE PHENOMENA, p. 770, FALSE PREGNANCY, p. 845, ARTIFICIAL INSEMINATION IN DOGS, p. 786, and other headings in this chapter. In the bitch, endocrine disturbances resulting in infertility may be of several varieties and it is impossible to make sharp distinctions between them. The prolonged and excessive production of estrogen usually coincides with the presence of ovarian cysts. Ovariohysterectomy is the best method of treatment, but chorionic gonadotropin (℞ 167) or progesterone (℞ 165) therapy may be attempted.

Hypoestrinism sometimes results in continuous anestrus, or in "silent heat" with absence of gross proestrual bleeding. For this condition, estrogens (℞ 163) may be helpful. However, they should be used with care or serious repression of ovarian function may result. Some bitches have abnormally long anestrus and may respond to equine gonadotropin (℞ 168).

Hypoprogesteronism, leading to failure of implantation or early abortion, is believed to be the cause of infertility in some instances. In these, progesterone, in doses of 5 to 25 mg, IM, 2 or 3 times weekly during the early stages of pregnancy, may be helpful.

Hypoandrogenism in males may result in impotence. The desire for coitus may be increased by the administration of testosterone (R 178) 1 or 2 days before breeding.

Congenital defects or **tumors** of the reproductive system of either sex may result in breeding failures. **Infections** of the female genital system, such as vaginitis, acute and chronic metritis and pyometra, may result in infertility. Similarly, in the male, balanitis, orchitis, epididymitis and prostatitis may result in reduced fertility. Brucellosis (q.v., p. 353) has been shown to produce sterility following orchitis.

Psychologic and environmental factors also influence fertility. House pets may be reluctant to breed and rough handling or distractions during supervised breeding may affect the conception rates. Close confinement of male dogs may result in temporary sterility. Inanition and obesity may affect reproduction, but the influence of nutrition is apparently not of great importance. Senile changes affect the reproductive capacity of both sexes. The senile dog may be completely infertile.

The following suggestions may be helpful in improving fertility in dogs: (1) Both male and female should be in a good state of health and in good, lean, physical condition. (2) The breeding should take place in an atmosphere free from unnecessary distractions. (3) The correct breeding time should be accurately determined. The best conception rates usually occur when bitches are bred twice, within 48 hours, during the first 4 days of true estrus. The examination of daily vaginal smears may help to define more accurately the optimum time for breeding (see ARTIFICIAL INSEMINATION IN DOGS, p. 786). (4) The reproductive organs of the male should be examined and, if necessary, a specimen of semen collected for assessment of quality (see SEMEN QUALITY AND MALE FERTILITY, p. 775). (5) Artificial insemination may be used when physical or psychic abnormalities preclude successful natural mating.

INCONTINENCE OF URINE DUE TO HYPOESTRINISM

Inasmuch as the disease is seen principally in spayed bitches, the cause is thought to be hypoestrinism.

Clinical Findings and Diagnosis: Involuntary urination usually occurs when the animal is relaxed or asleep. Urine is frequently found where the animal has been sitting, or the animal may unconsciously dribble urine when in motion. The perineal hair often is urine-soaked and the skin scalded. In addition to intermittent incontinence, the animals will urinate normally.

That the animal is a spayed female and that the passage of urine is an unconscious act are important. Differential diagnosis includes unilateral ureterovaginal fistula, neoplasm of the bladder neck and bladder atony. The mechanism of this condition is unknown. Other causes of incontinence such as ectopic ureters and neurologic causes of incontinence must be eliminated.

Treatment: Diethylstilbestrol is administered at the rate of 0.1 to 1.0 mg daily to effect. Large dogs may be started on a high initial oral or parenteral dose of up to 5 mg the first day or two. Oral dosage is as effective as parenteral and has the advantage of being adaptable to home administration. When the animal is no longer incontinent, the dose is gradually reduced to the minimum maintenance dose. It is important that the clinician take time to explain to the owner that the disease will require lifelong treatment, that the animal can be a pleasant house pet with the cooperation of the owner, and that signs of estrus and a bleeding tendency can result from prolonged or unecessarily high doses of diethylstilbestrol. Minor accidental or surgical wounds bleed excessively when animals are given continual high doses of diethylstilbestrol. It should also be noted that excessive doses of estrogens will cause depression of bone marrow activity and possibly an aplastic anemia.

In a few instances the dosage required to control incontinence may be great enough to produce estrus. In such cases, combining stilbestrol with testosterone may control the incontinence and suppress the signs of estrus. In some spayed females, stilbestrol does not control the incontinence. In such cases, a possibility exists that a postoperative adhesion between the uterine stump and the bladder may be responsible for the incontinence.

FALSE PREGNANCY IN DOGS
(Pseudopregnancy, Pseudocyesis)

The appearance of the signs of pregnancy and lactation in the bitch at approximately 60 days after estrus. The syndrome can follow the first or any estrus and tends to recur during subsequent estrus cycles. It may be complicated by uterine lesions. False pregnancy is associated with persistent corpora lutea but the mechanisms responsible are unknown. The role of the hypothalamus and pituitary is uncertain. Prolonged activity of the corpora lutea is thought to be responsible for the clinical signs.

The signs are those of intensified and prolonged metestrus and vary in intensity from slight distension of the abdomen and hyperplasia of the mammary glands to those of impending parturition. A serous secretion may appear at the nipples or lactation may begin, sometimes complicated by mastitis. Changes in temperament are frequent. Some bitches make a nest in a dark area, "mother" a toy or shoe, etc., and refuse to eat or come when called. Digestive disturbances and mild hypothermia or hyperthermia may also occur. The history, abdominal palpation and radiographs can serve to exclude the possibility of true pregnancy.

Mild cases need not be treated. Pregnancy may lessen the intensity of subsequent episodes. Ovariohysterectomy can be performed once lactation ceases. Testosterone (R 178), or estrogens, particularly diethylstilbestrol (R 162) or a combination of both have been employed with variable results. The combination may be superior and tends to avoid the signs of estrus caused by estrogens. Hormones should not be used in breeding bitches as they probably increase the severity of concurrent endometrial pathology. Progesterone (R 165) has also been used. Self-nursing should be prevented through the use of suitable restraints.

DISEASES OF THE PROSTATE GLAND
BENIGN OR CYSTIC HYPERPLASIA

This is the most common disease of the prostate gland of dogs. Sixty percent of all dogs over 6 years of age have some degree of prostatic hyperplasia, although the majority of these animals show no signs. Prostatic hyperplasia in dogs is usually of a cystic type; these cysts may reach an enormous size. The etiology of the condition is unknown, but it may be the result of endocrine imbalance.

Clinical Findings: The principal signs are tenesmus and constipation. Urinary signs, such as frequent attempts to urinate, hematuria, distension and atony of the bladder occur infrequently. Alteration of the gait of the animal frequently accompanies prostatic enlargement. There may be a definite lameness in a hind leg, or weakness may be evident in the hindquarters.

Perineal hernia may occur in association with prostatic enlargement. Although all dogs with perineal hernia do not have enlarged prostates and vice versa, the association between the 2 conditions is so frequent that prostatic enlargement should always be suspected in cases of perineal hernia.

Diagnosis: While an idea of the size of the prostate can be obtained by simultaneous rectal and abdominal palpation, the only accurate determination of its size is by radiography. The introduction of contrast material (radiopaque substance or air) into the bladder will provide sufficient contrast to outline the prostate. Radiographs, while showing definite abnormalities of size and shape of the gland, cannot differentiate all the disease conditions of the prostate.

Treatment: Castration is the most simple and direct treatment. Reduction in the size of the prostate may be expected in most cases within 2 months. Prostatic atrophy may be hastened by the administration of small (0.1 mg) doses of diethylstilbestrol, given intermittently. Continuous administration of large doses of synthetic estrogens in dogs may result in squamous metaplasia or cystic enlargement of the prostate.

Benign hyperplasia with large cyst formation is not likely to respond to diethylstilbestrol. In these cases and in those that do not respond to castration and estrogen therapy, prostatectomy may be considered.

Cystic Uterus Masculinus

This condition is part of the complex of conditions that result in enlargement of the prostate gland.

The size of these cysts, which often exceeds 5 cm, suggests that they are not merely dilations or confluency of smaller cysts but vestiges of the müllerian ducts, the uterus masculinus, that have become activated to secrete.

Unlike the reaction of the enlarged acini of cystic hyperplasia to estrogens, i.e., to become smaller, these cysts of the uterus masculinus enlarge and may become massive. It is imperative, therefore, if estrogen therapy is employed to reduce the size of a hyperplastic gland, that the dosage be minimal and that the patient be closely observed for untoward reaction.

The cyst is most easily identified radiographically. The urine should be cultured to determine the sensitivity of any organisms. The urine should also be examined for the presence of malignant epithelial cells.

The treatment is surgical. Estrogen therapy is contraindicated.

SUPPURATIVE PROSTATITIS
(Prostatic abscess)

Inflammation of the prostate is not uncommon in dogs. Whether suppuration occurs will depend upon the type of organism involved in the inflammatory process.

The route of infection may be ascending or descending. It is presumed that most prostatic infections are secondary to urinary-tract infections.

The signs of prostatitis are similar to those previously described for benign prostatic hyperplasia. In addition, however, these animals show an elevation of temperature and pain upon abdominal or rectal palpation of the prostate. If the finger can reach the inflamed gland, the prostate is found to be warm, sensitive and fluctuant. A blood count may reveal leukocytosis, and white blood cells as well as bacteria are found in the urine. By rectal massage of the prostate, exudate can usually be collected for microscopic examination. Not only does this procedure confirm the site of the inflammatory reaction, but it allows one to characterize the exudate.

The diagnosis is based upon the clinical signs and upon radiographic evidence of prostatic enlargement.

PROSTATIC CYSTS

Blockage of prostatic ducts may result in accumulation of secretions and cyst formation.

The development of clinical signs usually occurs when the cyst is of sufficient size to cause pressure on adjacent organs. The syndrome may resemble benign prostatic hyperplasia or, if the cyst becomes infected, the signs may be similar to those of prostatic abscess. Some cysts attain a huge size and are readily detected by abdominal palpation in the posterior abdomen. They must then be distinguished, both by palpation and by radiography, from the urinary bladder. A pneumocystogram or the use of a radiopaque catheter may be helpful in making this distinction.

Aspiration of the contents of the cyst has been recommended, but this technique is frequently followed by recurrence. Some cysts are attached to the prostate gland by a relatively small stalk, making surgical removal easier. Marsupialization of the cyst has been reported to be of benefit in a few instances. Castration may be of some benefit. If the cyst is infected, antibiotics should be used as indicated by culture and sensitivity testing.

PROSTATIC NEOPLASMS

Several types of primary neoplasms have been encountered in the prostate gland. The prostate may also be the site of metastatic tumors, e.g., lymphosarcoma.

Primary carcinoma of the prostate is not rare and it is to be expected that with increasing numbers of older dogs there will be a corresponding increase in prostatic neoplasms.

The signs of prostatic neoplasm parallel those of the other prostatic diseases. True urinary incontinence may be present. Together with the usual signs of prostatic disease, radiographic studies give the best diagnostic evidence. Prostatic carcinomas frequently spread to the bony pelvis and extend into the bladder or ureters. Metastasis has usually occurred before a diagnosis is established. The animal should be examined very carefully for metastasis before surgery is attempted. Castration and treatment with estrogens has been recommended as a palliative treatment for prostatic carcinoma.

PROSTATIC CALCULI

This is relatively rare; when it does occur, it is often in conjunction with cystic calculi. The cause of primary prostatic calculi is poorly understood. The calculi consist of bacteria, tissue debris and mineral deposits. The signs associated with prostatic calculi are those common to other prostatic and urinary-tract diseases, e.g., hematuria, pain, frequent urination and constipation. Radiography provides diagnostic confirmation since the calculi are obvious. Surgical removal of the calculi from the prostatic parenchyma, followed by suitable antibiotic or chemotherapeutic measures, is the only treatment.

CANINE TRANSMISSIBLE VENEREAL TUMOR

Tumors usually found on or near the genitalia. Occasionally they occur on the face, shoulders and other regions. It is a venereal disease, with most evidence suggesting that the transmission is by cell transplantation. There is little evidence to date to support the viral etiology that has been proposed.

Spontaneous regression of the tumor may occur. Metastasis is occasionally reported, most often to the regional lymph nodes, but infrequently to internal organs and to the eye. Transmission readily occurs through coitus, and dogs of all ages are susceptible. The tumors are first noted as small hyperemic nodules which gradually increase in size. There is usually a broad base of attachment with the surface being lobulated or ulcerated. During rapid growth, the tumor has a bright-red color. Later when ulceration occurs, a serosanguineous discharge, possibly accompanied by some suppuration, is present. In the male, the tumors are located most frequently on the penis or prepuce, less often on the scrotum or perineum. The vulva and vagina are the usual sites of the tumor in the female.

The recommended treatment is surgical removal, preferably by electrocautery to minimize chances of reinoculation. Radiotherapy has been used with apparent benefit at doses of 1000 to 2000 r in 2 to 4 divided doses. Additional evaluation of this approach to treatment is needed. Whole blood or serum from recovered dogs has also been advocated.

DISEASES OF THE URINARY SYSTEM (SM. AN.)

CYSTITIS

This common bladder disease is usually caused by bacterial infection, most commonly by ascension of *E. coli* or *Proteus* from the lower urinary tract. In cats, the disease has been transmitted by inoculating other cats with a bacteria-free filtrate of urine from affected cats and also by the inoculation of a virus isolated from affected animals. Urinary stasis, neurologic derangements of micturition and acquired or congenital defects of the bladder wall are often predisposing factors. Iatrogenic infection by catheterization is not unknown.

Clinical Findings: Cystitis is characterized by frequent urination, hematuria, dysuria, straining and unproductive attempts to urinate. Frequency is less obvious to the owner of the male dog because of its natural tendency to urinate often. Housetrained pets often will signal their desire to go out more frequently than before. However, mild chronic cystitis frequently causes a housebroken animal to violate its training without showing urgency. Hematuria is most evident in the last part of the voided sample. The bladder often is in a state of spasm, or the wall may be thickened.

In chronic cystitis, the signs are similar, but not as pronounced except that the incidence of hematuria is greater and the bladder wall thicker.

Diagnosis: The history usually is revealing, although an unobservant or embarrassed owner may confuse the animal's attempts to urinate with attempts to defecate, and hence interpret the condition as constipation or diarrhea. Palpation disclosing a distended bladder suggests urethral obstruction.

Palpation of a thickened, or a small, firm contracted bladder suggests cystitis. Examination of the prostate in male dogs should be routine to eliminate or confirm the possibility of complicating prostatic disease. The prostate may be examined by digital and abdominal palpation; however, radiographic studies are necessary for accurate diagnosis. A pneumocystogram or injection of a 5% solution of a contrast medium into the bladder is particularly helpful in detecting abnormalities of the bladder. The passage of catheters may reveal the presence of urethral calculi or strictures. Urine sediment contains white blood cells, red blood cells, bacteria and transitional epithelial cells. Common invading organisms are *E. coli, Pseudomonas aeruginosa, Proteus,* streptococci and staphylococci.

Treatment: Urinalysis, especially pH determination, is desirable as a prerequisite to rational therapy. In cystitis, the urine is frequently alkaline. Altering the pH to acid has a useful bacteriostatic effect and also tends to halt precipitation of crystalline sediment. Acidification is usually attempted with any one of several agents (℞ 541, 542, 596, 600), the dose to be increased until urine tests by litmus or nitrazine paper indicate a constantly acid urine. A high-protein (meat) diet will assist in keeping the urine acid. In the absence of antibiotic sensitivity tests, a fairly successful empirical procedure is to treat the patient with one of the proven urinary bacteriostatic agents, such as sulfisoxazole (℞ 91) or nitrofurantoin (℞ 98) and to change the treatment, if necessary, after a few days' trial. Chemotherapeutic agents, such as the sulfonamides, nitrofurantoin, and the antibiotics, such as streptomycin (℞ 54), chlortetracycline (℞ 11) and chloramphenicol (℞ 7) that are eliminated by way of the urinary tract, may have therapeutic value. Chloramphenicol appears to be particularly effective. Some of the new semisynthetic penicillins such as ampicillin (℞ 3) are highly effective against gram-negative bacteria. Occasionally, bladder irrigations with nitrofurazone solution (1:9) are useful in treating chronic cystitis. Sufficient solution should be injected slowly through a catheter to achieve only a moderate dilatation of the bladder. Ordinarily, infections infrequently ascend from bladder to kidney, but inept irrigation technique can force infection into the ureters.

If additional bacteriostatic therapy is desirable, a urinary antiseptic that functions in an acid medium, such as methenamine mandelate (℞ 543), may be administered. In all cases of cystitis, the treatment should be continued for at least a few days after signs subside; animals with persistent cases may require several weeks of therapy.

Urethritis: This is rarely diagnosed as a separate entity; it is usually a complication of other diseases.

ATONY OF THE BLADDER

Loss of tone of the muscular coat of the bladder wall is common in male dogs and cats, usually as a sequela to interference with urination by urethral obstruction. Urine retention with distension and atonicity of the bladder is a common and grave sequela to posterior paralysis (q.v., p. 630) (trauma of the spinal cord). Acute or chronic distension of the bladder fatigues the muscle fibers of the bladder wall so muscle contractility is lost for varying periods or permanently.

Frequent, and mostly unsuccessful, attempts to urinate characterize a recently developed case of atony and may be misinterpreted as a sign of cystitis. More commonly, there are few if any attempts to urinate, but a more or less constant dribbling from an inert, overloaded bladder.

Diagnosis is based on the presence of a large, full bladder from which the urine can be easily expressed. When empty, the organ feels like a collapsed balloon, the walls failing to contract as in a normal bladder. The diagnosis is easily confirmed by radiography.

Constant or, at least, frequent emptying of the bladder is required and the primary cause of the condition (urethral obstruction) must be eliminated if possible. Existing bladder infection should be appropriately treated. Distension of the bladder must be prevented for a period sufficient to allow the muscles to regain their tone (usually 5 to 10 days). Bethanechol chloride (℞ 635) may be useful. In refractory cases where muscle tone does not return, frequent manual expression is necessary or surgical urinary diversion is used.

HYDRONEPHROSIS

Hydronephrosis is characterized by a dilatation of the renal pelvis caused by partial or complete obstruction to outflow of urine in one or both kidneys. When the obstruction is acute, complete and bilateral, less extensive changes in the kidneys occur because the period of survival is too short. In unilateral or partial obstruction the animal survives long enough to have severe pressure atrophy of the renal parenchyma and cystic enlargement of the kidney. Hydro-ureter is a common accompaniment and is seen when the obstruction occurs lower in the tract. The condition is not infrequent and occurs in all species.

Urinary outflow obstruction may result from infections with inflammation of the pelvis, ureter, bladder or less often the urethra. Mechanical obstruction of the urinary tract may be produced by calculi or tumors, or by external pressure on the ureters, urethra, or neck of the bladder by an abdominal tumor, a gravid uterus, or by prostatic enlargement.

Swine may be predisposed to hydronephrosis by the conformation of the bladder. In cattle, a distended rumen may displace the left kidney and cause sharp curvature of, or pressure on, the corresponding ureter. Prostatic disease in the dog may cause enough obstruction of the urethra to result in hydronephrosis. Calculi are important etiologically.

The condition which is unilateral commonly goes undiagnosed by virtue of compensatory hypertrophy of the other kidney, which maintains renal function. Signs of vomiting, pain upon palpation and anorexia may be seen in cases of acute and complete obstruction. Infection may supervene and complicate the diagnosis. The fluid pressure produces atrophy of the functional kidney tissue and there is chronic inflammation of the interstitial tissue with fibrosis and lymphocytic infiltration. The papillae of the medulla disappear first; later, even the cortex may atrophy, leaving only interlobular connective tissue, persistent glomeruli and blood vessels. The affected kidney eventually becomes a grossly enlarged, functionless sac filled with urine or serous fluid. The enlarged kidney may become palpable through the abdominal wall in small animals or per rectum in large animals. Bilateral hydronephrosis produces renal insufficiency and terminal uremia. X-ray examination and IV pyelograms are useful to grossly determine the residual renal mass.

The primary objective is to reestablish the flow of urine by removing the obstruction or alleviating its cause.

GLOMERULONEPHRITIS

An inflammatory lesion of the glomerulus and associated vasculature, more common than had been assumed earlier. The cause is unknown, but it has been hypothesized that there is an immunologic basis for the disease. Histologically it is characterized by diffuse inflammation and thickening of the glomerular capillary basement membranes. This condition commonly leads to progressive renal failure.

Glomerulonephritis may be asymptomatic. Classical signs, when associated with the nephrotic syndrome, include loss of lean body mass, edema, ascites and anorexia. Laboratory findings may include massive proteinuria, hypoalbuminemia, lipemia and anemia. In the later stages, all the signs and laboratory findings of chronic renal failure may be present. The nephrotic syndrome is not always associated with glomerulonephritis. Urine specific gravity is usually normal early in the disease. In late stages, the specific gravity is usually low. The finding of massive proteinuria should suggest the possibility of a glomerular lesion. A renal biopsy is necessary to determine the cause.

Treatment is aimed at relieving the nephrotic syndrome by correcting the fluid balance and elevating plasma-protein concentrations. In the absence of severe renal failure a high-protein diet should be fed. A low-sodium diet and intermittent diuretic therapy (℞ 519, 520, 523) is helpful to control the edema and ascites. Corticosteroids may be used in an attempt to minimize glomerular changes; however, their usefulness in the dog and cat has not been proved.

PYELONEPHRITIS

An inflammatory disease of the renal pelvis and parenchyma. It may be acute or chronic, focal or diffuse, arrested or active. The most common bacterial organisms associated with this infection are the gram-negative organisms, *E. coli* and *Proteus*. It is usually considered an ascending urinary-tract infection and may be associated with chronic obstruction, calculi, cystitis or congenital defects. Also, it may occur in the absence of any other urinary-tract infection.

Because pyelonephritis may be subclinical, the incidence is unknown. Its presence should always be considered in cases of calculi and lower urinary-tract infection. Signs may include depression, anorexia, polydipsia and polyuria. When the condition is advanced, renal pain, intermittent fever and vomiting may be seen in cases associated with renal calculi. Examination of the urinary sediment usually reveals many white blood cells, bacteria, microscopic hematuria and cellular casts.

Urinary culture and antibiotic sensitivity tests are essential; long-term antibiotic therapy, several months in duration, is usually necessary. In addition, urinary acidifiers, as ammonium chloride (℞ 541), and urinary antiseptics (℞ 543) are helpful. High-protein diets and high-fluid intake should also be encouraged. Eradication of the infection can be confirmed by repeated negative urine cultures.

ACUTE INTERSTITIAL NEPHRITIS

This disease in dogs is attributable to a number of infectious disorders, but chief among these appears to be that caused by *Leptospira canicola* or *L. icterohaemorrhagiae*. It has, therefore, been classified as an infectious bacterial disease and is discussed under LEPTOSPIROSIS IN DOGS (q.v., p. 347).

CHRONIC RENAL FAILURE

A condition resulting from prolonged and significant loss of functional renal tissue. Its causes include: pyelonephritis, renal amyloidosis, chronic obstructive uropathy, congenital lesions, glomerulonephritis and genetic renal diseases as well as unknown causes. The term *chronic interstitial nephritis* has been used to describe this condition but since this term is essentially a pathologist's term to describe the morphologic appearance of kidneys of dogs and cats affected with chronic, progressive and irreversible renal disease, it does not contribute to the understanding of the underlying cause.

Clinical Findings: Polydipsia, polyuria and occasional vomiting are the early signs. As renal failure ensues over a period of weeks or months, anorexia, dehydration, nonregenerative anemia, renal osteodystrophy, depression and weight loss are commonly seen. In the terminal stages, oral ulcerations, diarrhea or constipation, severe dehydration, continual vomiting, convulsions and coma lead to death.

Diagnosis: The diagnosis is established by laboratory findings including an inability to alter urine specific gravity from a range of 1.008 to 1.012; there may be abnormal elements in the urine sediment, including white cells and casts. The BUN, plasma creatinine and inorganic phosphorus are elevated. A moderate to severe nonregenerative anemia is commonly present. In terminal uremia, hyperkalemia and acidosis may be present. In order to determine the cause and severity of renal failure, IV pyelograms, renal biopsy, urine culture and specific renal-function tests are generally required.

Differential Diagnosis: This condition must be distinguished from acute nephritis and renal failure which is potentially reversible. This can usually be accomplished with a very careful history and the laboratory findings listed above. The polydipsia and polyuria of chronic renal failure may be confused with diabetes insipidus, diabetes mellitus, pyometra, pyelonephritis without renal failure, and several other obscure polyuric states. Adrenal insufficiency may be confused with renal failure, since many of these animals are vomiting and azotemic. The prevalence of chronic renal failure is equally high in dogs and cats.

Prognosis: Severe loss of renal tissue is a permanent disabling condition. However, animals can survive for long periods with a small fraction of their renal tissue, due to compensatory hypertrophy and hyperplasia. The prognosis of an individual animal depends upon the severity of the metabolic defects associated with uremia, cause of the renal failure, number of surviving nephrons and concurrent infections.

Treatment: The first step in therapy is to break the vomiting-dehydration cycle that further diminishes renal function. All fluid and some caloric requirements are met by parenteral fluid administration, either subcut. or IV. The severity of dehydration should be estimated (mild—5% of body wt, moderate—6 to 8%, severe—12%) and a quantity of a balanced electrolyte solution, based on this estimate, should be administered. After rehydration, an osmotic diuresis, using either dextrose or mannitol (℞ 522), should be induced. The response of the patient should be monitored by frequent clinical evaluations, rate of urine flow, frequent weighing and repeated measurements of the BUN or plasma creatinine concentration. Lactated Ringer's solution (℞ 565) should be used if hyperkalemia is not present. Sodium bicarbonate infusion or tablets (℞ 475) may be given to correct acidosis. Vomiting may be eased by treating the gastritis with protectants such as aluminum hydroxide (℞ 478). Vomiting may be suppressed with specific antiemetic drugs, antihistamines, or one of the tranquilizers (℞ 363). Under no circumstances should fluid restriction be imposed.

Dietary therapy which restricts protein intake will sometimes relieve the uremic signs. A very low-protein intake of only high-quality proteins such as egg and meat is used. The use of such a diet commonly requires a major change in the animal's dietary habits. A high-caloric intake should always be encouraged. The dietary therapy is generally the same for dogs and cats. Cats are notoriously averse to dietary change and must be induced to eat a variety of nonprotein foods.

Additional therapeutic considerations include: multiple-B-vitamin preparations; a high-calcium intake; vitamin D; sodium chloride, 2 to 10 gm/day in divided doses; sodium bicarbonate, 1 to 6 gm daily; bone-marrow stimulants; and in some cases periodic blood transfusions. Animals in chronic renal failure require additional sodium chloride and sodium bicarbonate for the remainder of their lives.

RENAL ABSCESS, PERINEPHRITIC ABSCESS AND PARALUMBAR ABSCESS

These are grouped under one heading because they are often interrelated.

Etiology: Trauma resulting in disturbance of kidney circulation, hematoma, or damage to the perirenal fat can cause necrosis which results in abscess of the renal cortex or perirenal tissue. The existence of infection in the presence of renal calculi or kidney worms may also cause abscess formation. Septic ligatures that have been used to tie off the ovarian artery are a common cause of perinephritic abscess. The infection, by subperitoneal extension from the kidney area, frequently erupts in the paralumbar fossa and becomes a paralumbar fistula. Penetrating foreign bodies of the intestine, osteomyelitis of the transverse lumbar process and foreign bodies in the lumbar area likewise can cause abscess and fistula formation.

Diagnosis: Palpation of a large tender mass in the renal area is a suggestive sign. Fever, lumbar pain and elevated leukocyte count point to abscess formation. Urinalysis may reveal evidence of active infection. Renal failure may be present if the process involves both kidneys. Roentgenograms, particularly dorsoventral films, often reveal shadows of enlarged kidneys or abscesses. The roentgenogram also should reveal radiopaque foreign bodies and osteomyelitis if they exist. Culturing the exudate from a paralumbar fistula may be helpful. *Nocardia* are isolated at times.

Treatment: Animals suspected of having renal or perinephritic abscesses should be submitted to surgical exploration. The abscess usually is encapsulated so the removal of the entire mass is feasible. Paralumbar abscesses and fistulas present a somewhat different problem, as they do not always arise in the kidney. When local examinations, bacteriologic cultures and radiographs fail to reveal the exact cause and location of the abscess, the final step is abdominal exploration. When radiographic examination for foreign bodies and osteomyelitis are unproductive, local exploration of the abscess or fistula should be undertaken. By this means, foreign material not otherwise detectable may be discovered. *Nocardia* infections respond at times to high doses of penicillin and sulfadiazine.

CONGENITAL RENAL DEFECTS

Renal Dysplasia and Hypoplasia: These defects are present most commonly in the dog. The kidneys may be unilaterally or bilaterally small, firm and pale. Some kidneys have a uniformly diminished renal cortex. At histologic examination such kidneys demonstrate primitive and bizarre tubules and glomerular structures, and excessive fibrous tissue.

Affected animals usually have signs of polydipsia and polyuria which precede signs of uremia. Dwarfing will occur if the onset of renal failure occurs within the first few months of life. Changes in the urinalysis, hemogram and blood chemistry are the same as in other chronic, progressive renal diseases. Severe renal failure is usually present at 6 months to 3 years of age. The diagnosis can be suspected on the basis of breed and age of onset. A renal biopsy may be helpful in confirming the diagnosis. Treatment is the same as for any other chronic renal failure.

Ectopic Ureter: This defect has been most commonly reported in the dog (usually females) and is usually first noticed at 3 to 6 months of age. Urinary incontinence with continual dripping of urine is the classic sign. A low-grade vaginitis or vulvitis may be present due to urine scalding. The ureter or ureters involved may open into the urethra, prostate, or vagina. Diagnosis may be confirmed by IV pyelogram which traces the course of the ureter. The most successful treatment is surgical removal of the affected kidney and ureter when the defect is unilateral, or by transplanting the affected ureters into the bladder when the disease is bilateral or when the opposite kidney is abnormal.

Unilateral Renal Agenesis: This is relatively frequent in the cat and quite rare in the dog. One kidney and its associated ureter are usually absent. This is usually an incidental finding in the cat and renal function is usually normal.

Polycystic Kidneys or Solitary Cysts: Also known as congenital cystic kidneys, the term polycystic kidney applies when the renal parenchyma is largely replaced by multiple-cyst formation. It is relatively uncommon in both dog and cat. Such kidneys are usually found to be grossly enlarged by palpation. Polycystic kidneys may cause no clinical signs or may lead to progressive renal failure. The diagnosis is usually made on the basis of physical and radiographic findings or by exploratory laparotomy. Pyelonephritis is a common finding in such kidneys and may precipitate renal insufficiency.

Miscellaneous Anomalies: Double or multiple renal arteries are seen in approximately 5% of dogs. Other congenital defects, including renal fusion, persistent urachus, congenital changes in position, and congenital hydronephrosis and hydro-ureter, are relatively infrequent in both the dog and cat.

RENAL AMYLOIDOSIS

Amyloidosis is an idiopathic disease characterized by intercellular deposition of an amorphous, eosinophilic, hyaline-appearing substance in many organs and body tissues. In dogs and cats the kidneys are sites where amyloid deposition frequently assumes major clinical importance. While this condition occurs in many species, it has been most frequently reported in the dog.

Early signs usually include heavy proteinuria, weight loss, polydipsia and polyuria. As the condition progresses, azotemia, anemia, and the classic signs of renal failure are seen. In some cases, renal failure appears very late following the chronic debilitating course. The nephrotic syndrome may be present with ascites and peripheral edema.

Diagnosis is made on the basis of progressive renal failure, hypercholesteremia and persistent proteinuria. The 24-hour urine-protein excretion may range from 0.5 to 15.0 gm in the dog and lead to hypoproteinemia. A renal biopsy is necessary to confirm the presence of amyloid deposition in the glomeruli.

There is no known treatment; however, symptomatic and supportive treatment of the accompanying progressive renal failure may be beneficial. A high-protein diet may be used before severe renal failure is present and may retard hypoproteinemia and the nephrotic syndrome. A diuretic (R 519, 520) may be used in alleviating signs associated with excessive fluid accumulation in the nephrotic syndrome.

ACUTE TUBULAR NECROSIS

Acute tubular necrosis is the result of a major insult to the kidney parenchyma which results in acute renal failure. In general, 2 broad groups of etiologic factors may be identified. In the first are the many situations associated with vascular collapse and hypotension with resultant ischemia of renal tissue. This may be seen in severe hemorrhage, burns, major surgery, overwhelming infections, hypersensitivity, shock, and severe water and electrolyte depletion. The second is the group caused by the ingestion of nephrotoxic substances. Mercuric chloride, phosphorus, carbon tetrachloride, amphotericin B, arsenicals and ethylene glycol are the most common nephrotoxins.

The signs of acute renal failure include: vomiting, anorexia, dehydration, oral ulceration, hypothermia and oliguria or anuria. Laboratory results are similar to those found in chronic renal failure, except anemia is not commonly present and hyperkalemia is usually found. A renal biopsy is most useful in confirming a diagnosis and in helping to establish a prognosis.

Immediate and adequate attention must be given to the restoration of deficits of blood volume, extracellular fluid and electrolytes. This must be done with some caution in the oliguric animal and with awareness that correction of the fluid deficit itself may not correct the renal dysfunction. Repeated blood chemistry determinations and measurement of urine flow must be monitored for several days. The use of mannitol (℞ 522) or a potent diuretic (℞ 519, 520, 521) to stimulate diuresis may be helpful if the animal is treated early in the course of acute renal failure.

Metabolic acidosis may be a life-threatening factor in this situation and is treated with sodium bicarbonate infusions. If renal function is not immediately reversible within 48 to 72 hours, peritoneal dialysis may be used to maintain the animal until the extent of renal injury is known.

MISCELLANEOUS GENITOURINARY DISEASES (SM. AN.)

VULVITIS AND VAGINITIS

Etiology: Although common, inflammation and infection of the vulva or vagina are often overlooked. Entire adult, adolescent or spayed females may be affected. In entire females, vaginitis may result from injury during breeding or parturition. Contamination of the perineal area may result in ascending infection. Foreign bodies and bacterial infection are the most common causes in the dog. Chronic vulvovaginitis may be of endocrine origin, e.g., in the hyperestrinemia of cystic ovaries. Many cases are associated with urethritis (bacterial) or a chronically infected or inflamed cervix following spaying.

Clinical Findings: The common signs are increased licking of the vulva, blood-tinged mucoid discharge, or yellowish purulent discharge. The labia may or may not be swollen. Spayed females may attract males as the discharge emits an odor attractive to them. This condition is often inaccurately described as constant heat. (*See* HYPERESTRINISM, p. 839.)

Diagnosis: Diagnosis is made on the finding of a persistent discharge emanating from a reddened and sometimes swollen vaginal mucosa. Close examination, with good light and magnification (an electric otoscope with a large ear speculum makes a convenient and efficient instrument for examining the vagina) discloses small red nodules, pustules or hypertrophied lymph follicles covering the mucous membrane. The area most commonly affected and most apt to be overlooked is the small cul-de-sac on the floor of the vagina formed by the folding of its walls. In severe cases, the entire vaginal mucosa may be affected.

The clitoris is often engorged and sensitive. Visual examination is seldom helpful because the focus of infection may be in the cervix, uterine body, or even a uterine horn that was not removed at the time of surgery. In these animals, contrast radiography using air or positive contrast material to outline the vagina and cervix is required. After ovariohysterectomy, granulomas of the stump of the uterus occur on rare occasions and will present similar signs.

Treatment: Good hygiene, clipping of the perineal hair, bathing, douching with isotonic saline or antibiotic solutions, or introduction of antibiotic suppositories is often effective. Some clinicians prefer astringent treatment, such as swabbing, or douching with 1% copper sulfate solution or application of 2% copper sulfate ointment. Stubborn or severe cases require systemic as well as local antibiotic therapy and often the simultaneous administration of stilbestrol sufficient to induce estrus. The estrogen is given daily in fairly large doses (1 to 5 mg), until vulvar hypertrophy and a bloodstained discharge appear.

Antibiotic sensitivity tests are needed in persistent and chronic infections. Good results usually follow oral administration of antibiotics e.g., potassium penicillin V, 20,000 u/lb of body wt daily in 3 divided doses; chloramphenicol 15 to 25 mg/lb daily in 3 doses or sulfisoxazole, 30 to 60 mg/lb daily in 3 divided doses. Treatment should be continued for several days after the visible signs subside. Adolescent puppies may be treated conservatively inasmuch as the vaginal infection often subsides spontaneously after estrus.

FISTULA

Genitourinary fistulas in small animals vary from urethrocutaneous fistulas in male animals to rectovaginal, ureterovaginal, vesiculoureterocervical, vaginal and vesiculorectal fistulas in females. Except for the few cases of congenital fistulas, the condition is acquired. Penetrating wounds, particularly bite wounds into the urethra, are seen only occasionally in the male, and rectovaginal fistulas from the same cause rarely are seen in the female. The most common cause of acquired fistulas is surgical error. The persistence of the fistula usually is due to the presence of a foreign body, such as a calculus or suture that has remained in the surgical wound. The presence of a stricture below the wound will help perpetuate the fistula. The uncomplicated wound or fistula usually will heal spontaneously.

Treatment consists of removing the obstruction to healing, e.g., calculus or suture, whereupon the fistula usually heals.

STRICTURE

Aside from stricture of the urethra, the only other genitourinary stricture, rarely seen in small-animal practice, is that of the ureter. It is discussed under HYDRONEPHROSIS (q.v., p. 852). Some narrowing or lack of distension of the urethra normally occurs in male dogs and cats: in dogs (1) proximal to the os penis, (2) at the ischial arch and (3) sometimes at the prostatic groove; in cats (1) at the tip of the penis and (2) at the ischial arch. Most cases of urethral stricture occur as a result of surgery or trauma to the extrapelvic part of the urethra. In the pelvic part of the urethra, strictures arise from trauma caused by pelvic fractures, and from prostatic disease. Urethral strictures develop in cats from the inflammation caused by the passage of calculi or repeated or unskilled catheterization.

Signs consist of frequent urination, dribbling, straining to urinate, hematuria and licking of the external urethral orifice. If the urethra is occluded, retention of urine and distension of the bladder result.

Prompt relief of the obstruction caused by the stricture is imperative. Catheterization is the simplest procedure, with use of successively larger sounds to distend the constricted area after the bladder distension has been relieved. Placement of an indwelling catheter is sometimes successful, although dogs and cats are adept at removing catheters no matter how carefully restrained. When passage of a catheter is not advisable or possible, temporary relief may be provided by cannulating the bladder through the abdominal wall with a small-bore (22-gauge) hypodermic needle and withdrawing the urine by means of an attached syringe. Painful catheterization is resisted and repeated dilatation of the urethra under anesthesia is obviously a dangerous procedure in animals suffering from incipient uremia, hence one of the most successful procedures in difficult cases is the surgical creation of an artificial fistula proximal to the stricture.

PHIMOSIS

Narrowness of the orifice of the prepuce. This may be congenital, but often results from or accompanies balanitis, especially in adolescent puppies. Dysuria or a preputial discharge and licking of the part will call attention to the difficulty.

In congenital phimosis, the orifice may be so small that

urine is expressed only with difficulty and the sheath in such cases often is distended with urine. The phimosis occurring in adolescent puppies often corrects itself as the dog becomes sexually mature. If balanitis is the cause, and does not respond to therapy, surgery is required. Prompt surgical relief is imperative if dysuria is present.

PARAPHIMOSIS

Constriction of the prepuce posterior to the glans penis. The usual cause is a partial phimosis that prevents retraction of the engorged glans into the sheath following erection. The venous circulation in the organ is impaired by the constricting prepuce. The edematous glans then cannot be withdrawn into the sheath. Cold packs may aid in reducing the edema. Liberal lubrication may then facilitate reducing of the prolapsed organ by manipulation. Severe paraphimosis is treated surgically. Usually the erection will subside when the animal is sedated or anesthetized. If this does not happen, one of the veins draining the penis may be thrombosed. Prolonged strangulation of the penis may result in necrosis.

RESPIRATORY SYSTEM

EPISTAXIS
(Nosebleed)

Trauma is the most common cause of epistaxis in domestic animals. Foreign bodies, neoplasms, parasitic infections, inflammation or ulceration of the nasal cavities also are frequent causes. Prior respiratory infection and excessive use of antiinflammatory drugs may predispose to epistaxis.

Trauma of the cranial vault may cause epistaxis and signs of concussion. In horses, the careless or rough passage of a stomach tube may result in bleeding from the nose. Racehorses of all ages may be affected with epistaxis of unknown cause while racing. Infections of the guttural pouches (q.v., p. 112) with erosions of the venous sinuses or branches of the internal carotid artery may produce severe epistaxis in horses. Sporadic idiopathic epistaxis may occur in any species.

Diagnosis: Epistaxis may be differentiated from hemoptysis by the character of the blood. In epistaxis, the blood has the character of venous blood, is not heavily mixed with air and does not have the frothy appearance of blood coming from the lower respiratory tract. Blood of gastrorrhagia may appear at the nostrils and is characterized by hemolysis and a mixture of ingesta. Epistaxis may be bilateral.

Treatment: All treatment should be aimed at removing the cause, if known. Where the cause is obscure, cold packs may be placed over the nose. Tampons may be inserted into the affected nostril. It is unwise to pack both nostrils. Vasoconstrictor drugs, e.g., epinephrine (R 509), may be used in association with the tampon, but their action is temporary. Topical thrombin (R 552) will quickly arrest bleeding if the bleeding point can be determined.

Calcium (R 585), tolonium chloride (R 553) and vitamin K (R 554) may contribute to decreasing the blood-clotting time. Several hemostatic preparations (R 170, 544, 545, 548) are used in racehorses with a history of bleeding. The drugs are given before the race to reduce the incidence of epistaxis. After severe episodes of epistaxis, blood transfusions may be necessary.

HEMOPTYSIS

Hemorrhage from the respiratory tract beyond the larynx, but usually from the lungs. Causes include trauma, parasites, neoplasms, infectious processes that erode capillaries, pulmonary infarction and cardiac dilatation in the horse. Diagnosis is made from the appearance of blood-tinged saliva or nasal discharge or free blood coming from the nostrils. There may or may not be respiratory embarrassment. Complete rest is important. Little else will be useful but blood transfusions, oxygen and coagulants may help (R 549, 585).

RHINITIS

An inflammation of the nasal mucous membrane, producing a serous, mucoid or mucopurulent discharge.

Etiology: The most frequent cause of a bilateral nasal discharge in domestic and pet animals is infection. In dogs the cause is often canine distemper (q.v., p. 311), in cattle, IBR (q.v., p. 268), while in cats it may be panleukopenia (q.v., p. 320) or other respiratory diseases (q.v., p. 321). Other causes are extensions of oral infections via the nasopharynx; traumatic or congenital palate defects; poor nutrition, often accompanied by severe parasitism; projectile vomiting, with resulting nasal contamination; and sinusitis.

The most common causes of unilateral rhinitis are nasal foreign bodies (most often plant matter); extension of an alveolar infection; and nasal or sinus tumors (especially in horses), with secondary infection.

Rhinitis accompanied by a serous nasal discharge is often seen with acute allergic reactions. The role of rhinitis in chronic allergic conditions, such as allergic dermatitis, is difficult to evaluate.

Clinical Findings and Diagnosis: The nasal mucosa first becomes very dry and hyperemic. This is followed by a serous discharge which later becomes mucoid or mucopurulent. In simple rhinitis, there are no other signs and the animal appears to be in good condition generally. There may be some sneezing or a slight cough. Excoriation of the skin about the nose may occur. Later, encrustation of the discharge around the nose may lead to difficulty in breathing.

Treatment: An effort should be made to find and eliminate the primary cause of rhinitis. Identification of the infectious agent is of value in treating chronic bacterial rhinitis which is often accompanied by sinusitis. The proper drug should be used in high doses. It may be necessary to trephine the affected sinuses in chronic infections. Culture, sensitivity testing and experience will assist the selection of appropriate antibacterial agents. Other medications may be of value (R 59, 62, 70, 455, 535).

Infections caused by gram-positive bacteria often respond to penicillin parenterally administered (R 44); gram-negative organisms usually respond to streptomycin (R 54); a penicillin-streptomycin combination (R 41), administered parenterally, may be helpful in controlling secondary bacterial infection when the organism is not identified.

The nose should be cleaned daily with a warm boric acid solution and the nostrils and surrounding areas coated with petrolatum to prevent excoriation. Proper care and hygiene are essential.

NECROBACILLOSIS

The term necrobacillosis is used to describe any disease or lesion with which *Sphaerophorus* (*Fusiformis*) *necrophorus* is associated. It includes calf diphtheria, necrotic rhinitis of pigs, foot rot of cattle (panaritium), foot abscess of sheep, post-parturient necrosis of the vagina and uterus, and focal necrosis of the liver of cattle and sheep, quittor of horses, and numer-ous other necrotic lesions in ruminants and, less commonly, pigs, horses, fowls and rabbits. It is probably a secondary in-vader rather than a primary cause and is usually part of a mixed infection. However, its necrotizing endotoxin undoubt-edly plays a role in the production of characteristic lesions.

S. necrophorus is part of the normal flora of the mouth, in-testine and genital tracts of many herbivores and omnivores, and is widespread in the environment. It is thought to gain entry to the body through wounds in the skin or mucous mem-branes.

CALF DIPHTHERIA

An infectious disease of calves affecting the larynx (necrotic laryngitis) or the oral cavity (necrotic stomatitis) charac-terized by fever and ulceration and swelling of the affected structures.

Etiology: *Sphaerophorus necrophorus* has long been considered the cause of this disease. However, other factors or agents may also be involved.

Clinical Findings: Calf diphtheria usually occurs as necrotic stomatitis in calves less than 3 months of age and as necrotic laryngitis in older calves. The calf with necrotic stomatitis has difficulty in nursing, the appetite is depressed and temperature may rise to 104°F. In calves with necrotic laryngitis, the most prominent sign in severe cases is loud wheezing. The early signs may include a rise in body temperature to 106°F, rapid respiration, and salivation. Later, protrusion of the tongue and a nasal discharge may be noted. Calves may develop both necrotic stomatitis and necrotic laryngitis, and may develop a cough as the lungs often become involved. Dehydration and emaciation are also prominent signs. The course of the disease usually is short, the untreated patient succumbing to toxemia and pneumonia within 2 to 7 days.

Lesions: The chief lesions are necrotic ulcers of varying depth on the oral and pharyngeal mucous membranes. The occurrence of croupous or diphtheritic membranes is common. The parts most often involved are the tongue, particularly its borders, the inner surface of the cheeks and the lining of the pharynx. In the more severe cases, the lesions extend into the nasal cavity, the larynx, the trachea and even the lungs.

Diagnosis: The signs are usually sufficient for establishing a prompt and accurate diagnosis. Difficulties may be encountered in outbreaks where an older calf is the first to become ill, or in herds where the disease affects only 1 or 2 calves. A careful study of the signs and the lesions should be made under all circumstances. Contributing etiologic factors include excessive moisture, dirty barns and feed lots, and warm weather.

Prophylaxis and Treatment: Affected animals must be isolated from healthy ones. Cleaning and disinfecting the stables and sheds are important steps in preventing spread of the disease. Daily physical examination of all young calves is recommended for early recognition of new cases. Sulfonamide and antibiotic therapy is recommended. The sulfonamides of choice are sulfamerazine (℞ 75), sulfamethazine (℞ 82) and sulfapyridine (℞ 86). Penicillin (℞ 44), the tetracyclines (℞ 11, 29), or penicillin and streptomycin (℞ 41) may prove beneficial, and also chloramphenicol (℞ 7) where its use is permitted. Supplemental feeding with milk, eggs and nutritious gruel is advisable.

NECROTIC RHINITIS OF PIGS
(Bull-nose)

A disease of young growing pigs characterized by suppuration and necrosis, arising from wounds of the oral or nasal mucosa. Confusion exists in the literature because of the use of the misnomer "bull-nose" to also describe atrophic rhinitis (*see* below).

Etiology: *Sphaerophorus necrophorus* is commonly isolated from the lesion and undoubtedly contributes to the disease, but many other types of organisms are frequently present. They gain entry through damage to the roof of the mouth, often as a result of clipping the needle teeth too short.

Clinical Findings: Swelling and deformity of the face, occasionally hemorrhage, snuffling, sneezing, foul-smelling nasal discharge, sometimes involvement of the eyes with lacrimation and purulent discharge, loss of appetite and emaciation are signs of bull-nose. Generally, only 1 or 2 pigs are affected in the herd.

   Lesions: The facial swelling usually is hard, but incision reveals a mass of pinkish-gray, foul-smelling, necrotic tissue or greenish-gray tissue debris, depending on the age of the lesion. The nasal and facial bones become involved in the process and as a consequence the facial deformity may be marked.

Diagnosis: Necrotic rhinitis is readily differentiated from atrophic rhinitis by the bulging type of facial distortion observed in bull-nose. Atrophic rhinitis causes no swelling other than that due to the upward or lateral deviation of the snout. The character of the exudate and its location within the tissue of the snout or face are distinctive of bull-nose.

Prophylaxis and Treatment: Prevention is directed towards avoiding injuries to the mouth and snout and improved sanitation. Where the disease occurs repeatedly, great care should be taken in clipping needle teeth.

   If the condition is advanced, it is doubtful whether treatment is advisable. Early surgical intervention and packing the cavity with sulfonamide or tincture of iodine may be useful. In young pigs, sulfamethazine (℞ 82) and antibiotics (℞ 11, 29) given orally are of value.

ATROPHIC RHINITIS OF SWINE

A disease characterized by sneezing followed by atrophy of the turbinate bones and distortion of the nasal septum which may be accompanied by shortening or twisting of the upper jaw.

Etiology: The etiology is probably complex and not fully understood. A variety of infectious and noninfectious agents can cause enough inflammation of the upper respiratory tract to stimulate sneezing. An important primary cause of atrophic rhinitis in the U.S.A. appears to be *Bordetella bronchiseptica*. This bacterium is not host-specific and may be harbored for long periods in the nasal cavities of other animals as well as pigs. The viruses of inclusion-body rhinitis and of pseudo-rabies cause a very acute transient rhinitis in young pigs, but in uncomplicated infections, do not usually lead to atrophy and distortion.

Clinical Findings: The disease is widespread and usually mild. Mild forms have little effect on the general health or profitability of the pigs, but in severe outbreaks, growth rate and efficiency of feed conversion may be affected, particularly if pneumonia is present.

Acute signs usually appear between 3 and 8 weeks of age and in severe cases, nasal hemorrhage may occur. The lacrimal ducts may become occluded and tear stains then appear below the medial canthus of the eyes. As the disease progresses, some affected pigs may develop lateral deviation or shortening of the upper jaw but others may suffer atrophy of the turbinates with no outward distortion apparent. The degree of distortion can be judged from the relationship of the upper and lower incisors if breed variations are taken into account.

The severity of *Bordetella*-caused rhinitis in a herd depends largely on (1) the age of the pig when infected (severe turbinate damage results when infection occurs before 4 weeks of age); (2) the virulence of the strain of organism involved; (3) the presence of other infectious agents (e.g., simultaneous infection with *Pasteurella multocida* results in increased turbinate atrophy); and (4) the immune status of the pigs.

Lesions: The degree of atrophy and distortion is best assessed by examining the cut surface of a transverse section made with a saw at the level of the second premolar tooth (the first cheek tooth up to 7 to 9 months of age); additional parallel sections are recommended in some areas. In the active stages of inflammation, the mucosa will have a blanched appearance and there may be purulent material present on the surface. In later stages the nasal cavities may be clear, but there may be variable degrees of softening, atrophy, or grooving of the turbinates, deviation of the nasal septum, and asymmetrical distortion of the surrounding bone structure.

Diagnosis: The characteristic signs and lesions are commonly used as the basis for diagnosis. The implications of such a diagnosis, particularly in individual pigs at necropsy, must be carefully weighed. Atrophic rhinitis may have no economic effect on the herd, particularly if no pneumonia is present. A specific diagnosis of *B. bronchiseptica* infection can only be made by laboratory culture. Culture of nasal swabs from 6- to 8-week-old pigs is an effective method of determining infection in a herd. Atrophic rhinitis must be differentiated from necrotic rhinitis (q.v., p. 868).

Prophylaxis: The incidence and severity of atrophic rhinitis in growing pigs may be reduced by good sanitation and management practices and by using sulfonamides at the level of approximately 100 gm per ton in the ration. The maintenance of a closed herd helps to reduce the chances of exacerbation through the introduction of additional agents. When pigs are introduced into a rhinitis-free herd, the health status of the donor herd should be checked. Repopulation with specific-pathogen-free pigs is usually an effective method of establishing herds free from serious forms of atrophic rhinitis. It is rarely possible, however, to keep herds entirely free from mild outbreaks of sneezing, and a low level of aberrant turbinates and nasal bones at necropsy is common even in herds which show no clinical signs of rhinitis.

B. bronchiseptica-free herds may occasionally be established by sulfonamide treatment of all swine in a herd. However, a combination of drug therapy and repeated nasal culture is more effective in removing all carrier animals from a breeding herd. Since species other than swine may be carriers of this organism, it is advisable to keep dogs, cats and rodents away from the herd.

Treatment: Sulfonamides may be effective in treating *Bordetella*-caused rhinitis, however the incidence of sulfonamide-resistant *B. bronchiseptica* is increasing. Treatment results in a low level of sulfonamide being eliminated in the nasal secretions. Sulfamethazine in the feed at the level of 100 gm/ton may clear the carrier state in 3 to 5 weeks. Higher levels do not hasten the process. Sodium sulfathiazole at the level of 0.5 to 0.66 gm/gal. of drinking water is also effective.

LARYNGITIS

An inflammation of the larynx. Although laryngitis may be caused by irritation of the larynx by the inhalation of dust, smoke, irritant gases, the lodging of a foreign body or excessive vocalization, more often it is caused by one of the upper respiratory tract diseases. Laryngitis may accompany infectious tracheobronchitis and distemper in dogs, infectious rhinotracheitis and the other various influenzas of cats, infectious rhinotracheitis and calf diphtheria in cattle, strangles, infectious viral rhinopneumonitis, viral arteritis and infectious bronchitis in horses. Laryngitis occurs in sheep because of *Sphaerophorus necrophorus* or *Corynebacterium pyogenes* infections and in pigs as a part of influenza.

Clinical Findings: A cough is the principal sign. It is at first harsh, dry and short but later becomes soft and moist and may be very painful. It may be induced by pressure on the larynx, exposure to cold or dusty air, the swallowing of coarse food or by attempts to administer medicines. A fetid odor may be detected on the breath. Difficult noisy breathing may be evident and the animal may stand with head lowered and mouth open. Swallowing is difficult and painful. Cats may have vocal changes. Systemic signs are usually attributable to the primary disease as in calf diphtheria where temperatures of 105°F may occur. Death due to asphyxiation may occur especially if the animals are exerted.

Diagnosis: Diagnosis is made on the clinical signs. In dogs and cats it may be possible to examine the larynx, but the pain will make this difficult unless anesthesia or analgesia is first induced. The history and signs of the primary disease will usually quickly identify the cause of the laryngeal problem.

Treatment: Identification and treatment of the primary disease is essential. In addition, certain palliative procedures such as the inhalation of steam, the confining of the animal to a warm, clean environment, the feeding of soft or liquid foods and the avoidance of dust will speed recovery and give comfort to the animal. The cough may be suppressed with antitussive preparations (℞ 392, 395) and bacterial infections controlled with antibiotics (℞ 59) or sulfonamides (℞ 75, 82). Control of pain with judicious use of an analgesic (℞ 588), especially in cats, will allow the animal to eat and thus speed recovery. Tracheotomy may be necessary if obstruction of the larynx is severe enough to cause cyanosis.

LARYNGEAL EDEMA

Edema of the mucosa and submucosa of the larynx, particularly the aryepiglottic folds and vocal cords. The course is acute or peracute, depending on the cause and severity of the disease. Obstruction of the larynx may result.

Etiology: Laryngeal edema develops because of allergy, inhalation of irritants, injuries to the mucosa, or in the course of the insertion of a tracheal tube or operations on the larynx. In cattle, laryngeal edema has been observed in the course of blackleg, respiratory infections, urticaria and serum sickness. In swine, it may occur as a part of edema disease.

Clinical Findings: Edema of the larynx may develop within hours. It is characterized by a rapidly increasing inspiratory, sometimes expiratory, dyspnea accompanied by laryngeal stenotic sounds of a roaring, whistling or rattling type. There is a severe cough, the visible mucous membranes are cyanotic and the pulse rate increased. In severe cases in horses, there is profuse sweating. The temperature is increased. Laryngoscopic examination reveals a severe swelling of the laryngeal mucosa, with little space between the vocal cords. Prognosis is favorable if treatment, particularly surgical intervention, is performed in the early stage; otherwise it should be guarded.

Treatment: In severe cases, first aid consists of tracheotomy as soon as possible. Local treatment consists of spraying astringents directly on the affected areas. Cold packs around the neck may be helpful. Systemic treatment depends on the cause. In cases of infectious and inflammatory laryngeal edemas, antibiotics should be administered systemically. In severe cases, epinephrine (℞ 509) may also be given. In allergic laryngeal edema, antihistamines (℞ 535, 538, 539) and corticosteroids (℞ 149) are administered.

LARYNGEAL HEMIPLEGIA
(Roaring)

A chronic, unilateral or occasionally bilateral paralysis of the intrinsic muscles of the larynx causing audible inspiratory dyspnea. The condition is most common in Thoroughbred and other light horses and occurs less frequently in draft horses. It is rare in other species.

Etiology: The immediate cause is degeneration of one or both of the recurrent laryngeal nerves, giving rise to partial or complete paralysis of the intrinsic muscles of the larynx. As a result, the arytenoid cartilages fail to rotate outward on inspiration, causing reduction in the size of the lumen of the larynx and consequent inspiratory dyspnea. Paralysis occurs on the left side in 92% of the recorded cases, on the right side in 6% and on both sides in 2%; this observation has led to the theory that the degeneration is related in some way to constant irritation produced by the pulsations of the aorta as the left recurrent laryngeal nerve passes around it. Accidental injury to the nerve by overextension of the head must be considered as a possible cause. Some cases of roaring presumably can be traced to previous infectious or debilitating diseases, ingestion of lead or certain plants or to hereditary predisposition to the disease.

Clinical Findings and Diagnosis: The obvious sign is a whistling or roaring sound heard on inspiration. In mild or recent cases, the sound may be produced only after strenuous exercise, while in advanced cases, it may become obvious after light exercise or even in the resting animal. The roaring usually subsides within 10 minutes after exercise is stopped. Affected animals are unfit for work and tire quickly as a result of the dyspnea. Many horses in the early stages of the disease may emit a characteristic grunt when frightened or when struck a sudden blow over the ribs. Experienced clinicians may be able to detect a pit between the arytenoid and thyroid cartilages on laryngeal palpation. Some animals show respiratory difficulty when the head is pulled to the side or when eating grain.

The characteristic respiratory signs may be sufficient for diagnosis; it may be confirmed by endoscopic examination of the larynx.

Treatment: Spontaneous remissions are rare. Ventriculectomy of the larynx is successful in restoring about 70% of affected horses to usefulness while surgical retraction of the arytenoid cartilages has proven effective in some cases that have not responded to ventriculectomy.

INFECTIOUS TRACHEOBRONCHITIS OF DOGS
(Kennel cough)

A mild, self-limiting disease, involving the trachea and bronchi of dogs of any age. It spreads rapidly among animals that are closely confined as in hospitals or kennels.

Etiology: The specific cause is unknown, but since the disease is highly contagious and apparently transmitted via the airborne route, viral etiology is probable, and both a herpesvirus and a complex of adenoviruses are suspect. Many bacterial species have been isolated, but these are undoubtedly opportunists. Environmental factors, such as cold, drafts and high humidity, apparently play a part in susceptibility to the disease.

Clinical Findings: The incubation period is 5 to 10 days. The outstanding sign is a harsh, dry cough which is aggravated by activity or excitement. The coughing occurs in paroxysms, followed by retching or gagging in attempts to clear small amounts of mucus from the throat. Paroxysms of inspiratory dyspnea (reverse sneeze) are noted in some cases. The cough is easily induced by gentle pressure over the larynx or trachea.

The body temperature is normal in the early stages, but may be moderately elevated as secondary bacterial invasion takes place. Blood counts are normal initially, but may show slight neutrophilia with a left shift in the later stages.

Diagnosis: A history of exposure to other dogs, a profound cough in the absence of other findings, and apparent localization of the condition in the trachea and bronchi should lead to a tentative diagnosis of infectious tracheobronchitis. Trauma to the trachea produces somewhat the same clinical picture, but signs are generally not as severe as in infectious tracheobronchitis.

The primary disease is self-limiting. The most severe signs are noted during the first 5 days, but continue in some degree for 10 to 20 days. A longer course suggests secondary bacterial complications. Stress, particularly of adverse environmental conditions, may cause relapse during the later stages.

Treatment: Because of the highly contagious nature of the disease, animals should be treated as out-patients if possible. Individual cases are best treated with mild expectorants containing codeine (℞ 395). Expectorants containing antihistamines may also be used (℞ 540). While antibiotics have no effect on the primary disease, they may be used to good effect in controlling secondary bacterial infection (℞ 7, 11). Corticosteroids (℞ 145, 152) may alleviate signs but should not be used in the absence of an antibacterial agent. The use of nitrofurantoin (℞ 98) is reported to provide relief from the clinical signs. Proper hygienic measures, good nutrition and good nursing all contribute to recovery.

BRONCHITIS (SM. AN.)

Acute or chronic inflammation of the bronchi. The primary site most commonly is in the bronchioles, but may extend to the lung parenchyma.

Etiology: Bronchitis frequently is secondary to other disease, such as heart disease, enteritis and parasitism. Initiating factors include bacterial infection, aspiration of smoke, irritating gases or other chemicals and sudden changes in atmospheric temperature. Foreign bodies in the airway and developmental abnormalities such as laryngeal deformities may lead to bronchitis.

Clinical Findings: Spasms of coughing are the outstanding sign. They are most severe in the morning, and the animal may cough up large quantities of mucus. On auscultation, the respiratory sounds may be essentially normal. In advanced cases, sonorous rales are heard. The temperature is slightly elevated. The acute stage of bronchitis passes quickly—in 2 or 3 days. The cough, however, may persist for 2 or 3 weeks. In severe cases, it is difficult to differentiate bronchitis from pneumonia and the process frequently extends into the lung parenchyma, resulting in pneumonia.

Lesions: The mucous membrane of the bronchi and bronchioles is inflamed. Their lumina contain frothy serous or mucopurulent exudate. The act of coughing is an attempt to remove the exudate from the respiratory passages.

Diagnosis: The diagnosis is made on the signs and by the fact that the disease, in the acute form, is mild and self-limiting. Older dogs with bronchitis should be examined for heart disease. Radiographs will show an increase in density in bronchial areas of the lung and this may be difficult to distinguish from pneumonia.

Treatment: Palliative treatment usually is effective, however treatment of concurrent disease is indicated. Rest, warmth and proper hygiene are important. Parenteral fluids (℞ 556) may be indicated during the course of the fever. The persistent cough is best controlled by expectorants containing codeine (℞ 395), or similar antitussives. A mucolytic agent (℞ 391) may be helpful. Some relief may be afforded by medicated inhalations (℞ 393). Antibiotics, such as penicillin and streptomycin combinations (℞ 41), chlortetracycline (℞

11) or chloramphenicol (℞ 7) are indicated if the fever persists for more than 3 days or if the infection extends to the lung parenchyma. The use of oxygen may be considered in severe cases.

BRONCHIECTASIS

A chronic disease of the bronchi and bronchioles characterized by irreversible cylindrical or saccular dilatation and complicated by secondary infection. Clinically, it is difficult to differentiate from chronic bronchitis. The differential diagnosis can only be accomplished reliably by bronchography, although a diagnosis may usually be made from plain radiographs in chronic cases. Animals with early cases may respond to surgical intervention, i.e., resection of the affected lobe, but most cases, when seen by the practitioner, are too far advanced for this. Treatment as for chronic bronchitis offers the best chance of a comfortable existence.

PNEUMONIA (SM. AN.)

Acute or chronic inflammatory change of the lungs and bronchi, characterized by disturbance in respiration and hypoxemia, and complicated by the systemic effects of toxins absorbed from the involved area.

Etiology: This condition usually results from primary viral involvement of the respiratory tract followed by secondary bacterial invasion. Components of the feline respiratory complex, canine distemper and infectious tracheobronchitis may predispose to it. Canine and feline herpesvirus may cause severe reactions, especially in young animals. Classical pneumonia is usually the disease as noted in the bacterial invasion phase. Any interference with immune and protective mechanisms may predispose to pneumonia. Many different bacteria have been isolated from animals with this disease. Parasitic invasion of the bronchi, as by *Filaroides, Aelurostrongylus* or *Paragonimus,* may cause pneumonia. Protozoan involvement, usually caused by *Toxoplasma* (q.v., p. 456) is seen rarely. Mycotic bronchopneumonia may result from *Aspergillus, Histoplasma* (q.v., p. 417) or *Coccidioides* (q.v., p. 418) invasion. *Cryptococcus* pneumonia has been described in cats.

Injury to the bronchial mucosa and the inhalation or aspiration of irritating materials may cause pneumonia directly and predispose the tissues to secondary bacterial invasion.

Clinical Findings: The initial signs are usually those of the primary disease. Lethargy and anorexia are usual. A deep cough of low amplitude is noted. Progressive dyspnea, "blowing" of the lips and cyanosis are evident. Body temperature is usually increased moderately and blood counts show a leukocytosis. Auscultation of the thorax usually reveals consolidation which may be patchy, but usually is diffuse. There is progression towards liquefaction, which is signaled by the occurrence of moist rales. Radiographic examination reveals very little early in the disease, but as inflammation progresses there is evidence of increased density and peribronchial consolidation. Complications such as pleuritis, mediastinitis, or perhaps invasion by opportunist organisms such as *Nocardia* may occur.

Diagnosis: Diagnosis of pneumonia may not be difficult but determination of the specific cause will require laboratory examination of exudate, mucus, etc. Viral involvement usually results in an initially high body temperature of 104° to 106°F. Leukopenia is usual with the exception of infectious tracheobronchitis. Mycotic pneumonias are usually chronic in nature and respond poorly or not at all to routine antibacterial therapy. Protozoan pneumonia may be acute or chronic. Acutely affected animals may die within 24 to 48 hours of the onset. Miliary nodules in the lungs may lead to a suspicion of protozoan pneumonia on necropsy. Those chronically affected typically fail to respond to antibacterial therapy. Skin and serologic tests have proven of little value in diagnosis. A history of recent anesthesia or severe vomiting might lead one to suspect aspiration pneumonia.

Treatment: The animal should be placed in warm, dry quarters. Anemia should be corrected if it is present. Oxygen therapy should be used if cyanosis is severe. This is best applied by means of a tent, using an oxygen concentration of 30 to 50%. Antibiotic therapy (℞ 6, 41, 58) should be instituted as early as possible. Antitussive agents should be used only if the cough is severe (℞ 592). Expectorants should be employed only with extreme caution, and probably never in the acute case. Supportive therapy should be used where indicated. Fluid infusion, particularly when administered IV, can be dangerous in the pneumonia patient and should be used with caution.

Animals treated as outpatients should be re-examined 4 to 6 days later. The chest should be radiographed again even though the animal may have improved clinically since consolidation of the lungs may still be present.

PNEUMONIA (LG. AN.)

Economic losses due to pneumonia are greatest in cattle and swine but also occur in horses and sheep. For details see THE BOVINE RESPIRATORY COMPLEX, p. 385, and THE EQUINE RESPIRATORY COMPLEX, p. 246, and consult the index for the specific pneumonias of each species.

ENZOOTIC PNEUMONIA OF CALVES
(Virus pneumonia)

An infectious, nonparasitic, enzootic pneumonia of calves that may be initiated by any one of several independent etiologic agents. It is primarily a problem in housed calves from 1 to 4 months of age but can affect week-old calves. Calves over 6 months of age and mature cows usually do not show clinical signs but may act as carriers.

Etiology: Enzootic pneumonia of calves may be caused by a number of agents, including parainfluenza-3 virus, adenovirus, reovirus, rhinovirus, respiratory syncytial virus, chlamydiae (*Bedsonia*, psittacosis-lymphogranuloma-venereum group) and *Mycoplasma* spp. Experimentally, each of the above agents is capable of producing lesions in the lungs of calves, but they are seldom as severe as those seen in natural cases of the disease. The duration of the illness and the fact that in fatal cases secondary bacterial infections (notably *Pasteurella* spp. and *Corynebacterium pyogenes*) are commonly present may account for this discrepancy. Further investigation is required before the relative importance of each of these agents is known.

Clinical Findings: The earliest clinical signs include a harsh, dry cough and serous nasal discharge. Affected calves are bright, alert and are not anorectic. Temperatures range from 103° to 105°F and there is a moderate increase in respiratory and heart rates. On auscultation, bronchial tones and heart sounds are increased over the anterior ventral third of the lung.

Affected calves may recover without treatment in 10 to 14 days, although broad-spectrum antibiotics may aid this process, depending on the etiologic agent and the extent of secondary infection. Some calves, particularly those under 2 weeks of age, will exhibit acute respiratory distress and may require extensive antibiotic and fluid and electrolyte therapy.

Most cases of enzootic pneumonia are not seen by a veterinarian until they have secondary bacterial pneumonia: these calves have the clinical signs of pasteurellosis (q.v., p. 385) and should be treated accordingly. A high percentage of these calves will recover completely but a few will remain permanently stunted because of extensive lung damage.

Lesions: The lesions are those of bronchopneumonia with characteristic dark-red areas of partial alveolar collapse (atelectasis). The atelectasis is confined to the anteroventral aspects of the lung in early cases and consolidation also occurs as the disease progresses. Terminal cases often have evidence of bacterial infection and lung abscesses are common.

Treatment: Calves that are anorectic and depressed can be treated with a broad-spectrum antibiotic for 4 to 5 days. The initial treatment should be given IV and can be continued by IM injections. Secondary bacterial pneumonia may also be treated with sulfonamides or penicillin-streptomycin (*see* PASTEURELLOSIS, p. 385).

Control: The raising of dairy calves in complete isolation from older cattle and other affected calves will aid in control. These calves should receive colostrum but should be removed from their dams at birth and raised in a separate area until they are 4 to 6 months of age. Housing requires a draft-free ventilation system and a constant room temperature of 60° to 65°F at a relative humidity of 65 to 75%. The control of enzootic pneumonia in nursing beef calves may be assisted by correct ventilation or by raising the cows and calves outside.

PROGRESSIVE PNEUMONIA OF SHEEP

Apparently related diseases are the conditions known in France as la bouhite, in Iceland as maedi, in the Netherlands as zwoegerziekte, and in South Africa as Graaf-Reinet disease. A distinction should be made between progressive pneumonia and jaagsiekte or pulmonary adenomatosis (q.v., p. 882).

Progressive pneumonia is a slowly developing, chronic disease of the lungs, characterized clinically by gradually increasing dyspnea, emaciation and eventual death. In the U.S.A., progressive pneumonia is primarily a disease of range sheep, where affected animals are commonly known as "lungers".

Etiology: Characteristic lesions have been reproduced by inoculation of bacteria-free filtrates. A virus has been isolated from the lungs of affected sheep and has been shown to be related to the virus which causes maedi. However, it has yet to be proved that the virus isolated is the cause of progressive pneumonia. Zwoegerziekte is also caused by a virus which is closely related to maedi virus.

Clinical Findings: Clinical signs rarely occur in sheep under 2 years and are most common in sheep more than 4 years old. The disease may last from 2 to 18 months. Affected animals have a progressively increasing dyspnea and a double expiratory effort. There is progressive loss of condition and, surprisingly, no significant bronchial exudate and little coughing.

Lesions: The lesions are confined to the lungs and the associated lymph nodes. The lungs do not collapse normally when the thorax is opened, and they weigh 2 or 3 times the normal weight. They are a dull color which is best described as beige. The basic changes are typically diffuse, involving the entire lung. On palpation the tissue is firmer than normal, but retains some elasticity. In advanced cases there are consolidated areas in which secondary infections are usually involved. The mediastinal lymph nodes are enlarged and somewhat edematous. The primary microscopic lesion is interalveolar and peribronchial infiltration of lymphocytes, monocytes and macrophages, with nodular accumulations of lymphoid cells. This distinguishes progressive pneumonia from pulmonary adenomatosis, in which the primary lesion is papilliform epithelial proliferation.

Differential Diagnosis: The clinical diagnosis of progressive pneumonia cannot be made with certainty. In pulmonary adenomatosis there is often a copious mucous nasal exudate but in some instances this sign may be absent. Verminous pneumonia and pulmonary caseous lymphadenitis are other conditions requiring differentiation. Necropsy will rule out the latter 2 and, in most cases, pulmonary adenomatosis also. In flocks experiencing progressive pneumonia for the first time, the diagnosis should be confirmed histologically.

Control: There is no effective treatment. Three methods of control are possible: 1) slaughter of all suspects as soon as they are detected; 2) slaughter of the entire flock and replacement with "clean" sheep after a suitable interval; and 3) a 2-flock system whereby sheep from the affected flock are slaughtered as soon as possible and "clean" sheep are purchased and kept strictly isolated from the affected flock.

PULMONARY ADENOMATOSIS
(Jaagsiekte)

A chronic pneumonia of sheep characterized by adenomatous growth of the alveolar epithelium (*see also* PROGRESSIVE PNEUMONIA, p. 880). It has been reported from Europe, Asia, Africa and South America, and seems likely to become important wherever sheep are raised intensively.

The cause is not yet established but appears to be viral. The incubation period is long (4 months to several years) and the course chronic but relentless. Spread is probably by inhalation of infected droplets. Early signs of panting after exercise and occasional coughing are followed by progressive emaciation, dyspnea and nasal discharge. In advanced cases moist rales can be heard at a distance from affected sheep. Forcible lowering of the head is followed by discharge of copious watery mucus from the nostrils, a sign considered to be pathognomonic. Appetite and body temperature are unaffected unless complicated by a secondary bacterial infection which is common in the terminal stages.

Lesions are confined to the thorax, and consist of consolidation, excessive bronchial fluid and sometimes abscesses and pleuritis. The characteristic alveolar adenomata are seen histologically.

There is no treatment. Field trials of a formalized vaccine have yielded conflicting results. Incidence can be lowered by slaughter of clinically affected sheep; eradication requires slaughter of all sheep in affected areas.

MYCOTIC PNEUMONIA

A chronic inflammation of the lungs caused by fungi and yeasts. (It has been customary to include the lung infections caused by *Actinomyces* and *Actinobacillus*.)

Etiology: *Cryptococcus, Histoplasma, Coccidioides, Blastomyces* and *Aspergillus,* along with other fungi and yeasts have been incriminated as causative agents in this condition in domestic animals (*see* SYSTEMIC FUNGUS INFECTIONS, p. 416). The tissues and secretions of the respiratory passages are an excellent environment for the multiplication of these organisms. Fungal infections are often concurrent with bacterial infections.

Clinical Findings: A short, moist cough is characteristic. As in other types of pneumonia, a thick mucoid nasal discharge may be present. As the disease progresses, dyspnea, emaciation and generalized weakness become increasingly evident. Respiration becomes abdominal, resembling that seen in diaphragmatic hernia. On auscultation, harsh respiratory sounds are heard. In advanced cases, the normal sounds of breathing are decreased or almost inaudible. Leukocytosis and periodic elevation of the temperature occur, probably in conjunction with aggravation of the bacterial infection. Pathologic changes in the eyes, e.g., corneal ulcer, blindness and purulent discharge, are not uncommon in cases of blastomycosis.

Lesions: Focal lesions of chronic inflammation are present in the lungs. Abscess formation and cavitation may be seen in conjunction with yellow or gray areas of necrosis. Some animals show numerous miliary nodules which can be seen on roentgenograms.

Diagnosis: A tentative diagnosis of mycotic pneumonia may be made if an animal with chronic pneumonia exhibits the signs described and does not respond to antibiotic therapy. However, a positive diagnosis will require laboratory assistance, and radiography may be useful. Some antigens, e.g., histoplasmin and blastomycin, have been developed and are an aid to diagnosis. Culture of the sputum which is expelled in spasms of coughing may reveal the infective organism. The clinical diagnosis can be confirmed at necropsy by appropriate cultural and histopathologic techniques.

Treatment: There is no entirely satisfactory method of treating systemic mycotic infections, but stilbamidine (℞ 358) and amphotericin (℞ 350) may be helpful.

ASPIRATION PNEUMONIA
(Foreign-body pneumonia, Inhalation pneumonia, Gangrenous pneumonia)

A form of pneumonia characterized by pulmonary necrosis and caused by the entry of foreign material into the lungs.

Etiology: Faulty administration of medicines is the most common cause of aspiration pneumonia. Liquids administered by drench or dose syringe must not be given faster than the animal can swallow, and drenching is particularly dangerous when conducted with the animal's tongue drawn out, when the head is held high, or when the animal is coughing or bellowing. Administration of liquids by nasal intubation is not without risk, and careful technique is especially necessary in debilitated animals. Cats are particularly susceptible to pneumonia caused by aspiration of mineral oil. Inhalation of food sometimes occurs in calves and swine. Attempts by animals to eat or drink while partly choked may result in aspiration pneumonia. Disturbances of deglutition, as in anesthetized or comatose animals (e.g., cows in lateral recumbency with milk fever) or in those suffering from vagal paralysis, acute pharyngitis, abscesses or tumors of the pharyngeal region, esophageal diverticula and encephalitis, are frequent predisposing causes. In sheep, inexpert dipping may cause aspiration of fluid. Inhalation of irritant gases or smoke is an infrequent cause.

Some anesthetics, such as ether and the thiobarbiturates, stimulate salivation. Atropine sulfate (R 489) will help to control salivation, while the use of an endotracheal catheter with an inflatable cuff will prevent fluid aspiration during surgery.

Clinical Findings: A history disclosing an event within the previous 1 to 3 days when foreign-body aspiration could have occurred, is of great diagnostic value. In the horse, the temperature usually rises to 104° or 105°F during the first few days and then becomes remittent. Pyrexia is also observed in cats, dogs and cattle, but sometimes cattle develop little or no fever. The pulse is accelerated and respiration rapid and labored. A sweetish, fetid breath characteristic of gangrene may be detected, the intensity of which increases as the disease progresses. This is often associated with a purulent nasal discharge that sometimes is reddish brown or green. Occasionally, evidence of the aspirated material can be seen in the nasal discharge or in expectorated material, e.g., oil droplets. On auscultation, typical bubbling rales and occasional splashing sounds over one or both sides of the chest are heard early in the condition, and these are followed by dry rales, pleuritic friction rubs and the crackling sounds of emphysema. A course of 1 to 5 days is usual. Cattle and swine recover more frequently than horses, but in all species, the mortality is high. In outbreaks following dipping of sheep, losses rise from the second day to about the seventh and then decrease gradually.

Lesions: The pneumonia is usually in the anterior ventral parts of the lungs and may be unilateral or bilateral. In the early stages, the lungs are markedly congested, with areas of interlobular edema. The bronchi are hyperemic and full of froth. The pneumonic areas tend to be cone-shaped with the base toward the pleura. There usually is an acute fibrinous pleuritis, often with pleural exudate. Suppuration and necrosis follow, the foci becoming soft or liquefied, reddish brown and foul smelling.

Treatment: The animal should be kept quiet. A productive cough should not be suppressed. Broad-spectrum antibiotics should be used in animals known to have inhaled a foreign substance, whether it be a liquid or an irritant vapor, without waiting for signs of pneumonia to appear. Care and supportive treatment are the same as for infectious pneumonia. In small animals, oxygen therapy may be beneficial. Mortality is high despite all treatments.

HYPOSTATIC PNEUMONIA

A condition arising from failure of the blood to pass readily through the vascular structures of the lungs.

Etiology: This condition is a result of passive congestion of the lungs and is seen most commonly in old or debilitated animals. It is usually secondary to some other disease process, e.g., congestive heart failure. Paralyzed dogs or animals recovering from anesthesia that are unable to move voluntarily sometimes develop hypostatic pneumonia if they are not moved regularly.

Diagnosis: Any primary disease must be determined and treated. Coughing is not always a prominent sign, but as the condition progresses, dyspnea and cyanosis become apparent. Secondary bacterial infection is common. A roentgenogram will reveal increased density of the lung and the mediastinal space may be shifted to the atalectic side.

Treatment: The position in which the patient lies must be changed regularly, at least once every hour. Horses or cattle in lateral recumbency for several hours must not be turned suddenly as the weight of blood in the congested lung may cause death by asphyxia. Exercise must be encouraged insofar as it is compatible with the condition of the patient. If a primary cause can be determined, specific therapy, e.g., digitalis

(℞ 507) for congestive heart failure or chlorothiazide (℞ 519) for edema, may be instituted.

Narcotics and sedatives should be kept to a minimum to encourage mobilization and to avoid depression of the cough reflex. Maintenance of proper hydration is also important.

PULMONARY EMPHYSEMA

Abnormal distension of the lung with air (overinflation of the lung). In the majority of cases, emphysema first affects the alveolar ducts and alveoli and hence the term **alveolar emphysema.** If alveolar walls are disrupted, air leaks into the interlobular and subpleural connective tissue and is termed **interstitial emphysema.** The latter occurs more commonly in cattle and pigs than in horses. In interstitial emphysema of cattle, it is not uncommon for air in the interstitial tissue of the lung to dissect a path beneath the pleura, into the mediastinum and via the fascial planes to beneath the skin of the back to cause **subcutaneous emphysema.**

The pathogenesis of emphysema is variable and not completely understood. In general, the complete or partial occlusion of airways may lead to overdistension of some alveoli because air is forced in at inspiration or by collateral flow but fails to evacuate at expiration. The lesion depends upon the nature and rate of occlusion of the air passages and is often present along with edema and atelectasis which also may follow occlusion of airways.

Animals that die slowly from many diseases have a gasping, forced inspiration that can overdistend the alveoli; consequently, emphysema is a common postmortem finding. This lesion is considered to be an agonal change. Pulmonary emphysema may also occur without primary lung lesions when there is a laryngeal obstruction with an anaphylactic reaction. Not all horses with heaves have emphysema but they do have a degree of inflammation of small bronchioles that may lead to emphysema.

Regardless of the cause and pathogenesis, emphysema produces inefficient evacuation of pulmonary air space, normal gaseous exchanges cannot occur and the elastic recoil of the lung is reduced. This produces the characteristic clinical sign of pulmonary emphysema, an expiratory dyspnea, due to the failure of this elastic recoil.

Examples of the clinical features, treatment and control of pulmonary emphysema are discussed under specific diseases such as acute atypical interstitial pneumonia of cattle (*see* below) and chronic alveolar emphysema (heaves) of horses (q.v., p. 889).

It should be emphasized that emphysema can occur in various tissues unrelated to pulmonary emphysema. Some examples include the emphysema associated with gas-forming bacteria, e.g., *Clostridium chauvoei,* and emphysema surrounding traumatic lesions and surgical incisions.

ACUTE BOVINE PULMONARY EMPHYSEMA (ABPE)
(Atypical interstitial pneumonia of cattle, Fog fever)

Atypical interstitial pneumonia is one of the more important pulmonary disorders of cattle in North America, and also occurs elsewhere at varying levels of incidence. The disease is a recognizable clinical and pathologic entity but the etiology has not yet been clarified. The acute form occurs chiefly in pastured cattle in the late summer and fall, and is associated with a change in forage.

Etiology and Incidence: Clinical evidence suggests that the condition is an acute allergic reaction, and a number of possible allergens have been suggested. Pastured cattle are thought to obtain sensitizing substances directly or indirectly from many lush green plants such as alfalfa, rape and kale; DL-tryptophan (an amino acid) has been used to reproduce the condition experimentally. The larvae of the lungworm *Dictyocaulus viviparus* may be a sensitizing agent. In stabled animals, the allergens are thought to be dust and fungal spores from fodder. Many students of the disease(s) regard the particular syndrome related to forage change (ABPE) as an entity separate from the other manifestations of interstitial pneumonia.

While the seasonal incidence of the acute syndrome in pastured animals is well known, its occurrence in any particular year is unpredictable. A herd may be affected one year only, or for several years in succession, or 2 or more years may elapse between outbreaks. Severity varies between herds and between affected individuals of the same herd. There is a distinct but not exclusive age incidence, usually only older animals being affected; lactating cows seem to be most susceptible. Morbidity may be as high as 50%. Characteristically, several animals in a group develop clinical signs at about the same time.

The disease has an acute and a chronic form based on clinical and pathologic observations. The chronic form does not commonly follow the acute form as in many infectious diseases. It has been postulated that the clinical and pathologic differences in the acute and chronic forms are a manifestation of the type of allergen and duration of exposure.

Clinical Findings: In the acute disease, which most often occurs within hours or a few days following a change in forage, the sudden onset of severe expiratory dyspnea is characteristic. Respirations are accelerated and labored, the neck often extended and the tongue protruded. The pulse is rapid and weak. The temperature may rise briefly to 103° to 104°F or higher, but temperature increase is most often related to exertion of the distressed animal. On auscultation, moist and dry rales with crackling sounds of emphysema may be heard over extensive areas of the lungs. Crepitus along the back indicates subcut. emphysema. Affected animals tend to remain standing. Death may occur within a day of onset of clinical signs but animals which survive for 48 hours usually recover. The initial prognosis is always guarded as the mortality rate may reach 50% of affected animals. Young animals seem less susceptible.

In the chronic disease, the usual history is of gradual loss of appetite, gradual drop in milk production and gradual increase in respiratory rate. This usually happens over a 4- to 5-day period, but may take as long as 3 to 4 weeks. Body temperature is variable, and there is an absence of nasal discharges and signs of toxemia. On lung auscultation, there is little to hear early in the condition except increased bronchial tones. As the disease progresses, grossly abnormal lung sounds may be heard. These include increased bronchial tones, moist rales, dry rales, crackling sounds of emphysema and pleuritic friction rubs. Mortality is virtually 100% in a period ranging from 2 weeks to 6 months from the onset of clinical signs.

Lesions: The significant lesions are found within the respiratory tract. The lungs are pale, heavy and do not collapse when the thorax is opened. The normal lobular pattern of the lung is distinct due to the distension of the interlobular spaces by edematous fluid and gas (interstitial emphysema). The lobules are pink to tan and most lobes of the lung are affected. Affected areas have a rubbery consistency. The extensive involvement of the diaphragmatic lobe helps to distinguish the lesions from most other acute pneumonias of cattle. Emphysema is quite variable and may be extensive or minimal. The disease should not be diagnosed on the basis of emphysema alone because this lesion is a common agonal change in cattle and is not the primary or main lesion in atypical interstitial pneumonia.

Histologically, the acute syndrome is characterized by thickened alveolar walls as well as the flooding of aveoli and alveolar ducts with pink-staining proteinaceous material. The chronic form is characterized by a glandular appearance of alveolar lining cells and thick alveolar walls.

Prophylaxis: While there is no known method of preventing the condition other than avoidance of inciting forage, the incidence and severity can be greatly reduced as follows: On farms where the disease has occurred in previous years, the periods during which the herd is turned onto suspect pasture should initially be short and gradually increased over about 10 days, after which the herd may be pastured permanently. Adequate ventilation systems will help control the chronic form of the disease. More exact preventive measures will require more knowledge of the etiology.

Treatment: All animals should be removed from the pasture when acute atypical pneumonia occurs, and usually can be returned to the pasture in 10 to 14 days if observed closely. Death may supervene rapidly if affected animals are roughly handled or excited. Antihistaminics (℞ 538, 539) in double the usually recommended dosage, given IM in conjunction with 10 ml of epinephrine (1:1,000) and repeated every 6 to 8 hours to effect, have come to be the treatment of choice. Corticosteroids have also been used. However, there is little clinical evidence that treatment affects the outcome and this is supported by recent experimental evidence suggesting that histamines are not important in allergic conditions affecting the lungs of cattle.

HEAVES
(Chronic pulmonary emphysema)

A respiratory disease of horses characterized by an expiratory dyspnea, chronic cough, unthriftiness, and lack of stamina. The signs may be aggravated by exercise, dusty surroundings and feeding of certain roughages, particularly alfalfa hay.

Etiology: The primary cause of the expiratory distress is rupture of the alveolar walls with or without escape of air into the interstitial tissue. The exciting causes are multiple: allergic reactions to certain feeds, exposure to dust or molds, infections of the respiratory tract causing a chronic bronchitis. Extreme exertion, particularly if the animal has coexisting respiratory disease, may be a cause.

Clinical Findings: The disease is usually progressive in nature, and may appear to be periodic. In most cases, respiratory distress is greater during hot and dry weather, or when the animal is exposed to dusty surroundings.

Inspiration is hurried with the nostrils dilated. In advanced cases the elbows may be abducted. The expiratory phase of the respiratory cycle is prolonged with forcible contraction of the abdominal muscles resulting in the formation of a ridge (heave line) along the costal arch. In severe cases, the anus may protrude, the ribs may be permanently rolled forward, and the animal may appear to have an enlarged chest cavity. A short, weak, persistent cough and a nasal discharge commonly are present. The cough often occurs on or following feeding of the grain ration. Dry or moist rales may be present. Percussion may reveal hyperresonance in advanced cases.

Lesions: The lungs are pale and fail to collapse when the thorax is opened. Imprint of the ribs upon the lungs may be noted. Microscopic examination reveals alveolar and interstitial emphysema. The normal pulmonary architecture is lost, the alveolar walls being thinner than normal. Rupture of alveoli results in formation of large and irregular air sacs. A diffuse bronchitis is usually present.

Diagnosis: The diagnosis of heaves is made upon the basis of clinical signs and the history. The early stages may present some difficulty because of similarity of signs accompanying other respiratory diseases such as bronchitis and pharyngitis. Once established, the disease is readily recognized by the characteristic expiratory distress.

Treatment: There is no specific cure; treatment is palliative. The affected animal should be kept in dust-free surroundings. Legume hays should be avoided. Keeping the animal on green pasture may be of considerable benefit. Complete pelleted feeds, particularly those containing beet pulp as the roughage, may be quite effective in certain cases. Those cases due to allergic causes may respond to bronchial dilators (℞ 639, 648) or to the steroids.

PULMONARY EDEMA

An effusion of serous fluid from the capillaries into the interstitial tissue and alveolar spaces of the lung. Edema of the lungs may occur in conjunction with circulatory disorders, occasionally in anaphylaxis and allergies, and in infectious diseases such as malignant edema and bovine pleuropneumonia. Brain injury in dogs may cause pulmonary edema.

Discomfort, respiratory embarrassment, dyspnea and openmouth breathing are evident. Animals will stand in preference to lying down or will lie only in sternal recumbency or may assume a sitting position. Auscultation of the chest may reveal wheezing and fluid sounds. Radiographs will reveal increased density. If the cause is removed, the fluid will be resorbed. If not, the course may be fatal.

The lungs are pale, heavy, doughy in consistency, pit on pressure and do not collapse. Fluid oozes from the cut surface and foam fills the bronchioles and bronchi. The interlobular septa are widened.

The cause should be removed and the animal kept quiet. Antihistamines (R 539) may be useful for allergies, digitalis (R 507) for cardiac insufficiency and antibiotics and sulfonamides for infections. A diuretic (R 519) may be indicated.

PLEURITIS (SM. AN.)
(Pleurisy)

Inflammation of the pleura.

Etiology: Pleuritis may be primary or secondary, acute or chronic. It may be caused by any pathogenic organism which gains entrance to the pleural cavity but often is an extension of other respiratory infections.

Clinical Findings: Pleuritis causes pain. Respirations are shallow and abdominal. The rectal temperature may be elevated. Auscultation of the chest discloses friction sounds which diminish with pleural effusions. Effusions also ease the pain. The lungs may be partially collapsed from pressure of the fluid.

Lesions: Acute pleuritis is characterized by hyperemia and swelling of the membrane. After about 48 hours serous exudate appears, which may progress to a fibrinous or purulent state. Fibrin attaches to the surface in the form of threads or bands or elevated patches. The fibrin may form an attachment between the visceral and parietal surfaces of the pleura and if it is not resorbed it becomes organized by fibroblasts and permanently ties the 2 surfaces together. If the inflammatory process heals early, no adhesions form and no permanent damage is done.

Diagnosis: A history of prior respiratory infection, elevated temperature and thoracic pain are suggestive of pleuritis. Ausculation will reveal friction sounds and radiographs will reveal the line of effusion along the chest wall.

Treatment: Rest and relief of cough, if present, are important. Meperidine (R 590) repeated every 8 hours will control the pain. Fluid may be aspirated by thoracentesis to relieve respiratory distress. Antibiotics (R 11, 41) should be given to control the infection. An enzyme (R 572) may be mixed with the antibiotic or injected IM.

EMPYEMA
(Purulent pleuritis, Pyothorax)

Pus in the pleural cavity. Empyema is caused by pyogenic bacteria or fungi reaching the thoracic cavity by way of the blood or by extension of a pneumonic infection or traumatic gastritis or by penetrating wounds of the chest. In dogs with empyema, nocardiosis (*Norcardia asteroides*) should be suspected.

Empyema usually is a secondary infection and the signs may be masked by the primary disease. Cough, fever, pain and dyspnea in combination may be present. Lung sounds will be heard above the fluid line and percussion will reveal loss of resonance in the lower chest cavity. Thoracentesis and radiographs are useful diagnostic aids.

Prognosis is guarded. All pus should be aspirated from the pleural cavity, cultured for bacteria and the bacteria checked for drug sensitivity. One half of the calculated dose of antibiotic (R 11, 41) dissolved in sterile water should be given through the same (aspirating) needle, and the other half given IM. This is repeated daily until the animal is afebrile and the exudate sterile. Proteolytic enzymes (R 570, 572) may be mixed with the antibiotic and given IM or injected in the pleural cavity to hasten lysis and resorption of pus.

HEMOTHORAX, HYDROTHORAX AND CHYLOTHORAX

Hemothorax is most commonly caused by trauma to the thorax. It may also occur rarely in association with neoplastic disease. Hydrothorax is the accumulation of transudate in the thoracic cavity and in nearly every instance is caused by some interference with blood flow or lymph drainage. Chylothorax is a relatively rare condition. The cause is rupture of the thoracic duct.

The signs of all 3 conditions include respiratory embarrassment and weakness if bleeding is severe. Diagnostic aids include examination of fluids, radiographs and auscultation. Treatment is designed to remove or correct the cause whenever this is possible. Surgery may be indicated either to correct the basic condition or to provide relief.

PNEUMOTHORAX (SM. AN.)

Air in the pleural cavity. This may be traumatic or spontaneous in origin. Air enters the pleural cavity through penetrating wounds of the thoracic wall or traumatic or spontaneous rupture of the lung. If the body of air is large, the lung will collapse. Respirations are painful, dyspneic and abdominal. The animal may be in a state of collapse. Mucous membranes may be cyanotic. There may be puncture wounds of the chest or evidence of fractured ribs. Radiographs reveal a pocket of air in the dorsal thoracic cavity and rib fractures if present. Traumatic wounds of the chest wall may be evident.

Any penetrating wound must be closed. Mildly affected animals recover and the air is slowly absorbed. Lung function gradually returns. In severe cases, air can be removed by thoracentesis and use of a 3-way valve. Oxygen therapy may be indicated. If wound infection is a possibility, antibiotics (R 41) should be administered.

SKIN AND CONNECTIVE TISSUE

DERMATITIS

Dermatitis can be produced by direct and indirect causes involving a wide variety of agents, including external irritants, burns, allergens, trauma, and infections that may be bacterial, parasitic or fungal in origin. Dermatitis can be associated with a concurrent disease and an hereditary predisposition to dermatosis has been suspected. Allergies form an important group of etiologic factors, especially in small animals (q.v., p. 4).

Clinical Findings: The most common sign is scratching, followed by the appearance of the skin lesions which progress from edema and erythema to papules, vesicles, oozing and crusting. Secondary infection is common, with pustules or purulent lesions. As the disease becomes chronic, the erythema decreases and there are fewer vesicles or papules; but infiltration and thickening of the skin increases, the lesions are dryer and the skin may crack. The clinical picture may vary considerably with the species affected and with the causal agent of the skin lesions.

Treatment: Once the underlying cause is determined, its elimination will effect a prompt recovery. However, the numerous possible origins of dermatitis can at first necessitate establishing therapy on an empirical basis. In the choice and application of local treatment, certain general principles should be observed. Treatments of moist skin areas will differ from those of dry lesions. Internal and external therapy may be indicated.

The corticosteroids are often of great value in reducing the acute phase of dermatitis and in relieving pruritus. Dosage of adrenocortical steroids must be established individually. Corticosteroids, at times with antibiotics, can be used as topical ointments or lotions in erythematous, edematous and pruritic dermatitis and are usually effective (℞ 537, 539).

Local treatment of each type of lesion should be considered individually. Clipping of the haircoat of the affected area and surrounding the lesion is highly advantageous. To prevent scratching and licking, sedatives and various protective devices (as stuffed, pneumatic or cardboard collars, hobbles, or, when necessary, bandages) should be employed.

Preparations with a tar base (℞ 412, 426) are commonly used in the local treatment of dry, scaly, or crusted dermatitis; wet dressings (℞ 401) are useful in weeping or moist lesions. Certain dressings with a stimulating effect on the epithelium (℞ 430, 439) are useful in inactive cases. A chlorquinaldol-steroid ointment (℞ 136) can be used for local treatment of chronic dermatitis. Where it is desirable to remove scurf and epithelial debris thoroughly, a selenium sulfide shampoo (℞ 432), or nonirritating oily preparations are quite effective. Indirect causes of dermatitis, e.g., imbalanced nutrition, concurrent disease or infections, must be treated accordingly.

PYODERMA
(Pyogenic dermatitis, Acne, Secondary pyoderma)

A pyogenic infection of skin, which can be primary or secondary, superficial or deep.

Microorganisms commonly isolated from pyodermas include *Staphylococcus aureus*, coagulase-positive (found most often); *Staph. epidermis*, coagulase-negative; streptococci (both hemolytic and nonhemolytic); corynebacteria and *Proteus vulgaris*. Short-haired breeds and young animals are more often affected. Metabolic disorders, endocrine imbalance or various intoxications may, in some cases, predispose to the development of pyogenic dermatitis.

Clinical Findings: In horses, lesions of folliculitis often develop in the saddle and lumbar region (*see also* SADDLE SORES, p. 921), particularly in summer. The affected area is first swollen and very sensitive. This is followed by formation of papules and pustules. These may become confluent or rupture, forming plaques and crusts. Severe folliculitis may develop over large areas of the body, especially on the neck, sides of the thorax, inner surface of the thighs or on the prepuce. At times, deeper parts of the skin are involved and ulcers may be formed. In cattle, folliculitis which may proceed to necrosis develops mainly on the lower part of the tail. In dogs, superficial and deep pyoderma are recognized. Superficial pyogenic infection (impetigo) develops mostly on the abdomen, groin and medial surfaces of the thighs. It may also be seen on the head, nose, lips, in vulvar folds and between the toes.

Deep pyogenic dermatitis is characterized by a penetrating suppurative inflammation of skin, hair follicles, sebaceous glands and deeper parts of the cutaneous and subcut. tissues. Thus, folliculitis, furunculosis and abscesses are successive stages. Deep suppurative lesions may fuse, especially in the subcutis, forming ulcerated fistulous tracts discharging pus. These involvements are most commonly noted on the extremities and rump. Animals suffering from extensive deep pyoderma may have elevated temperature, anemia, leukocytosis and enlargement of the regional lymph nodes.

In long-haired dogs, deep pyogenic dermatitis involves the trunk, lips, vulvar folds and interdigital skin and, occasionally, the posterior portion of the abdomen and axillae. In puppies, secondary pyogenic infection occasionally develops during the course of an infectious disease.

Prognosis: The prognosis for pyoderma is more favorable in horses than in other animals. In horses, the lesions may disappear spontaneously within several weeks. The prognosis for secondary pyoderma in severely affected animals, particularly dogs, may be unfavorable.

Treatment: Irritation of the affected areas should be avoided. In the early stage, bathing in warm antiseptic solutions such as hexachlorophene (℞ 423) is useful. Choice of therapy depends upon the type of the lesions. Superficial pyogenic dermatitis is relatively easy to treat. Among the topical preparations for superficial conditions are: STA (salicylic acid 8, tannic acid 8, 70% alcohol 100 parts), 5% alcoholic solution of crystal violet (gentian violet) and a number of other lotions and sprays containing a variety of proprietary antibacterial agents (℞ 398, 404, 524).

It is essential to treat deep pyogenic dermatitis both topically and systemically. Deep pyodermas should be incised for drainage before local application of antibiotic ointments (℞ 398, 417, 420). In undetermined cases, nitrofurans, antibiotics or sulfonamides along with enzyme preparations may be injected through a blunt needle directly into the fistulous tracts. If possible, cultures should be made and sensitivity tests done to determine the most effective antibiotic. Pyoderma of lip or vulvar folds is treated topically by antiseptic drying preparations such as 10% silver nitrate. When the lesions become dry, an antiseptic ointment is rubbed into the affected areas which are then dusted with a powder (antibiotic, sufonamide, iodoform, tannoform).

Juvenile pyoderma lesions are cleansed with a mild antiseptic solution. Crusts covering the skin are softened with lukewarm mineral oil or with antibiotic compresses (neomycin 1:1,000) and gently removed. Mild antiseptics are then applied, preferably by spraying.

For systemic treatment, sulfonamides (℞ 75, 82), antibiotics (℞ 25, 41), autogenous vaccines, bacterins and enzymes may be used. In stubborn cases, X-ray therapy should be considered by those experienced in this technique.

RHABDITIC DERMATITIS

An acute dermatitis of dogs and cattle caused by the nematode *Rhabditis strongyloides*. *R. strongyloides* is saprophytic, living in moist soil and decaying organic matter. Lesions are confined to areas of the body soiled by urine and feces, or in contact with moist, filthy bedding.

The condition is infrequent and occurs sporadically in dogs, but may assume epizootic forms in cattle. It is characterized by pruritus, acute dermatitis followed by pustules, crusts and alopecia. The worms can be found in skin scrapings or expressed from pustules. The larva is cylindrical, approximately 600 μ in length and 38 μ in width.

Rhabditic dermatitis can be prevented and controlled by providing clean dry bedding and disinfecting the surroundings. Improving the hygiene usually results in spontaneous recovery. Exposure to sunshine is also beneficial. Recovery may be hastened by cleaning of the areas involved and application of astringent and disinfectant preparations (℞ 620).

DERMATOPHILUS CONGOLENSIS INFECTION

(Dermatophilosis, Cutaneous actinomycosis, Cutaneous streptotrichosis, Lumpy-wool disease)

An epidermal infection of Herbivora including deer, horses, cattle, sheep and goats, characterized by the formation of horny crusts which adhere firmly to the infected skin. It was formerly thought to be several related but distinct diseases, i.e., mycotic dermatitis, proliferative dermatitis of the legs in sheep and streptotrichosis of cattle, horses and goats.

Etiology: *Dermatophilus congolensis* (*dermatonomus, pedis*), an aerobic actinomycete, is the only species in the family Dermatophilaceae. It forms a branched mycelium that divides transversely and then longitudinally to produce thick bundles of very small cocci. These enlarge and mature into flagellated ovoid "zoospores", 0.6 to 1 μ in diameter. When the crusts are wetted, the zoospores emerge to the surface where they are available for the transmission of infection. The organism has no resistant stage and transmission is presumably fairly direct.

There is evidence that plant and insect vectors serve as a mechanical means of transfer. In some cases spiny plants and insects also facilitate infection by disrupting the lipid and keratinous covering of the skin, thus providing the zoospores with access to the living epidermal layer. Infection may also be associated with skin damage by other agents including heavy rain.

The distribution of lesions usually corresponds to the predisposing skin damage. Thus, in the presence of spiny plants, sheep may be infected on the lips or brisket, or on the legs and feet ("strawberry foot rot") whereas infections following heavy rain are mainly on the dorsal areas of the body ("lumpy-wool"). In infected cattle ("cutaneous streptotrichosis") the lesions are often generally distributed suggesting the possible involvement of insects that attack all parts of the body surface.

Clinical Findings: The hyphae of *D. congolensis* invade the living epidermal cells, especially in the hair or wool follicle sheaths, inducing local acute inflammation and rapid cornification of the infected epidermis. Alternate layers of dried exudate and cornified epidermis accumulate on the skin where they are bound by the hair or wool fibers into a compact amber crust.

From a clinical point of view the lesions vary in 2 important qualities—extent and persistence. The extensive confluent infection sometimes seen in lambs and calves proves fatal in many cases. Less extensive infections usually have little effect on the general health of the animal, apart from severe lesions on the lips, which may lead to death from starvation. Death may also follow secondary blow-fly strike or screwworm infestation.

In most individual animals the infection is overcome and the crusts are separable from the skin within about 3 weeks. However, in a number of sheep (particularly Merinos) and cattle the infection becomes chronic and the crusts are built up into large horny masses. In sheep this produces the typical "lumpy-wool" condition. Chronic infection prevents the shearing of sheep and detracts seriously from the value of the hides of cattle.

Diagnosis: *D. congolensis* is usually demonstrable in stained smears and cultures made from finely chopped macerated crusts. It is gram-positive and grows well on nutrient agar at 37°C, especially in an atmosphere of 10% CO_2. There is complete hemolysis around colonies on sheep but not horse blood agar. Isolation from material that is heavily contaminated or poor in viable *D. congolensis*, is facilitated by passage in sheep or guinea pigs. The material should be wetted and applied to lightly scarified skin.

In sheep, dermatophilosis may be distinguished from contagious ecthyma by the lack of infectivity of bacteria-free filtrates made from suspensions of crust material. The lesions usually differ from those of ringworm and scabies in their greater tendency to accumulate hard crust, but must sometimes be differentiated by microscopic and cultural examination.

Prophylaxis: Because small, almost inapparent lesions are widely widespread among herbivorous animals, quarantine measures are of little or no value. Vaccination induces a good immunologic response but has very little effect on the extent or duration of infection. The application of disinfectants should decrease the spread of infection if applied at times when transmission is likely; in sheep, shear-cut infections have been successfully prevented by spraying with 0.5% zinc sulfate. In other circumstances the correct time to spray would be more difficult to predict.

Treatment: In acute cases the duration of infection is short and treatment is usually unwarranted. Healed lesions, in which the crusts are held in place by the hair fibers, are sometimes mistaken for active infections and treated. This has led to erroneous claims for local treatments involving the removal of crusts prior to disinfectant applications. External treatments have no curative value because many hyphae are inaccessible in the follicle sheaths.

Persistent infections may be rapidly and effectively cured with a single large injection of streptomycin and procaine penicillin combined. Although ineffective alone, penicillin greatly potentiates the action of streptomycin. A dose rate of 20 mg streptomycin plus 20,000 u procaine penicillin per pound of body weight IM is recommended. Sheep with lumpy-wool can be shorn 2 months after treatment. An insecticide may have to be applied to control secondary blow-fly strike.

DERMATOMYCOSES
(Ringworm)

Infections of keratin-bearing tissues (skin, hair and nails) caused by fungi called dermatophytes. Most domestic animals are susceptible although swine and sheep seem to be less commonly infected than other animals. Anthropophilic dermatophytes infect man primarily and lower animals only rarely. Zoophilic dermatophytes are animal pathogens mainly but can cause disease in man. Geophilic dermatophytes are free-living soil fungi that parasitize man or animals under certain conditions. The infection starts in the stratum corneum where thread-like hyphae develop from spores. The hyphae grow about halfway down the hair follicles and then enter the hairs. They grow down the hair to the first layer of keratinized cells where growth stops. The hyphae may produce spores within the hair (endothrix type) or produce spores in rows or mosaics along the outer surface of the hairs (ectothrix type). The lesion usually spreads in a circular manner from the original point of infection giving rise to the term "ringworm".

The clinical signs of ringworm are not pathognomonic. Diagnosis must be arrived at by (1) examination using Wood's lamp (cobalt-filtered ultraviolet), (2) direct microscopic examination of hairs or scrapings, or (3) culture.

1. The Wood's lamp is primarily useful for the diagnosis of *Microsporum canis* infections in animals and *M. audovini* infections in man. Infected hairs or lesions fluoresce with a yellowish-green color. The examination should be made before medication is started because certain medicaments, mineral oil for example, will cause pseudofluorescence, while others, such as iodine, may block fluorescence in infected hairs.

2. Direct microscopic examination of hairs or skin scrapings is an effective office or field procedure for the rapid diagnosis of ringworm infection. Hairs or scrapings from a suspected area of infection are put on a slide in a drop of 10% potassium hydroxide and covered with a cover slip. After gentle heating to clear the specimen, it is examined for the presence of hyphae or spores.

3. Culture on Sabouraud's agar plates takes the longest time but is the most effective and specific means of diagnosis. It frequently shows infections that may have been missed by the

first 2 procedures, and also aids in the identification of the specific etiologic agents. Hairs or scrapings are placed on the agar and the Petri dish is sealed with adhesive tape to reduce evaporation. Addition of 0.5 mg of cycloheximide per milliliter is necessary to prevent rapid growth of other contaminating molds. The plate can be kept at room temperature. It should be incubated at least one week and may require as much as 4 weeks to produce sufficient growth for identification.

RINGWORM IN CATTLE

Trichophyton verrucosum is the most frequent cause of ringworm in cattle, but *T. mentagrophytes* is occasionally isolated. Although cattle of all ages may be affected, the disease is most common in calves. After an incubation period of 2 to 4 weeks, the hair in the infected area breaks off or falls out and, by 2 to 3 months, round, sharply circumscribed, thick, asbestos-like plaques are seen. Lesions expand at the periphery and frequently are 12 to 75 mm in diameter. Sites of predilection include the skin around the eyes, ears, muzzle and neck; but few areas escape infection if the condition is left untreated. The disease is more commonly seen during the winter months in stabled animals, but may occur at any time. The fungus is resistant and may survive up to 4 years in dry scales. Infection is transmitted readily from animal to animal and from animal to man by direct or indirect contact.

Diagnosis: The appearance of round, scaly or encrusted, alopecic patches or plaques strongly favors a diagnosis of ringworm. The diagnosis can be readily confirmed by demonstration of the fungus on the affected hairs by microscopic examination of specimens cleared by potassium hydroxide. Chains of spherical, rather large (4 to 6 μ) spores surround the hair shaft.

Treatment: When thick crusts are first removed with a brush and mild soap, ringworm usually responds to local application of fungicidal drugs, but persistent treatment may be required. Daily applications of a mixture of equal parts tincture of iodine and glycerin or a 20% solution of sodium caprylate to the lesion until it disappears often is effective. All parts of the lesion should be soaked thoroughly at each application. Tincture of iodine or Lugol's solution applied every other day also is effective. Cattle with widespread infection may be given 2 IV treatments one week apart consisting of 30 gm of sodium iodide in 250 ml of water. Oral administration of griseofulvin has given good results, but may not be used in animals kept for food purposes, and may not be economically feasible for most large animals. The antifungal activity of topically applied thiabendazole may provide a useful treatment.

RINGWORM IN HORSES

Trichophyton equinum is the primary cause of ringworm in horses. *T. mentagrophytes* is found occasionally. The infection is characterized by a focal edematous lesion with piloerection and finally alopecia and formation of a thick crust. Microscopic examination of cleared hairs reveals spores arranged in chains around the hair.

Ringworm in horses usually occurs at sites where the skin comes in contact with infected animals or contaminated saddle blankets, harness and grooming tools.

Treatment: After working, the horse should be washed with a solution of 30 gm of captan (Vangard 45) in 3 gal. of water. This should be repeated every 4 days until clinical cure is obtained. A mixture of equal parts of iodine and glycerin applied daily to the lesion is effective.

RINGWORM IN DOGS AND CATS

Approximately 70% of ringworm in dogs is caused by *Microsporum canis,* 20% is due to *M. gypseum* and 10% is due to *Trichophyton mentagrophytes*. In cats, 98% is caused by *M. canis,* while *M. gypseum* and *T. mentagrophytes* each account for about 1%. Because of the high percentage of *M. canis* infections, the Wood's lamp becomes a valuable diagnostic tool when examining these species. It must be kept in mind, however, that *M. gypseum* and *T. mentagrophytes* do not fluoresce and a negative Wood's lamp examination does not rule out ringworm.

The clinical appearance of ringworm is more variable in cats than in dogs. There may be no clinically apparent lesions or there may be only a few broken hairs around the face and ears. Other lesions may be scaly and alopecic or, in more severe cases, there may be alopecic crusted lesions involving a large part of the body. In general, older rather than younger cats are more likely to be carriers with clinically inapparent infections. The clinically normal carrier dog is seen less frequently.

Lesions in dogs usually appear as circular scaly patches with broken stubs of hair within the lesions or they may be completely alopecic inside the ring. The lesion is most active at the periphery where there may be vesicles and pustules. In severe infections, large areas of the dog's body may show alopecia, scaling, erythema or crust formation. *M. canis* is transmissible to man and it is not uncommon for the owner and the animal to have similar lesions.

Treatment: Griseofulvin (R 352) is the treatment of choice. It inhibits fungal growth at the point of lowest penetration on the hair shaft. Spread of the infection to other parts of the body or other animals or man can be reduced or eliminated by the use of antifungal dips, such as a 1:200 solution of 45% captan, or iodine shampoos applied to the whole body on the 7th and 14th days of griseofulvin therapy. After clinical recovery there may still be active fungal elements in the portions of the hairs above the skin surface and when possible, it is usually wise to clip the hair to remove the infected terminal ends.

Lesions that become infected secondarily should be treated with suitable antimicrobial agents (R 398, 406, 420).

MANGE (LG. AN.)

A contagious skin disease caused by one of several species of mites which may spread by direct contact with diseased animals or from various objects which have been in contact with diseased animals, e.g., harnesses, blankets, grooming utensils, bedding, stables or attendants. The incubation period for the development of clinical mange depends on the mode and the place of the infection and the susceptibility of the host. Usually, 2 to 6 weeks elapse before the first visible skin lesions develop. Mites of similar appearance occurring in different host species are regarded as being different mite species or as varieties of the same species; they are specific to their respective hosts.

MANGE IN HORSES

Sarcoptic mange (*Sarcoptes scabiei* var. *equi*) is the most severe type. It spreads very quickly in infected animals, as well as to other individuals. Early lesions appear on the head, neck and shoulders. Regions protected by long hair and lower parts of the extremities usually are not involved.

The disease is first characterized by intense pruritus. Small papules and vesicles develop into an acute dermatitis, scale formation increases rapidly and later crusts form. The bald and encrusted patches enlarge and the skin thickens, forming folds, particularly in the neck region. In advanced cases, the lesions may extend over the entire body, leading to emaciation, general weakness and loss of appetite. The course is nearly always chronic. The prognosis is the most unfavorable of all the types of horse mange, particularly in severe infestations and in animals in poor condition.

For treating individual cases, acaricidal preparations are applied by spraying, rubbing, or dipping. For groups of animals, dipping is the most convenient and effective method of treatment. Lime-sulfur (℞ 312) can be used if the dip is heated to 90° to 95°F and the animals are dipped 4 to 6 times at intervals of 10 to 12 days. Nicotine sulfate dip (℞ 315) usually gives control with one application. Lindane at 0.06% concentration (℞ 313) can be used as a spray or dip, where local laws permit its use.

Psoroptic mange (caused by *Psoroptes equi* var. *equi*) produces skin lesions on sheltered parts of the body, particularly those covered with long hair, e.g., beneath the forelock and the mane, at the root of the tail and in the submaxillary region; it also occurs in the axilla and on the prepuce and udder. Sometimes, the mites may also be found in the external auditory meatus. The cutaneous lesions are similar to the sarcoptic type, but usually have larger and thicker crusts, the skin is less folded, the itching is less, and the mites can be found in the crusts more easily. The course is chronic and the prognosis is more favorable. The treatment corresponds to that used for the sarcoptic type.

Chorioptic mange, often known as "leg mange", is caused by *Chorioptes bovis* var. *equi.* Cutaneous lesions are found chiefly on the lower parts of the hind legs. In severe cases, skin lesions may spread to the flank region, shoulder and neck. The disease is characterized by intense itching, scales, crusts, thickening of the skin and, in neglected cases, a moist dermatitis in the fetlock region. The signs subside in summer; however, with the return of cold weather, they develop again. The chorioptic mites are easily found in scrapings collected from the affected area. The course as a rule is chronic; the prognosis for "leg mange" is favorable. Treatments recommended for other mange mites also are effective against chorioptic mange.

Demodectic mange is seldom diagnosed in horses. The mites live in the hair follicles and in the sebaceous glands, the tissues being damaged mechanically or by the toxins produced. Clinical signs are characterized by papules and ulcers, particularly around the eyes and on the forehead. Subsequently the lesions spread to the shoulder region and finally over the entire body. The affected skin is covered with scales. Pruritus is absent.

Successful treatment with sulfur preparations, such as 3 to 5% flowers-of-sulfur ointment has been reported.

MANGE IN CATTLE
(Barn itch)

All types of mange occur in cattle; but, the chorioptic type usually is predominant. Identification of the type of mange present and its differentiation from other dermatoses can only be achieved microscopically. At times mange and ringworm occur simultaneously or as intercurrent infections in herds and individual animals.

Scabies (*Sarcoptes scabiei* var. *bovis*) shows lesions first on the head and neck, and then spreads to other parts. Sometimes, the lesions appear in the perineal region and between the thighs. The skin eruptions are similar to those in horses. They are characterized by a squamous, crusted appearance; the skin itself thickens, forming large folds. The lesions may heal spontaneously during the summer, particularly when the animals are kept on pasture.

Psoroptic mange is due to *Psoroptes equi* var. *bovis* and occurs rather seldom in cattle. It appears first on the neck, at the base of the horns and, in severe cases, spreads to the legs.

Chorioptic mange caused by *Chorioptes bovis* var. *bovis* is the most common type of mange in cattle. The skin lesions develop chiefly in the tail region spreading to other parts of the body. Sometimes, the lesions start on the legs and the disease is called "leg mange". The treatment of cattle mange is similar to that described for horses. Lime-sulfur dips (℞ 312) are very effective, if the full course of 6 treatments is given—one treatment every 7 to 10 days. Dips or sprays containing 0.06% lindane (℞ 313) are effective where use of this drug is permitted.

Demodectic mange sometimes occurs epizootically and causes considerable damage to hides. The disease has been found most often in cattle between the ages of 4 and 8 years, or in younger animals. Bovine demodectic mites differ from those found in other animals. The skin lesions generally appear on the neck, the shoulder region and the trunk. Occasionally, they develop on the muzzle and, in rare instances, over the entire body surface. First small papules and nodules develop. Sometimes, they have a red color, and a thick, white material, having a waxy consistency, can be expressed from them. This caseous and greasy material contains numerous mites. In rare cases, the nodules are filled with pus and may coalesce, forming abscesses covered with small scales. In some cases, cutaneous lesions consist of thick crusts and the skin thickens forming heavy folds. The course of bovine demodectic mange generally is mild, but may extend over many months. Recovery is usually spontaneous.

In cattle, the remedies recommended for sarcoptic mange have been used, but the therapeutic effect is doubtful. In valuable animals the best therapeutic results have been achieved with incisions of the nodules and painting with tincture of iodine.

MANGE IN SHEEP AND GOATS

In sheep, the disease is caused by *Sarcoptes scabiei* var. *ovis*, *Psoroptes equi* var. *ovis,* or *Chorioptes bovis* var. *ovis*.

Sarcoptic mange in sheep occurs only on the nonwooly skin, starting as a rule on the head as "head mange".

Psoroptic mange (sheep scab) is the most frequent type in sheep. It occurs almost exclusively on the thickly wooled areas where it produces large scaly, crusted lesions. Intense itching is generally the first sign. When larger skin areas are involved, the animals show gradual emaciation, anemia and cachectic hydremia. The psoroptic mites may be found even in the ear canal ("ear mange"). Psoroptic mange in sheep is a notifiable disease and affected flocks are subject to quarantine regulations.

Chorioptic mange in sheep is also called "leg mange", producing lesions most often on the hind legs, and on the scrotum of rams.

Since large numbers of animals usually are affected, dips are the most common treatment. A single dipping in 0.06% lindane (℞ 313) controls psoroptic mange, where use of this drug is permitted. Other mange infestations may require a second treatment. Nicotine, arsenic, sulfur and creosote also have been used in treating mange, but are less efficient.

Demodectic mange has also been reported in sheep, causing skin lesions similar to those in other large animals.

In **goats, demodectic mange** is similar to that described for cattle. The cutaneous lesions are found on the skin of the neck, shoulder, thorax and flank. The nodules, ranging in size from a pinhead to a hazelnut, contain a thick, grayish material of waxy consistency which can be easily expressed. Numerous demodectic mites are found in this material. The nodules of demodectic mange in goats appear as cysts with mild inflammation in the surrounding tissue. This infection in goats may be a very stubborn condition causing, in some countries, great damage to the hides. The treatments recommended for sarcoptic mange have been used, but the results are doubtful. In valuable goats, incision of the nodules and painting with tincture of iodine gives the best therapeutic results.

"ITCH MITE" INFESTATION

An infestation of sheep by *Psorergates ovis* in which the pruritus induced by the mite caused the host to bite and rub the affected areas damaging the fleece. The disease has been reported from Australia, New Zealand, South Africa, the U.S.A., Argentina and Chile. As control measures can be carried out before the infestation becomes serious, the disease is not regarded as of major economic importance.

The life cycle (6 stages—egg, larval, 3 nymphal and male and female adult) is completed in 4 to 5 weeks. The development of all stages occurs in the stratum malpighii of the epidermis, where the mites are considered to feed on cell fluids.

The first signs often occur about 2 to 3 years after arsenical dips are abandoned in favor of the newer insecticides. The incidence increases slowly in the flock until, after 3 or 4 years, 10% of the older sheep may be actively biting or rubbing. Characteristic signs are few. A damaged fleece, alopecia, crusting or chronic dermatitis resulting mainly from self-inflicted trauma (in the absence of *Psoroptes*, lice, keds, mycotic dermatitis, fleece rot or grass seeds) are suspicious signs. The withers and sides of the trunk are usual sites of involvement.

Demonstration of the mites in skin scrapings is the only positive diagnosis (*see* CLEARED, UNSTAINED SMEAR METHOD, p. 1386). Several skin scrapings may be necessary.

Dipping in 1% lime sulfur or 0.2% arsenic is considered to give satisfactory results. This need not be done annually, but only as the incidence on the flock warrants.

MANGE IN SWINE

The sarcoptic type caused by *Sarcoptes scabiei* var. *suis* is the only form of any importance in swine. The lesions usually start on the head, spread over the body, the tail and the legs. The skin is thickened, rough and dry, covered with grayish crusts and thrown into large folds. Itching is intense, and growth is stunted. Deep skin scrapings should be examined as swine also suffer from other kinds of skin disease, including ringworm. Spraying with lindane at a concentration of 0.05 to 0.1% or malathion 0.5% (R 273) is effective; 0.25% chlordane solution can also be used. (Use of some or all of these for food-producing animals is prohibited in some countries.)

Demodectic mange occurs also in swine, causing skin lesions similar to those seen in other large animals. Treatment with remedies used in sarcoptic mange has been attempted, but the results appear unreliable.

MANGE (SM. AN.)

CUTANEOUS ACARIASIS

A skin disease caused by parasitic mites of either the sarcoptic or demodectic type. Sarcoptic mange is highly contagious while demodectic mange is noncontagious.

Etiology: Sarcoptic mange of dogs is caused by a *Sarcoptes scabiei* var. *canis*. The body of the mite is almost circular with 4 pairs of legs, all, except the posterior pair, extending beyond the margin of the body. Eggs are laid in tunnels as the female burrows into the skin. Eggs hatch in the tunnels. The larvae have only 3 pairs of legs. The species infesting the cat, *Notoedres cati,* is smaller and more circular than the one in the dog. The transition from ova to adult usually takes 10 to 14 days.

Demodectic mange is caused by *Demodex canis*. The mites have vermiform bodies and the elongated abdomen is marked with transverse striations. Adult and nymphs have, on the anterior portion of the body, 8 legs, each divided into 5 segments, while larvae have only 6 legs. The mites inhabit the skin and usually are found in the sebaceous glands or hair follicles where eggs, larvae, nymphs and adults may be found. The complete life cycle is not known. *D. cati* is occasionally found on cats where it may cause lesions similar to those in the dog.

Clinical Findings: The sarcoptic mite causes intense pruritus as it burrows in the skin and the animal scratches and rubs persistently. The skin becomes dry, thickened and wrinkled. Crusts are formed in the involved areas. Usually, the lesions first appear on the head around the eyes, ears or muzzle and then spread to the neck, abdomen and extremities.

In cats, mange usually starts at the tips of the ears, spreads to the face and then to the whole head. It also may extend to involve the rest of the body and legs.

The *Demodex*-infected animal may show a variety of lesions from slight small patches of alopecia around the eyes or over the body to extensive hemorrhagic or pyodermic lesions completely covering the body. Skin lesions can be classified as squamous or pustular. In the squamous type, there is only a mild inflammatory change with absence of hair in the affected region and a slightly thickened skin with a fine scaly appearance. The skin may be erythematous or hyperpigmented to varying degrees.

In the pustular type, the skin is highly reddened, with blood and serum oozing from affected areas, along with purulent material resulting from bacterial invasion (usually *Staphylococcus aureus*). The skin may be thickened and often appears to have been excoriated. Lesions may cover the entire body. Occasionally, the entire skin is markedly reddened with little or no pustule formation ("red mange"). In severe cases, the mites may invade the lymph nodes and other tissues.

Diagnosis: Since the sarcoptic mites are in tunnels in the skin and the demodectic mites are in the hair follicles and sebaceous glands, deep scrapings of infected areas are best. A 6 to 10% solution of potassium hydroxide, placed on the slide with the skin scraping, dissolves the debris and the mites are seen more easily under the low power of the microscope.

Treatment: Clipping the dog, especially if long-haired, is important, for many lesions will be uncovered. A soap and water or mineral-oil bath to soften and remove crusts and scurf assists the acaricide in reaching the mites. Vigorous application of the medication is necessary since most of the mites are below the surface of the skin. A sound nutritional program should be established.

In treating sarcoptic mange, lime and sulfur dips and washes (℞ 312) have been successful, but several treatments always are necessary before all of the mites are destroyed. This is the safest treatment for puppies. Sulfur ointments (℞ 316) are useful, especially in localized lesions or in cases where dipping would not be practical. Benzyl benzoate emulsions or solutions also are practical; either a 25 or 50% emulsion (℞ 309) is excellent for topical application. Benzyl benzoate in combination with other acaricides (℞ 310) also gives excellent results. Dips containing lindane (℞ 314) have been widely used. A single and thorough dipping and scrubbing is often all that is necessary. Chlordane dips (℞ 318) given 7 days apart also are used successfully. Since the disease is so often generalized, dips are usually far more practical than the use of ointments.

The chlorinated hydrocarbon acaricides are toxic for cats. Lime and sulfur washes (℞ 312), sulfur ointments or rotenone compounds are successfully used. Good results can be obtained by using an ointment of sulfur (℞ 316) applied to affected areas.

Demodectic mange is one of the most persistent diseases and

often responds poorly to treatment. Benzyl benzoate emulsions
(℞ 309), or an emulsion of lindane and benzyl benzoate (℞
310) have been used successfully. These emulsions should be
thoroughly massaged into the skin daily for a week and the
animal then should be rested for another week before further
applications are made, or treatment can be carried out every
third day until the lesions heal. Not more than 30% of the
body should be treated at any one time. Rotenone preparations, such as Canex (℞ 311), also are very useful. The use
of organophosphates both orally and topically has given good
results (℞ 284). Demodectic mange in cats can be treated
locally with Canex.

In cases where secondary infection has become established,
vigorous antibiotic therapy is recommended, especially penicillin in combination with ointments of neomycin or bacitracin.
Reports indicate that griseofulvin (℞ 352) may be used successfully as systemic therapy.

NASAL ACARIASIS
(Nasal mites)

An infestation of the nasal cavity and paranasal sinuses of
dogs by the mite *Pneumonyssoides* (*Pneumonyssus*) *caninum*
usually without, or with only mild, signs. The adult mite has
a pale-yellow body. The gravid female contains a fully developed embryo that almost fills the abdomen. The method
of transmission of the parasite is unknown.

Except for an accumulation of mucus and a mild hyperemia
of the mucous membranes, no signs or lesions are usually
attributed to the infestation. Signs of a severe rhinitis may
occasionally be seen. Most infestations are found on postmortem examination. A few cases have been reported where
the mite was found on the nose of sleeping dogs. Treatment
has not been attempted.

OTOACARIASIS
(Otodectic mange, Ear mange, Parasitic otitis externa)

An infection of the ears with parasitic mites, e.g., *Otodectes
cynotis* in dogs and cats. (*See* PARASITIC OTITIS EXTERNA, p.
220. *See also* DISEASES OF RABBITS: EAR MITE INFESTATION, p.
1134.)

CHEYLETIELLA PARASITIVORAX (*YASGURI*)
INFESTATION

Acarid infestations by *Cheyletiella parasitivorax* (*yasguri*)
have been reported in dog, cat, rabbit, fox and man. The dis-

ease is highly contagious and cross-infestations between species occur. The causative agent, commonly known as the rabbit fur mite, inhabits the pelage and skin surface of animals; it also can live free in nature. It is a large mite (388 X 266 μ) easily identified microscopically by its large palpal claws, numerous feathered bristles and cones on the tarsi.

Two clinical forms, exfoliative and crustose, have been recognized in the dog. In the first, a scaling process (mimicking dandruff) occurs primarily on the dorsal trunk, and is most evident on the skin, with a few scales in the pelage. Alopecia and inflammatory changes are usually present only secondary to scratching. The degree of pruritus varies from moderate to intense. In the second form, multiple discrete, circular, alopecic crusts (2 to 5 cm in diameter) are observed on the dorsal and lateral trunk. The lesions may expand or enlarge and appear similar to ringworm; however, no inflammatory border is evident and no dermatophytes can be demonstrated. The lesion also resembles the crustose form of seborrhea which occurs so commonly in Cocker Spaniels.

Though cats may have the exfoliative form, most have the crustose variety. The lesions strongly resemble ringworm except that most of them occur on the neck and trunk.

Diagnosis depends upon identification of the organism in skin scrapings. Deep scrapings are unnecessary. Material removed for microscopic examinations should be placed in 10% potassium hydroxide and viewed under 25X magnification.

Successful treatment may be achieved with derris washes or dustings, or the topical application of a variety of insecticides including 0.02% lindane (B 243), organophosphorus compounds (B 293) benzyl benzoate-lindane solution (B 244) or Thionium shampoo with lindane (B 303). Topical applications should be repeated until clinical cure is achieved and neither the organism nor its eggs can be demonstrated by microscopic examination. It may be necessary to treat the environment simultaneously.

ACANTHOSIS NIGRICANS

Dermatosis characterized by hypertrophy of the papillae, superficial hyperakeratosis and increased pigmentation. It occurs in dogs, particularly Dachshunds, Airedale and other terriers and German Shepherd Dogs.

Etiology: Dogs with this disease may have a significant decrease in thyroid activity, and the thyroid gland, the gonads and adrenal cortex also could be involved in the development of this condition. Thyrotropic hormone exerts a highly favorable effect, possibly indirectly, on the skin lesions. The frequent appearance of lesions in friction areas indicates that mechanical influence may also play a role.

Clinical Findings: Lesions usually are found on the inner side of the thighs, the scrotum, abdomen, flanks, axillae, the ventral surface of the neck and tail, around the lips and eyelids, and on the extensor surfaces of the toes. As a rule, the lesions are bilaterally symmetrical. In the initial stages, the affected skin becomes swollen. Excessive shedding of hair takes place and within a few days a grayish blue-black pigmentation appears. The skin gradually becomes thickened and rough. Later the skin becomes covered with scales and many folds are formed. The color deepens until it is black. Occasionally, a case of acanthosis occurs without pigmentation. In some cases, the pathologic changes may extend to the mucous membranes of the mouth, conjunctiva, vagina and anus. As a rule, there is no pruritus.

The course of the disease is usually chronic. Since the advent of hormone therapy the prognosis has become favorable, and many cases of acanthosis nigricans can be controlled, but it frequently recurs.

Treatment: Thyroid extract is given orally in tablets. A medium-sized dog should receive 180 mg daily for 4 days, then 120 mg daily for 4 days and then 60 mg daily for 20 days. In severe cases, this treatment can be repeated after 14 days. Triiodothyronine is also effective as thyroid therapy. The dose is 0.5 mcg/lb of body wt daily for 28 days. It can be repeated after 2 weeks of rest.

It is also helpful if thyrotropic hormone, 1 or 2 USP units daily, is given during the first week of therapy. Propylthiouracil or methylthiouracil, 50 mg twice a day for 21 days, decreases circulating thyroxin, thus stimulating the anterior pituitary gland to produce more TSH. Sex hormones may be used, especially, in aged dogs, in the same way as described in hormonal eczema (see MISCELLANEOUS DERMATOSES, p. 914). Corticosteroids (R 154) are especially useful in dogs with severe hyperpigmentation.

Other internal therapy includes potassium and sodium iodide (R 579) and nonspecific proteins. For external therapy, sulfur ointment (R 440), therapeutic shampoos and ichthammol ointment (R 412) have been used.

MISCELLANEOUS DERMATOSES

A number of systemic diseases produce varying lesions in the skin as part of their clinical manifestation. These are most often noninflammatory and commonly display alopecia as part of their syndrome. In some instances the cutaneous changes are characteristic of the particular disease. Often, however, the dermatosis is not obviously associated with the underlying condition and careful differentiation must be made to separate a primary skin disorder from the secondary signs of an apparently unrelated or undiagnosed ailment. Some of these are mentioned briefly below, and are also described in the chapter on the specific disorder.

Dermatosis may be associated with nutritional deficiencies, especially those of vitamins, proteins, fats, minerals and trace elements. Dermatitis is sometimes observed in the course of chronic disorders of internal organs, such as nephritis, hepatitis, pyometra or diseased anal glands. A variety of skin changes may also develop in the course of poisoning, e.g., hyperkeratosis in cattle, poisoning by thallium sulfate (rat poisons), ergotism, mercurialism and iodism.

In dogs, dermatosis can develop as a result of hormone imbalance. In males, dermatoses may be associated with underdevelopment of the testicles, especially Sertoli cell tumors. Skin disorders caused by imbalance of sexual hormones are more common in female than in male dogs. Skin lesions may also develop in dogs and cats after spaying and castration at a premature age. These dermatoses assume, as a rule, a special location and character. Alopecia or a squamous eczema with crusted accumulations of skin debris characteristically develops around the base of the tail, the anus and the vulva, between the hind legs and on the posterior part of the abdomen. In advanced cases, the lesions spread to other parts of the body.

Dermatoses have also been observed in disorders of the thyroid gland. In hypothyroidism, the skin lesions are characterized by diminished hair growth and alopecia. In rare cases, cutaneous signs of myxedema develop. The skin of the hypothyroid patient is dry, scaly, thickened and folded. Acanthosis nigricans and seborrheic disorders also may be found.

Faulty production of hypophyseal hormones also may cause dermatoses. Hypopituitarism is characterized by loss of hair, especially in the axillary region and on the sides of the thorax and abdomen. Disorders of the adrenal glands also are manifested by skin changes. In the course of a deficient activity of the pancrease (hypoinsulinism), diabetic pruritus may be a sign.

The treatment of all these conditions depends on differential diagnosis. Once this is established and dealt with, the skin lesions usually need only symptomatic care (e.g., control of scratching) until they disappear with the resolution of the primary disease.

If a hormonal deficiency is present, substitutional therapy is indicated. In gonadal hormone deficiencies, androgens and estrogens are used. In male dogs, from 5 to 50 mg testosterone is given daily, depending on the size of the animal. Where skin lesions are caused by testicular tumors, castration is the most effective treatment. In females, with eczema associated with hypoestrinism, 0.1 to 0.5 mg of diethylstilbestrol is given daily. For the treatment of hypothyroidism associated with skin conditions, thyroid extract (R 182) is given orally.

ALOPECIA
(Baldness, Atrichia)

Local or general loss of hair, fur or wool. True alopecia is baldness without other visible skin disease. However, the term alopecia is also associated with many inflammatory skin disorders.

Etiology: Alopecia may be congenital or acquired. The former has been described in cow, horse and dog. Hairlessness invariably accompanies congenital goiter in pigs farrowed by iodine-deficient sows. Acquired alopecia is due to a variety of diseases and intoxications, e.g., gastroenteritis, pneumonia, dietary deficiencies and general infectious diseases, particularly those causing febrile reactions or epithelial destruction, and poisoning as by mercury, iodine or formalin. Disorders of the thyroid, pituitary and gonads have caused hair loss, especially in dogs, as have large doses of estrogens. Temporary alopecia in horses, sheep and dogs is sometimes seen in advanced pregnancy or lactation. Localized hair loss may result from repeated local friction, the continued application of chemicals or irritants, the presence of ectoparasites and X-rays.

Clinical Findings: Alopecia in veterinary medicine is a frequent sign of a specific skin disease, e.g., ringworm and mange. The loss of hair in acquired alopecia usually starts as localized areas of baldness, which then may increase in size, coalesce with adjacent lesions, or remain static. Pruritus is variable. In neurogenic and endocrine alopecia, the lesions are confined to local areas or show a symmetric pattern of development. The course of alopecia is chronic and the prognosis unfavorable, unless the primary cause is identified and treated.

Treatment: The primary cause of the alopecia must be diagnosed and treated for satisfactory recovery to take place. The extent of recovery depends on the duration of the disease and the amount of damage to the hair follicles. Particular attention should be given to diet and skin cleanliness. In alopecia arising from endocrine hypofunction, substitution therapy is indicated. In other cases removal of obviously diseased glands may be helpful. Dogs affected with a hypothyroidism characterized by alopecia respond well to thyroid therapy (Ŗ 181). Local treatment of alopecia is of questionable value. However, if local medication is used, the agents should be nonirritating, rapid-drying lotions containing ingredients such as resorcinol (Ŗ 427) or salicylic acid (Ŗ 429).

ECZEMA NASI OF DOGS
(Collie nose)

A congenital, abnormal reaction of the skin to sunlight, mostly in Collies, Shetland Sheepdogs, German Shepherd Dogs and mixed breeds closely related to these. The disease primarily affects the nose, the eyes and the adjacent areas.

Clinical Findings: The disease runs a slow, insidious course. The onset is mild; as the condition progresses, the skin on the bridge of the nose becomes markedly irritated and the lesion may extend from the dorsum of the nose to the periorbital skin, with an associated conjunctivitis and blepharitis. Exfoliation of the skin of the nose becomes progressive with encrustation, ulceration and bleeding. Depigmentation occurs and the skin becomes pink to bright red and sore. The lesions are most intense in the summer months and subside during the winter.

Treatment and Propyhlaxis: The condition can be treated merely by keeping the dog away from sunlight or by the administration of para-aminobenzoic acid (PABA) (Ŗ 633). This is the active principle in sun-screening preparations which are usually applied topically. Other sun-screening drugs that may be used are quinacrine hydrochloride (Ŗ 644) or chloroquine diphosphate (℞ 636). Topical application of a corticosteroid ointment can also be used (e.g., ℞ 450). Unfortunately, on cessation of treatment, the signs often reappear, so the therapy must be more or less continuous during the season in which signs are obvious. Tattooing the nose with a mechanical device manufactured for that purpose has been reported to be helpful in some animals.

URTICARIA
(Nettle rash, Hives)

A skin disorder characterized by multiple plaquelike eruptions, which are rounded in outline, elevated and flat-topped. The urticarial skin eruptions, formed by a localized edema in the dermis, often develop and disappear suddenly.

The disease occurs in all domestic animals, but most often in horses and pigs. Allergic urticaria may be either exogenous or endogenous. Exogenous hives may be produced by toxic, irritating products of the stinging nettle or by the bites of insects and occurs most during the summer season, in horses, dogs and swine. Some chemicals such as carbolic acid, turpentine, carbon disulfide, or crude oil also may cause the condition.

Sensitive animals, particularly short-haired dogs and purebred horses, exhibit a phenomenon called dermographism, wherein rubbing or whipping produces urticaria-like skin lesions. It is of no clinical significance.

Endogenous or "symptomatic" urticaria may develop after absorption of ingested allergens and has been mostly seen in horses and dogs. In horses, it has been noted in the course of gastrointestinal conditions, particularly severe constipation or inflammation of the intestinal mucosa. Sensitive animals may develop urticaria as an allergic reaction after feeding on various plants, foodstuffs, or after parenteral administration of foreign proteins, particularly serums, vaccines and bacterins (see ALLERGY OF THE SKIN, p. 4). Urticaria has been observed in cows being dried off and in bitches during estrus. In young horses, dogs and pigs, urticaria has been associated with intestinal parasites.

Clinical Findings: The wheals or plaques appear within a few minutes or hours. In severe cases, the cutaneous eruptions are preceded by fever, loss of appetite, or dullness. The skin lesions are of a rounded shape, flat-topped, varying in diameter from ½ to 8 in., and may be slightly depressed in the center. They can develop on any part of the body, but mainly on the back, flanks, neck, eyelids and the legs. In advanced cases, they may be found on the mucous membranes of the mouth, nose, conjunctiva, rectum and vagina. As a rule, the lesions disappear as rapidly as they arise, usually within a few hours.

In sheep, the urticarial skin lesions usually develop on the udder and on the hairless parts of the abdomen. In pigs, the eruptions have been observed around the eyes, on the snout, the abdomen and between the hind legs, as well as on the back.

In general, the prognosis for urticaria in animals is favorable. A fatal outcome is rare and then probably due to anaphylactoid effects.

Treatment: Acute urticaria usually disappears spontaneously without treatment. In especially severe cases, epinephrine (R 511) or corticosteroids may be given subcutaneously. The lesions promptly disappear, but will return rapidly if the allergen is not eliminated. Antihistamines (R 535, 539), adreno-cortical hormones (R 149, 154) and anterior pituitary hormones (R 137) have also been found effective. Usually local treatment of the urticarial skin lesions is not necessary. In especially severe cases, cold packs of water, vinegar or alcohol (70%) may be applied; a corticosteroid (R 154) should be given parenterally.

PARAKERATOSIS IN SWINE

A nutritional deficiency disease, characterized by skin lesions involving the superficial layers of the epidermis, frequently affecting young pigs between the ages of 6 and 16 weeks. The incidence may reach 60% in some herds.

Etiology: Parakeratosis is a metabolic disturbance resulting from a relative deficiency of zinc (q.v., p. 1330) and an excess of calcium in the diet. The disease is most prevalent in pigs receiving diets containing mainly vegetable proteins and excess calcium supplements.

Clinical Findings: Signs are limited to the changes in the skin; mild lethargy and slight anorexia may be associated with increased severity of the lesions.

Lesions: Excessive growth and keratinization of skin epithelium with the formation of horny crusts and fissures are the outstanding lesions. Brown spots or papules are first seen on the ventrolateral areas of the abdomen, and on the pastern, fetlock, hock and tail, coalescing to involve larger areas until the entire body may be covered. The crusts are horny and dry on exposed surfaces and are usually easily removed. Occasionally, secondary infection of the cracks and fissures causes them to fill with a dark, sticky exudate and debris which may tend to confuse the condition with exudative dermatitis of an infectious nature.

Treatment: Highly satisfactory results can be obtained by adjusting the intake of calcium and zinc. The calcium level in the diet should be maintained between 0.65 and 0.75% and supplemental zinc added at the rate of 25 to 50 ppm (equivalent to an addition of 0.4 lb of zinc sulfate or carbonate per ton of feed). For pigs that have developed the disease as a result of improper diets, access to succulent, green pasture forage will shorten their convalescence and hasten recovery.

EXUDATIVE EPIDERMITIS (XE)
(Greasy pig disease)

An acute, generalized dermatitis of pigs which occurs from 5 to 35 days of age, characterized by sudden onset, with morbidity of 10 to 90% and mortality of 5 to 90%.

Etiology: The lesions of exudative epidermitis are caused by *Staphylococcus hyos* but the bacterial agent is unable to penetrate the intact skin. Abrasions on the feet and legs or lacerations on body frequently precede infection. In acute cases a vesicular-type virus may be the predisposing factor.

Clinical Findings: The first signs are listlessness, apathy, and dullness of the skin and hair coat, followed by a dandruff-like condition. Later the pig becomes more depressed and refuses to eat. The body temperature remains near normal. The skin thickens and reddish-brown spots appear from which serum exudes. There is often purulent inflammation of the external ear, and catarrhal inflammation of the eyes.

Vesicles, possibly caused by a virus, develop on the skin, burst, and become infected. The body is rapidly covered with a moist, greasy exudate of sebum and serum, and later heavy crusts, and an obnoxious odor develops. Vesicles and ulcers also form on the nasal disk and tongue. The feet are nearly always involved with erosion of the coronary bands and heel, and the hoof may be lost. Death occurs within 3 to 5 days.

In some animals the disease may be milder with lesions developing slowly. The mortality usually is low but many affected pigs recover slowly and growth is retarded.

Lesions: Necropsy of severely affected pigs reveals marked dehydration, congestion of the lungs and inflammation of the peripheral lymph nodes. Other lesions that may be present usually do not have specific diagnostic value.

Treatment: The causative organism is inhibited by most antibiotics. Early treatment may reduce the severity of the disease, but treatment is less effective as the disease progresses. Treatment should include isolation of infected litters and administration of a broad-spectrum antibiotic to infected pigs, as well as to those not yet showing clinical signs. The treatment of pigs with no signs should be continued for several days. Pigs gain resistance with increasing age. Litters farrowed for some time after clinical signs have subsided should receive antibiotics prophylactically. The **farrowing areas** should be disinfected.

PITYRIASIS ROSEA IN PIGS

A specific noninfectious hereditary skin disease **of young** pigs which occurs in many countries.

In general, lesions are confined to the abdomen and groin in pigs 4 to 8 weeks old, rarely before 10 days of age. They resemble ringworm, and consist of small, raised, erythematous swellings with distinct borders. As they extend peripherally as purplish wheals, the skin, at the center, resumes a more normal appearance. The lesions may coalesce and in severe cases may affect most of the underside of the pig. Fully developed lesions are easily identifiable, but early or complicated cases should be differentiated from ringworm and other dermatoses. Spontaneous healing is the rule; most lesions resolve within 3 to 6 weeks, but may take as long as 10 weeks to disappear.

Treatment will not alter the course in uncomplicated disease, but infected lesions may benefit from antibacterial therapy.

The condition is chiefly of importance because of the blemish which may interfere with sales of pedigreed stock. It is recommended that all animals believed to be carrying the genetic factor should be removed from the breeding herd.

INTERDIGITAL CYSTS

Inflamed, multiform nodules involving the interdigital webs of dogs. Difference of opinion exists on their etiology; the most probable main causes are: (1) foreign bodies, ingrowing hairs, awns and grains of sand which cause granulomatous reactions, and (2) bacterial infections, mainly staphylococcal, which cause suppurative reactions.

Clinical Findings: In its early stage, the interdigital cyst appears as a small papule, but later it progresses to a nodular stage. The nodule will be between 1 and 2 cm in diameter, reddish purple, shiny, and fluctuant, and may rupture when palpated, to exude a thick bloody material. There may be one or more nodules on one or more feet. Those caused by foreign bodies are usually solitary and often on a front foot. Recurrence is not common in these cases. If caused by bacterial infection, there may be several nodules with new lesions developing as others dry up. Pain may or may not be apparent, but is more common in nodules that are about to rupture and which contain foreign bodies.

Treatment: Foreign-body granulomas may respond to heat for 15 to 20 minutes 3 to 4 times a day, and removal of the foreign object. One or 2 weeks are required for the lesion to resolve. If hot foot baths are not effective, surgical excision is the most practical approach.

Bacterial granulomas: Antibiotic or immunologic treatment of these lesions will depend upon identification of the etiologic agent and determination of its antibiotic sensitivity. It may be necessary to tranquilize the dog or to bandage the feet to prevent licking until the lesions have healed.

SADDLE SORES

The saddle region of riding horses frequently is the site of injuries of the skin and of the deeper soft and bony tissues. Clinical signs vary according to the depth of injury and the complications caused by secondary infection.

Sores affecting only the skin are characterized by inflammatory changes that may range from erythematous through papular, vesicular, pustular and finally necrotic. Frequently the condition starts as an acute inflammation of the hair follicles and progresses to a purulent folliculitis. The affected areas show loss of hair and are swollen, hot and painful. The serous or purulent exudate dries, forming crusts. Advanced lesions are termed "galls". In cases of more serious damage of the skin and underlying tissues, abscesses may develop. They are characterized by hot, fluctuating, painful swellings from which serosanguineous fluid can be aspirated. Severe damage to the skin and subcutis or deeper tissues results in dry or moist necrosis. Chronic saddle sores are characterized by a deep folliculitis (hard nodules) or a localized indurative and proliferative dermatitis.

Treatment: Excoriations and inflammations of the skin of the saddle and harness regions are treated as any other skin inflammations. Absolute rest of the affected parts is necessary. During the early or acute stages, astringent packs (Burrow's solution or 2% lead acetate) are indicated. Chronic lesions and those superficially infected may be treated by hot applications and massage with stimulating ointments (iodine), or antibiotic ointment (R 417). For the treatment of purulent saddle sores, systemic antibiotics may be useful (R 44) in conjunction with local treatment. Hematomas should be aspirated or incised. If tissue necrosis occurs, the devitalized tissue should be surgically removed. A skin astringent and antiseptic of value in some cases, consists of 500 ml of 0.1% alcoholic sublimate, 30 gm tannic acid and 1 gm gentian violet.

FOOT ROT OF CATTLE
(Necrotic pododermatitis, Foul of the foot)

A necrotizing infection of tissues within and immediately surrounding the hoof, occasionally complicated by arthritis and synovitis of the adjacent joints and tendon sheaths, caused by the infective organisms penetrating through surface injuries. The disease is worldwide and all breeds of cattle are susceptible. Throughout the U.S.A., it is common in cattle confined in pens or on pasture.

Etiology: The sole infectious agent has long been thought to be *Sphaerophorus necrophorus* but recently a gram-negative bacillus and spirochete have also been incriminated. These organisms closely resemble the causative agents of foot rot in sheep, *Fusiformis nodosus* and *Spirochaeta penortha*, although they have not been positively identified. It is possible that all 3 organisms are involved.

Before the infectious agents can gain entry, some break in the continuity of the skin or horn of the foot must occur. Injury to the skin in the interdigital space and around the coronet is commonly caused by sharp objects, by maceration from continuous exposure to mud or manure, and possibly by other primary infectious agents. Cracks in the horny integument may also permit entry of infection.

Clinical Findings: Once established in the injured epithelium, the organisms invade connective tissue, causing a coagulative necrosis. Rarely, the infection may spread proximally in the limb and metastasize to the lungs and other viscera and to joints other than those of the foot. One or more feet may be infected. In the acute stage, inflammation usually extends to the fetlock joint. Interdigital tissues are necrotic and covered with a dry exudate; the surrounding tissue is edematous and hyperemic. The necrotic process may extend deep into connective tissue and occasionally into the interphalangeal joints; such chonically infected joints discharge exudate continuously through tracts that open into the interdigital space or around the coronet. Healed feet show thickening from scar tissue, which may bulge into the interdigital space. Healed coffin joints usually exhibit ankylosis and exostoses of the second and third phalanges.

The patient is acutely lame. In severe cases, anorexia and fever are present, weight is lost and milk yield falls. Occasionally death occurs as a result of the spread of infection to internal organs. The course is short for uncomplicated cases and prolonged if joints become arthritic or other complications develop. Healing may occur at any stage.

Diagnosis: This is based on history and the presence of the typical signs and lesions. Thorough cleaning and trimming of the hoof is essential to permit a complete inspection. The disease is to be differentiated from deep penetration of the foot by foreign bodies, mechanical injuries and sprains of various kinds, vesicular lesions from viral diseases and hematogenous infections of the feet. Radiographs occasionally are of value in identifying foreign bodies, arthritis, exostoses and other skeletal changes.

Treatment: Early treatment is essential to shorten the course of the disease and prevent sequelae such as suppurative arthritis and bacteremia. The kind of treatment is usually determined by the class of cattle affected, housing method and stage of the disease. Valuable breeding stock are usually treated individually. The animal is closely confined and the foot is cleaned, trimmed and debrided if necessary. When an open lesion is present an antibacterial ointment (R 435) or 5%

copper sulfate is applied and the foot is bandaged. If given early in the course of the disease, a single therapeutic dose of either penicillin (R 44) or sulfonamide (R 75, 82) is usually curative.

Commercial cattle of lesser value are usually treated orally. Individual treatment with a long-acting sulfonamide such as sulfabromomethazine (R 65) is satisfactory when only a few animals are affected. When numerous animals are affected, sulfonamides (e.g., R 65) placed in the feed and copper sulfate foot baths (2 to 5%) are frequently used. The whole herd is driven through a foot bath once or twice daily for several days. Walking animals through a 1:20 mixture of powdered copper sulfate and slaked lime is useful around water holes or where a foot bath is not practical.

When suppurative arthritis occurs, the affected claw may be amputated through the first phalanx or by disarticulation of the pastern joint with curettage of the distal end of the first phalanx to destroy the secreting joint surface. A third method, disarticulation through the infected coffin joint distal to the coronary band, is less commonly performed. Animals can usually function well with one claw removed, if a sound claw and strong pastern remains.

Prophylaxis: Avoidance of sources of injury to the feet is of primary importance. Barn lots should be cleaned frequently and be smooth, level and free of sharp objects, especially cinders. Mud holes and stagnant pools that act as reservoirs for the infective organisms should be eliminated. Routine foot trimming should be practiced when cattle are confined on soft footing. If concrete is so rough that it will cause excessive hoof wear, generous amounts of bedding should be provided. Foot injuries should be treated promptly. Ethylenediamine dihydroiodide is commonly added to salt in an attempt to prevent foot rot. Although controlled experimental evidence of its effectiveness is lacking, the practice finds wide support among cattlemen.

INFECTIOUS FOOT DISEASES OF SHEEP

(Foot rot)

Apart from the foot lesions of diseases that also affect other parts of the body (e.g., foot-and-mouth disease, contagious ecthyma, bluetongue and dermatophilosis) there is a group of infectious diseases specific to the feet. These diseases are all due to mixed infections with combinations of bacteria including the gram-negative anaerobe *Sphaerophorus* (*Fusiformis*) *necrophorus*, and they are all initiated by a bacterial invasion of the interdigital skin. This invasion is mainly due to penetration of the interdigital epithelium by *S. necrophorus* and *Fusiformis nodosus*, which are the only organisms capable of penetrating the intact skin. Penetration by *F. nodosus* produces little tissue reaction, but penetration by *S. necrophorus* produces a severe reaction. It appears that *F. nodosus* requires the assistance of *S. necrophorus* to induce clinical foot rot.

OVINE INTERDIGITAL DERMATITIS (OID)

A necrotizing condition of the interdigital skin due to a mixed infection with *S. necrophorus* and *Corynebacterium pyogenes*. Cold weather and heavy stocking on damp pastures are considered to be predisposing causes. A similar condition in sheep grazing on stubble has been attributed to mechanical damage inflicted by the short, stiff stubble; similarly, injuries to the interdigital epithelium frequently result from "clay balling", a condition in which hardened balls of clay mold themselves into the shape of the interdigital space, and become difficult to dislodge causing constant irritation and great lameness. The bacteriology of these cases requires clarification.

Clinical Findings: Lameness may be seen in more severe cases. The interdigital skin is usually red and swollen, and covered with a moist film of necrotic tissue that tends to erode in patches. At the skin-horn junction the hoof may be separated slightly from the underlying tissue. The disease is often transient but may persist while pastures remain wet; most lesions heal rapidly with the advent of dry conditions. Where the disease is associated with stubble, there is usually improvement on removal to ordinary pastures.

Diagnosis: The clinical appearance is characteristic but similar conditions involving other organisms must be excluded. In the case of foot rot (q.v., pp. 926-8) microscopic examination of stained smears will reveal the presence of *Fusiformis nodosus*. Strawberry foot rot (*D. congolensis* infection) (q.v., p. 898) affects the hairy skin of the coronet and pastern. Virus diseases such as contagious ecthyma and foot-and-mouth disease must be diagnosed by reference to flock history and appropriate virologic methods.

Control and Treatment: Healing may be assisted by the external application of disinfectants such as 5% formalin (℞ 409), and by removal to drier pastures if available. Sheep on stubble should be transferred to ordinary pasture.

VIRULENT FOOT ROT

A specific necrotizing disease affecting the epidermis of the interdigital skin and hoof matrix. The disease is chronic and progressive. It commences as an interdigital dermatitis and extends to involve large areas of the hoof matrix. The infected tissue is destroyed so that the hoof loses its anchorage and becomes detached. Foot rot is a contagious disease and under wet conditions with heavy stocking the incidence may approach 100%. The infection is also found in other ruminants including cattle, goats and deer.

Etiology: Foot rot is due to a mixed infection with 2 gram-negative anaerobic bacteria, *Fusiformis nodosus* and *Sphaerophorus necrophorus*; neither organism alone can cause the disease. *S. necrophorus* is a normal resident of the sheep's environment and is thus always available. Infection, therefore, depends on the presence of *F. nodosus*, a strict parasite that does not survive for more than about a week in the soil or pastures; hence, its availability depends on the presence of infected animals. *F. nodosus* is accordingly regarded as the transmissible and specific causal agent of foot rot, although its contribution to the disease process is not necessarily greater than that of *S. necrophorus*.

The transmission of foot rot to healthy animals requires a warm, moist environment. Under these conditions the interdigital stratum corneum becomes macerated; filaments of *S. necrophorus* superficially invade the epidermis and induce a slight subclinical hyperkeratosis. If *F. nodosus* makes contact with the skin at this stage its association with *S. necrophorus* is initiated and foot rot results. If *F. nodosus* comes into contact with a lesion of ovine interdigital dermatitis (q.v., p. 925) foot rot will similarly ensue.

Clinical Findings: The most obvious sign is lameness, which may be very severe. Some animals remain recumbent or on their brisket and knees, which tend to become depilated and inflamed. Affected animals lose condition. Rams infected in the hind feet may be unable to serve and similarly ewes with hind-feet lesions may be unable to bear the weight of a ram at service. In early cases, examination of the feet may reveal nothing more than an interdigital dermatitis of similar appearance to OID. In slightly more advanced cases, where the infection has begun to extend into the hoof matrix, there is slight detachment of the hoof at the skin-horn junction. As the disease progresses the epidermal necrosis and separation of horn spread to the heel and sole, and finally the outer wall, so that the hoof is eventually attached only at the coronet. The necrotic tissue has a very characteristic unpleasant odor. The lesions often become flyblown.

The disease persists for years in some sheep. Under dry conditions the infection may be hidden in small pockets within the foot where it is detectable only on paring. Sheep so affected act as subclinical carriers. Recovery from foot rot is not followed by appreciable immunity.

Diagnosis: Although slight or early cases may be confused with OID or benign foot rot, the extensive underrunning and separation of the horn in more advanced cases is diagnostic of the virulent form. To the experienced observer the characteristic odor of the necrotic tissue is a valuable aid to diagnosis. In the laboratory the diagnosis may be confirmed by the presence of *F. nodosus* which is seen in stained smears as a fairly large gram-negative bacillus with swollen ends.

Control and Treatment: Topical treatment requires the paring away of all underrun horn to expose the infected tissue. This is followed by the application of a bactericidal agent such as 5% formalin (℞ 409) or 10% copper sulfate (℞ 613) or by spraying with 10% chloramphenicol. For use on a flock basis, topical treatment has the disadvantage that it is much less than 100% efficient; a single lesion left uncured is enough to re-infect the flock.

Less arduous and more effective, but more expensive, is parenteral chemotherapy. A mixture of procaine penicillin G and dihydrostreptomycin is given as a single IM injection at the dose rate, for each agent, of 70 mg/kg body wt or 70,000 u/kg. For best results this treatment should be combined with minimal paring of overgrown or loose, detached horn, and should immediately be followed by a walk through a disinfectant foot bath (℞ 409 or 613). The sheep should then be held on a dry surface overnight, or returned to a fresh, clean pasture when conditions are suitable.

Although recovery from foot rot is not followed by any appreciable immunity, a useful degree of protection can be induced with vaccines containing *F. nodosus*. Vaccination is performed mainly for prevention, but there is also a therapeutic effect which is manifested usually as a tendency of vaccinated sheep to recover more rapidly than others left un-vaccinated. Vaccination is best used as a means of minimizing the incidence of infection and the amount of therapeutic work required to control it. Vaccines have recently been marketed in the United Kingdom and New Zealand and should soon be more widely available. They are of 2 kinds: One is an emulsion of antigen in mineral oil, given in single annual doses. The other is an alum-treated vaccine that requires a primary course of 2 injections at an interval of at least 6 weeks, and single boosting injections once or twice per year as needed.

Whichever methods of treatment and prevention are used, best results will be obtained if the healthy sheep are segregated on an uninfected pasture, i.e., one that has been free of sheep for at least 2 weeks. The healthy flock may be increased by the addition of previously infected sheep that have remained cured after treatment, or of new sheep that have proved to be healthy after a suitable period of observation. Entry to the healthy flock should always be through a disinfectant foot bath. Contact should not be allowed with other ruminants that may harbor the infection.

Eradication: Owing to the considerable economic losses foot rot causes in the flock, it is best to attempt total eradication. This can be effected by a combination of topical and parenteral therapeutic treatments, not forgetting that any cattle or goats present on the farm can be carriers of the disease and should be segregated from the sheep.

BENIGN FOOT ROT
(Foot scald)

A form of foot rot in which the infection is confined largely to the interdigital skin, with minimal underrunning of the adjacent horn even under continuously wet conditions. Lameness is common but less severe than in virulent foot rot. The etiology is the same as in the virulent disease but the causal strains of *Fusiformis nodosus* are less virulent. The same control measures are required although there is very little underrun horn to be pared.

INFECTIVE BULBAR NECROSIS (IBN)
(Heel abscess, Digital suppuration)

A necrotizing disease of the deeper connective tissues of the foot, especially the digital cushion. Infective bulbar necrosis (IBN) usually has a sporadic incidence but may affect up to 15% of ewes in late pregnancy. IBN develops as a complication of disease causing interdigital dermatitis and is not itself communicable.

Etiology: IBN is due to a mixed infection with *Sphaerophorus necrophorus* and *Corynebacterium pyogenes*. These 2 organisms invade the deeper connective tissues of the foot as an extension of infection from the epidermal lesions of OID, virulent or benign foot rot or, possibly, contagious ecthyma. It has been suggested that anoxia, due to an interference with blood supply to the foot, may be a factor facilitating invasions of deeper tissues.

Clinical Findings: IBN develops most often in cool weather when the soil and pastures are wet. It appears during or following outbreaks of the interdigital infections from which it arises. The disease may affect any foot of any sheep but is most common in the medial digits of the hind feet of ewes in late pregnancy. It is commoner in fat rams than in other dry sheep.

IBN causes severe lameness. The infected digit is usually hot and the bulb of the heel swollen. In the early stages it may be possible to express necrotic material through an opening in the interdigital skin via the channel left by the bacterial invasion. With healing of the interdigital lesions this opening usually closes to be replaced by one or more sinuses opening through the skin above the coronet. The lesions usually heal spontaneously, but slowly. This may leave the foot deformed or with its function affected and the sheep permanently lame, especially in cases where the necrotizing process has extended from the digital cushion into tendon sheaths or joints.

Diagnosis: The swelling of the heel and discharging sinuses are diagnostic.

Control and Treatment: There is no known surgical or chemotherapeutic treatment of any value. The incidence may be limited by measures to control the initial cause of interdigital dermatitis.

LAMELLAR SUPPURATION
(Toe abscess)

An acute infection of the laminar matrix of the hoof, usually restricted to the toe and abaxial wall. The disease is sporadic and the bacterial etiology variable, but cases due to *Sphaerophorus necrophorus* and *Corynebacterium pyogenes* are usually more severe and extensive than those involving streptococci or other organisms. Infection probably enters through fissures in the bearing surface between the wall and sole. It is sometimes, but not always, assisted by impaction with mud and feces where there is overgrowth of the hoof or where there is separation of the wall following laminitis.

Lameness is severe and the affected digit hot and tender. There may be a sinus above the lesion at the coronet. Affected sheep recover rapidly after paring of the horn to provide dependent drainage.

FOOT ROT OF SWINE

An ulcerative, granulomatous, infectious disease of pigs, observed wherever pigs are reared on concrete floors. The abrasive effects of concrete plus dampness apparently provide an entrance for the spirochete and fusiform organisms associated with this disease. It occurs in adult breeding stock as well as in feeder pigs.

Clinical Findings: Affected pigs are extremely lame and reluctant to get up to feed. The characteristic lesion appears as a necrotic sinus on the lateral wall of the hoof where it joins the sole. This lesion progresses to the coronary band where the horn adjacent to affected areas becomes blackened. Further progression leads to a series of necrotic sinuses with surface ulceration and the formation of granulation tissue. In advanced cases, the infection can involve the tendon sheaths and extend into the bone and the joints of the foot to produce osteomyelitis and arthritis. These severe infections are often referred to as "bush foot" or "bumble foot" of pigs.

Diagnosis: Careful clinical examination will usually establish the diagnosis. This condition should be differentiated from the lesions of the foot caused by the vesicular virus diseases and other causes of arthritis in swine. In addition, the condition must be differentiated from a lameness in pigs caused by an excessive growth of horn on the bulb of the heel, with eventual ulceration. (This condition also occurs with pigs on concrete, and is more common in North America than foot rot; it responds to foot trimming and a copper sulfate foot bath.)

Control and Treatment: Since intensive swine rearing dictates that pigs be raised on concrete, the condition is difficult to completely prevent. Adequate bedding will lower the incidence. Early detection and forcing pigs to walk through a foot bath of 5% copper sulfate once a day for 5 to 10 days usually will control the condition. Antibiotic therapy can also be attempted but the results are often disappointing. Pigs with advanced arthritis and osteomyelitis will not respond to standard therapy and should be salvaged. Claw amputation can be attempted on valuable breeding animals.

PART II
TOXICOLOGY

ARSENIC POISONING

In describing arsenic poisoning and its treatment, a sharp distinction must be made between inorganic and organic compounds.

INORGANIC COMPOUNDS

These include arsenic trioxide, arsenic pentoxide, sodium and potassium arsenate, sodium and potassium arsenite, and calcium and lead arsenate.

Etiology of Inorganic Arsenic Poisoning: Due to the diminishing use of these substances, poisoning is now seen relatively infrequently. The sources of poisoning usually are preparations used as rodenticides, weed killers, and baits and insecticides. Often these are discarded or long-forgotten materials stored on the premises. Arsenites are used to some extent as dips for the eradication of ticks. Lead arsenate is sometimes used as a teniacide in sheep.

Clinical Findings: Inorganic arsenic poisoning is usually an acute disease whose major action is on the gastrointestinal tract. Profuse, watery diarrhea, often tinged with blood is characteristic. This condition is accompanied by severe dehydration, weakness and depression. The pulse is weak and abdominal pain often is evident. The underlying cause of these effects is increased capillary permeability and cellular necrosis. Animals inadvertently sprayed with soluble arsenites may exhibit massive skin necrosis.

The onset usually is rapid and the course from hours to several weeks. Although inorganic arsenicals are not highly cumulative, chronic poisoning is recorded in man with the major effects being dry, exfoliative dermatitis with cracking of the skin. Animals are rarely subjected to the long-term exposure conditions required for this form to develop.

Lesions: The principal effects are observed in the gastrointestinal tract. Inflammation of the intestine is followed by edema, rupture of the blood vessels and necrosis of epithelial and subepithelial tissue. The necrosis may progress to perforation of the gastric or intestinal wall. The contents of the gut are usually fluid, tinged with blood and may contain shreds of epithelial tissue. Generally, there is a diffuse inflammation of the liver and other abdominal viscera.

Laboratory Diagnosis: The chemical determination of arsenic in tissues and ingesta provides adequate confirmation. Liver and kidney of normal animals rarely contain more than 1 ppm arsenic (wet wt) and poisoning usually is associated with concentrations in excess of 3 ppm in these organs. The determination of arsenic in ingesta is of value if exposure occurred within the previous 24 to 48 hours.

Treatment: The only specific antidote of proven value is dimercaprol (℞ 601). Supportive therapy may be of even greater value, particularly where cardiovascular collapse is imminent, and should be directed toward restoration of blood volume and correction of the massive dehydration. Electrolyte solutions of the extracellular type are indicated for this purpose.

ORGANIC COMPOUNDS OF ARSENIC

These include several phenylarsonic acid derivatives used in swine and poultry for the purpose of improving production and, in the case of swine, to treat dysentery. The major compounds in this class are arsanilic acid, roxarsone (3-nitro-4-hydroxyphenylarsonic acid), nitarsone (4-nitro-phenylarsonic acid) and carbarsone (4-ureidophenylarsonic acid).

Etiology of Organic Arsenic Poisoning: This form of poisoning almost always results from the use of excessive amounts in the diet of swine and poultry. Severity and rapidity of onset are dose-related. Visible signs of poisoning may be delayed for weeks following incorporation of 2 to 3 times the recommended levels or may occur within days when the excess is 10-fold or more over recommended levels.

Clinical Findings: The earliest sign of poisoning, usually not detected, is reduction in weight gains. This is followed by motor incoordination and posterior paralysis in swine. Animals remain alert and retain good appetites. Blindness is characteristic of arsanilic acid intoxication, but this property apparently is not shared by the other compounds listed.

Laboratory Diagnosis: An analysis of the feed for either total arsenic or the suspect compound is indicated if any doubt exists as to the cause of illness.

Treatment: There is no specific treatment of demonstrated value but the neurotoxic effects of these compounds are usually reversible. Blindness due to arsanilic acid is irreversible, but the animals still retain good appetites and make good weight gains if competition for food is eliminated. Some doubt exists as to the reversibility of the other neurotoxic effects when the onset of intoxication is very slow and the exposure is prolonged.

LEAD POISONING

Lead causes a common form of metallic poisoning in animals, in part because of the extensive use of lead preparations in agriculture. Since it is a cumulative poison, repeated small doses may prove toxic. Swine and goats are relatively resistant.

Etiology: Paint containing lead, and discarded storage batteries are among the commoner sources of poisoning. Weathering does not alter the toxic properties of lead. Vegetation in the vicinity of lead smelters may accumulate enough lead by atmospheric deposition to cause poisoning in livestock. A few instances of poisoning in animals have occurred where the residue resulting from the evaporation of leaded gasoline was the suspected source. Animals are sometimes poisoned by consuming forage which has been sprayed or dusted with lead arsenate. If an animal consumes a large amount of lead arsenate in a short time, the toxic action of arsenic supersedes that of lead.

Lead is sparingly soluble in the gastrointestinal tract, and its rate of absorption is limited. Repeated ingestion of small quantities may cause systemic toxicity, as may a large single dose. Wild ducks frequently are poisoned by ingested lead shot. The shot are retained among the gizzard contents (*see* p. 1087).

Clinical Findings: These vary with the species and age of the animal and the time over which the lead is ingested. Animals affected with **acute lead poisoning** rapidly become depressed, walk in circles and often walk into fences because of blindness, stand with the head pressed against a firm object, grind the teeth and sometimes bellow. Muscular twitching, "snapping" of the eyelids, staggering and convulsive seizures are common. Often, an animal may be unable to rise after 2 or 3 convulsions. The temperature may be elevated in severe cases, the pulse is fast and weak, and respiration is rapid, shallow and somewhat labored. Sheep may show similar signs, but usually those of depression predominate. Dogs show similar signs except that they do not walk in circles. In the horse, acute lead poisoning produces acute gastritis, and diarrhea usually develops if the animal survives more than 36 hours. Muscular weakness, blindness, prostration and convulsions are other signs.

In **chronic lead poisoning** the accumulation of a toxic burden of lead in cattle as a sequela to long-term intake usually results in sudden development of the acute syndrome described above. A distinct syndrome of chronic lead poisoning in cattle has never been adequately documented.

Chronic lead poisoning in the horse results in paralysis of laryngeal muscles with inspiratory dyspnea in addition to the other signs. Pneumonia may develop following the laryngeal paralysis.

The "lead line" on the gums is seldom observed in animals. In most cases of chronic lead poisoning, examination of the blood reveals anemia and basophilic stippling of erythrocytes.

Lesions: Gross lesions in **acute lead poisoning** are inconstant. Subepicardial and subendocardial petechial and ecchymotic hemorrhages are often seen but are of little diagnostic value. The lesions of **chronic lead poisoning** are likewise few and nonpathognomonic. Horses chronically affected often die as a result of aspiration pneumonia secondary to the laryngeal paralysis associated with lead poisoning in this species.

Laboratory Diagnosis: The chemical determination of the concentration of lead in the kidney cortex and liver or in unclotted blood provides adequate confirmation of suspected abnormal lead accumulation. Values greater than 4, 4 and 0.2 ppm (wet wt) for these tissues, respectively, indicate abnormal accumulation.

Treatment: Effectiveness of treatment depends on the extent of injury to the liver, kidneys and brain. Extensive injury to these tissues makes treatment of little value. Intestinal lavage or a cathartic, such as magnesium sulfate (℞ 606), may be employed to remove lead remaining in the digestive tract. Administration of calcium disodium ethylenediaminetetraacetate (℞ 604) is indicated since it will combine with the lead rendering it nontoxic and more rapidly excreted. Calcium (℞

605) is perhaps of some benefit when given IV because it relieves intestinal spasm and suppresses mobilization of lead from bone, although the therapeutic significance of this action is questionable.

STRYCHNINE POISONING

Strychnine poisoning of a deliberate or malicious nature occurs occasionally. Accidental poisoning from rodenticides occurs less frequently than in the past, and from excessive (or cumulative) intake of nux vomica or other strychnine-containing medicaments only rarely.

Clinical Findings: Although the syndrome may be confused with tetanus, the dramatic signs of strychnine poisoning are quite suggestive. Liquid strychnine sulfate may produce a response within a few minutes after ingestion, but more often signs are delayed for at least an hour, the interval varying with the type of compound ingested, the dose, and the nature and amount of the stomach contents. Strychnine is usually oxidized and excreted from the body within 10 hours after absorption.

The initial signs of anxiety and increased respiration are frequently overlooked. These progress rapidly to constant panting, muscular tremors and extreme response to sensory stimulus, particularly to touch or sound. Tonic convulsions become evident, initially keyed by the above stimulus, later with no apparent external stimulus, and progressive worsening is evident. Death results from respiratory paralysis.

Treatment: In suspected malicious administration of strychnine to the dog, prior to the appearance of signs, the stomach may be evacuated through the use of apomorphine (℞ 460). Gastric lavage, using warm hypertonic saline solution, or better, potassium permanganate, 1:1,000, or strong tea (or 2% tannic acid solution), can be attempted, but is difficult to perform. High enema with warm saline may be advantageous.

If convulsions are present or imminent, pentobarbital sodium is the drug of choice in small animals; chloral hydrate may be used in larger animals; both must be given to effect and repeated as necessary. At this stage, morphine or apomorphine are contraindicated as they further depress medullary center activity and may cause early death of the patient. The administration of 5% dextrose in isotonic saline helps to maintain kidney function.

Throughout, it is important to minimize stimulation of the patient.

CYANIDE POISONING

Cyanide inhibits oxidative enzyme systems and causes death from anoxia.

Etiology: Cyanides are sometimes used in fumigants, soil sterilizers, fertilizers and rodenticides. Livestock loss may occur as a result of improper or malicious use of these compounds. The most important cause of cyanide poisoning among domestic animals is the ingestion of cyanogenetic plants. Such plants grown in the U.S.A. include arrow grass (*Triglochin* sp.), Johnson grass (*Sorghum halepense*), Sudan grass (*Sorghum vulgare* var. *sudanensis*), common sorghum (*Sorghum vulgare*), wild black cherry (*Prunus serotina*), chokecherry (*Prunus virginiana*), pincherry (*Prunus pennsylvanica*) and flax (*Linum usitatissimum*). These plants contain cyanogenetic glycosides that, when hydrolyzed by an enzyme during digestion, yield hydrocyanic (prussic) acid. Cyanogenetic glycoside content is increased by heavy nitrate fertilization and by wilting, trampling and plant diseases. Very young, rapidly growing plants also contain greater quantities of the glycoside. Freezing does not ordinarily increase the glycoside content of these plants, but it does tend to increase the quantity of free hydrocyanic acid that the plants contain, thus resulting in a temporary increase in their toxicity. Spraying of cyanogenetic plants with a herbicide may increase the toxic hazard.

Clinical Findings: The signs are caused by tissue hypoxia since hydrocyanic acid inhibits the enzyme system necessary for transport of oxygen from blood to the tissue. Signs observed will depend on the size of the dose and the time over which it is absorbed.

If large doses are consumed rapidly, generalized convulsions develop and animals die within a few minutes. If smaller doses are consumed over a long period, the more common clinical course is observed. The onset of this form is sudden and characterized by salivation and a gradual increase in respiratory rate. Marked dyspnea develops in 5 to 15 minutes. The heart beat is rapid and weak. Muscle fasciculation occurs early and progresses into generalized spasms with opisthotonos just prior to death. Most animals stagger and struggle before they go down. The mucous membranes are bright red, but may become cyanotic at terminus. Death from respiratory paralysis occurs during severe convulsions. The heart continues to beat for several minutes after struggling ceases and breathing stops. Blood often passes from the nostrils and the mouth near the time of death. The course usually does not exceed 30 to 45 minutes; most animals that live for 2 hours after the onset of signs will recover.

Lesions: In peracute intoxication the venous blood may be bright red (cyanhemoglobin), but more commonly it is dark. The blood clots slowly. Congestion and hemorrhage may be found in the trachea and lungs and the skeletal muscles are dark red. Congestion of the liver and distension of the veins are commonly observed. Hemorrhages may be found on the serous surfaces. The rumen is often distended with gas and the odor of "bitter almonds" may be detected when the cadaver is opened. If the dose of cyanide is especially high, prolonged preservation of the carcass may occur. If the dose is low and death is delayed, an acute gastroenteritis is likely.

Diagnosis: The history, signs, postmortem findings and demonstration of the presence of hydrocyanic acid in the stomach contents permits a diagnosis. Tests for hydrocyanic acid should be made at the time of necropsy. Several reliable field-test kits designed for this purpose are available commercially. If it is necessary to submit specimens to a laboratory for analysis, 150 to 250 gm of stomach contents should be collected soon after death, sealed in an airtight container, refrigerated and submitted immediately. Suspected plant material can also be tested.

Prophylaxis: Efforts to prevent the occurrence of poisoning from cyanogenetic plants must be directed toward avoiding their use for grazing when factors that increase the toxic hazard are present. There is little danger from feeding well-cured hay made from these plants. The risk of cyanide poisoning may also be decreased by the heavy feeding of ground cereal grains before animals are turned out to graze. Carbohydrates tend to inhibit the action of the enzyme that hydrolyzes the glycoside.

Treatment: Since hydrocyanic acid combines more readily with methemoglobin than with hemoglobin, the first objective in therapy is to produce a degree of methemoglobinemia by the IV administration of sodium nitrite. Second, the cyanide moiety of cyanmethemoglobin is converted to thiocyanate by using sodium thiosulfate as a sulfur donor. Because of the importance of speed, sodium nitrite and sodium thiosulfate usually are administered together (℞ 610). If a single dose of this mixture does not result in prompt relief of signs, it may be repeated only once or twice because of the danger of excessive methemoglobinemia, which can itself cause death of the animal. Sodium thiosulfate alone (℞ 611) is relatively free from toxic effects and may be repeated if necessary.

CHRONIC FLUORIDE POISONING
(Fluorosis)

Toxic quantities of fluorides occur naturally in a few products used in feeding animals, e.g., certain raw rock phosphates, the superphosphates produced from them, partially defluorinated phosphates and the phosphatic limestones. In certain areas, the drinking water, usually from deep wells, contains high levels of fluorides. Fluorine-containing gases and dusts from some chemical factories have contaminated forage crops. Among such factories are those engaged in producing acid phosphate from rock phosphates, the electrolytic production of aluminum, the manufacture of bricks from fluorine-bearing clays, the calcining of ironstone and certain enameling processes. Contamination of the surrounding area, particularly in the direction of the prevailing wind, may extend 5 to 6 miles. Furthermore, forage crops grown on high-fluorine soils have elevated values due to mechanical contamination with soil particles.

Laboratory tests rate sodium fluoride the most toxic, and calcium fluoride the least toxic of the common fluorides. The fluorides of rock phosphates and most cryolites are intermediate between these two, whereas those in hay contaminated by industrial residues approach sodium fluoride in toxicity. A re-evaluation of the fluorine hazard suggests 50 to 100 ppm of fluorine in the total dry ration as maximal safe level for dairy and beef cattle, 100 to 200 ppm for sheep and swine, and 300 to 400 ppm for chickens. These data are based on fluorides as they exist in rock phosphates. Where the fluorides are in the form of soluble fluoride or originate from industrial fumes or dusts, the tolerance levels are approximately two-thirds these values. In the case of breeding animals whose usefulness exceeds 5 to 8 years, the lower figure given in each range should be used.

Clinical Findings: Inasmuch as teeth are seldom examined, the first sign of fluorosis detected may be exostoses, usually with apparent lameness. Other signs have been associated with fluorosis, e.g., dryness and stiffness of the hide, poor condition, abnormal hoof growth, diarrhea, decreased appetite and lowered milk yield.

Lesions: The most sensitive clinical index of fluoride poisoning is the mottling, staining and excessive wearing of the permanent teeth formed during the time of excessive fluoride ingestion. Teeth that are fully formed before exposure to fluorides are not noticeably affected. A more advanced stage of fluorosis is marked by abnormalities of the skeletal system. The bones become chalky white, soft, thickened and, in the extreme, develop exostoses that may be palpated, especially along the long bones and on the jaw. Degenerative changes in the kidneys, liver and several endocrine organs, and anemia, have been reported, but none of these latter lesions is pathognomonic.

Most of the fluoride retained by the body is deposited in the bones and teeth, the fluoride content of which increases in proportion to the amount and duration of the intake. Normal, dry, fat-free bone may contain up to approximately 1,000 ppm of fluorine. Fluorine contents of bones as high as 3,000 ppm are encountered in animals in which effects of fluorosis are slight and limited to early mottling of the teeth. In chronic fluorosis bone values may exceed 8,000 ppm. Normal urine contains less than 5 ppm of fluorine, whereas high intakes produce values in excess of 10 ppm.

Diagnosis: Casual observation of animals suffering from fluorosis may suggest osteoporosis or deficiency of calcium, phosphorus, or vitamin D. The lameness in advanced cases may be wrongly attributed to any number of accidents. The nonspecific staining of teeth often seen in cattle may be confused with incipient fluorosis. Accurate diagnosis depends on observing their elevated fluorine content and ultimately discovering the source of the element.

Treatment and Control: Control, other than by the removal of animals from affected areas, is difficult. It has been suggested that affected areas may be utilized for the production of animals having a relatively short economic life, e.g., pigs, poultry or finishing cattle and sheep. The feeding of aluminum sulfate reduces fluorine absorption by about a third and thus offers some control of chronic fluorosis.

MERCURY POISONING

The toxic effects of organic and inorganic compounds of mercury are sufficiently dissimilar to require separate discussion.

INORGANIC COMPOUNDS

These include mainly mercuric chloride (corrosive sublimate), a disinfectant; mercurous chloride (calomel), a cathartic; and elemental mercury. Poisoning in animals is usually due to the accidental ingestion of mercuric chloride or solutions thereof. Elemental mercury may cause poisoning by inhalation of its vapor. Mercurous chloride may be toxic when retained in the gastrointestinal tract for prolonged periods.

Clinical Findings: In cases of overwhelming doses death may occur very rapidly due to ventricular fibrillation. More commonly the severe corrosive gastrointestinal effects, such as vomiting, bloody diarrhea and necrosis of the alimentary mucosa, are evident. In such cases severe renal damage also occurs, with anuria, or polyuria in less severe cases. In the rare case of chronic poisoning due to inorganic mercury the major action is on the CNS and resembles organic mercury poisoning (see below).

Lesions: In acute poisoning due to oral intake of inorganic salts of mercury, severe degenerative and inflammatory lesions of the gastrointestinal tract are observed at all points of contact.

Laboratory Diagnosis: Careful laboratory analysis should readily differentiate between normal concentrations of mercury in tissues and feed (<1 ppm) and concentrations associated with acute poisoning. The organ of choice for toxicologic examination is the kidney, which selectively accumulates mercury.

Treatment: The specific antidote for mercury is dimercaprol (R 601). Binding of mercury still in the gastrointestinal tract with proteins such as eggs and milk is advisable. A gastric lavage with sodium formaldehyde sulfoxalate (100 to 250 ml, 5% solution) also is useful. This serves to reduce divalent mercury to the less toxic monovalent form. The use of electrolyte solutions to combat dehydration should be monitored carefully to avoid overhydration in the presence of anuria.

ORGANIC COMPOUNDS

These include various fungicides used mainly to treat seeds stored for planting, and mercurial diuretic drugs. The fungicides are either phenyl or alkyl mercurials. This usually results from the inadvertent use of treated seed as livestock feed. Recently concern has been expressed that the general human population may be exposed to excessive amounts of methyl mercury from contaminated fish because methyl mercury is readily formed from inorganic mercury by aquatic microorganisms and fish accumulate the methyl mercury.

Clinical Findings: Phenyl mercurials have toxic properties very much like those of inorganic mercury compounds, except that they are not corrosive. Alkyl mercurials, by contrast, usually cause neurologic effects. These include ataxia, head-pressing (in the case of cattle), tetanic spasms, opisthotonus and paralysis. Overdosage of mercurial diuretics may cause ventricular fibrillation, stomatitis, emesis, diarrhea, nephritis and hepatitis. Laboratory diagnosis is as for inorganic mercury.

Treatment: The neurologic signs associated with alkyl mercurials are almost invariably accompanied by degenerative lesions of the CNS. Treatment in such circumstances is useless. In the case of poisoning by phenylmercurials, dimercaprol (℞ 601) may be of some benefit if neurologic signs are absent. Dimercaprol is an effective antidote for mercurial diuretics.

MOLYBDENUM POISONING
(Molybdenosis)

While molybdenum appears to be an essential nutritive element, its significance as a dietary constituent arises mainly from the toxic effects it produces in ruminants when ingested in excessive amounts. The relationship of molybdenum to copper is complex and is influenced by the sulfate content of the diet. Because supplements containing copper prevent or alleviate molybdenosis, molybdenosis and copper deficiency should be considered as interrelated phenomena. Non-ruminants are much more resistant to molybdenum toxicity.

Etiology: The tolerance of ruminants to a high intake of molybdenum depends upon a number of factors: (1) the copper content and intake of the animal—the tolerance decreases as the content and intake fall (see NUTRITIONAL DEFICIENCIES IN CATTLE AND SHEEP: COPPER, p. 1322), (2) the inorganic sulfate content of the diet—increasing levels of sulfate intensify toxicity associated with low copper intakes, (3) the chemical form of the molybdenum, (4) the presence of certain sulfur-containing amino acids, (5) the species of animal—cattle are less tolerant than sheep and (6) the age—young animals are most susceptible.

Molybdenum poisoning associated with copper deficiency has been observed in regions having peat or muck soils. In parts of the San Joaquin Valley of California and on some of the Eocene shales of the Western U.S.A., the forage may contain up to 100 ppm of molybdenum. In other areas the metal is used in fertilization and while normal applications of molybdenum for this purpose do not ordinarily increase the level in the forage above 1 ppm, extra quantities may result in forage with 4 or 5 ppm or more.

In the presence of high molybdenum and low copper intakes, liver copper in cattle, sheep and goats may decrease to 30 ppm or less of the dry weight. The blood copper may reach levels as low as 0.06 ppm. The presence of molybdenum in the liver at levels of 5 to 100 ppm is indicative of an abnormal molybdenum intake. A hypochromic anemia, with hemoglobin concentrations as low as 6 gm per 100 ml of blood, is observed in severe cases. Serum calcium and inorganic phosphorus values usually remain normal, even when rarefaction is present in the bones.

If the copper content is below 5 ppm in rapidly growing pastures, 1 ppm molybdenum on a dry-weight basis may be hazardous. Levels of 100 ppm copper and 0.05% sulfur and above usually prevent toxic signs with molybdenum concentrations as high as 3 to 4 ppm. With extremely high levels of molybdenum, up to 150 ppm in the dry matter, a total daily intake of copper, equivalent to between 0.5 to 2.0 gm of $CuSO_4 \cdot 5H_2O$ may be required to protect cattle.

Clinical Findings: The signs of molybdenum toxicity are nonspecific and vary from an apparently poor performance, particularly in young animals, to serious conditions which include severe diarrhea ("peat scours"), anemia, emaciation, joint-pain and fading of the haircoat. Emaciation and anemia are the only conditions observed at necropsy. Diagnosis may be established on the basis of abnormal concentrations of molybdenum and copper in blood or liver.

Other signs of toxicity attributed to molybdenum with an associated low copper intake include:

1. An abnormal pacing gait ("pacing disease"). The animal moves with obvious pain and is reluctant to rise.

2. In young animals the lesions resemble those of rickets, with beaded ribs and swollen ends of the femur and cannon bones especially noticeable. In older animals, the bones become progressively more rarefied due to increased loss of phosphorus from the body and fractures frequently occur. There is also a loss of milk yield in cows.

3. Severe molybdenum poisoning causes permanent sterility in the bull, while in the cow there is a failure of estrus.

Prophylaxis and Treatment: In areas where the molybdenum content of the forage is below 5 ppm, the use of 1% copper sulfate ($CuSO_4 \cdot 5H_2O$) in salt has provided satisfactory control of molybdenosis. With higher levels of molybdenum, 2% copper sulfate has been successful. Up to 5% has been used in a few regions where the molybdenum levels are very high. In areas where, for various reasons, cattle do not consume mineral supplements, the required copper may be supplied as a drench, as parenterally administered repository copper preparations, or as a top-dressing to the pasture.

One gram of copper sulfate and 1 mg of cobalt carbonate in water solution per 100 lb of body weight, given at weekly intervals, has been the most effective treatment for molybdenum poisoning. Response usually is noted within 4 to 6 weeks and often within 2 weeks' time. Supplementary phosphorus feeding has proved to be valuable supportive treatment.

COPPER POISONING

The condition occurs in cattle and swine but these are more resistant than sheep, in which most cases appear. The meat breeds and their crosses are more susceptible than the wool breeds. Acute poisoning, usually the result of accidental ingestion of copper salts, is relatively straightforward; chronic poisoning, whether primary or secondary, is complicated by a variety of interacting factors. Primary chronic copper poisoning remains completely subclinical until the system is overloaded in some incompletely understood fashion; then blood levels of copper are suddenly elevated and the animal dies rapidly of acute IV hemolysis.

Secondary chronic copper poisoning may be phytogenous, usually in sheep pasturing subterranean clover (*Trifolium sub-*

terraneum), **or** hepatogenous, following liver damage, usually from ingestion of alkaloids (*see* SENECIO POISONING, p. 1003). Although chronic poisoning is most common where soil copper levels are high, many factors, including the levels of molybdenum, sulfate and protein in the diet, may be involved.

Death from acute poisoning may follow intakes of 20 to 110 mg/kg of body wt in sheep and young calves, and 220 to 880 mg/kg in mature cattle. Daily intakes of 3.5 mg/kg, pasture containing 15 to 20 ppm (dry matter), and pelleted feeds containing 50 ppm have caused chronic poisoning of sheep. Copper is commonly used as a feed additive for swine, at 125 to 250 ppm of copper in the diet; levels above 250 ppm are dangerous —although as for sheep, other factors may be protective, e.g., high levels of protein, zinc or iron.

Clinical Findings: Most animals that develop clinical signs will die.

Acute poisoning: Severe gastroenteritis is marked by abdominal pain and scouring. Monogastric animals may vomit. Feces and vomitus have a green to bluish color. Shock and death follow. Dysentery and icterus become apparent in the few that live more than 24 hours.

Chronic poisoning: The manifestation is quite acute, but gastroenteritis is absent. Appetite fails, thirst and depression are marked and there is severe hemoglobinuria, pallor and icterus. Most animals die within 1 to 2 days of the onset of signs.

Lesions: In the acute disease, gastroenteritis predominates; there is erosion and ulceration, particularly of the abomasum, which may rupture. In those that live long enough, the evidence of hemolysis is present as it is in the chronic disease. Icterus; a swollen, yellow liver; soft, friable spleen; dark, bluish, swollen kidneys and the hemoglobinuria are evident.

Diagnosis: The signs and lesions, especially the blue-green ingesta, are quite suggestive but require laboratory confirmation. In chronic cases, blood levels of copper will be 5 or more times increased above the normal 100 mcg/100 ml. Normal liver levels (dry matter basis) are less than 350 ppm; in chronic poisoning these are markedly elevated. In acute cases, feces may contain as much as 8,000 to 10,000 ppm of copper.

Treatment: The prognosis is always grave. Treatment of the shock and use of calcium versenate and penicillamine may be worth trying for valuable individuals.

Control: For phytogenous and hepatogenous outbreaks, ingestion of the plants involved must be prevented. Because their effect is cumulative, hepatotoxic plants may lead to outbreaks after more than one pasture season. When the problem is related to grazing of subterranean clover, encouragement of grass in the pasture and top-dressing with molybdenized superphosphate (4 oz Mo per acre) are useful. The use of a mineral lick composed of 240 lb finely ground gypsum and 187 lb coarse common salt, sprinkled and *mixed thoroughly* with 2 gal. water containing 1 lb sodium molybdate, is also protective. In an outbreak in sheep, deaths stopped within 3 days of providing ammonium molybdate, 50 to 100 mg/head daily, and sodium sulfate, 0.3 to 1.0 gm/head daily.

SELENIUM POISONING

Although selenium is highly toxic in overdoses, the element is required in trace amounts to maintain life and to prevent such conditions as exudative diathesis in chicks (q.v., p. 1349) and muscular dystrophies in many species (*see* MYOPATHIES AND RELATED CONDITIONS IN DOMESTIC ANIMALS, p. 575).

Etiology: Chronic selenium poisoning ("alkali disease") results when animals consume naturally seleniferous forages and grains which contain 5 to 40 ppm of selenium. Soils capable of supporting seleniferous plants have been found only in regions where the mean annual rainfall is less than 20 in. Certain plants known as "accumulators" require selenium for growth and often contain several thousand ppm of selenium. When consumed by animals, these accumulator plants may produce an acute type of poisoning called "blind staggers". Seleniferous plants which are not removed from the land may decay, be incorporated in the topsoil and become a source of selenium for non-seleniferous plants. These plants may then be a toxic hazard. Whether seleniferous *Astragalus* plants may contain other toxic substances has not been definitely determined. There are many *Astragalus* spp. which are not seleniferous but contain toxins poisonous to animals.

Seleniferous vegetation containing over 50 ppm of selenium has been found growing in all of the states west of the Mississippi River except those adjoining the river and the State of Washington. Such vegetation also has been found in Alberta, Saskatchewan and Manitoba in Canada, and in Mexico. Since the selenium in soils comes from certain geologic formations, the areas producing highly seleniferous vegetation are spotty and localized. Most of the cases of selenium poisoning in livestock have been reported from Colorado, Nebraska, South Dakota and Wyoming. Selenium poisoning in livestock has also been reported from Ireland, Israel and northern Queensland in Australia. Occasionally, the condition develops in dogs following the use of selenium-containing shampoos.

CHRONIC SELENIUM POISONING

"ALKALI DISEASE" TYPE

Gross lesions in chronic selenium poisoning of the "alkali disease" type usually include erosion of the joints of the long bones, atrophy and cirrhosis of the liver, atrophy of the heart, anemia and ascites. Hemoglobin concentrations decrease in the early stages and can be an aid in early diagnosis. The selenium in hair clippings may be used as an indication of previous intake of this element.

Clinical Findings: Chronic selenium poisoning in cattle, horses and swine develops within a few weeks when seleniferous grains or forages are consumed. The signs common to these species include cracking of the hoofs, lameness, stiffness of joints, dullness and lack of vitality, emaciation and loss of hair. In horses, the loss of long hair from the mane and tail usually is the first clinical sign and is followed by cracking of the hoof at the coronary band. New growth of the hoof pushes the dead tissue downward and, if the growth interruption has been prolonged, the old portion of the hoof may separate and slough. In cattle, a series of interruptions of growth may result in deformed hoofs, 6 to 7 in. long and turned upward at the ends. Swine fed seleniferous feeds show breaks in the hoof similar to those in cattle. Sows have a lowered conception rate and an increase in the number of pigs born dead. Chronic selenium poisoning of the "alkali disease" type is not common in sheep. Death losses occur from acute poisoning soon after sheep are moved onto seleniferous range forage. Consumption of seleniferous feeds for extended periods results in anorexia, emaciation, weakness, anemia and the birth of weak, blind lambs with bone deformities.

Control: A high-protein ration will help to control selenium poisoning. The use of salt containing 37.5 ppm of arsenic may reduce the incidence of chronic selenium poisoning in cattle on seleniferous range. The use of arsanilic acid (0.005 to 0.01%)

in the ration also seems to reduce the effects of high-selenium intake in calves and pigs.

Stiffness in cattle and horses may be relieved by the oral administration of compounds, such as naphthalene and bromo-benzene, which form mercapturic acids. The usual treatment is to give 4 or 5 gm of naphthalene daily for 5 days and repeat the dosage after a 5-day interval.

"BLIND STAGGERS" TYPE

This develops in animals grazing on ranges where highly seleniferous plants are growing. In cattle, blind staggers is manifested in 3 stages: First, there is a tendency to wander and the animal may walk into objects in its path. The temperature is normal, but there is impairment of vision and poor appetite. In the second stage, the wandering increases and the front legs become weak. Vision becomes further impaired. Third, the throat and tongue become paralyzed, temperature is subnormal, and death follows from respiratory failure. In sheep, the 3 stages are not as clearly differentiated as in cattle. Congestion and necrosis of the liver, congestion of the renal medulla, epicardial petechiae, hyperemia and ulceration in the abomasum and small intestine, and erosion of the articular surfaces, particularly of the tibia, are the usual lesions observed at necropsy. There is no specific antidote: supportive therapy (e.g., forced fluids) may be useful.

ACUTE SELENIUM POISONING

Acute selenium poisoning occurs in cattle and sheep as a result of consuming, at one time, sufficient highly seleniferous (accumulator) plants to cause severe intoxication. Death usually occurs within a few hours. The gait is uncertain, the temperature elevated, the respiration labored with frothing from the nostrils, and the pupils dilated. Prostration occurs before death from respiratory failure. Losses in sheep grazing on seleniferous vegetation may be high. One outbreak is recorded in which 340 mature sheep died within 24 hours of consuming highly seleniferous *Astragalus bisulcatus*.

There is no known treatment for acute selenium poisoning.

SALT POISONING

Salt (sodium chloride) may be toxic when excessive quantities are consumed. Deaths have been attributed to salt poisoning in cattle, swine, sheep, horses, dogs and poultry in various parts of the world. In the U.S.A., swine and sheep are the most frequently affected species.

Etiology: There is disagreement regarding the toxicity of salt to animals. Usually, to cause clinical signs and death, the dose rate must be high. In one study in swine and sheep, 1 to 2 gm of salt per pound of body weight given in water with a stomach tube, regularly produced poisoning. Drinking of chloride water with 1.3% salt has led to reduction in lambing percentage and weight gain of lambs and to diarrhea and increased mortality. A profound eosinophilic dermatitis in swine can be caused by topical application of sodium chloride.

Availability of water is the most important factor influencing the appearance of signs of salt poisoning. Those that have an unlimited supply of fresh drinking water available can tolerate much larger quantities of salt than those that do not. A high percentage of all cases of salt poisoning result from the ingestion of brine or whey that has been contaminated with salt. Most animals appear to be more susceptible during very hot weather. Animals that have been on a low intake of salt are more likely to ingest toxic levels. Range cattle fed concentrate supplements, to which salt had been added to control the feed intake, have developed signs of salt poisoning when the supply of water was limited by excessively cold weather.

A syndrome identical to that of salt poisoning has been produced by the administration of excessive quantities of sodium acetate to cattle, or of sodium propionate to pigs. These facts, together with negative results in experiments in pigs where high concentrations of the chlorine ion were used, suggest that salt poisoning is primarily due to an excess of the sodium ion.

Clinical Findings: At necropsy the organs are dehydrated but otherwise usually appear quite normal. Mild or acute gastroenteritis may be present. Histologically, eosinophilic meningoencephalitis and encephalomalacia characterize the disease in swine.

The onset of signs is sudden and in acute cases usually occurs within an hour or 2 after ingestion of the salt. The first signs are hyperesthesia and extreme nervousness. Muscle twitching and fine tremors are commonly observed at the onset. Afflicted animals gradually become ataxic and often blind. Most animals become progressively weaker until they go down. The temperature is normal, the pulse rapid but weak, but the breathing very rapid and shallow. Diarrhea often develops after a few hours. Polyuria may occur. The course is rapid; many die within a few hours, others within 36 to 48 hours.

Convulsions seldom occur, except in pigs. In subacute sodium salt poisoning in these animals, the most frequent and certainly the most striking phenomenon is the occurrence of epileptiform convulsions. These episodes are always heralded by twitching of the snout, with tonic and clonic spasms involving progressively the muscles of the face, neck, trunk, forelegs and finally the hind limbs. The pig may move backwards rapidly and assume a sitting-dog position or even fall over backward. Each convulsion lasts up to a minute and, in typical cases, ends with profuse salivation, complete exhaustion and collapse. Experimentally and clinically affected animals have been observed to convulse at regular 7-minute intervals. The animal may die during a seizure (respiratory arrest) or the fits may suddenly cease with permanent recovery after a period of readjustment.

Treatment: The foremost consideration is to provide fresh water, in small amounts at frequent intervals at first, to all animals. Those that can and do drink seldom need additional treatment. Severely affected animals sometimes cannot find water and often are unable to drink if they do find it. Water should be given to these animals via stomach tube. Calcium gluconate (℞ 506) administered IV or IP to effect (normal heart rate) to all severely affected animals has been recommended as supportive treatment.

NITRATE AND NITRITE POISONING

Consumption of large doses of nitrate may result in severe gastroenteritis and death in any of the domestic animals. More commonly nitrates are reduced in the rumen to nitrite, then to hydroxylamine and finally to ammonia. The rate at which this reduction takes place is an important factor affecting toxicity.

Etiology: Nitrite poisoning may occur in any species as a result of accidental ingestion of nitrites. It is seen occasionally in dogs following accidental consumption of antirust tablets, or the ingestion of dog foods containing excessive quantities of nitrite. Nitrite poisoning in ruminants usually occurs as a result of consumption of nitrate fertilizer or of forages of high nitrate or nitrite content. Few plants ordinarily have high nitrate content but under certain conditions, plants have the ability to accumulate large quantities of nitrates. Toxic levels of nitrate are sometimes found in common pasture species, such as the rye-grasses, during rapid growth. Crops grown on summer fallow may have a nitrate content in excess of crops grown on land in continuous crop production. Most losses occur in the Great Plains States when oats, barley or wheat are fed as hay, particularly if the hay is fed several days after it has been moistened by rain, snow or excessive dampness. A variety of common weeds growing on marshy or muck soils that have high nitrogen and relatively low phosphorus and potassium contents accumulate abnormal quantities of nitrates. Low temperatures, limited sunlight, poor mineral sources and applications of plant hormone herbicides contribute to increased nitrate levels. The most commonly incriminated plants have been the redroot pigweed (*Amaranthus retroflexus*) and lamb's-quarters (*Chenopodium album*), although many other plants can accumulate nitrates. Ruminants fed rations containing grains or concentrates can metabolize and utilize considerably more nitrate than ruminants maintained on roughage alone.

Water from shallow wells in certain areas of the Great Plains may contain nitrates in concentrations toxic for cattle. Losses have occurred during freezing weather due to an increase in nitrate concentration in the stock tanks.

The nitrite ion in blood converts hemoglobin to methemoglobin. Nitrites are also vasodilators which cause peripheral circulatory failure. The signs which appear and death are the result of hypoxia.

Clinical Findings: The signs of nitrite poisoning appear suddenly. Dyspnea becomes progressively more severe until signs of marked respiratory distress characterized by mouth breathing, violent respiratory movements and extreme apprehension are noted. Rapid, weak heart beat, subnormal body temperature, muscular weakness, ataxia and cyanosis rapidly develop. The patient may die in convulsions within an hour but in the usual case, death results after a clinical course of 3 to 4 hours. Of the animals that develop marked dyspnea but recover, some develop interstitial pulmonary emphysema and continue to suffer respiratory distress after disappearance of the methemoglobinemia. Most of these animals fully recover within 10 to 14 days. Pregnant females frequently abort following recovery from nitrite poisoning. Low daily intake of nitrate or nitrite has been reported to cause no clinical evidence of disease except abortion. In such cases methemoglobin has not been demonstrated in blood. Although it has been contended that nitrite caused avitaminosis A in animals, it appears probable that some other factor was responsible for this condition.

Lesions: The blood is colored chocolate brown from its methemoglobin content. The submucosa of the rumen, reticulum and omasum, and the mucosa of the abomasum usually are congested. Petechial hemorrhages on the serous surfaces are commonly observed.

Diagnosis: Methemoglobinemia is sometimes difficult to detect, especially if the necropsy is delayed. On the other hand, unless samples of blood sent for laboratory diagnosis are assayed within a few hours of being drawn, they are likely to contain a large proportion of spontaneously formed methemoglobin.

Perhaps the most sensitive and reliable simple test for nitrites is the diphenylamine blue (DPB) test. To test for nitrite, 0.5 to 1.0 ml of a 1% solution of diphenylamine in concentrated sulfuric acid is placed on a glass or porcelain plate and 1 or 2 drops of a solution or suspension of the suspect material is placed to one side, but in contact with the reagent. A blue color diffusing from the test material into the reagent indicates the presence of nitrite. The 2 solutions should not be mixed, as faint reactions may be obscured. Water used to suspend materials to be tested should be free of all metallic salts. The DPB test is useful not only for testing blood or serum (either fresh, citrated or preserved), but can also be readily used in the field for testing drinking water, plant material and stomach contents. While it is not specific for nitrites, a positive reaction can be very helpful in arriving at a diagnosis of nitrite poisoning.

Treatment: Administration of a 2% solution of methylene blue (R 607) aids in the reduction of methemoglobin to hemoglobin. Mineral oil or mucilaginous substances may be given orally to protect the irritated mucous membranes.

———————————

PITCH POISONING
(Clay pigeon poisoning, Coal tar poisoning)

An acute, highly fatal disease of swine characterized clinically by depression and pathologically by striking liver lesions.

Etiology: This disease often results from the ingestion of clay pigeons of the old type. It has been shown experimentally that small quantities of clay pigeons (15 gm) consumed over a period of 5 days will kill swine. Pastures contaminated with this material are dangerous for long periods; deaths from pitch poisoning have been reported 35 years after the last known time that a pasture was contaminated with clay pigeons. The same disease has been produced by the consumption of other pitch- or bitumen-containing products such as roofing material, certain types of tar paper, tarred building boards and plumbers' pitch. The phenols in tar have been shown to have a higher toxicity than the other constituents. Coal-tar derivatives, e.g., creosote, have been shown to induce stillbirth in sows, skin lesions in baby piglets and to interfere with vitamin A storage by the sow.

Clinical Findings: The onset usually is sudden and the course so rapid that few signs are observed. Occasionally an animal may be ill for several hours to several days before it dies. The first sign of disease is depression and weakness, followed by marked ataxia and, finally, affected animals assume a position of sternal recumbency and die in coma. The only other prominent clinical findings are tenderness to deep palpation over the abdomen, anemia and icterus during the latter stages.

Lesions: The carcass is usually icteric with excessive quantities of fluid in the peritoneal and occasionally the pleural and pericardial cavities. The most characteristic lesion is a markedly swollen liver which has a mottled appearance; the lobules are clearly outlined by a light-colored zone. Their centers contain deep-red dots the size of a pinhead. This rather characteristic change usually involves the entire liver in the most acute cases. In those that live longer, the lesions may be confined to the periphery of the organ. Liver lesions are absent in a very small percentage of cases.

There is no known treatment.

BOVINE HYPERKERATOSIS
(X-disease)

A toxicosis resulting from the ingestion of, or contact with, highly chlorinated naphthalenes which were found in certain lubricants and wood preservatives. An early sign is a watery discharge from the eyes and nose. This is followed by depression, anorexia, salivation, intermittent diarrhea and a loss of condition. Prior to the appearance of the visible signs, there is a rapid fall in the plasma vitamin A. As the disease progresses, there is an accumulation of hard keratin-like material on the skin which makes it thick, inelastic and wrinkled. The areas of the skin most frequently involved are the neck, shoulders and withers. Papillary proliferations appear on the gums, tongue, dental pad, hard palate, oral mucosa, muzzle, margins of the nostrils and esophagus and omasum. Secondary infections, such as enteritis, pneumonia and abscesses, may develop.

Cystic nodules often occur on the mucosa of the large bile ducts and the gallbladder. Degeneration and fibrosis of the liver may be evident and microscopic examination reveals degeneration, fibrosis and proliferation of the bile ducts. The kidneys, in some cases, are enlarged, pale in color with white streaks in the cortex. Degeneration of tubule cells, fibrosis and dilatation of the tubules of the renal cortex are common changes. Squamous metaplasia occurs in various portions of the reproductive tracts of both sexes as well as in the salivary glands. The pancreas may become fibrotic and the acini cystic. Frequently, the gastric and intestinal glands and the mucous glands of the gallbladder undergo cystic dilatation. There may be enteritis and the abomasal mucosa, especially near the pylorus, often shows reddened areas, flat erosions and small ulcers. At the present time bovine hyperkeratosis is primarily of historic interest. However, there is a recent report of a herd outbreak, presumably caused by the presence of chloronaphthalenes and polychlorobiphenyls (PCBs) in second-hand rubber floor mats used in the cow stable. Ordinarily, if the toxic substance is removed while the appetite is good, many animals will recover. There is no specific treatment.

POISONING BY HERBICIDES

Many of the chemicals used to control undesirable plants are highly toxic to domestic animals, while others are relatively non-toxic. The majority of livestock losses associated with herbicides are directly related to their improper or careless use. Very few losses occur when these chemicals are used properly. This discussion includes some of the more commonly used herbicides and those with which livestock losses most frequently have been associated.

Ammonium Sulfamate (Ammate): Ammonium sulfamate has not been found to be toxic to many species of animals when it is fed experimentally. Ruminants, including deer, apparently can metabolize this chemical and, in some experiments, have made better gains than control animals not fed Ammate. Reports have appeared from various parts of the country, however, which indicate that sudden deaths have occurred among cattle and deer gaining access to plants treated with ammonium sulfamate. Additional field and experimental observations must be made in order to clarify the matter of the toxicity of ammonium sulfamate.

Borax is used both as a herbicide and as a soil sterilant and is toxic to animals of it is consumed in moderate to large doses. No cases of boron poisoning are known to have occurred when this chemical has been used properly for either of these purposes. Cases of poisoning have occurred, however, when borax has been accidentally included in rations for livestock. The chief signs of acute boron poisoning are diarrhea, rapid prostration and convulsions. There is no known effective treatment. The IV injection of large quantities of balanced electrolyte solutions may be beneficial.

Dinitro Compounds: The dinitrophenol and dinitrocresol compounds are highly toxic to all classes of animals. They are readily absorbed through the skin and lungs and, therefore, poisoning can occur if animals are sprayed accidentally or have immediate access to herbage that has been sprayed. Dinitro-compounds produce a marked increase in oxygen consumption and a resultant depletion of glycogen reserves. The chief clinical signs are fever, dyspnea, acidosis, tachycardia and convulsions, followed by coma and death with a rapid onset of rigor mortis. Cataracts may occur in chronic cases of dinitrophenol intoxication. Exposure to dinitro-compounds can very often be recognized by yellowing of the skin around the mouth and of the hair around the nose and hoofs. No effective antidote is known. Affected animals should be sheltered in a shady place and cooled with water. Chlorpromazine may help control the hyperthermia. Infusion of large quantities of carbohydrate solutions and parenteral administration of vitamin A may also be useful. Residues of the dinitrocompounds that remain on foliage which has been properly treated with these chemicals are not dangerous to livestock.

Pentachlorophenol is used both as a herbicide and as a wood preservative. It is highly toxic when ingested and, like the dinitro compounds, it can be absorbed through the intact skin and by way of the lungs. It is an intense irritant to the skin and mucous membranes. Animals should be kept away from enclosures to which this chemical has been recently applied.

Animals fed in troughs made of lumber treated with penta-chlorophenol may show salivation and irritation of the oral mucosa. The chief clinical signs of pentachlorophenol poison-ing are nervousness, restlessness, rapid pulse and respiratory rates, weakness, muscle tremors and clonic convulsions, fol-lowed by death. No effective treatment or antidote is known. Pentachlorophenol-treated foliage is not dangerous to animals when the herbicide has been properly handled.

The plant hormone herbicides, 2,4-D (2,4-dichlorophenoxy-acetic acid), **2,4,5-T** (2,4,5,-trichlorophenoxyacetic acid) **and MCP** (2-methyl-4-chlorophenoxyacetic acid), and their salts and esters, are by far the most common chemicals used to control undesirable plants. Many millions of acres of field crops and pasture have been treated with these chemical weed killers. Livestock have grazed most of these pastures and have been fed feeds produced from many additional acres of field crops so treated with few if any authenticated instances of poisoning. As a group, these chemicals have been shown to be nontoxic to experimental and farm animals under practical conditions. When large doses are fed experimentally, general depression with loss of appetite, accompanied by loss of weight, general tenseness and muscular weakness, particularly of the hindquarters, are noted. Large doses in cattle may interfere with rumen function. Certain hazards to livestock may, how-ever, arise as a sequence of an alteration in the chemical composition of the plant induced by these herbicides (*see* NITRATE AND NITRATE POISONING, p. 951).

Sodium Chlorate is an old but still rather widely used herbi-cide. One of the greatest hazards associated with its use is that of fire. Treated plants and clothing that have been con-taminated are highly combustible and constitute real fire hazards. Many cases of chlorate poisoning of livestock have occurred both from the ingestion of treated plants and from accidental consumption of feed to which it was mistakenly added for salt. Cattle sometimes are attracted to sodium chlorate-treated foliage. Considerable quantities of this chemi-cal must be consumed before signs of toxicity appear. The minimum lethal dose of sodium chlorate is 500 mg/lb of body wt for cattle, 700 to 1300 mg/lb for sheep and 2300 mg/lb for poultry.

Ingestion of sodium chlorate results in the conversion of hemoglobin to methemoglobin. The signs that result are due to methemoglobinemia. Treatment with methylene blue (R 607) must be repeated frequently because, unlike the nitrites, the chlorate ion is not inactivated in the conversion of hemoglobin to methemoglobin and is capable of producing an unlimited quantity of methemoglobin as long as it is present in the body. The IV administration of isotonic salt solution in large quantities may hasten the elimination of the chlorate ion.

Arsenicals: Some of the inorganic arsenicals (sodium arsenite and arsenite trioxide) still are used as herbicides, although the high incidence of livestock losses which frequently follow their use for this purpose has made them somewhat unpopular. Cattle sometimes readily consume toxic quantities of treated foliage. Deer often are attracted to trees poisoned with arsenite and apparently lick the chemical from the trees. The highly soluble arsenicals sometimes are concentrated in pools after a rain has washed them from recently treated plants. Animals that consume this water frequently develop arsenic poisoning (q.v., p. 933).

Organic arsenical herbicides (cacodylic acid and derivatives, MSMA, DMSA) produce signs and lesions resembling, in general, those found in inorganic arsenical poisoning. Toxic single oral doses for cattle and sheep range from 10 to 25 mg/lb. Poisoning may be expected from much smaller doses consumed on successive days.

Chlorobenzoic Acids: 2,3,6-TBA (Trysben), dicamba (Banvel D): These herbicides are toxic to cattle and sheep in single oral doses in the range of 100 to 200 mg/lb of body wt. Such dosages can be obtained by these animals only through carelessness in handling and storage. The signs and lesions follow the pattern described for hormone type herbicides (*see* p. 957).

Phenylurea Compounds: Diuron (Karmex), linuron (Lorox), monuron (Telvar), fenuron (Dybar): For cattle and sheep these herbicides are toxic in single oral doses of 100 to 200 mg/lb of body wt. Such dosages can be obtained only through carelessness in handling and storage. Signs and lesions follow the pattern described for hormone type herbicides (*see* p. 597).

Triazine Compounds: Atrazine (Aatrex, Atratol, Gesaprim, Primatol A), promazine (Gesamil, Primatol P), simazine (Gesatop, Primatol S), prometone (Primatol, Gesafram), pyrometryne (Caparol, Primatol, Gesagard), Lambast: These compounds are toxic to sheep and cattle in single oral doses ranging from 10 to 100 mg/lb of body wt. Cumulative action is not remarkable. The signs and lesions follow the pattern described for the hormone type herbicides (*see* p. 957).

Amide Compounds: Diphenamid (Dymid, Enide), CDAA (Randox): Diphenamid is much less toxic than CDAA, the toxic oral doses for cattle and sheep being in the range of 200 mg/lb and 10 mg/lb of body wt respectively. The signs and lesions follow the pattern described for hormone type herbicides (*see* p. 957).

Thiocarbamate Compounds: Diallate (Avadex), triallate (Avadex B W, Far-go): The single oral doses of these compounds for cattle and sheep are in the range of 100 to 200 mg/lb of body wt, quantities unlikely to be available except through spillage or careless handling. Signs and lesions are as for the hormone type herbicides (*see* p. 957).

POISONING BY RODENTICIDES

A large group of poisons have been used against rodent pests. Farm animals, pets and wildlife often gain access to these poisons via the baits or the destroyed pests. Rodenticides sometimes are used maliciously to kill animals. This discussion covers only the rodenticides that are in most common use. Strychnine poisoning is discussed separately (*see* p. 937).

Red Squill produces convulsions which alternate with paralysis, and is a rather potent emetic. The rat is incapable of vomiting and, therefore, red squill is more toxic to that species than to most other animals. However, swine, dogs and cats occasionally have been poisoned despite the unpalatability of the squill for these species. The chief clinical signs are vomiting, depression, weakness, ataxia, paresis which may progress to posterior or generalized paralysis, bradycardia, cardiac arrhythmias, dyspnea, cyanosis and sometimes cutaneous erythema. Vomiting does not always occur in swine and complete paralysis seldom develops in dogs. The clinical course seldom exceeds 24 to 36 hours. Death occurs suddenly as a result of cardiac arrest.

Treatment consists of complete isolation to prevent undue exertion which might result in cardiac embarrassment. Emetics and gastric lavage should be used if vomiting has not occurred. Saline cathartics may aid in elimination of unabsorbed glycoside. Atropine sulfate (℞ 489) administered subcut. at 6- to 8-hour intervals may prevent cardiac arrest.

Phosphorus: Prior to the introduction of more recent products, phosphorus, in its white (or yellow) form, was used widely in preparations employed in the extermination of rodents and rabbits. These preparations were, and to a lesser extent still are, a hazard to domestic animals. The onset of signs of phosphorus poisoning is sudden. The early signs include vomiting, severe diarrhea, which often is bloody, marked signs of abdominal distress and a peculiar garlic-like odor to the breath. On the third or fourth day of illness, additional signs, which are largely due to acute liver damage, develop. They include hemorrhage, severe abdominal pain and generalized icterus. The patient rapidly becomes prostrate and dies in convulsions. Postmortem findings include severe gastroenteritis, a fatty liver, multiple hemorrhages, black tarry blood that fails to clot, and the cadaver may be phosphorescent.

To be successful, treatment must be instituted early. The judicious use of emetics may be beneficial if vomiting has not already emptied the stomach. A 1% solution of copper sulfate is an effective emetic, and also forms a copper phosphide complex that is not absorbed. Gastric and gastrointestinal lavage using a 0.01 to 0.1% solution of potassium permanganate or a 1% solution of copper sulfate should be used in an attempt to oxidize the toxic allotrope. Gastric lavage should be followed by a saline cathartic. Any form of fat in the diet must be avoided for at least 3 to 4 days because fats favor the absorption of phosphorus. No treatment has been successful after signs of acute liver damage have appeared.

Thallium Sulfate is now infrequently used as a rodenticide. It has proved to be toxic to all species to which it has been fed. Mature animals are more susceptible than young ones. The signs of poisoning include vomiting, anorexia, excessive salivation, abdominal distress, severe diarrhea, ulcerative stomatitis, dyspnea, weakness, blindness, hyperesthesia, convulsions and loss of hair or wool after clinical recovery. The most prominent necropsy findings are those of marked ulcerative gastroenteritis and cutaneous erythema.

Treatment of acute thallium poisoning comprises the use of emetics, gastric lavage with a 1% solution of sodium iodide, and IV administration of a 10% solution of sodium iodide (R 609). Diphenylthiocarbazone (Dithizon) orally at 10 mg/lb body wt, t.i.d., for 3 to 4 days is reported to be a useful antidote. Symptomatic treatment of the diarrhea and convulsions is indicated with particular attention to fluid and electrolyte balance.

ANTU (alpha naphthylthiourea): All animals that have been studied have proved to be susceptible to ANTU poisoning. Most cases, however, have occurred in dogs and swine. There is a marked variation in susceptibility with age, older animals being most susceptible. An important consideration is the degree of fullness of the stomach; animals with an empty stomach readily vomit after ingestion of ANTU and seldom are poisoned, while those with a full or partially filled stomach usually absorb fatal quantities of the chemical before vomiting occurs.

The onset of signs is sudden and usually characterized by vomiting. Progressive weakness rapidly develops. Affected animals become ataxic, later exhibit a propensity to sit and finally remain recumbent. Marked signs characteristic of pulmonary edema—dyspnea, dullness and flatness on percussion and moist rales—rapidly appear, and coughing is common. The pulse rate is rapid but weak; heart sounds are faint. The temperature gradually becomes subnormal. Diarrhea develops late in the course of the disease. Patients gradually become comatose and die from hypoxia. The course is rapid, many poisoned animals dying within an hour, the majority within 2 to 4 hours. Animals that survive 12 hours may recover.

The lesions are suggestive: The most striking finding is edema of the lungs with hydrothorax. Hyperemia of the tracheal mucosa, moderate to acute gastroenteritis, marked hyperemia of the kidneys and a pale mottled liver are found in most cases. A 10% solution of sodium thiosulfate, IV, has been reported beneficial. Positive-pressure oxygen therapy may help to relieve the pulmonary edema.

Sodium Fluoroacetate: This colorless, odorless, tasteless, water-soluble chemical has been found to be highly toxic to all animals to which it has been fed. Fluoroacetate is not toxic in itself, but it is metabolized to fluorocitrate, which blocks the tricarboxylic acid cycle—a mechanism necessary for energy production by cells. It produces its effects by 2 general mechanisms: (1) overstimulation of the CNS resulting in death in convulsions, and (2) alteration of cardiac function which results in myocardial depression, cardiac arrhythmias, ventricular fibrillation and circulatory collapse. Both effects occur to a certain degree in all animals. The CNS stimulation is the main reaction in dogs, while the cardiac effect is predominant in the horse, sheep and chicken. Swine, however, appear to be about equally affected by both.

The onset is rapid and occurs between 15 minutes and several hours after ingestion of the chemical, depending on the dose. Most species exhibit an initial period of nervousness and restlessness. This is followed in all species, except the dog and pig, by marked depression and weakness. Patients rapidly become prostrate, the pulse is weak and 2 to 3 times the normal rate. Death occurs as a result of cardiac failure. Usually, dogs and swine rapidly develop tetanic convulsions. Many exhibit evidence of severe pain. The clinical syndrome displayed is reminiscent of strychnine poisoning in these species. Vomiting is a prominent clinical finding in swine. The course is rapid, affected animals dying between 15 minutes and several hours after signs have appeared. Few animals that develop marked signs recover. The most common necropsy finding is the presence of subepicardial hemorrhages on a heart that has stopped in diastole. The blood is usually dark and tarry in appearance.

Treatment consists of administering emetics and gastric lavage. Intravenous administration of phenobarbital sodium or pentobarbital sodium within ½ to 3 hours after ingestion of a median lethal dose of the poison has saved experimental animals. The amount of barbiturate given in such cases has been as high as 15 to 20 mg/lb of body wt. Glyceryl monoacetate (monacetin) serves as a competitive antagonist of fluoroacetate. The recommended dose is 0.25 ml/lb, IM every half hour for several hours. This compound also may be administered IV in 5 parts of sterile isotonic saline solution.

Warfarin and **Pindone** have potent antiprothrombin activity and are potentially dangerous to all classes of mammals and birds. Intoxications in domestic animals have been largely the result either of contamination of feed with warfarin concentrates or with malicious use of the chemical. Swine have been poisoned by feed mixed in equipment used immediately beforehand to prepare rodent bait. The clinical signs and treatment are as for sweet clover poisoning (q.v., p. 990).

TOXICITY OF ORGANIC INSECTICIDES AND ACARICIDES

There has been criticism from many quarters against certain of the pesticides to be discussed in this section. There are changes proposed in State and Federal legislation, changes expected as the result of executive interpretation, changes as one ecologic interest challenges another. For these reasons, it is important that every user of pesticides make a particular effort to always read and follow current label directions—not just once, but each and every time a new container is purchased. (*See also* PROTECTION OF PERSONS HANDLING INSECTICIDES, p. 976 and GENERAL PRECAUTIONS, p. 977.)

The day-to-day and month-to-month changes that will occur will be the result primarily of pressure from environmentalists, consumers and others, rather than toxicologists concerned with the safety of livestock and other domestic animals, since the safety of these compounds for these animals has been rather carefully established in the past. It is of utmost importance that changing recommendations and regulations be treated with respect and full compliance. Prosecution of individuals, including veterinarians, has already occurred and will continue, for failure to follow label directions or to heed label warnings and for failure to warn the animal owner of the precautions to be taken. At all times, read and follow the label instructions of current products.

Poisoning by the organic insecticides and acaricides may be caused by their direct application to animals, by the ingestion of the compounds on feed or forage treated for the control of plant parasites, or by accidental exposure. It is not within the scope of this section to cover all materials currently used as insecticides or acaricides. For this reason, discussion is limited to those organic compounds known to be most frequently hazardous as toxicants to livestock or as residues in animal products.

An ideal insecticide or acaricide should be efficacious without the risk of injury to livestock or the person making the application and without leaving residues in the tissues, eggs or milk. While many compounds meet some of these requirements, few of those presently available satisfy all of them.

Under present regulations, labels must carry warnings against use of many compounds on certain animals or under certain circumstances. These warnings may be concerned with acute or chronic toxicity or with the avoidance of residues in meat, milk or other animal products. In either case it is imperative that label instructions be followed to the letter.

PETROLEUM PRODUCTS

Petroleum fractions have been used as insecticides and acaricides for many years, either alone or as part of more-or-less complex formulations. Certain light mineral oils, kerosene and xylene may be applied to the skin in small quantities without harmful effects other than perhaps transitory erythema or discomfort. In general, such materials should not be used on cattle in excess of 60 gm per adult. When larger quantities are used, severe reactions may occur, such as drying, cracking, or blistering of the skin, inappetence, depression, dyspnea, salivation and, occasionally, death. Xylene irritates the skin of cattle, and in sheep, excessive amounts produce dramatic signs, including dizziness, trembling and narcosis. The toxic effects of xylene are observed within a few minutes of exposure and may last for several hours, depending upon the degree of exposure. The effects of oils and fractions of petroleum are observed within the first few days after application and may be seen for several days or weeks thereafter. Through failure to recognize their toxic effects, many cases of poisoning or injury following the use of these substances have been wrongly attributed to the insecticide dissolved in them.

Treatment of poisoning or damage due to petroleum products should be directed to the removal of the material from the skin with the aid of soap or detergents and copious quantities of water. Further treatment is dependent upon the clinical signs.

SOLVENTS AND EMULSIFIERS

Solvents and emulsifiers are required in most liquid preparations of insecticides. These compounds may or may not be toxic; usually they are of very low toxicity, but like the petroleum products (which many are), they must be given consideration as possible causes of poisoning. In direct treatment there must be excellent emulsification, with an average droplet size of approximately 5 μ (preferably smaller), or excessive deposits will be made on the animals treated. Treatment should be as for the petroleum products.

PURITY OF PRODUCT

In all syntheses of chemicals, the reactions rarely yield 100% of the product of interest. In any synthesis, be it a natural crop or man-made, there will be present, in infinitely variable proportions, related compounds which may have different biologic effects from the compound sought. A prime example of this is to be found with TDE (Rothane, DDD). The p,p'-isomer is an effective insecticide of low toxicity for most mammals. The o,p-isomer has rather remarkable effects upon the adrenal glands of at least the human and the dog and is employed as a drug in human medicine to treat certain adrenal malfunctions. Recent publications indicate p,p'-DDT and o,p-DDT have a similar relationship.

Final purity may often rest with the consumer. Storage of products under extremes of temperatures may lead to deterioration as may the holding of partially emptied containers for unusually long periods. Although the practice is declining, some consumers continue to "mix their own" combinations, often to the disadvantage of the animals treated.

INSECTICIDES DERIVED FROM PLANTS

Most of the insecticides derived from plants have traditionally been considered safe for use on animals. Derris (rotenone) and pyrethrum are examples of such materials. Nicotine in the form of nicotine sulfate (Black-leaf 40) is an exception. Unless it is carefully used, poisoning may result. Animals poisoned by nicotine sulfate show tremors, incoordination, nausea and disturbed respiration, and finally become comatose and die.

Necropsy lesions of nicotine poisoning include pale mucous membranes, dark blood, hemorrhages on the heart and in the lungs, and congestion of the brain. Treatment of nicotine poisoning consists of removing the material by washing or by gastric lavage, applying artificial respiration, and providing the usual measures for cardiac arrest and shock. Mildly affected animals recover rapidly and spontaneously.

SULFUR AND LIME-SULFUR

Sulfur and lime-sulfur are 2 of the oldest insecticides. Elemental sulfur is practically devoid of toxicity, although poisoning has occurred occasionally when very high proportions were mixed in the feed of cattle. Specific toxic dosages are not known, but probably exceed 2 gm/lb of body wt. Lime-sulfur, which is a complex of sulfides, may cause irritation, discomfort, or blistering, but rarely causes death. Treatment consists of removing the residual material and applying bland protective ointments plus any supportive measures that may be indicated.

CHLORINATED HYDROCARBON COMPOUNDS

Those most commonly used (or that may have been used) on animals and in their environment are DDT, Rothane (TDE), methoxychlor, lindane, benzene hexachloride (BHC), chlordane, toxaphene, dieldrin, aldrin and heptachlor.

Acute Toxic Doses

DDT poisoning of cattle, sheep, goats, hogs, horses and dogs is not observed, except under the most unusual circumstances.

Poisoning of poultry and cats occurs occasionally. Cattle tolerate applications of sprays containing as much as 8% DDT. Sheep, goats, hogs and horses are not harmed by sprays or dips containing 1.5% of DDT, even when applied every 4 days for 4 applications. Dogs tolerate 1% dips and sprays. Cats have been reported to be highly susceptible to DDT, although exact toxic doses have not been presented. Chickens have been poisoned by 1% dips of DDT.

When administered orally, DDT is definitely toxic to cattle, sheep and goats in doses of 225 mg/lb of body wt. The minimum acute toxicity level for DDT is 110 mg/lb. Single doses of 45 mg/lb are tolerated by sheep, goats, cattle and horses. Horses have been given as much as 110 mg/lb without producing clinical signs.

When applied as a 0.5% spray to lactating cows, an average of 0.5 ppm appears in the milk with a peak of about 1.5 ppm 2 days after spraying. DDT appears in the milk of cows occupying barns sprayed with DDT unless precautions are taken to prevent contamination of the feed and contact between the animals and the treated walls and stanchions. DDT is not recommended for use on animals producing milk for human consumption.

DDT is stored in the fat of cattle that are sprayed with it or are consuming it in treated or contaminated feeds. A single spraying with 0.5% DDT produces a residue in the fat of cattle of about 11 ppm. Additional spraying at 2- or 3-week intervals gradually increases the residue. Six applications of DDT at 3-week intervals have produced a residue of 35 ppm in the fat of cattle, while 31 applications at 2-week intervals produced from 80 to 100 ppm. After the cessation of treatment, an interval of at least 24 weeks is required for the elimination from the fat tissue of a residue of 35 ppm. Cattle fed a diet containing 10 ppm of DDT for 28 days have shown a residue of 7 ppm in the fat. Sheep so fed had a residue of 3 ppm. The fat of meat in interstate (U.S.A.) commerce must not contain more than the officially established tolerance for DDT; therefore, judgment must be used in the treatment of animals ultimately destined for slaughter so that this limit is not exceeded.

Rothane (TDE) is chemically related to DDT and its toxicity is of approximately the same order. Residues in the tissues and the amounts excreted in milk are also similar. Statements relating to DDT, therefore, apply in general to this compound.

Methoxychlor is one of the safest available chlorinated hydrocarbon insecticides. Young dairy calves tolerate 120 mg/lb of body wt; 220 mg/lb is mildly toxic. While 450 mg/lb produces rather severe poisoning in young calves, sheep are not affected. One dog was given 450 mg/lb daily for one month without showing signs. The extent of absorption and storage of methoxychlor is less than with DDT or rothane, but the duration of storage is about the same. About 0.4 ppm of methoxychlor may be found in milk one day after spraying a cow with a 0.5% spray. Because of this excretion, sprays of methoxychlor are no longer recommended for use on animals producing milk for human consumption. Six applications of a 0.5% spray at 3-week intervals will produce a residue in the fat of cattle of 2.4 ppm. Cattle and sheep store essentially no methoxychlor when it is fed to them at the rate of 25 ppm in the total diet for 112 days. The established tolerance for methoxychlor in fat will not be exceeded, provided it is used only as recommended.

Benzene hexachloride (BHC, hexachlorocyclohexane) is a very useful insecticide for large animals and for dogs, but is highly toxic to cats in the concentrations necessary for parasite control. Only the **gamma isomer** of this compound is insecticidal. Unfortunately, the same isomer accounts for its acute toxicity. The commercial name "lindane" is used for a product that contains 99% or more of the gamma isomer.

Cattle in good condition tolerated 0.2% applications, but in stressed, emaciated cattle poisoning has resulted from spraying or dipping in 0.075% material. Horses and hogs appear to tolerate 0.2 to 0.5% sprays, thereby leaving an adequate margin of safety for these species. Ordinarily, sheep and goats tolerate 0.5% applications. Emaciation and lactation are known to increase the susceptibility of animals to poisoning by the gamma isomer of BHC; therefore, such animals should be treated with extreme caution. Very young calves are poisoned by a single oral dose of lindane at 2 mg/lb of body wt. Mild signs appear in sheep given 10 mg/lb and death occurs at 45 mg/lb. Adult cattle have been given 6 mg/lb without producing signs. BHC is stored in the fat of the body and excreted in the milk. While all the isomers behave in this manner, the gamma isomer is eliminated rapidly, while the other isomers are excreted more slowly. Cattle sprayed or dipped in 0.075% lindane showed 23 ppm in their fat. This residue declined to zero over a period of 12 weeks. Because isomers, other than the gamma, are stored excessively and for long periods, it is best that lindane be used in preference to the technical BHC, which contains several isomers. Chickens are susceptible to lindane poisoning to about the same extent as young calves, 0.05% dips producing about 10% mortality.

Chlordane: Livestock become exposed only through consumption of treated plants or through carelessness and accidents. Very young calves have been killed by doses of 20 mg/lb, and the minimum toxic dose for cattle is about 40 mg/lb. Sheep have been poisoned by 45 mg/lb and killed by 60 mg/lb. Cattle fed chlordane as 25 ppm of their diet for 56 days showed 19 ppm in their fat at the end of the feeding. Emulsions and suspensions have been used safely on dogs at concentrations not exceeding 0.25%, provided freshly diluted materials were used. In dry powders, it has been safely used in concentrations up to 5% on dogs. No injury resulted to pigeons, Leghorn cockerels and pullets that had been subjected for 30 to 60 days to vapors emanating from chlordane-treated surfaces.

Toxaphene can be used with reasonable safety if recommendations are followed, but can produce poisoning when applied or ingested in excessive quantities. Dogs and cats are particularly susceptible to toxaphene poisoning and it should never be used on these animals. Young calves have been poisoned by 1% toxaphene sprays, while all other farm animals except poultry can withstand 1.0% or more as sprays or dips. Chickens have been poisoned by dipping in 0.1% emulsions and turkeys have been poisoned by spraying with 0.5% material. Toxaphene is primarily an acute toxicant and does not persist unduly in the tissues of treated animals. Adult cattle have been mildly intoxicated by 4%, and definitely harmed by 8%, sprays. Poisoning of adult cattle has resulted from dipping in emulsions which contained only 0.5% of toxaphene, an amount ordinarily safe. After considerable study, it was found that such poisoning was due to the emulsions breaking down and allowing the fine droplets to coalesce. The large droplets readily adhere to the hair of cattle and the resultant dosage becomes equivalent to that obtained by spray treatments of much higher concentration. Toxaphene is lethal to young calves at 4 mg/lb but not at 2 mg/lb. The minimum toxic dose for cattle is about 15 mg/lb, and for sheep between 10 and 15 mg/lb. Spraying Hereford cattle 12 times at 2-week intervals with 0.5% toxaphene produced a maximum residue of 8 ppm in the fat. Cattle fed 10 ppm of toxaphene in the diet for 30 days had no detectable toxaphene tissue residues, while steers fed 100 ppm for 112 days stored only 40 ppm in their fat. This amount was eliminated in 2 months after the feeding of toxaphene had been suspended.

Dieldrin has not been recommended for use on livestock in the U.S.A., with the exception of sheep, because of the residues that appear in meat and milk. In sheep, the material has given outstanding results in controlling the sheep ked when used as a 1.0 to 1.5% dust. While residues limit its application, dieldrin is actually an insecticide of moderate toxicity. Young dairy calves are poisoned by oral doses of 4 mg/lb but tolerate 2 mg/lb, while adult cattle tolerate 4 mg/lb and are poisoned by 10 mg/lb. Pigs tolerate 10 mg/lb and are poisoned by 20 mg/lb. Horses are poisoned by 10 mg/lb. Because of its high effectiveness against insect pests on crops and pasture and consequent low dosage per acre, dieldrin is not likely to produce poisoning of livestock grazing the treated areas. Diets containing 25 ppm of dieldrin have been fed to cattle and sheep for periods of 16 weeks without producing any harmful effect other than a residue in their fat. Residues in animal fat are slow to disappear. Considerable judgment must be exercised in the marketing of animals grazing treated areas or consuming products from previously treated areas to avoid violation of regulations as the tolerance for such residues is zero in the U.S.A.

Aldrin is a potent insecticide and a near relative of dieldrin. It is of the same order of toxicity and the statements pertaining to dieldrin may be considered to apply in general to aldrin. It is not recommended for use on livestock because of its tendency to produce considerable residue in the tissues of animals. The animal body converts aldrin to dieldrin and stores the material as dieldrin. Specific analyses for aldrin will, therefore, usually yield negative results, while dieldrin analyses reflect the true level of storage.

Heptachlor has not been recommended for use on livestock in the U.S.A. It is a very effective insecticide against certain plant-feeding insects and, therefore, is encountered from time to time in areas grazed by livestock. Heptachlor is tolerated by young dairy calves in doses as high as 6 mg/lb of body wt but is toxic to them at 10 mg/lb. Sheep tolerate 10 mg/lb but are poisoned by 20 mg/lb. Diets containing 60 ppm of heptachlor have been fed to cattle for 16 weeks without producing any harmful effect other than the residues in the fat tissues. Heptachlor must, therefore, be considered as another chlorinated hydrocarbon of moderate toxicity. It is converted by animals and stored in the body fat as heptachlor epoxide. For this reason, a specific analysis performed for heptachlor will usually yield negative results, while the epoxide method will reveal storage.

Clinical Findings: The chlorinated hydrocarbon insecticides are general stimulants to the CNS. They produce a great variety of signs, most of which are neuromuscular manifestations. The affected animal generally is first noted to be more alert. Twitching of the muscles is then observed, the process commencing in the facial region and extending backward until all the body musculature is involved. In poisoning by DDT, rothane and methoxychlor, progressive involvement leads to trembling or shivering movements which are followed by convulsions and death. With the other chlorinated hydrocarbons, the muscular twitchings are followed by convulsions, usually without the intermediate trembling. Convulsions may be clonic, tonic, or both and may last from only a few seconds to several hours or may be brief and frequent. Abnormal postures, such as touching the sternum to the ground while maintaining the standard position with the hind limbs, or keeping the head down between the forelegs, are often seen. Some animals stand with their heads pressed against a wall or fence. Many animals exhibit almost continual chewing movements. Occasionally, an affected animal becomes belligerent and will attack other animals or moving objects. There usually is a copious flow of thick saliva and incontinence of urine. Outcries of various sorts also are common. During the convulsive states, high fevers may occur. Some affected animals show none of these active signs, but are depressed, almost oblivious to their surroundings and do not eat or drink. Such animals may live several days longer than those showing the more violent manifestations. In certain cases, there is an alternation of clinical signs, the animal first being extremely excited and then severely depressed. The severity of the signs observed at a given time is not a sure prognostic index. Some animals have only a single convulsion and die, while others suffer innumerable convulsions but subsequently recover. The signs of poisoning by these insecticides are highly suggestive, but are not sufficiently definitive to be diagnostic. Encephalitis or meningitis often present signs similar to those observed in insecticide poisoning.

Signs of acute intoxication by chlordane in birds are nervous chirping, collapse on hocks or side, excitability and mucous exudates in the nasal passages. Signs of subacute and chronic intoxication are molting, dehydration and cyanosis of the comb, loss of body weight and cessation of egg production. Molting and cyanosis of the comb are nonspecific signs.

Lesions: If death has occurred suddenly, there may be nothing more than cyanosis. More definite lesions occur as the duration of the intoxication increases. There is usually congestion of various organs, particularly the lungs, liver and kidneys, plus a blanched appearance of all organs if the body temperature was high before death. The heart generally is in systole, and there are usually many hemorrhages of varying size on the epicardium. In some cases, the appearance of the heart and lungs suggests a peracute pneumonia, and, if the animal was affected for more than a few hours, there may be edema of the lungs. The trachea and bronchi may contain a blood-tinged froth. Cerebrospinal-fluid volume is excessive in many cases, and the brain and spinal cord frequently are congested and edematous.

Treatment: At this time, there are no known specific antidotes for poisoning by the chlorinated hydrocarbon insecticides. When exposure has been by spraying, dipping or dusting, a thorough bathing, using detergents (if possible, otherwise soap) and copious quantities of water, is recommended. If the material was taken internally, gastric lavage is indicated, together with saline purgatives. The use of oils for this purpose is contraindicated because they may increase, rather than decrease, absorption.

Regardless of the manner of exposure, the signs exhibited by the animal should be controlled. When these are of the excitatory type, the use of barbiturates or chloral hydrate is indicated. All disturbing elements of the environment should be reduced or removed. If the animal shows marked depression, anorexia and dehydration, therapy should be directed toward supplying appropriate nourishment and fluids by the use of IV injections and, if necessary, introduction of food and water through a stomach tube.

ORGANOPHOSPHORUS COMPOUNDS

A large number of organophosphorus compounds have been developed for plant and animal protection. They vary greatly in toxic effect, and each has its own characteristics in regard to tissue storage and excretion in milk. In general, however, this family of compounds offers a distinct advantage by producing little or no tissue residues.

Tetraethyl pyrophosphate (TEPP) probably is one of the most acutely toxic of all insecticides. It is calculated that as little as one drop in the conjunctival sac of man would lead to severe poisoning if not death. Although it is not used on animals, they may occasionally be exposed to it accidentally. As an example, a herd of 29 cattle ranging in age from calves to adults were accidentally sprayed with 0.33% TEPP emulsion. The entire herd died within 40 minutes of the time of application.

Parathion, a widely used material for control of plant pests, is approximately one-half as toxic as TEPP. It has been used as a dip and spray on cattle in some countries, but not in the U.S.A. The majority of the cases of human poisoning (occupational) by insecticides thus far reported have been attributed to parathion or its degradation products. As a spray, it produces definite signs of poisoning in young calves at a 0.02% concentration and occasional transitory signs at 0.01%. Orally, parathion is toxic to sheep at 10 mg/lb of body wt, but not at 5 mg/lb. Young dairy calves are poisoned by 0.2 mg/lb, while 20 mg/lb is required to poison older cattle. Parathion is used extensively in the control of mosquitoes and insects in the orchard and on truck crops. Normally, because so little is used per acre treated, it presents no particular hazard to livestock. Because of its potency, particular care should be taken to prevent accidental exposures to the compound. Parathion is not stored in animal tissues in appreciable amounts.

EPN is related to parathion, but is approximately one-half as toxic when externally applied. When given orally, it is of approximately equal toxicity.

Malathion is one of the safest of the organophosphorus compounds and is roughly equivalent to toxaphene, 0.5% sprays not being toxic to young calves while 1% sprays are. Adult cattle tolerate 2% sprays. Given orally, malathion is toxic at 45 mg/lb, but not toxic at 25 mg/lb of body wt. Young calves tolerate 5 mg/lb, but are poisoned by 10 mg/lb. Malathion appears in the milk of dairy cattle.

Ronnel produces mild signs of poisoning in cattle at 60 mg/lb of body wt, but severe signs do not appear until the dose is increased to about 200 mg/lb. Concentrations as high as 2.5% in sprays have failed to produce poisoning of cattle, very young dairy calves or sheep. Poisoning by ronnel usually occurs in 2 stages: The animal first becomes rather weak and, although moving about normally, may be very placid. Diarrhea also may appear at this time, the feces often being flecked with blood. Later, salivation and dyspnea appear if the dose is high. At the lower dosages, the salivation and dyspnea will probably not be seen. Blood cholinesterase activity declines slowly over a period of 5 to 7 days. Ronnel produces residues in meat and milk, therefore strict adherence to label restrictions is essential.

Coumaphos is used against cattle grubs (*Hypoderma* spp.), *Dermatobia hominis* and a number of other ectoparasites and for treatment of premises. The maximum concentration which may be safely used on adult cattle, horses and hogs is

0.5%. Young calves and all ages of sheep and goats must not be sprayed with concentrations higher than 0.25%. For them, the drug may be lethal at 0.5% concentrations. Adult cattle may show mild signs at 1.0% concentrations.

Diazinon: When sprayed, young calves appear to tolerate 0.05%, but are poisoned by 0.1% concentrations. Adult cattle may be sprayed repeatedly at weekly intervals with 0.1% concentrations without inducing poisoning. Orally, diazinon appears to be tolerated by young calves at 0.2 mg/lb. of body wt but poisoning results at 0.4 mg/lb. Adult cattle tolerate 4 mg/lb orally, but are poisoned by 10 mg/lb. Sheep tolerate 8 mg/lb, but are poisoned by 12 mg/lb.

Trichlorfon: As a spray, the material is tolerated by adult cattle at a 1.0% concentration. When administered orally, this compound is tolerated by young dairy calves at 2 mg/lb of body wt, but it produces poisoning at 4 mg/lb. In adult cattle, 20 mg/lb appears to be tolerated, while 40 mg/lb produces poisoning. Sheep and horses are poisoned by 40 mg/lb, but appear to tolerate 20 mg/lb. Dogs were unaffected by the feeding of 1,000 ppm of trichlorfon for 4 months. Trichlorfon is metabolized very rapidly.

Ciodrin is a compound of rather low toxicity. A notable exception is that Brahman cattle are markedly more susceptible to poisoning than are the European breeds. Cattle (except as above), sheep, goats and pigs all tolerate sprays containing Ciodrin at 0.5% levels or higher. The toxic dose appears to be in the 2% except for Brahmans where 0.144% to 0.3% may be toxic.

Dichlorvos is a rapidly metabolized and excreted compound. The compound has many uses on both plants and animals. Residues in meat and milk are not a problem if label directions are followed. Dichlorvos is of moderate toxicity. Orally the minimum toxic dose is about 4 mg/lb in young calves and 10 mg/lb in sheep and horses.

Dioxathion is a mixture of cis- and trans-isomers (70%) and reaction products (30%). It is used for both plant and animal protection. It is rapidly metabolized and is not likely to produce residues in meat greater than the 1 ppm official tolerance. Concentrations of 0.15% or less are generally employed on animals. Dioxathion has killed cattle at 0.8% and dairy calves at 0.5% when applied as a full wet-spray. Sprays of 0.1 to 0.25% may be occasionally toxic for very young dairy calves. Sheep and Angora goats seem to be unharmed by 0.25% concentrations. Orally, dioxathion has killed young calves at 4 mg/lb and produced intoxication at 2 mg/lb.

Ruelene is active both as a systemic and contact insecticide in livestock, has some anthelmintic activity, and is of rather low toxicity. Dairy calves have been poisoned by oral doses of 20 mg/lb and above, while adult cattle required 40 mg/lb for the same effect. Sheep have shown moderate intoxication by 80 mg/lb while Angora goats were about twice as sensitive. Pigs have been poisoned by 5 mg/lb and horses by 20 mg/lb. As a topical spray most livestock tolerate concentrations of 2%.

Carbophenothion: Dairy calves under 2 weeks of age sprayed with water-based formulations showed poisoning at 0.05% and higher concentrations. Adult cattle have been poisoned by concentrations of 1.0% and higher. Sheep and goats have been poisoned by oral doses of 10 mg/lb and higher but not at 4 mg/lb. The LD_{50} for rats is about 14 mg/lb; a daily dosage of 1 mg/lb for 90 days produced poisoning. Dogs were not poisoned when fed a diet containing 32 ppm for 90 days.

Supona: Adult cattle were poisoned by sprays containing 0.5% and above, while young calves were poisoned only when the concentration was raised to 2%. The minimum oral toxic dose appears to be about 10 mg/lb for all ages of cattle.

Dimethoate: When administered orally, the minimum toxic dose for young dairy calves was about 22 mg/lb, while 10 mg/lb was a lethal dose for cattle one year of age. Daily doses of 4.5 mg/lb for 5 days in adult cattle lowered blood cholinesterase activity to 20% of normal but did not produce signs of poisoning. Horses have been poisoned by oral doses of 27 to 36 mg/lb. When applied topically, sprays of 1% concentration have been tolerated by calves, cattle and adult sheep.

Phorate: The maximum nontoxic oral dose for young calves was 0.04 mg/lb; for cattle and sheep, 0.2 mg/lb; for goats 0.1 mg/lb. Higher doses produced poisoning.

Disulfoton: The maximum nontoxic oral dose is 0.4 mg/lb for young calves, for cattle and goats 1 mg/lb, and for sheep 2.2 mg/lb.

Oxydemetonmethyl: Maximum nontoxic oral dose was 0.4 mg/lb for young calves, 1 mg/lb for cattle and 2.2 mg/lb for sheep and goats.

Azinphosmethyl: The maximum nontoxic oral dose for calves was 0.2 mg/lb, for cattle and goats 1 mg/lb, and for sheep 2.2 mg/lb.

Clinical Findings: The organophosphorus compounds have in common a widely variable ability to inhibit cholinesterase activity. For some compounds, this appears to be the primary mechanism of poisoning, while for others, the inhibition is secondary. Not all of the actions of these materials are understood. When cholinesterase inhibition is the primary mechanism of intoxication, the clinical syndrome is associated with cholinergic signs such as mild-to-profuse salivation, dyspnea, signs of abdominal pain, ataxia, frequently diarrhea and, occasionally, convulsions. When given in small, repeated doses, these compounds may progressively lower blood cholinesterase activity until no activity can be detected, yet no signs appear. In other cases, when the activity is lowered to 20% or less of normal, signs are noted. Sometimes poisoning may appear while the blood activity is rather high. In this respect, is must be remembered that signs are observed when nerve cholinesterase is inhibited and that the enzyme in the blood reflects only in a general way, the levels in the nerve tissues. Onset of signs after exposure may be within 5 or 6 minutes or may be delayed for 2 days or more. The course of intoxication is influenced principally by the dosage. Malathion, trichlorfon, parathion and TEPP produce poisoning of short duration, followed by death or full recovery within 24 hours. Ronnel and coumaphos produce their effects over a much longer period, in extreme cases signs of intoxication may be seen for as long as 30 days. In acute poisoning death appears to be immediately preceded by paralysis of the respiratory center.

Lesions: In most cases of acute poisoning with organophosphorus compounds the necropsy findings are essentially negative. In the more prolonged cases, there may be visceral changes usually associated with anoxia. Diagnosis of organophosphorus poisoning cannot be based solely upon necropsy lesions. Blood and tissue cholinesterase levels may not fluctuate proportionately; therefore, determination of blood cholinesterase levels is not an accurate index of the presence or degree of poisoning.

Treatment: Organophosphorus insecticide poisoning can usually be treated successfully with atropine sulfate, using the following amounts as average initial doses: cattle—30 mg/100 lb of body wt, sheep—50 mg/100 lb, horses—6.5 mg/100 lb, dogs—2 to 4 mg total. One-fourth to ⅓ of the dose should be given slowly IV, the remainder subcut. or IM. It is important that atropinization be reached and maintained over several hours. The dosage may be repeated, judging time and amount by the response of the patient.

An improved treatment combines atropine with 2-PAM (2-pyridine aldoxime methyl chloride); the latter encourages the regeneration of cholinesterase.

Treatment for removal of the poison from the animal, as suggested for the chlorinated hydrocarbons (p. 971) should also be given. Rest and quiet surroundings are indicated. Artificial respiration or the administration of oxygen is advantageous. The use of phenothiazine-derived tranquilizers should be avoided. The use of succinylcholine should be avoided for at least one week following the administration or use of any of the organophosphorus compounds.

CHEMICAL ANALYSIS IN DIAGNOSIS

Chemical analyses are of very little value in establishing a diagnosis of poisoning by organic insecticides; most chlorinated hydrocarbon insecticides leave an easily detectable residue even when the health of the animal is unimpaired, while others, particularly the organic phosphorus compounds, may not leave detectable residues even when the true cause of death. The analytical methods available for these compounds are of a tedious and specialized nature, therefore expensive. In all cases it is essential to confirm the identity and quantity of each suspected compound by at least 2 different types of analysis. The validity of chemical analysis is highly dependent upon the care exercised by the collector of the tissues to avoid contamination with the compound from the skin or the environment.

PROTECTION OF PERSONS HANDLING INSECTICIDES

Absorption of insecticides occurs in man as it does in animals. Each exposure, no matter how brief or small, results in some of the compound being absorbed and perhaps stored. Repeated short exposures may eventually result in intoxication. Every precaution should be taken to minimize exposure. This may include the use of rubber gloves, respirators, rain gear or frequent changes of clothing, with bathing at each change. Such measures are generally sufficient to guard against intoxication. Overexposure to chlorinated hydrocarbon insecticides is difficult to measure except by the occurrence of signs of poisoning.

The cholinesterase-inhibiting property of the organophosphorus compounds may be used to indicate degree of exposure if frequent determinations of the activity of the blood enzyme are made. Serum esterase is usually inhibited first and, in the absence of declining erythrocyte activity indicates a recent exposure of only moderate degree. Depression of the erythro-cytic-enzyme activity indicates a very severe acute exposure or a chronic exposure over a long period. Generally, depression of erythrocytic activity to 60 to 70% of normal is not cause for concern, but depressions beyond this must be viewed as pertinent warnings. It is important to remember that normal cholinesterase activity values vary from individual to individual and that a determination of activity has significance only when it can be compared with the normal value for that particular individual.

GENERAL PRECAUTIONS

Organic pesticides may have deleterious effects upon fish and wildlife as well as upon domesticated species. In no event should amounts greater than those specifically recommended be used, and maximum precautions must be taken to prevent drift or drainage to adjoining fields, pastures, ponds, streams or other premises outside the area in which the treatment is essential.

BRACKEN FERN POISONING

Bracken fern (*Pteridium aquilinum*, *Pteris aquilina*) is widely distributed in North America and in many other parts of the world.

Ingestion of the plant produces a cumulative type of poisoning which requires 1 to 3 months to develop, depending on the quantity consumed, time of year, condition of animal and other factors. It is sometimes difficult to convince farmers that the plant is poisonous because the disease can appear 2 or more weeks after removal of livestock from the fern-infested area. Most cases develop in the summer and early fall following periods of drought. Even when present as a contaminant in hay, the plant is toxic and cases have been observed in stable-fed animals. The disease occurs in horses, cattle, sheep and, possibly, in swine.

Etiology: Two toxic principles are involved: a thiaminase, which inactivates thiamine and is apparently not toxic to cattle and only partially so to sheep; and second, the so-called aplastic-anemia or radiomimetic factor, which depresses bone marrow function in cattle. Thiamine or other B-complex vitamins are ineffective in treating cattle. Both the leaves and rhizomes of the fern contain the toxic principles, their concentration varying with the season.

In the rat and horse, bracken fern poisoning is manifested in a thiamine deficiency. In an affected horse, thiamine decreases from an average normal of 8.5 mcg/100 ml of blood to a low of 2.8 mcg and increases to 11.5 mcg during thiamine therapy. At the same time, the pyruvic acid content of the blood increases from a normal of 2.2 mg/100 ml to a high of 8.5 mg with a decrease to 2.1 mg upon treatment. This response is evident in 2 days.

Clinical Findings: Affected horses exhibit anorexia, incoordination, circumduction of the limbs and a crouching stance with arched neck and feet planted wide apart. When the signs are severe, tachycardia is present as contrasted to bradycardia at the onset. The animal dies in a clonic spasm with typical opisthotonos. In most cases, the rectal temperature is normal, but in some instances it reaches 104°F.

Affected cattle present 2 different syndromes described as the enteric and laryngitic types. The **enteric type** is the most common and is marked by the passage of large clots of blood in the feces due to hemorrhage in the abomasum and intestines. The cecum and colon are often filled with clots of blood. The animals are depressed, anorectic, pyretic (106° to 110°F), weak, and have anemic mucous membranes with petechiae. There is often bleeding from the natural body orifices. The blood frequently fails to clot normally and, during the season when tabanid flies are abundant, the skin of affected cattle is marked by numerous streaks of blood where these insects have been feeding. Poisoned cattle often try to hide and may be aggressive when efforts are made to drive them. The **laryngitic type** is most frequent in younger animals and is marked by edematous swelling of the throat region that may interfere with breathing. The signs of the enteric type of disease are also observed with this syndrome.

The physiologic processes in the bone marrow, and possibly elsewhere, are greatly affected as shown by the reduction of leukocytes and blood platelets. Once developed, this condition is not reversed by any currently used nutritional factor. A carcinogenic factor becomes evident in long-term and low-level feeding of bracken to cattle, resulting in enzootic hematuria associated with bladder tumors. Blindness caused by progressive degeneration of the neuroepithelium of the retina was seen in sheep grazing bracken in Yorkshire ("bright blindness").

Differential Diagnosis: The widespread hemorrhages are an important diagnostic aid in cattle, although the above signs easily can be confused with several infectious diseases and other poisonings marked by hematologic changes. Chief among these are leptospirosis, anaplasmosis, bacillary hemoglobinuria and *Crotalaria* or sweet-clover poisoning.

The morbidity in affected herds varies from 5 to 10% and occasionally is higher. Animals which develop acute signs seldom recover. The onset is sudden and death may occur in 12 to 72 hours, although chronically affected animals may linger for 4 to 10 days.

Prophylaxis: Bracken and other poisonous plants are usually grazed for the want of more suitable food. The disease has been prevented in cattle and horses by an alternative grazing plan whereby they are allowed on a bracken-contaminated pasture for 3 weeks and then are removed for 3 weeks. The fern growth is retarded by close grazing or trampling and the stand in a pasture can gradually be brought below dangerous levels by this alternative grazing system. Weed killers developed to date, or burning of pastures, are not effective in the control of bracken.

Treatment: In horses, thiamine usually is given subcut. at a dose of 100 mg in the morning and afternoon of the first day of treatment and 100 mg daily for 7 days thereafter. In extreme cases, 200 mg of thiamine has been administered for 14 days before the animals completely recovered.

In acutely affected cattle, the mortality rate is usually above 90%. Treatment with DL-batyl alcohol (℞ 602, 603) and antibiotics has been used with equivocal results. The herd should be removed from bracken-contaminated pasture. A feed high in protein and energy is indicated. If animals are anemic, blood transfusions (2 to 4 L) from a donor not grazing bracken may help prevent the development of acute signs. Injections of antibiotics will assist in combating secondary infection resulting from the leukopenia.

POISONOUS PLANTS OF TEMPERATE

Dangerous Season	Scientific Name	Common Name	Habitat and Distribution	Affected Animals
SPRING	*Hymenoxys* spp.	Bitterweed, Rubberweed, Pingue	Roadways, lakebeds, flooded areas, overgrazed range; western.	Sheep, also cattle
	Nolina texana	Sacahuista, Beargrass	Open areas on rolling hills and slopes; southwest.	Sheep, cattle and goats
	Cicuta spp.	Water hemlock	Open, moist to wet situations.	All
	Delphinium	Larkspurs	Either cultivated or wild. Usually in open foothills or meadows; mostly western.	All grazing animals, mostly cattle
	Phytolacca americana	Pokeweed, Poke	Recent clearings, pastures, waste areas; eastern.	Cattle, swine
(and occasionally fall)	*Xanthium* spp.	Cocklebur	Fields, waste places, exposed shores of ponds or rivers.	All animals, more common in swine
	Peganum harmala	African rue	Arid to semi-arid ranges; southwest.	Cattle and sheep
	Sarcobatus vermiculatus	Greasewood	Alkaline or saline bottom soils, not in higher mountains; western.	Sheep
	Veratrum spp.	False hellebore	Low, moist woods and pastures, and high mountain valleys.	Cattle, sheep and fowl
	Tetradymia spp.	Horsebrush	Arid foothills and higher desert and sagebrush ranges; western.	Sheep
	Zygadenus spp.	Death camas	Foothill grazing lands, occasionally boggy grasslands, low open woods.	Sheep, cattle and horses

NORTH AMERICA

Important Characteristics	Toxic Principle and Effects	Remarks and Treatment
Much-branched annual or perennial up to 2 ft high. Yellow flower head. Leaves divided into narrow glandular segments.	Depression, loss of appetite, abdominal pain, green nasal discharge, salivation, prostration.	Fresh or dry. Remove from pasture. Avoid overgrazing.
Perennial with many clustered, long, narrowed leaves. Several flower stems with many small white flowers in clusters.	Toxin in buds, flowers and fruit. Photosensitization. Anorexia, icterus, prostration.	Remove animals from range during blooming season. (*See* PHOTOSENSITIZATION, p. 6.)
White flower, umbels. Veins of leaflets ending at notches. Stems hollow except at nodes. Tuberous roots from chambered rootstock.	A higher alcohol—excessive salivation, violent convulsions, dilation of pupils, diaphragm contractions, pain.	Death usually rapid. Use sedatives to control spasm and heart action. Intestinal evacuation followed by astringents may help.
Annual or perennial herbs. Flowers each with one spur, in racemes. Perennial with tuberous roots. Leaves palmately lobed or divided.	Alkaloid delphinine and others —straddled stance, repeated falling, nausea, rapid pulse and respiration, constipation, bloating.	Use ℞ 486.
Tall, glabrous, green, red-purplish perennial herbs. Berries black-purple, staining, in drooping racemes.	More than one—vomiting, spasms, respiratory paralysis, ulcerative gastritis.	Roots most poisonous. 10 ml nikethamide (cattle).
Coarse annual herb. Fruit one solid mass, 2 beaked, with 2 cavities, armed with hooked spines.	Hydroquinone—anorexia, depression, incoordination, twitching, paralysis, inflammation of mucous membranes.	Only cotyledons poisonous. Eaten after emerging from seed. Milk, vegetable oil and fats may be beneficial.
Much-branched, leafy, perennial, bright green, succulent herb; leaves divided; flowers white.	Alkaloids—weakness of hind limbs. listlessness, subserous edema and hemorrhage of small intestine.	Unpalatable. Eaten only under drought conditions.
Large shrub with spiny stems; fleshy, alternate cross-section. Flowers inconspicuous.	Oxalates—kidney lesions, weakness, depression, prostration, coma.	Poisoning occurs only on steady diet of greasewood leaves. Provide other forage.
Erect herbs; leafy throughout, leaves large and plaited. Flowers small and white or greenish.	Steroid alkaloids—salivation, prostration, depressed heart action, dyspnea; "Monkeyface" in lambs.	Remove animals from range. Provide other forage.
Shrubs with yellow flowers in spring, not later. Leaves spiny, silvery white, early deciduous.	Resinous substances—weakness, "bighead" photosensitization; liver injury, death.	Cumulative. Remove animals from range and light. Antihistaminics. (*See* PHOTOSENSITIZATION, p. 6.)
Perennial bulbous herbs with basal flat grass-like leaves; flowers greenish, yellow or pink, in racemes or panicles. No onion odor.	Steroid alkaloids of the veratrum group—salivation, vomiting, staggering or prostration, coma and death.	Hay with dried camas is poisonous. 2 to 3 subcut. injections of 2 mg atropine sulfate and 8 mg picrotoxin in 5 ml of water per 100 lb body wt.

POISONOUS PLANTS OF TEMPERATE

Dangerous Season	Scientific Name	Common Name	Habitat and Distribution	Affected Animals
SPRING and SUMMER	Aesculus spp.	Buckeyes	Woods and thickets; Eastern U.S.A. and California.	All grazing animals
	Amianthium muscaetoxicum	Fly-poison, Staggergrass	Open woods, fields, and acid bogs; eastern.	All grazing animals
	Lantana spp.	Lantana	Ornamentals and wild in lower coastal plain of southeast, and southern California.	All grazing animals
	Quercus spp.	Oaks	In most deciduous woods.	All grazing animals
SUMMER and FALL	Prosopis juliflora	Mesquite	Dry ranges, washes, draws; southwest.	Cattle
	Centaurea solstitialis	Yellow star thistle	Waste areas, roadsides, pastures; mostly western.	Horses
	Oxytenia acerosa	Copperweed	Arid, alkaline soils in foothills, and sagebrush plains; western.	Cattle, also sheep
	Eupatorium rugosum	White snakeroot	Woods, cleared areas, waste places, usually the more moist and richer soils; eastern.	Cattle and sheep
	Solanum spp.	Nightshades, Jerusalem cherry, potato, Horsenettle	Fence rows, waste areas, grain and hay fields.	All
FALL or WINTER	Haplopappus heterophyllus	Rayless goldenrod	Dry plains, grasslands, open woodlands and along irrigation canals; western.	Cattle, sheep and horses

NORTH AMERICA

Important Characteristics	Toxic Principle and Effects	Remarks and Treatment
Trees or shrubs. Leaves opposite and palmately compound. Seeds large, glossy brown, with large white scar.	Glycoside, aesculin and possibly others—depression, incoordination, twitching, paralysis, inflammation of mucous membranes.	Young shoots and seeds especially poisonous. Use stimulants and purgatives.
Bulbous perennial herb. Leaves basal, linear white flowers in a compact raceme, the pedicels subtended by short brownish bracts.	Alkaloid, of the veratrum group—salivation, vomiting, rapid and irregular respiration, weakness, death by respiratory failure.	No practical treatment. Especially dangerous for animals new to pasture. Keep animals well fed.
Shrubs. Young stems 4-angled. Leaves opposite. Flowers in flat-topped clusters. Berries black.	Lantadene A, a polycyclic triterpenoid—erythema, pruritus, edematous suffusions and usually sloughing of skin, gastroenteritis, bloody watery feces.	Remove plants from pasture. Keep animals out of light sources after eating plant.
Mostly deciduous trees, rarely shrubs, with 2 to 4 leaves clustered at tips of all twigs.	Tannic acid—anorexia, constipation, dry muzzle, black pelleted feces followed by diarrhea with blood and mucus, frequent urination, thin rapid pulse.	Remove animals from oak source. Treat symptomatically.
Deciduous shrub or small tree with smooth or furrowed gray bark, paired spines; leaves divided. Legume pod long, constricted between seeds.	Malnutrition, excessive salivation, stasis of rumen; sublingual or submaxillary edema, loss of weight.	Believed that high-sucrose content of beans alters bacterial flora to extent that cellulose cannot be digested and B-vitamins synthesized.
Annual weed. Leaves densely covered with cottony hair. Terminal spreading cluster of bright yellow flowers with spines below. Branches winged.	Involuntary chewing movements, twitching of lips, flicking of tongue. Mouth commonly held open. Unable to eat. Eventual death from starvation or thirst.	Force food far back into mouth.
Tall, perennial herb with leaflets; flowers in many heads resembling goldenrod.	Stupor, loss of appetite, coma, death without struggling.	Supplement diet.
Perennial herb; leaves 3-nerved, taper-pointed, opposite; flowers small, white, many.	An alcohol, tremetol—trembling, depression, vomiting, labored respiration, death.	"Milk sickness." "Trembles." Cathartics and stimulants may help.
Fruits small, when ripe yellow, red, or black; structurally like tomatoes; clustered on stalk arising from stem between leaves.	Glycoalkaloids—weakness, trembling, dyspnea, nausea, constipation or diarrhea, death.	Leaves, shoots and berries may be poisonous. In cattle repeated doses of 2 to 3 mg carbachol or of injection of 15 mg strychnine may be useful.
Bushy perennial 2 to 4 ft tall, with many yellow flower heads. Leaves alternate, sticky.	An alcohol, tremetol—trembling, depression, vomiting, labored respiration, coma, death.	"Milk sickness." Keep animals away by fencing.

POISONOUS PLANTS OF TEMPERATE

Dangerous Season	Scientific Name	Common Name	Habitat and Distribution	Affected Animals
	Halogeton glomeratus	Halogeton	Deserts, overgrazed areas, winter ranges, alkaline soils; western.	Sheep, also cattle
	Sophora secundiflora	Mescal bean	Hills and canyons, limestone soils; southwestern Texas into Mexico.	Cattle, also sheep and goats
	Notholaena sinuata var. *cochisensis*	Jimmy fern, Cloak fern	Dry rocky slopes and crevices, chiefly limestone areas; southwest.	Sheep, goats and cattle
	Glottidium vesicarium, *Sesbania* spp.	Bladder pod, Rattlebox, Sesbane, Coffeebean	Mostly open low ground, abandoned cultivated fields; southeast.	All
	Daubentonia punicea	Rattlebox, Purple sesbane	Cultivated and escaped in waste places; southeastern coastal plain.	All
FALL, WINTER and SPRING	*Melia azedarach*	Chinaberry	Fence rows, brush, waste places; southeast.	Swine, cattle
ALL SEASONS	*Baccharis* spp.	Silverling, Baccharis, Yerba-de-pasmo	Open areas, often moist; eastern and southwestern.	All grazing cattle
	Pteridium aquilinum	Bracken fern	Dry poor soil, open woods, sandy ridges.	All grazing animals
	Prunus spp.	Chokecherries, Wild cherries, Peaches	Waste areas, fence rows, woods, orchards, prairies, dry slopes.	All grazing animals
	Acacia berlandieri	Guajillo	Semiarid range lands; southwestern Texas into Mexico.	Sheep, also goats

NORTH AMERICA (Continued)

Important Characteristics	Toxic Principle and Effects	Remarks and Treatment
Annual herb. Leaves fleshy, round in cross-section, tip with stiff hair. Axillary flowers inconspicuous. Fruits bracted and conspicuous.	Oxalates—dyspnea followed by rapid death.	Alfalfa hay or dicalcium phosphate, fed free-choice when added to 3 parts salt, is effective preventive in sheep. Avoid dense growths of weeds.
Evergreen shrub or small tree. Leaves alternate, divided and leathery; flowers violet-blue, fragrant; seeds large and bright red with hard seed coat, in legume pod.	Alkaloid sophorine—trembling, stiff gait, falling after exercise; recumbent for few minutes, then arise alert and fall again if exercised.	Not cumulative. Provide supplemental feed.
Evergreen, perennial, erect fern with divided leaves, folding when dry.	After exercise by walking, will have arched back, stilted movement of hind legs, and usually increased respiration. Continued walking induced violent trembling and death if not allowed to rest.	Avoid driving during danger period. Provide ample watering, placed to avoid long walks.
Tall annual. Legume pods flat, tapered at both ends, 2-seeded. Leaves pinnate-divided. Flowers yellow.	Saponins—intense inflammation of gastrointestinal tract, yellowish diarrhea, frequent urination, shallow and accelerated respiration, death.	Seeds poisonous. Remove plants from pasture. Keep animals off pasture after seed pods form.
Shrub. Flowers orange. Legume pods longitudinally four-winged.	A saponin—rapid pulse, weak respiration, diarrhea, death.	Seeds poisonous. Keep seeds from animals. Use saline purgative followed by stimulants and soft food.
Tree. Leaves 2 to 3 pinnate; fruit cream or yellow with a furrowed globose stone, persisting on tree through winter.	Nausea, constipation, excitement or depression, often weakened heart action and death.	Fruit most poisonous. Use stimulants and cathartics followed by easily digestible diet.
Shrubs; numerous small, whitish flowers; leaves resin-dotted, and persistent southward.	Glucosidal saponin having digitaloidal properties—paralysis and death soon after ingestion. Depression and weakness in chronic cases.	Most dangerous during new growth in spring or root sprouts in fall.
Leaves firm, leathery, thrice pinnate.	(See BRACKEN FERN POISONING, p. 977.)	
Large shrubs or trees. Flowers white or pink. Cherries or peach. Crushed twigs with strong odor.	Prussic acid—slobbering, increased respiration rate, dyspnea, rapid weak pulse, convulsions, rapid death.	(See CYANIDE POISONING, p. 938.)
Deciduous shrub or small tree; leaf divided; flowers white to yellowish in dense heads; fruit a legume with margins thickened.	Amine, N-methyl beta phenylethylamine—after eating for 6 to 9 months, may have locomotor ataxia called "limber leg." Mortality as high as 50% in extreme drought.	Dominates vegetation in some areas. Valuable to sheep industry due to high nutritive value and dominance. Supplemental feeding.

POISONOUS PLANTS OF TEMPERATE

Dangerous Season	Scientific Name	Common Name	Habitat and Distribution	Affected Animals
(especially spring)	*Agave lecheguilla*	Lechuguilla	Low limestone hills, dry valleys and canyons; southwest.	Sheep and goats, rarely cattle
	Asclepias spp.	Milkweeds	Dry areas, usually waste places, roadsides, streambeds.	All
(especially spring)	*Astragalus* spp. *Oxytropis* spp.	Locoweeds, Poison vetch	Nearly all habitats; mostly western.	All
(especially spring)	*Stanleya pinnata*	Prince's plume	Foothills or deserts; western.	All
	Drymaria pachyphylla	Inkweed, Drymary	Heavy alkaline clay soil in low areas or dry overgrazed pastures; southwest.	Cattle, sheep; also goats
	Gutierrezia microcephala	Broomweed, Snakeweed, Slinkweed, Turpentine weed	Widespread over dry range and desert; overgrazed lands; western.	Cattle, sheep, goats and swine
	Psilostrophe spp.	Paperflowers	Open range lands and pastures; southwest.	Sheep
	Senecio spp.	Groundsel, Senecio	Grassland areas; mostly western.	Cattle, horses and sheep
(especially dry season)	*Triglochin* spp.	Arrowgrass	Salt marshes, wet alkaline soils, lake shores.	Sheep and cattle
	Hypericum perforatum	St. Johnswort, Goatweed, Klamath weed	Dry soil, roadsides, pastures, ranges.	Sheep, cattle, horses and goats
	Agrostemma githago	Corn cockle	Weed, grain fields and waste areas.	All

NORTH AMERICA (Continued)

Important Characteristics	Toxic Principle and Effects	Remarks and Treatment
Perennial stemless, with thick fleshy tapered leaves having sharply serrated margins. Flowering infrequently with tall terminal panicle.	A photodynamic agent; also a saponin that is hepatonephrotoxic—photosensitization, generalized icterus, listlessness, progressive weakness, coma, death.	Remove animals from range and provide shade. (See PHOTOSENSITIZATION, p. 6.)
Perennial herbs with milky sap; seeds very silky-hairy from elongated pods.	Resinoid and others—loss of control, spasms, bloating, pulse rapid and weak, rapid breathing, coma, death.	Mainly due to drought or overgrazing.
Perennial stemmed or stemless herbs. Leaves with many small leaflets. Flowers like garden peas, in racemes.	Selenium or "locoine" in different species. Weakness, trembling, ataxia, or paralysis.	Cumulative. (See SELENIUM POISONING, p. 947 as one type.)
Perennial herb, woody at base and coarse; leaves divided; flowers yellow in showy spike.	May not be eaten but does accumulate selenium.	(See SELENIUM POISONING, p. 947.)
Much-branched, succulent, prostrate annual with opposite leaves and small white flowers.	Diarrhea, lack of appetite, arched back, coma, death.	Occurs after rain. Avoid overstocking to improve range.
Much-branched, perennial, resinous shrub, with many yellow-flowered heads.	Saponin. Loss of appetite, listlessness, hematuria in severe cases. Abortion with retained placenta in cattle.	Supplement diet.
Perennial composite with erect, woolly stems branching from base. Many small heads of yellow flowers.	Sluggishness, stumbling, coughing, vomiting, depression, death.	About 2 weeks of grazing before signs appear. Pasture rotation, or placing animals on other feed.
Perennial or annual herbs; heads of yellow flowers with whorl of bracts below.	Alkaloids—aimless walking, slight staggering, staring expression, and running into fences or other objects. Hepatic cirrhosis, edema of visceral peritoneum and distension of gallbladder.	Cumulative, fresh or dry. Supplemental feeding. Treat symptoms. (See SENECIO POISONING, p. 1003.)
Grass-like, except leaves are thick; heads of fruits globular on erect raceme. Flowers inconspicuous.	Prussic acid in leaves—abnormal breathing, trembling, and jerking, convulsions. Rapid poisoning.	(See CYANIDE POISONING, p. 938.)
Perennial herb or woody below; leaves opposite, dotted; flowers many, yellow, with many stamens.	Primary photosensitizer; skin lesions in white skin, itching, blindness, convulsions, death.	Fresh or dry. Remove animals from infested areas. (See PHOTOSENSITIZATION, p. 6.)
Green winter annual with silky white hairs, opposite leaves, purple flowers, black seeds.	Sapogenin, githagenin—irritation of mucosa, vomiting, vertigo, diarrhea.	Toxin in seeds. Avoid grain screenings containing seed. Give oils, demulcents, cardiac stimulants.

POISONOUS PLANTS OF TEMPERATE

Dangerous Season	Scientific Name	Common Name	Habitat and Distribution	Affected Animals
	Helenium hoopesii	Sneezeweed	Moist slopes and well-drained mountain meadows; western.	Sheep, also cattle
	Lupinus spp.	Lupines, Bluebonnet	Dry to moist soils, roadsides, fields, and mountains; mostly western.	Sheep, also cattle, goats, horses and swine
	Conium maculatum	Poison hemlock	Roadside ditches, damp waste areas, especially northward.	All
	Crotalaria spp.	Crotalaria, Rattlebox	Fields and roadsides; Eastern and Central States.	All
	Datura stramonium	Jimsonweed	Fields, barn lots, trampled pastures, and waste places on rich bottom soils.	All
	Gelsemium sempervirens	Yellow jessamine	Open woods, thickets; eastern.	All
(especially winter and spring)	*Kalmia* spp.	Laurel, Ivybush, Lambkill	Rich moist woods, meadows; or acid bogs; eastern and northwestern.	All, often sheep
	Nerium oleander	Oleander	Common ornamental in southern regions.	All
(especially winter and spring)	*Prunus caroliniana*	Laurel cherry, Cherrylaurel	Woods, fence rows and often escaped from cultivation; southern regions.	All grazing animals
	Ricinus communis	Castor bean	Cultivated in southern regions.	All
	Sorghum vulgare	Sorghum, Sudan grass, Kafir, Durra, Milo, Broomcorn, Schrock, etc.		

NORTH AMERICA (*Continued*)

Important Characteristics	Toxic Principle and Effects	Remarks and Treatment
Perennial herb with orange sunflower-like heads or yellow flowers. Leaves alternate.	Glycoside dugaldin—salivation, "spewing sickness," vomiting, weakness.	Cumulative. Cathartics may help. Avoid dense areas of weed.
Perennials; leaves simple or palmately divided; flowers in terminal raceme.	Alkaloids D-lupanine, sparteine and others, nervousness, convulsions or coma.	Fresh or dry. Eating of pods with seeds frequent cause of poisoning. Not cumulative. (*See* MYCOTOXIC LUPINOSIS, p. 998.)
Purple-spotted hollow stem; leaves resemble parsley, parsnip odor when crushed; tap root; flowers white, in umbels.	Alkaloid coniine and others —loss of appetite, salivation, bloating, feeble pulse, paralysis.	Vegetative parts, later the seeds most poisonous. Give stimulants.
Annual legume with yellow flowers in racemes; pods inflated; bracts at base of pedicels of flowers and fruits persistent; leaves simple or divided.	Alkaloid monocrotaline—diarrhea, abnormally light or dark comb in fowl. Diarrhea, stupor alternating with apparent improvement, walking in circles in horse and mule. Bloody feces, anorexia, weakness in others. In all death.	Cumulative. All parts, especially seeds, poisonous. Seeds often found in combined corn. No treatment known. Keep plant from fields and hay.
Leaves wavy; flower large (4 in.) white, tubular; fruit a spiny pod, 2 in. long.	Alkaloids atropine, hyoscyamine and hyoscine—nausea, vertigo, thirst, dilated pupils convulsions, death.	Rapid death. KI or tannic acid per os; cardiac and respiratory stimulants.
Climbing or trailing vines with evergreen, entire, opposite leaves; yellow tubular flowers, very fragrant.	Alkaloids gelsemine and gelseminine—weakness, convulsions rigid extremities, lowered respiration and temperature, death; "limp-neck" in fowl.	Use relaxing agents, sedatives; repeat as required.
Woody shrub with evergreen glossy leaves; flowers pink to rose, showy.	Andromedotoxin—salivation, nasal discharge, emesis paralysis, coma, death.	Laxatives, demulcents nerve stimulants.
Evergreen shrub. Leaves whorled and prominently finely pinnately veined beneath. Flowers showy, white to deep pink.	Cardiac glucosides—nausea, depression, increased pulse rate, mydriasis, bloody diarrhea. Later weak and irregular heart beat, death.	Fresh, clipped or dried leaves most dangerous.
Leaves evergreen, shiny, leathery. Broken twigs with strong cherry bark odor.	Prussic acid—slobbering, increased respiration rate, dyspnea, rapid weak pulse, convulsions, rapid death.	Wilted parts most poisonous. (*See* CYANIDE POISONING, p. 938.)
Large palmately lobed leaves; seeds resembling engorged ticks, usually 3 in somewhat spiny pod.	Ricin, irritant blood poison—nausea, vomiting, diarrhea, thirst, cessation of rumination, death.	Seeds and "press-cakes" most dangerous. Gastric lavage, warmth, sedation.
Coarse grasses with terminal flower cluster. Some to 8 ft tall.	Prussic acid—slobbering, increased respiration rate, dyspnea, rapid weak pulse, convulsions, rapid death.	Dark green, short (2 ft) second growth or stunted by dry weather most dangerous. (*See* CYANIDE POISONING, p. 938.)

POISONOUS PLANTS OF TEMPERATE

Dangerous Season	Scientific Name	Common Name	Habitat and Distribution	Affected Animals
	Sorghum halepense	Johnson grass	Weed of open fields and waste places in south; scattered north to New York and Iowa.	All grazing animals
ALL SEASONS (especially winter)	*Pinus ponderosa*	Western yellow pine	Coniferous forests of Rocky Mountains at moderate elevations; western.	Cattle

SWEET CLOVER POISONING

An insidious hemorrhagic disease occurring in animals that consume toxic quantities of spoiled sweet clover hay or silage.

Etiology: During the process of spoiling, the harmless natural coumarins in sweet clover are converted to dicoumarol (bishydroxycoumarin). When toxic hay or silage is consumed by animals, hypoprothrombinemia results, presumably because dicoumarol combines with the proenzyme to prevent formation of the active enzyme required for the synthesis of prothrombin. It probably also interferes with synthesis of Factor VII, and other coagulation factors (*see* HEMOPHILIA AND OTHER HEMOSTATIC DISORDERS IN DOMESTIC ANIMALS, p. 29). The toxic agent passes through the placenta in pregnant animals. All species of animals studied have been shown to be susceptible, but instances of poisoning have involved mainly cattle and, to a very limited extent, sheep, swine and horses.

Clinical Findings: All clinical signs are referable to the hemorrhages which result from faulty blood coagulation. The time of appearance of clinical disease after consumption of toxic sweet clover varies greatly and depends to a large extent on the dicoumarol content of the particular specimen of sweet clover fed and the age of the animals. If the dicoumarol content of the ration is low or variable, animals may consume it for months before signs of disease appear.

Initial signs of disease may be stiffness and lameness, due to bleeding into the muscles and articulations. Hematomas, epistaxis or gastrointestinal bleeding may be observed. Death sometimes occurs suddenly with little preliminary evidence of disease and is caused by spontaneous massive hemorrhage or bleeding after injury, surgery or parturition. Absorptions,

NORTH AMERICA (Continued)

Important Characteristics	Toxic Principle and Effects	Remarks and Treatment
Coarse grass with large rhizomes and white midvein on leaf. Topped by large, open panicle.	Prussic acid—slobbering, dyspnea, increased respiration rate, rapid weak pulse, convulsions, rapid death.	Dark green second growth or stunted by dry weather most dangerous. (See CYANIDE POISONING, p. 938.)
Tree, 150 to 180 ft; leaves in groups of 3, yellowish green, 7 to 11 in. long; barky platy, reddish orange.	Toxin in leaves; browsing cattle predisposed to abortion.	Remove from western yellow pine stands in later stages of gestation.

stillbirths and neonatal deaths may occur, rarely without signs in the dams.

Lesions: Hemorrhage is the characteristic necropsy finding. It may occur anywhere in the body, but the subcut. and IM tissues are common sites.

Diagnosis: This requires a history of continuous consumption of sweet clover hay or silage over relatively long periods, compatible signs and lesions, and markedly prolonged blood clotting time or demonstration of reduced prothrombin content of the plasma. Most other diseases with hemorrhagic manifestations, such as blackleg, pasteurellosis, bracken fern poisoning and aplastic anemia, can be readily differentiated on the basis of clinical, pathologic and hematologic findings.

Prophylaxis: Cultivars of sweet clover that are low in coumarin content, and hence safe to feed, have been developed. If one of these is not available, the only certain way to prevent the disease is to avoid feeding sweet clover hay or silage. Although well-cured sweet clover in good condition is not dangerous, the absence of visible spoilage is insufficient evidence of safety. There is no chemical test for dicoumarol that can be quickly performed. Suspected feed may be fed to rabbits; a shorter feeding period is required to produce fatal hemorrhage, and determination, at intervals, of prothrombin time in the rabbits further reduces the test period.

Treatment: The objectives are to prevent further hemorrhage, and to correct the anemia. Immediate correction of the hypoprothrombinemia as well as the anemia can be accomplished to a degree by the IV administration of 2 to 4 liters of whole blood per 1,000 lb body wt (from an animal that has not been fed sweet clover). This procedure should be employed in all animals with marked signs, and repeated if necessary. In addition, parenteral administration of synthetic vitamin K (menadione—℞ 549), repeated if necessary, will permit increased prothrombin production. All severely affected animals should receive this drug until their blood clotting time returns to normal. Either the administration of synthetic vitamin K or a blood transfusion is sufficient to correct mild cases of intoxication if feeding of the incriminated diet is stopped.

MYCOTOXICOSES
(Fungal or Mold toxicoses)

Acute or chronic intoxications due to the ingestion of feed contaminated with toxins produced during growth of various saprophytic or phytopathogenic fungi or molds. The toxins may be produced on hay, cereals, pastures or fodder, or may be present in constituents used in the manufacture of meals or pelleted animal diets. Some animal diets, especially those containing grains or nuts, may contain several toxigenic species of molds which may produce a number of mycotoxins having different toxic or pharmacologic properties. Under these circumstances clinical effects and lesions found in disease outbreaks may not conform to the usual descriptions of outbreaks or to experimental findings in animals dosed with mycotoxins isolated from pure mold cultures.

Treatment of mycotoxicoses is ineffective but some animals recover if the source of toxin is removed; others are stunted or die. Since toxigenic molds are ubiquitous the aim should be to prevent damage to, and mold spoilage of, cereals, groundnuts and fodder by correct harvesting and proper storage. High relative humidity is a growth requirement for all molds but temperature requirements vary considerably.

Mycotoxic diseases which occur throughout the world are summarized in the table on pages 994 to 997.

AFLATOXICOSIS

This disease, recognized in many parts of the world, is caused by toxigenic strains of *Aspergillus flavus*. Aflatoxins are produced on groundnuts, soy beans, corn and other cereals in the field or during storage as seeds, processed meals and cakes when moisture content and temperatures are sufficiently high for mold growth.

Aflatoxins likely have been partly responsible for other previously recognized mycotoxic diseases such as Moldy Corn Toxicosis, Poultry Hemorrhagic Syndrome and "Aspergillus Toxicosis".

Epizootiology: The disease affects growing poultry, especially ducklings and turkey poults. Young swine, pregnant sows, calves and dogs are highly susceptible. Adult cattle, sheep and goats are also susceptible when fed toxic diets over longer periods. The toxin is excreted in the milk. Experimentally, all species of animals tested have shown some degree of susceptibility to aflatoxins. Their potent carcinogenic effects upon the liver have been demonstrated in several species.

Clinical Findings: In all animals the first signs in an outbreak are inappetence, reduced growth rate or loss of condition. Other signs are rarely seen until about 7 to 14 days before death. Icterus, apathy and hemorrhagic enteritis may be evident.

Lesions: In all species, in acute cases, the liver shows severe fatty degeneration, is friable and may show small hemorrhages under the capsule. Icterus is often present. The kidneys are enlarged and may also show small hemorrhages. In chronic cases the liver is mottled and firm due to cirrhosis. In cattle, swine, sheep and dogs, a hemorrhagic enteritis with ulceration may also be present.

Diagnosis: The history of the outbreak, the necropsy findings and the histologic examination of liver tissue should establish the diagnosis. Aflatoxicosis may be confused with phosphorus poisoning (q.v., p. 960) in dogs, and with *Senecio* poisoning (q.v., p. 1003) and mycotoxic lupinosis (q.v., p. 998) in cattle and sheep.

If available, samples of the feed should be forwarded for laboratory examination. Testing for toxicity of extracts by dosing ducklings will also give positive evidence within 7 days.

MOLDY CORN TOXICOSIS

A hemorrhagic disease observed in swine, cattle and dogs that have consumed diets containing moldy field corn (maize). The exact cause has not been determined but *Aspergillus flavus* and *Penicillium rubrum,* isolated from toxic moldy corn, have been shown to produce lesions and signs in mice, swine and cattle similar to the toxicosis observed in field cases. Depending on the individual outbreak other fungi may also be involved. This toxicosis has been observed in late summer and fall in the Southeastern U.S.A. Mortality ranged from 5 to 55% in affected herds.

Gross icterus and tissue hemorrhages are the most constant findings at necropsy. In acute cases, massive hemorrhages are observed in most tissues. In chronic cases extensive icterus and

FUNGI & MOLDS TOXIC TO DOMESTIC ANIMALS

Disease	Fungi or Molds	Toxins (where known)	Countries where reported	Contaminated Toxic Foodstuff	Animals Affected	Signs and Lesions
Aflatoxicosis	*Aspergillus flavus*, possibly other aspergilli & some penicillia	Aflatoxins	widespread	Moldy peanuts, Soybean, Cottonseed, Rice	All poultry, Swine, Cattle, Sheep, Dogs	(*See* AFLATOXICOSIS, p. 992 and POULTRY MYCOTOXI- COSIS, p. 1065.)
"Aspergillus toxicosis"	*A. chevalieri* *A. clavatus* *A. fumigatus* *A. flavus*					This name was used before the discovery of aflatoxin. (*See* AFLATOXICOSIS, p. 992, POULTRY HEMORRHAGIC SYNDROME, p. 1085, and MOLDY CORN TOXICOSIS, p. 993.)
Dendrodochio- toxicosis	*Dendrodochium toxicum*	Dendrodochins I and II	U.S.S.R.	Moldy straw	Horses	Affects central nervous and cardiovascular systems— rapid death.
Diplodiosis	*Diplodia zeae*	Unknown	Southern Africa	Moldy corn	Cattle	CNS hypersensitivity fol- lowed by paresis. Recovery usual on removal from source.
Ergot	*Claviceps purpurea*	Ergot alkaloids	widespread	Seedheads of many grasses	Cattle, Horses	(*See* ERGOTISM, p. 1001.)
	C. paspali	Ergot alkaloids	widespread	Seedheads of paspalum grasses	Cattle, Horses, Sheep	(*See* PASPALUM STAGGERS, p. 1000.)
Facial eczema (Pithomyco- toxicosis)	*Pithomyces chartarum*	Sporidesmins	New Zealand, Australia, South Africa, probably U.S.A.	Toxic spores on pasture	Sheep, Cattle	(*See* FACIAL ECZEMA, p. 9.)

Fusariotoxicosis	Fusarium tricinctum, F. culmorum, F. equiseti, F. scirpi & other fusaria	Diacetoxyscirpenol & other epoxides	U.S.A., U.S.S.R., Australia	Overwintered cereal crops, Growing maize, Tall fescue grass	Cattle	Loss of appetite and milk production, diarrhea and staggers; recovery upon removal from crops. (Possibly also associated with FESCUE LAMENESS, p. 999.)
Leucoencephalomalacia	Fusarium moniliforme	Not known	Egypt, U.S.A.	Moldy corn	Horses	Dependent on degree and specific site of brain lesion.
Mold Nephrosis	Penicillium viridicatum	Not known	Denmark	Moldy barley	Swine	Subcut. edema of perineum, perirenal edema, renal hemorrhages, proteinurea, occasionally posterior paresis.
Moldy corn toxicosis	Probably Penicillium rubrum Aspergillus flavus and other fungi.	Probably Rubratoxins A & B, Aflatoxins and other mycotoxins	U.S.A.	Moldy corn, Peanuts	Horses, Swine, Cattle, Poultry, Dogs	(See MOLDY CORN TOXICOSIS, p. 993 and AFLATOXICOSIS, p. 992.)
Mushroom Poisoning	(a) Amanita verna, (b) A. muscaria	(a) Amanitins (b) Muscarine	U.S.A	Eaten from pastures	Cattle	(a) Severe inflammation of intestinal tract. In severe cases, convulsions and death. (b) Parasympathomimetic stimulation.
Mycotoxic Lupinosis (as distinct from lupine alkaloid poisoning)	Phomopsis leptostromiformis	Not known	widespread	Moldy seed, pods, stubble and haulm of several Lupinus spp. affected by Phomopsis stem blight.	Sheep, occasionally cattle and horses	Lassitude, inappetence, stupor, icterus, marked liver injury—usually fatal termination.

continued on next page

FUNGI & MOLDS TOXIC TO DOMESTIC ANIMALS (Continued)

Disease	Fungi or Molds	Toxins (where known)	Countries where reported	Contaminated Toxic Foodstuff	Animals Affected	Signs and Lesions
Myrothecio-toxicosis	*Myrothecium verrucaria* *M. roridum*	Verrucarins Roridins	U.S.S.R.	Moldy rye stubble	Sheep, Cattle	Acute: diarrhea, respiratory distress, hemorrhagic gastro-enterocolitis, death. Chronic: ulcerations of intestinal tract, unthriftiness, gradual recovery.
Poultry hemorrhagic syndrome	Probably *Aspergillus flavus* *A. clavatus* *Penicillium purpurogenum* *Alternaria* sp.	Probably aflatoxins and others	U.S.A.	Toxic grain and meal	Growing chickens	Depression, anorexia, no gain in weight, death. Widespread internal hemorrhages, sometimes aplastic anemia. (*See* HEMORRHAGIC SYNDROME, p. 1085.)
Slobbers	*Rhizoctonia leguminicola*	Alkaloid Slaframine	U.S.A.	Blackpatch-diseased legumes (notably red clover) eaten as forage or hay	Sheep, Cattle	Salivation, bloat, diarrhea, sometimes death—recovery usual when removed from clover.
Stachybotryo-toxicosis	*Stachybotrys atra*	Unknown	U.S.S.R.	Toxic pastures or roughage, other contaminated feed	Horses, Cattle, Sheep, Swine	Stomatitis and ulceration, anorexia, leukopenia. (Horses may also show incoordination and blindness.) Extensive hemorrhages in many organs, inflammation and necrosis in the gut.
Vomiting syndrome in swine	*Fusarium roseum* (= *F. graminearum*) Sexual stage: *Gibberella zeae* other fusaria	Unknown emetic principle	U.S.A., U.S.S.R., Korea	Scabbed barley	Swine, Dogs	Vomiting and diarrhea. Recovery when diet is changed.

Vulvovaginitis of swine	Fusarium roseum (= F. graminearum) Sexual stage: Gibberella zeae	Zearalenone (estrogen)	U.S.A.	Moldy corn and pelleted feeds	Swine	Swollen vulva, prolapse of vagina, hypertrophy of mammary glands. Recovery when diet is changed.

cachexia are the predominant gross findings. Acute signs occur within 8 to 12 hours after the ingestion of toxic corn or may extend over a period of 1 to 3 days. They may include depression, incoordination, anorexia and icterus. Chronically affected animals show general depression, anorexia and cachexia.

As in aflatoxicosis, early diagnosis of moldy corn poisoning may be difficult. There is no treatment.

MYCOTOXIC LUPINOSIS

Lupines (*Lupinus* spp.) cause 2 distinct forms of poisoning in domestic animals, viz., lupine poisoning and lupinosis. The former is a nervous syndrome caused by alkaloids present in bitter lupines. Lupinosis is an icteric disease caused by a mycotoxin of as yet undetermined structure and has been reported from Europe, Australia, New Zealand and South Africa. Sheep, cattle and occasionally horses are affected when they graze infested lupine material especially after rain when saprophytic growth has occurred.

The causal fungus is *Phomopsis leptostromiformis,* a phytopathogen causing *Phomopsis* stem-blight especially in white and yellow lupines, blue varieties being very resistant. It produces sunken linear stem lesions containing black stromatic masses and also affects the pods and seeds. It is also a saprophyte and under favorable moisture and temperature conditions grows well on dead lupine material, e.g., haulm, pods and stubble. It can also be grown artificially on other substrates, e.g., corn.

The fungus produces a potent hepatotoxin and the syndrome may be confused with aflatoxicosis. In acute poisoning, lethargy, anorexia and ruminal stasis are the first signs encountered after a latent period of 2 to 3 days and this is followed by intense icterus and constipation. At necropsy the characteristic finding is a severe fatty degeneration of the liver. In more chronic cases varying degrees of cirrhosis are encountered and in sheep almost complete cirrhosis may be seen, producing a "boxing glove" liver the size of a man's fist.

The diagnosis is confirmed by histopathologic examination of liver tissue and by the identification of the causal fungus on lupine material. Mycotoxic lupinosis can be avoided by growing lupine varieties (e.g., blue lupines) which are resistant to *Phomopsis* blight.

VULVOVAGINITIS IN SWINE

Fusarium roseum (*graminearum*), the sexual stage of which is known as *Gibberella zeae,* produces 3 types of toxic metabolites: an emetic principle, a feed-refusal factor and zearalenone or F2 toxin. The latter is a potent estrogen which causes vulvovaginitis in swine, and the syndrome is produced when moldy corn infested with certain strains of this fungus, or even pelletted feed produced from such corn, is fed. *Fusarium* is almost exclusively a field fungus and the toxin is especially produced during fluctuating temperatures in spring and fall.

The condition cannot be distinguished from excessive estrogen administration and the signs encountered are especially evident in young gilts. Conspicuous tumefaction of the vulva (with occasional prolapse of the vagina and rectum) and enlargement of the mammary glands due to ductular proliferation are the most obvious signs. There is hypertrophy of the uterus and a decrease in size of the ovaries. Abortion and fetal resorption may be encountered and reproductive performance may be influenced. In young boars, arrest in the development of the genitalia may be seen.

The condition can usually be rectified by removing the contaminated feed.

FESCUE LAMENESS
(Fescue foot)

A condition, resembling ergot poisoning, caused by a toxic substance in tall fescue (*Festuca arundinacea*). It commences with lameness in one or both hind feet and may progress to necrosis of the distal part of the affected limb. The tail and ears also may be affected.

Etiology: The cause of fescue lameness is a toxic substance of tall fescue grass, which has actions similar to those produced by sclerotia of *Claviceps purpurea,* but which is not localized in the seed heads. Tall fescue is a coarse, aggressive and rank-growing grass which becomes dominant in moist pastures and on ditch banks or waste areas where pasture control is poor. This species is commonly referred to as reed, giant or ditch-bank fescue. In Australia, it is called Williams grass.

Reliable reports of occurrence of fescue lameness have come from Kentucky, Tennessee, Florida, California, Colorado and Missouri as well as from New Zealand, Australia and Italy. "Alta" and "Kentucky 31" strains of tall fescue may, under some conditions, cause lameness.

Ergot poisoning (q.v., p. 1001) probably is not the cause of fescue foot. Ergot toxicosis is seasonal in its occurrence, whereas fescue foot occurs at all seasons of the year in animals which graze on tall fescue grass. Typical fescue foot has been produced in cattle by feeding dried grass free of seed heads and ergot. Recent work indicates that the fungus *Fusarium tricinctum* produces a metabolite (toxin I) that produces the clinical signs of fescue lameness and it is probable this condition is a mycotoxicosis.

Clinical Findings: In cattle, the first signs develop within 10 to 14 days of grazing on tall fescue grass. There is local heat, swelling, severe pain and lameness of one or more feet. Usually, one hind foot is affected first. With continued feeding on fescue, an indented line appears at some point, usually between the hock and the claws. Dry gangrene affects the distal part, which eventually may be sloughed. Experimental feeding has caused dry gangrene of the tip of the tail. Low environmental temperature is thought to contribute to the lesions. At necropsy, there are no lesions other than those associated with the swelling or dry gangrene.

Horses are reported not to be affected. Sheep may or may not become lame, but lose condition. There may be interference with fetal development which reduces lambing percentage by 60 to 70%.

Control: Removal to other food will result in recovery if the lesions have not progressed to dry gangrene, and the animals are kept warm. Risk of fescue lameness is reduced by maintaining legumes in the sward since tall fescue has proved to be one of the least palatable of our cultivated or wild grasses and, therefore, will not be consumed in large amounts when other forage is available. Most reports indicate an increased incidence of fescue lameness as the age of the stand increases. This may be due to an increased fungal infestation. Severe droughts may be followed by an increased number of cases of fescue foot. Tall fescue tends to survive protracted droughts more sucessfully than other commonly grown forage plants.

PASPALUM STAGGERS

An incoordination of animals resulting from eating paspalum. The life history of this fungus is similar to that of *C. purpurea* (*see* ERGOTISM, p. 1001). The sclerotia, which mature in the seed heads in the autumn, are round, 2 to 4 mm in diameter annd yellow-gray in color. Ingestion of sclerotia causes nervous signs in cattle most commonly, but horses and sheep also are susceptible. Guinea pigs can be affected by experimental feeding.

The nature of the active principle is not yet known, but it is not the same as the alkaloids of *C. purpurea*. A sufficiently large single dose will cause signs which persist for several days. Animals display continuous trembling of the large muscle groups. If they attempt to move, their action is jerky and limb movements are incoordinated. If they attempt to run, they fall over in awkward attitudes. Condition is lost after prolonged exposure and complete paralysis can occur. The time of onset of signs depends on the degree of the infection of seed heads and the grazing habits of the animals. Experimentally, early signs appear in cattle after about 100 gm of sclerotia per day have been administered for more than 2 days. Young sclerotia may be more toxic than mature ones.

Recovery follows removal of the animals to feed not contaminated with sclerotia of *C. paspali*. Topping of the pasture to remove contaminated seed heads has been effective in controlling this condition.

ERGOTISM

A disease of cattle and other farm animals resulting from the continued ingestion of sclerotia of the parasitic fungus *Claviceps purpurea* that replaces the grain or seed of rye and other small grains or forage plants, such as the bromes, bluegrasses and ryegrasses. The sclerotia may contain varying quantities of ergot alkaloids of which the levorotatory alkaloids, ergotamine and ergonovine(ergometrine), are pharmacologically most important.

Etiology: Ergot causes vasoconstriction by direct action on the muscles of the arterioles, and repeated dosages injure the vascular endothelium. These actions result initially in reduced blood flow and eventually complete stasis with terminal necrosis of the extremities due to thrombosis. In addition, ergot has a potent oxytocic action and also causes stimulation of the CNS, followed by depression.

Clinical Findings: Cattle may be affected by eating ergotized hay or grain or occasionally by grazing seeded pastures that are infected with ergot. Lameness is the first sign and may appear 2 to 6 weeks or longer after commencement of feeding, the length of time depending on the concentration of alkaloids in the ergot and the quantity of ergot in the day's feed. Hind limbs are affected before forelimbs, but again the extent of involvement of a limb and the number of limbs affected depend on the amount of ergot eaten in each day's feed. A high body temperature and increased pulse and respiration rates accompany the lameness.

Associated with the lameness are swelling and tenderness of the fetlock joint and pastern. Within about a week, sensation is lost in the affected part, an indented line appears at the limit of normal tissue and dry gangrene affects the distal part. Eventually, one or both claws or any part of the limb up to the hock or knee may be sloughed. In a similar way, the tip of the tail or ears may become necrotic and be sloughed. Exposed skin areas, such as teats and udder, appear unusually pale or anemic.

Lesions: The only constant lesions at necropsy are in the skin and subcut. parts of the extremities. The skin is normal to the indented line, but in advanced cases is cyanosed and hardened beyond. Subcut. hemorrhage and some edema occur proximal to the necrotic area.

Sheep given the alkaloid experimentally had ulceration in the mouth and gastroenteritis; the legs were not affected. A convulsive syndrome in sheep has been associated with the ingestion of ergot.

A syndrome of agalactia in sows, characterized by complete absence of hypertrophy of mammary glands in the preparturient period and subsequent starvation of the piglets, has followed the ingestion of ergot-infested grain. Piglets from such sows are often weak at birth.

Control of ergotism consists of the immediate change to an ergot-free diet. Under pasture feeding conditions frequent grazing or topping of pastures prone to ergot infection during the summer months to allow few or no flowering heads to develop should control the disease. Grain with any sign of ergot infection should not be fed to pregnant or lactating sows even if the degree of infection is low (i.e., less than 0.6% infected grain).

RYEGRASS STAGGERS

A condition affecting sheep, cattle or horses during late summer and autumn, when the pasture is dry with some slow growth. Pastures in which perennial ryegrass (*Lolium perenne*) or perennial Italian crosses predominate are most commonly involved. The condition has not been reported when pastures are thoroughly dry, but it sometimes occurs following grazing of green ryegrass or hay-aftermath growth, 6 to 8 in. long.

The condition is characterized by tetanic muscle spasms following exercise.

Etiology: The cause is unknown, although sclerotia of *Claviceps purpurea* are frequently present in quantity on the ryegrass during outbreaks. It is suspected that alkaloids associated with the pasture may be responsible. This condition is neither associated with cobalt deficiency as in the case of "phalaris staggers", nor any vitamin or mineral deficiency. The serum calcium, magnesium, phosphate, glucose and ketone concentrations are normal in affected animals.

Clinical Findings: Signs occur following sudden or rigorous exercise and vary from slight spasm and stiffness of the limbs to complete tetany. In severe cases, animals remain prostrate and may starve.

Sheep and calves walk with their heads erect and in rigid extension. Locomotion occurs in stiff, bounding movements as the legs become rigidly extended. The animal falls in lateral recumbency with opisthotonos, nystagmus, stiffly extended limbs and fasciculation of muscle groups. The attack subsides within a short time, the animal sits with a dazed appearance and rejoins the flock when recovered. Signs recur if animals which have recently recovered from an attack are forced to run. Calves have more violent spasms than sheep. Adult cattle graze with legs spread and avoid rapid movements. Horses often walk with a reeling gait.

Improvement of pasture due to rainfall or removal of animals from ryegrass pasture results in complete recovery. Outbreaks have not persisted for more than a few weeks even when animals remained on ryegrass pasture.

Morbidity ranges from 5 to 75%. Mortality is low and death is usually accidental. No constant gross or microscopic lesions are found at necropsy. The muscle dystrophy observed in some cases has been regarded as secondary in origin.

Control: There is no known effective treatment. Affected animals should be fed other fodder and disturbed as little as possible.

SENECIO POISONING
(Pyrollizidine Alkaloidosis, Seneciosis, Ragwort, Ragweed Poisoning)

A chronic poisoning caused by many toxic plants found most commonly in the genera *Senecio*, *Crotalaria* and *Heliotropium* but also in *Amsinckia*, *Echium*, *Cynoglossum* and *Trichodesma*. These plants grow mainly in temperate climates, but some (e.g., *Crotalaria*) require tropical or subtropical climates. Overall, their distribution is worldwide and it is likely that their toxic effects are unique. The plants most commonly responsible for losses are ragwort (*S. jacobaea*), woolly groundsel (*S. riddelli*, syn. *S. longilobus*) and seeds of yellow tarweed (*A. intermedia*).

The toxic factors common to these plants are a number of pyrollizidine alkaloids which affect mainly the liver. Cattle, horses and swine are the species most susceptible to intoxication. Sheep are much less susceptible because the toxic alkaloids are largely degraded in the rumen before absorption. Individual susceptibility varies greatly within species and may be influenced by sex, age and diet. Young growing animals are most susceptible as the alkaloids have a marked antimitotic effect on liver cells.

Under normal conditions these plants are unpalatable and are avoided by grazing animals. During drought conditions the growing plants may be eaten. Animals are also poisoned by eating the plant material in hay or silage. Seeds from *Crotalaria* and *Amsinckia* which have been harvested with grain have been responsible for the disease in horses, cattle, swine and poultry.

Clinical Findings: The clinical signs and the pathologic effects are similar in all animal species affected regardless of the species of plant responsible or the toxic pyrollizidine alkaloids it contains. The acute form of the disease, characterized by sudden death from acute hemorrhagic liver necrosis and visceral hemorrhages, is rare. The effects upon the liver of repeated low intake of toxic plants are cumulative and progressive; clinical signs may not be seen for several weeks (often after consumption of the plant has ceased). In *Heliotropium* spp. poisoning severe losses are produced in sheep only after the plants have been grazed for a second season.

In horses and cattle some of the following signs are seen: loss of condition, anorexia, dullness, and constipation or diarrhea. Tenesmus and passing of bloodstained feces may be followed by rectal prolapse, especially in cattle. Ascites and icterus may be present and cattle sometimes show intermittent photosensitization. Some animals may become progressively weaker and rarely move while others wander aimlessly with an awkward gait, either stumbling against or actively pushing headlong into fences or other structures. Still others may become frenzied and dangerously aggressive. Pica may be observed in some individuals. Death may occur suddenly or following prolonged recumbency with hepatic coma and high blood ammonia levels.

Lesions: In acute cases the liver may be enlarged, hemorrhagic and icteric. In chronic cases the liver is atrophied, fibrous, misshapen, and usually pale with a glistening surface due to fibrous thickening of the capsule. Other livers are markedly icteric. The gallbladder is often edematous and grossly distended with thick mucoid bile. Edema of segments of the bowel, mesentery and associated lymph nodes is common and much ascitic fluid may be found in the abdominal cavity. In some cases numerous small hemorrhages are present in the abdominal serous membranes.

Characteristic histologic changes are found in the liver. Irreversible enlargement of individual hepatocytes (megalocytosis) is unique, and is conspicuous in the horse and sheep, but less pronounced in cattle. In cattle, marked perivenous fibrosis of sublobular veins is usually present, but this is not a consistent finding in the horse and sheep. In all species there are marked increases in connective tissue both within and around the lobules.

Diagnosis and Treatment: Factors of importance in diagnosis are history of outbreaks, clinical signs and gross necropsy findings. Confirmation can usually be obtained from histologic examination of liver tissue obtained by biopsy or at necropsy.

Further intake of toxic plant material must be prevented. Animals showing clinical signs rarely recover and lesions present in asymptomatic animals may progress and result in further losses over several months. Since high-protein intake may prove harmful, diets with a high-carbohydrate ratio are indicated. Intravenous administration of methionine in 10% dextrose solution is claimed to be of value in treating horses.

The diminished ability of the liver to regenerate after pyrollizidine alkaloid poisoning suggests that a guarded prognosis should always be given. Factors in preventing further outbreaks should be stressed.

ALGAL POISONING

A usually acute and highly fatal condition caused by drinking water containing high concentrations of toxic blue-green algae. Fatalities and severe illness of livestock, pets, wild animals, and people have been associated with algal blooms in the northern half of the U.S.A., Texas, Canada, Russia, Argentina, Australia and South Africa.

Poisoning usually does not occur unless there is a dense bloom of toxic algae. The factors leading to such blooms include warm, sunny weather, ample nutrients (especially nitrates), and a gentle prevailing wind which drifts and collects the algae against the windward shore where it produces a blue-green scum. Such conditions commonly occur during the summer months in drainage ponds and lakes used for watering livestock.

Etiology: Early studies indicated the primary toxic principle to be an alkaloid which affected the CNS and liver. A secondary toxic principle was believed to be algal phycobilin pigments which accumulated in the skin of animals and produced photosensitization. More recent research has discounted the alkaloidal nature of the toxic principle and incriminated a 7-amino acid cyclic polypeptide, which rapidly produced toxic signs.

Strains of *Microcystis aeruginosa* (*toxica*), *M. flos-aquae* and *Anabaena flos-aquae* algae are most commonly responsible for algal intoxication, although certain bacteria associated with the algae may also produce toxins, which are less potent.

Clinical Findings: Toxic signs usually appear within 15 to 45 min. after ingestion of the poisonous material. Death may occur in less than 24 hours and often within 1 or 2 hours after ingestion of the toxin. The most commonly reported sequence of events is rapid prostration, convulsions and death. Abdominal pain, muscular tremors, dyspnea, cyanosis and excessive salivation are commonly reported. Some show severe gastrointestinal manifestations which include diarrhea, bloody feces and icterus. Photosensitization frequently occurs in animals which survive for several days.

Control: Removal of animals from the affected water supply is essential. Algal growth may be suppressed with copper sulfate or other algicide treatment, but this does not remove the toxin already present in the water. If no other water supply is available, animals should be allowed to drink from the clearest water at the leeward shore.

Animals dying from algal poisoning must not be used for food as the toxic principle is stable and consistently produces toxic symptoms in the consumer.

Treatment: Following removal from the contaminated water supply, affected animals should be placed in a protected area out of direct sunlight. Ample quantities of water and good quality feed should be made available. Cathartics or emetics may be used to remove toxins from the gastrointestinal tract. (CAUTION: Affected animals are usually very weak, and violent procedures should not be employed.)

Even though the alkaloidal nature of the toxin has been discounted, 1 to 2 oz of sodium thiosulfate in solution given IV or orally seems to be of benefit. In surviving animals, a long recuperative period is to be expected.

SNAKE BITE

Venomous snakes fall into 2 classes: the elapine snakes, which include the cobra, mamba, and coral snake, and the viperine snakes, which comprise 2 families—the true vipers, e.g., puff adder, Russell's viper and common European adder, and the pit vipers, e.g., rattle snakes, cottonmouth moccasin, and fer-de-lance. Elapine snakes have short fangs and tend to hang on and "chew" their victims. Their venom is mainly neurotoxic, and kills by paralyzing the respiratory center; in cases of recovery there are seldom any subsequent ill-effects. Viperine snakes have long, hinged fangs; they strike once and then withdraw. Their venom is mainly hemotoxic, causing pronounced local damage; subsequent necrosis may lead to the loss of a limb even if the victim recovers. However, all snake venoms contain both neurotoxic and hemotoxic factors.

The severity of any snake bite depends on the toxicity of the venom and the amount injected, as well as the location of the bite, the size and species of the victim, and its age and general condition of health. Experimental work suggests that the order of decreasing sensitivity is horse, sheep, ox, goat, dog, pig, cat.

The active principles of venom include hyaluronidase, cholinesterase, proteolytic enzymes, phosphates and neurotoxins. The latter have been shown to be basic polypeptides.

Since the lethal dose of a poison is based upon the quantity of poison introduced per unit of body weight, horses and cattle seldom die as a direct result of snake bite, but lack of medical attention may result in serious secondary damage. Fatalities in horses and cattle have resulted however from bites on the muzzle, head or neck.

Undoubtedly, the death rate from snake bite in all parts of the world is higher in dogs than in any other domestic animal. Due to the relatively small weight of the dog in proportion to the amount of venom injected, the bite of even a small snake is frequently fatal.

Clinical Findings and Diagnosis: Usually, horses and cattle are bitten on the legs or head, especially the latter; sheep have been bitten on the udder or scrotum. Dogs are frequently bitten on the legs but the most common site is probably the head with the shoulders and thighs next in order. The presence of hair may obscure the typical fang marks, though a close examination should reveal the point of entry of the venom.

Venoms from viperine snakes may produce prolonged intense pain, muscular weakness, impaired vision, nausea, paralysis, edema, shock, cyanosis, hemolytic anemia, necrosis of tissue and bleeding tendencies. The venom of the rattlesnake causes an almost immediate reaction in the form of extensive swelling around the wound. When horses and cattle are bitten about the head, their lips, face and submaxillary region become grossly swollen which results in pronounced dyspnea. Sloughing of the skin in the region of the wound may follow a bite. If a limb has been struck, the swelling usually causes lameness. In the case of an elapine snake bite the pain and local swelling may be absent, but the systemic signs are more pronounced.

Shock, in all its classical elements, accompanies all severe snake bites. Body temperature is frequently lowered. Lassitude and somnolence usually ensue. If a dog has been exercising violently, as is frequently the case, and if the venom is deposited in a highly vascular area, death commonly occurs in a matter of 5 to 10 minutes. Severe bacterial infections are sometimes sequelae to snake bites.

Treatment: In the treatment of snake bite, speed is essential. As exercise increases the rate of absorption of the venom, the patient should be carried to the veterinarian, or kept quiet and still until his arrival. Should there be any delay in obtaining expert help, the following first aid treatment may be useful in the case of a bite by a viperine snake. It would be of little value in the case of an elapine bite. The animal should be placed at rest and the hair clipped from the wound. If the bite is on a limb, a wide tourniquet should be placed 2 in. above the site of the bite. The tourniquet must not be so tight as to arrest arterial circulation. It should be released every 15 or 20 minutes for a period of 1 or 2 minutes. After injection of antivenin, the tourniquet should be discarded.

In the case of a bite from a dangerous snake, such as a rattlesnake, the fang wounds should be enlarged with lineal incisions paralleling the blood supply. Suction should be applied to the incisions for at least 30 minutes. Ordinary rubber suction cups have been shown to remove significant quantities of venom from FRESH VENOM SITES in 15 minutes. Oral suction should never be employed.

Early injection of polyvalent antivenin is most desirable; in fact, it is the only lifesaving measure in cases of bites from dangerous snakes, and for this reason is indicated in all cases of poisonous snake bites regardless of the interval between bite and institution of treatment. It has proved beneficial when administered for head bites of horses as late as 24 hours after the bite.

The smaller the animal, the more antivenin is required. The initial dose for dogs may be as high as 100 ml; 1 to 5 ampules (15 ml each) should be administered to an average-sized dog, depending upon the kind and size of the snake and the condition of the victim. All antivenin should be given IV, but the subcut. or IP route is preferred for first-aid use in the field. A minimum of 3 vials of antivenin should be administered at once except in the case of a small snake such as the European adder, where a single vial will probably be enough. For a cow, 50 ml of antivenin may suffice. It is advisable to administer additional doses at 1- to 3-hour intervals as the patient's condition warrants. A little antivenin may be injected locally at the site of the bite.

Corticosteroids are indicated. They exert a beneficial effect on the shock that invariably accompanies snake bite. Although not lifesaving in lethal cases, they do prolong survival time and help minimize tissue destruction. Broad-spectrum antibiotics should be administered. Infusions of isotonic saline and dextrose solutions, in addition to blood transfusions, are beneficial. Incision wounds should be kept open and draining until the animal shows marked improvement.

Calcium gluconate is a time-honored treatment of doubtful value. Tetanus antitoxin should be given in prophylactic doses. Sedatives, analgesics and ataractics should be employed with care and should not be given in doses that will mask important clinical signs.

If antivenin is not available, if the animal is seen by the veterinarian within an hour and if the bite is located in an area to which tourniquets cannot be applied, then excision of an area of skin 7 cm in diameter, including the associated subcut. tissue, may be lifesaving in the case of a bite by a viper or pit viper.

Contrary to former opinion, the use of excessive heat or cold is contraindicated in the treatment of the lesion. Since antihistamines have been shown to potentiate the effect of snake venom, their use is contraindicated. Certain cobras are capable of "spitting" their venom at the eyes of their victim from a distance of several feet, causing severe pain and often temporary blindness. Treatment consists of washing the eye with water or diluted serum.

PART III
POULTRY

THE AVIAN LEUKOSIS COMPLEX

A complex of 3 groups of neoplastic diseases which primarily affect the hemopoietic system of chickens. Recently the complex has been referred to as the **Avian Reticuloses**. The **leukosis-sarcoma group** mainly affects the hemopoietic system and is caused by a ribonucleic acid (RNA) virus infection. It includes lymphoid leukosis, erythroblastosis, myeloblastosis, myelocytomatosis and several other etiologically related conditions, including sarcoma, nephroblastoma, endothelioma and osteopetrosis. **Marek's disease** in its "classical" manifestation predominately affects the nervous system and is caused by a deoxyribonucleic acid (DNA) virus infection. In the acute form of Marek's disease, however, the viscera are more extensively involved. At present, **reticuloendotheliosis,** the third group, is essentially an experimentally induced disease caused by an RNA virus, and will not be discussed.

The provisional classification of the avian leukosis complex is based on pathologic and etiologic differences among the disease groups. It differs from earlier classifications by dissociating the lymphoid lesions occurring in lymphoid leukosis from those occurring in Marek's disease. The term **"visceral lymphomatosis"** of previous classifications referred to the visceral lesions of both lymphoid leukosis and Marek's disease; to avoid confusion this term will not be used (except to note its use as a synonym for Lymphoid Leukosis, q.v., p. 1015).

The disease complex is a serious economic problem in domestic chickens, and sporadic occurrences have been recorded in other avian species. The economically important members of the complex are Marek's disease and lymphoid leukosis. The other forms usually occur sporadically, although rare flock outbreaks of myelocytomas, osteopetrosis, sarcomas and erythroleukosis have been described.

Diagnosis: Differentiation of the entities in the leukosis-sarcoma classification of the avian leukosis complex can often be made by gross inspection of lesions. In uncertain cases, histologic sections of tissues, bone marrow and blood smears are needed for definitive diagnosis.

Differential diagnosis between lymphoid leukosis and Marek's disease requires skill and experience because of their similar appearance and the lack of routine diagnostic tests.

Nonneoplastic disease characterized by the development of tumor-like inflammatory granulomas, such as tuberculosis and pullorum disease, must be differentiated from the neoplastic

TABULAR COMPARISON OF LESIONS AND SIGNS

Feature	Lymphoid Leukosis	Marek's Disease
Age	Over 16 weeks	Any age after 3 weeks, most common from 12 to 24 weeks
Paralysis	Rare	Characteristic
Enlargement of peripheral or autonomic nerves and ganglia	Rare (if ever)	Common
Bursa of Fabricius	Nodular tumors are common	Atrophy or diffuse involvement
Neoplasia of ocular and feather follicular tissue	Rare	Common
Characteristic cells	Lymphoblastic tumors	Infiltrating pleomorphic lymphocytes

diseases in which discrete tumors develop. Inflammatory nodules can be differentiated from neoplasms by tissue distribution, color, consistency, texture and association with other inflammatory and degenerative lesions. In questionable cases, tissue smears or sections will reveal the presence of definitive microscopic characteristics such as bacteria, fungi, or cell type.

The neural involvement of Marek's disease must be differentiated from other diseases of the nervous system, such as Newcastle disease, encephalomyelitis and riboflavin deficiency.

Control: *See* p. 1020.

THE LEUKOSES

Etiology: Lymphoid, erythroid and myeloid leukosis, myelocytomatosis, the related soft-tissue neoplasms, and osteopetrosis are caused by closely related RNA-containing viruses, most of which are able to produce more than one type of neoplasm. The viruses all have a common group-specific antigen which can be demonstrated by the complement-fixation test for avian leukosis viruses (COFAL test). The group can be divided into at least 4 subgroups on the basis of host genotype range, interference and major antigenic properties. Virus neutralization is type-specific and if cross-reactions occur, they do so only between viruses of the same subgroup.

The leukosis viruses have the ability to act as "resistance-inducing factors" (RIF) which interfere with the neoplastic transformation of cell cultures of genetically susceptible chick-embryo fibroblasts by Rous sarcoma virus. This property is the basis of the RIF test for detecting leukosis viruses. A leukosis virus will only interfere with a sarcoma virus belonging to the same subgroup.

Certain sarcoma viruses are defective. Cells infected by them become morphologically transformed but do not produce infectious virus. When such nonproducer (NP) cells are super-infected with a leukosis virus the cellular genome is activated and infectious sarcoma virus is produced in addition to the helper leukosis virus. The phenomenon is the basis of the NP activation test.

The COFAL and NP activation tests are group-specific, the RIF test is subgroup-specific and the neutralization test is type-specific. The tests are useful for detecting the presence of infection in a flock and for identifying viral types. Marek's disease virus and reticuloendotheliosis virus do not react in any of the described tests.

LYMPHOID LEUKOSIS
(Visceral lymphomatosis, Big-liver disease)

A contagious malignancy of lymphoid cells caused by an RNA virus-induced neoplastic transformation of lymphocytes within the follicles of the bursa of Fabricius. Metastases of malignant lymphocytes subsequently occur to cause diffuse or focal involvement of the liver, spleen and other organs. The disease affects birds which are 4 months of age or older.

Transmission: The virus is widespread in poultry operations and is excreted in the feces and saliva of both diseased and carrier birds. Birds are most susceptible to contact infection during the hatching and brooding periods. Chicks from immune hens have maternal antibodies which provide a temporary passive immunity to contact infection during the first few weeks of life. In the absence of maternal antibodies, exposed birds develop specific antibodies which may or may not eliminate the virus. Some of the infected birds develop lesions of leukosis and others become asymptomatic carriers. Hens which continue to carry the virus pass the infection to some of their offspring through the egg. The infected embryos become immunologically tolerant to the virus which results in a persistent viremia, a lack of antibody production, and a lack of lesions after hatching. Tolerant adult hens transmit the virus to all of their offspring in contrast to nonviremic carrier hens which only transmit the virus intermittently. Infected birds of both sexes may transmit the infection horizontally by contact, but the male has no known role in vertical transmission to the embryo.

Clinical Findings: There are no characteristic signs; affected birds may be in good or poor condition, the comb is often pale and shrunken and an enlarged liver may be palpable.

Lesions: The initial lesions are focal tumors of the bursa of

Fabricius which may progress to cause massive enlargement of the whole organ. The neoplastic cells metastasize to other organs such as the spleen, kidneys, bone marrow, gonads and especially the liver. Gross lesions may vary from single or sparsely scattered discrete large gray-white nodular lymphomas to diffusely disseminated miliary foci of tumor cells. Often the lesion is manifested as a uniform enlargement and grayish discoloration of the affected organ. The initial metastatic lesion is comprised of a microscopic extravascular focus of homogeneous lymphoblasts. The microscopic foci subsequently enlarge and coalesce to form the grossly apparent lesions. Occasionally a concomitant leukemia develops.

Diagnosis: *See* p. 1013.

Control: *See* p. 1020.

ERYTHROID LEUKOSIS
(Erythroblastosis)

A leukemia characterized by neoplastic proliferation of immature erythroid cells. Intravascular accumulations of tumor cells cause enlargement of the liver and the spleen.

Erythroid leukosis occurs sporadically in the field, usually in birds 6 months of age or older. A specific viral etiology is supported by isolation of strains of virus from natural infections that are able to induce erythroid leukosis in young chicks within 2 weeks after exposure. Some strains of lymphoid leukosis virus also appear to be able to induce erythroid leukosis under appropriate conditions.

Clinical Findings: Birds become listless, cyanotic and die suddenly in the acute proliferative form of the disease. Chronically affected birds may survive several months during which signs of anemia (pallor or a yellowish discoloration of unfeathered parts), emaciation and diarrhea may develop.

Lesions: The characteristic gross lesions in fresh specimens are a diffuse bright cherry-red discoloration and enlargement of the liver, spleen and kidneys. The carcass is pale, and petechial hemorrhages may be apparent in various tissues. The marrow is hyperplastic and has a "currant-jelly" consistency. Leukemia is produced by the release of neoplastic basophilic erythroblasts from the bone marrow into the peripheral blood. The primitive cells accumulate in the sinusoids of the liver, spleen and other organs and they characteristically predominate in blood smears.

A chronic, anemic form of erythroid leukosis occurs in which excessive proliferation of erythroblasts and organ enlargement do not occur. In such cases the liver contains small groups of erythroblasts with foci of lymphoid and granulocytic reactive hyperplasia.

Diagnosis: Tissue sections, and blood and bone marrow smears contain characteristic neoplastic immature erythroid cells.

Control: *See* p. 1020.

MYELOID LEUKOSIS
(Myeloblastosis, Granuloblastosis)

Essentially an extravascular growth of malignant granulocytes and a concomitant striking granulocytic leukemia. It usually occurs sporadically in mature birds. A specific viral etiology is supported by the existence of virus strains that predominantly produce myeloid leukosis, and the inability of lymphoid leukosis viruses to produce the disease.

Clinical Findings: These are similar to those associated with erythroid leukosis (*see above*).

Lesions: The liver, spleen and kidneys are diffusely enlarged. The liver may have a granular appearance and is discolored grayish yellow. The marrow is hyperplastic and pale. Leukemia results when neoplastic immature granulocytes pass from the bone marrow into the general circulation. These cells invade extravascular sites of the liver, spleen and other organs where they continue to proliferate.

Diagnosis: Tissue sections, and blood and bone marrow smears contain a predominance of neoplastic myeloblasts and myelocytes.

Control: *See* p. 1020.

MYELOCYTOMATOSIS
(Knothead, Chloroma)

A virus disease characterized by myelocytic tumors of the skull, ribs and long bones. It occurs sporadically in immature birds.

Clinical Findings: Occasionally, birds have protuberances of the skull which may be hard, soft, or have a very thin layer of brittle bone overlaying the tumor.

Lesions: Soft, yellowish-white tumors develop on the cranium, long bones and the pleural surface of the thoracic cage. Occasionally, muscular invasion, visceral metastasis, or a concomitant leukemia occurs. The tumors and leukemic cells are proliferating myelocytes with characteristic eosinophilic granules.

Diagnosis: The presence of neoplastic heterophils in smears or sections of tumors is diagnostic.

Control: *See* p. 1020.

OSTEOPETROSIS

(Osteopetrotic lymphomatosis, Marble bone, Thick-leg disease)

Osteopetrosis is regarded as a dysplastic skeletal disease rather than a neoplastic disease. It is included in the avian leukosis complex because of its high frequency in transmission experiments with some strains of leukosis virus. It occurs sporadically in the field in birds of all ages, more often in males than in females. Virus strains have been isolated that usually produce the lesions of osteopetrosis alone, but it appears that the disease is also produced by some strains of lymphoid leukosis virus.

Clinical Findings: Most bones of the skeleton can be affected, but the most pronounced changes occur in the long bones. Enlargement of the metatarsi is obvious and thickening of other bones is evident on palpation. The affected bones are warm and skeletal involvement is usually bilateral.

Lesions: The dysplasia principally involves the diaphyses of the long bones. Abnormal bone is formed by hyperplastic activity of subperiosteal and endosteal osteoblasts that produces a thickened bony cortex and results in obliteration of the marrow cavity. Osteopetrosis may be accompanied by the lesions of lymphoid leukosis or may occur alone in which case splenic atrophy usually occurs.

Diagnosis: Bilateral skeletal dysplasia is characteristic of the disease.

Control: *See* p. 1020.

MAREK'S DISEASE

(Fowl paralysis, Neurolymphomatosis gallinarum, Acute leukosis)

A highly infectious disease of poultry characterized by gross enlargements of the nerves and tumors of the visceral organs, skin and muscle produced by infiltration and proliferation of pleomorphic lymphoid cells. Atrophy of the follicles and interfollicular infiltration of the bursa of Fabricius may also occur.

Etiology and Epizootiology: Marek's disease is caused by a DNA virus belonging to the cell-associated or B group of herpesviruses. The virus produces characteristic syncytial cytopathic effects in cell cultures of chicken kidney and duck embryo fibroblasts. Nuclei of such cultured cells and the nuclei of cells of infected feather follicular epithelium, develop eosinophilic Cowdry Type A inclusion bodies which are outlined by a halo of marginated nuclear chromatin. Antigens are produced in the cell cultures and in the feather follicles, which will react with serum from infected birds in the agar gel precipitation and fluorescent antibody tests.

Transmission of the virus through the egg is not important. Infectious cell-free virus is not present in large quantities in the blood, visceral organs or tumors. The virus matures to its infectious form in the feather follicular epithelium and is disseminated in the dander from infected chickens. The virus spreads readily over long distances and infection of new hosts is thought to occur primarily by inhaled aerosols of infectious dander. Nearly all flocks of chickens are infected by the time they reach sexual maturity. Clinical disease, however, is an exceptional sequela to virus infection. Most birds develop antibodies which are passed to offspring as a form of temporary passive protection. The occurrence of disease depends on the genetic resistance of the chicken, the age at which the bird becomes infected, the dose of virus received and the pathogenicity of the virus strain.

Clinical Findings: Most commonly, the disease occurs in 12- to 24-week-old birds. Exceptional cases have occurred as early as 3 weeks and as late as 18 months of age. Birds classically develop lameness or paralysis of the legs, wings, neck, eyelids or other parts of the body. Occasionally, dyspnea, dilatation of the crop, diarrhea and emaciation occur. Young birds affected by the acute form may only show signs of anorexia and depression. Neoplastic lesions of the viscera, skin and muscle are the predominant lesions in such birds. When the eyes are involved, the iris is discolored gray and the pupillary margin becomes irregular. Light accommodation is eventually lost and blindness results.

Lesions: Birds commonly have enlargements of one or more of the peripheral or autonomic nerves. The brachial, sciatic, celiac and vagus nerves are most frequently involved. The thickened nerves lack striations and are grayish and edematous. Lymphomas are frequent in the ovary, but may also develop in the testis, liver, lung, skin, muscle, kidney, proventriculus and other organs. Lesions of the viscera (acute leukosis) are most common in young chickens. In sexually mature chickens, visceral lesions may appear very similar to those of lymphoid leukosis. The bursa of Fabricius usually undergoes atrophy in Marek's disease, but occasionally it is diffusely involved in the neoplastic process.

Microscopically, the nerve infiltrations and lymphomas are a mixture of large, medium and small lymphocytes. In some nerves the lesion appears as an edematous inflammation. The involved iris is infiltrated by the pleomorphic lymphocytes which can also be found in some optic nerves and eye muscles.

Diagnosis: *See* p. 1013.

CONTROL OF THE AVIAN LEUKOSIS COMPLEX

There is no known treatment for any of these diseases. Currently, vaccine is available to aid the control of Marek's disease only. Control of all members of the complex is based on hygienic rearing techniques and breeding for resistance.

Hygienic control is based on prevention of introduction of disease by infected embryos or chicks, and prevention of contact infection between infected and uninfected stock. The RNA viruses of the leukosis-sarcoma group of diseases are perpetuated by vertical transmission through the egg in contrast to the DNA virus of Marek's disease. Eggs or chicks from different strains or hatcheries, therefore, should not be hatched or brooded together because a congenitally infected chick can contaminate others. Moreover, chicks in immunologic balance with other diseases endemic in their parent flock may not have resistance to the endemic diseases of another flock. Hens which are not shedding RNA leukosis viruses must be identified to obtain clean eggs. A minimum of 9 eggs comprising 3 pools must be tested from each hen before it can be regarded as a noncarrier. Chicks from such sources must then be raised in hygienic isolation to prevent exposure to oncogenic viruses as well as other pathogens.

Premises should be thoroughly cleaned and disinfected before the introduction of new stock. All-in, all-out brooding should be practiced for any one location. Effectiveness of disinfection depends on the thoroughness of technique. Insect control must be practiced because both the larvae and adults of the darkling beetle, *Alphitobius diaperinus,* have been incriminated as carriers of acute leukosis. Birds should be maintained in isolation away from sources of Marek's disease, including aerosols of dust and dander, for the first 3 months of life. During this time they are extremely susceptible to the disease and a filtered air supply under positive pressure within the house is necessary to insure the benefits of absolute isolation procedures.

Genetic composition influences the response of birds to the viruses of the leukosis complex. Available evidence indicates that selection for resistance to one group of diseases is not likely to result in resistance to the others. At the cellular sites, genetic resistance appears to be specific for each subgroup of virus. In contrast, suppression of tumor growth implies a broader type of resistance. Response to virus exposure is used as the final criterion for selection regardless of the method used for identifying genetic resistance including sib-, progeny- and line-testing, or longevity.

Live-virus vaccines have recently been developed to control Marek's disease. While the mechanism of protection is incompletely understood, it is evident that the development of lesions is prevented. Birds are vaccinated at one day of age because of the constant danger of exposure to ubiquitous virulent strains of virus if vaccination is delayed. Conscientious attention to manufacturer's recommendations for vaccine use is imperative for adequate protection. In the U.S.A., a cell-culture propagated turkey herpesvirus is used, usually given IP or subcut. at one day of age. Elsewhere a cell-culture propagated Marek's disease herpesvirus originating in chickens is utilized; this may be either a naturally occurring mild strain, or an attenuated virulent strain. Chick-embryo vaccines have also been utilized but are reported to be less effective.

FOWL POX

A relatively slow-spreading virus infection of chickens and turkeys characterized by the formation of nodules in the skin progressing to heavy scab formation, and of diphtheritic membranes in the upper digestive and respiratory tracts. The disease is world-wide and usually most prevalent during periods of large mosquito populations.

Etiology and Epizootiology: Fowl pox virus, a large DNA virus, is highly resistant and may survive for years in dried scabs. Although some characteristics of the virus from turkeys differ from that of chickens, they may be considered together for most practical purposes. The virus is present in abundance in the lesions and is slowly transmitted to penmates through minor wounds and abrasions of the skin. Affected birds are viremic. A number of mosquitoes including *Aedes aegypti, A. vexans, Culex pipiens* and *Stegomyia faciata* serve as major vectors. Demonstrated capability of transmitting infection for at least 39 days suggests that mosquitoes serve as more than mechanical carriers. Transmission within flocks is rapid when mosquitoes are plentiful. Apparently no carriers remain following clinical recovery.

Clinical Findings: Lesions are prominent prior to significant disturbance in flock performance. Cutaneous lesions usually occur only on the unfeathered parts of the head of the chicken and head and upper neck of the turkey; generalized skin infection is rare. The lesion is initially a raised blanched nodular area that enlarges, becomes yellowish in color, and progresses to a heavy, dark scab. Multiple lesions usually develop which often coalesce. Lesions in various stages of development can often be found on the same bird. Localization around the nostrils may produce nasal discharge. Lesions on the eyelids may result in lacrimation, closing of the lids, large caseous exudative accumulations in the conjunctival sac and sometimes eventual loss of the eye.

Lesions may also occur in the buccal mucosa or in the larynx and trachea (wet pox or fowl diphtheria). Occasionally lesions occur almost exclusively in one or more of these sites. Caseous patches firmly adherent to the mucosa of the larynx and mouth develop. Tracheal lesions may be diffuse and progress to a heavy, brown pseudomembrane.

Usually the course of the disease in a flock is protracted. Extensive infection in a flock results in a slowly developing but marked decline in egg production with some loss of fertility. Cutaneous infections usually cause little mortality. Flocks generally return to normal production upon recovery.

Diagnosis: Cutaneous infections usually produce characteristic lesions. Appropriately stained sections or scrapings of affected areas usually reveal characteristic intracytoplasmic inclusion bodies. A few isolates have been found which produce few or no inclusion bodies. Isolation may be accomplished on the chorioallantoic membrane of embryonating eggs. The disease is readily reproduced by applying ground lesions to scarified skin or denuded feather follicles of the same species. Particular care is necessary to distinguish laryngeal and tracheal lesions from infectious laryngotracheitis.

Prophylaxis and Treatment: In areas where pox is prevalent, vaccination of chickens and turkeys with live embryo-propagated virus is practiced. The most widely used vaccine is a pigeon-pox virus isolate with high immunizing ability and low pathogenicity. In high-risk areas, vaccination should be done in the first few weeks of life; revaccination at 12 to 20 weeks is often sufficient. Because the infection spreads slowly, vaccination is often useful in limiting spread in affected pens if less than 20% of the birds have lesions.

Vaccinated birds should be examined in one week for swelling and scab formation at the vaccination point. Lack of such a reaction indicates impotent vaccine, previously existing immunity, or careless vaccination. Revaccination is indicated, possibly with another serial lot of vaccine.

Birds in which caseous deposits interfere with breathing may be helped by removal of the material and swabbing the site with tincture of iodine.

POX IN OTHER AVIAN SPECIES

Infections with pox virus have been recorded from a large variety of avian species. Some isolates are infectious for only the host species, whereas others are infectious for one or more additional species. Gross immunity is also unpredictable. Classification is usually based on host origin. Canary pox is usually severe with mortality sometimes approaching 100%. Cutaneous lesions may develop as well as systemic infection with cytoplasmic inclusion bodies in the salivary glands, liver, pancreas and other organs of epithelial origin. No effective vaccine is available for this species.

INFECTIOUS LARYNGOTRACHEITIS

An acute, highly contagious respiratory disease of chickens and pheasants characterized by severe dyspnea, coughing and rales; or subacute disease with lacrimation, tracheitis, conjunctivitis and mild rales.

Etiology: The disease is caused by a virus and has been reported from most of the intensive poultry-rearing sections of the U.S.A. and many other countries.

Clinical Findings: In the acute form, gasping, coughing, rattling and extension of the neck during inspiration are seen from 6 to 12 days after natural exposure. Reduced productivity is a varying factor in laying flocks. Affected birds lose their appetite and become inactive. The mouth and beak may be bloodstained from the tracheal exudate. Mortality varies but may reach 50% in adults. Signs usually subside after about 2 weeks, although some birds may cough for a month.

The subacute form has a low mortality, a more protracted course, and is characterized by milder respiratory signs, lacrimation and conjunctival edema.

A small percentage of recovered birds remain carriers and may serve as sources of infection. Infection also may be spread by mechanical transfer.

Diagnosis: The presence of the clinical signs indicated above, and finding blood, mucus and yellow caseous exudate in the trachea or a hollow caseous cast in the trachea or, in the subacute form, punctiform hemorrhagic areas in trachea and larynx, and conjunctivitis with lacrimation permit a presumptive diagnosis. In uncomplicated cases, the air sacs are not involved. A conclusive diagnosis may be made by (1) demonstrating intranuclear inclusion bodies in the tracheal epithelium early in the course of the disease; (2) isolation and identification of the specific virus in chick embryos, tissue culture, or chickens; (3) infraorbital sinus or vent inoculation of known immune and susceptible birds. Neutralization of virus is less dependable but has been used. Microscopically, a desquamative necrotizing tracheitis is characteristic.

Prophylaxis and Treatment: Some relief from the effects of the disease is obtained by keeping the birds quiet, lowering the dust level and using mild expectorants, being careful that the latter do not contaminate feed or water. Vaccination should be practiced in enzootic areas or farms where a specific diagnosis is made. Immediate vaccination of adults in the face of an outbreak will shorten the course of the disease. Vaccination is currently being done with modified strains of lower virulence applied by drop to the eye (conjunctiva). The use of so-called virulent strains applied by brush or drop method to the vent mucosa is now limited to California. Broiler flocks in some areas must be vaccinated when young, but protection is not likely to be solid when done under 4 weeks of age. Some vaccine producers recommend revaccination when birds are to be held to maturity.

INFECTIOUS BRONCHITIS

An acute, rapidly spreading, viral, respiratory infection of chickens, characterized by rales, coughing and sneezing, without the accompaniment or subsequent development of nervous signs.

Etiology and Incidence: Infectious bronchitis is caused by a virus which, so far as is known, infects only chickens. It is widespread in the U.S.A. and Canada and has been reported from other parts of the world.

The virus is resistant to the action of antibiotics and can be cultivated readily in 9- to 11-day-old chick embryos. Embryonic mortality is variable. Six days after injection into the allantoic sac, living embryos should be examined for stunting or tight curling of the embryo or urate deposits in the mesonephros. Similar embryonic changes have been observed with the B_1 strain of Newcastle disease virus.

Epizootiology: Recovered birds are immune and do not remain carriers. The virus can be spread by droplet infection through the air, by contamination of feed sacks, equipment, clothing and shoes of caretakers. In the Northeastern U.S.A., the virus does not persist on premises more than 4 weeks after signs have ceased. Although bronchitis virus has been isolated from eggs laid by fowls in the acute stages of the disease, chicks that hatch from such eggs are not infected. Parentally conferred immunity protects the chick for a short period.

Clinical Findings: Coughing and rattling are manifest from 18 to 48 hours after exposure. Slight nasal discharge is seen occasionally in young chicks only. There is occasional facial swelling. Wet eyes are commonly seen. Spread to other birds in the same pen takes place in 24 to 48 hours and usually all susceptible birds on a farm become infected within a short time. The morbidity is practically 100%, although the severity of the signs may vary considerably. Respiratory signs cease in 2 or 3 weeks.

Mortality is highest in very young chicks and may reach 60%. The mortality is negligible in birds older than 5 or 6 weeks. Feed consumption and egg production in laying fowls drop sharply. A decrease of 20 to 50% in egg production, with many misshapen, thin- or soft-shelled eggs of poor internal quality is not uncommon. Frequently, egg quality is impaired permanently.

Mortality may be reduced in young chicks by providing good environmental conditions. In older growing chickens, the prognosis is excellent and recovery is uneventful. On the other hand, laying birds may never reach their former egg production level even months after recovery from the respiratory infection. Such flocks should be marketed.

Diagnosis: The isolation of the virus in chick embryos, with the production of embryonic lesions, is the most certain procedure. A history of an acute, rapidly spreading, respiratory disease, which is not Newcastle disease (negative to the hemagglutination-inhibition test) with typical changes in the eggs of producing birds, is good presumptive evidence. Serum neutralization tests (3 weeks after onset or later) will yield significant antibody titers. After recovery, birds are refractory to challenge with virulent bronchitis virus.

Postmortem examination reveals a catarrhal tracheitis, bronchitis and, occasionally, slight thickening and clouding of the air sac membranes. In fatal cases, caseous plugs may be found in primary and secondary bronchi. Ova in producing birds are flaccid. Yolks and eggs with shells are often found in the abdominal cavity.

Treatment: No medication is available that will alter or shorten the course of the disease. Increasing the temperature in the room and under the hover by 5° to 10°F may lower mortality. Food consumption should be stimulated by all possible means.

Immunization may be carried out by the use of live-virus vaccines which produce relatively mild respiratory signs. These vaccines are usually given in the drinking water, or as a dust or spray. Such products should be used according to the manufacturer's specific recommendations.

A new problem in immunization and diagnosis of infectious bronchitis has been posed by the recognition of variant strains of the virus. Several of these have been found in flocks experiencing vaccine breaks. They were not of the Massachusetts or Connecticut serotypes although they share some antigenic components with some of the previously recognized standard strains. In Australia and the U.S.A. several of these variant strains have been associated with mortality due to nephritis in chickens.

NEWCASTLE DISEASE
(Avian pneumoencephalitis)

An acute, rapidly spreading virus disease of domestic poultry and other birds in which the respiratory signs (coughing, sneezing, rales) are often accompanied or followed by nervous manifestations.

Etiology and Occurrence: Newcastle disease virus is a hemagglutinative paramyxovirus, with strains varying from nonpathogenic to extremely pathogenic. American isolates, even though highly pathogenic, produce no distinctive gross lesions, whereas European isolates often do. Virus isolates kill 9-day-old chicken embryos in 1 to 6 days. The disease occurs all over the world in a wide variety of domestic and wild birds, and occurs in man as a mild influenza-like disease with conjunctivitis.

Epidemiology: Recovered birds rarely are carriers. Egg transmission to chicks is uncommon. Respiratory exudates and the dejecta of infected birds are the chief means of spread. These may contaminate tools, boots, and clothing of caretakers and visitors. Carcasses of birds slaughtered and eviscerated for food may serve to spread the virus, as may raw garbage containing material from such carcasses. Wild birds may spread the virus. Poultry vaccines have been found to be contaminated. Parental antibodies in the yolk are found in the chick for 2 to 4 weeks after hatching, serving to protect against severe disease.

Clinical Findings: Signs are respiratory or nervous or both, and appear almost simultaneously throughout the flock 2 to 15 days after exposure, the average being about 5 days. Respiratory signs are gasping and coughing. Nervous signs, which may accompany but usually follow the respiratory signs, are: drooping wings, dragging legs, twisting of head and neck, circling, walking backward (particularly after drinking water), and complete paralysis. Clonic spasms are seen in moribund birds. Depression and inappetence are seen. Laying flocks may have partial or complete cessation of production, which may be permanent. Eggs abnormal in color, shape, or surface, and with watery albumen, are produced. (Some poisonings produce similar changes, e.g., thiram.) Mortality depends on the virulence of the virus strain, the environmental conditions, and the condition of the flock. In general, mortality is higher in very young flocks (but 100% mortality may occur in adult flocks).

Lesions: Lesions are highly variable, reflecting the variation in tropism and pathogenicity of the virus. Petechiae of the serous membranes may be seen, as may (European strains) hemorrhages of the proventricular mucosa and hemorrhages of the intestinal serosa with accompanying branny, necrotic areas on the mucosal surface. Congestion and mucoid exudates may be seen in the respiratory tract, with opacity and thickening of the air sacs. Sometimes cloudiness of the eye is seen.

Diagnosis: Tentative diagnosis of a rapidly spreading, respiratory-nervous disease may be confirmed by isolation of the hemagglutinating virus, identified by inhibition with known Newcastle disease antiserum. Paired serum samples showing a rise in HI antibodies also serve to identify the disease.

Prophylaxis and Treatment: Vaccination with a live-virus vaccine is widely used. Lentogenic strains (notably the B-1) are most commonly used, often combined with infectious bronchitis vaccine. Mass methods of administration—drinking water (most common), dust, spray—are effective. To use chlorinated drinking water, ½ lb of skim milk powder per 10 gal. of water must be added to prevent virus inactivation. Chicks may be vaccinated at a day of age or at 2 weeks of age (low parental antibodies at that time). Vaccination should be repeated every 2 to 3 months.

Mesogenic strains are used as vaccines by wing-web, IM, or feather follicle inoculation. These may cause post-vaccination paralysis in some birds, and should not be used on young chicks (under a month) nor in laying birds, unless the manufacturer's directions specifically advise such use. On the other hand they engender a more permanent immunity.

Inactivated virus vaccines may be given by IM or intratracheal injection. Immunity is not permanent, but these are safe to use in laying flocks, baby chicks, and in flocks affected by other problems. Some countries prohibit the use of live virus.

Nursing care, including increased temperature of the house, is helpful in reducing losses from the disease.

The regulatory status of the disease should be ascertained from the responsible officials (state or federal).

AVIAN INFLUENZA
(including Fowl plague)

An acute virus disease of birds, sometimes characterized by extremely high mortality among birds of all ages. Incubation period is 3 to 7 days.

Etiology, Epidemiology and Distribution: The causal agents are myxoviruses of the Influenza A group. A number of serologically distinct subgroups are known, each with further subdivisions. The hemagglutinative viruses grow readily in chicken embryos, and less readily in avian and mammalian tissue cultures. Avian influenza virus will cause pneumonia in mice. Spread occurs by virus discharged from infected birds, and possibly by mammals and man. Virus has been recovered from birds 2 months after inoculation. Apparently recovered birds develop increased HI antibodies after stress. Influenza has been found in all parts of the U.S.A. (except the South) especially the North Central and Western Regions; in Canada, Great Britain, Europe and South Africa.

Clinical Findings: Respiratory signs are most common, mild and transitory in lightly affected birds but progressing to moist rales with cyanosis and edema of the head in severely affected birds. Bloodstained oral and nasal discharges are common in the latter. A drop in egg production and poor fertility have been noted in turkeys.

   Lesions: Petechiae, ecchymoses, and congestion of serous and mucous membranes, and of body fat, are found along with consolidation of the lungs, often with caseation of the air sacs.

Diagnosis: Isolation of the virus in embryonated eggs yields amnioallantoic fluid which repeatedly agglutinates the same erythrocytes after resuspension. Newcastle disease antiserum does not inhibit the agglutination. Gel-diffusion precipitation tests with Influenza A antigen reveal past infection. In its severe forms the disease resembles acute fowl cholera, severe Newcastle disease, ornithosis and erysipelas. In milder forms it resembles mycoplasmosis, infectious bronchitis and tracheal pox.

   (N.B. Laryngotracheitis has also been called chicken influenza. Goose influenza is a bacterial disease.)

Prophylaxis and Treatment: In areas of endemic fowl plague, vaccines have been used with variable success. Since any Influenza A virus might cause fowl-plague-like disease, monovalent vaccines are likely to have failures. Treatment of affected flocks with broad-spectrum antibiotics and increased house temperatures help control mortality. Suspected outbreaks should be reported to State and Federal authorities.

AVIAN ENCEPHALOMYELITIS (AE)
(Epidemic tremor)

A viral disease marked by ataxia and tremor of head, neck and limbs, which occurs worldwide in chickens, pheasants,

Japanese quail and turkeys. As other species are susceptible to artificial inoculation, they are likely, also, to have the natural disease.

Etiology: The causative picornavirus can be grown in chicken embryos from nonimmune hens. It is transmitted through eggs laid by infected hens for about a month after infection.

Clinical Findings: Signs, sometimes present at hatching or delayed until several weeks of age, commonly appear at 7 to 10 days of age. The chief signs are unsteadiness, sitting on hocks, paresis, and even complete inability to move. Muscular tremors are best seen after exercising the bird; holding the bird on its back in the cupped hand helps in detection. Even completely ataxic birds are conscious. About 5% of the flock may be affected, although much higher morbidity and mortality may occur. The disease in adult birds is inapparent, except for a transient drop in egg production and flock activity in some cases. The disease in turkeys is often milder than in chickens.

Lesions: No gross lesions of the nervous system are seen. Lymphocytic accumulations in the gizzard muscle may be visible as grayish areas. Lens opacities occur, usually weeks after infection. Infected embryos have poorly developed voluntary muscles.

Microscopic lesions are lymphocytic foci in pancreas, liver, gizzard, proventriculus, and CNS (perivascular cuffing), along with neuronal degeneration and endothelial hyperplasia.

Diagnosis: AE must be differentiated from avian encephalomalacia, calcium deficiency, Newcastle disease, arbovirus encephalitis, Marek's disease, mycotic encephalitis, brain abscess and hereditary tremor (inbred flocks). Diagnosis is based on history, signs and histologic study of brain, proventriculus, gizzard and pancreas. Virus isolation in AE-antibody-free eggs is sometimes necessary to confirm the diagnosis. Lesions are not present in infected adults.

Prophylaxis and Treatment: Immunization of breeder pullets with a locally-isolated virus or a commercial vaccine is advised. Vaccination should be repeated at time of molt if flocks are to be held for a second laying year. Vaccination of table-egg flocks is sometimes advisable. Affected chicks and poults are ordinarily destroyed as few recover. Asymptomatic chicks may develop lens opacities months later.

INFECTIOUS BURSAL DISEASE (IBD)
(Gumboro disease)

An acute, highly contagious viral disease of young chickens characterized by edema and swelling of the bursa of Fabricius, necrosis of lymphoid elements, vent picking, prostration and mortality. The disease has been confused with a nephritis or nephrosis syndrome caused by aberrant or variant strains of infectious bronchitis virus. IBD has been diagnosed in most major poultry producing areas of the U.S.A. and is widespread globally. It includes the disease formerly known as **infectious avian nephrosis.**

Etiology and Transmission: Infectious bursal disease virus (IBDV), has been isolated from the bursa of Fabricius, kidneys, spleen, thymus, liver, intestinal tract, lungs and blood. Suspensions of these organs, infective feces and the embryo-propagated virus have been used to reproduce the disease. The virus is probably transferred from farm to farm by fomites. IBDV is difficult to eradicate from the premises since it apparently survives for a considerable length of time.

IBDV may be isolated in 8- to 11-day-old chicken embryos that are obtained from "clean" breeder flocks after inoculation with material from affected birds in the early stages of the disease. The chorioallantoic membrane route is somewhat more sensitive to infection than allantoic sac inoculation. Embryo deaths generally occur within 3 to 7 days after inoculation. Virus titers of 10^2 to 10^6 may be obtained. In early transfers of IBDV, embryo-tissue suspension should be employed. Upon subsequent adaptation to embryos, allantoic fluids can then be used. The virus is neutralized by specific IBD antiserum only. All isolates, to date, have appeared antigenically similar and possess no relationship to infectious bronchitis virus strains including those which cause severe kidney damage.

Clinical Findings: Onset is sudden, with severe prostration, dehydration, incoordination, diarrhea, soiled vent feathers, straining to void droppings, vent picking and inflammation of the vent. Clinical signs are usually seen between 3 and 6 weeks of age, but the disease has been diagnosed in younger and older birds. Infections vary from subclinical to those causing losses in excess of 20%. The growth of broilers to market weight may be delayed by 3 to 5 days. The incubation period is usually 3 to 4 days and the recovery period short, often within a week. Clinical signs may not be observed in some pens of an affected house or other houses in close proximity. Parentally conferred immunity may alter the clinical pattern since passive antibodies may persist as long as 5 to 6 weeks. Recovered birds have a high degree of resistance. The disease tends to occur repeatedly on the same farm, regardless of complete depopulation procedures. Persistence of the causative agent on the premises is one of its most important characteristics.

Lesions: In the early stages the bursa will be swollen, gelatinous in appearance and sometimes hemorrhagic, and occasionally the kidneys will be swollen and show degenerative changes. Muscle congestion occurs often and IM hemorrhages sometimes. Light breeds appear to be affected more severely than meat-type chickens.

Prophylaxis and Treatment: There is no treatment. Limited success has been achieved on contaminated farms in eliminating the problem through depopulation and disinfection. The virus is resistant to environmental conditions found on most poultry farms, and possibly unknown reservoirs of infection exist.

IBD vaccines, of chick embryo origin, low in virulence and of sufficient potency, induce satisfactory protection when given at 1 to 7 days of age by eye drop and drinking water routes. Although high parental immunity sometimes neutralizes the effectiveness of the vaccine, it appears the best means of minimizing the severe clinical effects in problem flocks.

EASTERN ENCEPHALITIS IN PHEASANTS

An acute virus disease of pheasants, characterized by neurologic signs, high morbidity and often high mortality. The disease is responsible for serious economic loss to producers unless adequate control measures are taken. The infective agent is the virus of the Eastern type of encephalitis (q.v., p. 251). Infection is normally transmitted by mosquitoes, but once established in a flock, transmission is facilitated by the birds pecking at one another. Serologic and other data clearly indicate that many other species of birds carry an inapparent infection. The virus has been isolated from mice, rats, fox, dogs and other mammals.

Clinical Findings and Diagnosis: The lesions are typical of the viral encephalitides. Signs include inappetence, staggering and paralysis. Recovered birds may be blind, have unilateral or bilateral paralysis of various muscle groups and have difficulty in holding the head up. The morbidity may reach 90% and, in some outbreaks, the mortality in individual pens has been as high as 90%. It is of interest to note that, while birds in some pens are affected, those in adjacent pens may show no signs. Diagnosis may be confirmed by inoculation of guinea pigs or mice, or by chick-embryo tissue culture methods. **Prophylaxis** may be accomplished in some instances by effective control of the mosquito population and by husbandry practices designed to reduce injuries from pecking, e.g., debeaking of the birds at regular intervals and the provision of adequate space for exercise. Preventive vaccination reduces mortality to less than 5%. It is recommended in enzootic areas, particularly in flocks with a history of previous outbreaks. A dose is 1/10 the equine dose of either an Eastern or Bivalent Eastern and Western vaccine injected into the pectoral muscles, preferably at 5 to 6 weeks of age, or when the birds are released from breeder houses. Efforts should be made to have most birds vaccinated by the first week in July, since in Northeastern U.S.A., outbreaks usually commence some 2 weeks later.

PSITTACOSIS-ORNITHOSIS
(Chlamydiosis)

An acute or chronic disease of wild and domestic birds, characterized by respiratory and systemic infection, transmissible to other animals and man. The disease in man and psittacine birds is called psittacosis, that in other birds, ornithosis.

Etiology and Occurrence: The cause is any avian strain of *Chlamydia psittaci*. Other closely related mammalian strains cause polyarthritis and reproductive disorders in sheep and cattle. All chlamydial strains contain identical group-specific antigens but may differ in the antigenic specificity of their cell-wall antigens.

The disease occurs worldwide, being particularly important in colonially nesting species, in domestic poultry (turkeys, pigeons, ducks) exposed to wild birds, and in caged birds passing through dealers' collecting houses.

Epizootiology: Aerosols and dusts from respiratory discharges or digestive dejecta are infective. Nestlings in colonies or breeding farms become infected and may become carriers if they survive. Such carriers, under environmental stress, may have a recurrence and transmit the infection. Chlamydial strains of unusually high virulence that cause high mortality have been found in gulls, egrets and turkeys. Strains of less virulence are usually found in psittacine birds, pigeons, ducks and chickens.

Clinical Findings: Nasal discharge, diarrhea, dullness, weakness, inappetence and loss of weight are often seen.

Lesions: Thickened, inflamed air sacs coated with yellowish-white exudate, with occasional perihepatitis, pericarditis and hepatosplenomegaly are found in acute cases. Chronic infections, which are common in psittacine and columbidan species, may only have an enlarged spleen or an enlarged, discolored liver.

Diagnosis: Tentative diagnosis may be made by detection of intracytoplasmic groups of chlamydiae in impression smears of diseased organs stained by the Giemsa or Machiavello method. Confirmation should be made by a laboratory competent to isolate and identify chlamydiae. Freshly collected liver, spleen, kidney and lungs should be shipped frozen. Cloacal excretions may also be sent for chlamydial isolation attempts if it is necessary to preserve the life of a valuable bird. Serologic tests (agglutination, hemagglutination, complement-fixation, etc.) are also best performed by specialists.

Thyroid enlargement (from iodine deficiency), or *Sternostoma* mites are often causes of respiratory difficulty in pet birds. Swollen spleen and severe respiratory distress may result from haemosporidial infections (*Plasmodium, Leucytozoon, Haemoproteus*). Aspergillosis is common in birds. Influenza and mycoplasmosis produce respiratory signs and lesions. Chickens may have air sac disease.

Prophylaxis and Treatment: Chlamydiosis is relatively rare in food birds. Reasons for the sporadicity of outbreaks are not clear. Preventive measures, such as screening houses against wild bird entry, are justified, but drug prophylaxis, in the absence of cases in the area, is not warranted. Effective vaccines are not available.

Pet birds should come from breeding establishments free of the infection. If the infection status is not known, tetracycline-impregnated seed should be fed to the birds to reduce the possibility of infection during transport and during stays in pet stores.

On tentative diagnosis, treatment with tetracycline antibiotics (400 gm/ton of feed, 2 gm/gal. of water, 5 mg/2 oz bird), continued for at least a week, should be initiated.

Public Health Significance: The disease in man usually follows heavy exposure to infective aerosols or dusts. Some individuals are more susceptible than others.

A simple preventive measure for the veterinarian examining dead birds is the use of a detergent disinfectant to wet the feathers. This also drowns lice and mites, helps prevent spread of other infective agents, and keeps feathers from floating in the air or sticking to the hands. Other protective measures in examining live birds include: dust masks, plastic face shields, fan-exhausted examining hoods or glove boxes.

Outbreaks should be reported to public health and regulatory officials.

VIRAL ENTERITIS OF DUCKS
(Duck plague)

A contagious disease of waterfowl characterized by weakness and sudden death, caused by a herpesvirus that kills duck embryos but not chicken embryos. Originally reported in Holland, it also occurs in India and China and an outbreak occurred in commercial ducks on Long Island (U.S.A.) from 1967 through 1968. It has been diagnosed in the Northern U.S.A. in wild waterfowl and in aviculturists' flocks.

Experimentally, the incubation period is 3 to 7 days. The onset is sudden with early signs of weakness and lethargy accompanied by thirst and watery diarrhea. Early in the course of the disease a catarrhal-hemorrhagic enteritis is often found. Petechial and ecchymotic hemorrhages are found in the heart, pancreas and mesentery. In older breeder ducks, in addition to these findings, muscular hemorrhages are seen on longitudinal mucosal folds of the esophagus, at the junction of the esophagus and proventriculus, in the cloacal mucosa, and in the thymus and liver. Later yellowish-white elongated plaques occur particularly in the esophagus and cloaca. Petechia and pinpoint white spots are observed in the liver.

The typical lesions permit a field diagnosis. Confirmation is obtained by use of specific serum or virus-neutralization tests.

A modified live-virus vaccine is effective in preventing excessive losses but its use is restricted. The disease is reportable. Quarantine and slaughter procedures adopted under this program have been successfully employed in commercial flocks in the U.S.A.

VIRAL HEPATITIS OF DUCKS

An acute, highly contagious, viral disease of young waterfowl, particularly ducklings, characterized by a short incubation period, sudden onset, high mortality and the development of rather characteristic liver lesions. It is found in all duck-raising areas of the world.

Etiology: A virus, readily propagated in chick and duck embryos, is the cause. It does not produce hemagglutination. Experience in the field indicates the absence of egg transmission. Experimentally, infection can be transmitted by parenteral or oral administration of infected tissues. A variant virus exists that is more difficult to isolate and replicate.

Clinical Findings: The incubation period is from 18 to 48 hours. Affected ducklings become lethargic, paddle spasmodically with their feet and die within a few minutes with typical opisthotonos. Clinical evidence of the disease has not been seen in ducks over 4 weeks of age. Mortality may be as high as 90%. Practically all deaths occur within a week after the onset of the disease.

Lesions: The liver is slightly enlarged and covered with hemorrhages from pinpoint-size to 1 cm in diameter.

Diagnosis: A presumptive diagnosis may be based on the history and pathognomonic lesions. Virus isolation or serum neutralization tests may be used for positive identification.

Prophylaxis and Treatment: Antibody therapy (antiserum or yolk) at the time of initial loss is the only effective flock treatment. Immunization of breeder ducks using modified live-virus vaccine provides parenteral immunity that effectively prevents the high losses in ducklings. Modified live or inactivated virus will also prevent high losses when products serologically similar to the infection are administered a week before exposure.

VIRAL HEPATITIS OF TURKEYS

An acute, highly contagious, frequently subclinical infection of turkeys which produces hepatic and pancreatic lesions.

Etiology and Incidence: The causal agent is isolated without difficulty from the liver or other tissues of poults, but is isolated less consistently from older birds. It grows readily in the yolk sac of 5- to 7-day-old chick or turkey embryos. It is thermostable, ether-, phenol- and Creolin-resistant, but is susceptible to a high, but not low pH. There is evidence that the infection is geographically widespread and it is common in some areas. Mortality has been reported only in poults.

Clinical Findings: The liver exhibits foci of necrosis which range from 1 to 3 mm in diameter and may be confluent. Hemorrhage or congestion may nearly obscure the degenerative changes. Occasionally, the liver is bile-stained. The liver lesions resemble those of blackhead, but the absence of cecal lesions in hepatitis helps to distinguish the 2 diseases. The pancreas frequently exhibits relatively large gray areas of degeneration.

In the subclinical form, the lesions are less extensive and hepatic hemorrhage or congestion is seldom prominent. Affected tissues return to normal in 3 to 4 weeks.

Most flock infections appear to be subclinical. Perhaps only under conditions of additional stress or other undetermined factors do morbidity or mortality occur. Clinical cases usually occur in poults between 1 and 3 weeks of age, but may be seen also in older birds. In these clinical infections, slight morbidity signaled by depression may be observed, but death is usually sudden. Losses may range from 2 to 20% with an average of 5%.

Diagnosis: Paratyphoid and paracolon infections produce necrotic areas in the liver that may be confused with those of virus hepatitis. These and other bacterial and mycotic infections must be eliminated by appropriate culturing techniques. Granulomas may be identified grossly or histologically. Blackhead usually produces concurrent cecal lesions unless modified by medication. In the latter case, histopathologic examination or demonstration of the respective etiologic agents is necessary.

Prophylaxis and Therapy: There is no known treatment. Secondary bacterial invasion does not appear to be important, but if it does occur it should be treated on the basis of specific etiology. Although recovered birds possess demonstrable resistance to reinfection, no circulating antibodies have been found. Sanitation may be of value in preventing dissemination of the agent.

THE SALMONELLOSES

Infections caused by *Salmonella* spp. may be divided into those caused by (1) two species highly host-adapted to the chicken and turkey (*Salmonella pullorum* and *S. gallinarum*), and (2) the remaining nonhost-adapted species comprising some 1300 species. The latter group (paratyphoid) may infect and be transmitted among almost all animals. (*See also* SALMONELLOSIS, p. 377). They have major public health significance because of possible infection of man from contamination of food.

A quite similar group of pathogens, important in turkeys, which are commonly called paracolons or *Arizona* spp., are now grouped as *Arizona hinshawi* and will be considered separately (p. 1041).

PULLORUM DISEASE

Infections by *S. pullorum* usually cause high mortality in young chickens and turkeys and occasionally in adult chickens. The disease in other avian species usually occurs only if these are maintained in close contact with infected chickens or turkeys. Infections in mammals are rare. Once common, the disease now has been eradicated from most commercial stock.

Transmission is chiefly by direct egg transmission, but may also occur by direct or indirect contact. Egg- or hatchery-transmitted infection usually results in mortality during the first few days of life and continues to 2 to 3 weeks of age. Affected birds huddle near a source of heat, do not eat, appear sleepy and show whitish fecal pasting around the vent. Survivors frequently become asymptomatic carriers with localized infection of the ovary. Some of the eggs laid by such hens hatch and produce infected progeny.

Lesions: Lesions in young birds usually include unabsorbed yolk-sacs, focal necrosis of the liver and spleen, and grayish nodules in the lungs, heart and gizzard muscle. Firm cheesy material in the ceca and raised plaques in the mucosa of the lower intestine are sometimes seen. Occasionally synovitis is prominent. Adult carriers sometimes have no gross lesions but usually they have pericarditis, peritonitis or distorted ovarian follicles with coagulated contents. Acute infections in mature chickens produce lesions that are indistinguishable from those of fowl typhoid.

Diagnosis: Lesions may be highly suggestive, but diagnosis should be confirmed by isolation and identification of *S. pullorum*. It is readily isolated by direct plating on most non-selective solid aerobic media. Infections in mature birds can be identified by serologic tests followed by necropsy and culturing for confirmation.

Treatment and Control: Several sulfonamides, antibiotics and other antibacterials are effective in reducing mortality but none eliminate the infection from a flock. Furazolidone at a level of 0.022% in the feed is one of the most effective treatments.

Control is based on a regular testing program of breeding stock to assure freedom from infection. Chickens are tested by a tube agglutination or whole-blood method. The latter method is not dependable for testing turkeys, and either a tube agglutination or serum plate test is used. Variant or polyvalent antigens are sometimes necessary.

FOWL TYPHOID

The causal agent, *S. gallinarum*, is very similar to *S. pullorum*, and some European workers consider them as one. Infection is now chiefly confined, in the U.S.A. and Canada, to a few areas. Although *S. gallinarum* is egg-transmitted and produces lesions in chicks and poults, similar to those produced by *S. pullorum*, it has a much greater tendency to be transmitted among growing or mature flocks. Mortality at all ages is usually high.

Lesions in the older bird consist of dehydration, swollen, friable and often bile-stained liver with or without necrotic foci, enlarged spleen and kidneys, anemia and enteritis. Diagnosis is accomplished by isolation and identification of the causal agent by standard bacteriologic methods.

Treatment and control are the same as for pullorum disease. The standard serologic tests for pullorum disease are equally effective in detecting fowl typhoid.

PARATYPHOID INFECTION

Paratyphoid infections may be caused by any one of the many nonhost-adapted salmonellae. Frequently several species infect a bird or flock concurrently. *S. typhimurium* is most common, but the prevalence of other species varies widely by geographic location and strain of bird. In the U.S.A., most infections are produced by 10 to 20 species. Probably all birds are susceptible, and infections are common in all species of domesticated birds. Usually the incidence in infected young flocks is high, but declines to a low percentage by maturity. Efforts to control paratyphoid infections in domestic poultry are chiefly stimulated by public health considerations.

Clinical Findings: Infections are often substantially subclinical. Mortality is chiefly confined to the first few weeks of age, and is higher in ducks and turkeys than in chickens. Some species or strains are more pathogenic than others. The stress of shipping, delayed feeding, chilling or overheating increases mortality. Clinical signs are not distinctive. Depression, poor growth, weakness, diarrhea and dehydration may occur. Lesions may include an enlarged liver with or without areas of focal necrosis, unabsorbed yolk sac with coagulation, and cecal cores. Occasionally infections localize in the eye or synovial tissues.

Diagnosis: Isolation and identification of the causal agent is essential. Direct culture from liver and yolk sac onto almost any standard type of aerobic media is adequate for isolation. Either a selenite or tetrathionate enrichment broth, transferred in 24 to 48 hours to brilliant green agar, may be used to isolate the organism from intestinal or environmental samples.

Treatment and Control: Several antibacterial agents are of value in preventing mortality; none is capable of eliminating flock infection. Furazolidone at 0.022% in the feed is commonly used. Turkeys, in particular, are commonly injected with one or more antibiotics after hatching.

Control methods have not been developed to the point of dependability. Strict sanitation in all hatching processes is helpful in preventing transmission between successive lots of birds in a house. Early fumigation of hatching eggs is recommended to prevent penetration by salmonellae on the shell surface. Washing should be done only if conditions are strictly controlled. No method has been devised to destroy the pathogens in the egg as a result of true egg transmission, although apparently such infection is relatively rare. The heat of pelleting is reasonably effective in destroying salmonellae in feed ingredients. Maintenance of poultry in confinement and exclusion of all pets, wild birds and rodents helps prevent introduction of infection. The water source should be free of contamination.

Several methods of determining the salmonella status of breeding flocks have been devised. Periodic cultural examination of environmental samples from litter, dust, and water and culturing samples of hatchery debris and cull chicks can be reasonably accurate for detecting infection. Serologic tests are not highly dependable but have been of value in detecting *S. typhimurium* infection in turkey flocks.

ARIZONA INFECTION
(Paracolon infection)

An acute or chronic egg-transmitted infection, chiefly of turkeys, by any of the serotypes of *Arizona hinshawii* (*Paracolobactrum arizonae*).

Etiology and Incidence: More than 100 serotypes have been identified from a variety of birds, mammals and reptiles. Two serotypes, 7:1,7,8 and 7:1,2,6, account for most isolates from turkeys; food-borne infections of man occur occasionally, but usually are produced by other serotypes. One or more *Arizona* serotypes are present in a large percentage of turkey flocks. Reptiles captured in the vicinity of turkeys are frequently infected and are thought to act as a reservoir of infection. Clinical infections in other birds and mammals are relatively rare.

Clinical Findings: Neither signs nor lesions are distinctive. Mortality is usually confined to the first 3 to 4 weeks of age. Poults are unthrifty, and in some flocks a considerable percentage develop eye opacity and blindness.
  Lesions: Yolk sacs are slowly absorbed and livers may be enlarged and mottled. Some flocks are extensively infected without developing appreciable mortality. Infection usually persists in a flock. Some birds develop peritonitis, salpingitis, or local ovarian infections, but infections of the intestinal tract are more common.

Diagnosis: A diagnosis must be based on isolation and identification of the organism. The same culture methods as those used for paratyphoids are satisfactory. Environmental samples may also be used for detecting infection. Egg transmission levels are often high so cultural examination of dead embryos, egg shells and cull poults may be used to identify infected breeding stock.

Treatment and Control: A variety of drugs are used to minimize mortality in poults. Streptomycin, spectinomycin or other antibiotics are commonly injected at the hatchery. Furazolidone at 0.011 to 0.022% in the feed is also often used during the first few weeks. Early fumigation of hatching eggs and rigorous hatchery sanitation are aids to reducing transmission.

FOWL CHOLERA

An acute or chronic, generalized or local, infectious disease of domestic poultry and wild birds, often of sudden onset with high morbidity and mortality, with enteritis, submucous and subserous hemorrhages, and vascular congestion.

Etiology and Incidence: *Pasteurella multocida,* the cause of fowl cholera, is a small, pleomorphic, gram-negative, nonmotile, aerobic rod which can infect a wide variety of birds and mammals, including man. Waterfowl seem particularly susceptible. It may survive at least 3 months in contaminated soil or in a decaying carcass. Drying and direct sunlight kill it. Sick or carrier birds and mammals contaminate feed, air, water and soil. Improper disposal of carcasses may allow spread by rodents and other scavengers. Birds on range are exposed to infected wild birds and mammals. Cold wet weather favors outbreaks.

P. haemolytica and *P. gallinarum* (considered by some as variants of *P. multocida*) and *Yersinia (Pasteurella) pseudotuberculosis* may be isolated from birds with cholera-like disease.

The disease is found universally, but it is not common in commercial chicken flocks in the U.S.A., except in crowded areas and where ranging is practiced. It is enzootic in some breeding hen flocks. The disease is rarely diagnosed in chickens younger than 12 weeks. Ranged turkey flocks are more likely to be exposed.

Clinical Findings: These vary greatly, depending on acuteness and localization. Often, birds will die suddenly. During an outbreak birds will be seen with cyanotic combs and wattles, difficult breathing, and copious watery diarrhea. Lameness and swollen joints are seen. Chronically infected birds may have swollen wattles or torticollis. In waterfowl, the disease is often peracute. Affected canaries are weak and comatose, puffed-out in appearance, with red or purple abdominal skin. More chronically affected canaries may survive for a time, having a depraved appetite and bloody or ocher droppings.

Lesions: Peracutely affected birds may have no visible lesions, acute ones may show petechiated mucous and serous membranes; in less acute cases there are usually small foci in a light-colored liver. Lung nodules may be found. Pus may be present in joints, tendon sheaths, middle ear, turbinates, infraorbital sinus, air passages, wattles and peritoneal cavity. The pus is initially fluid, later cheesy. The spleen occasionally is swollen and congested (more frequently in ducks and geese). There is usually a catarrhal enteritis. Canaries may have a "mulberry" liver and blood-tinged exudate in the peritoneal cavity. Edematous wattles, often unilateral, may be seen in the chronic form of the disease.

Diagnosis: Chickens and turkeys: Cholera must be distinguished from the salmonelloses, vibrionic hepatitis, staphylococcal infections, Newcastle disease, erysipelas, colibacillosis, ornithosis, fowl pox, and the purely respiratory diseases. The rabbit is the test animal of choice and will die in 12 hours when injected IP with infective materials.

Ducks and geese: Fowl cholera should be the first disease suspected in waterfowl. Botulism may be distinguished by lack of bacteremia. Birds suffering accidental deaths present evidence of trauma and have no bacteremia. Blockage of the digestive tract by fibrous material may cause cholera-like deaths.

Yellow foci are found in the liver and spleen of canaries with pseudotuberculosis. Ornithosis is distinguished by examination of Giemsa-stained smears of spleen surface. Streptococcosis is detected by the cocci in blood or exudates.

Prophylaxis: Polyvalent bacterins are effective in preventing the disease in chickens, turkeys and rabbits. These are best given as 2 or more doses subcut. at intervals of a month. Injection high on the neck may cause swollen heads. Vaccination after exposure is less satisfactory. Precautions to be taken are: complete separation of age groups, use of wire or concrete floors, screening against wild birds, keeping domestic pets out of houses, avoidance of ranging and use of proper disposal methods for carcasses. Depopulation and thorough clean-up is the most effective method of eliminating the infective agent from the premises.

Treatment: Drug therapy in the field is often handicapped by cold, damp weather which favors the disease and reduces water consumption. Since the appetite is usually poor in sick birds, the drug intake may be below effective levels. Sulfaquinoxaline sodium (Ŗ 87) in feed or water usually controls mortality, as do sulfamethazine (Ŗ 81) and sodium sulfamerazine (Ŗ 77). (Use sulfas with caution in breeders.) High levels (400 gm/ton) of tetracycline antibiotics in the feed or parenterally may be useful.

AVIAN STREPTOCOCCOSIS

An acute or chronic bacterial infection of chickens, turkeys and other birds of all ages, caused by various streptococcal species. Any one of *Streptococcus faecalis, Str. zooepidemicus,* or *Str. gallinarum* causes this disease. It occurs sporadically worldwide but is a relatively minor cause of disease loss. The natural means of spread is unknown but carriers may exist. In acute cases, death occurs with no premonitory signs. In more chronic cases, depression and debility are seen. The liver, lungs and other organs exhibit congestion and enlargement, with necrotic foci. Fibrinous peritoneal exudate with catarrhal enteritis is common. Finding and identifying the responsible organisms is the only definite means of diagnosis. Lesions may resemble those of pullorum disease, fowl cholera and other infectious diseases.

Therapy should be based on antibiotic sensitivity tests but is likely to be disappointing. General procedures, such as depopulation and thorough clean-up, may be necessary.

NEW DUCK SYNDROME
(Anatipestifer infection, Coliform septicemia)

A contagious respiratory disease, primarily of young ducks, characterized by a fibrinous pericarditis and peritonitis. It is probably the most important disease problem facing the duck industry in the U.S.A. The causal agent, *Pasteurella anatipestifer,* is fastidious and may be difficult to isolate. *Escherichia coli* may produce lesions similar to *P. anatipestifer* and can be isolated in pure culture.

Affected ducks have a mild cough, greenish-white diarrhea and show varying degrees of incoordination. Many birds have a head tremor. Others lie on their back and paddle with their feet. Dehydration often is the cause of death. Fibrinous pericarditis, perihepatitis, peritonitis and airsacculitis are the most constant lesions. The liver and spleen are swollen. Caseous pneumonia, salpingitis and fibrinous meningitis often visible grossly, may be present. A presumptive diagnosis may be made on the basis of the lesions and signs. Cultures of any isolated organism should exclude *P. multocida,* the causative agent of fowl cholera.

Sulfaquinoxaline (R 88) is recommended to prevent high mortality due to *P. anatipestifer.* Careful management has been most rewarding in controlling losses caused by *E. coli.*

TUBERCULOSIS

A slow-spreading, usually chronic, granulomatous bacterial infection of birds, usually mature, characterized by gradual weight loss.

Etiology and Occurrence: *Mycobacterium avium* is the usual cause, although *M. tuberculosis (hominis)* or *M. bovis* may also infect birds, especially parrots. *M. avium* is very resistant, surviving in the soil for as long as 4 years, in 5% phenol up to 24 hours, in 3% HCl for 2 hours or more, and in 4% NaOH for 30 min or more. The disease occurs worldwide, most commonly in small barnyard flocks with birds of several years running together, and in zoos; it is rarely found in large commercial flocks. Wild birds, such as starlings and raptors, have been found infected.

Infected birds excrete the organism in their feces. Cadavers and offal may infect predators and cannibalistic flockmates. Rabbits, swine and mink are readily infected. Cattle may be sensitized to tuberculin and johnin. Man is highly resistant but has been infected in a few instances.

Clinical Findings: Usually there are no signs until the disease has progressed to where the bird is thin and sluggish. Lameness may be observed. Granulomatous nodules of varying size are found in many parts of the body. In chickens, these are usually in the liver, spleen, bone marrow and intestine. Raptors usually have liver and spleen lesions, without intestinal involvement. Large pultaceous lesions may be found in body cavities. Bone marrow nodules and small mesenteric nodules may be found. Lesions are not calcified.

Diagnosis: The finding of acid-fast bacteria, usually present in large numbers, in impression smears from lesions permits a diagnosis. Live birds may be tested with avian and mammalian tuberculins, or serologically. False reactions due to exposure to other mycobacteria may occur.

Treatment and Control: Treatment is uneconomic in commercial poultry. It is probably inadvisable, and in some countries is illegal, even in valuable individuals, because of the possible danger to human health. In any case isoniazid is less effective against *M. avium,* and said to be toxic to birds. Streptomycin may also be toxic in the levels required to be effective.

Commercial poultry flocks are rarely affected. Relatively

rapid turnover of populations, together with improved general sanitation, has largely eliminated the once common infection. Infected poultry should be destroyed. If housed, the house should be thoroughly cleaned and disinfected. Dirt-floored houses should have several inches of the floor removed and replaced with dirt from a place where poultry have not ranged. All openings should be screened against wild birds. It is best not to reuse ranges where tuberculous poultry have been. The incidence of avian tuberculosis in zoos may be reduced by a regular program of tuberculin testing of new birds in quarantine and of all birds once a year.

ERYSIPELOTHRIX INFECTION

An acute or subacute septicemic disease of turkeys, particularly males, caused by *Erysipelothrix insidiosa* and characterized by multiple diffuse hemorrhages in the large muscle masses and under the serous surfaces of the visceral organs. Outbreaks of economic importance have also occurred in ducks and, occasionally, in geese. It occasionally causes disease in the domestic chicken.

Etiology: In the acute septicemic infection of poultry, *E. insidiosa* can be found in almost any part of the body including the blood. Contaminated soil probably is the source of infection and the organism probably enters the body through skin lesions. Uncooked fish meal or meat scraps in the feed are suspected as occasional sources of infection. In an outbreak the affected birds provide ample infective material for other members of the flock.

Clinical Findings: The disease usually appears in the fall and affects growing birds on range. Toms are more often affected than hens because of greater transmission during fighting. Affected birds lose their appetite, become listless and develop a greenish-yellow diarrhea. They may show dyspnea and a nasal discharge. A red-purple swelling of the caruncle is highly suggestive (but not pathognomonic) of *Erysipelothrix* infection. In untreated flocks, the mortality may reach 40%. The most characteristic lesions are diffuse hemorrhages in the abdominal, pectoral and femoral muscles as well as in the fascial sheaths. Subserous hemorrhages in viscera are also common. The liver and spleen are usually congested and enlarged and may present hemorrhagic infarcts. There may be a catarrhal exudate in the intestines.

Diagnosis: A tentative diagnosis may be made on the basis of lesions and clinical signs, but this should be confirmed by isolation and identification of *E. insidiosa*. A gram-stained smear from a lesion may enable an experienced diagnostician to recognize the organism by its size, shape, and usual occurrence in a paired "V" arrangement.

Prophylaxis: Bacterins prepared from immunogenic strains of *E. insidiosa* are widely used prophylactically. Immunity does not provide complete protection against severe artificial exposure but is usually adequate under field exposure. Occasionally, vegetative endocarditis and myocarditis develops from chronic local infection in vaccinated birds.

Treatment: All birds in affected flocks should be treated with penicillin, at 5,000 u/lb of body wt by subcut. or IM injection, and simultaneously injected with *E. insidiosa* bacterin. Penicillin alone will suppress infection for only 4 to 7 days. Parenterally administered streptomycin is also effective as well as orally administered tetracyclines at 400 to 500 gm/ton of feed.

LISTERIOSIS

This infection in birds occurs most frequently as a septicemia, but localized encephalitis similar to that seen in ruminants has been reported in chickens and turkeys, and encephalitis combined with septicemia has been observed in young geese. Chickens, geese, ducks and canaries appear to be the most commonly affected birds.

Etiology and Epizootiology: *Listeria monocytogenes* has been isolated from at least 22 avian species, including zoo specimens and game birds, indicating that the bacterium is widely distributed among fowls. Since it has been isolated from apparently normal birds and from birds dying from causes other than uncomplicated listeriosis, it is possible that birds may play an important role in the spread or perpetuation of the disease, not only in birds but also in mammals (including man). There is evidence that the bacterium may survive for at least 4 years in a chicken flock without manifestation of active disease. Further evidence incriminating birds as carriers is the frequent occurrence of relatively high agglutinating-antibody titers against *L. monocytogenes* in apparently normal birds and the common association of *L. monocytogenes* with other diseases, such as salmonellosis, Newcastle disease, worm infections, lymphomatosis and devitalization due to other causes.

Conjunctivitis due to *L. monocytogenes* in people employed in poultry-processing plants has been traced to the handling of apparently normal, but infected, chickens. There is strong circumstantial evidence that other forms of listeric infection, particularly listeric abortion in women, may result from contact with infected or carrier birds.

Clinical Findings and Diagnosis: Young birds appear to be more susceptible. In listeric septicemia among domestic birds, outbreaks are sporadic and mortality in the individual flock may vary within wide limits. Adult birds usually die suddenly with few clinical signs, while young birds waste slowly before death. At necropsy in uncomplicated listeric infection, the most striking lesion may be either massive necrosis of the myocardium with pericarditis and an increased amount of pericardial fluid, or focal hepatic necrosis, or both. The gram-positive *L. monocytogenes* may be found in the myocardial fibrils, and within or adjacent to the hepatic cells. There may be generalized edema, splenomegaly, peritonitis, enteritis and salpingitis. These lesions may be absent when listeric infection is associated with other disorders. The bacterium is most easily cultivated from the blood or from the affected organs. In some instances it may be necessary to refrigerate the tissue to be cultured before the bacterium can be isolated.

In listeric encephalitis, the signs are marked torticollis, a tendency to walk in circles and coarse tremors of the skeletal muscles. No gross lesions have been reported for this form of the disease, and *L. monocytogenes* can be isolated only from the brain.

Control: Recommended control includes rigid sanitation and culling and isolation of affected birds. The present widespread use of poultry feeds containing antibiotics may be an effective prophylactic measure against listeric infection.

SPIROCHETOSIS

An acute or chronic, febrile, bacterial disease of birds, characterized by listlessness and leg weakness.

Borrelia anserina, the causal organism, is thin (0.4 μ), actively motile, spiral, and of variable length (6 to 30 μ). It may be cultivated in complex culture media containing serum, in chicken embryos, or in chicks. The disease occurs in many parts of the world, generally in tropical or temperate regions, including several of the Southwestern States. It affects gallinaceous birds, waterfowl and a wide variety of other birds. The disease is transmissible through droppings or other moist materials containing the organism, or indirectly through blood-sucking arthropods, notably *Argas persicus*.

Clinical Findings: Affected birds are droopy, weak in the legs, feverish, thirsty and have a yellow-green diarrhea with increased urates. Incoordination or complete paralysis may be seen. The spleen is often enlarged or mottled, the heart may be enlarged and pale, and the liver is usually enlarged and congested, with many small foci. There is catarrhal enteritis, with large amounts of yellow-green urates in the posterior gut.

Diagnosis: Dark-field microscopic examination of a thin wet smear of the blood reveals actively motile spirochetes, usually in great numbers. At crisis, late in the disease, agglutinins appear which clump the spirochetes in large round masses. Later still, they may be very scarce. Since it is possible to mistake filamentous protoplasmic extrusions from erythrocytes or motile haemosporidial microgametes for spirochetes, stained smears must be examined with care. Clumped organisms resemble smudged leukocytes, and it is easy to miss the occasional spirochete in late stages. Following crisis an agglutination test may be used for diagnosis.

Treatment and Control: Penicillin (1000 u/lb body wt), neoarsphenamine (5 mg/lb), and oxytetracycline (1 mg/lb) are among the drugs effective parenterally. Bacterins are used successfully in many parts of the world to prevent losses. A coccidiostat containing an arsenical, roxarsone, at levels used for controlling coccidiosis, is said to prevent development of the disease in artificially infected birds. Screening of houses and insecticide applications help reduce the level of exposure by vectors.

NECROTIC DERMATITIS
(Clostridial dermatomyositis, Gangrenous dermatitis, Gangrenous cellulitis)

An infectious disease of chickens characterized by sudden onset, a sharp increase in mortality and gangrenous necrosis of the skin over the thighs and breast. This disease occurs sporadically in growing chickens from 4 to 16 weeks of age and affects both broiler and layer replacement stock.

Etiology: *Clostridium septicum* is the most commonly isolated pathogen but other clostridia, notably *Cl. perfringens*, Type A, and *Cl. novyi* (*oedematiens*) have been reported. Other bacteria almost always accompany the clostridia in culture, particularly *Staphylococcus* spp. and *Escherichia coli*. In addition, numerous environmental factors appear to be involved. These include: skin trauma from surgical procedures, mechanical devices or cannibalism; heavily contaminated, moist built-up litter; and devitalization of the skin as occurs in staphylococcal infections and in selenium deficiency. The disease has been produced by subcut. or IM inoculation of *Cl. septicum* in conjunction with a chemical irritant (calcium chloride). Inoculated chickens develop gangrenous necrosis of the skin and underlying musculature and death frequently occurs within 12 to 48 hours.

Clinical Findings: The first sign is usually a sudden drastic increase in mortality in the affected flock; overall mortality ranges from 10 to 60%. Affected chickens die within 8 to 24 hours after showing signs of extreme depression, lameness and prostration. Externally, there are patches of red to black gangrenous skin over the breast or thighs and frequently feather loss or sloughing of the epidermis are noted. Palpation of the affected areas often reveals crepitation owing to gas bubbles in the subcutis and musculature. At necropsy, there is accumulation of bubbly serosanguineous fluid in the subcutis and the underlying musculature has a cooked appearance. The liver and spleen are enlarged and may contain large areas of necrotic infarcts. The kidneys are usually swollen and the lungs are congested and edematous.

Diagnosis: The most definitive diagnostic procedures are histopathologic demonstration of gas gangrene and numerous large filamentous bacilli in the skin, musculature and liver, and isolation of the causative clostridia. These procedures coupled with the history and clinical findings will differentiate this condition from exudative diathesis (selenium deficiency), staphyloccal infection and other diseases involving the skin.

Control: This disease can usually be prevented by maintaining proper litter condition, minimizing mechanical injury and controlling cannibalism through effective debeaking or other procedures. The causative organisms are sensitive to a wide variety of antibiotics *in vitro*. Administration of oxytetracycline or chlortetracycline at 200 gm/ton of feed has produced a rapid decline of mortality in field outbreaks.

AVIAN VIBRIONIC HEPATITIS
(Avian infectious hepatitis)

A usually chronic, sometimes subacute or acute, disease of chickens characterized chiefly by parenchymal degeneration and necrosis of the liver. The disease has been recognized in most of the poultry-raising areas of North America, in Northern Europe and in South America. It is found most often in mature stock, although birds as young as 4 weeks of age may become infected.

Etiology: Avian vibrionic hepatitis is caused by a *Vibrio*. Once the disease becomes established on a farm, it tends to recur. The organism is isolated most easily from the bile, but can also be isolated from the liver, heart, blood, spleen and kidneys. It grows readily when inoculated into the yolk sacs of 6-day-old chick embryos where it causes mortality within 3 to 6 days. Reducing oxygen tension enhances growth in a variety of enriched media. The organisms remain viable in bile samples for 5 to 7 days when stored at 4°C, and for at least 2 years when kept frozen at −70°C. Turkey poults (only very young poults), rabbits, pheasants, ducks and mice can be experimentally infected, but hamsters appear to be refractory.

Clinical Findings: Vibrionic hepatitis has an insidious onset, and usually only a few birds in a flock appear affected at any one time. Occasionally the disease is acute, with sudden deaths. In subacutely affected pullet flocks, egg production lags, while in older flocks, egg production may decrease as much as 35% over extended periods. Severely affected birds lose weight and are listless and roost or stand apart from the rest of the flock. Their combs usually become shriveled, dry and scaly. Birds less severely affected may appear normal, but their egg production pattern is intermittent. Both light and heavy breeds are susceptible.

Lesions: The most striking features of the disease in older chickens are the variable hemorrhagic and necrotic changes in the liver. Some livers have many small hemorrhages, but occasionally there are bubble-like hematocysts under the capsule. Severe hemorrhage sometimes ruptures the capsule, releasing blood into the body cavity. Other livers have a few pinhead-sized grayish-white necrotic foci, or are enlarged and mahogany-brown, or may be firm and friable with irregular asterisk- or cauliflower-shaped necrotic areas up to 1 cm in diameter distributed throughout. Often the liver is bile-stained. Ascites and hydropericardium are seen; the kidneys are enlarged and pale. A catarrhal enteritis is often present. In young chickens, the heart lesions are more severe and consistent than in mature birds.

In mild or early infections, lymphocytic and heterophilic portal triad infiltration is seen. Fatty metamorphosis, congestion, vascular dilatation and hemorrhage are observed in the liver. In more severe cases, lymphocytic and granulocytic foci, focal degeneration and irregular areas of necrosis are the predominant changes. The liver capsule may be thickened by edema and inflammatory cells. The kidneys have focal areas of heterophils and lymphocytes, often in interstitial areas. The bone marrow has increased numbers of large immature myelocytes. Blood examinations indicate an increase in the heterophil, thrombocyte and total leukocyte counts and a decrease in the hemoglobin content, packed cell volume, and erythrocyte and lymphocyte counts.

Parasitic infections and other stressor agents appear to enhance pathogenicity of the *Vibrio* and may be necessary to allow important pathogenic expression.

Diagnosis: A presumptive diagnosis of hepatitis can be made from a typical history of low egg production, an increased number of culls and careful postmortem examination of multiple specimens. In most cases, the lesions can readily be distinguished from those of leukosis.

Heavy seeding of blood-agar plates with bile followed by 18 to 24 hours incubation under reduced oxygen tension (10% CO_2) allows sufficient growth so that the vibrios can be demonstrated in stained smears or by phase-contrast microscopy. The inoculation of embryos is a more sensitive method for isolating *Vibrio*, but is more expensive and time-consuming than agar inoculation. Histologic examination of tissues can be used as an aid in diagnosis if attempts to isolate the *Vibrio* fail.

Treatment: Dihydrostreptomycin sulfate (25 mg/lb of body wt, one injection IM) or furazolidone (200 gm/ton of mash on an all-mash diet for 14 days and 100 gm/ton for a further 14 days) gives good control, if given early in an outbreak. Since exposure apparently leads to little immunity, reinfection sometimes occurs. The only recourse is to treat again.

AVIAN MYCOPLASMOSIS

Several *Mycoplasma* spp. have been isolated from avian hosts. Only 3 of these fastidious bacterial species (*M. galli-*

septicum, M. meleagridis and *M. synoviae*) have been demonstrated to be important pathogens of poultry. Each has significantly distinctive epizootiologic and pathologic characteristics.

MYCOPLASMA GALLISEPTICUM
INFECTION (MG)
(PPLO infection, Chronic respiratory disease,
CRD, Infectious sinusitis of turkeys)

A chronic primary infection of the respiratory tract of chickens, turkeys and occasionally other avian species which is often complicated by other infectious agents.

Etiology and Incidence: The causative agent, *Mycoplasma gallisepticum*, can be isolated and propagated in embryonating chicken embryos and in a variety of artificial media. The infection has been identified in all major chicken- and turkey-producing areas of the world. Until recently a majority of flocks were infected.

Clinical Findings: Spread is usually slow both within and between pens; although aerosol transmission can be important during the clinical disease, most birds are infected through the egg. Such infected progeny commonly carry the infection in a latent form for weeks or months before clinical signs become evident. Clinical disease is often precipitated by stresses such as crowding, onset of egg production, infections from live-virus vaccines, or field infection with infectious bronchitis or Newcastle disease.

Affected chickens show varying degrees of respiratory distress. In uncomplicated cases, signs may be so minor that rales are only heard at night. Mortality is significant only if there are complicating infections. Feed conversion, rate of lay, hatchability, and chick and poult quality are adversely affected. Turkeys are likely to develop severe sinusitis.

Clinical recovery of the flock occurs after several weeks or months, but the infection remains and egg transmission can be expected to continue, though with decreasing frequency, for the remainder of life.

Lesions: Uncomplicated MG infections in chickens result in relatively mild sinusitis, tracheitis and airsacculitis. In broilers in particular, *Escherichia coli* infections are often concurrent and result in severe air-sac thickening, turbidity, and exudative accumulations together with fibrinopurulent pericarditis and perihepatitis. Localization in synovial tissues sometimes occurs. Turkeys develop severe mucopurulent sinusitis, and varying degrees of tracheitis and airsacculitis.

Diagnosis: Agglutination reactions with MG antigen are most commonly used for diagnosis. Occasional cross-agglutination from *M. synoviae* antibodies occurs. Isolation from affected tissues can be accomplished in MG-free embryos or chicks or in appropriate artificial media. Isolates must be identified as several different *Mycoplasma* spp. are found in birds. Intercurrent infections with Newcastle disease, infectious bronchitis, influenza, chlamydiae and other respiratory pathogens offer the major problem of differential diagnosis.

Treatment and Control: Many antibacterial agents have been shown to be useful in the control of this disease—chlortetracycline, erythromycin, carbomycin, oxytetracycline, spiramycin, streptomycin and tylosin. The last seems to be most effective. In chickens there are often complicating infections, and variations in treatment response occur that are due to the differences in susceptibility of the secondary invaders.

The usual recommendation in handling field cases is to use an injectable antibiotic if the disease is severe, followed by feed or water treatments for 3 to 5 days. In milder infections feed or water administration is usually sufficient.

Eradication of MG from both chicken and turkey breeding stock is well advanced in the U.S.A. and several other countries. Control has been based on identifying isolated groups of breeders which are not infected as indicated by agglutination tests, or by treating hatching eggs, usually with tylosin or by heating, to destroy the infecting organism. Progeny are hatched and maintained in isolation from infected stock and tested periodically.

MYCOPLASMA MELEAGRIDIS INFECTION (MM)

A widespread infectious disease of turkeys chiefly affecting the respiratory tract of young birds but commonly present in the reproduction tract of breeding hens.

Etiology and Incidence: *Mycoplasma meleagridis,* the causal agent, was recognized as a major pathogen of turkeys following the widespread elimination of *M. gallisepticum* from breeding stock. Infection is currently present in all major turkey bloodlines and in most flocks.

Epizootiology: Transmission of *M. meleagridis* among adult turkeys and between generations is unique among avian diseases in being closely related to genital contact. Early infections usually become quiescent by sexual maturity. The phallus and adjacent area of the tom retain infection and contaminate semen, which serves as a vehicle for infecting the vagina of the hen. Hens may also retain infection in the bursa of Fabricius which serves as a source of infection of the reproductive tract following rupture of the cloacal-vaginal occluding membrane at puberty. Such infections ascend the reproductive system and may reach the surface of the ovary. The high rate of egg transmission of *M. meleagridis* that results from infection of the reproductive tract of the hen is not true transovarian infection but rather infection incorporated during the formation of the egg following ovulation. Transmission also occurs between birds chiefly in young flocks with active infections of the respiratory tract.

Clinical Findings: Egg infection appears to reduce hatchability and poult quality. In stressful conditions poult mortality may be considerable during the first few weeks. Growth rates may be reduced. It appears that infections of the periarticular tissues of the hock joints and of the cervical vertebrae as well as adjacent bone during early rapid growth can produce major bone deformities resulting in crooked necks and hocks. Rales may develop in flocks at 3 to 8 weeks of age and persist for several weeks without significant mortality or serious interference with growth rate.

Lesions: Poults have airsacculitis with thickening, turbidity, and sometimes marked caseous exudative accumulations. Respiratory signs are seldom evident in the young bird. Tracheitis and airsacculitis may develop and produce clinical signs after a few weeks. Lesions often recede with advancing age but may be present at slaughter and cause considerable condemnation.

Treatment and Control: No practical method of eradicating infection from flocks has been developed. Dipping hatching eggs in or injecting them with tylosin is effective in reducing the incidence of egg transmission and subsequent bone deformities. Procedural precautions to minimize contamination during semen collection and artificial insemination help prevent infecting the female genital tract. Several serologic tests have been used experimentally to detect infection. Such tests are dependable during periods of active infection but often fail to show a reaction when the pathogen is quiescent.

INFECTIOUS SYNOVITIS
(Infectious arthritis)

An infectious disease of poultry, characterized by inflammation of the synovial membranes. It occurs most frequently in chickens 4 to 10 weeks of age, and has been found in turkeys. The condition has also been called enlarged hock condition, arthritis and tendovaginitis. It has been reported from all of the important poultry-growing areas in the U.S.A., as well as from Canada and Great Britain.

Etiology: The causative agent, *Mycoplasma synoviae*, has fastidious growth requirements. The incubation period following artificial infection varies from 5 to 10 days; the disease usually is clearly evident in 7 days. Older birds are usually more resistant. The natural mode of transmission is not clear, although experimental studies indicate that the organism is egg-borne or inhaled.

Clinical Findings and Lesions: The liver is enlarged and sometimes discolored green. The spleen is enlarged and the kidneys are enlarged and pale. These lesions are particularly characteristic early in the disease and are less apparent as the disease progresses. A yellow, viscid exudate is present in almost all synovial structures; most commonly observed in the keel bursa, hock and wing joints, it is also seen in the mandibular, costal and digital articulations. In chronic cases, this exudate may become inspissated and orange in color.

Although the disease has been reported in older birds, those between 4 and 8 weeks of age are more commonly affected. The first sign is lameness and swelling of the hock and other joints. Green droppings are also a constant early feature. In field outbreaks, although mortality may be very low, the disease produces up to 30% of cull and crippled birds.

Diagnosis: A field (presumptive) diagnosis can be made based on the lesions and clinical signs described above. The green discoloration of the liver must be differentiated from that seen in fowl typhoid and staphylococcal infection in turkeys. The synovial exudate may be similar to that seen in staphylococcal arthritis, but in synovitis its yellowish color and sticky homogeneous consistency are different. The fact that all synovial structures tend to be involved in infectious synovitis helps to differentiate it from a staphylococcal infection. Pullorum disease may cause swellings of the joints clinically simulating synovitis. Agglutination and hemagglutination-inhibition tests have been developed, but there is evidence of cross-reaction with *M. gallisepticum* when either infection produces a high titer of agglutinins.

Treatment and Control: Serologic testing and isolation similar to the *M. gallisepticum* program should eventually control this infection. The most effective treatment at present is the administration of chlortetracycline in the feed at the rate of 200 gm per ton. Oxytetracycline also gives beneficial results. The IM injection of 200 mg streptomycin per bird very early in the course of the disease is quite effective in operations where individual birds can be treated and witholding times can be met. The condition has been prevented experimentally by the administration of 100 gm of one of the tetracycline antibiotics per ton of feed. Field use indicates similar results under natural conditions. Some differences in the susceptibility of isolates to various medicaments have been noted, which may explain the variable response in treating field cases.

INFECTIOUS CORYZA

An acute or chronic disease of chickens, characterized by nasal discharge, sneezing and swelling or edema of the face and, less frequently, by lower respiratory tract infection.

Etiology and Epizootiology: *Haemophilus gallinarum,* the causative agent, is a hemophilic, gram-negative, pleomorphic, nonmotile bacterium. The disease has been found throughout the U.S.A. and has been reported from many other parts of the world. Its incidence varies greatly from area to area and at the present time is not a problem except in certain endemic locations such as California. Acute, uncomplicated infectious coryza is characterized by rapid onset, the nasal discharge appearing on the first or second day following artificial inoculation. This type is of relatively short duration in the laboratory, but usually runs a longer course under natural conditions.

Introduction of the disease into the flock results in rapid spread and high morbidity. The course in a flock may be as short as 10 to 14 days, or extend as long as several months. The mortality may be negligible, but adverse effects on body weight and egg production may be considerable. Complications with other infections are common, resulting in more severe chronic disease. Chickens that recover may be carriers for months and are the most common source of new outbreaks. Transmission takes place by airborne infective droplets and by contamination of drinking water and equipment.

Clinical Findings: In its mildest form, the only sign is a serous nasal discharge, either persistent or of short duration, with little or no systemic effect. In the more severe form, there is edema of the face that may extend, especially in males, to the intermandibular space and wattles. In chronic cases the adjacent sinuses become distended with a yellow caseous exudate. Other complications may be conjunctivitis, tracheitis, bronchitis and airsacculitis.

Diagnosis: Reproduction of the typical disease by contact or intranasal inoculation and demonstration of *H. gallinarum* is the most reliable procedure. A history of a nasal discharge which affects a large percentage of the chickens and persists in a flock for weeks or months is good presumptive evidence. Swelling of the face and wattles must be differentiated from fowl cholera. Other diseases that must be considered are mycoplasmosis (CRD), laryngotracheitis, fowl pox, infectious bronchitis, Newcastle disease and vitamin A deficiency.

Prophylaxis and Treatment: In endemic areas, all replacements should be made with day-old chicks unless the bird source is known to be free of infectious respiratory diseases. Survivors of an outbreak should be completely and permanently separated from all other chickens either by segregation in a separate house or removal from premises. Recurrence may be ascribed to carrier birds and the fact that the infection engenders only a transient low-grade immunity.

Early treatment is important, therefore water is medicated immediately and until it can be replaced with medicated feed. Erythromycin (R 20) has been reported to be beneficial in some cases. Various sulfonamides (e.g., R 77, 81) have been used and streptomycin has been found to be effective when used IM at a dosage of 200 mg per bird. In more severe outbreaks, treatment may result in improvement, but the disease may recur when medication is discontinued.

Autogenous bacterins have been reported to be beneficial in protecting against a decrease in egg production and lesions in the lower respiratory tract. Some states have licensed bacterins, however their regulatory status is uncertain.

OMPHALITIS
(Navel ill, "Mushy chick" disease)

A specific condition characterized by infected, unhealed navels in chicks, poults and other young fowl.

Etiology: This noncontagious disease is associated with excessive humidity and marked contamination of the incubator. The navels fail to close. Opportunist bacteria (coliforms, staphylococci, *Pseudomonas* and *Proteus*) are often recovered. Proteolytic anaerobes are prevalent in outbreaks. Losses may be increased by chilling or overheating during shipment.

Clinical Findings: The affected chicks or poults usually appear normal until a few hours before death. Depression, drooping of the head and huddling near the source of heat usually are the only signs. The navel is found inflamed and a scab may be present. The yolk sac is not absorbed and is often highly congested or broken, with extensive peritonitis. Edema of the sternal subcutis may occur. Mortality often begins with hatching and continues to the 10th to 14th day of age, with losses to 15% in chickens or 50% in turkeys. Persistent unabsorbed, infected yolks often produce stunted chicks or poults.

Prophylaxis: Careful control of temperature, humidity and sanitation in the incubator will prevent the disease. Only clean, uncracked eggs should be set. If eggs are washed, a sanitizing detergent must be used according to directions. Time, temperature and frequent changes of water are equally as critical as the concentration of sanitizer in both wash and rinse water. The rinse should be warmer than the wash water but not over 140°F.

The incubator should be thoroughly cleaned and fumigated between hatches and prior to the start of the hatching season. Fumigation must be carried out with closed vents at high temperature and humidity. Thirty milliliters of formalin (40% formaldehyde) and 15 gm of potassium permanganate should be used per 20 cu ft, or paraformaldehyde in a heating device should be used in strength recommended by the manufacturer. Contamination of the machines may readily occur following fumigation unless care is taken to clean and disinfect the exterior of the machines and the rooms in which they are located.

There is no specific treatment.

ULCERATIVE ENTERITIS
(Quail disease)

An acute or chronic infection, primarily of the lower intestine, which is particularly severe in quail but also occurs in chickens, turkeys, pheasants, grouse, pigeons and probably other species.

Etiology: The infectious agent is a gram-positive bacillus with subterminal spores; there is considerable evidence that it is a *Clostridium,* usually *Cl. perfringens* type A. Particularly in species less susceptible than the quail, it appears likely that some predisposing factor or factors are necessary to produce the disease.

Clinical Findings: Susceptible quail may suffer an explosive disease with virtually 100% mortality in a few days. In other species, clinical signs are usually less dramatic and mortality usually does not exceed 10% and may be much lower during the clinical course of 2 to 3 weeks or more. Affected birds may die without obvious premonitory signs with little weight loss. Infected quail discharge characteristic droppings that are streaked with urates and have a watery ring. Chronically affected birds are listless, anorectic and humped up, with retracted neck and partially closed eyes. Recovered birds are resistant to reinfection but may act as carriers.

    Lesions: The primary lesions are in the ceca and intestine. Acute lesions are punctate hemorrhages in the wall of the lower intestine accompanied by enteritis. Chronic lesions appear as necrotic ulcers in the mucosa surrounded by an inflammatory zone or as large ulcers with yellow diphtheritic membranes with depressed centers and raised edges. Perforating ulcers may result in local or diffuse peritonitis. Hepatic changes appear as yellow foci or irregularly shaped yellow areas in the parenchyma. The spleen may be enlarged and hemorrhagic.

Diagnosis: Although histomoniasis and the hemorrhagic syndrome may superficially resemble ulcerative enteritis, coccidiosis causes the greatest problem of differential diagnosis. Often both infections occur simultaneously. The spore-forming rods can be demonstrated in Gram's stains of blood, liver and spleen from septicemic specimens. Histopathologic lesions of the affected intestine show severe tissue destruction and massive invasion by these bacteria. Isolation can be accomplished by injecting liver and spleen suspensions into the yolksac of 5-day-old chicken embryos. Heating the inoculum at 70°C for 10 minutes prior to inoculation helps assure freedom from contaminating bacteria.

Prophylaxis and Treatment: The etiologic agent apparently is a frequent environmental contaminant and in common with other spore-forming bacilli is highly resistant to an adverse environment. It is particularly useful to maintain quail on clean ground or on porches with wire or slat floors. Ground that has been contaminated with the organism should not be used for quail for at least 2 years. As recovered birds may act as carriers, strict isolation should be maintained between young stock and recovered birds.

The drugs of choice are bacitracin and streptomycin. Streptomycin can be used prophylactically or therapeutically in the drinking water (R 57) and in the feed at the rate of 30 mg/lb (60 gm/ton). Bacitracin is used in the feed at the rate of 50 to 100 gm/ton or in the drinking water at the same rate as streptomycin (R 57). The tetracyclines (R 15, 36), and furazolidone at the rate of 200 gm/ton of feed are also effective.

Birds exposed to natural infection without treatment develop some immunity, but medicated flocks often have little resistance against reinfection. Therefore, contaminated litter should be removed and it may be necessary to continue or repeat treatment periodically.

BLUECOMB DISEASE OF CHICKENS

(Pullet disease, Avian monocytosis,
Summer disease, Housing disease)

An acute or subacute condition primarily of young laying chickens, of nonbacterial origin, but otherwise suggestive of an infectious disease. The demonstrable changes are in the nature of a hepatonephrosis.

Etiology: The true cause of the disease and its status as a distinct entity have not been established. Absence of significant cultivable bacterial organisms is characteristic. Predisposing factors are assumed to be hot weather, dehydration, abrupt changes in feed or environment, delayed vaccination procedures and, in general, factors leading to faulty adaptation. It occurs predominantly during the warm season, especially 3 to 4 days after temperatures exceed 85°F. However, experimental exposure to high ambient temperatures, with or without adequate water supply, has failed to reproduce the disease. A filterable, nonhemagglutinating agent has been isolated from the intestinal contents of acutely affected birds, suggesting a viral etiology.

Clinical Findings: Although the various names attached to the syndrome suggest a preferential incidence as to sex, age and season, exceptions are noted. Usually, the onset is sudden and characterized by decreased feed consumption, lowered egg production, depression and whitish or watery, often fetid, diarrhea. Individual birds may exhibit crop distension, cyanosis, sunken eyes and terminal fever. Initial mortality may be high, but the total rarely exceeds 5%. The course of the disease is about 2 weeks. Hematologic examination usually reveals hemoconcentration with increased coagulability and hemoglobin, and absolute and relative monocytosis. The cells are mostly of the mature type. Biochemical studies of blood may disclose a uremia.

Lesions: Bluecomb disease is characterized by dehydration, circumscribed pale areas of degeneration in the skeletal musculature, sparse petechiation of serous membranes, delicate, evenly spaced, yellow foci in the liver, mucoid enteritis, chalky appearance of the pancreas, degenerative ovarian follicles and various renal changes from edema to uric nephritis. Histopathologically, affected muscle is characterized by Zenker's degeneration, and liver by focal necrosis. A catarrhal enteritis may be present with obstructive mucoid casts, while the gross pancreatic changes correspond to cloudy swelling of the acinar tissue. Renal lesions vary from glomerular tuft swellings and tubular casts with pseudo-giant-cell formation to crystalloid uric acid foci.

Diagnosis: The common infectious and neoplastic conditions, such as fowl cholera, pullorum disease and leukosis, must be excluded. Hematologic examinations, especially differential counts, are of value in birds that show no gross lesions.

Control: Chlortetracycline (B 12) or oxytetracycline (B 31) have given good results. Good management practices are important. Grain feeding should be reduced. Black-strap molasses, perhaps because of its high-potassium content, is used either in the drinking water (2%) or in an intermittently administered crumbly wet mash (up to 30%). Since birds often refuse food, medication in the drinking water is preferable, either with 0.5% potassium chloride, or with soluble preparations of chlortetracycline (B 16), or oxytetracycline (B 32) at rates of 2 to 10 gm/10 gal. After a week, the water treatment may be replaced by either 1.5% potassium chloride in the feed, or by high-level antibiotic mashes for 2 weeks (B 15, 36).

For prevention of the syndrome, poultry operations should be planned carefully so as to avoid stress factors, such as vaccinations near commencement of lay, insufficient shade or ventilation, inadequate water supply and abrupt changes in feeding and management.

TRANSMISSIBLE ENTERITIS OF TURKEYS
(Bluecomb, Mud fever)

An acute highly infectious disease of turkeys characterized by anorexia, diarrhea, weight loss and mortality, particularly in poults.

Etiology: Although the disease is readily reproduced by feeding bacteria-free filtrates of intestinal contents from infected turkeys to susceptible poults, the etiologic agent has not been clearly defined. It is thought to be either a reo- or picornavirus. Multiple agents could be responsible for the syndrome.

Clinical Findings: A short incubation period, often 48 to 72 hours, is followed by general depression, anorexia and diarrhea in the flock. Discolored fluid droppings with mucoid threads or casts, dehydration, and marked weight loss is evident. Body temperature is subnormal. Mortality may approach 100%, but is greatly influenced by environmental conditions and age of the flock.

Lesions are chiefly confined to the intestines, which show some inflammation, contain fluid, and sometimes foamy material often with gelatinous or mucoid casts. Dehydration is prominent. The spleen is often reduced in size.

Diagnosis: Although clinical findings and lesions are highly suggestive of transmissible enteritis, caution in diagnosis is necessary because of lack of pathognomonic lesions and a demonstrable infectious agent. Other disorders producing similar signs should be eliminated. Hexamitiasis in young poults and lack of feed and water at any age can produce similar signs.

Prophylaxis and Treatment: Infection is not egg-transmitted but infected birds shed the agent for a considerable time. Poults should be raised in isolation from infected or recovered stock.

Affected flocks should be protected from adverse environmental conditions; elevating brooding temperatures, providing supplemental heat, and sheltering ranged flocks is helpful. Antibiotics appear to be useful, probably by indirect effect. Water medication is preferred as sick birds drink more than they eat. The antibiotics which may be effective at 1 gm per gal. are neomycin, streptomycin, penicillin, bacitracin, oxytetracycline and chlortetracycline; however, such treatment for 5 to 10 days often results in serious *Candida* infections.

MYCOTIC DISEASES

ASPERGILLOSIS

(Brooder pneumonia, Mycotic pneumonia, Pneumomycosis)

A disease, usually of the respiratory system, of chickens and turkeys and less frequently of ducklings, pigeons, canaries, geese and many other wild birds. In chickens and turkeys, the disease may be epizootic on some farms, whereas, in wild birds, it appears to be sporadic, frequently affecting only an individual bird.

Etiology: It is generally agreed that *Aspergillus fumigatus* is the cause of the disease. However, several other species of *Aspergillus,* as well as other genera, such as *Penicillium,* may be incriminated.

Clinical Findings: Dyspnea, gasping, accelerated breathing and signs of nervous involvement may be observed. Somnolence, inappetence, emaciation and increased thirst are also present. The encephalitic form appears most commonly in turkeys.

Lesions: In young chicks or poults up to 6 weeks of age, the lungs are most frequently involved. Pulmonary lesions are characterized by cream-colored plaques from a few millimeters up to several centimeters in diameter. Such lesions may also be found in the syrinx, air sacs, and systemically, in the liver, intestines and occasionally the brain. An ocular form of the disease has been observed in chickens and turkeys in which large plaques may be expressed from the medial canthus.

Diagnosis: The fungus can be demonstrated by cultural methods or by microscopic examination of fresh preparations. One of the plaques teased apart and placed on a Petri dish of suitable fungus media usually results in a pure culture of the organism. Histopathologic examination using a special fungus stain, reveals granulomas containing mycelia. Confirmation of pathogenicity of the isolate is accomplished by injecting it into the air sacs of susceptible 3-week-old chicks.

Differential diagnosis from infectious bronchitis, Newcastle disease and laryngotracheitis is important. Aspergillosis is usually seen in birds 7 to 40 days old.

Prophylaxis and Treatment: The avoidance of moldy litter or feed serves to prevent outbreaks. Treatment of affected individuals is considered useless. The organism is frequently found in wet hay or sawdust litter. Often infection will clear up in young birds if the flock is culled, the house thoroughly cleaned and fresh litter from a different source used. All moldy litter should be removed and burned. The pen should be sprayed with 1% copper sulfate and all equipment cleaned and disinfected.

MYCOTOXICOSIS
(Turkey X disease, Aflatoxicosis)

Disease caused by ingestion of aflatoxin, which is produced by *Aspergillus flavus* growing on the feed—groundnut (peanut) meal, cereals, etc. *See also* pp. 992-997.

Clinical Findings: Depression, inappetence and reduced growth rate, together with loss of condition and mortality, are common. Turkey poults and ducklings are particularly susceptible and pheasant chicks are to a lesser degree. Ataxia, convulsions and opisthotonos are common signs.

Lesions: There may be a membranous glomerulonephritis and hyaline droplet nephrosis, and some degree of ascites and visceral edema may be apparent. The liver is pale and mottled with widespread necrosis. Excessive bile production is common. A marked catarrhal enteritis, especially in the duodenum, is characteristic. Diagnosis can be confirmed by histopathologic examination of the bile duct in which hyperplasia is common. The hepatic cells are enlarged with some necrotic foci.

Control: No specific treatment is known. The ingredients of the diet should be examined for the presence of peanut meal. *A. flavus* may be isolated but without further tests it is not confirmatory of the disease. Biologic assays for the toxin are available in which ducklings or poults are used. Chemical methods, using fluorescent techniques and chromatographic tests, are available. 8-Hydroxyquinoline, at 500 ppm in the mash, has been suggested as an antimycotic to prevent the growth of *A. flavus* in the feed. The successful use of thiabendazole (45 mg/lb of grain) for this purpose has also been reported.

THRUSH
(Moniliasis, Oidiomycosis, Sour crop)

A mycotic disease of the digestive tract of chickens and turkeys caused by *Candida* (*Monilia, Oidium*) *albicans*.

Lesions are most frequently found in the crop and consist of a thickened mucosa and whitish, raised, circular ulcer formations. The mouth and esophagus may show these same lesions. Hemorrhagic spots, necrotic debris and pseudomembranes are not uncommon. Depression and emaciation may be the only clinical signs. An accurate diagnosis may be established by demonstrating tissue invasion histologically and by culture of the offending organism. Young chicks and poults are most susceptible to infection.

A satisfactory treatment is not known. All sick birds should be removed from the flock and a program of disinfection carried out. Copper sulfate at a dilution of 1:2,000 in the drinking water has been recommended. Nystatin at the level of 50 mg/lb fed in the diet has shown significant protection against moniliasis.

FAVUS
(White comb)

An uncommon cutaneous mycotic disease of chickens and sometimes of turkeys caused by the fungus *Trichophyton (Achorion) gallinae.*

The condition is characterized by grayish-white, scurfy areas on the comb, wattles and unfeathered portions of the body. Clinical signs of weakness, cachexia, emaciation, depression and icterus have been reported. The feathers of the neck may be lost, leaving a honeycomb appearance of the skin surface. Necrotic foci, nodules and yellowish caseous deposits on the mucosa of the upper respiratory tract may be found. The disease spreads slowly, but may eventually infect a large proportion of the flock.

Recommended treatment is the local application of 5% formaldehyde in vaseline. Other treatments that have been used are mercury bichloride (corrosive sublimate) (1:500), 5% phenol solution, green soap, or a mixture of iodine and glycerin (1:6).

AVIAN COCCIDIOSIS

A parasitic disease caused by one or more species of coccidia. Found in a wide variety of avian hosts, these protozoan organisms are host-specific, each species usually occurring in a single host species. Because some hosts support several species of coccidia there are as many types of coccidiosis as there are coccidial species. Except for renal coccidiosis in geese, all coccidia of domestic fowl involve the digestive tract.

Etiology: The life cycle of the genus *Eimeria,* responsible for most infections of poultry, is summarized under MAMMALIAN COCCIDIOSIS (q.v., p. 450). Coccidia are almost universally present in poultry-raising operations, but clinical disease occurs only after ingestion of relatively large numbers of sporulated oocysts by a susceptible host. Both clinically infected and recovered birds shed oocysts in droppings, which serve as means of contaminating feed, dust, water, litter and soil. Oocysts may also be transmitted by mechanical carriers such as equipment, clothing, insects and other animals. Sporulation under optimum conditions (temperature 70° to 90°F, plus moisture and oxygen) varies from 1 to 2 days for the various species. The prepatent period varies from 4 to 7 days. Sporulated oocysts may survive for long periods dependent upon environmental conditions such as pH, temperature and moisture.

Pathogenicity of coccidia varies among strains of the species and by genetic susceptibility of the host. Markedly pathogenic species invade the mucosa, tunica propria and sometimes the submucosa; less pathogenic strains produce more superficial lesions. Acquired immunity of a portion of the flock from earlier subclinical infection can greatly moderate the disease. Flock management techniques are often designed to allow development of immunity without clinical disease by controlling infection. Birds are susceptible at all ages but disease is less frequent in older birds because of immunity from earlier exposure.

Clinical Findings: Chickens: In *E. tenella* infection, involvement of the ceca rather than the small intestine is a distinguishing characteristic. Clinically, the infection can be recognized by the accumulation of blood in the ceca and bloody droppings. Cecal cores, which are accumulations of clotted blood, tissue debris and oocysts, may be found in birds that are past the acute stage of the disease.

E. necatrix produces major lesions in the anterior or midportion of the small intestine, recognizable by the spotted appearance of the unopened intestine. Small white spots usually are intermingled with rounded, bright- or dull-red spots of various sizes. In severe cases, the intestinal wall is thickened, the involved area is dilated to 2 or 2½ times the normal diameter, and there may be blood in the lumen. Fluid loss may result in marked dehydration; crops are often concurrently distended with water. While the damage is in the small intestine, the sexual phase of the life cycle is completed in the ceca; thus *E. necatrix* oocysts are not found in the small intestine. Oocysts of all other species develop in the area of major lesions.

E. acervulina and *E. mivati* infections, characterized by numerous gray or whitish transverse patches in the upper half of the small intestine, are not easily distinguished on gross examination. The clinical course in a flock is usually protracted. Poor growth and the development of culls are often observed with a low mortality. *E. maxima* causes dilatation and thickening of the small intestine, which may contain a grayish, brown, or slightly pink mucous exudate. The oocysts are large.

E. brunetti occurs in the lower small intestine, rectum, ceca and cloaca. In moderate infections, there is catarrhal enteritis and thickening of the intestinal wall. A severe infection may cause an extensive coagulation necrosis and sloughing of the mucosa throughout the entire intestine. Oocysts are sometimes difficult to demonstrate.

E. hagani occurs mainly in the upper half of the small intestine. Numerous round, small hemorrhagic spots, visible through the serosa, may be seen in the duodenum. Pathogenicity is relatively low. *E. mitis* parasitizes the mucosa of the small intestine and is usually concentrated in the upper half. This species, not seriously pathogenic, is characterized by very small oocysts. *E. praecox* parasitizes the mucosa of the upper third of the small intestine, but is considered relatively nonpathogenic.

Signs of coccidiosis are highly variable in flocks and range from decreased growth rate to a high percentage of visibly sick birds and high mortality. Usually there is decreased feed intake with an increase in water consumption. Weight loss, the development of culls, decreased egg production in hens, and increased mortality are observed in clinical infections. Survivors of severe infections recover in 10 to 14 days but may require more time to return to normal production. The course of infection in a flock is unpredictable. The degree of acquired immunity of the host population prior to the development of clinical disease may also greatly influence the clinical severity and course of a flock infection.

Turkeys: Only 3 of the 8 coccidia of turkeys (*Eimeria adenoeides, E. gallopavonis* and *E. meleagrimitis*) are considered to be pathogenic. *E. dispersa, E. eimeridae, E. innocua, E. meleagridis* and *E. subrotunda* are said to be relatively nonpathogenic. Oocyst sporulation occurs in 1 to 2 days; the prepatent period varies from 4 to 6 days.

E. adenoeides and *E. gallopavonis* infect the lower ileum, ceca and rectum. The developmental stages are found in the epithelial cells of the villi and crypts. The affected portion of the intestine may be dilated and have a thickened wall. Thick creamy material, or caseous casts containing enormous numbers of oocysts are found. *E. meleagrimitis* chiefly infects the upper small intestine. The lamina propria or deeper tissues may be parasitized and result in a necrotic enteritis. The 5 nonpathogenic species occur either in the upper or lower portion of the intestine.

The common signs seen in infected flocks include a drop in feed consumption, rapid loss of weight, droopiness and ruffled feathers. Mortality is variable but may be very high. Bloody droppings do not occur. Clinical infections are seldom observed beyond the age of 8 weeks.

Ducks: A large number of specific coccidia have been reported in both wild and domestic ducks but there is a question of the validity of some of the descriptions. The following have been reported in the domestic duck: *Eimeria battakhi, E. danailovi, E. saitamae, Wenyonella anatis, W. philiplevinei* and *Tyzzeria perniciosa. T. perniciosa* is known to be a pathogen; members of the *Eimeria* species have also been described as pathogenic while the other coccidia of domestic ducks are considered relatively nonpathogenic.

Infrequent but dramatic outbreaks occur in ducklings between 2 and 5 weeks old. Morbidity and mortality may be high. *T. perniciosa* produces ballooning of the entire small intestine with mucohemorrhagic material that later becomes caseous. Other species apparently produce a hemorrhagic enteritis with an anatomic distribution characteristic of the species.

A variety of coccidia have been reported from wild ducks.

Geese: The most striking coccidial infection of geese is that produced by *Eimeria truncata*, in which the kidneys are enlarged and studded with poorly circumscribed yellowish white streaks and spots. The tubules are dilated with masses of oocysts and urates. Mortality may be very high. At least 5 other species of *Eimeria* have been described as parasitizing the intestine of geese.

Diagnosis: The presence of coccidial infections is usually readily established by the demonstration of oocysts in feces or in intestinal scrapings. Responsible diagnosis of coccidiosis as a clinical problem in poultry sometimes demands a high order of skill as the observation of oocysts has little necessary relationship to current or impending clinical disease.

Knowledge of flock appearance, morbidity, mortality, feed intake and growth rate or rate of lay are often of critical importance for diagnosis. Necropsy of several representative specimens is advisable. Severe classical lesions of *E. tenella* and *E. necatrix* may be diagnostic. Familiarity with the lesions, and the size, shape and location of oocysts allows a reasonably accurate differentiation of the coccidial species in most instances. Mixed coccidial infections are common.

A diagnosis of coccidiosis is warranted only if oocysts, merozoites or schizonts are demonstrated and if lesions and flock history are compatible with the diagnosis. The frequency of subclinical coccidial infections in some individuals in a population demands care in eliminating other possible flock disorders.

Control: Complete prevention of infection cannot be expected by practical methods of management. Maintaining poultry at all times on wire floors to separate birds from droppings is usually adequate to prevent all but minor infections. Only rarely is clinical coccidiosis observed under such circumstances. Other methods of control are designed to allow development of immunity from infection, or to minimize infection if no immunity is necessary. As chickens may experience serious problems from coccidiosis throughout life, methods to control the disease in this species will be discussed in detail.

Immunity: A species-specific immunity develops, the degree of which is largely dependent upon the extent of parasitism that occurs following exposure. Repeated infection with small numbers of oocysts produces greater immunity than from the same numbers given at one time, and is less damaging to the host.

"Vaccines" in the form of standardized doses of sporulated oocysts of the various coccidial species are available. The "vaccine" is administered in the drinking water during the first 14 days of age. As the "vaccine" serves only to introduce infection, litter must be managed to allow sporulation and recycling of the coccidia. Usually a portion of the litter is sprayed as necessary to keep it moist but not wet. Drugs are sometimes used to moderate the infection.

Drug use when immunity needed: A great variety of coccidiostatic drugs are available for use in preventing clinical infections. Ideally, the environmental conditions interacting with the suppressing effect of the drug should allow sufficient infection to produce a gradual development of immunity without clinical disease. Although this objective is often achieved, failures occur either by overly suppressing infection, which results in little or no immunity, or by inadequate suppression and the development of clinical infection. Moistening litter is sometimes necessary to allow oocyst sporulation needed for adequate exposure and infection.

Drug use when no immunity needed: No immunity is necessary in chickens reared for meat production or in floor-reared layers to be moved to cages. Under these circumstances it is desirable to minimize coccidial exposure and infection. Litter should be dry to minimize oocyst sporulation, and highly effective coccidiostatic drugs at relatively high levels may be used continuously to minimize infection. Drug withdrawal is only necessary (as required by the specific drug used) to avoid residues in meat or eggs.

Coccidiostatic Drugs: A large variety of drugs are available for use as feed additives for preventing or controlling coccidiosis in chickens. Dosage varies among the drugs as does relative effectiveness against coccidial species. Some of the drugs are recommended for use at different levels for different circumstances. Relatively low levels are to be used if immunity is desired or if low exposure is expected, higher levels are used if no immunity is needed or if a high level of exposure is anticipated.

Examples of drugs currently in wide use are: aklomide (Aklomix), amprolium (Amprol), amprolium and ethopabate (Amprol Plus), buquinolate (Bonaid), monensin (Coban), clopidol (Coyden), decoquinate (Deccox), nequinate (Statyl), nicarbazin, sulfadimethoxine and ormetoprim (Rofenaid), sulfachloropyrazine (Esb₃), and sulfaquinoxaline (S.Q.). These products are provided by the manufacturer in premixes with detailed instructions for use.

Treatment: Many of the coccidiostats which are effective in preventing infection have little value in treatment. The sulfonamides, including sulfamethazine (R 342), sulfaquinoxaline (R 343, 344), and various combinations of those and other sulfonamides as well as amprolium (R 325) are the most commonly used drugs for treating infected flocks. The drugs may be administered in either feed or water, but water medication is often preferred because severely affected birds continue to drink after they have ceased eating feed. Sulfonamides are contraindicated in fowl with aplastic anemia.

E. acervulina, in particular, often persists as a flock problem for a protracted period. It is often advisable to follow a course of treatment in such flocks by a period of 2 to 4 weeks of prophylactic medication.

Increased levels of vitamins A and K are sometimes used extemporaneously in the ration to help minimize mortality and to improve the rate of recovery.

Drug Resistance: Coccidial strains of all species parasitizing chickens, and to a lesser extent those of turkeys, have developed that are resistant in some degree to one or more coccidiostats. In some cases the resistance is relatively high and is a fixed characteristic of the strain. It is a common practice to periodically change coccidiostats when drug resistance reaches a point that clinical coccidiosis develops. Resistance to some coccidiostats develops more rapidly than to others.

HISTOMONIASIS
(Infectious enterohepatitis, Blackhead)

A protozoan disease affecting turkeys, chickens, peafowl, ruffed grouse and quail. Turkeys of all ages are susceptible, but greatest mortality occurs in birds under 12 weeks old.

Etiology: Histomoniasis is probably the result of dual etiology, one being the protozoan *Histomonas meleagridis* and the other any one or more of a group of common bacterial inhabitants of the intestinal tract of chickens and turkeys. Some bacteria seem capable of acting with the protozoan to produce disease in gnotobiotic animals while others do not. The protozoan does not seem capable of producing the disease in the absence of bacteria. As a rule both the liver and ceca of infected birds are involved. In the lumen of the ceca, *H. meleagridis* has from 1 to 4 flagella and tends to rotate in a counterclockwise direction. In the tissues of both the ceca and liver, it assumes an ameboid form.

This disease has traditionally been thought of as affecting turkeys, while doing little damage to chickens. This is not entirely true. The disease in chickens has an early cecal involvement. Liver involvement occasionally occurs in a mild form. Mortality is low but morbidity can be high in young chickens, especially those of broiler age. Tissue responses to infection may be gone in 4 weeks but the bird may be a carrier for another 6 weeks.

Under certain conditions, *H. meleagridis* may be transmitted directly from one bird to another by ingestion of infected feces, but it is more often transmitted by ingestion of the embryonated eggs of the cecal worm, *Heterakis gallinarum*, which can harbor *H. meleagridis*. A large percentage of chickens harbor this worm which, in itself, is not pathogenic, but is very important as a transmitter of histomoniasis. Its eggs are very resistant and may remain viable in the soil for months or even years. Studies have also shown that 3 species of earthworms can harbor *Heterakis* larvae containing *H. meleagridis* and that they are infective to both chickens and turkeys.

Clinical Findings: Listlessness, drooping wings, unkempt feathers and sulfur-colored droppings are the chief signs. The head may be cyanotic, hence the name "blackhead". Young birds have a more acute type of the disease and die within a few days after signs appear. Older birds may be sick for some time and become very emaciated before death. The incubation period is 15 to 21 days. On rare occasions, acute histomoniasis in chickens may cause cecal bleeding. This may lead to confusion of the disease with cecal coccidiosis.

Lesions: The most important lesions occur in the liver and ceca. The primary lesions are in the ceca, and exhibit marked inflammatory changes and ulcerations causing a thickening of the cell wall. Occasionally these ulcers erode through the cecal wall, causing a peritonitis and involvement of other organs. The ceca contain a yellowish-green caseous exudate or, in later stages, a dry cheesy core. The liver lesions are circular, yellowish green and characteristically depressed. In the turkey, they may be 4 cm in diameter.

The lesions in the liver and ceca are pathognomonic. However, the liver lesions must be carefully differentiated from those of tuberculosis, leukosis, avian trichomoniasis and mycosis, which are raised and grayish or gray-yellow. In some cases, especially in chickens, histopathologic examination is very helpful. Histomonads are intercellular, although the parasites may be so closely packed between cells as to appear intracellular. The nuclei are much smaller than those of the host cells, and the cytoplasm less vacuolated. Scrapings from the liver lesions or from the ceca may be placed in isotonic saline solution for direct microscopic examination. It is important in such examinations to differentiate *Histomonas* from other cecal flagellates and from *Blastocystis*.

Prophylaxis and Treatment: Strict sanitation is indicated. The use of large wire platforms for feeders and waterers reduces the danger of receiving an infective dose. As healthy chickens often carry infected cecal worms, the practice of ranging chickens with turkeys should be avoided. Grouse and quail also may be carriers capable of bringing the infection to the turkey yards. Since *H. gallinarum* ova can survive in soil for many months, turkeys should not be put on ground contaminated during the past 12 to 24 months. A rotation system, in which the turkeys are moved every 3 to 5 weeks, helps to reduce the chances of infection.

The following drugs have been found to be effective in the control of this disease: 2-amino-5-nitrothiazole (℞ 324); 2-acetylamido-5-nitrothiazole (℞ 348); nitarsone (℞ 334);

furazolidone (℞ 330); carbarsone (℞ 347); dimetridazole (℞ 327). Phenothiazine and tobacco dust are used to remove cecal worms, but have no direct effect on *Histomonas* itself.

HEXAMITIASIS

An acute, catarrhal enteritis of turkey poults, young pheasants, quail and peafowl. Formerly it was known as **infectious catarrhal enteritis.** The highest mortality occurs in birds from 1 to 9 weeks of age.

Etiology: The disease is caused by the protozoan parasite *Hexamita meleagridis.* This flagellate is spindle-shaped, averages 8 μ long by 3 μ wide and has 6 anterior and 2 posterior flagella. It has not yet been cultured in artificial media.

Hexamita meleagridis is transmitted directly from one bird to another by ingestion of infected feces. Many of the survivors of an outbreak become carriers and hexamitae are shed in the droppings from time to time. Pheasants, quail, chukar partridges and peafowl also are susceptible to the disease and may be the source of infection in poults. Natural infection has not been observed in chickens. Pigeons are susceptible to another species of *Hexamita.*

Clinical Findings: There are no specific signs. There is watery diarrhea (never hemorrhagic) and the feathers are dry and unkempt. The birds are listless, tend to huddle together, and lose weight rapidly, even though they continue to eat. They may die in convulsions, probably because of the low blood sugar levels.

Lesions: There is catarrhal inflammation with atony in the small intestine, especially the duodenum and upper jejunum. Bulbous dilatations of the intestine filled with watery contents are characteristic. Microscopically, the crypts of Lieberkühn contain myriads of hexamitae which attach themselves to the epithelial cells by their posterior flagella.

Diagnosis: Diagnosis depends on finding hexamitae upon microscopic examination of scrapings of the duodenal and jejunal mucosa. Hexamitae move with a very rapid, darting motion in contrast to the jerky motion of trichomonads. In order to avoid contamination of the instruments with other cecal protozoa, the duodenum should be opened first. Hexamitae may be demonstrated in poults which have been dead for several hours if the scrapings are placed in a drop of warm (40°C) isotonic saline on the slide. A few hexamitae in birds more than 10 weeks old do not justify a diagnosis of hexamitiasis.

Prophylaxis and Treatment: Since at least one-third of the survivors of an outbreak remain carriers, breeder turkeys and poults should if possible be raised on separate premises. When breeder birds are present, there should be separate attendants and equipment for the poults. Wire platforms should be used under feeders and waterers. Pheasants and quail may be carriers and sometimes bring the infection to turkeys.

Furazolidone (℞ 330), nithiazide (℞ 335), oxytetracycline (℞ 36) or chlortetracycline (℞ 15) are used to prevent and treat hexamitiasis. Treatment does not substitute for adequate sanitation and management programs.

TRICHOMONIASIS

A disease of domestic fowl, pigeons, doves and hawks, characterized, in most cases, by caseous accumulations in the throat, usually accompanied by loss of weight. It has been termed "canker", "roup" and, in hawks, "frounce". Falconers have known the disease for many centuries.

Etiology: The causative organism is a flagellated protozoan, *Trichomonas gallinae*, which lives in the head sinuses, mouth, throat, esophagus and other organs of birds. It is more prevalent among domestic pigeons and wild doves than among chickens or turkeys, although severe outbreaks have been reported among domestic fowl. Some strains are highly fatal in pigeons and doves. Hawks, which may become diseased after eating infected birds, commonly show liver lesions, with or without evidence of throat involvement. Parent pigeons and doves transmit the infection to their offspring in contaminated pigeon milk. Contaminated water is probably the most important source of infection for chickens and turkeys.

Clinical Findings: The course of the disease is rapid and the terminal lesions are extensive. The first lesions appear as small, yellowish areas on the oral mucosa. They grow rapidly in size and coalesce to form masses which frequently completely block the esophageal passage, and may prevent the bird from closing its mouth. Much fluid may accumulate in the mouth. There is a rapid weight loss and the bird becomes weak and listless. Death usually ensues within 8 to 10 days.

Eye involvement is evidenced by a watery discharge and, in more advanced stages, the production of exudate about the eyes may finally result in blindness. In chronic infections, the bird appears healthy, although trichomonads usually can be demonstrated in scrapings from the mucous membranes of the throat.

Lesions: On necropsy, the bird may be riddled with caseous necrotic foci. The mouth and esophagus are a mass of necrotic material which may extend into the skull and sometimes through the surrounding tissues of the neck to involve the skin. In the esophagus and crop, the lesions may take the form of yellow, rounded, raised areas, with a central conical caseous spur, often referred to as "yellow buttons". The crop may be covered by a yellowish diphtheritic membrane which may extend to the glandular stomach. There is no involvement of the gizzard or intestine.

Lesions of internal organs are most frequent in the liver. They may vary from a few small areas of yellow necrosis to almost complete replacement of liver tissue by caseous necrotic debris. Adhesions and involvement of other internal organs appear to be contact extensions of the huge liver lesions.

Diagnosis: While the lesions of *T. gallinae* infection are quite characteristic, they are not pathognomonic; pox and other infections can closely simulate the signs of trichomoniasis. Diagnosis should be confirmed by laboratory demonstration of the causative trichomonad. This is readily accomplished by microscopic examination of a smear containing mucus or fluid from the throat. The organisms can be readily cultured on a variety of artificial media; 0.2% Loeffler's dried blood serum in Ringer's solution or in saline-bicarbonate solution provides a good medium, or a 2% solution of pigeon serum in isotonic salt solution may be employed. Good growth is obtained at 37°C. Antibiotics may be used to reduce bacterial contamination.

Control: Because *T. gallinae* infection in pigeons is so readily transmitted from parent to offspring in the normal feeding process, chronically infected birds should be removed at once.

In pigeons, recovery from infection with a less virulent strain of *T. gallinae* appears to be accompanied by some protection against subsequent attack from a more virulent strain.

Aminonitrothiazole has proved effective against several strains of *T. gallinae*. It may be administered in gelatin capsules, at the rate of about 20 mg/lb body wt daily for 7 days. Nithiazide is also active against this disease in squabs, when given to the adults at the rate of 30 gm of 16.7% soluble powder to each 4 gal. of drinking water. Metronidazole when given orally at 60 mg/kg of body wt prevented mortality. Dimetridazole given orally at 50 mg/kg of body wt or in the drinking water (0.05% for 5 to 6 days) suppressed the disease.

TOXOPLASMOSIS

The etiology and general characteristics of toxoplasmosis are discussed under this heading on p. 456. In poultry, the first signs are apathy, unsteady gait and a pale and shriveled comb. The birds walk in circles, and exhibit torticollis, muscular spasms, paralysis and blindness. The course is generally protracted, lasting from 2 to 3 weeks, and is often fatal. Characteristically there are either lesions of the CNS, such as necrosis of the midbrain and optical chiasm, and defects of the retina, or changes in the heart and gastrointestinal tract. The pericardial sac is distended and contains reddish serous fluid; subpericardial nodules may be present. The proventriculus and the intestines are ulcerated.

Since the dye test is negative, or only slightly positive, the diagnosis is confirmed by histologic examination and isolation trials. Treatment has not been established, but a sulfonamide-pyrimethamine combination (q.v., p. 458) may be of use.

LEUCOCYTOZOON DISEASE

A disease of birds, caused by protozoan parasites similar to those that cause malaria. The parasites invade various tissues as well as the blood cells. Many species have been described from different kinds of birds. Acute outbreaks of the disease have been reported in chickens, geese, turkeys and ducks.

Etiology: Several species of the parasites have been described from various wild and domestic birds, but few are known to cause serious disease. Those recorded from domestic birds are: *Leucocytozoon simondi* and *L. anseris* from ducks and geese, *L. neavei* from guinea fowl, *L. smithi* from turkeys, and *L. sabrazesi*, *L. caulleryi* and *L. andrewsi* from chickens. Domestic birds originally acquired the infection from wild birds and, depending on the circumstances, the latter may be responsible in certain areas for initiating the transmission each year.

Chronic infections may persist in birds from one year to the next with certain ornithophilous black-flies (Simuliidae) and biting midges (*Culicoides* spp.) serving as vectors and infecting healthy birds. (*L. caulleryi* is the only one transmitted by the *Culicoides* spp.)

Black flies deposit their eggs on rocks, vegetation, logs or other objects, in or near the edge of rapidly flowing streams, or occasionally in shallow lake margins. The larvae attach themselves to an object in the stream and food is carried to them in the flowing water. Adult flies emerge in late spring and early summer. They fly, or may be carried by winds, for some distance from the streams in which they develop but are more numerous close to their breeding places. Biting midges breed in wet ground.

Clinical Findings: Acute disease occurs when there is a high parasitemia; otherwise, the infection is subacute or chronic. The disease has a relatively sudden onset with anemia, leukocytosis, splenomegaly and hypertrophy of the liver commencing about one week after infection. Fatalities usually occur within a week after infection has appeared in the blood. Birds with heavy infections show lack of appetite, dullness, loss of equilibrium, lameness and weakness. Chickens with acute infections with *L. caulleryi* are anemic; some vomit and die from hemorrhage; some excrete green feces. Retarded growth and lowered egg production occur in those surviving. Death may be due to severe anemia, to pathologic changes in the liver and brain resulting therefrom, and to respiratory embarrassment caused by the presence of large numbers of gametocytes in the lung capillaries.

Outbreaks of the disease occur during the late spring and summer when black flies and biting midges are present. Lowgrade chronic infections may be found in birds at other times. Highest mortality (up to 100% in ducks) has been reported in young birds, especially in operations where new stock is continually introduced. The disease in ducks is characterized by sudden onset and mortality usually of up to 35%. Death due to *L. caulleryi* is reported in 10 to 80% of infected older chickens.

Diagnosis: Laboratory diagnosis is based on an examination of thin blood films that have been stained with Wright's or Giemsa stain to reveal the sexual stages of the parasite in the peripheral blood cells. Red blood cells as well as lymphocytes may be invaded. The degree of alteration in the host cell varies with the different species of parasite. The typical elongated cells, with attenuated ends, are observed in ducks, geese and turkeys, and in chickens affected with one species. Two other species in chickens occur in round cells only; *L. caulleryi* is often free from the host cell.

Control: Pyrimethamine, 0.00005% in the diet, sulfadimethoxine, 0.0025% or sulfaquinoxaline, 0.005% in the diet or drinking water continuously, prevents infection with *L. caulleryi*. No satisfactory treatment is presently available for other species.

A method of preventing the disease in young turkeys is to dispose of all adults several weeks before the young birds are exposed to black flies. This method fails in areas where wild turkeys are also carrying the parasite. Tightly screening the houses is effective, but is practical only on a limited scale. Keeping ducks and turkeys inside may give some protection as the flies seldom feed inside buildings. Chickens cannot be protected this way as biting midges will feed inside buildings.

The large-scale rearing of ducks in areas where ornithophilous black flies are prevalent is to be avoided. It is difficult to eradicate the biting midges from paddy fields and swampy areas where they breed.

BLOOD SPOROZOA OF BIRDS

Aside from *Leucocytozoon*, birds may be infected with other malarial parasites. These belong to the genera *Haemoproteus* and *Plasmodium*. Physical signs are similar to those observed in infections with *Leucocytozoon* (q.v., p. 1077). Diagnosis is made by examination of stained thin blood smears and demonstration of the causative organisms in the red blood cells. During the acute stages of the disease, the liver and spleen are enlarged and dark in color.

Haemoproteus is common in pigeons, doves, quail, ducks and many species of wild song birds. It has been reported on a few occasions from turkeys. Fatalities have been observed among pigeons, doves and quail. The parasites are transmitted by bloodsucking flies of the genus *Lynchia*. In ducks, the vector is a *Culicoides*.

Plasmodium gallinaceum has not been observed in domestic poultry in North America, although it occurs in other parts of the world. *P. durae* has been reported as a severe pathogen in turkeys in East Africa. An unidentified *Plasmodium* has been reported in chickens in Wisconsin. Turkeys, but not chickens, are experimentally susceptible to *P. circumflexum* isolated from wild Canadian geese. A number of other species occur in a variety of wild birds, but chickens and turkeys are not susceptible to these species.

DISORDERS OF THE REPRODUCTIVE SYSTEM

Ruptured Egg Yolks: A sporadic condition causing death in laying hens, in which the yolk-filled ova rupture into the abdominal cavity. This disturbance is common in flighty pullets. Yolk material covers the viscera and often results in peritonitis. Rupture may be accompanied by severe hemorrhage, but whether this or the escape of yolk into the abdominal cavity is the cause of death is not known. The condition is frequently associated with chronic *Pasteurella multocida* or acute *Escherichia coli* infection.

Internal Laying: An aberration of the oviduct in which the fully formed egg is forced out of the infundibulum by reverse peristalsis or some unknown physical process, and comes to lie in the abdominal cavity. Such eggs act as foreign bodies and may become surrounded by inflammatory tissue resembling a tumor. Careful culling can eliminate many internal layers. No control or treatment is known.

Prolapse of the Oviduct ("Blowouts"): A displacement of the oviduct characterized by a large mass protruding from the vent. While the exact cause is unknown, the following factors may be involved: (1) sex hormone imbalance, (2) hereditary predisposition, (3) laying at too early an age, (4) laying eggs of an unusually large size and (5) starting production when overly fat.

If the condition is observed early, affected birds should be removed from the flock, the prolapsed part washed and replaced by gentle pressure. If the tissues are swollen, dirty and injured, the bird should be destroyed. The condition invites cannibalism.

Salpingitis (Oviductitis): An inflammation of the oviduct characterized by distension of this structure with a foul-smelling exudate. A great variety of bacteria may cause salpingitis, but enteric species are most commonly encountered. The infection arises in some cases as a result of invasion from the intestinal tract. In young growing pullets, the infection is often associated with mycoplasmosis or infectious bronchitis.

At necropsy, a severe peritonitis is usually found. The

oviduct is enlarged and filled with white or yellow, thick, tenacious exudate. In cases of longer standing, the exudate may be firm, caseous or inspissated.

The disease accounts for much of the mortality in laying flocks. Since so many different organisms seem involved, bacteriologic examination is of little value. Treatment is not practical and the affected bird should be destroyed.

ARTIFICIAL INSEMINATION IN POULTRY

In contrast to its use in farm animals, artificial insemination in turkeys is used most commonly as a means of improving fertility rather than of dispensing the superior germ plasm of proven sires. Low fertility in the turkey, caused by deficient mating resulting from large, heavy muscled birds or reduced sex drive, is a serious and costly problem in the production of hatching eggs. In overcoming this problem, artificial insemination is now widely accepted. In chickens, the practice has not found wide application, but is routinely used in special breeding work.

Chicken and turkey semen is collected by stimulating the male to protrude its copulatory organ by massaging the under side of the abdomen and the back over the testes. This is followed quickly by pushing the tail forward with one hand and, at the same time, using the thumb and forefinger of the same hand to "milk" semen from the ducts of this organ. Ejaculation is more rapid in the chicken than in the turkey. The semen is usually collected in a glass tube or sometimes with an aspirator. The volume of semen averages about 0.20 to 0.25 ml in the turkey, with a spermatozoon concentration of 6 to 10 million or more per cubic millimeter. In the chicken, semen volume is 2 or 3 times, and the spermatozoon concentration approximately one-half, that in the turkey.

Chicken and turkey semen cannot yet be stored for longer than about an hour without considerable loss of fertilizing capacity. Similarly, semen from either of these species is not normally diluted before being used for insemination. However, it has been shown that freshly collected turkey semen diluted 1:1 with 1.024% saline, having a freezing point depression of $-0.65°C$, gives as good fertility as undiluted semen when used immediately. This applies early in the season but fertility decreases rapidly later in the season. Further dilution tends to reduce drastically the fertilizing capacity of the semen.

For insemination, pressure is applied to the abdomen around

the vent. This causes the cloaca to evert and the oviduct to protrude so that a syringe or the plastic straw on the insemination gun can be inserted about an inch into the oviduct and the correct amount of semen delivered. Due to the high sperm concentration of turkey semen, 0.025 ml of undiluted pooled semen gives optimum fertility. However, amounts as small as 0.01 ml have also been shown to give excellent results. For maximum fertility, turkeys must be inseminated at regular intervals of 10 to 14 days. In the chicken, due to the lower spermatozoon concentration and shorter duration of fertility, 0.1 ml of undiluted pooled semen, at intervals of 5 to 7 days, is required to maintain fertility at a high level.

DISSECTING ANEURYSM IN TURKEYS
(Aortic rupture, Internal hemorrhage)

A fatal disease of turkeys, and less frequently of chickens, characterized by massive hemorrhage resulting from rupture of aneurysms formed in various parts of the blood vascular system by blood being forced between the coats of the arterial wall. The frequency with which the posterior aorta is affected has given rise to the term "aortic rupture".

The disease has been reported in the U.S.A., Canada and Great Britain. The largest and most rapidly growing male turkeys, between 8 and 24 weeks of age, in the best-managed flocks, are most often affected. The disease also occurs in females, but the incidence is lower. It is seldom observed in poorly managed flocks. The disease has been observed in most breeds of turkeys raised in the U.S.A. Dissecting aneurysms also occur in chickens, but the incidence is extremely low.

Etiology: The exact cause is still unknown. Three factors probably must be present before fatal dissecting aneurysms will occur: The birds must be fed and managed in such a way that they are growing rapidly, there is some evidence that the birds must have a genetic susceptibility, and there must be a prolonged lipemia during the period of rapid growth. The lipemia may result from a high dietary intake of fat or the effects of hormonal factors, such as high levels of estrogens. Although beta aminopropionitrile, the toxic agent in *Lathyrus odoratus,* is capable of producing dissecting aneurysms in turkeys, there is no evidence that the nitriles are responsible for the occurrence of dissecting aneurysms under natural conditions.

Clinical Findings: Affected birds are found dead with no premonitory signs of disease. Occasionally, a caretaker will observe an apparently healthy bird die within a few minutes. The incidence is usually less than 1%, but may rise to 10%. Formerly, when male turkeys were implanted with stilbestrol, the incidence was as high as 20%.

Lesions: Necropsy reveals markedly anemic cadavers with large quantities of clotted blood in the peritoneal or pericardial sac. Occasionally, massive hemorrhage into the lungs, kidneys and leg muscles occurs. The rupture in the wall of the posterior aorta at about the position of the testes, or in the atrium, can readily be located by carefully washing away the clot. Ruptures in smaller blood vessels are more difficult to locate.

Histologic examination reveals that the aortic rupture is caused by an intramedial hemorrhage of the dissecting type. In almost every instance, there is either intimal thickening or a large, fibrous plaque in the region of the rupture. Staining for fats reveals that there is a marked accumulation of lipids in the thickened intima and in the fibrous plaques.

Treatment: There is no known treatment; the use of coagulants and vitamin K is useless, since there is no defect in the clotting mechanism. Losses sometimes may be reduced during the critical period between 16 and 20 weeks of age by limiting feed intake. High-fat diets should not be fed during this period. There is some evidence that continuous, low-level feeding of reserpine after 4 weeks of age reduces losses from this disease. The dose recommended by the manufacturer is 0.0001% in the ration for not more than 5 days or 0.00002% continuously.

BOTULISM
(Limberneck, Western duck sickness)

A type of intoxication due to ingestion of food materials containing toxins of *Clostridium botulinum*.

Etiology: Type A and Type C toxins of *Cl. botulinum* are the most common causes of botulism in poultry and wildfowl. This organism occurs commonly in the soil and may contaminate foodstuffs. In order to produce botulism, the organism must have multiplied and formed its toxin in the food before it is ingested. The principal causes are improperly sterilized, home-canned vegetables and occasionally other home-canned foods, improperly processed and spoiling foods of animal origin, such as sausages and hams, and decomposing carcasses and the fly maggots living in them.

"Western duck sickness" or "alkali disease" occurs in the Western U.S.A. and Canada, and kills millions of wild waterfowl in certain years. It occurs around lakes or marshes where flooding has occurred and where there is relatively shallow water containing decaying vegetation. Anaerobiosis results in such cases and *Cl. botulinum* can multiply in the decaying organic material and form toxins. Waterfowl become affected when they feed in these areas.

Clinical Findings and Diagnosis: No characteristic lesions can be seen. There may be a slight enteritis and an enlarged spleen. The toxin affects the nervous system, causing a flaccid paralysis which is well described by the name "limberneck," given to the disease. In addition, the feathers are characteristically loose and come out easily. Death usually is due to respiratory paralysis.

A presumptive diagnosis of botulism can be made from the physical appearance and a history of eating spoiled food, carcasses, or maggots. A positive diagnosis can be made only by injection of a filtrate from the suspected food or the intestinal contents of affected birds into 2 sets of mice or guinea pigs, of which one set receives simultaneously injections of bivalent Type A and Type C botulinum antitoxin. Isolation of *Cl. botulinum* from the feed or intestine is valueless, since it may occur in them normally.

Control: Chickens should not be fed spoiled foods which are considered unfit for human consumption. Carcasses should be picked up from chicken yards and buried deeply or burned. Laxatives, such as Epsom salts (℞ 481) are of value in treating exposed birds which have not shown signs of the disease. No feed should be given. *Cl. botulinum* antitoxin (℞ 104) may be of some value. It has been used successfully in treating wild waterfowl with signs of western duck sickness, but relatively few birds can be handled in this way. It has been reported that dilute solutions of potassium permanganate (1:3,000) as a crop lavage or in drinking water are useful. Recently, much greater success has been obtained by herding ducks away from affected areas with pyrotechnics, airplanes or boats, by draining such areas and by distributing feed for the birds elsewhere.

HEMORRHAGIC SYNDROME
(Aplastic anemia, Hemorrhagic anemia)

A disorder of growing chickens characterized by fatty bone marrow, increased blood clotting time, anemia, hemorrhage and variable mortality.

Etiology and Incidence: The cause is unknown but evidence indicates that it is not infectious. Somewhat similar disorders have been produced by administering sulfonamides, by feeding trichloroethylene-extracted soybean oil meal and by feeding extracts of several commonly occurring molds. Aflatoxin produced by *Aspergillus flavus* in peanut meal and high-moisture corn has been involved (*see*, p. 1065). A variety of antibiotics and other compounds are also capable of disturbing hemopoiesis.

The syndrome was first generally recognized in the U.S.A. during 1951–52 and was considered of major economic importance. The incidence has since declined and the disease is now relatively infrequent. As a clinical problem, it has been recognized in many of the intensive poultry-producing areas of the world.

Clinical Findings: Affected flocks first manifest depression, accompanied by pale combs and wattles. The most thrifty birds in a flock are often most severely affected. Hemorrhage in various tissues is an inconstant finding. Occasionally, blood is observed in the droppings. Hemorrhage into the anterior chamber of the eye, in the subcutis of the legs and shanks and from the nostrils may be prominent. Mortality, which usually does not extend over more than a 14-day period, rarely exceeds 20% and is usually less than 5%; most birds recover spontaneously.

Lesions: Fatty infiltration of the bone marrow appears to be a basic change in the disorder. The change may be relatively slight or may progress to a true aplastic anemia. Hemorrhages may be found in the heart, proventriculus, intestines and skeletal musculature. Hemoglobin values range from low to very low in severely affected birds. An initial leukocytosis may occur which is followed by terminal leukopenia. Clotting time is increased, but is difficult to determine accurately in the chicken.

Diagnosis: Diagnosis is based on demonstrating the general lesions associated with this condition and by elimination of specific infections. Coccidiosis and ulcerative enteritis may offer a problem in differential diagnosis. Schizonts or oocysts are usually demonstrable in considerable numbers in coccidiosis. Although hemorrhage may occur from the intestinal mucosa in both coccidiosis and hemorrhagic syndrome, only in the former does the mucosa usually show extensive thickening. Ulcerative enteritis seldom produces hemorrhage from the intestinal mucosa. Fatty metamorphosis of the bone marrow is not prominent in either coccidiosis or ulcerative enteritis.

Treatment: No specific treatment is at present available. Fortifying the ration with compounds such as vitamin K, B-vitamins or trace minerals is thought by some to be helpful. Sulfonamides are contraindicated because of their marked ability to aggravate the syndrome. Other compounds capable of suppressing hemopoiesis and blood clotting should be avoided.

If the condition is a fungal toxicosis, practices which reduce fungal proliferation, such as keeping the litter and feed dry, should be helpful. Moldy, high-moisture grain or damaged grain should also be avoided.

POISONINGS

Inorganic Sources

Carbon monoxide: This poisoning commonly arises from exhaust fumes when chicks are being transported by truck. Fumes from anthracite or oil heaters also may be responsible. The mortality may be high unless fresh air is provided immediately. At necropsy, the beak is found to be cyanotic and a characteristic bright pink color is noted throughout the viscera, particularly the lungs. Diagnosis can be confirmed by a spectroscopic analysis of the blood.

Arsenic: Rat poisons, Paris green, lead arsenate and other arsenical compounds are common sources of poisoning in birds. Chickens are quite tolerant to arsenic and, unless large amounts are consumed, few deaths occur. Poisoned birds become restless and show spasmodic jerking of the neck. There may be a depraved appetite and loss of equilibrium. Large doses cause submucous inflammation of the crop and gizzard and a catarrhal enteritis. Severe kidney degeneration may be noted.

Copper: Copper sulfate in single doses above 1.0 gm is fatal. The signs are a watery diarrhea and listlessness. A catarrhal gastroenteritis accompanied by a greenish seromucous exudate throughout the intestinal tract is found at necropsy.

Lead: Lead poisoning usually is caused by paint or orchard spray material. Amounts of 7.2 mg of metallic lead per pound of body weight are lethal. Clinical signs are depression, loss of appetite, emaciation, thirst and muscular weakness. Greenish droppings are commonly observed within 36 hours. As poisoning progresses, the wings may be extended downward. Young birds may die within 36 hours after ingesting lead. Diagnosis of acute lead poisoning may be made from the history and necropsy findings of a greenish-brown color of the gizzard mucosa, enteritis and degeneration of the liver and kidney. Chronic poisoning produces emaciation, and atrophy of the liver and heart. The pericardium is distended with fluid and the gallbladder is thickened and enlarged. Urate deposits are usually found in the kidneys. Ingestion of lead shot often occurs in wild waterfowl on heavily gunned feeding grounds. The retention of only a few shot in the gizzard can kill a duck.

Mercury: Poisoning occurs from mercurial disinfectants and fungicides, including mercurous chloride (calomel) and bichloride of mercury (corrosive sublimate). Clinical signs are progressive muscular weakness and incoordination. Diarrhea may occur, depending on the amount of chemical ingested. In some cases, the caustic action of the chemical produces gray areas in the mouth and esophagus, which usually ulcerate if the bird lives for more than 24 hours. Catarrhal inflammation of the proventriculus and intestines occurs in some birds. If a large amount of mercury is ingested, extensive hemorrhage may occur in these organs. The kidneys are pale and studded with small white foci. The liver shows fatty degeneration.

Selenium: The ingestion of feeds containing more than 5 ppm of selenium decreases the hatchability of eggs because of deformities of the embryos, which are unable to emerge from the shell because of beak anomalies. Eyes may be missing and feet and wings may be deformed or underdeveloped.

Selenium in a concentration of 10 ppm as in seleniferous grains, in the laying ration, usually reduces hatchability of fertile eggs to zero. Mature birds seem to tolerate more selenium in their feed than swine, cattle or horses, without exhibiting signs of poisoning other than poor hatchability of the eggs. Starting rations containing 8 ppm of selenium have reduced the growth rate of chicks, but 4 ppm had no noticeable effect on growth rate. The feeding of rations containing as little as 2.5 ppm to poultry has resulted in meat and eggs containing concentrations of selenium in excess of the suggested tolerance limit in foods.

Sodium arsenite and some of the organic arsenicals, when

administered to laying hens with selenium, have given some improvement in hatchability.

Salt: The addition of 0.5% salt (NaCl) to the ration of chickens and turkeys is recommended, but amounts in excess of 2% are usually considered dangerous. Rations for chicks have contained as much as 8% without injurious effect, but rations containing 4% were harmful to poults and levels of 6 to 8% have resulted in mortality. The addition of 2% sodium chloride to the feed, or 4 parts per thousand in the water, will depress growth in young ducks and lower the fertility and hatchability of the eggs in breeding stock.

Salt levels high enough to produce salt poisoning may be reached when salty protein concentrates are added to rations already fortified with salt or when the salt is poorly incorporated in the feed. Sporadic poisoning has also been reported from the accidental ingestion of rock salt or salt provided for other livestock. Necropsy findings are not diagnostic. Enteritis and ascites are common findings. Watery droppings and wet litter are often suggestive of a high-salt intake.

Boric acid: This is quite toxic for birds, resulting in depression, diarrhea and progressive weakness. Necropsy findings include severe crop thickening, gastroenteritis and degenerative kidney changes.

Organic Sources

Various organic chemicals, especially those used to treat seed grain, are dangerous.

Thiram: This substance, used to treat seed corn, is toxic to chicks at 40 ppm and goslings at 150 ppm, causing leg deformities and loss of weight. Turkey poults tolerate up to 200 ppm.

EDB (ethylene dibromide): Certain grains treated with fumigants containing this chemical are toxic to laying hens. Egg weights are significantly reduced with as little as 0.5 mg of EDB per bird daily.

BAPN (beta aminopropionitrile): This substance is toxic for turkeys. In diets containing *Lathyrus odoratus* seeds, BAPN at 0.06% produced massive internal hemorrhage, particularly of the aorta in turkeys. BAPN at 0.03 and 0.06% of the diet of laying hens produced soft-shelled and malformed eggs, and egg production and hatchability were significantly reduced.

DDT (dichlorodiphenyl-trichloroethane): This chemical, once much used for fly and insect control, is toxic to birds if consumed at levels above 0.03% of the diet. The clinical signs are dyspnea, tremor, convulsions and prostration. Death may occur. There are no significant lesions found at necropsy.

Crotalaria: Many species of *Crotalaria* seeds are toxic to chickens. Concentrations above 0.05% in the feed produce signs of toxicosis. There is a marked reduction in weight gain at 0.2%, and 0.3% will cause death in 18 days. Lesions consist of ascites, swelling or atrophy of the liver, and hemorrhages. Resistance to the toxin increases with age.

Common vetch: The seed of the common vetch, *Vicia sativa*, will cause high mortality when fed at levels of 30 to 40% of the rations.

Nicotine: The usual source of poisoning from nicotine is "Black Leaf 40" which contains 40% of nicotine sulfate. Amounts of 0.5 to 1.0 ml are fatal. This solution is used for the control of external parasites by painting it on the roosts. It is volatile at high temperatures. Affected birds show uneasiness, wing paralysis, dilated pupils, and often vomit. Ecchymoses in the heart and lungs are seen at necropsy.

Toxic fat: An unidentified "toxic fat" factor in some feed produces hydropericardium and ascites in young chickens. In young pullets it reduces growth, retards sexual development and increases mortality. Hatchability is lowered. Turkeys and ducks are less susceptible than chickens. The chemical nature of the toxin is unknown. The signs of intoxication include ruffled feathers, droopiness and labored breathing. Lesions include ascites and hydropericardium, necrosis of liver, subepicardial hemorrhage and bile duct hyperplasia. Although the amount of toxin varies in feeds from different sources, 0.25 to 5% fed for 35 to 150 days produced typical lesions.

Carbolineum: Fumes resulting from this chlorinated coal-tar poultry house spray produce burns of the face, wattles and feet, together with gasping, ascites, and acute swelling and degeneration of the liver.

Gossypol: Cottonseed meal contains appreciable amounts of gossypol which produces severe cardiac edema resulting in dyspnea, weakness and anorexia.

Polychlorinated biphenyl: PCB residues have recently been reported in chicken and turkey meat in excess of the 5 ppm permitted in edible tissue, and in egg products in excess of the permitted 0.5 ppm. The product has been traced to such sources as heat-exchange fluid and plastic wrappers from bakery goods which have been ground and included in poultry feed. Presently, spectrographic methods have been developed to clearly distinguish between PCBs and chlorinated pesticides such as DDD and DDT.

The product depresses egg production and markedly reduces hatchability. PCBs are found in the fatty tissue of birds. Up to 40 ppm in tissue does not produce changes that are evident in birds by gross necropsy.

Autointoxication

Self-poisoning due to the retention of the waste products of metabolism or the absorption of products of decomposition including bacterial toxins which occur within the intestine. Signs include cyanosis, sluggishness and diarrhea. Congestion of the muscles and viscera with kidney congestion, swelling and blockage may be noted. A catarrhal enteritis is usually present. Antibiotics (e.g., chlortetracycline, oxytetracycline) given at the rate of 100 gm/ton of mash may be helpful together with a laxative (℞ 482).

DIGESTIVE-TRACT HELMINTHIASIS

Etiology: Some 60 species of worms occur in poultry in the U.S.A. Injury to the host results from direct destruction of tissues, and the amount of destruction is directly related to the total number of worms in the infections, which comprise a number of species. Damage from the parasitisms is best measured in terms of reduced or delayed production, i.e., weight gains and eggs. In the highly specialized broiler plants of today, parasites are seldom of importance; the parasites mainly affect pullets and hens in laying and supplying flocks. Small farm flocks can have large numbers of parasites.

Clinical Findings: The signs are: general unthriftiness, retarded growth, inactive "colorless" birds with depressed appetite in an environment where sanitation has broken down. Specific lesions have not been associated with every parasite. Generally they are nodules, irritations, minute hemorrhages where worms may be attached, and ulceration when fine-bodied worms are accumulated beneath the mucosa.

Diagnosis: The worms must be separated from ingesta. A real knowledge of numbers present cannot be obtained when the digestive tract is opened and examined directly. The tract is scraped, and it and its contents put into separate containers of water. A good light source is essential. Many worms are not actively motile. The esophagus and crop are removed in one piece, the inner surfaces stretched taut and capillarids looked for "sewn" into the mucous membrane. The outer surface of the proventriculus is examined for female *Tetrameres*. The gizzard lining must be removed to find the gizzard worms. The ceca are split separately to find the cecal worms; the cecal contents and scrapings are examined closely for the capillarids which are thin and without active movement. The rest of the digestive tract is opened from the posterior end. It is slit and scraped forwards to loosen tapeworms.

Control: Control of worm parasites of all domestic animals is dependent upon sanitation, management and treatment. In the case of poultry, however, treatment plays a lesser part than does either sanitation or management. When anthelmintics are used, there are generally various proprietary forms of phenothiazine for cecal worms, and nicotine sulfate or piperazine salt, generally citrate, for the large roundworm, *Ascaridia galli*. The antibiotic hygromycin is available for treatment of the above 2 roundworms and for specific treatment of intestinal capillariasis caused by the threadworms. A new anthelmintic "Meldane-2", a coumaphos preparation, has been shown to have high efficacy for removal of capillarids. Control of cecal worms is related to prevention of infectious enterohepatitis in turkeys (q.v., p. 1072). Tapeworm infection can be treated with dibutylin dilaurate (Butynorate) or dichlorophen. Dosage instructions issued by the manufacturer should be followed since poultry usually are treated on a flock basis utilizing medicated feed or drinking water.

In the average small farm flock, poultry parasite control can be accomplished if farmers will undertake to follow the procedures of the all-pullet flock system.

WORMS COMMONLY PRESENT IN DIGESTIVE TRACT OF CHICKENS AND TURKEYS

Intestine
    Nematodes
        Ascaridia galli (in chickens) to 11.5 cm   below duodenum
        Ascaridia columbae (in pigeons)
        Ascaridia dissimilis (turkey)
        Capillaria obsignata to 1.8 cm   ileum
        Capillaria caudinflata   ileum
    Cestodes
        Hymenolepis carioca   duodenum
        Raillietina cesticillus   jejunum
        Raillietina tetragona   ileum
        Raillietina echinobothrida   ileum

Ceca
    Nematodes
        Heterakis gallinarum to 1.5 cm
        Capillaria anatis (chicken) to 1.5 cm

Crop
    Nematodes
        Capillaria annulata to 12 cm
        Capillaria contorta to 12 cm

GAPEWORM INFECTION

The gapeworm, *Syngamus trachea,* inhabits the trachea and lungs of many domestic and various wild birds. Infection may occur directly by ingestion of infective eggs or larvae; however, severe field infection is associated with the ingestion of transport hosts, such as earthworms, snails, slugs and arthropods such as flies. Many gapeworm larvae may encyst and survive within a single invertebrate for years. Range infection is favored by seasonal climatic abundance of specific invertebrate hosts, e.g., great numbers of earthworms brought to the surface by spring rains. Although gapeworms are not a problem in confinement-reared poultry, serious economic losses occur in range-reared pheasants and turkeys.

Clinical Findings: Young birds suffer most. Sudden death and verminous pneumonia characterize early outbreaks. Later, signs of gasping, choking, shaking of the head, inanition, emaciation and suffocation may follow. Necropsy reveals adult gapeworms obstructing the lumina of the trachea, bronchi and lungs. Respiratory inflammation may be present. The blood-red female gapeworm is usually found attached to a much smaller, paler male whose head becomes permanently embedded deep in the host tissue. The joined pair have a "Y"-shaped, or forked appearance. The female worm may become detached from the male and feed freely within the lumen, or be coughed up and discharged from the body.

Prophylaxis and Treatment: To prevent wild birds from introducing infection, pens should be isolated by overhead and lateral screening. After infection occurs, pens should be rested and preferably rotated with crops; however, poultry and game birds should not be placed on newly plowed fields. Earthworm populations can be reduced prior to introduction of range-reared birds by soil treatments such as Shell D-D, ethylene dibromide, rotenone and chlordane. Various molluscacides, such as copper sulfate or pentachlorophenate, will destroy slugs and snails.

Administration of thiabendazole at 0.1% in the feed continuously for 10 days to 2 weeks is highly effective in eliminating gapeworms, and 0.05% feed medication when given continuously for 4 days or longer helps prevent and control infections. Poultry treated while larvae are migrating in the body will develop immunity to gapeworms even though therapy may abort infection.

MANSON'S EYEWORM INFESTATION

Manson's eyeworm, *Oxyspirura mansoni*, is a slender thread-like nematode, 12 to 18 mm in length, which occurs beneath the nictitating membrane of chickens and other fowl in various tropical and subtropical regions. The worm eggs are washed down the nasolacrimal duct into the pharynx and swallowed. The eggs are passed in the feces and are ingested by the intermediate host, the Surinam cockroach, *Pycnoscelus surinamensis.* Under favorable conditions, the larvae reach the infective stage within the body of the roach in about 50 days. The roaches are readily eaten by fowl and the liberated larvae migrate up the esophagus to the mouth and thence to the eye through the nasolacrimal duct.

Irritation of the eye produced by the parasite causes inflammation, lacrimation, blinking, corneal opacity and disturbed vision according to the degree of infestation. The affected bird may rub its head against the wings and scratch at the eye as if to dislodge a foreign body.

Strict sanitary measures and disinfection of premises, plus the use of approved insecticides on roach-infested premises provide the most efficient control. Surgical removal of the nictitating membrane is reported in some countries to be a useful prophylactic measure.

The eye is anesthetized with a local anesthetic and the worms are exposed in the lacrimal sac by lifting the membrane. One or 2 drops of a 5% cresol solution placed in the sac kills the worms immediately. The eye then should be immediately irrigated with pure water to wash out the dead worms and excess cresol solution. Within 48 to 72 hours after treatment, the eyes show improvement and gradually become clear if the destructive process caused by the parasite is not too far advanced.

FLUKE INFECTION IN POULTRY

Although trematodes continue to be of importance in some production systems, and as parasites of certain wild birds, they are of diminished importance where modern poultry production methods are used.

***Prosthogonimus macrorchis* Infection:** This pyriform fluke (about 7 mm by 5 mm) develops to maturity in the bursa of Fabricius except in those birds, such as chicken, turkey and pheasant, which do not have a functional bursa; in these it develops in the oviduct. Birds become infected by eating mature or immature dragonflies (secondary host) bearing the metacercariae. Development to adults requires about 14 days. The primary host is a snail.

In ducks and other birds with a functional bursa, only light infections are found, and no clinical signs are observed. In gallinaceous birds, where the parasites develop in the oviduct, heavy infections may occur. Such birds go off feed, become droopy, lose weight and lay fewer eggs. The eggs are soft-shelled and, in extreme cases, egg laying ceases. A calcareous discharge, presumably from uterine glands, soils the cloacal feathers. The lesions range from mild inflammation of the oviduct to distension and even rupture of the oviduct with exudate and egg material. Death may occur.

Since the fluke eggs appear in the bird's droppings only periodically, fecal examination is diagnostically unreliable. Necropsy may disclose flukes in the oviduct.

Infection can be prevented by keeping birds away from aquatic situations where they can feed on dragonflies. Installation of 2 to 5 ml of carbon tetrachloride directly into the crop may be beneficial in heavy infections.

Collyriclum faba Infection: This parasite is found in subcut. cysts in turkeys, chickens and other birds. The life cycle is unknown; probably it involves snails and insects such as dragonflies or mayflies. The cysts, about 4 to 6 mm in diameter, and usually containing 2 adults, may occur anywhere on the body, but most are found near the vent. Young birds may have locomotor difficulty and poor appetite; heavy infection may be fatal. The cysts ooze exudate, attract flies, and may become infected with bacteria. The worms can be removed surgically. Prevention is by keeping birds away from aquatic insects.

ECTOPARASITISM

LICE

Biology: Chickens are infested with at least 7 species of biting lice but no sucking lice. They live on bits of skin, feathers, etc., but consume blood if it is available. The entire life cycle is usually completed on the body of the original host. Man can harbor chicken lice but usually only as a temporary carrier.

The common lice of chickens are the chicken body louse *Menacanthus stramineus* (on the skin), the shaft louse *Menopon gallinae* (on feather shafts), the chicken head louse *Cuclotogaster heterographus* (mainly on the head and neck) and the wing louse *Lipeurus caponis* (mainly on the wing feathers, rather inactive). Less commonly found on chickens are the fluff louse *Goniocotes gallinae* (very small, in the fluff), the brown chicken louse *Gonoides dissimilis* (brownish, on feathers, southern in distribution) and the large chicken louse *Gonoides gigas* (bluish gray, very large and strongly marked).

Turkeys, geese and ducks sometimes harbor chicken lice when raised with chickens but, more commonly, turkeys are infested with the large turkey louse *Chelopistes meleagridis* and the slender turkey louse *Oxylipeurus polytrapezius*. Geese and ducks are infested with *Anatoecus dentatus,* whereas only ducks are infested with *Anaticola crassicornis* and *Trinoton querquedulae* (*luridum*). *Anaticola anseris*, which also occurs in ducks, and *Trinoton anserinum* are encountered on geese and swans. Ducks and geese seldom are heavily infested with lice.

Other domesticated and cage birds are infested with species of Mallophaga which are usually specific for each host.

Clinical Findings: The irritation produced by the lice causes reduced egg production and rate of weight gains. Examination of birds particularly around the vent and under the wings, but also elsewhere, will reveal eggs on the feathers or moving lice on the skin or feathers.

Control: Lice and other ectoparasites of poultry must be considered as any other infectious disease; isolation from all possible means of contamination must be maintained.

Birds are seldom treated individually but a thorough dusting with sodium fluoride, if done twice about 10 days apart, is effective for most lice. Malathion (℞ 320) is effective, or the roost can be painted with nicotine sulfate (℞ 322). Where the birds or the litter or both have to be treated, a 4% dust of malathion (℞ 321) or a 0.5% dust of coumaphos (℞ 250) can be used. These 2 products may also be used as a spray.

THE FOWL TICK
(*Argas persicus*)

Biology: The fowl tick occurs worldwide in tropical and subtropical countries. The tick is active in poultry houses throughout the year whenever temperatures are high enough. The adults and nymphs rarely are seen feeding on the birds, as they attack at night and hide in cracks and crevices during the day. The larvae may be found on the birds, as they frequently remain attached for as long as 2 days in taking their first blood meal. After feeding, the larvae molt into the nymph stage.

Nymphs may feed and molt many times before reaching the adult stage. The adults feed repeatedly, with the females laying 50 to 100 eggs after each feeding. In warm weather, the eggs may hatch in 10 days, but cool weather prolongs the incubation period as much as 3 months or longer.

Clinical Findings: The fowl tick produces anemia and toxemia, with the anemia being of greater importance. Affected birds lose weight, appear anemic, are depressed and their egg production decreases. Red spots can be seen on the skin where the ticks have fed. Since the ticks are nocturnal, the birds may show some uneasiness when roosting. Death losses are rare, but production may be seriously depressed.

Control: The fowl tick is difficult to eradicate because the adults and nymphs are usually not on the birds in the daytime. Therefore the first efforts to control this pest must be isolation to prevent infestation, well-constructed housing to reduce hiding places, plus cleanliness in the poultry house.

Malathion (R 320) affords good control if applied at least 1 gal. to each 1,000 sq ft of surface. Malathion does not produce residues in the tissues of birds maintained in close contact with the treated areas and may be used where poultry houses cannot be depopulated.

For areas and buildings from which the birds can be removed, sprays or paints containing 0.5% lindane (R 319—use ½ strength), chlordane (R 318) or toxaphene (R 304) applied at a rate of at least 1 gal./1,000 sq ft of surface, should effect control. Since these materials may appear as residues in the flesh and eggs of birds that come in contact with them, treated areas must be kept empty for periods as set forth by the manufacturer.

THE RED MITE
(*Dermanyssus gallinae:* Roost mite, Nocturnal mite)

Biology: The red mite attacks chickens, pigeons, canaries and various wild birds. It is less than 1 mm long and gray in color until it engorges with blood and becomes red. These common pests are nocturnal feeders and during the day hide in the cracks and crevices of the chicken house where they lay their eggs. They propagate very rapidly during the warm months and more slowly in cold weather. The life cycle may be completed in as little as a week. Transmission is accomplished by contact or through the use of infested equipment. A house may remain infested for 6 months after birds are removed.

Clinical Findings: In laying flocks, egg production is lowered. Young birds become emaciated and death occasionally results. Birds may be uneasy on the perches at night. Examination of birds at this time, or of roosts during the day, particularly cracks and where roost poles touch supports, will disclose grayish accumulations.

The mites can produce a serious anemia, and may transmit diseases such as spirochetosis and fowl pox. Severe irritation of the skin is common.

Control: Sanitation and isolation so that birds do not become infested must be stressed. Carbolineum or creosote diluted with equal parts of kerosene applied to roosts and supports and nests once a year when the pens are empty will prevent infection. The recommendations given for the use of malathion, coumaphos and nicotine sulfate for the control of lice (*see* p. 1095) will also control the red mite.

FEATHER MITES
(*Ornithonyssus sylviarum:* Northern feather mite)
(*Ornithonyssus bursa:* Tropical feather mite)

Biology: Feather mites are common on chickens, robins, swallows and sparrows throughout the U.S.A. and Canada. Slightly smaller than the red mite, they differ from it in that they occur continuously on the birds and the surroundings both day and night. They are quick to crawl onto a person handling birds.

Clinical Findings: Infestation commonly leads to lowered egg production and emaciation, and can be severe enough to cause death. Examination of the birds reveals the mites which are often only recognized because the small dust-like particles move. They are voracious blood suckers and may produce scabs.

Control: Feather mites are extremely difficult to control. Many compounds have been tried with varying degrees of success. The following treatments are recommended: (1) nicotine sulfate (R 322) as a roost paint; (2) a 0.25% wettable powder spray of coumaphos (R 247), used at the rate of 1 gal. per 100 birds directly on the birds. Do not contaminate feed or water or use in conjunction with other organic phosphates. Do not use within 10 days of vaccination or other stress influences. (3) 4% malathion dust (R 321) or spray application to the roosts, droppings, nests and over litter.

THE SCALY LEG MITE
(*Cnemidocoptes mutans*)

This small mite usually tunnels into the epithelium under the scales of the legs, and the resulting irritation and exudation cause the legs to become thickened, encrusted and unsightly. It also may attack the comb and wattles. Under modern systems of sanitation it is not common. If possible the first cases should be culled. The roosts and nests should be painted with carbolineum. The legs may be dipped in 1 part of kerosene plus 2 parts of raw linseed oil.

THE DEPLUMING MITE
(*Cnemidocoptes laevis* var. *gallinae:* Body mange mite)

This microscopic mite causes intense irritation at the base of the feathers. The wing and tail feathers are usually lost. To control this mite isolate affected birds and treat with an ointment of caraway oil and petrolatum (℞ 317) or dip in 1 gal. water plus 2 oz wettable sulfur and 1 oz of soap.

THE SUBCUTANEOUS MITE
(*Laminosioptes cysticola*)

The subcut. mite is a small parasite which is most often diagnosed by observation of white-to-yellowish caseocalcareous nodules about 1 to 3 mm in diameter in the subcutis, perhaps a reaction of the bird's tissue to enclose a foreign body after death of the mite. Careful examination of the skin and subcutis of birds under the dissecting microscope may more frequently reveal the mite. No attempts are made to control this parasite except to destroy the bird.

THE AIR-SAC MITE
(*Cytodites nudus*)

The air-sac mite occurs in bronchi, lungs, air sacs and bone cavities of several species of birds. Opinions vary as to the amount of damage done to the host. It will be recognized as whitish dots on the surface of the air sacs. Control has been the recommendation to destroy the affected birds.

CHIGGERS
(*Trombicula alfreddugesi:* Red bugs, Harvest mites)

These small mites are parasitic on chickens, turkeys, man and wild animals. Chiggers are prevalent in the Southern U.S.A., particularly on heavy soil. They breed on the ground in waste areas, such as fence rows. Young birds may be severely affected, become emaciated, droopy and die. A vesicle or abscess may form at the point of attachment of the chigger.

Control is partly accomplished by keeping the grass on the range cut short. Dusting the range with about 50 lb of sulfur, 40 lb of 1% malathion, ⅓ gal. of 45% chlordane, or ½ gal. of toxaphene per acre will control chiggers. One part of sulfur to 5 parts of petrolatum may be applied to the skin lesions.

BEDBUGS
(Cimex lectularius)

These reddish-brown, oval, flattened, wingless insects are about 6 mm in length. They are bloodsucking parasites and can subsist on the blood of wild and domestic animals and man. They can live without food for at least a year. Bedbugs have been known to become troublesome in old henhouses and in poultry-fattening cages. They may cause considerable trouble in pigeon lofts. The life cycle takes about 4 to 6 weeks. Control is best accomplished by thorough cleaning of the houses and reducing hiding places such as cracks, to which these insects retire during the day. Usually, spraying with malathion or with carbolineum or creosote oil diluted with kerosene, after removing birds from premises, is quite a satisfactory control measure. Most methods of control for mites are equally effective for bedbugs.

MOSQUITOES

Perhaps the most common mosquito in the Southern U.S.A., and in the same latitude around the world, is *Culex pipiens* sp. *quinquefasciatus*. This mosquito feeds readily on poultry. Swarms of this and other species feeding on chickens have been known to be responsible for a marked drop in egg production and even death. Several viral diseases of birds are transmitted by them. The usual control measures are employed, such as oily preparations on nearby pools and other breeding places, and spraying of the walls and ceilings of evacuated chicken houses with 1% malathion water emulsion every 5 to 7 days.

FLIES AND GNATS

The pigeon fly (*Pseudolynchia canariensis*) is a small, flat, brownish fly which causes most trouble in pigeon lofts. The flies suck blood, move rapidly through the birds' feathers and may cause heavy losses in squabs. Most prevalent in the Southern U.S.A., it is the transmitter of *Haemoproteus columbae,* which causes pigeon malaria. The pigeon loft especially should be thoroughly cleaned every 20 days. Squabs can be dusted with pyrethrum powder. Derris powder (℞ 323) also is effective as a dust.

Black flies (members of the family Simuliidae), known as buffalo gnats or turkey gnats, are bloodsuckers and transmit *Leucocytozoon* disease (q.v., p. 1077). These small flies are less than 6 mm in length and breed in running water. They are most common in the north temperate zones, but may occur in the South. They often attack in swarms and can cause anemia and death of birds. Control is exceedingly difficult since these flies breed in streams. The range may be treated with a 1% DDT dust (where lawful) and all poultry houses should be screened.

FLEAS

The sticktight flea (*Echidnophaga gallinacea*) is most common in the Southern U.S.A. After mating, the female burrows into the skin, causing ulcers on the bird. The eggs hatch and the larvae drop to the ground where they feed and the life cycle is complete in 60 days. Other birds and mammals may become infested.

The "western" hen flea (*Ceratophyllus niger*) seems to be confined to the Pacific coast area. This flea actually breeds in the droppings and only feeds on birds occasionally.

The "European" chick flea (*C. gallinae*) is widespread in the U.S.A. It breeds in the nests and litter, and only goes on the birds to suck blood. It is known to attack many other birds besides chickens.

Control is accomplished by cleaning the houses and dusting the birds and treating the infected premise with malathion (℞ 321).

MISCELLANEOUS CONDITIONS AFFECTING POULTRY

BREAST BLISTERS

A large abscess, usually found on the carinal apex of the sternum, containing a clear or blood-tinged fluid or thick, white-to-yellow pus. The condition in market chickens and turkeys causes serious financial loss when birds are sold.

The etiology is obscure, but direct trauma and heritable predisposition have been suggested. In birds eating from sharp-edged troughs, injuries may occur as early as 6 weeks of age. Staphylococci are commonly recovered from these lesions. Heavy turkeys raised on wire, or older roosting birds are also occasionally affected. Frequently the condition is not noticed until the birds are marketed.

Provided the blisters have not reached an advanced stage, the fluid can be removed surgically. To be economically successful, this treatment must be carried out at least one month prior to marketing. Simple breast blisters should be differentiated from infectious synovitis (q.v., p. 1056), which usually affects other synovial structures.

BUMBLEFOOT
(Abscess of the foot pads)

A sporadic local infection of the feet of chickens and turkeys characterized by enlargement and lameness in one or both feet. The condition usually appears after an injury to the foot pad. Various bacteria may be present, but staphylococci are most commonly found. A fowl cholera (*Pasteurella*) organism of low virulence and *Mycobacterium avium* have also been reported. The condition is more common in the heavy breeds. Lameness is associated with a localized bulbous swelling of the foot pad. A superficial wound may or may not be present. In advanced cases, the entire leg may be involved. Although the condition may be obvious, it should be differentiated from infectious synovitis (q.v., p. 1056). The latter disease occurs usually in birds up to 12 weeks of age, whereas bumblefoot is more prevalent in older, heavier birds.

Incidence may be reduced by removal of high roosts and other objects which allow birds to jump from high places to concrete floors. Equipment should not have sharp projections or protruding nails as these may injure the feet. If treatment is elected, the hard core or pus in the swelling should be evacuated, bleeding controlled, and the resulting cavity thoroughly cleaned and painted with tincture of iodine, or packed with ammoniated mercurial ointment. Sulfathiazole ointment has also proved satisfactory.

GOUT
(Acute toxic nephritis)

A condition of low incidence usually found in adult hens, characterized by the presence of urates in the viscera or joints. Two types of the disease occur, visceral and articular. The cause is unknown. Vitamin A deficiency and high-protein diets have both been suggested as of etiologic significance, but there is little evidence to support these views. It is most common in laying flocks. Affected birds become dull and listless, and eventually die. The condition must be distinguished from thallium poisoning.

At necropsy, the visceral type shows a white, flakelike, material (uric acid crystals) covering all abdominal organs. This material may also be present in the pericardial sac. In the articular type, which is uncommon, the joints may be enlarged and swollen. When opened, these joints exude a thick, white, tenacious fluid, composed almost entirely of synovia and uric acid crystals.

No specific treatment or control is known.

KERATOCONJUNCTIVITIS

A condition of chickens, ducklings and turkeys characterized by a severe conjunctivitis, keratitis and ulceration of the cornea, commonly leading to blindness in one or both eyes. The morbidity in turkeys may reach 40% and in chickens it may approach 100%. The condition should be differentiated from a clouding of the lens which is frequently found in avian encephalomyelitis.

The specific cause is unknown. However, the condition is generally associated with a high atmospheric concentration of ammonia which arises from the litter under circumstances of poor ventilation and unsanitary surroundings. It can usually be controlled by changing to fresh, dry litter and improving the ventilation. Supplementing the ration with vitamin A may be helpful. Affected birds should be isolated to avoid cannibalism and treated individually with antibiotic eye ointments and vitamin A concentrates.

PENDULOUS CROP
(Crop bound, Sour crop, Impacted crop, Sagging crop)

A disease of both chickens and turkeys characterized by a greatly enlarged, dependent crop which becomes distended with food. The cause is unknown, but hereditary factors, impaction due to coarse, long-fibered food, or paralysis of the crop may be of etiologic importance. No treatment is completely satisfactory. Flooding the crop with isotonic salt solution or mineral oil through a dose syringe, to loosen the mass, may effect a cure. In valuable birds, surgical removal of the contents and reduction of the crop size is reasonably successful.

PART IV

FUR, LABORATORY
AND ZOO ANIMALS

FUR-ANIMAL MANAGEMENT

MINK

The ranch should be located on well-drained soil, well away from urban areas. There are no practical means of reducing the odor of a mink farm. A guard fence around the ranch, although not essential, may prevent the escape of mink from the ranch, and keep out stray dogs or skunks.

Mink are housed individually in wire mesh pens raised above the ground. A nest box with a hole for entry is attached outside or placed within the pen. Soft marsh hay free from awns, or fine wood-wool makes suitable nest material. Nest boxes should be cleaned and nest material replaced as required, especially before a female whelps, and during cold weather.

Sheds, which have been used to house mink for pelting, are used increasingly for breeding stock and throughout the year, provided lighting is adequate to supply the usual daylight hours and there is plenty of air circulation in the warmer months. If mink are housed outdoors, nest boxes must have waterproof lids and pens must have some shade during the summer and autumn.

Mink are fed by placing a day's ration of a meat-cereal-water mixture on top of the wire. Most ranchers place food on pans inside the run for small kits which cannot reach the food on top of the pen. Mink require an ample supply of fresh water. Watering cups fastened to the outside of the pen with a lip protruding inside are commonly used. Automatic watering systems with individual nipples are used in sheds, until the temperature drops to freezing. Cold storage facilities are necessary to freeze and store the meat portion of the ration. A day's supply of meat and meat by-products is thawed, cereal is added and the combined ration is mixed with water to a consistency that will remain on the wire of the pen without dropping through. Ready-mixed feeds are available in some areas. This may be delivered daily, ready to feed, or may be in frozen blocks, which are kept in cold storage and thawed as required. Dry diets are used on some ranches for part of the year.

Mink are normally pelted in November or December. Several methods of killing are used, depending on the preference of the rancher. Cervical dislocation is commonly used. Magnesium sulfate, nicotine sulfate, ether or strychnine may be injected into the heart.

Ranchers usually keep one male for each 5 female breeders. March is the mating season. Mink are much more active at this time, and a clucking sound is characteristic, but there are no external signs of estrus. After a male is placed in a female's pen, mating should occur within an hour. If fighting ensues they should be separated. Ovulation is induced by coitus. Females may ovulate 2 or 3 times and 2 matings are usual to ensure a high conception rate but there should be an interval of 6 to 8 days between matings. Ova from 2 ovulations have been known to contribute to the same litter. There is delayed implantation of the fertilized ova, so the apparent gestation period varies from 40 to 75 days.

Mink have one litter a year of 1 to 12 kits (average 4). Most litters are born during the last week in April and the first 2 weeks in May. Kits are blind, hairless and weigh about 10 gm when born, but grow rapidly throughout the summer to reach a weight of about 800 gm (females) or 1600 gm (males) by October. Kits are weaned at about 6 to 8 weeks of age, and may be separated shortly thereafter into singles, twos or threes. Complete separation is delayed until later in the season, on some ranches.

CHINCHILLA

The chinchilla is a small rodent with large, almost bare ears, prominent tactile hairs protruding from the upper lip, and well-developed hind limbs. The fur, which is very soft and normally grayish in color, is produced in tufts of several strands from each hair follicle. The female, weighing about 1½ lb, is slightly larger than the male. The color and marking of both sexes are the same. There are now 3 recognized species, the Peruvian *Chinchilla chinchilla chinchilla*, the Bolivian, *C. boliviana* (both formerly *C. brevicaudata*), and the Chilean, *C. villidera* (formerly *C. laniger*). The differences are minor, the former 2 species being slightly larger and darker.

Although chinchillas originated from the Andes mountains of South America, they can be raised almost anywhere in temperate zones. Ranchers with a smaller number of animals may keep them in dry and well-ventilated basements. If a special building is planned for chinchilla raising, it should be situated so that its length runs north and south, to allow the animals access to a maximum of sunlight.

Pens are usually constructed of wire mesh for easy cleaning and adequate circulation of air. A nest box may be used. Water is usually supplied from bottles or by an automatic system. A pan or box containing a mixture of Fuller's earth and white sand should be placed in the pan each day, to provide a dust bath. A hayrack and a self-feeder for pellets should be included as part of the equipment for each pen.

The pens must be cleaned; the interval is dependent on the type of pen. Most mild disinfectants can be used. Cresol compounds should be avoided since they may cause a severe inflammation of the feet. Water bottles should be cleaned and disinfected at frequent intervals.

The breeding unit should have an area designated for the storage of hay and pellets. Some feed rooms have a solid bale-sized bin for hay. Garbage cans may be used to store pellets. Rodents, dogs and other animals must be kept away from feeds that the chinchillas are to consume.

Chincillas may breed when they are 7 to 9 months old. Either pair-mating, or the controlled access of one male to a battery of 4 or 5 pens each containing a female, may be used. Mating often occurs at night and may be preceded by a fight. One of the best indications of a successful breeding is the finding of a "stopper" or plug-like structure in the bottom of the pen. This structure is formed in the vagina and is expelled at the time of breeding, but it may not be found because frequently it is consumed by one of the chinchillas. The gestation period varies with the species; for *C. villidera*, the average is 111 days, while for the other 2 it is 128 days. If the female has conceived, the mammary glands will enlarge soon after the 60th day. A litter consists of 1 to 4 young, the average being 2. The female comes in estrus within a few hours of parturition. The male is sometimes left in the pen during littering so that a mating may take place shortly thereafter, however the female may be aggressive at this time. A second estrus occurs within about 28 days.

Newborn chinchillas are furred and active at birth but should not be subjected to drafts. Heat (e.g., a small electric light bulb) should be provided in the nest box, especially in cold, damp weather. The young should be kept under observation for the first few days, to be certain that they are being nourished adequately. If the female is weak or the young are orphaned, a lactating guinea pig may be substituted for the mother. Dry fortified cereal such as that used for babies makes a satisfactory supplement for young chinchillas. Occasionally, one may hear unusual noises in the nest box. This may indicate that the young chinchillas' teeth are so sharp that the dam will not allow them to nurse. Such teeth can be filed with a small emery board. The young are weaned at about 60 days.

Tattoo marks are made in the ears so that individual animals can be identified. The pelt becomes prime from December to February, depending on local climatic conditions. The most convenient way to handle chinchillas is by grasping them gently at the base of the tail. If they become excited, the hair comes out in patches. Chinchillas may bite, but they are not considered vicious.

DISEASES OF MINK

DISEASES OF KNOWN OR SUSPECTED VIRAL ETIOLOGY

PLASMACYTOSIS
(Aleutian disease)

A slowly progressive disease of mink, characterized by poor reproduction, gradual weight loss, increased susceptibility to bacterial infections, and high mortality due to terminal renal failure. All color types of mink are susceptible. The causative agent is thought to be a virus or virus-like. Transmission may occur *in utero* by direct or indirect contact with infected mink.

Gross pathologic changes include enlargement of the spleen, kidney changes varying from swelling and petechiation to atrophy and pitting, and enlargement of mesenteric lymph nodes. Histopathologically, the most characteristic findings include proliferation of plasma cells in the kidneys, liver, spleen, lymph nodes and bone marrow; bile duct proliferation in the liver; hyaline changes in renal glomeruli and tubules; and fibrinoid arteritis.

Serum protein abnormalities (hypergammaglobulinemia and depression of albumin) are present in all mink with plasmacytosis (except in early or terminal cases) but these changes may be caused also by other chronic infections. The iodine agglutination test (R 649) detects these serum changes, and is useful in the control of plasmacytosis.

Mink that are to be kept for breeding stock are tested in the late fall (before selection of breeding stock and pelting) and in January or February (before breeding). New introductions to the herd should be tested. Because there is no vaccination or effective treatment, all positive reactors should be pelted.

The infective agent is present in the saliva, urine, feces, and blood of infected mink, and care should be taken to disinfect equipment after handling, vaccinating, or testing mink on infected ranches.

DISTEMPER

Mink of all ages are susceptible to canine distemper. The incubation period varies from 9 to 14 days. The virus may be recovered from infected mink 5 days before the appearance of clinical signs. Mink that have apparently recovered may continue to excrete the virus for several weeks.

Transmission may be direct (through contact or aerosol) or indirect (the virus may persist for 20 minutes or more in the environment). Clinical signs may be dermatotropic (hyperemia, followed by swelling, wrinkling, thickening and crustiness of the skin on the face, feet and ventral abdominal wall), neurotropic (convulsions and "screaming fits") or a combination of these.

At necropsy, organs usually appear to be normal, but in most cases, histopathologic examination reveals eosinophilic intracytoplasmic or intranuclear inclusions in epithelial cells of the urinary bladder, kidney, liver, intestine, lung or trachea. Similar inclusions may be seen in mink with Aleutian disease, but distemper inclusions are negative with the periodic acid-Schiff stain.

Treatment is not recommended; all mink showing signs of distemper should be destroyed. All apparently normal mink should be vaccinated prophylactically at 10 to 12 weeks of age (10 days after weaning) and breeding stock should be vaccinated annually, in January or February. Aerosol vaccines may be advantageous, since handling subclinically infected mink is avoided and thus the possibility of transmission of distemper or other diseases by handling the mink or by using contaminated needles, syringes or other equipment, is minimized.

VIRUS ENTERITIS
(Fort William disease)

A highly contagious, feline-panleukopenia-like disease of mink, caused by a virus related to that of feline panleukopenia. All ages are susceptible, but the disease is most common in kits. Transmission usually occurs by the fecal-oral route, and the incubation period varies from 4 to 8 days. Clinical signs include anorexia, depression, and the passage of pale, mucoid, unformed feces, often containing blood and intestinal casts. Characteristic gross pathologic findings are flaccid dilation and marked hyperemia of the small intestine, with liquid, fetid content, but these changes are not present in all affected mink. Histopathologic examination usually reveals severe enteritis, with hydropic degeneration of epithelial cells in the intestinal mucosa; these cells may contain inclusion bodies similar to those of feline panleukopenia.

All mink showing signs of virus enteritis should be destroyed, and all clinically normal mink should be vaccinated with a formalized mink-tissue vaccine as soon as the diagnosis is made. After an outbreak, breeders should be revaccinated in January or February, and annual vaccination of kits is recommended in enzootic areas. Because some inadequately formalized mink-tissue vaccines have been suspected of containing Aleutian disease virus or the mink encephalopathy agent, live feline panleukopenia-attenuated-virus vaccines have been used in some areas. Although the viruses of mink and feline enteritis are cross-immunogenic, they do not appear to be cross-infective under natural conditions.

AUJESZKY'S DISEASE
(Pseudorabies)

Aujeszky's disease is occasionally reported in mink fed contaminated pork products. Mortality may be high, and clinical signs are referrable to the CNS (tonic and clonic convulsions, excitement alternating with depression and, in some cases, self-mutilation). The diagnosis is confirmed by inoculation of brain tissue from suspect mink into rabbits. Since contaminated pork is usually the source of infection, suspect pork should be cooked before it is fed to mink.

TRANSMISSIBLE MINK ENCEPHALOPATHY

This scrapie-like disease has caused high mortality in adult mink. The incubation period in experimental infections is 8 months or longer, and clinical signs are similar to those of scrapie (hyperirritability, ataxia, compulsive biting, somnolence, coma and death). Histopathologic findings in brains of affected mink are similar to those of scrapie in sheep. Although mink have been experimentally infected by intracerebral inoculation of brain material from scrapie-infected sheep, and by the feeding of tissues from infected mink, the means of natural transmission is unknown. Control measures cannot be suggested, therefore, except to suggest exclusion of sheep by-products from the ration in endemic areas.

BACTERIAL DISEASES

BOTULISM

Botulism occasionally causes heavy losses in unvaccinated mink consuming food containing botulinus (Type C) toxin. Usually, many mink are found dead within 24 hours of exposure to the toxin, while others show varying degrees of paralysis and dyspnea. Postmortem findings are nonspecific and are related to death from respiratory paralysis.

Toxic feed should be removed, and stored feed or ingredients examined for the presence of toxin. Antiserum therapy is of questionable benefit, and recovered mink are not immune to further challenge. Annual vaccination of kits and breeders with botulism (Type C) toxoid is recommended to prevent outbreaks. Mink are usually vaccinated subcut. with a combined virus enteritis-botulism vaccine. This may be administered at the same time as distemper vaccine, but must be injected at a different site, since the formalin from this vaccine may inactivate the modified live virus distemper vaccine.

HEMORRHAGIC PNEUMONIA

This disease, caused by *Pseudomonas aeruginosa,* has caused serious losses on mink ranches. Mink of all ages are affected and the disease is most common in the autumn. Clinically and at necropsy, the disease may resemble heat stroke, but history and bacteriologic culture establish the diagnosis. Vaccination with *Pseudomonas* bacterin appears to be the most successful means of control. Losses usually stop within a few days of vaccination.

TUBERCULOSIS

Mink are susceptible to infection with avian, bovine, human and perhaps other tubercle bacilli. Infection is usually foodborne, and the disease may become endemic on some ranches. Clinical signs include weight loss, and in some cases, abdominal distension. At necropsy, the mink is severely emaciated and has an enlarged spleen and lymph nodes; in many cases, there is miliary involvement of lungs, liver and other organs. The diagnosis is confirmed on the basis of acid-fast stains of smears of affected tissues. Treatment of affected mink is ineffective and impractical, and control consists of culling visibly affected mink, and using meat products from inspected processing plants for feed. Tuberculin tests are generally ineffective in detecting infected mink.

URINARY INFECTIONS AND UROLITHIASIS

Urinary tract infections cause serious losses in female mink in late spring (during pregnancy and lactation) and in male mink in late summer and autumn (during the rapid-growth and furring period). Several predisposing factors have been suggested, including avitaminosis-A, diethylstilbestrol toxicity, and contamination of food, cages or nest boxes by pathogenic bacteria.

Affected mink usually die without showing clinical signs. Gross postmortem findings include acute hemorrhagic cystitis or pyelonephritis or both, usually associated with urinary calculi (magnesium ammonium phosphate) in the bladder or kidneys. A variety of organisms, including staphylococci, coliforms and *Proteus,* are commonly isolated.

In severe outbreaks, bacteriologic culture and sensitivity tests should be done to determine the causative organism, and the treatment of choice added to the feed. Where a continual problem exists, feed grade (75%) phosphoric acid may be added to the feed (0.8 lb/100 lb of feed) from March to October, to reduce the pH of the urine, since magnesium ammonium phosphate calculi are soluble in solutions of pH 6.0 or less.

MISCELLANEOUS BACTERIAL DISEASES

Various diseases, including septicemia, pneumonia, pleuritis, abscesses, cellulitis and enteritis occur sporadically on mink ranches, but occasionally they may become herd problems. Many bacteria have been isolated from these diseases, including *Proteus, Klebsiella,* coliforms, streptococci, staphylococci and salmonellae.

Antibacterial sensitivity tests should be done to determine the treatment of choice in individual mink, or the herd if several mink are involved. Drugs may be administered orally or parenterally and if many mink are to be treated drugs should be added to the feed. Dosage can be estimated on the basis of body weight—female mink weigh 1½ lb, and males from 4 to 4½ lb. Dosage levels recommended for dogs should be used and adjusted for weight. However, certain drugs, such as sulfonamides and streptomycin, are not recommended for mink.

Whenever possible, the source of infection should be determined and eliminated. For example, enteritis is often caused by spoiled feed, and abscesses by injury from wire or splintered wood in the pens, awns in hay or straw used for bedding, or spicules of bone in the feed. Outbreaks of tularemia, anthrax, brucellosis and clostridial infections have been caused by the feeding of contaminated feed, often containing tissue of animals that have died or are carriers of these infections. Careful selection of feed ingredients, and disinfection of equipment and pens are very important in the prevention and control of many infections of mink.

NUTRITIONAL DISEASES

Steatitis (yellow-fat disease) is common in young, rapidly growing mink as a result of excessive rancid unsaturated fatty acids in the diet. Affected mink may be found dead, or they may exhibit slight locomotor disturbances followed by death. Necropsy findings include yellow, edematous internal or subcut. fat that contains an acid-fast pigment. Control consists of removal of the source of the rancid fats, and proper storage of feed. Stabilized vitamin E may be administered in the feed (2 to 5 mg/mink) for 2 weeks, and affected kits should be injected parenterally with 10 to 20 mg for several days.

Chastek paralysis (thiamine deficiency) results from feeding certain raw fish containing thiaminase. These include whitefish, freshwater smelt, carp, goldfish, creek chub, fathead minnow, buckeye shiner, sucker, channel catfish, bullhead and minnow, white bass, sauger pike, burbot and saltwater herring. Affected mink gradually lose their appetite and weight, and die after terminal convulsions and paralysis. Thiaminase-containing fish should be cooked, or fed raw only on alternate days. Affected mink may be injected IP with 1 mg/lb of body wt of thiamine hydrochloride, and adequate thiamine (brewer's yeast) should be present in the ration.

Because of the rapid growth of mink kits, **rickets** is common where rations are deficient in vitamin D, calcium or phosphorus. Affected kits usually crawl unsteadily in a frog-like posture, have rubbery bones, and are smaller than normal. The diet should be supplemented as required, and severely affected kits may be treated on an individual basis.

Nursing sickness occurs in lactating female mink. Affected females become thin and weak, stop eating and wander about aimlessly, ignoring their kits and sometimes carrying food in their mouths without eating it. Death occurs within a few days of onset of clinical signs. Gross postmortem lesions are nonspecific, but include lipidosis and dehydration. Kits from affected females must be weaned or fostered as soon as possible, and affected females should be tempted to eat with liver, freshly killed sparrows, etc. To control this condition, kits should be encouraged to start eating solid food as early as possible by placing trays containing soft feed in the pen. Salt may be added (0.5% of ration, if it is not already present in the commercial cereal) and plenty of fresh water and feed should be available to nursing females at all times.

Cotton underfur usually indicates **anemia** in mink, and may be caused by certain fish (Pacific hake, coalfish, whiting) which interfere with iron retention in the mink. This condition can be prevented by cooking the offending fish, or by feeding it on alternate days.

Gray underfur occurs when high levels of turkey offal or uncooked eggs are fed to young mink. Avidin, a factor present in eggs, inactivates biotin, a vitamin required for pigmentation. Affected mink may be injected with 1 mg biotin twice weekly for 4 weeks, and turkey offal should be cooked or biotin added to the ration.

POISONINGS

Lead poisoning is common in mink that have ingested lead-containing paints from wire or other equipment. Affected mink gradually lose weight and die within 1 or 2 months. Dicalcium phosphate or calcium gluconate and vitamin D should be added to the ration on affected ranches.

Insecticides other than pyrethrum, piperonyl butoxide and rotenone may be highly toxic to mink. The above insecticides should not be used on mink under 8 weeks of age, or where these mink can contact them (nest boxes, etc.). Other insecticides should be avoided whenever possible.

Wood preservatives (chlorinated phenols, cresols) cause mortality of kits in the first 3 weeks of life, and occasionally, in older mink. They should not be used where mink can chew on treated wood (pens or nest boxes).

Diethylstilbestrol-containing products cause reproductive failure and a high incidence of urinary tract infections in mink, and care should be taken not to include them in the ration. Similarly, **thyroids** and **parathyroids** included in meat trimmings may result in reproductive failure if present at high levels.

Chlorinated hydrocarbons and **polychlorinated biphenyls** (PCB) contained in the ration have been suspected of causing reproductive failure in mink.

DMNA: The addition of sodium nitrite as a preservative to stale herring meal results in the formation of dimethylnitrosamine (DMNA) which is very hepatotoxic in mink, causing hepatic degeneration, ascites and extensive internal hemorrhage.

Sulfaquinoxaline upsets normal blood-clotting mechanisms of mink and causes extensive internal hemorrhage resulting in serious losses. **Streptomycin** is very toxic to mink and the use of this antibiotic should be avoided whenever possible.

MISCELLANEOUS DISEASES

Fur-clipping and **tail-biting** are common vices of mink, and may be related to abnormal behavior patterns of captivity. Fur-clipping decreases the value of the pelt, and tail-biting frequently results in fatal hemorrhage. There is no effective treatment, but it may be advisable to avoid using affected mink for breeding purposes.

Urinary incontinence (wet-belly disease) is a nonfatal condition usually affecting male mink in the late summer and autumn, characterized by dribbling of urine and staining of the pelt around the urinary orifice. Since affected areas of the pelt must be discarded, the condition is of economic importance. Although the cause of this condition is unknown, recent work suggests that the feeding of high levels of fresh raw chicken waste or fish may be a cause, and that cooking these ingredients may prevent the disease.

Starvation and **chilling** are common causes of death in mink fed inadequate fat or too little feed during the winter and early spring. Affected mink are very thin, and may run until they collapse and die, or they may be found dead in their cages. Such deaths are most common after sudden decrease in environmental temperature, especially in the early spring. Postmortem examination reveals emaciation and an absence of body fat, in some cases accompanied by lipidosis and gastric ulceration. This disease must be differentiated from plasmacytosis and other chronic diseases on the basis of gross postmortem and histopathologic examination.

Gray diarrhea in mink resembles chronic pancreatitis in dogs, and is characterized by a ravenous appetite and the passage of large amounts of gray, fetid feces. Affected mink appear to die of starvation. No pancreatic abnormalities, viruses, bacteria or parasites have been demonstrated as possible causes. Treatment is of questionable value although some mink have responded to long-term therapy with nitrofurazone.

Pregnancy disease occurs in female mink in late pregnancy, and is characterized by death of affected mink with extensive placental hemorrhage. The cause of this condition is unknown, but fresh feed, fresh water and good bedding in nest boxes may be effective in preventing the disease.

Gastric ulcers, and **lipidosis** are common in mink, and are usually associated with other diseases or with a period of inappetence.

Hereditary diseases (hydrocephalus, hairlessness, "screw neck", "bobbed tails", Ehlers-Danlos syndrome, hemivertebra) are occasionally seen in mink and must be controlled by pelting of the sire, dam and liter mates of the affected mink.

Coccidiosis is no longer important since nest boxes are off the ground.

Flesh-fly infestation: Flies of the genus *Wohlfartia* are the most important external parasites of mink. The only satisfactory measure of control is to use 5% ronnel dust in the nest boxes beginning a few days prior to the occurrence of the flies in an area. One heaping teaspoonful is placed in the nesting hay of each nest box. It should not be used for kits less than 3 days old. Treatment may be repeated once after a 14-day interval. (*See Cuterebra* INFESTATION OF SMALL ANIMALS, p. 750.)

VACCINATION OF EXOTIC MAMMALS

Rabies: Wild-caught animals, even when young, may have been exposed to rabies virus. Although they appear to be normal, a short observation period is inadequate as incubation may be prolonged. Because of the potential danger of rabies, the keeping of wild animals as pets should be discouraged. There are, of course, other excellent reasons for discouraging this practice.

Most exotic pets presumably are closely confined, minimizing danger of being exposed to rabies in free-living animals. Rabies vaccination of exotic pets should be undertaken with great caution; it must be emphasized that there is marked variation between species and among individuals in their response to vaccines. Clinical disease and death are common sequelae when "modified" live-virus vaccines, safe for domestic Canidae and Felidae, are used for "wild animals" in captivity.

If vaccination is considered to be necessary, only inactivated rabies virus vaccine should be used; inactivated nervous tissue vaccine, caprine or ovine origin, or inactivated tissue-culture vaccine (20% tissue suspension) is administered subcut., preferably in 2 sites at the rate of 5 ml for up to 25 lb of body wt and an additional 1 ml for each additional 5 lb of body wt up to a total of 15 ml. Young animals are vaccinated at 3 to 4 months of age. Vaccination must be repeated annually.

Distemper: All members of the Canidae, Procyonidae, Mustelidae and Hyaenidae, and some members of the Viverridae, are considered to be susceptible to distemper. There is some doubt about the susceptibility of the Ursidae. Distemper in exotic animals generally resembles that in the dog but may also cause the affected animal to lose its fear of man, thus resembling rabies.

Caution is advised in vaccinating wild-caught species, because of the danger that they may have been exposed to the virus, and thus may be incubating the disease. There is marked variation between species and individuals in their reaction to modified live-virus vaccines, therefore only inactivated virus vaccines should be used unless there is a precedent. Most of the information available is from the experience of zoo veterinarians and there are differences in reports of apparent safety and efficacy of immunizing products; therefore recommendations can be made only as a guide and with the reservations above. Annual revaccination is recommended.

Killed tissue vaccines: Inactivated canine-distemper virus vaccine: Young should be vaccinated shortly after weaning, 2 doses of 2 ml each at 14- to 21-day intervals. For larger adult animals, the initial dose should be doubled.

Modified live-virus vaccines: (*See* DISTEMPER IN MINK, p. 1111.) Mink distemper vaccine (chick-embryo or cell-culture origin) is given subcut. (1 to 2 ml, or according to the manufacturer's directions and size of the animal). Modified canine-distemper live-virus, chick-embryo or cell-culture origin is also given subcut. (2 ml or according to the manufacturer's directions and size of the animal).

Panleukopenia: All Felidae, most of the Mustelidae and some of the Procyonidae and Viverridae are believed to be susceptible to panleukopenia (feline distemper) virus infection (*see* VIRUS ENTERITIS OF MINK, p. 1111). Caution should be exercised when undertaking prophylaxis, and inactivated virus vaccines are recommended (*see* DISTEMPER IN EXOTIC MAMMALS, above). Booster doses are recommended when animals are handled or moved, and also annually. Inactivated virus feline-distemper vaccine (mink- or feline-tissue origin): for small species, 1 ml (IM or subcut.); for large cats, 2 ml/10 lb body wt (maximum 40 ml), or 2 to 4 ml, and repeated at 10-day intervals for 2 to 4 times (depending on the size of the cat).

Infectious Hepatitis: Canidae are susceptible (the disease in foxes is called **encephalitis**, as the chief manifestations are nervous signs). A modified live virus combination, canine distemper-hepatitis vaccine has been used in cases where the use of a modified live virus vaccine is advisable (*see* DISTEMPER). Annual booster doses are given.

Canine distemper-hepatitis vaccine (modified live virus, tissue culture origin or combined chick embryo-tissue culture origin) is given subcut., 2 ml, repeated in 14 days. Canine-hepatitis vaccine, modified live virus (porcine-tissue culture origin), is given subcut., 2 ml.

Leptospirosis: When they are at risk, Canidae, Procyonidae and Mustelidae may be vaccinated with *Leptospira canicola-icterohaemorrhagiae* bacterin. Young are vaccinated at 6 to 8 weeks of age (4 ml subcut., repeated in 14 days). Booster doses are given every 6 months.

DISEASES OF CHINCHILLAS

Many diseases of chinchillas are herd problems and are diagnosed on the basis of postmortem examination. Because several diseases may produce identical or similar pathologic lesions, they must be differentiated on the basis of bacteriologic culture. Clinical signs may be vague, nonspecific or nonexistent, although certain conditions such as dermatomycosis and malocclusion can be detected in the living animal.

Treatment is usually administered on a herd basis by medication of the drinking water or feed. If chinchillas appear reluctant to drink medicated water, sugar may be added in small amounts until water intake is normal. Individual treatment by oral or IM routes is traumatic and impractical, except in clinically ill individuals. Often treatment must be repeated several times at weekly intervals to control disease outbreaks. No more than one treatment should be administered at a time; when more than one disease co-exist, each disease should be treated individually (e.g., first listeriosis, then pseudomoniasis, then giardiasis).

Whenever possible, antibacterial treatments should be selected on the basis of bacteriologic culture and sensitivity. Certain antibiotics such as penicillin, streptomycin and lincomycin may cause severe inappetence and impaction if administered orally. Broad-spectrum antibiotics may seriously upset the intestinal microflora if administered for prolonged periods, therefore 3- to 5-day treatments, repeated at weekly intervals if necessary, should be used. Since secondary disease outbreaks are common in chinchillas, all animals dying during an outbreak should be examined to determine the need for continuing or changing treatment.

Many diseases of chinchillas are transmissible to man, and chinchilla owners should be made aware of this.

Pseudomonas aeruginosa is an important pathogen of chinchillas, causing conjunctivitis, otitis, pneumonia, enteritis, metritis or septicemia. Focal typhlocolitis is a characteristic postmortem finding, but diagnosis must be confirmed by bacteriologic culture. Bacterins are the treatment of choice and can be prepared easily by the practitioner or diagnostic laboratory. Supplementary chlorination of the drinking water is recommended during outbreaks.

Chinchillas are very susceptible to infections caused by *Listeria monocytogenes.* Mortality is high, and losses may continue for long periods in spite of treatment. Focal hepatic necrosis is the most common postmortem finding, but direct smears and bacteriologic culture are required to establish the diagnosis. Water-soluble chloramphenicol in the drinking water is the treatment of choice, and may have to be repeated several times. Treatment is given for 3 consecutive days at weekly intervals until losses cease.

Salmonellae occasionally cause outbreaks in chinchilla herds and must be differentiated from listeriosis on the basis of bacteriologic culture. **Streptococci** and **staphylococci** may cause conjunctivitis, pneumonia, metritis and death in chinchillas. *Pasteurella (Yersinia) pseudotuberculosis* infections may resemble listeriosis in many respects. *Pasteurella multocida* and *haemolytica* cause pneumonia or sudden death, and usually are readily detectable on bacteriologic culture or blood or tissue smears. *Proteus* are often isolated from metritis, and occasionally from conjunctivitis, otitis and enteritis, but, except in metritis, are of questionable pathogenic significance. Several other bacterial species are occasionally isolated from chinchillas, but are not considered to be important pathogens in this host.

Toxoplasma gondii has caused serious outbreaks in chinchilla herds. Clinical signs are nonspecific. Necropsy findings may include straw-colored fluid in the body cavities, pulmonary congestion, splenomegaly and enlargement of lymph nodes. Inoculation of susceptible laboratory animals and careful histopathologic examination of affected chinchillas must be done to establish the diagnosis. Sulfonamides (R 67) administered to the herd for 10 to 14 days may be effective in controlling outbreaks.

Giardia cysts and trophozoites are seen frequently in large numbers on intestinal scrapings and smears from chinchillas that have died after a period of intermittent watery diarrhea, impaction, or without clinical signs. Mortality may be high in such outbreaks, and often no other cause of death can be found. Fresh, unrefrigerated carcasses must be examined soon after death. Occasionally trophozoites or cysts can be seen in the feces of living chinchillas. Giardiasis often is secondary to other diseases, therefore bacteriologic culture should be done to eliminate this possibility. Treatment is done on a herd basis (R 339) and may have to be repeated if losses continue. Long-term therapy with thiabendazole may be useful.

Trichomonads are occasionally seen on intestinal smears of dead chinchillas, but are of questionable pathogenicity in this host.

Trichophyton mentagrophytes is the most common cause of ringworm in chinchillas. Affected individuals usually have loss of hair and reddening in lightly furred areas (nose, around eye, at base of tail) but direct microscopic examination or culture on Sabouraud's agar are required to confirm the diagnosis. Ringworm should not be confused with fur-chewing which is characterized by large patches of clipped fur. Topical ringworm treatments are of questionable value. Affected animals should be isolated and treated with griseofulvin (R 352). If several chinchillas are affected, herd treatment should be considered.

Fur-chewing is a common vice of chinchillas characterized by clipping of the fur on the flanks and other parts, leaving patches of short fur. Numerous causes have been proposed, but the condition probably is an abnormal behavior pattern precipitated by confinement, boredom or nervousness. The herd incidence, which may be high, has been reduced in some cases by the elimination of affected animals from the breeding herd, decreasing the environmental humidity and temperature and supplying good-quality hay free-choice to the animals.

Malocclusion is a common dental deformity of chinchillas, characterized by overgrowth and angularity of molar and incisor teeth. Affected animals are usually over a year of age, lose weight rapidly and salivate profusely (slobbers). Death results from starvation or secondary diseases. Examination of the mouth with an otoscope reveals overgrown, angular teeth. Since the condition is thought to be hereditary (caused by a recessive gene), and because it recurs after surgical correction, euthanasia of affected chinchillas should be recommended.

Metritis is a common cause of infertility in chinchillas and is characterized by a white or creamy discharge seen upon opening the vagina. Bacteriologic culture and sensitivity tests are required to determine the treatment of choice. After the infection has been controlled, estrogenic compounds may be injected to re-establish estrus in affected females. The value of hormone treatments of sterile chinchillas is questionable, however, since many of these do not conceive in spite of induced estrus.

Intestinal impaction, intussusception and **rectal prolapse** are seen commonly in chinchillas and often are secondary to pseudomoniasis, listeriosis or other infections. Impaction is characterized by the passage of small hard droppings, which decrease in numbers until none is passed. Sometimes it can be relieved by oral administration of 0.5 to 2 ml of equal parts of mineral oil and milk of magnesia b.i.d., until the droppings are normal. Subcut. fluids may be administered to offset dehydration. Rectal prolapse or intussusception or both are associated with diarrhea or impaction. These conditions usually recur after surgical correction, thus a poor prognosis should be given in affected animals. In all cases, the initial cause of these conditions must be determined to rule out the possibility of concurrent bacterial or parasitic infection.

Surgical procedures are occasionally required in chinchillas (e.g., cesarean, rectal prolapse) although the prognosis for life or reproductive capacity following surgery often does not make such procedures economically attractive. Ether, halothane or methoxyfluorane can be used as inhalation anesthetics, but chloroform is toxic to chinchillas and other rodents. Pentobarbital sodium (35 mg/kg) or thiopental sodium (40 mg/kg) can be administered IP for surgical anesthesia.

RABBIT MANAGEMENT

The **housing** required for rabbits raised outdoors is dependent on the climate and should be located on nearly level, well-drained soil. Shade should be provided over a portion of the hutch. All construction should be simple and allow for ventilation and light. In general, hutches should be 2½ ft deep and 4 ft in length. Large breeds should have hutches 6 ft long. The bottoms of hutches can be made of ½-in. hardware cloth for the small breeds, but for the medium and heavier breeds, ⅝ in. should be used. In northern regions, the sides and back of the hutch should be of solid construction, whereas in warmer climates, only a roof is required.

The hutch should be equipped with feed hoppers for pellets, water containers and nest boxes. The hoppers should be constructed so as to prevent contamination. Heavy, flat-bottomed ceramic crocks holding a day's supply of water are good receptacles. Automatic watering systems are used on large farms. The nest box should be so constructed that it can easily be removed from the hutch for cleaning and disinfecting between litters. It should be of a size sufficient to prevent crowding, but small enough to keep the young warm. Apple boxes make excellent nest boxes. Straw or wood shavings make good bedding in either warm or cold weather. The hutches should be thoroughly cleaned each week.

Over 30 million pounds of domestic rabbit meat is consumed annually in North America. Increasing numbers of rabbits are used in research and teaching, probably about 700,000 yearly. For this purpose, many rabbits are raised indoors in more controlled environments, using more easily sanitized materials such as stainless steel and plastics.

The **selection of breeding stock** is dependent upon the purposes of the raisers. The wool breeds include the English and French Angora. American Chinchilla, Checkered Giant, Rex, Satin, and Silver Marten are fur breeds, while those bred for meat are the White New Zealand, Red New Zealand, Californian and Flemish Giant. The white breeds, the White New Zealand and the Californian, are the most popular, as they produce a white pelt. Of the 28 rabbit breeds recognized in America, most laboratory usage is of the White New Zealand, Dutch and various mixed breeds, usually white.

Rabbits are sexually mature from 7 months for the medium breeds to 9 to 12 months for the giant breeds. The small breeds, such as the Polish and the Dutch, mature at about 5 months. Rabbits do not have a regular estrous cycle. The receptiveness of the doe, which is an induced ovulator, is established by excitement or close proximity to other rabbits. A ratio of 10 does to one buck is considered to be maximum, with 4 or 5 matings per week for the buck occasionally employed, and 2 to 3 matings a week with continuous use. The breeding program should be carried on throughout the year. The gestation period is 31 to 32 days. The pregnant doe will make her own nest in the nest box 3 or 4 days before parturition (kindling). The does should be left as quiet as possible during this period. The young may be examined on the second or third day. Considering a nursing period of 8 weeks, one doe can produce 4 litters a year if breeding failures do not occur. By rebreeding the doe when the young are 6 weeks old, 5 litters per year are obtained in many commercial rabbitries. A false pregnancy may occur as a result of infertile mating or one female riding another. These females cannot conceive for 17 days (the period of false pregnancy); therefore, test matings to determine whether the doe will accept the buck are routine on the 18th day after mating. If the doe has conceived, the fetuses can be palpated on the 12th day after breeding.

Rabbits should be carried by grasping the loose skin over the withers with one hand and placing the other under the rump to support the weight from beneath. If they are not held properly and securely, fractures or luxations of thoracic and lumbar vertebrae may follow struggling. The claws on the rear limbs are capable of inflicting severe lacerations on unprotected arms of handlers. Some breeders tattoo their animals for identification purposes. The right ear is reserved for registration marks.

The sex of the rabbit may be determined when the rabbit is 3 days of age; however, it usually is done at weaning time. By depressing the external genitalia, the mucous membrane can be exposed. In the male, the mucous membrane protrudes and forms a circle, whereas, in the female, it will extend and form a slit. Castration has no advantage for meat-type rabbits, as the growth for males and females is about the same until after market age. Angora rabbits raised longer than 6 months are sometimes castrated. The technique is similar to that of castrating cats, although it should be noted that the testes in the scrotum are lateral-to-anterior to the penis, as in marsupials, and unlike most other placental mammals.

When they are unobserved, usually in the early morning or at night, rabbits re-ingest part of their feces by contorting themselves so that the mouth touches the anus. They feed only on the soft matter that has passed through the tract but once. This trait of rabbits, which is normal and not a sign of nutritional deficiency, is often called pseudorumination. This coprophagy serves an important nutritional function by supplying the animal with intestinally synthesized B-vitamins, particularly thiamine. Stability of the normal intestinal microflora may depend on normal coprophagy; wire-mesh cage or hutch flooring does not prevent coprophagy.

Feeding rabbits (q.v., p. 1280 has been greatly aided by commercially available pelleted diets, most of which are nutritionally adequate.

DISEASES OF RABBITS

Although most techniques suitable for dogs and cats may be applied to rabbits for physical examination and restraint, general anesthesia of rabbits with barbiturates is often accompanied by significant mortality. Inhalation agents such as halothane are often safer to use.

VIRAL DISEASES

With the exception of rabbit pox, and a herpesvirus infection (Virus III), viral diseases in rabbits are restricted to the infectious fibromas and papillomatosis. The former are tumors composed of connective tissue and consist largely of fibroblasts and their products. They are located under, rather than in, the skin, in which respect they differ from the papillomas. There are 2 types of known infectious fibrotic tumors which occur under natural conditions, the tumor of infectious myxomatosis and the Shope fibroma. Both are viral and restricted to rabbits, the former to the domesticated species only, in the U.S.A., and the Shope fibroma to the cottontail.

INFECTIOUS MYXOMATOSIS

Infectious myxomatosis is a fatal disease of the ordinary domestic rabbit, Angoras, Belgian hares, Flemish Giants and the European wild rabbit. The cottontail and the jack rabbit are quite resistant, as are man, dog and other animal species tested. The virus causing the disease is transmitted by mosquitoes, biting flies and direct contact.

In the U.S.A., myxomatosis is restricted largely to the coastal area of California and Oregon, where epizootics occur every 8 to 10 years during the months of May to August, which correspond to the height of the mosquito season. These areas are limited to the geographic distribution of the California brush rabbit (*Sylvilagus bachmani*), the reservoir of the infection. In the rabbitries involved, losses range from 25 to 90%. During intervening years, only sporadic outbreaks occur. Rabbits of all ages are susceptible, although the young up to the age of a month appear more resistant than the adult animals.

The first characteristic sign observed is a conjunctivitis that rapidly becomes more marked and is accompanied by a milky discharge from the inflamed eyes. The animal appears listless, is anorectic and the temperature frequently reaches 108°F. In severe acute outbreaks, some of the animals may die within 48 hours after showing signs. Those that do not die at this stage become progressively depressed, develop a rough coat, and the eyelids, nose, lips and ears become edematous, giving a swollen appearance to the head. The vent becomes inflamed and edematous and, in the male, swelling of the scrotum occurs. A very characteristic sign at this stage is the drooping of the edematous ears. A purulent nasal discharge invariably appears, the breathing becomes labored and the animal goes into a coma just before death, which usually occurs within 1 to 2 weeks after the appearance of clinical signs. Occasionally, an animal will linger on for several weeks before death ensues. In these cases, fibrotic nodules appear on the nose, ears and forefeet. Animals inoculated experimentally with laboratory strains of the virus invariably develop small nodules at the point of injection several days thereafter and these are followed by the development of similar nodules on other parts of the body, particularly the ears.

No characteristic lesions are found at necropsy. The spleen is occasionally enlarged and black in color.

The seasonal incidence of the disease, the clinical appearance of the infected animals and the high mortality are all of diagnostic significance.

A live vaccine prepared from an attenuated myxomatosis virus has been shown to protect both field- and laboratory-infected animals, and is available commercially.

THE SHOPE FIBROMA

The Shope fibroma occurs under natural conditions in the cottontail only, although the domestic species of rabbits can be infected by the inoculation of virus-containing material. The disease is not of economic importance, but is of considerable scientific interest.

Experimentally, it has been found possible to protect domestic rabbits against the virus of myxomatosis by the inoculation of living fibroma virus, but this has several drawbacks: The virus fails to immunize consistently, the resultant immunity is short-lived, and fibromas appear at the site of inoculation.

PAPILLOMATOSIS

Papillomas are benign tumors consisting of small, grayish-white, pedunculated nodules on the under surface of the tongue or the floor of the mouth, occasionally seen in domestic rabbits. Individuals are not treated, but the balance of the herd may be vaccinated with an autogenous vaccine: To a 10% suspension of papilloma tissue in isotonic salt solution, 0.4% formalin is added and allowed to stand at 5°C for a week. Then it is cultured and, if bacteriologically sterile, inoculated subcut. in 0.5-ml quantities at 7-day intervals for 3 weeks. This virus (Papova virus) is distinct from the Shope papilloma virus seen in wild rabbits.

RABBIT POX

An acute, generalized disease of laboratory rabbits, pox is characterized by pyrexia, nasal and conjunctival discharge and skin rash. The mortality rate varies, but is always high. The disease has not been recognized in wild rabbits.

The causative virus is closely related to vaccinia virus and some outbreaks may have been caused by a virulent strain of vaccinia. The virus may be isolated and identified by methods appropriate to vaccinia (see POX DISEASES, p. 238).

Spread of this disease through a rabbitry or an animal house is very rapid, but rabbits which have been inoculated with smallpox vaccine (vaccinia virus) are immune.

BACTERIAL AND FUNGUS DISEASES

PASTEURELLOSIS

A highly contagious disease, common in domestic rabbits, transmitted either by direct or indirect contact. Apparently, rabbits develop little immunity following infection. Some animals are healthy carriers and probably perpetuate the disease in the rabbitry. An indirect fluorescent-antibody test for use on nasal swabs has been found effective in identifying carriers, which may constitute up to 90% of apparently healthy rabbits in conventional colonies. *Pasteurella multocida* infections may be manifested in the following conditions:

Snuffles or nasal catarrh: An acute, subacute or chronic inflammation of the mucous membranes of the air passages and lungs. The signs are a thin or purulent exudate from the nose and eyes. The fur on the inside of the front legs just above the paws will be matted and caked with dried exudate from the rabbits pawing at their noses. The infected animal usually sneezes and coughs. Snuffles, in general, occurs when the resistance of the rabbit is low or at kindling time. Those animals that recover may become carriers. *Bordetella bronchiseptica* may play a role in some cases also. Pneumonia (q.v., p. 1129) can ensue.

Abscesses caused by *Pasteurella* may be found in any part of the body or head. Rabbits of all ages are susceptible. When bucks are penned together, their fight wounds frequently develop into abscesses. In most instances, it is advisable to eliminate rather than to treat the affected rabbit. The condition may terminate in a septicemia, the animal dying within 48 hours. Necropsy reveals bronchial congestion, tracheitis, splenomegaly and subcut. hemorrhages.

A troublesome **genital infection** is often caused by *Pasteurella* but several other organisms also may be involved. It is manifested by an acute or subacute inflammation of the reproductive tract. This condition most frequently is found in adults, more often in does than bucks. If the condition is bilateral, the does often become sterile, but if only one horn is infected, a normal litter may develop in the other. In the female, a pyometra is produced, of which the vaginal discharge of a thick, yellowish-gray pus may be the only sign noted. The buck may exhibit a discharge of pus from the penis, but usually an orchitis is noted. A chronic infection of the prostate and seminal vesicles is most likely if the animal is not culled, and venereal transmission may ensue. It is best to eliminate the animal as a source of infection. The infected hutch and its equipment should be thoroughly disinfected. For a valuable breeder, antibiotics (℞ 11, 31, 36) may be used in combating the infection; however, a poor prognosis should be given.

PSEUDOTUBERCULOSIS

Nodules resembling the tubercles of tuberculosis, and caused by *Pasteurella pseudotuberculosis,* may be observed in the parenchyma of the liver, lungs, spleen and the intestinal wall. There is evidence that suggests that the organisms enter the host through contaminated food or water. The signs are lassitude, anorexia, emaciation and dyspnea. These rabbits should be destroyed, since man is susceptible, and should not be marketed. The contaminated hutches should be cleaned and disinfected with a strong, hot lye solution.

LISTERIOSIS

Young rabbits are most frequently affected. The losses occur chiefly in the spring and fall. The animals become very emaciated during the course of the disease. Some affected rabbits exhibit a typical torticollis. At necropsy, one can notice many small, white foci scattered through the hepatic parenchyma. Affected individuals should be destroyed.

MASTITIS
(Blue Breasts)

Mastitis is occasionally observed in domestic rabbits. The cause is believed to be streptococci or staphylococci. The malady may spread through the rabbitry, rapidly attacking lactating does. The mammary glands become hot, reddened and swollen; later, the glands may become cyanotic, hence the common name. The doe will not eat, but may crave water. A temperature as high as 105°F, or higher, is often noted. The condition may be treated by the parenteral injection of penicillin (℞ 44). Treatment of does where the inflammation is extensive is not advocated and euthanasia of both does and young is recommended; hand-raising infant rabbits is difficult.

PNEUMONIA

Pneumonia is not uncommon in domestic rabbits. It may occur in adult animals or may infect the young while they are in the nest box. Frequently, it is a secondary and complicating factor in the enteritis complex. The cause is bacterial with *Pasteurella* accounting for the greatest number of cases. Other bacteria involved may be *Klebsiella pneumoniae, Bordetella bronchiseptica* and pneumococci. Drafty, damp, unsanitary hutches and inadequate bedding are predisposing causes. The animals usually succumb within 4 days after the first signs have been noted. Affected rabbits are off feed and show elevated temperature (104°F), dyspnea, diarrhea and lassitude. Necropsy reveals a bronchopneumonia, pleuritis, or pericardial petechial hemorrhages. Treatment consists of a course of oxytetracycline (℞ 25), chlortetracycline (℞ 11) or penicillin (℞ 44). Combinations of penicillin and streptomycin (℞ 41) are also useful and effective for such mixed infections.

CONJUNCTIVITIS
(Weepy eye)

Mature bucks and young rabbits seem particularly susceptible. The affected rabbits rub their eyes with their front feet. There is an exudate which may vary in consistency and color. Any of the common ophthalmic ointments containing sulfonamides (℞ 389, 390), antibiotics (℞ 375) or antibiotics and a steroid (℞ 387) are satisfactory for treatment. In cases of deep-seated infections, injections of penicillin (℞ 44) should be given. A conjunctivitis also accompanies rabbit pox (q.v., p. 1127) and myxomatosis (q.v., p. 1126).

SPIROCHETOSIS
(Vent disease)

A true venereal disease of domestic rabbits characterized by appearance of denuded or scab-covered areas about the external genitalia and caused by the spirochete *Treponema cuniculi*. It is found in both sexes and is transmitted by coitus. It is not transmissible to other domestic animals or man. Small vesicles or ulcers are formed which ultimately become covered with a heavy scab. These lesions are usually confined to the genital region, but in some cases the lips and eyelids may be involved. Infected animals should not be mated. Penicillin in daily doses of 50,000 units appears to be specific therapy. Lesions usually heal within 10 to 14 days and recovered animals can be bred without danger of transmitting the infection.

HUTCH BURN
(Vent disease, Urine burn)

Hutch burn is often confused with spirochetosis or true vent disease. It affects the vent and external genitalia and is caused by wet and dirty hutch floors. Constant exposure to urine splashes and soiled corners chap the membranes of the vent and genital region, allowing the area to become secondarily infected. Brownish crusts cover the area and a bleeding and purulent exudate may be present. Keeping hutch floors clean and dry, and the application of antibiotic ointment to the lesions will hasten recovery.

SCABBY NOSE

Similar to hutch burn in many respects, this infection causes a chapping and cracking of the skin on the nose and lips. Most cases are contracted from infected vents. When secondary infections develop, large brown scales are produced on the nose and lips. Cases of hutch burn should be dealt with first and those with scabby nose should be treated with an injection of 50,000 units of penicillin, repeated on the third day.

DIARRHEAS

These conditions, which comprise one of the most important disease complexes of rabbits, are often referred to as bloat, scours, or diarrhea. Not only do many rabbits die, but the young animals that have been affected fail to regain lost weight by weaning time. The disease may occur sporadically or as an epizootic. The greatest mortality occurs in the age group between 5 and 9 weeks, just before or after weaning. As the animals become older, the mortality decreases. An attack of the disease does not confer immunity. The cause is unknown.

The signs, which may be acute in onset, include anorexia, lassitude and a rough hair coat; the ears droop and the eyes have a squinty appearance. The temperature may be subnormal. Affected individuals sit in a "humped" position and grind their teeth. They may be constipated or exhibit a profuse diarrhea. The feces may consist of clear, viscid, mucoid material. Occasionally there is great thirst, but at other times the rabbits refuse to drink. There are no significant findings at necropsy. The stomach and anterior part of the intestine may contain liquid, gas and some undigested food; the colon usually is filled with a jelly-like mucous material. The mucous membrane of the cecum and intestine may be reddened. Ulcers are not uncommon. Pellets containing antibiotics, such as the tetracyclines, may lower the mortality during the sucking period. However, the results are unpredictable.

Tyzzer's disease is now known to occur in rabbits and a hemorrhagic enteritis and typhlitis results. The causative organism, *Bacillus piliformis,* has been cultivated in chick embryos. Treatment with oxytetracycline in the drinking water at the dosage prescribed for poultry has been successful (*see* ULCERATIVE ENTERITIS, p. 1059).

Probably most diarrheas of young rabbits, however, are not associated with specific pathogens, but with undesirable changes in the intestinal microflora associated with weaning.

RINGWORM

The lesions may occur on any area of the rabbit's skin, with a loss or thinning of the fur. These affected areas usually are circular, raised, reddened and are capped with white, bran-like, flaky material. The lesions may fluoresce under the Wood's lamp. The most common cause is *Trichophyton mentagrophytes* var. *granulare,* which also affects man, guinea pigs, mice and rats. For proper control, the animals should be disposed of. A degree of control can be obtained with the continual application of powdered sulfur to all nest boxes prior to kindling or by the use of topical agents such as those containing salicylic and benzoic esters of propylene glycol, aqueous solutions of sodium caprylate, and tinctures containing tannic, benzoic and salicylic acids. The drug of choice is griseofulvin at an individual dose of 25 mg/kg body wt daily for 14 days or in the feed at 375 mg/lb of feed (*see* RINGWORM IN DOGS AND CATS, p. 903).

MISCELLANEOUS

Salmonellosis (*S. typhimurium*) occurs occasionally in rabbits. Systemic mycoses due to *Nocardia, Aspergillus* and *Candida* have been reported.

PARASITIC DISEASES

COCCIDIOSIS

One of the most common diseases of rabbits is coccidiosis. Those animals that do recover from this protozoan infection frequently become carriers and perpetuate the malady. There are 2 forms, hepatic coccidiosis as caused by *Eimeria stiedae,* and intestinal coccidiosis, the cause of which may be *E. magna, E. irresidua, E. media,* or *E. perforans.* So-called "nasal coccidiosis" is the result of the rabbits contaminating the mucous membrane of their nose while practicing coprophagy (*see* RABBIT MANAGEMENT, p. 1123).

Hepatic coccidiosis: The severity of the signs is dependent on the number of oocysts ingested. There may be an infection with no apparent signs or the infection may cause death after a short course. Young rabbits are the most susceptible. Affected animals exhibit diarrhea, anorexia and a rough hair coat. Growing rabbits fail to make normal gains. The animals usually succumb within 30 days after a severe experimental exposure.

At necropsy, in most cases, the lesions are easily recognized. Small, grayish-white nodules or cysts are found throughout the parenchyma of the hepatic tissue. They may be sharply demarcated in the early cases, while in the later stages, they coalesce with other affected areas. The early lesions have a milky content, whereas older lesions may have a more cheese-like consistency. Microscopically, the nodules are composed of hypertrophied bile ducts. A large number of oocysts are seen. This form of coccidiosis is diagnosed from the gross and micro-scopic changes along with demonstration of the oocysts in the bile ducts.

Sulfaquinoxaline administered continuously in the drinking water in a concentration of 0.025% for 30 days prevents the development of the clinical signs of hepatic coccidiosis in rabbits heavily exposed to *E. stiedae*. Sulfaquinoxaline may also be given in the feed at 0.025% for 20 days, or for 2 days out of every 8, until marketing. The rabbits acquire an immunity to subsequent infections. Lower concentrations of the drug are not satisfactory. The maximum prophylactic effect is obtained by 3 weeks of administration. A concentration of 0.10% of sulfaquinoxaline in the feed, or 0.05% in the feed and 0.04% in the drinking water, given continuously for 2 weeks, is recom-mended for therapeutic control of naturally occurring out-breaks. The drug should not be given within 10 days of slaugh-ter of the rabbits for food. The above treatments will be of no avail unless a sanitary program is simultaneously instituted. The feed hoppers and water crocks should not become con-taminated with feces. The hutches should be kept dry and the accumulated feces removed at frequent intervals. Sulfametha-zine, sulfamerazine, or succinylsulfathiazole in the feed at 0.5% concentration have also been used during outbreaks.

Intestinal coccidiosis: This form of the disease will occur in rabbits receiving the best of care, as well as in rabbits raised under unsanitary conditions. Inability to gain, anorexia and "pot belly" are prominent signs. The lesions are inconsistent: The early cases show few changes, while in the advanced cases, the intestine may be thickened and pale. All of the responsible coccidia develop in the small intestine. While losses due to liver coccidiosis may be held to a negligible level through a sanitary program, and will permit profitable production, the same program will not eliminate intestinal coccidiosis. It is im-portant that any diseased rabbit be removed from the rabbitry and its feces examined for coccidia. Sulfaquinoxaline fed con-tinuously for 2 weeks at 0.1% of the feed has been used for treatment.

LARVAL TAPEWORM INFECTION

Rabbits are intermediate hosts for 2 tapeworms of the dog, *Taenia pisiformis* and *T. serialis*. The larval forms are found in the viscera of the rabbit. If the cysts develop under the skin, they can be surgically removed. The rabbit is also the intermediate host for the cat tapeworm, *T. taeniaeformis*. The larval stage, a segmented worm, is found in a white cyst in the liver. Dogs and cats should not be allowed near the rabbits' feed, water, bedding or feeding utensils as they may transmit tapeworm eggs in their feces, nor should dogs and cats eat the viscera of rabbits, as they may become infected and perpetuate the cycle.

EAR MITE INFESTATION

Ear mites, *Psoroptes equi* var. *cuniculi* or *Chorioptes bovis* var. *cuniculi,* are the most common external parasites of rabbits. Head shaking and ear flapping, along with scratching at the ears with the hind feet are common signs. Torticollis and spasms of the eye muscles may be observed. Affected rabbits lose flesh, fail to produce and succumb to secondary infections. These infections frequently damage the inner ear and may reach the CNS. The mites irritate the lining of the ear, causing serum and thick crusts to accumulate. Under good restraint or even general anesthesia, the brown, crumbly exudate should be removed with cotton soaked in dilute hydrogen peroxide. After cleaning, the ears are swabbed with 1 part Canex (℞ 311) in 3 parts mineral or vegetable oil. The medication should be applied around the external ear and down the side of the head and neck as well. The application has to be repeated after 6 to 10 days. Additional treatments may be necessary. The hutches used by the affected rabbits must be carefully cleaned and disinfected.

MANGE MITE INFESTATION

Not infrequently, rabbits are infected with either *Sarcoptes scabiei* or *Notoedres cati.* The rabbits scratch themselves almost continually. There is a loss of hair on the chin, nose, head, base of the ears and around the eyes. The condition is extremely contagious. It is difficult to eliminate the parasites on domestic rabbits. The owner should be advised to destroy the animals unless they are valuable breeders. They may be dipped in a lime-sulfur preparation, or Canex (℞ 311) may be rubbed into the lesions.

NOSEMATOSIS

Nosema (Encephalitozoon) cuniculi is a widespread protozoal infection of rabbits and occasionally of mice, guinea pigs, rats and dogs. It involves the brain and kidneys, mainly, but usually no clinical signs are produced. It is mildly contagious in a rabbitry or colony and is believed to be spread via urine or transplacentally. At necropsy, the lesions must be differentiated from those of *Toxoplasma gondii* (q.v., p. 456) by morphologic and staining criteria. It may be possible to eliminate carriers from a colony by examining brains of younger rabbits and then culling the dams of positive subjects. **Toxoplasmosis**, which is not as common in rabbits as nosematosis, may be diagnosed by available serologic methods.

PINWORMS

Passalurus ambiguus, the rabbit pinworm, usually is not economically or medically important. If necessary, it can be controlled by phenothiazine in the feed (1 gm/50 gm of molasses-treated feed).

NONINFECTIOUS CONDITIONS

WET DEWLAP

Some rabbits have a heavy fold of skin on the ventral aspect of the neck. As the rabbit drinks, this skin may become wet and soggy, leading to inflammation of the area. The hair may slip and the area may be attacked by blow flies. To prevent the occurrence of wet dewlaps, the water receptacles should have small openings or be set on low, flat boards. The hair in the affected area must be clipped and an antiseptic dusting powder applied.

CANNIBALISM

Many times, young does will kill and consume their young. Although the exact causes are not known, cannibalism has been attributed to nervousness, lack of water, or a poor ration. Does that are prone to kill their young should be disposed of. The young should not be examined too soon after kindling as this will excite the doe.

WOOL-EATING

In many instances, the stomach contents of rabbits contain small amounts of hair but impaction results only if a habit of wool-eating is formed. Rabbits may pull wool from the back of another rabbit or eat their own wool. It often is difficult to break this habit. Occasionally, wool balls will occlude the pyloric opening.

HEAT EXHAUSTION

Hot, humid weather along with poorly ventilated hutches may lead to death of many rabbits, particularly pregnant does. Affected rabbits lie on their sides and breathe rapidly. They should be immersed in a bucket of lukewarm water. Hutches should be constructed so that they can be sprinkled in hot, humid weather. Free access to water and salt blocks should be provided. Where it is possible to control the environment optimum criteria are: temperature 60° to 70°F, relative humidity 40 to 60%, with 10 to 20 air changes per hour.

KETOSIS (PREGNANCY TOXEMIA)

It has been suggested that ketosis may cause the death of many does at kindling or a day or 2 before they are due to kindle. Predisposing factors include obesity and lack of exercise. The most significant finding at necropsy is fatty liver and kidneys. To prevent the condition, the daily intake of pellets of all pregnant does should be restricted prior to kindling.

MILKWEED POISONING

This type of poisoning is caused by feeding hay containing woolly pod milkweed, *Asclepias eriocarpa,* reported only from the Pacific Southwest. It sometimes is called "head-down disease", inasmuch as the affected rabbits develop paralysis of the neck muscles and loss of coordination. If the animal has not consumed too much of the weed and the paralysis has not progressed too far, an attempt may be made to treat it. The head of the rabbit is held so that it can drink water and consume food. Leafy greens and carrots should be fed. Hay and bedding must be free of this weed in order to prevent the condition. The poisonous principle is a resinoid; consumption of approximately 0.25% of an animal's weight of green plant produces death. The use of rice straw or wood shavings for bedding will eliminate this hazard.

DYSTOCIA

The gestation period of the rabbit rarely exceeds 32 days. If a pregnant doe is overdue and is straining or in distress, an injection of oxytocin (℞ 172) is generally effective, providing presentation, normally anterior or posterior, is acceptable.

SORE HOCKS

Bruised or chafed hocks may become infected with a variety of bacteria. The lesions should be treated locally with a sulfonamide powder and the rabbit can be given an injection of penicillin. For prevention, the hutch floors should be kept clean and dry. Since excitement causes stamping which may lead to sore hocks, the animals should be kept as quiet as possible.

DENTAL MALOCCLUSION

The incisors, premolars and molars of rabbits grow throughout life. Normal length is maintained by constant grinding of opposing teeth. Incisoral malocclusion resulting from prognathism, brachygnathism, or broken opposing teeth, can result in anorexia. Temporary correction can be effected by cutting, from time to time, the overgrown teeth. Occasionally, the cheek teeth overgrow, causing severe tongue or buccal lesions. Observations suggest a hereditary basis for those cases of overgrowth resulting from congenital malformations, and this trait can be selected against in the breeding program.

CONGENITAL MALFORMATIONS

Some common malformations of rabbits, the genetics of which are poorly known, include variation in the number of ribs (12 or 13 pairs), degree of sternebral ossification, craniofacial abnormalities, missing or misshapen gonads and ventral body wall defects.

MUSCULAR DYSTROPHY

Nutritional muscular dystrophy in the rabbit is characterized by high neonatal mortality at 3 to 10 days of age with no prior signs. Occasional deaths occur in surviving young up to the age of 2 to 3 months. Breeding females undergo decreases in fertility. Gross lesions are absent; acute degenerative and inflammatory changes are present in sections of skeletal muscle. Dietary vitamin E deficiency is believed to be causal. Breeding females can be treated with oral DL-alpha tocopherol acetate (25 to 60 mg orally 3 times weekly for 8 weeks) or by feeding a diet containing about 9.0 mg alpha tocopherol per 100 mg of diet (see also, MYOPATHIES AND RELATED CONDITIONS IN DOMESTIC ANIMALS, p. 575).

SPECIFIC-PATHOGEN-FREE (SPF) RABBITS

It is possible to obtain neonatal rabbits by hysterectomy and raise them behind an environmental barrier in the laboratory, to serve as a nucleus for an SPF colony. To be truly SPF, regular monitoring with reliable techniques must be carried out. Pasteurellosis, coccidiosis, ear mites and pinworms have been practically eliminated under such programs. General mortality from all causes can be drastically reduced.

In Britain, the 3 most frequently diagnosed rabbit diseases in conventional colonies are the diarrheas, coccidiosis and respiratory diseases. In North America, they are the diarrheas, pasteurellosis and genetic maladies such as dental malocclusion.

DISEASES OF LABORATORY ANIMALS

This chapter deals with the more important diseases of those animals used in the largest numbers for research purposes: mice, rats, guinea pigs, hamsters, as well as various primates and amphibians. Diseases of other domestic species that are also widely used research animals, such as dogs, cats, rabbits and chickens, are dealt with elsewhere in the MANUAL.

The *Guide for the Care and Use of Laboratory Animals*: (USPHS Pub. No. 1024, 1972) is a primary reference for information on the basic principles and standards for the care and use of laboratory animals.

DISEASES OF MICE AND RATS

A program is essential to prevent or limit infectious disease in rat and mouse colonies. Its elements should include: production of animals free of their common pathogens; prophylactic or therapeutic medication; immunization; strict sanitation and husbandry; isolation; and test and slaughter procedures.

BACTERIAL DISEASES

Chronic murine pneumonia is a disease complex characterized by inflammation of the respiratory tract and middle ear. Signs include chattering and dyspnea in mice, and nasal discharge, snuffling, rales, dyspnea, head tilt, incoordination and circling in rats. Lesions include suppurative bronchitis and bronchopneumonia, mucopurulent rhinitis, and otitis media and interna. The primary etiologic agent is *Mycoplasma pulmonis;* however, *Pasteurella pneumotropica, Corynebacterium kutscheri, Bordetella bronchiseptica,* streptococci, pneumococci and viruses may act in concert with the primary agent. Diagnosis depends on lesions and isolation of the etiologic agent. The condition may be prevented by keeping a cesarean-derived colony behind a microbiologic barrier. Acute outbreaks of the disease may be controlled to a limited extent by oxytetracycline in the drinking water (℞ 30, 37).

Tyzzer's Disease: This enzootic disease is widespread in laboratory mice in Europe and Japan; outbreaks have been reported in rats, mice, hamsters, gerbils and rabbits in the U.S.A. The causative organism is a slender gram-negative rod, *Bacillus piliformis,* which can be propagated in tissue culture but not on ordinary microbiologic media. Stress or cortisone injections may precipitate an epizootic in colonies where the organism is present. Signs are diarrhea, humped back, poor haircoat, or sudden deaths, especially in young animals. Lesions usually include focal necrosis of the liver and inflammation of the terminal ileum. Diagnosis depends on histologic demonstration of the bacilli in bundles within the hepatocytes surrounding the focally necrotic areas, and negative cultures for *Salmonella, Corynebacterium* or other pathogens. The organisms stain well with Giemsa stain. Outbreaks may be controlled by isolation of affected animals, strict hygienic procedures and oxytetracycline in the drinking water (℞ 30, 37).

Salmonellosis (Paratyphoid): Organisms of the genus *Salmonella*, usually *S. typhimurium* or *S. enteriditis*, may cause enteritis and septicemia with focal necrosis of the liver or spleen in rats and mice. Antibiotics may ameliorate the acute infection (*see* SALMONELLOSIS, p. 377).

Pseudomonas Infection: Pseudomonads are part of the normal intestinal flora, but may cause early deaths in stressed or X-irradiated mice. *Ps. aeruginosa* may be isolated from the heart blood of dead animals or from the feces of carriers. Prevention and control are best accomplished by using 0.005 N hydrochloric acid (pH 2.5) as drinking water or by chlorination (10 to 16 ppm) of the drinking water.

Pasteurella Infection: Pasteurellae may cause localized inflammatory lesions and septicemia in rats and mice. *P. pneumotropica* infection may be latent; but when host defenses are reduced, bronchopneumonia, conjunctivitis, metritis, cystitis, or dermatitis may occur. Oxytetracycline (℞ 30, 37) has been used successfully in treating infections caused by this organism. *P. pseudotuberculosis, P. multocida,* or *P. pestis* rarely cause disease in laboratory rats and mice. Diagnosis depends on characteristic lesions and isolation of the organism.

Bordetella bronchiseptica Infection: *B. bronchiseptica* is a normal inhabitant of the respiratory tract of rats and may be associated with chronic murine pneumonia as a secondary invader. Its role as a primary pathogen in rats and mice is uncertain. Infected animals may show head tilt, dyspnea and conjunctivitis. Lesions include otitis media, purulent bronchopneumonia and purulent conjunctivitis. Diagnosis depends on isolation of the organism. Animals with clinical signs should be removed from the colony. Infection may be controlled with oxytetracycline in the drinking water (℞ 30, 37).

Corynebacterium kutscheri Infection (Pseudotuberculosis): *C. kutscheri* (*murium*) is an opportunistic pathogen of rats and mice. Infection may be inapparent, or result in nasal and ocular discharge, dyspnea, arthritis, or skin abscesses. Lesions are variable, but usually include focal caseous abscesses in the viscera and lymph nodes, and occasionally purulent arthritis. Diagnosis depends on characteristic lesions and isolation of the organism or serology (agglutination). Treatment with penicillin or tetracycline (℞ 30, 37) may prevent clinically apparent disease but will not eliminate the carrier state.

MISCELLANEOUS BACTERIAL INFECTIONS

Klebsiella pneumoniae may rarely cause bronchopneumonia, pleuritis, and abscesses in various organs of mice. *Diplococcus pneumoniae* may cause bronchopneumonia, pleuritis, pericarditis, meningitis and splenic infarcts in rats. *Streptobacillus moniliformis,* a gram-negative, highly pleomorphic bacillus, may rarely cause arthritis, pericarditis, and focal necrosis of the liver and spleen. It also causes rat-bite fever or Haverhill fever in man. Group A streptococcus or Type D enterococcus may rarely cause clinical disease in mice. Group A streptococcus causes cervical lymphadenitis, fibrinopurulent pneumonia, pleuritis, pericarditis and peritonitis. Type D enterococcus causes focal enteritis and focal hepatic necrosis. Diagnosis of these infections depends on isolation of the organism. Therapy is governed by the specific antibacterial sensitivity of the organisms.

VIRAL DISEASES

Ectromelia (Mouse Pox) is a devastating disease of laboratory mice caused by *"Poxvirus muris"*. It may remain latent or cause low-grade enzootic disease or violent epizootics. In the acute systemic form, there can be deaths with no lesions. In more chronic cases there may be facial swelling, conjunctivitis with a secondary rash, and ulcerating or scaly lesions of the head, tail or extremities. Occasionally, extremities become necrotic and slough. Other lesions include focal necrosis of the liver, spleen, pancreas and lymph nodes, and intestinal hemorrhage. Eosinophilic cytoplasmic inclusion bodies may be found in hepatocytes, pancreatic acinar cells or in swollen epidermal cells in areas of cutaneous inflammation. Diagnosis is based on characteristic lesions and serology (hemagglutination inhibition using vaccinia antigen, serum neutralization, indirect immunofluorescence). A single positive animal indicates that a colony is infected. Effective control is gained by vaccinating all susceptible animals every 6 months. A drop of vaccinia virus vaccine is placed near the base of the tail, and the skin is lightly scarified beneath the drop. A small papule occurs at the site of injection. Ectromelia-free colonies should be well isolated from wild and newly received rodents. Newly received mice should be isolated and observed for 2 to 3 weeks before they are introduced into the colony.

Epizootic Diarrhea of Infant Mice: EDIM is characterized by high morbidity and diarrhea in mice 5 to 15 days of age. Death occurs late in the disease due to constipation or secondary bacteremia. Recovered animals may be stunted. Lesions include distension of the colon with light mustard-colored feces and vacuolation of epithelial cells at the tips of small intestinal villi. These vacuolated cells may contain small acidophilic intracytoplasmic inclusions. Diagnosis is based on characteristic clinical and pathologic findings. The disease can be controlled and eliminated from most colonies by using filter-top cages and culling infected mice.

Lethal Intestinal Virus of Infant Mice: LIVIM is characterized by high mortality, diarrhea, emaciation, and death in mice, usually after 10 days of age. The colon is usually empty and the small intestine greatly distended by gas and fluid. Microscopic lesions include blunting of intestinal villi and multinucleate giant cells within the lumen. Affected epithelial cells may contain intracytoplasmic inclusions. Diagnosis is based on the pathologic findings. This disease may be controlled by using filter-top cages and culling infected mice.

Rat Virus Infection (Hemorrhagic Encephalopathy): Rat virus infection may be latent in wild and laboratory rats. Experimental inoculation causes runting, paralysis and sometimes death in nursing rats. Lesions include hemorrhagic necrosis of the brain and spinal cord and intranuclear inclusion bodies in reticuloendothelial cells. Diagnosis is based on lesions, animal inoculation (nursing hamsters or newborn rats) and serology (hemagglutination).

Sialodacryoadenitis: The virus which causes severe inflammation and necrosis of salivary and Harderian glands of rats is as yet unclassified. Infection may be latent, or animals may exhibit enlarged salivary glands and exophthalmos. Lesions include necrosis of the ductal epithelium of the submaxillary and parotid salivary glands, and necrosis with squamous metaplasia of the tubulo-alveolar epithelium of the Harderian gland. Diagnosis is based on pathologic findings and inoculation of susceptible rats.

Latent Viral Infections of Mice: A number of viruses can be isolated from clinically normal laboratory mice. These viruses do not usually pose significant clinical disease problems in laboratory colonies. However, they may seriously disrupt research by causing disease in animals whose resistance has been diminished by experimental procedures. The TABLE (p. 1142)

LATENT VIRAL INFECTIONS OF MICE

Disease	Agent	Lesions	Diagnosis	Comments
Adenovirus Infection	Adenovirus	Focal necrosis: heart.	Serology: CF[4], SN[9]; intranuclear inclusions: heart, kidney, adrenal.	Stunting lethargy, death in suckling mice only.
K-Virus Infection	Papovavirus	Interstitial pneumonia with proliferation of endothelial cells.	Serology: HI[8], SN; intranuclear inclusions; endothelial cells.	Labored breathing and death in suckling mice.
Lactic Dehydrogenase (LDH) Virus Infection	Unclassified virus	None.	Elevation of plasma LDH.	Causes elevated plasma enzyme levels. Contaminates transplanted tumors.
Lymphocytic Choriomeningitis	RNA virus	Lymphocytic choriomeningitis; necrosis: liver and lymphoid tissue.	Guinea pig or LCM-free mouse inoculation. Serology: I[4],	Clonic convulsions, transplacental infection. Transmissible to man.
Mammary Carcinoma	Bittner agent; RNA virus	Mammary adenocarcinomas, adenoacanthomas, carcinosarcomas.	Lesions.	Virus in milk of infected dam.
Minute Virus of Mice	Parvovirus	Encephalitis; choriomeningitis.	Serology: SN, HI.	Contaminates transplanted tumors.
Mouse Encephalomyelitis (Theiler's Disease)	Picornaviruses	Necrosis: brain stem, spinal cord.	Serology: HI. Neonatal hamster inoculation.	Flaccid posterior paralysis, virus carried in intestine.
Mouse Hepatitis	RNA virus	Focal necrosis: liver, lymph nodes, brain.	Serology: CF, Mouse inoculation.	Hepatotropic and neurotropic viral stains; occ. jaundice & neurologic signs.
Mouse Papule Disease	Unclassified virus	Papules in skin.	Intracytoplasmic inclusions: epidermis.	Differentiate from ectromelia.

Disease	Agent	Lesions	Diagnosis	Remarks
Mouse Pneumonitis (Nigg Virus Inf.)	Chlamydia sp. (Miyagawanella)	Interstitial and bronchopneumonia.	CF. Elementary bodies: bronchial epithelium.	Latent infection may be activated by intranasal instillations.
Mouse Thymic Agent Infection	Unclassified virus	Focal thymic necrosis.	Inoculation of newborn mice.	Affects newborn only.
Murine Leukemia	RNA viruses	Lymphocytic, granulocytic, or erythrocytic leukemia.	CO Mu L[5] and XC[6] tests.	Several viral strains cause several different types of tumors.
Pneumonia Virus of Mice Infection	RNA virus	Interstitial pneumonia; pulmonary edema.	Serology: HI, SN. Inoc. of PVM-free mice.	May affect rats also.
Polyoma Virus Infection	Papovavirus	Tumors in various sites.	Serology: HI, SN.	Stunted growth and tumor development 1-6 months after inoculation.
Reovirus Infection (Hepatoencephalomyelitis)	Reovirus Type 3	Necrosis: liver; myocardium, pancreas; neuronal degeneration; encephalitis.	Serology: HI, II[7].	Jaundice, yellow feces, oily hair and skin, neurologic signs.
Salivary Gland Virus (Cytomegalovirus) Infection	Herpesvirus	Intranuclear inclusions; salivary-duct epithelium.	Lesions.	May cause generalized infection and death in young mice.
Sendai Virus Infection	Myxovirus Parainfluenza Type I	Interstitial pneumonia.	Serology: HI.	May affect rats also.

1. Complement Fixation; 2. Serum Neutralization; 3. Hemagglutination Inhibition; 4. Immunofluorescence; 5. Complement Fixation for Murine Leukemia; 6. XC Cell Cytopathogenicity Test; 7. Indirect Immunofluorescence.

presents a summary of several of the more common latent viral infections of mice.

PARASITIC DISEASES

Protozoa: At least 4 species of coccidia (*Eimeria* spp.) may infect the intestinal tract of laboratory rats, and 8 species may infect mice. In addition, one species (*Cryptosporidium muris*) occurs in the stomach. Diagnosis is based on identification of oocysts after fecal flotation, or by finding organisms in the epithelial cells of the intestinal tract. Renal coccidiosis due to *Klossiella muris* occurs in mice. Oocysts are passed in the urine. Coccidial infection of the intestine, stomach, or kidney rarely causes lesions or clinical signs.

Other generally nonpathogenic protozoa, such as *Entamoeba muris, Giardia muris. Trichomonas muris* and *Chilomastix bettencorti* may occur in the intestines of rats and mice. *Hexamita muris,* a flagellated protozoan, may cause diarrhea, weight loss and sporadic deaths in mice. Lesions include duodenitis with crypts dilated by numerous hexamitae. Diagnosis is based on microscopic lesions and demonstration of organisms in saline mounts and fixed smears from duodenum.

Hepatozoon muris occurs in the hepatic cells of rats and mice. One stage in the life cycle occurs within the leukocytes of the blood stream. A mite, *Echinolaelaps echidninus,* serves as the intermediate host. *Pneumocystis carinii,* an organism of uncertain classification may be found in the lungs of rats; respiratory signs may result from stress or immunosuppression. This organism may be transmissible to human beings. *Toxoplasma gondii* is an intracellular parasite (q.v., p. 456) with a wide host range including rat, mouse and man. It may cause encephalitis, pneumonitis, or enterocolitis. It must be differentiated from *Encephalitizoon (Nosema) cuniculi* which may cause focal encephalitis in rats, mice, guinea pigs, rabbits, dogs and human beings. *Sarcocystis muris,* a protozoan parasite of muscle, is occasionally an incidental necropsy finding. Treatment of rats or mice with clinically apparent protozoan infections is not considered feasible.

Blood Parasites: Several blood parasites have been reported in rats and mice. These include *Plasmodium berghei, P. vinckei, Trypanasoma lewisi, T. cruzi, Hepatozoon muris, Babesia muris, Haemobartonella muris* (rats only), and *Eperythrozoon coccoides* (mice only), which is now classified as a rickettsia although formerly considered to be a protozoan. These organisms do not normally cause clinically apparent disease unless animals are splenectomized or severely stressed. Blood-sucking ectoparasites may transmit the disease.

Nematodes: *Heterakis spumosa* is found in the cecum and colon of rats and mice. No lesions have been reported. Diagnosis is based on identification of ova in the feces. *Nippostrongylus muris* occurs in the small intestine of rats and mice. Clinical signs include unthriftiness, diarrhea and dyspnea. Lesions include pneumonia and pulmonary hemorrhage due to larval migration through the lungs. Characteristic eggs are passed in the feces. *Gongylonema neoplasticum* occurs in the epithelium of the stomach, esophagus and tongue. There is little tissue reaction; infection does not produce neoplasms. The intermediate host is the cockroach. Embryonated eggs are passed in the feces. Adult *Trichinella spiralis* (q.v., p. 696) are found in the duodenum of rats and many other animals. The pinworms, *Aspiculuris tetraptera* and *Syphacia* spp., occur in the cecum and colon of rats and mice. Impaction by worms, colonic intussusception, or rectal prolapse may result. *Aspiculuris* eggs are passed in the feces; *Syphacia* eggs are deposited on the perianal region by the female worm. Diagnosis can be made by fecal flotation (*Aspiculuris*) and by the cellophane-tape method (*Syphacia*). Control is difficult because of reinfection due to the presence of eggs on fomites and in air currents. An effective treatment is trichlorfon plus atropine (Dyrex R, 2.5 gm/L of distilled water), in the drinking water for 2 weeks, combined with strict sanitation of equipment and facilities. *Capillaria hepatica* occurs in the liver parenchyma of mice and rats. Eggs cause yellow streaks and patches in liver due to the local chronic inflammatory response. Eggs are liberated only when the liver is eaten by some other animal. The eggs are then passed in the feces to develop on the ground to become infective. The nematode, *Trichosomoides crassicauda*, lives in bladder, kidney, pelvis and ureters of rats. Operculated eggs are passed in the urine. Larvae migrating through the lungs may cause focal granulomas.

The adult lungworm, *Angiostrongylus cantonensis*, occurs in the pulmonary artery of rats. The life cycle is complex and involves a snail or slug as an intermediate host and 2 moults within the brain of the definitive host. It has little pathologic significance for the rat but is transmissible to, and causes meningoencephalitis in man.

Acanthocephala: The thorny-headed worm, *Moniliformis moniliformis*, inhabits the small intestine of rats, mice and other rodents. The thorn-like hooks on the head may cause enteritis, ulceration and occasionally intestinal perforation with subsequent peritonitis.

Cestodes: The dwarf tapeworm, *Hymenolepis nana,* occurs in the small intestine of rats and mice, and is transmissible to man. The life cycle may be either direct or indirect. The tapeworm, *Hymenolepis diminuta,* occurs in the anterior ileum of rats and mice. A flea, beatle or cockroach may act as an intermediate host. *Oochoristica ratti* is a rare tapeworm of mice and is usually of little importance in laboratory mice. The treatment of choice for tapeworms is niclosamide (℞ 225). Rats and mice may also harbor the intermediate forms of *Taenia taeniaeformis (Cysticercus fasciolaris)* in the liver and *Taenia serialis (Coenurus serialis)* in the connective tissue. Their presence indicates probable fecal contamination of the food supply by the definitive host(s).

Ectoparasites: The mites, *Myobia musculi* and *Radfordia affinis,* in mice cause loss of hair, and scabby lesions over the head, neck and shoulders. Breeding males seem to be most severely affected. *Myocoptes musculinus* and *M. romboutsi* cause hair loss and dermatitis, usually in lactating females and unweaned young. *Psorergates simplex* causes chronically inflamed epidermal cysts which are visible on the inner surfaces of the skin. Mites affecting rats are *Bdellonyssus bacoti* and *Radfordia ensifera* which cause dermatitis, and *Notoedres muris* which causes vesicles, papules and wart-like projections on the ears, nose, tail, feet and external genitalia. Lice and superficial mites are most easily and consistently diagnosed by killing a suspect animal and observing it with a magnifying glass or dissecting microscope, periodically over 24 hours, for the presence of mites as they migrate up the hair shafts. Migration may be hastened by placing the carcass or skin in the refrigerator, followed by examination of the carcass after removal to room temperature. The burrowing mite, *P. simplex,* may be diagnosed by examining for the subcut. pinpoint, white focal lesions.

Rats and mice may be infected with a variety of fleas. *Polyplax spinulosa* (rat) and *Polyplax serrata* (mouse) may cause loss of hair and pruritus.

Ectoparasites may be effectively treated by whole-body immersion in 2% malathion, using 2 dippings with a 2-week interval. This treatment is drastic and 2 to 5% mortality may result. A more innocuous but still effective treatment is immersion in a 2% suspension of Aramite in water containing a wetting agent such as 0.1% sodium alkyl aryl sulfonate (Nacconal). Animals over 2 weeks of age may be dusted thoroughly with 0.1% lindane powder. After any treatment, animals should be moved to clean cages, preferably with filter caps.

Mycotic Diseases

Ringworm (*see* Ringworm in guinea pigs, p. 1149).

Histoplasmosis, coccidioidomycosis, sporotrichosis, cryptococcosis and phycomycosis do not usually pose significant problems in laboratory colonies, but they may seriously disrupt research because of an overwhelming effect on animals whose resistance has been diminished by radiation or immunosuppressive drugs.

Noninfectious Diseases

Fighting: Trauma due to fighting is often a significant cause of morbidity and mortality in male mice. Fighting usually occurs at night and results in bite and scratch wounds over the head, perineum and lower abdomen. Frequently, these lesions become septic. A high incidence of secondary amyloidosis has been reported in animals that have lesions stemming from fighting. Fighting can be prevented by separating males, or preferably, by grouping males at the time of weaning rather than later.

Chloroform Toxicity: Mature male mice of some inbred strains (C_3H, CBA, A, HR) are exquisitely sensitive to low levels of chloroform vapor in the air. A chloroform spill may result in the death of large numbers of mature males while immature males and females are unaffected. Lesions include necrosis of convoluted renal tubules. There is no practical treatment once signs have become apparent.

Ringtail is a condition of young rats and mice characterized by annular constriction and later edema, necrosis, and spontaneous amputation of the tail. The condition in rats can be experimentally produced by lowering the ambient relative humidity. The disease can be controlled by providing a relative humidity of at least 50% in breeding colonies.

Nutritional Diseases

Highly standardized balanced rations for rats and mice are commercially available. Most manufacturers provide separate diets for maintenance, breeding and other specific purposes. The importance of these diets are set out in detail in their labeling. The rations should be stored properly and used promptly since nutritional quality falls during storage. Ideally, rations should be fed within 12 weeks of the milling date. If colonies are fed fresh diets manufactured by a reputable company, the possibility of clinically apparent nutritional deficiency is remote.

DISEASES OF THE GUINEA PIG

Antibiotic Toxicity: Guinea pigs and hamsters are highly susceptible to the toxic effects of many of the commonly used antibiotics. Toxicity results from overgrowth of the normal gram-positive cecal flora by gram-negative rods. This causes fatal enterocolitis, with diarrhea and death in 3 to 7 days. Antibiotics with an activity spectrum directed primarily against gram-positive organisms (e.g., penicillin, lincomycin, erythromycin, tylosin) should not be used in guinea pigs and hamsters. Broad-spectrum antibiotics should not be used orally because of their direct effect on the intestinal flora, but may be used parenterally with caution.

Metastatic calcification occurs most often in male guinea pigs over a year of age. Signs include slow weight gains, stiff joints and high mortality. At necropsy, calcium deposits are seen in the lung, liver, heart, aorta, stomach, colon, kidney, joints and skeletal muscles. There are conflicting reports concerning the etiology; however, most investigators agree that when animals are fed diets low in magnesium and potassium, the calcific lesions increase with the phosphorus content of the ration. It is believed that hyperphosphatemia results from the inability of the guinea pig to conserve fixed bases by excreting ammonia in the urine; thus, the low-base reserve impairs normal urinary excretion of phosphorus. The condition may be aggravated by increasing the vitamin D content of the ration beyond 6 IU/gm. The condition may be minimized or prevented by feeding diets that contain adequate magnesium (0.35%), a calcium:phosphorus ratio of 1.3 to 1.5:1, and not more than 6 IU of vitamin D per gram.

Scurvy: (Vitamin C Deficiency): Guinea pigs require a dietary supply of ascorbic acid (vitamin C) because they lack the enzymes necessary for conversion of L-gulonolactone to L-ascorbic acid. Signs of vitamin C deficiency are unsteady gait, painful locomotion, hemorrhage from gums, swelling of costochondral junctions and emaciation. Lesions include hemorrhages in the subcutis, around joints and on all serosal surfaces. Microscopically, there is disarray of cartilage columns and fibrosis of the marrow in areas of active osteogenesis. The condition may be prevented by providing 1 to 3 mg ascorbic acid per 100 gm body wt daily. Commercial guinea pig diets contain vitamin C which is stable for 3 months after milling. Marginal diets should be supplemented with greens or vegetables high in vitamin C.

Muscular Dystrophy: Guinea pigs are exquisitely sensitive to dietary deficiency of vitamin E. Signs are stiffness, lameness and refusal to move. Microscopic lesions include coagulative necrosis, inflammation and proliferation of sarcolemmal nuclei in skeletal muscle. Diets should contain 3 to 5 mg of vitamin E per 100 gm.

Pregnancy toxemia in guinea pigs is a metabolic disorder similar to that observed in sheep prior to parturition (q.v., p. 508). Predisposing factors are obesity and any stress that might induce temporary anorexia during the late stages of pregnancy. Clinical findings are anorexia, adipsia, muscle spasms, coma within 48 hours of onset, and death within 4 to 5 days unless the course is interrupted by parturition. Laboratory findings are aciduria, proteinuria and hyperlipemia. Microscopically, there is fatty degeneration of parenchymatous organs and hyperlipemia. Control may be achieved by prevention of obesity, avoidance of stress during late pregnancy and provision of a high-quality ration during pregnancy. Early treatment of affected animals with oral propylene glycol, IP calcium gluconate, or parenteral corticosteroids may be helpful although the prognosis remains poor.

Ringworm is a common mycotic infection in guinea pigs, usually caused by *Trychophyton mentagrophytes* or *Microsporum gypseum*. It causes characteristic, crusty, flaking lesions on the skin. Facial lesions are usually prominent. Diagnosis is based on characteristic lesions and cultural and microscopic identification of the causative organism. The disease is usually self-limiting if good husbandry and sanitation are maintained. Long-term feeding of griseofulvin (℞ 353) is effective. Isolated skin lesions may be treated effectively with tolnaftate cream (℞ 360). The disease is contagious to man.

BACTERIAL AND VIRAL DISEASES

Lymphadenitis: Inflammation and enlargement of the cervical lymph nodes is a common finding in guinea pigs. The causative organism is usually *Streptococcus pyogenes* although other bacteria may also cause the condition. The organisms may gain entry to the lymphatics from abrasions of the oral mucosa or from the upper respiratory tract. Clinical findings are large, often unilateral, swellings or abscesses in the ventral region of the neck. Microscopically, there is suppuration of the cervical lymph nodes. Diagnosis is based on clinical signs and isolation of the causative organism. Feeding of abrasive materials should be avoided. In addition, upper respiratory tract infections should be prevented and controlled. Affected animals should be culled since organisms from the draining abscesses may infect other animals in the colony. Antibiotic therapy is generally unrewarding because of toxicity (q.v., p. 1148).

Pneumonia in the guinea pig may be viral or bacterial (*Streptococcus pyogenes, Diplococcus pneumoniae, Klebsiella pneumoniae, Pasteurella pneumotropica, Bordetella bronchiseptica*). Clinical signs are those of respiratory distress. Diagnosis is based on signs, pneumonic lesions and isolation of the causative organism. Prevention and control depend on maintenance of good husbandry procedures and culling of affected animals. Treatment with antibiotics should be approached cautiously since most commonly used antibiotics are toxic for the guinea pig (q.v., p. 1148). Treatment with tetracycline orally (℞ 37) or parenterally (℞ 26), or chloramphenicol (℞ 8) may be helpful.

Salmonellosis in guinea pigs is similar to the disease in other animals (*see* p. 377).

PARASITIC DISEASES

Several protozoa (*Toxoplasma gondii, Eimeria caviae, Encephalitizoon [Nosema] cuniculi*), nematodes (*Paraspidodera uncinata*), and lice (*Gyropus ovalis, Gliricola porcelli*) may infect guinea pigs. (*See* p. 1145 et seq. for control and treatment of nematodes and ectoparasites.)

DISEASES OF THE HAMSTER

BACTERIAL DISEASES

Hamsters are susceptible to infection by a number of common bacterial pathogens. These include streptococci, pneumococci, salmonellae, leptospires, staphylococci and pasteurellae.

Clinical signs and lesions are similar to those seen in other animals. Antibacterial therapy should be given with the utmost caution since hamsters are highly susceptible to the toxic effects of many antibiotics (*see* p. 1148).

PARASITIC DISEASES

Helminths: Many hamster colonies are infected by the tapeworm, *Hymenolepis nana*, and the pinworm, *Syphacia obvelata*. (*See* p. 1146 et seq. for lesions and therapy.)

External Parasites: Many external parasites, including *Notoedres, Sarcoptes,* and the tropical rat mite, *Ornithonyssus bacoti*, may infect hamsters. (*See* p. 1146 et seq. for lesions and therapy.) Two *Demodex* species, *D. criceti* and *D. aurati*, are commonly found on hamsters; there are no associated lesions unless animals are debilitated from other causes.

NUTRITIONAL DISEASES

Hamsters are very sensitive to vitamin E deficiency which leads to skeletal muscular dystrophy. Balanced diets formulated specifically for hamsters are commercially available; however, hamsters also thrive on commercially available rat and mouse diets.

OTHER DISEASE PROBLEMS

Antibiotic Toxicity: (*see* p. 1148).

Proliferative Ileitis (wet tail, regional enteritis) is a specific, apparently infectious, disease syndrome of uncertain etiology. The disease is enzootic in many laboratory and commercial colonies and may reach epizootic proportions. Clinical signs are diarrhea (wet tail), dehydration, anorexia and depression. Weanling animals are often affected. Lesions include ileitis or typhlitis or both, and colitis with marked hyperplasia of the ileal epithelium. This epithelial hyperplasia results in marked thickening and rigidity of the ileal wall with partial stenosis of the lumen. The condition responds to oral therapy with neomycin sulfate (15 mg/animal/day in divided doses). After initial oral dosing, the drug may be administered in the drinking water for 4 to 5 days. It is advisable to isolate affected animals and maintain strict sanitation in contaminated rooms.

DISEASES OF PRIMATES

The following primates are among the most widely used for research purposes:

Old World Origin	New World Origin
Tupaia glis (tree shrew)	*Saimiri sciureus*
Macaca mulatta	(squirrel monkey)
(rhesus monkey)	*Aotus trivirgatus*
Cercopithecus aethiops sabeus	(owl monkey)
(African green monkey)	*Cebus* spp.
Papio spp. (baboon)	(capuchin monkey)
Macaca fascicularis	*Ateles* spp. (spider monkey)
(crab-eating monkey)	*Saguinus, Callithrix* spp.
Macaca arctoides	(marmoset)
(stump-tailed monkey)	
Macaca nemestrina	
(pig-tailed monkey)	
Pan spp. (chimpanzee)	

Although some of these species are being bred in captivity in increasingly significant numbers, most are imported. They usually arrive at the laboratory within 30 to 45 days after initial capture, at which time they may be carrying, or be highly susceptible to, numerous infectious diseases. Accordingly, they should be held in quarantine before use for at least another 30 to 60 days, to provide for adequate evaluation of their health status and adaptation to the laboratory environment.

BACTERIAL DISEASES

Tuberculosis: All primates are susceptible to tuberculosis, although species differences exist. For example, rhesus monkeys (*Macaca mulatta*) are exquisitely sensitive, while crab-eating macaques (*Macaca fascicularis*) appear to be relatively resistant. Clinical signs are not a reliable indication of the extent of tuberculosis in the rhesus monkey. A vigorous appearing animal may have extensive miliary disease involving thoracic and abdominal organs; signs of debilitation may only appear shortly before death. A testing program is essential, and tuberculin tests on all newly received primates should be considered mandatory. The tests should be performed at the time of arrival and at 2-week intervals thereafter until at least 3 consecutive negative tests have been recorded for the entire group. After their release from quarantine, all primates should be skin-tested at least quarterly. The test consists of injecting Koch's Old Tuberculin (15 mg in 0.1 ml of water) intradermally in the upper eyelid or in the abdominal skin. The subject is examined at 24, 48 and 72 hours. A positive hypersensitivity reaction is marked by edema, induration or erythema, which may be subtle in some species such as the squirrel monkey (*Saimiri sciureus*). Roentgenographic examination of the chest may aid diagnosis of well-established cases, but the tuberculin skin test should be considered the primary diagnostic method for routine surveillance. All positive reactors should be destroyed. The presence of tuberculosis should then be confirmed by necropsy. Semi-annual skin tests or chest radiographs for personnel working in primate facilities should also be provided.

Isoniazid (INH) is an effective tuberculostat. It should not be administered during the quarantine period because it may suppress the skin test reaction, and thus prevent detection of positive reactors before the animals are released from quarantine. However, once animals are released, routine maintenance on isoniazid will effectively prevent development of tuberculosis. Despite a possible suppressing effect of isoniazid on the hypersensitivity reaction, skin testing should be performed regularly on all primates maintained on isoniazid. An effective daily dose of isoniazid is 5 to 10 mg/kg of body wt administered in a sugar cube or incorporated in the feed. There is no evidence that the continuous use of isoniazid will lead to the development of isoniazid-resistant mycobacteria.

Dysentery: The organisms most commonly associated with primate dysenteries are *Shigella, Salmonella,* and occasionally, *Escherichia coli, Pseudomonas aeruginosa* and *Aerobacter aerogenes*. Apparently healthy primates may be carriers of any of these organisms. Routine stool cultures for *Shigella* to identify carriers are of questionable value inasmuch as the identification, isolation and treatment of carrier animals has not been shown to prevent subsequent outbreaks of shigellosis in primate colonies.

Dysentery is a major problem in primates undergoing conditioning. Clinical signs include watery or mucoid blood-tinged feces, and rapid dehydration, emaciation and prostration. Rectal prolapse is an occasional sequela. The presence of helminths or protozoa may be a complicating factor. Mortality can be extremely high in acute outbreaks unless prompt treatment is instituted to restore and maintain normal fluid and electrolyte balance. The most common pathologic lesions at necropsy are hemorrhagic enteritis, enterocolitis, or simply colitis.

Affected primates should be treated individually. A nasogastric tube can be passed readily in most primates; it is indispensable for direct therapy. Fluid mixtures containing electrolytes, antibacterial agents, protectives and antispasmodics can be administered in this way (℞ 474). Broad-spectrum antibiotics may also be given (℞ 4, 8, 26). If circumstances prevent individual therapy, mass treatment of a colony for shigellosis or salmonellosis can be accomplished by incorporating furazolidone in the food (℞ 93), However, this is less satisfactory than individual treatment.

Pneumonia: Upper respiratory disease and pneumonia of bacterial origin can cause widespread illness and mortality, particularly in newly imported primates. Causative agents include *Diplococcus pneumoniae, Klebsiella pneumoniae, Bordetella bronchiseptica, Haemophilus influenzae,* and various species of streptococci, staphylococci and pasteurellae. Pneumonia may accompany or follow primary disease elsewhere; for example, pneumonia and dysentery often occur together. Clinical signs may include coughing, sneezing, dyspnea, mucoid or mucopurulent nasal discharge, lethargy, anorexia and unthriftiness. The principal lesions seen at necropsy are those of broncho- or lobar pneumonia.

Antibiotic therapy is generally helpful in treating primate pneumonias. Cultures from pharyngeal swabs are most useful in isolating the causative agent and determining the specific antibiotic sensitivity. Various penicillins, chloramphenicol, lincomycin, or cephalothin should be administered (℞ 5, 8, 23). Intensive nursing and other supportive therapy, such as fluid administration, may also aid recovery in selected cases.

VIRAL DISEASES

Herpesvirus Infections: At least 7 herpesviruses have been isolated from primates. They exist as latent or subclinical infections in reservoir hosts; at least 3 have caused fatal infections when transmitted naturally to other hosts. Herpesvirus B is generally innocuous in *Macaca* spp., but in man it causes a highly fatal encephalitis and encephalomyelitis. Transmission may occur through a monkey bite or by contamination of a superficial wound with infected saliva; aerosol transmissions of the virus may also occur. Herpesvirus T causes mild herpetic lingual ulcers and stomatitis in squirrel monkeys (*Saimiri sciureus*); but fatal epizootics have followed natural transmission to owl monkeys (*Aotus trivirgatus*) and marmosets (*Saguinus*). "*Herpesvirus hominis*" occurs as a mild infection in man and certain primates, but owl monkeys are highly susceptible and may die of the infection. Similar fatalities have occurred in tree shrews (*Tupaia glis*). Manifestations of infection may include mucous membrane or skin ulcerations, conjunctivitis, meningitis, or encephalitis.

Marburg Agent Disease (Vervet Monkey Disease): A highly fatal generalized disease occurred in European laboratory workers after handling tissues of *Cercopithecus aethiops pygerethrus* (vervet monkeys) from Uganda. Subsequently, a virus was isolated from human patients and infected monkey tissues. The virus was transmitted experimentally to vervet, squirrel and rhesus monkeys, all of which developed uniformly fatal illness within 2 weeks. A petechial skin rash was often seen late in the course of the experimental disease. Because of the danger to laboratory personnel, special care should be exercised in handling vervet monkeys or monkey tissues of Ugandan origin.

Hepatitis: Newly imported chimpanzees may carry and transmit to man the virus of infectious hepatitis. Elevated SGOT and SGPT values in chimpanzee sera are of diagnostic significance.

Inasmuch as vaccines are not available to protect primate colony personnel or the primates themselves against these virus infections, efforts should be made to prevent exposure. This is best accomplished by careful training of personnel in the handling of primates; by use of protective clothing, face masks and gloves; by separating primates in species-specific rooms; and by strict attention to hygienic standards.

Miscellaneous Viral Diseases: Several other viruses produce clinical disease in primates. **Rubeola** (measles) infection can assume epizootic proportions. The virus causes a nonpruritic, exanthematous rash on the chest and lower portions of the body; it may also cause interstitial, giant-cell pneumonia, rhinitis and conjunctivitis. There is no specific treatment. The efficacy of human measles vaccine in protecting nonhuman primates against rubeola is unknown. **Monkey pox** may occur in primate colonies. It is characterized by a maculopapular rash and variolous pustules. Affected monkeys usually survive. After recovery, animals are immune to challenge with vaccinia virus. Another pox virus, **Yaba virus**, produces histiocytomas with growths usually most prominent about the face. Some of the tumors may become very large, but spontaneous regression usually occurs.

PARASITIC DISEASES

Newly imported primates harbor numerous parasites. Some are commensal; others can be made self-limiting by strict sanitation and good husbandry. However, some parasites can cause serious disease or debilitation and should be removed by specific treatment.

Helminths: *Oesophagostomum* may cause characteristic granulomatous nodules in the large bowel associated with development of the worms and with an immune reaction of the host. The nodules sometimes rupture and thus cause peritonitis. *Strongyloides* and *Trichostrongylus* are invasive; adults may cause enteritis and diarrhea; larvae may cause pulmonary lesions during migration. These helminths, as well as *Trichuris* can be treated effectively with thiabendazole (100 mg/kg of body wt), administered orally at 2- to 4-week intervals. *Prosthenorchis* are filarid worms, common in Central and South American primates, that burrow into the mucosa of the ileocecal junction and sometimes perforate the bowel, or cause obstruction when present in large numbers. Cockroaches are intermediate hosts; their elimination, along with strict sanitation, is essential to freeing infected monkeys of these acanthocephalan worms. *Dipetalonema* and *Tetrapetalonema* occur in the peritoneal cavity. They may be present in large numbers without apparent harm to the host.

Protozoa: Primates may serve as hosts of various intestinal amoebae. *Entamoeba histolytica* is the principal pathogenic form in nonhuman primates as it is in man. In a heavy infection it may cause severe enteritis and diarrhea, and cysts may be demonstrated in the feces in large numbers. Chloramphenicol (R 8), oxytetracycline (R 26) and furazolidone (R 93) have been used successfully to control amebiasis in conjunction with strict sanitary measures.

Blood parasites, such as *Plasmodium, Leishmania* and *Trypanosoma,* also are common. There is generally an equilibrium between the parasite and the natural host, but serious reactions may result from cross-infections. Transmission of simian malarias to man has occurred in areas where the appropriate mosquito vectors are present. The disease does not usually pose a clinical problem in primate colonies, but the presence of blood parasites may render infected primates unsatisfactory for some types of research; however, some primate species, such as owl monkeys, are excellent models for malaria research.

Naturally occurring toxoplasmosis (*T. gondii*) has been reported more frequently in Central and South American primates than in African or Asian primates. Clinical signs of infection tend to be nonspecific (lethargy, anorexia, diarrhea). Hepatic focal necrosis and fibrinous pneumonia with edema are common histologic findings. Toxoplasma can be demonstrated in blood smears in acute cases.

Arthropods: Pulmonary acariasis (*Pneumonyssus*) occurs commonly in wild-caught Asian and African primates, particularly rhesus monkeys and baboons. Infection is rare in laboratory-raised primates. The life cycle of *Pneumonyssus* is not well understood. Infections do not usually produce serious disease, although they may stimulate sneezing and coughing. Lesions include dilatation and focal chronic inflammation of terminal bronchioles. The gross lesions of mite infestation may occasionally be confused with tuberculous granulomas.

Mange mites (*Psorergates* spp., *Sarcoptes scabiei*) or sucking lice (*Pedicinus longiceps*) are seen occasionally and may produce dermatoses. Topical treatment of affected animals with pyrethrin-containing compounds is recommended (℞ 298). Use of more toxic parasiticides should be avoided because of the possibility of ingestion during grooming.

MYCOTIC DISEASES

Microsporum and *Trichophyton* are known to affect primates. Topical treatment of ringworm with undecylenic acid ointment or tolnaftate (℞ 360), or oral administration of griseofulvin (℞ 353) is recommended. *Candida* are common saprophytes of the skin, alimentary tract and reproductive tract of primates, and act as facultative pathogens in debilitating conditions. Ulcers or white, raised plaques may be seen on the tongue or mouth; the fungus may also attack fingernails. Oral lesions must be differentiated from those of trauma, monkey pox, or herpesvirus infections. A topical cream containing chlordantoin (℞ 357) is effective in superficial infections. Oral nystatin (℞ 354) is effective for digestive tract candidiasis. Cutaneous streptothricosis caused by the actinomycete, *Dermatophilus congolensis*, has been reported in owl monkeys (*Aotus trivirgatus*). Papillomatous lesions are seen in the face and extremities. The infection is transmissible to man. Aspergillosis may occur in various primate species, and is usually a facultative pathogen. It is significant because it may be secondary to or predispose to tuberculosis.

NUTRITIONAL DISEASES

All laboratory primates are susceptible to vitamin C deficiency. Vitamin-C-deficient animals usually succumb to infectious diseases before clinical signs of the deficiency appear. Commercial monkey diets contain vitamin C which is stable for 3 months after the diet is packaged. Supplemental sources are citrus fruits. Orally administered pediatric vitamin preparations containing ascorbic acid are readily accepted. Daily intake of approximately 4 mg of ascorbic acid per kilogram of body weight will prevent scurvy.

Nutritional bone disease is particularly common in Central and South American primates. They are unable to utilize vitamin D_2, which is of plant origin and adequate to prevent rickets and osteomalacia in Asian and African primates. The New World primates require vitamin D_3, without which they develop osteodystrophia fibrosa (q.v., p. 562). Animal proteins provide an adequate source of vitamin D_3; or as little as 1.25 IU of crystalline vitamin D_3 per gram of diet can be added to the ration.

DISEASES OF AMPHIBIANS

The most widely used amphibians are leopard frogs (*Rana pipiens*), bullfrogs (*Rana catesbiana*), African clawed toads (*Xenopus laevis*), marine toads (*Bufo marinus*), salamanders (*Ambystoma* spp.) and Mexican axolotls (*Seridon mexicanum*). The vast majority are caught wild for use in laboratories; relatively few breeding colonies exist. Malnutrition, parasitism, and certain bacterial and virus diseases are common. These problems have not been studied systematically from the perspective of veterinary medicine. Good husbandry and adequate feeding are key elements in managing amphibians intended for laboratory use. However, individual or mass treatment of diseased animals can be used selectively in overcoming certain disease states.

BACTERIAL DISEASES

Most amphibians are carriers of *Aeromonas hydrophila*, a facultative pathogen that is the most common cause of the infection commonly called "red leg". Malnourished, newly received amphibians are particularly susceptible. Clinical signs may include lethargy; emaciation; ulcerations of the skin, nose and toes; and characteristic cutaneous pinpoint hemorrhages of the legs and abdomen. Hemorrhages may also occur in skeletal muscle, tongue and nictitating membrane. In acute cases, these signs may be absent. Histologic evidence of systemic infection may include inflammatory or necrotic foci in the liver, spleen and other coelomic organs. Individual treatment with oxytetracycline (150 mg/kg of body wt, b.i.d.) or chloramphenicol (50 mg/kg of body wt, b.i.d.) is effective. The antibiotics should be administered in a small volume of distilled water (0.2 ml to a 30-gm frog) by stomach tube (No. 5 French) for at least 5 consecutive days. Treatment of groups of frogs can be attempted by placing them in holding tanks containing oxytetracycline in the water (1 mg/ml). Cutaneous absorption may not be adequate to provide therapeutic systemic levels; however, this procedure may help to control or limit the spread of infection.

Amphibian tuberculosis is generally less devastating than mammalian tuberculosis. It is seen most commonly in debilitated animals; healthy amphibians normally are resistant, even though *Mycobacterium* spp. are widely present in aquaria. The usual route of infection is by ingestion or by direct entry of mycobacteria through skin abrasions. Accidental infection from unsterile parenteral injections may also occur. Primary pulmonary tuberculosis is less common. Affected animals may exhibit typical tuberculous granulomas in the liver, kidney, spleen, lungs and other coelomic organs. Specific treatment is not feasible.

VIRAL DISEASES

Renal adenocarcinomas (Lücke tumors) are relatively common in wild-caught *Rana pipiens* originating in the Northeastern and North-Central U.S.A. Few tumor-bearing frogs are seen in the summer; but the incidence may exceed 8% in the winter. The difference presumably is due to the effects of temperature on the causative agent, thought to be a herpes-type virus. Metastasis of the tumor to liver, lungs and other organs is common; both the primary and metastatic tumors can become very large. There is no treatment, but the Lücke tumor is an excellent model for research on viral oncogenesis.

PARASITIC DISEASES

Helminth parasites, protozoa and ectoparasites are extremely common in wild-caught amphibians; but heavy parasite loads are often well tolerated. Inflammatory reactions to parasitism are often imperceptible. Laboratory-reared animals have a strikingly lower incidence of helminths than those collected in the field. The parasite loads of wild-caught amphibians can be reduced strikingly by maintaining them under good conditions of husbandry and nutrition in the laboratory.

NUTRITIONAL DISEASES

Long-term laboratory maintenance of amphibians requires live food. Rickets is one example of a nutritional deficiency that may occur in *Rana* spp. Live food such as crickets, sow bugs, meal worms, or flies should be fed. Coating of the insects with powdered multiple-vitamin preparations, including vitamin D, is one way to supplement a natural diet.

SOME PHYSIOLOGIC DATA

Species	Approx. Gestation Period* (days)	Approx. Litter Size	Age (Weight) when Mature	Total RBC ($\times 10^6/mm^3$)	Total WBC ($\times 10^3/mm^3$)	Average Body Temp. (C°)	Approximate Water Consumption** (per day)
Mice	19	6-10	6 wk (20-30 gm)	7-11	4-12	37	4-7 ml
Rats	21	6-14	3 mo (0.2-0.3 kg)	7-10	5-15	38	30 ml
Guinea Pigs	68	1-4	3-4 mo (0.4-0.5 kg)	5-7	7-14	39	0.15 L
Hamsters, golden	16	4-10	2 mo (0.1-0.2 kg)	6-7	7-10	38	0.1-0.2 L
Gerbils	25	2-9	3 mo (60-100 gm)	7-8	8-11	39	4.0 ml
Rabbits	30	4-12	5-6 mo (3-4 kg)	5-7	6-12	40	0.3-0.7 L
Squirrel Monkeys	170	1	3-5 yr (0.6-1.1 kg)	8.3	8.2	39	0.07-0.11 L
Rhesus Monkeys	165	1-2	3-5 yr (5-11 kg)	4-6	10-20	38	0.2-1.0 L
Chimpanzees	225	1	8-12 yr (40-50 kg)	4-6	6-14	37	0.6-1.5 L
Opossums	12-13	8-18†	1 yr (2-6 kg)	3-6	15-29	36	0.1-0.2 L
Baboons	154-183	1	3-6 yr (11-30 kg)	4-5	5-9	39	0.3-0.5 L

* See also REPRODUCTIVE PHENOMENA, p. 770
** Varies with no. of animals per cage, moisture in feed, temperature, etc.
† Seven survive pouch life.

MANAGEMENT OF CAGED BIRDS

Many of the conditions encountered in bird practice are fairly obvious and quite simple to treat. In establishing a diagnosis, it is necessary to ascertain the length of time the owner has had the bird in his possession, as sickness in a newly acquired bird may be due to a lack of knowledge of the proper method of care and feeding.

Caged birds should not be subjected to sudden variations of temperature. They seem especially susceptible to heat, particularly if accompanied by prolonged low humidity. If suddenly subjected to it, they may go into a premature molt. Healthy birds can withstand cold far better than excessive heat and it is essential that the cage be placed in the section of the room which has an even temperature and is well protected from drafts. Birds maintained in outdoor aviaries year-round, with adequate shelter for protection against severe winds and rains, exhibit vastly superior plumage.

After placing a newly acquired bird in the cage, it is best to stay away from it for the first few hours until the bird settles down. Extreme patience is needed in caring for certain high-strung individuals, which flutter hysterically when approached.

Feeding: New owners should be advised to feed finches and parakeets the packaged seed mixtures prepared by reliable bird-seed firms. In addition, small amounts of celery tops, spinach, endive, carrot tops, apple, orange or banana may be fed twice a week. These foods should be discontinued temporarily if diarrhea develops.

For parrots, it is preferable to provide a mixture containing oat groats, cracked corn, hemp, large millet and canary seed. A small quantity of sweet apple, lettuce, or watercress may be given, but frozen or wilted foods should be scrupulously avoided. Commercially prepared pigeon feed pellets are a nutritionally balanced diet. It may take several days to adapt the bird to the new food, therefore care should be taken to first offer a mixture of seed and pellets, gradually reducing the seed content. Prepared "Monkey Biscuits" may be offered to large macaws. Oven-dried eggshells or cuttlebone are necessary to supply the bird's calcium requirement. Commercially prepared bird gravel sprinkled on the floor of the cage provides the grit needed for digestion and assists in keeping the bird's feet clean. Obesity in caged birds is undesirable and can be overcome by decreasing the quantity of food and increasing the flight space. Owners, however, should be warned against allowing the bird to fly about indoors without any restriction, as many freak accidents have been known to result from this practice. Concussions are common in birds that fly into window panes or mirrors and severe burns have resulted from flying into open flames or hot liquids.

Molting is the normal loss of feathers which occurs once or more a year. Parrots and budgerigars have no regular molting season and require no special treatment at that time. In finches, the molt usually starts in July and lasts almost 3 months. During this period, the birds evidence a lowered vitality and should receive supplemental nutrients, such as the mashed yolk of hard-boiled eggs, toasted bread crumbs and B-complex vitamins. In the absence of external parasites, feather-plucking is believed to be due to a deficient diet or boredom and this condition occasionally is corrected by the addition of freshly crushed bone meal to the diet; boredom may be overcome by providing additional space, a companion bird, or both. In most instances, however, this habit is a vice that cannot be overcome. The profuse hemorrhage that occurs when a new young feather is broken can be controlled only by removing the entire root. Spiral and other abnormal feathers may be eliminated by binding a silk or nylon suture around the base and allowing the ligature to remain in place until the feather drops out.

Upon first opening the cage door, the bird will naturally become disturbed and flutter excitably. However, if the hand is held still, the bird eventually will settle in one spot where it can easily be captured by cupping the palm of the hand over the bird's back, holding the wings close to the body. Any fatigue from fluttering or unnecessary struggling during handling may further aggravate a bird's illness. Parakeets can be prevented from biting while being examined by enclosing the neck of the bird between the index and middle fingers. While the bird is thus restrained, it is well to palpate the pectoral muscles. The plumpness of the breast is an indication of the bird's general condition. In chronic disorders, these muscles will atrophy and cause the carinate portion of the sternum to become quite prominent. Overgrown beaks and claws can be trimmed with cuticle nippers or podiatrists' toenail nippers. If the toe is held up to the light, the blood vessel in the nail can be seen and cutting the nail too short can be avoided. If bleeding should occur, it can be controlled by the application of a styptic, such as tincture of ferric chloride.

Macaws, cockatoos and the large Amazon parrots have powerful beaks capable of inflicting serious wounds and it is not always possible to restrain and treat such a bird single-handedly. An assistant, wearing heavy gloves, should grasp the bird around the neck and place the bird's body up under his arm. Another simple method is to wrap the bird in a heavy bath towel leaving the head uncovered. It is preferable that the owner does not witness the procedure as the raucous screeching and screaming of a restrained parrot is quite distracting. In cutting the beaks of these large birds, the bill is held closed with the left hand and the right used to pare down the overgrowth. If one mandible is misshapen or longer than the other, the excessive growth must be cut away, bringing the mandibles into normal alignment, with the tip of the upper overhanging that of the lower. Chewing pieces of natural branches or wooden spools will help prevent a recurrence.

General anesthesia may be accomplished by use of ketamine, Equithesin, ether or methoxyflurane. The anesthetist may wish to use the agent with which he is most familiar. Ketamine is given at the rate of 6 to 12 mg/lb. It is excellent for use in larger birds such as macaws, hawks and owls. Ketamine is administered in the pectoral muscle or thigh. Equithesin (chloral hydrate, magnesium sulfate, pentobarbital) is administered IM at 0.2 to 0.22 ml/100 gm of body wt using a half-inch, 26 to 27 gauge needle.

Volatile anesthetic may be administered by placing the bird's head into a standard anesthetic cone or glass jar. Cotton saturated with anesthetic is placed at the end of the cone. The excess space around the bird's head may be sealed off with towels. The patient should be monitored frequently until anesthetized. It may be necessary to place small birds into an anesthetic chamber. A wooden box with a small window is suitable for this purpose. Ether or methoxyflurane may be applied to a cotton pad in one corner of the box. The bird must be closely observed and removed promptly when anesthetized. If additional anesthesia is needed it may be administered by use of a gauze square saturated with the anethestic and placed over the nares. For large birds endotracheal intubation may be utilized.

Setting **fractures** of the tiny bones in birds requires a certain amount of patience and ingenuity. Anesthesia may be necessary if the bird struggles. Splints made from adhesive tape, sometimes with toothpicks or quills, have been found to be fairly satisfactory. The technique of applying these must be adapted to the location of the break. They should be left in place for 14 to 21 days. Intramedullary pins may be used in larger birds. Deformed or crippled toes usually do not respond to treatment and should be amputated if they interfere with normal activity. **Sore feet** and **scaly legs** in caged birds usually are the result of neglect in keeping perches well cleaned and can be remedied by frequent soaking of the legs with a warm solution of boric acid, followed by the application of olive oil. Multiple abscesses may occur on the feet; they may be drained surgically and antibiotics given in full doses.

Gouty deposits in the feet may be confused with abscesses. **Gout** usually occurs in the tarsophalangeal joint and the ventral surface of the toes. There is no treatment for gout in birds.

A sick bird, regardless of the cause, will appear listless and sit huddled on the perch with its feathers puffed out and the eyes half closed. Many **respiratory infections** in birds present much the same signs, such as labored breathing, gaping, wheezing and nasal discharges. A solution made by dissolving a 50-mg soluble chlortetracycline tablet in 1 oz of water is useful in respiratory diseases. Two to 5 drops should be given orally with an eye dropper 3 times a day until the bird improves. Tetracycline pediatric drops are equally satisfactory. The bird should be held in an upright position and the drops given slowly, giving the bird time to swallow. If the owner is sure the bird is drinking, the medication can be put in the drinking water. One hundred milligrams of the soluble tetracycline antibiotics may be added to the drinking cup. Sulfamethazine (2 oz of 12.5% solution in a gallon of water) is especially useful in cases where the causative organisms are resistant to antibiotic therapy. Ten drops of the 12.5% solution may also be added directly to the drinking cup. It is important to keep sick birds warm, a temperature of 80°F not being excessive. A swelling on the face below the eye usually indicates empyema of the infraorbital sinus and the accumulation of cheeselike pus must be carefully removed under anesthesia and the area bathed with a mild antiseptic solution.

When **diarrhea** is observed, it is important to question the owner regarding the bird's diet. In parrots, all food should be withheld for a period of 24 hours. With finches and parakeets, green and rich foods should be discontinued. Bread crumbs moistened with Kaopectate or dilute paregoric can be added to the diet or administered directly by mouth until the condition subsides. If the feathers around the vent have become matted and form an obstruction, they should be trimmed away. Antibiotics may be given orally or by IM injection if the diarrhea is believed to be due to a systemic infection, and the dosage should be calculated in proportion to body weight. Adult parakeets weigh 25 to 55 gm, finches about 15 gm and large macaws seldom exceed a weight of 1.5 kg.

New owners may be unfamiliar with the normal courtship behavior and believe the female to be ill when they see the male bird feeding her. Occasionally, a female will become **egg-bound** and is found crouching on the floor of the cage, trembling and apparently in pain. Simply increasing the cage temperature to 90 to 95°F will often result in delivery of the egg. If this fails, the bird is turned on its back and warm lubricant is placed in the cloaca. After the bird is anesthetized, the egg is propelled backward by constant and gentle pressure. A small amount of lubricant is applied to the egg as it comes into view and a blunt sterile probe is rotated around the egg. Pressure applied again will deliver the egg. If prolapse of the cloaca occurs following severe straining, local anesthetic should be applied and the protruded portion gently replaced with a blunt instrument, such as a rectal thermometer. A bird in this condition should be caged alone until recovery takes place as other birds will peck at the inflamed tissue.

The incubation period of finch eggs is 12 to 14 days. After the young birds have hatched, the parent feeds them regurgitated food for the first few weeks. A good commercial nestling food should be supplied until the baby birds are old enough to crack their own seeds (6 weeks). If the breast feathers of the hen appear moist as if she were sweating, it is due to fecal contamination from diarrhea in the chicks and this should be treated by adding Kaopectate to the food.

The spontaneous occurrence of malaria and other protozoan infections has been reported occasionally. Unfortunately, the signs of psittacosis, aspergillosis, *Salmonella* and *Pasteurella* infections usually are not distinct from other systemic disorders and a positive diagnosis can be made only after cultures have been examined. When psittacosis (q.v., p. 1033) is suspected, public health agencies should be consulted and the complement-fixation test used to verify the diagnosis.

Parakeets are very subject to **tumor** formation. Lipomas occur most frequently on the breast, perineum and the region of the uropygial glands. Many of these tumors can be removed surgically. Tumors found on the wings, legs and beak are frequently fibrosarcomas and will often recur if excised surgically. Internal tumors most frequently involve the kidneys and testicles. An internal tumor may be evidenced by a gradual loss of condition, diarrhea, dyspnea and swelling of the perineum. Since most abdominal tumors in small caged birds are malignant, they are usually inoperable.

The following **parasitic diseases** are of rather common occurrence: *Trichomonas gallinae* causes "canker" in pigeons and "frounce" in falcons and hawks, characterized by necrosis of the esophageal and crop epithelium. It may also affect canaries. Signs are inappetence, diarrhea and dyspnea. Treatment consists of 1 gm of Enheptin in 1 liter of water for 6 days.

Coccidiosis causes diarrhea, anorexia and death. It may be treated with 10 drops of 10% solution of sulfamethazine in 1 oz water for 3 days, 2 days without, then 3 days additional.

Gapeworms in the trachea cause severe dyspnea, anorexia, anemia and gasping. Thiabendazole (44 mg/kg of body wt) and mechanical removal of worms with forceps may be effective. *Capillaria* and ascarids may cause loss of weight and death. Piperazine, 50 mg/ml in water, 1 ml/100 mg body wt by stomach tube is fairly effective.

Swiftly moving, biting lice can be seen with a magnifying glass. They cause irritation, loss of condition and ruffling of feathers. Pyrethrin, 0.5% powder, is the treatment of choice. Feather mites or red mites (*Dermanyssus gallinae*) are nocturnal feeders. They may be detected by placing a cloth cover over the cage at night. Mites are found on the underside of the cloth in the morning. After removal of the birds, the cages are scalded and washed with soda, and sprayed with lindane. The birds are dusted with pyrethrin powder.

Scaly face and leg disease of budgerigars is caused by the mite *Cnemidocoptes pilae.* Signs are scaly epithelial proliferation of the cere, deformed beak, scaly legs and crusty lesions around eye and vent. A 10% emulsion of benzyl benzoate for 3 days or 0.2% lindane in soft paraffin is effective.

CARE OF ZOO ANIMALS

The immediate surroundings and the management of captive wild animals have a direct and important bearing on their well-being. The appropriate "furniture" should be provided to prevent development of undesirable stereotyped behavior (pacing, circling, self-mutilation, etc.). Cages should be carefully designed to ensure ease of cleaning by using impervious materials. Constant emphasis must be placed on vigorous sanitation measures, such as prompt removal of feces, daily cage washings and thorough scrubbing and disinfection at frequent intervals. The choice of disinfectants and insecticides is important.

Except for tropical specimens, healthy captive mammals and birds do not require a great deal of heat. Reptiles require access to temperature gradients of up to 95°F, but must not be kept in direct sunlight on hot days for prolonged periods of time. A moderate temperature of 65° to 68°F is adequate for most species, although there are species variances. Some mammals and birds native to warmer climates adjust surprisingly well when allowed access to their outdoor cages during the winter months, and often show improvement in the appearance of pelage or plumage during the cold weather. Local experience regarding climatic needs for different species is valuable information, and each zoo should keep records in order that they can more appropriately care for the animals in their possession. The simple fact that certain animals will endure extremes of climate is no license to subject them to adverse conditions. Proper shelters and close observation are always indicated. During cold weather it is recommended that the floor of sleeping quarters for mammals be insulated, heated or covered with clean bedding to prevent excess loss of body heat.

The treatment of disease conditions in captive wild animals does not differ substantially from that of domestic species, except in the method of restraint. Most zoo animals resent being handled and will usually fight manual restraint. Struggling with an animal in order to administer medical or surgical treatment may do more harm than can be offset by the treatment. It is therefore advantageous to conceal medication in the food or drinking water, whenever possible, without arousing the animal's suspicion; this method eliminates the anxiety of both animal and caretaker.

The squeeze cage or chute is frequently used in the modern zoo. While the dimensions and construction may vary, all operate on the same principle, having one side or end, or the top, which can be moved to restrain the animal against the opposite side, end or bottom of the cage. A top-to-bottom type of squeeze cage is preferable for large cats. Only a few procedures can be accomplished on an unanesthetized animal under such circumstances, but the method is fairly satisfactory for physical examination, administering injections, trimming ingrown claws or applying topical medication. Animals in squeeze cages can usually be adequately restrained for vaccination procedures. Squeeze cages may be improvised in the animal's regular quarters. Whenever possible, patients should be enticed into the cage rather than forcibly compelled to enter it. Tranquilizers (℞ 369) can be administered IV or IM, with the aid of a squeeze cage.

A useful instrument for administering drugs to wild animals is a gun to propel a projectile syringe. Intramuscular injections can be made accurately at a distance up to approximately 35 yards. Injectable preparations such as antibiotics, tranquilizers and anesthetics can readily be administered by such guns. Tranquilizers, anesthetics and agents producing muscular relaxation, such as succinylcholine (℞ 533) are given according to body weight, hence accurate data of weights for various species are of critical importance in the safe use of the gun. It may be possible to administer some vaccines in this way, but vaccination procedures will be limited if the vaccinating dose is small.

Many zoos install small nest boxes or catch pens within the exhibit enclosures. Such retreats are equipped with doors that can be operated remotely, and are used to trap or catch animals on exhibit. From these catch pens, the confined animal can readily be transferred to a squeeze cage, anesthetic chamber, or into a shipping crate if the animal is to be moved any great distance.

Smaller mammals and birds may be caught and restrained in a long-handled loop net. These nets must be sufficiently deep so that when the animal is caught and drops into the blind end of the net, the upper part can be twisted to prevent escape. The operator doing this work should wear gloves as a protection against bites or scratches.

Safe immobilization and anesthesia in wild animals is of special concern. Many procedures, routinely accomplished on domestic animals with minimal restraint, will require chemical immobilization of the zoo specimen, for the welfare of both the patient and the handler.

Phencyclidine (Sernylan) at a dosage of 0.25 to 1.0 mg/lb of body wt is usually predictable in primates, Ursidae, Felidae and Canidae. A combination of fentanyl and droperidol (Innovar) produces marked sedation and analgesia in the Canidae, Ursidae and primates, when administered IM at a dosage level of 0.05 ml/lb of body wt, with variable results. M99 (etorphine) administered in combination with acetylpromazine and hyoscine, has been extensively used for immobilization and analgesia in many ungulates, elephants and rhinoceros. The user, however, must be aware of the necessity of understanding the interrelationship of the pharmacologic action of these drugs when given in combination. Artiodactyla subjected to prolonged stress and excitement may be a bad risk for M99. One advantage of M99 is that a rapidly-acting antidote, M-285 (cyprenorphine), is available for IV injection. Other immobilizing agents, such as xylazine (Rompun), have shown promise for some exotic mammals.

Where anesthesia is desired and sedation has been achieved, barbiturates can be used either IV or IP. If IV administration is possible, the anesthesia should be given to the desired effect. In IP administration, about one-half the usual dosage is sufficient to render the animal tractable after administration of the ataractic drugs. Only examination of the individual animal will reveal if the jugular, caudal, femoral, saphenous, brachial or radial vein is prominent enough for IV injection.

Anesthetic chambers have long been used for administration of ether or chloroform. They vary in size from those suitable for laboratory animals to large metal-lined wooden boxes for lions and tigers with sliding lift doors in each end. Ample plexiglass viewing area is necessary. If the chamber is airtight and a suitable vaporizer is used, sufficient concentrations of methoxyflurane or bromochlorotrifluoroethane (Fluothane) can be vaporized to induce anesthesia. After removal from the chamber, patients can be intubated or anesthetized by other methods.

All newly acquired specimens should be quarantined to help prevent the introduction of infectious diseases. Isolation quarters should be separate from exhibit areas and serviced by separate caretakers. These facilities should be so constructed that they can be easily disinfected and cleaned. Death losses of zoo animals are often greatest during the initial acclimation period. Special care is therefore required in noting dietary intake, stool formation, signs of disease or any abnormal behavior. Adjusting animals to new feeds and feeding schedules is frequently a difficult procedure. Some specimens may require forced feeding.

Wild animals are vulnerable to a wide variety of endo- and ectoparasitic infestations, somewhat parallel to those found in domestic animals. The impact of the parasites on individual animals is variable, but is probably greatest at the time of the animal's shipment and arrival at the zoo. During this period of extreme stress, many normally commensal parasites, especially protozoa, appear to be capable of establishing pathogenic processes. Acute diarrhea may result from massive infestations of *Trichomonas, Giardia* or *Balantidium*. Amebiasis is fairly common in primates and reptiles and may terminate in death. Paromomycin, 4.5 mg/lb of body wt twice daily, is effective against *Entamoeba* and has the advantage of being effective against *Salmonella* and *Shigella* in higher dosages.

Periodic examination of skin and pelage and fecal specimens should be made during the quarantine period for ecto- and endoparasites, and appropriate treatment regimens should be instituted. Parasites with indirect life cycles will less frequently pose a health problem if the exhibit area is clean and free of intermediate hosts. If ectoparasites are found on newly received animals, proper spraying of the shipping crate and its contents is recommended before the crate leaves the quarantine area. Some zoos routinely use an organophosphate spray for such purposes.

Diagnostic tests should be routine. Tuberculosis is a potential threat in primates, and especially old-world primates; it may spread rapidly if introduced into a primate colony. For this reason no primate should be added to the collection without first having been tuberculin-tested (q.v., p. 365). Chest X-rays are also recommended.

Vaccination programs should also be done during the quarantine period to protect animals against disease to which they are known to be susceptible (*see* VACCINATION OF EXOTIC MAMMALS, p. 1118).

Newly arriving specimens require caution and patience during uncrating and release since they are often frightened and fatigued. Ungulates have been fatally injured when released from shipping crates by suddenly running directly into barriers. Birds often try to fly through the glass fronts. Canvas, or colored plastic drop cloths, suspended from fences or cage walls, or the opaquing of the glass windows with soap, offers some measure of protection against such occurrences.

Though the new arrival may appear famished, it is preferable to limit the quantity of food and especially water supplied at the first feeding. Later the frequency and volume of feed should be increased. More often the new arrival refuses to eat for the first few days. This is particularly true of wild animal pets that appear to be despondent over the loss of their former owners or companions.

Such individuals must be pampered and fed their former diets, only gradually weaning them to the standard zoo diet (*see* EXOTIC AND ZOO ANIMAL NUTRITION, p. 1281) for the species. Despite elaborate precautions, a number of new animals fail to adapt to the zoo environment and die.

With larger numbers of birds or mammals, and especially when several species are housed in one exhibit or flight cage, it is often recommended that several feeding and watering stations be established. Multiple feeding areas at appropriate elevations will help reduce traumatic injuries and death resulting from territorial invasions. If different types of feed are offered to mixed groups in one enclosure, it may be beneficial to feed these types of feed separately. It does appear that multiple feeding stations will actually help reduce the size of individual territories.

Zoo personnel working with wild animals must develop their observation skills in order to adequately recognize general condition of the animals and normal and abnormal behavioral patterns. The health of the collection is substantially dependent upon the interest, alertness and power of observation of the keepers. These individuals should be familiar with the normal appearance of their charges; they should be encouraged to report any uncommon behavior at once. Overzealous reporting of inconsequential observations is preferable to indifference.

All zoos should be conservation-minded and interested in animal reproduction. It is therefore important that the nature of the animal and its behavioral pattern be understood. During the breeding season it is often preferable to have only one male with the females, depending, of course, upon the species involved. In mixed groups of Artiodactyla it is possible to establish estrous cycles by species and thus have only one male in the enclosure at a time. The other males can be rotated to coincide with the estrous periods of their species. Such measures often will reduce traumatic injuries. At parturition it is often advisable to remove the males for several weeks to prevent attack on the postpartum female or her offspring.

Bone fractures are best repaired under general anesthesia. Since maintaining a splint on a wild animal is often a difficult problem, appropriate internal fixation combined with a light cast is preferable wherever possible. When a cast is applied, freedom of movement and a minimum of discomfort to the patient must be assured, as the cast must be left as applied for 3 to 4 weeks. In fractures of the metacarpus in small ruminants where reasonable apposition exists and no other problems are foreseen, leaving the animal undisturbed is preferable and less dangerous than attempts to capture and restrain it.

In birds and small animals, potassium penicillin G should be used, as procaine penicillin is not well tolerated. Massive doses of 45,000 to 90,000 units/lb of body wt in small animals are often indicated rather than smaller doses and more frequent handling.

Dentistry in zoo animals may present unique problems. The root of the canine tooth in monkeys and carnivores is more extensive than the exposed crown, and it is not possible to remove such a tooth intact by simple traction and rotation; dislodging with a dental elevator is essential. A small electric drill or bone chisel may have to be used to remove a section of the maxilla around the labial margin of the root. The incisor teeth of rodents, such as a beaver, porcupine and capybara grow continuously throughout life, and unless these animals are supplied with coarse feed or logs to gnaw on, their incisors will grow excessively long and interfere with the animal's ability to feed.

Routine procedures include trimming of beaks and nails of birds. Pinioning of birds to prevent flight is readily accomplished by amputating one wing just distal to the radiocarpal joint. Other pinioning methods are also used and can be found in the literature. Large, adult birds should be given a local or general anesthetic. Ligation for control of hemorrhage is important, indeed it is vital in mature birds of large species. Pinioning of young birds is commonly easier and more successful than the same procedure on the adults.

Much can be learned about diseases affecting zoo animals if a complete necropsy is made following death of an animal. The prosector should constantly be aware of the variations in anatomy as such observations may aid in disease diagnosis and treatment.

FISH DISEASES

Fish diseases are similar in many respects to those found in any vertebrate group. Pathologic changes include hyperemia, anemia, hemorrhage, edema, inflammation, atrophy, hypertrophy, hyperplasia, neoplasia and necrosis. Histologic and cytologic evidence has been established for disturbances of fat, carbohydrate, protein, pigment and mineral metabolism. These manifestations may be caused by infectious or parasitic agents or be due to nutritional deficiencies, hormonal imbalances, embryologic abnormalities, hereditary factors, aging, abnormal chemical and physical conditions, injury or environmental stresses. The infectious and parasitic agents are similar to those found in diseases of warm-blooded animals. In addition, since each species of fish is adapted to specific temperature and pH ranges, any sudden change in one or both factors may result in derangement of the homeostatic mechanisms, resulting in death by shock. A decrease in dissolved oxygen or an increase in carbon dioxide concentration may result in death by asphyxiation. Supersaturation of oxygen or increased concentration of nitrogen or other gases frequently produces emboli resulting in serious tissue damage. Sewage, farm or industrial pollution, algal growth or decomposition processes in tank, hatchery or pool may also cause a reduction in oxygen below the minimum requirement. Death may also be due to toxic substances released by phytoplankton "blooms" (e.g., "red tide"), to agricultural pesticides or industrial wastes.

BACTERIAL DISEASES

The bacterial diseases described below are the most commonly encountered among cultured fishes. However, if fish are placed under severe stress conditions, many of the saprophytic bacteria present in the aquatic environment may produce disease and death.

The major pathogenic bacteria of fish are classified in the order Pseudomonadales in the genera *Pseudomonas*, *Aeromonas* and *Vibrio*. They produce bacteremic infections with hemorrhage, ascites and enteric disorders. Identification of the pathogen is necessary for accurate diagnosis. *Pseudomonas fluorescens* or *P. putida* produce disease in trout, aquarium fish, catfish and other pondfish and are treated with antibiotics (℞ 35). The best known aeromonad pathogen is the nonmotile *Aeromonas salmonicida,* the cause of **furunculosis** of salmon, trout and other fish throughout most of the world. Furunculosis can be treated with sulfonamides (℞ 76, 92), antibiotics (℞ 35), or nitrofurans (℞ 95). Other aeromonad pathogens include 3 closely related motile species, *A. liquefaciens, A. punctata* and *A. hydrophila,* which many investigators consider one species. They cause **hemorrhagic septicemia** of trout, pondfishes and European carp; **fin rot** and **tail rot** in aquarium fishes; **red leg** of frogs; and **ulcerative stomatitis** of snakes. These bacteria, on occasion, produce disease in humans. Treatment is the same as for the pseudomonad pathogens. Diseases caused by *Vibrio anguillarum,* and to a lesser extent *V. parahaemolyticus,* affect principally marine and estuarine fishes. Freshwater species may become diseased, especially if fed a diet containing marine fish or fish products containing vibrios. For prevention of vibriosis in fishes, oral vaccines appear to be promising. Oxytetracycline (℞ 35), sulfamethazine (℞ 83), or a combination of a sulfamethazine and furazolidone (℞ 94) are useful in prevention or treatment of outbreaks of vibriosis.

Myxobacteria (Myxobacteriales) are long, thin (2 to 10 μ by 0.5 to 0.75 μ) gram-negative rod-shaped bacteria with gliding motility, which produce several diseases in fishes. **Columnaris disease** caused by *Chondrococcus columnaris* was the first described disease of any animal caused by a myxobacterium. The disease affects warm- and cold-water, freshwater fishes when temperatures are above 15°C (60°F). It begins as an external infection producing grayish-white areas on the head, lips or fins. These areas superficially resemble a fungus infection. The lesions gradually spread and become necrotic. A localized necrotic lesion often develops on gill tissue. If untreated, the disease usually becomes systemic. In early stages external treatment with diquat (℞ 638) is beneficial. For systemic infection, oxytetracycline (℞ 35) and nifurpirinol (℞ 97), a new nitrofuran, are effective. Lowering water temperature below 15°C (60°F) is effective in prevention.

Peduncle disease, also known as coldwater disease, caused by *Cytophaga psychrophila* affects juvenile salmonids, particularly fry and fingerling coho salmon and fingerling brook trout, in water temperature below 10°C (50°F). The disease begins as an external infection in the caudal area and then becomes systemic.

Benzalkonium chlorides (℞ 400) are useful in controlling external infection, and sulfisoxazole (℞ 92) and oxytetracycline (℞ 35) are used for systemic infections; best results may be obtained by using both. Raising water temperature above 12°C (53°F) is also effective if the disease has not progressed too far.

Bacterial gill disease is a serious problem with cultured juvenile salmonids. It is characterized by hyperplasia of gill lamellae and the presence of masses of myxobacteria on swollen lamellae. Several types of myxobacteria and other bacteria have been isolated from diseased fish but none have been found to be the etiologic agent. It is probable that infection occurs after trout are exposed to stress factors. External disinfectants (℞ 400, 638) are used for prevention and treatment. Bacterial gill disease also occurs among warm-water pondfish. The most promising control measures appear to be addition of copper sulfate (℞ 407) or diquat (℞ 638), both at 1.0 ppm, to pond water. Myxobacterial infection among saltwater fish are generally associated with *Sporocytophaga*. The infections are external and disinfectants (℞ 400, 638), antibiotic baths (℞ 9) or nitrofuran baths (℞ 97) may be beneficial.

Kidney disease of salmonids is a chronic, and at times acute, disease caused by a *Corynebacterium*. The disease is characterized externally by exophthalmos and blebs or blisters on flanks. Internally the kidney may be swollen and may contain grayish-white areas. Hemorrhages may occur in reproductive organs. Microscopic examination of gram-stained material from external lesions or kidney lesions show small gram-positive diplobacilli, the causative agent. The disease is treated with erythromycin (℞ 19). **Ulcer disease** of trout is caused by *Haemophilus piscium* and is treated with oxytetracycline (℞ 35). Mycobacterial infections occur in many marine and aquarium species causing multiple foci of infection in internal organs. An enteric organism, as yet unclassified and designated as the "RM" bacterium, causes a condition known as **red-mouth** in rainbow trout in the Western U.S.A. Oral immunization with a killed cell bacterin has been successful on a small scale. The disease is treated with a combination of sulfamerazine and an antibiotic (℞ 79). Epizootics among fish have also been attributed to bacteria classified as *Nocardia, Pasteurella, Flavobacterium, Streptomyces, Streptococcus* and *Achromobacter.*

On occasion it may become necessary to treat a nonspecific bacterial disease in small tropical fish. In such instances addition of nifurpirinol (℞ 97) or chloramphenicol (℞ 9) to the water for several days is useful and may constitute specific treatment.

VIRAL DISEASES

The development of cell and tissue culture of cold-blooded vertebrates resulted in the establishment of the etiology of several viral diseases of fishes which are described below.

Infectious pancreatic necrosis (IPN) is a severe disease of very young salmonids caused by a rhabdovirus. Epizootics occur among hatchery-reared salmonids in the U.S.A., Canada and Europe and are characterized by fish frantically whirling on their long axis then lying quietly on the bottom. Affected fish become dark, show swollen abdomens, exophthalmos and hemorrhagic areas on the ventral surface. Food is not present in the stomach or gut. Histologically, necrosis occurs in acinar and islet cells of the pancreas and in cells of adjacent adipose tissue. Survivors of epizootics become carriers and shed virus in feces, eggs and sperm. Diagnosis is based on isolation of the virus and identification of the agent by a serum neutralization test.

Infectious hemopoietic necrosis (IHN) is the name applied to diseases formerly known as Sacramento River Chinook disease (SRCD) and Oregon Sockeye disease (OSD). IHN is an acute disease principally affecting the fry and fingerlings of rainbow trout, Chinook and Sockeye salmon raised in the U.S.A. and Canada. The disease is caused by a rhabdovirus. Affected fish may have long fecal casts, ascites, exophthalmos; and hemorrhages at the base of fins, in the peritoneum, air bladder, lateral body wall and membranes covering brain and heart. Histologically, extensive degeneration and necrosis occurs in the hemopoietic tissues of kidney and spleen. Fish which recover become carriers, and virus may be isolated from ovarian fluid of mature females. At present, diagnosis of IHN depends on isolation of the virus and determination of certain of its characteristics to distinguish it from the IPN virus.

Viral hemorrhagic septicemia (VHS) is probably the most important disease of rainbow trout in Europe, affecting both fingerling and larger trout. VHS is caused by a rhabdovirus, and affected trout show alternate periods of frantic swimming and quiescence. There are several forms of the disease: the acute, characterized by reduced appetite, erratic swimming, multiple hemorrhages in skeletal muscle and viscera, and hyperemic and swollen kidney and liver; the chronic, in which trout seek quiet areas, show exophthalmos, swollen abdomen, and anemia; and the nervous form, which may be the last stages of an epizootic and in which trout usually show frenzied swimming and leaping. Transmission may occur through water, and virus is probably shed through water, feces, urine and eggs. Diagnosis is based on isolation of virus and identification by means of a serum neutralization test.

Channel catfish virus disease (CCVD), caused by one of the herpesvirus group, was first described in the late 1960s and affects channel catfish and to a lesser degree white and blue catfish. The disease occurs mostly in the Southern and Southwest States, but may occur wherever catfish are propagated. Affected catfish whirl on their long axis, or swim convulsively and lie quietly on the pond bottom. Characteristically, just before death fish hang vertically in water with their heads at the surface. Diseased specimens show hemorrhages at the base of fins and abdomen, distended abdomen, pale or hemorrhagic gills, ascitic fluid and pale and swollen kidneys. Histologically, necrosis and edema occur in the kidneys and gastrointestinal tract. As for other viral diseases, positive diagnosis is based on isolation of virus and serologic identification.

Spring viremia of carp (SVC) is a recently described viral disease of fish. Caused by a rhabdovirus, it is limited at present to Europe and affects cultured carp. SVC is probably a form **of infectious dropsy of carp** (IDC), a disease with complex syndromes. Affected carp may show distended abdomen, exophthalmos and bleeding in the anterior eye chamber, protruding and inflamed anus, petechiae in kidneys, liver, pericardium, heart, intestine, gas bladder, skeletal muscles, and edema of all internal organs.

Lymphocystis is a benign disease of worldwide distribution which affects freshwater and marine teleosts. Nodular masses resembling warts occur on the fins and body. The masses are composed of hypertrophied cells which may undergo a 50,000 to 100,000-fold increase in cell volume. The causative agent is a polyhedral virus. Although the virus can be isolated in cell culture, diagnosis of lymphocystis is usually based on the gross examination of the lesion.

Stomatopapilloma of eels (formerly known as cauliflower disease) may be of viral etiology in that a viral agent has been isolated from some diseased specimens. There are no published reports on infectivity or transmission of the disease with the isolated virus.

Diseases in which viruses have been seen by electron microscopy include fish pox of cyprinids, walleye epidermal hyperplasia, walleye sarcoma, lymphosarcoma in pike, and pleuronectid papillomas.

Diseases of possible viral etiology include: contagious stomatitis of South American cichlids; malignant kidney tumor in an aquarium cyprinodont; Atlantic salmon papilloma; brown bullhead papilloma; ulcerative dermal necrosis of Atlantic salmon; swim-bladder disease of carp.

There is no specific chemotherapy useful in the treatment of viral fish diseases. Temperature manipulation as a means of control is apparently effective in contagious stomatitis and IHN. However, strict hygiene, avoidance of known diseased carriers or eggs from carrier fish are the only means of general control of viral fish diseases.

PROTOZOAN DISEASES

The protozoan subphyla and the genera most responsible for diseases of fishes are: Sarcomastigophora (*Amyloodinium, Costia, Cryptobia, Hexamita, Oodinium* and *Trypanosoma*); Ciliophora (*Brooklynella, Chilodonella, Cryptocaryon, Ichthyophthirius, Trichodina, Trichodinella* and *Trichophrya*); Sporozoa (*Eimeria* and *Haemogregarina*); Cnidospora (*Ceratomyxa, Henneguya*, and *Myxosoma* of the Myxosporidia and *Glugea, Nosema* and *Plistophora* of the Microsporidia).

The most pathogenic are the ectoparasitic protozoa of the Sarcomastigophora and Ciliophora, with the most common and widely distributed ones being the Myxosporidia of the Cnidospora. All degrees of host-specificity exist from tissue- and species-specificity to none at all. The ectoparasitic forms can be readily treated by addition of drugs and chemicals to the water. Knowledge of systemic treatment of the tissue-inhabiting forms is minimal.

Amyloodinium and *Oodinium* are dinoflagellates responsible for **velvet disease** of aquarium fish. *Amyloodinium* invades primarily the gills and in heavy infections also the skin. *Oodinium* normally invades both gills and skin. Transmission of both is by the motile infective-dinospore stage. Low concentrations of copper sulfate or acetate (B 407) eliminates these protozoa from the water. The dinospores of *Amyloodinium* are not formed under 10°C.

Costia, Cryptobia and *Hexamita* are parasitic flagellates. *Costia,* an external parasite, is the most ubiquitous and troublesome, but is controlled easily with dilute formalin (B 410). It invades the skin and gills and has direct transmission. *Cryptobia* is a hemoflagellate, and *Hexamita* lives within the intestinal tract. Both have been implicated in salmonid epizootics, but are not major problems.

Brooklynella and *Chilodonella,* marine and freshwater forms, respectively, are ectoparasitic ciliates. *Chilodonella* can be a serious pathogen in freshwater fishes, and *Brooklynella* can produce severe lesions on gills of marine fish kept in aquaria. Dilute formalin (B 410) or acetic acid (B 396) will usually remove these protozoa from the fish.

Two of the most ubiquitous pathogenic ciliates are *Ichthyophthirius* of freshwater fishes and *Cryptocaryon* of marine fishes. *Ichthyophthirius* has caused epizootics in nature, while *Cryptocaryon* has not been recorded as causing epizootics in nature, but does so in aquarium conditions. Both of these ciliates invade and burrow under the epidermis causing white spots. Once under the epidermis, they feed on host cells, cause irritation as evidenced by the fish flashing and rubbing against the aquarium, cause hypersecretion of mucus and loss of osmoregularity.

The visible white spots contain mature trophozoites. Upon maturation these burrow out of the fish, settle upon some substrate, encyst and undergo successive divisions within the cyst until the infective unit, the tomite, is formed. As many as 1,000 tomites can be produced from a single cyst. Tomites are free-swimming but die if they do not make contact with a host within 24 hours (depending on water temperature).

The free-swimming tomite is easily eliminated with formalin (B 410). Treatment of the tissue-inhabiting stage cannot be recommended as controlled experimental treatment data are not available. Both *Ichthyophthirius* and *Cryptocaryon* cause heavy economic losses, with *Ichthyophthirius* alone causing an estimated $1,000,000 loss per year.

Trichodina and *Trichodinella* are also external ciliates which occasionally cause epizootics in cultured and aquarium fishes. They are easily controlled by formalin (B 410).

Eimeria and *Haemogregarina* are coccidian parasites. *Eimeria* is found in both freshwater and marine fish. In freshwater fish it is found within the intestine and visceral mass, and believed to be pathogenic. *Eimeria* of marine fish are known to be pathogenic, producing liver lesions, parasitic castration, and partial or total occlusion of kidney and air bladder.

Ceratomyxa, Henneguya and *Myxosoma* are histozoic myxosporidians which are serious pathogens of fish. *Ceratomyxa* affects anadromous and freshwater salmonids and has been responsible for total losses of rainbow trout. *Myxosoma* species parasitize many species of fishes. The most important species is *Myxosoma cerebralis,* the causative agent of **whirling disease** of salmonids. The disease is most severe to trout during their first year of life. The mode of transmission is unknown. Upon gaining entrance, the parasite localizes in cartilage and starts its vegetative growth, which produces lesions. The sign of whirling is caused by damage to the cartilaginous capsule of the organ of equilibrium. The blacktail condition is caused by degradation of affected cartilage of the vertebral column posterior to the 26th vertebra where the sympathetic nerves controlling caudal pigment cells have their origin. It is probable that the weakened skeleton in this area causes pressure on the caudal nerves and pigment-cell control is lost. Since there is no effective treatment once fish become infected, control involves thorough disinfection of all hatching and fish-rearing facilities and destruction of infected fish. The use of ultraviolet irradiation on contaminated water is a promising method of control.

Henneguya, a myxosporidium of warm-water fishes, has its greatest effect on catfish culture, producing cysts within the skin and gills. It has caused mortalities of small fingerling catfish. As with *Myxosoma* and all the myxosporidia, there is no known effective treatment once fish become infected. Prevention is aided by general disinfection.

The mode of infection of fish by microsporidians is unknown. These protozoa are obligate cytozoic parasites which reproduce within individual host cells, sometimes producing cell-hypertrophy tumors called xenomas. These can range in size from several microns to nearly a centimeter, e.g., *Nosema hertwigi* in smelt and *Plistophora cepedianae* in gizzard shad. Other important fish microsporidians are *Plistophora ovariae* in ova of golden shiners, *P. salmonae* in gills of trout, *P. hyphessobryconis* in body muscle of neon tetras, *Nosema lophii* in ganglion cells of cranial and spinal nerves of various marine fish and *N. stephani* of various species of flounder.

MYCOTIC DISEASES

The most abundant and troublesome fungal diseases of fishes reared by fish culturists and tropical-fish fanciers are caused by members of the genus *Saprolegnia*. Fungi in *Achlya, Branchiomyces* and *Ichthyophonus* also may occur on, and in, fish and fish eggs.

Life cycles of many fungi are complex and unknown. The sex organs, which at times are necessary for taxonomic differentiation, are produced only on special media. Transmission of *Saprolegnia* is by the flagellated zoospores which are produced within sporangia. *Saprolegnia* are known to be primary invaders of fish and fish eggs while many other fungi are saprophytic opportunists taking advantage of necrotic tissue associated with physical injury, virus-, bacteria- and parasite-induced lesions. Treatment consists of the addition of malachite green (℞ 416) to the water.

Branchiomyces is known to invade the gills of warm-water fish in Europe, North America and other areas of the world causing necrosis of gill tissue. Control is by pond disinfection using calcium oxide (℞ 402).

Ichthyophonus is a well-known fungus causing recurring epizootics in Atlantic herring, mackerel and yellowtail flounder with a 2 to 80% infection incidence in these species. Similar infections have been found in hatchery-reared salmonids, and in tropical freshwater fish in various parts of the world. The organism causes granuloma-like lesions of the heart, brain, liver, kidney and other tissues and organs. No chemotherapy is known. Control consists of prophylaxis and not feeding contaminated raw-fish products without first freezing or heat-treating.

PARASITIC WORMS

Worm parasites are common in fish and include representatives of all the major groups. In many instances, however, they do not appear to injure the host seriously, unless exceptionally abundant. Many species of ectoparasitic flukes or monogenetic trematodes, e.g., *Gyrodactylus* and *Dactylogyrus* of fresh- and brackish-water fish, *Benedenia* and *Microcotyle* of marine fish, may multiply rapidly under favorable conditions. A few of these species are viviparous, but most lay eggs. The latter hatch into ciliated larvae (onchomiracidia) which swim about freely for a time, but must make contact with the fish host within a definite period or die. When contact with the fish is made, the parasite anchors itself to skin or gills by its posterior hooks, sheds the ciliated epidermis and begins to grow at the expense of the host. Treatment with formalin (℞ 410) is usually effective. The marine forms (*Benedenia* and *Microcotyle*) are easily dealt with by immersing the fish in fresh water for 1 to 5 minutes.

The internal flukes or digenetic trematodes have a much more complicated life history involving 2 or 3 hosts, usually a snail and often a fish-eating animal, in addition to the fish. The larval forms (cercariae) are released from the snail and become encysted in the muscle and skin where they may form yellow or black bodies, commonly called "grubs" by the fisherman. Other flukes in fish may encyst in the eyes, brain, heart, liver, kidney, spleen, gonads, mesenteries and walls of vessels. Infections of the gonads by these immature trematodes often result in parasitic castration; exceptionally heavy infections affect the proper functioning of the specific organs involved.

Tapeworms, nematodes and spiny-headed worms (*Acanthocephala*) are also common parasites of fishes; sexually mature adults are usually found in the gastrointestinal tract of fishes and fish-eating animals, while the immature worms occur in the flesh (e.g., *Diphyllobothrium latum,* the broad fish tapeworm of man) and other parts of the body. Kamala (R 220) in the diet is the treatment of choice for tapeworms of fish.

Leeches are important transmitting agents for the numerous blood parasites of fishes (e.g., *Trypanosoma, Cryptobia, Haemogregarina* and certain hemosporidia related to the *Babesia* of cattle) and since they are bloodsuckers, they may on occasion cause severe anemia.

PARASITIC COPEPODS

Copepods form another large group of parasites which may be found on, or partially in, the body and gills of freshwater and saltwater fish. All are highly specialized for a parasitic life and, in some cases, this has been carried so far that they resemble worms more than crustaceans. When abundant on the gills, they may cause serious injuries. These parasites are controlled by spraying a solution of lindane (where its use is permitted) on the surface of ponds at the rate of 1 gm for each 2,500 gal. of water.

NUTRITIONAL DISEASES

In the last decade substantial progress has been made in development of proper diets for fishes and thus eradication of many of the nutritional diseases. On the basis of research, diet formulations have been developed and used to prepare dry-pelleted diets which have replaced the practice of feeding raw fish, liver, spleen and similar foods.

Nutritional fish diseases have plagued fish culture in the past and continue to be a problem. Trout hepatoma caused severe losses in rainbow trout in Europe and the U.S.A. in the early 1960s. It was found that the disease was caused by the presence of aflatoxin, which was produced by *Aspergillus flavus* and other molds growing on improperly stored fish food. Feeding fish diets containing rancid fats have resulted in lipoid degeneration of the liver and a diabetic condition called "sekoke" in carp raised in Japan. Although diseases caused by vitamin deficiencies were greatly reduced through research into vitamin requirements of fishes, new information is constantly being found. It was thought, until recently, that fish do not require ascorbic acid. However, deficiencies of this vitamin cause scoliosis, lordosis and poor regeneration of damaged tissues. Nutritional problems in fish culture today include anemia and low plasma protein caused by improper balanced or deficient diets. To detect these conditions, microhematocrit determinations, refractometric measurement of serum protein and electrophoretic methods have been developed and standardized for hatchery-reared fish. **Visceral granuloma** of brook trout and **nephrocalcinosis** of rainbow trout are important diseases of hatchery-reared fish. Both are chronic, degenerative inflammatory diseases which affect primarily the stomach and kidney. Both conditions are diet-associated: visceral granuloma with the presence of cottonseed meal in the diet and nephrocalcinosis with impaired calcium metabolism. However, the etiology of these diseases still remains unexplained.

NOTICE.—If fish are to be used for human or animal food, treatment should be in accordance with current laws and regulations.

DIAGNOSTIC SERVICES

The addresses of several laboratories from which information may be obtained on fish disease problems are given below. Specimens may be sent for diagnosis if prior permission is obtained.

Eastern Fish Disease Laboratory, U.S. Fish and Wildlife Service, Leetown, Route No. 1, Box 17, Kearneysville, West Virginia 25430

Fish Pathology Laboratory, Michigan Department of Natural Resources, P.O. Box 507, Grayling, Michigan 49738

Fish Pathology Laboratory, N.Y. State Department of Environment Conservation, 8314 Fish Hatchery Road, Rome, N.Y. 13440

New York Aquarium, N.Y. Zoological Society, Seaside Park, Coney Island, Brooklyn, New York 11224

Western Fish Disease Laboratory, Building 204 Naval Support Activity, Seattle, Washington 98115

Western Fish Nutrition Laboratory, Cook, Washington 98605

PART V
NUTRITION

DAIRY CATTLE NUTRITION

NUTRITIONAL REQUIREMENTS

The specific dietary needs of dairy cattle are greatly modified by rumen activity. For the first 4 to 6 weeks after birth, dairy calves have dietary requirements similar to those of swine and dogs. They need high-quality, easily digested feeds to supply available energy, essential amino acids and all of the vitamins and essential minerals. Soon after a month of age, as the amount of roughage and grain consumption increases, microbiologic activity in the rumen becomes increasingly active in synthesizing essential amino acids and the B-vitamins, and in digesting cellulose. Mature dairy cattle, therefore, can thrive, largely independent of a dietary supply of essential amino acids or high-quality protein and the B-vitamins. In common with other ruminants, they utilize coarse feeds, high in cellulose, which are less useful for non-herbivores such as man.

The nutrient requirements of dairy cattle were published by the Committee on Animal Nutrition of the National Research Council in 1971. These requirements are summarized in TABLE 1. Specific requirements are shown for total feed, total and digestible protein, total digestible nutrients, digestible energy, metabolizable energy, calcium, phosphorus, carotene and vitamins A and D. Other essential nutrients are mentioned solely in the text since often their specific requirements are not known for each of the physiologic functions such as growth, reproduction and lactation.

WATER

Dairy cattle will suffer more quickly from an inadequate water intake than from deficiency of any other nutrient. Milk production will be depressed if they are not allowed all the water they wish. Water should be clean and free from contaminants at harmful levels.

Cows will consume 3 to 4 lb of water for each pound of dry matter consumed and another 3 to 4 lb/lb of milk produced. Thus, cows yielding 80 lb of milk may drink over 300 lb per day. On succulent feeds, water consumption is less. In winter, cows will drink more water if it is warmed slightly.

Calves during the latter part of the milk feeding period, heifers and bulls should also receive all the water they will drink.

ENERGY

The principal use of feed by the body is as a source of energy. All organic nutrients, e.g., protein, carbohydrates and fats, supply energy. Thus, the energy values of the organic components of a feedstuff are combined and expressed as total digestible nutrients (TDN), digestible energy (DE), metabolizable energy (ME) or net energy (NE). TDN and DE account for energy losses in the feces, ME from the feces, urine and combustible gases in the gut, and NE equals ME minus the heat increment or energy losses from the metabolism of feed nutrients. The latter 2 connotations reflect a truer value of the feedstuffs for productive purposes and more accurately compare concentrates with roughages.

Insufficient intake of energy is a more frequent cause of retarded growth, delayed puberty and depressed milk production than all other nutrient deficiencies combined. The energy requirements (TABLE 1) serve primarily as guides. Lower intakes than suggested will reduce growth rates and milk yields; larger intakes will increase growth rates and may increase milk production or fat deposition or both in lactating cows.

Under extreme experimental conditions, calves have been shown to require the essential fatty acids. Under usual feeding conditions, even when low-fat milk replacers are used, the deficiency does not occur. A specific dietary fat requirement,

TABLE 1. DAILY NUTRIENT REQUIREMENTS OF DAIRY CATTLE

Body Wt kg	Body Wt lb	Daily Gain lb	Feed[6] kg	Feed[6] lb	Protein Total gm	Protein Digestible gm	Energy DE[7] Mcal	Energy ME[7] Mcal	Energy TDN kg	Energy TDN lb	Ca gm	P gm	Carotene mg	Vitamin A 1000 IU	Vitamin D IU
Growth of Heifers for Herd Replacement															
25[1] (5)[3]	55	150	0.4[2]	0.9	90	80	1.8	1.5	0.4	0.9	1.5	1.1	2.6	1.0	165
55 (10)	121	400	1.2	2.6	180	145	4.0	3.3	0.9	2.0	4.5	3.5	5.8	2.3	360
75 (15)	165	750	2.1	4.6	330	245	6.6	5.4	1.5	3.3	9.1	7.0	7.9	3.2	495
100 (34)	220	750	2.9	6.4	370	260	8.8	7.2	2.0	4.4	10.9	8.4	11	4	660
200 (53)	441	750	5.3	11.7	500	330	15.0	12.3	3.4	7.5	18	14	21	8	1320
300 (72)	661	750	7.5	16.5	640	395	19.8	16.2	4.5	9.9	24	18	32	13	—
400 (93)	882	750	9.3	20.5	800	465	22.9	18.8	5.2	11.5	26	20	42	17	—
500 (133)	1102	600	9.5	20.9	935	505	23.4	19.2	5.3	11.7	27	21	53	21	—
600	1323	150	8.6	19.0	810	405	23.3	15.5	4.3	9.5	24	18	64	26	—
Maintenance of Mature Lactating Cows[4]															
400	882	—	5.5	12.1	521	245	13.6	11.2	3.1	6.8	17	13	42	17	—
500	1102	—	6.5	14.3	638	300	16.3	13.4	3.7	8.2	20	15	53	21	—
600	1323	—	7.5	16.5	734	345	18.9	15.5	4.2	9.3	22	17	64	26	—
700	1543	—	8.5	18.7	830	390	21.1	17.3	4.8	10.6	25	19	74	30	—
800	1764	—	9.5	20.9	915	430	23.3	19.1	5.3	11.7	27	21	85	34	—
Maintenance of Mature Breeding Bulls															
600	1323	—	9.6	21.2	735	345	23.8	19.5	5.4	11.9	22	17	64	26	—
800	1764	—	12.0	26.5	915	430	29.5	24.2	6.7	14.8	27	21	85	34	—
1000	2205	—	14.1	31.1	1075	505	34.8	28.6	7.9	17.4	32	25	106	42	—
1200	2646	—	16.1	35.5	1235	580	39.7	32.5	9.0	19.8	38	29	127	51	—

Maintenance and Pregnancy (Last 2 Months of Gestation)

400	882	—	7.2	15.9	650	355	17.2	14.1	4.0	8.8	23	18	76	30	—
500	1102	—	8.6	19.0	780	430	21.1	17.3	4.8	10.6	29	22	95	38	—
600	1323	—	10.0	22.0	910	500	24.6	20.2	5.6	12.3	34	26	114	46	—
700	1543	—	11.3	24.9	1000	555	27.7	22.7	6.3	13.9	39	30	133	53	—
800	1764	—	12.6	27.8	1150	630	31.2	25.6	7.1	15.6	44	34	152	61	—

Milk Production (Nutrients Required per kg of Milk)[5]

%Fat									
3.0	70	45	1.23	0.99	0.280	0.617	2.5	1.8
3.5	74	48	1.34	1.06	0.305	0.672	2.6	1.9
4.0	78	51	1.46	1.13	0.330	0.728	2.7	2.0
4.5	82	54	1.57	1.21	0.355	0.783	2.8	2.1
5.0	86	56	1.68	1.28	0.380	0.838	2.9	2.2

1 Small breed.
2 Based on milk replacer.
3 Large breeds (weeks of age).
4 Figures are for mature cows; to allow for growth add 20% for first-lactation and 10% for second-lactation heifers.
5 The energy requirement is presented as the actual amount required with no adjustment required for any reduction in feed value at high levels of feed intake. To account for depressions in digestibility, which occur at high planes of nutrition with certain types of rations, such as corn silage, coarse-textured grains or forages with high cell-wall content (e.g., Bermuda grass, sorghum, etc.), an increase of 3% feed should be allowed for each 20 lb of milk produced above 44 lb/day.
6 Estimates, since total amount depends upon the forage:concentrate ratio; as fed (90% dry matter) basis.
7 Assumes that 1.0 kg TDN contains 4.409 Mcal DE and that 82% of DE (except from milk) is available as ME; plus TDN ×
3.616=ME. (Adapted from Nutrient Requirements of Dairy Cattle, Fourth Revised Edition, National Research Council, 1971.)

for ruminating cattle does not appear to exist or is at least met by normal feedstuffs.

PROTEIN

The digestible-protein values in TABLE 1 represent the approximate minimum requirements. However, it is important to recognize that when high-protein feeds are cheap, they can safely be used to furnish more than the amounts recommended. The requirements are expressed as crude protein ($N \times 6.25$), although it is recognized that dairy cattle, except young calves, can also make use of nonprotein-nitrogen sources such as urea and ammonium compounds. Bacteria in the rumen are able to convert the nonprotein nitrogen into true protein, which is then digested by the host. When urea and ammonium salts are appreciably cheaper than protein-rich feeds or when protein supplements are not available, it is a good nutritional practice to use the nonprotein feeds to balance the ration of dairy cows and heifers. Urea can furnish one-fourth of the nitrogen in concentrate mixtures if care is taken to ensure that it is carefully mixed to prevent an excessive intake, which may prove toxic. Palatability may be a problem if over 1.5% of the total concentrate is urea. Since rumen bacteria need to adjust to urea, such feeds should be gradually introduced over a 3-week period. Dairy cattle thrive on protein from a single feed source. It is unnecessary to use feeds from a wide variety of sources, since protein quality is relatively unimportant for ruminating dairy cattle.

MINERALS

Dairy cattle need a dietary source of calcium, phosphorus, magnesium, sulfur, potassium, sodium, chlorine, iron, iodine, manganese, copper, cobalt, zinc, selenium and molybdenum. Of these elements, sodium and chlorine (as common salt), calcium, phosphorus, iodine, cobalt and copper are the ones that are generally known to present problems in the practical feeding of dairy cattle. In special cases the others could be of nutritional significance.

Salt (sodium chloride) is not supplied by ordinary feeds, with the possible exception of good pasture, in amounts large enough to meet the needs of dairy cattle. Allowing animals free access to salt is the most satisfactory way of meeting the requirement. Block salt licks are adequate. It is also desirable to add 1 to 1.5% of salt to concentrate mixtures for growing calves, young stock, milking cows and bulls. Milk furnishes adequate salt to young calves. Excessive salt is not harmful when adequate water is available.

Calcium and Phosphorus: Care must be taken to supply adequate amounts of calcium and phosphorus. The calcium and phosphorus contents of certain feeds and supplements are shown in TABLE 2. It will be observed that alfalfa and clover

TABLE 2. SOME GOOD SOURCES OF CALCIUM
AND PHOSPHORUS (AS FED)

Feed	Calcium %	Phosphorus %
Alfalfa hay	1.48	0.23
Clover hay	1.24	0.25
Dried skim milk	1.31	1.02
Dried whey	0.87	0.79
Wheat bran	0.14	1.17
Cottonseed meal	0.15	1.10
Distillers' solubles	0.35	1.37
Bone meal	28.98	13.59
Defluorinated rock phosphate	32.00	18.00
Dicalcium phosphate	27.00	19.07
Limestone	33.84	0.02

hays are rich in calcium but somewhat low in phosphorus. This is true for most legumes. Nonlegume forages are moderately low in calcium and phosphorus.

All concentrate feeds used for dairy cattle are relatively deficient in calcium. Wheat bran, distillers' solubles and cottonseed meal are the common feeds richest in phosphorus, but they are low in calcium. Bone meal, defluorinated phosphates and dicalcium phosphate are the most common supplements of calcium and phosphorus. Limestone (feeding grade) is the cheapest source of calcium. It is recognized that both the ratio of calcium to phosphorus and the presence of vitamin D affect calcium and phosphorus utilization. The new NRC recommendations (TABLE 1) call for calcium:phosphorus ratios of 1.3 to 1.4:1 for growth, maintenance and milk production. For growth, somewhat wider calcium:phosphorus ratios are not detrimental. A wise practice is to keep ratios under 2.5:1 for springing cows to minimize problems from milk fever. Use of mineral supplements containing only phosphorus may be advisable on high-alfalfa diets. It is a recommended practice to allow animals free access to either bone meal, dicalcium phosphate or defluorinated rock phosphate in a sheltered box. When necessary, other mineral elements may be added as well. A surer method to guarantee satisfactory intakes is to combine the supplements in the concentrate ration. This is especially true for high-producing cows.

Iodine is required by the animal for the synthesis by the thyroid gland of iodothyroglobulin and the hormone thyroxine, by which the thyroid exercises a degree of control over the basal metabolic rate and the functions of growth, reproduction and lactation. In the neonatal calf, simple goiter (q.v., p. 188) is evident when maternal intake is deficient. The iodine requirement is increased by the presence of goitrogenic substances in feeds, such as raw soybeans and some soybean products, linseed, certain clovers and cruciferous crops generally. Pasture plants vary greatly in their ability to take up iodine from the soil. The only feeds naturally rich in iodine are the saltwater fish meals and dried kelp, so that any deficiency is more readily treated with stabilized iodized salt containing 0.007% iodine (0.01% KI) or as a part of a trace-mineral mixture in the concentrate.

Since the thyroid can store iodine, the daily requirement does not have to be met each day. Excessive quantities, however, fed over short periods will give rise to signs of iodism. Iodine deficiency, which occurs on deficient soils such as around the Great Lakes and westward to the Pacific Coast, is discussed under NUTRITIONAL DEFICIENCIES IN CATTLE AND SHEEP: IODINE (q.v., p. 1321).

Cobalt is required by ruminants for the normal functioning of the ruminal microflora. When the intake of cobalt is inadequate, the bacterial population in the rumen is altered and the synthesis of vitamin B_{12} greatly lowered. The animal requires the vitamin per se.

In many areas, the forages are deficient in cobalt. Usually the legumes are richer than the grasses. Corn appears to have a low content, while linseed meal is a rich source. When the forage contains less than 0.07 ppm of cobalt (dry basis), signs of deficiency may occur in cattle. Effective supplementation of the ration of dairy cattle can be achieved by adding 2 gm of cobalt sulfate to each ton of concentrate mixture. Details of cobalt deficiency are given under NUTRITIONAL DEFICIENCIES IN CATTLE AND SHEEP: COBALT (q.v., p. 1322).

Copper is required by the animal as a constituent or activator of certain enzyme systems concerned with hemoglobin synthesis, melanin production, hair growth and the functional integrity of bone and nervous tissues. Except in very general terms, it is not possible to set a uniform copper requirement for all areas because it is markedly influenced by the level of other dietary constituents, particularly molybdenum, inorganic sulfate and phosphorus. The levels of these minerals being normal, the daily requirement of copper for dairy cattle is about 50 mg, which may be satisfied by forage that contains not less than 5 ppm (dry basis).

There are many areas in the U.S.A. where, either because of a low copper content of the herbage or the presence of complicating factors such as high molybdenum, the copper content of the ration must be supplemented to maintain normal health, growth, production and reproduction in dairy cattle (*see* NUTRITIONAL DEFICIENCIES IN CATTLE AND SHEEP: COPPER, p. 1322).

Sulfur usually is supplied by proteins as a constituent of the amino acids cystine and methionine. All plant materials also contain sulfur as inorganic sulfates. It has been shown experimentally that rumen bacteria cannot utilize urea nitrogen to synthesize protein unless the ration also contains sufficient sulfur to form the cystine and methionine. Sulfur is also essential for the bacterial synthesis of the vitamins thiamine and biotin. From a survey of the sulfur content of the common dairy feeds it appears doubtful that extra sulfur would be beneficial in dairy rations except where large amounts of urea or other nonprotein nitrogen sources are used. A ratio of nitrogen to sulfur of 10:1 is recommended. Rumen bacteria apparently are able to utilize all forms of sulfur, even the elemental yellow flowers of sulfur.

VITAMINS

Young calves up to 4 to 5 weeks of age should receive all of the known vitamins in their feed except niacin and ascorbic acid. Niacin is synthesized from dietary tryptophan and normal tissue synthesis of ascorbic acid is adequate.

As bacterial function develops in the rumen, the B-vitamins are synthesized in large amounts and need not be supplied in the diet thereafter. Milk, cereal grains and other feeds consumed by young calves contain sufficient of the B-vitamins to meet their needs before rumen synthesis begins. Thus, supplying the B-vitamins is not an important practical problem in cattle.

Vitamins A, D and E: A deficiency of any of these vitamins is relatively rare in practice, although it is known that vitamins A and D at times are deficient in the rations of dairy calves. White muscle disease (q.v., p. 578) due to a deficiency of vitamin E or selenium is uncommon in dairy cattle although not infrequent in beef cattle and sheep.

When cows are fed poor-quality, bleached roughage for long periods, they may show reproductive failure from vitamin A deficiency, or they may give milk low in vitamin A. The best assurance against vitamin A deficiency in dairy cattle is to provide abundant pasture in summer and high-quality, properly cured hay or silage in winter. When adequate good-quality forage is not available, vitamin A supplements may be desirable. Most commercial concentrates now contain at least 2,000 IU of vitamin A per pound, as a cheap insurance against a deficiency.

All natural feeds, except sun-cured hay, have a low vitamin D content. Animals that are exposed to sunlight for as little as an hour a day synthesize ample vitamin D and do not require high levels in their feed. Vitamin D deficiency may be observed in young calves which are closely confined and do not consume sun-cured roughage. Whole milk and skim milk are always low in vitamin D. Concentrate mixtures are also naturally low in the vitamin. As little as 200 IU of vitamin D per pound of calf feed is adequate. Feeding sun-cured hay *ad libitum* to young calves will prevent vitamin D deficiency. Under normal conditions, wilted legume silage furnishes ample vitamin D for dairy calves and dairy animals receive enough vitamin D from ordinary roughages and from exposure to sunlight. Feeding 20 million IU of vitamin D per cow per day starting 5 days before expected calving date and continuing through the first day post partum (maximum feeding period 7 days) has markedly reduced the incidence of milk fever in milk fever-prone cows.

Vitamin E is being added to dairy concentrates to help preserve the flavor of milk. In spite of the widespread use of vitamins A, D and E in dairy concentrates, the appearance of a frank deficiency in the field is unlikely.

Vitamin K is synthesized in the rumen in ample quantities.

FEEDING AND MANAGEMENT PRACTICES

Dairy cattle will require some concentrates until the age of 8 to 10 months, although forage will supply an increasing percentage of the ration after about 4 months. In addition, concentrates will be needed for cows in lactation and when forage quality or consumption is low.

In determining the amount and kind of concentrate mixture needed, it is essential to know what type of roughage is available; then a concentrate can be selected that will supply the amounts of additional nutrients needed at lowest cost. As an aid in formulating concentrate mixture, the nutrient requirements stated as amounts per kilogram of feed are shown in TABLE 3. NOTE: These data are for total feed, including forage and concentrates.

The approximate amounts of nutrients furnished by some of the common dairy cattle feeds are listed in TABLE 4. Hays and silages of the same species vary greatly in composition depending upon the stage of maturity at the time of cutting and the curing and preservation methods. Thus, although the precise value of a hay or silage cannot be known without a chemical analysis (or even a feeding experiment), its approximate value can be estimated from TABLE 4, and a concentrate mixture of appropriate composition can be made or purchased to balance the roughage available.

High-protein feeds, such as soybean meal, cottonseed meal, linseed meal and coconut meal usually are higher in price than the cereal grains. Therefore, it is generally good economy to use concentrate mixtures as low in protein as will supply an adequate amount of digestible protein. Simple mixtures are as effective as complex ones, although feed companies pass on significant economies by using by-product feeds in complex mixtures.

Palatability and nutrient content rather than the number of ingredients in a mixture largely determine the value of feeds for dairy cattle.

Calves should receive colostrum for at least the first 3 days and then milk at the rate of 10% of body weight during the first few weeks after birth or a milk replacer at an equivalent level. They usually can be weaned from milk at 4 to 6 weeks of age or when they are regularly consuming hay and 1 to 2 lb starter ration daily. During the first week, starter containing at least 18% protein and hay should be placed before calves. The calf should be allowed all the starter it will eat up to a maximum of 5 lb a day. Calves do not like finely ground and dusty feeds. They will readily consume coarsely cracked or rolled grains or feeds in which the "fines" are pelleted. Early-cut, green, leafy, soft-stemmed hay is the best kind for calves. They should be offered all they will eat. After 4 to 6 months of age the calf starter may be replaced with a cheaper type of grower ration or regular milk-cow ration containing 16% total protein.

Heifers and **young stock** which are well-grown will normally not need concentrates after 8 months of age if fed fine quality forage. More rapid gains or improved conditions, if desired

TABLE 3. NUTRIENT CONTENT OF RATIONS FOR DAIRY CATTLE

QUANTITY PER KILOGRAM OF DRY MATTER

Nutrients	Calf Starter Mn[1]	Heifer Grower Ration Mn	Dry Cow Ration Mn	Lactating Cow Rations Daily Milk Production[2]		Mature Bull Ration Mn
				<20 kg Mn	>30 kg Mn	
Protein, gm	160.0	100.0	85	140	160	77
Digestible, gm	120.0	62.0	51	105	123	36
Energy, Mcal						
Digestible (DE)	3.2	2.9	2.3	2.7	3.1	2.5
Metabolizable (ME)	2.6	2.4	1.9	2.1	2.5	2.0
TDN, gm	720	660	530	600	700	560
Ether extract, gm	25	20	20	20	20	20
Crude fiber, gm	(150)	150	150	130	130	150
Calcium, gm	4.1	3.4	3.4	4.3	5.3	2.4
Phosphorus, gm	3.2	2.6	2.6	3.3	3.9	1.8
Magnesium, gm	0.7	0.8	0.8	2.0	2.0	0.8
Potassium, gm	7.0	7.0	7.0	7.0	7.0	7.0
Sodium, gm	1.0	1.0	1.0	1.8	1.8	1.0
Sodium chloride, gm	2.5	2.5	2.5	4.5	4.5	2.5
Sulfur, gm	2.0	2.0	2.0	2.0	2.0	2.0
Iron, mg	100.0	100.0	100.0	100.0	100.0	100.0
Cobalt, mg	0.1 (10)	0.1 (10)	0.1 (10)	0.1 (10)	0.1 (10)	0.1 (10)
Copper, mg	10.0 (100)	10.0 (100)	10.0 (100)	10.0 (100)	10.0 (100)	10.0 (100)
Manganese, **mg**	20.0	20.0	20.0	20.0	20.0	20.0
Zinc, mg	40.0 (500)	40.0 (500)	40.0 (1000)	40.0 (1000)	40.0 (1000)	40.0 (1000)
Iodine, mg	0.1	0.1	0.6	0.6	0.6	0.1
Molybdenum, **mg**	(6)	(6)	(6)	(6)	(6)	(6)
Fluorine, **mg**	(30)	(30)	(40)	(40)	(40)	(40)
Selenium, mg	0.1 (5)	0.1 (5)	0.1 (5)	0.1 (5)	0.1 (5)	0.1 (5)

Carotene, mg	4.2	4.0	8.0	8.0	8.0	8.0
Vitamin A equiv., IU	1600	1500	3200	3200	3200	3200
Vitamin D, IU	250	250	300	300	300	300
Vitamin E, mg						

[1] Minimum suggested. (Maximum suggested.)

[2] Interpolation is adequate between 20 and 30 kg of milk production. (Adapted from *Nutrient Requirements of Dairy Cattle,* Fourth Revised Edition, 1971.)

TABLE 4. THE ESTIMATED NUTRIENT CONTENT OF SOME COMMON FEEDS FOR DAIRY AND BEEF CATTLE

Feed	Total protein	Dig. prot.	TDN	DE	Calcium	Phosphorus	Carotene
	%	%	%	Mcal/kg	%	%	mg/kg
Dried Roughages (90% Dry Matter Basis)							
Alfalfa hay							
Good (early bloom)	16.2	10.8	60	2.25	1.25	0.23	114.3
Poor (late bloom)	12.24	8.55	48	2.18	1.20	0.20	33.3
Lespedeza hay	14.13	6.39	45	1.98	1.07	0.23	43.0
Other legume hays	8.0	12.0	55	2.20	1.20	0.20	40.0
Grass hays							
Early cut	10.0	4.5	58	2.25	0.59	0.31	40.0
Late cut	7.2	3.6	48	2.20	0.40	0.20	10.0
Weathered range grass	4.0	0.2	41	1.80	0.30	0.08	—
Corn stover	5.3	2.0	53	2.3	0.44	0.08	—
Cottonseed hulls	3.9	0.2	39	1.7	0.14	0.09	—
Silages (30% Dry Matter Basis)							
Corn silage	2.5	1.5	21	0.93	0.08	0.06	3.0
Sorghum silage	1.9	0.5	17	0.77	0.11	0.06	3.0
Grass silage	3.1	1.7	18	0.77	0.12	0.06	7.7
Legume silage	5.6	3.4	16	0.70	0.42	0.10	15.0
Concentrates (90% Dry Matter Basis)[1]							
Beet pulp (dried)	9.0	4.1	65	2.86	0.68	0.10	—
Barley	11.7	8.8	75	3.29	0.08	0.42	—
Brewers grains (dried)	25.3	18.7	59	2.62	0.26	0.49	—
Citrus pulp (dried)	6.6	3.5	69	3.06	2.14	0.12	—
Corn	9.0	6.8	82	3.61	0.02	0.32	2.0
Corn gluten feed	25.3	21.8	74	3.26	0.46	0.77	7.0
Cottonseed meal	40.3	32.7	68	2.98	0.15	1.18	—
Distillers grains with solubles	26.8	21.1	79	3.49	0.09	0.36	4.0
Linseed meal	34.7	30.6	68	3.02	0.40	0.82	—
Milk, whole[2]	3.1	3.0	15	0.69	0.12	0.10	—
Milo (sorghum)	11.3	6.4	75	3.24	0.05	0.32	—
Molasses, cane[2]	3.2	1.8	68	3.00	0.89	0.08	—
Oats	11.9	8.9	68	3.02	0.10	0.35	—
Soybean meal	46.4	39.4	73	3.21	0.32	0.68	—
Wheat	12.9	10.1	79	3.49	0.05	0.37	—
Wheat bran	16.2	12.6	63	2.78	0.14	1.19	—

[1] Except for whole milk; cane molasses.
[2] As fed; milk—12% dry matter; molasses—75% dry matter.

TABLE 5. POUNDS OF CONCENTRATES TO BE FED DAILY

Daily Milk Yield	Fat Percentage of the Milk			
	3.5%		5.0%	
	Excellent Roughage	Poor Roughage	Excellent Roughage	Poor Roughage
lb	lb	lb	lb	lb
20	—	9	—	11
25	—	11	3	14
30	—	13	6	17
35	3	16	9	20
40	5	18	11	22
45	8	22	14	26
50	10	25	17	29
55	13	28	22	33
60	16	31	26	37
65	19	35	31	
70	24	38	35	
75	29			
80	33			
90				
	Feed to maximum appetite			

or needed, will result with daily feeding 2 to 3 lb of concentrates. It is advisable to feed 5 to 6 lb daily if the forage is of poor quality or scanty.

Pregnant cows and **heifers** should receive some additional feed during the last 2 months of gestation (TABLE 1). Two weeks before freshening cows may be "lead-fed" by offering concentrates in increasing amounts up to 1 lb/100 lb of body wt. During early lactation cows will respond to an increasing amount of concentrate (1.5 lb/day) to about 30 to 36 lb. This helps offset the general observation that high-producing cows cannot eat enough to satisfy their nutritional needs during early lactation. Greater intakes are possible if cows are fed concentrates more often, e.g., 3 times a day. After the peak of lactation, the concentrate level should gradually be adjusted to that needed for the amount and fat percentage of the milk produced and the quality of the forage available. Suggested daily intakes of concentrates for cows of the high- and low-testing breeds receiving good or poor roughage or pasture are shown in TABLE 5. The condition of the cow and her ability to handle concentrates without going "off feed" should also be considered in determining actual allowances. Protein levels of concentrates that will meet the requirements for different forage qualities are: nonlegume, including all corn silage, 20%; mixed legume-nonlegume 16%; all legume 12 to 14%.

BEEF CATTLE NUTRITION
NUTRITIONAL REQUIREMENTS

Beef cattle production, whether on range, improved pasture or in the feed lot, is most economical when the most effective use is made of roughages. Young growing grass or other pasture crops usually can be depended upon to supply ample nutrients needed by beef cattle, and on good-quality mixed pasture, mature cattle can consume enough such food for normal growth and maintenance. However, when pasture matures and weathers, or good pasture and other crops are harvested in such a fashion that excessive losses occur due to shattering, leaching or spoilage, the nutritive value, particularly with regard to protein, phosphorus and vitamin A content, may be so reduced that the feed is suitable only as a maintenance ration for adult cattle. Such feeds must be supplemented if they are to be used for other than maintenance.

Furthermore, the major- and trace-mineral content of pasture and forage crops may be influenced by corresponding levels in the soil. Normally, supplemental minerals are supplied in a free-choice mineral mix. Certain nutrients are required by beef cattle in the daily ration. Others can be stored in the body in rather large amounts and a deficiency is improbable over short periods. When body stores are high (vitamin A, for example), dietary supplementation is not necessary until these stores become reduced.

The daily nutrient requirements for various classes of beef cattle, according to the Committee on Animal Nutrition of the National Research Council, 1970, are shown in TABLE 6 (p. 1204).

The following dietary constituents are required for successful growth, fattening and reproduction in beef cattle:

WATER

Beef cattle must have an abundant supply of good water at least once daily. Range cows consume a minimum of 2.5 gal. of water in winter and up to 12 gal. per head in summer. When salt is fed with a protein concentrate to control the protein intake, more water is needed to aid in excreting the excess salt. Breeding cows, yearlings, and 2-year-old steers need about 10 gal. of water daily and fattening calves will drink 6 to 8 gal. With fresh, succulent feeds, less water is required.

ENERGY

Beef cattle, with the exception of young calves, can meet their energy requirements for maintenance from roughage, provided they have the capacity to handle such feed and it is sufficiently palatable. A shortage of energy occurs on overstocked pastures, with inadequate feed allowance or during a drought. For performance above the maintenance level, additional energy from concentrates is necessary.

For maintenance, especially in cold weather, roughages of varying quality may have similar energy values. The heat released during the digestion and assimilation of feeds contributes to the maintenance of body temperature for wintering stock cattle where little productive energy is required. For fattening, reproduction and lactation, however, much productive energy is needed, thus the necessity of good-quality feeds.

The energy requirement for wintering of mature beef cattle ranges from 130 to 180 Kcal digestible energy per 100 lb of body wt. For growing calves, lactating cows, or fattening cattle, the requirement is much greater.

PROTEIN

Since protein quality is relatively unimportant, except in young animals, beef cattle can thrive on protein from a single feed source. Nevertheless, a certain amount of digestible protein in the daily ration is essential and, except for an overall scarcity of feed, a shortage of this constituent is the most common factor limiting growth, weight gains and reproductive performance. Protein deficiencies of long duration eventually will lead to a depression of appetite with consequent weight loss and unthriftiness even though ample energy is available.

Feeds vary greatly in the digestibility of their protein fraction. For example, the protein of common grains and most protein supplements is about 75 to 85% digestible, that of alfafa hay about 70%, while that of the grass hays usually varies from 35 to 50%. The protein of feeds such as weathered grass hay and cottonseed hulls is very poorly digested. Thus, total protein intake may be "adequate" but digestible protein insufficient to meet the animal's needs.

Lack of protein in the ration also affects adversely the bacterial population in the rumen and this, in turn, reduces the digestibility of low-protein feeds. Much of the potential nutritive value in roughages may, therefore, be lost if protein levels are not adequate. There is very little storage of protein in the body and thus it must be present in the daily ration for best results.

Digestible-protein requirements vary with body weight, growth, fattening and reproduction. Growing beef calves require about as much digestible protein as mature, nonpregnant beef cows. Steers on a full feed of grain, making maximal gains, have a much higher requirement than cattle of the

TABLE 6. NUTRIENT REQUIREMENTS OF GROWING AND FINISHING BEEF CATTLE[1]
(Nutrient Concentration in Ration Dry Matter)

Body Wt	Daily Gain	Daily Dry Matter[2]	Total Protein	Digest. Protein	Energy			Ca	P	Vitamin A
					ME[3]	TDN[4]				
lb	lb	lb	%	%	(Mcal/lb)	%		%	%	IU/lb
Finishing Steer Calves										
330	2.0	7.7	12.8	8.6	1.28	78		0.60	0.43	1000
660	2.4	15.7	12.2	8.1	1.21	74		0.37	0.27	1000
990	2.3	20.7	11.1	7.1	1.21	74		0.22	0.22	1000
Finishing Yearling Steers										
550	2.9	15.9	11.1	7.1	1.18	72		0.40	0.28	1000
660	2.9	18.3	11.1	7.1	1.18	72		0.35	0.25	1000
880	2.9	22.7	11.1	7.1	1.18	72		0.27	0.22	1000
1100	2.7	25.4	11.1	7.1	1.18	72		0.23	0.22	1000
Finishing 2-Year-Old Steers										
770	3.1	22.7	11.1	7.1	1.16	71		0.29	0.22	1000
880	3.1	24.9	11.1	7.1	1.16	71		0.27	0.22	1000
1100	3.1	29.5	11.1	7.1	1.16	71		0.22	0.22	1000
1200	2.9	30.2	11.1	7.1	1.16	71		0.22	0.22	1000
Finishing Heifer Calves										
330	1.8	7.7	12.8	8.6	1.29	78		0.51	0.37	1000
660	2.2	16.1	12.2	8.1	1.21	74		0.31	0.25	1000
880	2.1	19.2	11.1	7.1	1.21	74		0.26	0.22	1000

Finishing Yearling Heifers

550	2.6	16.8	11.1	7.1	1.18	72	0.36	0.26	1000
660	2.6	19.0	11.1	7.1	1.18	72	0.31	0.23	1000
880	2.6	23.6	11.1	7.1	1.18	72	0.28	0.22	1000
990	2.4	24.3	11.1	7.1	1.18	72	0.22	0.22	1000

Growing Steers

330	1.1	7.1	12.2	8.1	1.18	72	0.38	0.31	1000
440	1.6	7.1	13.3	9.0	1.29	78	0.53	0.41	1000
	1.6	10.8	11.1	7.1	1.04	63	0.27	0.20	1000
660	1.6	11.0	10.0	7.1	1.14	69	0.36	0.28	1000
	1.6	17.6	11.0	6.1	0.94	57	0.21	0.18	1000
880	1.1	21.4	8.9	5.2	1.04	63	0.18	0.18	1000
	1.6	21.8	8.9	5.2	1.04	63	0.18	0.18	1000

Growing Heifers

330	1.1	7.1	12.2	8.1	1.19	72	0.38	0.31	1000
440	1.6	7.3	13.3	9.0	1.28	78	0.52	0.39	1000
	1.1	11.0	11.1	7.1	1.04	63	0.26	0.20	1000
660	1.6	11.9	10.0	7.1	1.14	69	0.33	0.26	1000
	1.1	18.1	11.0	6.1	0.94	57	0.18	0.18	1000
880	1.6	22.5	8.9	5.2	1.04	63	0.20	0.18	1000
	1.6	23.4	8.9	5.2	1.04	63	0.18	0.18	1000

Dry Mature Pregnant Cows

990	—	15.0	5.9	2.8	0.82	50	0.16	0.16	1000
1100	—	16.8	5.9	2.8	0.82	50	0.16	0.16	1000
1210	—	17.6	5.9	2.8	0.82	50	0.16	0.16	1000

(continued on next page)

TABLE 6. (Continued)

Body Wt	Daily Gain	Daily Dry Matter²	Total Protein	Digest. Protein	Energy		Ca	P	Vitamin A
					ME³	TDN⁴			
lb	lb	lb	%	%	(Mcal/lb)	%	%	%	IU/lb
Cows Nursing Calves (First 3 to 4 months)									
880	—	20.5	9.2	5.4	0.91	57	0.28	0.23	1800
990	—	21.8	9.2	5.4	0.91	57	0.28	0.22	1800
1100	—	23.1	9.2	5.4	0.91	57	0.27	0.22	1800
Bulls, Growth & Maintenance (moderate activity)									
600	2.2	19.2	13.9	9.6	1.00	65	0.26	0.21	1800
880	0.9	22.0	13.3	9.0	1.00	65	0.19	0.18	1800
1100	0.7	26.5	13.3	9.0	1.00	60	0.18	0.18	1800
1320	0.5	25.6	12.2	8.1	1.00	60	0.18	0.18	1800
1540	0.3	28.0	11.1	7.1	0.91	57	0.18	0.18	1800

1 A modification of Table 2, National Academy of Sciences Publication 1137, Nutrient Requirements of Beef Cattle, 1970.
2 Feed intake was calculated from the net energy requirements and average net energy values for the kind of ration fed.
3 Metabolizable energy (ME) requirements for growing and finishing cattle were calculated from the net energy for maintenance and net energy for gain requirements for weights and rates of gain.
4 TDN was calculated from ME by assuming 3.1655 Kcal of ME per gram of TDN.

same age and weight that are making only moderate gains. The digestible-protein requirement for maintenance in beef cattle is about 0.6 lb/1,000 lb of body wt daily, and for rapid growth and fattening, it is nearly double this amount. Cows nursing calves need about 70% more digestible protein than dry cows.

Urea is commonly used in commercial protein supplements to supply one-third or more of the total nitrogen. It is well utilized at this level, provided the ration has ample phosphorus, trace minerals, sulfur and soluble carbohydrate (starches and sugars). The amount of crude protein ($N \times 6.25$) supplied by nonprotein nitrogen must be stated on the feed tag. Toxicity is not a serious problem where urea is fed at the recommended levels and thoroughly mixed with the feed. The rapid ingestion of urea at levels above 20 gm/100 lb body wt may, however, lead to toxic effects. Several urea-molasses mixtures, which may contain nearly 10% urea, are now being sold as feed supplements for beef cattle. Caution should be exercised when cattle are started on these supplements. Biuret may also be used as a nonprotein-nitrogen source.

MINERALS

Qualitatively, the mineral requirements of beef cattle are essentially the same as those of dairy cattle; quantitatively, however, they generally are much lower than for high-producing dairy cows. In practice, the minerals most likely to be deficient in beef cattle rations are sodium and chlorine (as salt), calcium and phosphorus. (*See* NUTRITIONAL DEFICIENCIES IN CATTLE AND SHEEP, p. 1317.) Natural feeds usually contain adequate amounts of the other required mineral elements, i.e., potassium, magnesium, sulfur, iodine, iron, copper, cobalt, manganese, selenium and, probably, zinc. Under certain circumstances, however, feedstuffs may not provide adequate amounts of some essential minerals and it becomes necessary to supplement the diet. The actual method used is determined very largely by the type of husbandry. Under intensive systems of stocking, calcium, phosphorus, potassium and magnesium are best applied as fertilizer to the pasture, since, in addition to supplying the necessary minerals to the animal, this practice may well increase the total yield of forage. Copper and cobalt also may be added to the fertilizer mixture. Perhaps the most economical and widely used methods of supplementation in the U.S.A. are to add a calcium and phosphorus source to trace mineral salt, preferably in the loose form, or to purchase a commercial mineral supplement.

The salt (NaCl) requirements of beef cattle are unknown.

Beef calves wintered on dry roughage and a small amount of protein supplement made slower and more expensive gains than others receiving salt. In contrast, fattening calves full-fed grain gained as rapidly and efficiently with no salt as others fed salt. Similar comparisons have not been made in the U.S.A. with grazing cattle, but, when salt is provided free-choice, cattle on pasture consume more salt than those in dry lot.

Range cattle usually consume 2.0 to 2.5 lb of salt per head per month when the feed is succulent and 1.0 to 1.5 lb per month with dryer feed. When salt is added to protein feeds to limit the protein intake, beef cows often obtain more than 1.0 lb a day over long periods without injury, if they have plenty of water.

In Australia and New Zealand, cattle grazing on good pasture are rarely fed salt and there is some question whether the amounts provided in the U.S.A. are really necessary. Salt is usually fed free-choice, but the salt requirements of finishing cattle fed high-grain rations can be met by 0.5% salt in the total ration.

Calcium is relatively high in most roughages, but low in cereal hays, corn silage, and sorghum grains and other concentrates. Legume hay is a richer source of calcium than grass hay or straw, but even nonlegume roughages will often supply the amount necessary for maintenance. When the roughage is produced on soil exceptionally low in calcium, or when cattle are full-fed grain with only a limited amount of nonlegume hay, corn or sorghum silage, a calcium deficiency may arise. Calves may not obtain enough from their ration to make normal growth. Since the beef cow produces less milk than the dairy cow and usually is consuming more roughage, a deficiency of calcium is unlikely. However, it is good husbandry to supply a free-choice mineral mix at all times. This may consist of two-thirds dicalcium phosphate and one-third iodized or trace mineral salt. In addition, iodized or trace-mineralized salt should be supplied free choice. A commercial mineral supplement can also be used in the total ration. A calcium: phosphorus ratio of about 2:1 in the total ration is thought to be most desirable, although it appears that wider ratios can be tolerated if the minimum requirement for each element is met and adequate vitamin D is available.

Phosphorus is much more apt to be deficient in ordinary beef cattle rations, since it is often low in roughages. Many soils in the beef-producing areas of the world are low in available phosphorus. Further, when weathered native range grass is the only roughage, or when such feeds as cottonseed hulls, stover or cobs are fed, the phosphorus level may drop precariously low. When the phosphorus content of forages drops below 0.16%, maximum performance is not attained. For best digestibility of feeds, the minimal phosphorus level in the rations should be approximately 0.2%. Most protein feeds are relatively good sources of phosphorus; therefore, when such feeds are given in amounts necessary to supplement poor-quality roughage, adequate phosphorus intake is assured. However, a mineral mix offered free-choice is recommended. Steamed bone meal, dicalcium phosphate, defluorinated rock phosphate, monosodium phosphate, sodium tripolyphosphate and ammonium polyphosphate are good sources of phosphorus. Since most grains are good sources of phosphorus, fattening cattle usually obtain their requirement from the grain. A phosphorus intake of 2 to 3 gm/100 lb body wt is considered ample for fattening cattle.

A specific deficiency of **cobalt** in beef cattle usually arises from a low level in the forage as a consequence of a regional soil deficiency. Such soils are known in many parts of the world. With some of the other minerals, e.g., **iodine and copper**, and possibly **zinc** and **selenium**, the explanation is not so clear. There may be a simple deficiency in the soil and, therefore, in the plant. Further, the level in the food may be reasonably high, but the animal unable to utilize the particular element because of the presence, in unusual amounts, of other substances in the diet. Therefore, induced deficiencies develop, which fortunately can be overcome by suitable supplements. These conditions are described under NUTRITIONAL DEFICIENCIES IN CATTLE AND SHEEP, p. 1317.

VITAMINS

While cattle probably require all the known vitamins, a dietary source of vitamin B complex and vitamins C and K is not necessary, because, in all but the very young animal, the vitamin B complex and vitamin K are synthesized in the required amounts by the ruminal microflora, and vitamin C is synthesized in the tissues of all cattle. If, however, rumen function is impaired or the bacterial population is inhibited by starvation, shortage of protein, cobalt deficiency or excessive levels of antibiotics or medicaments, synthesis of these vitamins may not occur at a normal rate.

Vitamin A: Since most beef cattle are produced in range and semiarid regions and are fattened on large amounts of grain and limited quantities of roughage, a shortage of vitamin A is always a potential danger. Many stock cattle and pregnant cows are wintered on low-quality roughages low in carotene.

With the exception of newly harvested yellow corn, grain and other concentrates are almost devoid of vitamin A precursors. Since cattle on green pastures have the ability to store large quantities of vitamin A and carotene in their bodies the length of time elapsing before a deficiency becomes apparent varies considerably. Thus, depending on the amount of green feed obtained during the previous grazing season, weaned calves may have sufficient liver stores to last 80 to 140 days on low-carotene rations before showing evidence of deficiency yearling cattle about 100 to 150 days and mature cattle about 6 to 8 months. Newborn calves have very small liver stores of vitamin A and, therefore, must depend on colostrum and milk to meet their needs. These sources may not be sufficient if the dam is fed a ration low in carotene during gestation and while nursing the calf. Therefore, severe signs may become apparent in the young suckling calf within 2 to 4 weeks of birth while the dam appears normal.

It is sound practice to supply from 2 to 5 lb of good legume hay, or 0.5 to 1.0 lb of dehydrated alfalfa meal, in the daily ration of stocker cattle and pregnant cows as assurance against a vitamin A deficiency. Many commercial protein and mineral supplements may be economically fortified with dry, stabilized vitamin A. When certain trace minerals are added, vitamin A must be protected against destruction. Access to green pasture, even for short periods, is the ideal method of alleviating a deficiency. The daily requirement for beef cattle appears to be approximately 5 mg of carotene or 2,000 IU of vitamin A per 100 lb body wt. Lactating cows may require considerably more than this in order to maintain high vitamin A levels in the milk.

Vitamin A deficiency under feed lot conditions has caused considerable loss to cattle feeders, especially where high-concentrate and corn silage rations have been fed. Destruction of carotene during storage or in the digestive tract, or the failure to convert carotene to vitamin A may all be involved in increasing the vitamin A requirement of these cattle. Growing and finishing steers and heifers fed these rations for several months will require 1,000 IU of vitamin A per pound of air dry ration. Commercial vitamin A supplements are not expensive and should be used when such rations are fed and any danger of a deficiency exists.

Vitamin D deficiency is comparatively rare in beef cattle since they usually are outside in direct sunlight and fed sun cured roughage. In northern latitudes, during long winters, or in purebred herds where show calves are kept in the barn or turned out only at night, a vitamin D deficiency is possible

Direct exposure to sunlight, feeding sun-cured roughage or supplementary vitamin D, 300 IU/100 lb of body wt, are considered adequate to protect against a deficiency.

The interrelationships of vitamin E and selenium in reproduction and in the etiology of various myopathies of calves are discussed under MYOPATHIES AND RELATED CONDITIONS IN DOMESTIC ANIMALS (p. 575).

FEEDING AND MANAGEMENT PRACTICES

Feeds for beef cattle vary widely in quality, palatability and essential nutrient content. The composition of some common feeds for beef cattle is shown in TABLE 4 (p. 1200). To be most effective, any supplement must be patterned to fit the kind and quality of roughage available. Under certain systems of management, beef cattle are wintered as economically as possible on low-quality roughages and thus may not receive the recommended nutrient requirements for optimum performance. This may not be undesirable if no severe deficiency develops and the cattle can make up for poor winter gains on abundant summer pasture. However, where maximum performance is desired (cows nursing calves, rapid growth of calves, steers on full feed), an attempt should be made to meet or exceed the nutrient requirements as shown in TABLE 6 (p. 1204).

Feeding and management practices for the 3 systems of beef production are discussed separately.

THE BREEDING HERD

In most areas, a spring calving program is followed (February to May) depending on the available feed, growth of early spring pasture and prevailing climate. Fall calving is on the increase, particularly in the South, and wintering the lactating cow presents a much greater nutritional problem than wintering pregnant cows. Beef cattle are commonly weaned at 6 to 8 months of age; their dams are bred again while on summer pasture. Heifers may be bred to drop their first calves as 2-year-olds (24 to 27 months of age) if good winter feeding is practiced to assure maximum development and prevent high death losses at parturition. Heifers should weigh at least 600 to 650 lb at breeding time and should be fed well thereafter to allow for continued growth, good milk production and early conception.

Older cows have greater body reserves and less critical requirements than heifers; therefore, they can be wintered on poorer rations. They usually are fed all the hay, fodder, silage or dry grass they will consume. This roughage ration should provide a minimum of 5.9% total protein. If it does not, then

1.0 to 2.0 lb of 20 to 30% protein supplement or its equivalent should be fed daily. A mineral mix should be provided.

Mature beef cows may lose 150 lb or more of body weight from fall to spring. This weight loss does not impair reproductive performance if spring and summer pastures are adequate. Under most profitable systems of management, a cow will maintain her weight from fall to fall. Lactation is a much more severe strain than gestation. Feeding beef cows more than is necessary for satisfactory production, such as frequently occurs in purebred herds, is unnecessary. Large accumulations of body fat may lead to difficulty in conception and at calving, a lower calf crop and a shorter life span.

Beef calves are castrated and dehorned before 3 months of age. At this time, they may be vaccinated for blackleg and malignant edema. Spaying heifers depresses gain and is seldom profitable. Often, a system of "creep-feeding" is practiced whereby suckling calves are allowed access to grain mixture in an enclosure or feeder. A typical creep-feed mixture contains 6 parts of corn, 3 parts of oats and 1 part of protein supplement. The mixture should preferably be ground as coarse as possible.

Most beef cows are pasture-bred, and in the better herds the bulls remain with the cows for a 2-month period. Bulls for pasture mating should be at least 15 months of age and well developed. Not more than 12 to 15 females should be mated to a yearling bull, while mature bulls can safely settle 30 to 35 cows. Where pastures are large, or the terrain is rough and mountainous, 1 bull per 15 to 20 cows may be necessary. Growing bull calves and yearlings should receive about 2 lb of protein supplement, 3 to 5 lb of grain and good-quality roughage. Mature bulls are commonly wintered in the same manner as the cow herd, with a greater feed allowance during the late winter. Highly fitted show bulls may have to be "let down" by gradual reduction in the ration and much exercise before they are suitable for pasture mating.

STOCKER CATTLE

It is common practice to winter calves or yearlings to make moderate gains, with faster and cheaper gains on summer pasture. Such cattle may be sold as feeders or fattened out in dry lot the following fall. The cost of winter gain on harvested feeds is invariably higher than summer gain on grass; hence, it is advisable to winter cattle so as to make the greatest possible gain on grass. In order to maintain good health, weanling calves should gain at least 1 lb per day. Two pounds of grain plus 1 to 2 lb of protein supplement are recom-

mended, in addition to nonlegume roughage. If legume roughage is fed, no protein supplement will be needed. Other cattle,
particularly if they enter the winter in fleshy condition, may
do well to maintain their fall weight. A free-choice mineral
mix and trace-mineralized salt should be supplied. Limited
amounts of grain fed to older cattle on pasture during the late
summer may increase their market value.

FATTENING CATTLE

This phase of beef production consists of full feeding grain
and limited amounts of roughage until slaughter condition is
attained. Older cattle may fatten on pasture alone, or with a
few pounds of grain to improve market grade. Weanling calves
are commonly shipped direct to the feed lot and commonly
on a warm-up program for 120 to 150 days followed by finishing ration for 100 to 150 days; yearlings require about 150
days and older steers from 100 to 125 days. Grain consumption
of cattle on full feed is approximately 2.0 to 2.5 lb/100 lb of
body wt. Roughage consumption usually is limited to about
one-fourth to one-third of the total grain intake after cattle are
on full feed. Cattle self-fed mixed rations will consume about
3% of their body weight daily. For calves, about 1.5 to 2.0
lb of 30 to 35% protein supplement are required daily for best
gains and market grades where nonlegume roughage is fed.

The grain allowance for fattening cattle should be increased
gradually. Feeding too much grain early in the period may
lead to lactic acidosis, founder, severe scouring and cattle that
go "off feed". About 4 to 6 weeks are required to get calves
on a full feed of grain, while a shorter time is necessary for
older cattle. Self-fed, mixed rations should contain at least
50% roughage as cattle are started on feed.

Corn or sorghum silage is a very palatable roughage for fattening cattle, and plain cattle of lower grade may be fattened
principally on silage supplemented with protein. Alfalfa or
grass silage is relatively high in protein, carotene and minerals,
but is somewhat lacking in available energy. This is especially
true when no grain or molasses is added as a preservative.
Alfalfa hay is an excellent roughage, but may cause bloat in
calves if fed as the only roughage. Grains for fattening cattle
have about the same relative value as is indicated by their
TDN content. Soybean and linseed meals, or protein mixtures
containing them, are equal or slightly superior to cottonseed
meals for fattening cattle. Commercial protein supplements
can also be fed. They are also fortified with minerals, vitamins and feed additives. A small amount of molasses (1 lb
per head daily) may improve rations containing low-quality

roughages, such as corn cobs, weathered hays or cottonseed hulls.

A number of nonfeed hormone or hormone-like supplements are used to increase gains in fattening cattle, either as feed supplements or as injectable implants. The use of these, e.g., diethylstilbestrol, and of certain of the antibiotics, commonly result in appreciable improvement in rates of gain and feed efficiency, but the uncertainty of official regulations governing their use preclude the inclusion of specific recommendations here. Strict compliance with the manufacturer's use directions is the safest course.

The use of tranquilizers to reduce stress and weight loss during weaning or shipment has not proved consistently beneficial. Various means of processing rations, such as pelleting, flaking and high-moisture ensiling, have been shown to be beneficial, at least in some situations.

CONDITIONING FEEDER CATTLE AFTER SHIPMENT

Research results from university experiment stations have confirmed the value of therapeutic oral dosages of a combination of chlortetracycline (CTC) and sulfamethazine (SMZ) for feeder cattle from 14 to 21 days immediately following shipment. Both drugs, when fed in combination at a daily dose of 350 mg each for this period, will lower significantly the incidence of the shipping fever syndrome and also will result in more rapid regain of shrinkage suffered during shipping. Size of the animal as related to levels of CTC and SMZ is not critical. Some animals may not respond to this treatment and should be isolated for individual attention. The nutritional program which is recommended for such cattle is a full feed of medium-quality roughage plus 1 to 2 lb per head daily of a 32% protein supplement which derives at least two-thirds of its protein from natural sources. The prescribed daily dose of CTC and SMZ for one animal may thus be incorporated into each 1 to 2 lb of the protein supplement.

SHEEP NUTRITION

The economical and efficient production of lamb and wool is contingent on maximum production per unit of feed. Economical maintenance of breeding animals, a high percentage lamb crop weaned, continuous and rapid growth of lambs, heavy weaning weights and a heavy fleece weight are important to efficiency; all are based largely on adequate nutrition.

Definition of the nutritional requirements for maintenance,

reproduction, growth, finishing and wool production of sheep is complicated because sheep are maintained under a wide variety of environmental conditions. Not only do farm and feed lot conditions differ markedly from those in range areas, but there is also considerable variation from farm to farm and from ranch to ranch.

NUTRITIONAL REQUIREMENTS

An adequate diet for sheep should include water, feeds containing energy (carbohydrates and fats), proteins, minerals and vitamins.

TABLE 7 contains the daily nutrient requirements suggested by the National Research Council, 1972. These amounts are sufficient to promote optimum growth and production. They are designed to meet the needs of individuals within a group that have higher than average requirements and, to this extent, should provide a margin of safety for animals whose requirements are average or below. There may be occasions, under field conditions of particular stress, when additional nutrients should be provided.

WATER

The usual recommendations are approximately 1 gal. of water per day for ewes on dry feed in winter, 1½ gal. per day for ewes nursing lambs and approximately ½ gal. per day for fattening lambs.

In many range areas, water is the limiting nutrient and even when present may be unpotable because of dirt, filth or high mineral content. For best production, range sheep should be watered once a day during warm weather. However, the cost of supplying water sometimes makes it advisable to water range sheep every other day. When soft snow is available, range sheep do not need additional water. If the snow is crusted with ice, the crust should be broken to allow access to the supply. When dry feeds, such as alfalfa hay and pellets are fed, sheep may not obtain sufficient water from snow.

ENERGY (TDN)

The provision of adequate energy is perhaps the most important problem in sheep nutrition. This is because so much of the diet depends on grass and forage which is either sparse or of poor quality. Poor forage, even in abundance, may not provide sufficient digestible energy.

TABLE 7 shows that the energy requirement of the ewe is greatest during the first 8 to 10 weeks of lactation. Since milk production declines after this period and the lambs are for-

TABLE 7. DAILY NUTRIENT REQUIREMENTS OF SHEEP (MOISTURE-FREE BASIS)

Body Wt (kg)	Body Wt (lb)	Wt Gain or Loss (gm)	Wt Gain or Loss (lb)	Dry Matter Per Animal (kg)	Dry Matter Per Animal (lb)	Dry Matter Percent Live Wt	Energy TDN (kg)	Energy DE² (Mcal)	Energy ME (Mcal)	Total Protein (gm)	DP³ (gm)	gm DP per Mcal DE (gm)	Ca (gm)	P (gm)	Carotene (mg)	Vit A (IU)	Vit D (IU)
EWES⁴—Maintenance																	
50	110	10	0.02	1.0	2.2	2.0	0.55	2.42	1.98	89	48	19.8	3.0	2.8	1.2	850	278
60	132	10	0.02	1.1	2.4	1.8	0.61	2.68	2.20	98	53	19.8	3.1	2.9	1.5	1020	333
70	154	10	0.02	1.2	2.6	1.7	0.66	2.90	2.38	107	58	20.0	3.2	3.0	1.8	1190	388
80	176	10	0.02	1.3	2.9	1.6	0.72	3.17	2.60	116	63	19.9	3.3	3.1	2.0	1360	444
Nonlactating: first 15 weeks gestation																	
50	110	30	0.07	1.1	2.4	2.2	0.60	2.64	2.16	99	54	20.5	3.0	2.8	1.9	1275	278
60	132	30	0.07	1.3	2.9	2.1	0.72	3.17	2.60	117	64	20.2	3.1	2.9	2.2	1530	333
70	154	30	0.07	1.4	3.1	2.0	0.77	3.39	2.78	126	69	20.3	3.2	3.0	2.6	1785	388
80	176	30	0.07	1.5	3.3	1.9	0.82	3.61	2.96	135	74	20.5	3.3	3.1	3.0	2040	444
Last 6 weeks gestation or last 8 weeks lactation suckling singles⁵																	
50	110	175(+45)	0.39	1.7	3.7	3.3	0.99	4.36	3.58	158	88	20.2	4.1	3.9	6.2	4250	278
60	132	180(+45)	0.40	1.9	4.2	3.2	1.10	4.84	3.97	177	99	20.5	4.4	4.1	7.5	5100	333
70	154	185(+45)	0.41	2.1	4.6	3.0	1.22	5.37	4.40	195	109	20.3	4.5	4.3	8.8	5950	383
80	176	190(+45)	0.42	2.2	4.8	2.8	1.28	5.63	4.62	205	114	20.3	4.8	4.5	10.0	6800	444
90	198	195(+45)	0.43	2.3	5.1	2.6	1.33	5.85	4.80	214	120	20.5	5.0	4.7	11.2	7650	500

First 8 weeks lactation suckling singles or last 8 weeks lactation suckling twins[5]

50	110	−25(+80)	−0.06	2.1	4.6	4.2	1.36	5.98	4.90	218	180	21.7	10.9	7.8	6.2	4250	278
60	132	−25(+80)	−0.06	2.3	5.1	3.9	1.50	6.60	5.41	239	143	21.7	11.5	8.2	7.5	5100	333
70	154	−25(+80)	−0.06	2.5	5.5	3.6	1.63	7.17	5.88	260	155	21.6	12.0	8.6	8.8	5950	388
80	176	−25(+80)	−0.06	2.6	5.7	3.2	1.69	7.44	6.10	270	161	21.6	12.6	9.0	10.0	6800	444

First 8 weeks lactation suckling twins

50	110	−60	−0.13	2.4	5.3	4.8	1.56	6.86	5.63	276	173	25.2	10.9	7.8	6.2	4250	278
60	132	−60	−0.13	2.6	5.7	4.3	1.69	7.44	6.10	299	187	25.1	11.5	8.2	7.5	5100	333
70	154	−60	−0.13	2.8	6.2	4.0	1.82	8.01	6.57	322	202	25.2	12.0	8.6	8.8	5950	388
80	176	−60	−0.13	3.0	6.6	3.7	1.95	8.58	7.04	345	216	25.2	12.6	9.0	10.0	6800	444

Replacement lambs and yearlings[7]

30	66	180	0.40	1.3	2.9	4.3	0.81	3.46	2.91	130	75	21.7	5.9	3.3	1.9	1275	166
40	88	120	0.26	1.4	3.1	3.5	0.84	3.58	3.03	133	74	20.6	6.1	3.4	2.5	1700	222
50	110	80	0.18	1.5	3.3	3.0	0.83	3.69	2.97	133	73	19.9	6.3	3.5	3.1	2125	278
60	132	40	0.09	1.5	3.3	2.5	0.83	3.61	2.97	133	72	19.9	6.5	3.6	3.8	2550	333
70	154	10	0.02	1.4	3.1	2.0	0.78	3.52	2.78	129	70	19.9	6.5	3.6	4.4	2970	388

RAMS—Replacement lambs and yearlings[7]

50	88	250	0.55	1.8	4.0	4.5	1.17	5.15	4.22	184	108	21.0	6.3	3.5	2.5	1700	222
60	132	200	0.44	2.3	5.1	3.8	1.38	6.07	4.98	219	122	20.1	7.2	3.8	3.8	2550	333
80	176	150	0.33	2.8	6.2	3.5	1.54	6.78	5.56	249	134	19.8	7.9	4.4	5.0	3400	444
100	220	100	0.22	2.8	6.2	2.8	1.54	6.78	5.56	249	134	19.8	8.3	4.6	6.2	4250	555
120	265	50	0.11	2.6	5.7	2.2	1.43	6.29	5.16	231	125	19.8	8.5	4.7	7.5	5100	666

(continued on next page)

TABLE 7 (Continued)

Body Wt		Wt Gain or Loss		Dry Matter[1]			Energy			Nutrients per Animal							
				Per Animal		Percent Live Wt	TDN	DE[2]	ME	Total Protein	DP[3]	gm DP per Mcal DE	Ca	P	Carotene	Vit A	Vit D
(kg)	(lb)	(gm)	(lb)	(kg)	(lb)		(kg)	(Mcal)	(Mcal)	(gm)	(gm)		(gm)	(gm)	(mg)	(IU)	(IU)
							LAMBS—Fattening[8]										
30	66	200	0.44	1.3	2.9	4.3	0.83	3.65	2.99	143	87	23.8	4.8	3.0	1.1	765	166
35	77	220	0.48	1.4	3.1	4.0	0.94	4.14	3.39	154	94	22.7	4.8	3.0	1.3	892	194
40	88	250	0.55	1.6	3.5	4.0	1.12	4.92	4.03	176	107	21.8	5.0	3.1	1.5	1020	222
45	99	250	0.55	1.7	3.7	3.8	1.19	5.24	4.30	187	114	21.8	5.0	3.1	1.7	1148	250
50	110	220	0.48	1.8	4.0	3.6	1.26	5.54	4.54	198	121	21.8	5.0	3.1	1.9	1275	278
55	121	200	0.44	1.9	4.2	3.5	1.33	5.85	4.80	209	127	21.7	5.0	3.1	2.1	1402	305
							Early—Weaned[9]										
10	22	250	0.55	0.6	1.3	6.0	0.44	1.92	1.58	96	69	35.9	2.8	1.7	1.2	850	67
20	44	275	0.60	1.0	2.2	5.0	0.74	3.21	2.63	160	115	35.8	5.0	3.0	2.5	1700	133
30	66	300	0.66	1.4	3.1	4.7	1.02	4.49	3.68	196	133	29.6	7.2	4.3	3.8	2550	200

[1] To convert dry matter to an as-fed feed basis, divide dry matter by percentage dry matter.

[2] 1 kg TDN = 4.4 Mcal DE (digestible energy). DE may be converted to ME (metabolizable energy) by multiplying by 82%.

[3] DP = digestible protein.

[4] Values are for ewes in moderate condition, not excessively fat or thin. For fat ewes feed at next lower weight; for thin ewes feed at next highest weight.

[5] Values in parentheses for ewes suckling singles last 8 weeks of lactation.

[6] Values in parentheses for ewes suckling twins last 8 weeks of lactation.

[7] Replacement lambs (ewe & ram) requirements start at time they are weaned.

[8] Maximum gains expected—if lambs are held for later market, they should be fed similar to replacement ewe lambs. Lambs capable of gaining faster than indicated need to be fed at higher level; self-feeding permits lambs to finish most rapidly.

[9] 40 kg early-weaned lamb fed same as finishing lamb of equal weight.

(From *Nutrient Requirements of Sheep*, National Research Council, 1972) aging for themselves, the requirement of the ewe is reduced to a level equivalent to that of ewes one month before lambing. This is of considerable economic importance.

PROTEIN

Even though wool is chiefly protein, sheep do not need more of this nutrient, per unit of feed, than other farm animals. As with other ruminants, quantity of protein is a more critical factor than quality. Good-quality pasture and forage will provide the necessary protein for mature sheep. It should be emphasized, however, that sheep do not digest the protein of poor-quality, mature and weathered forage as efficiently as cattle and that there are instances when a protein supplement should be fed with grass, hay and winter range.

Sheep can convert nonprotein nitrogen, such as urea and biuret, into protein in their rumen. This source of nitrogen can provide all the necessary supplemental nitrogen in high-energy diets containing a nitrogen:sulfur ratio of 10:1. In lamb finishing diets, the inclusion of alfalfa and diethylstilbestrol enhances nitrogen utilization.

MINERALS

It has been demonstrated that sheep require sodium, chlorine, calcium, phosphorus, iodine, iron, cobalt, copper, magnesium, sulfur, potassium, manganese, molybdenum, zinc and selenium. Excesses of fluorine, selenium and molybdenum in natural feeds sometimes cause toxic signs in sheep; similarly, excessive amounts of copper in the feed or supplements can cause copper poisoning, especially where molybdenum content is low. Trace mineralized salt, commonly fed to sheep, contains 8 of these necessary minerals and provides an economical method of preventing deficiencies. These are sodium, chlorine, iodine, manganese, cobalt, copper, iron and zinc. Since sheep diets usually contain sufficient potassium, iron, magnesium, sulfur and manganese, no discussion of these minerals will be presented.

Salt: Except on certain alkali areas of the western winter range and along the seacoast where forage and soil are high in salt, sheep are provided with common salt (sodium chloride). Sheepmen in the U.S.A. and Canada believe that sheep need salt to remain thrifty and make economical gains. However, salt supplements are rarely fed to sheep on good pasture in New Zealand and Australia.

Mature sheep will consume 0.02 lb of salt daily and lambs

one-half this amount. Range operators commonly provide from 0.5 to 0.75 lb of salt per ewe per month.

Calcium and Phosphorus: In plants, generally, the leafy parts are relatively high in calcium and low in phosphorus, whereas the reverse is true of the seeds. Legumes, in general, have a higher calcium content than grasses. As grasses mature, phosphorus is transferred to the seed (grain). Furthermore, the phosphorus content of the plant is markedly influenced by the available phosphorus in the soil. Low-quality pasture, devoid of legumes, and range plants tend, therefore, to be naturally low in phosphorus, a situation which is accentuated as the forage matures and the seeds fall, and by a deficiency of phosphorus in the soil, which is characteristic of much range country. Consequently, sheep subsisting on mature, brown, summer forage and winter range sometimes develop a phosphorus deficiency (q.v., p. 1320). Sheep kept on such forages or fed low-quality hay with no grain should be provided with a phosphorus supplement.

On the other hand, since most forages have a relatively high calcium content, particularly if there is an admixture of legumes, natural feeds usually supply the required amounts of this element. However, when corn silage or other feeds from the cereal grains are fed exclusively, each sheep should be fed 0.02 to 0.03 lb of ground limestone daily.

Sheep seem to be able to tolerate wide ratios as long as they contain more calcium than phosphorus. Range ewes do well on ratios as wide as 12:1. On the other hand, an excess of phosphorus may be conducive to development of urinary calculi; a Ca:P ratio of 1.5:1 is appropriate for feed lot lambs.

For pregnant ewes, the diet should contain not less than 0.18% of phosphorus and, for lactating ewes, not less than 0.27%. A content of 0.20 to 0.40% of calcium is considered adequate.

Iodine: Sometimes, either as a consequence of a low available iodine content of the soil or the presence in the food of goitrogenic substances which interfere with the utilization of iodine by the thyroid, the iodine requirements of sheep are not met in the natural diet and iodine supplements must be fed. Regions naturally deficient in iodine are known throughout the Western U.S.A., in the Great Lakes area and in many other parts of the world. A deficiency of iodine (q.v., p. 1321) can be prevented by feeding iodized salt to the pregnant ewe.

Cobalt: An intake of 0.1 mg daily for a 120-lb sheep is considered adequate; this amount will be obtained in the daily ration, provided the forage contains not less than 0.07 ppm of cobalt. Normally, legumes have a higher content than grasses. Where it becomes necessary to supplement the ration to avoid cobalt deficiency (q.v., p. 1322), it may be done by feeding trace mineralized salt.

Copper: Pregnant ewes require approximately 5 mg of copper daily and this amount is provided, under normal conditions, when the forage contains not less than about 5 ppm. However, the amount of copper in the diet necessary to prevent a copper deficiency (q.v., p. 1322) in the animal is influenced by the intake of other dietary constituents, notably the level of molybdenum and inorganic sulfate. High intakes of molybdenum in the presence of adequate sulfate increases the copper requirement of the animal. When necessary, additional copper may be supplied in the salt mixture. Since sheep are more susceptible than cattle to the toxic effects of copper, care must be taken to avoid copper toxicosis. This is particularly true where the molybdenum content in the soil and feed is low.

Selenium: Interest in selenium for many years was confined to its toxic effects upon animals. It has now emerged as an essential trace element for sheep and has been effective in the control of nutritional muscular dystrophy (q.v., p. 578). Areas east of the Mississippi River and in the Northwestern U.S.A. appear to be low in selenium.

Zinc: The requirement of growing lambs for zinc is approximately 30 ppm. The requirement for normal testicular development is somewhat higher. Since many feeds do not contain this much zinc the possibility of a deficiency is real. Furthermore, a high calcium intake will increase the need for zinc.

VITAMINS

Sheep diets usually contain an ample supply of vitamins A, D and E. Under certain circumstances, however, supplements may have to be provided. The B-complex vitamins and vitamin K_2 are synthesized by the rumen microorganisms and, under practical conditions, supplements are unnecessary. However, polioencephalomalacia sometimes occurs in sheep. This condition is apparently due to destruction of thiamine in the rumen, and animals respond to thiamine administration. Vitamin C is synthesized in the tissues of sheep.

On diets rich in carotene, such as high-quality pasture, sheep have the ability to store large quantities of **vitamin A** in the liver, sufficient often to meet their requirements for 6 to 12 months. Daily supplies are, therefore, unnecessary and deficiencies are rarely a problem. (*See* NUTRITIONAL DEFICIENCIES IN CATTLE AND SHEEP: VITAMIN A, p. 1325.)

Vitamin D supplies are derived both from the feed and by exposure of the skin to ultraviolet light. When the exposure of the skin to sunshine is reduced by prolonged cloudy weather or confinement rearing and when the vitamin D content of the diet is low, the amount supplied may be inadequate for the animal's needs. The requirement for vitamin D is increased when the amounts of either calcium or phosphorus in the diet are low or when the ratio between them is wide. Fast growing young lambs kept in sheds away from intense sunlight or maintained on green feeds (high carotene) during the winter months (low irradiation) may show slow growth rate and other signs of vitamin D deficiency (q.v., p. 1327). Normally, however, sheep on pasture seldom need vitamin D supplementation.

The major sources of **vitamin E** in the natural diet of sheep are green feeds and the germ of seeds. A deficiency of this vitamin, therefore, is uncommon in mature sheep but does occur, among lambs 2 to 8 weeks of age. The interrelationship of vitamin E and selenium is interesting (*see* p. 576).

FEEDING FARM SHEEP

The nutrient requirements as outlined in TABLE 7, with the tables on feed composition (p. 1362 *et seq.*), can be used to calculate adequate rations for sheep. Using these data and the results of practical experience, suggestions for the feeding of sheep are outlined below.

Specialized Sheep Production: There has been much information compiled in recent years concerning larger sheep units under a confined system of management. Such innovations as early weaning or artificial rearing of lambs, slotted floors, accelerated lambing, synchronization of breeding, production testing and chemical shearing have been tested and are being used. It is questionable if the extensive use of pasture for lambs in the Midwest and Eastern U.S.A. will expand or even continue.

Use of Forage: Good hay is a highly productive feed; poor hay, no matter how much is available, is suitable only for maintenance. Hay quality is determined primarily by (1) its botanic composition, e.g., a mixture of palatable grasses and legumes—brome, alfalfa or bluegrass, clover, (2) the stage of maturity when cut, e.g., the grass before heading and alfalfa before one-tenth bloom, (3) method and speed of harvesting as it affects loss of leaf, bleaching by sun and leaching by rain and (4) by spoilage and loss during storage and feeding. In general, the same factors influence the quality of silage. Sheep make excellent use of high-quality roughage stored either as hay or low-moisture, grass-legume silage, or occasionally chopped green feed.

FEEDING EWES

Research results now indicate that the period from weaning to breeding of the ewe is more critical than was previously thought. It appears that the "flushing" period should occur during this time rather than for only a few weeks prior to turning in the ram. Ewes should not be allowed to become excessively fat but they should make a very slight daily gain from weaning to breeding. The rate of gain depends on the desired weight gain. If pasture production is inadequate, ewes may be confined and fed high-quality hay and if necessary, a very little grain to make this desired weight increase.

There is evidence that breeding on legume pastures tends to depress the size of the lamb crop. Mixed pasture 2 weeks before and during breeding is, therefore, preferred.

After mating, ewes can be maintained on pasture, thus allowing feed to be conserved, if necessary, for other times of the year. Good pasture for this period will put the ewes into the winter feeding period in good condition. One of the rations outlined in TABLE 8 may be used when pasture is unavailable.

During the last 6 to 8 weeks of pregnancy, intra-uterine growth of the lamb is rapid and, from a nutritional viewpoint, this is the critical period. Commencing 6 to 8 weeks before lambing, therefore, the plane of nutrition should be increased gradually and continued without interruption by the addition of supplements such as those described in TABLE 9. The amount offered will depend on the condition of the ewes. If ewes are in fair to good condition, 0.5 to 0.75 lb is usually sufficient. The roughage of the ration should provide all the protein required by ewes for most efficient feeding of the farm flock. If necessary, the ewes may be classified according to age and condition and divided into groups for differential treatment.

TABLE 8. RATIONS FOR PREGNANT EWES UP TO 6 WEEKS BEFORE LAMBING

Feed	Ration No.			
	1	2	3	4
	lb	lb	lb	lb
Legume hay, such as alfalfa, clover, or lespedeza	3.0-4.5	1.5-2.0	—	—
Corn or sorghum silage	—	4.0-5.0	—	6.0-8.0
Legume grass, low-moisture (50%) silage	—	—	6.0-8.0	—
Cottonseed, soybean, linseed, or peanut meal 90%; limestone 10%	—	—	—	0.25

TABLE 9. GRAIN MIXTURE FOR PREGNANT EWES

Feed	Mixture No.			
	1	2	3	4
	lb	lb	lb	lb
Whole barley, corn or wheat	60	75	75	50
Whole oats	30	—	25	50
Beet pulp, dried	—	25	—	—
Wheat bran	10	—	—	—

Lactating Ewes: Succulent pasture furnishes plenty of energy, protein, vitamins and minerals for ewes and lambs; no added grain is necessary. When pasture is not available or not used under confinement rearing, ewes should be fed one of the rations outlined for pregnant ewes in TABLE 8, and 1.0 to 1.5 lb of one of the grain mixtures in TABLE 9. Ewes should have access to trace mineralized salt and dicalcium phosphate as previously discussed. Ewes with twin lambs should be separated from those with single lambs and fed more grain. Ewes nursing twin lambs produce 20 to 40% more milk than those with singles. Under confinement rearing or accelerated lambing, it is a common practice to wean lambs at 2 months of age. The ewe's milk production declines rapidly after this period and since the lambs are consuming feed from a creep it results in more efficient use of feed.

FEEDING LAMBS

At about 2 weeks of age, the lambs should have free access to a creep except if they are born on succulent pasture. If pasture is to be used later they should be creep-fed for 1 or 2 months until it is available. If it will not be available until the lambs are 3 or 4 months of age, they should be finished in dry lot. The grain should be ground coarse or rolled at first, but may be fed whole later. At first, small amounts are fed and the feed is kept clean and fresh. The amount is gradually raised until the lambs are on full feed.

Feeding lambs from birth to market in dry lot together with early weaning at 2 to 3 months of age is becoming increasingly popular throughout the U.S.A. A complete diet of hay, grain and supplement is ground, mixed, and either fed in this form or made into a 3/16- or ⅜-in. pellet. These lambs usually reach market weight in 3½ to 4 months. Some examples of creep ration used in dry-lot feeding are shown in TABLE 10.

TABLE 10. CREEP RATION FOR YOUNG SUCKLING AND EARLY-WEANED LAMBS

Feed	Mixture No.			
	1	2	3	4
	lb	lb	lb	lb
Alfalfa hay, leafy ground	25	30	40	—
Dehydrated alfalfa leaf meal	—	—	—	35
Corn, shelled	54.5	—	20	48
Corn or wheat	—	55	—	—
Oats or barley	—	—	20	—
Soybean, linseed or cottonseed meal	19	10	10	10
Molasses	—	3.5	8.5	5.5
Bone meal or dicalcium phosphate	1	1	1	1
Limestone	1	—	—	—
Trace mineralized salt	0.5	0.5	0.5	0.5
Antibiotic (mg/lb)	10	7.5	20.0	20.0
Vitamin A (IU/ton)	2,000,000	—	5,000,000	5,000,000
Vitamin D (IU/ton)	800,000	—	625,000	625,000
Vitamin E (IU/ton)	80,000	—	10,000	10,000

Rearing Lambs on Milk Replacer: In today's intensified type of sheep production, lambs such as orphans, extras or those from poor milking ewes should be raised on milk replacers. They should first receive colostrum, if not from a ewe then from a supply that has been frozen. Milk replacers designed specifically for lambs are currently available. They contain approximately 30% fat and 25% protein and a high level of antibiotic. It is advisable to inject lambs with iron-dextran, vitamins A, D and E and a combination of penicillin and streptomycin.

Multiple nipple pails or containers are used and the milk should be offered cold. Cold milk replacer can be used by older lambs, which will nurse more often, and the milk will not sour as quickly. The lambs should be given water to drink in addition to the milk when a creep ration is offered to them at 9 to 10 days of age. They can be weaned from the milk abruptly at 4 to 5 weeks of age if consumption of creep feed is at a reasonable level.

FINISHING FEEDER LAMBS

Preconditioning before the lambs leave the producer's property should be encouraged. This would include starting on feed, vaccination, worming and under some conditions shearing. If this is not done, then the lambs should be rested for several days and fed dry, average-quality hay. Following this rest the above-mentioned practices should be performed. Vaccination should be against enterotoxemia and possibly contagious ecthyma.

Feeding Method: There is no best method or diet for finishing lambs. They may be finished on alfalfa or wheat pasture with no grain. They may be started on pasture or crop aftermath and fed grain later. When fed in dry lot they are usually self-fed. These diets may be either completely pelleted, ground and mixed, a mixture of alfalfa pellets and grain or a high-concentrate type. Self-feeding means more efficient use of labor and this provides the opportunity to increase size of operation. Self-feeding usually results in maximum feed intake and gain. Hand-feeding can be mechanized with an auger system or self-unloading wagon. It involves feeding at regular intervals so that the lambs clean up the feed before they are fed again. Feed consumption and gain can be controlled. Corn silage should be hand-fed.

Starting on Feed: Feeders who feed lambs the year around or feed heavy lambs usually prefer to place the lambs on full feed as rapidly as possible. This means full feeding within 10 to 14 days. Lambs can be safely started on self-fed, ground or pelleted diets containing 60 to 70% hay. Within 2 weeks the hay is reduced to 30 to 40%. Other roughages such as cottonseed hulls or silage can be used in a similar manner. Lambs can be started and finished on pelleted rations that contain less grain than needed for non-pelleted rations. Digestive disturbances are usually reduced also. Cost may be relatively higher.

Two practices are helpful in starting lambs on feed more rapidly and in feeding diets that may be entirely of a concentrate nature. These are vaccination against enterotoxemia and feeding tetracyclines at a level to supply 25 to 30 mg per lamb daily.

Feeds: Corn, sorghum or alfalfa silage can replace about half the hay with hand-feeding but finish and yield will be decreased to some extent. About 3 lb of silage is equal to 1 lb of hay. Grain mixtures used in self-feeding are given in TABLE 11. Corn, barley, milo or wheat, or a mixture of these grains

TABLE 11. RECOMMENDED FORMULAS FOR FINISHING LAMBS
(lb/ton basis)

	Starter 10-day period	Alfalfa hay	Dehydrated alfalfa	Pelleted
No. 2 shelled corn	500	600	—	815
Ground ear corn	—	—	1230	—
Milo	—	700	—	—
Hay	1280	500	—	—
Dehydrated alfalfa	—	—	400	400
Molasses	100	150	175	150
Oat hulls	—	—	—	500
Urea	—	—	—	15
Soybean meal	—	130	—	100
Linseed meal	100	—	175	—
Feeding limestone	10	10	10	10
Trace mineral salt	10	10	10	10
Vitamin D	—	—	200,000 IU	200,000 IU
Tetracycline	50 gm	20 gm	20 gm	20 gm

are also satisfactory. If these grains are used, 0.5% salt and 0.5% bone meal or equivalent should be added to the grain. Pelleting of the rations for fattening lambs is beneficial, especially when low-grade roughages are used. Caution should be used when feeding large amounts of wheat; lambs not adapted to it are more apt to develop acute indigestion than if on grains such as corn, sorghum or barley.

Mineral supplements including salt should be offered separately whether or not they are included in the grain mixture. The use of the hormone diethylstilbestrol (where its use is permitted) increases growth rate 10 to 15% and feed efficiency 8 to 10% but tends to decrease carcass quality.

FEEDING MATURE BREEDING RAMS

Mature breeding rams should be grazed on pasture when available, or fed rations 1, 2 or 3 outlined in TABLE 8. If rams are in a thrifty condition at breeding time and the ewes are on a good flushing pasture, it should not be necessary to grain-feed the ram while with the ewes. In warm climates, rams should be shorn prior to mating and turned with the ewes at night only, if the daytime temperature is above 90°F.

FEEDING RANGE SHEEP

The condition of the sheep, the amount and kind of forage on the range and the climatic conditions will determine the kind and amount of supplement to feed. Supplements usually consist of high-protein pellets or cottonseed meal and salt, medium-protein pellets, low-protein pellets or corn, alfalfa hay and minerals.

When the diets of sheep on the western winter range are properly supplemented, the lamb crop can be increased 10 to 15% and wool production increased about 1 lb per ewe. Each operator will need to determine if this increased production will more than cover cost of supplementation. One recommended practice is to feed about 0.25 lb of high-protein (36%) supplement or 0.33 to 0.5 lb of medium-protein (24%) pellet about 3 weeks before the breeding season, during the breeding season, during extremely cold weather and for about 30 days before green feed starts in the spring (TABLE 12). In addition, small lambs, small yearling ewes, old ewes with poor teeth and thin ewes should be separated from the large band and fed one of the above supplements from about December 1 until shearing time. In many instances, the old ewes, lambs and yearlings from more than one band can be herded together in a special flock.

When sheep are unable to obtain a full ration of forage because of deep snow, 1 to 3 lb alfalfa hay and 0.2 to 0.3 lb of a low-protein pellet mixture (TABLE 12) or corn should be fed. If alfalfa hay is not available, 0.5 to 1.0 lb per head of a low-protein pellet mixture should be fed daily for emergency feeding periods.

Deficiencies of Range Forages: Deficiencies most apt to occur among range forages are protein, energy, phosphorus and carotene (vitamin A). These are most prevalent as the forages approach maturity or are dormant and they may appear singly or in combination. Range sheep often travel long distances and are exposed to cold weather. This results in a higher energy requirement. Protein supplements such as soybean or cottonseed meal increase digestibility and utilization of forage as well as providing needed protein and phosphorus. Most ranges used for winter grazing are considered adequate in carotene because most browse species, even in the dormant stage, furnish as much carotene as sun-cured alfalfa hay. However, when sheep are required to graze dry-grass ranges for periods longer than 6 months without intermittent periods of green feed, vitamin A supplements are recommended.

TABLE 12. PATTERN FOR RANGE SUPPLEMENTS FOR SHEEP

Main Groups	Sub-groups	Feedstuff	Suggested Maximum	Proportions of Individual Feeds — Recommended Amount of Protein		
				high	medium	low
			%	%	%	%
Energy feeds	Grains	Barley	75		33.0	57.5
		Corn	60	5.5	10.0	15.0
		Wheat	60			
		Milo	60			
		Oats	15			
		Screenings No. 1	10			
	Mill feeds	Wheat mixed feed	10			
		Shorts	10			
		Molasses	15	5.0	5.0	10.0
		Beet pulp	10			10.0
Protein supplements	30–40% Protein feeds	Cottonseed meal	75	62.5	32.5	5.0
		Linseed meal	25			
		Soybean meal	75	10.0	10.0	
		Peanut meal	25			
	20–30% Protein feeds	Corn gluten feed	15			
		Corn distillers' dried grains	10			
		Wheat distillers' dried grains	10			
		Brewers' dried grains	5			
		Safflower meal	25			
		Cull beans	15			
Mineral supplements		Bone meal or defluorinated phosphate		4.0	3.0	2.0
		Dicalcium phosphate				
		Disodium phosphate				
		Monocalcium phosphate				
		Monosodium phosphate				
		Salt or trace mineralized salt		0.5	0.5	0.5
Vitamin supplements		Dehydrated alfalfa meal	20	12.5	6.0	
		Sun-cured alfalfa meal	20			
		Vitamin A and carotene concentrates				
Total				100.0	100.0	100.0
Suggested composition						
Total crude protein %				36.0	24.0	12.0
Phosphorus %				1.5	1.0	0.5
Carotene mg/lb				15.6	7.8	—
Rate of feeding, lb/day—ewes				0.25	0.33 to 0.50	0.20 to 1.0

Mineral Mixtures: On the range, portable mineral boxes are convenient for sheep. Suggested mineral mixtures high in phosphorus are given in TABLE 13. One of these mineral mixtures should be fed free choice along with salt in a 2-compartment mineral box. Mixture 1 is used if there are no iodine or trace mineral deficiencies, Mixture 2 where an iodine deficiency exists and Mixture 3 if deficiencies of trace minerals are present.

TABLE 13. SUGGESTED MINERAL MIXTURES FOR SHEEP

Ingredient	Mixture No.		
	1	2	3
	lb	lb	lb
Salt	50	—	—
Iodized salt	—	50	—
Trace mineralized salt	—	—	50
Bone meal or phosphorus supplement	50	50	50

Under winter range conditions, the amount of phosphorus supplement which should be added to range pellets will vary with the type of range forage available, the rate of feeding and the ingredients used in the pellets. It is suggested that 36%, 24% and 12% protein pellets contain 1.5%, 1.0% and 0.5% phosphorus, respectively. It is assumed that the 36% protein pellets will be fed at the rate of 0.25 lb per head daily, the 24% protein pellets at the rate of 0.33 to 0.5 lb and the 12% protein pellets at a rate of 0.2 to 0.5 lb, together with alfalfa or clover hay.

SWINE NUTRITION

NUTRITIONAL REQUIREMENTS

Advanced technology contributes to the many phases of modern swine production. This is most evident in nutrition as formulation of diets becomes more precise and economical as synthetic nutrients, by-products and new feeds become available.

The nutrient requirements for swine, given in the following tables, are from the report issued by the Committee on Animal Nutrition of the National Research Council, entitled *Nutrient Requirements of Swine,* revised in 1968. Requirements are given for nutrients for which there are reasonably reliable quantitative data. These requirement values have not been increased by any intentionally added amounts for specific nutrients to provide overage. Factors such as stress conditions, availability of nutrients or variability in animals may dictate increased levels of some nutrients to optimize performance. These requirements should be distinguished from therapeutic doses of many times the normal needs, which may be administered singly or over short periods, to correct deficiencies. Natural diets may contain more of some nutrients than the table recommends, but the effect is minimal except in extreme cases of imbalance. Ingredient concentration should be modified to prevent serious imbalances from occurring. Data on the composition of feedstuffs for swine are presented in TABLE 47, p. 1368.

Quantitative data for some of the nutrients required by swine are known. This is particularly true for older animals and for functions such as reproduction and lactation. The nutrients required by swine may be classified as water, energy (chiefly carbohydrates and fat), protein (amino acids), minerals and vitamins. In TABLES 15 and 16 nutrient requirement values are expressed per kilogram of total diet. Certain antibiotics and arsenicals are added to swine diets to increase the rate and efficiency of gain, but are not considered to be nutrients.

WATER

This constituent can be best supplied by allowing the pigs free and convenient access to it. The water allowances for full-fed pigs are given in TABLE 14. The water consumption

TABLE 14. WATER ALLOWANCES FOR FULL-FED PIGS

WEIGHT OF PIG	WATER CONSUMPTION FREEWILL, DAILY PER PIG			
	Spring Pigs		Fall Pigs	
lb	lb	gal.	lb	gal.
50	5.5	0.69	4.5	0.56
100	9.0	1.12	7.5	0.94
150	10.0	1.25	9.0	1.12
200	9.0	1.12	9.6	1.20
300	6.0	0.75	6.0	0.75
400	5.2	0.65	5.2	0.65

(From Evvard, J. M., 1929. *Iowa Agricultural Experiment Station Research Bulletin* 118)

in kilograms of growing-finishing pigs can be estimated fairly closely by multiplying by 2 the amount (in kilograms) of air-dry feed consumed. Yearling brood sows on experiment consumed about 1 gal. (4 kg) of water daily during the winter gestation period. For maximum milk production, lactating sows should be given all the water they will consume.

ENERGY

The amount of feed consumed by growing pigs fed *ad libitum* is controlled principally by the energy content of the diet. If diets contain excessive amounts of fiber (exceeding 5 to 7% without commensurate increases in fat, the rate and efficiency of gain are adversely affected. Energy requirements of swine are expressed in terms of calories either as digestible energy (DE) or metabolizable energy (ME). The ME values increasingly are finding favor for use by swine nutritionists as values for more and more feedstuffs are determined.

FEEDING LEVELS

Daily feed intake estimates may be obtained from the figure on p. 1233 for growing-finishing pigs. Such information is useful as a guide in projecting total feed requirements or prescribing medication via the feed.

The feeding levels set forth by the National Research Council provide a daily intake of 2 kg (4.4 lb) for pregnant gilts and sows. Sows and gilts need little more energy during pregnancy than is required for maintenance of body weight and good health. The diets upon which these recommendations are based would be classified as high-energy diets (corn-soybean meal type) with no oats, alfalfa meal or other energy diluent. The voluntary intake of pregnant swine is difficult to control even with a high-fiber level and invariably both excessive intake and weight gain occur.

A feeding method for pregnant gilts and sows receiving wide acceptance is that of feeding only one day out of 3, the total quantity of feed offered being the same (e.g., 6 kg every third day instead of 2 kg daily). The feed is spread out to allow opportunity for individuals to eat simultaneously.

For feeding during lactation the National Research Council recommends 5 kg (11 lb) and 5.5 kg (12.3 lb) of feed daily for first-litter and mature sows, respectively. High-energy diets are usually fed during lactation. Many producers are restricting the feed offered to sows during the last half of lactation (i.e., beyond 3 weeks) or are offering feed to sows based on the number of nursing pigs.

PROTEIN AND AMINO ACIDS

Amino acids normally incorporated into proteins long have been recognized to be essential for maintenance, growth, ges-

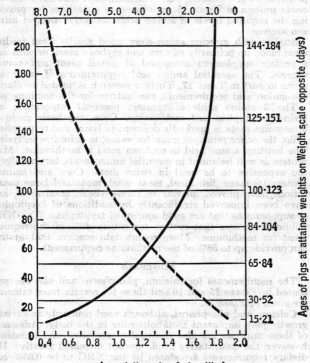

**DAILY FEED, DAILY GAINS, AND INCLUSIVE
AGE RANGES OF MARKET PIGS
ACCORDING TO ATTAINED WEIGHTS**

- - - - Ave. daily feed (air dry basis)(lbs)

Attained weight of pigs (lbs)

Ages of pigs at attained weights on Weight scale opposite (days)

Ave. daily gain of pigs (lbs)

**STANDARD CURVES ON GAINS AND FEED INTAKE OF PIGS
AT VARIOUS WEIGHTS**

(From *Nutrient Requirements of Swine*, National Research Council, 1964)

tation and lactation of swine. Many amino acids are synthesized in the animal, however, the essential amino acids cannot be synthesized at a sufficiently rapid rate to permit normal growth and must be provided in the diet. The amino acids arginine, histidine, isoleucine, leucine, lysine, methionine, phenylalanine, threonine, tryptophan and valine are indispensable to the growing pig. The suggested feeding levels for crude protein in TABLE 15 are offered as guidelines for providing the required levels of amino acids and other needed nitrogen sources.

Studies with growing swine show good results from feeding diets made up primarily of corn and soybean meal, or corn and a protein supplement composed of mixed plant and animal sources. The essential amino acid requirements of swine are given in part in TABLE 17. Further research is needed to clarify the amino acid requirements, particularly for the finishing pig.

The 3 amino acids of greatest practical importance are lysine, tryptophan and methionine. Corn, the basic grain in most swine diets, is markedly deficient in lysine and tryptophan. Milo, the other principal grain for swine, is quite low in lysine. The limiting amino acid in soybean meal is methionine. Milk protein is well balanced in essential amino acids, but usually is too expensive to be used in swine diets. Corn and animal-protein (tankage, fish meal, meat meal, meat and bone meal) rations have proved inferior to corn-soybean meal diets, and have been improved significantly by additions of tryptophan or supplements that are good sources of tryptophan. The NRC publication states that cystine can satisfy 40% of the requirement for methionine. More recent data confirm that cystine can provide up to 56% of the methionine requirement.

MINERALS

The requirements for calcium, phosphorus and salt are presented in TABLES 15 and 16 and those for certain trace minerals are given in TABLE 18.

Calcium and **phosphorus,** although used primarily in skeletal growth, play important metabolic roles in the body. Adequacy of these minerals are also essential to gestation and lactation; however, the quantitative needs are not increased greatly. The dietary requirements are stated by the NRC to be 0.65% calcium and 0.50% phosphorus for the growing pig and 0.50% calcium and 0.40% phosphorus for the finishing swine. These levels were established with more purified diets and would be inadequate for phosphorus in diets containing phytate phosphorus such as corn-soybean meal diets. The usual recommendation for such diets is the continued feeding of 0.50%

TABLE 15. NUTRIENT REQUIREMENTS OF GROWING AND FINISHING SWINE: PERCENTAGE OR AMOUNT PER KILOGRAM OF DIET

NUTRIENTS		Full-fed on Cereal Grains			Full-fed on Corn		Full-fed on Wheat, Barley, Oats	
		5-10	10-20	20-35	35-60	60-100	35-60	60-100
		Requirements						
Protein and energy								
Crude protein	%	22	18	16	14	13	15	14
Digestible energy	Kcal	3,500	3,500	3,300	3,300	3,300	3,100	3,100
Inorganic nutrients								
Calcium	%	0.80	0.65	0.65	0.50	0.50	0.50	0.50
Phosphorus	%	0.60	0.50	0.50	0.40	0.40	0.40	0.40
Sodium	%	—	0.10	0.10	—	—	—	—
Chlorine	%	—	0.13	0.13	—	—	—	—
Vitamins								
Beta carotene	mg	4.4	3.5	2.6	2.6	2.6	2.6	2.6
Vitamin A	IU	2,200	1,750	1,300	1,300	1,300	1,300	1,300
Vitamin D	IU	220	200	200	125	125	125	125
Thiamine	mg	1.3	1.1	1.1	1.1	1.1	1.1	1.1
Riboflavin	mg	3.0	3.0	2.6	2.2	2.2	2.2	2.2
Niacin[2]	mg	22.0	18.0	14.0	10.0	10.0	10.0	10.0
Pantothenic acid	mg	13.0	11.0	11.0	11.0	11.0	11.0	11.0
Vitamin B6	mg	1.5	1.5	1.1	—	—	—	—
Choline	mg	1,100	900	—	—	—	—	—
Vitamin B12	mcg	22	15	11	11	11	11	11

DIET, LIVEWEIGHT CLASS (kg)[1]

[1] The following shows expected daily gain (in kilograms) for each of the liveweight classes (left to right): 0.30, 0.50, 0.60, 0.75, 0.90, 0.70 and 0.80.

[2] It is assumed that all of the niacin in the cereal grains and their by-products is in bound form and largely unavailable.

(From *Nutrient Requirements of Swine*, National Research Council, 1968)

TABLE 16. NUTRIENT REQUIREMENTS OF BREEDING SWINE: PERCENTAGE OR AMOUNT PER KILOGRAM OF DIET

Nutrients		Bred Gilts and Sows[1]	Lactating Gilts and Sows[2]	Boars (Young and Adult)[3]
Protein and energy				
Crude protein	%	14	15	14
Digestible energy	Kcal	3,300	3,300	3,300
Inorganic nutrients				
Calcium	%	0.75	0.6	0.75
Phosphorus	%	0.50	0.4	0.50
NaCl (salt)	%	0.5	0.5	0.5
Vitamins				
Beta carotene	mg	8.2	6.6	8.2
Vitamin A	IU	4,100	3,300	4,100
Vitamin D	IU	275	220	275
Thiamine	mg	1.4	1.1	1.4
Riboflavin	mg	4.1	3.3	4.1
Niacin	mg	22.0	17.6	22.0
Pantothenic acid	mg	16.5	13.2	16.5
Vitamin B_{12}	mcg	13.8	11.0	13.8

[1] Liveweight range (kg): 110 to 160.
[2] Liveweight range (kg): 140 to 200.
[3] Liveweight range (kg): 110 to 180.

TABLE 17. ESSENTIAL AMINO ACID REQUIREMENTS OF SWINE[1]

Amino Acids	Growing Pigs Weighing		Finishing Pigs	Bred Sows and Gilts
	5-10 kg	20-35 kg		
Arginine	—	0.20[2]	—	—
Histidine	0.27	0.18	—	0.20[2]
Isoleucine	0.76	0.50	0.35	0.43
Leucine	0.90	0.60	—	0.66[2]
Lysine	1.20	0.70	0.50	0.49
Methionine[3]	0.80	0.50	—	0.35
Phenylalanine[4]	—	0.50	—	0.52[2]
Threonine	0.70	0.45	—	0.42
Tryptophan	0.18	0.13	0.09[2]	0.08[2]
Valine	0.65	0.50	—	0.46

[1] Each requirement is expressed as a percentage of the diet. Requirements are based on the protein and digestible-energy-level requirements shown in TABLES 15 and 16.
[2] This level is adequate; the minimum requirement has not been established.
[3] Cystine can satisfy 40% of the need for methionine.
[4] Tyrosine can satisfy 30% of the need for phenylalanine.
(From *Nutrient Requirements of Swine*, National Research Council, 1968)

phosphorus to market weight. The use of feedstuffs such as tankage, meat meal, meat and bone meal and fish meal that are rich sources of calcium and phosphorus, may preclude the need of adding a phosphorus supplement.

Calcium sources normally used in swine diets, limestone and oyster shell, have a high biologic availability. Steamed bone meal, defluorinated phosphate, soft phosphate or dicalcium phosphate may be used to increase both dietary calcium and phosphorus. There is some variation in the biologic availability of the phosphorus in these supplements.

TABLE 18. TRACE MINERALS FOR SWINE

Mineral Element	Requirement mg/kg Diet	Tolerance Level mg/kg Diet	Toxic Level mg/kg Diet
Copper	6[1]	100	250
Iron	80[1]	1,000	5,000
Iodine	0.20	—	—
Magnesium	400	—	—
Manganese	40	80	4,000
Zinc	50[2]	1,000	2,000
Selenium	0.10	—	5

[1] Baby pig requirement.
[2] Higher levels may be needed if excess calcium is fed.
(From *Nutrient Requirements of Swine*, National Research Council, 1964, 1968)

Sodium chloride: The recommended salt allowance is 0.5% of the total diet. Animal and fish by-products as well as certain cereal by-products contribute appreciable amounts of salt.

Iodine is used by the thyroid gland to produce thyroxine, which affects cell activity and the rate of metabolism in the body. The iodine requirement of pregnant sows is approximately 0.44 mg/100 kg of body wt daily. Growing swine probably require somewhat less than this. Stabilized iodized salt containing 0.007% iodine, fed to meet the salt requirement, will meet the iodine needs of swine.

Iron and **copper** are necessary for hemoglobin formation and to prevent nutritional anemia. Fifteen milligrams of iron per pig daily for the first 3 weeks after birth will maintain normal levels of hemoglobin. The requirement for copper is listed by the NRC as 6 mg/kg total diet. It has been reported that pigs receiving 11 mg or more of copper per kilogram of body weight daily do not show copper deficiency signs.

Iron, which is severely deficient in milk, can be supplied orally to the suckling pig by mixing ferric ammonium citrate with water in a baby pig waterer or periodically dropping a mixture of iron sulfate and a carrier, such as corn, on the floor of the farrowing cage. Baby pig anemia (q.v., p. 19) can also be prevented with injectable iron compounds. Feeding iron and copper salts to pregnant or lactating sows or injecting iron dextran into these sows has not resulted in sufficient placental transfer or mammary uptake of these minerals to prevent anemia in baby pigs.

Cobalt is present in the vitamin B_{12} molecule and if the diet contains adequate vitamin B_{12} a growth response to cobalt is unlikely. The requirement for this mineral has not been definitely established.

Manganese is essential for normal reproduction and growth, but the quantitative requirement is unknown. It appears that 40 ppm (18 mg/lb) is adequate for growth, gestation and lactation.

Potassium: When practical diets are fed, no deficiency is encountered because natural feedstuffs contain adequate amounts of potassium to meet the pig's needs.

Magnesium is a dietary essential for growing swine. The requirement has been established at 400 ppm (181 mg/lb) in the complete diet. Because of the content of this mineral in ordinary feedstuffs, a deficiency is unlikely under practical conditions.

Zinc is interrelated with calcium in swine nutrition. Supplemental zinc is recommended at the rate of 50 to 70 ppm (45 to 64 gm/ton) to prevent the occurrence of parakeratosis (q.v., p. 918), particularly when diets contain excessive calcium (i.e., 1% or more).

Selenium: The selenium content of soils and ultimately crops is quite variable. Areas generally west of the Mississippi contain considerable amounts of selenium while soils east of the river tend to yield crops deficient in selenium. The requirement of 0.1 ppm is low, but the need is well documented (*see* WMD AND RELATED DISEASES IN SWINE, p. 581).

VITAMINS

Requirements for 9 vitamins are given in TABLES 15 and 16.

Vitamin A: The use of stabilized vitamin A has become commonplace in manufactured feeds and in vitamin supplements or premixes. Concentrates containing natural vitamin A (fish oils for the most part) may be used to fortify diets, but both natural vitamin A and carotene, a precursor of vitamin A from plants, are rather easily destroyed in the presence of air, light, high temperatures, rancidity, and certain mineral elements. Since the potencies of vitamin A sources are expressed on an International Unit (IU) basis, it is convenient to place carotene on this basis also. The National Research Council has eclared 1 IU vitamin A equal to 0.30 mcg of crystalline vitamin A alcohol, 0.344 mcg vitamin A acetate, 0.55 mcg of vitamin A palmitate or 2.0 mcg beta carotene. The pig is considerably less efficient in converting carotene to vitamin A, so that approximately 3 times more beta carotene is required by the pig than the rat in meeting an equivalent vitamin A requirement. Green forage is an excellent source of carotene, as are high-quality legume hays. Dehydrated alfalfa meal is available as a standard feed ingredient and can be purchased with a guaranteed carotene content. Corn is not a reliable source.

Vitamin D: This antirachitic fat-soluble vitamin is necessary for proper bone growth and ossification. Vitamin D_2 (irradiated plant sterol) and vitamin D_3 (irradiated animal sterol) can be used by the pig to meet the vitamin D requirement. The requirements given in TABLES 15 and 16 are 200 to 220 IU of vitamin per kilogram of diet for growing pigs weighing 20 kg and less, while the requirement for heavier swine is 125 IU/kg, when the diets contain recommended amounts of calcium and phosphorus. Vitamin D needs can be met by exposing pigs to direct sunlight for a short period each day. Sources of vitamin D include irradiated yeast, sun-cured hays, activated plant or animal sterols, fish oils and vitamin A and D concentrates.

Vitamin E (tocopherol) is required by swine of all ages. It is interrelated with selenium in nutrition of swine and is included at 11 to 22 IU per kilogram of a diet where selenium and vitamin E deficiencies have been reported. Vitamin E supplementation can only partially obviate a selenium deficiency. Green forage, legume hays and meals, cereal grains and especially the germ of cereal grains contain appreciable amounts of vitamin E.

Vitamin K, the antihemorrhagic fat-soluble vitamin, is necessary to maintain normal blood clotting time. A hemorrhagic condition has recently been reported in growing swine, perhaps indicating a deficiency of vitamin K in swine fed practical diets. It may be important to include supplemental vitamin K (100 mcg/kg diet is at least adequate) in problem areas.

Thiamine: This water-soluble vitamin is not of practical importance in diets commonly fed to swine because grains and other feed ingredients supply ample amounts to meet the requirement of about 1.1 mg/kg of total diet.

Riboflavin: The requirement of breeding stock and of lightweight pigs is 2.6 to 3.0 mg of riboflavin per kilogram of diet. For 22 kg or heavier growing pigs, 2.2 mg/kg diet is required. Riboflavin is a constituent of several enzyme systems in the

body. Swine diets are normally deficient in this vitamin ar
the crystalline form is added in premixes. Natural sources i
clude green forage, milk by-products, brewer's yeast, legun
meals and some fermentation and distillery by-products.

Niacin (nicotinic acid): The requirement for niacin is
mg/kg diet for the 10-kg pig, 14 to 18 mg/kg diet for the 20-k
pig and 10 mg for heavier pigs. Niacin is a component of c
enzymes concerned with utilization of carbohydrates. The p
can convert some tryptophan to niacin. Corn contains 9
10 mg of niacin per pound, but the niacin from corn and oth
cereal grains appears to be unavailable to swine. Swine die
are normally deficient in this vitamin and the crystalline for
is added in premixes. Natural sources of niacin include fish ar
animal by-products, brewer's yeast, peanut meal and distiller
solubles.

Pantothenic acid: The requirement for pantothenic acid p
kilogram of diet is 13 mg for 5- to 10-kg pigs, and 11 mg f
pigs of other weights, and about 16 mg for breeding animal
Pantothenic acid is especially important in the female, sin
it is necessary for reproduction. Swine diets are normally d
ficient in this vitamin and the crystalline form is added in pr
mixes. Natural sources of pantothenic acid include green fo
age, legume meals, milk products, brewer's yeast, fish soluble
wheat bran, peanut meal and rice polishings.

Pyridoxine (vitamin B₆): The requirement for pyridoxine
1.1 mg/kg diet for 10- to 20-kg pigs. The requirement of old
pigs has not been determined. This vitamin is important
amino acid metabolism in the body. It is present in plentif
quantities in the feed ingredients usually fed to swine.

Choline is essential for the normal functioning of the liv
and kidneys. The pig can synthesize some choline fro
methionine in the diet. The requirement for choline is list
as 900 mg/kg diet for the 10- to 20-kg pig. Quantitative nee
for older pigs have not been determined. Swine diets a
normally deficient in this vitamin and the crystalline form
added in premixes. Natural sources of choline include fish sol
bles, fish meal, soybean meal, liver meal, brewer's yeast, tan
age and meat meal.

Vitamin B₁₂: The requirement for vitamin B₁₂ is 15 mcg/l
diet for the 10- to 20-kg pig and 11 mcg for swine of heavi
weights and for breeding stock. Vitamin B₁₂ is needed by tl
young pig for growth and normal hemopoiesis. It is present
animal, marine and milk products, but the B₁₂ potency
natural feed sources is quite variable. Swine diets are ofte
deficient in this vitamin and the crystalline form is added
premixes.

Biotin, folic acid and ascorbic acid: Biotin and folic acid are essential for pig growth. Ascorbic acid apparently is synthesized by the pig at a rapid enough rate to meet its needs. There is no evidence to indicate the need to supplement practical swine diets with biotin, folic acid and ascorbic acid.

FEEDING AND MANAGEMENT PRACTICES

Swine Feeding Plan: A fundamental principle of economic pork production is the feeding of a diet in which the nutrient deficiencies of economically available cereal grains are corrected by supplementation. Dependable manufactured supplements that supply the necessary amino acids, minerals and vitamins are available.

A plan of feeding swine of all ages is outlined in TABLES 19 and 20. With the exception of bred sows and gilts, this plan may be used for self-feeding the hogs. The grain may be ground and mixed with the appropriate supplement according to ratios given in TABLES 19 and 20, or the grain and appropriate supplement may be given free-choice For bred sows and gilts, the mixed ration may be hand-fed daily or fed periodically as described previously to promote the desired rate of gain and condition.

TABLE 19. AMOUNT OF CRUDE PROTEIN AND SUPPLEMENT RECOMMENDED IN SWINE RATIONS FED IN DRY LOT[1]

Liveweight (lb)	Average Daily Feed (lb)	Percent Crude Protein	Ratio of Supplement to Grain	Supplement per Hog per Day (lb)[2]
Growing swine				
25	2.0	18	1:2.25	0.6
50	3.2	16	1:3.14	0.8
100	5.3	14	1:4.80	0.9
150	6.8	13	1:6.25	0.9
200	7.5	12	1:8.67	0.8
250	8.3	12	1:8.67	0.8
Pregnant females				
300	4.4	14	1:4.80	0.75
500	4.4	14	1:4.80	0.75
Lactating sows				
350	11.0	15	1:3.83	2.2
450	12.5	15	1:3.83	2.5

[1] Based on the protein requirements set forth by the National Research Council (1968) and on the assumption that grain (corn and small grains) averaging 9% protein is mixed or fed with commercial dry-lot supplements containing 38% protein.

[2] Values in this column may be used as a check on pigs fed supplement free-choice to determine whether overconsumption or underconsumption is occurring and may be used as a guide in hand-feeding supplement on a daily basis.

The consumption of creep-feed prior to 3 weeks of age is minimal. Litters nursing beyond this age should be self-fed a palatable starter diet until weaning. Supplemental feed is needed for optimum performance since milk production peaks at 3 to 4 weeks of age while the pig's demands are increasing rapidly.

Preparation and Feeding of Farm Grains: Corn: An improvement in gain and particularly feed efficiency can be expected from grinding corn. The older the pig the greater the response that can be expected from grinding. The grain should be reduced to a medium-fine particle size. The necessity of grinding corn has been increasingly obvious with the trend to artificial drying of corn. The vitamin A in corn is so subject to oxidation that this vitamin should be added to corn diets as if the corn contained none.

TABLE 20. AMOUNT OF CRUDE PROTEIN AND SUPPLEMENT RECOMMENDED IN SWINE RATIONS FED ON GOOD PASTURE

Liveweight (lb)	Average Daily Feed (lb)	Percent Crude Protein	Ratio of Supplement to Grain	Supplement per Hog per Day (lb)[2]
Growing swine				
25	2.0	16	1:3.75	0.5
50	3.2	14	1:5.6	0.5
100	5.3	12	1:10	0.5
150	6.8	11	1:14.5	0.4
200	7.5	10	1:30	0.25
250	8.3	10	1:30	0.25
Pregnant females				
300	3.5	12	1:10	0.32
500	3.5	12	1:10	
Lactating sows				
350	10	13	1:7.25	1.2
450	11.5	13	1:7.25	1.2

[1] Based on the assumption that the protein requirements set forth by the National Research Council (1968) can be reduced by 2 percentage points when swine are on good pasture and that grain (corn and small grains) averaging 9% protein is mixed or fed with a commercial pasture supplement averaging 42% protein.
[2] See footnote 2 on TABLE 19.

Oats: Because of the relatively low-energy content of oats they should not account for more than 20% of the cereal grain in the diet. On that basis finely ground oats can replace corn on a pound-for-pound basis.

Wheat contains 2 to 3% more protein than corn, but little or no increased substitutive value is gained since lysine content in wheat is only slightly greater than that of corn. The metabolizable energy values of wheat and corn are nearly identical. Wheat should be coarsely ground before feeding.

Barley: For hogs, ground or rolled barley has about 90% the feeding value of corn. Barley is about equal to corn when it makes up one-third to one-half of the grain mixture. Grinding increases the value of barley about 15%. Scabby barley should not be fed. Pelleted barley diets containing adequate amounts of all required nutrients are nearly equal to diets based on ground yellow corn and the necessary supplements.

Milo (grain sorghum): This has become a significant energy source for swine in the Western and Southwestern parts of the U.S.A. The protein content will vary from 6 to 12% depending upon whether the crop is grown on irrigated or nonirrigated land and whether the soil was fertilized. In general, milo may be substituted for corn on an equal-weight basis in formulation procedures, being similar in metabolizable energy and lysine content. Since milo contains little or no carotene, vitamin A must be supplied. For most efficient use, milo should be ground and fed in a complete mixed diet.

Management of Sows and Litters: Preventing baby pig fatalities increases profits in the hog enterprise. About one-fourth of all pigs die before reaching weaning age. The following are management tips that will help reduce this loss:

1. The more vigorous a pig is at birth, the better are its chances of survival. To produce healthy pigs, the gestation diets need to be adequate in all nutrients.

2. The condition of the sow at farrowing and the need for using a laxative feed at farrowing is primarily a reflection of feeding during gestation. Constipation problems are minimal if the sow is limit-fed (2 kg/day) throughout gestation. After farrowing, the sow should be allowed to return to appetite as she chooses. Some form of limit feeding is recommended in late lactation beyond peak milk production.

3. As the pigs are born, the navel should be daubed with tincture of iodine. The value of daubing the navel is lost once the cord dries. Needle teeth should be clipped, taking care not to injure the gums. The tails may be docked to preclude the possibility of tail biting at some subsequent time.

4. Care should be taken to see that each pig has nursed. If necessary the milk flow (or "let-down") may be stimulated in some sows (R 173). If the sow is slow in coming to milk, weak pigs may gain from receiving artificial milk. Extra pigs or orphan litters can be raised on artificial milk, but success depends on good management and sanitation. Greater returns

may be gained by dividing pigs evenly among litters. Ear-notching pigs helps to identify the more productive litters at a future date.

5. An effective nutritional anemia-prevention program is essential to a successful swine production system (*see* p. 1238).

6. A palatable pig starter ration should be available from 3 weeks of age until time of weaning.

7. Boar pigs should be castrated at 4 weeks of age or earlier.

8. The use of some type of farrowing stall generally results in reduced baby pig mortality. The time of moving sow and litter to a nursing area (if this is part of the system) and the age of weaning vary with the physical facilities. Pigs are normally weaned between 3 and 6 weeks of age. With proper management and facilities pigs are often weaned in groups as they reach 12 to 15 lb starting at about 3 weeks of age.

9. Parasite control programs should be established for both external (q.v., p. 725) and internal parasites (q.v., p. 667).

Management of Growing Swine: The nutritional needs of growing-finishing pigs are best met by a program of full-feeding. Limited feeding will reduce the rate of gain considerably but may improve feed efficiency and the carcass quality of finishing pigs. If feed wastage is a problem with self-fed pigs, a feed saving would possibly be realized in a limited-feeding system. However, it is more desirable to adjust feeders to allow what is conveniently cleaned up.

TABLE 21 indicates space needs of growing swine. The management recommendations for growing pigs given herein are

TABLE 21. SPACE NEEDS OF GROWING-FINISHING SWINE

Items	Weaning to 75 lb	75 lb to 125 lb	125 lb to Market Size
Sleeping-space or shelter per pig, square feet			
Summer	4	5-6	8
Winter	4	5-6	8
Pigs per linear foot of self-feeder space (or per hole)			
On dry lot	4	3	3
On pasture	4-5	3-4	3-4
Percent of feeder space for protein supplement			
On dry lot	25	20	15
On pasture	20-25	15-20	10-15
For hand-feeding or hand-watering, running feet of trough per pig[1]	¾	1	1¼

[1] Access from one or both sides.

adapted from a report by the Nutrition Council of the American Feed Manufacturers Association. Recommendations for housing and space needs of swine are rapidly changing. It is currently recommended that growing-finishing swine be provided 4 sq ft of floor space from 50 to 125 lb, and 8 sq ft from 125 to 200 lb body wt, when the pigs are maintained on slatted or partially slatted floors. This assumes adequate ventilation.

Where high summer temperatures are a problem, installation of sprays or fogging nozzles may be profitable.

One automatic watering cup should be provided for every 20 pigs (an automatic waterer with 2 openings is considered equivalent to 2 cups). Pigs varying widely in weight should not be raised together. Ordinarily, the range in weight should not exceed 20% above or below the average.

Growth Stimulants: Antibiotics and arsenicals are commonly added to swine diets to promote growth. Antibiotics in general have resulted in a larger and more consistent response than the arsenicals when added to growing-pig rations. The levels of antibiotics fed to various-age swine should be in accordance with the recommendations of the manufacturers. Efficacy and approval for feeding is based on prescribed levels. The following statements summarize the research results dealing with antibiotics:

1. The inclusion of effective antibiotics in diets for growing swine tends to increase the rate of gain by about 10% on the average. This has been observed for both pasture and dry-lot feeding.

2. The average increase in feed efficiency due to antibiotic feeding of growing pigs is approximately 5%.

3. The antibiotics commonly used are penicillin (alone or in combination with streptomycin), chlortetracycline, oxytetracycline, bacitracin and tylosin. There are now legal restrictions on this use of some antibiotics.

4. For best results, the antibiotic should be left in the diet throughout the growing-finishing period.

5. The feeding of antibiotics causes pigs to increase their daily consumption of feed.

6. It may help to reduce the number of runts and unthrifty pigs and cause such pigs to make more rapid and efficient gains.

7. It helps in preventing and controlling scours and certain forms of enteritis. (This advantage may be lost if resistant strains of enteritis-causing organisms develop.)

8. Results of several studies indicate that feeding antimicrobial agents at breeding time and at farrowing result in improved reproductive performance.

9. There is considerable variability in the response from adding antibiotics to pig starters fed to suckling pigs. The inclusion of antibiotics in pig starters is recommended because of the possible value in controlling scours and in increasing feed consumption of the pigs.

10. The feeding of antibiotics to swine will not substitute for: (a) A good feeding program. The necessary protein, minerals and vitamins must be supplied in the proper dry-lot or pasture supplement to balance the cereal grains. (b) A good sanitation program. All steps of an effective swine sanitation system should be followed. (c) A good disease-control program. (d) A good breeding program.

HORSE NUTRITION

Feeding the horse is both art and science, and much of the current knowledge of horse nutrition is based on the observations of practical husbandry. The feeding recommendations given below are drawn both from experience and research. It is important to remember that horses are kept for a much longer time than most farm animals, and feeding programs must support the development of sound feet and legs which will sustain a long, useful and highly athletic life.

NUTRITIONAL REQUIREMENTS

Although horses obviously utilize hay and other roughage more efficiently than do other nonruminants, such as poultry or swine, the arrangement of the equine digestive tract limits this ability as compared with the ruminant. The site of fermentation in the horse is the cecum and large intestine, where large numbers of microorganisms digest hemicellulose and cellulose, utilize protein and nonprotein nitrogen and synthesize certain vitamins. Some of the products of fermentation such as volatile fatty acids and vitamins are absorbed and used. The microbial protein synthesized from nitrogen entering the cecum and colon undergoes only limited proteolysis, and the supply of essential amino acids from an unbalanced dietary nitrogen source is not satisfactorily balanced by microbial amino acids for optimum growth. The horse, therefore, is more dependent upon the quality of the diet than the ruminant.

WATER

Water requirements are dependent largely upon environment, amount of work being performed, the nature of the feed and the physiologic status of the horse. Daily consumption may vary from 5 to 12 gal. The working horse should be watered at least 3 to 4 times during the day. If the horse is hot, it should be cooled out first before being given unlimited access to water. If a horse is not being worked, it may be provided water *ad libitum*.

ENERGY

Energy requirements may be classified into those needed for maintenance, growth, pregnancy, lactation and work. Recent studies with light horses have resulted in prediction equations for estimating energy requirements. These equations permit the calculation of energy needs at any state of performance or production. Such estimates are provided in TABLES 22 and 23. It should be noted that individual differences of considerable magnitude exist in the need for energy, and some horses are "easy keepers", while others require prodigious amounts of feed. Thus, while these formulas provide a sound basis for estimating energy needs, the horseman should be aware of his responsibility to make a personal judgment of the energy needs of any individual horse.

Maintenance: To maintain body weight and support normal activity of the nonworking horse, digestible energy (DE) needs in Kcal/day equal $155W^{0.75}$, where W equals weight of the horse in kilograms.

$$DE \text{ (Kcal/day)} = 155 \, W_{kg}^{0.75}$$

WEIGHT CONVERSION TABLE

lb	kg	$kg^{0.75}$
100	45.4	17.5
200	90.7	29.4
300	136.1	39.8
400	181.4	49.4
500	226.8	58.4
600	272.2	67.0
700	317.5	75.2
800	362.9	83.1
900	408.2	90.8
1000	453.6	98.3
1100	499.0	105.6
1200	544.3	112.7
1300	589.7	119.7
1400	635.0	126.5

Growth: The DE requirements for growth (to be added to that for maintenance) can be estimated from the following equation in which Y equals the Kcal DE/day/gm of gain and X equals the fraction of adult weight.

$$Y \text{ (Kcal DE/day/gm gain)} = 3.8 + 12.3X - 6.6X^2$$

Pregnancy: There are few data on energy needs of pregnancy. Most of the tissue growth occurs during the last 90 days of gestation. The National Research Council has estimated that the increase in DE needs above maintenance during this period is 963 Kcal/day for a 500-kg (1,100 lb) mare.

Lactation: The National Research Council has estimated that 792 Kcal of DE/kg of milk produced per day should be added to maintenance needs to support lactation. Some data on average milk production of mares are shown below.

Months after foaling	average/Daily Milk Production (kg)		
	Draft horse	Light horse	Shetland pony
0 to 1	15.4	13.9	10.3
1 to 2	16.8	14.7	11.8
2 to 3	18.2	16.9	12.5
3 to 4	17.0	15.1	9.5
4 to 5	14.7	10.9	9.1

Work: Many factors such as type of work, condition and training of the horse, fatigue, environmental temperature and the skill of the rider or driver can influence the energy requirements of work. A guide to the amount of DE required above maintenance for various activities of light horses is shown below.

Activity	DE (Kcal/hr/kg body wt)
Walking	0.5
Light (slow trot, some cantering)	5.1
Medium (fast trot, cantering, some jumping)	12.5
Heavy (cantering, galloping, jumping)	24.0
Severe (strenuous effort, competitive racing)	39.0

PROTEIN AND AMINO ACIDS

Although some amino acid synthesis occurs in the cecum and large intestine, the entire amino acid needs of the growing, working or lactating horse cannot be met in this way. For this reason, the protein quality of the feeds used for horses is important. While dietary amino acid requirements have not been established, the feed recommendations presented in TABLE 24 contain an adequate distribution of those amino acids considered essential for the nonruminant.

Nitrogen needs expressed as crude or digestible protein are presented in TABLES 22 and 23. The young growing horse has a considerably greater need for protein than the mature horse. Also, the protein requirements of growing horses of the heavier breeds are higher at the same body weight than those of the lighter breeds. Fetal growth during the last fourth of pregnancy increases protein requirements slightly, while lactation increases requirements still further. Work apparently does not increase the protein requirement very much, providing the increased energy requirements are met. If a horse is ridden or driven hard without being fed enough to meet the increased demands for energy, body fat and then muscle will be metabolized, resulting in a net nitrogen loss.

MINERALS

Because the skeleton is of such fundamental importance to the performance of the horse, its mineral requirements deserve careful attention. However, excessive intakes of certain minerals may be as harmful as deficiencies. For this reason mineral supplements should be based on the consumption of the basic feeds in the diet. For example, if the horse is consuming mostly roughage with little grain, phosphorus is more likely to be in short supply than is calcium. However, if little roughage and much grain is being consumed, a shortage of calcium is most likely. Perhaps the largest problem in evaluating the adequacy of mineral intake is the availability of the minerals in the total ration. Aside from actual feeding trials, no suitable test for availability of minerals now exists. Some caution is necessary in interpreting mineral requirements.

Calcium and **phosphorus:** The requirements for these 2 elements are given in TABLES 22 and 23. The need during early growth is much greater than for maintenance of the mature animal. Work may increase requirements slightly, particularly for phosphorus. The last fourth of pregnancy and lactation increase the need appreciably. Aged horses may require 30 to 50% more calcium and phosphorus than is required for maintenance of younger horses. However, excesses of dietary calcium will interfere with the utilization of magnesium, manganese, iron and probably zinc. The calcium:phosphorus ratio should be maintained at not less than 1.1:1. A desirable ratio is about 1.5:1 although, if adequate phosphorus is fed, foals will tolerate a ratio of 3:1 and mature horses a ratio of 5:1.

Sodium and **chlorine:** Salt requirements are markedly influenced by perspiration losses. Fifty to 60 gm of salt may be lost daily in the sweat and 35 gm in the urine of horses at moderate work. Supplemental salt may be provided at the rate of 1% of the grain ration plus extra salt *ad libitum* to replace the losses during hard work and hot weather. If more convenient, the entire salt needs may be provided *ad libitum;*

TABLE 22. DAILY NUTRIENT REQUIREMENTS OF GROWING HORSES[1]
(100% dry matter basis)

Age	Body Weight		Percent of Mature Weight	Daily Gain		Daily Feed[2]		Digestible Energy	Daily Nutrients per Animal					
									Total Protein	Digestible Protein	Ca	P	Vitamin A[3]
Mo	kg	(lb)		kg	(lb)	kg	(lb)	Mcal	gm	gm	gm	gm	IU (thousands)
Growing Horses 200 kg (441 lb) Mature Weight													
3	50	(110)	25.0	0.70	(1.5)	2.94	(6.5)	7.43	526	383	17.4	10.9	2.0
6	90	(198)	45.0	0.50	(1.1)	3.10	(6.8)	8.53	462	315	16.6	10.4	3.6
12	135	(298)	67.5	0.20	(0.4)	2.89	(6.4)	7.95	338	206	12.0	7.5	5.4
18	165	(364)	82.5	0.10	(0.2)	2.94	(6.5)	8.08	314	181	10.4	6.5	6.6
42	200	(441)	100	0	(0)	3.00	(6.6)	8.24	300	160	8.0	6.0	5.0
Growing Horses 400 kg (882 lb) Mature Weight													
3	85	(187)	21.3	1.00	(2.2)	3.80	(8.4)	10.44	741	553	26.1	16.4	3.4
6	170	(375)	42.5	0.65	(1.4)	4.51	(9.9)	12.41	640	430	35.0	21.9	6.8
12	260	(573)	65.0	0.40	(0.9)	4.96	(10.0)	13.63	600	370	22.0	14.8	10.4
18	330	(728)	82.5	0.25	(0.6)	5.13	(11.3)	14.10	575	339	18.0	13.8	14.2
42	400	(882)	100	0	(0)	5.04	(11.1)	13.86	505	268	16.0	12.0	10.0
Growing Horses 500 kg (1102 lb) Mature Weight													
3	110	(243)	22.0	1.10	(2.4)	4.39	(9.7)	12.07	834	618	30.5	19.1	4.4
6	225	(496)	45.0	0.80	(1.8)	5.60	(12.3)	15.40	800	536	46.0	28.7	9.0
12	325	(716)	65.0	0.55	(1.2)	6.11	(13.5)	16.81	750	472	26.0	17.4	11.0
18	400	(882)	80.0	0.35	(0.8)	6.24	(13.8)	17.16	700	418	23.0	16.1	16.0
42	500	(1102)	100	0	(0)	5.96	(13.1)	16.39	597	317	20.0	15.0	12.5

Growing Horses 600 kg (1323 lb) Mature Weight

3	140 (309)	23.3	1.25	(2.8)	5.15	(11.4)	14.15	958	705	52.0	32.2	5.6
6	265 (584)	44.2	0.85	(1.9)	6.26	(13.8)	17.21	870	582	51.2	32.0	10.6
12	385 (849)	64.1	0.60	(1.3)	6.86	(15.1)	18.86	837	524	32.9	20.6	15.4
18	480 (1058)	80.0	0.35	(0.8)	6.98	(15.4)	19.20	775	458	31.3	19.6	19.2
42	600 (1323)	100	0	(0)	6.83	(15.1)	18.79	684	364	24.0	18.0	15.0

[1] Adapted from *Nutrient Requirements of Horses*, National Research Council, Revised 1972.
[2] Based on 2.75 Mcal DE/kg 100% dry feed.
[3] One mg of beta carotene equals 400 IU of vitamin A.

TABLE 23. DAILY NUTRIENT REQUIREMENTS OF MATURE HORSES[1]
(100% dry matter basis)

| Body Weight | | Daily Feed[2] | | Daily Nutrients per Animal | | | | | |
kg	(lb)	kg	(lb)	Digestible Energy Mcal	Total Protein gm	Digestible Protein gm	Ca gm	P gm	Vitamin A[3] IU (thousands)
Mature Horses at Rest (Maintenance)									
200	(441)	3.00	(6.6)	8.24	300	160	8.0	6.0	5.0
400	(882)	5.04	(11.1)	13.86	505	268	16.0	12.0	10.0
500	(1102)	5.96	(13.1)	16.39	597	317	20.0	15.0	12.5
600	(1323)	6.83	(15.1)	18.79	684	364	24.0	18.0	15.0
Mature Horses at Light Work (2 hr/day)									
200	(441)	3.80	(8.4)	10.44	383	202	8.0	6.0	5.0
400	(882)	6.68	(14.7)	18.36	672	355	16.0	12.0	10.0
500	(1102)	7.96	(17.5)	21.89	803	424	20.0	15.0	12.5
600	(1323)	9.23	(20.3)	25.39	930	491	24.0	18.0	15.0
Mature Horses at Medium Work (2 hr/day)									
200	(441)	4.79	(10.6)	13.16	483	255	9.2	7.0	5.0
400	(882)	8.65	(19.1)	23.80	871	460	17.2	13.0	10.0
500	(1102)	10.43	(23.0)	28.69	1047	553	21.2	16.0	12.5
600	(1323)	12.22	(26.9)	33.55	1229	649	25.2	19.0	15.0

Mares, Last 90 days of Pregnancy

200	(441)	3.16	(7.0)	8.70	364	216	10.4	8.0	10.0
400	(882)	5.41	(11.9)	14.88	613	375	19.5	15.0	20.0
500	(1102)	6.31	(13.1)	17.35	725	434	24.0	18.0	25.0
600	(1323)	7.25	(16.0)	19.95	837	502	28.0	21.0	30.0

Mares, Peak of Lactation

200	(441)	5.54	(12.2)	15.24	750	480	34.0	23.4	10.0
400	(882)	8.91	(19.6)	24.39	1181	748	42.0	35.6	20.0
500	(1102)	10.04	(22.1)	27.62	1317	829	47.0	38.6	25.0
600	(1323)	10.92	(24.1)	30.02	1404	876	64.0	43.4	30.0

[1] Adapted from *Nutrient Requirements of Horses*, National Research Council, Revised 1972.

[2] Based on 2.75 Mcal DE/kg 100% dry feed.

[3] One mg of beta carotene equals 400 IU of vitamin A.

TABLE 24. LIGHT-HORSE FEEDING GUIDE

Kind of Horse	Daily Allowance	Kind of Hay[1] (In season, any good pasture can replace part or all of the hay except for horses at work or in training.)	Suggested Grain Rations[1] (With all rations and for all classes and ages of horses, provide free access in separate containers to (1) salt [iodized or trace mineral salt in iodine-deficient areas] and (2) a mixture of ⅓ salt and ⅔ dicalcium phosphate or steamed bone meal.)		
			Ration No. 1	Ration No. 2	Ration No. 3 (alone)
Stallions in breeding season (weighing 900 to 1,400 lb)	0.75 to 1.5 lb grain/100 lb body wt, together with a quantity of hay within same range.	Grass-legume mixed (or ⅓ to ½ legume hay, with balance grass hay.)	Oats 55lb Wheat 20lb Wheat bran 20lb Soybean meal 5lb	Corn 35lb Oats 35lb Wheat 15lb Wheat bran 15lb	Oats
Pregnant mares (weighing 900 to 1,400 lb)	0.75 to 1.5 lb grain/100 lb body wt, together with a quantity of hay within same range.	Grass-legume mixed, or ⅓ to ½ legume hay, with balance grass hay (straight grass hay may be used first half of pregnancy.)	Oats 80lb Wheat bran 20lb	Barley 45lb Oats 45lb Wheat bran 10lb	Oats 95lb Soybean meal 5lb
Foals before weaning (weighing 100 to 350 lb with projected weights of 900 to 1,400 lb)	0.5 to 0.75 lb grain/100 lb body wt, together with a quantity of hay within same range.	Legume hay.	Oats 50lb Wheat bran 40lb Soybean meal 10lb (Rations balanced on the basis of the following assumptions: (1) Mares of lighter breeds [about 900 lb mature weight] will give foals about 4½ gal. milk daily; (2) mares of heavier breeds [about 1,400 lb/mature wt] will give foals about 6 to 6½ gal. milk daily.	Oats 30lb Barley 30lb Wheat bran 30lb Soybean meal 10lb	Oats 80lb Wheat bran 20lb
Weanlings (weighing 350 to 450 lb)	1 to 1.5 lb grain and 1.5 to 2 lb hay/100 lb body wt.	Grass-legume mixed (or ⅓ to ½ legume hay, with balance grass hay).	Oats 30lb Barley 30lb Wheat bran 30lb Soybean meal 10lb	Oats 70lb Wheat bran 15lb Soybean meal 15lb	Oats 80lb Soybean meal 20lb

Class of horse	Good luxuriant pastures²	Roughage	Suggested grain rations¹
Yearlings 2nd summer (weighing 450 to 700 lb)		Grass-legume mixed (or ⅓ to ½ legume hay, with balance grass hay).	Oats 80 lb, Wheat bran 20 lb — — Barley 35 lb, Oats 35 lb, Bran 15 lb, Soybean meal 15 lb — — (alone) / Oats
Yearlings or rising 2-year-olds; 2nd winter (weighing 700 to 1,000 lb)	0.5 to 1 lb of grain and 1 to 1.5 lb hay/100 lb body wt.	Grass-legume mixed (or ⅓ to ½ legume hay, with balance grass hay).	Oats 70 lb, Corn 30 lb — — Oats 70 lb, Barley 30 lb
Light horses at work, in riding, driving and racing (weighing 900 to 1,400 lb)	*Hard use:* 1.25 to 1.5 lb grain and 1 to 1.25 lb hay/100 lb body wt. *Medium use:* 0.75 to 1 lb grain and 1 to 1.25 lb hay/100 lb body wt. *Light use:* 0.4 to 0.5 lb grain and 1.25 to 1.5 lb hay/100 lb body wt.	Grass-legume mixed (or ⅓ to ½ legume hay, with balance grass hay).	Oats (alone) — — Oats 70 lb, Barley 30 lb — — Oats 70 lb, Corn 30 lb
Mature idle horses; stallions, mares, and geldings (weighing 900 to 1,400 lb)	1.5 to 1.75 lb of hay/100 lb body wt.	Pasture in season; or grass-legume mixed hay.	(With grass hay, add 0.75 lb daily of a high-protein supplement.)

¹ Good-quality oats and grass-legume hay are the standard feeds for light horses. However, feeds of similar nutritive properties can be interchanged in the ration as price relationships warrant. This makes it possible at all times to obtain a balanced ration at the lowest cost. Some of these feeds are: (a) the grains (oats, corn, barley, wheat and sorghum); (b) the protein supplements (linseed meal, soybean meal and cottonseed meal); (c) hays of many varieties.

² If in training or for other reasons without access to pastures, the ration should be intermediate between the adjacent upper and lower groups.

salt poisoning is unlikely unless a salt-starved animal is suddenly exposed to an unlimited supply of salt, or water is not available.

Magnesium: The daily magnesium requirement has been variously estimated at 14 to 34 mg/kg (6.4 to 15.4 mg/lb) of body wt. Outbreaks of tetany that respond to magnesium therapy have been reported from humid grassland areas. The addition of 5% MgO to the salt mixture has been protective.

Potassium: Forage-eating animals generally require about 0.6% potassium in their rations. Any horse ration that does not contain forage, molasses or oil meals may be limited in potassium. Any ration containing at least 50% of forage can be expected to meet the potassium needs.

Sulfur: It is doubtful that sulfur beyond that in methionine is a dietary essential. If the protein requirement is met, the sulfur intake of horses will usually be at least 0.15%—a level which is apparently adequate.

Iodine: Most iodized salts will provide the dietary iodine requirement which has been estimated to be 0.1 ppm. The iodine should be in a stable but available form. Pentacalcium orthoperiodate, calcium iodate, cuprous iodide, ethylenediamine dihydroiodide (EDDI) and stabilized potassium iodide are generally satisfactory. Diiodosalicylic acid is not recommended because of poor iodine availability. Iodine toxicity has been noted in pregnant mares consuming as little as 40 mg of iodine per day. Goiter due to excess iodine was noted in both mares and their foals, and several cases were associated with use of large amounts of dried seaweed (kelp) in the diet.

Cobalt: The dietary requirement for cobalt is apparently less than 0.05 ppm. It is undoubtedly incorporated into cyanocobalamin (vitamin B_{12}) by the microorganisms in the cecum and colon. Absorption of the synthesized vitamin is probably sufficient to obviate any need for preformed vitamin B_{12}.

Copper: The dietary copper requirement for horses probably does not exceed 8 ppm. The presence of 5 to 25 ppm of molybdenum in forages has interfered with proper copper utilization.

Iron: The maintenance requirement for iron is probably less than 40 ppm. For rapidly growing foals the requirement is estimated to be 50 ppm. Work with other species suggests that ferric oxide and ferrous carbonate are not effective iron supplements, and ferrous sulfate is the compound of choice.

Manganese: The requirement for the horse has not been established. The amounts found in the usual forages are considered sufficient.

Zinc: Based on work with other species, the zinc requirement is estimated at 50 ppm of the ration. This mineral is relatively innocuous and intakes several times the requirement are considered safe.

Fluorine: Fluorine has been shown to retard dental caries in humans, but the effects of excessive ingestion are of much more concern in horse nutrition. Rock phosphates, when used as mineral supplements for horses, should contain no more than 0.1% fluorine. Fluorine intake should not exceed 50 ppm in the diet or 1 mg/kg (0.45 mg/lb) of body wt.

Molybdenum: Although an essential cofactor for xanthine oxidase activity, no quantitative requirement for the horse has been demonstrated. Excessive levels may interfere with copper utilization.

Selenium: The requirement for selenium is inversely related to the alpha tocopherol content of the diet. The dietary requirement probably does not exceed 0.2 ppm, but there are regions of the world (including the lower Great Lakes states and part of New Zealand) where soils are deficient. In other areas (including parts of North and South Dakota) feeds may contain from 5 to 40 ppm of selenium, producing a characteristic toxicity (q.v., p. 947).

Perhaps the most satisfactory method of providing supplementary calcium, phosphorus and salt for horses is to furnish trace mineral salt on one side of a double-compartment box and a mixture of one-third trace mineral salt and two-thirds dicalcium phosphate on the other. If relatively more phosphorus than calcium is desired, a mixture of mono- and dicalcium phosphate is appropriate. The mineral box should always be protected from rain.

VITAMINS

Carotene and vitamin A: The vitamin A requirement of the horse can be met by carotene, a precursor of vitamin A in plants, or by the vitamin itself. Fresh green forages and good-quality hays are excellent sources of carotene. However, because of instability to oxygen and light, the carotene content decreases with storage, and hays that are a year old or more may not furnish sufficient vitamin A activity to meet requirements. Dietary beta carotene is converted to vitamin A by horses so that 1 mg is equivalent to approximately 400 IU. Horses that have been consuming fresh green forage will usually have sufficient liver vitamin A stores to maintain adequate plasma vitamin A levels for 3 to 6 months. The National Research Council has estimated that the vitamin A requirements for maintenance, growth, pregnancy and lactation are 25, 40 and 50 IU/kg (11.3, 18.1 and 22.7 IU/lb) of body wt, respec-

tively. These requirements expressed per pound of feed may
be found in TABLES 22 and 23. Prolonged feeding of excess
vitamin A may cause bone fragility, hyperostosis and epithelial
exfoliation.

Vitamin D: It is normally assumed that grazing horses or
horses which exercise regularly in sunlight and consume sun-
cured hay will have their requirements for vitamin D met in
this way. However, if exposure to sunlight is restricted by
confinement, hay may not always supply the requirement. It
has been estimated from other species that 6.6 IU of vitamin
D per kilogram (3 IU/lb) of body wt should be sufficient.
Vitamin D toxicity is characterized by general weakness, loss
of body weight, calcification of the blood vessels, heart, other
soft tissues, and bone abnormalities. Dietary excesses as small
as 10 times the requirement may be toxic and will be aggravated by excessive calcium intake.

Vitamin E: No research has provided unequivocal proof of
the beneficial effects of supplemental vitamin E, and certainly
no minimum requirement has been established. It seems quite
likely that selenium concentration in the feed is related to the
need for this vitamin. Based on work with sheep and cattle,
evidence of vitamin E deficiency might be most likely to appear in the foal nursing a mare on dry winter pasture or given
only low-quality hay unsupplemented with grain. Horses
forced to exert severe physical effort are also likely to develop
the deficiency if they are fed diets grown in low-selenium areas.
If selenium intakes are 0.15 ppm of the diet, it is likely that
5 to 10 IU of vitamin E per kilogram (2.3 to 4.5 IU/lb) of diet
would be adequate. (*See also* p. 1257.)

Vitamin K: This vitamin is synthesized by the microorganisms of the cecum and colon, probably in sufficient quantities
to meet the normal requirements of the horse.

Ascorbic acid: Ascorbic acid is synthesized by the tissues of
the horse, and this synthesis has been shown to be adequate for
maintenance of mature horses.

Thiamine: Although thiamine is synthesized in the cecum
and colon by bacterial action and about 25% of this may be
absorbed, thiamine deficiency has been observed in horses fed
poor-quality hay and grain. While not necessarily a minimum
value, 55 mcg of thiamine per kilogram (25 mcg/lb) of body
wt per day will maintain peak food consumption, normal gains
and normal thiamine levels in skeletal muscle. Occasionally,
horses are poisoned by consuming certain plants that contain
thiaminases or antithiamines (*see* BRACKEN FERN POISONING,
p. 977).

Riboflavin: Under certain conditions, riboflavin may be required in the diet. A number of reports have implicated riboflavin deficiency in periodic ophthalmia. One report indicates that the riboflavin requirement may be met by supplying 44 mcg/kg (20 mcg/lb) of body wt per day.

Cyanocobalamin (vitamin B₁₂): Intestinal synthesis of this vitamin is probably adequate to meet ordinary body needs, provided sufficient cobalt is present in the diet. Absorption of vitamin B_{12} from the cecum has been established, and the feeding of a B_{12}-free diet had no effect on the normal hematology of adult horses. Parenteral injections of vitamin B_{12} into race horses has been shown to result in rapid and nearly complete excretion of the injected dose. In cobalt deficient areas, the presence of the vitamin B_{12} in the ration may be useful.

Niacin: This vitamin is probably synthesized in adequate quantities by the bacterial flora of the cecum and colon.

Pantothenic acid: Bacterial synthesis in the intestinal tract probably meets the requirements for this vitamin. Although not necessarily a minimum figure, Shetland ponies appeared healthy when provided with 39.7 mcg/kg (18 mcg/lb) of body wt daily. The National Research Council has estimated that 2 mg/kg (0.9 mg/lb) of diet should be sufficient.

Folic acid, biotin and **vitamin B₆:** All these vitamins are probably synthesized in adequate quantities in the intestine.

FEEDS AND FEEDING PRACTICE

The horse is an athlete and to produce top performance it must be properly nourished and appropriately trained. Proper nourishment implies more than a simple provision of essential nutrients. The master horseman not only provides the essential nutrients, but provides them in an appropriate form at the proper time. Horses do best when regularly fed and, because they have a relatively limited capacity for roughage at any one time, they may need to be fed frequently. For a hard-working horse in harness or under saddle, this may mean feeding 3 or more times a day. Under these circumstances, the principle of "feeding a little at a time and often" is a good one. A horse should not be worked on a loaded stomach and if 3 meals a day are offered, the daily roughage ration should be split between the morning and evening meals and should be offered at least 1 to 2 hours before work starts. The noon meal should be light and 2 to 3 ears of corn might suffice. An alternative to this plan would be to feed one-fourth of the hay ration in the morning, a second fourth at noon and the remaining half at night.

Hot horses should be offered only small amounts of water

until they are cooled out. This water should be clean and fresh.

Because horses are particularly sensitive to toxins found in spoiled feeds, all grains and roughages should be of good quality and free from mold. Likewise, dusty feeds should not be fed because of their tendency to initiate or aggravate respiratory problems.

FEEDS

Pasture: The use of good pasture makes an ideal feeding program because it provides both nutrients and the opportunity to exercise. The pasture should be managed in such a way as to keep it free of weeds. Old, excessively mature growth should be clipped. A legume-grass mixture is ideal because it offers the advantages of good nutrient supply, a long grazing season and a long-lived stand. Alfalfa and smooth bromegrass make a good combination for many parts of the world, although many choices exist. Most grasses are improved by the presence of legumes.

Hay: The same species which make a good pasture usually make a good hay. Exceptions are low-growing plants, such as bluegrass and ladino clover. Legume-grass mixtures are generally high yielding and contain considerably more protein, minerals and vitamins than do grasses alone. However, they may be more difficult to cure in a humid climate, and moldy hay should be avoided.

Concentrates include the grains and by-product feeds high in energy or protein. In many instances it may be desirable to process them before feeding to improve nutrient availability and to increase their bulkiness (increase their volume per unit of weight). The bulkier concentrates are less apt to produce intestinal impaction and colic. Also the speed of digestion in the upper digestive tract is very important. Should any large volume of undigested grain reach the lower gut, the consequences can be serious. Excessive fermentation of such grain can result in founder.

Oats, perhaps the grain of choice, may be fed whole but rolling or crimping will increase its bulk 20 to 30% and will improve digestibility. Newly harvested oats may be dangerous due to the development of molds if their moisture content exceeds 14%.

Barley is a good grain for horses, which is higher in energy than oats but lower than corn. It may be fed as the only grain to horses that have a high energy need. It should be rolled or crimped.

Corn is a high-energy feed, useful for horses that are working hard or which are being fattened. It is low in bulk and more prone to produce colic than oats or barley if carelessly used. A good method of feeding is on the cob. This promotes salivation and the horse cannot bolt the grain. To maximize digestibility shelled corn may be cracked or rolled, but the moisture level should be low enough to avoid spoilage during storage.

Sorghum grain and *wheat* may be fed to horses with care to avoid colic. These grains should be cracked or rolled.

Wheat bran is a bulky, mildly laxative feed that is well liked by horses. It is a good feed on idle days and may be substituted for part or all of the regular concentrate ration on those days when a hard-working horse is not under saddle or in harness.

Soybean meal is a palatable protein supplement with good amino acid balance for use with grains. It might be fed when pastures or hay are low in protein and are of poor quality or when protein requirements are greatest, such as during early growth or lactation.

Linseed meal is also a very useful protein supplement. Its mucin content gives it a mildly laxative effect which may be helpful in certain feeding programs. The amino acid balance is not as good as that of soybean meal, being particularly low in lysine.

Cane molasses is frequently used to stimulate the appetite of poor eaters. It is low in dry matter but does supply appreciable energy due to its high sugar content. The sugar also increases the desire for water.

Corn oil may occasionally be useful in improving the appearance of the hair coat when the diet is of poor quality and the intake of dietary essential fatty acids is low. Approximately 50 ml (2 oz) of corn oil per day, placed on the feed, is quite effective. An excess should not be used because it may markedly increase the need for vitamin E.

Limestone of a high grade (38% calcium) may be used as a supplementary source of calcium when this element alone is needed. Such a situation might prevail when poor-quality grass pasture or grass hay is the only roughage provided. Grains, being low in calcium, will not help much. When both supplementary calcium and phosphorus are needed, *dicalcium phosphate, steamed bone meal,* or *defluorinated rock phosphate* is recommended. Dicalcium phosphate is particularly good because it is low in cost per unit of phosphorus, odorless, the elements are quite available and there is no danger of anthrax. *Monocalcium-dicalcium phosphate* mixtures will supply relatively more phosphorus than calcium, when the need for supplemental phosphorus is greater than that for calcium.

A supplement of both calcium and phosphorus might be needed when poor-quality grass pasture or grass hay is provided without grain. Grain containing appreciable phosphorus would tend to correct any deficiency of this element.

Salt (NaCl) should be provided in a block or in loose granular form *ad libitum*. It may be desirable to use a "trace mineralized" salt containing added iodine, iron, copper, cobalt, manganese and zinc. The need for these additional minerals will vary with the locality, but trace mineral salts are readily available and not costly. They may provide some nutritional insurance in areas where trace element deficiencies are a problem.

Succulent feeds: These feeds are high in water, are somewhat laxative and tend to stimulate the appetite. They should be introduced gradually when offered for the first time. Carrots are the safest and most satisfactory. A daily allowance of 1 to 3 lb is a desirable feeding rate. An artificial succulent feed can be made by soaking dried beet pulp in water sweetened with cane molasses. Well-preserved silage of good quality and free from mold affords a highly nutritious succulent forage during the winter months. As horses are much more susceptible to mold botulism and to digestive disturbances than are cattle and sheep, none but choice fresh silage should ever be fed. Various types of silages may be successfully used but corn silage and grass-legume silage are the most common. Mechanical silo unloaders may blend good and spoiled silage together and the spoilage may go undetected until digestive disturbances develop. Thus, the use of silage for horses is fraught with considerable danger.

Silage should not replace more than one-third to one-half of the roughage ration, considering that 3 lb of wet silage is approximately equivalent to 1 lb of hay. Thus, the silage allowance does not usually exceed 10 to 15 lb daily for a mature animal, although in some instances much larger amounts have been fed satisfactorily.

RATE OF FEEDING

Individual differences in the need for energy and nutrients make it difficult to generalize about the amount of feed to provide. The following rules of thumb will serve as guides and will usually satisfy the requirements. However, there is no substitute for observation and good judgment.

Horses at light work: Allow about 0.5 lb of concentrate and 1.25 to 1.5 lb of hay per 100 lb of body wt.

Horses at medium work: Allow about 1 lb of concentrate and 1 to 1.25 lb of hay per 100 lb of body wt.

Horses at hard work: Allow about 1.25 to 1.5 lb of concentrate and 1 lb of hay per 100 lb of body wt.

As will be noted from these recommendations, the total allowance of concentrates and hay will generally fall within the range of 2 to 2.5 lb daily per 100 lb of body wt. No grain should be left from one feeding to the next and all edible forage should be cleaned up at the end of each day.

The need for grain while on pasture depends on pasture quality, but is more important for young than for mature horses. It is desirable to creep-feed nursing foals and they will frequently eat good-quality hay even when on pasture. They may be given free access to a concentrate mixture if accustomed to this regime gradually.

SUGGESTED RATIONS

A light horse feeding guide is presented in TABLE 24 with suggested rations. While these will generally meet the needs of the horses for which they were designed, many other choices exist. It is logical to use feeds which are locally available and in certain areas of the world several of the feeds suggested are not grown or are too high in price. Alternatives should be chosen on the basis of nutrient composition, palatability and general suitability for the horse.

Today many complete pelleted feeds, incorporating both concentrate and roughage, are being used for horses. They have proved generally satisfactory, although some horses may develop the habit of cribbing when meal-fed. As all ingredients in a pelleted feed are ground before being pelleted, the problems connected with incomplete chewing are thus reduced, especially in older horses with dental problems. If properly compounded, some complete pelleted feeds can be fed *ad libitum* without danger, horses will tend to regulate intake to energy needs and few problems with cribbing will develop.

DOG NUTRITION

Although classified as a carnivore, the dog utilizes a wide variety of foodstuffs efficiently. This ability enables the dog to meet his nutritional requirements from a remarkable diversity of diets.

NUTRITIONAL REQUIREMENTS

Dogs regulate their food intake to meet their energy requirements, not to meet their requirements for any nutrient. The ideal way to provide a dog with its nutrient needs, therefore, is to balance the exact daily quantity of nutrients it needs into exactly the amount of food it will eat each day to obtain the energy it needs. A series of tables listing the energy and nutrient requirements for average-sized dogs has been prepared by the Subcommittee on Canine Nutrition of the National Research Council. Modifications of several of these tables are used in this discussion (TABLES 25 and 26). For those interested in a more detailed account of the dog's nutritional requirements, the bulletin *Nutrient Requirements of Dogs*, published by the National Research Council, 2101 Constitution Ave., Washington, D.C., provides an excellent source of material.

PROTEIN

The dog's protein requirements usually are met by commercial dog foods having a minimum of 20 to 28% mixed, good quality protein, on a dry-matter basis. This protein should constitute approximately 20% of the diet's total calories. A protein's ability to meet a dog's requirements depends on its quality and digestibility. The quality of a protein is related to its ability to supply amino acids in the correct quantity and proportion. The higher the quality of protein fed, the lower the percentage of total protein needed in the diet. Eggs, dairy products, muscle meats and the less tendinous organs are all sources of good-quality protein. Some vegetable proteins are also satisfactory sources of amino acids for dogs.

High protein intakes, to help maintain milk production, are indicated for lactating bitches. The appearance of high mortality among newborn pups has been associated with the protein composition of the bitch's diet. These losses can be stopped by feeding raw liver to the bitch during the gestation period.

CARBOHYDRATES

The dog utilizes carbohydrates with about the same efficiency as man. Carbohydrates are economical sources of energy and help spare proteins from being used for energy. To insure adequate amounts of proteins, fats, minerals and vitamins in the diet, carbohydrates should not constitute more than 60% of the calories in the diet. Starches are poorly digested raw, and should be cooked. Lactose (milk sugar) is poorly digested by some adult dogs and ferments in their intestinal tract, producing diarrhea. Bitch's milk contains less than one-fourth the amount of lactose of cow's milk. Sucrose (table sugar) can also produce intestinal disturbances.

FATS

Dietary fat supplies concentrated energy, essential fatty acids, and improves palatability. While only 2% fat is needed to supply essential fatty acids, fat levels of 12 to 14%, on a dry-matter basis, are more realistic to supply adequate energy. Although most dogs can tolerate rations containing more than 50% fat, some are nauseated at such levels. High-fat rations are undesirable, also, because the concentrated intake of calories produces a proportionate reduction in total food intake, with a resultant reduction of protein, mineral and vitamin intake.

Highly unsaturated fats (e.g., corn oil) will alleviate dry, scaly coats produced by an unsaturated fatty acid or total energy deficiency; 1 ml/10 lb of body weight daily will usually produce an improvement in such cases. The opened oil should be kept refrigerated.

Fats added during the manufacture of dry dog foods are stabilized with antioxidants to retard rancidity. Rancid fats destroy fat-soluble vitamins and may contribute to vitamin deficiencies.

VITAMINS

Dogs require at least 13 vitamins. One, ascorbic acid (vitamin C), can be synthesized by most dogs. The exact requirements for some vitamins are not precisely known, but it is possible to suggest levels which are adequate under most circumstances. TABLE 25 (p. 1266) presents a summary of currently estimated vitamin requirements.

Adding vitamin supplements to adequate commercial rations for healthy dogs is unnecessary. There are some diseases where specific vitamin requirements are increased and well-regulated supplementation may be useful. (*See* NUTRITIONAL DEFICIENCIES IN DOGS, p. 1338.)

MINERALS

The dog requires a number of dietary minerals for health (TABLE 25). Most balanced commercial foods contain these minerals in ample amounts. The metabolism of most minerals is interrelated and they are best utilized when provided in the proper ratio to one another. Calcium and phosphorus, for example, are best utilized when provided in a ratio of 1.2:1. Supplemental calcium should not be added to adequate rations. Excessive amounts of ingested calcium increase the requirement for phosphorus, manganese, zinc and other nutrients. Excess absorbed calcium may be deposited in soft tissue and

TABLE 25. NUTRIENT REQUIREMENTS FOR GROWTH OF DOGS
(In percentage or amount per kg of food)

Dog Food	Dry Basis	Dry Type	Semi-moist	Canned or Wet
Moisture level, %	0	10	25	75
Dry Matter Basis, %	100	90	75	25
Protein, %	22	20	16.5	5.5
Carbohydrate (maximum), %	71.5	65	54	18
Fat, %	5.5	5.0	4.0	2.0
Linoleic/arachidonic acid, %	1.6	1.4	1.8	0.4
Calcium, %	1.1	1.0	0.8	0.3
Phosphorus, %	0.9	0.8	0.7	0.25
Potassium, %	0.6	0.5	0.45	0.2
Sodium chloride, %	1.1	1.0	0.8	0.3
Magnesium, %	0.05	0.04	0.03	0.01
Iron, mg/kg	60	54	45	15
Copper, mg/kg	7.3	6.5	5.5	1.8
Cobalt, mg/kg	8.4	2.2	1.8	0.61
Manganese, mg/kg	5.0	4.5	3.6	1.2
Zinc, mg/kg	20	18	15	5.0
Iodine, mg/kg	4.8	4.4	3.6	1.2
Vitamin A, mg/kg	1.5*	1.4	1.2	0.4
Vitamin D, mg/kg	0.007**	0.006	0.005	0.002
Vitamin E (alpha tocopherol) mg/kg	48	43	36	12
Vitamin B12, mg/kg	0.02	0.002	0.017	0.006
Folic acid, mg/kg	0.18	0.17	0.13	0.04
Thiamine, mg/kg	0.73	0.65	0.55	0.18
Riboflavin, mg/kg	2.2	1.9	1.6	0.5
Pyridoxine, mg/kg	1.0	0.9	0.75	0.25
Pantothenic acid, mg/kg	2.2	1.9	1.6	0.54
Niacin, mg/kg	10.6	10	7.5	2.5
Choline, mg/kg	1200	1100	900	300

* The vitamin A quantity of 1.5 mg crystalline A = 5,000 IU/kg of ration;
1 mg vitamin A alcohol = 3,333 IU of vitamin A.
1 mg beta-carotene = 1,667 IU of vitamin A activity.
For dogs carotene is approximately one-half as valuable as vitamin A alcohol.
** This amount of pure vitamin D corresponds to 264 IU vitamin D/kg of feed.

joints producing arterial plaques and arthritis, or excreted in the urine where it may become a constituent of urinary calculi.

DOG FOODS

Commercial dog foods can be found in 4 general types—dry, canned, soft-moist and frozen—according to their processing method and water content. Since all of their energy and nutrients are in their dry matter, dog foods should be reduced to a dry-matter basis when they are compared. This can be done by eliminating the water mathematically (i.e., subtracting the percentage of moisture from 100%). To obtain the percent that each nutrient contributes to the total dry matter, the percentage of each nutrient is divided by the total dry-matter percentage. Other things that should be compared are the ingredient limitations and nutrient degradation inherent in each processing method, the relative digestibility of nutrients, the caloric density and the economics of each food.

Dry dog foods are available as biscuits, meals or expanded pellets. The latter form has become the most popular, and is made by combining meat and meat by-products, cereal grains, fats, vitamins and minerals; subjecting the mixture to heat and pressure, then forcing the resultant doughy mass through an extruder. The heat of processing converts starches into a more easily digestible form and destroys undesirable enzymes in soybean meal. But, heat also adversely affects heat-labile members of the B-complex vitamins and vitamin A. Because dry foods contain less than 10% moisture, more nourishment is available from them, pound for pound, than from any other type. They require no refrigeration and partially emptied containers can be returned to the shelf. Dry foods may become rancid or infested with insects or vermin with prolonged storage. The overall digestibility of most dry foods will average between 65 and 75%, and they will contain between 1,500 and 1,600 cal/lb.

Canned dog foods are available as a mixed ration, as the so-called "all meat" foods or as a stew. The fundamental differences between the 3 are the quantities of animal tissue used and the amount and nature of the plant foods incorporated into each. Ration-type foods contain a mixture of meat and meat by-products, cereal grains, vitamins and minerals. "All meat" foods contain almost nothing but meat and meat by-products such as liver, udder, lung, spleen and hollow viscera. Most are fortified with added vitamins and minerals. Stews contain meat and meat by-products along with vegetables such as carrots and peas and usually a gravy made from meat juices and starches or malto-dextrins. They too are frequently fortified with vitamins and minerals.

Canned foods contain between 62% (ration) and 78% ("all meat") water, but processing at temperatures of at least 250°F and air-tight sealing prevents them from spoiling. The heat of processing destroys some nutrients, particularly vitamins. The acceptability of canned foods usually exceeds that of dry foods. The digestibility of the total dry matter in canned foods averages 75 to 85% and they will contain approximately 500 cal/lb of ration-type or 600 cal/lb of "all meat".

Soft-moist foods are available as patties, pellets, extruded ribbons and simulated hamburger. Because they contain about 25% moisture, soft-moist foods must contain bacteriostats, fungistats and humectants to aid in preservation. Soybean meal, fresh meat by-products and sucrose constitute the major ingredients. Vitamins and minerals are added. The processing method destroys few, if any, nutrients. Although soft-moist foods do not require refrigeration, once the package is opened the food deteriorates quickly. The digestibility of the ingredients in soft-moist foods usually runs 80 to 85%. An average food contains 1,300 to 1,350 cal/lb. They are somewhere between dry and canned foods in acceptability.

Frozen foods are available as a mixture of fresh ingredients, or as a single ingredient such as a meat or a meat by-product. The quantity of moisture can be quite variable, depending upon the water content of the prefrozen product. Freezing destroys few, if any, nutrients, but the food must be kept frozen or it spoils quickly. Frozen meat and meat by-products vary from 1,200 to 1,600 cal/lb, while the mixed rations vary even wider, depending on their formula. Most frozen foods have a digestibility between 80 and 90%, and are probably the most palatable of all the food types.

DRUGS AND CONTAMINATING SUBSTANCES IN DOG FOODS

Various drugs and chemicals may find their way into dog foods, by accident, or as a means of easy medication. Several anthelmintics are available for adding to food as a means of reducing parasites in dogs. Chemicals used in the control of plant and animal parasites may find their way into feeds and cause injury to dogs. Such dogs usually recover if they are changed to an uncontaminated diet.

Dry dog foods occasionally become moldy, infested with insects or grain mites. The owner may be puzzled when his dog suddenly refuses to eat a food previously highly acceptable. Mite eggs pass in the feces of dogs consuming such foods and must be differentiated from true parasite ova. Occasionally the mites, themselves, are found in the feces. Moldy or spoiled foods should never be fed to dogs.

GENERAL CONSIDERATIONS IN FEEDING DOGS

When evaluating the nutritional problems of dogs, consider: 1) The conditions under which the dog lives. 2) The role the owner plays in dog nutrition is of as much practical importance as the dog's actual requirements. Owners may indulge their animals with foods that subject them to careless and haphazard feeding practices. 3) Extraneous substances may find their way into the diet. 4) The water content of the foods. 5) The limitations of the published chemical and biologic analyses of foodstuffs.

Neither the guarantees on a label nor the conventional chemical analysis tells much about the true nutritive value of a food. Protein, for example, is determined by analysis for nitrogen, which then is multiplied by a constant and expressed as protein. (No information is given regarding that protein's digestibility or biologic value.) Many of the large commercial producers of dog foods maintain elaborate research facilities designed to help evaluate and improve their products. During recent years many foods on the market have improved remarkably, and tampering with their formulation may do more harm than good.

Whenever supplementation is necessary, it should always be calculated on a dry-matter basis. For example, the addition of 4 oz of corn oil to 1 lb of canned food (which contains about 4 oz of dry matter) results in a 100% addition of fat. However, if 4 oz of corn oil are added to 1 lb of dry food (which contains about 14.4 oz of dry matter) the fat content is increased only 27%. While both of these examples probably represent excessive fat additions, that amount might be tolerated by the dog when added to the dry food. The same amount, added to canned food, however, would lower the intake of protein, minerals and vitamins to the extent that serious nutritional deficiencies would develop. Diets, marginal in one or more nutrients, having their fat level, hence their caloric density, increased, often produce a deficiency due to the decrease in the actual quantity of food eaten. Pets that are fed mostly table scraps often have an excess of fat in their diet.

TABLE 26 gives average caloric intakes needed to maintain dogs at various weights. Such a table only serves as a starting place, however. It is necessary to consider each dog individually and adjust each diet to the case at hand. A variety of things affect the dietary needs of a dog; these are:

Stages of the life cycle: Growth requires about twice the intake of nutrients, per pound of body weight, that adult maintenance does. Gestation may require an increase of 10 to 20% in food intake during the last weeks. Lactation requires as much as 300% increase in energy (hence food intake) by the fifth or sixth week of lactation.

Environment: Seasonal variations in environmental temperatures influence dietary intake, which varies inversely with the temperature. The winter-energy requirement may double over the summer requirement in cold climates. Dogs confined to

TABLE 26. ESTIMATED DAILY FOOD INTAKES REQUIRED BY DOGS OF VARIOUS SIZES

| Weight of Dog | | Requirements for Maintenance | | | | Requirements for Growth | | | |
| | | Dry-type food[1] | | Canned dog food[2] | | Dry-type food[1] | | Canned dog food[2] | |
kg	lb	per kg body wt gm/kg	per dog kg	per kg body wt gm/kg	per dog kg	per kg body wt gm/kg	per dog kg	per kg body wt gm/kg	per dog kg
2.3	5	40	0.09	120	0.27	80	0.18	240	0.54
4.5	10	33	0.15	101	0.46	66	0.30	202	0.92
6.8	15	28	0.19	85	0.58	54	0.38	190	1.29
9.1	20	27	0.25	81	0.74	54	0.49	160	1.45
13.6	30	25	0.34	77	1.05	50	0.68	154	2.10
22.7	50	25	0.57	75	1.70	50	1.13	150	3.40
31.8	70	25	0.79	75	2.38	50	1.60	150	4.80
49.9	110	24	1.20	74	3.69	38	2.40	—	—

[1] Dry food contains 6 to 12% moisture. Calculations of the amounts of dry food have been based upon energy supplied by food containing 90% dry matter, 77% protein plus carbohydrate, 5% fat and 10% ash, fiber and other material. This supplies a calculated 1,580 and 3,480 Kcal/lb and kg, respectively, of which 80% is digestible. On this basis digestible Kcal would be 1,264 and 2,784, respectively.

[2] Calculated on the basis of 25% dry matter and the same nutrient ratios as in [1] above, with the total and available energy calculated as 439 and 413 (85% of the total) Kcal/lb and 966 and 821/kg, respectively.

The daily food intake for soft-moist diets will depend on the precise moisture level, acceptability and caloric content. Individual soft-moist products vary in moisture levels.

Data adapted from NAS-NRC Publication 989, *Nutrient Requirements of Dogs*, 1962 Revision.

small pens or apartments have lower energy needs than dogs permitted to exercise in large pens or yards.

Exercise: Hard-working dogs, such as hunting dogs, racing dogs, and herding dogs may have their energy requirement increased as much as 50 to 70% above maintenance. High-energy concentrated rations are available for dogs with high-energy requirements. When increased energy is not provided, the animal may continue to work for a time, but only at the expense of body reserves, resulting in weight loss and debilitation. While extra exercise helps promote good muscular condition, it is not necessary for normal health. Dogs receiving limited exercise should be given a restricted diet to avoid undesirable gains in body weight.

Increased metabolism: Theoretically, hyperthyroidism, tissue injury and fever increase the basal metabolic rate and produce increased nutritional demands. It has been estimated that each 1°F of fever increases the calorie demand by 7%.

Malnutrition and corrections of weight deficiency: Neglect, the lost dog, and convalescence following severe blood loss, debilitation or parasitism are some of the common circumstances that necessitate diets high in protein, calories and vitamins. Protein levels of 1 to 2 gm/lb of body wt, a 50 to 70% increase in calorie intake above maintenance, and a daily dose of a multivitamin preparation calculated to provide at least the dog's minimum daily requirement, are good principles to follow when feeding such animals. It is better to bring these patients along slowly than to force gains too rapidly. Frequent daily feedings may help to increase the total food intake.

Obesity and correction of excessive weight: City dogs (which get little exercise) and those which are mature or approaching old age are often indulged by their owners. Because of the "treats" such dogs often receive, they are fed poorly balanced diets, high in sugars and fats. Discontinuation of all snacks and restriction of the amount of total food consumed to that amount which supplies only 60% of the calories needed to maintain the dog's normal body weight is indicated. An adequate vitamin and mineral intake is important. It may be desirable to provide a high level of protein intake (i.e., 1 to 2 gm/lb of body wt daily). Such animals usually are more content and have better bowel action if a fairly high level of fiber (e.g., 8% on a dry-matter basis) is included in their daily ration. The veterinarian's efforts to correct obesity are often undermined by lack of cooperation from owners, which may prove an insurmountable problem.

Disease: Many diseases respond favorably to dietary modification. Notable among these are chronic renal disease, congestive heart failure and gastrointestinal disorders. The primary objective in the dietary management of any disease should be to provide the dog with adequate nourishment while simultaneously compensating for metabolic or organic dysfunctions.

CAT NUTRITION

NUTRITIONAL REQUIREMENTS

Since the body weights of cats are more uniform than those of dogs, nutrient recommendations can be given either as a percent of the calories in the diet or a percent of the dry matter of the diet. Like the dog, the cat is able to meet its nutritional needs from a wide variety of diets. The nutritional requirements of the cat are given in TABLES 27 to 29.

PROTEIN

The cat has a uniquely high protein requirement. Healthy adult cats need at least 1.0 gm of a protein having a biologic value of 100, per pound of body weight per day, about twice that needed by the dog. Optimal diets for cats should contain at least 30% of the calories from protein. This amounts to 20% or more protein on a dry-weight basis. For growing kittens this amount should be increased to 33% or more. Protein suitable for cats must supply amino acids in the proper ratio and quantity. The more a protein is able to do this, the less of it is required to provide the cat's requirements. Animal proteins are, in general, more suitable for cats than plant proteins.

TABLE 27. GUIDE TO AVERAGE DAILY CALORIC REQUIREMENTS OF CATS

Age	Expected Wt lb	Daily Calorie Requirements Kcal/lb body wt	Total Daily Calories
Newborn-1 wk	0.25	190	50
1-5 weeks	1	125	125
5-10 weeks	2	100	200
10-20 weeks	4.5	65	290
20-30 weeks	6.5	50	325
Adult Tom	10	40	400
Adult Queen (pregnant)	7.5	50	375
Adult Queen (lactating)	5.5	125	690
Neuter { Male	9	40	360
Female	5.5	40	220

TABLE 28. RECOMMENDED VITAMIN ALLOWANCES
FOR THE CAT

Vitamin	Daily Dietary Allowance	Comment
A	1,000-2,000 IU (300-600 mcg)	Cannot utilize carotene
D	50-100 IU	May synthesize and lick from coat.
Essential fatty acids	1% total F.A.	Tolerate high saturated F.A. intake.
K	Not normally needed in diet	Intestinal synthesis supplies needs.
E (alpha tocopherol)	0.4-4.0 mg	Avoid diets high in α-poly-unsaturated F.A.
Thiamine (B₁)	0.2-1.0 mg	Increase during lactation, fever.
Riboflavin (B₂)	0.15-0.2 mg	Increase during lactation, fever and on high-fat diet.
Niacin	2.6-4.0 mg	Increase during lactation, fever.
Pyridoxine (B₆)	0.2-0.3 mg	Increase during lactation, fever.
Pantothenic acid	0.25-1.0 mg	
Biotin	0.1 mg	
Choline	100 mg	
Inositol	10 mg	
Folic acid	Levels not determined.	Intestinal synthesis occurs.
B₁₂ (cobalamins)	Levels not determined.	
C (ascorbic acid)	Not normally needed in diet.	Metabolic synthesis usually supplies cat's needs.

TABLE 29. RECOMMENDED MINERAL
ALLOWANCES FOR THE CAT

Element	mg/day
Sodium (minimum)	20-30
Sodium chloride	1,500
Potassium	80-200
Calcium*	200-400
Phosphorus*	150-400
Magnesium	8-10
Iron	5
Copper	0.02
Iodine	0.01-0.02
Manganese	0.2
Zinc	0.25-0.3
Cobalt	0.16

* Ca:P ratio—0.9-1.1.

FATS

As much as 60% of the calories in a cat's diet can come from fat, but diets containing between 14% and 40% on a dry-matter basis have been used most successfully. Diets containing the upper limits tend to produce obesity. If there is insufficient vitamin E in the diet, too much fat may lead to steatitis. Whatever the level of fat in the diet, it should contain not less than 1% linolenic or arachidonic acids. Fat has an important effect on the palatability of a cat's diet, and a small addition may materially improve a diet's acceptability.

CARBOHYDRATES

Although carbohydrates may not be essential in the cat's diet, they offer a less expensive calorie source than fat. Starches must be cooked or they will be digested poorly. Except for an occasional case of lactose or sucrose sensitivity, most carbohydrates are well tolerated by the cat, but will be poorly accepted unless incorporated into a diet properly formulated to appeal to the cat palate.

VITAMINS

Cats require at least 13 vitamins to maintain health. TABLE 28 presents the currently recommended vitamin allowances for the cat. Most commercial cat foods are fortified with vitamins making supplementation unnecessary. Such supplementation can even be dangerous.

MINERALS

While most vitamin requirements of the cat are greater than those of the dog, the mineral requirements are generally less. The current dietary requirements for minerals are listed in TABLE 29. The ratio of one mineral to another is as important as their dietary level. Injudicious supplementation with one or more minerals is more likely to do harm than good.

CAT FOODS

Commercial cat foods can be obtained in 3 different types: canned, dry and soft-moist. Like dog foods, cat foods should be reduced to a dry-matter basis for comparison (q.v., p. 1266). Most dog foods are not satisfactory for cats.

Canned cat foods are available as either ration-type or meat and meat by-product ("gourmet") foods. The latter may contain only a single ingredient, such as liver, shrimp or fish, and with or without fortifying mineral and vitamin mixes. Others may contain the full range of animal by-products seen in dog foods. Canned cat foods contain from 72% (ration) to 78% (meat) water. Heat, used in processing, may destroy some of the vitamin potency in any canned food. They are probably among the most palatable foods available for the cat.

Dry cat foods are available as expanded nuggets that may be molded into various shapes. The heat of processing can destroy some nutrients. Because of their processing limitations, some dry foods may contain too little fat to supply an adequate amount of energy daily. Most dry cat foods contain between 7 and 9% water. One of the most essential husbandry practices for cats eating dry foods is maintaining a constant water supply. The acceptability of dry cat foods ranges from very high to very low.

Soft-moist cat foods are available in several shapes. Their advantages and disadvantages are similar to soft-moist foods for dogs. The inability to incorporate fat above certain levels may cause some soft-moist cat foods to be marginal in energy for cats. Soft-moist foods contain about 25% water and their nutrients are between 75 and 85% digestible by the cat. Their acceptability is variable, but some are so palatable that their feeding must be restricted or the cat will become obese.

DRUGS AND CONTAMINATING SUBSTANCES IN CAT FOODS

The ingredients used in manufacturing cat foods may become contaminated in many ways. The levels of many of these contaminating substances are restricted by law, but usually at levels considered hazardous for humans. Generally speaking, cats become intoxicated at much lower levels than either humans or dogs. Consequently, cats may react to foods containing "safe" levels of contaminants. In particular, such substances as estrogens, chlorinated hydrocarbons and those with phenyl and cresyl bases are likely to be injurious.

GENERAL CONSIDERATIONS IN FEEDING CATS

Cats are not "finicky" eaters; healthy cats eat a variety of foods, and with the same enthusiasm as any other mammal. Being occasional feeders by nature, however, cats prefer to eat only about once every 24 hours. If fed more often, or continuously, they often become highly selective in what they eat. While odor, consistency, taste and learned dietary habits will determine which food a cat selects, such things as noises, lights, food containers, the presence or absence of man or other animals, and disease will determine how much of that food the cat will eat. Conditions requiring dietary modifications are:

Stages of the life cycle: Growth requires about twice as great a nutritional intake as maintenance does. Lactation also requires greatly increased nutrient intake. Because growing kittens and lactating queens cannot, physically, consume enough at one feeding to furnish their daily needs, they must be fed several times a day.

Environment: Seasonal variations in temperature may require a cat to eat twice as much during winter months as during summer months. This is especially true of cats that remain outdoors year-round or at night.

Alterations in optimum body weight: Both underweight and overweight cats may be seen. The diet must supply a balanced nutrient intake and a properly augmented or reduced energy intake given if either condition is to be improved.

Disease: Numerous diseases may require dietary changes. Any time the diet is so deficient as to cause disease the diet must, obviously, be changed to an adequate one. Diseases unrelated to deficiency may produce a more subtle, but equally important, dietary need. Among these are parasitic diseases, renal diseases, pancreatic diseases, hepatic diseases, gastrointestinal diseases and most metabolic disorders. (*See* FEEDING THE SICK CAT, p. 1315 and NUTRITIONAL DEFICIENCIES IN CATS, p. 1340.)

FUR ANIMAL NUTRITION

MINK

Although he wants optimum growth, quality fur development and top reproduction-lactation performance of his mink, the mink rancher must consider feedstuff availability and cost as well as nutritional balance of the diet. Modern ranch diets are formulated with a combination of fortified cereal, liver, muscle meats (horsemeat, nutria, rabbits, whole poultry), cooked eggs, packing house by-products (lung, rumen, spleen), poultry by-products (heads, feet, entrails) and fish (whole or fillet scrap). The fortified cereal provides digestible carbohydrates, vitamin concentrates and trace minerals.

The exact content of the practical ranch diet will vary from region to region depending upon the availability and economics of feed ingredients. However, nutritional rations within the final dietary mixture will be relatively similar throughout the industry. Ash levels of 7 to 8% on a dry-matter basis provide ample calcium and phosphorus for the mink. Protein levels should be consistent with the energy concentration of the diet, i.e., a good 10 percentage points above the level of fat present (e.g., minimum of 35% protein with a diet containing 25% fat).

It is important to stress fresh and frozen products which have been properly prepared and stored. Bacteria in the finished feed must be kept to a minimum if top performance is to be expected. Spoiled, off-odor feed products cannot be tolerated by the mink.

Proper nutritional balance in terms of protein, fat and minerals is essential for top performance and minimum feed volume per pelt produced—thus feed analyses during each phase of the year are important (low-energy diets can be very expensive in terms of feed volume while excessive-energy diets can provide suboptimum performance).

There should be ample water at all times for the mink and ample feed provision. Feed may be restricted in late February and March to keep animals trim for breeding and whelping but throughout the rest of the year the amount fed should be determined by the appetite of the animal. Mink may consume (on the average) as much as 8 to 10 oz of wet-mixed feed per day in the period from weaning to pelting. In the critical months of May and June they may be fed 2 to 3 times per day to meet the high nutritional demands for lactation and fast early growth. Twice daily feeding in July and August is common while once a day feeding is practical during the fur production months of September to December. The Sunday feeding may be omitted after the last week of September if the mink are in good condition.

A typical ranch diet would contain 20% fortified cereal, 80% of fresh or frozen meat products and enough water to provide a hamburger-like consistency. Common diets contain about ⅓ dry matter (feed solids) when fed to the mink on wire netting.

Nutrient requirements for the mink are given in TABLE 30. Water must be made available at all times via water cups, troughs or automatic pressure nipples. Feed for the young kits being started on feed (about 3 weeks of age) should be like porridge with a high water content.

Although the National Research Council (NRC) recommendation for the postweaning protein allowance is 25% on a dry-matter basis, most practical diets provide 35 to 40% protein in combination with 20 to 25% fat and 25 to 35% carbohydrate. A lean, high-protein diet with emphasis on cooked eggs, liver and muscle meats is used for the breeding-reproduction period from January into late April. Higher energy levels may be used during the lactation-early growth period (May–June) with higher levels of protein in the high caloric density diets. For the late growing period of July and August, good growth and minimum feed volume may be achieved with a diet containing 20% fortified cereal in combination with 25% fat and 35 to 37% protein on a dry-matter basis. For the fur production period (September–December), many ranchers use a "leaner" diet (20 to 22% fat on a dry-matter basis) and place a stronger emphasis on quality proteins like cooked eggs and muscle meats.

TABLE 30. NUTRIENT REQUIREMENTS FOR MINK
(In percentage of dietary dry matter, or amount per kilogram of dry matter fed)

Nutrient	Growth (Weaning to pelting)	Maintenance (Mature)	Pregnancy	Lactation
Energy (Kcal ME/kg dry diet)	5,300	4,250	5,300	*
Protein, %	25			
Vitamins				
Vitamin A, IU	3,500			
Vitamin E, mg	25			
Thiamine, mg	1.2	1.1		
Riboflavin, mg	1.5			
Pantothenic acid, mg	6.0			
Niacin, mg	20			
Pyridoxine, mg	1.1			
Folic acid, mg	0.5			
Minerals				
Salt (NaCl), %	0.5	0.5	0.5	0.5
Calcium, %	0.4	0.3	0.4	0.6
Phosphorus, %	0.4	0.3	0.4	0.6
Ca:P ratio	1:1 to 2:1	1:1 to 2:1	1:1 to 2:1	1:1 to 2:1

* Energy requirements for lactation increase sharply with (a) number of young produced and (b) growth of the young. The recommended level for growth may be taken as basal and increased according to the above criteria.

From *Nutrient Requirements for Mink and Foxes*, National Research Council, 1968.

More recently, rancher interest has centered on fortified cereal products containing fish meal or poultry meal which can be fed at levels as high as 35 to 70% of the diet (in combination with 30 to 65% fresh or frozen meat, poultry or fish products or a mixture of these). Recently 100% dry diets (mixed with water prior to feeding) and pellets have been made available for year-round practical mink nutrition.

In the planning of diets, consideration must be given to a number of factors in addition to nutritional content of the feedstuff. Ranchers must avoid products containing diethylstilbestrol residues and must be careful to exclude thyroid and parathyroid tissues from the mink's diet. Many freshwater fish such as carp, bullheads and smelt as well as ocean herring (but not freshwater herring) contain a thiaminase enzyme which destroys vitamin B_1 and causes Chastek paralysis in the mink. High levels of Pacific hake and Atlantic hake or whiting should not be used inasmuch as their formaldehyde content may inhibit iron absorption and lead to the development of "cotton fur". Eggs must be cooked to denature the avidin which would inhibit biotin absorption and lead to suboptimum fur development.

Fresh or frozen liver is an essential for top reproduction-lactation performance of the mink and should be fed at a 5 to 10% level (preferably the latter) during the period from February 1st into early June.

Commercial fortified cereal products are quite digestible for the mink inasmuch as they contain high proportions of cooked or toasted cereal grains. It is important to emphasize the fact that most raw grains except for oat groats must be cooked prior to incorporation in the diet inasmuch as the starches present in raw grains are relatively indigestible for mink.

The quality of fat used is important throughout the year. Fish or horse fat can bring about a disease known as "yellow-fat disease" unless the diet contains high levels of vitamin E. High levels of fat in the fall fur production months may contribute to a problem known as "wet-belly disease" (q.v., p. 1117), in which soiling of the inguinal region with urine may cause pelt damage. The use of a lean diet in September and higher levels of fortified cereal in late fall (late October and November) will minimize "wet-belly disease" problems on the ranch.

Mineral supplementation of the diet is not required if the rancher is using a quality, fortified cereal product. Diets containing 35 to 40% of bone-in products provide more than ample calcium and phosphorus for the needs of the mink. Extra salt supplementation (0.5% NaCl) may be used in the period from May 15th to late June to prevent the dehydration problem known as nursing anemia.

With the use of a quality fortified cereal, there is no need for extra vitamin supplementation unless the rancher is using high levels of fish scrap or rancid fish or horsemeat; such diets require a higher level of vitamin E. If the rancher is making his own cereal formulation, he may use commercial vitamin supplements with vitamin concentrations in the diet similar to those recommended by the NRC Sub-Committee on Fur Animal Nutrition. Vitamin A must be provided as the vitamin and not as beta carotene, which is inefficiently utilized by the mink.

CHINCHILLA

In their native habitat, chinchillas live at high elevations in the Andes Mountains of South America. The flora in this region consists of coarse grasses. The chinchilla, a herbivore, developed a highly efficient digestive system in order to survive in those regions. It is said to have the largest cecum of any animal in proportion to its size. The gastrointestinal tract is more than 10 ft long.

Diets containing large amounts of grains, nuts, meals, succulent grasses and other easily digested carbohydrates may cause bloat, diarrhea, prolapse or other digestive disturbances.

Chinchillas usually feed early in the evening or during the night and can be raised successfully on a diet consisting of a good grade of rabbit pellets and hay. They should be given just the quantity they will clean up in one 24-hour period—about 10 to 15 gm of pellets a day. It is believed that chinchillas require from 14 to 16% plant protein in their diet. Variations from this level may lead to difficulty.

The animals should have hay before them at all times to supply the large quantity of roughage they require. The more hay they consume in proportion to the amounts of pellets, the better. There is some diversity in opinion regarding the most satisfactory type of hay. At least 4 different kinds are being fed: alfalfa, timothy, bean straw and orchard or prairie hay. Although the chinchillas prefer alfalfa, there have been no controlled experiments to show which is superior. All of the hays should be fed dry and must not be moldy. The alfalfa and timothy hay should be clean, bright-green, and with pliable stems. Alfalfa hay is prone to absorb moisture and will mold rapidly at the temperatures occurring in many chinchilla houses. Dietary changes in hay should be gradual. The hay should not have been sprayed with commercial insecticides, such as chlordane. The chinchillas can tolerate only small quantities of such chemicals.

Only weak, debilitated animals require supplementary feeding. Such feeding to the entire herd may result in obesity in many of the animals. Wheat germ meal is a satisfactory supplement; it must, however, be stored in a cool place or it will become rancid. Raisins, apples and prunes may stimulate the appetite. Small quantities of succulent green feeds, such as dandelion leaves, lawn clippings and garden trimmings, may also be used. These foods must be collected from areas where dogs have not trespassed. Salt spools containing trace minerals may be provided. Animal protein or pellets containing cod or other fish oils should not be fed.

RABBIT NUTRITION

Pelleted rabbit feeds have largely supplanted home-grown feeds and provide good nutrition at low cost. TABLE 31 helps to summarize the information on nutritional requirements of rabbits at various productive phases.

The more nearly optimum the balance of the amino acids in the diet, the lower is the requirement for dietary protein.

TABLE 31. SOME MAJOR NUTRIENT REQUIREMENTS FOR RABBITS

| | Protein | | Fat | Fiber | Digestible Carbo-hydrates | Total Digestible Nutrients |
	Total %	Digestible %	%	%	(NFE), %	%
Maintenance	12	9	1.5-2.0	22-25	40-45	50-60
Growth and Fattening	16	12	2.0-4.0	16-20	45-50	60-70
Pregnancy	15	11	2.0-3.0	18-22	45-50	55-65
Lactation (with litter of 7 or 8)	17	13	2.5-3.5	15-20	45-50	65-75

Coprophagy, which is common in the rabbit, serves as a bacterial predigestion in the cecum. The bacteria can then be digested by the rabbit when reingested to supply protein, B-vitamin and improve the availability of some carbohydrates and minerals.

High-performing rabbits will consume about 3 times as much water as dry feed and should have free access to fresh, clean water. Rabbits require salt in their ration or free choice (blocks), as well as a supply of calcium, phosphorus, magnesium, manganese, potassium and other minerals in lesser or trace amounts. A trace mineral mixture is recommended.

The fat-soluble vitamins A, D, E and K are necessary. The dietary requirement is highest for vitamins A and E. Also, these vitamins may be more rapidly destroyed through oxidation than the others. Bacteria in the gut help to form vitamin K. Good rabbit feeds will supply a source of most B-vitamins although the dietary needs depend upon the performance rate desired. Disease and stress increase the need for daily vitamin intake.

EXOTIC AND ZOO ANIMAL NUTRITION

Fish, birds and rodents are the most common exotic pets purchased by private individuals and among the more successful inhabitants of zoos. Small initial investment, low maintenance costs and readily available commercial diets that guarantee success of such species are perhaps major factors in the popularity of such species.

Zoos have historically been moderately successful in maintaining the large herbivores as these animals adapt readily to a variety of roughages and grain supplements. In contrast, captive carnivores (mammals and birds), primates and reptiles have suffered gross nutritional abuse. Such problems are ag-

TABLE 32. SUGGESTED DIETS FOR ZOO ANIMALS

MAMMALS

Animal	Prepared or Additional Feeds	Meat	Egg	Milk	Greens	Bread	Apple	Orange	Banana	Sweet Potato	Carrot	Oatmeal	Corn	Bone Meal	Meal Worms	Alfalfa Hay	Timothy Hay	Apricots, Grapes, Prunes, Raisins
Monotremes																		
Echidna		+	R	+														
Marsupials																		
Virginia Opossum	Dog meal, pellets or canned dog food		+	+	+	+	+		+									
Tasmanian Devil	Canned dog food, young mice																	
Wombat	Equine pellets, rabbit pellets																	
Phalanger	Canned dog food, monkey pellets				+	+	+	+	+	+	+							
Kangaroo and Wallaby	Equine pellets, rabbit pellets															+		
Tree Kangaroo	Equine pellets, rabbit pellets						+		+	B	+	+						+
Insectivores																		
Hedgehog	Canned dog food, earthworms	B		+											+			

Animal									R/B	Diet
Philippine Tree Shrew	+		+	+				+	B	Canned marmoset diet
Mole	+					+			B	Canned marmoset diet
Solenodon	+		+	+	+	+		+	R	Crushed fruits and carrots, canned marmoset diet
Carnivores										
Cats										Canned feline diet, feline or carnivore sausage
Hyena		+								Canned feline diet, feline or carnivore sausage
Ringtail or Cacomistle				+	+	+			R	Dog pellets, canned feline diet
Raccoon, Kinkajou and Coatimundi			+	+	+.	+	+		R	Canned or semimoist dog food, dog pellets
Genet, Civet, Skunk				+		+			R	Dog pellets, canned feline food or feline sausage
Fox, Wolf										Dog pellets, semimoist dog food
Fennec Fox										Dog pellets, semimoist dog food
Badger				+		+				Dog pellets, semimoist dog food
Otter										*

R = raw   B = boiled
* See SPECIAL MIXTURES FOR MAMMALS, p. 1295.

continued on next page

MAMMALS (Continued)

Animal	Prepared or Additional Feeds	Meat	Egg	Milk	Greens	Bread	Apple	Orange	Banana	Sweet Potato	Carrot	Oatmeal	Corn	Bone Meal	Meal Worms	Alfalfa Hay	Timothy Hay	Apricots, Grapes, Prunes, Raisins
Giant Panda	*																	
Lesser Panda	*																	
Bear	Dog pellets; fish, omnivore diets	+				+	+				+							
Sea Lion	Fish (mackerel, herring; butterfish)																	
Rodents Squirrel, Marmot, Prairie Dog	Rabbit pellets, laboratory animal pellets, nuts, oats, sunflower seed				+	+	+	+	+		+		+			+		
Palm Squirrel	Rabbit pellets, laboratory animal pellets, sunflower seed, chopped fruits, dog pellets				+	+							+					
Kangaroo Rat, Pack Rat	Chopped fruits, dog pellets, rabbit pellets, laboratory animal pellets				+	+							+			+		

	Food											
Jerboa	Oats, millet seed, monkey pellets, laboratory animal pellets	+		+			+		+	+		
Beaver	Twigs and willow branches, rabbit pellets, laboratory animal pellets		+	+			+		+	+		
Porcupine	Dog pellets, branches (evergreen for American porcupines), rabbit pellets, laboratory animal pellets				+							
Hutia-conga	Rabbit pellets, laboratory animal pellets		+	+	+	+	+	+	+		+
Agouti	Laboratory animal pellets, monkey pellets, rabbit pellets		+		+	+					
Paca	Oats	+			+	+	+	+		+
Capybara	Oats, rabbit pellets, monkey pellets, laboratory animal pellets				+	+			+
Edentates											
Anteater	*	+	+	+	+	+	+	+		+
Armadillo	Canned dog food; meat, eggs and milk, mixed	+	+	+	+	+	+	+		+
Sloth	Leaves and twigs	+	+	+	+	+	+	+		+
Aardvark	*								R	+

R = raw   B = boiled
* See SPECIAL MIXTURES FOR MAMMALS, p. 1295.

continued on next page

MAMMALS *(Continued)*

Animal	Prepared or Additional Feeds	Meat	Egg	Milk	Greens	Bread	Apple	Orange	Banana	Sweet Potato	Carrot	Oatmeal	Corn	Bone Meal	Meal Worms	Alfalfa Hay	Timothy Hay	Apricots, Grapes, Prunes, Raisins
Even-Toed Hoofed Animals Antelope	Herbivore pellets or dairy conditioner (morning and evening feeding)															+	+	
Deer	Moose and deer pellets																	
Camel	Herbivore pellets and dairy conditioner				+		+				+					+	+	
Llama, Alpaca, Vicuna	Herbivore pellets and dairy conditioner				+		+				+					+	+	
Giraffe	Oats, dairy conditioner				+	+	+				+					+	+	
Hippopotamus	Equine pellets, dairy conditioner (equal parts)				+	+	+		+		+					+		
Odd-Toed Hoofed Animals Zebra, Ass	Equine pellets, herbivore pellets				+		+				+						+	
Rhinoceros	Equine pellets, dairy conditioner				+	+					+					+	+	

Animal	Food											
Tapir	Equine pellets, dairy conditioner					+		+			+	
Elephant	Equine pellets, dairy conditioner		+									
Hydrax	Rabbit pellets, barley	+	+	+		+		+			+	
Primates									+		+	
Lemur	Monkey pellets (moistened), leaves, berries and flowers, small stems	+	+	+		+		+	+		+	
Slow Loris, Galago	Monkey pellets (moistened)							B			B	
Gibbon, Baboon, Woolly Monkey, Macaque, Colobus, Grivet, Spider Monkey, Squirrel Monkey, Capuchin, Mangabey		+			+	+		+	+		+	
Marmoset	Monkey pellets, semi-moist dog food	+			+	+		+	+		+	
Tarsier	Boiled egg, monkey pellets, canned marmoset diet, lizards	+	+	+	+	+		+	+		+	
Gorilla, Orangutan	Grasshoppers, chameleons (Anolis); young mice, canned marmoset diet / * monkey pellets					+		+	+	+	+	

R = Raw   B = boiled
* See SPECIAL MIXTURES FOR MAMMALS, p. 1295.

Birds

Bird	Prepared or Additional Feeds	Greens	Apple	Banana	Orange	Sweet Potato	Bread	Scratch Feed*	Millet, Canary, Wild Grass Seeds	Mackerel	Smelts	Minnows	Herring	Soft Food Mixt. I*	Carnivorous Bird Diet	Soft Food Mixt. II*
Koel			+	+	+											+
Owl	Whole small rodents occasionally														+	
Frogmouth	Whole mice														+	
Nighthawk	Must be hand-fed														+	
Trogon, Quetzal	Quetzal food*		+	+	+						+	+				+
Kingfisher	Mice														+	
Laughing Jackass	Mice														+	
Motmot, Hornbill	Mice														+	+
Barbet, Toucan	Mice, meal worms, insects		+	+	+										+	+
Cock of the Rock	Young mice		+	+	+											+
Manakin, Pitta, Old World Oriole	Canned dog food for Pittas		+	+	+											+

Animal	Food
Crow, Magpie, Jay	Young mice
Bower Bird, Bird of Paradise	Insects, grapes, young mice
Babbling Thrush	
Tyrant Flycatcher	Insects
Bulbul, Mockingbird, Thrasher, Thrush	Insects
Shrike	
Starling, Mynah	Mynah bird pellets
Honey Eater	Liquid food*
Sugar Bird	Liquid food*
Warbler	Many insects
Finch, Waxbill, American Oriole, Blackbird	Soft Food Mixt. II for orioles; insects, thistle seed
Tanager	Liquid food*
Grosbeak, Finch	Seeds including sunflower seeds
Ostrich, Rhea, Emu, Cassowary	Game bird pellets, chopped alfalfa, ratite pellets, laboratory animal pellets, young mice
Tinamou	Game bird pellets

C = chopped   B = boiled
* See SPECIAL MIXTURES FOR BIRDS, p. 1295.

continued on next page

Birds *(Continued)*

Bird	Prepared or Additional Feeds	Greens	Apple	Banana	Orange	Sweet Potato	Bread	Scratch Feed*	Millet, Canary, Wild Grass Seeds	Mackerel	Smelts	Minnows	Herring	Soft Food Mixt. I*	Carnivorous Bird Diet	Soft Food Mixt. II*
Penguins Emperor, King	2 drops of saturated solution KI and one 000 capsule cod-liver oil every other day. Also butterfish									+						
Humboldt, Ringed, Galapagos, Fairy											+					
Loon, Grebe	Butterfish										+	+				
Pelican	Butterfish										+					
Cormorant, Snake Bird	Butterfish										+		+			
Heron, Bittern, Stork	Butterfish									+	+		+			
Ibis, Spoonbill	Kibbled dog biscuit, ground carrots										C	+				
Flamingo	Flamingo mix*															
Screamer	Game bird pellets	+						+								
Duck, Goose, Swan	Game bird pellets, duck pellets	+						+								

Bird	Food	Rats, mice, rabbits	Game bird pellets, ground peanuts for quail	Game bird pellets	Chopped boiled egg	Pigeon pellets	Grapes, pigeon pellets	Cut butterfish	Carrots, sunflower, hemp, canary seeds, large millet seeds, oats, peanuts, parrot pellets, pigeon pellets, monkey pellets	Liquid food*, canary seed, parrot pellets, pigeon pellets	Millet, oats, pigeon pellets	Canned dog food, whole mice for some Cuckoos
Secretary Bird, Vulture, Hawk	Rats, mice, rabbits	+										
Galliformes including Guan, Grouse, Quail, Pheasant, Peacock	Game bird pellets, ground peanuts for quail		+	+								
Crane, Rail	Game bird pellets			+								
Gallinule, Sun Bittern	Chopped boiled egg				C							
Pigeon, Dove	Pigeon pellets					+						
Fruit Pigeon	Grapes, pigeon pellets						+					
Gull, Teru, Avocet, Stilt, Plover	Cut butterfish							+				
Parrot, Macaw, Cockatoo	Carrots, sunflower, hemp, canary seeds, large millet seeds, oats, peanuts, parrot pellets, pigeon pellets, monkey pellets								+		+	
Lory, Lorikeet	Liquid food*, canary seed, parrot pellets, pigeon pellets									+		
Parakeet	Millet, oats, pigeon pellets								+		+	
Touraco, Cuckoo	Canned dog food, whole mice for some Cuckoos											+

C = chopped   B = boiled

*See SPECIAL MIXTURES FOR BIRDS, p. 1295.

REPTILES

Animal	Prepared or Additional Feeds	Canned Dog Food (all meat)	Fish	Smelt	Egg	Bread	Lettuce	Carrots, grated	Greens, chopped	Tomatoes (canned)	Apple	Banana	Melon
Alligator	Insects for immature; whole rodents for adults		+										
Crocodile	Insects for immature; whole rodents for adults		+										
Caiman	Insects for immature; whole rodents for adults		+										
Turtle, Tortoise Snapping Turtles	Insects	+	+										
Alligator Snapper			+										
Mud Turtle	Earthworms	+	+										
Box Turtle		+	+			+	+			+	+	+	+
Giant Tortoise		+				+	+		+	+	+	+	+
Snakes	Mice, rats, guinea pigs, rabbits, toads, frogs, lizards												

Animal	Food
King Cobra	Eats only other snakes in captivity, e.g., water snakes
Lizards	
Iguanas	Mice, dandelions
Gecko	Live insects
Basilisk Lizard	Live insects
Monitor	Day-old chicks
Skink	Tomatoes occasionally
Chameleon	Flies, grasshoppers, spiders (must be alive)
Salamander	Meal worms, earthworms
Electric Eel	

gravated by the biochemical and microbiologic instability of fresh diet ingredients and may be reduced by substitution of canned, dried or frozen feedstuffs in nutritionally adequate mixtures. The results of inadequate nutritional programs were advanced nutritional disease, physical deformities and early death in 25 to 75% of the exotic carnivorous species imported as pets or for zoological display.

More recently, numerous commercially prepared diets have been specifically designed for exotic species (monkey pellets, marmoset diet, feline canned diet or sausage and carnivore sausages, pellets for moose, deer and other herbivores as well as rodents, parrot pellets, mynah bird pellets, and omnivore foods). Such specific prepared diets and commercial diets developed for the domestic or laboratory animal trade have virtually eliminated the excuse for widespread nutritional disease in exotic pets or zoological specimens formerly fed mixtures of fresh foods cafeteria style. Commercially available human milk substitutes, bitch's milk, queen's milk, milk replacer, and whole cow's milk may be used as diets in sucklings of appropriate species.

Trace mineral salt blocks or spools (95% NaCl) should be made available *ad libitum* to all species of terrestrial and arboreal mammals and psittacine birds. The block should be securely affixed to the outside of the cage of large primates to prevent them from using it as a missile.

Branches and small limbs from unsprayed willow, poplar, mulberry, maple, or eucalyptus should be made available daily to gnawing forms of mammals (capybara, beaver, porcupine and small rodents) to maintain proper occlusion of the ever-growing incisors. Such material may also be offered to all species of primates as a form of low calorie constructive occupation. Alfalfa hay may be offered if continuous access to branches is not possible.

Some species of fish fed to exotic mammals, birds and reptiles (smelt, herring and minnows) have high tissue levels of thiaminase. Either such fish should be cooked before mixing with other diet ingredients, or diets containing such fish should be supplemented with thiamine at 10 mg/lb of fish to prevent the appearance of clinical thiamine deficiency (q.v., p. 1115 and in cats, p. 580).

A source of potable water should be available 24 hours per day. Accidental dehydration occurs often in winter when water sources freeze over and during the heat of late summer when higher intakes are required.

Recommended foodstuffs for preparing a dietary program for an exotic pet or zoological specimen are listed in TABLE 32.

SPECIAL MIXTURES FOR MAMMALS

Otter

Daily:
- 2 lb fish
- ½ lb raw meat
- ⅔ lb mixture of ground meat, dog or mink food and bone meal, with vitamin-mineral concentrate added (minimum 10 mg thiamine/lb of fish).

Lesser Panda

Morning:
- 1 cup Pablum
- ⅓ cup evaporated milk
- ½ tsp. honey
- 1 raw egg
- Vitamin-mineral concentrate

Evening:
- Cut fresh fruits
- Fresh bamboo sprays

Giant Panda

Morning:
- Formula as for Lesser Panda, increased quantity.

Evening:
- 6 apples   6 carrots
- 4 bananas   2 loaves of bread
- Greens (green soybean, cornstalks in season and fresh bamboo sprays)
- 1 qt dog biscuits

Anteater, Aardvark, Aardwolf

Mix together:
- 4 boiled eggs
- 8 oz ground meat
- 8 oz evaporated milk
- 16 oz water
- 2 oz Pablum or canned dog food
- 8 oz dog pellets
- Multivitamin-mineral concentrate
Mix in blender for best acceptability.

Gorillas, Orangutans
(4 to 6 years of age)

Morning:
- 1 to 2 pints skim milk and cereal (whole grain)
- 1 orange, 1 banana and 1 apple
- 2 tsp. multivitamin-mineral preparation
- 2 cups gelatin dessert

Noon:
- 1 to 2 pints skim milk
- ½ cup cottage cheese
- 1 banana, 1 apple, 1 boiled sweet potato, 1 orange

Evening:
- 4 oz canned or ground meat
- 4 slices bread
- 2 bananas
- 4 apples
- 3 oranges
- Greens
- Sugarcane
- 3 prunes or dried apricots
- 6 raw carrots
- 3 boiled sweet potatoes
- 1 hard boiled egg
- 1 to 2 pints skim milk

SPECIAL MIXTURES FOR BIRDS

Scratch Feed

- Oats
- Cracked Corn
- Kafir
- Wheat

Quetzal Food

- 2 tbsp. zwieback crumbs
- 2 tbsp. steamed brown rice
- 2 tbsp. grated carrot
- 1 tbsp. grated hard boiled egg
- 1 tbsp. cottage cheese

- 1 tbsp. Pablum
- ½ tbsp. brewers' yeast
- 15 drops cod-liver oil
Mix well and make into marble-sized pellets. Also feed diced bananas, grapes, cherries and raisins.

Soft Food Mixture I:

- Puppy meal
- Grated carrot
- Dried flies
- Powdered shrimp
- Finely ground cooked meat

Soft Food Mixture II:

A. ¾ gal. puppy meal finely ground.
   Mix 1 oz cod-liver oil with the
   meal.
   ¼ gal. dried flies.
   Mix with the above 6 lb diced
   bananas, ⅓ lb grated apple
   and ½ head finely chopped
   lettuce or escarole.
B. 5 grated hard boiled eggs
   1 cup steamed brown rice
   1 cup grated carrot
C. Ground scalded heart.
Place a small portion of each on each
feeding dish.

Liquid Food:

A.M.
   2 tsp. honey
   1 tsp. Pablum

1 tsp. condensed milk
Beef extract
3 drops vitamin concentrate
Water (q.s. ad 8 oz)
P.M.
Water } Equal parts
Honey }

Flamingo Diet

2 lb mixed, precooked cereal
9 lb trout Chow no. 4
1 cup oyster shell flour
1 tbsp. iodized salt
1¼ cup brewer's dried yeast
3 lb shrimp meal, dried
8 cups Super Caradee
4 cups laying mash
Mix well with 4 gal. water to soupy
consistency. (1 day's ration for
25 birds)

It should be stressed that a complete prepared product should
be supplemented with only minimal amounts (10 to 15% of
the total diet) of fresh foods. To reverse this, i.e., to offer
the prepared diet only as a supplement to a great mound of
fresh food, will produce poor results.

POULTRY NUTRITION

NUTRIENT REQUIREMENTS

In the sixth revision of the Nutrient Requirements of
Poultry published by the National Academy of Sciences
(1971), nutrient requirement figures were not increased by
"margins of safety" as had been customary in the past. The
values are actual requirements derived from experimentally
determined levels found by various research workers to be adequate for normal growth, health and productivity. The requirement figures should cover most populations; however,
such factors as varying nutrient composition of feed ingredients and differing feed mixing and storage conditions may
reduce nutrient levels to below those intended. Because of
this and since such factors as high environmental temperature
may increase nutrient needs, the feed formulator may wish to
add "margins of safety" by increasing the levels suggested in
the nutrient requirement TABLES, 33 to 38, shown below. These
requirements for chickens, turkeys, ducks, pheasants, bobwhite
quail and Japanese quail are in terms of percentages or units
per kilogram of feed, which accords with customary practice.

ENERGY, PROTEIN AND AMINO ACIDS

The metabolizable energy requirement values are corrected to nitrogen equilibrium as most poultrymen and feed manufacturers express available energy for poultry diets on this basis. It is difficult to establish energy requirements per unit of feed since birds adjust their feed intake in an attempt to satisfy energy needs. Also, protein requirements can be stated only in relation to the energy level of the diet and degree of fat deposition desired. This calorie:protein ratio concept extends also to amino acids. Some of the amino acid requirement figures in TABLES 33 and 34 were established by direct experimentation while other values were calculated, assuming the amino acid requirements to be proportional to protein requirements.

The 13 amino acids shown in TABLE 33 are considered to be essential for poultry. While glycine can be synthesized by poultry there must be enough dietary serine present to provide for this need. Cystine and tyrosine are considered essential even though they can be replaced by methionine and phenylalanine, respectively. There are 2 important relationships between individual amino acids and vitamins in practical feed formulation; methionine can spare choline as a methyl donor, and tryptophan can be used to synthesize niacin. These are practically important interrelationships since the 2 vitamins can be supplied in diets more economically than the 2 amino acids.

A number of feeding programs have been devised to restrict energy, protein and amino acid intakes of replacement pullets to retard growth and to delay the onset of sexual maturity to give optimum results in the laying and breeding periods. These systems are particularly important for broiler-strain pullets.

VITAMINS

Vitamin requirements are presented in TABLES 35, 36, 37 and 38 in terms of milligrams per kilogram of diet except in the case of vitamins A, D and E, which are given in International Units (IU) or International Chick Units (ICU).

One IU of **vitamin A** activity is equivalent to 0.6 mcg of beta carotene; 1 mg of beta carotene = 1,667 IU of vitamin A. In the chicken, as in the rat, 0.6 mcg of beta carotene is equivalent to one USP unit of vitamin A, except when the carotene intake provides vitamin A activity greatly in excess of the requirement. The vitamin A requirements recommended herein are based on the use of stabilized vitamin A preparations and are thus somewhat lower than previously recommended levels.

Requirements for **vitamin D** are expressed in ICU. Birds use vitamin D_3 from fish oils and irradiated animal sterol quite effectively, but vitamin D_2 from irradiated ergosterol is less efficacious for birds than for rats and other mammals. One ICU of vitamin D represents the vitamin D activity of 0.025 mcg of pure vitamin D_3. With low levels of phosphorus there may be a difference in the efficacy of vitamin D_3 and vitamin D derived from fish oils, particularly with turkeys. However, this should not be a consideration with the levels of calcium and phosphorus recommended herein.

One IU of **vitamin E** is equivalent to 1 mg of synthetic DL-alpha-tocopherol acetate. The requirements of vitamin E will vary depending upon the type and level of fat in the diet, the level of selenium, the levels of trace minerals and the presence or absence of antioxidants other than vitamin E.

The growing chicken can use betaine as a methylating agent, but betaine cannot replace choline in preventing perosis. Betaine is widely distributed in practical feedstuffs and may be important as a sparer of choline. Vitamin B_{12} can also reduce the requirement of the chick for choline. The choline requirement values presented are applicable to diets containing the specified levels of vitamin B_{12}.

MINERALS

The calcium requirement of laying hens is difficult to define. Adding too much calcium to diets interferes with the utilization of several other minerals and fat, and tends to reduce the palatability of the diet and to cause roughening of the egg shells. The recommended level of 2.75% for laying birds is adequate for most conditions but hens subjected to environmental temperatures of 85° to 90°F or more for prolonged periods require a level of 3.0 to 3.5% calcium.

UNIDENTIFIED NUTRIENTS

The chick is known to have a quantitative requirement for 39 nutrients, including metabolizable energy. There is evidence that there are still some unidentified growth and hatchability factors present in such ingredients as dried whey, marine by-products, distillers' solubles and green forages.

ANTIBIOTICS

Antibiotics have been used in poultry feeds since 1950 as a means of increasing growth rate and improving feed efficiency. They are still effective for this purpose and are used at a level of 2 to 10 mg/kg of feed depending on the antibiotic used.

However, in some countries regulations now restrict this usage for certain antibiotics, and care should be taken to comply.

FEED REQUIRED FOR GROWTH AND EGG PRODUCTION

Data on the amounts of feed required and the time required to attain certain weights in chicks and turkeys are presented in TABLES 39 and 40. The values are typical for the breeds under consideration.

Data showing the approximate quantities of feed required by chickens of different live weights for maintenance and for the production of various numbers of eggs per annum are shown in TABLE 42.

The figures in TABLES 39, 40 and 42 are intended merely as a guide in estimating the amount of feed required for a particular purpose. Considerable variation from the figures presented may result from differences in the nutrient density of feed, the strain or breed used, the amount of feed wasted, and the environmental temperature.

FEEDING AND MANAGEMENT PRACTICES

Most of the diets used in feeding poultry are commercially mixed rather than home-mixed; in general they are prepared by feed manufacturing companies, most of which employ trained nutritionists. The formulation and mixing of poultry feeds is a highly technical job involving the use of an increasing amount of knowledge and experience in purchasing ingredients, the use of computers, experimental testing of formulas and laboratory control ingredients. Improper mixing can result in vitamin and mineral deficiencies, lack of protection against disease or chemical or drug toxicity. Laboratory control is needed to insure good-quality feed.

The physical form of the feed exerts an important bearing on the results to be expected. More and more feeds for starting and growing birds are being sold in the form of crumbles or pellets. The pelleting process involves treating the mash with steam and then passing the hot, moist mash through a suitably sized die under pressure. The pellets are then cooled quickly and dried by means of a forced air draft. The conditions used in pelleting have an important bearing on the nutritional quality of the pellets, or the crumbles which result from rolling the pellets.

METHODS OF FEEDING

"All-mash" rations, or so-called "complete" feeds are, in general, those which are to be used without supplementation

TABLE 33. ENERGY, PROTEIN AND AMINO ACID REQUIREMENTS OF CHICKENS

	Broilers			Replacement Pullets (Egg- or Meat-Type)			Laying and Breeding Hens (Egg- or Meat-Type)
	0-6 weeks	6-9 weeks	0-6 weeks	6-14 weeks	14-20 weeks		
Metabolizable energy (Kcal/kg)	3,200	3,200	2,900	2,900	2,900	2,850	
Protein (%)	23	20	20	16	12	15	
Arginine (%)	1.4	1.2	1.2	0.95	0.72	0.8	
Glycine and/or serine (%)	1.15	1.0	0.8	0.8	0.6	?	
Histidine (%)	0.46	0.4	0.4	0.32	0.24	?	
Isoleucine (%)	0.86	0.75	0.75	0.6	0.45	0.5	
Leucine (%)	1.6	1.4	1.4	1.1	0.84	1.2	
Lysine (%)	1.25	1.1	1.1	0.9	0.66	0.5	
Methionine (%)	0.86	0.75	0.75	0.6	0.45	0.53	
Methionine (%) or Cystine (%)	0.46	0.4	0.4	0.32	0.24	0.28	
	0.40	0.35	0.35	0.28	0.21	0.25	
Phenylalanine (%)	1.5	1.3	1.3	1.05	0.78	?	
Phenylalanine (%) or Tyrosine (%)	0.8	0.7	0.7	0.55	0.42	?	
	0.7	0.6	0.6	0.5	0.36	0.4	
Threonine (%)	0.8	0.7	0.7	0.55	0.42	?	
Tryptophan (%)	0.23	0.2	0.2	0.16	0.12	0.11	
Valine (%)	1.0	0.85	0.85	0.7	0.5	?	

TABLE 34. ENERGY, PROTEIN AND AMINO ACID REQUIREMENTS OF TURKEYS

	Male 0-4 Female 0-4	4-8 4-8	8-12 8-11	12-16 11-14	16-20 14-17	20-24 17-20	Mature Breeders
Metabolizable energy (Kcal/kg)	2,750	2,810	2,930	3,020	3,095	3,170	2,850
Protein (%)	28	26	22	19	16.5	14	14
Arginine (%)	1.6	1.5	1.3	1.1	1.0	1.0	?
Glycine and/or serine (%)	1.0	0.95	0.8	0.7	0.6	0.8	?
Histidine (%)	0.55	0.5	0.45	0.35	0.3	0.25	?
Isoleucine (%)	1.1	1.0	0.85	0.75	0.7	0.55	?
Leucine (%)	1.9	1.8	1.5	1.3	1.1	0.95	?
Lysine (%)	1.5	1.4	1.2	1.0	0.9	0.75	?
Methionine (%)	0.87	0.8	0.7	0.58	0.52	0.43	?
or							
Methionine (%)	0.52	0.48	0.4	0.35	0.31	0.26	?
Cystine (%)	0.35	0.32	0.3	0.23	0.21	0.17	?
Phenylalanine (%)	1.80	1.65	1.4	1.20	1.10	0.90	?
or							
Phenylalanine (%)	1.00	0.95	0.8	0.67	0.60	0.50	?
Tyrosine (%)	0.80	0.75	0.65	0.53	0.50	0.40	?
Threonine (%)	1.00	0.95	0.8	0.70	0.60	0.50	?
Tryptophan (%)	0.26	0.24	0.2	0.17	0.15	0.13	?
Valine (%)	1.2	1.1	0.95	0.80	0.70	0.60	?

TABLE 35. VITAMIN, MINERAL AND LINOLEIC ACID
REQUIREMENTS OF CHICKENS[1]
(In percentage or amount per kilogram of feed)

	Starting Chickens (0-8 weeks)	Growing Chickens (8-18 weeks)	Laying Hens	Breeding Hens
Vitamin A activity (IU)[2]	*1,500*	*1,500*	4,000	4,000
Vitamin D (ICU)[3]	*200*	*200*	500	500
Vitamin E (IU	*10*	?	?	?
Vitamin K1 (mg)	0.53	?	?	?
Thiamine (mg)	1.8	?	?	0.8
Riboflavin (mg)	3.6	1.8	2.2	3.8
Pantothenic acid (mg)	10	10	2.2	10
Niacin (mg)	27	11	10[4]	10[4]
Pyridoxine (mg)	3	?	3	4.5
Biotin (mg)	0.09	?	?	0.15
Choline (mg)[5]	1,300	?	?	?
Folacin, starch diet (mg)	0.55	?	0.25	0.35
Folacin, sugar diet (mg)	1.2	?	?	?
Vitamin B12 (mg)	0.009	?	?	0.003
Linoleic acid (%)	?	?	1.0	1.0
Calcium (%)	1.0	0.8	2.75[6]	2.75[6]
Phosphorus (%)[7]	0.7	*0.4*	0.6	0.6
Sodium (%)[8]	0.15	0.15	0.15	0.15
Potassium (%)	0.2	0.16	?	?
Manganese (mg)	55	?	?	33
Iodine (mg)	0.35	0.35	0.30	0.30
Magnesium (mg)	500	?	?	?
Iron (mg)	80	?	?	?
Copper (mg)	*4*	?	?	?
Zinc (mg)	*50*	?	?	*65*
Selenium (mg)	*0.1*	?	?	?

[1] These figures are estimates of requirements and include no margins of safety. Italicized figures are tentative.

[2] May be vitamin A or provitamin A.

[3] See text, page 1298. These levels of vitamin D are satisfactory when levels of calcium and readily available phosphorus conform to this table.

[4] In diet that contains 0.15% of tryptophan.

[5] See text, page 1297.

[6] This amount of calcium need not be incorporated in the mixed feed because calcium supplements fed free-choice are considered part of the ration.

[7] At least 0.5% of the total feed of starting chickens should be inorganic phosphorus. All the phosphorus of nonplant feed ingredients is considered to be inorganic. Approximately 30% of the phosphorus of plant products is non-phytin phosphorus and may be considered part of the inorganic phosphorus required. A portion of the phosphorus requirement of growing chickens and laying and breeding hens must also be supplied in inorganic form. For birds in these categories, the requirement for inorganic phosphorus is lower and is not as well defined as for starting chickens.

[8] Equivalent to 0.37% of sodium chloride.

TABLE 36. VITAMIN AND MINERAL REQUIREMENTS
OF TURKEYS[1]

(In percentage or amount per kilogram of feed)

	Starting Poults (0-8 weeks)	Growing Turkeys (8-16 weeks)	Breeding Turkeys
Vitamin A activity (IU)[2]	4,000	4,000	4,000
Vitamin D (ICU)[3]	900	900	900
Vitamin E (IU)	10	?	25
Vitamin K₁ (mg)	0.7	?	?
Thiamine (mg)	2.0	?	?
Riboflavin (mg)	3.6	?	3.8
Pantothenic acid (mg)	11	?	16
Niacin (mg)	70	?	?
Pyridoxine (mg)	4	?	?
Biotin (mg)	0.3	?	?
Choline (mg)	1,900	?	?
Folacin (mg)	0.9	?	0.8
Vitamin B₁₂ (mg)	0.003	?	?
Calcium (%)	1.2	0.8	2.25[4]
Phosphorus (%)[5]	0.8	0.7	0.75
Sodium (%)[6]	0.15	0.15	0.15
Potassium (%)	0.4		?
Manganese (mg)	55	?	33
Magnesium (mg)	500	?	?
Iron (mg)	60	?	?
Copper (mg)	6	?	?
Zinc (mg)	70	?	?
Selenium (mg)	0.2	?	?

[1] These figures are estimates of requirements and include no margins of safety. Italicized figures are tentative.

[2] May be vitamin A or provitamin A.

[3] See text, page 1298. These levels of vitamin D are satisfactory when levels of calcium and readily available phosphorus conform to this table.

[4] This amount of calcium need not be incorporated in the mixed feed because calcium supplements fed free-choice are considered part of the ration.

[5] At least 0.5% of the total feed of starting poults should be inorganic phosphorus. All the phosphorus of nonplant feed ingredients is considered to be inorganic. Approximately 30% of the phosphorus of plant products is nonphytin phosphorus and may be considered part of the inorganic phosphorus required. Presumably, a portion of the requirement of growing and breeding turkeys must also be furnished in inorganic form.

[6] Equivalent to 0.37% of sodium chloride.

with whole grain. As intimated above "all-mash" may in fact be in the form of crumbles or pellets and not mash so that the designation "complete" feeds is perhaps more correct. For newly hatched or starting birds of any species, the use of a "complete" feed in crumble form is the program of choice regardless of other considerations. The use of "complete" feed programs for growing stock, and particularly for laying and breeding stock, is also highly recommended. Among the advantages of the complete-feed program over the "mash and grain" system are the simplicity of feeding, accuracy of medi-

TABLE 37. NUTRIENT REQUIREMENTS OF PHEASANTS
AND QUAIL[1]
(In percentage or amount per kilogram of feed)

	Pheasants	Bobwhite Quail		Japanese Quail	
	Starting and Growing	Starting and Growing	Breeding	Starting and Growing	Breeding
Total protein (%)	30[2]	28	?	*24*[3]	*24*
Lysine (%)	?	?	?	*1.4*	?
Methionine and cystine (%)	?	?	?	*0.75*	*0*
Vitamin A activity (IU)[4]	?	13,000	?	?	?
Vitamin D (ICU)[5]	*1,200*	?	?	*480*	?
Riboflavin (mg)	*3.5*	?	?	?	?
Pantothenic acid (mg)	*10*	10	?	*30*	?
Niacin (mg)	*60*	?	?	?	?
Calcium (%)	?	?	2.3	0.8	?
Phosphorus (%)	1.0	?	1.0	*0.65*[6]	?
Sodium (%)	0.085[7]	0.085[7]	?	?	?
Chlorine (%)	0.11	0.11	?	?	?
Iodine (mg)	0.30	0.30	?	?	?
Zinc (mg)	?	?	?	*25*	?

[1] These figures are estimates of requirements and include no margins of safety. Italicized figures are tentative.
[2] At energy level of 2,300 Kcal of metabolizable energy per kilogram of feed.
[3] May be reduced to 20% at 3 weeks of age.
[4] May be vitamin A or provitamin A.
[5] See text, page 1298.
[6] At least 0.3% of the total feed should be inorganic phosphorus as defined in footnote 7, Table 35.
[7] Equivalent to 0.21% of sodium chloride.

TABLE 38. NUTRIENT REQUIREMENTS OF DUCKS[1]
(In percentage or amount per kilogram of feed)

	Starting and Growing Ducks
Total protein (%)	17
Vitamin D (ICU)[2]	220
Riboflavin (mg)	4
Pantothenic acid (mg)	11
Niacin (mg)	55
Pyridoxine (mg)	2.6

[1] These figures are estimates of requirements and include no margins of safety.
[2] See text, page 1298.

cation, improved balance of dietary nutrients, and superior feed conversion efficiency.

Where an economical supply of local grain is available, the mash and grain system may, however, prove to be more profitable. On the other hand, with the increased use of bulk bins and automatic feeders, the saving in labor costs with the simplified, "complete" system of feeding makes it attractive to many poultrymen in spite of other considerations.

Regardless of the system of feeding employed, the poultryman should follow the recommendations of the feed manufacturer with regard to the feeding of extra calcium, grit or whole grain. Plenty of fresh, clean water should be available at all times.

MANAGEMENT OF GROWING CHICKENS

In cold weather, a solid chick guard is used around the hover to keep the chicks from straying and to prevent floor drafts. In warm weather a wire guard may be used. The guard is initially placed 2 to 3 ft from the edge of the hover; gradually it is expanded, and removed at the end of a week. Feeder trays and waterers should be evenly distributed in the area between the hover edge and the chick guard.

At least 3 in. of suitable litter, spread to an even depth, is provided at the start. Litter must be free from mold; it should be able to absorb moisture without caking, be nontoxic and of large enough particle size to discourage its being eaten. It is stirred and fresh litter added as needed. Clean litter should be used for each brood. Chicks are started with 24 hours light, and thereafter given at least ½ hour of darkness each 24 hours to get them used to lights going out. Both length of day and intensity of light are important considerations. In rearing, length of day should never be decreased. This fundamental principle has no exception but feeding in the rearing period combines with day-length control to influence the rate at which birds mature. Where light intensity cannot be controlled in rearing, pullets should be debeaked at 4 to 7 days of age. In controlled environment housing, with dim lights, this job may be delayed until later in the growing period.

Pullets should be treated for external and internal parasites as required. Vaccination can control many diseases and should be utilized for the problem diseases of the area (*see* the infectious diseases portion of the poultry section, p. 1010 et seq. for details).

MANAGEMENT OF LAYING CHICKENS

The sooner the pullets are housed in their laying quarters the better (plan to have them there no later than 2 weeks before egg production commences). Beaks should be retrimmed as necessary and culls removed at time of housing.

Feeders should be of the proper type and size for the stock and management system. If the lip of the feeder is level with the backs of birds there will be less feed wastage. Feeders which are too shallow, too narrow or lack a lip or flange on the upper edge may permit excessive wastage of feed.

Artificial Lights: Sufficient light should be used to provide an average 13- to 14-hour light period daily for both market egg and hatching egg layers. An intensity of at least one footcandle of light at the feed trough (10.76 lux) should be provided; this is approximately equal to one 60-watt light bulb to each 100 sq ft (about 9 sq meters), hanging 7 ft (2.13 meters) above the birds. Production may be impaired if light intensity is reduced during the laying period. With cage systems of all types, more even illumination is achieved by using smaller wattage bulbs closer together rather than large bulbs. Ceiling and wall surfaces should be light in color and bulbs suspended over the center of each aisle. With 2- or 3-tiered cages, the bulbs are suspended at a height 6 to 7 in. (15 cm) above the level of the top cage.

Record Keeping: To be successful in intensive poultry keeping, records should be kept of everything that happens to the flock including such things as batch date, regular body weights, quantity and type of feed given, mortality (so that amount of feed to give can be accurately calculated), disease history, medications, vaccination dates, light program and pen temperatures.

Floor Space, Feeding and Watering Requirements: There is a trend to house egg-production and even broiler stock in cages right from the start. For broiler breeders, buildings with up to ⅔ slatted floor area have distinct advantages over all-litter types. For egg strain pullets reared from day of age to end of egg-production cycle in cages, there is little chance of altering the feeding and watering space available, but periodic checks are necessary to ensure that feed and water are being continuously supplied. With the success of nipple and cup-type waterers and the various types of automatic feeding arrangements it becomes more difficult to give specific recommendations for feeding and watering space. Floor space allotments will vary with such factors as the selling price of eggs and the cost of feed. The poultryman must make the decisions as to proper floor space and feeding and watering requirements based on advice from equipment manufacturers, careful observation and past experience as to profitability.

The space requirements for egg-strain and meat-strain birds set forth in TABLES 41 and 43 will serve as a useful guide.

TABLE 39. FEED REQUIRED AND TIME REQUIRED TO OBTAIN CERTAIN AVERAGE LIVE WEIGHTS OF CHICKENS

Average Live Weight (kg)	Kind of Chicken and Quantity of Feed (kg) Required per Bird				Kind of Chicken and Age (weeks) at Which Certain Live Weights Are Reached			
	White Leghorns		Broiler Strains		White Leghorns		Broiler Strains	
	Females	Males	Females	Males	Females	Males	Females	Males
0.25	0.5	0.45	0.40	0.35	3.2	2.9	2.4	2.0
0.5	1.15	1.0	0.85	0.80	5.8	5.0	3.8	3.6
0.75	1.85	1.6	1.35	1.30	8.2	6.8	5.0	4.4
1.0	2.65	2.35	2.0	1.85	10.6	8.3	6.0	5.3
1.25	3.8	3.15	2.7	2.4	13.3	9.7	7.0	6.0
1.5	5.3	4.1	3.5	3.0	16.4	11.3	8.0	6.9
1.75	8.2	5.3	4.4	3.7	19.8	13.0	9.0	7.8
2.0	—	—	5.4	4.5	—	—	10.4	8.5

TABLE 40. FEED REQUIRED AND TIME REQUIRED TO OBTAIN CERTAIN AVERAGE LIVE WEIGHTS IN BROAD-BREASTED BRONZE AND WHITE TURKEYS

Average Live Weight (kg)	Quantity of Feed (kg) Required per Bird		Age (weeks) at Which Certain Live Weights Are Reached	
	Females	Males	Females	Males
0.25	0.3	0.3	2.0	1.8
0.5	0.75	0.75	3.5	3.3
1.0	1.75	1.6	5.6	5.2
1.5	3.0	2.6	7.0	6.9
2.0	4.25	3.9	8.3	7.6
2.5	5.6	5.1	9.7	8.7
3.0	7.2	6.35	11.0	9.6
4.0	10.6	9.1	13.5	11.2
5.0	15.0	12.35	16.3	13.1
6.0	20.45	15.8	19.2	14.9
7.0	26.65	19.25	23.1	16.8
8.0	—	23.15	—	18.6
9.0	—	27.2	—	20.5
10.0	—	31.75	—	22.3

TABLE 41. SPACE REQUIREMENTS FOR EGG-STRAIN BIRDS

CAGES

Age in Weeks	Floor Area per Bird		Straight Trough Feeder Space per Bird Not Less Than		Birds per Nipple	Birds per Cup	Trough Space per Bird	
	sq in.	sq cm	in.	cm			in.	cm
0-6	25	156	1.0	2.5	15	25	1.0	2.5
7-18	43	277	2.0	5.0	8	12	1.0	2.5
19 onward	60	388	3.0	7.5	8	12	2.0	5.0

LITTER AND SLATS

Age in Weeks	Floor Area—Litter Only or Combined With Slats		Straight Trough Feeder Space per Bird		Pans (15" Dia.) per 100 Birds		Drinkers	Trough Space per Bird	
	Sq ft/bird	Birds/ sq meter	in.	cm	Full Fed	Restricted	Birds per Fount	in.	cm
0-6	0.5	20	1.0	2.5	3	—	100	1.0	2.5
7-13	1.0	10	2.0	5.0	4	5	50	1.0	2.5
19 onward	1-1.5	7-10	3.0	7.5	4	—	30	2.0	5.0

TABLE 42. FEED REQUIRED BY CHICKENS OF DIFFERENT LIVE WEIGHTS FOR MAINTENANCE AND FOR VARYING LEVELS OF EGG PRODUCTION

Average Live Weight		Average Total Feed Required per Bird per Year for Maintenance and the Production of the Indicated Number of Eggs			
kg	lb	0 Eggs per Year (kg)	100 Eggs per Year (kg)	200 Eggs per Year (kg)	300 Eggs per Year (kg)
1.36	3.0	21.5	28.0	34.0	40.5
1.59	3.5	23.5	30.5	36.5	43.0
1.81	4.0	25.5	32.5	38.5	45.0
2.04	4.5	27.5	34.0	40.5	47.0
2.27	5.0	29.5	36.0	42.5	49.0
2.50	5.5	31.5	38.0	44.5	51.0
2.73	6.0	33.5	40.0	46.5	52.5
2.95	6.5	35.5	42.0	48.0	54.5
3.18	7.0	37.0	43.5	50.0	56.5

TABLE 43. SPACE REQUIREMENTS FOR MEAT-STRAIN BIRDS

Age	Floor Space	Feeder Space*	Cups or Founts* (per 1,000 birds)
From Day 1	Heated area 5 sq ft (0.46 sq meter) of brooder per 100 chicks	10 trays per 1,000 (feed little and often)	8
From Week 1	1 sq ft per bird (10-11 birds per sq meter)	2 in. (5 cm) per bird	20
From Week 8	2 sq ft per bird (5-6 birds per sq meter)	4 in. (10 cm) per bird	30
Mated Adults	All litter: 3 sq ft per bird (3.6 birds per sq meter)	4 in. (10 cm) per bird	30 (60 in hot weather)
	½ to ⅔ slats: 2 ¼ sq ft per bird (4.3 birds per sq meter)		

* For feeder and drinking trough space, count both sides of the trough. Drinking trough space (all ages) is 1 in. (2.5 cm) per bird, except double this for adults in hot weather.

Pen Size: The smaller the pen population the better the average flock performance. The ideal flock size depends on several factors, including labor and cost and can only be determined by the individual poultryman.

NUTRITION OF SICK ANIMALS

The response of sick animals to certain rations or specific nutrients will depend on the nature and duration of the illness. Two basic aspects must be considered: (1) determining and eliminating the cause of the illness, and (2) supplying the necessary nutrients which will facilitate, as rapidly as possible, a return to health and efficient production. Nutrition of sick animals requires clinical wisdom, knowledge of disease processes and applications of the principles of medicine and nutrition.

Basic Considerations: In general, well-fed animals are more resistant to bacterial and parasitic infections but are probably more susceptible to viral infections. Good nutrition is of value during the recovery phase of any disease process, whether it be of viral or bacterial origin. Diseases that precipitate inappetence, diarrhea and high fever cause the greatest depletion of nutrients from the body. Efforts should be directed to minimizing nutritional depletion. Feeds and nutrients that improve appetite and restore losses from the digestive tract are most important. Specific therapeutic diets should be considered in distinct entities such as a low-sodium diet in cardiovascular disease, a low-fat diet in pancreatic disturbances and the use of lipotrophic nutrients such as choline and methionine in liver diseases. It is also important to understand the "cause and effect" relationship characterizing nutritional therapy. Even though a nutrient markedly influences recovery from an illness, it may be erroneous to conclude that the original disturbance was due to a nutritional deficiency.

General Principles: Nutritional therapy consists of providing a normal ration modified to provide for the nutrients lost during the course of the disease, and if necessary, to increase its palatability.

The oral route is the method of choice for administering nutrients. If there is complete anorexia, nutrients may be given in warm water by stomach tube. Parenteral therapy to provide immediate nourishment is indicated in prostrate animals. Depending on the nature of the illness some general principles to consider are:

Restoration of appetite: Because inappetence accompanies many illnesses, palatability assumes a particular importance. Ruminants will often eat good-quality roughage, including green forage, when they will not consume concentrate mixtures. Rations high in urea not only tend to be unpalatable but may also be toxic in sick animals. Also in ruminants, factors required in rumen fermentation such as the mineral elements, especially cobalt, should be fed. Inoculation of the rumen with cud material may be helpful in chronic disturbances of the rumen. Sweetening rations with a small amount of molasses will often induce feed consumption. Small amounts of fresh feed every few hours is better practice than a large amount at one feeding. Most feed not readily consumed should be removed before the next feeding as it may become stale and unpalatable. Housing sick animals in close proximity to animals eating normally will often encourage feed consumption. Parenterally administered glucose, protein hydrolysates, vitamin B_{12} and other vitamins aid in stimulating the appetite and supply immediate supportive treatment.

Readily available energy: This is especially important in animals in which digestion and metabolism are impaired or reduced. Energy is required to meet the normal requirements of body functions. During fever, requirements are estimated to be increased by 5 to 7% with each increase of 1°F in body temperature. Low blood glucose values may produce serious neurologic disturbances. Administration of glucose aids the liver in detoxifying toxic products. Meeting energy requirements minimizes tissue nitrogen catabolism. In addition to parenteral glucose, to correct an acute weakness, a low-fiber, appetizing type of ration should be fed. In cold environments, body heat loss should be minimized by providing heated stabling or covering the animal with blankets.

Quality and quantity of protein: It may be important to supply an improved quality of protein for sick animals. This may be accomplished by feeding proteins of high biologic values such as milk or eggs. Vital tissue protein must be replaced, as well as proteins associated with other vital substances, such as enzymes and hormones, and those needed to form immune substances to resist infection. In most diseases, the quantity of protein may be increased 4 to 5% to replace the losses due to increased catabolism. High levels of protein are not indicated during impaired renal function because of the threat of accumulating nitrogenous end products in the blood.

Fat: Good-quality fat has merits in some therapeutic diets. In the monogastric animal it increases palatability, is a concentrated source of energy, and aids in the metabolism of the fat-soluble vitamins. It also supplies the essential fatty acids that may aid in correcting skin disturbances.

Fluids, electrolytes and minerals: Fluid and electrolyte imbalance are deterrents to organ function. Proper extra- and intracellular electrolyte composition must be maintained. During enteric disturbances, large volumes of water and electrolytes, especially sodium and potassium, may be excreted. Alkalosis or acidosis will dictate the choice of electrolyte solutions to be used in therapy. Caution should be exercised in potassium administration as indiscriminate use may be harmful. Fresh clean water should always be easily available. Anemia is present in many illnesses due to either increased loss of blood or deficient synthesis of hemoglobin. The diet of anemic animals should be carefully balanced, and the presence of adequate amounts of vitamins K and B_{12} and iron should be assured.

Vitamins and unidentified growth factors: In sickness the requirement for vitamins and possibly for unidentified growth factors is increased. The depletion of water-soluble vitamins is relatively rapid, that of fat-soluble vitamins is much slower. In therapy, a 5- to 10-fold increase in the intake of water-soluble vitamins over the normal requirements is suggested. Vitamins A and E are indicated in chronic illness and during stress. Lesions of the gastrointestinal tract and liver may also interfere with the synthesis and metabolism of vitamins. Liver and milk are suggested as good sources of unidentified growth factors.

A balanced ration: In sick, as in normal animals, a balanced ration should be fed. The vitamins and minerals are required together with other substances in metabolizing the energy and protein portion of the diet. The use of a specific nutrient in the treatment of an illness may be only temporarily helpful. An effort should be made to supply all the nutrients in their proper proportions at the same time. Under field conditions this can sometimes be accomplished by substituting rations formulated for species having higher and more critical nutritional requirements. For example, weanling pigs recovering from an enteric infection might be fed a chick starter ration for a few days.

FEEDING SICK AND HOSPITALIZED DOGS

The best planned diet is useless unless eaten, and anorexia is a major problem in hospitalized dogs. It is often difficult to tempt sick dogs to eat anything, especially foods to which they are unaccustomed. Food, casually offered, may be avidly accepted by a healthy kennel inmate, but ignored by a sick pet. Intangible factors, such as talking to the dog when the food is presented, scratching his ears or hand-feeding the first portion of food, often induce the dog to eat. Warming the food may be helpful. Chicken fat, garlic powder, meat broth and raw or cooked liver added to the diet may increase taste appeal.

Infection and nutritional status influence each other. Nutrition influences both the resistance of the host to infection, and the ability to resist consequences of infection. For some diseases, obesity may be as disabling as deficiency. Infection affects the nutritional status of the host, the amount of food consumed and the dietary needs of specific animals.

Central-nervous stimulants (strychnine), vitamins (thiamine and riboflavin), digestives and hormones (androgens, corticosteroids) are sometimes employed in the hope they may increase the animal's food intake. Dogs also have marked individual preferences for the consistency of their food. Some prefer food wet, others just moistened, and some completely dry. It is well not to attempt sudden changes in the diet if it can be avoided.

Hospitalized dogs should be fed familiar types of food (if not contraindicated by the illness) by attendants who like dogs and will cater to them as the occasion demands.

The basic dietary requirements of healthy dogs (q.v., p. 1263) may have to be modified rather drastically in the face of altered physiology or disease. Some changes may be temporary (as the intake of lactating bitches) and some relatively permanent (as in diets for chronic disease, such as nephritis or diabetes). Many disease conditions respond well to diet modifications. Often the diets needed are difficult to prepare, but commercial diets are available to fill the needs for most common maladies. The best of these dietary foods are more expensive than regular maintenance dog foods, but are effective and convenient. Where such foods are not suited to the particular patient, the veterinarian must formulate a diet. By keeping in mind the basic nutritional requirements of normal dogs and using the following principles as guides, diets which enhance other therapeutic measures can be produced.

Parasitism: Parasites and nutrition are bound together. Certain families of dogs tend to succumb to demodectic mange when fed poor diets. No diet has been found that will alleviate this condition after it has developed, however. Dogs fed an excellent diet rich in vitamins, minerals and protein, will succumb to hookworm infection if the total feed intake is so restricted that the dog remains thin; but when fed adequate amounts of the same diet, dogs do not succumb to hookworms. Puppies fed high-energy, high-protein diets can also ward off massive roundworm infections.

Renal disease: One of the main functions of the kidney is the excretion of nitrogenous waste products. It is important during renal insufficiencies to provide low, but adequate, quantities of dietary protein. The aim should be to keep the dog barely in nitrogen balance. This can be done by providing approximately 0.6 gm of high-quality protein per pound of body weight daily. Additional amounts will be needed in cases where urinary protein losses are high. Fats and carbohydrates should be increased to make up the normal caloric requirement and other ingredients supplied as in the normal diet. Patients can advantageously be kept on a high-sodium intake (by using sodium bicarbonate or bouillon cubes as supplements) and should be allowed liberal quantities of water. Many of these animals have polydipsia and polyuria and total water consumption is high. Water intake should not be restricted under any circumstances.

Gastrointestinal and digestive disease: Both inflammatory and functional disorders of the alimentary tract call for a diet which is nonstimulating (soft consistency, low residue). Eggs, dairy products, potatoes, chicken breasts, white bread and cooked rice are especially useful in such cases. Generally the best practice is to feed small amounts frequently. Constipation may be seen in older, overindulged house pets that have restricted opportunities for exercise. Such patients are often helped by feeding high-residue or bulky diets. Cooked oatmeal, bran and fibrous vegetables, such as squash, may be used to add bulk to the diet. It is important to be certain that adequate protein is supplied. An increased fluid intake may also be helpful.

Pancreatic disease can sometimes be managed by diet control alone. A diet high in carbohydrates and calcium but low in fat and protein is desirable. Supplemental enzyme therapy may be necessary.

Hepatic disease: What to feed the dog with liver disease is a controversial subject. Some advocate low-fat, high-protein diets. Others suggest low-protein, moderate-fat diets. Probably more important than either the level of fat or protein is the assurance that adequate amounts of readily available carbohydrates are included in the diet of the dog with liver disease.

Diabetes mellitus: Diabetic patients can usually be maintained in satisfactory condition for several years when insulin and intelligent diet therapy are coordinated. Uniformity of day-to-day treatment is desirable in each individual case. A constant daily dose of insulin requires uniform exercise and a consistent dietary intake. A high-protein, high-fat diet with carbohydrates provided in nonconcentrated form is most desirable. After the quantity of protein and carbohydrates is established, the necessary calories are provided by adding fats. It is best to feed diabetic patients small amounts frequently in order to maintain a relatively stable blood glucose level.

Heart failure: Many older dogs develop congestive heart failure. In such cases, restriction of the sodium intake is an important part of therapy. Low-sodium dietetic foods for dogs work well. Rations should be prepared without the use of salt, baking soda or baking powder. Generally, muscle-meat, freshwater fish, whole-grain cereals, rice and macaroni products, salt-free yeast bread, fresh or frozen vegetables and cooking oils or lard are desirable ingredients to use in low-sodium diets. Proprietary dog foods, regular bread, most processed foods and canned meats and vegetables are usually high in sodium because of added salt.

Food-induced allergy: Dogs may become allergic to almost any dietary protein. It is essential to the diagnosis of dietary allergy to have the dog sign-free. This is most successfully accomplished in 1 of 3 ways: 1) by withholding all food for several days, 2) by feeding a special elimination diet, 3) by feeding a hypoallergenic diet. Once sign-free, the dog should be fed one food at a time, for 5 days. If signs do not recur, the food can be considered nonallergenic. The object is not to determine to what foods the dog is allergic, but to determine a sufficient number of foods to which the dog is not allergic to formulate an adequate diet. If a dog should develop a response to a food, withdraw that food and allow the dog to become sign-free again before proceeding further. Food-induced allergies are among the most difficult to handle because owners may "cheat" or dogs may accidentally eat foods to which they are allergic.

Surgery: Pre-operative feeding is dictated by the surgical procedure scheduled. Generally, an empty gastrointestinal tract is desired, but excessive fasting, either before or after surgery, may be contraindicated since it may weaken the animal or deplete its glycogen reserves. The most successful pre- and postoperative diet is one that is known to be capable of supporting puppy growth.

FEEDING THE SICK CAT

Virtually all sick cats are anorectic. As a consequence, and because of their high metabolic requirements, sick cats rapidly become dehydrated and emaciated if they are not nourished. Sick cats have an imperative need for water, electrolytes, calories and B-vitamins.

For cats that refuse to eat, the best method of artificially feeding them is with a stomach tube and a concentrated, high-calorie, liquid food. This practice should not be continued any longer than needed, the cat being encouraged to eat on its own as soon as possible. Often just a little food in the stomach will revive the dormant appetite. Offering tuna, liver or kidney, or other special foods the cat is known to enjoy, often tempts the difficult cat to start eating.

Proper feeding can be an important factor in the therapy of several diseases of the cat. While there are but a few diets available commercially for specific diseases of the cat, many special diets can be formulated by the veterinarian and made by the cat owner. Even the commercial diets may need to have special foods added in small amounts to improve their acceptance by the sick cat.

Parasitism: Cats, like dogs, can withstand much greater loads of both external and internal parasites when fed a diet containing adequate amounts of protein, energy and vitamins.

Renal disease: The cat's protein requirement is over twice that of the dog, but the by-products of protein metabolism are excreted in the same manner, via the kidneys. During renal disease, therefore, protein must be restricted in the cat's diet, but not to the degree that it is for the dog, otherwise, hypoproteinemia results. The barest minimum which will keep a cat in positive protein balance is between 1.0 and 1.4 gm of protein (of BV 100) per pound of body weight per day. Since few common protein sources for the cat have a biologic value of 100, more realistic figures are probably 2.0 to 2.25 gm of protein per pound of body weight per day.

Gastrointestinal disease: Most cats with gastrointestinal disease can be fed in a manner similar to other monogastric animals with such a condition. One disease syndrome is worthy of note, however: chronic constipation caused by megacolon or Hirschsprung's disease should be managed, not with the bulk and roughage conventionally fed during ordinary constipation, but with highly digestible, low-residue foods. Since denervation is associated with the syndrome, the stimulatory effects of bulk and roughage are lost and such foods merely tend to further fill and stretch an already atonic colon and rectum.

Urolithiasis: While high-ash diets do not cause urolithiasis in cats, diets with restricted levels of magnesium may prevent the recurrence of urethral plugging. Since both urinary magnesium concentrations and urinary specific gravity seem to be factors, the following steps should help prevent recurrence of urethral plugging: 1) Restrict the diet of ingredients low in magnesium. Since about 70% of the magnesium in an animal's body is in its skeleton, foods containing whole fish, whole ground chicken or ground bone should be avoided. 2) Increase in the cat's water intake. Since dry foods contain only about 10% water and soft-moist foods only about 25%, neither should be fed to cats prone to urolithiasis. Fresh water should be available to cats at all times. The addition of ¼ to ½ teaspoonful of table salt to the cat's food each day will often increase the water intake noticeably.

NUTRITIONAL DEFICIENCIES IN CATTLE AND SHEEP

Nutritional deficiencies involving energy, protein, certain minerals, and vitamins A, D, E and K have been reported for ruminants under natural conditions. Experimentally, it has been possible to produce and study deficiencies of thiamine, riboflavin, biotin, choline and pantothenic acid in young dairy calves, deficiencies that may never occur in the field.

A simple, uncomplicated deficiency, as observed in carefully controlled experiments, is rarely if ever seen in the field. More likely, a deficiency of several nutrients contributes to the signs observed. Many of the signs of nutrient deficiencies are nonspecific and are often the total result of a low plane of nutrition. Further, the interactions of one nutrient to another and to other dietary constituents, in the development of deficiencies, are not always clearly defined. This is well illustrated by the interrelationship of copper, molybdenum and sulfate, of vitamin E and selenium, of zinc, copper and calcium, and of iodine and the various goitrogens.

ENERGY

It is generally agreed, that given a balanced, high-energy ration, ruminants will consume feed until they satisfy some physiologic need for energy. In the strict sense most ruminants are energy-limited (for maximum performance) since they are not fed *ad libitum,* e.g., growing heifers, mature cattle or sheep on "satisfactory" pasture or stovers, and dry cows, etc. Veal calves, cows in high production or fattening steers, on the other hand, are fed *ad libitum.* The most common energy deficiency is the inappropriate allotment of feed with a resulting reduced production efficiency. Generally this is unintentional or thought to be "economical" or it may be forced on the feeder by drought, poor pastures or low-quality, highly lignified, unpalatable forage.

A frank caloric deficiency is often subclinical in nature, resulting in lowered production, retarded growth, delayed puberty and lowered reproductive performance. In severe cases it is often complicated with other deficiencies particularly of vitamin A, protein and phosphorus. Appetite remains good. Young ruminants may be temporarily or permanently stunted and mature animals become thin and unthrifty. Milk production rapidly decreases in proportion to the deficiency and nonfat milk solids decrease. Pregnant animals will likely produce weak young and milk production will be inadequate to support the newborn. Surviving calves and lambs will often not do well and be unthrifty at weaning time if continually underfed.

Livestock in poor physical condition are more susceptible to the ravages of weather and parasites, and more likely to consume toxic plants if grazing poor pastures.

Research has shown that a reduced growth rate to puberty will extend the life span. Excessive feeding in early life is contraindicated because of the development of unnecessarily fat animals. Since the onset of puberty is a function of body size, a better energy parameter is to supply an adequate amount, such that the females will be big enough to breed at the proper time for effective management, e.g., 12 to 15 months for dairy and beef cattle. When cattle were underfed to 2½ years of age they were able to recover all of the loss in size when fed thereafter. Under current U.S. livestock conditions, however, dramatic underfeeding by design is not justified; growing animals should be "kept coming" but not allowed to become too fat.

The energy requirement for maintenance is 24 to 100% greater when grazing than for stall feeding.

PROTEIN

A deficiency of protein often goes hand in hand with an energy shortage and may be the first limiting factor in practical cattle and sheep feeding when these animals are on poor pasture. Roughages commonly fed are often too low in protein for optimum performance. Adequate amounts of protein (or nitrogen) are required, not only by the animal itself, but also by the rumen microflora whose composition and function may be markedly altered on a low-protein diet. Intake of low-protein feeds is depressed and growth is seriously retarded. Other signs may be similar to those encountered with insufficient energy. Weight gains and the condition of fattening cattle and sheep are reduced, milk production is lowered and, if severe or prolonged, the animals become thin and emaciated. Weight losses may occur even though ample energy is available. In addition, with sheep, the growth of the wool fiber is restricted and "breaks" occur in the fleece.

Pregnant cows or ewes on a low-protein diet may lose considerable body weight and become thin and weak. Estrus may become irregular and conception delayed. Such females may have difficult parturition, be troubled with retained placenta, milk poorly and produce offspring that have poor chances of survival or, at best, are small and thin at weaning. Such unthrifty stock lack resistance to adverse weather, infections and parasites.

MINERALS

Sodium Chloride: Salt is an essential component of the acid-base mechanism in the body and is needed for the maintenance of proper osmotic relationships. Animals promptly adjust to low-salt diets by reducing sodium excretion in the urine. Continued deprivation results in an intense craving for salt in which animals chew and lick various objects such as wood, metal and dirt. Feed consumption declines, loss of body weight and a drop in milk production occur. Feed efficiency is poor. As death approaches, milking cows shiver, show incoordination, weakness and cardiac arrhythmia.

The animal can best judge its need for salt, which should be available throughout life. Following a salt deficiency it should be offered back to the animal gradually. Salt intoxication is unlikely if adequate water is available.

Calcium: The bones and teeth contain about 99% of the body calcium in their structure and serve as a reserve of this element. The 1% remaining is found in the soft tissues and body fluids and is essential for proper nerve function, cardiac and other muscular activity and blood clotting. A dynamic equilibrium exists between these 2 pools.

A calcium deficiency in the young prevents normal bone growth and retards general growth and development. Frank rickets may occur. If bone reserves are substantial in the adult, it requires a lengthy depletion period before bone mineral loss is sufficient to result in fragile bones. Under these conditions milk yield is depressed but not its calcium content. Blood calcium will be low only after an extended period of deficient intake. For positive diagnosis, the calcium content of the feed should be checked.

In practical feeding conditions, calcium deficiency is always suspected except where milk and legume forage are used extensively; almost all concentrates and nonlegume forages, including corn silage, require supplementation. Heavily lactating animals have the greatest need due to significant secretion in the milk. During early lactation, a high-producing cow will always be in negative calcium balance but will restore her reserves in late lactation if fed adequate levels. Young animals absorb calcium much more efficiently than older ones, hence a need to provide adequate levels throughout life. Animals heavily fed on concentrates with little forage, will need supplemental calcium. Milk fever is characterized by a reduced blood calcium but is not due to a calcium deficiency.

Ground limestone, steamed bone meal and dicalcium phosphate are excellent sources of calcium. Addition of lime to fields can increase the calcium content of the forage produced.

Phosphorus: About 75% of the body phosphorus is present in the bones and teeth. The remaining 25%, in the soft tissues, is found in phosphoprotein, nucleoprotein, phospholipids and hexose phosphate, which are essential in organ structure, nutrient transport and energy utilization.

A deficiency of phosphorus in the young results in slow growth, poor appetite, unthriftiness and has produced a knock-kneed condition in lambs. Energy utilization is reduced. In the adult, milk production declines, bones become fragile and feed intake is poor. The animals may become lame and stiff. Anestrus and low conception rates may occur. The phosphorus content of the milk does not decline. While a depraved appetite (chewing of wood, dirt, etc.) has long been recognized as often occurring with a phosphorus deficiency, this sign is not specific. Many animals engage in this vice on perfectly balanced diets, or with other deficiencies.

Blood-phosphorus content is closely allied to the phosphorus content of forages and availability in the soil. Over much of North America, pasture and especially range forage have a low phosphorus content. Most of the winter range areas of the West are deficient in phosphorus, particularly those ranges characterized by a predominance of dry, leached grass and shad scale. Forages produced on deficient, unfertilized soils may be marginal in phosphorus content and deficiencies occur when these roughages form the entire ration. Use of phosphorus fertilizers markedly increases crop yields in these areas and may also raise the percentage of phosphorus in the forage. Fortunately, grains, protein supplements and by-product feeds usually are adequate in phosphorus and may supplement low-phosphorus roughages effectively.

Phosphorus deficiency can be corrected or prevented most easily by feeding phosphorus supplements, such as bone meal, dicalcium phosphate or defluorinated rock phosphate. Bone meal contains approximately 14% phosphorus, while dicalcium phosphate and defluorinated rock phosphate normally contain 20.5 and 18.0% phosphorus, respectively. Rock phosphates should contain less than 0.1% fluorine to avoid toxicity from this element. Colloidal clay phosphates (so-called "soft" phosphates) contain phosphorus in a relatively unavailable form and also may have a considerable fluorine content. Wheat bran, cottonseed meal, linseed meal and soybean meal are rich in phosphorus and their use in concentrate mixtures will insure adequate intakes. While the ratio of calcium to phosphorus may vary widely in natural feeds, a ratio between 1:1 and 2:1 is considered most favorable. A ratio of more phosphorus than calcium is highly undesirable. Vitamin D is essential for the absorption and utilization of both calcium and phosphorus. In cows prone to milk fever, a ratio of approximately 2:1 is recommended before parturition.

Iodine: About 80% of the body iodine is stored in the thyroid gland in the form of thyroglobulin, thyroxine and trace quantities of other iodinated amino acid derivatives including triiodothyronine. Iodine apparently exerts its total physiologic role as a component of the thyroid hormones which control cellular energy exchange, metabolic rate and tissue growth and development.

A simple iodine deficiency results in an enlargement of the thyroid gland, or goiter, with a reduction of thyroxine secretion. Pregnancy is the most critical period. In cattle and sheep the newborn are goitrous and weak. Lambs may be woolless. Mortality is high especially shortly after birth. Lambs which survive for more than a week usually recover spontaneously and make normal gains.

Iodine deficiency occurs in areas in which soil, and hence plant and water, iodine is low such as around the Great Lakes and in the Northwestern U.S.A. Some plants such as cabbage, soybeans and yellow turnips may promote goiter development because they contain substances (goitrogens) which inhibit thyroxine production. The goitrogenic effect of raw soybeans is only partially destroyed in processing.

Iodized salt is an effective source of iodine and is widely used. If iodized salt is used, care should be taken that the iodine is stabilized since weathering can reduce the iodine content below that which is needed. The same is true for trace-mineralized salt. In both types of salt, 0.007% iodine (0.01% KI) is usually added. Neither iodized nor trace-mineralized salt should be added to a concentrate supplement to limit feed intake.

Cobalt: While cobalt is considered a dietary essential, the tissues actually require vitamin B_{12} which contains cobalt as an integral part of its molecule. Rumen microorganisms utilize dietary cobalt to synthesize vitamin B_{12} which then is the source of supply for the animal. Vitamin B_{12} will alleviate signs of a cobalt deficiency.

Deficient animals show a normocytic, normochromic anemia with a concomitant loss of appetite, retarded growth, general emaciation, rough hair coat and a loss of milk production. While herbage and liver analyses are helpful in diagnosing the deficiency, the proof positive is the prompt improvement in feed intake following the feeding of cobalt.

Natural forages containing less than 0.07 ppm of cobalt are usually considered deficient for sheep and cattle. Regions where, from time to time, these minima are not reached are known to exist in the states of Florida, Michigan, Wisconsin, New Hampshire and New York, in Western Canada, Scotland, South Africa, Australia and New Zealand.

Drenches of about 1.0 mg of cobalt, given twice a week, have corrected the deficiency syndrome in sheep. In cattle, feeding 5 to 15 mg of cobalt daily will cure cobalt deficiency and as little as 1 mg will prevent its occurrence. The inclusion of 15 to 30 gm of cobalt chloride or sulfate per 100 lb of salt is usually adequate to prevent deficiency in both cattle and sheep. The use of such trace-mineralized salt is the most common method of supplying cobalt to ruminants in the U.S.A. In New Zealand and in other intensively farmed areas, cobalt is applied to the soil annually at the rate of 5 oz of cobalt sulfate per acre, either as a spray or included in the phosphate fertilizer. A cobalt "bullet" (90% cobalt oxide baked hard in 10% clay) which can be given orally and comes to rest in the rumen has been developed. It dissolves slowly over many months and has been used with success as a preventive. This "bullet" is used quite extensively under some range conditions where other methods of oral administration are not practical. However, in about 5% of sheep, the bullet is regurgitated and lost, and in a further small percentage, a deposit forms over the bullet which prevents solution of the cobalt. Injections of cobalt are not effective since the site of B_{12} synthesis is in the rumen. Extremely large doses of cobalt may be toxic, but this level is about 100 times the requirement.

Copper and Molybdenum: Copper is involved at the functional level in the formation of the porphyrin nucleus of hemoglobin and in maintaining the function of bone osteoblasts. It is also essential in melanin production and in keratin (wool) formation. General signs of a deficiency include anemia, brittle or fragile bones, loss of hair or wool color and, in sheep, poor wool growth characterized by a loss of crimp (steely wool). Specifically in cattle, poor growth, anemia, bone fragility, diarrhea and a myocardial fibrosis occur. Ends of leg bones become enlarged and the hair loses its color. Milk production and body condition are poor and fertility is low and calves may show congenital rickets. With sheep, anemia and depressed growth are less common. Demyelination of certain tracts in the fetal and neonatal CNS results in incoordination, which leads to immobilization, blindness and death. The disease is known as "swayback" or "enzootic ataxia". Bone fragility may also occur.

In many areas, copper deficiency can be a simple deficiency of the element (primary). In other areas where excessive molybdenum and sulfate exist in the feed, these substances act to reduce copper solubility in the digestive tract and induce a copper deficiency (conditioned deficiency).

A normal level of sulfate in the diet counteracts the effects of molybdenum toxicity by increasing its rate of excretion. Higher sulfate levels, however, appear to enhance molybdenum intoxication with a detrimental effect on copper utilization. Frank cases of molybdenum toxicity on "teart" pastures, which are characterized by profuse scouring, can be alleviated by copper at levels of 0.25 gm of copper sulfate per 100 lb of body wt daily.

The requirement for copper is about 5 ppm of the dry diet. Adequate intakes can be met if feeds have this level or by providing 0.5% copper in a trace-mineralized salt. Toxic levels are about 10 times the minimum requirement.

Iron: Normal hemoglobin formation requires iron as a component of the heme molecule. A microcytic normochromic anemia develops in calves on an iron-low diet (milk). Most feedstuffs contain adequate iron and a deficiency in adult cattle is not a problem. Young calves or lambs confined to a milk diet will develop anemia. Providing 30 mg of iron per day will prevent anemia in milk-fed calves. On normal feeding regimes where dry feeds are offered from birth, no special iron supplements are needed.

Magnesium: About 50 to 75% of the tissue magnesium is found in the bones where it is relatively difficult to mobilize. The normal calcium:magnesium ratio is about 55:1. A variable (15 to 50%) is bound to serum proteins. It plays a vital role as an activator of many enzyme systems involving energy exchange. It is also involved in maintaining normal nerve irritability and function. Signs of a magnesium deficiency are always accompanied by a low blood magnesium level (1.0 mg/100 ml) but low levels may occur without manifestation of signs.

By feeding experimental rations deficient in magnesium or by giving whole milk as the only food for 8 to 10 months, magnesium deficiency has been produced in calves (see HYPOMAGNESEMIA, p. 508). Throughout the world, adult cattle, most especially lactating cows turned to early spring pasture, may develop signs of "grass tetany" or "grass staggers" (q.v., p. 506). Pastures fertilized to provide sward containing 0.2% magnesium will prevent the condition.

Sulfur: All ruminants require sulfur to synthesize the sulfur-containing amino acids, cystine and methionine. A deficiency results in poor growth and in sheep a marked impairment of wool growth. If the diet is adequate in natural proteins, the sulfur intake will be satisfactory, but if high levels of nonprotein nitrogen such as urea are used, sources of sulfur such as elemental sulfur or inorganic or organic sulfur should be added. A nitrogen-to-sulfur ratio of 10:1 is recommended for cattle. This element is a cofactor of many enzymes and an integral part of others. It is essential in bone formation in as yet an unknown way.

Manganese: Manganese has been less extensively studied in ruminants. In beef cattle, a deficiency resulted in delayed estrus, reduced fertility, abortions and deformed young. The calves had deformed legs with "over knuckling" and enlarged joints, and grew poorly. Dairy heifers were slower to exhibit estrus and conceive.

Most feeds are adequate in manganese, precluding a need for supplementation. As corn is relatively low, beef cattle on high-concentrate diets may need attention. A level of 20 to 30 mg/kg of diet is adequate.

Zinc: Many enzymes which are widely distributed throughout the body, such as carbonic anhydrase, many dehydrogenases and alkaline phosphatase, contain zinc. It is probable that zinc is intimately related to the processes of cell division.

Zinc deficiency signs have been produced experimentally with highly specialized diets. In lambs, such a diet produced slipping of wool, swelling and lesions around the hooves and periorbital regions of the eyes, hypersalivation, anorexia, wool-eating, general listlessness and reduction of growth. Beef calves develop parakeratosis, and the mouth becomes inflamed. They are stiff in the joints and unthrifty in appearance. In dairy calves, alopecia and a general dermatitis of the neck and head, which are exacerbated by trauma, are seen. Wounds fail to heal properly. In practice, zinc deficiency is uncommon, but when in question, zinc may be provided in a trace-mineralized mix or in the mineral portion of a concentrate.

Selenium: The nutrition of selenium is inextricably entwined with that of vitamin E. Both have been shown to prevent nutritional muscular dystrophy (q.v., p. 575) in calves and lambs. In sheep, selenium but not vitamin E alone prevented dystrophy when fed to ewes. It is probable that these 2 nutrients are interrelated at the cellular level.

A deficiency of selenium is a geographic one, found in many parts of the world due to inadequate soil levels. Striking responses to selenium therapy by lambs suffering unthriftiness have been reported in New Zealand. Selenium therapy has also been effective in the treatment of a number of myopathies both experimentally produced and naturally occurring in lambs and calves. The addition of selenium to feed in inorganic form has been prohibited. A dietary level of 0.1 ppm is adequate for ruminants.

Levels of 5 ppm are toxic and result in loss of appetite, loss of hair from the tail, sloughing of hoofs and eventual death. Some plants and soils contain toxic levels of selenium.

VITAMINS

Vitamin A serves to maintain the integrity of all epithelial tissues including germinal epithelium. Thus, a deficiency, besides reducing the efficiency of the epithelium *per se*, permits much of this tissue to be exposed to a secondary invasion of indigenous pathogens. Most signs of a deficiency can be traced to this single function. Since vitamin A is related to epithelium, the requirements are generally related to body weight.

Tissue vitamin A may be derived from either provitamin A (carotene, a green pigment in plants, which is converted in the intestinal wall to vitamin A), or from preformed vitamin A *per se*.

Carotene is destroyed when roughage is dried and bleached, hence a deficiency may occur in cattle and sheep under drought conditions or when they are fed weathered roughage for long periods. Carotene is abundant in growing pasture, silage and well-cured hay that has been stored less than 6 months. Grains (with the exception of yellow corn) and cereal by-products contain little or none of this vitamin.

Usually, the first signs of vitamin A deficiency are excessive lacrimation, thin or watery diarrhea, nasal discharge, coughing and pulmonary involvement. Night blindness may develop in the early stages; in fact, this sign has been used experimentally to establish minimum carotene requirements. Vitamin A levels in the blood decline to less than 8 to 10 mcg/100 ml of plasma in calves and below 12 to 15 mcg in yearlings and older cattle. Considerable individual variation, however, is often observed in plasma vitamin A levels; carotene blood levels of cattle are consistently low in a deficiency and are indicative of insufficient carotene intake. Sheep circulate only traces of carotene in the blood.

Calves and lambs have very low vitamin A blood levels at birth and depend on colostrum, a rich source of vitamin A, to protect them against deficiency until a sufficient supply can be obtained from other sources.

Calves and lambs from females with vitamin A deficiency may be born dead or so weak that they die within a few days; females may abort during the latter stages of pregnancy. Injury to the optic nerve as a result of stenosis of the optic foramen may occur in growing animals. Cerebrospinal-fluid pressure is elevated and, as a result, staggering gait, muscular incoordination and convulsions ("fainting" of feed-lot cattle) have been frequently reported. Anasarca is often observed in fattening cattle, and opacity and cloudiness of the cornea and xerophthalmia with subsequent infection and blindness may result.

Young bulls and rams may become sterile as a result of failure of spermatogenesis. Vitamin A-deficient mature bulls show muscular incoordination which makes them unable to mate. This occurs before spermatogenesis is altered.

While there is little difference in normal plasma carotene levels among the major beef breeds, there is considerable difference among dairy breeds because of the variations in their ability to metabolize carotene to vitamin A. The liver can store large quantities of vitamin A. Most animals off good pasture can live 200 days on their liver reserves.

With the exception of irreparable changes in the eye or bony tissues, signs of vitamin A deficiency can be rapidly corrected by high intakes in vitamin A. At this point, treatment should be by injection of preformed vitamin A. The requirement is about 2000 IU/100 lb of body wt. Up to 100 times this level is not detrimental for a therapeutic dose. Changing to diets adequate in carotene or vitamin A is imperative. The rate of conversion of carotene to vitamin A by ruminants is lower than in monogastric animals. It also fluctuates widely and unpredictably. Therefore, many commercial feeds are now fortified with dry, stabilized vitamin A and supplements are used to fortify home-grown rations. Such a source of vitamin A may be more economic and dependable than carotene from natural feeds.

Vitamin D: Calcium, phosphorus and vitamin D are closely related in metabolism. Vitamin D aids in the absorption and deposition of calcium and phosphorus. An absolute or relative deficiency of any one will cause rickets in growing animals. Experimental rickets is usually brought about by a deficiency of both vitamin D and phosphorus and an excess of calcium. Young ruminants, especially dairy calves, on milk alone may suffer from rickets as a consequence of a deficiency of vitamin D, even in the presence of calcium and phosphorus. Similarly, a vitamin D deficiency under conditions of prolonged cloudy weather or indoor feeding, especially in the case of fast-growing lambs and calves is a possibility. On the other hand, older sheep and cattle on pasture do not need additional vitamin D.

Evidence of vitamin D deficiency begins with a drop in the organic phosphorus level in the plasma and an increase in alkaline-phosphatase value. Serum calcium may also decline, but this effect is usually less consistent. For signs, *see* RICKETS, p. 564.

Rickets due to lack of vitamin D can be cured in the early stages by feeding irradiated yeast or other vitamin D supplements. For calves or lambs, a single dose of 5,000 IU or more followed by the use of feed containing 200 IU of vitamin D per pound of body weight, and daily exposure to sunlight, is recommended. Either vitamin D_2 or D_3 is effective in ruminants. Sun-cured forage is the best natural source of vitamin D. Even grass silage and corn silage have sufficient dead leaves (thus sun-cured) to provide ample vitamin D to growing calves that are housed indoors and are thus more than adequate for cows.

Vitamin E: Most natural feeds contain vitamin E, but oxidation rapidly destroys it so that old hay or ground grain may be poor sources. A deficiency of vitamin E or selenium is recognized as a common cause of muscular dystrophy in calves and lambs. Vitamin E does not seem to be associated with reproductive failures in ruminants and so it is of practical importance only with the young. Details of muscular dystrophy are described under MYOPATHIES AND RELATED CONDITIONS IN DOMESTIC ANIMALS, p. 575.

Vitamin K: A deficiency is seen only in the presence of dicoumarin from moldy sweet clover. This results in the so-called "sweet clover disease" (q.v., p. 990). This vitamin is synthesized by rumen bacteria and is widely distributed in green, leafy forages.

B-complex vitamins: Deficiencies have not been observed in ruminants past 1 to 2 months of age except where they have been restricted to special diets. Rumen bacteria have the ability to synthesize all the B-complex vitamins if other factors necessary for their synthesis are present (e.g., cobalt in B_{12} synthesis). Niacin (nicotinic acid) is also synthesized from tryptophan within the tissues of even young calves. This, together with that synthesized in the rumen, fully meets the needs of ruminants. Most of the other B-vitamins have been shown to be essential in the diet of very young calves before rumen function becomes established. However, milk and other natural feeds contain adequate amounts to meet the needs of young calves and lambs.

It must be borne in mind that the ruminant is dependent upon bacterial synthesis for B-complex vitamins and might actually undergo a shortage of these if it goes "off feed" for long periods. Further, low-protein rations or mineral-deficient feeds may depress the number of bacteria or the synthesis mechanism of the rumen microflora. The practice of administering certain B-complex vitamins or yeast preparations to ruminants that have been off feed for a considerable period has been tried with apparent success in the field and may have some logical basis.

The precise relationships between diet and polioencephalomalacia (q.v., p. 644) have yet to be determined, but the disease is related to thiamine deficiency.

Vitamin C (ascorbic acid): Since it is synthesized in the tissues even of young ruminants, deficiencies of this vitamin do not occur and it is not required in the diet.

NUTRITIONAL DEFICIENCIES IN SWINE

The diagnosis of nutritional deficiencies by outward observation of signs in swine is difficult. Quite often, the clinical signs observed are due to a complex of poor management, infectious diseases and parasitism, as well as malnutrition. For most nutrient deficiencies, the signs are not specific. For example, poor appetite, reduced growth and unthriftiness are common to most nutrient deficiencies. A deficiency of a single nutrient may bring about inanition; the subsequent starvation may cause multiple deficiencies. Then, too, a nutritional deficiency may exist without the appearance of definite signs. In the field, the deficiency may be only slight or borderline, making the diagnosis difficult.

The diagnosis of a nutrient deficiency by observing the response to nutritional therapy is not always clear cut. The 1968 report by the Committee on Animal Nutrition of the National Research Council in the bulletin entitled *Nutrient Requirements of Swine* states:

> "Some acute conditions that are produced in the laboratory by omitting an essential constituent from the diet can be dramatically reversed by supplying the missing constituent. It does not follow, however, that long-standing conditions can be made to recede in the same way. Many functional and anatomical lesions resulting from inadequate diets are irreversible."

A positive diagnosis of a nutritional deficiency should be made only after the following: (1) observance of several of the clinical signs expected and (2) a careful review of the dietary, disease and management history of the animals.

The usual clinical signs of dietary deficiencies are outlined in TABLE 44. A brief discussion of each along with related matters follows.

PROTEIN

Feeding a suboptimum level of protein to pigs results in reduced gains, fatter carcasses and poorer feed conversion. Protein deficiency may result from a suboptimal feed intake or from an imbalance of one or more of the essential amino acids. For optimum utilization of protein, all essential amino acids must be liberated during digestion at rates commensurate with needs. Therefore, protein supplement should not be hand-fed at infrequent intervals, but should be mixed with the grain or be available at all times with grain on a free-choice basis.

No evidence has been presented to support the theory of "protein poisoning". Rations containing as much as 34 to 51% protein have proved laxative, but not harmful and no toxic effects were noted.

FAT

A semipurified ration containing 0.06% fat produced such deficiency signs as loss of hair, scaly dermatitis, necrotic areas on the skin of the neck and shoulders, and an unthrifty appearance in growing pigs. However, a level of 1.0 to 1.5% fat in the diet appeared ample to furnish the essential fatty acids required by swine. With practical rations, a specific fat deficiency is unknown.

MINERALS

The clinical signs of deficiencies of the more important mineral elements are briefly discussed under the headings below.

Calcium and Phosphorus: Deficiencies of calcium and phosphorus result in rickets in growing pigs and osteomalacia in mature swine. Signs include deformity and bending of long bones, and lameness in young swine and fractures and posterior paralysis in older swine. Deficient sows produce weak pigs, and usually show a posterior paralysis, sometimes as a result of fractures in the lumbar region resulting in posterior paralysis. Sows with a marginal deficiency often give birth to strong and vigorous pigs that grow normally. However, after nursing the pigs for 3 or more weeks, the sows develop a posterior paralysis. A lack of vitamin D also will cause these signs if the dietary calcium or phosphorus differs markedly from the recommended feeding level. (*See* RICKETS, p. 564.)

Sodium and Chlorine: Pigs fed low-salt diets show slow growth, reduced appetite and poor hair and skin condition.

Iodine: Bred females fed rations deficient in iodine produce pigs that are weak or stillborn, and hairless at birth. With a borderline deficiency, the newborn pigs may only be weak at birth, but on necropsy, enlarged thyroids are found together with histologic abnormalities of these glands. (*See also* GOITER, p. 188.)

Iron and copper: Deficiency of these 2 elements reduces the rate of hemoglobin formation and produces typical nutritional anemia. Signs of nutritional anemia in suckling pigs include low hemoglobin and red blood cell count, pale membranes, enlarged heart, an edematous condition of the skin about the neck and shoulders, listlessness and "thumps".

Zinc: A relative lack of this element results in parakeratosis (q.v., p. 918) in growing swine, particularly when diets contain more than the recommended amount of calcium. The exact mode of action of zinc in the prevention of parakeratosis is not known, nor has its role in the support of other life processes yet been fully elucidated.

Selenium/Vitamin E: The delineation of individual deficiencies of these 2 nutrients is not evident at this time. Debilitating conditions have occurred in many swine herds in recent years that have responded to either 22 IU of vitamin E per kilogram of body weight or 0.15 ppm of selenium in the diet (*see* CARDIAC AND SKELETAL MYOPATHIES AND HEPATOSIS DIAETETICA IN SWINE, p. 581).

VITAMINS

Signs resulting from deficiency of the vitamins of greatest practical importance are briefly discussed below.

Vitamin A: A vitamin A deficiency results in disturbances of the eye and of the epithelial tissues of the respiratory, reproductive, nervous, urinary and digestive systems. Reproduction is impaired in sows and vitamin A-deficient sows may farrow blind, eyeless, weak or malformed pigs. Herniation of the spinal cord in the fetal pig is reported as a unique sign of vitamin A deficiency in the pregnant sow. Growing pigs, deficient in vitamin A, show incoordinated movements and develop night blindness and respiratory disorders.

Vitamin D: Deficiency signs include rickets, stiffness, weak and bent bones, and posterior paralysis.

Riboflavin: In riboflavin-deficient swine, reproduction is impaired. Deficient sows exhibit anorexia and farrow dead pigs from 4 to 16 days prematurely. The stillborn pigs have very little hair, often are partially resorbed and may have enlarged forelegs. Growing pigs fed low-riboflavin rations gain very slowly, have poor appetite, exhibit a rough haircoat and an exudate on the skin, and may have cataracts.

Niacin: Niacin-deficient pigs have inflammatory lesions of the gastrointestinal tract. The pigs exhibit diarrhea, weight loss, rough skin and haircoat, and a dermatitis on the ears. Enteric conditions may be due to niacin deficiency, bacterial infection, or both. Deficient pigs respond readily to niacin therapy, but infectious enteritis is not benefited. However, adequate dietary niacin probably allows the pig to maintain its resistance to bacterial invasion.

Pantothenic acid: Growing pigs and pregnant sows develop a typical "goose-stepping" gait and show incoordination and a noninfectious bloody diarrhea when maintained on pantothenic acid-deficient diets. When the deficiency becomes severe, anorexia develops.

TABLE 44. CLINICAL SIGNS OF DIETARY DEFICIENCIES

Deficient Nutrients	Slow or Interrupted Growth	Reduced Appetite	Poor Hair and Skin Condition	Lameness and Stiffness	Diarrhea	Impaired Reproduction	Dead or Weak Offspring at Birth	Weakened Bone Structure	Anemia	Other Effects
Energy	+	-	-	-	-	+	-	-	-	Reduced fatness in proportion to body wt.
Protein level	+	+	+	-	-	+	+	-	+	Poor feed efficiency; overfat carcass.
Protein quality (essential amino acids)	+	+	+	-	-	-	-	-	-	
Essential fatty acids	+	+	+	-	-	-	-	-	-	Loss of hair; scaly, dandruff-like dermatitis, especially of feet and tail.
Calcium	+	+	+	+	-	+	+	+	-	Severe cases may show reduced serum calcium and tetany, rickets.
Phosphorus	+	+	-	+	-	+	+	+	-	Reduced blood phosphorus, poor feed efficiency, rickets.
Potassium	+	+	+	-	-	-	-	-	-	Decreased feed efficiency; cardiac impairment.
Sodium (as common salt)	+	+	+	+	-	-	-	-	-	Depraved appetite.
Magnesium	+	+	+	+	-	+	+	+	-	Hyperirritability and tetany, weak pasterns.
Manganese	-	-	-	+	-	+	-	+	-	Reduced skeletal growth, increased backfat and irregular estrus.
Iodine	-	-	+	-	-	+	+	-	-	Birth of hairless pigs, goiter.
Iron	+	+	+	-	-	+	+	-	+	High mortality, susceptibility to parasitic invasion, "thumps."

Nutrient										Description
Copper	+	−	−	−	−	+	+	−	+	Lack of rigidity of leg joints, hocks excessively flexed, forelegs crooked, use of forelegs impaired.
Zinc	−	+	−	−	+	+	+	+	+	Severe dermatosis; parakeratosis.
Vitamin A	−	−	+	+	−	+	−	−	+	Incoordination of movement, head tilted, extreme weakness of back, brown greasy exudate, night blindness and constriction of optic nerve.
Vitamin D	−	−	+	+	−	+	−	−	+	Rickets, enlarged joints, weak bones.
Vitamin E/Selenium	−	+	−	−	−	+	+	+	−	Brownish yellow discoloration of adipose tissue, waxy degeneration of muscle tissue. Sudden death, hepatic necrosis.
Thiamine	−	−	+	+	+	−	−	−	+	Slow pulse, low body temperature, flabby heart.
Riboflavin Niacin	+−	−−	+−	++	++	+−	++	+−	++	Crooked legs, stillborn pigs. Occasional vomiting, foul-smelling feces, pig pellagra.
Pantothenic acid	−	−	+	+	+	+	+	+	+	Incoordinated wobbly gait (goose-stepping).
Pyridoxine	+	−	−	−	+	+	+	+	+	Epileptiform fits, slowing of growth after first convulsion.
Choline	−	−	+	+	−	+	−	+	+	Lack of coordination, improper rigidity of joints, fatty livers, renal glomerular occlusion and tubular epithelial necrosis.

continued on next page

TABLE 44. *(Continued)*

Deficient Nutrients	Slow or Interrupted Growth	Reduced Appetite	Poor Hair and Skin Condition	Lameness and Stiffness	Diarrhea	Impaired Reproduction	Dead or Weak Offspring at Birth	Weakened Bone Structure	Anemia	Other Effects
Vitamin B_{12}	+	+	-	-	-	-	-	-	+	Hyperirritability, posterior incoordination, voice failure, pain in rear quarters.
Biotin	+	+	+	-	-	-	-	-	-	Alopecia, cracking of feet.

In general, all applicable symptoms marked + for a given nutrient deficiency should be observed in the sick animal before a positive diagnosis is made that deficiency of that nutrient in fact exists or is the cause of the ill health of the pig.

(From *Nutrient Requirements of Swine*, National Research Council, 1964, 1968)

Choline: Choline-deficient pigs exhibit incoordinated movements and an abnormal shoulder conformation. At necropsy, they have fatty livers and kidney damage (renal glomerular occlusion and tubular epithelial necrosis).

Vitamin B$_{12}$: Baby pigs fed synthetic diets low in vitamin B$_{12}$ show hyperirritability, voice failure, pain in the hindquarters and posterior incoordination. Histologic examination of the bone marrow reveals an impairment of the hemopoietic system. Under farm conditions, weanling pigs fed practical diets low in vitamin B$_{12}$ do not show the above signs, but merely gain more slowly than pigs receiving an adequate allowance of this vitamin.

NUTRITIONAL DEFICIENCIES IN HORSES

Descriptions of uncomplicated nutrient deficiencies in the horse are rare. The natural feeds typically consumed are most likely to be deficient in protein, calcium, phosphorus, sodium, chlorine and iodine, depending on the age and productive level of the horse and the geographic area. Dried, weathered forages may be very low in carotene and where these are fed for long periods, vitamin A deficiency may develop. New Zealand workers have described a myopathy in foals which has been attributed to a selenium deficiency (q.v., p. 578). An anemia which responded to parenteral cyanocobalamin (vitamin B$_{12}$) therapy has been described. Thiamine and riboflavin deficiencies have been produced experimentally.

Signs of deficiency are frequently nonspecific and diagnosis may be complicated by a simultaneous shortage of several nutrients. The consequences of increased susceptibility to parasitism and bacterial infections may superimpose still other clinical signs. In the following paragraphs, signs of deficiency noted in the horse will be recorded where these are available. Where they are not, the most likely signs which might be expected from research with other species will be described.

ENERGY

Many of the nonspecific changes found in deficient subjects are related to caloric deficiency and result from inadequate intake of a well-balanced diet or from poor utilization of the diet which follows the development of a specific deficiency. In partial or complete starvation most internal organs exhibit some atrophy. The brain is least affected, but the size of the gonads may be strikingly decreased. Hypoplasia of lymph nodes, spleen and thymus leads to a marked reduction in their size. The adrenal glands are usually enlarged. The young skeleton is extremely sensitive and growth slows or may completely stop. In the adult, the skeleton may become osteoporotic. A decrease in adipose tissue is an early and conspicuous sign, not only in the subcutis, but in the mesentery, around the kidneys, uterus and testes, and in the retroperitoneal area. Low fat content of the marrow in the long bones is a good indicator of prolonged inanition. The ability to perform work is impaired, and endogenous nitrogen losses increase as muscle proteins are metabolized for energy.

PROTEIN

A deficiency of dietary protein may represent either an inadequate intake of high-quality protein or the lack of a specific essential amino acid. It is doubtful that synthesis by microorganisms in the gut plus proteolysis of microbial protein is adequate to meet the essential amino acid needs of the horse. The deficiency effects are generally nonspecific and many of the signs differ in no respect from the effects of partial or total caloric restriction. In addition, there may be depressed appetite, decreased formation of hemoglobin, erythrocytes and plasma proteins. Edema is sometimes associated with the hypoproteinemia. Milk production is decreased in lactating mares. Decreased activity of the following liver enzymes has been noted: pyruvic oxidase, succinoxidase, succinic acid dehydrogenase, D-amino acid oxidase, DPN-cytochrome C reductase and uricase. Corneal vascularization and lens degeneration have been noted in some species. Antibody formation is impaired.

MINERALS

Calcium: The young growing horse or the lactating mare being fed on poor-quality grass hay or pasture are most likely to develop calcium deficiencies. Serum calcium levels may be depressed while serum inorganic-phosphorus levels may be elevated; however, single samples of blood are generally not diagnostic. Serum alkaline-phosphatase activity is usually elevated. Clotting time may be prolonged slightly. Young, growing bone is frequently rachitic and brittle. Fractures may be common and poor healing follows. Adult bone may be osteoporotic.

Phosphorus: A deficiency is most likely in horses being fed poor-quality grass hay or pasture without grain. Serum inorganic-phosphorus levels may be depressed and serum alkaline-phosphatase activity increased. Occasionally, serum calcium levels may be elevated. Bone changes resemble those described for calcium deficiency.

Sodium and **chlorine:** Horses are most likely to develop signs of sodium chloride (salt) deficiency when worked hard in hot weather. Perspiration and urinary losses are appreciable. Horses deprived of salt tire easily, stop sweating and exhibit muscle spasms. Anorexia and pica may be evident. It is to be noted, however, that pica is not a specific sign of NaCl deficiency. The milk production of lactating mares will seriously decline. Hemoconcentration and acidosis may be expected.

Iodine: Deficiency is an enzootic problem in many areas (*see* GOITER, p. 188).

Cobalt: Deficiency is apparently rare in horses; they have been known to thrive on pastures so low in cobalt that sheep and cattle dependent upon them wasted and died. The normal feedstuffs of horses generally contain very little vitamin B_{12}. It has been demonstrated, however, that the horse can synthesize this vitamin in the gut and that it is absorbed. Certain anemias have been reported in horses which responded to vitamin B_{12} therapy. Supplementary cobalt was not tried.

Selenium: Although not definitely known to be responsive to selenium administration, due to lack of controlled studies, a white muscle disease has been observed in foals (q.v., p. 578).

VITAMINS

Vitamin A: A deficiency may develop if dried, poor-quality roughage is fed for a prolonged period. If body stores are high, several months may pass before signs appear. The deficiency is characterized by nyctalopia, lacrimation, keratinization of the cornea, susceptibility to pneumonia, abscesses of the sublingual gland, incoordination, impaired reproduction, capricious appetite and progressive weakness. Hooves are frequently deformed, the horny layer unevenly laid down and unusually brittle. Metaplasia of the intestinal mucosa and achlorhydria have been reported. Genitourinary mucosal metaplasia may be expected. Bone remodeling is defective. The foramina do not enlarge properly during growth and skeletal deformities are evident.

Vitamin D: If sun-cured hay is consumed or the horse is exposed to sunlight, it is doubtful that a deficiency of vitamin D would develop. Prolonged confinement of a young, growing horse offered only limited amounts of sun-cured hay may result in reduced bone calcification, stiff and swollen joints, stiffness of gait, irritability and reduction in serum calcium and phosphorus.

Thiamine: The signs of deficiency, which have been produced experimentally in the horse, include anorexia, loss of weight incoordination, lowered blood thiamine and elevated bloo pyruvate. At necropsy the heart is dilated. Similar signs hav been observed in bracken fern poisoning (q.v., p. 977). Unde normal circumstances the natural diet plus synthesis by micro organisms in the gut probably meet the thiamine need.

Riboflavin: Although natural feeds plus synthesis within th gut should normally provide adequate riboflavin, limite evidence indicates an occasional deficiency when the diet is o poor quality. The first sign of acute riboflavin deficiency i the appearance of catarrhal conjunctivitis in one or both eyes This is accompanied by photophobia and lacrimation. Ther may be a gradual deterioration of the retina, lens and ocula fluids, resulting in impaired vision or blindness. Periodi ophthalmia, which has been linked to riboflavin deficiency, i possibly one of the sequelae of leptospirosis (q.v., p. 353), o of onchocerciasis (q.v., p. 692).

Cyanocobalamin (vitamin B_{12}): The need for vitamin B_{12} i probably met by synthesis in the gut. One observation of a anemia (low erythrocyte and hemoglobin concentration which responded to vitamin B_{12} therapy has been reported. I is thought that an extremely low cobalt level in the diet wa the prime cause.

NUTRITIONAL DEFICIENCIES IN DOGS

Most cases of deficiency disease in dogs are multiple de ficiencies. The accurate diagnosis of such a disease is difficul and invariably uncertain. In addition to the lack of specificit of signs, poor husbandry, infectious diseases and parasitism frequently complicate diagnosis.

ENERGY

The most insidious deficiency in dogs is that produced by diet deficient in total calories. Energy is the first use to which all food is put. Multiple deficiencies develop with energy deficient diets, even when otherwise adequate quantities o nutrients are present, because the nutrients are metabolized fo energy rather than being used to meet the nutrient require ment.

PROTEIN

Diets consisting almost entirely of carbohydrates, such a corn meal mush and molasses, are rarely fed today and pro tein deficiency is now seldom seen. When it is, it usually i the result of a deficiency of one or more specific amino acids rather than a total protein deficiency. The signs of protein deficiency include anorexia, anemia, weight loss, unthriftiness and reduced immunity. Extreme cases of hypoproteinemia are characterized by edema, ascites, reduced enzyme activity and the impairment of antibody synthesis.

FAT

Because fat is the most concentrated source of energy, a deficiency of fat usually results in a total energy deficiency before it produces a deficiency of essential fatty acids. While 2% of the correct fats (e.g., lard, horse fat or corn oil) will supply the daily need for essential fatty acids, it cannot provide enough energy to make any diet adequate. In fact, most dermatoses attributed to fatty acid deficiencies are probably due to a total energy deficiency.

VITAMINS

Cases of true dietary vitamin deficiency are rare because of the availability of vitamins in natural ingredients and vitamin-fortified foods. More likely, but still uncommon, are cases produced by reduced consumption due to anorexia or unpalatable diets. These latter deficiencies are invariably multiple in nature, with the accompanying complexity and overlapping signs. The vitamins most apt to be associated with deficiency are A, D, and the B-complex.

Vitamin A: Poor quality growth, reproductive failures and eye problems characterize vitamin A deficiency. Abscesses, blindness and paralysis may occur in advanced cases. When seen, the deficiency usually is due to diets in which vitamin A has been destroyed by poor processing, improper storage or rancid fats.

Vitamin D: A deficiency producing rickets in young dogs and osteoporosis in adults. It is extremely difficult, clinically, to distinguish it from deficiencies of calcium, phosphorus, magnesium and several other minerals. Hypervitaminosis D is a far greater threat to dogs because of injudicious supplementation, under the mistaken notion that the clinical signs are of vitamin D deficiency when they are actually produced by an energy or mineral deficiency or imbalance.

B-complex: Under most clinical circumstances it is preferable to consider the B-complex vitamins as a single entity. The primary signs associated with B-complex deficiencies are anorexia, anemia and CNS disorders. As in diagnosis, therapy with B-complex vitamins should always be accomplished by administering as a single entity, in multiples of the minimum daily requirement.

MINERALS

Like vitamins, minerals are readily available, inexpensive and rarely deficient in good-quality dog foods. The occasional mineral deficiency seen usually appears as a skeletal or hemapoietic abnormality.

Calcium and **phosphorus** are the principal minerals involved in nutritional skeletal disease. However, deficiencies of copper, magnesium and manganese also produce bone lesions. These conditions are virtually impossible to differentiate, etiologically. Fortunately, such differentiation is unnecessary clinically. Regardless of the cause, the appearance of nutritionally related skeletal lesions indicates the diet is deficient and must be replaced with one that is adequate if the condition is to be reversed.

Iron, copper and **cobalt:** Collectively or individually, a deficiency of any of these minerals will produce an anemia. The type will depend on the mineral(s) involved, but the effective solution is the same in every case—replace the deficient diet with one that is adequate.

NUTRITIONAL DEFICIENCIES IN CATS

WATER

Dehydration is a serious problem in disorders of the alimentary and respiratory tracts and kidneys. During anorexia, 1% glucose-saline or similar solutions, 20 to 30 ml/lb of body wt per day (30 to 40 ml/lb in kittens), given orally or parenterally, will help maintain fluid balance and urine flow.

Insufficient fluid intake may precipitate urolithiasis. Fluid intake is increased substantially by adding 1% sodium chloride and mixing additional water in the food. Excessive thirst and frequent urination may indicate diabetes mellitus, diabetes insipidus or kidney damage. The cat with polydipsia, or having salt added to its diet, should never be denied drinking water.

PROTEIN AND ENERGY

Unless there is sufficient energy in a cat's diet, protein needed for other body functions will be converted to energy. Consequently, the ratio of protein to calories is probably more important than the actual quantity and makeup of the energy sources. Feedstuffs too low in fat, containing too much indigestible carbohydrate or not enough B-complex vitamins all can result in an energy-deficient diet. Too little animal protein, too much fat or too much carbohydrate can cause a protein-deficient diet.

The signs produced by an improper protein-calorie ratio may include any or all of the following: weight loss; dull, unkempt haircoat; anorexia; reproductive problems; persistent, unresponsive parasitism; persistent, unresponsive, low-grade infection; unexplained "breaks" in the vaccination program; rapid, precipitous weight loss after injury or during disease; failure to respond properly to injury or disease—and should suggest modification of the diet.

FAT-SOLUBLE VITAMINS

Vitamin A: Liver and fish liver oils and synthetic vitamin A are the principal sources of vitamin A for cats since they cannot utilize carotene. Classical xerophthalmia, follicular hyperkeratosis, and retinal degeneration occur rarely, usually associated with concomitant protein deficiency. Borderline deficiency is more common, especially in chronic ill health. Plasma vitamin A levels below 30 mcg/100 ml indicate deficiency. Hypovitaminosis A affects reproduction, causing stillbirths, congenital anomalies (hydrocephaly, blindness, deafness, ataxia, cerebellar dysplasia, intestinal hernia) and resorption of fetuses. Overdosing with vitamin A must be avoided. Hypervitaminosis A may produce forelimb lameness, with or without hyperesthesia, associated with radiologic evidence of scoliosis, ankylosis and exostosis.

Vitamin D: Classical signs of rickets (q.v., p. 564) are rare in kittens and confined to those born in winter, kept permanently in dark quarters, or from queens fed vitamin D-deficient rations. It is important to avoid hypervitaminosis D through overdosing.

Vitamin E: Steatitis (q.v., p. 580) results from a diet high in polyunsaturated fatty acids, particularly from marine fish oils. Kittens develop anorexia and muscular dystrophy; depot fat becomes discolored by brown or orange pigment. Lesions occur in cardiac and skeletal muscles.

WATER-SOLUBLE VITAMINS

Apart from thiamine and pyridoxine deficiency, water-soluble vitamin deficiencies are usually the result of disease processes which limit alimentary synthesis and absorption, or increase metabolic requirement or kidney loss. In such circumstances oral or parenteral administration of multiple B-vitamin preparations may prevent the onset of "feline pellagra" which is characterized by ulcerative stomatitis, especially of the tongue, and by conjunctivitis.

Thiamine deficiency rarely occurs on a fresh-meat or good commercial diet. Thiaminase from uncooked fish can produce a deficiency. Destruction of thiamine may also result from treatment of food with sulfur dioxide or heating during drying or canning. Cats eating a thiamine-deficient diet develop anorexia, an unkempt coat and a hunched appearance. Convulsions follow, becoming more severe, leading in a few days to prostration and death-signs often described by owners as indicative of "poisoning". Diagnosis can be confirmed in the early stages by giving thiamine orally or IM. Recovery occurs in a matter of hours. If the diet is not supplemented following this treatment, a relapse can be expected. At necropsy, small petechial hemorrhages may be found in the cerebrum and midbrain.

The pyridoxine-deficient cat loses weight, becomes anemic and suffers kidney damage due to the accumulation of oxalate. A severe form of calcium oxalate urolithiasis ensues.

MINERALS

The requirement for dietary calcium in kittens and queens is increased. Insufficient supplies result in the condition referred to as nutritional hyperparathyroidism (q.v., p. 562). Signs of irritability, hyperesthesia and loss of muscle tone appear with temporary or permanent paralysis. Rarefaction of the skeleton, particularly the pelvis and vertebral bodies, can be confirmed radiologically, and is a valuable diagnostic aid. There is often a history of diet confined almost wholly to meat. The condition can be corrected by replacing the current diet with one that is known to be capable of supporting kitten growth.

Iodine deficiency may occur on meat diets but rarely on diets containing saltwater fish or on good cat rations. The deficient kitten will show signs of hyperthyroidism in the early stages, with increased excitability, followed later by hypothyroidism and lethargy. The condition can be confirmed by size (over 12 mg/100 gm of body wt) and histopathology of the thyroid gland at necropsy.

Iron and copper in meat can be utilized efficiently by cats. Occasionally deficiencies probably result from alimentary disorders. Excess dietary manganese may darken coat color in partial albinos such as Siamese, and also reduce fertility.

NUTRITIONAL DEFICIENCIES IN POULTRY

A nutritional deficiency may be either simple or multiple, that is, the total feed consumed may not contain an adequate quantity of one or more indispensable nutrients. A given deficiency may be borderline, marked, or absolute. About the only observable result of a borderline deficiency is slightly retarded growth, slightly decreased egg production, or slightly reduced hatchability. An absolute deficiency of any indispensable nutrient causes death. A marked deficiency of one or more indispensable nutrients leads to the development of a deficiency disease.

In many deficiency diseases, the same general signs, such as retarded growth, poor feathering and weakness, are observed. Thus, it is not always possible to recognize the cause from the signs. In most instances, a correct diagnosis can be made only by obtaining complete information about the diet and management of the birds, in addition to observing the signs in the affected living birds and making necropsies of at least a few birds soon after death. Because they are difficult to diagnose, chronic deficiencies may be more injurious in the long run than acute ones.

In assessing a diet, it is well to keep in mind that the composition of the individual ingredients is variable and that some nutrients are comparatively unstable and some are unavailable as they occur naturally in feeds. A diet that appears to contain just enough of one or more nutrients may actually be deficient to some degree in those nutrients. Conditions of stress (bacterial, parasitic and viral infections; high or low temperatures; low humidity; drugs) may either interfere with the absorption of a nutrient or increase the quantity required. Thus, conditions of stress may, in effect, cause an otherwise adequate diet to be deficient.

Only deficiencies occurring on practical diets in the field are discussed herein.

PROTEIN AND AMINO ACID DEFICIENCIES

Etiology: The optimum level of protein intake for the young growing chick appears to be about 20 to 21% of the diet, for the young growing poult and gallinaceous upland game birds, about 26 to 30% and for young growing ducklings, about 22%. When the protein content of the diet is reduced below these levels, the birds tend to grow more slowly. Small reductions in the protein content of the diet, however, often may be compensated for by an increased feed intake unless the diet is unusually bulky.

Even though a diet contains the above specified quantities of protein, satisfactory growth will not result without sufficient amounts of all the indispensable amino acids. A deficiency of protein causes an increased deposition of fat in the bird since productive use cannot be made of the energy consumed if protein intake is suboptimum.

Clinical Findings: Except in the case of lysine, the only apparent indication of amino acid deficiency is retarded growth. In the turkey poult (particularly the Bronze variety), a deficiency of lysine inhibits the pigmentation of the feathers; some of the feathers on the wings are white or have a white bar. Normal pigmentation of new feathers takes place as soon as adequate diet is fed, but the unpigmented portion of an already existing feather remains colorless.

MINERAL DEFICIENCIES

Calcium and Phosphorus Deficiencies

A deficiency of either calcium or phosphorus in the diet of young growing birds results in an abnormal development of the skeleton even though the diet contains a fully adequate quantity of vitamin D (*see* VITAMIN D DEFICIENCY, p. 1351). The abnormal development is neither prevented nor stopped by increasing the intake of vitamin D, if the deficiency of either calcium or phosphorus is marked.

This abnormal condition of the skeleton commonly is referred to as rickets, but some writers distinguish between the condition that results from a deficiency of calcium (osteoporosis) and that which results from a deficiency of phosphorus (rickets). Osteoporosis may be observed in adult as well as in young growing birds, whereas rickets is observed only in the latter.

Etiology: The newly hatched bird is essentially osteoporotic as its bones have a much lower calcium:phosphorus ratio than they do later on if the diet is fully adequate. Hence, the newly hatched bird requires an immediate supply of calcium in its diet. If the diet is markedly deficient in either calcium or vitamin D, the osteoporotic condition becomes more pronounced. If, however, the diet contains sufficient calcium, but is deficient in either phosphorus or vitamin D, rickets develops. One means of producing rickets experimentally is to feed a diet high in calcium, but low in phosphorus.

Clinical Findings: The first signs of a deficiency of calcium or phosphorus, or both, in young growing birds are very similar to those of vitamin D deficiency. Typical of all 3 deficiencies (calcium, phosphorus and vitamin D) are a lame, stiff-legged gait, retardation of growth and ruffled feathers. In calcium deficiency, the leg bones are springy, but in phosphorus or in vitamin D deficiency, they are rubbery and the joints tend to be enlarged. In calcium, but not in phosphorus deficiency, some of the birds may become paralyzed.

If a bird in heavy egg production does not obtain enough calcium from its feed, the skeleton is depleted and becomes osteoporotic; a few thin-shelled eggs and also eggs with low hatchability are produced and then production ceases. If there is a very marked deficiency of calcium, a paralytic condition may develop. If calcium is not supplied, death follows within 1 to 3 days after the onset of the paralysis.

Laboratory Findings: In both rickets and osteoporosis, there is a decreased ash content of the bones. The changes in the content of calcium and phosphorus in the blood depend on the content of calcium and phosphorus in the diet. If the dietary calcium level is low, the blood may have an approximately normal calcium and a high phosphorus content. If the diet is deficient in both calcium and phosphorus, the blood may contain less than the normal quantities of these elements.

Prophylaxis and Treatment: For the prevention of calcium and phosphorus deficiencies, it is sufficient to provide diets with adequate quantities of these 2 elements. In the case of the growing bird, it is particularly desirable not to have a gross excess of calcium in the diet because rickets will tend to occur on a diet normally adequate in phosphorus and vitamin D if a gross excess of calcium is added to it. Feeding diets containing more than 2.5% calcium during the growing period produces a high incidence of nephrosis, visceral gout, calcium urate deposits in the ureters and high mortality.

An improvement in egg-shell strength can be achieved by feeding about two-thirds of the calcium supplement in the form of oyster-shell flakes or coarse limestone, with the remaining one-third as ground limestone. At no time should oyster shell or any other form of calcium supplement be added without an equivalent reduction in the amount of limestone as feeding too much calcium reduces shell quality. Offering the coarse supplement permits the birds to pick out their requirements when they need it most.

If paralysis resulting from calcium deficiency should develop, an effective treatment—if started very soon after the paralysis occurs—is to give orally 1 gm of calcium carbonate in a gelatin capsule daily for 2 or 3 days and to feed a fully adequate diet. Treatment of experimental calcium deficiency usually causes disappearance of the paralysis within 48 hours.

MANGANESE DEFICIENCY

A deficiency of manganese in the diet of young growing chickens is one of the causes—the first to be recognized—of perosis; in the diet of laying chickens, it is one of the causes of thin-shelled eggs and poor hatchability (*see* CALCIUM AND PHOSPHORUS DEFICIENCIES, p. 1344, *also* VITAMIN D DEFICIENCY, p. 1351).

Etiology: Many of the feedstuffs used in feeding poultry do not contain enough manganese to meet the requirement for this element. This is especially true of corn, and diets based on corn usually are deficient in manganese unless they contain a special source, such as manganese sulfate or manganese oxide. Manganese deficiency is now much less common because virtually all commercial feeds contain added manganese. For that reason, it is well to consider the other possible causes when perosis is encountered.

Clinical Findings: Perosis is a malformation of the hock joint. The signs usually found are swelling and flattening of the hock joint, sometimes followed by slipping of the Achilles tendon from its condyles. The tibia and the tarsometatarsus may exhibit bending near the joint and lateral rotation. One or both legs may be affected. A shortening and thickening of the long bones of the legs and wings is also apparent. Perosis caused by manganese deficiency is exacerbated by excessive amounts of calcium and phosphorus in the diet. Birds reared on wire or slatted floors are more susceptible to perosis than those reared on litter.

The signs of perosis in poults, ducklings and goslings are similar to those observed in chicks. Perosis has been observed in various wild birds, including pheasants, grouse, quail and sparrows.

When adult chickens are fed a diet deficient in manganese, no observable changes in their leg joints occur, but the shells of their eggs tend to become thinner and less resistant to breakage. If the deficiency is sufficiently marked, both egg production and hatchability are reduced. The reduced hatchability results from an increase in the embryonic mortality that occurs after the 10th day of incubation. The embryonic mortality reaches its peak at about the 20th and 21st days.

The embryos that die after the 10th day usually are chondrodystrophic; they have short, thickened legs, short wings, "parrot beaks", a globular contour of the head, protruding abdomen and, in the most severe cases, retarded development of the down. The few chicks that sometimes hatch usually have very short leg bones (micromelia) and in some cases, the bones may be deformed as in the chicks in which perosis develops after hatching.

Prophylaxis and Treatment: The only way to prevent perosis is to feed a diet adequate in all indispensable nutrients, especially manganese, choline, niacin, biotin and folic acid. After deformities have occurred, they cannot be corrected by feeding an adequate diet. Effects of manganese deficiency on egg production are fully corrected by an adequate diet that contains 33 to 40 mg/kg of manganese, provided that the diet does not contain excessive quantities of calcium and phosphorus. It would be very unusual to find a commercial feed for laying chickens that contained an excessive quantity of calcium; however the intake may be excessive where calcium supplements are provided free choice. When meat scrap or meat-and-bone scrap is used as the principal source of protein, the feed may contain an excessive quantity of phosphorus.

IRON AND COPPER DEFICIENCIES

A microcytic, hypochromic anemia can be produced by iron or copper deficiency. However, there is no change in the number of red blood cells. Both copper and iron deficiencies will cause depigmentation in the feathers of Rhode Island Red or New Hampshire chickens. Copper deficiency in chicks produces dissecting aneurysms of the aorta and various bone deformities. Copper is needed in elastin formation. Most practical diets for poultry will contain enough iron and copper to prevent deficiencies. Some feed manufacturers add small amounts as an insurance measure.

IODINE DEFICIENCY

Very few cases of goiter, or enlarged thyroids, have been observed in poultry, probably because it is difficult to observe the glands. Goiter has been produced experimentally in chickens by feeding a diet exceedingly low in iodine (about 0.025 ppm) to laying hens. The possibility of an iodine deficiency in poultry may easily be obviated by adding as little as 0.35 mg of iodine per kilogram of feed.

MAGNESIUM DEFICIENCY

Magnesium deficiency does not occur in poultry fed practical diets. It may be produced experimentally by feeding a diet of highly purified feedstuffs. When such a diet is fed to young chicks, one observes poor growth and feathering, decreased muscle tone, ataxia, progressive incoordination and convulsions followed by death.

POTASSIUM DEFICIENCY

A great majority of the natural feedstuffs and many of the by-product feedstuffs used in feeding poultry contain much more potassium than is needed. Deficiencies of this mineral, therefore, are not seen in commercially raised poultry.

SALT DEFICIENCY

The salt requirement of chickens, and presumably other kinds of poultry, is rather low. Of the 2 chemical elements in salt, sodium is required in appreciably larger quantity than chlorine. Diets containing less than 0.15% of sodium retard growth in young chicks and depress egg production and hatchability in laying chickens. A high level of potassium appears to increase the requirement of sodium and a high level of sodium appears to increase the requirement of potassium. Most practical poultry diets require the addition of 0.25 to 0.5% of sodium chloride to prevent a deficiency.

Inasmuch as nearly all feedstuffs contain some salt and a few contain from 1 to 4.5% or more (e.g., whey, fish meal, meat scrap, condensed fish solubles), an excess of salt is possible. An excess causes the droppings to be loose and watery. Chickens may be raised on diets that contain as much as 3% of salt, but growth is retarded and efficiency of feed utilization is reduced. The same percentage—or even less—of salt in the drinking water is very toxic.

ZINC DEFICIENCY

With a diet deficient in zinc, growth is retarded and feather development is poor. The hock joints become enlarged and the long bones are shortened and thickened. Slipping of the tendons does not occur. On occasion the skin on the foot pads becomes dry and thickened with fissures and hyperkeratosis developing.

In mature hens, zinc deficiency reduces egg production and hatchability. Embryos show a wide range of skeletal abnormalities including micromelia, curvature of the spine, and shortened, fused thoracic and lumbar vertebrae. It is usual practice to include a zinc supplement in all practical poultry diets.

SELENIUM DEFICIENCY

A deficiency of selenium in growing chickens causes exudative diathesis. The early signs (unthriftiness, ruffled feathers) usually occur between 5 and 11 weeks of age. The subcut. edema results in weeping of the skin which is often seen on the inner surface of the thighs and wings. The birds bruise easily, with large scabs often forming on an old bruise. In laying hens, the tissue damage is unusual but egg production and feed conversion are adversely affected.

Despite the widespread occurrence of selenium deficiency in practical diets, it is illegal in some countries for the manufacturer to add inorganic selenium supplements to feeds; when exudative diathesis occurs, a veterinarian may prescribe the use of a supplement such as sodium selenite in the drinking water. Where permitted and where deficiency is likely to occur, it is advisable to add selenium to the feed. Otherwise, feeds grown on high-selenium soils are good sources of selenium and may be incorporated in poultry rations. Fish meal and dried brewer's yeast are also good sources. There is considerable variation in the availability of selenium in different feedstuffs.

Even in the presence of adequate levels of vitamin E, poultry rations must contain 0.15 to 0.2 mg of selenium per kilogram of feed. As little as 8 to 10 mg/kg is toxic to poultry.

VITAMIN DEFICIENCIES

VITAMIN A DEFICIENCY

Vitamin A is required for the normal development and repair of all epithelial structures and for the normal development of the bones. Although vitamin A has not been found to be of value in building immunity, it is of value in maintaining the "first line of defense", the epithelial structures.

Etiology: Vitamin A and its several precursors (alpha-, beta-, and gamma carotene and cryptoxanthin) are relatively unstable.

Feeds stored for a long time before being fed may contain too little vitamin A activity to meet the requirements of birds to which they are fed, especially if they contain meat scrap or fish meal from particular lots.

Clinical Findings: When young chicks are fed a diet markedly deficient in vitamin A activity, their rate of growth becomes subnormal after about 3 weeks and then declines very rapidly.

The first characteristic signs, other than decline in rate of growth, are droopiness, ataxia and a ruffled appearance of the feathers. If the chicks survive more than a week after they become droopy, the eyes may become inflamed and there may be a discharge from the nostrils; in some chicks, there is swelling around the eyes and an accumulation of a sticky exudate beneath the lids. When the diet is not markedly deficient in vitamin A, the first signs may not appear until the chicks are 5 to 6 weeks old, in which case a larger proportion of the chicks eventually develop eye lesions and marked nervousness.

The signs of vitamin A deficiency in the poult are similar to those in the chick, but tend to be more acute.

In mature chickens and other poultry, the signs of vitamin A deficiency develop more slowly than in young birds, but the inflammation of the nose and eyes is much more pronounced. A borderline deficiency of vitamin A results in decreased egg production and reduced hatchability.

Lesions: In mature birds, vitamin A deficiency produces lesions resembling pustules in the mouth, pharynx and esophagus; in young growing birds, these lesions are found less frequently. Often there are white or grayish-white deposits of urates in the kidneys and ureters. Such deposits, however, occur more frequently in young chickens than in young turkeys. Sometimes, there are deposits of urates on the surface of the heart, liver and spleen. Usually, urate or urate-like deposits are found in the thickened folds of the bursa of Fabricius.

In general, there is keratinization of the epithelial cells of the olfactory, respiratory, upper alimentary and urinary tracts. In severe cases, especially if the birds are mature, virtually all organs may be affected. Also, there are degenerative changes in both the central and peripheral nervous systems.

In very marked vitamin A deficiency in the chicken, the uric acid content of the blood may increase to 8 or 9 times its normal value. The accumulation of uric acid in the blood and the previously mentioned occurrence of deposits of uric acid in the ureters, kidneys and elsewhere probably are the result of failure of repair of the epithelial structures, especially those of the kidneys.

The nasal structures apparently may be used in diagnosing borderline deficiencies. In all degrees of vitamin A deficiency, there are true squamous metaplasia of the secretory and glandular epithelium, and secondary inflammatory or obstructive changes. In absolute vitamin A deficiency, there are atrophy, squamous metaplasia and hyperkeratinization.

Prophylaxis and Treatment: While the naturally occurring vitamin A precursors tend to be unstable in storage, most feed manufacturers include an antioxidant in feed which is to be stored for an appreciable length of time. This coupled with the fact that stabilized, dry vitamin A supplements are almost universally used today, makes it unlikely that vitamin A deficiency will be encountered in practice.

However, if vitamin A deficiency does develop through inadvertently omitting the vitamin A supplement or because of poor mixing, feed containing 3 to 4 times the normally recommended level can be fed for about 2 weeks. The dry, stabilized forms of vitamin A are the supplements of choice for the feed. There are also water-dispersible forms of vitamin A which can be administered through the drinking water; when feasible, this will usually give faster recovery than medication of the feed.

VITAMIN D DEFICIENCY

Abnormal development of the bones has been discussed under calcium and phosphorus deficiencies (p. 1344) and manganese deficiency (p. 1346). Vitamin D is required for the normal absorption and metabolism of calcium and phosphorus. A deficiency of vitamin D always produces rickets in young growing chickens and other poultry, even when the diet contains calcium and phosphorus in adequate quantities.

Etiology: The rickets and osteoporosis encountered in the practical production of poultry most frequently are the result of a deficiency of vitamin D. When poultry are reared in strict confinement, they require more vitamin D, as such, than when they have access to sunshine.

Clinical Findings: The first signs in young growing chickens and turkeys are a tendency to rest frequently in a squatting position, a disinclination to walk and a lame, stiff-legged gait. These are distinguished from the clinical signs of vitamin A deficiency in that birds with a vitamin D deficiency are alert rather than droopy and walk with a lame rather than a staggering gait (ataxia). Other signs, in the usual order of their occurrence, are retardation of growth, enlargement of the hock joints, beading at the ends of the ribs and marked softening of the beak. As in many other nutritional diseases of poultry, the feathers soon become ruffled.

In breeds of chickens that are red or buff in color, a deficiency of vitamin D causes an abnormal black pigmentation of some of the feathers, especially those of the wings. If the deficiency is very marked, the blackening of the feathers becomes pronounced and nearly all the feathers may be affected. When vitamin D is supplied in adequate quantity, the new feathers and the newer part of the older feathers are normal in color; the discolored portion remains black.

When laying chickens are fed a diet deficient in vitamin D, the first sign of the deficiency is a thinning of the shells of their eggs. If the deficiency is marked, there is a rather prompt reduction of both egg production and hatchability. After a time, the breast bones become noticeably less rigid and there may be beading at the ends of the ribs.

Lesions: In young chickens and turkeys, a deficiency of vitamin D produces marked changes in the bones and the parathyroid and thyroid glands, and variable changes in the calcium and phosphorus content of the blood (*see* CALCIUM AND PHOSPHORUS DEFICIENCIES, p. 1344). The bones may be quite soft or only moderately so. The epiphyses of the long bones usually are enlarged. The parathyroid becomes enlarged, sometimes to about 8 times its normal size, as a result of an increase in both the size of the cells and the number of epithelial cells.

In adult chickens, a deficiency of vitamin D eventually produces changes in the parathyroid similar to those produced in young chicks. The bones tend to become rarefied (osteoporotic) rather than soft.

Treatment: There is no need to change the feeding program being used. Enough extra vitamin D is added to the mash to provide 3 times the normally recommended level for a period of about 3 weeks. It is suggested that dry, stabilized forms of vitamin D_3 be used for feeding to poultry.

VITAMIN E DEFICIENCY

Chicks fed a diet deficient in vitamin E may show one or more of 3 classical deficiency disorders, namely, encephalomalacia, exudative diathesis and muscular dystrophy. Various dietary changes unrelated to the vitamin E content of the diet can completely prevent any one of these diseases without affecting the course of the other two. Thus, synthetic antioxidants can prevent encephalomalacia, inorganic selenium can prevent exudative diathesis while cystine can prevent muscular dystrophy. It would appear that no common metabolic defect can account for all 3 disorders.

Vitamin E is required for normal reproductive performance in the hen and for normal fertility in the mature male.

Etiology: Although both selenium and antioxidants can spare the requirements of vitamin E for certain functions, practical poultry diets must still contain sufficient vitamin E. Encephalomalacia has been a field problem for many years. It occurs with diets borderline in vitamin E that also contain polyunsaturated fats such as cod-liver oil or soybean oil in the process of undergoing oxidative rancidity. Since it is correlated with peroxidation of fats it may be prevented with vitamin E or a suitable antioxidant such as ethoxyquin. Exudative diathesis is a frequent occurrence on corn and soybean meal diets when these are grown on soils deficient in selenium. Both vitamin E and selenium are necessary to prevent the disease. Nutritional muscular dystrophy, not ordinarily a commercial problem, is found only when the diet is deficient in both vitamin E and sulfur amino acids. Because of the importance of sulfur amino acids for growth and feed efficiency they are usually present in adequate levels in practical diets.

Clinical Findings: Signs of encephalomalacia are sudden prostration, with legs outstretched and toes flexed, and retraction of the head. In the early stages the gait is incoordinate. Upon necropsy, lesions are found in the cerebellum and sometimes in the cerebrum. In some birds necrotic reddish or brownish areas can be detected on the surface of the cerebellum.

Exudative diathesis is a severe edema produced by a marked increase in capillary permeability (see SELENIUM DEFICIENCY, p. 1349). Broilers are often severely downgraded because of the yellow staining inside the thighs caused by leakage of plasma into the subcut. tissues in this area.

Nutritional muscular dystrophy in chicks is characterized by degeneration of the muscle fibers, especially of the breast but also occurring occasionally in the leg muscles. There is perivascular infiltration, with marked accumulation of eosinophils, lymphocytes and histocytes. These cells, along with the degenerated muscle fibers, present a picture of degeneration, with large numbers of free nuclei in evidence.

In mature chickens no outward signs of vitamin E deficiency are apparent even after a prolonged period. However, degenerative changes in the testes may occur, leading to loss of fertility. Egg production appears not to be affected by a vitamin E deficiency, but hatchability is markedly reduced. During incubation of the eggs, growth and differentiation are slow with many embryos dying during the first 2 days of incubation due to circulatory failure.

Vitamin E deficiency in poults causes nutritional myopathy. This disorder is characterized by lesions in the muscular wall of the gizzard which appear as circumscribed gray areas that often are of firmer texture than normal muscle and are not unlike scar tissue.

Prophylaxis and Treatment: Only stabilized fat should be used in feed. Where feed is to be stored for more than 2 weeks a chemical antioxidant should be used. Storage at high environmental temperatures and high humidity accentuates destruction of vitamin E.

Signs of exudative diathesis and muscular dystrophy, when caused by lack of vitamin E, can be reversed if seen in time, by administration of vitamin E by oral dosing or through the feed. Oral administration of a single dose of 300 IU of vitamin E per bird will usually cause remission of the diseases. Old feed should be removed and replaced by a fresh supply, amply fortified with vitamin E.

Vitamin K Deficiency

A deficiency of vitamin K causes a reduction in the prothrombin content of the blood and, in the chick, may reduce the quantity in the plasma to less than 2% of normal. Since the prothrombin content of the blood of normal, newly hatched chicks is only about 40% of that of adult birds, very young chicks are readily affected by a deficiency of vitamin K.

Etiology: Until about 1952, cases of vitamin K deficiency seldom, if ever, were encountered in poultry. Since 1952, however, there have been many reports of a hemorrhagic disease in young growing chickens that often may be cured by adding vitamin K—sometimes both vitamin K and vitamin E—to the feed. One of the probable causes of this rise of hemorrhagic disease, which became a cause for concern in 1953, may lie in the changes that have been made in poultry feeds since then. Alfalfa meal is one of the better sources of vitamin K (and usually of vitamin E as well) among feedstuffs. Between about 1946 and 1952, there was a growing tendency to reduce greatly its quantity in poultry feeds. There has also been a trend toward the use of solvent-extracted soybean meal and other seed meals and a trend toward the use of better quality but less putrefied fish meals, which are lower in vitamin K than the original expeller meals and putrid fish meals. It has been suggested that this so-called "hemorrhagic syndrome" (q.v., p. 1085) is not a vitamin K deficiency, but probably caused by certain toxic substances elaborated by molds normally found on grains and corn and in feeds made from such grains.

Clinical Findings: In very young chicks deficient in vitamin K, blood coagulation time begins to increase after about 5 to 10 days and becomes greatly prolonged in 7 to 12 days. After about a week, hemorrhages often occur in any part of the body, either spontaneously or as the result of an injury or bruise. The only external signs are the resulting accumulations of blood under the skin. Postmortem examination usually reveals accumulations of blood in the various parts of the body; sometimes there are petechial hemorrhages in the liver and almost invariably there is erosion of the gizzard lining.

When hemorrhagic disease is encountered under practical conditions, the signs usually are observed after the age of 3 weeks.

Prophylaxis and Treatment: Vitamin K deficiency usually can be prevented by including about 2.5% of alfalfa meal in the feed. The inclusion of menadione in the feed, at the rate of 1.0 gm/ton, is effective, and is now a common practice.

There are a number of stress factors which increase the requirements for vitamin K. Dicumarol, sulfaquinoxaline and warfarin are antimetabolites of vitamin K. Coccidiosis and other intestinal parasitic diseases also increase the need for this vitamin.

When signs of vitamin K deficiency are encountered, the feed should be changed immediately to one that contains about 5% of alfalfa meal, or menadione and vitamin E may be added to the feed at the rate of 1.0 gm and 10,000 IU, respectively, per ton.

VITAMIN B_{12} DEFICIENCY

The vitamin B_{12} requirement of poultry is exceedingly small; an adequate allowance is only a few mcg/kg of feed. Vitamin B_{12} is produced by many bacteria and, in general, is present in feedstuffs of animal origin and in feces. Vitamin B_{12} is now included in most commercial poultry feeds, thus making a deficiency unlikely. It is required for growth and hatchability.

Marked vitamin B_{12} deficiency is difficult, if not impossible, to produce in birds that have free access to their droppings. However, such birds may not receive optimum vitamin B_{12} levels and may fail to achieve growth at a maximum rate. No truly characteristic signs of vitamin B_{12} deficiency have been reported, except for an increased incidence of gizzard erosion. A deficiency of vitamin B_{12}, however, is one of several causes of retarded growth, decreased feed efficiency and reduced hatchability. Vitamin B_{12} deficiency is easily prevented and cured by feeding a diet containing feedstuffs of animal origin or a commercial cobalamin supplement.

CHOLINE DEFICIENCY

Choline has several physiologic functions in poultry. In addition to being necessary for the prevention of perosis, it plays a role in growth, methylation and the regulation of the synthesis and transport of lipids. A deficiency of choline in the diet, even when there are adequate quantities of manganese, biotin, folic acid and niacin, results in the development of perosis (see MANGANESE DEFICIENCY, p. 1346) and the retardation of growth. There is some evidence that choline is required for the maintenance of maximum egg production and high hatchability. However, the laying hen has considerable ability to synthesize choline and practical diets may provide sufficient for their needs.

Prophylaxis and Treatment: Diets containing appreciable quantities of soybean meal, wheat bran and wheat middlings are not likely to be deficient in choline because soybean meal is a good source of choline, and wheat bran and middlings are good sources of betaine, which is able to perform the methyl-donor function of choline. Other good sources of choline are distillers' grains, fish meal, liver meal, meat scrap, distillers' solubles and yeast. A number of commercial choline supplements are available and choline is routinely added to a number of poultry feeds.

NIACIN (NICOTINIC ACID) DEFICIENCY

Etiology: There is good evidence that chickens—even chick and turkey embryos—are able to synthesize niacin, but that the rate of synthesis may be too slow for optimum growth. It has been claimed that before there can be a marked deficiency of niacin in the chicken, there must first be a deficiency of tryptophan. In any case, tryptophan serves as a precursor of niacin.

Niacin deficiency has been observed in chicks, ducks, geese and turkey poults when certain practical-type diets were fed. Diets high in corn and soybean meal are particularly amenable to improvement by inclusion of supplementary niacin. Ducks and geese have a considerably higher requirement for niacin than chicks. Most of the niacin present in practical feedstuffs such as corn is unavailable to poultry. Mature birds have considerably more ability to synthesize niacin than young birds.

Clinical Findings: In the case of a borderline deficiency of niacin in the diet of chicks, the only sign is retarded growth. Chicks and turkey poults fed a diet deficient in niacin develop a hock disorder similar in appearance to perosis, with swollen hocks and bowed legs. Both goslings and ducklings develop abnormalities of the legs. The condition in goslings has been referred to as perosis and that in ducklings as "bowed legs". When laying chickens are fed a diet deficient in niacin, there is a loss of weight and both egg production and hatchability are reduced. (*See also* MANGANESE DEFICIENCY, p. 1346.)

Prophylaxis and Treatment: Niacin deficiency in chickens may be prevented by feeding a diet that contains about 27 mg/kg, but a number of nutritionists recommend 2 to 2½ times as much. An allowance of 55 to 70 mg of niacin per kilogram of feed appears to be satisfactory for ducks, geese and turkeys. It is good economics to provide ample niacin in poultry diets so that the birds do not have to synthesize it from tryptophan, which is difficult to supply.

PANTOTHENIC ACID DEFICIENCY

Etiology: Although most feedstuffs used in feeding poultry are fairly good sources of pantothenic acid, diets composed largely of cereal grains and containing some meat scrap or fish meal, or both, may not contain enough of this vitamin. Corn that has been kiln-dried tends to have a lowered content and in general, pantothenic acid in feedstuffs is destroyed by dry heat.

Clinical Findings: When chicks are deficient in pantothenic acid, their growth is retarded and their feathers acquire a ragged appearance. Within 12 to 14 days, the margins of the eyelids become granulated and frequently a viscous exudate causes the eyelids to stick together. Crusty scabs appear at the corners of the mouth; the skin on the bottoms of the feet often becomes thickened and cornified. In chronic pantothenic acid deficiency, after a period of 4 to 5 months, there is a loss of feathers from the head and neck. Depigmentation of the feathers has been reported.

The signs of pantothenic acid deficiency in young turkeys are similar to those in young chickens and include general weakness, keratitis and sticking together of the eyelids. Young ducks do not show the usual signs seen in chickens and turkeys, except retarded growth; however, their mortality is very high.

When the diet of laying chickens is deficient in pantothenic acid, the concentration of this vitamin in their eggs decreases and hatchability is greatly reduced. The few chicks that hatch grow slowly and their mortality is high.

Lesions: Lesions of the spinal cord, characterized by myelin degeneration of the medullated fibers, occur in chicks fed a diet deficient in pantothenic acid. Degenerating fibers may be found in all segments of the spinal cord down to the lumbar region. Involution of the thymus, a fatty liver and an acute nephritis have also been reported.

Prophylaxis and Treatment: While it is easy to formulate feed mixtures that are fully adequate in pantothenic acid, it is often more economical to add calcium pantothenate (at the rate of about 5.0 to 5.5 mg/kg of feed).

Sometimes, half-grown chickens fed practical diets develop a scaly condition of the skin. The exact cause of this condition is not known, but it has been treated successfully in some instances by putting both calcium pantothenate and riboflavin in the drinking water (2.0 gm of calcium pantothenate and 0.5 gm of riboflavin in 50 gal. of water) for a few days.

RIBOFLAVIN DEFICIENCY

Etiology: Only a few of the feedstuffs fed to poultry contain enough riboflavin to meet the requirement of the young growing chick, poult, or duckling. Hence, if the ingredients of a poultry feed are not carefully selected or if a special supplement is not included, it may be deficient in riboflavin. Riboflavin is available commercially. It is generally added to practical rations so that riboflavin deficiency is now relatively uncommon.

Clinical Findings: The characteristic sign of riboflavin deficiency in the chick is "curled toe" paralysis. It, however, does not develop when there is an absolute deficiency, or when the deficiency is very marked, because the chicks die before it appears. Three degrees of severity of "curled toe" paralysis have been described. The first is characterized by a tendency of the chicks to rest on their hocks and a slight curling of the toes; the second, by marked weakness of the legs and a distinct curling of the toes on one or both feet; and the third, by toes that are completely curled inward or under and a weakened condition of the legs that compels the chicks to walk on their hocks.

Other signs of riboflavin deficiency are stunting, diarrhea after 8 to 10 days and high mortality after about 3 weeks. There is no apparent impairment of the growth of the feathers;

on the contrary, the main wing feathers often appear to be disproportionately long.

Signs of riboflavin deficiency in the poult and duckling differ from those in the chick. In the poult, a dermatitis appears in about 8 days, the vent becomes encrusted, inflamed and excoriated, growth is retarded or completely stopped by about the 17th day and deaths begin to occur about the 21st day. In the duckling, there usually is diarrhea and cessation of growth.

When laying hens are fed a diet deficient in riboflavin, egg production is decreased and hatchability reduced, roughly in proportion to the degree of the deficiency. The embryonic mortality has 2 typical peaks and often a third peak. These are, respectively, on the fourth and 20th days and on the 14th day of incubation. Most of the embryos are dwarfed and exhibit pronounced micromelia; some of the embryos are edematous. The down fails to emerge properly, thus resulting in a typical abnormality, termed "clubbed" down, which is most common in the areas of the neck and around the vent.

Lesions: Riboflavin deficiency in young poultry produces specific changes in the main peripheral nerve trunks. In acute cases, there are hypertrophy of the nerve trunks and readily observable changes in their appearance. Degenerative changes also appear in the myelin of the nerves. Congestion and premature atrophy of the lobes of the thymus may also be observed.

Prophylaxis and Treatment: By formulating the diet to contain about 3.6 to 4.0 mg of riboflavin per kilogram, riboflavin deficiency is easily prevented.

THIAMINE (VITAMIN B₁) AND VITAMIN B₆ DEFICIENCIES

Most of the feedstuffs used in feeding poultry contain more than adequate quantities of thiamine and vitamin B₆. Accordingly, deficiencies of these vitamins rarely, if ever, occur when practical diets are fed.

FOLIC ACID (FOLACIN) DEFICIENCY

Etiology: Until recently it was believed unlikely that folic acid deficiency would occur in chicks or turkeys under field conditions. However, modern solvent-extracted soybean meal appears to be lower in the vitamin than the old expeller meal and today much of the folic acid in alfalfa is destroyed by pelleting. Also, fish meal and meat meal are rather poor sources. While much of the folic acid is present in feedstuffs in conjugated form, the young chick can utilize it well.

Clinical Findings: In young chicks the chief signs are retarded growth, poor feather formation, feather depigmentation in colored breeds and excessive mortality. The outward signs are accompanied by a macrocytic hyperchromic anemia. In turkey poults, growth rate is reduced and a characteristic cervical paralysis develops in which the birds extend their necks and appear to gaze downwards. Since field cases have usually appeared in young poults, it is possible that the breeder hens were fed diets deficient in the vitamin. In breeding chickens, folic acid deficiency reduces egg production and hatchability. Deficient embryos show bending of the tibiotarsus, mandible defects, syndactyly and hemorrhages.

Prophylaxis and Treatment: Where fish meal or solvent-extracted soybean meal are used as a major source of protein or the feed is pelleted, it may be advisable to supplement the turkey breeder hen diet with synthetic folic acid. For normal livability of poults, turkey breeder diets should contain about 0.8 mg/kg of feed. Many feed manufacturers are now supplementing turkey breeder and starter diets with folic acid at the rate of about 0.5 to 1.0 gm/ton. Where signs occur in young poults, the vitamin may be added to the drinking water at the rate of 150 to 200 mg/gal. In birds that are down, injection of 150 mg of folic acid per bird usually results in recovery within a few days.

BIOTIN DEFICIENCY

Etiology: Good sources of biotin include liver, dried brewer's yeast, molasses and green leafy plants. Cereals, meat meal and fish meal are poor sources. Some of the biotin in natural feeds occurs in bound form which is poorly available to the bird. An abnormal intestinal flora can increase the requirement of birds for the vitamin. It is possible for practical poult diets to be deficient. The vitamin is necessary to prevent perosis in chicks and poults.

Clinical Findings: In poults the typical signs include broken flight feathers, bending of the metatarsus and a dermatitis affecting the bottoms of the feet, the corners of the mouth and the edges of the eyelids. In mature turkeys and chickens, biotin deficiency causes reduced egg hatchability. Signs in embryos include "parrot beak", chondrodystrophy, micromelia and syndactyly. Dermatitis of mature birds similar to that in chicks and poults has not been reported.

Prophylaxis and Treatment: A number of factors increase biotin requirements, including oxidative rancidity of feed fat, competition by intestinal microorganisms and a lack of carry-over into the newly hatched poult. Since the best feed sources of biotin are often expensive or difficult to obtain and not completely available to the bird, it is good practice to add 150 to 200 mg of synthetic biotin to turkey breeder and starter diets. Certain antibiotics added to the feed will spare the need for biotin, presumably by fostering a less competitive intestinal flora. Practical diets for chickens appear to contain an adequate level of biotin without the addition of the synthetic vitamin.

Raising the feed level of such materials as dried brewer's yeast or adding synthetic biotin to the feed or water are effective means of counteracting existing cases of biotin deficiency.

COMPOSITION OF FEEDSTUFFS

At times, it may be necessary to calculate the nutrient composition of a feed to determine whether the feed is deficient in one or more nutrients. It also may be necessary to formulate a special feed from locally available feedstuffs, or add a supplement which is particularly rich in a specific mineral, vitamin, or amino acid. In view of this, the nutrient composition of a wide variety of grains, concentrates, roughages, silages and other feeds are shown in the several tables following.

The trace mineral contents of basic feedstuffs are listed in TABLE 45. For calculation of ruminant diets, the composition of grains, hays, silages, roots and tubers is given in detail in TABLE 46. Because of the unique nutritional requirements of poultry and swine, the composition of feedstuffs commonly used for these species is given in TABLE 47. The amino acid composition of most of these feedstuffs is given in TABLE 48.

The values presented in these tables represent averages, of course, and local conditions may cause certain components to vary considerably. When rations are being calculated, such variation should be determined or a reasonable margin must be allowed in the composition of the particular ration at hand.

TABLE 45. TRACE MINERAL CONTENT OF BASIC FEEDSTUFFS*

Feedstuffs	Chlorine %	Cobalt ppm	Copper ppm	Iodine ppm	Iron ppm	Magnesium %	Manganese ppm	Potassium %	Selenium ppm	Sodium %	Zinc ppm
Alfalfa meal, 17% protein	0.37	0.18	10	0.5	200	0.3	43	1.8	0.05-0.45*	0.18	35
Barley	0.15	0.1	7.5	0.05	50	0.12	16	0.6	0.1-0.3	0.02	17
Beet pulp, dried	—	0.1	12.5	—	300	0.25	35	0.2	—	—	1
Blood meal	0.27	0.1	9	—	3800	—	5	0.09	0.07	0.3	—
Bone meal, steamed	0.02	—	—	—	800	0.6	30	0.2	—	0.45	—
Citrus pulp, dried	—	—	6	—	200	0.16	7	0.6	—	0.04	—
Coconut oil meal	0.03	0.1	19	—	680	0.25	55	1.1	—	0.01	425
Corn, dent, yellow, No. 2	0.05	2.0	4.5	0.05	35	0.12	5	0.3	0.03-0.38	0.1	14
Corn gluten feed	0.22	0.1	50	—	500	0.3	25	0.6	—	0.01	—
Corn gluten meal	0.07	0.1	30	—	400	0.05	7	0.03	—	0.04	10
Cottonseed meal	0.03	0.1	20	0.12	100	0.55	20	1.3	0.2	0.2	—
Distillers' dried corn grains	0.17	—	45	—	200	0.06	19	0.8	1.15	0.3	—
Distillers' dried corn solubles	0.26	—	80	—	600	0.64	74	1.7	0.06	0.3	—
Fish meal, menhaden	1.20	—	8	—	270	—	36	0.7	—	0.5	85
Fish meal, herring	1.00	—	20	—	300	0.1	10	0.5	0.50	3.0	150
Fish solubles, 50% solubles	2.7	—	48	1.0	300	0.2	25	1.8	1.7	0.14	110
Hominy feed, white or yellow	0.05	—	2	—	10	0.24	14	0.2	—	—	38
Linseed oil meal	0.2	0.1	25	0.07	300	0.6	37	1.3	1.0	—	—
Meat and bone scrap, 50% protein	0.75	0.2	12	1.3	500	1.13	19	0.55	1.1	0.7	—
Milk, cow's	0.1	—	0.3	0.04	2	0.01	0.06	0.14	0.1-0.8	0.05	100
Milo	0.07	—	—	0.02	50	0.13	13	0.35	0.04	0.01	4
Molasses, beet	1.3	0.1	14	1.6	100	0.23	5	4.75	—	1.15	17
Molasses, cane	2.8	0.4	18	1.6	100	0.35	42	2.4	—	0.17	—
Oats	0.12	0.9	60	0.06	70	0.17	38	0.37	0.05-0.22	0.06	—
Oyster shell, ground	—	—	6	—	2900	0.3	130	0.1	0.01	0.2	—
Peanut oil meal	0.03	0.06	—	—	20	0.24	25	1.15	0.28	0.07	20
Rice bran	0.07	—	30	—	190	0.95	200	1.7	—	0.07	30
Rye grain	—	—	13	0.05	45	0.12	35	0.7	0.2	—	35
Sesame meal	0.06	—	6	—	—	0.75	48	1.2	—	0.04	100
Skim milk	0.9	—	3	—	30	0.11	2	1.5	0.08-0.15	0.5	40

Soybean meal, 44% protein	0.04	0.1	20	0.13	150	0.27	35	2.0	0.05-1.0	0.01	27
Soybean meal, dehulled	0.03	0.1	20	0.1	150	0.25	40	2.0	0.05-1.0	0.01	45
Wheat bran	0.08	0.1	12	0.07	150	0.55	115	1.2	0.6	0.06	80
Wheat grain	0.08	0.08	7	0.04	50	0.16	20	0.5	0.05-0.8	0.06	15
Wheat standard middlings	0.03	0.1	22	0.1	100	0.37	118	1.0	0.28-0.88	0.02	150
Whey, dried	0.7	0.1	45	—	7	0.13	5	1.2	0.08	0.5	3
Yeast, dried brewers'	0.12	0.2	30	0.01	50	0.23	6	1.7	0.11-1.1	0.07	40
Yeast, dried torula	0.02	0.04	13	—	90	0.13	13	1.9	0.03-0.05	0.01	100

* The trace element content of most feedstuffs varies over a wide range, depending largely upon the trace element content of the soil upon which the crops were grown. This is especially true of selenium.

TABLE 46. AVERAGE COMPOSITION OF FEEDSTUFFS FOR CATTLE, HORSES AND SHEEP
Grains, Seeds and By-Product Concentrates

Feedstuffs	Dry Matter	Crude Protein	Digest. Protein	TDN	Fat	Fiber	Calcium	Phosphorus	Carotene
	%	%	%		%	%	%	%	mg/lb
Barley	89	11.5	10.0	71	1.9	5.0	0.1	0.4	—
Beet pulp, dried	91	9.0	4.3	62	0.6	19.0	0.68	0.1	—
Blood meal or dried blood	91	80.0	56.5	60	1.5	1.0	0.3	0.22	—
Bone meal, steamed	95	12.0	9.0	10	3.0	2.0	29.0	13.5	—
Brewers' grains, dried	92	25.0	20.7	60	6.2	15.0	0.27	0.5	—
Buttermilk, dried	93	32.0	28.8	83	6.0	0.3	1.35	0.9	—
Citrus pulp, dried	90	6.5	2.9	75	5.4	13.0	2.0	0.1	—
Coconut meal	93	20.0	17.3	77	6.6	12.0	0.2	0.6	—
Corn, dent, yellow, No. 2	86	8.7	6.7	81	3.8	2.0	0.03	0.27	1.3
Corn, flint	89	9.9	7.5	83	4.3	2.0	0.02	0.2	—
Corn gluten feed	90	25.0	21.8	75	2.4	8.0	0.46	0.77	3.8
Corn gluten meal	91	43.0	36.5	80	2.3	4.0	0.15	0.4	7.4
Cottonseed meal	91	41.5	33.0	63	1.6	12.0	0.1	1.1	1.4
Distillers' dried corn grains	92	27.0	19.8	84	9.0	12.0	0.1	0.4	1.7
Distillers' dried corn grains with solubles	92	27.0	19.8	82	9.0	9.0	0.1	0.4	0.3
Distillers' dried solubles	93	27.0	21.0	78	9.0	4.0	0.35	1.4	—
Fish meal, menhaden	92	61.0	50.0	58	7.5	1.0	5.5	2.8	—
Fish meal, sardine	93	65.0	53.5	71	4.5	1.0	4.9	2.8	—
Flaxseed screenings	91	15.8	8.8	56	9.5	12.0	0.37	0.43	—
Hominy feed, white or yellow (y)	91	10.7	7.5	84	6.5	5.0	0.05	0.5	4.0 (y)
Kafir grain	90	11.8	9.5	80	3.0	2.0	0.04	0.33	—
Limestone	—	—	—	—	—	—	30-38	—	—
Linseed meal	91	35.0	30.5	75	4.5	9.0	0.4	0.9	—
Meat and bone scrap, 50% protein	94	53.0	43.8	67	10.0	2.0	10.6	5.1	—
Milk, cow's	12	3.1	2.9	16	3.7	0	0.12	0.09	0.4
Milo	89	11.0	8.6	84	2.8	2.0	0.04	0.29	—
Molasses, beet	77	6.7	3.5	61	—	—	0.15	0.03	—
Molasses, cane	75	3.2	—	72	—	—	0.9	0.1	—
Oats	**89**	**11.8**	**9.4**	**60**	**4.5**	**11.0**	**0.1**	**0.35**	**—**

Feedstuff									
Oyster shell, ground							38.0	—	
Peanut meal, solvent-extracted	92	47.5	42.0	77	1.2	13.0	0.2	0.65	
Phosphate, defluorinated rock	100						32.0	18.0	
Phosphate, dicalcium	96						27.0	19.0	
Potato meal, or dried potatoes	90	6.0	2.1	70	0.4	2.0	0.07	0.02	40
Oat hay	88	8.0	4.9	57	2.7	27.5	0.25	0.20	0.1
Oat millfeed	92	4.5	2.7	35	1.8	30.0	0.1	0.2	
Oat straw	90	4.0	0.7	47	2.0	37.0	0.3	0.1	
Pea hay, field	89	13.5	10.6	55	2.5	25.0	1.2	0.25	21
Peanut hay	91	11.0	7.0	58	5.0	24.5	1.15	0.15	13
Prairie hay, western, moderately green	92	6.3	0.9	50	2.4	29.0	0.5	0.17	4
Prairie hay, western, mature	92	4.2	5.0	44	2.3	31.0	0.35	0.08	
Reed canarygrass hay	91	8.0	2.8	42	2.0	28.0	0.30	0.25	
Ryegrass hay	88	8.4	0	50	2.2	36.0	0.45	0.28	8
Ryegrass straw	91	3.5	3.5	50	1.1	22.0	0.28	0.1	14
Sorghum fodder	86	6.8	9.7	49	2.7	29.0	0.35	0.15	3
Soybean hay	89	14.5	12.0	46	3.0	27.0	1.15	0.2	
Soybean hay, in bloom	90	15.0	1.4	51	1.2	39.0	1.2	0.20	2
Soybean straw	88	4.8	5.5	37	2.0	26.0	1.4	0.05	5
Sudan grass hay	88	11.3	3.1	54	2.3	30.0	0.50	0.30	2
Timothy hay, all analyses	88	6.8	4.2	45	2.3	29.0	0.30	0.17	
Timothy hay, early bloom	86	7.6	1.8	47	2.2	31.0	0.55	0.23	
Timothy hay, mature	88	5.1	13.5	35	2.3	25.0	0.15	0.15	
Vetch hay	86	17.5	3.4	52	1.7	24.0	1.2	0.30	44
Wheat hay	90	6.4	0.3	44	1.5	37.0	0.15	0.18	
Wheat straw		3.2		43			0.15	0.07	
SILAGES, ROOTS, TUBERS									
Alfalfa silage, wilted	36	6.4	4.4	21	1.2	11.0	0.5	0.1	9
Alfalfa, not wilted, no preservative	26	4.6	2.6	14	1.0	9.2	0.5	0.10	12
Alfalfa silage, molasses added	32	5.6	3.7	18	1.1	9.5	0.6	0.07	14
Beet top silage, sugar	32	3.8	2.5	15	0.6	3.9	0.31	0.07	5
Clover, ladino, silage	25	5.3	3.8	21	1.4	7.5	0.36	0.06	15
Corn silage, well-matured	27	2.2	1.2	20	0.8	7.0	0.1	0.05	2
Corn silage, dough stage	26	2.2	1.0	15	0.8	7.0	0.10	0.05	4
Corn stover silage (ears removed)	27	2.0	0.6	14	0.7	8.5			

continued on next page

TABLE 46. (Continued)

Feedstuffs	Dry Matter	Crude Protein	Digest. Protein	TDN	Fat	Fiber	Calcium	Phosphorus	Carotene
Cowpea silage	26	3.7	1.8	13	1.2	7.0	0.4	0.1	—
Mangels	9	1.3	0.9	7	0.1	0.8	0.02	0.02	—
Orchardgrass silage	24	3.4	2.0	20	1.0	7.5	0.3	0.1	18
Potato, tubers	21	2.2	1.3	17	0.1	0.4	0.01	0.05	—
Sorghum silage, sweet	27	2.1	0.8	15	0.7	7.5	0.08	0.05	2
Soybean silage, not wilted	25	4.0	2.9	15	0.7	7.5	0.35	0.18	10
Rice bran	91	13.5	9.2	55	15.0	11.0	0.06	1.82	—
Rice, rough	89	7.3	6.0	70	1.9	9.0	0.04	0.26	—
Rice polishings	90	11.8	9.0	78	13.0	3.0	0.04	1.4	—
Rye	89	11.9	9.4	78	1.6	2.0	0.06	0.35	—
Sesame meal	93	48.0	43.5	72	5.0	5.0	2.0	1.3	—
Skimmed milk, dried	94	33.5	30.0	80	1.0	0.2	1.3	1.0	—
Soybean meal, 44% protein	89	45.8	42.0	73	1.0	6.0	0.3	0.65	—
Soybean meal, dehulled	88	49.5	46.3	78	0.8	3.0	0.25	0.6	—
Wheat, hard, winter	89	13.5	11.5	77	1.8	3.0	0.05	0.4	—
Wheat, soft	89	10.8	8.3	78	1.7	2.3	0.09	0.3	—
Wheat bran	90	16.0	13.0	63	4.1	10.0	0.15	1.15	1.2
Wheat flour middlings	90	18.0	15.4	81	4.2	5.0	0.75	0.75	0.08
Wheat screenings	89	15.0	10.8	65	3.0	7.0	0.08	0.35	—
Wheat standard middlings	90	17.0	14.5	62	4.5	8.0	0.15	0.9	1.4
Whey, dried	94	13.8	11.8	78	0.8	—	0.9	0.8	—
Yeast, dried brewers'	93	45.0	38.5	73	5.0	3.0	0.15	1.4	—
Yeast, dried torula	93	48.0	41.5	70	5.0	2.0	0.55	1.7	—
DRY ROUGHAGES									
Alfalfa hay, average	89	15.5	11.0	50	1.9	28.0	1.48	0.23	20
Alfalfa hay, ¾ to full-bloom	88	14.0	10.0	48	1.6	30.0	1.15	0.15	15
Alfalfa leaf meal, good	89	21.0	16.5	58	2.8	14.6	2.10	0.25	80
Alfalfa meal, dehydrated, 17% Protein	92	17.5	12.2	47	2.6	25.0	1.3	0.25	45
Alfalfa straw	90	9.5	4.9	41	1.2	40.0	0.8	0.2	6

Barley hay	87	7.8	4.3	49	1.8	23.0	0.18	0.25	—
Barley straw	88	3.6	0.7	47	1.6	37.5	0.30	0.1	—
Bromegrass hay, all analyses	90	11.0	5.6	47	2.3	28.5	0.40	0.25	26
Clover hay, alsike, all analyses	88	12.9	8.6	48	2.5	26.0	1.15	0.22	75
Clover hay, crimson	88	14.8	10.2	55	2.0	28.0	1.25	0.15	67
Clover hay, ladino	91	21.0	16.2	60	3.0	17.5		0.35	15
Clover hay, red	88	13.0	7.9	48	2.6	26.5	1.4	0.2	—
Corn cobs, ground	90	2.5	0	46	0.5	32.5	0.1	0.04	—
Corn fodder, all analyses	82	7.3	3.8	53	2.0	21.0	0.4	0.2	16
Corn stover, all analyses	79	5.0	2.1	51	1.2	27.0	0.38	0.07	1.4
Cowpea hay	91	16.5	12.3	51	2.6	25.0	1.20	0.30	—
Kafir fodder	89	8.2	4.3	50	2.4	25.0	0.35	0.1	8
Kafir stover	82	4.8	1.9	51	1.6	27.0	0.35	0.15	1
Lespedeza hay, all analyses	91	13.0	5.6	45	2.5	28.0	1.0	0.20	19
Lespedeza hay, in bloom	93	12.5	6.1	46	2.9	29.0	1.0	0.20	19
Soybean silage, wilted	35	6.7	3.7	19	0.9	9.0	0.45	0.12	10
Sudan grass silage	23	2.4	1.5	15	0.7	8.0	0.15	0.05	—
Timothy silage, all analyses	38	3.8	1.9	19	1.2	13.0	0.20	0.10	13

TABLE 47. AVERAGE COMPOSITION OF FEEDSTUFFS FOR POULTRY AND SWINE*

Feedstuffs	Metabolizable Energy (Kcal/lb)	Protein (%)	Fat (%)	Fiber (%)	Calcium (%)	Phosphorus (%)	Niacin (mg/lb)	Riboflavin (mg/lb)	Pantothenic Acid (mg/lb)	Choline (grm/lb)
Alfalfa meal, dehydrated, 17% protein	620	17.5	2.6	25	1.3	0.3	16	5.0	12.0	0.72
Barley, adequate rainfall	1290	11.5	1.9	5	0.1	0.4	26	0.8	3.0	0.45
Blood meal	1300	80	1.5	1	0.3	0.22	14	0.7	0.5	0.13
Bone meal, steamed	—	12	3	2	29.0	13.5	2	0.4	0.45	—
Buttermilk, dried	1240	32	6	0.3	1.35	0.9	4	14.0	13.5	0.80
Citrus pulp, dried	—	6.5	4.5	13	2.0	0.1	10	1.0	6.0	0.42
Corn, dent, yellow	1560	8.7	3.8	2	0.03	0.27	10	0.5	2.2	0.20
Corn gluten meal	1510	42	2.3	4	0.15	0.4	23	0.7	4.7	0.15
Cottonseed meal, solvent process	920	41	1.6	11	0.15	1.1	20	2.3	8.0	1.3
Crab meal	850	31	1.8	11	15.5	1.6	20	3.0	3.0	0.9
Distillers' dried corn solubles	1320	27	9	4	0.35	1.4	52	7.7	9.5	2.2
Fats:										
Animal tallow	3230	—	100	—	—	—	—	—	—	—
Lard	3980	—	100	—	—	—	—	—	—	—
Vegetable oils	4050	—	100	—	—	—	—	—	—	—
Feather meal	1050	84	2.5	1.3	0.2	0.8	14	1.0	5.0	0.4
Fish meal	1350	61	7.5	1	5.5	2.8	26	2.4	4.0	1.4
Fish oils	3660	100	—	—	—	—	—	—	—	—
Fish solubles, 50% solids	670	30	4	0	0.1	0.7	110	4.5	17.0	1.2
Hominy feed, 5% fat	1300	11	6.5	5	0.05	0.5	23	1.0	3.5	0.45
Liver and glandular meal	1300	65	16	2	0.7	1.1	73	18.0	48.0	4.8
Meat and bone scrap, 50% protein	900	53	10	2	10.6	5.1	18	1.1	1.2	0.75
Molasses, beet	900	6.7	0	0	0.15	0.03	19	1.2	2.1	0.4

Molasses, cane	890	3.2	0	0	0.9	0.1	16	1.5	17.5	0.4
Oats	1190	11.8	4.5	11	0.1	0.35	7	0.7	6.0	0.49
Oatmeal, feeding	1420	16.9	6	3	0.09	0.45	5	0.9	6.6	0.57
Peanut meal	1200	47.5	1.2	13	0.2	1.82	77	5.0	24.0	2.0
Rice bran	740	13	15	11	0.06	0.65	130	1.2	10.5	0.57
Rice polishings	1300	11.8	13	3	1.30	1.4	240	0.8	26.0	0.6
Skimmed milk, dried	1140	33		0.2	0.04	1.0	5	9.1	15.0	0.7
Sesame meal	870	48	1	5	2.0	1.3	14	1.7	2.5	0.2
Sorghum kafir	1480**	11.8	5	2	0.04	0.33	18	0.5	5.7	0.3
Sorghum milo	1480	11	3	2	0.04	0.29	19	1.5	5.0	1.2
Soybean meal, 44% protein	1020	45	2.8	6	0.3	0.65	12	1.4	5.0	1.2
Soybean meal, dehulled	1150	49.5	1	3	0.25	0.6	10	3.0	6.6	1.9
Sunflower seed meal	900	47	0.8	11	0.3	1.2	132	0.5	18.0	0.45
Wheat, hard	1480	13.5	3		0.05	0.4	23	0.5	6.0	0.45
Wheat, soft	1480	10	1.8	2.3	0.09	0.3	27	1.4	5.0	0.46
Wheat bran	590	15	1.7	10	0.15	1.15	95	0.9	13.0	0.83
Wheat shorts	1200	17	4.1	5	0.10	0.75	44	0.4	8.0	0.8
Wheat red dog flour	1240	17	4.2	4	0.07	0.5	24	0.9	6.2	0.8
Wheat middlings	820	17	4.5	8	0.15	0.9	45	0.9	9.0	1.1
Whey, dried	870	13.8	0.8	0	0.9	0.8	5	14.0	22.0	1.1
Yeast, dried brewer's	840	45	5	3	0.15	1.4	200	16.0	50.0	1.75
Yeast, dried torula	840	48	5	2	0.55	1.7	230	20.0	38.0	1.3

* *See* TABLE 48 for amino acids in feedstuffs.
** Estimated value.

TABLE 48. IMPORTANT AMINO ACIDS IN FEEDSTUFFS FOR POULTRY AND SWINE

Feedstuffs	Arginine %	Lysine %	Methionine %	Cystine %	Tryptophan %	Glycine %
Alfalfa meal, dehydrated, 17% protein	0.8	0.9	0.29	0.32	0.21	0.9
Barley	0.53	0.53	0.18	0.18	0.21	0.36
Blood meal	3.5	6.9	0.9	1.4	1.1	3.4
Buttermilk, dried	1.1	2.4	0.7	0.3	0.5	—
Citrus pulp, dried	0.2	0.2	0.08	0.11	0.06	—
Corn, dent, yellow	0.45	0.2	0.18	0.18	0.1	0.5
Corn gluten meal	1.4	0.8	1.0	0.7	0.2	1.5
Cottonseed meal, solvent process	3.3	1.6	0.5	1.0	0.5	2.4
Crab meal	1.7	1.4	0.6	—	0.3	—
Distillers' dried corn solubles	1.0	0.9	0.6	0.6	0.2	1.1
Feather meal	5.9	2.0	0.6	3.0	0.5	—
Fish meal	4.0	5.3	1.8	0.94	0.6	4.4
Fish solubles, 50% solids	2.4	2.7	1.0	1.7	0.8	4.9
Hominy feed	0.5	0.4	0.18	0.18	0.1	0.5
Liver and glandular meal	4.1	4.8	1.3	1.0	0.6	5.6
Meat and bone scrap, 50% protein	3.5	3.5	0.7	0.6	0.7	7.5
Oats	0.7	0.4	0.18	0.18	0.18	0.5
Oatmeal, feeding	1.0	0.5	0.20	0.20	0.2	0.2
Peanut meal	5.9	2.3	0.4	0.7	0.5	2.5
Rice bran	0.5	0.5	0.2	0.1	0.1	—
Rice polishings	0.5	0.5	0.2	0.1	0.1	—
Skimmed milk, dried	1.2	2.8	0.9	0.4	0.4	0.2
Sesame meal	4.3	1.2	1.2	0.6	0.6	—
Sorghum milo	0.4	0.3	0.16	0.18	0.09	—
Soybean meal, solvent-extracted	3.2	2.9	0.67	0.75	0.60	2.6
Soybean meal, dehulled	3.6	3.2	0.74	0.83	0.65	2.9
Sunflower seed meal	3.2	1.3	0.65	0.4	0.6	—
Wheat, hard	0.7	0.45	0.18	0.22	0.15	0.7
Wheat, soft	0.4	0.3	0.13	0.2	0.12	0.5

Wheat bran				0.17	0.5	0.8
Wheat shorts	0.9	0.3	0.2	0.18	0.7	0.9
Wheat red dog flour	0.4	0.19	0.2	0.15	0.6	1.0
Wheat middlings	0.4	0.2	0.2	0.17	0.6	0.9
Whey, dried	0.3	0.2	0.4	0.2	1.2	0.5
Yeast, dried brewer's	1.7	0.5	0.55	0.75	3.1	2.3
Yeast, dried torula	2.7	0.5	0.6	0.8	3.8	2.6

PART VI
ADDENDUM

DIAGNOSTIC PROCEDURES FOR THE OFFICE LABORATORY

Procedures suitable for the veterinarian's office are included in this chapter. Emphasis is given to those which may be carried out with simple equipment and a minimum of technical skill. However, an enlarging spectrum of packaged kits for chemical diagnostic tests makes it increasingly feasible to do tests hitherto thought difficult or cumbersome.

PARASITOLOGIC EXAMINATIONS

EXAMINATION OF FECES

Feces should be fresh or refrigerated whenever possible, since the results are more difficult to interpret on samples in which development of embryos or deterioration of oocysts or eggs has occurred. Only fresh feces must be examined for lung-worm larvae, since other larvae may be found in older feces. *Strongyloides* are passed as larvae or as eggs that hatch shortly thereafter in dog feces. Specimens of feces to be mailed to a diagnostic laboratory should be fixed in 5% formalin (suitable for all parasitologic examinations).

Examination by Flotation: A saturated salt (NaCl) solution is prepared by dissolving as much granulated table salt as possible in water at room temperature. The saturated salt solution does not require a preservative, is neither sticky nor attractive to flies, and is replacing sugar solution as the better flotation solution.

About 2 gm of feces are placed in a waxed paper cup and approximately 15 ml of the salt solution is added. This is stirred with a wooden tongue depressor until the entire sample is in suspension, then strained through a clean gauze square into a test tube, using enough solution to fill it to within one-quarter of an inch from the top. The tube is placed in a centrifuge and run at low speed (1,000 to 2,000 rpm) for approximately 6 minutes. When centrifugation is completed, a large drop is lifted from the surface film by means of a beaded glass rod and transferred to a microscope slide, covering a circular area approximately 1 cm in diameter.

Drops from several samples may be placed on one slide to achieve economy of effort. The floated debris is examined by means of a compound microscope, using the low-power lens for scanning and the high-dry for further study if necessary for identification. Reduced illumination from a good light source is used so that the relatively transparent eggs and oocysts are well defined. Paper cups, tongue depressors and gauze are discarded after each sample.

Quantitative Examination: This procedure utilizes both flotation and quantitation and requires not only an aliquot of a uniform specimen but also a special counting chamber, the McMaster slide. This is available commercially, and is sold complete with directions for use. The number of eggs per gram of feces, coupled with the presence or absence of clinical signs will indicate the degree of infection and the measures to be taken.

EXAMINATION OF BLOOD FOR PARASITES

Dirofilaria immitis in the dog and occasionally in the cat and other carnivores, and *Dipetalonema reconditum* in the dog and possibly other carnivores, spend part of their life cycles in the blood stream. (*See* HEARTWORM INFECTION, p. 686.) Certain protozoan parasites are also found in the peripheral blood, for example, the nonpathogenic *Trypanosoma theileri* (*americanum*) may be seen occasionally in cattle blood. These protozoa are found free in the plasma. Other parasites, which may be seen on or inside the red blood cells, are *Piroplasma* (*Babesia*) in the dog and horse, *Haemobartonella* in the dog and cat, *Eperythrozoon* in pigs, *Anaplasma* in cattle, *Leucocytozoon* in ducks and *Haemoproteus* in pigeons. *Ehrlichia canis* may be found occasionally in mononuclear cells of the peripheral blood in dogs. They may also be found rarely in the neutrophils. *Histoplasma capsulatum* organisms can also be seen occasionally in peripheral monocytes in the dog and perhaps the cat.

Examination of the Erythrocytes for Parasites: Several blood smears (q.v., p. 1381) of varying thicknesses are made on clean slides; the smears are fixed for at least 2 minutes with absolute methanol; stained with Wright's or, perhaps better, with Giemsa stain (q.v., p. 1387) and carefully examined by means of the oil-immersion objective. Confusing artifacts are usually refractive as compared with the parasites. New methylene blue (q.v., p. 1382) may also be used to visualize red cells and contents.

URINALYSIS

Strip Test and Tablet Procedures: The commercial availability of many strip tests and tablets for urinalysis has simplified the procedures considerably. These test strips have as many as 6 tests on the one plastic strip (glucose, pH, bilirubin, ketone bodies, protein and blood). Test tablets are available for reducing substances, bilirubin and blood. A test strip is also available for urobilinogen. These strips are sufficiently reliable to be most useful, especially in the small laboratory. The rapidity with which the various abnormal constituents can be detected precludes their determination by more cumbersome methods.

Collection of the Specimen: A specimen is obtained as voided or by catheterization. Unless tests can be run within an hour, the urine specimen is placed in the refrigerator. If urine is to be kept longer or sent through the mail, toluene (2 ml/100 ml of urine) is added as a preservative. Other preservatives may be used; however, it is recommended that the preservative be identified as some interfere with subsequent tests.

Specific Gravity: If a Goldberg refractometer is unavailable, the specific gravity may be determined as follows: The urinometer cylinder is filled approximately two-thirds full with urine and the float is placed into the tube, being careful that it does not adhere to the sides of the cylinder. The specific gravity is read at the bottom of the meniscus on the stem of the float. If the temperature of the urine differs appreciably from that at which the urinometer was standardized, 0.001 is added for each 3°C above the temperature standard or subtracted for each 3°C below it. The approximate normal range (all species) is 1.015 to 1.050. (Since normal plasma has a specific gravity of about 1.018, the size and shape of red blood cells in urine of similar specific gravity will appear normal. Specific gravities above 1.018 will crenate the cells and below 1.018 will hemolyze or swell them.)

Color: The color of the freshly voided urine is noted in a standard container, either the collection bottle or the urinometer cylinder. The normal color may range from very pale yellow (practically colorless) to dark amber. Abnormal colors of red or green may denote the presence of blood, blood pigments, pigmented drugs or their breakdown products. Urine may change color on standing, especially horse urine, which becomes dark brown.

Transparency: Normal freshly voided urine usually is clear, but may be turbid due to crystalline precipitates. Horse urine is normally turbid due to the presence of calcium carbonate crystals and mucin. A fine, diffuse cloudiness may be due to bacteria. Increased turbidity usually is the result of pus cells.

Reaction: A strip of indicator paper (Nitrazine or pHydrion) is dipped into fresh urine; the color change is noted and the pH is read by comparing it with the color standard included with the paper. The pH of urine of dogs and cats may range from 4.5 to 7.5. The urine of herbivorous farm animals usually is neutral to pH 8.0, becoming more alkaline upon standing. Sucking calves, because of their high-protein diet, will have an acid urine until their rumens develop.

Protein: If the urine is not clear, it should be cleared by centrifugation before performing the test. A few drops of 20% sulfosalicylic acid are added to 1 or 2 ml of urine in a test tube. Development of a milky precipitate is a positive reaction. Commercially available indicator-impregnated paper strips are available for detecting proteinuria. These require only a drop of urine. A small amount of protein is filtered normally by the kidney; however, the detection methods are not sensitive enough to indicate its presence. Sexually mature male dogs may show a trace to 1+ reaction due to sexual secretions.

Glucose: A reagent strip moistened in fresh well-mixed urine gives a color reaction if glucose is present. The color is checked against the chart provided, at 10 seconds after moistening. Glucosuria usually indicates a blood glucose level exceeding 160 mg/100 ml of blood, although rarely kidney tubular damage will lead to loss at "normal" blood levels.

Ketone Bodies: An approximate level of ketone bodies is easily determined by means of Acetest tablets or powder, used as directed by the manufacturer. Commercially available reagent-impregnated paper strips (or multi-test dip sticks) are possibly more practical for small-animal practice. Ketone determination is of limited practical interest in species other than the cow and sheep (*see* KETOSIS, p. 497). However, in extreme instances of diabetes in any species, a positive reaction may sometimes occur, as it may with starvation, persistent diarrhea or vomiting, or with febrile or cachectic diseases.

Bilirubin (Bile Pigment): A piece of filter paper is soaked in urine, spread out and allowed to dry partially; a drop of concentrated nitric acid is placed on the most discolored portion of the paper. A play of bluish-green color indicates the presence of bile pigments and varies from faint green (1+) to very dark green (4+). Alternatively, a tablet available commercially detects conjugated bilirubin in a drop of urine. This test is specific and sensitive.

In most species, the detection of conjugated bilirubin in the urine is an indication of impaired biliary excretion, and serves to differentiate obstructive from hemolytic icterus. However, many healthy dogs and possibly 1 in 4 normal cattle have bilirubinuria.

Blood: The presence of blood usually can be detected grossly by the color and turbidity of the specimen. Blood causes the urine to appear red or pink and opaque, whereas hemoglobin yields a red or pink and clear solution. Centrifugation at 1,500 rpm for 5 minutes will differentiate between red blood cells (hematuria) and hemoglobin (hemoglobinuria). Both blood and hemoglobin have a brownish color in very acid urine. Test tablets for blood in urine are available commercially.

Microscopic Examination of Urinary Sediment: A sample of whole urine is centrifuged at slow speed (approximately 600 to 1,000 rpm) for about 6 minutes. The supernatant fluid is poured off into another tube to be used for the chemical tests and a small amount of sediment is placed on a slide; a cover glass is applied and the sediment is examined microscopically. The sediment may consist of formed materials (epithelial cells, leukocytes, erythrocytes, tube casts and bacteria) and crystals which vary in amount and variety, according to the reaction and concentration of the urine. In alkaline urines, triple phosphates and carbonates are the most common. In acid urines, oxalates, calcium sulfate and various urate crystals appear. In dogs, other than Dalmations, crystals of uric acid or other urates seldom appear. Recently the Sternheimer-Malbin staining technique has replaced the examination of unstained urinary sediment. The various constituents stain characteristically with the dye thus making identification relatively simple. The presence of crystals in the urinary sediment is frequently of little diagnostic significance; however, oxalate crystals suggest oxalate or ethylene glycol poisoning, and quantities of cystine crystals suggest congenital cystinuria.

HEMATOLOGY

Counting the cellular elements in the blood of animals is valuable in assessing conditions of health and disease. The variation from animal to animal of the same species is considerable and depends in part on the sex, nutrition, age, diurnal and sexual cycles, and stresses such as strenuous exercise and excessive environmental heat or cold. For these reasons, the values given in TABLE 1 must be considered as guides rather than as rigid criteria. With malnutrition, iron deficiency or chronic disease, the animal may develop an anemia expressed as a reduction in the number of circulating red blood cells or in the content of hemoglobin in each cell. (*See* ANEMIA, p. 14.)

The white blood cell count usually rises well above its normal range in acute bacterial infections and also in such conditions as neoplasia, chemical or metabolic intoxication and traumatic states. However, the same conditions can on occasion lead to lowered white cell counts; e.g., overwhelming bacterial septicemias may cause profound neutropenia. In acute viral infections, the white blood cell count usually decreases from its normal level. The response varies depending on the nature of the invading microorganism and the species of animal. With most pus-forming organisms, the number of neutrophils (polymorphonuclear leukocytes) increases markedly. A marked rise also is seen in anthrax, encephalitis and meningitis. Increase in monocytes and lymphocytes usually indicates a more chronic process or the end stage of an acute infectious process. A rise in eosinophils may represent an allergic response, sometimes due to parasitic infection. Abnormal or immature cells in the blood may present evidence for a disease of the blood-forming organs (bone marrow, liver, spleen, lymph nodes) as in leukemia and certain toxic states.

Collection of the Specimen: Blood should be collected by means of venipuncture with a dry needle and syringe. (If the equipment is wet-sterilized, it should be thoroughly rinsed in isotonic saline solution before the venipuncture.) Dogs are usually bled from the cephalic vein, although when large amounts of blood are to be collected, the jugular vein may be employed. Pigs are best bled by puncture of the anterior vena cava, and the larger animals by jugular puncture. Samples for hemoglobin and cell counts may be collected from kittens and other small animals by shaving an ear and nicking the external ear vein, or by clipping a toenail. Blood collected by

TABLE 1. SOME NORMAL LEUKOCYTE VALUES*
(Approximate ranges—in 10^3/cu mm)

	Leukocytes	Neutrophils	Immature Neutrophils	Lymphocytes	Eosinophils	Monocytes
Horse	5-15	3-7	0-0.1	1.5-5.5	0-0.5	0-0.8
Ox	5-13	0.6-4	0-0.12	2.5-7.5	0-2.4	0.25-0.84
Sheep	5-13	0.7-6	rare	2-4	0-1	0-0.75
Goat	5-13	1.2-7.2	rare	2-9	0.05-0.65	0-0.55
Pig	7-20	3.2-10	0-0.8	4.5-13	0.5-2	0.25-2
Dog	8-18	3-12	0-0.3	1-4.8	1-1.3	0.15-14
Cat	8-25	2.5-13	0-0.3	1.5-7	0-1.5	0-0.85
Rabbit	6-13	2-6	rare	0.2-0.5	0-0.5	0.1-1
Rat	5-25	0.001-5	rare	7-13	0-0.5	0.1-1
Mouse	4-12	0.5-4	rare	3-9	0-1	0-1
Chicken	9-56	3-17	—	10-30	0-0.5	0-1
					0.05	0-5

* For erythrocyte counts, hematocrit values (PCV, %) and hemoglobin levels *see* ANEMIA, p. 14.

venipuncture into vials containing KEDTA (potassium ethyl-enediamine tetraacetic acid) is satisfactory for the various procedures if done within a few hours of collection. The specimen should be mixed thoroughly before taking samples from the container. Ideally, smears for differential cell counts should be made from blood before the use of an anticoagulant; however, this is not always possible. KEDTA is the anticoagulant of choice for most hematologic procedures.

Packed Cell Volume (Hematocrit): One of the easier and more useful tests for the small laboratory, this determination has largely superseded the erythrocyte count and hemoglobin determination as a practical means of evaluating the red cell status. The microhematocrit procedure is most suitable. Blood is drawn into the capillary tube (containing an anticoagulant) directly from a venous or capillary puncture, sealed and centrifuged. A reading is obtained by placing the centrifuged tube against a special hematocrit chart.

Leukocyte Count: The "Unopette", a system utilizing disposable pipettes, is satisfactory for determination of total leukocyte counts, and also for erythrocyte (*see* PACKED CELL VOLUME, above) and thrombocyte counts. Directions for use are supplied by the manufacturer along with the necessary materials.

Differential Leukocyte Count: New, "electronically cleaned", dry slides are used for making blood smears. A medium-sized drop of blood is placed near one end of a slide placed horizontally on a table; another slide held at an angle (approximately 30°) is pulled back until it touches the drop. As the drop spreads along the acute angle so formed, the spreader slide is pushed quickly and smoothly toward the opposite end, spreading a thin film on the slide; the slide is then waved in the air to obtain quick drying of the smear. Rapid drying of the smear prevents crenation and other distortions of the cells. When preparing blood smears in cool or humid stables or kennels or outdoors in winter, the slide should be warmed beforehand and if possible, warm air should be blown over the film to prevent crenation of the erythrocytes. Unstained smears should be stored in a dry dust-free box until staining (never in the refrigerator).

The smears are stained with Wright's or Giemsa stain (q.v., p. 1387), washed thoroughly in flowing water and permitted to dry. The smear is scanned with the low-power lens to ascertain adequacy of staining and distribution of the leukocytes. Then the slide is examined by oil-immersion microscopy and 100 or 200 cells are classified and the values expressed as percent. This relative value when multiplied by the total count gives the differential count in absolute values. The absolute values are less subject to error in interpretation than are relative values.

Reticulocyte Count: A few drops of blood are mixed with an equal volume of a solution composed of 1% new methylene blue (℞ 650) in isotonic salt solution and permitted to stand in a stoppered tube for 15 minutes or longer at room temperature. A drop of the mixture is placed on a slide, smeared and air-dried. The oil-immersion objective is used, noting the percent of reticulocytes as compared with the total number of erythrocytes seen. Reticulocytes in dogs and cats vary from 0 to 1%, while in hoofed animals they are rarely seen. Counting the number of reticulocytes seen per 1,000 red blood cells is the standard procedure and the value is expressed as a percent.

Platelet Count: While the error in counting platelets is high, the accuracy is usually sufficient to be useful. An estimate may be obtained (1) by using the "Unopette" system, or (2) in conjunction with a total leukocyte count, by counting the number of platelets per 100 white blood cells in a blood film. From this, the number of platelets per cubic millimeter is obtained by dividing 100 into the number of platelets multiplied by the white cells per cubic millimeter. A count of 5 to 25 may be taken as normal. Because of the likelihood of error, 10 fields should be counted and the result averaged. Counts are elevated following stress, including surgery. The cause of primary thrombocytopenia is unknown. The secondary condition follows disease of the bone marrow or spleen, and in a number of the diseases of the blood and reticuloendothelial systems.

BLOOD CHEMISTRY

Blood-chemical determinations are useful in the diagnosis of animal diseases. They should be used sparingly and wisely chosen. Attention must be given to relatively simple tests that will assist in improved diagnosis and prognosis. Also, the choice of the test should be governed by findings in the clinical examination and in preliminary urine and blood studies. The technique used is not important and may differ according to the facilities of the office laboratory. The easiest and cheapest methods, where only a few types of tests are to be run, are those for which commercial laboratory kits have been prepared containing all the apparatus and reagents necessary for a single test. The tests usually depend on titration or visual colorimetry, by means of blood color standards.

For example, a rapid, simply conducted yet reasonably accurate chromatographic method for the determination of urea nitrogen, the "Urograph" technique, is obtainable. (If many kinds of procedures are planned, it is more economic to purchase a photoelectric colorimeter that may be used for all the determinations and is adapted to methods of greater accuracy.) The techniques recommended by the distributors of these kits should be followed, since they are adapted to the particular instrument. The recommended reagents should be purchased ready-mixed.

Recently there have become available many office-laboratory diagnostic systems, some of them include ancillary equipment as a centrifuge, colorimeter, heating unit, and some are based on prepackaged reagent kits. The various systems are basically similar and have many procedures in common for the more frequently determined blood constituents. The reagents and equipment such as test tubes and pipettes are disposable. Although each differs in some respect, and they are highly competitive, the test results are sufficiently reliable to have practical value in the small laboratory. Very small amounts of serum or plasma are used for the analyses, thus eliminating the necessity of a protein-free filtrate. Procedures must be followed precisely or very variable results will be obtained.

Blood Glucose: A simple and reliable colorimeter "field" test ("Dextrotest") is available making it possible to estimate blood glucose at 100, 150 or 200 mg/100 ml of blood. This has an obvious limitation for diagnosis for bovine ketosis, but is useful in detecting abnormally high levels as in diabetes mellitus or chronic pancreatitis. (That even simpler tests will detect above normal ketone levels in milk or urine removes much of the shortcoming of this test.)

LIVER FUNCTION TESTS

Serum Bile Pigments: The quantitative Ehrlich reaction (van den Bergh test) measures both the total bilirubin and the bilirubin glucuronide in the blood. The difference is free bilirubin. High levels of bilirubin glucuronide (direct-reacting pigment) indicate an obstructive lesion either in the liver or in the bile duct system. High levels of mainly free bilirubin (indirect-reacting pigment) suggest a hemolytic process. An exception is the horse, in which nearly all bilirubin in the blood reacts indirectly irrespective of cause. A careful corre-

TABLE 2. BLOOD CHEMISTRY
SOME NORMAL VALUES (Approx. ranges)

	Urea Nitrogen	Glucose	Ca++	PO4---	Mg++	Na+	K+	Cl-
		Values in mg/100 ml				in mEq/L*		
Dog	10-20	70-100	8-12	2-5	2-5	135-150	3.5-5.5	100-115
Cat	20-30	70-100	8-12	4-8	2-5	145-155	3.5-5.5	100-115
Ox	10-20	40-60	8-12	4-8	2-5	130-150	3.5-5.5	100-115
Sheep	8-20	30-60	8-12	4-8	2-5	150-160	3.5-5.5	100-115
Pig	8-20	75-150**	8-12	4-8	2-5	140-160	3.5-5.5	100-115
Horse	10-20	60-110	8-12	3-6	2-5	145-150	3.5-5.5	100-115

* For conversion of mEq/L to mg/L, see p. 1455.
** Baby pig.

lation of the clinical and laboratory findings is quite important. Specific clinical tests for bilirubin must be used in the horse.

Urobilinogen: Strip tests are now available commercially for the determination of urobilinogen. The presence of anaerobic bacteria in normal dogs' livers make the interpretations of this test difficult since these organisms are capable of producing urobilinogen in the liver when the bile duct is completely obstructed. The absence of urobilinogen in the urine, when associated with clay-colored feces, indicates obstruction of the bile duct. Increased levels are observed in both hemolytic and hepatocellular diseases.

Fecal Stercobilin and Urobilin: These pigments impart color to the normal feces; clay-colored feces suggest bile-duct obstruction. Light-colored feces also occur following the ingestion of bones and antibiotics, as well as in some pancreatic diseases. Many dietary substances contribute substantially also to the color of feces.

Bromsulfophthalein (BSP) Excretion Test: This dye test is primarily helpful in detecting latent hepatic disease without icterus. BSP is injected IV into dogs at 5 mg/kg, and large animals at approximately 2 mg/kg. Normal dogs exhibit less than 10% retention at 30 minutes. A BSP clearance test is recommended in large animals in which the percentage of dye removed per minute from the blood is calculated. Mature horses and cattle remove at least 20% per minute.

PANCREATIC FUNCTION TESTS (DOG)

Acute Pancreatitis: If it is associated with acute abdominal signs, the finding of an elevated activity of serum lipase, which is liberated from a necrotic pancreas, is usually diagnostic. Serum lipase activity as measured by conventional techniques is usually less than 1 unit in normal dogs.

Chronic Pancreatic Fibrosis or Atrophy: Two tests (*see* below) may be used: Test 1 is simple and is tried first but since it may yield 25% false negative results, Test 2 should be tried if no digestion of film occurs in Test 1.

Test No. 1 (X-ray film test): Nine milliliters of 5% sodium bicarbonate solution are made up to 10 ml total volume by adding feces and stirred. A drop of the mixture is placed on X-ray film (undeveloped film or dark portion of developed film). This is incubated at 37.5°C for 1 hour or for 2½ hours at room temperature. (Caution: if drop dries, test is unreliable.) The material is washed off under a gentle stream of tap water. A cleared area under the drop indicates the presence of trypsin. In the absence of trypsin, the film is only watermarked.

Test No. 2 (gelatin tube test): Nine milliliters of water are made up to 10 ml total volume by adding feces and mixed. A tube containing 2 ml of 7.5% gelatin is warmed to 37.5°C until the gelatin is liquid, and then 1 ml each of the fecal dilution and 5% sodium bicarbonate are added. This is well mixed and then incubated at 37.5°C for 1 hour or at room temperature for 2½ hours, followed by refrigeration for 20 minutes. Failure of the mixture to gel indicates the presence of trypsin (proteolytic enzyme).

CLINICAL MICROBIOLOGY

Bacteriologic methods adapted to the office laboratory are the study of stained and unstained smears, preparation of simple cultures and antibiotic sensitivity tests. Stains, culture media and test disks for the various antibiotics are available. It is useful to examine smears of urinary sediment (especially if the sample can be obtained without catheterization) or of various exudates stained by Gram's method.

Gram Stain: This technique serves the purpose of indicating the presence of bacteria as well as being a basic differential stain. A moderately thin film is prepared and fixed by heating gently over a flame. The smear is covered with Gram's gentian or crystal violet for 1 minute, washed briefly with water and covered with Gram's iodine for 1 minute. It is decolorized 5 to 10 seconds with acetone-alcohol, immediately flooded with water, drained and counter-stained with safranine or basic fuchsin for 1 minute. It is then washed, dried and examined by oil-immersion microscopy. Gram-positive organisms, such as cocci, appear dark-blue or black, and gram-negative organisms, such as the coliforms and pseudomonads, appear pink. The nuclei of leukocytes stain pink. All fungi are gram-positive.

The Cleared, Unstained Smear Method: The technique is employed to demonstrate ringworm fungi, molds and the "ray fungi" of actinomycosis. Mange mites, if present, may also be detected. For ringworm, a recent lesion is selected and hair and skin scales are secured by scraping the periphery of the lesion with a scalpel. If the lesion is dry or scaly the scalpel blade may be moistened with oil or glycerol. Scrape deeply (to blood). For actinomycosis or molds growing in tissue, pus or tissue debris must be used. The material is placed on a slide, and a few drops of 10 to 40% sodium hydroxide solution are added. It is allowed to stand for 30 minutes (or heated gently for 5 minutes), and a cover glass is carefully pressed on the preparation. Examination is with the low- and high-power objectives using reduced illumination, looking for spores within or along the hair shafts or in epidermal cells in the case of ringworm. "Ray fungi" and mycelial segments are diagnostic of actinomycosis or tissue mold infection.

Wright's Stain: Commercial Wright's stain may be purchased in liquid form, and is used with phosphate buffer (B 651). The slide is placed on a staining rack and sufficient Wright's stain is added to cover the slide. After 1 minute an equal amount of the phosphate buffer is added and mixed by blowing on the slide until a metallic sheen appears. Time for stain to react must be determined for each batch of stain; 3 minutes is suggested as a trial period. Scum and stain are quickly floated off with neutral distilled water (see B 651), and the slide is air-dried.

Giemsa Stain should be purchased in liquid form. The film is fixed in absolute methanol for 3 to 5 minutes and is dried. A Coplin jar is filled with staining solution prepared by adding one drop of the Giemsa stain to each milliliter of neutral distilled water (see B 651). The air-dried slide is left in this for 30 minutes, washed in neutral distilled water and again air-dried.

Cultures: Cultures may be prepared by inoculating media (thioglycollate broth or transport media) in the office or field and sending them to a diagnostic laboratory for identification, or by submitting specimens of aseptically collected exudates and other materials. Appropriate culture media can be purchased in screw-capped vials and kept in the refrigerator until needed. Thioglycollate broth supports both aerobic and anaerobic growth, hence it is ideal for initial culture. This is either submitted to a diagnostic laboratory or incubated for 24 hours at 37°C. If growth occurs, it may be subcultured, stained or spread on blood agar for sensitivity testing.

Sensitivity Testing: Paper disks, impregnated with various antibiotics, are available commercially for detecting sensitivity of organisms. These disks are applied to the surface of blood agar plates which have been streaked with the suspect organism. After incubation for 24 hours at 37°C the inhibition of growth of the organism is determined by the colony-free zone around the disk. It is the presence or absence of a colony-free zone, not its width, which is significant. For more accurate results, Trypticase Soy Agar plates should be used.

CLINICAL PROTOZOOLOGY

As an office procedure, clinical protozoology is confined to collection of samples and identification of the organism, as culture of protozoa is beyond the capability of most small laboratories.

For the direct examination of fecal or vaginal material for trophozoites of *Entamoeba, Giardia* or trichomonads, the sample must be fresh and kept warm as the trophozoites are very fragile. The specimen may be mixed with warm 0.9% NaCl for ease of examination. The smear can also be stained with an aqueous (1:10) dilution of 1% iodine in 2% KI. This solution will bring out some of the morphologic features of the protozoa. More satisfactory protozoan stains are demanding in terms of technique, and perhaps best done only in laboratories that handle enough volume to allow reliable competence.

If immediate examination is not possible or necessary, prepared fixed smears may be submitted to a diagnostic laboratory. It is possible to obtain slides with a fixative already on them. It is then only necessary to make a smear on these pre-processed slides and mail them, a procedure suitable for detecting both intestinal and vaginal protozoa.

CLINICAL CYTOLOGY

These techniques may be used to study the cellular character of tumors and tissues from various disease processes to obtain a diagnosis without tissue sectioning. Smears may be prepared from material obtained by punch or aspiration biopsy or by imprinting blocks of tissue. As an example: A fresh surface on a piece of liver tissue is prepared at necropsy and imprints made by touching the cut surface to a slide, stained with Wright's, Giemsa or new methylene blue stain (q.v., p. 1382) and examined for the presence of intranuclear inclusions. These are diagnostic of infectious canine hepatitis (q.v., p. 313); however, the possibility of infection with other organisms, such as bacteria, *Toxoplasma,* or *Histoplasma* should not be overlooked. As another example, *Erlichia canis* is more readily detected in impression smears of the lung than in peripheral blood.

SOME PHYSIOLOGIC VALUES

BODY TEMPERATURE

The body temperature is determined by the balance between the production and loss of heat. Heat production results from oxidation of energy stores, especially in the muscles and large glands, such as the liver. The rate of production is increased by exertion, shivering, or excessive thyroid activity. In herbivores, bacterial fermentation in the alimentary tract is an additional source of heat.

Heat is lost by radiation (60%), evaporation (30%) and convection (10%). Losses are accelerated by exposing more surface area and by bringing more blood to the body surfaces. Animals exposed to excessive heat will spontaneously seek a cooler environment where heat losses are accelerated.

Heat dissipation mechanisms vary from species to species. For example, the panting of the dog evaporates water from the respiratory tract and tongue with considerable loss of heat. In species with large specialized surfaces, such as the ears of the rabbit and the elephant, heat loss increases with the surface area. Fur reduces the ability to lose heat. As a consequence, furry animals are specially vulnerable to high environmental temperatures. Ruminants have only a limited ability to sweat, hence their evaporative heat loss is not efficient.

Temperatures are taken by deep insertion of an appropriate mercury thermometer into the rectum for at least 3 minutes. Electronic thermometers which record temperatures in a few seconds are now in use. Basal temperature may be obtained early in the morning after a period of rest, without exciting the animal. The body temperature of various animals in health varies considerably. As can be seen from TABLES 1 and 2 on pp. 1391, 1392, normal temperature may vary from as low as 95°F to as high as 110°F depending on the species.

Normal Variation: The body temperature of healthy animals is subject to slight diurnal variations. The temperature rises during the day and falls during the night. Large animals, such as the horse, cow and elephant, show small diurnal variations of about 1°F. Certain animals, such as the camel, which are adapted to large variations in environmental temperature and restricted availability of water, have diurnal fluctuations of body temperature of as much as 11°F. In very small animals, the balance between heat production and loss is easily disturbed, and the variations are greater, of the order of 5° or 10°F.

Exertion, excitement, or prolonged exposure to warm or humid environments, may cause a rise of several degrees in the body temperature. Hyperthermia due to reduced heat loss may seriously affect normal functions. For example, cows subjected to excessively high environmental temperatures reduce their food intake, lose weight and fail in milk production. Heat loss is associated with water loss. When water is not available, dehydration leads to inhibition of sweating and fever may develop. This form of hyperthermia is treated readily by the administration of water.

Seasonal variations in body temperature are related to environmental stresses and to the reproductive cycle. In cold weather, the rectal temperature may be recorded 1° to 2°F below the summer levels. Prior to ovulation, the basal temperature may be 1°F below the level of the preceding days. During estrus, the level is somewhat higher. It is slightly above the normal range during the first half of pregnancy.

Young animals have more labile temperature levels than older animals, with somewhat greater diurnal fluctuations; the young respond to infection with a much higher temperature elevation than do older animals. In very old animals, even severe infection may produce little or no change in the body temperature.

Fever is an abnormally high body temperature. In diurnal fever, which may indicate chronic infection, the temperature levels may rise several degrees during the day, returning to normal each night. In acute infections, the temperature may remain several degrees above the normal level for a few days, sometimes with a superimposed diurnal fluctuation. The relapsing fever of some chronic infections (e.g., brucellosis) is characterized by several days of elevated body temperature, followed by several days of normal temperature.

A chill usually heralds a febrile episode. The episode begins with extreme irritability, shivering, the seeking out of a warm environment and the reduction of body surface area from which heat can be lost, as by curling up. At the time of the chill, the body temperature is already above normal; shivering produces more heat and causes the temperature to rise further. These responses may be seen after the injection of foreign proteins, such as vaccines and sera.

Metabolic disturbances occur as a result of fever. The most striking of these is due to excessive loss of water leading to dehydration. Severe dehydration may produce a rise in body temperature which is resolved on the administration of fluids. Persistent fever can lead to a loss of sodium chloride and

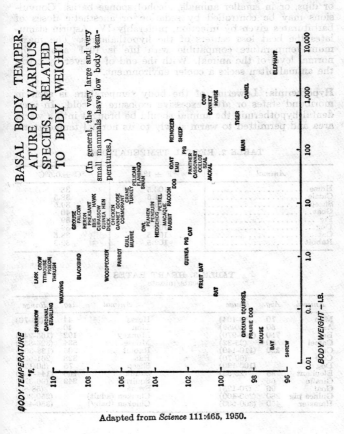

BASAL BODY TEMPERATURE OF VARIOUS SPECIES, RELATED TO BODY WEIGHT

(In general, the very large and very small mammals have low body temperatures.)

Adapted from *Science* 111:465, 1950.

bring about muscular twitching or even generalized convulsions. Disturbances in acid:base and salt:water balances, associated with prolonged fever or hyperthermia, may lead to acidosis. During hot weather and after fever, horses and cattle should have salt available to replenish losses.

If fever persists, convulsions may ensue. These must be stopped since they lead to excessive heat production. The fever may be treated by cooling the animals with cold soaks or dips, or in smaller animals, alcohol sponge baths. Convulsions may be controlled by sedation or anesthetic doses of barbiturates given by injection, preferably IV. Aspirin stimulates the heat loss centers of the hypothalamus. The maximum temperature compatible with life is 10°F above the normal level of the animal. With the end of a fever by crisis, the animal often seeks a cooler environment.

Hypothermia: Lowering of the body temperature is seen in moribund states or after excessive exposure to cold. In accidental hypothermia the animal should be brought into a warm area and permitted to warm slowly to its normal temperature.

TABLE 2. RECTAL TEMPERATURES

Animal	°F ± 1°F	°C ± 0.5°C
Horse	100.5	38
Cattle	101.5	38.5
Sheep	103	39.5
Goat	104	40
Pig	102	39
Dog	102	39
Cat	101.5	38.5
Rabbit	102.5	39.3

TABLE 3. HEART RATES
beats/minute

Animal	Avg.	Range	Animal	Avg.	Range
Man	70	(58-104)	Horse	44	(23-70)
Ass	50	(40-56)	Lion	40	
Bat	750	(100-970)	Monkey	192	(165-240)
Camel	30	(25-32)	Mouse	534	(324-858)
Cat	120	(110-140)	Rabbit	205	(123-304)
Cow		(60-70)	Rat	328	(261-600)
Dog		(100-130)	Sheep	75	(60-120)
Elephant	35	(22-53)	Skunk	166	(144-192)
Giraffe	66		Squirrel	249	(96-378)
Goat	90	(70-135)	Swine		(58-86)
Guinea pig	280	(260-400)	Chicken (adult)		(250-300)
Hamster	450	(300-600)	Chicken (baby)		(350-450)

TABLE 4. RESPIRATORY RATES
breaths/min

Animal	Resp. rate	Animal	Resp. rate
Hamster	74	Horse	12
Rat	97	Chicken: Male	12-20
Guinea pig	90	Female	20-36
Rabbit	39	Duck: Male	42
Monkey	40	Female	110
Cat	26	Goose: Male	20
Dog	22	Female	40
Sheep	19	Pigeon	25-30
Man	12	Turkey: Male	28
Cow	30	Female	49

TABLE 5. DAILY FECAL OUTPUT

Animal	Pounds
Horse	30-50
Sheep	2-6.5
Swine	1-6.5
Dog	0.06-0.09 when fed flesh
	0.3-0.9 moderate amount of bread
	2 large amount of bread
Dairy cow	60/1000 lb of body wt
Ox	30-75 maintenance & low production
	80-100 fattening

TABLE 6. DAILY URINE VOLUME

Animal	ml/kg of body wt
Cat	10-20
Cattle	17-45
Dog	20-100
Goat	10-40
Horse	3-18
Sheep	10-40
Swine	5-30
Man	8.6-28.6

The data in the above tables, (TABLES 2 through 6), were adapted in part from *Duke's Physiology of Domestic Animals*, 8th ed., M. J. Swenson, Ed., © 1970, by permission of Cornell University Press, and from other sources.

VETERINARY RADIOLOGY

RADIOGRAPHY

Equipment: The basic equipment for satisfactory veterinary radiography is a diagnostic-type X-ray machine with adequate protective housing. In small animal practice such a machine should have a capacity of 100 kVp (kilovolt peak) and 100 mA (milliamperes). A machine of greater capacity, in a well-planned fixed installation is necessary for use on large domestic animals. However, a light, mobile unit with a highly flexible, well-shielded head, with a capacity of 85 kVp and 30 mA is satisfactory for radiography of the extremities of large animals.

A filter in the useful beam of not less than 2.5 mm of aluminum and an interval timer that can be used at 1/60th of a second with the larger unit and 1/10th of a second with the mobile unit are essential.

All units must be equipped with a coning device to reduce scatter and limit stray primary radiation. A collimator with adjustable lead shutters and an illuminated field effectively limits the primary beam thereby reducing the radiation hazard and improving the technique.

Whenever the part to be radiographed exceeds 10 cm in thickness, the use of a grid markedly improves detail. A grid with a 6:1 ratio and 60 lines per inch is satisfactory for most diagnostic needs in large- and small-animal radiography. Additional equipment should include at least two 10 by 12 in. and two 14 by 17 in. cassettes with par- or high-speed screens, film hangers, a film-marking device, calipers to measure the part thickness, a tape for measuring source to tabletop or focal-film distance, 2 film illuminators and darkroom supplies. Protective aprons and gloves of at least 0.5 mm lead equivalent should be provided for 2 or more persons.

Darkroom: The darkroom must be lightproof and so designed as to provide separate wet and dry working surfaces. The room should be equipped with a 3-compartment tank for developer, water rinse and fixer and with a capacity to handle 14 by 17 in. films. The temperature of the solutions must be maintained between 60° and 74°F, preferably at 68°F, by running water or refrigeration. Since the rate of development varies directly with the temperature of the developer, the temperature of the solutions should be checked before use and a time-temperature chart should be consulted at temperatures other than 68°F. Manufacturer's instructions should be followed, but as a rule the developing time for screen film is 5 min and fixing requires 10 min. Films should be washed for 30 min in running water prior to drying in a dust-free atmosphere.

During processing, films should be removed from the solutions quickly and the excess solution not be permitted to drain back into the tank. This loss is replaced by replenishing from stock solutions, thereby maintaining the strength of the developer and fixer. Replenishing cannot be continued indefinitely, and the solutions should be discarded when the volume of replenisher used equals 3 times the original quantity of developer. In any event, the solutions should be discarded at the end of a 3-month period due to oxidation. Developing solutions must not be replenished while films are being processed.

Essential Factors in Radiography: The following factors contribute to the production of a satisfactory radiograph: (1) correct kVp for satisfactory penetration, (2) sufficient mA/s to ensure proper density, (3) time of exposure short enough to stop motion, (4) proper target-to-film distance to obtain maximum photographic detail, (5) close approximation of the part radiographed to the film, (6) immobilization of the part, (7) uniform sensitivity of screens and films, (8) standard darkroom technique, (9) standard positions for exposure.

The **kilovolt peak (kVp)** is the crest-value measurement of the pulsating potential generator. It indicates a measurement of the energy level in the X-ray beam and when the value is high the penetrating power of the beam is greater, the contrast on the film is diminished and the "quality" of the beam is said to be "hard". When the kVp is lower, the beam is said to be "softer" and, because absorption is greater, contrast is improved while penetration is diminished. Good radiologic technique requires the selection of a beam sufficient to penetrate the thickness of the tissue examined while providing contrast sufficient for the examination of the various tissues involved.

Milliamperage is a measurement of current flowing across the X-ray tube. The milliamperage per second (mA/s) directly determines the total film exposure or density. Good technique requires the proper selection of time and amperage to give the density required under the condition of the examination. The mA/s required to produce a given radiographic density is directly proportional to the square of the local-film distance when other factors are constant.

The use of a higher kVp with a reduction in mA/s results in less radiation exposure to the patient without significantly detracting from film quality.

In order to reduce the loss of detail by motion of the patient, short exposure times are desirable. Motion may be further reduced or eliminated by sedation or anesthesia. To minimize image distortion caused by divergence of the X-rays, the part to be radiographed should be in close contact with the cassette. As previously recommended, par- or high-speed screens increase the photographic effect with little loss of detail.

To accomplish the best radiography, a technique chart should be developed using thickness of the part measured in centimeters, relating each change in thickness to a corresponding change in kVp to mA/s. A handy rule for determining a technique is as follows: Two times the thickness of the part in centimeters plus 40 equals the kVp. Using the calculated kVp and 3 mA/s with par-speed screens, the films should be of diagnostic quality. For parts exceeding 10 cm, a 60 line, 6:1 grid should be employed and the mA/s must be increased to 6.

Positioning: Correct positioning of the patient is essential for good radiography, and 2 views should always be taken at right angles to each other. Whenever possible, positioning should be accomplished by the use of foam rubber blocks, leg ties, etc., always striving to reduce human exposure. Rotation of the part is to be avoided, particularly in radiographs of the thorax, skull and canine pelvis.

Whenever a joint is to be examined, the beam should be projected directly across the articular surface so that the intra-articular space and articular facets can be assessed. The beam should be perpendicular to the film to minimize distortion.

Standard lateral projections utilizing a horizontal beam are useful in demonstrating free fluid in the thoracic cavity or the multiple fluid levels and gas caps seen in stasis of the bowel.

Radiographic Interpretation: Immediately following processing, the films should be examined for technical quality and a preliminary diagnosis may be made. A definitive diagnosis should await a thorough study of the dried radiograph.

In assessing the image for pathologic changes a systematic step-by-step analysis is made of each anatomical part. Gross pathologic changes usually fall into one or more of the following categories: 1) Alteration in the position of an organ or part. Such alterations may be the result of a congenital anomaly, inadequate support, passive displacement by enlargement of adjacent viscera and rotation of viscera as in gastric torsion.

2) Alteration in size. Increase in size of an organ may be indicative of hypertrophy, hyperplasia, neoplasia, congenital anomaly, etc. Reductions in size occur with atrophy, hypoplasia, scarring, maldevelopment, etc.

3) Alterations in contour. Contour changes may affect a lo-

calized portion or the entire organ silhouette. Contour changes result from maldevelopment, trauma, cicatrization, loss of tone, neoplasia, necrosis, etc.

4) Alteration in density. Increases in density of tissues which are normally radiolucent are frequently due to calcification of soft tissues. Such calcium deposits are commonly indicative of poorly nourished or necrotic tissue, precipitation due to altered tissue pH or around a nidus and metaplasia or neoplasia. Other dense mineral concrements include renal and cystic calculi and fecal concretions. Decreases in the density of soft tissues usually are due to the abnormal presence of air or gas in tissues as in gangrene, subcut. emphysema or ileus of the small intestine.

In assessing osseous structures with diminished radiographic density 2 major causes should be considered: disturbance in mineralization and disturbance of osteoid formation. The former includes rickets and related nutritional deficiency states, whereas the latter is osteoporosis and may be due to endocrine disturbances, disuse atrophy, protein deficiency, etc.

Increases in bone density may be the result of increased mineral deposition within the substance of the bone proper or by periosteal proliferation. The pattern of periosteal new bone may be classified as layer-like, lace-like or spiculated and may be indicative of the cause.

On occasion, productive and destructive changes may occur in the same bone, as in osteomyelitis and neoplasia.

5) Alteration in architecture. To determine the presence of architectural changes requires familiarity with normal anatomy and its aberrations. When in doubt about a particular radiologic finding, comparison with a film of a similar part in another patient is often helpful.

6) Alterations in alignment or function. Alignment of bones and joints is usually demonstrable in plain films and dynamic phenomena may be studied by means of fluoroscopy.

Contrast Media: Selective delineation of an organ or body cavity may be accomplished by use of contrast media. Basically there are 2 types of contrast media: (1) negative media such as air, CO_2 and O_2 which outline the structure by increasing blackness on the film, and (2) positive media such as insoluble salts of heavy metals or inorganic iodides which are opaque and appear white on the film.

Negative media are commonly used in pneumocystograms, pneumoperitoneums and pneumocolons. Barium sulfate, a positive medium, is ideal for visualization of all parts of the gastrointestinal tract. The urinary bladder can be defined by introduction of 10% sodium iodide and when used in conjunction with air, the double contrast effect is excellent in defining intraluminal lesions. Numerous commercially prepared media with organic soluble iodides as the base are available for urography, cardioangiography, angiography, etc., and the selection of the medium is left to the discretion of the veterinarian. For detailed instructions on the radiographic technique of contrast studies, the reader is referred to texts on radiology.

FLUOROSCOPY

Fluoroscopy is an excellent means of studying the dynamic phenomena of an organ or part, but it must be used judiciously. Unfortunately the diagnostic units in most veterinary hospitals are not designed for safe operation as fluoroscopes and in such cases the technique should be avoided. For details of equipment standards the National Council on Radiation Protection, Publication No. 36, should be consulted.

The eyes of the fluoroscopist should be dark-adapted for 20 minutes before the examination of the patient and protective aprons and gloves must be worn. Only persons actively participating in the procedure should be in the room, and if possible the patient should be anesthetized or sedated to expedite the procedure.

RADIATION PROTECTION

While it is possible to use X-rays and radioactive material with safety, few private veterinary establishments are equipped to provide the necessary protection for the veterinarian, his assistants and clients. The veterinarian is legally responsible for the protection of his assistants and may be liable for injury following careless or unintentional exposure of others. Because of the large amounts of radiation required, it is questionable whether the general practitioner should attempt radiation therapy of neoplastic or even inflammatory lesions in his patients. Since radiation therapy centers, with qualified veterinary radiologists, are becoming established, the general practitioner might well refer patients requiring this form of therapy to such specialists.

According to the recommendation of the National Council on Radiation Protection and Measurements, maximum exposure to X-ray or gamma radiation from external sources for radiation workers is 100 milliroentgens per week. All persons using equipment producing such radiation should wear film-badges routinely and the degree of exposure should be checked regularly. Hands and other parts of the body always should be kept out of the primary beam and leaded gloves and aprons hould be worn routinely for protection against stray radiation. Users of ionizing radiation are referred to the National Council on Radiation Protection, Publication No. 36, "Radiaion Protection in Veterinary Medicine" and reports numered 17, 22, 33, 34 and 35.

ROUTES FOR MEDICATION

Selection of a drug and its route of administration is determined by assessment of several factors. The diagnosis of the disease process and the disease status of the patient will dictate the treatment needed. The species or breed of the patient, its size, temperament, tractability and idiosyncrasies will influence the form, frequency and manner in which the drug is administered. The treatment of an out-patient may vary considerably from that of a hospitalized patient. The ability and willingness of an owner to treat the patient often s the ultimate determinant of a treatment regime. With all actors considered, it is essential that the clinician's decision complement the indications, properties and optimal therapeutic efficacy of the drug selected.

Topical medication applies primarily to treatment of ocular, otic, dermatologic and nasal disorders. Topical preparations are available in ointments, aqueous solutions, aerosols and powders. The use of aqueous forms requires frequent administration (e.g., every 2 hours); ointments act over a longer period and should be applied in small amounts at longer intervals. Ocular preparations should be limited to ointments and aqueous solutions; probably the same should apply to the ears. Topical treatment of skin lesions can be frustrating in some species, requiring concurrent use of restraint collars or sedatives. Only thin layers of a medicament should be applied, and it should be gently worked into the lesions. Aqueous solutions and aerosols can be used in the nasal passages; oily preparations are generally contraindicated because of the chance of causing lipid pneumonia. Some propellants are also hazardous. Since absorption of topical medication can occur, the toxic potential of any medicament must be respected.

Oral administration of drugs is a popular method of treatment. Its efficacy is dependent on the condition of the gastrointestinal system, and in some instances the tolerance of the system to the drug administered. Vomiting or diarrhea are obvious reasons for unsuccessful attempts to attain therapeutic drug levels. Coated drug preparations (e.g., enteric-coated sodium chloride) have on occasion passed undissolved in fecal material. A patient that has recently eaten may retain medication in the stomach long enough to diminish optimal therapeutic effect.

Oral preparations are available in tablets, pills, capsules or liquid mixtures. To insure that a particular drug reaches the lower bowel before it disintegrates, it is often coated with a substance that is resistant to the acid medium of the stomach. Depending upon the situation and the type of patient, administration of a drug may be "easier said than done" (e.g., the owner's inability to treat his cat is a common complaint) and requires patience, ingenuity and persistence to be successful. If the patient is reliably consuming food or water, the drug may be administered in either of these. Palatability must be taken into consideration; animals that chew their food (e.g., cats, monkeys) can detect pills readily. Manual administration of pills or capsules allows visual assurance of drug intake in cats and dogs; forceps may be used in difficult patients. "Balling guns" are used in large animals. Liquid preparations should be given carefully to avoid the complication of aspiration pneumonia. Stomach tubes, passed through mouth or nostril may be used in most species; the size of tubing depends upon the age, species, purpose and route selected. Many patients can be drenched with special syringes. A convenient pouch for deposition can be created in the dog by drawing the cheek outward at the outer commissure of the mouth. Fortunate is the clinician whose patient voluntarily drinks its medication.

Parenteral administration of drugs implies injection of drugs into a patient's body. With few exceptions (subconjunctival, intrauterine, rectal) this requires preparation of the skin; hair is clipped or parted and the exposed skin is cleansed with pHisohex and an antiseptic solution or both. The drug container cap is also sterilized. Particular care is exercised in preparing vials containing modified live virus so as not to destroy immunologic properties. The use of sterile needles and syringes is imperative and is accomplished by autoclaving, boiling or antiseptic soaks; disposable sterile units are very popular. A respect for the anatomic relationships of muscle, nerve and vascular channels, and proper restraint of the patient allows correct injection technique. Before deposition of medication, withdrawal of the syringe plunger is important, regardless of the tissue involved; aspiration of blood into the syringe is acceptable only in IV injections.

Injection therapy is not without its complications and the following are a few of the situations that may result: Sterile as well as bacterial abscesses form occasionally. Anaphylactic or allergic reactions occur with biologics and antibiotics. Extravascular spillage of irritant drugs can lead to skin sloughs. The tonicity of drugs (i.e., isotonic, hypertonic) can be a factor abused in the selection of route of administration. Sciatic palsy has resulted from poor injection technique. Arterial administration, instead of by IV routes, while sometimes useful, may be catastrophic in some situations (e.g., tranquilizers in horses). Pyrogen-contaminated fluid units can cause febrile reactions. Transfusions of incompatible types can result in severe systemic reactions.

Intravenous (IV) injection offers several advantages. The rapid availability of a drug, or use of larger volume of solutions, is possible. Irritating drugs or hypertonic drugs can be given with fewer problems. Induction anesthesia is controlled effectively by this route. Generally, medication is given slowly; increased rate of flow is indicated in cases of recent blood loss. When large volumes of a solution, or increased rate of flow, are necessary the patient should be monitored closely, particularly cardiovascular patients. Should restraint of a patient be a problem, or if a patient is being monitored in an intensive care situation, the use of indwelling IV catheters of inert plastic tubing is advantageous.

Subcutaneous (subcut.) and intraperitoneal (IP) injections are often referred to as the "pool routes"; depots of fluid in these areas allow slower but sustained absorption benefits. Should a vascular channel not be accessible, blood transfusions can be given IP. However, a very debilitated patient, or a patient in shock, will not pick up these "pool" fluids. Irritating drugs should not be administered by these routes; if given subcut., such drugs should be administered in small amounts at several sites. Dialysis in uremic patients and cases of intoxication has been done by IP lavage techniques.

Intramuscular (IM) injections benefit from good blood supply and rapid absorption. Drugs should be given in small amounts. Pain and lameness may occur with this route of administration. "Kapture" guns loaded with special syringes containing tranquilizers or paralyzing drugs are available for catching or treating untamed large animals.

Other routes of injection include **intradermal** (TB testing); **intraruminal** via the left flank region in cattle and sheep (antifoaming agents in bloat); and **intramammary** (infectious mastitis of cattle and sheep). **Intrathoracic** injection may be used as in cases of exudative pleurisy of cats where enzymes

and antibiotics might be helpful. **Rectal** injection has pri
marily been limited to suppositories and enemas, although it
application to fluid therapy and anesthesia is appreciated
Epidural injection of local anesthesia is a common techniqu
in obstetrical procedures in cattle, and has been used in othe
species. **Implantation** is a form of subcut. injection whereb
repository pellets of certain substances are slowly absorbe
over a given period (e.g., stilbestrol in feeder cattle, desoxy
corticosterone acetate in dogs with hypoadrenocorticalism)
Inhalation administration is practiced with gas anesthetic
nebulization therapy and oxygen therapy (see OXYGEN THEF
APY, below).

Administration of gases is done by use of masks, speciall
adapted cages or containers, and endotracheal tubes. Al
though induction anesthesia can be accomplished with mask
or closed containers, the more popular method is to anesthe
tize the patient with IV administration of an ultrashort-actin
anesthetic and then intubate the trachea; the method chose
obviously depends on the species dealt with (e.g., rat, do
horse). Maintenance anesthesia can be administered by a ga
anesthetic machine or a drop method into a cone or mask.

Nebulization therapy is finding more application in veter
inary medicine, particularly in situations where oxygen
being given. The procedure can be as simple as adding ce
tain volatile substances to hot water (tincture of benzoin o
oil of eucalyptus); the resulting steam carries these vaporize
substances into the treatment environment. Certain drug
such as ephedrine, epinephrine and penicillin can be directl
atomized into an oxygen supply line. Sophisticated equipmer
uses compressed air or oxygen to deliver antifoaming agent
(e.g., ethyl alcohol) to patients with pulmonary edema, an
detergent materials (Tergemist or Mucomist) to patients wit
bronchial exudates.

OXYGEN THERAPY (SM. AN.)

Oxygen therapy is a supportive measure rather than a sp
cific treatment. It is designed to prevent anoxia or to limit
so that serious or perhaps irreparable damage does not de
velop before treatment has become effective. Oxygen therap
bolsters the patient and acts as an adjunct to other trea
ments in such conditions as pneumonia and heart weaknes
When anoxia occurs, the inhalation of oxygen-enriched a
mosphere (oxygen concentrations of 50 to 100%) enables th
blood to absorb and transport increased quantities of oxyge

Pathologic Physiology of Anoxia: There are 4 recognized types of anoxia:

Anoxic anoxia is desaturation of the arterial blood below the normal oxyhemoglobin concentration of about 97%. It results from an insufficient delivery of oxygen by the lungs to the blood. It develops in respiratory deficiency and in various forms of pulmonary disease and asphyxia. Interference with gaseous exchange through the lung alveoli prevents normal saturation of the arterial blood, even though the alveolar oxygen pressure is normal. Insufficient oxygen exchange during anesthesia leads to this type of anoxia.

Anemic anoxia results from inability of the blood to transport sufficient amounts of oxygen. It occurs in anemia from any cause, following severe hemorrhage, and in carbon monoxide and nitrite poisonings.

Stagnation anoxia indicates circulatory deficiency as in passive congestion, cardiac failure, shock or embolism. Respiration is not primarily affected; the blood has access to oxygen in the lungs, but transportation to the tissues is retarded owing to interference with movement of blood through the capillaries.

Histotoxic anoxia results from an inability of the tissues to utilize oxygen. It is brought about by chemicals, such as cyanide, alcohol, some of the narcotics, tetrachloroethylene and the barbiturates.

Fluid Balance: Anoxia, or any other injury to the capillary walls, increases capillary permeability and produces capillary atony which results in local blood stasis. This blood is out of circulation as effectively as if lost by external hemorrhage. At the same time, tissue function is reduced or lost. This permits the liberation of abnormal metabolites, which, in turn, further disturb the circulation.

The 2 major factors, capillary atony and anoxia, are reciprocal in action; either of them will bring the other into action. Anoxia is thus one of the chief factors in the dynamics of shock.

Equipment and Methods: The basic oxygen therapy unit consists of a cylinder, a regulator and a length of tube. To this basic unit can be attached any number of appliances, some fairly simple, some extremely complicated, to effect any required oxygen concentration. So many methods and so much equipment have been developed exclusively for veterinary use that almost any need can be met. Information about the various types of oxygen cylinders, regulators, tubing and standard oxygen equipment available is best obtained from a reliable commercial oxygen supply house.

Oxygen is available in high-pressure cylinders of various sizes. A pressure-reducing valve must be attached to the cylinder valve outlet before such cylinders can be safely used.

Cautions: 1. Although oxygen itself is not explosive, it strongly supports combustion. Protection from fire depends on keeping all hazards such as cigarettes, open flames, electric connections or heating pads away from any concentration of oxygen.

2. Oxygen is explosive in combination with certain other substances such as cyclopropane and oil. Therefore, valves or any of the threads or equipment through which oxygen is to be passed should not be oiled.

3. Oxygen cylinders contain the gas under high pressure and, therefore, must be handled with particular care. Obsolete or makeshift regulators should not be used. When a new cylinder is opened, pressure should be released gradually and the valve pointed, as a gun would be, away from persons or animals.

Oxygen Administration: Inhalation therapy can be administered by: (1) holding a tube to the nose with or without a mask over the nose and mouth (this is generally not a satisfactory method); (2) passing a tube into the pharynx; (3) intratracheal intubation with or without an inflation cuff; (4) placing the patient's head or the entire patient in an oxygen chamber; or (5) inserting a tracheal tube via a tracheostomy. The gases used can be any of the following: (1) pure oxygen; (2) oxygen in various mixtures with room air, ranging from 50 to 95% oxygen; (3) oxygen with nebulized drugs, such as neomycin and polymyxin B or a mucolytic agent such as 10 or 20% acetylcysteine (which may be given by aerosol or local instillation); or (4) oxygen mixed with gaseous anesthetics, such as halothane or nitrous oxide.

Inhalation therapy is an excellent supportive measure for any patient that is seriously ill, but the cost may become prohibitive for patients requiring treatment for more than a few days. However, it is entirely practical in acute cases, such as septicemia, and in patients with high fever where the critical state would not be expected to last more than 2 or 3 days.

EMERGENCY OXYGEN DEFICIENCY

Emergency conditions benefited by inhalation therapy include shock, acute hemorrhage, any acute respiratory difficulty and severe anaphylactic reactions, in all of which a type of anoxia exists.

Oxygen can be administered in a matter of seconds and is utilized immediately by the patient. Therefore, it is of prime importance as one of the most quickly effective emergency measures. In emergencies, it is used only for a short time as a supportive measure until other treatments can become effective.

Acute Dyspnea: Hypoventilation of this type occurs in association with overheating, and the labored breathing indicates an oxygen demand beyond the patient's capacity. If simple overheating, such as sunstroke, is treated before permanent damage is done, oxygen alone is often adequate therapy. It should be administered as cold as possible.

Strangulation: Foreign-body aspiration usually only partially occludes the trachea. Partial occlusion may cause death if atmospheric air is breathed, but administration of 100% oxygen often will support life long enough for the patient to cough and dislodge the foreign body, or it will maintain life long enough for the foreign body to be removed.

Anoxia of the Newborn: Newborn animals that have been subjected to prolonged or difficult delivery, or weak newborns, nearly always have respiratory distress. Prompt aspiration and administration of oxygen by inhalation and sodium bicarbonate by IV injection to combat acidosis will save animals which otherwise would be lost.

Suffocation: One of the common causes of so-called "anesthetic deaths" is obstruction or occlusion of the upper air passages. This occurrence is particularly common in the short-nosed breeds of dogs, in which it usually results from a collapse of the epiglottis behind the soft palate. Forced inspiration of the type which occurs whenever such obstruction is encountered only tends to seal tighter the union between the lips of the epiglottis and the palate and to insure asphyxiation by self-strangulation. This can be prevented by the insertion of any stiff-walled tube into the trachea as soon as anesthesia is accomplished. One of the simplest, yet most effective methods of administering oxygen for a short time to a patient exhibiting respiratory distress is through such an intratracheal tube.

DISEASES OF THE RESPIRATORY AND BLOOD-VASCULAR SYSTEMS

Diseases of the lungs, heart and blood that can be benefited by inhalation therapy include:

1. pulmonary involvements such as hyperemia, edema, pneumonia, interstitial emphysema, asthma, filarial embolism, bronchitis and contusion;

2. cardiac asthenia, dilatation, valvular insufficiencies and filarial infection;

3. shock, extensive hemorrhage and extreme anemia.

Lungs: Acute pulmonary involvements, such as hyperemia, edema, pneumonia and interstitial emphysema, have in common a decrease in the oxygenation of the hemoglobin, and their treatment with oxygen is similar. The oxygen chamber is used and duration of treatment will vary from an hour or 2 to several days. The oxygen must be cooled and humidified. The rate of flow should be controlled according to the requirements of the patient. During the early stages of severe anoxia, the oxygen requirement is greater than after the patient has improved. The oxygen flow serves 2 purposes: (1) to supply the patient and (2) to remove excess carbon dioxide. Therefore, the oxygen is not supplied according to any fixed formula, but in sufficient quantity to give relief. An oxygen concentration above 70% without interruption becomes harmful after 2 days. If, however, the patient is removed occasionally from 70% concentration to room air, this concentration can be maintained indefinitely without ill effect.

Filarial embolism accompanying treatment for heartworms (q.v., p. 686) or occurring spontaneously in heavily infected dogs causes a severe transitory dyspnea which can be relieved by oxygen therapy. Chronic pulmonary involvements, such as passive hyperemia from cardiac insufficiency and chronic bronchitis, are accompanied by varying degrees of dyspnea and a tendency to cough. Many of these dogs are in danger of asphyxia. Owners of seriously ill patients can be supplied with simple oxygen equipment and instructed in its home use.

Heart: An acute heart weakness (neurocirculatory asthenia) is frequently seen in dogs that have become overheated, as by confinement in a closed car in the hot sun, and in fat, phlegmatic dogs following unaccustomed exercise, such as swimming. The diagnosis usually is obvious and the history revealing. The patient shows typical circulatory insufficiency in the form of marked dyspnea, cyanosis and accelerated and weakened pulse. Unless effective treatment in the form of an abundant supply of pure oxygen is given promptly, convulsions and death may result from cerebral anoxia. Shock is frequent sequela to this condition and should be prevented by appropriate treatment.

Chronic heart weakness is characterized by frequent attacks of vertigo and loss of consciousness. These signs are due to defective circulation to the brain with venous stasis. Other less obvious, but important, results of the stasis are respiratory involvements, such as bronchitis, interference with nutrition and elimination and anuria.

Blood: Diseases of the blood which are relieved by the use of oxygen are: (1) a relative decrease in the blood volume as in shock, (2) an absolute decrease in the blood volume as in hemorrhage and (3) anemia. In all cases, oxygen is an intermediate measure to sustain or resuscitate the patient until the specific treatment, such as fluid administration, hemorrhage control and blood transfusion, can become effective. Labored breathing is the clinical evidence that absolute decrease in blood volume has developed to the point where oxygen will be of benefit. In these cases, a high concentration of oxygen is administered by means of a mask or with only the head in the small oxygen chamber so that the rest of the body is accessible for the specific therapy required.

ROUTINE IMMUNOLOGIC PROCEDURES

Vaccination is an important adjunct in the control of many livestock diseases, but the immunity is relative and may be overcome by massive exposure, by moderate contact with a highly virulent strain of the infecting agent or by stress, such as poor environmental conditions. Vaccination should not be considered a panacea in disease control and it should be supplemented with sanitary and management measures designed to prevent the introduction and spread of infection.

When an effective immunizing agent is injected, the tissues react to form immune bodies against the agent. This reaction may be accompanied by signs of distress, and these signs may be exaggerated if the animal is not in a state of good health when vaccinated. If a live vaccine is employed in an unhealthy animal, it may actually produce the disease it was intended to prevent.

Effective active immunization can be accomplished only by vaccines that are high in specific antigen content, or in the case of passive immunization, serum rich in antibody. Improved methods for virus culture have resulted in vaccines that contain a high concentration of antigen. Newer methods of attenuation, particularly by passage through unnatural hosts, have further improved the virus vaccines. Employing heterotypic viruses as vaccines has provided cross-protection in some cases without exposing the patient to the actual causal agent.

The following is a description of the various biologics used routinely to immunize livestock including poultry:

Vaccines: In common usage, the term vaccine has come to mean all types of biologic agents used to produce active immunity.

Toxoids: Toxoids are prepared from potent toxin which is detoxified with formalin and the active antigenic fraction precipitated with alum and resuspended in isotonic salt solution. It has the antigenic but not the poisonous properties of the toxin.

Bacterins: These are bacterial suspensions inactivated by physical and chemical means. A formalized whole culture of bacteria is called anaculture. These agents will not produce disease, but their immunizing power usually is lower than that of living agents. The maximum duration of the immunity ordinarily is not more than 12 months.

Live bacterial suspensions: These produce a more solid and lasting immunity than the bacterins. They may, however, cause the disease and should be given either in the form of attenuated strains or at an age when the effects would be the least harmful. Their effectiveness is dependent on the number of viable organisms in the suspension. Careless handling, such as failure to keep under refrigeration and permitting contamination, lowers the viable count and results in ineffective vaccination. Brucellosis vaccine Strain 19 is an example of an attenuated live bacterial suspension.

Spore vaccines: Against anthrax, suspensions of spores are used, the virulence of which has been lowered by cultivation at a higher than optimal temperature. The culture is allowed to sporulate, the cells washed from the media and the resultant suspension heated to destroy vegetative forms. Such a vaccine provides a more solid immunity than the bacterin, but is only good for a year. Because it is living, this vaccine should be used only in areas where anthrax is enzootic.

Live unmodified viruses: These confer, if properly handled, an effective and lasting immunity. They must be used with caution and given with antiserum if the virus is one that may cause an acute fatal disease like hog cholera. Otherwise, they may be given at an age when they cause only a mild form of the disease from which animals or birds recover prior to going into production. This type of immunization is called premunizing and the result premunition. Fowl pox vaccine is an example.

Modified viruses: Such viruses are modified by serial passage through unnatural hosts. During these passages, the virus loses virulence for the natural host and becomes adapted to growth on the new host. Although losing virulence, the virus retains its antigenic properties and acts as a vaccine. These are effective and produce lasting and solid immunity. Hog-cholera-modified virus is a vaccine of this type, as are the viruses that have been adapted to grow in the embryonated egg and are used in the living state.

Inactivated viruses: These have been inactivated by chemicals, usually formalin, phenol, or chloroform. Their effectiveness depends on the quantity of antigen present. Most are grown in the embryonating egg and are rich in antigen. The immunity produced is strong in most instances, but vaccination should be repeated annually. In some cases, 2 injections are recommended.

Antisera: These are hyperimmune sera originating from a variety of sources depending on the specific antigen. Some are homologous because the antigen is active in only one species. When other than homologous serum is used, anaphylactic reactions may occur. Included in this group are the antitoxins. Immunity is present immediately following the administration of an antiserum but is of brief duration. Antisera are used prophylactically and therapeutically in certain viral and bacterial diseases.

HANDLING VACCINES

Biologics produced under license are free from contaminants. Care should be taken to maintain that condition. Containers with multiple doses should be discarded when partially used unless they are opened in an aseptic manner and stored under refrigeration. When lyophilized products are reconstituted with diluent, they should be used immediately or they will deteriorate rapidly. Vaccines have varying expiration dates, depending on the particular product. They should not be used beyond the stated time. This date is based on holding the vaccine under optimum conditions, such as keeping it in a cool place, or preferably refrigerated. Vaccines that are outdated have lost part of their antigenic properties and are ineffective as immunizing agents. Empty live-virus containers should be burned or immersed in strong disinfectant. Carelessly discarded virus bottles can result in outbreaks of disease.

The degree of sanitation practiced during vaccination varies with the extent of the operation. It varies from the vaccination of a single dog where complete asepsis is possible, to the vaccination of a thousand or more head of cattle passing through a chute in a dusty corral. In the latter operation, cleanliness can be obtained without sacrificing efficiency. A liberal supply of needles maintained in disinfectant and exchanged periodically is advisable. Disease can be transmitted in mass vaccinations.

Biologics are administered in accordance with the producer's directions; some are given intradermally, others subcut. or IM. In most instances, the material is inoculated in one place. Where the amount is large, as in the case of antiserum in large animals, it is advisable to inject the material in several places.

Active immunity should not be considered to be established until at least 10 days following vaccination. It is not the purpose of an immunizing agent to protect an animal that is inoculated while in the incubation stage of a disease. Antiserum should be administered simultaneously with the vaccine if the individual has been exposed to the etiologic agent.

When live, unmodified, fully virulent viruses are used, it should be remembered that the vaccinated animal may become a carrier and shed the virus for varying periods. This means that susceptible stock should not have contact with vaccinates until the period of elimination has passed. This varies with each virus.

PASSIVE IMMUNITY IN THE NEWBORN

In certain species, antibodies are transferred to the fetus through the placenta or the yolk sac. In others, such transfer does not occur. The newborn from the latter lack passive immunity. This is compensated for, usually, by high-antibody concentration in the colostrum. Horses, cattle, sheep, goats, pigs and dogs are species in which passive immunity in the newborn is acquired by way of the colostrum. Antibodies from the colostrum are readily absorbed from the intestinal tract of the newborn, in most cases during the first 24 hours of life only. Because it is essential that the newborn animal receive all the passive immunity available to protect it during early life, efforts should be made to provide the necessary colostrum as soon as possible after birth; antibodies are absorbed at a decreasing rate even during the first 24 hours. The newborn animal is subject to infection until the antibodies are absorbed.

COMMON IMMUNIZING AGENTS

The following list includes vaccination procedures commonly carried out on most of the domestic animals in the principal livestock-raising areas of the world. Only those agents and measures are listed which are regarded as producing reliable and effective immunity for specific diseases. Autogenous vac-

CATTLE

Disease	Agent	Procedure
1. Anaplasmosis (*Anaplasma marginale*)	Virulent blood that contains the organism (not permitted in the U.S.A.)	Give to calves less than 1 year old during winter months—Premunition.
	Vaccine, inactivated	Give 2 injections, 4 weeks apart, with last dose preceding vector season by at least 2 weeks. Annual booster injections recommended.
2. Anthrax (*Bacillus anthracis*)	Spore vaccine, attenuated	Used each spring where anthrax is enzootic.
	Avirulent vaccine	Used each spring where anthrax is enzootic.
	Anaculture	Used each spring in areas where the disease is not enzootic, but may occur.
3. Blackleg (*Clostridium chauvoei*)	Anaculture	Used on animals 6 to 12 months of age.
4. Botulism (*Clostridium botulinum*)	Toxoid (Types C & D)	Used before turning cattle on pasture in areas where the disease is prevalent.
5. Brucellosis (*Brucella abortus*)	Strain 19 vaccine, lyophilized	Administer to calves at 3 to 8 months of age.
6. Contagious pleuropneumonia (*Mycoplasma mycoides*)	Vaccine, chick embryo-adapted	Administer to young cattle in infected areas.
7. Dysentery (*Clostridium perfringens*)	Anaculture (Types B & C)	Used to immunize dams before calves are born.
	Antiserum (Types B, C & D)	Used for immediate protection of newborn calves.
8. Black disease (*Clostridium novyi* [*oedematiens*], *sordelli*)	Anaculture	Administer in early spring. Yearly booster doses recommended in problem areas.
9. Foot-and-mouth disease (Virus)	Tissue culture vaccine, formalin-treated	Used only in areas where FMD is present.
10. Infectious bovine rhinotracheitis (IBR-IPV virus)	Tissue culture vaccine, modified	Produces active immunity for about 12 months.
	Vaccine, inactivated bovine tissue culture	Two injections at a 14-day interval. Can be used on pregnant cows.
11. Bacillary hemoglobinuria (*Clostridium haemolyticum*)	Anaculture	Protects for a full pasture season.

CATTLE (Continued)

Disease	Agent	Procedure
12. Leptospirosis (*Leptospira pomona*)	Anaculture or chick embryo vaccine, inactivated	Protects for 6 to 12 months.
13. Malignant edema (*Clostridium septicum*)	Anaculture	Usually produces life-long immunity.
14. Pasteurellosis (*Pasteurella multocida*)	Bacterin	Administer 10 to 14 days before animal is to be subjected to a stress.
15. Parainfluenza 3, SF-4 Strain	Vaccine, inactivated virus	Administer 2 doses at least 3 weeks apart prior to stress.
TELC Strain	Intranasal vaccine, porcine tissue origin	Spray nasal cavity 3 weeks prior to stress.
	Antiserum	Used to produce immediate passive immunity.
16. Piroplasmosis (*Babesia bigemina*)	Infected ticks	Place 1 or 2 on calf several weeks before turning out on pasture.
17. Rinderpest (Virus)	Goat-, rabbit-, or egg-adapted vaccine	Protects up to 1 year.
	Antiserum	Produces immediate immunity.
18. Salmonellosis (*Salmonella dublin*)	Bacterin, formalized and alum-precipitated	Administer to cow to protect newborn calf or to the calf.
19. Papillomas (warts) (Virus)	Bovine tissue vaccine	Produces only fair immunity.
20. Bovine virus diarrhea (Mucosal disease) (Virus)	Vaccine, modified, tissue culture origin	Long-term immunity
21. Staphylococcal mastitis (*S. aureus*)	Toxoid	Administer prior to calving. Protection is questionable.
22. Vibriosis (*Vibrio fetus*)	Bacterin	Administer 2 injections at least 2 weeks apart prior to breeding season.
23. Rabies (Virus)	Modified live virus, porcine tissue culture origin	Can be used in 6 species (dog, cat, horse, cattle, sheep and goat). Long-term immunity.
24. Lungworms (*Dictyocaulus viviparus*)	Irradiated larvae	Administer irradiated larvae twice, with a 6-week interval.

HORSES

1. African horse sickness (Virus)	Mouse brain-adapted vaccine	Annual vaccination.

continued on next page

HORSES (Continued)

Disease	Agent	Procedure
2. Equine encephalomyelitis (Virus)	Chick embryo vaccine, inactivated 1) Eastern 2) Western 3) Mixed	Administer each year in spring using type or types prevalent.
3. Venezuelan equine encephalomyelitis (Virus)	Guinea pig heart-adapted vaccine	Duration of immunity 1 to 3 years.
4. Equine rhinopneumonitis (Equine virus abortion)	Hamster-adapted virus	Intranasal vaccination during summer and fall of each year—Premunition.
5. Equine influenza	Tissue culture vaccine	Administered to young horses annually before beginning training, or when an epizootic threatens.
6. Malignant edema (*Clostridium septicum*)	(See cattle, above)	
7. Strangles (*Streptococcus equi*)	Bacterin, 4- to 5-hour-old culture killed in virulent phase	Administer to foal about 2 weeks before weaning. Be cautious about administering during or immediately following an outbreak.
8. Tetanus (*Clostridium tetani*)	Toxoid	Produces active immunity that can be maintained by yearly booster doses.
	Antitoxin (equine)	Used to produce immediate immunity.

SHEEP

Disease	Agent	Procedure
1. Anthrax (*Bacillus anthracis*)	(See cattle, above)	
2. Black disease (*Clostridium novyi* [*oedematiens*])	Anaculture	Several doses needed to produce solid immunity.
3. Blackleg (*Clostridium chauvoei*)	Anaculture	Vaccinate before turning out to pasture.
4. Bluetongue (Virus)	Vaccine, chick embryo-adapted	Immunize lambs shortly before weaning.
5. Botulism (*Clostridium botulinum*)	Toxoid (Type C)	Used in areas where the disease is common, before putting animals on pasture.
6. Contagious ecthyma (Virus)	Vaccine, dried scab material.	Vaccinate lambs each spring before pasture season begins.

SHEEP (Continued)

Disease	Agent	Procedure
7. Enterotoxemia (*Clostridium perfringens*)	Anaculture (Type D)	Administer to lambs about 2 weeks before entering feed lot, or to ewes 3 weeks prior to lambing.
8. Enzootic ovine abortion (*Chlamydia sp.*)	Vaccine, oil emulsion of alum-precipitated material from infected fetal membranes	One injection gives adequate protection for a year.
9. Epididymitis (*Brucella ovis*)	*B. abortus* Strain 19 vaccine plus bacterin of formalized *B. ovis*	Administer to rams at 9 to 12 months of age, or before start of breeding season.
10. Johne's disease (*Mycobacterium paratuberculosis*)	Bacterin, heat-killed suspension in light mineral oil	Lambs are vaccinated subcut. at 6 to 7 months of age with 1 ml of bacterin.
11. Lamb dysentery (*Clostridium perfringens*)	Anaculture (Type B)	Administer to pregnant ewes about 3 weeks prior to lambing.
	Antitoxin	Administer to lambs at birth.
12. Louping ill (Virus)	Vaccine, formalized nerve tissue	Administer to young lambs at weaning time.
13. Malignant edema (*Clostridium septicum*)	(See cattle, above)	
14. Pasteurellosis (*Pasteurella multocida*)	(See cattle, above)	
15. Rift Valley fever (Virus)	Vaccine, chick embryo-adapted	Administer to non-pregnant ewes.
16. Struck (*Clostridium perfringens*)	Anaculture (Type C)	Administer to lambs at weaning time.
17. Tetanus (*Clostridium tetani*)	(See horses, above)	

SWINE

Disease	Agent	Procedure
1. Hog cholera (Virus)	Vaccine, modified by serial passage in rabbits or tissue culture	Administer with or without serum to produce active immunity.
	Vaccine, inactivated	Used to produce active immunity in swine in areas where disease is not common.
	Antiserum, homologous	Administer at the onset of an outbreak or simultaneously with virus to immunize healthy pigs.

continued on next page

SWINE (Continued)

Disease	Agent	Procedure
2. Leptospirosis (*Leptospira pomona*)	Bacterin	Protects young swine.
3. Swine erysipelas (*Erysipelothrix insidiosa*)	Vaccine, virulent	Used only in areas where simultaneous method authorized.
	Vaccine, lyophilized	Administer to weanling pigs.
	Bacterin, alum-absorbed, formalized	Administer to weanling pigs.
	Antiserum	Administer at onset of outbreak.
4. Jowl abscesses (Group E *Streptococcus*)	Vaccine, live culture, avirulent (oral vaccine)	Use in healthy swine at least 10 weeks of age. Apply to posterior portion of hard palate and tonsillar area.

FOWL

Disease	Agent	Procedure
1. Infectious bronchitis (Virus)	Vaccine, chick embryo, lyophilized	Administer to chicks by placing in the drinking water, eye, or nasal passages at 7 to 14 days of age and repeat at 4 to 5 weeks and again at 14 to 16 weeks.
2. Laryngotracheitis (Virus)	Vaccine, chick embryo, or tissue-culture origin	Drop in eye of healthy birds over 6 weeks of age.
3. Fowl pox (Virus)	Vaccine, chick embryo, lyophilized	Administer in feather follicle or skin puncture to healthy birds at least a month before the start of egg production.
	Pigeon pox vaccine, chick embryo, lyophilized	Same as fowl pox.
4. Newcastle disease (Virus)	Vaccine, chick embryo	Same as infectious bronchitis.
5. Pasteurellosis (fowl cholera) (*Pasteurella multocida*)	Bacterin	Used to control fowl cholera in birds.
6. *Erysipelothrix* infection	Bacterin, alum-absorbed, formalized	Used especially to vaccinate turkey poults before placing on range.
7. Marek's disease	Vaccine, turkey herpesvirus	One day of age. Subcut. or IP.

DOGS

Disease	Agent	Procedure
1. Canine distemper	Vaccine, chick embryo-modified, lyophilized	Pups of unknown immune status should be given a dose of vaccine if older than 3 months. If younger than 3 months, 2 or more doses should be administered; the first dose should be given after the pup is weaned and the last dose at 12 to 16 weeks of age. Administration of a dose of vaccine at 2-week intervals more nearly approaches the ideal.
	Vaccine, tissue-culture origin, modified live virus	
	Antiserum and concentrated antiserum	There is increasing evidence that routine prophylactic use of agents that will passively immunize against canine distemper in pups has less merit than multiple doses of attenuated live virus vaccines. To avoid blocking of active immunization, the use of antiserum or concentrated antiserum for short-term protection is to be discouraged.
		Antiserum or concentrated antiserum is of questionable value in the treatment of dogs with clinical signs of distemper.
2. Infectious canine hepatitis (Virus)	Vaccine, tissue-cultured, modified	Administer to young dogs. (Simultaneous vaccination with modified distemper and infectious canine hepatitis virus is effective.)
3. Rabies (Virus)	Vaccine, chick embryo, lyophilized	For active immunization of dogs. Confers lasting immunity. Subject to state laws.
	Modified live virus, porcine tissue culture origin	Can be used in 6 species (dog, cat, horse, cattle, sheep and goat). Long-term immunity.
	Antiserum	Used to obtain immediate protection. Not readily available.

FOXES

1. Canine distemper (Virus)	(See dogs, above)	

continued on next page

FOXES (Continued)

Disease	Agent	Procedure
2. Epizootic fox encephalitis (Infectious canine hepatitis)	(See dogs, above)	
	Antiserum	Used to stop outbreaks.

MINK

1. Botulism (Clostridium botulinum)	Toxoid (Type C)	Administer to young mink to produce active immunity.
2. Canine distemper (Virus)	(See dogs, above)	

CATS

1. Feline panleukopenia (Virus)	Vaccine, formalized tissues of infected cats	Used to immunize healthy kittens.
	Antiserum	Used to protect susceptible kittens.
2. Feline pneumonitis (Chlamydia psittaci)	Vaccine, live, modified, egg origin	Vaccinate at 12 to 14 weeks, and every 6 months thereafter

FERRETS

Canine distemper	(See dogs, above)	

GUINEA PIGS

Pseudotuberculosis (Pasteurella pseudotuberculosis)	Vaccine, avirulent	Administer to guinea pigs at weaning time.

See also VACCINATION OF EXOTIC MAMMALS, p. 1118.

cines and mixed bacterins containing a number of antigens are not included, although both mixed bacterins and vaccines are known to be effective. Certain of the procedures listed are not practiced in North America because the diseases are unknown or have been eradicated. Nevertheless, they are included in the table for guidance for veterinarians who may find themselves confronted with unusual disease problems in other areas. More detailed instructions regarding each specific agent will be found in the chapter dealing with the disease in question. The directions of the manufacturer, regarding dosage, administration and cautions, should be followed strictly.

RUMEN INOCULATION

Inoculation of rumen contents from a healthy ruminant animal into the rumen of another animal for the purpose of initiating or restoring normal rumen function. The procedure has been used almost exclusively in cattle.

Functions of Rumen Microorganisms: The healthy rumen performs important digestive and nutritional functions because of the presence of enormous numbers of bacteria and ciliated protozoa. These microorganisms collectively produce enzymes capable of digesting cellulose and other plant constituents. They also synthesize many essential amino acids which are made available to the host by the subsequent digestion of the bacteria and protozoa in the abomasum and intestine. In addition, the rumen bacteria synthesize vitamins of the B-group plus vitamin K. Sufficient numbers and balance between species of these microorganisms are, therefore, important for the efficiency of the ruminant animal, and if they are upset by inadequate or abnormal food intake, drugs, poisons, or disease, rumen function is impaired.

Procedure: Rumen inoculum can be obtained at a local abattoir if there is need for a large quantity. For most purposes, however, the inoculum can be taken from a healthy animal by passing a stomach tube and siphoning some of the liquid from the rumen. The administration of approximately 4 gal. of lukewarm water will allow removal of greater quantities of rumen juice. One quart of fresh rumen contents usually is sufficient for one inoculation and is given to the recipient animal by stomach tube or drench. To facilitate administration, coarse material can be removed. Fresh rumen material is far superior to frozen or processed products.

Clinical Use: Any disease or condition that alters rumen function is detrimental to the normal flora present and this in turn may delay the return to normal of the convalescent animal. Cattle recovering from any gastrointestinal disorder, or diseases which have required administration of sulfonamides, antibiotics or other drugs may show anorexia due to rumen dysfunction and will benefit from rumen inoculation.

EXAMINATION OF ANIMALS
PRIOR TO SALE

This examination is requested of a veterinarian by the prospective buyer of an animal and is welcomed by the honest seller. Occasionally, the seller will request an examination of a limited nature, certifying one or more of the animal's soundness of body, health of udder, stage of pregnancy, semen quality or freedom from evidence of disease as determined by diagnostic tests or clinical examination. The results of these latter examinations usually are put into writing in the form of certificates and are used to assist in the sale and to serve as a measure of protection to the seller.

When examining an animal for a buyer, however, the examination usually is wider in scope and more complete, as advice is often sought on minor defects or blemishes, conformation, past diseases and injuries to the animal, its recent environment and record as well as precautions to be taken in introducing the animal into the client's herd or flock. The results and findings of all examinations should be recorded and reported accurately, particularly in cases of valuable animals that may be transported long distances. Then, if any disagreement should arise between the buyer and seller, the examination record is available and hopefully complete enough to satisfy both parties. The completeness of the examination may vary with the type and value of the animal. In making the examination, several steps should be taken.

History: It is desirable to get the history as completely as possible by questioning the seller, examining his records and even examining the rest of the herd and conditions under which they are quartered. The animal's breed, sex, age and markings should be noted and checked with the registration papers if the animal is registered. Consideration should also be given to the records of the sire and dam of the animal in question; for example, their breeding ability; the possibility of heritable defects in the strain to which each belongs, particularly if the animal is to be used for breeding; and, if they are dead, the cause of their deaths.

Inquiry or examination of records should be made as to whether the animal has had any previous diseases, injuries, or surgical operations and how severe these conditions had been. Any previous preventive inoculations should be noted, as well as their type and time of administration.

If the animal to be sold is to be used for breeding purposes, breeding records should be reviewed to determine if the animal is fertile, relatively fertile, or infertile. Breeding records of the herd from which the animal came should be examined to obtain evidence of diseases likely to affect reproduction. If the animal is an adult breeding female, the service dates should be noted.

The health of the herd of origin and possible contacts with other animals before the sale should, if possible, be determined as a protection to the purchaser. Animals at the time of sale, if so exposed, could be in the incubation period of the disease. If a complete history cannot be obtained, the client should be advised of the possibility of such diseases either being present in the incubative stage. Animals may have been given drugs such as tranquilizers or glucocorticoids that could alter the animals normal state. A suitable withdrawal period of several days to a month or more may be required for the animal to return to its original state.

Clinical Examination: General examination of the animal consists of noting the signalment including the breed, sex, age and color markings. The physical attitude, condition, conformation and temperature should be observed carefully. Conformation is of importance as certain types may predispose the animal to defects or diseases. The gait, especially in horses, should be observed at various speeds for evidence of lameness. The skin and coat should be examined for evidence of alopecia, ringworm, mange and pediculosis. It is also an indication of general health. The temperature should be taken as this may detect a febrile disease in its early or incubative stage. This general examination should be made carefully as suggestive signs of internal diseases or abnormalities often are found at this time, especially diseases of the nervous system, such as "wobbles", chorea, spastic signs and blindness.

Specific examination: Any abnormalities in pulse rate, nature or type of pulse or heart sounds should be carefully assessed, particularly in the horse used for heavy work. The size and fullness of the external veins are noted. Any edema of dependent portions of the body or ascites is noted and its cause determined. After examining the animal at rest, it should be exercised and the pulse and heart checked again. This is particularly important with horses. The external lymph nodes are then palpated.

The respiratory system is examined by noting the respiratory rate at rest and after work, as well as by auscultation of the lungs for evidence of bronchitis, heaves or chronic pneumonia. The trachea should be pinched near the larynx to see if a cough can be elicited. Horses usually have to be worked vigorously to bring out any evidence of heaves or roaring. In cases of difficult breathing, the nasal passages and sinuses may be examined for evidence of obstruction. Sneezing and bleeding from the nose is common in swine with atrophic rhinitis. Atrophy of the turbinates with distortion of the face and obstruction of the nasolacrimal duct occurs in the more advanced cases. Evidence of any abnormal nasal discharge should be noted and its cause ascertained if possible. External palpation of the pharynx, larynx and trachea may reveal defects or abnormalities.

In examining the digestive system, the animal should be observed while eating and drinking to note abnormalities in appetite, chewing, or swallowing. The teeth should be inspected to check for age and the presence of abnormal teeth. The tongue and mouth should be examined at the same time and the size of the salivary glands noted. In the ruminant, the act of rumination should, if possible, be observed. Auscultation of the abdominal cavity will reveal the degree of peristalsis of large and small intestine and rumen activity. The consistency, color and odor of the feces should be observed.

Examination of the urinary system in large animals may be done by rectal examination, palpating the kidneys, ureters and bladder. The urine should be examined for color and evidence of any abnormality, such as the presence of blood, pus, or excessive albumin. If possible, the animal should be observed urinating.

In large animals to be used for breeding, the genital system in the female should be carefully checked by external, vaginal and rectal examination. If the female is not pregnant, abnormalities or infections of the vulva, vagina, cervix, uterus, oviducts and ovaries that might prevent conception should be noted. The mammary glands and teats must be examined and palpated for evidence of disease or defects. If the animal is lactating, the milk should be examined. In young animals, the number and distribution of mammae and teats should be noted. If the female is pregnant, rectal findings should correlate with the breeding history. In the male, the external genital organs, penis, sheath, testicles and epididymides, should be inspected and palpated for abnormalities. Rectal examination of the male accessory sex glands and vasa deferentia should be made. The male should be observed in the act of copulating to note his libido and ability to mate. Examination of a semen sample is often required (q.v., p. 776).

The sensory organs, especially the eyes, should be carefully examined. Visual examination employing a flashlight in a dark stall or room is necessary to detect certain diseases of the eye that interfere with vision. The ophthalmoscope is useful to locate certain kinds of eye lesions. (See VETERINARY OPHTHALMOLOGY, p. 202.) The ears should be examined and impairment or lack of hearing noted.

In the horse particularly, further careful examination at various gaits, and while backing and turning, is required to determine abnormalities in coordination and postural reflexes, or lamenesses. Evidence of laminitis or soreness should be noted.

The limbs, feet and hoofs or claws should be carefully inspected for any unsoundness or blemish. The severity and possible future importance of such abnormalities should be assessed.

Special or Diagnostic Tests: Certain special diagnostic tests are routinely performed at the time of sale; others may be desired by the buyer. Tests may be indicated by the findings of the clinical examination. If the animal is to be shipped into another state or country after purchase, the required tests or inoculations have either to be performed before the sale or the sale may be subject to the satisfactory passing of these tests by the animals. The regulations of the state or country to which the animal is to be sent must, therefore, be thoroughly understood.

Commonly, serologic tests are carried out for brucellosis and leptospirosis. Diagnostic inoculations also are usually made to test for the presence of certain diseases, such as tuberculosis and Johne's disease. Fecal examinations may be made for the presence of parasites. Urine examinations to indicate the presence of blood, albumin, sugar or low specific gravity may be desirable.

Cultural tests may be conducted on samples of milk to determine the presence and type of infection in the udder, on urine specimens for evidence of urinary infection, on cervical or vaginal swabs from mares or cows for the presence of pathogenic organisms causing genital diseases, such as streptococcal and *Klebsiella* infections in mares, and vibriosis or trichomoniasis in cows. For the latter infections in bulls, culturing of the semen or preputial samples, or even test-mating with virgin heifers, may be indicated.

In certain abnormalities or diseases of the circulatory system, hemograms and blood chemistry tests may be employed. In lamenesses and lesions of the limb, roentgenographs or nerve blocks may be desirable. It may be advisable to collect one or more semen samples from prospective breeding males and have them examined for quality.

It must be emphasized that these special tests merely supplement the information obtained from the history and physical examination. Rarely do they provide data for an absolute statement of freedom from disease. The limitations of each procedure should, therefore, be drawn to the client's attention, so that there is no misunderstanding later. Certificates should be written with the greatest care and in such a fashion that they cannot be misinterpreted and should contain such qualifications as may be necessary.

The exhaustiveness of the examination is usually determined

by the wishes of the client and the value of the animal in question. Even after the most elaborate examination and testing, however, the client is well advised to isolate his newly purchased animal from the rest of his stock for a period of 3 weeks.

MEAT INSPECTION

Meat inspection is an important part of food hygiene. An effective meat inspection program must prevent the transmission of disease via carcasses, parts and meat products, and must assure the consumer that the meat supply is safe, wholesome and unadulterated. The inspection consists of antemortem, postmortem and processing inspection.

Antemortem Examination

The examination should be conducted on the day the animals are slaughtered and be made on the premises of the establishment. Animals suspected of being sick or diseased should be penned separately and apart from the healthy animals and be examined by the veterinary inspector prior to slaughter. They should be slaughtered apart from the regular kill and given a careful and thorough postmortem examination. The purpose is to eliminate all unfit animals and to segregate for more thorough examination all animals suspected of being affected with a condition that might influence their disposition on postmortem inspection. Dead or condemned animals should not be permitted to enter the slaughtering department or any other edible-products department of the plant. Hogs showing a temperature of 106°F or over, or cattle, sheep and goats with a temperature of 105°F or more should be condemned, or isolated until the temperature falls or specific diagnosis of the disease is established. Carcasses of animals slaughtered while suffering from high fever are red and congested. This appearance may result in a condemnation that could have been avoided.

Antemortem inspection is also of inestimable value to the local part-time inspector who is interested in the diseases that occur in his general vicinity. Many diseases of a toxic or infectious nature are difficult to detect in the slaughtered animal's carcass and organs. It is of particular value in conditions such as septic metritis, mastitis, tetanus, rabies and tuberculous meningitis, for in such conditions, postmortem findings are of little diagnostic value. Food poisoning outbreaks have been traced to the consumption of meat from animals slaughtered while obviously ill, but whose carcasses and organs showed little noticeable change on postmortem examination.

Postmortem Examination

Postmortem examination should be made at the time the animals are slaughtered. Inspection should consist of examination of the cervical and skeletal lymph nodes, the viscera and organs with their lymph nodes, and all exposed surfaces of the carcasses. "Cold inspections" lack value and permit the possibility of confusion of organs and other practices which lead to lessening of the inspection efficiency. For optimum results, the examination should be conducted during the slaughtering operations. In all cases where the inspector is not present to examine organs and parts separated from the carcasses, the parts and organs must be securely identified with tags in order to eliminate improper diagnosis due to confusion of parts.

The routine postmortem examination should consist of at least the following procedures:

Cattle: 1. Examination of the incised mandibular, suprapharyngeal and parotid lymph nodes. 2. Examination of the 2 layers of the incised masseter muscles. Examination and palpation of the tongue. 3. Examination of the incised mediastinal and bronchial lymph nodes of both sides. Palpation of the lung. 4. Incision of the heart to expose completely its internal surfaces. Careful examination of all surfaces of that organ. 5. Examination of the incised hepatic lymph nodes. Examination and palpation of the liver, including opening of the bile duct longitudinally. 6. Examination of the spleen. 7. Examination of the exposed surfaces of the carcass and linings of the thoracic, abdominal and pelvic cavities.

Calves and Veal: 1. Examination of the incised suprapharyngeal lymph nodes. 2. Examination of the external surface of the heart. 3. Palpation of the mediastinal and bronchial lymph nodes of both sides, and palpation of the lungs. 4. Palpation of the hepatic lymph nodes and the liver. 5. Examination of the exposed surfaces of the carcass and the linings of the thoracic, abdominal and pelvic cavities.

Lambs and Sheep: 1. Examination of the external surface of the heart. 2. Palpation of the mediastinal and bronchial lymph nodes and palpation of the lungs. 3. Examination and palpation of the liver. Opening of the bile duct transversely. 4. Examination of the spleen. 5. Examination of the exposed surfaces of the carcass and the linings of the thoracic, abdominal and pelvic cavities. Palpation of the prefemoral, superficial inguinal and prescapular lymph nodes.

Hogs: 1. Examination of the incised mandibular lymph nodes. 2. Palpation of the mediastinal and bronchial lymph nodes of both sides and palpation of the lungs. 3. Examination of the external surface of the heart. 4. Examination of the liver and palpation of the hepatic lymph nodes. 5. Examination of the spleen. 6. Palpation of the mesenteric lymph nodes and incision of all suspicious nodules. 7. Examination of the exposed surfaces of the carcass, the joints, and the lining of the thoracic, abdominal and pelvic cavities.

All of the above procedures should be performed routinely for each species. The identity of the heads, plucks and other viscera of each carcass should be maintained until such time as the carcass has been passed by the inspector.

When evidence of disease is found in any particular part, a more extensive examination should be given to determine the extent and degree of the condition. Suspects also should be given a more careful and more thorough postmortem examination.

Poultry: 1. A complete visual examination of the viscera and of the exterior and interior of the carcass, including palpation and other procedures necessary for proper identification and evaluation of disease processes, tissue changes, or other conditions that affect the fitness of the poultry for human use. 2. No viscera or any part should be removed from any dressed poultry except at the time of evisceration and postmortem inspection. 3. The carcass should be opened to expose the organs and the body cavity for proper examination.

Dispositions

Carcasses and animals should be disposed of with the following considerations in mind:

1. Whether the disease is transmissible to man.

2. Whether the disease process has so altered the normal characteristics of the meat as to cause it to be inedible or adulterated.

3. Whether the condition is so repugnant solely from the esthetic point of view as to require the carcass to be condemned in whole or in part.

Antemortem dispositions should be as follows:

1. Animals unfit for slaughter for food and to be immediately condemned.

    (a) Those with temperatures over 106°F (hogs) or 105°F (cattle, sheep, goats) (*see also* 2).

    (b) Those affected with rabies, tetanus, hog cholera, cancer eye, anthrax, extensive anasarca, generalized edema, severe emaciation, acute swine erysipelas, septicemia and any other condition rendering animals moribund or comatose.

2. Animals unfit for slaughter may be treated or rested if, in the opinion of the veterinarian, such action may result in an edible carcass as in the case of pregnancy, some high fevers and some "downers".

3. Animals suspected of a disease process, if passed for slaughter, should be given special examination post mortem.

4. Animals fit for straight slaughter.

Postmortem dispositions of carcasses will in general result in:

1. Passage of the entire carcass for food.

2. Condemnation of a part or organ system.

3. Passage of the entire carcass for special processing in order to eliminate disease transmission to humans and animals.

4. Condemnation of the entire carcass as in the case of animals affected with anaplasmosis, anthrax, bacillary hemoglobinuria in cattle, blackleg, hemorrhagic septicemia, icterohematuria in sheep, malignant catarrhal fever, babesiasis, pyemia, septicemia, unhealed vaccine lesions (vaccinia), carcasses affected with generalized anasarca, edema, neoplasms, melanosis and those with a urine or sexual odor that remains after chilling. Carcasses also may be condemned for excessive infection of parasites as for example with *Cysticercus bovis*. In addition, carcasses of all hogs affected with acute hog cholera, generalized erysipelas, or arthritis and polyarthritis, particularly those showing suppurative lesions in more than one joint, should be condemned.

Food Poisonings: All carcasses of animals so infected that consumption of the products thereof may give rise to food poisoning should be condemned. This includes all carcasses showing signs of: 1. Acute inflammation of the lungs, pleura, pericardium, peritoneum or meninges. 2. Septicemia or pyemia, whether puerperal, traumatic or without any evident cause. 3. Gangrenous or severe hemorrhagic enteritis or gastritis. 4. Acute diffuse metritis or mastitis. 5. Phlebitis of the umbilical veins. 6. Septic or purulent traumatic pericarditis. 7. Any acute inflammation, abscess or suppurating sore, if associated with acute nephritis, fatty and degenerated liver, swollen soft spleen, marked pulmonary hyperemia, general swelling of lymph nodes, diffuse redness of the skin, cachexia, icteric discoloration of the carcass, or the like, either singly or in combination.

Tuberculosis: The following principles should be used for guidance in passing on carcasses affected with tuberculosis:

1. No meat should be passed for food if it contains tubercle bacilli, or if there is a reasonable possibility that it may contain tubercle bacilli, or if it is impregnated with toxic substances of tuberculosis or associated septic infections.

2. Meat should not be destroyed if the lesions are localized and not numerous; if there is no evidence of distribution of tubercle bacilli through the blood or by other means to the muscles or to parts that may be eaten with the muscles and if the animal is well nourished and in good condition, since in this case there is no proof, or even reason to suspect, that the flesh is unwholesome.

3. Evidences of generalized tuberculosis are to be sought in such distribution and number of tuberculous lesions as can be explained only upon the supposition of the entrance of tubercle bacilli in considerable number into the systemic circulation. Significant of such generalization is the presence of numerous, uniformly distributed tubercles throughout both lungs, also tubercles in the spleen, kidneys, bones, joints and sexual glands, and in the lymph nodes connected with these organs and parts, or in the splenic, renal, prescapular, popliteal and inguinal glands, when several of these organs and parts are coincidentally affected.

4. Localized tuberculosis is limited to a single or several parts or organs of the body without evidence of recent invasion of numerous bacilli into the systemic circulation.

Facilities and Sanitation

All departments of the plant should be maintained in a clean and sanitary manner. The floors, walls and ceilings should be kept reasonably free of blood, fat, scraps and other debris during operations. Clean barrels for edible and nonedible items, properly marked, should be provided at convenient locations. Heads should be placed on suitable tables or on a head-inspection rack. The use of towels or other cloths for the washing of carcasses should not be permitted; spray nozzles should be kept for this purpose.

Employees should keep their hands and arms clean and, in all cases, after visiting the toilet, must wash their hands with soap and water before handling any product or implement. All implements, including knives, saws, cleavers and other instruments should be thoroughly cleaned and sterilized in water at a temperature over 180°F when contaminated or after being used on a diseased carcass or part of a carcass. Only clean garments should be worn by employees. Spitting on the floor or on whetstones, placing knives or skewers in the mouth and similar habits should be prohibited.

Floors, walls and ceilings in the various edible-product departments of the plant should be constructed of material that can be readily kept clean. The interior walls and, where practical, ceiling surfaces should be smooth and flat, and in edible-product departments, should be constructed of glazed tile, smooth Portland cement plaster, or other nonabsorbent material. The floors of the plant should be well drained; a slope of ¼ in. to the foot to drainage inlets is recommended. The floors should be smooth and impervious and in good repair; they should be free from cracks and depressions.

Drainage and sewage disposal should be adequate to maintain the plant and premises in a sanitary condition. Ventilation should be sufficient to ensure that the atmosphere in rooms where edible products are kept is free from obnoxious odors emanating from inedible-tank and offal rooms, catch basins, toilet rooms, hide cellars, refuse heaps, livestock pens and similar sources. Lighting should be adequately maintained in all rooms and sufficient for inspection and cleaning operations.

The plant should be provided with ample supplies of potable hot and cold water, with outlets conveniently located and equipped with faucets for hose connections, for ready use during slaughtering operations and for cleaning. Wash basins equipped with running hot and cold water, soap and towels should be placed in or near the dressing rooms and at such other places in the establishment as may be essential to ensure cleanliness of all persons handling products. Water for sterilizing purposes shall be maintained at a temperature of at least 180°F. All departments in the plant should have adequate protection against flies, rodents and other vermin. Equipment and utensils used in the plant should be made of such material and be so constructed as to be readily and thoroughly cleaned and should be kept clean and in sanitary condition. Shovels used for transferring ice or edible materials from one container to another should not be permitted to touch the floor.

Labeling of Raw Meat and Poultry

In the U.S.A., raw meat and poultry that pass requirements are labeled as inspected. It has been found, even after inspection in approved plants, that by the time it reaches the consumer, up to 50% of poultry, 27% of pork and 5% of beef is contaminated with salmonellae. This has given rise to a suggestion that the label now used should be enlarged to state clearly the need for refrigeration and protection from contamination.

DETECTION OF ILLEGAL MEAT

Meat should be examined, if possible, in good daylight with the help of a binocular loupe or a binocular dissecting microscope. Some of the large microscope lamps are useful for intense, spotlight illumination.

Foreign objects adhering to the surface, e.g., hair, feathers, or fibers, may be easily picked off and by their structure give valuable information as to the identity of the specimen. Fragments of parasites, insect larvae, or other abnormal small objects can be isolated and preserved.

Colors should be noted. The meat should be firm and its cut surface should be glossy. Gray or green discolorations indicate spoilage. Odors are important; the meat may smell stale, sour, moldy or rotten. Foreign odors from aromatic chemicals, urine, fish or other sources may be present. Some of these are accentuated by boiling or frying the meat. Tests employing these procedures and others for pH, NH_3, and H_2O are often revealing.

Histologic examination is a necessity in the investigation of sausage or similar meat products where the use of illegal parts of an animal is suspected. The detection of unacceptable components in ground-meat products can often be made by the histologist even after prolonged storage, curing and cooking. New methods in meat processing may require a histometric collagen determination to detect the inclusion of such adulterants.

Bacteriologic examination of meats suspected of being the cause of food poisoning outbreaks involves many different bacteriologic techniques and procedures, and identification of the known or suspected causative agent should be attempted by recognized appropriate methods.

From the point of view of organoleptic change, the bacteriology of meat spoilage is incompletely understood. In general, however, the types of organisms on any meat product are more important than are total numbers.

Bacteriologic evaluations of meat are made to: (1) demonstrate the presence or absence of pathogenic bacteria, (2) identify the type and number of spoilage organisms, (3) provide a clue as to the possible cause of spoilage, and (4) in the absence of a knowledge of the sanitary background of the product, to give the only indication of the sanitary background.

Serologic methods used to identify the origin of meat as to species are the precipitin and complement-fixation tests. The precipitin test has received the widest use because of its relative simplicity. There are 2 requirements for the use of the precipitin test: The meat to be tested must be fresh or at least only lightly cooked and potent specific antisera must be available. If the meat has been cooked to the point where the protein has completely coagulated, the test cannot be made.

The Precipitin Test: One or 2 oz of the meat to be tested are minced and mixed with about 50 ml of sterile isotonic salt solution. After agitation, it is kept for 3 hours at room temperature or overnight in a refrigerator. The mixture is filtered until a clear filtrate is obtained. Samples containing considerable fat should be defatted first with ether or chloroform and washed with distilled water. Pickled meat also should be washed first.

One-tenth milliliter of the antiserum is placed with a pipette in a small test tube (inside diameter 3.0 mm). Then, 0.2 ml of the meat extract to be tested is added carefully so that little mixing takes place at the interface of the 2 solutions. The formation of a white ring at the interface within 5 minutes indicates a positive test. In some cases, a positive reaction will only become visible after a longer period, i.e., 15 or 30 minutes. After an hour, the precipitate begins to settle out and the interface becomes poorly defined.

There is some diversity of opinion regarding the specificity of the precipitin test when attempting to distinguish between closely related species. Some workers have found that by using higher dilutions and giving the reactions up to 40 or 50 minutes to develop, differences can be brought out more distinctly. It has been found impossible by most workers to distinguish between such closely related species as the sheep and goat.

Spectrophotometric, chromatographic and electrophoretic techniques for differentiating proteins may be used in connection with the identification of meat. Electrophoresis has been of great value in meat products which had been boiled and where the precipitin test gave negative results.

COLLECTION AND SUBMISSION
OF SPECIMENS
FOR HISTOPATHOLOGIC EXAMINATION

Histopathologic examination is helpful in reaching a diagnosis; in some cases it is the most important single diagnostic aid; in others, it furnishes the only means of reaching a definitive diagnosis. Every clinician should investigate the existence, location and capacity of facilities for histopathologic diagnosis available to him and make use of this service.

Tissues for histopathologic examination should be collected as soon as possible after death to minimize the effect of autolysis. Tissues for histopathologic examination should *never be frozen* prior to fixation. Specimens should be less than one-half inch thick (preferably ¼ in.) and should be placed immediately into at least 10 times their volume of fixative. The thin slices or cubes will insure that the fixative will penetrate adequately. Concentrated formalin (formaldehyde solution, 40%) can be purchased at the drug store. If it is diluted, 1 part formalin to 9 parts tap water, a 10% formalin solution or 4% formaldehyde solution will result. This is adequate but not ideal. It is better to use phosphate-buffered 10% formalin at a pH of 7.5 to 8.0 and at room temperature. The tissues should be allowed to remain in this fixative, with some agitation, for 24 hours. The fixed tissues can then be removed from the fluid and placed in a plastic bag along with some cotton soaked in 10% formalin for mailing purposes.

For the brain, where the whole organ is often required, the following procedure is recommended: The brain is placed into concentrated formalin (formaldehyde 40%—in which it will float) and water added slowly with mixing until the brain just sinks below the surface but not to the bottom. It is allowed to remain in this solution for 24 hours or longer after which it may be removed and placed in a plastic bag with some cotton soaked in 10% formalin and mailed (suitably packed), or placed into 10% formalin until such time that processing is desired.

The specimen taken for examination should be representative of the lesion and, if possible, should include some of the apparently normal surrounding tissue. The mucosal surface of specimens from the gastrointestinal tract should be exposed before fixation. Autolytic changes occur very rapidly in the mucosa of the gastrointestinal tract. Ideally, sections of stomach and gut should be fixed within 1 to 2 minutes after death.

A covering letter with a detailed case history should be sent separately to permit tracing of delayed or lost samples and to assist the pathologist in arriving at a diagnosis. This report should identify the animal's species, breed (including morbidity and mortality), sex, age and owner; describe the clinical signs, gross appearance, size and location of the lesion or lesions; indicate whether the condition had been previously treated and if so, what type of treatment was given and the time of recurrence.

COLLECTION AND SUBMISSION OF SPECIMENS FOR TOXICOLOGIC EXAMINATION

When an animal dies from an unknown cause and poisoning is suspected, diligent attention should be given to securing the proper sample, complete history of signs, treatment, postmortem lesions and circumstances involved in the death. The practitioner who performs the necropsy and observes the animals and their environment firsthand may be able to suggest the toxic substance or group of substances involved. A complete history may enable the toxicologist to eliminate various poisons from further consideration and reduce the time and amount of analytic work required for results of diagnostic value. Cases of suspected poisoning should be carefully screened and samples submitted when the history, signs, lesions and the potential economic loss warrant it. Many lesions and signs of poisoning are similar to those of infectious diseases.

It should be emphasized that an adequate sample of the proper tissue is necessary. Tissues or fluids for chemical analysis should, if possible, be fresh and refrigerated. However, valuable information can sometimes be obtained if small sections (1 in. square by ¼ in. thick) of liver, brain, kidney and other organs preserved in formalin are also submitted for histopathologic examination.

Thought should be given to packing and subsequent transportation of samples. The container should be chemically clean and prepared beforehand. Refrigerator-type polyethylene bags or glass quart jars are very satisfactory. Jars which are closed with zinc or similar tops are undesirable, since tissues should not come in contact with any metal. Each sample must be placed in a separate container and in the case of the polyethylene bags, it is suggested that double bags be used. *Containers must be labeled with all information necessary to identify each specimen.*

If legal action is a possibility, the jar must be sealed to prove that there has been no tampering with the original contents. This is most easily done with common paper wrapping tape. The top of the jar is sealed with strips passed around the junction of the jar and its top as well as over the top itself. The junction of each piece of tape is then marked with ink, indelible pencil, or sealing wax; in this way the top cannot be removed and replaced without showing unmistakable signs of tampering. The jar should not be sealed with surgical tape or a similar type of tape as this can be removed and replaced without tearing. It is most desirable to have the samples pass through as few hands as possible while en route to the toxicologist.

It is best to pack the sample(s) with ice or solid carbon dioxide. A polystyrene refrigerator box, metal can, or stout cardboard box may be used for shipment. Packing must be done in such a way as to prevent breakage if all the ice melts. With dry ice, it is possible to preserve specimens for 72 hours.

When a chemical preservative is used, 95% ethyl alcohol, about 1 ml/gm of sample, is satisfactory. Denatured alcohol should not be used because of the chemical contamination that results from the presence of the denaturant. Formaldehyde is undesirable as it interferes with many tests. In cases of suspected cyanide poisoning, the liver, muscle and stomach contents should be preserved with a solution of 1% mercuric chloride and refrigerated. Adequate refrigeration is of special importance when submitting clean body fluids (readily obtained from an eye) and material for nitrate or nitrite analysis, since these salts are so rapidly metabolized by microorganisms that only low or insignificant levels may be found upon analysis.

In poison cases where a feed or water is suspected, samples of these and any descriptive feed tag should accompany the tissue specimens. It is especially important that a representative composite sample of the feed be submitted from the feed from the same lot or shipment. In many instances, the amount of feed involved is such that some of it may be fed to experimental animals in an effort to reproduce the signs and lesions observed in the field cases.

In collecting and submitting specimens for toxicologic examination, the following directions are useful:

1. Supply adequate information regarding the history, signs, postmortem lesions, environment and economic loss.

2. Collect an adequate sample of the proper tissue.

3. Give careful attention to using chemically clean containers and to proper sealing, labeling and preservation of samples.

4. Handle each case as if the evidence accumulated and the diagnosis made were to be used in court if there is any possibility of legal action.

Observation of the foregoing principles will facilitate the analysis and tend to eliminate the "test for all poisons" approach which is impractical if not impossible.

SUGGESTED SPECIMENS AND MINIMUM QUANTITIES TO SUBMIT FOR TOXICOLOGIC EXAMINATIONS

Type of Poison	Specimen for Analysis	Minimal Amount Required (or all available)
Alkaloids	Blood, urine	200 ml
	Liver, stomach content, kidney, brain	500 gm
All Poisons	Bait or feed	500 gm
Barbiturates	Blood	200 ml
	Brain, fat	500 gm
Chlorinated Hydro-carbons	Fat, liver, brain	500 gm
Chronic Arsenic	Skin, hair, stomach contents, liver, kidney	500 gm
Chronic Lead	Bone	200 gm
Fluoride	Bones, teeth	500 gm
	Urine, blood	200 ml
Heavy Metals	Urine, blood	200 ml
	Stomach contents, liver, kidney	500 gm
Hydrocyanic Acid	Blood, urine	200 ml
	Stomach contents, liver, muscle, (freeze immediately)	500 gm
Mycotoxins (e.g., aflatoxins)	Blood	200 ml
	Stomach contents, liver, kidney	500 gm
Nitrate, Nitrite	Blood	200 ml
	Stomach & gut contents (sealed air-tight containers)	500 gm
Organo-arsenicals	Hair, liver, kidney, stomach contents	500 gm
Organophosphates	Blood (for cholinesterase)	200 ml
	Brain, fat	500 gm
Oxalates	Urine	200 ml
	Kidney, stomach contents	500 gm
Selenium	Blood	200 ml
	Liver, kidney, hair	500 gm
Sodium Chloride	Stomach contents	500 gm
Strychnine	Urine	200 ml
	Stomach contents, liver, kidney	500 gm
Sulfonamides	Kidney	500 gm
	Urine	200 ml
Thallium	Urine	200 ml
	Kidney, stomach contents	500 gm
Warfarin	Blood	200 ml
	Stomach contents, liver	500 gm

DEAD-ANIMAL DISPOSAL AND DISINFECTION OF PREMISES

Animals that have died on farms, other than by slaughter for eventual consumption as food, may have died from traumatic injury, but usually death is caused by some type of disease process. The safest assumption is that all animals that have died on farms have some infectious agent present which should be prevented from further spread to the rest of the livestock.

The easiest way to dispose of carcasses is to have the animal picked up by a properly equipped rending establishment that will send a clean truck to the farm. The truck and operator should not further contaminate the premises with drippings of other dead; potentially dangerous disease vectors may be present on the truck. A renderer's truck should be sanitary and watertight, and the boots and equipment of the operator must be clean. When the trucker leaves a farm, he should again clean his boots and his person in order to preclude the possibility of spread to other farms.

Disposal of animals suspected of certain diseases is severely restricted by law. There usually are specific rules laid down by the proper supervising authorities for the disposal of carcasses of animals dead of infectious diseases. Veterinarians should bear this in mind prior to making recommendations for disposal of carcasses of animals that may have died from contagious diseases. In most instances, anthrax, blackleg, tuberculosis, vesicular exanthema, vesicular stomatitis and foot-and-mouth disease are all covered by appropriate regulations. These regulations normally call for cremation or burial in a trench at least 6 ft deep and covering of the carcasses with lime. A postmortem examination is necessary for the information of the owner and the veterinarian, except when anthrax or other such disease is suspected.

General Precautions: When handling carcasses suspected of containing infectious disease organisms, the anal, oral and nasal openings should be stuffed with wadding of material, such as clean toweling. This will prevent the spillage of any internal fluids. If a pit is used, once the carcass is in the pit, it may be advisable to cut slashes in the hide. If a contagious disease, such as anthrax, is suspected it is better if slashes are not made, for they increase the likelihood of bacterial sporulation. Anthrax bacilli do not normally sporulate in the absence of air. Removal of the skin of any animal that has died on a farm, other than one which is definitely known to have died from traumatic injury alone, is not advisable; the amount of money involved in recovery of the hide does not warrant the risk of further contamination of the farm with disease-producing organisms.

Dead animals should immediately be covered with kerosene or crude oil to keep flies, dogs, buzzards, crows and vermin away until they are disposed of. Carcasses are best cremated or buried where found, but should never be buried in low, swampy land or where drainage may result in contamination of other areas or water supplies. Weather conditions will necessarily limit the method used to dispose of the carcass, as for example, if the weather is wet, if it is dry, or if the ground is frozen. In severely wet weather, a trench should be dug around the carcass to avoid drainage and seepage which may spread infection. Should moving of the carcass be necessary, the greatest care must be taken to prevent discharges or hair from contaminating the soil over which the carcass is to be moved. It should never be dragged. A slide is best, improvised of an old wooden door or gate that can be burned or buried with the carcass. The slide should protect the carcass from becoming chafed and rubbed open from contact with the ground as it is moved. Everything that has come in contact with the dead animal should be burned, preferably, or thoroughly disinfected. Visibly contaminated soil should be removed with the carcass and treated as the carcass itself is handled. All workers should be informed of the risks of handling the carcass improperly and of the danger of contaminating other healthy animals. Each person should be impressed with the necessity of washing his hands and arms and avoiding the use of soiled clothing. Rubber boots should be worn in all such situations, and pails of disinfectant to clean them should be readily available, and used before leaving the place of disposal. Dogs and other pets should not be allowed to run loose and stray animals and wildlife of all sorts should likewise be discouraged from entering the area.

Cremation of Carcasses: Small animals, such as chickens, lambs, or pigs can be burned in a large open-pit furnace with a bed of coal. In the case of horses, cattle and sheep, however, which would have to be dismembered, cremation is the more advisable. There are 3 main methods of cremation:

1. The **cross-trench pit method** utilizes 2 dug trenches approximately 7 ft long, crossing each other at right angles to form a cross. Each cross trench should be 15 in. wide and at least 18 in. deep in the center, becoming shallower toward the extremities. In removing the soil for the trenches, it is placed in each angle of the cross so that there are 4 mounds of earth toward the center. Upon the mounds, pieces of iron or trunks of trees or large branches are placed to create a pyre on which the carcass is placed and underneath which straw, hay and kindling are placed. Green wood or coal then should be piled in a heap over the straw and kindling wood. A gallon or 2 of kerosene or used motor oil can be poured over the entire material and the straw then is ignited. In some instances, it has proved very helpful in properly cremating the entire carcass to use old rubber tires as fuel. The tires produce a high

temperature once they have ignited which aids considerably in the proper disposal of the carcass. Covering the carcass with green wood and semidry manure aids in raising the temperature to the ignition point.

2. The **oval-pit method** requires less digging than burial, but really is a combination of burial and cremation and is to be preferred where its use is possible. An oval pit 7 ft long and 4 ft wide should be dug to a depth of 3 to 4 ft and a crossed trench 9 x 9 in. dug in its floor. Upon the windward side of the pit, a ventilation trench 4 ft long and 1½ ft wide, and a foot deeper than the main pit, and at right angles to it, must be dug. A field drainpipe must be placed in a tunnel connecting the trench with the pit and this pipe stuffed with straw. Straw is laid in the bottom of the main pit, wood or coal is piled above it so that the pit is filled to three-quarters. Next, the carcass is placed in the pit. More wood or coal is piled around and above it, kerosene or motor oil is poured over the whole. The straw in the bottom of the ventilation trench is fired. A carcass cremated by this method takes about 8 to 10 hours to burn and requires little or no attention. When burning is complete, the soil is replaced and the ground leveled.

3. The **surface-burning method** is useful where there are numbers of animals to be burned. One long trench should be dug about 1½ ft deep and 1 ft wide, and about a 3 ft length allowed for each carcass. At intervals along each side, there should be placed side flues to coincide with each carcass. Straw, wood and coal are placed around the central trench and the carcasses are drawn to it. More fuel is heaped around and between them, and kerosene, motor oil or gasoline is sprayed over the whole. The straw is ignited. More fuel is added as required.

NOTE: Instead of the trench and side flues, logs of wood are sometimes laid on the ground and the carcasses are pulled over them. Fuel is piled around them and ignited; more fuel is added as required. This latter method is especially applicable where the ground is very wet, where there is rock immediately below the soil and digging is impossible, or where the ground is frozen.

Burial of Carcasses: The site selected should be one that will involve no danger of the pollution of streams, rivers, or other water supplies and where there is a sufficient depth of subsoil to allow 6 ft of soil above the uppermost limit of the carcass. The pit should be dug 8 to 9 ft deep, and it is important that the surface soil and subsoil not be mixed. When removing the dirt from the pit, it should be placed to allow for easy access to the edge. In some instances, shoring-up with lumber may be required; this is to allow the truck or carrier to be driven to the edge in order to dump the carcass into the pit with a minimum of surface contamination. As previously noted, the carcass should be transported to the pit on a wooden slide, such as a barn door or gate, and be so protected as to avoid contamination of the ground with blood and discharges from the animal. When the carcass has been treated with quicklime, the pit should be filled in with soil. Subsoil should be placed in first and then the topsoil. The owner should remember that this area will remain soft and his equipment or some of his other animals may sink into it. Therefore, it is advisable that the area be roped off or otherwise clearly marked and avoided. Such pits should not be plowed for at least 6 months after burial.

Disinfectants: In considering the use of disinfectants in connection with disposal of dead animals, it must be borne in mind that an effective job has to be done on a wide range of infectious agents from viruses to bacteria including spore formers. A number of useful and readily obtainable disinfectants are discussed below.

Sodium hydroxide in the form of commercial caustic soda or lye is the most suitable for general disinfection. The caustic soda or lye should contain at least 90% sodium hydroxide. The disinfecting solution is prepared by dissolving 2 lb of lye in 10 gal. of water. This solution can be used to disinfect objects contaminated by anthrax spores. Where whitewash is not objectionable, water-slaked lime (*not* air-slaked) may be added to the lye solution—5 lb/10 gal. The addition of lime to a solution of sodium hydroxide tends to prevent conversion of the active principle, sodium hydroxide, into sodium carbonate which is considerably less effective. The lime also is useful as an indicator to show where the solution has been applied.

Concentrated lye is a caustic poison. Care should be taken to avoid getting it into the eyes or breathing any of the fine dust that may arise where the dry material is handled. The comparatively weak solution employed for disinfection may be used safely, provided a reasonable degree of care is exercised. Washing with water usually will be sufficient to remove the lye solution should any get on the skin. If necessary, it may be neutralized by washing with vinegar. If any of the lye solution gets in the eyes, they should be washed with clean water, to be followed by a saturated aqueous solution of boric acid.

The dilute lye solution has little or no harmful effect on bare wood, rubber, or cotton. It is injurious to painted or varnished surfaces and to woolen or silk fabrics if allowed to remain in contact with them for a considerable period. Leather, even when oiled, will stand only limited exposure. Lye solution may be kept in containers made of bare wood, earthenware, enamelware, or any of the common metals except aluminum. The containers should be kept tightly covered to prevent the conversion of hydroxide into carbonate.

Sodium carbonate, commonly referred to as washing soda, is considerably less caustic and irritating than lye. It may be used in a 4% solution. This compound is more rapidly effective if the solution is hot or at least warm. It is more valuable as a cleansing agent than as a disinfectant.

Formaldehyde, which is used in a 3% solution, may easily be prepared from formalin. The latter is simply a 40% formaldehyde solution. As an example, to 3 gal. of formalin add sufficient water to make 40 gal.; this product will be 3% formaldehyde.

Saponated Cresol Solution USP, 3%, may be used or a similar cresylic disinfectant may be used by following manufacturer's directions. **Chloride of Lime USP** (30% available chlorine) may be made by adding 1 lb to 3 gal. of water, and is another useful disinfectant.

NOTE: The newer types of detergents are all of considerable value to aid in the removal of dirt, but in most instances do not disinfect.

SOCIAL BEHAVIOR AMONG DOMESTIC ANIMALS

Domestic animals exhibit specific behavior patterns among themselves and towards other creatures, and some of these interactions have been studied in detail both in wild and domestic conditions. Normally, a definite set of social relationships between males, females and the young can be seen in each species, but castration of either sex introduces new social behavior. The domestic animal's social interaction with man varies considerably from species to species depending on the farming systems used or whether the animal is a household pet.

With much of the herdsman's lore being lost with modern farming, more intensive conditions and the greater numbers of stock being handled, the actions of pets and farm livestock are sometimes poorly understood or even misinterpreted by their owners. Veterinarians having some basic knowledge of the underlying reasons for behavior can make an important contribution in this area. The following brief discussions outline some of the many elements of animal behavior.

THE RELATIONS BETWEEN MAN AND HIS ANIMALS

The removal of the young animal from its own species to be raised by hand leads to strong social attachments to man. However the optimum time for close relationships and the timing of developmental processes varies with the species. For example, in altricial species such as the dog, the optimum time is between 6 and 8 weeks of age, whereas with precocial species like the sheep, the corresponding time is from birth to 4 to 6 days. If the attachments to humans have been too exclusive, such hand-raised animals will tend to relate sexually to humans and some of the charm of caged birds is in their paying courtship to their human owners.

A domestic animal is dependent for some or all of its care and well-being on a human caretaker and man is thus woven in some way into the social reactions of his animals. A leader-follower relationship may occur in which the animal follows the human for food or companionship. In species which develop a dominance-subordination type of social structure it is important that the caretaker be dominant, particularly when the adult animals are dangerous. The dairy bull asserts increased dominance with maturity and growth. Dominance is best established at the appropriate time for the species, usually early in life when no punishment may be needed. As the social dominance interactions are specific for individuals, the fact that one person dominates an animal is no guarantee that another will be able to do so.

When animals are kept for specific purposes, for companionship or as a child substitute, unexpected social behavior may be encountered, having been reinforced by the close interaction with one owner. The early and complete isolation of an animal from its own kind not only leads to difficulties in later mating but increases the aggressiveness towards strangers and inhibits good mothering of the young.

On the other hand, overcrowding animals and poor management may lead to a considerable upset in normally expected social behavior and result in vice, injury or unthriftiness. A good stockman or veterinarian can predict these conditions from the social behavior of the animals concerned and take remedial steps before stock condition deteriorates further.

The basic behavior traits of each species do not alter through domestication, but the normal social behavior is transferred more or less to the human caretaker. Most dogs fit well into families because they react to man as they react to being a member of the pack. The approach to the master with attempts to lick the face is the normal greeting pattern of a subordinate wolf to its superior.

SOCIAL BEHAVIOR OF DOGS

The social behavior of dogs is similar to that of wolves. Wolves regularly travel over runways or hunting trails and urinate, defecate and scratch up the ground at "scent posts". Similarly, dogs let run freely, move over regular routes using "scent posts". Males travel more extensively than females and are more apt to use the posts. The stimulus for marking is scent of urine or feces of strange animals.

This "scent post" behavior keeps males informed of the sexual receptivity of females, as females in heat secrete a substance in urine which excites males, who then track them and attempt to mate. The female is attractive to the male a few days before bleeding begins, but is not receptive until it ends. With the exception of the Basenji breed, which comes into estrus once a year, close to the autumnal equinox, females come into estrus at 6-month intervals.

In wolves, both parents cooperate to feed the young when the pups are approximately 3 weeks old, by vomiting food. Weaning takes place at 7 to 10 weeks, and young wolves have been seen hunting at about 4 months, although not independently. The same general timing is followed in domestic dogs and vestiges of wild parental behavior is seen in the tendency for bitches to vomit food for their pups, and all dogs to bury bones and food.

Like the wolf, the dog is basically a pack-hunting animal. Either dogs or humans can satisfy this need for companionship. Isolation of a dog can act as a punishment during training. As pack animals, both wolves and dogs develop dominance-subordination relationships that permit them to live in groups in relative peace. A stable social order helps inhibit fighting in any competitive situation, such as those relating to food, living space and competition for human attention. Because size, strength and sex largely determine social dominance, these relationships are most effectively developed among young puppies. Strange dogs of the same breed are more often attacked and rejected from a closed social group than dogs of a different breed, though there are wide breed differences in the tolerance of strangers. There is little evidence that either wolves or dogs develop any strong system of leadership.

Man-Dog Relationship: Man and dog interact on at least 3 planes: The *first* is with care-dependency, beginning in early puppyhood. The adult dog, too, depends upon his master for food, shelter and companionship, and in relation to man, is a perpetual child. The *second* is within the social dominance structures, where the human being must be dominant or run the risk of being threatened or bitten in competitive situations. Dominance is best established by restraint rather than by severe punishment. If a smaller-breed dog challenges its owner's authority, it can be lifted off its feet by the loose skin of the neck and shaken into submission. The *third* interaction between man and dog is in a leader-follower relationship, which requires some training to produce in most dogs, even if a leash is used.

RAISING A PUPPY

House-Training: The bitch keeps her puppies clean by licking them and swallowing their excreta until they begin to eat solid food at about 3 weeks of age. A puppy avoids soiling its bed and will leave it to defecate and urinate but will not begin to use specific toilet areas until about 8 weeks. It must be kept under constant supervision from 7 weeks to prevent use of the wrong areas. The puppy can be tied on a short leash or kept in a small crate between hourly trips to the yard, and may soon be let loose in a room after being outside. During the day, most puppies cannot be continent for more than 2 hours before 12 weeks of age.

Social Development: In order to develop a strong relationship between dog and master, an attachment should begin from early puppyhood. As the most impressionable age is between 3 and 12 weeks, the new puppy should be selected at 5 weeks and taken home as near to 6 to 8 weeks as possible. Puppies raised in kennels away from much human association will become man-shy unless they are handled frequently from 4 to 5 weeks; if no handling is given until 4 months, they may become so shy that they will never be able to adapt themselves to human beings. Patience and careful training may partially overcome this shyness, but both the dog and owner are under a severe handicap. Such dogs frequently develop a "kennel-dog" syndrome when permanently shifted. They lack confidence and can be aggressive and show fear-biting. These signs may completely disappear if the dog is restored to its original kennel. Dogs kept too long in kennels form their strongest relationships with other dogs and do not make good pets. Dogs reared exclusively with human beings may be difficult to mate.

A dog's behavior is also determined by breed and strain. Proved temperament and trainability is as important as conformation or pedigree in the choice of a puppy.

Fundamentals of Training: All dogs should be taught obedience to commands such as: sit, stay, come, heel and no. A trained dog does willingly what its owner asks and as little as 10 minutes a day can produce a well-trained dog at 16 weeks if the training is begun at 7 weeks. These lessons should be uninterrupted and should start with simple tasks that the puppy can perform. Moderate repetition, consistency, praise for good performance and firmness towards misbehavior, with a relationship based on mutual trust and affection are the fundamentals of training.

PROTECTIVE AND TERRITORIAL BEHAVIOR

Adult dogs normally guard the territory around their homes and will attempt to keep out strangers by threat or attack. When off the home territory they seldom make trouble, and if moved to a new home, take up to 10 days to establish their new territory. Some control is necessary at this stage to prevent habits of chasing or biting.

Dogs are also likely to attack if the master is threatened by or threatens someone else. If a dog has developed this type of behavior, it must be kept under strict control.

The fact that one person dominates an animal is no guarantee that another will, and a dog owner must realize that although he dominates his pet, passersby may not and may be bitten if they do not submit. If a dog is allowed to successfully fight dogs or people, this becomes a habit and it makes him a danger and a nuisance. A severely threatened dog may bite from fear and in the typical "fear-biter" this has become a habit. A well-trained, well-controlled dog will seldom be a problem.

SOCIAL BEHAVIOR OF CATS

Although cats are solitary animals, some males form stable groups and roam. Fighting between members is rare once a social order has been established, though newcomers have to fight for a social position. Females and neutered males defend home territories more vigorously than entire males, which may wander extensively during the mating season.

Mating Behavior in the Cat: Best mating occurs when females are taken to males for the 3 days when the female is receptive. If the female will stand she may be held to aid the male mounting. The presence of a male heightens her sexual receptivity.

Sexual behavior begins in females between 6 to 8 months and during the breeding season the estrous cycle is repeated each 3 to 4 weeks. However, receptivity is confined to 4 to 10 days in this cycle. The 8-week breeding period of mature females in temperate zones falls in early spring and early fall, but occurs more often in the tropics. Males mature at about 11 months of age (range 6 to 18 months).

The female can be tested for receptivity by grasping the loose skin of her neck, rubbing her back and gently patting her anogenital area. Spontaneous signs of receptivity consist of the female approaching and crouching before the male, frequently treading and moaning. When fully aroused she twists from side to side, lifting the hind quarters as she crouches.

The mating act: Some males approach the female with a sharp howl. As the female crouches the male grips the loose skin of the neck with his teeth and mounts. He kneads her sides with his forepaws and because the penis is backward pointing he uses the hind legs to position himself for a series of rapid pelvic thrusts. Penetration is achieved within 3 minutes and is signaled by a loud cry from the female. After ejaculation the male releases or is thrown off the female as she turns on her side to roll her mouth, nose and face along the floor. She stops to lick her forelegs, body and genital area and will not allow the male to remount for at least 5 minutes.

Castration: No mating patterns develop in males castrated earlier than 4 months (puberty) and little is shown by mature, castrated and inexperienced males. After castration, experienced adult males show a gradual decline in sexual behavior after the first week or two, though some may persist for years. Ovariectomy leads to permanent loss of sexual behavior within 24 hours.

Parturition and Maternal Behavior: During birth, which usually lasts from 1 to 3 hours, the female changes position frequently. By licking each fetus she cleans them of birth membranes and stimulates breathing. The after-birth is eaten and the first nursing occurs within 2 hours of the birth of the litter. Licking of the anogenital region encourages urination and defecation in the kitten. Similar manual stimulation is required for hand-reared kittens.

Social Development of Kittens: Kittens approach and keep in contact with their mother and huddle at the home site. From less than a week of age they are disturbed when separated from mother, litter mates or home site. They cry and the female retrieves them. Until 3 weeks of age they use contact, smell and warmth to locate and grasp a nipple for suckling, though both eyes and ears open earlier. There is little competition for nipples after suckling positions have been adopted.

After the third week, kittens can leave the home site. Using hearing and sight they follow the mother when she goes to feed, and they begin to eat meat and other foods with her. She periodically permits them to suckle. They can be weaned after the sixth week if they can take milk and meat from dishes.

From the fourth or fifth week, kittens paw, chase, hug and roll together in play with little injury. A social order is formed within the litter. Lone kittens play with objects and their tails but are often frightened of other kittens. Play declines with sexual maturity but may reappear in castrated animals. Mature males play slightly more than females. Single male kittens are usually more aggressive when mature than those reared in a litter.

By the fifth week, kittens no longer huddle together but sleep singly or in pairs.

SOCIAL BEHAVIOR OF LIVESTOCK

As there are few studies of wild or feral sheep, pigs, cattle or horses, this discussion draws largely on observations of domestic stock.

Herd or Group Structure: Farm livestock associate together in groups, even under free-range farming systems. Sheep, cattle and horses maintain visual contact, and pigs, more a body-contact animal because of their poor vision, keep in auditory communication. If disturbed, sheep and horses first bunch and then run from the source of disturbance while pigs and cattle move in a looser group. Sheep orient themselves to one another at a visual angle of approximately 110°. During the bunching of animal groups in natural or high-density situations, individuals may be forced to violate the space of other species members. Social interactions at such close quarters depend on the position of the animals in the dominance order, where one adopts a dominant, and the other a subordinate posture. These orders, which are stable, require (1) a recognition of individual animals, (2) an initial encounter when the social position is first established and (3) a long-term memory that enables each animal to react to the other according to its social status. Aggressive behavior is most clearly seen when groups of pigs, cattle or horses are first formed. The frequent changing of group members should be avoided during husbandry practices. Production of milk and other physiological responses can be affected for several days while aggressive social interactions are taking place. Although sheep seldom show overt social dominance, rams compete at the start of each breeding season and sheep may show aggressive butting if intensive farming conditions increase the opportunity for competition over food or bedding areas. Butting in cattle and sheep, defined as the "butt or hook" order (depending upon whether the animal is polled or horned), biting of mane or withers in the horse, and pushing, biting and side-ripping with the tusks in boars are the common modes of fighting.

Development of Social Dominance: Piglets show some competitive fighting within a few days of birth for preferred nipples of the sow, but the other species do not develop a stable social order until some time after weaning. In semiwild cattle, bull calves stay in the cow herd and dominate the females by about 2½ years of age and then move into the bull group. Social-dominance effects can be very important in cases of high stock densities or poor farm layout. Inadequate trough space, narrow races, inadequate space in indoor housing or lack of feeders can mean that dominant animals command resources at the expense of subordinate animals. The latter will suffer and health and general production can be affected. Documented examples include the higher internal parasite load carried in some subordinate goats and the higher death rate during droughts when scarce food was commandeered by dominant stock.

There may be an upper limit to the number of group members that can be recognized or remembered by one individual. This number could be 50 to 70 in cattle and 20 to 30 in pigs.

The horse is very responsive to small changes in stance or skin pressures and these cues used during dominance-subordination interactions are utilized by the best horsemen in dealing with their animals. Sometimes tranquilizers have been used to aid social tolerance when strange pigs have to be penned together or when wild horses have to be broken.

Leader-Follower Relationships: Pigs are reluctant to lead and require to be driven, but sheep, cattle and horses are all subjected to a leader-follower order in free-range conditions. In sheep, the oldest ewe tends to lead naturally-constituted flocks while the mid-dominant animals lead groups of dairy cows. Some use is made by man of the "Judas" animal to lead flocks to slaughter, thus using the natural movement patterns of the species concerned. Sheep, cattle and horses can all be trained to lead, and cattle tied in pairs after weaning teach each other to lead. In the dairy cow, the movement order to milking is rather consistent over a season, though the rear animals are more fixed than the "leaders". The milking order is not necessarily the same as the leader-follower order when moving between grazing areas. Under free-range conditions the older stock can transfer information about seasonal pathways, good pasture areas, and watering points to their offspring if this bond is not disrupted before weaning. In this way, home-range areas can be established. Sheep in pastures of 100 hectares may establish up to 3 separate home-range areas. To this extent they can be considered territorial, and subgroups of the whole flock work with minimal overlap in these regions. In smaller pastures, dairy bulls set up small territories under set-stocking conditions between the age of 4 and 5 years but not before. The sudden attacks of dairy bulls on known handlers might be caused by this change to territorial behavior.

Sexual Behavior: The presence of the male at the beginning of the breeding season has an influence on the onset of the breeding cycle in both the sheep and the pig. Although the courtship procedures under free-range conditions are not as elaborate as in some species, male sheep and cattle spend considerable hours or even days in attendance on the pre-estral female. This interplay between male and female which aids reproductive success is not possible with artificial insemination programs. In the Asiatic buffalo, at least one dominant and one subordinate male are required for successful mating. In sheep, ewes at the peak of estrus attend the harem of the dominant male while the subordinate males mate with ewes before and after the maximal heat period. In many management systems the lack of libido or infertility of the most dominant male can greatly reduce the number of fertile matings.

Birth and Maternal Behavior: In feral sheep there is a strong tendency for the ewe to withdraw from the main flock for up to 3 days after giving birth before leading the lamb back into the group. Imprinting or the social bond is by then well established. Where possibilities do not exist for this withdrawal, other ewes a few hours off lambing may well steal the newly dropped lambs, being attracted by the presence of the birth fluids. Dominant cows can take calves from subordinate cows, but generally lose interest in them after producing their own young. The uninterrupted formation of the maternal-offspring bond within the first few hours after birth maximizes survival under free-range conditions. Bucket rearing of calves in competitive situations can influence later adult behavior, including mothering ability, and rapid drinking of milk from the bucket may lead to continued sucking of ears, testicles or other protuberances of fellow calves and establish undersirable habits of sucking in older stock. Some rams raised in all-male groups are reluctant to mate heterosexually in adulthood.

Man has domesticated his animals and become either a substitute maternal figure for the young captive animals or the dominant or near-dominant partner, as in the horse. With increasing mechanization in farming, care must be taken to foster empathy between man and animal if production is to be maintained.

SOCIAL BEHAVIOR OF CHICKENS

Development of Social Behavior: The chick shows social responses while still in the shell: it may give low-pitched distress calls if cooled, or rapid twitterings of contentment if warmed. Chicks hatched at slightly subnormal temperatures give distress calls as their moist down dries and they lose contact with the egg shell. Contact with a broody hen or other warm object prevents these calls. Newly hatched chicks are attracted to the hen by warmth, contact, clucking and body movements. This attraction is greatest on the day of hatching. They learn to eat, roost, drink and avoid enemies in the company of their mother.

The most sensitive period for imprinting in chicks is between 9 and 20 hours after hatching and fear is shown by the third day. The attachment to the mother is further strengthened as her voice and appearance are recognized. She rejects the chicks, however, as the down starts to disappear from their heads by pecking at them, and the clutch is dispersed.

Sexual Behavior: The testes secrete male hormones as the cockerel approaches maturity and these stimulate growth of comb and wattles and lead to crowing. Male courtship activities include "tid-bitting", a wing flutter and waltzing which leads to copulation. Crowing, which is rare in capons, advertises the location of the male and his territory to prospective mates and warns off other males. Interference by other males with copulation is common where several males are crowded into small pens with a few females.

In the pullet the ovarian medulla secretes enough male hormone for the growth of wattle and comb and some degree of aggressiveness. The ovarian cortex secretes female hormone which stimulates the growth of oviducts, inhibits male-type plumage and leads to the sex crouch when the cock places one foot on the back prior to mating.

Parental Behavior: Except in "nonbroody" breeds, incubation commences after a number of eggs have been laid. During sittings the eggs are turned, so preventing adhesions within the shell. A warm, defeathered, highly vascular brood-patch develops on each side of the breast. The broody hen clucks and ruffles her feathers if disturbed. Under feral conditions an elaborate approach behavior confuses predators and allows her to return to the nest undetected. During incubation, prolactin reduces ovarian activity and sexual behavior so that egg-laying ceases.

The hen uses brief, repetitive, low-pitched vocalizations to lead the chicks and indicate food sources. She warns them about ground or overhead predators, by cackling or by issuing a loud scream.

Flock Behavior: The clutch is the basis of flock organization and even after it has dispersed, chickens need company. A chick reared in isolation tends to stay apart from the flock. Flock birds eat more than birds kept singly.

Adult flock formation depends on mutual tolerance. Strangers are attacked and are only gradually integrated into the flock. Newcomers are relegated to positions near the bottom of the peck order. The peck order within each flock is stable and only active fighting will change it. Hens and cocks have separate peck orders as males in the breeding season do not peck hens. The male order is less stable than the female owing to their greater aggressiveness.

The peck order is most clearly seen in competition for food or mates, and subordinate hens may obtain so little food that they lay fewer eggs. Dominant hens mate less frequently than subordinate hens but dominant males mate more often than subordinate males. Birds in a flock kept in a state of social disorganization by the removal and replacement of birds eat less, may lose weight or grow poorly, and tend to lay fewer eggs than do birds in stable flocks. Additional feed and water troughs distributed about the pen enable subordinate hens to feed unmolested, and an adequate number of nesting boxes should be provided to ensure these birds the opportunity to lay. Flocks of over 80 birds tend to separate into 2 distinct groups and at least 2 separate peck orders will be established. If, through poor management, such groups are seriously disturbed, several hours may be required for individual birds to return to known pen positions.

Debeaking does not eliminate aggressiveness or prevent the development of the peck order but pecks by debeaked birds are often ignored by subordinates. Hens kept crowded on wire cannot exercise their normal pecking drive. They often attack other birds and feather picking may develop.

SOCIAL BEHAVIOR IN DOMESTIC TURKEYS

Social Organization: Domestic and wild turkeys have similar flocking patterns and social organization, but management practices determine the size and composition of domestic groups. Flock groups are organized according to a social dominance order which is less stable than that of chickens. In penned males some changes in rank may occur every few days. Certain varieties of turkeys tend to dominate others; e.g., Black over Bronze over Gray and in mixed sex groups, males dominate females.

The most common pair encounter is a simple threat, with one bird submitting to the other, otherwise both birds warily circle each other with wing feathers spread, tails fanned, and each emits a high-pitched trill. Then one or both turkeys will leap into the air and attempt to claw the other. The one that can push, pull or press down the head of the other will usually win the encounter. Bouts usually last a few minutes.

Much blood may be shed during a tugging battle since richly vascularized skin areas may be torn, but actual physical damage is slight and birds do not fight to the death. An injured lower ranking bird must be separated from the group until its wounds heal, as others will tend to peck and aggravate the wound.

Sexual Behavior: Turkeys are seasonal breeders with a peak occurring around March and April, but with the use of artificial light, they can be kept sexually active throughout the year. Turkeys are sexually mature in 8 months and breed the season after hatching.

Males initiate an elaborate courtship with postures and movements, but are ignored by all except receptive females. They crouch in response to the male's strutting, sitting down quietly with the head drawn in close to the body. The male slowly approaches, mounts, treads and makes cloacal contact with the everted oviduct of the female. The courtship process can take up to 10 minutes. Ejaculation follows swiftly, the male dismounts, and the female executes a postcopulatory feather ruffling and brief run. If the male fails to dismount she squirms out from under him. The receptivity of a female is terminated for 2 days on average, whether or not insemination has been achieved, but males often strut again immediately following copulation, and have been seen to mate with as many as 10 females in 30 minutes. No pair bonds are formed but range males often gather harems which they defend against other males. Only higher ranking males successfully complete a mating. Lower ranking females are mated more often than high ranking females but they lay fewer and smaller eggs.

Clutch size is from 8 to 15 eggs depending on the age of the females. After a single mating fertile eggs can be laid for 5 or 6 weeks, and when these are removed routinely, broody behavior is postponed.

Development of Social Behavior: Incubation takes 28 days and the poults move freely shortly after hatching. They normally become socially attached to the mother during the first day or two though occasionally they may imprint onto siblings, humans or other objects. Normally imprinted poults form tightly knit groups which may initially cluster for warmth but are cohesive even in fairly warm environments. Birds tend to "tidbit", feed or wander as a group, and if they are with the mother, she is the focus of activity, providing leadership and defense against intruders. Vocal and visual signals are used by both parents and young to stay in contact until the poults are at least 8 weeks old.

Fighting is rare prior to 3 months of age, but increases to a peak at 5 months, when social orders are formed. Males fight more vigorously among themselves than do females.

SOCIAL BEHAVIOR OF DUCKS

Most domestic ducks have originated from 2 species—the mallard (*Anas platyrhynchos*) and the muscovy (*Cairina moschata*). The muscovy has bare skin on the face of both sexes.

SOCIAL BEHAVIOR OF MUSCOVIES

Muscovies are promiscuous. The adult males, which are twice as heavy as females, are solitary and aggressive towards other males. Their displays are primitive and their calls are simple. The female, when alarmed, utters a weak quack. A hissing noise with tail-shaking, crest-raising and swinging of the males is both a threat to other males and a sexual display towards females. As females generally avoid displaying males, they may be chased to exhaustion before mating is possible. Following fertilization the female retires to her nest site and lays an egg a day. The nest is not occupied until incubation begins with the last or second last egg, and eggs are hatched after 35 days. As the male will attack sexually any female he may meet, he plays no part in the selection of the nest, incubation or care of the young. Males are avoided at all times.

SOCIAL BEHAVIOR OF MALLARDS

Wild mallards are monogamous and stay together from midwinter until the beginning of incubation, a period of 5 months. In domestic situations this may not be possible if sex numbers are not balanced.

Social Courtship: Social courtship begins after the summer molt of males. Sexually stimulated males display singly or in groups towards particular females, which in turn incite the males with a rather formalized display alternating between threatening and submissive gestures with a peculiar call. The threat is toward a strange male and submission is shown to the preferred male, who then swims ahead of the female and turns his nape towards her. Aquatic chases turn to aerial courtship flights as other males jockey for this favored position. Other courtship displays by competing males expose specific plumage towards the courted female. Fighting among males is typical but not crucial to pairing.

Paired birds leave the flock, but in domestic situations females cannot avoid attack by unpaired males and may be drowned or chased to exhaustion. The females are protected by mates until egg-laying is complete, and the male then deserts to molt. Thereafter incubation is often completely disrupted by the sexual attack of other males.

Incubation takes 28 days and the young leave the nest after the first day. The female undergoes her annual molt in the 6 to 8 weeks before the brood can fly.

Growth of Social Bonds: The young normally become firmly attached to their mother during a sensitive period in the first few days after hatching. A second, more gradual kind of imprinting helps them to respond sexually to their own species mates when mature. Males raised apart from their mothers tend to form homosexual pairs when mature, or when raised with females of another species attempt to mate with them. Female mallards respond sexually only to the visual and vocal stimuli of males of their own species.

READY REFERENCE GUIDES
WEIGHTS, MEASURES AND EQUIVALENTS
APOTHECARIES' SYSTEM

Weight	Volume
1 scruple (℈) = 20 grains (gr.)	1 fluid dram (ℨ) = 60 minims (♏)
1 dram (ℨ) = 60 grains	1 fluid ounce (℥) = 480 minims
= 3 scruples	= 8 fluid drams
1 ounce (℥) = 480 grains	1 pint (pt)* = 7,680 minims
= 8 drams	= 16 fluid ounces
1 pound (lb) = 5,760 grains	1 quart (qt)* = 2 pints
= 12 ounces	1 gallon (gal.)* = 4 quarts
(avoir.) = 16 ounces	

METRIC SYSTEM

Weight	Volume
1 microgram = 1,000,000 micro-	1 milliliter = 1,000 microliters
(mcg) micrograms	1 liter (L) = 1,000 milliliters
1 milligram (mg) = 1,000 micrograms	
1 gram (gm) = 1,000 milligrams	
1 kilogram (kg) = 1,000 grams	

EQUIVALENTS (ALL APPROXIMATE)
WEIGHTS

Metric	Apothecaries'	Metric	Apothecaries'
0.2 mg	= 1/300 grain	65.0 mg	= 1 grain
0.3 mg	= 1/200 grain	0.13 gm	= 2 grains
0.4 mg	= 1/150 grain	0.2 gm	= 3 grains
0.5 mg	= 1/120 grain	0.3 gm	= 5 grains
0.6 mg	= 1/100 grain	0.5 gm	= 7½ grains
1.0 mg	= 1/60 grain	0.7 gm	= 10 grains
3.0 mg	= 1/20 grain	1.0 gm	= 15 grains
6.0 mg	= 1/10 grain	4.0 gm	= 60 grains (1 dram)
10.0 mg	= 1/6 grain	6.0 gm	= 90 grains
15.0 mg	= ¼ grain	10.0 gm	= 2½ drams
25.0 mg	= ⅜ grain	15.0 gm	= 4 drams
30.0 mg	= ½ grain	31.0 gm	= 1 ounce

LIQUID MEASURE

Metric	Apothecaries'	Metric	Apothecaries'
0.06 ml	= 1 minim	30 ml	= 1 fl ounce
0.5 ml	= 8 minims	250 ml	= 8 fl ounces +
1.0 ml	= 15 minims	500 ml	= 1 pint +*
4.0 ml	= 1 fl. dram	1,000 ml	= 1 quart +*
		(1 liter)	

HOUSEHOLD MEASURES
(with approximate equivalents)

20 drops	≃	1 ml
1 teaspoon (tsp.)	=	4 ml = 1 fl dr
1 dessertspoon	=	8 ml = 2 fl dr
1 tablespoon (tbsp.)	=	15 ml = ½ fl oz
1 wineglass	=	60 ml = 2 fl oz
1 teacup	=	120 ml = 4 fl oz
1 tumbler	=	240 ml = 8 fl oz

COMPARATIVE APPROXIMATE LINEAR MEASURES

1 millimeter (mm) = 0.04 inch (in.)		1 inch (in.) =	2.54 centimeters (cm)
1 centimeter (cm) = 0.4 inch			
1 decimeter (dm) = 4.0 inches		1 foot (ft) =	30.48 cm
1 meter (m) = 39.37 inches		1 yard (yd) =	91.44 cm

* In the Imperial System, 1 pint = 20 fluid ounces, 1 quart = 40 fluid ounces, 1 gallon = 160 fluid ounces.

CENTIGRADE-FAHRENHEIT EQUIVALENTS

Conversion:

To reduce degrees F to degrees C, subtract 32, then multiply by 5/9.		To reduce degrees C to degrees F, multiply by 9/5, then add 32.	
Centigrade°	Fahrenheit°	Centigrade°	Fahrenheit°
Freezing (water at sea level):		Clinical Range:	
0	32	36.0	96.8
		36.5	97.7
Boiling (water at sea level):		37.0	98.6
100.0	212.0	37.5	99.5
		38.0	100.4
		38.5	101.3
−40	−40	39.0	102.2
		39.5	103.1
Pasteurization (Holding), 30 min at:		40.0	104.0
61.6	143.0	40.5	104.9
		41.0	105.8
Pasteurization (Flash), 15 sec at:		41.5	106.7
71.1	160.0	42.0	107.6

MILLIGRAM—MILLIEQUIVALENT
CONVERSIONS

The unit of measure of electrolytes is the milliequivalent (mEq), which expresses the chemical activity, or combining power, of a substance relative to the activity of 1 mg of hydrogen. Thus, 1 mEq is represented by 1 mg of hydrogen, 23 mg of Na, 39 mg of K, 20 mg of Ca, and 35 mg of Cl. Conversion equations are as follows:

$$mEq/L = \frac{(mg/L) \times Valence}{Formula\ Wt}$$

$$mg/L = \frac{(mEq/L) \times Formula\ Wt}{Valence}$$

(*N.B.:* Formula Wt = Atomic or Molecular Wt)

Milliosmols

The mEq is roughly equivalent to the milliosmol (mOsm), the unit of measure of osmolarity or tonicity. Normally, the body fluid compartments each contain about 280 mOsm of solute per liter.

ATOMIC WEIGHTS (APPROXIMATE) OF
SOME COMMON ELEMENTS

Hydrogen (H) = 1		Sodium (Na) = 23	
Carbon (C) = 12		Magnesium (Mg) = 24	
Nitrogen (N) = 14		Chlorine (Cl) = 35.5	
Oxygen (O) = 16		Potassium (K) = 39	
		Calcium (Ca) = 40	

CONVERSION FORMULAS

Gallons into Pounds: Multiply the specific gravity of the liquid by 8.33 * (weight in pounds of 1 gallon of water); then multiply this result by the number of gallons, to obtain the weight in pounds.

Pounds into Gallons: Multiply the specific gravity of the liquid by 8.33 * (weight in pounds of 1 gallon of water); then divide the number of pounds by the result, to obtain the volume in gallons.

Milliliters into Grams: Multiply the specific gravity of the substance by the number of milliliters, to obtain the weight in grams.

* 10 for Imperial gallons

Grams into Milliliters: Divide the number of grams by the specific gravity of the substance, to obtain its volume in milliliters.

Milliliters into Pounds: Multiply the number of milliliters by the specific gravity of the substance; then divide the product by 453.59 (equivalent in grams of 1 avoirdupois pound), to obtain its weight in pounds.

Pounds into Milliliters: Multiply the number of pounds by 453.59 (equivalent in grams of 1 avoirdupois pound); then divide the product by the specific gravity of the substance, to obtain the volume in milliliters.

Milliliters into Ounces: Multiply the number of milliliters by the specific gravity of the substance; then divide the product by 28.35 (equivalent in grams of 1 avoirdupois ounce), to obtain its volume in ounces.

Ounces into Milliliters: Multiply the number of ounces by 28.35 (equivalent in grams of 1 avoirdupois ounce); then divide the product by the specific gravity of the substance, to obtain its volume in milliliters.

Grains, Drams and Ounces into Grams (or ml): (1) Divide the number of grains by 15: or (2) multiply the number of drams by 4; or (3) multiply the number of ounces by 30. The result in each case equals the approximate number of grams (or ml).

Kilograms into Pounds: Multiply the number of kilograms by 2.2 or multiply the number of kilograms by 2 and add 10% to the product.

Pounds into Kilograms: Divide the number of pounds by 2.2.

PART VII
PRESCRIPTIONS

All the prescriptions referred to throughout the book ar
contained in this section. They are grouped in several larg
classes, mainly according to their chief pharmacologic or thera
peutic effect, but are numbered serially in the order of thei
listing, irrespective of classification. Thus, any prescription
number in the text (e.g., ℞ 123) allows the reader to refer directly to the corresponding prescription in this section.

Wherever possible, the drugs listed have been designated by their generic names. Where the specific preparation is perhaps better known by a single proprietary name, either the proprietary name alone (within quotation marks) is given, or is enclosed in parentheses, after the generic name. Where a drug is sold under 2 or more proprietary names, only the generic name is given. The pharmaceutical preparations set forth are those suggested by the authors of the various chapters. Where only one or a few of a number of possible preparations is given, those shown indicate only the preferences of the authors. Their appearance here does not constitute an implied or expressed warranty regarding specific products, nor does it imply endorsement of any one product over another by MERCK & CO., Inc. Every effort has been made to select representative drugs or preparations, but this should not be construed as restricting in any way the clinical judgment of the veterinarian in choosing related products or substituting other effective remedies at his discretion. Careful attention has also been given to the quantities and doses of the various agents listed, but personal experience, changes in manufacturer's formulations, or unusual conditions may make departures from those given necessary or desirable. Naturally, no guarantees can be made by the Editors regarding these recommendations.

Not only pesticide dips and sprays but most other drugs discovered in the past 25 years are now subject to federal regulations. These regulations have as their objective the protection of public health and welfare by establishing the safety and efficacy of drugs and tolerances for safe concentrations of drug residues in edible animal products. The latter requirement has necessitated the definition of specific withdrawal times and other warnings and cautions governing the use of certain compounds. Some products, for example, cannot be used on meat-producing livestock, while others cannot be used on poultry. The same precaution applies to such preparations as antibacterial compounds or other pharmaceuticals that may be given to dairy cattle in lactation. In some cases, suitable warnings have been included in the instructions accompanying each prescription. However, since the regulatory status of any specific drug is uncertain and subject to change at any time, the veterinarian should inform himself in detail regarding the conditions and cautions under which such agents are to be used. The manufacturer's instructions in this regard, which by law are placed conspicuously on the label, should be followed conscientiously and precisely.

Many of the prescriptions that appear throughout the text refer to various antibacterial agents. A detailed discussion of the uses, doses and administration of these substances is presented in the chapters titled SULFONAMIDE THERAPY (p. 460), ANTIBIOTIC THERAPY (p. 473) and NITROFURAN THERAPY (p. 493). Reading these chapters will provide the veterinarian with a much more complete picture of the usefulness of current and generally accepted anti-infectious agents than can be gained from the prescriptions alone. Corticosteroid therapy is also discussed, in the chapter beginning on p. 587.

In this edition of THE MERCK VETERINARY MANUAL, most of the doses of drugs or quantities of ingredients in prescriptions are given in metric measure. The few exceptions are where large quantities of a preparation must be made up (e.g., dips, medicated feeds) in which case avoirdupois measures are also given so that ordinary utensils may be used to measure the components. Body weight, when used as part of the dosage notation, is given in pounds. Conversion tables, given under the READY REFERENCE GUIDES (q.v., p. 1453), will quickly provide the reader with proper equivalents.

Antibiotics

1. ℞ Ampicillin injectable
suspension . . . . 200 mg/ml
1 to 3 mg/lb body wt, daily, subcut. or IM.

2. ℞ Antibiotic solution
Neomycin sulfate . . . . . 500 mg
Bacitracin . . . . 50,000 u
Polymyxin B sulfate . . . 100 mg
Water . . . . q.s. ad 100 ml
or Penicillin G (K or Na) 1,000,000 u
Dihydrostreptomycin . . . 1 gm
Water . . . . . q.s. ad 10 to 100 ml

3. ℞ Ampicillin
Dogs: 5 mg/lb of body wt, orally, b.i.d.

4. ℞ Ampicillin
100 mg/kg daily, IM, divided into 2 or 3
equal doses.

5. ℞ Cephalothin
50 mg/kg daily, IM, divided into 4 equal
doses.

Read introduction to prescriptions, pp. 1458 to 1460.
Note all warnings and cautions appearing on drug
labels and observe all local laws and regulations pertaining to drug usage.

6. ℞ Chloramphenicol

    15 to 50 mg/lb body wt, IM, in 3 or 4 divided doses.

7. ℞ Chloramphenicol

    Large animals: 2 to 5 mg/lb body wt, IM.
    Small animals: 25 to 50 mg/lb body wt daily, orally, divided into 3 doses
    or 5 to 15 mg/lb body wt, IM, once or twice daily.

8. ℞ Chloramphenicol

    50 mg/kg body wt, IV, b.i.d., or orally divided into 4 doses.

9. ℞ Chloramphenicol

    200 mg/gal. (50 mg/L) of water.
    Leave for several days.

10. ℞ Chloramphenicol

    Calves: 10 mg/lb body wt, IV or IM, repeated every 8 hours.
    Foals: 10 to 20 mg/lb body wt, IV or IM, repeated every 8 hours.
    Piglets: 15 mg/lb body wt, IM, repeated every 8 to 12 hours.

11. ℞ Chlortetracycline

    FOR STANDARD THERAPY: 15 to 50 mg/lb body wt orally daily, in divided doses
    or 2 to 5 mg/lb body wt IV daily in 2 equal doses. Administer until temperature has been normal for at least 24 hours after last dose.
    FOR SPECIFIC USES IN BOVINE ANAPLASMOSIS: *Destruction of carrier infection:* 5 mg/lb body wt parenterally daily for 10 consecutive days.
    Prevention by low-level feeding: 0.5 mg/lb body wt daily in feed for up to 60 days.
    Premunition: 2.5 mg/lb body wt parenterally in single dose when infected animals show first febrile response or approximately 3% of the erythrocytes contain anaplasms.
    FOR SPECIFIC USE IN PREVENTING UROLITHIASIS IN CATTLE AND SHEEP: 10 to 20 mg/lb daily, or mix 20 gm/ton of feed.

12. ℞ Chlortetracycline (capsule)

    50 mg per bird daily, orally.

For standard equivalents for measures, see pp. 1453 to 1456.

13. ℞ Chlortetracycline (boluses) . . 500 mg

Insert 2 to 4 boluses into uterus.

14. ℞ Chlortetracycline

400 gm/ton of feed, continued for 14 days.
NOTE: For porcine leptospirosis only.
100 to 200 gm/ton of feed. Useful only to
prevent development of additional abscesses.
NOTE: For jowl abscesses of swine only.

15. ℞ Chlortetracycline

200 to 400 gm/ton of mash for 2 weeks.

16. ℞ Chlortetracycline hydrochloride

Add 1 gm to each gal. of water, for 4 or 5
days.

17. ℞ Cloxacillin

All species: 1 mg/lb body wt, IM, 2 or 3
times daily.

18. ℞ Erythromycin

Orally: 2 to 5 mg/lb body wt, 3 or 4 times
a day.
IM or IV: 1 to 2 mg/lb body wt, only until
oral medication is possible.

19. ℞ Erythromycin

4.5 gm/100 lb (100 mg/kg) of fish, daily
for 21 days. Incorporate into ration.

20. ℞ Erythromycin

93 gm/ton of feed for broilers and replacement birds. Must be withdrawn 24 hours
before slaughter.

21. ℞ Erythromycin solution . . . . 200 mg/ml

1 to 2 mg/lb body wt, IV. Repeat in 12
hours.

22. ℞ Lincomycin hydrochloride monohy-
drate ("Lincocin")

Dogs: 10 mg/lb body wt, subcut. or orally,
b.i.d.

**Read introduction to prescriptions, pp. 1458 to 1460.
Note all warnings and cautions appearing on drug
labels and observe all local laws and regulations pertaining to drug usage.**

23. ℞ Lincomycin

  30 mg/kg daily, orally, divided into 4 equal doses
  or 20 mg/kg daily, IM, divided into 2 equal doses.

24. ℞ Neomycin sulfate

  Neonatal septicemias, all species: 5 mg/lb body wt, IM, b.i.d.
  Enteritis, small animals: 5 to 10 mg/lb body wt, orally daily, in divided doses.

25. ℞ Oxytetracycline

  Large animals: 3 to 5 mg/lb body wt, **IV** or IM daily.
  Small animals: 5 mg/lb body wt, IV or IM daily.
  Poultry: For spirochetosis, **1 to 5 mg/lb** body wt, IM as one dose.

26. ℞ Oxytetracycline

  5 mg/kg body wt, IM, b.i.d.

27. ℞ Oxytetracycline

  Swine, cattle: 5 to 10 mg/lb of body wt, IV or IM daily for 3 days.

28. ℞ Oxytetracycline

  5 to 15 mg/lb body wt, IV daily.
  30 to 50 mg/lb body wt, orally **in 3 to 4** divided doses daily.

29. ℞ Oxytetracycline (oral)

  15 to 50 mg/lb body wt orally daily, in **3** or 4 divided doses. (Oral administration limited to small animals and swine, and calves, foals or lambs not yet consuming roughage.)

30. ℞ Oxytetracycline (oral)

  50 mg/kg body wt daily (200 mg/pt of drinking water) prepared fresh 3 times weekly.

31. ℞ Oxytetracycline (capsule)

  50 mg per bird per day, orally.

For standard equivalents for measures, see pp. 1453 to 1456.

32. ℞ Oxytetracycline (water-soluble)

 3 gm/10 gal. water.

33. ℞ Oxytetracycline

 Cattle and horses (early stage): Initially **2** gm, IV or IM, followed by 1 gm daily for 3 or 4 days or until recovery.
 (Advanced stage): Initially 4 gm, IV or IM, followed by 2 gm at 12-hour intervals until recovery.
 Can be given in combination with penicillin.

34. ℞ Oxytetracycline (capsules) . . . **250 mg**

 Insert 4 to 8 capsules into uterus.

35. ℞ Oxytetracycline

 2.5 to 3.5 gm/100 lb (50 to 75 mg/kg) of fish, daily for 10 to 14 days.
 Incorporate into ration.

36. ℞ Oxytetracycline

 Swine: 400 gm/ton of feed, continued for **14** days.
 For prevention of additional jowl abscesses in swine: 100 to 200 gm/ton in feed.
 Calves: 500 gm/ton of feed. Feed 2-lb mixture daily for 3 to 5 days.
 Poultry: 200 gm/ton of mash for 2 weeks.

37. ℞ Oxytetracycline and vitamins ("Cosa-Terramycin" fortified soluble powder)

 50 mg oxytetracycline per pound of body weight daily (200 mg/pt of drinking water), prepared fresh 3 times weekly.

38. ℞ Penicillin . . . . 400,000 u/ml
 Streptomycin . . . . . . 0.5 gm/ml

 Into bursae: Inject 0.5 to 2.0 ml daily.
 Into anal gland: Inject 1.0 ml once or twice weekly.

39. ℞ Penethamate hydriodide injection

 3 to 5 million units, IM.

 Read introduction to prescriptions, pp. 1458 to 1460. Note all warnings and cautions appearing on drug labels and observe all local laws and regulations pertaining to drug usage.

40. ℞ Crystalline penicillin G . . 5,000,000 u
Dihydrostreptomycin . . . 5 gm
Isotonic salt solution . . . 100 ml

Infuse into uterus.
Cattle: 20 ml
Mares: 100 ml

41. ℞ Procaine penicillin G aqueous suspension

All species: 3,000 to 10,000 u/lb of body wt orally.

Streptomycin or Dihydrostreptomycin, aqueous

All species: 5 to 10 mg/lb of body wt daily. Mix drugs together and give in 2 or 3 divided doses, IM. Continue until temperature has been normal for at least 24 hours after last injection.

42. ℞ Procaine penicillin G . . 1,000,000 u
Dihydrostreptomycin . . 1.0 gm
Emulsifying vehicle* . . q.s. ad 100 ml

Instill 25 to 50 ml into the vagina. May be repeated at daily intervals as indicated.
* May also be used with water-dispersible ointment base, 15 gm.

43. ℞ Procaine penicillin G

Cattle: 12 to 20 million units, orally or intraruminally, preferably after neutralization of rumen contents.

44. ℞ Procaine penicillin G (in aqueous suspension)

Large animals: 3,000 to 10,000 u/lb body wt, daily.
Small animals: 10,000 to 20,000 u/lb body wt, daily.
NOTE: Where high blood levels are required rapidly, penicillin G potassium or sodium in aqueous solution (℞ 47) should be given either IV or IM at the same time as the initial dose of procaine penicillin.

45. ℞ Procaine penicillin
20,000 u/lb/day, IM.

For standard equivalents for measures, see pp. 1453 to 1456.

46. ℞ Benzathine penicillin G
   Procaine penicillin G . . āā 150,000 u/ml

   in aqueous suspension
   Up to 50 lb: 1 ml; *over 50 lb:* 2 ml, IM.
   Repeat every 3 to 5 days.

47. ℞ Penicillin G potassium or sodium

   Initial dose 3,000 to 10,000 u/lb body wt,
   IV or IM. Follow at once with a similar
   IM dose of procaine penicillin in aqueous
   suspension and repeat the latter every 24
   hours.

48. ℞ Penicillin G potassium . . . 250,000 u
   Sterile water . . . . . .   10 ml

   Inject 2.5 ml into joint space *twice daily*
   for 3 or 4 days.

49. ℞ Potassium penicillin . . . 5,000,000 u
   Dihydrostreptomycin . . .   2 gm
   Isotonic salt solution . . .   100 ml

   Flush into the guttural pouches daily for
   7 to 10 days.

50. ℞ Dihydrostreptomycin . . . .   1.0 gm
   Kaolin . . . .   10.0 gm
   Pectin . . . .   0.9 gm
   Water . . . .   100 ml

   1 teaspoon every 4 hours.

51. ℞ Dihydrostreptomycin

   Prophylaxis for newborn animals: 250 mg
   orally daily.
   Animals under 100 lb: 1.0 gm orally.
   Animals over 100 lb: 1.5 gm orally.
   The initial doses are followed by half doses
   every 12 hours for 3 or 4 days. The drug
   may also be given in the drinking water at
   the rate of 1.0 to 1.5 gm/gal.

52. ℞ Dihydrostreptomycin

   5 mg/lb, b.i.d., IM.

53. ℞ Dihydrostreptomycin

   5 to 10 mg/lb body wt, IM *once or twice*
   daily until at least 24 hours after apparent
   return to normal. Also intramammary infusion of 1 to 5 gm in aqueous vehicle.

Read introduction to prescriptions, pp. 1458 to 1460.
Note all warnings and cautions appearing on drug
labels and observe all local laws and regulations per-
taining to drug usage.

54. ℞ Streptomcyin or Dihydrostreptomycin

All species: 5 to 10 mg/lb body wt, IM daily in divided doses every 6 to 12 hours.
FOR LEPTOSPIROSIS: *Large animals:* 25 mg/kg body wt, IM in a single dose. May be repeated for 3 daily doses.
Small animals: 5 to 10 mg/lb body wt, IM every 12 hours.

55. ℞ Streptomycin or Dihydrostreptomycin . . . . 1 gm
Distilled water . . . . 10 ml

Inject 2.5 ml into joint space, b.i.d. for 3 or 4 days.
FOR VIBRIOSIS IN CATTLE: Infuse 10 ml of the solution into uterus with a suitable catheter.

56. ℞ Streptomcyin

Large animals: 0.5 gm/100 lb body wt, IM, b.i.d.

57. ℞ Streptomycin

Prophylaxis: 1 gm/gal. of drinking water continuously, or 5 to 10 gm/gal. for several days before and after suspected exposure.
Treatment: Depending on severity, 5 to 15 gm/gal. of drinking water for 5 to 10 days, then 1 gm/gal. for 5 days.

58. ℞ Tetracycline

Oral: (*large animals*) 5 to 10 mg/lb body wt; (*small animals*) 15 to 50 mg/lb body wt daily in 3 or 4 divided doses.
IM: 1 to 5 mg/lb body wt daily.
IV: 1 to 5 mg/lb body wt once or twice daily. Continue treatment until animal has been afebrile for 24 to 48 hours.

59. ℞ Tetracycline

Oral: 15 to 50 mg/lb of body wt daily divided into 2 or 3 doses.
Parenteral: 2 to 5 mg/lb of body wt daily divided into 2 doses.

60. ℞ Tetracycline

25 to 50 mg/lb body wt orally daily, in 3 or 4 divided doses. (Oral administration limited to small animals and swine, and calves and colts or lambs not yet consuming roughage.)
or 3 to 5 mg/lb body wt parenterally in 2 divided doses.

For standard equivalents for measures, see pp. 1453 to 1456.

61. ℞ Tylosin

> *Prophylaxis:* 100 gm/ton of feed for at least 3 weeks followed by 40 gm/ton of feed until swine reach market weight.
> *Treatment:* 0.25 gm/gal. water for 3 to 10 days followed by 40 to 100 gm/ton of feed for 2 to 6 weeks after drinking-water treatment.

62. ℞ Tylosin

> *Dogs:* Orally, 5 to 10 mg/lb of body wt, t.i.d.
> *Cattle:* IM, 1 to 2 mg/lb of body wt.

Sulfonamides

63. ℞ Phthalylsulfathiazole
("Sulfathalidine")

> 60 to 90 mg/lb body wt orally, daily for 3 or 4 days.

64. ℞ Salicylazosulfapyridine
("Azulfidine")

> 1.5 gm orally t.i.d. to a 40-lb dog.

65. ℞ Sulfabromomethazine
("Sulfabrom")

> *Foot rot of cattle:* 100 mg/lb body wt, in the feed daily for 2 consecutive days.

66. ℞ Sulfadiazine

> 30 mg/lb body wt orally or IV, b.i.d.

67. ℞ Sulfadiazine sodium
Sulfamerazine sodium . . . . āā 50 mg

> Given in the water or feed, daily for 10 to 14 days.

68. ℞ Sulfadiazine
Sulfamerazine
Sulfathiazole . . . . āā 150 mg

> 1 tablet per 7.5 lb body wt orally, in divided doses, for 4 days.

69. ℞ Sulfadimethoxine 10% solution

> 1 ml/8 lb body wt followed by 1 ml/16 lb every 24 hours IV, IM or subcut.

Read introduction to prescriptions, pp. 1458 to 1460. Note all warnings and cautions appearing on drug labels and observe all local laws and regulations pertaining to drug usage.

70. ℞ Sulfadimethoxine

> *Dogs:* 6 to 25 mg/lb daily.
> *Horses:* 12.5 to 25 mg/lb daily.

71. ℞ Sulfadimethoxine (tablets)

> 12.5 mg/lb body wt orally on the first day, then 6.5 mg/lb body wt for 5 days.

72. ℞ Sulfadimethoxine (tablets)

> 25 mg/lb body wt orally initially, then 2.5 mg/lb body wt for 3 to 5 days once daily.

73. ℞ Sulfaguanidine

> 0.75 to 1.00 gm/10 lb body wt orally, daily for 3 or 4 days.

74. ℞ Sulfaguanidine

> Mix with chopped hay or grain at the rate of 1 gm/lb feed.

75. ℞ Sulfamerazine

> 60 mg/lb body wt orally, followed by 30 mg/lb body wt every 12 hours for 4 days

> *or* **Sulfamerazine sodium**

> 30 to 60 mg/lb body wt, IV daily for 4 days.

76. ℞ Sulfamerazine

> 8 to 10 gm/100 lb (175 to 220 mg/kg) of trout, daily for 14 days.
> Incorporate into ration.

77. ℞ Sulfamerazine sodium

> 0.5% (10 lb/ton) in feed, given for 5 to 7 days.
> CAUTION: May be toxic.

78. ℞ Sulfamerazine sodium
Sulfapyridine sodium
Sulfathiazole sodium . . . . āā 20 gm
Sterile water . . . . . q.s. ad 500 ml

> 0.5 to 1.0 ml/lb body wt, IV or IP initially, then half the initial dose every 12 hours.

79. ℞ Sulfamerazine and oxytetracycline

> 9.1 gm sulfamerazine per 100 lb (200 mg/kg) of fish, daily for 5 days, followed by 2.5 gm of oxytetracycline per 100 lb (50 mg/kg) of fish, daily for 3 days.

For standard equivalents for measures, see pp. 1453 to 1456.

80. ℞ Sulfamethazine sodium

> 0.2% (8 gm/gal.) in drinking water for 5 days
>
> *or* 5 to 10 drops of a 25% solution orally, daily.

81. ℞ Sulfamethazine

> 0.4% (8 lb/ton) in feed, given for 3 to 5 days

> *or* Sulfamethazine sodium, 12.5% solution

> 30 ml/gal. of drinking water.

82. ℞ Sulfamethazine

> 60 mg/lb body wt orally or preferably IV followed by 30 mg/lb body wt orally every 12 hours for 3 or 4 days.

> *or* Sulfamethazine sodium

> 30 mg/lb body wt, IV or IP, daily for 4 days

83. ℞ Sulfamethazine

> *Prophylaxis:* 2 gm/100 lb (44 mg/kg) of fish daily, incorporated in a moist pellet.
> *Treatment:* 5 gm/100 lb (110 mg/kg) of fish daily for 10 days in a moist pellet, or 15 gm/100 lb (330 mg/kg) of fish daily for 10 to 15 days incorporated in dry starter diet.

84. ℞ Sulfamethizole (tablets)

> 125 to 500 mg orally, 4 times daily.

85. ℞ Sulfanilamide

> 60 mg/lb body wt orally on the first day, followed by 45 mg/lb body wt orally on succeeding days, until temperature has been normal for 48 hours.

86. ℞ Sulfapyridine

> 60 mg/lb body wt orally, followed by 30 mg/lb body wt orally every 12 hours for 4 days

> *or* Sulfapyridine sodium

> 30 mg/lb body wt, IV, daily for 4 days.

Read introduction to prescriptions, pp. 1458 to 1460. Note all warnings and cautions appearing on drug labels and observe all local laws and regulations pertaining to drug usage.

87. ℞ Sulfaquinoxaline sodium

For first 2 or 3 days, 0.04% in drinking water or 0.1% in the feed, prepared and given according to manufacturer's directions. If disease recurs, use 0.025% in the water or 0.05% in the feed for 2 days and repeat, if necessary, at 4-day intervals.

88. ℞ Sulfaquinoxaline

0.05% (1 lb/ton) in feed, given for a minimum of 5 days.

89. ℞ Sulfaquinoxaline

6 mg/lb body wt orally, daily for 3 to 5 days.
For therapy in cattle and sheep: 6 mg/lb body wt in the drinking water daily until signs subside.
For prophylaxis in cattle: 0.6 mg/lb body wt in the drinking water daily for 30 days, starting when animals are likely to be exposed to clinical infection.
CAUTION: In dogs, larger doses may produce hypoprothrombinemia which may be reversed or prevented by the use of menadione (℞ 549, 550) or vitamin K₁ (℞ 554).

90. ℞ Sulfathiazole

Horses and cats: 90 mg/lb body wt orally t.i.d.
Cattle, sheep, swine, dogs: 120 to 180 mg/lb body wt orally in equal fractional doses every 4 to 6 hours.

91. ℞ Sulfisoxazole

60 to 120 mg/lb body wt orally.

92. ℞ Sulfisoxazole

8 to 10 gm/100 lb (175 to 220 mg/kg) of trout, daily for 14 days.
Incorporate into ration.

Nitrofurans

93. ℞ Furazolidone

2 gm/kg of ration for 2 to 4 weeks.

94. ℞ Furazolidone and sulfamethazine

combine sulfamethazine, 3 gm/100 lb (66 mg/kg) of fish daily, and furazolidone, 2 gm/100 lb (44 mg/kg) of fish daily. Treat for 10 days.

For standard equivalents for measures, see pp. 1453 to 1456.

95. ℞ Furazolidone

4.5 gm/100 lb (100 mg/kg) of trout daily
for 14 days. This drug is to be mixed with
the ration and used immediately, as the
drug is rapidly inactivated by many ingredients of the diet.

96. ℞ Furazolidone suspension
("Furoxone")

Each milliliter contains 100 mg of furazolidone.
Piglets: Give 2 ml as initial dose and 1 ml
in 8 hours. Treatment may be continued
for 3 days. Treat all pigs in the litter.

97. ℞ Nifurpirinol ("Furpyrinol")

Expose fish to 1 ppm for 1 hour as a bath.

98. ℞ Nitrofurantoin

Tracheobronchitis: 2 mg/lb body wt orally,
every 8 hours for 4 to 7 days.
Urinary-tract infections: 2 mg/lb body wt
orally, every 8 hours for 7 to 14 days.

99. ℞ Nitrofurazone 0.2% solution

Introduce 20 to 60 ml into uterus with a
catheter.

100. ℞ Nitrofurazone 4.59% water-soluble
powder

Swine: 1 lb/50 gal. of drinking water for
7 to 10 days. Allow no other drinking
water. Solutions will deteriorate if in continuous contact with metal for over 7 days.

101. ℞ Nitrofurazone

Treatment: Dogs: 2 mg, t.i.d. for 10 days
orally, or until stools are normal.
Sheep and goats: 4.5 mg/lb body wt orally
daily for 7 to 10 days.
Swine: 0.44% in feed for 7 days.
Prophylaxis: Sheep and goats: 0.0165% in
feed for 21 days, starting when animals are
likely to be exposed to clinical infection.

102. ℞ Nitrofurazone

5 mg/lb body wt orally for 3 days.

**Read introduction to prescriptions, pp. 1458 to 1460.
Note all warnings and cautions appearing on drug
labels and observe all local laws and regulations pertaining to drug usage.**

Biologicals

103. ℞ *Brucella abortus* Strain 19 lyophilized
vaccine
5 ml subcut.

104. ℞ *Clostridium botulinum* Type A and
Type C antitoxin
2 to 4 ml, IP, depending on weight of bird.

105. ℞ *Clostridium chauvoei-septicum*
bacterin
Cattle, horses: 5 ml subcut.
Sheep, goats: 3 ml subcut.
For immunization against blackleg and ma-
lignant edema.

106. ℞ *Clostridium perfringens* Type D
bacterin
5 ml subcut.

107. ℞ Anti-canine-distemper serum
10 to 30 ml subcut.

108. ℞ Chemically inactivated canine-
distemper virus
Administer according to manufacturer's directions.

109. ℞ Modified canine-distemper live virus
(chick-embryo origin, lyophilized)
Administer according to manufacturer's directions.

110. ℞ Modified canine-distemper live virus
(tissue-culture origin, lyophilized)
Administer according to manufacturer's directions.

111. ℞ Feline-distemper vaccine, homologous,
killed tissue virus
Administer according to manufacturer's directions.

112. ℞ Feline-distemper vaccine, inactivated,
feline tissue culture origin
2 ml subcut. or IM. Repeat after 7 to 14
days. (Follow manufacturer's directions.)

For standard equivalents for measures, see pp. 1453 to 1456.

113. ℞ Chemically inactivated infectious-
canine-hepatitis virus

> Administer according to manufacturer's di-
> rections.

114. ℞ Anti-distemper-and-hepatitis serum

> 0.5 to 1.0 ml/lb body wt subcut., repeated
> at 7- to 10-day intervals if the animal is
> kept under conditions of exposure to the
> virus, and every 14 days if kept at home.
> (Follow manufacturer's directions.)

115. ℞ Chemically inactivated distemper
virus and chemically inactivated in-
infectious-canine-hepatitis virus
combination

> Administer according to manufacturer's di-
> rections.

116. ℞ Modified distemper live virus and infectious-canine-hepatitis live virus
combination

> Administer according to manufacturer's di-
> rections.

117. ℞ Canine immune globulin concentrate

> Administer according to manufacturer's di-
> rections.

118. ℞ Encephalomyelitis vaccine,
Eastern strain
  or Western strain
  or Eastern- and Western-strain mixture

> 2 doses of 1 ml each, intradermally, at 7-
> to 10-day intervals.

119. ℞ Mink enteritis vaccine, killed virus,
mink-tissue origin

> Administer according to manufacturer's di-
> rections.

120. ℞ "Flea Antigen" (Haver Lockhart)

> 3 injections of 0.5 ml intradermally at 7-
> day intervals.

**Read introduction to prescriptions, pp. 1458 to 1460.
Note all warnings and cautions appearing on drug
labels and observe all local laws and regulations pertaining to drug usage.**

121. ℞ Measles vaccine, modified live virus, canine tissue culture origin

Given IM according to manufacturer's directions.

122. ℞ Modified feline-pneumonitis live virus (chick-embryo origin, vacuum-dried)

Administer according to manufacturer's directions.

123. ℞ Feline homologous antiserum

Administer according to manufacturer's directions.

124. ℞ Equine rhinopneumonitis virus ("Pneumabort") (hamster-adapted live virus)

Immunization against viral rhinopneumonitis of horses: Administer 2-ml dose intranasally in July and October to farm horses. Use 2-ml dose once annually for horses in training and racing.

125. ℞ Canine kidney-tissue culture vaccine, HEP-Flury strain

Dogs, cats: 1 ml, IM.
Cattle: 2 doses, 1 ml each, IM, 6 weeks apart.

126. ℞ Chicken embryo vaccine, high-egg passage (HEP) Flury strain

Cats: 5 months or older, 1 ml, IM.
Cattle: 5 ml, IM.

127. ℞ Chicken embryo vaccine, low-egg passage (LEP) Flury strain

Dogs: over 3 months of age, 2 to 3 ml, IM.
CAUTION: Do not use in other animals.

128. ℞ Chicken embryo (fibroblast) tissue-culture vaccine, LEP-Flury strain

Dogs: 1 ml, IM.
CAUTION: Do not use in other animals.

129. ℞ Hamster kidney-tissue culture vaccine, fixed virus strain, phenolized or formalized

Cats, dogs: 3 to 5 ml, IM or subcut.
Sheep, goats: 10 to 15 ml, IM or subcut.
Cattle, horses: 50 ml.

For standard equivalents for measures, see pp. 1453 to 1456.

130. ℞ Hamster kidney tissue culture vaccine,
        LEP-Flury strain

> *Dogs:* 2 ml, IM.
> CAUTION: Do not use in other animals.

131. ℞ Feline panleukopenia vaccine modified
        live virus, tissue culture origin

> Administer according to manufacturer's di-
> rections.

132. ℞ Hamster kidney-tissue culture vaccine,
        fixed virus strain, with adjuvant,
        formalized

> *Dogs:* 2 ml, IM or subcut.
> *Cats:* 1 ml, IM or subcut.

133. ℞ Nerve tissue suspension vaccine,
        ovine or caprine origin, fixed virus
        strain, phenolized (Semple type)

> *Dogs, cats:* 3 to 5 ml subcut. or IM.
> *Sheep, goats, swine, cattle, horses:* 5 to 50
> ml subcut. or IM.

134. ℞ Porcine kidney-tissue culture vaccine,
        ERA strain

> *Dogs, cats, cattle, sheep, goats, horses:* 2
> ml, IM.

135. ℞ *Streptococcus suis,* modified live vac-
        cine ("Jowl-Vac")

> For prophylactic use only in healthy swine:
> Apply topically to the palatine tonsils and
> the pharyngeal mucosa when pigs are 10
> weeks old.

Corticosteroids and Anti-inflammatory Agents

136. ℞ Chlorquinaldol ("Sterosan")-hydro-
        cortisone ointment

Chlorquinaldol 3%
Hydrocortisone 1%

> Apply to lesions t.i.d.

137. ℞ Corticotropin (ACTH)

> *Dogs:* 1 u/lb body wt, IM, once or twice
> daily. Reduce dosage gradually over a 1-
> week period.

**Read introduction to prescriptions, pp. 1458 to 1460.
Note all warnings and cautions appearing on drug
labels and observe all local laws and regulations pertaining to drug usage.**

138. ℞ Corticotropin (ACTH)
200 USP units IM at day 110.

139. ℞ Corticotropin (ACTH) in gelatin or oil or other delayed-absorption vehicle
Large animals: 200 to 600 u, IM. Repeat after 2 or 3 days if necessary.
Small animals: 1 u/lb body wt, IM. Repeat after 48 hours.

140. ℞ Cortisone acetate (suspension or tablets)
Large animals: 0.5 to 1.5 gm, IM. Repeat on following day if necessary.
Small animals: 1 to 5 mg/lb body wt, IM or orally. Dose must be adjusted to response of animal to treatment.

141. ℞ Deoxycorticosterone acetate (DOCA)
Dogs: 1 to 2 mg, IM daily. Pellet implants, 125 mg, 1 to 2 pellets given each 6 to 12 months.

142. ℞ Dexamethasone
0.25 to 1.5 mg daily IM or orally.
Subsequent daily dose reduced.

143. ℞ Dexamethasone
Cattle: 1.0 to 1.5 mg/100 lb body wt, IM; concomitant antibacterial therapy outlasting the duration of glucocorticoid action is recommended.

144. ℞ Dexamethasone
Horses: 5 to 10 mg daily in single or divided doses. This dosage should be administered until a therapeutic effect is achieved or for 5 days.

145. ℞ Dexamethasone (tablets or suspension)
Large animals: 5 to 20 mg daily IM or orally.
Small animals: 0.125 to 1 mg daily IM or orally.
Subsequent daily dose to be reduced.

For standard equivalents for measures, see pp. 1453 to 1456.

146. ℞ Dexamethasone with aspirin and
aluminum hydroxide ("Decagesic")
(tablets)
Each tablet contains:
Dexamethasone . . . . 0.25 mg
Aspirin 500   mg
Aluminum hydroxide . . . 75   mg
1 or 2 tablets once or twice daily.

147. ℞ 9-Fluoroprednisolone acetate . . 2 mg/ml
Neomycin sulfate . . . . 5 mg/ml
of aqueous solution for infection
10 to 20 ml, IM, according to severity of
condition.

148. ℞ Hydrocortisone acetate (tablets or
suspension)
Large animals: 0.5 to 1.5 gm, IM. Repeat
if necessary.
Small animals: 1 to 2 mg/lb body wt
orally or IM.
Divide into 2 to 4 doses if given orally.
Adjust dose to patient's response and reduce to minimum effective maintenance dose.

149. ℞ Hydrocortisone solution 100 mg/ml
Large animals: 100 to 600 mg given by slow
IV infusion in 500 to 1,000 ml of 10%
dextrose or isotonic sodium chloride.
Small animals: 10 to 50 mg by slow IV infusion in 25 to 250 ml of 5% dextrose or
isotonic sodium chloride.

150. ℞ Phenylbutazone
Large animals: 1 to 2 gm/500 lb body wt,
for 3 to 5 days.
Small animals: 100 to 250 mg, t.i.d. Dosage
can be reduced after the 4th day.

151. ℞ Prednisolone
0.25 to 1.0 mg/lb body wt daily orally or
IM.

152. ℞ Prednisolone (tablets)
2.5 mg, b.i.d. for 3 days, then 1.25 mg,
b.i.d. for 3 days, followed by 1 mg, b.i.d.
for 1 week.

**Read introduction to prescriptions, pp. 1458 to 1460.
Note all warnings and cautions appearing on drug
labels and observe all local laws and regulations pertaining to drug usage.**

153. ℞ Prednisolone 5 mg and hydroxyzine
hydrochloride 10 mg ("Vetaraxoid")
(tablets)

Small animals: ½ to 1 tablet b.i.d. or t.i.d.

154. ℞ Prednisolone (tablets or suspension)

Cattle and horses: 100 to 400 mg, IM.
Dogs: 20 to 50 mg, IM daily for 3 to 5 days
until a response is noted; then tablets for
maintenance.
Orally: 10 to 25 mg daily in 2 or 3 doses.
Adjust dose to patient's response; then reduce gradually to minimum level needed
to maintain remission.
For allergy only: Dogs: 2.5 to 5.0 mg orally
2 to 4 times daily until the condition is
controlled and then adjust down to minimum maintenance level.

155. ℞ Prednisolone t-butylacetate

Arthritis and synovitis: Aspirate all fluid
from cavity and inject 2 to 5 ml.
Curb and sore shins: Inject 0.5 to 1.0 ml
in several sites over area of swelling.

156. ℞ Methylprednisolone acetate ("Depo-
Medrol") 20 or 40 mg/ml

Inject into the lesion or give parenterally
every 2 to 3 weeks.
Dogs: The average dose is 20 mg. In accordance with size and severity of the condition, dose may range from 2 mg in miniature breeds to 40 mg in medium breeds
and even as high as 120 mg in the largest
breeds or with severe involvement.
Cats: The average dose is 10 mg with a
range up to 20 mg.

157. ℞ Stanozolol (tablets) . . . . . . 2 mg

½ to 2 tablets, b.i.d.

158. ℞ Triamcinolone

0.05 to 0.1 mg/lb body wt orally or as a
single IM or subcut. injection. Oral dosage
should be reduced gradually within 2 weeks
to maintenance levels of 0.01 to 0.02 mg/lb
body wt.

For standard equivalents for measures, see pp. 1453 to 1456.

159. ℞ Triamcinolone acetonide . . 2 to 6 mg/ml

Aspirate all available fluid from the synovial cavity and inject 1 to 3 mg (dog), 6 to 30 mg (horse), depending on size of the cavity.

160. ℞ Dexamethasone

1 mg/lb body wt, IV.

Hormones

161. ℞ Chlorpropamide (tablets) . . . 100 mg

100 to 250 mg daily. Dosage must be adjusted individually.

162. ℞ Diethylstilbestrol

0.5 to 4.0 mg in oil, IM on the first day.
0.5 to 4.0 mg orally on the following 5 to 7 days

or Repository diethylstilbestrol 0.5 mg/lb, IM within 5 days of mating.

163. ℞ Diethylstilbestrol

Cattle and horses: 15 to 60 mg, IM, subcut. or orally daily.
Sheep and swine: 4 to 5 mg, IM, subcut. or orally daily.
Dogs: 0.2 to 1 mg/lb of body wt of the repository form, given IM, once, to a maximum of 25 mg/animal, *or* 1-mg tablet per dog (daily) for 5 days.

164. ℞ Estradiol 17-beta cypionate

0.5 to 2.0 mg, IM within 5 days of mating. In toy breeds the dose may be reduced to 0.25 mg.

165. ℞ Progesterone

Cattle and swine: 50 to 100 mg, IM daily.
Sheep: 10 mg, IM daily.
Dogs: 10 to 50 mg, IM daily until bleeding or signs subside.

166. ℞ Pituitary gonadotropin (LH)

Large animals: 25 mg (5 ml) IV. Repeat after 1 to 4 weeks if necessary.
Small animals: 1 mg (0.2 ml) IM or subcut. at weekly intervals as indicated.

Read introduction to prescriptions, pp. 1458 to 1460. Note all warnings and cautions appearing on drug labels and observe all local laws and regulations pertaining to drug usage.

167. ℞ Chorionic gonadotropin

    Large animals: 1,000 to 10,000 IU, IM
or 2,500 to 5,000 IU, IV.
    Dogs: 250 to 500 IU, IM or subcut. at
weekly intervals for 4 to 8 weeks.
    For hyperestrinism in bitches: 100 to 500
IU, IM daily until bleeding or signs subside.

168. ℞ Gonadotropic hormone (pregnant-
mare serum)

    Cows and mares: 1,000 IU subcut. for 2 or
3 consecutive days.
    Bulls and stallions: 500 IU subcut. weekly.
Repeat weekly if necessary.
    Ewes: 500 IU subcut.
    Bitches: 250 to 500 IU subcut. Repeat
after 9 days if necessary.
    Dogs: 375 to 750 IU subcut. Repeat when
necessary.

169. ℞ Pregnant-mare serum . . . . 15,000 IU
    Human chorionic
    gonadotropin . . . . . 10,000 IU
    Administer simultaneously in a single dose
by subcut. or IM injection.

170. ℞ Conjugated estrogens ("Premarin"
intravenous)

    Large animals: 20 mg, IV.

171. ℞ Insulin (protamine zinc)

    5 to 50 u per day depending on animal's
size and response.

172. ℞ Oxytocin

    Cows: 10 to 40 u, IV.
    Sows: 25 to 50 u, IM or subcut.
    Rabbits: 1 to 2 u, IM or subcut.

173. ℞ Purified oxytocin principle . . . 20 u/ml

    Small animals: 0.25 to 1.5 ml, IM or subcut.
    Sheep and swine: 1.5 to 2.5 ml, IM or sub-
cut.
    Cattle and horses: 2 to 5 ml, IM or subcut.
    Bovine mastitis: 1 to 2 ml, IV.

For standard equivalents for measures, see pp. 1453 to 1456.

174. ℞ Purified posterior pituitary injection
10 or 20 u/ml

Cattle and horses: 2 to 5 ml, IM, IV or
subcut.
Sheep and swine: 1 to 2 ml, IM, IV or
subcut.
Dogs: 0.1 to 0.5 ml, IM or subcut.

175. ℞ Vasopressin (ADH) tannate in oil

Dogs: 0.25 to 2 u, IM, once or twice daily,
adjusted to response.

176. ℞ Methyl prednisolone acetate ("Depo-
Medrol") 20 mg/ml

Aspirate all available fluid from the synovial cavity and inject 10 to 20 mg of the
drug.

177. ℞ Methyltestosterone (tablets)

0.5 to 1.0 mg/lb body wt orally, daily for 6
to 10 days.

178. ℞ Testosterone propionate

Large animals: 50 mg subcut., daily for 4
days.
Small animals: Depending on size and species, 10 to 50 mg, IM.

179. ℞ Testosterone propionate

1 mg/lb body wt, IM, to be given at 2-
to 8-week intervals.

180. ℞ Thyroid USP (tablets) . . . . 30 mg

1 tablet b.i.d., gradually increasing to 6 to
10 tablets per day, depending on the animal's size and the appearance of undesirable side effects.

181. ℞ Thyroid USP (tablets)

180 to 540 mg orally, daily in 2 or 3 divided
doses.

182. ℞ Thyroid USP

Ruminants: 2.5 to 5.0 gm/100 lb body wt
orally daily.
Dogs: 2.5 to 4.5 mg/lb body wt orally daily.
Dosage must be adjusted in terms of response.

**Read introduction to prescriptions, pp. 1458 to 1460.
Note all warnings and cautions appearing on drug
labels and observe all local laws and regulations pertaining to drug usage.**

183. ℞ Tolbutamide (tablets) . . . . 500 mg

0.5 to 3.0 gm daily. Dosage must be adjusted individually.

Intramammary Infusions

NOTE: For most of these, milk must be discarded for a period after the last treatment.

184. ℞ Sodium carbenicillin

5 gm as an infusion into the affected quarter. Repeat in 24 hours.

185. ℞ Chlortetracycline ointment

400 mg of active substance infused into the teat canal. Repeat at 24- to 48-hour intervals if necessary.

186. ℞ Sodium cloxacillin 200 mg in 3% aluminum monostearate base

Infuse on 3 occasions at 48-hour intervals into the infected quarter. Treated quarters may be milked out at normal milking.

187. ℞ Benzathine cloxacillin

500 mg in 3% aluminum monostearate base. Infuse into each quarter at drying off and leave without milking out.

188. ℞ Dihydrostreptomycin

0.25 to 1.0 gm in suspension, infused into the teat canal. May be repeated after 24 to 48 hours.

189. ℞ Erythromycin mastitis infusion . 300 mg

Infuse after each of 3 successive milkings.

190. ℞ Furaltadone and penicillin ("Altapen")

Infuse into teat canal at 12-hour intervals for 3 or more treatments.

191. ℞ Lincomycin hydrochloride . . . 200 mg

Infuse at 12- to 24-hour intervals on 3 occasions.

192. ℞ Neomycin mastitis ointment

500 mg of active substance infused into the teat canal. Repeat at 24- to 48-hour intervals if necessary.

For standard equivalents for measures, see pp. 1453 to 1456.

193. ℞ Oxytetracycline mastitis ointment

> 200 to 400 mg of active substance infused into the teat canal. Repeat at 24- to 48-hour intervals if necessary.

194. ℞ Penicillin mastitis ointment or suspension

> 100,000 u, 2 doses 24 hours apart, infused into the teat canal. (Continue regular milking.)

195. ℞ Procaine benzylpenicillin . . . 300 mg

> One infusion in each quarter at drying off.
> CAUTION: Not to be used in lactating cows.

196. ℞ Procaine benzylpenicillin . . . 300 mg
Novobiocin . . . . 250 mg

> Infuse into each quarter at drying off.
> CAUTION: Not to be used in lactating cows.

197. ℞ Penicillin and dihydrostreptomycin sulfate

> 100,000 u penicillin and 1 gm dihydrostreptomycin sulfate in emulsion-type vehicle, given by intramammary infusion. Repeat daily for 4 doses.

Anthelmintics

198. ℞ Arecoline hydrobromide

> *Dogs:* 0.75 to 1.25 mg/lb body wt orally, up to a maximum of 75 mg, after a 12-hour fast. If purgation does not occur within 1½ to 2 hours give a warm soapy enema.

199. ℞ Bephenium embonate (hydroxynaphthoate)

> *Sheep:* 125 mg/lb body wt in a single dose as a drench.
> *Dogs:* 15 mg/lb body wt orally, repeated after 6 to 10 hours.

200. ℞ Bunamidine hydrochloride

> *Dogs and cats:* 12.5 mg/lb orally after 12-hour fast. Repeat in 48 hours. In cases of *Echinococcus* infection double the dose. Vomiting or diarrhea may occur.

Read introduction to prescriptions, pp. 1458 to 1460. Note all warnings and cautions appearing on drug labels and observe all local laws and regulations pertaining to drug usage.

201. ℞ Bunamidine hydroxynaphthoate

Dogs and cats: 12.5 mg/lb orally just before feeding. Repeat in 48 hours. In cases
of *Echinococcus* infection double the dose.

202. ℞ n-Butyl chloride

For ascarids and hookworms: 1 ml/5 lb
body wt orally, up to 15 lb; 1 ml for each
additional 10 lb. Maximum dose 5 ml.
For whipworms: 0.6 to 1.0 ml/lb body wt
orally, following 18 hours' starvation.

203. ℞ Carbon disulfide

Horses: 2 ml/100 lb body wt orally, not to
exceed 20 ml.
Swine: 8 to 10 ml/100 lb body wt orally,
after 36 hours' starvation. Give in capsules
or via stomach tube.

204. ℞ Coumaphos

Cattle: Beef and dairy cattle feeds: 90 mg/
lb of body wt daily for 6 consecutive days.

205. ℞ Cyacetacide (cyanacethydrazide)

15 mg/kg subcut. or 17.5 mg/kg body wt
orally.
Maximum doses: cattle, 5 gm; *sheep, goats,
pigs,* 1 gm.
Effective against adult but not against immature lungworms.

206. ℞ Dichlorophen

Dogs and cats: 90 mg/lb body wt, given
immediately before feeding.

207. ℞ Dichlorvos

Mix into meal-type (nonpelleted) rations
just prior to feeding.
Swine: 13 to 18 mg/lb (15 to 40 mg/kg)
body wt.
Horses: 14 to 19 mg/lb.
Dogs: 15 to 24 mg/lb.
CAUTION: Do not administer to dogs having been treated with organophosphate insecticides or injectables without consulting
manufacturer's recommendations. Do not
administer in conjunction with teniacides
or n-butyl chloride or tetrachlorethylene.
Do not use in Greyhounds or Whippets.

For standard equivalents for measures, see pp. 1453 to 1456.

208. ℞ Diethylcarbamazine

For heartworm prophylaxis: Orally, daily:
2.5 mg/lb body wt from start of mosquito
season until 30 days after it ends; 5 mg/lb
for 30 days for limited exposure.

*For ascariasis (Sm. An.) and canine strongy-
loidosis:* 13 to 25 mg/lb body wt, orally
(tablets). Administer only after feeding.

For lungworms: 10 mg/lb body wt, parenterally, daily for 3 successive days or 20
mg/lb once. Effective against immature
but not against adult lungworms.

209. ℞ Disophenol

*For the common hookworm (Ancylostoma
caninum) of dogs:* 0.1 ml/lb of body wt,
subcut. once.

For Uncinaria stenocephala: 0.13 ml/lb
body wt, subcut.

210. ℞ Dithiazanine iodide

For large roundworms: 10 mg/lb orally for
5 days.

For microfilariae of heartworms: 5 mg/lb
orally 7 to 10 days.

For hookworm and whipworm: 10 mg/lb
orally for 10 days.

For intestinal threadworms: 10 mg/lb orally
for 3 weeks.

211. ℞ Dithiazanine iodide-piperazine citrate ("Dizan" solution)

Each milliliter contains 69 mg dithiazanine
iodide and 83 mg of piperazine base.

Horses: Administer via drench or stomach
tube, or mixed with daily ration as a
single dose. One ounce (30 ml)/100 lb body
wt for first 500 lb, ¾ oz/100 lb thereafter
up to 1,200 lb.

212. ℞ Arecoline acetarsol (tablets)

Dogs: 18 mg/8 lb body wt.

Cats: 18 mg/12 lb body wt. For best results give after a light meal.

CAUTION: Not recommended for puppies
under 3 months, for cats under 1 year, or
in the presence of febrile disease. Homatropine (5 mg) helps prevent vomiting.
An enema may help elimination.

**Read introduction to prescriptions, pp. 1458 to 1460.
Note all warnings and cautions appearing on drug
labels and observe all local laws and regulations pertaining to drug usage.**

213. ℞ Fenthion ("Talodex")

Use subcut. 40 to 70 mg (0.4 to 0.7 ml) per 10 lb body wt. Repeat at 2-week intervals for continuous control. Fenthion is a cholinesterase inhibitor. Do not use any drug, insecticide, pesticide or chemical having cholinesterase-inhibiting activity either simultaneously or a few days before or after treatment with fenthion.

214. ℞ Fenthion ("Talodex") 7% solution

7 mg/lb subcut.; repeat once or twice at 2-week intervals if needed.
Flea collars and other insecticides should not be used between 2 weeks before and after use of fenthion.

215. ℞ Gentian violet (enteric-coated)

30 to 60 mg, b.i.d. for 7 to 10 days. Repeat if necessary.

216. ℞ Glycobiarsol

100 mg/lb body wt, once daily, for 5 consecutive days. Tablets may be given orally or crushed in the feed.

217. ℞ Haloxon

Cattle and sheep drench: 16 to 32 mg/lb body wt (1½ oz/200 lb to 4 oz/1,000 lb).

218. ℞ Hexylresorcinol

Puppies: 0.2 to 0.4 gm.
Adult dogs: 0.6 to 1.0 gm.
Give in coated tablets or capsules after 12 hours' fast. Follow with saline cathartic after 24 hours.

219. ℞ Hygromycin

12 gm/ton of complete ration, fed continuously.

220. ℞ Kamala

Small- or large-mouth bass: 200 mg/lb (440 mg/kg) of fish for 3 days in diet.
Trout: 0.5 to 1.0% in diet (by weight) for 1 week.

For standard equivalents for measures, see pp. 1453 to 1456.

221. ℞ Lead arsenate

> *Calves:* 1 gm.
> *Mature cattle:* 2 gm.
> *Sheep:* 0.5 to 1.0 gm.
> Given orally and followed by castor oil.

222. ℞ Levamisole

> *Cattle, sheep and swine:* 2 to 5 mg/lb body wt, given as drench, bolus, pellet or water formulation.

223. ℞ Methyridine

> *Parenterally or orally:* 200 mg/kg body wt.
> *Maximum doses: cattle,* 54 gm; *sheep,* 9 gm.
> CAUTION: Toxic at twice the therapeutic dose; do not use for 2 weeks after treatment with any organophosphates.

224. ℞ Niclosamide

> *Cattle:* 22 mg/lb body wt as a drench.
> *Sheep:* 35 mg/lb body wt as a drench.
> *Dogs and cats:* 50 mg/lb body wt.
> Effective against all dog and cat tapeworms except *Echinococcus*, for which 125 mg/lb is claimed to have 50% efficiency.

225. ℞ Niclosamide

> 3 mg/gm of feed for 24 to 36 hours, to provide 450 mg/kg of body wt. Repeat in 8 to 10 days.

226. ℞ Phenothiazine

> *Cattle:* 10 gm/100 lb body wt, not to exceed 60 gm. May be fed prophylactically at the rate of 2 gm daily for 1 month following therapeutic dosing.
> *Sheep:* 12.5 gm for lambs under 50 lb, 25 gm for adults.
> *Horses:* 3 gm/100 lb body wt. Do not exceed 30 gm.

227. ℞ Phthalofyne ("Whipcide")

> 100 mg/lb body wt given once orally or IV.
> CAUTION: Use IV only when oral treatment is impractical or unfeasible. Do not use in animals with chronic nephritis, hepatitis, pancreatitis or cardiac insufficiency.

Read introduction to prescriptions, pp. 1458 to 1460. Note all warnings and cautions appearing on drug labels and observe all local laws and regulations pertaining to drug usage.

228. ℞ Piperazine salts

Salt	% Active Piperazine
Adipate	37
Chloride	48
Citrate	35
Dihydrochloride	50–53
Hexahydrate	44
Phosphate	42
Sulfate	46

Doses are given in terms of piperazine base (see above). For specific dosages, see product information.

Cattle, sheep, horses, swine, most large zoo animals: 50 mg/lb body wt.

Cats, dogs: 20 to 30 mg/lb body wt.

Laboratory rats & mice: 400 to 500 mg/100 ml drinking water.

229. ℞ Piperazine salt of niclosamide ("Mansonil")

Cattle: 28 mg/lb body wt as a drench.

Sheep: 42 mg/lb body wt as a drench.

Dogs, cats: 55 mg/lb body wt.

230. ℞ Piperazine hexahydrate

Growing pigs: 50 mg of piperazine base per pound body weight in drinking water (withhold all drinking water for the preceding 24 hours).

231. ℞ Piperazine—carbon disulfide complex with phenothiazine ("Parvex Plus")

Horses: Administer by stomach tube, 1 fl oz/100 lb body wt.

232. ℞ Piperazine—carbon disulfide complex ("Parvex")

Horses: Administer via stomach tube, 20 to 40 gm/500 lb body wt.

Swine: 60 mg/lb body wt, mixed in about one-fourth of the daily ration.

233. ℞ Pyrantel tartrate

Horses: 5 gm/100 lb body wt, given in the feed.

Swine: 10 mg/lb body wt, given in the feed.

For standard equivalents for measures, see pp. 1453 to 1456.

234. ℞ **Stibophen 6.3% solution**

> Administer according to manufacturer's directions.

235. ℞ **Tetrachloroethylene**

> *Dogs:* 0.1 ml/lb body wt in 1 dose orally (in capsule), after 12 hours' starvation.

236. ℞ **Tetramisole**

> *Orally:* 3.6 mg/lb body wt for the "L"-form, 7.3 mg/lb body wt for the "DL" mixture.

237. ℞ **Thiabendazole ("Thibenzole," "Equizole," "Omnizole")**

> *Cattle:* Routine worming: 3 gm/100 lb body wt orally; severe parasitism and infection with *Cooperia*: 5 gm/100 lb body wt orally.
> *Sheep:* Routine worming: 2 gm/100 lb body wt as a drench; severe parasitism: 3 gm/100 lb body wt as a drench.
> *Swine:* For *Strongyloides ransomi:* paste formulation, at 30 to 40 mg/lb body wt.
> *Horses:* 20 mg/lb body wt orally. Double the dose when treating for ascarids.
> *Laboratory animals:* 22 to 45 mg/lb body wt orally. Repeat after 2 weeks if severely infected.

238. ℞ **Thiabendazole—piperazine phosphate ("Equizole A")**

> Each ounce contains 6.67 gm thiabendazole and 8.33 gm piperazine base.
> *Horses:* 1½ oz/500 lb body wt.

239. ℞ **Arsenamide ("Thiacetarsamide") 1% solution**

> 0.1 ml/lb body wt, IV, b.i.d. for 2 days. Restrict exercise for up to 2 months. If pulmonary reaction occurs, give single dose of 20 mg prednisone IM followed by daily injections of antibiotics.
> NOTE: Avoid perivascular leakage since arsenamide is a sclerosing drug.

240. ℞ **Toluene**

> 0.2 ml/lb body wt orally in capsules or by stomach tube.

Read introduction to prescriptions, pp. 1458 to 1460. Note all warnings and cautions appearing on drug labels and observe all local laws and regulations pertaining to drug usage.

241. ℞ Trichlorfon 50% solution

Cattle: 1.5 ml (0.75 gm/100 lb body wt subcut). Maximum dose: 6.5 ml.
Horses: Doses vary with feed or stomach tube administration. Follow label instructions.

242. ℞ Trichlorfon, phenothiazine, piperazine mixture ("Dyrex T.F.")

Trichlorfon . . . . 3.64 gm
Phenothiazine . . . . . . 2.50 gm
Piperazine HCl* . . . . . 14.76 gm
* Equivalent to 8 gm of piperazine base.
Horses: Use total mixture for each 100 lb of body wt.

Insecticides and Acaricides

243. ℞ "Gammex" suspension

Gamma isomer of benezene
hexachloride 1%
Use by diluting 1:40 parts water as a wash, dip or spray. Repeat as indicated.
CAUTION: Not for use on cats or foxes. May be absorbed through the skin; user should wash with soap and water after use and wear mask if used as a spray.

244. ℞ "Mulzyl"

Benzyl benzoate . . . . . 20 %
Gamma benzene hexachloride 0.9 %
Chlorobutanol (chloral
derivative) . . . . 0.5 %
Phenylmercuric borate . . . 0.02%
Give 2 to 3 applications at intervals of 4 to 7 days. Do not get in the eye.
CAUTION: Do not apply to cats. Shake well before using. Wash hands thoroughly after using.

245. ℞ Carbaryl ("Sevin") 0.5% suspension

8 lb of 50% carbaryl wettable powder per 100 gal. water.
CAUTION: Do not use on lactating animals. Do not treat within 7 days of slaughter, nor more often than once every 4 days.

For standard equivalents for measures, see pp. 1453 to 1456.

246. ℞ Coumaphos 0.03 to 0.5% suspension

1 to 16 lb of 25% coumaphos wettable powder per 100 gal. water. As a spray or dip
for use on cattle, sheep, goats and swine.
Only 0.03% may be used on lactating dairy
cattle; 0.06 to 0.125% for use on beef cattle,
sheep, goats and swine. Only 0.5% for
grub control, combined with louse control
on beef or nonlactating dairy cattle.
CAUTION: Do not treat sick, convalescent or
stressed animals or those less than 3 months
old. Do not treat sheep or goats within 15
days of slaughter. Do not treat dairy dry
cows or heifers with 14 days of freshening.
Do not apply in conjunction with oral
drenches or other internal medication or
other organic phosphates. Do not treat
within 10 days of shipping, weaning or exposure to disease. 0.5% coumaphos will kill
cattle grubs, thus must not be on cattle
after the cut-off date for grub control unless these cattle have been treated earlier
with systemic insecticides. Do not re-treat
within 10 days.

**247. ℞ Coumaphos 0.25% suspension (dip or
spray)**

Mix 8 lb coumaphos 25% wettable powder
with each 100 gal. water in dipping vat.
Agitate dip suspension thoroughly prior to
each use to assure uniform suspension during use. Dip animals in standard fashion.
CAUTION: Do not dip dairy cattle within
14 days of freshening, or calves less than
3 months old.
For poultry: direct application: 1 gal. (of
wettable powder) per 100 birds: as a spray,
for northern fowl mite; for lice, twice this
amount is recommended.

**248. ℞ Coumaphos 0.375 to 0.5% suspension
(spray)**

Mix 12 to 16 lb coumaphos 25% wettable
powder with 100 gal. of water. Spray cattle,
wetting skin thoroughly. Spray pressures of
300 lb or higher recommended. Maintain
adequate agitation in spray tank to insure
uniform suspension during use. The higher
concentration needed in northern areas, or

**Read introduction to prescriptions, pp. 1458 to 1460.
Note all warnings and cautions appearing on drug
labels and observe all local laws and regulations pertaining to drug usage.**

for late fall application when long hair coats make thorough wetting of the skin difficult.
CAUTION: Do not treat dairy cattle within 14 days of freshening, or calves less than 3 months old.

249. ℞ Coumaphos 4% solution

Pour evenly along animal's backline ½ fl oz/100 lb body wt; maximum 4 fl oz per animal.
CAUTION: Do not treat lactating dairy animals or dairy cattle within 14 days of freshening, or calves less than 3 months old.

250. ℞ Coumaphos 0.5% dust

Use 1 to 2 oz per animal on sheep or goats.
CAUTION: Do not treat within 15 days of slaughter.

251. ℞ Coumaphos 1% oil solution

11.6% coumaphos emulsifiable
concentrate . . . . 1 gal.
No. 2 fuel oil or diesel oil . . 113 gal.

For saturating back rubbers at 1 gal./20 ft of cable.
CAUTION: Do not apply in conjunction with oral drenches or other internal medication, such as phenothiazine, or with other organic phosphates. Do not use with synergized pyrethrins, allethrin, or synergist. For dairy cattle suspend at a height that will prevent straddling.

252. ℞ Coumaphos 5% dust

CAUTION: Do not contaminate feed or water.

253. ℞ Crufomate ("Ruelene") 0.375% emulsion

1.5 gal. 25% crufomate emulsifiable solution per 100 gal. water. A spray for lice and grubs on cattle.
CAUTION: Must not be used after the area cut-off date for grub control with systemic insecticides. Treat only once. Do not apply within 28 days of slaughter. Do not treat lactating dairy cattle nor dairy dry cows or heifers within 28 days of freshening. Do not treat calves under 3 months old.

For standard equivalents for measures, see pp. 1453 to 1456.

Do not apply within 10 days before or after
shipping or weaning or after exposure to
contagious or infectious diseases. Do not
treat sick animals, nor animals under stress
from castration, dehorning, disease, overexertion, or excitement.

254. ℞ Crufomate ("Ruelene") 5% emulsion

1 gal. of 24% crufomate emulsifiable concentrate to 4 gal. water. Use as a pour-on
at 1 fl oz/100 lb body wt. Cattle over
800 lb, use 8 oz only.
CAUTION: Do not apply within 28 days of
slaughter. Do not treat lactating dairy
cattle nor dairy dry cows or heifers within
28 days of freshening. Use this treatment
only on cattle previously treated for grubs.
Do not use more often than every 28 days.
Do not treat calves under 3 months old
nor sick, convalescent or stressed livestock.
Do not treat within 10 days before or after
weaning or shipping or after exposure to
contagious or infectious diseases. Do not
apply in conjunction with oral drenches or
other internal medications or with other
organic phosphates.

**255. ℞ Crotoxyphos ("Ciodrin") 0.2%, di-
chlorvos ("Vapona") 0.05% emulsion**

2.5 pt 10% crotoxyphos, 2.5% dichlorvos
emulsifiable solution in 16 gal. water.
CAUTION: Do not use more than 1 gal. per
cow. Do not spray more often than every
7 days. Do not contaminate milk or milking utensils, nor feed hay or water.

**256. ℞ Crotoxyphos ("Ciodrin") 0.1 to 0.3%
emulsion**

1 to 3 qt of crotoxyphos emulsifiable solution (3.2 lb/gal.) in 100 gal. of water. Use
low concentration for high gallonage spraying, 2 to 3 gal. per cow; the high concentration for application of 1 to 2 qt per cow.
CAUTION: Do not apply more than once a
week.

**Read introduction to prescriptions, pp. 1458 to 1460.
Note all warnings and cautions appearing on drug
labels and observe all local laws and regulations pertaining to drug usage.**

257. ℞ Crotoxyphos ("Ciodrin") 0.8%,
dichlorvos ("Vapona") 0.2 % oil
solution

10% crotoxyphos, 2.5% dichlorvos
emulsifiable solution . . . . . 1 gal.
No. 2 fuel oil or diesel oil . . 16 gal.
For saturating back rubbers at 1 gal./20 ft
of cable. May be used for dairy cattle.

258. ℞ Crotoxyphos ("Ciodrin") 1% oil
solution

14.4% crotoxyphos emulsifiable
solution . . . . 1 qt
No. 2 fuel oil or diesel oil . . 4 gal.
For saturating back rubbers at 1 gal./20 ft
of cable. May be used for dairy cattle as
well as beef cattle.

259. ℞ Crotoxyphos ("Ciodrin") 3% dust

CAUTION: Avoid contamination of milk and
milking utensils. Do not place dust bags
where dairy cattle will be dusted coming
into the barn. Do not treat cattle under
6 months of age. Brahman cattle may exhibit hypersensitivity.

260. ℞. Crotoxyphos ("Ciodrin")—dichlorvos
("Vapona") oil-base spray

Crotoxyphos 1.00%
Dichlorvos 0.25%
Apply by hand or electric atomizer or automatic cattle sprayer at not over 2 oz per
animal daily.
CAUTION: Do not use in milk rooms. Do
not contaminate milk or milking utensils.

261. ℞ Diazinon 0.03% suspension or emulsion

1 pt 25% diazinon emulsifiable solution or
½ lb 50% diazinon wettable powder in 100
gal. of water.
CAUTION: Accepted only for use on sheep
(suspension) or dogs (emulsion). Do not
treat sheep within 14 days of slaughter. Do
not use on lambs less than 2 weeks old. No
longer approved for use as a barn spray or
in milk rooms in U.S.A.

For standard equivalents for measures, see pp. 1453 to 1456.

262. ℞ Diazinon 1% suspension or emulsion

4 gal. of 25% diazinon emulsifiable solution
or 16 lb of 50% diazinon wettable powder
per 100 gal. of water.
Residual spray for other fly resting places.
No longer approved for use as a barn spray
or in milk rooms in U.S.A.
CAUTION: Do not use on animals. Do not
contaminate feed, troughs or waterers. Do
not use around premises occupied by ducks
or other poultry.

263. ℞ Diazinon 2% dust

CAUTION: For use on sheep. Do not treat
within 14 days of slaughter.

264. ℞ Dichlorvos oil-base spray

Dichlorvos . . . . . . 0.5 to 1.0%

(May include pyrethrins and synergist also.)
Apply by hand or electric atomizer or automatic cattle sprayer at not over 2 oz per
cow daily.

265. ℞ Dimethoate 1% emulsion

2 gal. of 25% dimethoate emulsifiable solution per 100 gal. of water.
Residual spray for spraying of premises
only.
CAUTION: Do not use on animals. Do not
contaminate feed, mangers, waterers, milk
or milking utensils. All animals should be
out of the barn during spraying. Do not
spray in the milk house.

266. ℞ Dioxathion ("Delnav") 0.15% emulsion

2 qt 30% dioxathion emulsifiable solution
per 100 gal. of water.
CAUTION: Do not use on dairy cattle. Do
not reapply within 2 weeks. Do not treat
swine less than 3 months old.

**Read introduction to prescriptions, pp. 1458 to 1460.
Note all warnings and cautions appearing on drug
labels and observe all local laws and regulations pertaining to drug usage.**

267. ℞ Dioxathion ("Delnav") 1.5% oil
solution

30% dioxathion emulsifiable solution	**1 pt**
No. 2 fuel oil or diesel oil . . .	**19 pt**

For saturating back rubbers at 1 gal./20 ft of cable.
CAUTION: Do not use on lactating dairy cattle.

268. ℞ Famophos ("Famix")

Thoroughly mix 12 lb Famix Premix (33.3% famophos) per ton of feed supplement. Feed at ¼ lb/100 lb body wt per day for 10 days.
CAUTION: Do not treat beef within 4 days of slaughter, lactating dairy animals, or dairy cattle within 21 days of freshening.

269. ℞ Famophos ("Warbex") 13.2% solution
(pour-on)

Pour evenly along animal's backline ½ fl oz/100 lb body wt; maximum 4 fl oz/animal.
CAUTION: Do not treat calves under **3** months old, beef within 35 days of slaughter, lactating dairy animals, or dairy cattle within 21 days of freshening.

270. ℞ Fenthion ("Baytex") 1% emulsion

2 gal. of 45% fenthion emulsifiable concentrate per 100 gal. water.
Residual spray for premises spraying only.
CAUTION: All animals must be out of the barn. Avoid contamination of feed, water, milking utensils. Do not spray in the milk house. Wear respiratory and protective clothing during spraying.

271. ℞ Lindane 0.03% emulsion or suspension

20 oz 20% emulsifiable solution or 1 lb 25% wettable powder per 100 gal. of water.
CAUTION: Do not use on dairy cattle. Do not treat within 30 days of slaughter.

272. ℞ Lindane 0.5% dust

On large animals, up to double strength can be used.

For standard equivalents for measures, see pp. 1453 to 1456.

273. ℞ Malathion 0.5% suspension or emulsion

16 lb 25% wettable powder or 0.8 gal. 57%
emulsifiable solution per 100 gal. of water.
CAUTION: Do not use on lactating dairy
cattle. Do not apply to dairy dry stock
or heifers within 14 days of freshening. Do
not use on calves or swine less than a
month old.

274. ℞ Malathion 2% oil solution
57% malathion emulsifiable
solution . . . . 1 pt
SAE 30 motor oil . . . . . . 1 gal.
No. 2 fuel oil . . . . 3 gal.

For saturating back rubbers at 1 gal./20 ft
of cable.
CAUTION: Do not use on dairy cattle.

275. ℞ Malathion 5% dust
Malathion . . . . 1 lb
Diluent (clay, talc) . . . . . 19 lb

For hornfly control on dairy cattle use 3
tablespoons per animal, on the back only,
every 10 to 14 days.
CAUTION: Avoid contamination of mangers
and waterers, milk and milk utensils.

276. ℞ Methoxychlor 0.5% suspension or
emulsion

8 lb 50% wettable powder or 2 gal. of 25%
emulsifiable solution per 100 gal. of water.
For stable fly control by spraying of
premises only: Use double the above concentrations.
CAUTION: Do not use on lactating dairy
cattle, nor on dairy dry stock or heifers
within 14 days of freshening. Do not use
over 2 qt per animal nor more often than
once every 3 weeks.

277. ℞ Methoxychlor 5% oil solution
25% methoxychlor emulsifiable
solution . . . . 1 qt
No. 2 fuel oil or diesel oil . . . 4 qt

For saturating back rubbers at 1 gal./20 ft
of cable.

**Read introduction to prescriptions, pp. 1458 to 1460.
Note all warnings and cautions appearing on drug
labels and observe all local laws and regulations pertaining to drug usage.**

CAUTION: Do not use on lactating dairy cattle. Do not allow dairy dry stock or heifers access to back rubbers within 14 days of freshening.

278. ℞ Methoxychlor 10% dust

CAUTION: Do not use on lactating dairy cattle, nor on dairy dry stock or heifers within 14 days of freshening.

279. Methoxychlor 50% wettable powder

For hornfly control on dairy cattle, use 1 tablespoon per animal, on back only, every 3 weeks. For sheep keds and lice, use 1 tablespoon per animal after shearing.

CAUTION: Avoid contamination of mangers and waterers.

280. ℞ 0.025% Pyrethrins and 0.25% piperonyl butoxide emulsion

Prepare by diluting 2½ gal. of concentrate containing 1% pyrethrins and 10% piperonyl butoxide or MGK 264 to 100 gal. of water.

NOTE: For all birds and mammals.

281. ℞ Synergized pyrethrum emulsion
Pyrethrins 0.05%
Piperonyl butoxide . . . . 0.5 %

For emulsion spraying dilute a 1% pyrethrin concentrate with 9 parts of water and use about 1 qt per animal. Repeat application when fly annoyance recommences.

For automatic treadle sprayers use concentration to 0.5%, apply 2 ml twice daily. MGK 264 may be used instead of piperonyl butoxide.

For space spraying against adult mosquitoes, use Microsol Fog machine.

282. ℞ Synergized pyrethrum oil-base spray
Pyrethrins . . . . 0.05 to 0.1%
Piperonyl butoxide . 0.40 to 0.8%
Cattle spray base oil . 99.55 to 99.1%

Apply by hand or electric atomizer at milking time, not exceeding 2 oz per cow. Also useful on any mammal to repel and kill flies. May be used in the milk room, or residence at 2 oz/1,000 cu ft of space.

For standard equivalents for measures, see pp. 1453 to 1456.

283. ℞ Synergized pyrethrum and repellent spray

Pyrethrins	0.03 to	0.1%
Synergist	0.25 to	1.0%
Repellent	0.2 to	8.0%
Cattle spray base oil	99.52 to	90.9%

The repellent may be Stabilene, MGK 11 or MGK 326. The synergist may be piperonyl butoxide, MGK 264 or sulfoxide. For use on all mammals including dairy cows. Apply lightly with a hand or electric atomizer, wetting hair ends only, not over 2 oz per animal. Repeat as necessary.

284. ℞ Ronnel

Tablets	250 mg
Emulsifiable concentrate . .	33.3%

Demodectic mange: Both oral and topical treatment.
Orally: Tablets (in divided doses) at 25 mg/lb of body wt daily.
Topically: Diluted to 1% applied over entire body every 4 days. Both oral and topical application continued for a 30-day period.

285. ℞ Ronnel

Tablets	250 mg
Emulsifiable concentrate . .	33.3%

Orally: 25 mg/lb body wt daily.
Topically: Diluted to 0.25% as a dip or sponged over entire body.

286. ℞ Ronnel 0.25 or 0.5% emulsion

½ to 1 gal. of 41.2% ronnel, or 1 to 2 gal. of 24% ronnel, emulsifiable solution per 100 gal. of water for use as a spray or dip. Only 0.5% for wool maggots on sheep or goats.

CAUTION: Do not use on lactating dairy cattle nor on dairy dry stock or heifers within 21 days of freshening. Do not retreat within 2 weeks. Meat animals must not be treated within the following periods before slaughter; hogs—6 weeks, cattle—8 weeks, sheep and goats—12 weeks. Do not use other cholinesterase inhibitors simultaneously or within a few days before or after treatment with ronnel.

Read introduction to prescriptions, pp. 1458 to 1460. Note all warnings and cautions appearing on drug labels and observe all local laws and regulations pertaining to drug usage.

287. ℞ Ronnel 0.5% (topical)

> Mix 1 part of 5% ronnel smear with 9 parts
> of water. Apply as a wash on and around
> infested areas. Repeat as necessary.
> CAUTION: Do not slaughter within 21 days.
> Injurious to eyes, keep away. Wash from
> hands and skin after use.

288. ℞ Ronnel 1% emulsion

> 4 gal. of 24% or 2 gal. of 41.2% ronnel
> emulsifiable concentrate per 100 gal. water.
> Residual spray for premise spraying only.
> CAUTION: Do not use on animals. Do not
> contaminate feed, troughs, waterers, or
> milking utensils.

289. ℞ Ronnel 1% oil solution

> 1 gal. of 41.2% or 2 gal. of 24% ronnel
> emulsifiable solution, in No. 2 fuel oil or
> diesel oil, 55 gal.
>
> For saturating back rubbers at 1 gal./20 ft
> of cable.
> CAUTION: Do not use on lactating dairy
> cattle. Remove back rubbers at least 14
> days before cattle go to slaughter. Do not
> allow dairy dry stock or heifers access to
> back rubbers within 21 days of freshening.

290. ℞ Ronnel insecticidal mineral block or
granules (5.5% ronnel)

> Feed continuously free choice, summer and
> fall for a period of at least 75 days. Con-
> sumption should be 0.25 lb/100 lb body wt
> per month for effective grub control.
> CAUTION: Do not feed within 21 days of
> slaughter (beef) or freshening (dairy). Do
> not feed salt or other minerals when cattle
> are being fed this medication.

291. ℞ Ronnel 0.26% in feed

> Mix 1 lb insecticidal mineral granules (5.5%
> ronnel) with 20 lb other feed. Feed 0.3 lb of
> the medicated feed per 100 lb body wt
> per day for 14 consecutive days. Mix
> thoroughly with the daily feed ration. The
> balance of the daily ration should not in-
> clude ronnel-medicated feed.
> CAUTION: Do not feed within 28 days of
> slaughter (beef) or freshening (dairy). Do
> not feed salt or other minerals when cattle
> are being fed this medication.

For standard equivalents for measures, see pp. 1453 to 1456.

292. ℞ Ronnel 0.6% in feed

Thoroughly mix 30 lb, 40% ronnel with
1,970 lb of feed ingredients to make 1 ton
of medicated feed. Feed 0.3 lb of the
medicated feed per 100 lb body wt per day
for 7 consecutive days. Mix thoroughly
with the daily feed ration. The balance of
the daily feed ration should not include ronnel-
medicated feed.

CAUTION: Do not feed within 60 days of
slaughter (beef) or freshening (dairy). Do
not feed to lactating dairy animals.

293. ℞ Ronnel ("Ectoral") 33.3% emulsifiable concentrate

Use 1 oz emulsifiable concentrate to 1 qt
of water for 1% solution. May be sponged
on animals 3 times at 7- to 10-day intervals. For dogs only. For cats use 0.25%
solution.

CAUTION: Use rubber gloves for applying
sponging. Wash hands thoroughly after
each application. Do not use any drug,
insecticide, pesticide or chemical having
cholinesterase inhibiting activity either simultaneously or within a few days before
or after treatment.

294. ℞ Rotenone 0.0125% suspension*

1 lb cube- or derris-root powder containing
5% rotenone per 100 gal. of water; 20 lb
wettable sulfur may be added per 100 gal.
of water to increase ease of preparation of
the dip and effectiveness. For all animals
except swine.

* 0.5 lb detergent per 100 gal. of water
facilitates wetting and mixing.

295. ℞ Rotenone 0.5% suspension*

4 lb cube- or derris-root powder containing
5% rotenone per 5 gal. of water. For external application. Keep mixture well agitated.

* ½ oz detergent per 5 gal. of water facilitates emulsification.

**Read introduction to prescriptions, pp. 1458 to 1460.
Note all warnings and cautions appearing on drug
labels and observe all local laws and regulations pertaining to drug usage.**

296. ℞ Rotenone 1% dust

> 1 lb cube- or derris-root powder containing 5% rotenone per 4 lb or sulfur.
> For use on birds and mammals *except swine.*
> Cube or derris-root powder

297. ℞ Rotenone 1% dust

> Cube- or derris-root powder
>   containing 5% rotenone . . **20 lb**
> Diluent (talc, clay, etc.) . . . **78 lb**
> SAE No. 10 motor oil . . . . . **2 lb**
> For range flock sheep ked and louse control.

298. ℞ Rotenone powder

> Rotenone **1.00%**
> Other cube extractives . . . **1.66%**
> Pyrethrins **0.54%**
> Sprinkle on coat and rub thoroughly. Repeat after 3 days if necessary. Dusting bedding and quarters with this powder is advisable.

299. ℞ Ruelene 0.375% emulsion spray

> Mix 1½ gal. of 25% ruelene emulsion concentrate with 100 gal. of water.
> Spray cattle, wetting skin on back and sides thoroughly. Spray pressures of 300 lb or higher recommended.
> CAUTION: Do not treat within 28 days of slaughter (beef) or freshening (dairy).

300. ℞ Ruelene 8.3% emulsion (pour-on)

> Mix ½ gal. of 25% ruelene emulsion concentrate with 1 gal. of water. Pour evenly along animal's backline 1 fl oz/100 lb body wt up to 800 lb animal, but not more than 8 oz/animal.
> CAUTION: Do not treat within 28 days of slaughter (beef) or freshening (dairy). Do not apply in extremely hot or humid weather; the ruelene solvent may cause dermatitis under these conditions.

301. ℞ Ruelene 9.4% solution (pour-on)

> Pour evenly along animal's backline 1 fl oz/100 lb body wt, up to 800-lb animal, but not more than 8 oz/animal.
> CAUTION: Do not treat within 28 days of slaughter (beef) or freshening (dairy).

For standard equivalents for measures, see pp. 1453 to 1456.

302. ℞ Stirofos ("Rabon") 1% suspension or emulsion

> 16 lb 50% wettable powder or 4 gal. 25% Rabon emulsifiable concentrate per 100 gal. water. Residual spray for premises spraying only.
> CAUTION: All animals must be out of the barn. Avoid contamination of feed, water, milking utensils. Do not spray in the milk house.

303. ℞ "Thionium" shampoo with lindane

Potassium tetrathionate . . . 2.00%
Lindane 0.25%

> Use for routine shampooing of dogs.
> CAUTION: Do not use on cats or nursing puppies. Do not use more than once a week. Wash hands with soap and water after use.

304. ℞ Toxaphene 0.5% suspension or emulsion

> 10 lb 40% wettable powder or ⅔ gal. 60% emulsifiable solution per 100 gal. of water. For use on beef cattle, horses, sheep or swine.
> CAUTION: Highly toxic for dogs and cats. Do not use on dairy cattle. Do not treat within 28 days of slaughter.

305. ℞ Toxaphene 5% dust

> CAUTION: Do not contaminate feed or water. Do not use on dairy cattle or dairy goats. Do not treat within 28 days of slaughter, or allow cattle access to dust bags within 30 days of slaughter.

306. ℞ Toxaphene 5% oil solution

60% toxaphene emulsifiable
concentrate . . . . 1 gal.
No. 2 fuel oil or diesel oil . . 14 gal.

> For saturating back rubbers at 1 gal./50 ft of cable.
> CAUTION: Do not use on dairy cattle. Do not allow cattle access to back rubbers within 28 days of slaughter.

Read introduction to prescriptions, pp. 1458 to 1460. Note all warnings and cautions appearing on drug labels and observe all local laws and regulations pertaining to drug usage.

307. ℞ Trichlorfon 1% solution

Mix 10 lb of 80% trichlorfon soluble powder with 100 gal. of water. Spray cattle, wetting skin thoroughly. Spray pressures of 300 lb or higher recommended.

CAUTION: Do not treat beef cattle within 14 days of slaughter, calves under 3 months old, lactating dairy animals, or dairy cattle within 14 days of freshening.

308. ℞ Trichlorfon 8% solution

Pour evenly along animal's backline ½ fl oz/100 lb body wt; maximum 4 fl oz/animal.

CAUTION: Do not treat calves under 3 months old, beef within 21 days of slaughter, lactating dairy animals, or dairy cattle within 7 days of freshening.

309. ℞ Benzylbenzoate 25 or 50% emulsion

Dogs only: Apply thoroughly to affected areas.

310. ℞ Benzylbenzoate 25.0%
Lindane 1.0%

In emulsion or ointment base.
Dogs only: Apply thoroughly to affected areas daily on alternate weeks or every third day.

311. ℞ "Canex"
Chloroform . . . . 7.5 %
Rotenone 0.12%
Other ether extractives of
derris 0.38%
Inert ingredients 92.00%

Cats and dogs: Thoroughly massage into affected areas.

312. ℞ Lime and sulfur solution

(30 to 32% calcium polysulfide)
Dilute 1 qt with 4 gal. of water, and apply as dip or wash.
Large animals: Treatment repeated at 10- to 12-day intervals.
Dogs and cats: Treatment repeated at 5-day intervals.

For standard equivalents for measures, see pp. 1453 to 1456.

313. ℞ Lindane 0.06% emulsion or suspension

1¼ qt of 20% emulsifiable concentrate or 2 lb of 25% wettable powder per 100 gal. of water. Apply as dip, wash or spray.

CAUTION: Do not slaughter within 60 days of last treatment. Do not use on dairy cattle. Do not use on weak or emaciated sheep or very young lambs.

314. ℞ Lindane 0.1% suspension

Apply as dip or wash.

CAUTION: Not to be used on cats or their bedding.

315. ℞ Nicotine sulfate 0.04% solution

1 pt 40% concentrate per 125 gal. of water. Use as a dip or wash.

316. ℞ Sulfur Ointment USP

Apply thoroughly to affected areas once a day.

317. ℞ Caraway oil . . . . 1 part
Petrolatum . . . . 4 parts

Apply to affected areas of skin.

318. ℞ Chlordane 0.5% dip

Bathe animal or sponge on and let dry. Repeat after 7 days if necessary.

319. ℞ Lindane 1% emulsion

1 qt 20% lindane emulsifiable solution per 5 gal. of water.

As a roost paint: Apply 1 pt/150 ft of roost. Head lice are not controlled by this method. Effective for 1 month.

As a litter spray: Apply just enough to wet the surface of the litter. Effective for 3 months.

CAUTION: Use only when house is empty. Avoid contamination of feed, troughs and waterers. Do not use on market poultry.

Read introduction to prescriptions, pp. 1458 to 1460. Note all warnings and cautions appearing on drug labels and observe all local laws and regulations pertaining to drug usage.

320. ℞ Malathion 2% emulsion

> 4 fl oz 57% malathion emulsifiable solution per gallon of water.
> *As a roost paint:* 1 pt/150 ft of roost. Repeat after 10 days or as necessary. Head lice are not controlled by this method.
> *As house spray:* Apply liberally to walls, ceilings, roosts, litter, nests and adjacent areas. Will control poultry mites as well as lice.
> CAUTION: Do not contaminate feed, troughs or waterers.

321. ℞ Malathion 4% dust

> Liberally dust litter, floor space, nests, roosts, using approximately 1 lb/40 sq ft or use 2 lb per dusting box. A 2- by 3-ft box will care for 100 hens.
> Use a shaker can or rotary duster to treat individual birds—1 lb/160 birds. Repeat after 4 to 8 weeks or when necessary.
> CAUTION: Do not contaminate feed, troughs or waterers.

322. ℞ Nicotine sulfate 40%

> *As a roost paint:* Use 0.5 lb/100 ft of perch. Apply just before roosting time and provide adequate ventilation. Repeat after 10 days.
> NOTE: Head lice will not be controlled by this method.

323. ℞ Rotenone powder

> 5% rotenone, cube or derris . . 1 part
> Talc or sulfur . . . . 4 parts
> Dust all birds thoroughly using 1 lb/100 birds.

Antiprotozoan Agents

324. ℞ 2-Amino-5-nitrothiazole ("Enheptin" Soluble)

> *Turkeys: Prophylaxis:* 0.015% (1 oz/24 gal. of water).
> *Treatment:* 0.03% (1 oz/12 gal. of water) for 7 days.

325. ℞ Amprolium

> Given in enough drinking water to make a 0.024 or 0.012% solution, depending on severity. Continue for 5 to 7 days. Reduce to 0.006% for an additional 2 weeks.

For standard equivalents for measures, see pp. 1453 to 1456.

326. ℞ Sodium arsanilate or arsanilic acid

Prophylaxis: 0.01% (90 gm/ton) in feed.
Treatment: 0.025 to 0.4% in feed for **5 to 6** days for control of swine dysentery. Withdraw 5 days before slaughter for human consumption.

327. ℞ Dimetridazole

Soluble powder
Prophylaxis: 18.2 gm/50 gal. of water (0.01%).
Treatment: 36.4 to 72.8 gm/50 gal. of water (0.02 to 0.04%).
Tablets
Treatment: 125 mg per bird weighing **1 to 10** lb, 250 mg for sick birds over 10 lb.

328. ℞ Diminazene aceturate

For babesiasis in cow, horse, sheep and dog, and for *Trypanosoma vivax* and *T. congolense* infections, a single dose of 3.5 mg/kg body wt subcut. or IM will usually relieve clinical signs in 24 hours. For persistent trypanosome infections, 8 mg/kg body wt may be given. Maximum dose is 4 gm. Local reactions at site of infection may be severe in horses.

329. ℞ Ethidium bromide 1% aqueous solution

Active against *Trypanosoma congolense* and *T. vivax*; less active against *T. brucei*; inactive against *T. evansi*.
Treatment: 45 mg/100 lb body wt, subcut. or preferably IM.

330. ℞ Furazolidone

Prophylaxis: 100 gm/ton of ration. Feed continuously.
Treatment: 200 gm/ton of ration. Feed **2** or 3 weeks.

331. ℞ Homidium bromide ("Ethidium")

Horses and cattle: 0.45 to 0.7 mg/lb body wt, subcut., IV or IM.
Dogs: 0.45 mg/lb body wt subcut., IV or IM.

332. ℞ Imidocarb dihydrochloride 10% solution

0.45 ml/100 lb body wt, IM.

Read introduction to prescriptions, pp. 1458 to 1460. Note all warnings and cautions appearing on drug labels and observe all local laws and regulations pertaining to drug usage.

333. ℞ Isometamidium ("Samorin")

> *Treatment:* 1.0 to 2.0 mg/kg body wt (½ this dose in dogs), IM.
> *Prophylaxis:* 0.5 to 1.0 mg/kg, IM. Local reaction may be severe.

334. ℞ Nitarsone ("Histostat-50")

> 0.01875 to 0.025% (¾ to 1 lb/ton) in feed. Feed until 5 days before marketing.

335. ℞ Nithiazide ("Hepzide")

> *Prophylaxis:* Depending on severity of exposure, from 0.025 to 0.04% in the feed (1 lb 11 oz to 2 lb 11 oz of the 30% premix per ton), fed continuously until a day before marketing or 20 weeks of age.
> *Treatment:* 0.02% in the drinking water (1 lb of 16.7% soluble powder per 100 gal. of water) for 7 to 10 days. Tablets of 100 mg may be given to individual birds at the rate of 1 tablet per 5 lb body wt for 4 to 7 days.

336. ℞ Pamaquine naphthoate

> 0.22 to 0.45 gm/100 lb body wt, IM daily.

337. ℞ Phenamidine isethionate 2% solution

> 0.25 ml/lb body wt, subcut.

338. ℞ Phenanthridinium-pyrimidinium ("Prothidium")

> *Prophylaxis:* 2 mg/kg body wt provides protection for 3 to 5 months with no undesirable reactions except the local reaction from subcut. injection.

339. ℞ Quinacrine hydrochloride . . . 0.9 gm
Diiodohydroxyquin . . . . . . 0.9 gm
Water . . . . 100 ml

> Spray the solution with an atomizer onto the pellets and hay until the food ingredients are slightly damp. Approximately 0.5 ml are used per animal daily for 2 weeks. Fresh mixture should be prepared daily.
> NOTE: Diiodohydroxyquin is not soluble, hence the mixture must be thoroughly shaken to put this drug into suspension before spraying.

For standard equivalents for measures, see pp. 1453 to 1456.

340. ℞ Quinapyramine sulfate

Treatment: 4.4 mg/kg body wt in a 10% solution, subcut. Careful weight estimation is needed. Animals should be handled quietly at treatment time, and provided with shade and water. In horses, the dose should be divided and given in 2 or 3 sites, or better, give ½ dose and then a second ½ dose 5 to 6 hours later. There are occasional anaphylactic-type reactions in Equidae.

Prophylaxis: The soluble sulfate is combined (3:2) with the less soluble chloride. The dose is 0.025 ml/kg body wt of a solution containing 166 mg of the mixed salts per milliliter, given subcut. Must be repeated at 2- to 3-month intervals. A hard nodular swelling persists at the injection site for months or years.

341. ℞ Quinuronium sulfate ("Acaprin")

Cattle: 1 ml of 5% solution per 100 lb body wt, subcut. or IM.

Dogs: 1 ml of 0.5% solution per 45 lb body wt, subcut. or IM.

342. ℞ Sulfamethazine

For all species of coccidia in chickens and turkeys: Given either as 30 ml of a 12.5% solution in each gallon of drinking water or 0.4% (8 lb/ton of feed) in all-mash ration. Given for 3 days, followed by unmedicated feed or water for 3 days, then an additional 3 days of treatment. After 3 more days on plain feed or water, it may be necessary to repeat treatment for 1 or 2 days.

343. ℞ Sulfaquinoxaline sodium

For outbreaks of coccidiosis in chickens: 0.04% in drinking water or 0.1% in the feed, given for the first 48 or 72 hours, followed by 3 days on plain feed or water, then 0.05% in the feed or 0.025% in drinking water for two 2-day periods with a 3-day unmedicated interval.

Read introduction to prescriptions, pp. 1458 to 1460. Note all warnings and cautions appearing on drug labels and observe all local laws and regulations pertaining to drug usage.

344. ℞ Sulfaquinoxaline sodium

> *For all species of coccidia in turkeys:*
> 0.025% in the drinking water or 0.05% in
> an all-mash ration, given for 3 days, then
> nonmedicated water or feed for 3 days,
> then repeat treatment for 3 days. An ad-
> ditional 1 or 2 days of treatment following
> another 3 days' rest may be necessary.

345. ℞ Suramin

> *For trypanosomiasis:* Administer IV as a
> 10% solution. Care must be taken in cal-
> culating the doses for Equidae, especially.
> *Treatment:* Horses, 7 to 10 mg/kg, IV, 2
> or 3 times at weekly intervals; *cattle,* 12
> mg/kg; *camels,* 8 to 12 mg/kg, IV.
> *Prophylaxis:* to be repeated at 10-day in-
> tervals: *Horses,* 2 gm; *camels,* 1 to 2 gm.

346. ℞ Trypan blue 1% solution

> *Cattle:* 100 ml, IV.
> *Dogs:* 10 to 20 ml, IV.

347. ℞ Carbarsone

> *Turkeys: Prophylaxis:* 0.037% (2 lb/ton)
> in feed continuously until 5 days before
> marketing.

348. ℞ 2-Acetylamido-5-nitrothiazole
("Cyzine")

> *Turkeys: Prophylaxis:* 0.015% (0.1 lb/100
> lb feed).
> *Treatment:* 0.05% (0.33 lb/100 lb feed) for
> 14 days.

349. ℞ Amecarbalide isethionate 50% solu-
tion ("Diampron")

> *For babesiasis in cattle:* 5 mg/kg of body
> wt by IM, subcut. or slow IV injection.
> *For peracute cases in adult cattle:* double
> the dosage. If hemaglobinuria persists be-
> yond 24 hours, repeat the dosage.

Antifungal Agents

350. ℞ Amphotericin B

> 0.125 to 0.25 mg/lb body wt slowly IV in
> dilute (0.1%) solution, freshly prepared.
> Do not use isotonic saline.
> CAUTION: Reactions are common, see ℞ 351.

For standard equivalents for measures, see pp. 1453 to 1456.

351. ℞ Amphotericin B

0.1% solution in 5% dextrose. Administer IV slowly, at 0.125 to 0.25 mg/lb on alternate days or twice weekly. Total cumulative doses in excess of 5 mg/lb are associated with nephrotoxicity. Fever, chilling and nausea may be relieved with aspirin and antihistamines. BUN should be monitored and treatment suspended when levels exceed 75 mg% or when vomiting occurs.

352. ℞ Griseofulvin tablets

25 mg/lb body wt daily until skin or claws are negative for fungi (at least 3 to 4 weeks).

353. ℞ Griseofulvin

Guinea pigs: Feed in the daily diet at 2.5 mg/100 gm body wt.
Nonhuman primates: 25 mg/kg body wt, orally, for at least 3 to 4 weeks.

354. ℞ Nystatin ("Mycostatin") oral suspension 100,000 u/ml

1 ml, 4 times daily, orally. Continue for 48 hours after clinical recovery.

355. ℞ Nystatin tablets . . . . . 500,000 u

1 tablet t.i.d. for 10 or more days.

356. ℞ Nystatin ointment . . . . 100,000 u/gm

Apply to lesions 2 or 3 times daily.

357. ℞ "Sporastacin" cream

Chlordantoin 1.00%
Benzalkonium chloride . . . 0.05%
Apply to affected area once or twice daily as required.

358. ℞ Stilbamidine isethionate

0.5 to 1.0 mg/lb body wt, slowly IV in dilute (0.1 to 0.5%), freshly prepared solution only.
CAUTION: Reactions are common.

Read introduction to prescriptions, pp. 1458 to 1460. Note all warnings and cautions appearing on drug labels and observe all local laws and regulations pertaining to drug usage.

359. ℞ Thiabendazole

150 gm thiabendazole powder (containing 110 gm active ingredient) per 20 gal. of water per acre. Powder is to be thoroughly suspended in the water and evenly sprayed onto pastures by boom or aerial spray during dry, still weather conditions.

360. ℞ Tolnaftate cream 1% ("Tinactin")

Apply cream to each lesion and massage gently b.i.d. for 2 to 3 weeks.

Tranquilizers

361. ℞ Acepromazine maleate ("Acepromazine")

Horses: 2.0 to 4.0 mg/100 lb body wt, IV, IM or subcut.
Dogs: 0.25 to 0.5 mg/lb body wt, IV, IM or subcut.
Cats: 0.5 to 1.0 mg/lb body wt, IV, IM or subcut.

362. ℞ Chlormethazanone tablets . . . 100 mg

50 to 200 mg, 3 or 4 times daily.

363. ℞ Chlorpromazine

Large animals: 0.1 to 0.5 mg/lb body wt, IV or 0.5 to 1.5 mg/lb body wt, IM, 1 to 4 times a day.
Small animals: 0.5 to 3.0 mg/lb body wt orally or IM, 1 to 4 times a day. Dose and frequency of administration must be adjusted to response of animal.

364. ℞ Ethylisobutrazine

2 to 5 mg/lb body wt orally or IM *or* 1 to 2 mg/lb body wt, IV.

365. ℞ Mepazine

5 to 15 mg/lb body wt orally or parenterally. Dose depends on degree of tranquilization required and response of patient.

366. ℞ Meperidine hydrochloride . . . 50 mg/ml

5 mg/lb body wt, IM or subcut. Repeat as necessary.

For standard equivalents for measures, see pp. 1453 to 1456.

367. ℞ Meprobamate
>   *Dogs:* 200 to 400 mg orally, 2 to 3 times
>   daily.

368. ℞ Perphenazine
>   *Large animals:* 10 mg/100 lb body wt, IM
>   or IV.
>   *Small animals:* 4 mg/10 lb body wt orally
>   b.i.d. or 5 mg/20 lb body wt, IM or IV.

369. ℞ Promazine hydrochloride
>   *Large animals:* 0.2 to 0.5 mg/lb body wt,
>   IM or IV.
>   *Small animals:* 1 to 2 mg/lb body wt,
>   orally, IM or IV.
>   *Zoo species:* 2 to 4 mg/lb, IM.
>   Repeat after 4 to 6 hours if necessary.

370. ℞ Propiopromazine hydrochloride
     ("Tranvet")
>   *Large animals:* 0.05 to 0.1 mg/lb body wt,
>   IM or IV. The lower dose given IV is
>   preferred in the Thoroughbred and Stand-
>   ardbred.
>   *Small animals:* 0.1 mg/lb body wt, IM or
>   IV.

Ophthalmic Preparations

371. ℞ Atropine sulfate 1% aqueous solution
>   Instill into conjunctival sac every 30 minutes
>   until pupil is dilated.

372. ℞ Bacitracin ophthalmic ointment
     (500 u/gm)
>   *Large animals:* Apply inside lower lid of
>   affected eye b.i.d.
>   *Small animals:* Apply inside lower lid of
>   affected eye 3 or 4 times daily.

373. ℞ Butacaine sulfate 2% and nitromersol
     1:3,000 ophthalmic ointment
>   Apply to conjunctival surface following re-
>   moval of irritating agent.

374. ℞ Chloramphenicol 1% ophthalmic oint-
     ment or 0.25% ophthalmic solution
>   Apply to conjunctiva every 3 or 4 hours.

**Read introduction to prescriptions, pp. 1458 to 1460.
Note all warnings and cautions appearing on drug
labels and observe all local laws and regulations pertaining to drug usage.**

375. ℞ Chlortetracycline hydrochloride
ophthalmic ointment
Apply inside lower lid of affected eye 3 or
4 times daily.

376. ℞ Demecarium bromide 0.25% solution
1 drop into conjunctival sac daily.

377. ℞ Dexamethasone 0.1% ophthalmic solution
Instill 1 or 2 drops in eye every 2 to 4
hours.

378. ℞ Dichlorphenamide ("Daranide")
tablets
12.5 to 50 mg daily.

379. ℞ Diisopropyl fluorophosphate (0.1% solution in peanut oil)
1 to 2 drops into affected eye every 8 to
72 hours.

380. ℞ Hydrocortisone acetate 1.5% ophthalmic ointment
Apply 3 or 4 times daily.

381. ℞ Neomycin ophthalmic ointment
(5 mg/gm)
Apply inside lower lid of affected eye 3
or 4 times daily.

382. ℞ Nitrofurazone 0.2% solution
2 or 3 drops in conjunctival sac every 3
hours.

383. ℞ Penicillin ophthalmic ointment
(1,000 or 2,000 u/gm)
Apply inside lower lid of affected eye 3
or 4 times daily.

384. ℞ Prednisolone 1.5% ophthalmic ointment
Apply 3 or 4 times daily.

385. ℞ Prednisolone t-butylacetate
suspension . . . . 20 mg/ml
0.5 to 1.0 ml subconjunctivally.

For standard equivalents for measures, see pp. 1453 to 1456.

386. ℞ Prednisolone with neomycin ophthalmic ointment
Prednisolone acetate 0.25%
Neomycin sulfate 0.50%
Administer b.i.d.

387. ℞ Prednisolone 21-phosphate with neomycin ophthalmic solution and ointment
Prednisolone 21-phosphate . . . 5 mg/ml
Neomycin . . . . 5 mg/ml
Inflammation or infection of anterior eye:
Apply in conjunctival sac 2 or 3 times daily.
Otitis externa: Instill into ear canal with gentle massage: solution 3 to 4 times daily, ointment once or twice daily.

388. ℞ Sodium sulfacetamide 30% solution or 10% ophthalmic ointment
1 drop in conjunctival sac 4 times daily.
Ointment may be applied inside lower eyelid at night.

389. ℞ Sulfathiazole 5% ophthalmic ointment
Apply to conjunctival surface 2 or 3 times daily.

390. ℞ Sulfathiazole 5% and sulfanilamide 5% ophthalmic ointment
Apply to conjunctival surface 2 or 3 times daily.

Expectorants, Antitussives and Inhalants

391. ℞ Acetylcysteine 10 to 20% solution
Administer by direct application, intratracheal instillation or nebulization. May be used in combination with other drugs used in aerosol therapy.

392. ℞ Ammonium chloride
Ammonium carbonate . . . . āā 16 gm
Camphor . . . . 4 gm
Fluidextract Belladona . . . . 30 ml
Syrup . . . . q.s. ad 500 ml
Large animals: 15 to 30 ml orally every 4 hours.

**Read introduction to prescriptions, pp. 1458 to 1460.
Note all warnings and cautions appearing on drug labels and observe all local laws and regulations pertaining to drug usage.**

393. ℞ Compound Benzoin Tincture USP

Given in steam inhalations, **10 to 15 minutes,** several times daily.

394. ℞ Cresol

15 to 30 ml in a pail of steaming hot water. Allow animal to inhale vapor for 10 to 12 minutes, several times daily.

395. ℞ Terpin hydrate elixir with codeine

1 teaspoon every 3 hours.

Topical Dressings and Antiseptics

396. ℞ Acetic acid (glacial)

1:500 in water. Immerse fish for 1 minute.

397. ℞ 5% Methyl anthranilate and 5% titanium dioxide in neutral-tinted cream ("A-Fil")

Apply daily to affected areas.

398. ℞ Bacitracin . . . . **500 u**
Neomycin . . . . **5 mg**
Polymyxin sulfate . . . . . **5,000 u**

Anhydrous lanolin and hydrophilic ointment base.
Apply topically daily as indicated.

399. ℞ Benzalkonium chloride aqueous solution 1:1,000

Flush mouth freely as needed.

400. ℞ Benzalkonium chlorides

A. Alkyl benzalkonium chloride (10 or 50%) 1.0 to 2.0 ppm of active ingredient. For 1 hour for 3 consecutive days for epizootics and 1-hour exposure for prevention.
B. n-Alkyl dimethylbenzylammonium chloride (50%). Use in same way as benzalkonium chloride. Effective in hard-water areas.
C. Benzethonium chloride (98.8%). Use in same way as benzalkonium chloride.

For standard equivalents for measures, see pp. 1453 to 1456.

401. ℞ Burrow's Solution 1:20 (Aluminum Acetate Solution USP)

> Moisten 8 to 10 layers of gauze and wring out drip free. Apply to the affected area for 15 to 20 minutes 3 to 4 times daily, remoistening when the gauze reaches body temperature.

402. ℞ Calcium oxide

> 150 to 200 kg/hectare
> 132 to 176 lb (60 to 80 kg) per acre.

403. ℞ Calamine Lotion USP

> Apply under a bandage.

404. ℞ Calcium polysulfide ("Led-O-San")

> Apply topically daily until lesions begin to heal, then 2 to 3 times weekly until healing is complete.

405. ℞ Chlorhexidine . . . . 15 ml
     Water . . . . 2 qt

> Irrigate uterus with two-way flow catheter. Topically: apply undiluted as a spray as needed.

406. ℞ Chlortetracycline hydrochloride ointment (60 mg/gm)

> Apply to affected areas 2 to 4 times daily.

407. ℞ Copper sulfate

> 0.2 to 0.5 ppm in the water (depending on hardness of water—very toxic in soft water.)

408. ℞ Fibrinolysin (bovine) . . .   30 u
     Desoxyribonuclease . . . . 20,000 u
     In ointment base

> Use locally as directed.

409. ℞ Formalin 40% . . . . 200 ml
     Water . . . . 4 L

> Apply locally or use in a foot bath through which the sheep are driven.

Read introduction to prescriptions, pp. 1458 to 1460. Note all warnings and cautions appearing on drug labels and observe all local laws and regulations pertaining to drug usage.

410. ℞ Formalin
1:4,000 to 1:6,000. **Expose fish for 1 to 2** hours.

411. ℞ Gentian violet 1:500 aqueous solution
Stomatitis: Apply daily to ulcerated areas.
Vaginitis: Inject into vagina with catheter, or apply to mucosa with swab twice weekly.

412. ℞ Ichthammol
Salicylic acid . . . . . . āā 10 gm
Zinc oxide ointment . . . . 250 gm
Apply to affected areas once daily.

413. ℞ Tincture of iodine 2%
Apply freely to gums after scaling teeth.

414. ℞ Tincture of iodine 2% . . . . . 1 ml
Glycerin . . . . 30 ml
Apply to inflamed mucous membranes with a cotton swab.

415. ℞ Lawsone (0.035%) and dihydroxy-acetone (3%) and isopropanol (50%)
Spray affected areas once every 5 days.

416. ℞ Malachite green
Eggs: 5 ppm as a daily flush.
Live fish: 1:15,000 dilution, 10- to 30-second dip.
CAUTION: Should be chemically pure (zinc-free).

417. ℞ Neomycin 0.5% solution or ointment
Apply locally as wet dressings t.i.d.

418. ℞ Nitrofurazone Ointment NF XIII
Apply topically daily as indicated.

419. ℞ Nystatin . . . . 100,000 u
Neomycin . . . . 2.5 mg
Thiostrepton . . . . . . 2,500 u
Triamcinolone acetonide . 1.0 mg
In hydrocarbon gel
Apply daily as directed.

For standard equivalents for measures, see pp. 1453 to 1456.

420. ℞ Oxytetracycline ointment with poly-
  myxin B sulfate (topical)
  Oxytetracycline hydrochloride
  (30 mg/gm)
  Polymyxin B sulfate (10,000 u/gm)
  Apply topically to affected areas.

421. ℞ Paraffin
  Beeswax . . . . āā 60 gm
  Pine tar . . . . 120 gm
  Apply evenly over hoof wall.

422. ℞ Petrolatum white or amber
  Apply liberally over affected parts and on
  dressings.

423. ℞ Hexachlorophene 3%
  Use as a soap to wash lesions; rinse well.

424. ℞ Polyalkyleneglycol-iodine
  ("Weladol") shampoo (1% iodine)
  and cream (2% iodine)
  Pyoderma: Shampoo entire body, then massage cream thoroughly into skin. Repeat
  cream massage daily for 3 to 10 days, depending on degree and duration of infection. May be repeated as necessary.
  Otitis externa: Apply cream in ear canal
  daily.

425. ℞ Potassium permanganate 1:4,000
  solution
  Flush the mouth or sponge the gums as
  frequently as necessary.

426. ℞ "Pragmatar" ointment
  Cetyl alcohol-coal tar distillate 4%
  Near-colloidal sulfur 3%
  Oil-water emulsion . . qs. ad 100 gm
  Apply daily to affected areas.

427. ℞ Resorcinol
  Castor oil . . . . āā 5 ml
  Alcohol . . . . 200 ml
  Apply to affected skin and massage gently.

**Read introduction to prescriptions, pp. 1458 to 1460.
Note all warnings and cautions appearing on drug
labels and observe all local laws and regulations pertaining to drug usage.**

428. ℞ Sodium chloride
2.5% in the water for 2 to 4 days.

429. ℞ Salicylic acid . . . . 5 gm
Olive oil . . . . 50 ml
Peruvian balsam . . . . 3 gm
Apply to affected skin and massage gently.

430. ℞ Salicylic acid
Tannic acid . . . . āā 18 gm
Alcohol . . . . 600 ml
Apply daily to affected areas.

431. ℞ Salt solution
1 teaspoon table salt in a glass of warm
water to be used as mouth wash. Flush
mouth as needed.

432. ℞ Selenium sulfide 1% suspension
("Seleen")
Dogs: Shampoo the entire body. Flush off
residue thoroughly after use.
Cats: Apply only to affected areas.
CAUTION: This preparation is poisonous.
Protect eyes and normally hairless areas.

433. ℞ Sodium bicarbonate
1 teaspoon in a glass of warm water to be
used to flush mouth as needed.

434. ℞ Medicinal soft soap
Apply freely using gauze sponges until
wound is clean.

435. ℞ Sulfathiazole 5% ointment
Apply as wound dressing 2 or 3 times daily.

436. ℞ Sulfur iodide . . . . 1 part
Corn or olive oil . . . . 8 parts
Mix while very warm, cool and add 10 ml
formalin to 100 ml.
Apply daily to affected area.

437. ℞ Tyrothricin cream (0.5 mg/gm cream)
Apply topically daily as indicated.

For standard equivalents for measures, see pp. 1453 to 1456.

438. ℞ Zinc oxide . . . . 25.0 gm
      Precipitated calcium carbonate 25.0 gm
      Oleic acid . . . . 2.5 gm
      Linseed oil . . . . 25.0 gm
      Limewater . . . . 22.5 ml
        Apply daily to affected areas.

439. ℞ Peruvian balsam . . . . . . 5 gm
      Cresol . . . . 4 ml
      Alcohol . . . . q.s. ad 100 ml
        Apply topically.

440. ℞ Precipitated sulfur . . . . . 15 gm
      Lanolin . . . . 7 gm
      White ointment . . . . q.s. ad 100 gm
        Apply locally.

441. ℞ Zinc chloride solution
      Zinc chloride . . . . 2 gm
      Water . . . . q.s. ad 1 L
        Flush mouth with solution as needed.

Ear and Nasal Preparations

442. ℞ Alcohol . . . . 10 ml
      Glycerin . . . . 90 ml
      Salicylic acid . . q.s. ad saturation
      Boric acid . . . q.s. ad saturation
      Tannic acid . . . q.s. ad saturation
        Warm and apply in ear canal as drops,
        then massage gently.

443. ℞ Antibiotic-steroid ointment
      Neomycin base (as sulfate)   3 mg/gm
      Bacitracin . . . .   500 u/gm
      Polymyxin B sulfate . . . 10,000 u/gm
      Hydrocortisone acetate . .   10 mg/gm
      Lanolin-petrolatum base . .   q.s.
        Instill into ear canal with massage 1 to 2
        times daily.

**Read introduction to prescriptions, pp. 1458 to 1460.
Note all warnings and cautions appearing on drug
labels and observe all local laws and regulations pertaining to drug usage.**

444. ℞ "Canex"

Chloroform . . . . 7.5 %
Rotenone 0.12%
Other ether extractives of
   derris 0.38%
Inert ingredients . . . . . 92 %

Mix 1 part with 3 parts mineral oil and
instill into external ear as drops or apply
with cotton swab at 3-day intervals.

445. ℞ Ephedrine sulfate 1% solution

2 drops in each nostril every 3 hours.

446. ℞ Sodium and zinc caprylate ointment
("Naprylate")

Sodium caprylate 10%
Zinc caprylate 5%

Apply in ear canal with cotton swab.

447. ℞ "Cerumenex"

Triethylanolamine polypeptide
   oleate condensate 10.0%
Chlorobutanol 0.5%
Propylene glycol 89.5%

Partially fill the ear canal, massage for a
few minutes and clean.

448. ℞ Hydrocortisone-neomycin ointment or
solution

Hydrocortisone acetate . . . . 15 mg/gm or ml
Neomycin sulfate . . . . . . 5 mg/gm or ml

Instill 2 to 6 drops into ear canal with
gentle massage, 3 to 4 times daily. Instill
ointment into external ear canal with gentle
massage once or twice daily.

449. ℞ "Mercaptocaine Creme"

2-Mercaptobenzothiazole . . . 2 %
Benzocaine . . . . 5 %
2-Chloro-4-phenylphenol in
   emulsion base 0.2%

Apply in ear canal with cotton swab daily.

For standard equivalents for measures, see pp. 1453 to 1456.

450. ℞ "Metimyd" ointment with neomycin
Each ⅛-oz tube contains:

Prednisolone acetate	5 mg
Sodium sulfacetamide	100 mg
Neomycin sulfate	2.5 mg

After cleansing lesion, gently rub on ointment 3 or 4 times daily.

451. ℞ "Panalog" dermatologic ointment
Each milliliter contains:

Nystatin	100,000 u
Neomycin sulfate	2.5 mg
Thiostrepton	2,500 u
Triamcinolone acetonide	1.0 mg

Otitis: Clean ear of impacted cerumen and
foreign bodies. Instill 2 to 3 drops of ointment.
For mild cases: once daily to once a week;
For severe cases: as often as 2 to 3 times
daily.

452. ℞ "Pelene" drops

Resorcinol	5 %
Zinc oxide	4 %
Calamine	2 %
Oil of cade	1 %
Pyroligneous acid purified	0.4%
Zinc hydroxide	8 %

Instill 4 to 6 drops in cleaned ear canal
daily.

453. ℞ "Pellitol"

Resorcin	5%
Bismuth subgallate	1%
Bismuth subnitrate	9%
Zinc oxide	17%
Calamine	10%
Oil of cade	1%
Special ointment base	q.s.

Apply in cleaned ear canal with cotton
swabs or with special ear applicator tube.

454. ℞ Penicillin G sodium . . . . 100,000 u
Distilled water . . . . . 10 ml

Spray into each nostril with suitable atomizer as necessary.

**Read introduction to prescriptions, pp. 1458 to 1460.
Note all warnings and cautions appearing on drug
labels and observe all local laws and regulations pertaining to drug usage.**

455. ℞ Phenylephrine hydrochloride 1% solution

Small animals: nasal drops, use 2 to 4 times daily.

456. ℞ Phenylmercuric nitrate 1:5,000 (alcoholic solution)

Use saturated cotton swab to clean the ear canal.

457. ℞ "Ridamite"

Dimethyl phthalate 24%
Cottonseed oil 76%

Place 1 to 2 ml into the ear canal and massage gently. Also swab the pinnae of the ear and the feet. Repeat every 3 to 4 days until the condition is cleared.

458. ℞ Thymol . . . . 0.6 gm
Ethyl alcohol 70% . . . . . 30.0 ml

3 or 4 drops in ear canal every 2 days.

459. ℞ "Tresaderm" dermatologic solution

Each milliliter contains:
Thiabendazole . . . . . . 40.0 mg
Neomycin sulfate . . . . . 3.2 mg
Dexamethasone . . . . . . 1.0 mg

After cleaning the surface of the lesion of ceruminous or other material, apply topically 2 to 3 times daily. For otitis externa instill 5 to 15 drops. For surface lesions apply enough to moisten.

Emetics and Antiemetics

460. ℞ Apomorphine hydrochloride

Dogs: 3 to 6 mg subcut. May also be given by dropping a prepared tablet into the conjunctival sac.
Cats: 1 to 2 mg subcut.

461. ℞ Dicyclomine hydrochloride ("Spastyl") plus phenobarbital

Each capsule contains:
Dicyclomine HCl . . . . . 10 mg
Phenobarbital . . . . . . 15 mg

Dogs under 20 lb: 1 capsule b.i.d.
Dogs over 20 lb: 1 capsule 2 to 4 times daily as indicated.

For standard equivalents for measures, see pp. 1453 to 1456.

462. ℞ Dimenhydrinate tablets
0.5 mg/lb body wt.

463. ℞ Meclizine
1 mg/lb body wt per 24 hours.

464. ℞ Methylatropine nitrate (tablets) . 1 mg
2 to 5 mg, IM or subcut., or 1 to 2 tablets
30 minutes before trip.

465. ℞ Promethazine hydrochloride
0.5 mg/lb body wt.

466. ℞ Trimethobenzamide hydrochloride
Small animals: 100 to 200 mg, IV or IM,
1 to 4 times daily.

Antacids and Antidiarrheal Agents

467. ℞ "Anistat"
Each 8 oz contains:

Chloramphenicol	1.0 gm
Neomycin base (as sulfate)	1.0 gm
Sulfathiazole	6.0 gm
Sulfamethazine	2.0 gm
Absorbent demulcent base	q.s.

Calves and foals: 1st day: 3 oz, b.i.d.
morning and evening; 2nd day: 2 oz, b.i.d.
Pigs and lambs: Initial dose, 1 tsp/5 lb
body wt followed in 12 hours by 1 tsp/10
lb body wt and repeat as required.

468. ℞ Bismuth subnitrate or subcarbonate
(may be given with kaolin)
Dogs: 1 gm in 1 tbsp milk, t.i.d.
Cows and horses: 30 to 60 gm in capsule,
orally, t.i.d.
Calves: 10 to 20 gm in capsule, orally, t.i.d.
Lambs: 2 to 4 gm in capsule, orally, t.i.d.

469. ℞ Calcium carbonate, precipitated   360 gm
Warm water . . . . . . q.s. ad 1 gal.
Cattle: Administer in one dose by stomach
tube.

**Read introduction to prescriptions, pp. 1458 to 1460.
Note all warnings and cautions appearing on drug
labels and observe all local laws and regulations pertaining to drug usage.**

470. ℞ Cerium and benzocaine tablets

Cerium oxalate	120.0 mg
Benzocaine	30.0 mg
Calcium carbonate	0.3 mg

1 to 5 tablets daily.

471. ℞ Charcoal activated

1 to 3 gm orally.

472. ℞

Kaolin	200 gm
Pectin	4 gm
Water	q.s. ad 1 L

Adult cattle and horses: 180 to 300 ml every 3 hours.
Foals and calves: 90 to 120 ml every 2 to 3 hours.
Dogs and cats: 10 to 40 ml every 4 hours.

473. ℞ Nifuraldezone-bismuth ("Entefur")

Calves: 1-gm bolus, b.i.d. for 2 days.

474. ℞

Paregoric USP	4 ml
Pectin	50 mg
Kaolin	2 gm
Neomycin sulfate	125 mg
Potassium gluconate	23 mg
Water	50 ml

This is the dose for a 4- to 7-kg monkey, and should be adjusted proportionately for smaller or larger animals. Intubate via the nostril. Repeat dose b.i.d. for 3 to 7 days.

475. ℞ Sodium bicarbonate

For IV use: 3.75 gm/L of water (cannot be autoclaved).
For oral use: as powder or tablets.
Dosage: Horses: up to 60 gm.
Cattle: up to 120 gm.
Dogs & cats: up to 1.5 gm.

476. ℞

Tannic acid	0.6 gm
Water	30.0 ml

Dogs: 5 to 25 ml, orally.
Cats: 2.5 to 20.0 ml, orally.

For standard equivalents for measures, see pp. 1453 to 1456.

477. ℞ Calf scour powder

Sodium chloride	117 gm
Potassium chloride	130 gm
Sodium bicarbonate	168 gm
Potassium phosphate	135 gm
(dibasic salt K_2HPO_4)	

To prepare a liter of the solution, add 5.7 gm of the powder to a liter of water to which may also be added 50 gm of glucose. For 1 gal., add 1 oz powder and 0.5 lb glucose to 1 gal. of water. Give or feed 1 gal. of the final solution to a 100-lb calf in divided doses in 24 hours.

478. ℞ Aluminum Hydroxide Gel USP (suspension)

1 to 3 teaspoons (0.25 to 1.0 gm) 3 or 4 times a day.

Laxatives and Cathartics

479. ℞ Carbachol USP 1:1,000

2 to 4 ml subcut.

480. ℞ Dioctyl sodium sulfosuccinate (0.05% in water)

Small animals: Administer 90 ml rectally as a retention enema.

481. ℞ Epsom salt

1 lb mixed with bran in wet mash for 75 to 100 chickens. Withhold other feed until consumed.

482. ℞ Milk of Magnesia

1 pt mixed in 15 lb of wet bran mash for 500 birds; fed on top of the mash. Withhold other feed until consumed. Repeat the next day.

483. ℞ Milk of Magnesia

Magnesium hydroxide	1 to 2 lb
Water	q.s. ad 1 gal.

Administer in one dose by stomach tube.

Read introduction to prescriptions, pp. 1458 to 1460. Note all warnings and cautions appearing on drug labels and observe all local laws and regulations pertaining to drug usage.

84. ℞ Mineral oil

Cattle and horses: 2 to 4 L (2 to 4 qt)
via stomach tube.
Sheep and swine: 0.5 to 1.0 L (1 to 2 pt)
stomach tube.
Dogs: 1 to 4 tablespoons daily.

85. ℞ Mucilose flakes (purified psyllium)

Small animals: 1 to 2 tsp are sprinkled on
food, b.i.d.

86. ℞ Physostigmine salicylate . . . 60 mg
Pilocarpine hydrochloride . . . 120 mg

To be dissolved in 20 ml of water for
subcut. injection for 500- to 600-lb animal.
For cattle of 1,000 lb or more, double
quantities are to be used.

87. ℞ Psyllium hydrophilic mucilloid
("Metamucil" flakes)

Dogs: 1 tsp orally, t.i.d.

88. ℞ Surfactant laxative ("Doxidan")

Small animals: 1 capsule daily until the
stools become normal.

Antispasmodics

89. ℞ Atropine sulfate

Horses: 30 to 60 mg.
Dogs: 0.02 mg/lb.
Inject IM or subcut. 2 to 4 times daily.

90. ℞ Aminopropazine ("Jenotone")
solution . . . . 25 mg/ml

5 to 10 ml as needed, IM.

91. ℞ Belladonna Tincture USP . . . 6 ml
Deodorized Opium Tincture
USP . . . . q.s. ad 30 ml

50 drops in water orally every 4 hours.

92. ℞ Methampyrone 50%

Administer IV, IM or subcut.:
Horses: 10 to 20 ml.
Cattle: 5 to 15 ml.
Swine: 5 to 10 ml.
Dogs: 1 to 5 ml.
Cats: 0.25 to 2 ml.

For standard equivalents for measures, see pp. 1453 to 1456.

493. ℞ Methylatropine nitrate solution
(5 mg/ml) or tablets (1 mg)

Large animals: 5 to 15 mg, IM or subcut.
Small animals: 2 to 5 mg, IM or subcut.,
or 1 or 2 tablets before feeding, or 3 to 4
times daily.

494. ℞ Propantheline bromide ("Pro-
Banthine") 30-mg ampul

15 mg, IM every 8 hours.

Miscellaneous Digestants, Stomachics and Antiferments

495. ℞ Aromatic spirits of ammonia

Horses: 30 to 60 ml dissolved in 500 ml of
water, given via stomach tube.
Cattle: 30 to 120 ml dissolved in 1 L of
water, given orally.

496. ℞ Magnesium sulfate . . . . . 300 gm
Formalin . . . . 30 gm
Water . . . . 12 L (3 gal.)

Warm to body temperature and give slowly
via stomach tube.

497. ℞ Pancreatin granules or powder

Mix sufficient with each meal to keep stools
normal (approximately 1 to 1.5 gm).

498. ℞ Polysorbate 80

1 gm orally t.i.d.

499. ℞ Sodium sulfate . . . . 240 gm
Nux vomica . . . . 120 gm
Gentian . . . . 120 gm

15 gm orally, 2 or 3 times daily for mature
cattle.

Hematinics

500. ℞ Ferrous sulfate (tablets) . . . . 60 mg

Large animals: 1½ to 4 tablets.
Small animals: ½ to 1½ tablets.

**Read introduction to prescriptions, pp. 1458 to 1460.
Note all warnings and cautions appearing on drug
labels and observe all local laws and regulations pertaining to drug usage.**

501. ℞ Injectable iron solution

> (50 to 100 mg elemental iron per milliliter)
> *Prophylaxis:* 2 ml per pig at 2 to 4 days of age.
> *Treatment:* 2 ml per pig any time between 7 and 21 days of age.

502. ℞ Iron and ammonium citrate . . 1.2 gm
Copper gluconate . . . . . . 60.0 mg
Cobalt sulfate . . . . 15.0 mg
Honey or other flavored
base . . . . q.s. ad 30.0 ml

> *Cattle and horses:* 15 to 30 ml 2 to 3 times daily.
> *Suckling pigs:* Paint on udder of sow t.i.d. Individual pigs can be treated with 5 to 10 drops each daily.
> *Weaned pigs:* 60 ml per 100 animals daily, mixed in ration or drinking water.

503. ℞ Iron and sodium citrate
(capsules) . . . . 0.5 gm

> *Dogs:* 0.5 gm orally daily.

Cardiovascular Agents

504. ℞ Aminophylline

> 2.5 mg/lb body wt, t.i.d.

505. ℞ Atropine sulfate

> 0.05 mg/lb body wt subcut. every 8 hours.
> 0.5 to 2.0 mg orally every 8 hours.

506. ℞ Calcium gluconate 20% solution

> 5 ml/lb body wt, IV or IP until heart rate is normal. Repeat if necessary.

507. ℞ Digitoxin Tablets USP
or Digoxin Tablets
USP . . . . . 0.125, 0.25 or 0.50 mg
or Digoxin Elixir USP . . . . 0.05 mg/ml

> The total digitalization dose for the dog is 0.03 mg/lb body wt, orally, for 6 equal doses over 2 days. Maintenance dose is 0.01 mg/lb daily in 1 or 2 doses.

For standard equivalents for measures, see pp. 1453 to 1456.

508. ℞ Digitoxin Injection USP

> *Cattle: Total digitalization dose:* **1.4 mg/** 100 lb body wt IM in divided doses over a 24-hour period.
> *Maintenance dose:* 1/9 to 1/5 of the above dose.

509. ℞ Epinephrine Solution 1:1,000 USP

> *Horses and cattle:* 5 to 15 ml, IV or subcut.
> *Sheep and swine:* 2 to 4 ml, IV or subcut.
> *Dogs:* 0.5 to 2.0 ml, IV or subcut.

510. ℞ Epinephrine Solution 1:1,000 USP

> Dilute with 10 parts of isotonic salt solution.
> *Large animals:* 3 to 8 ml intracardially.
> *Small animals:* 0.1 to 0.5 ml intracardially.

511. ℞ Epinephrine Solution 1:1,000 USP

> *Cattle and horses:* 4 to 8 ml subcut.
> *Sheep and swine:* 1 to 3 ml subcut.
> *Dogs and cats:* 0.1 to 1.0 ml subcut. or 0.01 ml (or more) IV.

512. ℞ Isoproterenol tablets sustained action ("Proternol")

> *Dogs:* 15 to 30 mg every 4 to 6 hours.

513. ℞ Levarterenol Bitartrate Injection USP (2 mg/ml)

> 4 ml/L of 5% dextrose. Give IV at 0.5 ml/min.

514. ℞ Ouabain Injection USP . 0.25 or 0.5 mg

> *Cattle: Total digitalization dose:* 0.6 to 1.0 mg/100 lb body wt, IV divided into 4 doses and given over a 24-hour period.
> *Maintenance dose:* 1/8 to 1/5 the total digitalization dose.
> *Dogs:* 0.01 to 0.015 mg/lb body wt, IV or IM, repeated after 24 to 36 hours. For safety, divide the calculated amount in 2 equal doses and give 3 to 4 hours apart.

Read introduction to prescriptions, pp. 1458 to 1460. Note all warnings and cautions appearing on drug labels and observe all local laws and regulations pertaining to drug usage.

515. ℞ Quinidine sulfate (capsules) . . 10 gm

Horses:

1st day . . . . . 4 gm (test dose)
2nd day . . . . . 5 gm, t.i.d. at 3-hr intervals
3rd and 4th days . . 10 gm, q.i.d. at 2-hr intervals
5th and 6th days . . 10 gm, q.i.d. at 2-hr intervals

If necessary to give more than 40 gm daily, dosage may be increased cautiously in increments of 10 gm up to 90 gm (nine 10-gm doses at hourly intervals have been given in a single day). However, these higher doses are dangerous and extreme care must be taken to note the onset of toxic signs. Treatment should be stopped if obstructive swelling of nasal mucosa, laminitis, severe depression, restlessness or excessive sweating occur.

516. ℞ Quinidine Sulfate Tablets
USP . . . . 0.1, 0.2 or 0.3 gm

Dogs: 1 tablet initially as a test dose. After 3 or 4 hours, give 50 mg/10 lb body wt every hour until normal rhythm appears, toxic signs supervene or a total dose of 0.6 gm/10 lb body wt has been given.

517. ℞ Theobromine calcium salicylate
(tablets) . . . . 0.5 gm

1 tablet t.i.d. for a 35-lb dog.

Diuretics

518. ℞ Acetazolamide ("Diamox")

Dogs: 125 mg/30 lb, t.i.d.

519. ℞ Chlorothiazide

Cattle: 8 gm, once or twice daily.
Dogs: 5 o 10 mg/lb, two or three times daily.

520. ℞ Furosemide

Dogs and cats: 2 to 5 mg/lb body wt once or twice daily for 2 to 3 days, orally, IM or IV.
Horses: 250 to 500 mg once or twice daily for 2 to 3 days, orally, IM or IV.

For standard equivalents for measures, see pp. 1453 to 1456.

521. ℞ Hydrochlorothiazide

> *Cattle:* 125 to 250 mg (5 to 10 ml) IV or IM once or twice daily as required.
> CAUTION: Milk taken from dairy animals during treatment and for three days after latest treatment must not be used for human consumption.

522. ℞ Mannitol 20% solution or glucose 10% solution

> 1. Correct hydration with lactated Ringer's solution (℞ 565).
> 2. Administer 10% glucose or 20% mannitol solution IV slowly, and with careful monitoring of urinary output, state of hydration and BUN levels.
> 3. B-complex vitamins are necessary; tranquilization (℞ 363) and correction of acidosis may be required (℞ 475).

523. ℞ Mercurophylline Injection USP

> *Dogs:* 0.25 to 2.0 ml (50 to 200 mg) IM or IV. The IM route is somewhat safer and smaller doses should be used first to establish effective level. Use one dose every day for 3 to 6 doses and repeat if necessary after resting for 5 days, or 1 to 3 doses may be given every week as needed.

524. ℞ Trichlormethiazide 200 mg and dexamethasone 5 mg ("Nauqasone")

> *Cattle:* b.i.d. for 1 to 3 days. Use only after calving; if used earlier premature birth and retained placenta may result.

Sedatives and Anticonvulsants

525. ℞ Chloral hydrate

> 30 gm in capsule or dissolved in water via a stomach tube, daily.

526. ℞ Chloral hydrate

> 30 gm in 500 ml of sterile water, IV.
> *or* 45 gm in 500 ml of water, orally.

527. ℞ Diphenylhydantoin sodium

> 30 mg/15 lb body wt orally, every 6 to 8 hours.

> **Read introduction to prescriptions, pp. 1458 to 1460. Note all warnings and cautions appearing on drug labels and observe all local laws and regulations pertaining to drug usage.**

528. ℞ Meperidine hydrochloride

Large animals: 0.5 to 1.0 mg/lb, IV or 1 to 2 mg/lb, IM.

529. ℞ Mephenesin solution or tablets

Cattle: 400 to 600 ml of a 2% solution IV (single injection) or 10 gm, t.i.d. orally for 2 to 3 days.
Small animals: 0.5 to 1.0 gm orally t.i.d.

530. ℞ Pentobarbital sodium

Half the anesthetic dose, IV (ca. 6 mg/lb body wt).

531. ℞ Phenobarbital (tablets)

0.5 to 1.0 mg/lb body wt, orally, every 6 to 8 hours.

532. ℞ Primidone

Increase gradually from ½ tablet (125 mg) daily to 2 tablets (500 mg) per day over a 2-week period. Maintenance dose: 2 tablets daily.

533. ℞ Succinylcholine chloride

Ruminants: 3 to 5 mg/100 lb body wt, IM.
Equidae: 5 to 15 mg/100 lb body wt, IM.
Canidae: 0.5 mg/10 lb body wt, IM.
Large Felidae: 20 mg/100 lb body wt, IM.
Ursidae: 30 mg/100 lb body wt, IM.
CAUTION: All doses approximate. Not well tolerated by all species. Do not overestimate weights.

Antihistaminics

534. ℞ Chlorpheniramine maleate

Adult cats: 8 mg orally every 12 hours.
Kittens: 4 mg orally every 12 hours.

535. ℞ Diphenhydramine (capsules or solution)

0.2 to 1.0 mg/lb body wt orally or IV, 1 to 3 times daily.

536. ℞ Promethazine hydrochloride ("Phenergan") (solution, 25 mg/ml or tablets, 12.5, 25 or 50 mg)

0.1 to 0.5 mg/lb body wt, t.i.d.

For standard equivalents for measures, see pp. 1453 to 1456.

537. ℞ "Pyrahistine" with phenylephrine
Each milliliter contains:

Phenylephrine hydrochloride   2   mg
Methapyrilene hydrochloride   25   mg
Sodium bisulfite . . . .   0.2 %
Phenol as preservative . .   0.5 %

Cattle and horses: 1 ml/200 lb body wt, IV
or 1.6 to 2 ml/200 lb body wt, IM.
Dogs: 0.01 ml/lb body wt, or 0.02 to 0.03
ml/lb body wt, IM or subcut.

538. ℞ Pyrilamine maleate solution (2.5%)
or tablets, 12.5, 25 or 50 mg)

Large animals: 2 ml/100 lb body wt, IM,
or subcut.

539. ℞ Tripelennamine ("Pyribenzamine")
(2% solution or tablets)

Cattle and horses: 20 to 40 mg/100 lb body
wt, IV. May be repeated after 2 hours if
necessary.
Dogs: 2 mg/lb body wt, orally. Divide the
total daily dose into 3 or 4 parts and give
at 6- to 8-hr intervals.

540. ℞ Tripelennamine citrate . . . .   150 mg
Ammonium chloride . . . . .   400 mg
Ephedrine sulfate . . . . . .   50 mg
Syrup . . . . q.s. ad 20 ml

1 teaspoon every 4 hours.

Urinary Antiseptics and Acidifiers

541. ℞ Ammonium chloride

Dogs: 0.3 to 1.2 gm freely diluted with
water orally, 3 to 4 times daily.
Cattle and sheep: 4 to 30 gm/day.

542. ℞ Ethylenediamine dihydrochloride
("Chlor-Ethamine") (tablets) 90 mg

1 tablet t.i.d. Increase dosage if necessary
to make urine acid to litmus paper.

**Read introduction to prescriptions, pp. 1458 to 1460.
Note all warnings and cautions appearing on drug
labels and observe all local laws and regulations pertaining to drug usage.**

543. ℞ Methenamine Mandelate USP

Dogs: 0.25 to 1.0 gm orally, 1 to 4 times a day.

Hemostatics

544. ℞ Adrenochrome isonicotinic acid hydrazone ("Hemostop")

Large animals: 5 ml, IM.
Small animals: 0.25 to 1.0 ml, IM.

545. ℞ Carbazochrome salicylate

Large animals: 25 mg, IM.
Small animals: 1 mg/6 lb body wt, orally or IM.

546. ℞ Carbazochrome salicylate

2.5 to 10 mg every 3 hours.

547. ℞ "Gelfoam"

Saturate a small square of Gelfoam in isotonic salt solution or in thrombin solution and apply to bleeding areas, using mild pressure or leave in wound as a pack.

548. ℞ Hemostatic solution (aqueous emulsion of cephalin and lecithin)

Large animals: 10 ml, preferably IV.
Small animals: 1 to 5 ml, IV or IM.

549. ℞ Menadione

Large animals: 1 to 5 mg/lb of body wt, IM.
Swine: use small animal dose.
Small animals: 0.5 to 5 mg/lb of body wt, IM. Orally 3 to 10 mg/lb for 3 to 5 days.

550. ℞ Menadione Sodium Bisulfite Injection USP . . . . 2.5 mg/0.5 ml

0.5 to 1.0 ml injected IV. Repeat after 12 hours if needed. As much as 5 mg/lb body wt may be necessary when profound hypoprothrombinemia occurs (e.g., sulfaquinoxaline overdose).

551. ℞ Protamine Sulfate Injection USP

25 to 50 mg in 10 to 20 ml isotonic saline, IV.

For standard equivalents for measures, see pp. 1453 to 1456.

552. ℞ Thrombin NF XIII (solution)

> Spray on bleeding surface immediately following removal of excess blood by sponging.

553. ℞ Tolonium chloride

> 1 ml/10 lb body wt, IV, IM or subcut. Dosage may be repeated as needed.

554. ℞ Vitamin K₁ injection

> 0.5 to 3.0 mg/10 lb body wt, IV.

Parenteral Solutions

555. ℞ Dalton's oral electrolyte solution

Sodium chloride	117 gm
Potassium chloride	150 gm
Sodium bicarbonate	168 gm
Potassium phosphate (dibasic)	135 gm

> Add 1 oz to 1 gal. of water. *For calves:* Feed as warm solution or give by stomach tube at amount equivalent to 10% of body weight daily divided into 2 or 3 feeds.

556. ℞ Dextrose 5% and isotonic sodium chloride solution

> *Large animals:* 250 to 1,000 ml, IV daily.
> *Dogs:* 5 to 10 ml/lb body wt, by slow IV drip.

557. ℞ 5% Dextrose in lactated Ringers' solution (*see* ℞ 565)

> *Dogs:* 15 to 30 ml/lb body wt, by slow IV drip.

558. ℞ Electrolyte solution

Sodium chloride	5.50 gm
Calcium chloride	0.30 gm
Magnesium chloride	0.30 gm
Sodium acetate	6.10 gm
Potassium acetate	1.00 gm
Water for injections	q.s. ad 1 L

> *Calves:* Administer IV by continuous drip at the following rate:
> (A) Moderately dehydrated calves:

Read introduction to prescriptions, pp. 1458 to 1460. Note all warnings and cautions appearing on drug labels and observe all local laws and regulations pertaining to drug usage.

    (1) 25 ml/lb of body wt in first 4 to
       6 hours;
    (2) continue treatment for 20 hours at
       70 ml/lb body wt.
(B) Severely dehydrated calves:
    (1) 50 ml/lb body wt in first 4 to 6
       hours;
    (2) continue treatment for 20 hours at
       70 ml/lb wt.
Mature cattle: Give 25 to 50 ml/lb body
wt in first 4 to 6 hours and continue for
next 20 hours as required (e.g., at approximately 25 ml/lb for severe grain overload).

559. ℞ Ethoxyzolamide ("Cardrase")
    Dogs: 62.5 mg/30 lb, b.i.d.

560. ℞ Fluorescein 10% solution
    Fluorescein, soluble . . . . . 3 gm
    Isotonic salt solution . . . . 30 ml
    Dissolve, autoclave and use IV in one dose
    as the fluorescein test. The animal should
    be placed in a stall away from the sunlight.

561. ℞ Glucose 5% solution
    10 ml/lb body wt, subcut. or IV, once
    daily, preferably in divided doses.

562. ℞ Glucose 50% solution
    500 ml, IV.

563. ℞ Magnesium sulfate 25% solution
    Cattle: 400 ml, subcut.

564. ℞ Parenterin
    10 to 20 ml, IM or subcut.

565. ℞ Lactated Ringer's solution
    Sodium chloride . . . . . . 6.9 gm
    Potassium chloride . . . . . 0.3 gm
    Calcium chloride . . . . . . 0.2 gm
    Sodium lactate . . . . . . 3.0 gm
    Water for injections . . q.s. ad 1 L
    10 to 20 ml/lb body wt, IV daily, in divided
    doses.

For standard equivalents for measures, see pp. 1453 to 1456.

566. ℞ Ringer's solution

     Sodium chloride . . . . . . 90 mg
     Potassium chloride . . . . . 30 mg
     Calcium chloride . . . . . . 30 mg
     Water for injections . . q.s. ad 100 ml

Administer **5 to 15 ml/lb** body wt by slow IV drip.

567. ℞ Saline and dextrose solution

     Sodium chloride . . . . . 0.425 gm
     Glucose . . . . 2.5   gm
     Distilled water . . q.s. ad 100   ml

10 ml/lb body wt, subcut. or IV daily, preferably in divided doses, or as required.

568. ℞ Saline and sodium bicarbonate

     Mix equal parts of aqueous solutions:
     Sodium chloride 0.85%
     Sodium bicarbonate . . . . 1.3 %

Calves: Administer IV by continuous drip at the following rate:
(A) Moderately dehydrated calves:
     (1) 25 ml/lb of body wt in first 4 to 6 hours;
     (2) continue treatment for 20 hours at 70 ml/lb body wt.
(B) Severely dehydrated calves:
     (1) 50 ml/lb body wt in first 4 to 6 hours;
     (2) continue treatment for 20 hours at 70 ml/lb body wt.
Mature cattle: Give 25 to 50 ml/lb body wt in first 4 to 6 hours and continue for next 20 hours as required (e.g., at approximately 25 ml/lb for severe grain overload).

569. ℞ Isotonic saline with dextrose 6%

Piglets: Give 2 oz orally every 4 hours or 15 ml subcut. every 6 hours.

Read introduction to prescriptions, pp. 1458 to 1460. Note all warnings and cautions appearing on drug labels and observe all local laws and regulations pertaining to drug usage.

Parenteral Enzyme Preparations

570. ℞ Chymotrypsin suspension injectable
(5,000 u/ml)

> *Horses and cows (800 to 1,200 lb):* 5 ml
> daily. Adjust dose according to weight.
> *Dogs and cats: up to 10 lb:* 0.25 ml, b.i.d.
>   *10 to 50 lb:* 0.5 ml, b.i.d.
>   *over 50 lb:* 0.75 to 1.0 ml,
>   b.i.d.

571. ℞ Pancreatic dornase ("Dornavac")

> Dissolve 50,000 to 100,000 u alone or with
> antibiotics in a suitable volume of sterile
> water and inject into cavity or tract.

572. ℞ Streptokinase-streptodornase mixture
("Varidase")

> *All animals:* Dissolve 5,000 to 10,000 u in
> sterile water. Inject into pleural cavity or
> IM every 24 hours.

Systemic Iodine Preparations

573. ℞ Ethylenediamine dihydriodide

> 1 oz, b.i.d. in feed or capsule for 8 days,
> starting 10 days after estrus.

574. ℞ Ethylenediamine dihydriodide
(20 grains per oz)

> *Cattle:* ½ oz, b.i.d. for 8 to 10 days.
> *Calves:* 6 months old, 1 lb/300 head daily
> for 7 days, then 1 lb/500 head daily.
> *Adults:* 1 lb/100 head daily for 7 days, then
> 1 lb/300 head daily.
> CAUTION: Do not use in lactating dairy
> animals.

575. ℞ 4% Iodine in soybean oil
("Hypodermin")

> Inject subcut. in doses of 0.5 to 1 ml
> totaling no more than 6 ml. Repeat in 10
> days if necessary.

576. ℞ Lugol's solution

> Dilute with equal parts of distilled water
> and inject 2 ml into bursa.

For standard equivalents for measures, see pp. 1453 to 1456.

577. ℞ Lugol's iodine 5% . . . . **1 ml**
Isotonic salt solution . . . . . **9 ml**
> Using a fine gauge needle, make several
> 0.5 ml injections into the affected muscles.

578. ℞ Potassium Iodide Solution NF XIII
> 2 to 5 drops in water, daily for 2 or 3 days.

579. ℞ Potassium or sodium iodide
> *Horses:* 4 to 10 gm orally.
> *Cattle:* 10 gm/1,000 lb body wt orally.
> Daily doses for 2 to 4 weeks. Discontinue
> medication if signs of iodism appear.

580. ℞ Sodium iodide
> 0.75 gm/100 lb body wt, IV, repeated every
> 4 or 5 days. Discontinue medication if
> signs of iodism appear.

581. ℞ Sodium iodide 5 to 20% solution
> 3 gm/100 lb body wt, IV, injected slowly.
> Repeat after 7 to 10 days.
> CAUTION: Use cautiously in lactating dairy
> cows. Contraindicated in advanced preg-
> nancy.

582. ℞ Strong Iodine Solution USP (Lugol's
solution)
> 10 to 20 drops in water daily for 2 or 3
> days.

Calcium Preparations

583. ℞ Calcium borogluconate 25% solution
> *Cattle:* 250 to 500 ml, IV or IP.
> *Sheep:* 100 ml, IV or IP.
> *Horses:* 200 to 500 ml, IV.

584. ℞ Calcium borogluconate . . . . **250 gm**
Magnesium borogluconate or
sulfate . . . . **50 gm**
Distilled water . . . . q.s. ad 1 L
> *Cattle:* 400 to 800 ml IV, subcut. or IP.
> *Sheep:* 100 ml IV, subcut. or IP.
> *Horses:* 100 to 850 ml, IV.

**Read introduction to prescriptions, pp. 1458 to 1460.
Note all warnings and cautions appearing on drug
labels and observe all local laws and regulations pertaining to drug usage.**

585. ℞ Calcium gluconate

> *Cattle and horses:* 250 to 500 ml, IV, 20% solution, or half the dose IV and half sub-cut.
> *Sheep:* 50 ml, IV, 20% solution.
> *Dogs:* 5 to 20 ml, IV, of a 10% solution.
> *Cats:* 2 to 5 ml, IV, of a 10% solution.

586. ℞ Calcium gluconate
    (tablets) . . . . 0.5 to 1 gm

> 1 tablet t.i.d.

587. ℞ Calcium lactate
    Sodium lactate . . . . . . āā 250 gm
    Water . . . . 500 ml

> 250 gm orally, b.i.d. for 10 days.

Analgesics and Local Anesthetics

588. ℞ Acetylsalicylic acid
    (tablets) . . . . 300 mg

> 1 tablet t.i.d.
> CAUTION: Some cats are sensitive. Use with care in this species.

589. ℞ Dibucaine ointment

> Apply to rectum and anus every 4 hours.

590. ℞ Meperidine hydrochloride

> *Horses:* 250 to 500 mg, IV *or* 500 to 1,000 mg, IM.
> *Cattle:* 50 mg, IM daily.
> *Dogs and cats:* 5 to 10 mg/lb body wt, orally or IM. Repeated every 8 to 12 hours.

591. ℞ Methampyrone

> *Horses:* 10 to 20 ml, IV, IM or subcut.
> *Cattle:* 5 to 15 ml, IV, IM or subcut.

592. ℞ Morphine sulfate

> *Horses:* 60 to 90 mg, subcut.
> *Dogs:* 15 mg, subcut., repeated at 4- to 8-hour intervals if necessary.

593. ℞ Phenylbutazone
    Tablets NF XIII . . . . . . 100 mg

> *Horses:* 2 to 4 gm/1,000 lb body wt, not to exceed 4 gm daily.
> *Dogs:* 100 mg/5 lb body wt in 3 divided doses daily.

For standard equivalents for measures, see pp. 1453 to 1456.

594. ℞ Tetracaine hydrochloride 0.5% solution

> 1 drop into conjunctival sac every 2 to 3 hours.

Dietary Supplements

595. ℞ Amino acids 10% solution

> Administer IV, from 10 to 100% of the animal's own blood volume daily, depending on amount of other fluid intake.

596. ℞ Ascorbic acid

> *Dogs:* 100 mg, t.i.d., orally.

597. ℞ Ascorbic Acid Tablets USP . . 250 mg

> 1 tablet b.i.d.

598. ℞ Brewers' yeast dried

> *Cattle and horses:* 120 to 150 gm daily.
> *Sheep and swine:* 30 to 60 gm daily. Mix thoroughly with grain or ground feed.
> *Dogs:* 1 to 3 gm daily, as tablets or in food.

599. ℞ Choline chloride

> 0.5 to 2.5 gm added to diet daily.

600. ℞ DL-Methionine

> *Dogs:* 1 gm every 8 hours orally.

Detoxifying Agents

601. ℞ BAL (2,3-dimercaptopropanol)

> 2 to 3 mg/lb body wt, IM. Repeat at 8- to 12-hr intervals as necessary.

602. ℞ DL-Batyl alchohol 2% solution in 1% saline (brought into solution with 5% "Tween 80")

> 25 to 50 ml daily by slow IV injection.

603. ℞ DL-Batyl alcohol . . . . 5 gm
Olive oil . . . . 50 ml

> 10 ml subcut. daily for 5 days.

Read introduction to prescriptions, pp. 1458 to 1460. Note all warnings and cautions appearing on drug labels and observe all local laws and regulations pertaining to drug usage.

604. ℞ "Calcium Disodium Versenate" solution

Calcium disodium ethylene-
diaminetetra-acetate . . .   20 gm
Water . . . .   100 ml

1 to 2 ml/lb body wt, IV or subcut., daily.

605. ℞ Dicalcium-phosphogluconate
("C.G.P.")

Cattle and horses: 250 to 500 ml, IV.
Sheep and swine: 50 to 100 ml, IV. Repeat
after several hours.

606. ℞ Magnesium sulfate

Horses and cattle: 500 to 1,000 gm orally.
Swine: 50 to 200 gm orally.
Sheep: 20 to 50 gm orally.

607. ℞ Methylene blue . . . .   10 gm
Water . . . .   500 ml

20 ml/100 lb body wt, IV. Repeat if
necessary.

608. ℞ 2-PAM chloride (pralidoxime chloride)

20 mg/kg of body wt, subcut.

609. ℞ Sodium iodide 10% solution

30 to 45 mg/lb body wt, IV.

610. ℞ Sodium nitrite . . . .   20 gm
Sodium thiosulfate . . . . . .   30 gm
Sterile water . . . . .   q.s. ad   500 ml

20 ml/100 lb body wt, IV. To be given
slowly and repeated once only if necessary.

611. ℞ Sodium thiosulfate 20% solution

10 ml/100 lb body wt, IV. Repeat if
necessary.

Astringents and Escharotics

612. ℞ Alum . . . .   5 gm
Water . . . .   q.s. ad   100 ml

Apply topically to mucosa.

For standard equivalents for measures, see pp. 1453 to 1456.

613. ℞ Copper sulfate . . . . 450 gm
      Distilled water . . . . 4 L (1 gal.)

      Apply locally or use in a foot bath through
      which the sheep are driven.

614. ℞ Ferrous sulfate dried
      Copper sulfate dried
      Zinc sulfate dried . . . . . āā 10 gm

      Thrush: Apply to bottom of affected sulcus
      and retain with pledget of cotton or oakum.
      Canker: Apply to affected area and retain
      with bandage and foot pack.

615. ℞ Mandl's solution
      Iodine . . . . 0.60 gm
      Potassium iodide . . . . . 1.20 gm
      Peppermint oil . . . . . . 0.25 gm
      Glycerin . . . . . . q.s. ad 30 ml

      For topical application.

616. ℞ Picric acid 5%

      Saturate cotton pledget and pack.

617. ℞ Silver nitrate 2% solution

      Pharyngitis: Apply to inflamed mucous
      membranes with a cotton swab.
      Nonfunctional quarter: Infuse into teat ca-
      nal and milk out after 7 days. Repeat
      treatment after 2 or 3 weeks if necessary.
      NOTE: The total amount of chemical used
      should not exceed 1 gm (50 ml of a 2%
      solution) to avoid severe toxic reactions.

618. ℞ Silver nitrate 5% solution

      For topical use in cauterizing cysts, fistulas
      and mucosal lesions.

619. ℞ Tannic acid . . . . 1 ml
      Glycerin . . . . 30 ml

      Apply to inflamed mucous membranes with
      a cotton swab.

**Read introduction to prescriptions, pp. 1458 to 1460.
Note all warnings and cautions appearing on drug
labels and observe all local laws and regulations pertaining to drug usage.**

620. ℞ Tannic acid
Salicylic acid . . . . āā 5 gm
Alcohol 70% . . . . . q.s. ad 100 ml
Apply b.i.d. to the affected areas of the
skin after debridement and cleansing.

621. ℞ Zinc sulfate
Lead acetate
Copper sulfate . . . . . . āā 60 gm
Water . . . . q.s. ad 600 ml
Apply b.i.d. after washing the leg.

Counterirritants

622. ℞ Tincture of iodine 2%
Dilute with equal parts of distilled water
and inject 2 ml into bursa.

623. ℞ Tincture of iodine 2.5% . . . . 60 ml
Pine tar . . . . 240 gm
Soft soap . . . . 90 gm
Apply locally.

624. ℞ Tincture of iodine 5%
Rub well into coronet with brush. Repeat
daily for 4 or 5 days.

625. ℞ Tincture of iodine 7% . . . . 240 ml
Spirits of camphor . . . . . 60 ml
Turpentine . . . . 60 ml
Croton oil . . . . 0.6 ml
Mix and apply daily until a good blister is
formed. If the blister is to be used on a
very thin-skinned horse, 60 ml of glycerin
may be added to the mixture.

626. ℞ Tincture of iodine 7%
Glycerin
Spirits of camphor . . . . āā 180 ml
Isopropyl alcohol 95% . . q.s. ad 1 L
Apply to affected area, rub well and cover
with sheet cotton and bandage.

627. ℞ Red mercuric iodide
Cantharides powder . . . . āā 4 gm
Lard . . . . 30 gm
Rub in well and cover with wool bandage.
Remove bandage after 4 days.

For standard equivalents for measures, see pp. 1453 to 1456.

628. ℞ Red mercuric iodide . . . . . 20 gm

      Petrolatum . . . . 80 gm

> Mix thoroughly, clip hair from area to be blistered and rub in well for 5 to 10 minutes. Cover with sheet cotton and bandage. Remove dressing after 4 days.

Semen Diluters

629. ℞ Citrate buffer solution

    Sodium citrate

        ($Na_3C_6H_6O_7 \cdot 2H_2O$) . . .   3 gm

    Water distilled over glass and

        heated to 100°C . . . . .   100 ml

> Sterilize and store in darkness.

    Diluter

      Buffer solution

      Yolk from fresh eggs āā

      Penicillin . . . . 1,000 u/ml

      Streptomycin . . . . . .   1 mg/ml

> Mix on the day it is to be used to dilute semen.

630. ℞ For milk and glycerin diluter

> Place 500 ml of milk in double boiler and heat to 200°F for 10 minutes. Remove scum from top of milk. Cool and measure out 450 ml of milk in sterile flask. Add 500,000 u of penicillin and 500 mg of streptomycin. Measure out 200 ml of milk and add 50 ml of glycerol.
>
> Add semen to unglycerolated milk and cool to 40°F over a 3- or 4-hour period. Add similarly cooled glycerolated milk to semen-milk mixture in three equal portions at 10-minute intervals.

631. ℞ Phosphate buffer solution

    Potassium phosphate

      monobasic (KH_2PO_4) . .   0.2 gm

    Sodium phosphate dibasic

      dodecahydrate

      ($Na_2HPO_4 \cdot 12H_2O$) . . .   2.0 gm

    Water distilled over glass and

      heated to 100°C   100   ml

> Sterilize and store in darkness.

Read introduction to prescriptions, pp. 1458 to 1460. Note all warnings and cautions appearing on drug labels and observe all local laws and regulations pertaining to drug usage.

Diluter
 Buffer solution
 Yolk from fresh eggs āā
 Penicillin . . . . 1,000 u/ml
 Streptomycin . . . . . 1 mg/ml
Mix on the day it is to be used to dilute semen.

Miscellaneous

632. ℞ "Acetest" reagent tablets

A drop of urine is placed on tablet. Color reaction on tablet compared to color scale indicates amount of urinary ketones.

633. ℞ Para-Aminobenzoic acid (PABA)

Dogs: under 20 lb: 1 gm, t.i.d.
20 to 50 lb: 2 gm, t.i.d.
over 50 lb: 2 gm, 4 times daily.

634. ℞ Amphetamine sulfate

Cattle and horses: 0.1 to 0.3 gm subcut.
Dogs: 0.5 to 2.0 mg/lb body wt orally or subcut.

635. ℞ Bethanechol chloride

Dogs: 5 to 15 mg orally, 3 to 4 times a day.

636. ℞ Chloroquine diphosphate

125 to 250 mg orally daily.
CAUTION: May produce side reactions.

637. ℞ Diatrizoate sodium ("Hypaque") 50% solution

For IV urography: 5 to 40 ml, depending on size of animal.

638. ℞ Diquat ("Reglone")

18.4 to 16.8 ppm of formulated material (2 to 4 ppm diquat cation). One-hour exposure for 3 to 4 consecutive days for treatment. A single hour's exposure may be used for prevention.

639. ℞ Lobelia fluid extract . . . . . 60 ml
 Belladonna fluid extract . . . . 30 ml
 Fowler's solution . . . q.s. ad 500 ml
1 tablespoon on feed, t.i.d.

For standard equivalents for measures, see pp. 1453 to 1456.

640. ℞ Pentylenetetrazole injection
(100 mg/ml)

0.05 to 0.1 ml given slowly IV. (May also be given in electrolyte or dextrose infusion.)

641. ℞ Pilocarpine hydrochloride

5 to 10 mg subcut., t.i.d.

642. ℞ Prolipin ("Omnadin") solution

Large animals: 5 to 20 ml, IM or subcut. daily.
Small animals: 1 to 4 ml or subcut. daily.

643. ℞ Propylene Glycol USP

250 gm mixed with an equal volume of water, orally b.i.d. for 5 days.

644. ℞ Quinacrine hydrochloride
(tablets) . . . . 100 mg

½ to 1 tablet b.i.d. for 2 weeks, then ½ to 1 tablet once daily.
CAUTION: May produce side reactions.

645. ℞ Sodium morrhuate 5% solution

0.5 ml injected at 1-in. intervals into the tendon.

646. ℞ Sodium propionate

120 gm orally, b.i.d. for 10 days.

647. ℞ Sterile milk

Large animals: 5 to 25 ml, IM or subcut. Repeat at intervals of 1 to 5 days if indicated.
Small animals: 0.5 to 1.0 ml, IM or subcut. as an initial dose. Subsequent doses depend upon response and sensitivity of the patient.

648. ℞ Strychnine sulfate
Digitalin (soluble)
Atropine sulfate . . . . . āā 180 mg
Water . . . . 180 ml

1 teaspoon on feed, t.i.d.

Read introduction to prescriptions, pp. 1458 to 1460. Note all warnings and cautions appearing on drug labels and observe all local laws and regulations pertaining to drug usage.

649. ℞ Iodine agglutination test (IAT) for plasmacytosis

The iodine test solution is unstable and must be prepared weekly. It is stored refrigerated in amber bottles.

Iodine crystals	2 gm
Potassium iodide	4 gm
Distilled water	30 ml

Blood from a clipped toenail is collected in a nonheparinized capillary tube and centrifuged. The serum is mixed on a glass slide with fresh solution and stirred with a wooden applicator stick. Clumping or precipitation within a few seconds constitutes a positive reaction.

650. ℞ New methylene blue stain

New methylene blue	0.5 gm
Potassium oxalate	1.6 gm
Distilled water	100 ml

Filter before use.

651. ℞ Phosphate buffer

Disodium hydrogen phosphate	3.80 gm
Potassium dihydrogen phosphate	5.47 gm

Dissolve in 500 ml of distilled water and bring volume to 1 liter. The distilled water *must be neutralized* using hematoxylin as the indicator. Rinse clean test tube, add 5 ml of the distilled water and a few crystals of hematoxylin:

neutral—pale lavender in 10 seconds;
acid—becomes yellow and remains so for over 5 minutes;
alkaline—becomes red-purple at once or within a minute.

Adjust pH with 1% potassium hydroxide or 1% hydrochloric acid as necessary. Prepare neutral water daily or as necessary.

For standard equivalents for measures, see pp. 1453 to 1456.

INDEX

(Throughout the index, page numbers appearing in roman type indicate that the subject is identified in the text either as a heading or by boldface or italic type or by quotation marks. Page numbers in *italics* signify that the term occurs in the text merely as part of the discussion, without typographical emphasis.)

Amyloodinium spp., 1177
Anabaena flos-aquae (algal poisoning), 1006
  (photosensitization), 8
Anal atresia, 174
  fissure, 175
  fistula and sinus, 175
  prolapse, 173
  sac, impaction, suppuration, abscesses, 175
Anaphylaxis, 3
Anaplasma
  centrale, 279
  marginale, 279
  ovis, 279
Anaplasmosis, 279
Anas platyrhyncos, 1451
Anaticola
  anseris, 1095
  crassicornis, 1095
Anatipestifer infection, 1044
Anatoecus dentatus, 1095
Ancylostoma
  braziliense, 679
  caninum, 679
Anemia, (chapter), 14
  aplastic (poultry), 1085
  in baby pigs, *19 (see also p. 39)*
  bone marrow hypofunction, 18
  Coombs' positive, 20
  deficient heme synthesis, **18**
    globin synthesis, 19
  equine infectious, 254
  feline infectious, 324
  Heinz-body, *20*
  hemolytic, 21
    bacterial, 24
    chemical, 24
    hypersplenism and splenomegaly, 22
    increased RE removal, 22
    of newborn foals, 36
    of newborn pigs, 39
    physical agents, *22,* 25
    plant, 24
    red cell parasitism, 23
  hemorrhagic, poultry, 1085
  hypoplastic and aplastic, 17
  idiopathic autoimmune hemolytic, 21
  isoimmune hemolytic, foals, 36
  loss or lysis of normal red cells, 19, 22, 24, 25
    external parasitism, 25
    internal parasitism, 26
  due to marrow stem cell injury, 17
  in mink, 1116
  myelophthisic, 18
  nutritional, 17
  rape-induced, *20, 24*
  red cell, abnormal enzyme content, 19
    damage, 21
    defects, 20

Anemia *(cont'd)*
  reduction in hemoglobin synthesis, 18
Anencephaly, 627
Anestrus, and irregularities of estrus, 796
  cows, 796
  mares, 798
  sows, 799
Aneurysm, 65
  dissecting, turkeys, 1082
  verminous, horses, *162*
Angiostrongylus
  cantonensis, 1145
  vasorum, 641
Aniline, *8*
Anomalies, congenital, CNS, 627
  cardiovascular system, 56
  cysts and sinuses, neck, 118
  genitourinary tract, 790
  mouth, 91
  spinal, *632*
Anoplocephala spp., 678
Anorexia, 74
Anoxia, anemic, 1403
  anoxic, 1403
  fluid balance in, 1403
  histotoxic, 1403
  of the newborn, 1405
  pathologic physiology, 1405
  stagnation, 1403
Anthrax, 328
Antibiotic therapy, 473
  toxicity (chinchillas), *1120*
    (guinea pigs), 1148
    (hamsters), 1151
    (zoo animals), *1171*
ANTU poisoning, 961
Aortic body tumors, 609
  rupture (turkeys), 1082
  stenosis, 63
Aotus trivirgatus, 1152
Aplastic anemia (poultry), 1085
Apothecary system, and equivalents, 1453
Aphthous fever, 259
Appetites, in health and disease, 73
  restoration in sick animals, 1310
Aptyalism, 114
Argas persicus (fowl tick), 1095
  (tick infestation), 714
  (tick paralysis), 722
Argasidae, *714*
Arizona hinshawii, 1041
Arizona infection, 1041
Arrhythmias (heart), abnormal, **47**
  in normal animals, 46
Arrowgrass, *938, 986*
Arsenic poisoning, 933
  inorganic, 933
  organic, 934
    herbicide arsenicals, 953
  in poultry, 1086
Arteritis, equine viral, 248

Erodium spp., **7**
Eruption of teeth (ages, table), **79**
Erysipelas, swine, 370
Erysipelothrix insidiosa (rhusopa-thiae), 369
  (infectious arthritis, swine), 546
  (man), 374
  (neonatal septicemias), 395
  (nonsuppurative polyarthritis, lambs), 372
  (post-dipping lameness, sheep), **373**
  (swine), 370
  (turkeys), 1046
Erythremia, **27**
Erythroblastosis (poultry), 1016
Erythrocyte(s),
  count, 1381 (*see also* Hematocrit)
  examination of, for parasites, 1375
  values, normal ranges (table), 16
Erythrocytosis, apparent, *26*
  true, *27*
Erythroid leukosis (poultry), 1016
Erythromycin, 489
Escherichia coli, (abortion, horses), 802
  (bovine cystitis and pyelonephritis) 828
  (colibacillosis of weaned pigs), 148
  (equine respiratory disease), 250
  (cystitis, sm. an.), 851
  (diarrhea of newborn animals), 166
    (calves), 166
    (foals), 169
    (lambs), 170
    (piglets), 170
  (dysentery, primates), 1153
  (edema disease, swine), 148
  (infectious swine arthritis), 546
  (mastitis, cows), 812
    (goats), 816
    (sheep), 816
    (swine), 816
  (*Mycoplasma gallisepticum* infection), 1053
  (necrotic dermatitis, poultry), 1050
  (neonatal septicemias), *394*
  (new duck syndrome), 1044
  (pyelonephritis, sm. an.), *854*
  (pyometra, dogs), 841
  (ruptured egg yolks), 1080
Esophagism, 125
Esophagitis, lg. an., 124
  sm. an., 118
Esophagus, diseases of, lg. an., **122**
  sm. an., 118
Estrogens, extrinsic sources, 199
  growth effects, 199
Estrus, control, hormonal, 789
  irregularities of, cows, 796
  mares, 798
  sows, 799
Ethylene dibromide, poisoning (poultry), 1088
Eumycetomas, 428

Eumycotic mycetomas, 428
Eupatorium rugosum, 982
"European" chick flea, 1100
Examination of animals prior to sale, 1418
Exanthema, vesicular, 300
Extensor process disease, 544
Exudative diathesis (poultry), **1349,** *1352*
  epidermitis, 919
Eye, and ear (section), 201
  and optic nerve, congenital and inherited conditions, *212,* 629
  examination of, 202
  anterior chamber, 209
  lens, 210
Eyeball, 210
Eyelids, 202
Eyeworm, Manson's, infestation, **1093**

F

Face flies, 739
Facial eczema, 9, 994
  paralysis, 636
Fagopyrum esculentum, **7**
False distemper, 409
  hellebore, *980*
  pregnancy in dogs, 845
  quarter, *539*
Farcy, 388
  (bovine), *431*
Fasciola
  gigantica, 704
  hepatica, 702
Fascioloides magna, **704**
Fat
  deficiency, dogs, 1339
    swine, 1329
  necrosis, 176
  requirement, cats, 1273
    dogs, 1265
Fatty infiltration, muscle, **585**
Favus, 1066
Feather mites, 1097
Fecal output, daily, of various species (table), 1393
Feces, examination for parasites, **1374**
  stercobolin test, 1385
  urobilin test, 1385
Feeding
  beef cattle, 1211
    fattening cattle, 1213
    stocker cattle, 1212
  birds, *1231*
  cats, drugs and contaminating substances, 1275
    foods, 1274
    general considerations, 1275
  dairy cattle, 1196
    calves, 1197
    heifers and young stock, 1197
    pregnant cows and heifers, 1201

NOTES

GALEN

METHOD OF MEDICINE

I

LCL 516

GALEN

METHOD OF MEDICINE

BOOKS 1–4

EDITED AND TRANSLATED BY

IAN JOHNSTON

AND

G. H. R. HORSLEY

HARVARD UNIVERSITY PRESS

CAMBRIDGE, MASSACHUSETTS

LONDON, ENGLAND

2011

So YBP ¹²/₁₁ 24.00

First published 2011

LOEB CLASSICAL LIBRARY® is a registered trademark
of the President and Fellows of Harvard College

Library of Congress Control Number 2011921281
CIP data available from the Library of Congress

ISBN 978-0-674-99652-6

Composed in ZephGreek and ZephText by
Technologies 'N Typography, Merrimac, Massachusetts.
Printed on acid-free paper and bound by
The Maple-Vail Book Manufacturing Group

CONTENTS

For Reg

ACKNOWLEDGMENTS

A number of people have contributed significantly to bringing this translation project to what we hope is a satisfactory conclusion. We are very grateful to them for the considerable expenditure of time and effort they have been prepared to make. The following Greek scholars (the majority with a particular interest in ancient medicine and science) read individual books (in some cases two), commenting on and offering helpful criticism of the translation: Han Baltussen, Wayne Donaldson, Alan James, Geoffrey Lloyd, Bob Milns, Vivian Nutton, Ingvar Olsson, Niki Papavramidou, Owen Powell, Lars Rydbeck, John Vallance, and Philip van der Eijk. Their corrections and suggestions were much appreciated. We are grateful to two doctors, Michael Besser (a recently retired neurosurgeon) and Justine Johnston (a currently practicing GP), who between them read all the books apart from 1 and 2 and commented most helpfully from the viewpoint of the medical reader. We are grateful to Susan Collis, who not only read all the books in various stages of preparation and made numerous helpful suggestions, but also took responsibility for locating manuscripts, gathering materials, and carrying out various other tasks—her assistance has been invaluable. We are indebted to two people who commented on specific aspects of the work: Mathias Witt, who

ACKNOWLEDGMENTS

helped to clarify Galen's somewhat complex description of the surgical repair of the anterior abdominal wall (he has kindly allowed us to use his figures in the illustrations), and John Scarborough, for his comments on pharmacological matters. Finally, we would like to thank the Greek Book Fund (Australia) for their generous grant toward various expenses, including provision and preparation of the manuscripts. Our debt to all these people, and to others unnamed, is profound.

Ian Johnston
South Bruny Island

Greg Horsley
University of New England,
New South Wales

April 2010

INTRODUCTION

The basic aim of the practicing doctor most simply stated is to preserve the health of those who are healthy (*kata phusin*—"in accord with nature," in Galenic terms) and to restore to health those who have departed from it by suffering injury or succumbing to disease (*para phusin*—"contrary to nature"). Thus medicine has both prophylactic and therapeutic components, a point which Galen himself emphasizes in his *Method of Medicine* (*Methodus medendi*). And it is this *Method of Medicine* (*MM*), comprising fourteen separate books and occupying one whole Kühn volume, that is his systematic and comprehensive account of the therapeutic component. In it he details the principles of treatment of injury and disease following his own classification, illustrated by case reports and punctuated by various theoretical and polemical digressions and social comment. This great work is supplemented by the much shorter *Method of Medicine for Glaucon* (*MMG*), while the prophylactic limb is dealt with primarily in his *On the Preservation of Health*. The *MM* sits atop the theoretical edifice established by a number of Galen's other works, to which he refers repeatedly throughout his therapeutic magnum opus. These are his works on the basic structure of matter, those on physiology, those on anatomy, those on pathology and pathophysiology, those on the classification and causation of diseases and symptoms, and those on pharmacology.[1] These subjects—that is, basic science, anatomy, physiology, pathology, and pharmacology—have, more or less in this order, remained the components of the Western doctor's basic education to the present day. To them, Galen would, however, add philosophy, especially ethics and logic in the broad sense, components which he would undoubtedly see as unduly neglected in modern times.

Thus the full exposition of Galen's systematic approach to the treatment of the whole range of diseases, his *Method of Medicine*, became established as a work of very considerable and enduring influence for many centuries. It contributed significantly to the compendia prepared by the Western medical writers in the several centuries immedi-

---

[1] The main components of this foundation, which are considered in greater detail below, and which are available in Kühn, are as follows (references to English translations are given in parentheses where available): *De elementis secundum Hippocratem* (I.413–508K—P. H. de Lacy, 1996), *De naturalibus facultatibus* (II.1–214K—A. J. Brock, 1916), *De temperamentis* (I.509–694K—P. Singer, 1997), *De anatomicis administrationibus* (II.215–731K—C. Singer, 1956, W. H. Duckworth et al., 1962), *De usu partium* (II.1–939K, III.1–366K—M. T. May, 1967), *De locis affectis* (VIII.1–452K—R. E. Siegel, 1975), *De inaequali intemperie* (VII.733–52K—M. Grant, 2000), *De differentiis morborum*, *De morborum causis*, *De symptomatum differentiis*, *De symptomatum causis* (VI.836–80K, VII.1–272K—I. Johnston, 2006), *De simplicium medicamentorum temperamentis et facultatibus* (XI.379–892K, XII.1–377), *De compositione medicamentorum secundum locos* (XII.378–1007K, XIII.1–361K), *De compositione medicamentorum per genera* (XIII.362–1058K).

ately following Galen's death, men such as Oribasius and Paul of Aegina; it became foundational in the development of Arabic medicine; and, made available particularly by Linacre's Latin translation, it regained its influence in the West during the Renaissance, when Galenism again became the dominant medical philosophy. Peter English, in his 1656 translation of the *MM*,[2] which remains the only "complete" English translation prior to the present one, writes on the title page of his work, which he called Galen's *Method of Physick: Or, his Great Master-Peece, being the very Marrow and Quintessence of all his Writings*:

> Wherein He exceeds not only Himself, but also all others, on such a Subject, being not only sufficient thorowly to acquaint any judicious man with all the Principles of Physick or Medicine, but also it is absolutely necessary for directing all Practitioners in all their Physicall Applications and Cures.

So this substantial tome, written in the second century AD, was still, in effect, the therapeutic bible in Western medicine some fifteen centuries later.

Of course, the great development of scientific knowledge, which gathered pace from the seventeenth century on, had a major bearing on all the foundational areas of medical practice listed above. This development, still continuing at an astonishing pace, has rendered the conceptual basis of Galenic medicine obsolete. What has not become obsolete, however, is the method itself—that is, the

---

[2] Peter English, *Galen's Method of Physick* (Edinburgh, 1656). English concentrates on the practical elements of the work, omitting much of the polemic.

development of treatment based on an established theoretical and practical foundation. Nor has obsolescence affected the need to consider the means whereby knowledge of medical treatment is acquired and the ethical ramifications of its application. Both are factors to which Galen gives considerable attention in this work and elsewhere.

Galen's *MM* remains, then, a work of great interest, first as a detailed statement of the methodical approach to medicine in general and to treatment in particular and to other aspects of patient care which are not limited to any era; second, for the wealth of historical information it provides on medical practice during a period that saw marked development in this practice; and third as a reflection of social conditions at the time of its writing. Hence, it seemed worthwhile to add a modern English translation of Galen's "Great Master-Peece" to the highly polished and very accurate Latin version of Thomas Linacre and the much freer, incomplete paraphrastic version of Peter English.

1. GALEN'S LIFE

Apart from his final years, which remain something of a mystery, Galen's life is well documented and has been traced in a number of modern works, in a few instances as the sole topic[3] and in a greater number of instances as part

---

[3] Among these may be mentioned the books by G. Sarton, *Galen of Pergamon* (Lawrence, KA, 1954), and P. Moraux, *Galiene de Pergamene* (Paris, 1985), and the articles collected in V. Nutton in his *From Democedes to Harvey* (London, 1988), and the series of articles by J. Walsh published in the *Annals of Medical History*

of the introduction to a study of some aspect of his work. Much of the information comes from his own writings in which numerous anecdotes provide factual information as well as insights into the writer's character. The abbreviated account which follows is divided into a series of relatively well-defined periods.

The Early Years (129–146): Galen was born in Pergamum in Asia Minor in 129 into a well-to-do and highly respected family. His place of birth is of some relevance in that Pergamum was renowned for its shrine to Aesculapius and for its library, which acted as a considerable attraction to scholars. His father, Nikon, was a wealthy architect of the city, much respected both generally and by his son, in whose initial education he took an active role. His mother, now remembered through her son's unflattering portrayal, seems to have been notable for her intemperate and somewhat violent conduct. Galen himself gives the following contrasting descriptions of his two parents and of his attitude toward the behavior of each:

> I was extremely fortunate in having a father who was not in the least irascible, very civilized, very kindly and very courteous whereas my mother was so irascible that she sometimes bit the female servants, always bawling at, and fighting with, my father to an increasing extent—a Xanthippe to Socrates. For

between 1929 and 1939. For earlier studies, see Ackermann's *Historia Literaria Claudii Galeni* in Kühn, vol. I. Very recent accounts are those in *The Cambridge Companion to Galen*, ed. R. J. Hankinson (Cambridge, 2008), and by V. Nutton in his *Ancient Medicine* (London, 2004).

myself, seeing set side by side the virtues of my father's actions with the disgraceful affections of my
mother, there was an eager following and love of the
former but avoidance and hatred of the latter.[4]

Galen was initially schooled directly by his father in the
basic disciplines of geometry, mathematics, and arithmetic, as well as in logic and architecture.[5] He was then exposed to the teachings of the major philosophical schools,
his father arranging for him, from the age of fourteen, a series of teachers of philosophy. According to Galen's own
account these teachers included "a Stoic, a pupil of Philo-
pater," "a Platonist pupil of Gaius," "a pupil of Aspasius the
Peripatetic," and "an Epicurean from Athens."[6] Another
notable feature is Galen's description of his own aptitude,
which displays the high self-regard that seemingly remained intact throughout his life. Thus, in his early years,
what stands out is his comprehensive education in philosophy and related disciplines supervised by his father, and
the quite contrasting nature of his parents, one respected,
one reviled. One might, however, suspect that his mother's
intemperate nature found a reflection in Galen's own often
quite intemperate writings—it may be that his mother's
physical assaults found their counterpart in her son's verbal assaults![7]

[4] *De propriorum animi cuiuslibet affectuum dignotione et curatione*, V.40–41K.

[5] *De libris propriis*, XIX.40K.

[6] *De propriorum animi cuiuslibet affectum dignotione et curatione*, V.41K.

[7] Galen also expresses here his own uncertainty on this matter:
"Moreover, I do not know how I have the nature I have, for it is

Medical Training (147–157): The course of his education, and indeed of his life, was changed significantly in his seventeenth year by his father's dreams. In *On the Order of My Own Books*, Galen writes: "Then, persuaded by clear dreams, he made me, in my seventeenth year, train in medicine at the same time as philosophy."[8] There is the interesting question of the extent to which Galen continued his philosophical studies *pari passu* with his now primary study of medicine, both in the early years and throughout his life. This bears on his own repeated claim of the importance of philosophy to medicine and the significance of his knowledge of the former discipline in making him superior in the latter to many (all!) of his contemporaries. In fact, how important the continuing study of philosophy was to Galen and how significant his philosophical contributions were are matters of quite sharp disagreement among modern commentators. On the first point, Lieber provides the following quotation from a work surviving only in Arabic: "Since my youth I have studied logic. Then, when I started to study medicine, I renounced pleasure and disregarded worldly matters . . . I tried to give my whole time to the practice of medicine and to reflecting and meditating on it . . . He who can say that he has done as I did . . . may embrace that great science." On the basis of this, Lieber argues for the preeminence of medicine in Galen's life and studies, but does acknowledge an alterna-

---

difficult to say this in the case of adults, let alone children." (*De propriorum animi cuiuslibet affectuum dignotione et curatione*, V.40K).

8 *De ordine librorum suorum ad Eugenianum*, XIX.59K.

tive view, according philosophy and related matters a significant place.[9]

The initial years of Galen's medical education were spent in Pergamum. His first known teacher was the renowned anatomist Satyrus, who had come to the city and was apparently lodging with the Roman architect Rufinus, charged with the restoration of the shrine to Aesculapius. Among his other teachers while still in his home city were Stratonicus[10] and an unknown Pneumatist, as well as two other men about whom more is known: Ephicianus, like Satyrus a Rationalist, and the Empiric Aeschrion. On the former Galen writes: "Ephicianus was one who changed the training to something more Stoic."[11] On the latter he comments: "Aeschrion the Empiric, an old man most experienced in remedies . . . [was] my fellow citizen and teacher."[12]

Probably in 149 (the exact dates are unknown) two events occurred which had a major impact on the course of Galen's life. First, his father died, depriving him of his assiduous educational guide and supervisor. Although this did provide him with a substantial inheritance, it also left him more at the mercy of his irascible mother—factors which may have encouraged him to leave town. Second, his main teacher, Satyrus, returned to Smyrna. For what-

[9] See E. Lieber, "Galen: Physician as Philosopher. Maimonides: Philosopher as Physician," *Bulletin of the History of Medicine* 53 (1979): 262–85, esp. p. 272 (and nn. 18 and 19).

[10] *De atra bile*, V.119K.

[11] *De ordine librorum suorum ad Eugenianum*, XIX.58K.

[12] *De simplicium medicamentorum temperamentis et facultatibus*, XII.356K.

ever combination of reasons, Galen set out on his travels
to further his medical education. The actual date of his
departure from Pergamum is also uncertain, although
Nutton notes that his first surviving medical work was written in Smyrna in 149.[13] In these travels, which lasted until
157, his first port of call was Smyrna, a city also renowned
for learning and not far distant from Pergamum. It is probable that Galen spent about a year in Smyrna, studying under Pelops, a noted commentator on Hippocrates.[14] During this time he is said to have attended lectures by the
Platonist philosopher Albinus, himself a pupil of Gaius.
Galen is thought to have left Smyrna in search of instruction from Pelops' own teacher, Numisianus, possibly after a brief return to Pergamum for family reasons. It is
not clear whether Galen actually achieved his objective of
studying with Numisianus, either in Corinth or in Alexandria, where he subsequently went. It is likely that Numisianus had left Corinth before Galen arrived and died in Alexandria before Galen had moved on to that city.[15] Galen's
stay in Alexandria extended over the five years from 152
to 157. Regardless of whether he actually studied under
Numisianus or not, this was the major and culminating pe-

13 See V. Nutton in *The Western Medical Tradition*, ed. L. I.
Conrad et al. (Cambridge, 1995), p. 61.

14 See, for example, *De musculorum dissectione*,
XVIIIB.926K, and *De ordine librorum suorum ad Eugenianum*,
XIX.57K.

15 Opinions vary on whether Galen actually studied under
Numisianus, and if so, where. Apart from Nutton, *Western Medical Tradition*, see Sarton, *Galen of Pergamon*, p. 17, and Moraux,
Galiene de Pergamene, pp. 18, 61, as well as *In Hippocratis de
natura hominis librum commentarii*, XV.136–37K.

riod of his extended medical training. In particular, that city saw the refinement of his knowledge of anatomy—general, comparative, and surgical—and of pharmacology. Among Galen's teachers, or at least his associates in learning in Alexandria, was Numisianus' son, Heraclianus, whose views on anatomy were seen by Galen as similar to those of Satyrus, his first teacher on the subject. Other possible teachers in Alexandria were the Methodic Julianus and Lycus the Macedonian, against both of whom Galen subsequently wrote short treatises.[16] Finally, it should be noted that Galen is thought to have traveled widely while in Egypt, furthering his knowledge of medications.[17]

Initial Practice at Pergamum (157–161): Galen returned to Pergamum from Alexandria in his twenty-eighth year and was shortly thereafter appointed as the doctor to the city's gladiators, a post which was to provide him with many examples of "dissolution of continuity," a category of disease which he claims to have introduced to nosology. He thus completed his period of medical training, long and varied, and began the practice of medicine as his occupation. In this he combined his work among the gladiators with his other medical practice and with continuing study and research. By the time he entered medical practice on his return to Pergamum he had undergone a period of

[16] The treatises are *Adversus ea quae Iuliano in Hippocratis aphorismos enuntiata sunt*, XVIIIA.246–99K and *Adversus Lycum*, XVIIIA.196–245K.

[17] For detailed consideration of Galen's time in Egypt, see V. Nutton, "Galen in Egypt," in *Galen und das hellenistische Erbe*, ed. J. Kollesch and D. Nickel (Stuttgart, 1993).

training roughly equivalent to that required for specialist practice in English-speaking countries in modern times (i.e., around ten years) and his credentials were impressive.

Impressive also was his work during his sojourn in Pergamum. On his return from Alexandria, he records how he came to the notice of the Pontifex (High Priest of the Imperial Cult) through demonstrations of his method of treating tendon injuries, hence his appointment as doctor to the gladiator school. By his own account, he continued in this position for at least five seven-month periods.[18] This ongoing appointment afforded him a singular opportunity for the study of surgical anatomy and the management of all kinds of wounds and fractures, and may have contributed to the prominence he was subsequently to give "dissolution of continuity" in his system of disease classification.[19] Precisely why Galen left his apparently flourishing practice in Pergamum remains uncertain. Was it because of ambition, as Nutton suggests?[20] Was it because of unrest, personal or general, in Pergamum? Were other factors involved? Whatever the explanation, Galen left Pergamum around 161 and spent approximately four years, between 162 and 166, in Rome.

His First Period in Rome (162–166): Galen's journey to Rome was relatively rapid, although it may have in-

18 See *De compositione medicamentorum per genera*, XIII.599K et seq. A partial translation of this section is given by P. Moraux (1985), pp. 63–65.

19 See, for example, *De differentiis morborum*, XI.1 (VI.871–72K).

20 See Nutton, *Western Medical Tradition*, p. 62.

volved some study of medicinal plants en route, perhaps in Lemnos and Cyprus.[21] The precise date of his arrival in Rome is also uncertain but was probably either late 162 or early 163. The names of some of the more significant men he was associated with there are recorded in the introductory chapter to *On Anatomical Procedures* as follows:

> Then I went home, but not remaining there long, came to Rome where I made many dissections for Boethus. Present with him always were Eudemus the Peripatetic, Alexander of Damascus, now considered worthy to teach the Peripatetic doctrines at the public expense in Athens, and often other men in office like the one who is now Governor of the city of Rome, the Consul Sergius Paulus, a man altogether foremost in matters and doctrines of philosophy.[22]

Although his first stay in Rome was comparatively brief, lasting only until 166, it was eventful in several ways. Three aspects are of particular interest. First, he established himself as a student of the highly regarded Peripatetic philosopher Eudemus, who was in turn to benefit from his pupil's medical expertise, as recorded in detail in Galen's *On Prognosis for Epigenes*.[23] As Nutton remarks, "His cure of his old philosophy teacher Eudemus in the winter of

[21] Galen himself provides some information on these travels in *De alimentorum facultatibus*—see VI.507 and 617K.

[22] *De anatomicis administrationibus*, II.218K.

[23] *De praenotione ad Epigenem*, XIV.605K et seq.

162–163 was crucial in establishing him as a fashionable healer."[24] That, together with his triumph over doctors of opposing schools, redounded to his credit and was unquestionably of benefit in establishing his reputation. Second, there was his association with Boethus, flatteringly described in the opening sentences of his *On Anatomical Procedures*.[25] This was an association that encouraged and facilitated the continuation of Galen's own anatomical researches. The first part of one of his greatest works, *On the Use of the Parts*, was completed during this period and sent to Boethus, who had been appointed governor of Palestine in 165.[26] Two notable anatomical achievements made during the decade between 157 and 167 were his recognition of the recurrent laryngeal nerve and his demonstration that the arteries contained blood.[27] Third, as part of an active practice of medicine, he engaged in public demonstrations and debates with members of other sects and schools. While this must have furthered his reputation, it most certainly also made him some enemies.

His Return to Pergamum (166–168): In 166, he left Rome and returned to Pergamum, visiting various parts of Greece during his journey. The reasons for his departure, as in the case of those for his prior departure from Perga-

24 See Nutton, *Western Medical Tradition*, p. 62.

25 *De anatomicis administrationibus*, II.215–16K.

26 See M. T. May, *Galen on the Usefulness of the Parts of the Body*, 2 vols. (Ithaca, 1968), vol. 1, pp. 3–4.

27 The former was made during his time in Pergamum; see *De usu partium*, III.263–345K. For the latter, see *De anatomicis administrationibus*, II.641–50K.

mum, are not clear. Galen himself, in different works written at quite different times, cites two distinct reasons. The first was the difficulty he experienced with his rivals in Rome coupled with improved conditions in Pergamum. The second was the advent of plague in Rome.[28] It may also be that it was always his intention to return to Pergamum when the disturbances in his home city, thought to have contributed to his initial decision to depart, had settled.

His Second Period in Rome (168–200): His stay in Pergamum this time was to be very short. In 168 he was summoned by Marcus Aurelius to join the imperial army on campaign in northern Italy. An abandonment of the immediate military objectives resulted in the army's return to Rome in 169, Galen with it. He was to remain in Rome for at least the greater part of his remaining life. The years immediately after his return, specifically 169–176, were to prove most noteworthy in terms of his literary output, seeing the completion of a number of his major and other works, including the first six books of his *MM*. During this time Marcus Aurelius entrusted him with the responsibility for the medical care of his ill-fated son Commodus while the emperor was away from the capital. When Marcus Aurelius again returned to Rome in 176, Galen was made imperial physician, his crowning achievement in terms of gaining powerful patronage.

The Final Years (200–216/7?): The details of the final part of Galen's life become increasingly obscure, in no

---

[28] For the first, see *De praenotione ad Epigenem*, XIV.623 and 648K, and for the second, *De libris propriis*, XIX.15K.

small part because they are not chronicled by Galen himself with the same completeness as the earlier years. Nonetheless, his literary output continued apace, the final years of the century seeing the completion (i.e., the final eight books) of his enduringly influential major work on the practice of medicine, *The Method of Medicine*.[29] Also from late in the century are the two short works which provide valuable information about his own writings, *On My Own Books* and *On the Order of My Own Books*.[30] Earlier speculation had him leaving Rome somewhere around his seventieth year and returning home to his native Pergamum for the remainder of his life.[31] His death was said to have occurred at the age of seventy or seventy-one (i.e., 199–200), based on the Byzantine lexicon, the *Suda*. The thinking now is that he lived well into the third century. The latest date for any of his writings is that for his *On Theriac to Piso*, which, according to Nutton, could not have been earlier than 204 and may have been as late as 207.[32] Where he died is also unknown. He may have remained in Rome or returned to Pergamum for his last years. Nutton gives no credence to the story of his dying at Perama in Egypt while on a pilgrimage to Jerusalem—indeed, why would he make such a journey? In conclusion, what can be said at the present time is that he probably died in either 216 or 217 at the age of eighty-seven, but how and where he died remain unknown.

---

[29] *Methodus medendi*, X.1–1021K.   [30] *De libris propriis*, XIX.8–48K and *De ordine librorum suorum ad Eugenianum*, XIX.49–61K.   [31] See Sarton, *Galen of Pergamon*, p. 24.

[32] This is in keeping with the Arabic tradition; see Nutton, *Ancient Medicine*, p. 226.

2. PREDECESSORS AND
CONTEMPORARIES

By Galen's time a very considerable body of writing on science, medicine, and philosophy had been amassed by the Greeks and Romans. By his own account Galen had immersed himself deeply in this rich collection of material and regarded himself as proficient in all three forms of knowledge. In many respects his own work is a synthesis and systematic exposition of prior thought in which he espouses a position based on certain well-established theories and rejects other, conflicting views. In medicine he does the former strongly, consistently, and persuasively, the numerous and often convoluted digressions of his presentation notwithstanding. The latter he does with a somewhat intemperate vigor and scorn. Certain individuals he praises, one or two even unreservedly; others he castigates remorselessly.

In his *MM* Galen refers to over fifty individual doctors and philosophers. The writings of many of these men are no longer extant. Further, quite a number of them are mentioned only in Books 1 and 2 and often only in lists of worthies presented as supporters of Galen's polemic against Methodism. There is no specific consideration of their teachings. There is, however, a group of men whose teachings are examined in more or less detail. Some are men whose ideas form the basis of Galen's own theory and practice; others are men whose thinking Galen opposes, often very strongly. What follows is a brief account of the members of the group as a whole and their relevance to Galen's formulations as expressed in his *MM*. The order is chronological and without distinction between doctors, philosophers, and scientists—in the spirit, perhaps, of Galen's own concept of the doctor being also a philosopher and scientist. The dates given refer to the period of activity of each individual and are necessarily approximate in most cases.

Euryphon of Cnidos (460–440 BC) was an older contemporary of Hippocrates. He is said to have accompanied the latter to the court of the Macedonian king Perdikkas II in relation to the treatment of the king's son. The ancients, including Galen, attributed the preparation of the *Cnidian Sentences* and some other "Hippocratic" writings to Euryphon (VII.960K). He was renowned as an anatomist. Galen refers to his treatment of phthisis with women's milk in his *MM* (X.474K) and also in two other works: *On the Good and Bad Juices of Foods* (VI.775K) and *On Marasmus* (VII.701K).

Herodicus of Cnidos (440–400 BC) has been confused in a number of instances with Herodicus of Selymbria. The reference to him in the *MM* is, as with Euryphon, in relation to the use of women's milk in the treatment of phthisis (X.474K). Other treatments associated with his name are purging by vomiting and the use of steam baths. Both Euryphon and Herodicus attributed disease to a failure of the proper processing of food with the resultant creation of harmful residues. The former is sometimes credited with formulating the concept of diet.

Hippocrates of Cos (440–370 BC): It is now recognized that the Hippocratic corpus was completed over an extended period of time, most probably the two hundred years from approximately the middle of the fifth century BC to the middle of the third century BC, by various and in some instances unidentified hands.[33] However, setting aside the problems of authorship, authenticity, and uniformity of the doctrines expounded, there is no doubt that Hippocrates, at least as Galen identified him, was the major precursor of the latter's own views. On this point it is noteworthy that a considerable part of Galen's literary output was devoted to commentaries on Hippocratic texts; there are seventeen works in Kühn apart from those thought to be spurious.[34] Properly understood and interpreted—that is, according to Galen himself—Hippocrates provided the foundation for all that Galen embraced in the theory and practice of medicine. In areas of doubt, the uncertainties could be used to Galen's advantage in dismissing aspects with which he disagreed. In respect to Galen's overall attitude to Hippocrates, Lloyd speaks of "the importance of the almost unbounded admiration he [Galen] always expressed, throughout his life, for Hippocrates, his 'guide in all that is good.'"[35]

Three principles of primary importance to Galen were taken from Hippocrates. First, there was the humoral theory of the composition of the body, as expressed in Hippocrates' *Nature of Man*, with its stated opposition to the existing claims of a single basic substance, characteristic of much of pre-Socratic philosophy. Second, there was the

---

[33] Informative recent studies of the "Hippocratic question" include those of G. E. R. Lloyd, *Methods and Problems in Greek Science* (Cambridge, 1991) and J. Jouanna, *Hippocrates* (Baltimore, 1999).   [34] *De libris propriis*, XIX.33–37K.

[35] See G. E. R. Lloyd, "Galen on Hellenistics and Hippocrateans: Contemporary Battles and Past Authorities," in Kollesch and Nickel, *Galen und das hellenische Erbe*, p. 125.

view, whether implicit or explicit, that each individual disease had a causal explanation which should be sought and, if identified, would be of relevance to treatment. Third, and related to the second, there was the allopathic principle underlying treatment. Of more general importance were Hippocrates' perceived emphasis on ethics and his methodology, both of which prefigure Galen's own belief in the essential nexus between medicine and philosophy. To quote Lloyd again, Hippocrates "could be used as a perfect demonstration of how, in methodology, in natural philosophy, even in moral philosophy, the best doctor is also a philosopher."[36] It is also of no small significance that Hippocrates was held in high regard by the two philosophers most admired by Galen, Plato and Aristotle. Two additional points of note are, first, that Galen wrote a work (no longer extant) on the consistency of Hippocrates' views between his *Nature of Man* and his other writings, and second, that he included his short work on the best doctor also being a philosopher in the section under Hippocrates in Galen's *On My Own Books*.[37]

Plato (390–348/7 BC): The major figure among Galen's philosophical predecessors, to judge by Galen's own account, is undoubtedly Plato. The broad issues of Galen's debt to Plato, his assessment of the latter's contribution to both philosophy and medicine, and his interpretation and utilization of Plato's theories contain a number of subsidiary issues which are more or less controversial. There is no question, however, about Galen's attitude toward Plato, who enjoys the same preeminent place among his

36 Ibid., p. 140.
37 *De libris propriis*, XIX.37K.

philosophical predecessors as Hippocrates does among the medical. As de Lacy writes:

> Plato is repeatedly praised. He is first among philosophers, as Hippocrates is the best of all physicians. Like Hippocrates, he is "divine." He is a member of the "chorus" that is closest to God, whose members are devoted to the pursuit of the highest arts and sciences and are honoured equally with the gods.[38]

Galen undoubtedly made a detailed study of Plato's writings and was directly exposed to his theories through at least two of his teachers. This is apparent from the list in *On My Own Books* of nine works on Plato (only two survive in Kühn); the important *On the Opinions of Hippocrates and Plato* and the interesting *The Faculties of the Soul Follow the Mixtures of the Body*. Fortunately, several further works have been recovered, at least in part, from other sources.[39]

In summary, the matters on which Plato is of particular relevance to Galen include the following: the concept of the body as composed of the four elemental qualities (hot, cold, dry, and moist), as propounded in the *Timaeus*; the recognition of design in nature, involving the concept of the "Demiurge"; the tripartite division of the soul, involving consideration of the physical correlates of the psychical; and Plato's ideas on causation in general and in medi-

---

[38] See P. H. de Lacy, "Galen's Platonism," *American Journal of Philology* 93 (1973): 27–33, esp. pp. 32–33.

[39] See ibid., pp. 30–31, for a summary of these works and for the possible addition of a further work about Plato's views on the soul.

cine in particular, as expounded primarily in the *Timaeus* and the *Phaedo*.[40] On a somewhat more minor but nonetheless important issue, Galen's agreement and identification with Plato on the need to give primary attention to matters themselves rather than to terminology is revealed in the following statement from the former's *On Anatomical Procedures*:

> But if you are at least persuaded by Plato and myself you will always think little of names, whereas you will be attentive primarily and particularly to the knowledge of matters.[41]

These same sentiments, with or without reference to Plato, are repeatedly expressed by Galen both in the *MM* and elsewhere. Overall, the dialogues of particular relevance in tracing Galen's links to Plato are the *Timaeus, Phaedrus, Phaedo*, and *Charmides*, although, as de Lacy has pointed out, at least twelve dialogues are specifically mentioned and quoted from in Galen's writings.[42]

A further point of some significance is the degree of accord between the ideas of Plato and those of Hippocrates, especially on the issues listed. Related to this is the extent

---

[40] The four references to Plato are, respectively, *Timaeus*, 48B et seq.; *Timaeus*, 28A et seq.; *Timaeus*, 69C–71A, *Phaedrus*, 253 et seq.; and *Timaeus*, 82A, *Phaedo*, 97–100.

[41] *De anatomicis administrationibus*, II.581K. According to P. H. de Lacy, "Galen's Platonism," the reference to Plato is either "*Statesman* 261E" or "the conclusion of the *Cratylus*." C. Singer, in his translation of *De anatomicis administrationibus*, also mentions the *Republic* 533E and the *Sophist* 244.

[42] See de Lacy, "Galen's Platonism," p. 30.

to which Plato's ideas on purely medical matters themselves derive from Hippocrates, and also from Philistion of
Locri (*vide infra*). Galen certainly assumes a close correspondence between the ideas of Hippocrates and Plato, at
least as they bear on medical matters, and perhaps even a
significant dependence of the philosopher on the physician. This is a complex matter. It might be said that Galen's
view at least requires a somewhat imaginative reading of
Hippocrates if one is to see Plato's concepts clearly prefig-
ured there. An associated question concerns the degree to
which Plato's doctrines are differently interpreted when
refracted through the prism of later theories, Aristotelian
and Stoic in particular, by someone writing in the second
century AD.

Diocles of Carystus (4th century BC)**:** Although his
dates are very uncertain, it can be said that among doctors, he falls somewhere between Hippocrates and the two
great Alexandrians, Herophilus and Erasistratus. In some
quarters he is regarded as having been a pupil of Hippocrates. He may have been a contemporary of Aristotle and
certainly shared with the latter the cardiocentric view of
the *hegemonikon*, or soul. He is thought to have written
prolifically (around twenty titles are associated with his
name), but none of his writings have survived. Galen, however, had access to at least some of them, it would seem.
Diocles is classified among the Dogmatics and espoused
the concepts of *pneuma* and the four humors (blood,
phlegm, and yellow and black bile). He is widely referred
to by Galen on a variety of topics. On the matter of treatment, he held the Hippocratic view on the importance of
opposites. Particular remedies associated with his name
include diet, exercise, bathing, emetics, fomentations,

phlebotomy, and medications. In the *MM* he is mentioned along with a number of early doctors as holding a similar view of the structure of the body to those articulated by Galen in his *On the Elements According to Hippocrates* (X.462K).

Philistion of Locri (370–340 BC) is undoubtedly of importance in the early history of medicine and is mentioned twice in the opening two books of the *MM*. However, the degree and nature of his importance to Galen are difficult to assess, given the paucity of available information. There are no extant writings, and references to him in Galen's own works are very few.[43] Galen does, however, link him with the theories of Empedocles and to the so-called Sicilian school of medicine.[44] He is also held by some to have influenced Plato in the composition of the *Timaeus*, which would give him a particular relevance among Galen's antecedents. On the question of causation of disease, his views are probably recorded in the *Anonymus Londinensis* and bear a close resemblance to Galen's own. In summary, it can be said that Philistion related disease causation to the four elemental qualities, to the condition of the body, and to external factors. Of more general relevance are his concepts of innate heat and the important role of *pneuma*. Both are, of course, features of Galen's own physiological and pathological formulations.

---

43 See *De usu respirationis*, IV.471K, and *In Hippocratis librum de acutorum victu commentarii*, XV.455K.

44 See P. J. van der Eijk, *Diocles of Carystus: A Collection of Fragments with Translation and Commentary* (Leiden: E. J. Brill, 2000), introduction, p. ix, n. 2.

Mnesitheus of Athens (370–330 BC) is mentioned along with Dieuches on an Athenian votive inscription. Like Diocles, he is regarded as a Dogmatic who adhered to the concepts of humors, *pneuma*, and innate heat, all important factors in Galenic theory. In the *MM* he is mentioned along with Diocles and Dieuches as holding the same view of bodily composition as that described by Galen in *On the Elements According to Hippocrates*. Elsewhere in Galen he is described as skilled in anatomy, knowledgeable about foods and drugs, and believing in the use of phlebotomy.

Aristotle (355–322 BC)**: The place of Aristotle among Galen's predecessors is a somewhat complex one. Certainly he is not accorded the same unqualified respect as Plato and Hippocrates. For example, de Lacy has drawn attention to two passages which clearly display a less than reverent attitude. In the first, Aristotle is linked with Praxagoras as a target of criticism for their jointly held major misconception of the function of the heart—"they were either blind themselves or were addressing a blind audience"—while in the second, where his views are criticized in *On the Semen*, he is twice addressed patronizingly as "dearest Aristotle."[45] Nevertheless, it could be argued that an analysis of Galen's works overall would support the view

---

[45] See de Lacy, "Galen's Platonism," p. 33. The two passages referred to are to be found in *De placitis Hippocratis et Platonis*, V.187–188K, and *De semine*, IV.530 and 553K, respectively. As regards the latter, de Lacy remarks that the phrase "dearest Aristotle" "expresses a certain exasperation at the obtuseness of the person criticized."

that Aristotle's influence was the most significant, at least in matters other than the purely medical.

For example, in Galen's teleological views, which especially inform his major work *On the Use of the Parts*, it is Aristotle's immanent teleology rather than the Platonic "Demiurge" which is most discernible. In his methodology, Galen is clearly and profoundly influenced by Aristotle, particularly by the works of the *Organon*. In his conception of the structure of the body he was firmly committed to the theory of four elemental qualities, which, while not attributable to Aristotle, was held and developed by him. Further, in his formulations of structural levels, which are of considerable importance to the classifications of diseases and symptoms advanced in the four treatises on these subjects and restated in the *MM*, Galen followed Aristotelian concepts, especially the idea of *homoiomeres*. In his consideration of causation he is also clearly influenced by Aristotle, both in the assumption of the validity of the search for causal explanations and in the specific ideas. In his attention to taxonomy, Galen is obviously following Aristotelian principles. He was unquestionably influenced by the psychology of *De anima*, as indeed were almost all who came after Aristotle and grappled with the same subject matter. Finally, the empirical component of his studies and the use of observation of biological phenomena as the basis for theoretical formulation reveal an Aristotelian imprint.

A comparison of Galen's writings on Aristotle with those on Plato and Hippocrates finds that they are fewer and less well preserved. Counting all parts of a commentary on a single Aristotelian work as one book, there are eleven works listed in the section on Aristotle in *On My*

Own Books.[46] None of these is extant. Of particular interest are Galen's remarks about his works on logic generally,[47] where, having noted the relative lack of conflict in this subject among Peripatetics as compared to Stoics and Platonists, he makes the following observation, illuminating in terms of his relationship to Aristotle:

> I say the philosophers—the Peripatetics, the Stoics, and the Platonists—differ among themselves in logical theory, although these are again specific in each of the sects. It is surely the case that among the Peripatetics discord is slight, whereas among Stoics and Platonists it is great.[48]

Praxagoras of Cos (325–275 BC) came from a notable medical family, although relatively little is known about him and none of his works survive. He has been identified as a follower of Diocles of Carystus and perhaps a teacher of Herophilus,[49] giving him particular relevance in the early studies of anatomy. He espoused theories which attracted Galen's criticism. This was certainly justifiable in relation to the cardiocentric view of mental and emotional function, shared by other notables, including Aristotle, and also to his belief that the arteries carried *pneuma*, a concept developed by Erasistratus in his theories of disease causation. On the positive side, however, he is credited with having made the structural distinction

---

46 *De libris propriis*, XIX.47K.

47 *De libris propriis*, XIX.39–45K.

48 *De libris propris*, XIX.40–41K.

49 See F. Steckerl, *The Fragments of Praxagoras of Cos and His School* (Leiden: E. J. Brill, 1958), p. 34 on this matter.

between arteries and veins. His particular similarity to Galen, who identified him as a Dogmatic, was his belief in the importance of seeking a causal explanation for disease. Indeed, he is said to have written a book on the subject.[50] In addition, there are his early studies of the pulse and its abnormalities, another subject substantially developed by Galen, and his incorporation of *pneuma* into theories of physiology and pathology. Praxagoras also expanded on the concept of humors, subdividing the basic four on the grounds of color, taste, and other aspects to make ten. He particularly associated disease with alteration of the humors and specifically fever with putrefaction of humor. In the *MM* he is linked with Hippocrates and Pleistonicus among doctors and with Plato and Aristotle as a proponent of the Dogmatic method in respect of treatment (X.261K).

Pleistonicus (300–240 BC) was possibly also from Cos and was a pupil of Praxagoras, whose theories he embraced. Galen generally refers to him in conjunction with Praxagoras and others of the Dogmatic persuasion, as in the reference to the latter in the *MM* given above. Several views associated with him are that air enters the arteries not only from the heart but also from the whole body, that digestion involves putrefaction, and that water is preferable to wine as an aid to digestion.

Dieuches (300–200 BC) is linked with Mnesitheus and Diocles of Carystus particularly as one of the noted medical Dogmatics. Galen writes of him as an anatomist, as someone who wrote on medications, and as using phlebotomy. He is also referred to by Pliny the Elder and by Oribasius on matters of regimen and treatment.

[50] See ibid., p. 5.

Herophilus of Chalcedon (280–260 BC), along with his close contemporary Erasistratus (*vide infra*), has been classified as a Dogmatic, although with Herophilus at least this is not entirely uncontroversial.[51] Both have also been subjects of recent detailed studies and collections of *fragmenta*.[52] Although precise dates have not been established for either, it is probable that Herophilus was slightly earlier. His primary contribution was to anatomy, especially of the nervous system, liver, and heart. From the viewpoint of his importance for Galen, he subscribed to the same physiology based on the four elemental qualities with a significant role for *pneuma*, the latter being importantly implicated in neurological function by Herophilus. He also played a major part in establishing "pulse theory," a subject enthusiastically and extensively taken up by Galen. In terms of methodology, Herophilus argued for attention to be directed to phenomena but did, it is thought, accept the importance of causal explanation. It may be said that if he was indeed a Dogmatic, he had significant Empiric tendencies and was arguably less committed to detailed causal explanation than Galen was subsequently.

Erasistratus (260–240 BC) provides quite a contrast to his fellow Alexandrian in terms of Galen's later evaluation. While he too made significant contributions to anatomy, mainly with regard to the cardiovascular system and peripheral nerves, in a number of his theoretical formulations he was strongly criticized by Galen. First, in his phys-

---

[51] H. von Staden, *Herophilus: The Art of Medicine in Early Alexandria* (Cambridge, 1989), pp. 115–24.

[52] See ibid. for Herophilus and I. Garofalo, *Erasistrati Fragmenta* (Pisa, 1988) for Erasistratus.

iology and pathology he moved away from the concept of four elemental qualities, basing his physiology on a corpuscular theory following, it is said, Straton of Lampsacus. Longrigg writes that Erasistratus "conceived of his particles as very small imperceptible corporeal entities partially surrounded by a vacuum in a finely divided or discontinuous condition."[53] In his explanation of disease he gave particular importance to blood and *pneuma,* invoking the concepts of *plethora* and *paremptosis* (*vide infra*). In short, what was involved in these presumed pathological processes was an increase in blood in the veins to an abnormal level, causing a spillover into the arteries with a resultant displacement of *pneuma.* Other aspects of Erasistratus' theorizing to which Galen took exception were his concept of *horror vacui* (or "following toward what is emptied"), his theory of digestion, his departure from the idea of "complete" teleology, and some of his attitudes to therapy. Also, on the issue of causation there were certainly substantial differences, although it may be said that Erasistratus did clearly accept the need for causal explanation.

Chrysippus (250–205 BC**):** Galen's attitude to the Stoics in general may be characterized as ambivalent. He has recorded his own early exposure to Stoic doctrines, and indeed, his first written work was said to have been a commentary on a work by Chrysippus: "When I was still a boy and my father first handed me over to someone who taught the logical theory of Chrysippus and the notable Stoics, I prepared in relation to this, notes of the syllogis-

---

[53] J. Longrigg, *Greek Rational Medicine* (London, 1993), p. 214.

tic books of Chrysippus."[54] In fact, the five works on the Stoics which Galen lists in *On My Own Books* all bear on logic and related matters.[55] Of the Stoics, it is predominantly Chrysippus who is mentioned in Galen's writings, although his two predecessors, Zeno of Citium and Cleanthes, as well as the later Stoic Posidonius, are also mentioned.[56] The ambivalence referred to may be revealed by comparing Galen's observations on Chrysippus in the *MM* with those in *On the Opinions of Hippocrates and Plato*. In the former the Stoic is linked with Hippocrates, Plato, and Aristotle in espousing what Galen himself accepts as the correct explanation of matter, whereas in the latter he is roundly criticized in several passages.[57]

Asclepiades of Bithynia (120–90 BC) has been described by Frede as "a pivotal figure" in the Rationalist/ Empiricist debate,[58] but he is undoubtedly also pivotal in a

[54] *De libris propriis*, XIX.43K.

[55] *De libris propriis*, XIX.47–48K.

[56] All three early Stoics are mentioned together in *De placitis Hippocratis et Platonis*, V.283K. Posidonius is quoted contra Chrysippus in the same work (V.397K et seq.).

[57] The passage in the *Methodus medendi* (X.16K) is as follows: "For Hippocrates first put forward the hot, cold, dry and moist, while Aristotle demonstrated [these] after him. And the followers of Chrysippus took these up as already given and did not dispute, but said that all things are mixed from these, and that these affect and act on each other and that Nature is systematic. They accept all the other doctrines of Hippocrates about Nature, apart from there being some small differences between them and Aristotle." On the criticisms, see de Lacy, "Galen's Platonism," p. 33.

[58] See R. Walzer and M. Frede, *Galen: Three Treatises on the Nature of Science* (Indianapolis: Hackett, 1985), p. xxix.

wider sense. In essence, Asclepiades represented the culminating articulation of atomistic theories as applied to medicine up to the first century BC. This was a theory that could trace its heritage back through the somewhat disparate strands of Strato of Lampsacus, Heraclides of Pontus, and Epicurus to its origin with Democritus. As with a number of the significant figures already discussed, his writings have not been preserved, although the recent work by Vallance provides a detailed account of his views and intellectual progenitors.[59] Unfortunately, much of the information derives from Galen himself, who, being totally opposed to Asclepiades' key concepts, cannot be taken as an impartial source. Asclepiades based his physiology and pathology on the concept of fragile corpuscles (*anarmoi onkoi*) which traveled through channels (*poroi*) not anatomically definable but distributed throughout the body. Diseases occurred when this process was interfered with, in particular when there was impaction (*emphraxis*).

Themison of Laodicea (90–40 BC) is, in one place, credited by Galen as being the founder of the Methodic sect (XIV.684K) and as formulating the concept of "communities" (of diseases—X.35K). He may have studied under Asclepiades but may also have been linked with the Empiric Theodas of Laodicea, whom Galen mentions once in the *MM* (X.142K). Themison is credited with developing certain compound medications, particularly utilizing beeswax. Four books attributed to him (but no longer extant) are *Acute Diseases, Chronic Diseases, Rules of Health*, and *Letters*.

[59] J. Vallance, *The Lost Theory of Asclepiades of Bithynia* (Oxford, 1990).

Thessalus of Tralles (AD **20–70**): On Galen's description, Thessalus was a charlatan of base origins who practiced a highly dubious form of medicine. He is reviled throughout the *MM* but especially in the first two books. According to Thessalus himself, as revealed in a fragment of a letter to Nero which Galen quotes, he "established a new sect and, as all doctors who came before passed on nothing useful regarding either the preservation of health or the relief of disease, it is the only true sect."[60] He claimed that the craft of medicine could be learned in six months, and by anyone, without attention to the several other disciplines which Galen considered so important (logic, geometry, etc.). Methodism did, then, have a theoretical foundation, being based on the particle/void concept of the structure of matter derived from the Atomists ultimately and from Asclepiades in medicine. Diseases were described as due to either constriction/obstruction or dilatation/flux involving theoretical pores, or a combination of the two (*vide infra*). Moreover, diseases were divided into "communities" which were the basis of treatment. None of Thessalus' writings survive, but he is credited with a substantial body of work, including treatises on the "communities" and on method. These are quoted and referred to disparagingly by Galen, who repeatedly describes both Thessalus and his sect as "methodless" or "amethodical."

Athenaeus of Attaleia (AD **30–70**) was perhaps the founder of the Pneumatist school of doctors. He accepted the theory of the four elemental qualities (hot, cold, moist, and dry) but gave particular prominence to *pneuma* as

[60] *Methodus medendi*, X.8K.

a fifth "elemental" component of the body. He defined health as equilibrium between *pneuma* and the four elemental qualities and disease as a disequilibrium or imbalance of the five factors (i.e., a *dyskrasia*) rather than of the four only. His theoretical formulations were based on Stoic concepts, and he was linked by Galen with the Stoic Posidonius. Whether he was, in fact, a student of the latter is uncertain, even unlikely. It seems that Galen admired Athenaeus, although there were points of disagreement, both theoretical and practical.

Philippus of Rome (AD **45–95**) is often mentioned in conjunction with Archigenes, both identified as Pneumatists. Philippus is said to have written extensively on medications, although none of his writings survive. He is mentioned in the *MM* in relation to his ideas on bathing, which Galen opposes.

Soranus of Ephesus (AD **98–138**) is one of the most notable of ancient doctors, not least because one of his works survives complete (*On Gynecology*), along with fragments of another work (or works)—possibly his *Surgical Operations*. His methods were also detailed by Caelius Aurelianus in a surviving work. Although a Methodic, he does not come in for the same harsh criticism from Galen as other members of the sect (particularly Thessalus). He is briefly mentioned twice in the *MM*, once in a list of Methodics (X.53K) and once as the teacher of Attalus (X.910K).

Philippus of Egypt (AD **100–170**) is distinguished from Philippus of Rome, although only a single Philippus is listed in the Kühn index. Philippus of Egypt is associated with theories about holding back the advance of age, which is the context of the single reference in the *MM* (X.495K).

Quintus of Pergamum (AD 115–145) is described by Galen as a teacher of both Marinus (XV.136K) and Satyrus (II.225K), although in modern accounts he is said to have been a student of the former. Either way, he was a noted anatomist (*vir summe anatomicus*—XIX.22K). Galen also described him as the most outstanding doctor of his time, although recognizing that he diverged from Hippocrates in his views. Quintus was, in fact, banished from Rome on the grounds of malpractice, and apparently died soon after. Galen categorizes him as an Empiric.

Attalus (AD 130–170) is described by Galen as a student of Soranus and therefore a Methodic. In the *MM* he features in a case report involving the Cynic philosopher Theagenes. His treatment methods fail to save the patient and are strongly criticized by Galen (X.909–16K). It has been suggested that he may be the same person as Statilius Attalus, personal physician to Antoninus Pius and Marcus Aurelius.

Justus the Ophthalmologist (AD 160–180) is mentioned once by Galen in the *MM* (X.1019K), where he is described as treating hypopyon in a particular way. There is no reference to a written account of this technique, which Galen may have witnessed at first hand.

The Schools or Sects: The establishment of schools or sects of doctors in the Graeco-Roman world was a gradual development which had its origins in the fourth and third centuries BC and became a prominent feature in the two centuries prior to Galen and during his own time. However, it seems that the sects faded into insignificance in the centuries immediately following his death. Presumably this was in no small part due to Galen himself. The basic division into Rationalist/Dogmatic and Empiric depended on distinctly different theories as to how knowledge generally was acquired, and particularly how technical knowledge such as medical knowledge was acquired. The key issue was whether it was useful to attempt to explain phenomena on the basis of fundamental theories of the composition and structure of matter as applied to the human body and to incorporate theories of causation into such explanations. To the Rationalists it was. For the Empiric, however, knowledge was limited to observing phenomena, accumulating a body of experience through the observed phenomena, and applying this accumulated experience to the interpretation of new phenomena. Subsequently in medicine, subdivision of the Rationalist position arose based on the different theories of structure and function which underlay practice.

The basic tenets of Rationalism were as follows: (a) to formulate through reason or adopt a theory already so formulated of the structure and function of the human body and the nature of health and disease; (b) to accept the idea of causation, and in particular to accept that all observable phenomena have a cause but that the cause may be hidden from direct observation; (c) to work out what the appropriate remedies are for each disease on the basis of this theoretical foundation. To quote Celsus: "Therefore there are those who, professing to a rational medicine, put forward these things as necessary: a knowledge of hidden causes involving diseases; then of evident [causes]; after these of natural actions and last of inferior parts."[61]

The basic tenets of Empiricism were that there was no need to formulate any foundational theory of structure

---

[61] Celsus, *De medicina* I, Proemium 13.

and function and no need to accept causation generally or to look for underlying, hidden causes to explain phenomena. The doctor experienced the phenomena one by one, accumulated the experiences, and acted on this accumulated experience. The particular processes of acquiring the experience and applying it were identified as *peira* (experience), *teresis* (observation), *historia* (inquiry—or in medicine collected case histories), and *metabasis* (inference from analogy). On the negative side, what the medical Empirics opposed is summarized by Frede as follows:[62]

> What the Empiricists clearly wanted to reject were formal inferences, either deductive or inductive, in particular inferences by means of which people were supposed to get a grasp on the theoretical truths which underlie what they could observe, and more emphatically those inferences which were supposed to lead to theoretical truths concerning theoretical entities, like the atoms which can only be grasped by reason.

The main schools or sects that developed later were the Methodics and the Pneumatists. Both of these were essentially Rationalist in type, at least to begin with, differing from the existing Rationalists in the nature of their theoretical formulations. Thus Methodism as a medical sect might be said to begin with Asclepiades (*vide supra*), who did base his physiology and pathology on a theory dependent on reason—the previously mentioned view that the body is composed of fragile corpuscles (*anarmoi onkoi*) which move through channels or pores (*poroi*) postulated

[62] Walzer and Frede, *Galen,* p. xxiii.

by reason but not accessible to observation. In this theory disease was due to a disturbance of the normal situation secondary to abnormal constriction or dilatation of the channels or pores, existing either alone or in combination. These abnormal states were, it would seem, not accessible to observation and therefore could not be experienced, and neither could the causes of the changes. As Methodism evolved, however, through Themison to Thessalus (Galen's bête noire) in particular, the theoretical basis was lost sight of and the abnormal states, of which there were only three (constriction, dilatation, and a combination of the two) were regarded as directly observable. Moreover, the trainee doctor could become sufficiently familiar with their manifestations to launch himself into practice within a very short time—the notorious six-month training period. Thus Methodism shed its Rationalist foundation and became a form of Empiricism—truly the Methodics had become "methodless," as Galen so often states in the *MM*.

Relatively little is known about the Pneumatist school. There is agreement that its founder was Athenaeus of Attaleia, although his dates are unclear and no writings survive, as is the case with other known members, Archigenes of Apamea and Agathinus of Sparta.[63] Some of the writings of Aretaeus of Cappadocia, a contemporary of Galen's, do, however, remain. In adding the role of *pneuma* to that of the four elemental qualities in their considerations of the genesis of health and disease, they display definite links to earlier philosophical thought, particularly to Diogenes of Apollonia and to Stoic physics, as described above. Galen

---

63 See M. Wellman, *Die pneumatische Schüle bis auf Archigenes in ihrer Entwicklung dargestellt* (Berlin, 1895).

himself incorporated *pneuma* into his physiological and pathological formulations and was, it might be said, sympathetic toward the Pneumatists as a group. Certainly in terms of causation they might be seen as espousing the same basic principles, although differing in specifics, as would be expected. In classification, however, there would clearly be differences. The subjects of Galen's own relation to the Pneumatists, and the extent to which they were defined as a school, would undoubtedly bear further study.

Galen himself did not have any hard-line allegiance to one school or another. He was, he would claim, aware of the advantages and disadvantages of each. Certainly he followed Rationalist principles insofar as his method of medicine was based on a theoretical foundation formulated by reason—notions of the primary elements composing the body, of their anatomical arrangement and the purposes of this, of their physiological functioning, of the range of their various pathological alterations, of the clear definition of terms, of an understanding of the nature and importance of causation, and of the establishment of a comprehensive classification of diseases according to the principle of *diairesis*. He was, however, also aware of some of the pitfalls of Rationalism as a dogma, writing in his *MM* as follows:

> On the other hand, for those who make reason (*logos*) the principle of discovery and order, who propose that this is the one road leading to the goal, there is the necessity to begin from something primary, agreed upon by all men, and in this way then proceed to the rest. They do not in fact do this, but rather the majority take up disputed starting-points, not demonstrating them, and proceed to the rest in

the same way, laying down the law rather than demonstrating.[64]

Equally, Galen was aware of the importance of experience. In the opening paragraph of his work *On Medical Experience* he writes:[65]

> When I take as my standard the opinion held by the
> most skillful and wisest doctors and the best philos-
> ophers of the past, I say: The art of healing was origi-
> nally invented and discovered by *logos* (reason) in
> conjunction with experience. And today also it can
> be practiced excellently and done well by one who
> employs both of these methods.

Repeatedly in the *MM* Galen refers to the two ways of
gaining knowledge: through reason and through experience. Moreover, theoretical formulations, if they are not
verified by and in accord with experience, must be rejected, while experience that is not "organized" by reason
risks being unsystematic and irrational. One of Galen's major objections to Methodism, at least in the Asclepiadean
form, was that it was based on the wrong theoretical foundation. Further, according to Galen, Asclepiades despised
experience. The later developments of Methodism, culminating in the work of Thessalus, were clearly more of an
anathema to him. In essence the problem was that the
Methodics now had no method, as he recurringly states
in his *MM*. Somewhat curiously, given the virulence of
his criticism of the Methodic sect and Thessalus as its

---

64 *Methodus medendi*, X.32K.

65 See Galen, *On Medical Experience*, in Walzer and Frede,
Galen, translation after Walzer, p. 47.

self-styled champion, Galen seems to have had no quarrel with Soranus. Nor did he have any major difficulty with the Pneumatists—those differences that are recorded are largely with specific individuals (e.g., Athenaeus) on specific points. The same applies to his differences with the Erasistrateans, although in this case the points of difference are more fundamental. Galen might, then, be best categorized as a small-*e* eclectic, drawing what he saw as relevant from all the schools or sects, and molding it into a method of medicine which is comprehensively expressed in his great therapeutic treatise.

3. GALEN'S WRITINGS

Galen's written work is remarkable on at least three counts: its sheer volume, the broad range of its subject matter, and its enduring influence. On the first point, no ancient author of any genre surpasses, or even matches, Galen's prodigious output, although of course much ancient writing has been lost. Also, quantity alone is no guarantee of quality. Nevertheless, Galen's preserved writings account for about 10 percent of all surviving literature in Greek prior to AD 350—and these don't include the considerable proportion of his writings that were also lost, particularly in the fire near the Temple of Peace that occurred in 192.[66] The best early record of Galen's writings is to be found in two of his books, *On My Own Books* and *On the*

---

[66] See Hankinson, *Cambridge Companion to Galen*, p. 1, and Sarton, *Galen of Pergamon,* p. 23, regarding the fire. Galen himself refers to the fire in *De libris propriis*, XIX.19K.

Order of My Own Books, especially the former. In this, counting multivolume works on a single topic as single treatises, there are 187 separate treatises listed. It is, however, not always clear what constitutes a separate treatise, and not all Galen's writings are included anyway. There are also those works written after Galen wrote *On My Own Books* and works he may have omitted for some reason.

A major portion of Galen's extant writings is preserved today in Carl-Gottlob Kühn's edition of the *Galeni Opera Omnia*, first published in the 1820s and most recently reprinted in 1997 in 21 volumes (volumes 17 and 18 are divided into parts A and B; volume 20 is a Latin index separately prepared). In Kühn's edition there are 124 titles. A current listing of these titles marks 23 as spurious and a further 3 as questionable.[67] The genuine works range in length from 3 to 4 pages only (e.g., *On the Causes of Respiration*) to those in excess of 1,000 pages (e.g., *On the Use of the Parts* and the *Method of Medicine* itself).[68] In Ackermann's introduction to Kühn's Galen he lists 100 genuine works, 44 "*libri manifeste spurii*," 19 *fragmenta*, and 18 commentaries on works by Hippocrates.[69] There had been two previous complete Greek editions: the Aldine edition, published in Venice in 1525, and the edition of R. Chartier, published in Paris in 1679. There was also the Giunta edi-

---

[67] See Hankinson, *Cambridge Companion to Galen*, pp. 391–97.

[68] The references to these works in the Kühn edition are as follows: *De causis respirationis*, IV.465–69K; *De usu partium libri I–XI*, III.1–939K, and *libri XII–XVII*, IV.1–366K; *Methodus medendi*, X.1–1021K.

[69] See Kühn, vol. I, *Historia literaria Cl. Galeni*, pp. lxvii–clxxxvi.

tion of the Latin Galen, which was published in 1541–1542 with Giovanni Battista da Monte as the general editor. Bylebyl has described this as "perhaps the greatest landmark in the whole movement by Renaissance physicians to bring about a rebirth of ancient Greek medicine in their own time."[70] Other works are still being discovered, some from Greek and Latin manuscripts and some from Syriac and Arabic sources. López-Férez in 1991 listed 23 such works as well as 26 additional spurious works, while Hankinson in 2008 listed 16 genuine works.[71] The former list does not include all the same titles as the latter. Critical editions of a number of Galen's works, both those included in Kühn and those from other sources, have appeared in the slowly accumulating *Corpus Medicorum Graecorum* series, the first volume of which appeared in 1904 and the most recent in 2001.[72]

Second, the range of subjects covered in Galen's writings is equally extraordinary. From his first work, some notes on the writings of the Stoic Chrysippus,[73] to the very

---

[70] See J. J. Bylebyl in F. Kudlien and R. J. Durling, eds., *Galen's Method of Healing,* Proceedings of the 1982 Galen Symposium (Leiden: E. J. Brill, 1991), p. 173.

[71] J. A. López-Férez, *Galeno: Obra, Pensamiento e Influencia* (Madrid, 1991), pp. 326–29 ; Hankinson, *Cambridge Companion to Galen*, p. 397.

[72] K. Kalbfleisch, *Galen de Causis Contentivis, Scripta Minora*, vol. 1 (Leipzig, 1904) and D. Nickel, *Galeni de Foetuum Formatione* (Berlin, 2001).

[73] Described in *De libris propriis*, XIX.19K; neither Galen's notes nor Chrysippus' work are extant.

late, and possibly last, work, *On Theriac to Piso*,[74] he covered the entire range of practical medicine and its basic sciences and made important original contributions. He wrote extensively on the medical schools and sects and produced detailed commentaries on earlier works, particularly those of Hippocrates, as well as writing on theoretical and nonclinical aspects of medicine. On philosophical topics his range was also very wide, although he was particularly preoccupied with the works and ideas of Plato and Aristotle. There were also a number of works on Stoic and Epicurean philosophy as well as on other general philosophical topics. Finally, there was a miscellaneous group of writings which includes works on lexicography, linguistic matters, politics, comedy, education, and writing. Needless to say, such a prodigious output must have precluded detailed revision of individual works, while the nature of book production at the time and Galen's own somewhat itinerant way of life meant that he did not have all his previous works to hand when writing a new treatise. As a consequence, his writings display repetition, prolixity, and lack of accurate cross-referencing. In addition, given the scope of his work, the depth of the author's familiarity with and experience in the wide range of topics he covers is, not surprisingly, quite variable. Also, as many have remarked, his writing is strongly tinctured with his own high opinion of himself and a correspondingly low opinion of perceived adversaries on whatever topic. While his vigorous and col-

---

[74] See Kühn XIV.210–94K: this work is listed by López-Férez, *Galeno,* as spurious, although Nutton regards it as probably authentic; see Nutton, *Western Medical Tradition,* p. 63.

orful attacks on his opponents make for entertaining reading, they may come at the expense of reasoned argument. In his *MM* these verbal assaults are directed almost entirely at Thessalus and Methodics generally. All in all, however, his writings are of inestimable value, not only for the ideas they contain and the detailed account of the medical practice of the time which they provide, but also because they constitute an invaluable source of information on the no longer extant works of other writers.

Third, the influence of Galen's writings has been considerable and continuous, extending to the present day, albeit with inevitable peaks and troughs and also differences in how and on whom the influence was or is being felt. Only a few brief comments will be made here on what is a subject of considerable magnitude in its own right. In the later part of the second century, particularly as Galen's career evolved and his written output grew to the substantial proportions mentioned above, the conclusion must be that his was one of the dominant voices (if not the most dominant) on all matters medical throughout the wide area of the Roman Empire. A true evaluation of just how dominant is difficult or impossible to arrive at, given that the major (and almost only) source of information is Galen himself. What can be said is that a measure of the importance of his writings in the several centuries after his death is gained from the extensive inclusion of his ideas and methods in the works of the medical "encyclopedists" of the time that do remain extant—men such as Oribasius (ca. 350–400), Aetius of Amida (ca. 500–550), and Paul of Aegina (ca. 630–670).

By the sixth century Galen's core treatises on the theory

and practice of medicine had been gathered together in what became known as the Galenic or Alexandrian canon, comprising the following works:

1. On [Medical] Sects—*De sectis ad eos introducuntur* (I.64–105K)

2. The Medical Art—*Ars medica* (I.305–412K)

3. Synopsis on Pulses—*Synopsis de pulsibus* (IX.431–549K)

4. The Method of Medicine, to Glaucon—*Ad Glauconem de methodo medendi* (XI.1–146K)

5. Collection 1 (on anatomy)—On Bones for Beginners (*De ossibus ad tirones*, II.732–78K); On the Anatomy of Arteries and Veins (*De venarum arteriarumque dissectione*, II.779–830K); On the Anatomy of Nerves (*De nervorum dissectione*, II.831–56K); On the Anatomy of Muscles (*De musculorum dissectione*, XVIIIB.926–1026K)

6. On the Elements according to Hippocrates—*De elementis secundum Hippocratem* (I.413–508K)

7. On Mixtures (*Kraseis*)—*De temperamentis* (I.509–694K)

8. On the Physical Capacities (Natural Faculties)—*De naturalibus facultatibus* (II.1–214K)

9. Collection 2 (on diseases and symptoms)—On the Differentiae of Diseases (*De morborum differentiis*, VI.836–80K); On the Causes of Diseases (*De causis morborum*, VII.1–41K); On the Differentiae of Symptoms (*De symptomatum differentiis*, VII.42–84K); On the Causes of Symptoms (*De symptomatum causis*, VII.85–272K)

Around this time the ongoing process of translation began—a process that was critical for the preservation of a substantial percentage of Galen's remarkable output. At the risk of oversimplification, five stages may be identified in the history of the translation and preservation of Galen's works:

1. The translation of the components of the Alexandrian canon from Greek to Syriac by Sergius of Resaena in the sixth century.
2. The major program particularly attributed to the Christian doctor Hunain ibn Ishâq (died 873), which resulted in the translation of 129 works into Syriac and Arabic during the ninth century.

3. The progressive translation of the majority of Galen's extant works from Greek, Syriac, and Arabic into Latin which began in the eleventh century with men such as Constantine the African (fl. ca. 1080), Gerard of Cremona (d. 1187), and Burgundio of Pisa (d. 1193). This culminated in the veritable explosion of Latin translation which marked the period from the late fourteenth to the sixteenth century and involved such notable translators as Niccolò de Reggio (active 1304–1350), Niccolò Leoniceno (1428–1524), and Thomas Linacre (ca. 1460–1524).

4. The preparation of the two versions of the complete works with both Greek and Latin texts, the first by René Chartier in 1679 in Paris and the second by Carl-Gottlob Kühn in Leipzig from 1821 to 1833.

5. The preparation of critical editions of individual treatises and the translation of a goodly number into modern European languages, the latter starting particularly with Daremberg's French translations of 1854 and the former with the beginning of the *Corpus Medicorum Graecorum* at the start of the twentieth century. This movement has gathered considerable pace in the last fifty or so years, such that in the recent *Cambridge Companion to Galen* edited by Hankinson (2008) there are no fewer than 89 translations since 1950, although some are of the same work.[75]

---

[75] See Hankinson, *Cambridge Companion to Galen*, pp. 391–403.

Before giving a brief overview of the *MM* itself, it is useful to consider the key works which provide the theoretical basis for Galen's great practical text—works which for the most part (but not altogether) coincide with those comprising the Alexandrian canon listed above. In fact, Galen refers to over forty of his own works in the course of his *MM*. There is, however, a smaller subgroup, the constituents of which are frequently referred to. These are the works most pertinent to the theoretical basis of Galen's method or system of medicine generally and treatment in particular or, in the case of the works on medications and his *On the Preservation of Health*, to its application. These works, listed in note 1 above, include *On the Elements according to Hippocrates* (which details his views on the elemental composition of the body); the anatomical works, *On Anatomical Procedures* and *On the Use of the Parts*; the physiological works on *krasis* and its abnormalities and on the physical or natural capacities; and the work of pathology *On the Affected Parts*. The most frequently cited works are, however, those on medications—that on the composition and potency of a wide range of simple medications and the two long treatises on compound medications, one on the relationship to the parts to which they are applied and one on the classes of such medications. There is also mention of a probable earlier work on medications that has not survived. Reference to his work *On the Preservation of Health* is frequent and to the lost work, *On Demonstration*, infrequent. There are also several references to the work on medical nomenclature recovered from the Arabic.

In addition to these works, the four treatises on the

classification and causation of diseases and symptoms should also be regarded as important components of the theoretical foundation of his system of medicine and are frequently referred to. In fact, this group is perhaps the most important of Galen's other works as far as the *MM* is concerned, for two reasons. First, the key definitions (*vide infra*) which form a significant part of these four short treatises are of critical importance for his *MM* and are restated, albeit in a somewhat less systematic and more discursive manner, in the opening two books of that work. Second, the system of classification of diseases set out in his work *On the Differentiae of Diseases* forms the basis for the arrangement of the work on treatment. In summary, then, Galen makes quite clear, in the course of his *MM*, exactly which of his works the practitioner must be thoroughly familiar with if he is to put the method to use successfully in his own practice.

4. GALEN'S METHOD

In his *MM* Galen aims to establish a rational methodology which would allow the doctor to select the appropriate treatment for a particular disease in a particular patient and to modify this treatment in a rational manner according to the course of events. However, the *MM* is certainly not a therapeutic recipe book simply listing treatments for the whole range of diseases set out in an *a capite ad calcem* arrangement. And although it does contain anecdotal observations, case reports, and various polemical and other digressions, among all these "distractions" it does articulate a well-conceived methodology. This methodology is, moreover, necessarily based on a sound theoretical foundation—one which can only be established by a thoroughgoing knowledge of the basic medical sciences. To acquire this, the methodical practitioner must acquaint himself with a group of treatises, predominantly Galenic but also those of other notables, such as Hippocrates and Plato. Galen refers to the components of this group of treatises repeatedly in the course of his *MM*.

The initial requirement for the doctor who would practice this method is an understanding of the basic structure of the human body. This involves two levels: the fundamental components and their organization into recognizable structures. Galen is quite unequivocal in his position on the fundamental components. They are the four elemental qualities (hot, cold, moist, and dry), which are related on the one hand to the four elements (fire, water, air, and earth), and on the other hand to the four humors (blood, phlegm, yellow bile, and black bile) (see Figure 1). He espoused, then, a continuum theory of matter—a theory which can be traced back to Empedocles. Galen quite clearly identified the originators of his received concepts of basic structure as Hippocrates, Plato, and Aristotle, and especially the first. His own statement of the theory is to be found primarily in his *On the Elements according to Hippocrates* and *On Hippocrates' Nature of Man*. Both are works in which he elaborates on Hippocrates' own *Nature of Man*. In the opening paragraph of his work *On Mixtures* (*Temperaments; vide infra*) he writes: "Animal bodies are a mixture of hot, cold, moist, and dry and these qualities are not mixed equally in each case. In ancient times this was satisfactorily demonstrated by the best doctors and philosophers. There is also a work of mine covering the apparent

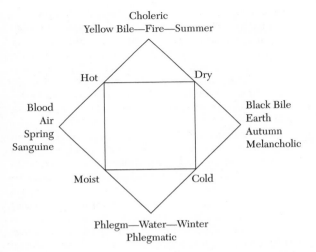

Choleric
Yellow Bile—Fire—Summer

Hot

Dry

Blood
Air
Spring
Sanguine

Black Bile
Earth
Autumn
Melancholic

Moist

Cold

Phlegm—Water—Winter
Phlegmatic

Figure 1. A diagrammatic representation of the Hippocratic humoral system based on his *On the Nature of Man*—following H. Sigerist, *A History of Medicine*, Oxford University Press, New York, 1961.

facts of the case. It is the one in which I investigate the elements according to Hippocrates."[76]

What Galen implacably opposed were Atomist theories, which postulated that matter in general was composed of minute discrete particles, all similar, existing and moving in an empty space or void—theories originating

[76] *De temperamentis*, I.509K.

with Leucippus (460–420 BC) and Democritus of Abdera (440–380 BC). These primary entities, the elements, were taken to be indestructible, immutable, and impassable in themselves, forming the identifiable structures of the world by their unending associations and disassociations. This was the theory first applied specifically to medicine by Asclepiades of Bithynia (ca. 120–90 BC). It was a theory unequivocally repudiated by Hippocrates, and so by Galen.

At the macroscopic level of the animal body, the four elemental qualities were conceived of as being inherent in the anatomical structures identifiable by dissection. In general, for Galen there were essentially two forms of organization of these anatomical structures—*homoiomeres*, or uniform parts, and organic (i.e., instrumental) parts or organs. Examples of the former are muscle, bone, and cartilage; examples of the latter are heart, liver, and lungs. The structure and arrangement of the bodily components, themselves composed of the four elemental qualities inherent in their substance, are set out in Galen's various major and minor anatomical treatises. In his *On the Use of the Parts* he considers not only the structure but also the function of all the organic parts and articulates his Aristotelian teleology. Specifically, and contrary to the Erasistratean position, his view is that every part of the body has a particular function.[77] On the subject of gross anatomy, although Galen made significant discoveries in his own right, he drew heavily on the prior work of Aristotle and the two great Alexandrian anatomists, Herophilus and Erasistra-

[77] See, for example, *De usu partium*, Book 4, chapter 15 (May, *Galen on the Usefulness of the Parts of the Body*, vol. 1, p. 232).

tus, however much he may have differed from the latter on the issue of the physiological functioning of the anatomical structures identified.

The key components of Galen's own physiological scheme are set out in three works multiply referred to in his *MM*: *On Mixtures* (*Kraseis*), *On the Natural Faculties* (*Physical Capacities*), and *On the Opinions of Hippocrates and Plato*. However, a full appreciation of Galen's views on physiology requires the study of quite a number of other, shorter treatises—for example, those on the pulse and respiration. The essential elements of his physiology, required for an understanding of his overall method of medicine, are as follows. All parts of the body, whether *homoiomerous* or organic, have a certain *krasis*, or mixture of the four elemental qualities. Although this *krasis* may vary from part to part and from individual to individual, there is an optimum "state" (or perhaps range of "states") in each case which is necessary for the healthy functioning of the part or the organism as a whole. This "state" may be described as a "condition" (*diathesis*), "constitution" (*kataskeue*), "state" (*hexis*), or "state" (*schesis*), and the homeostatic (to borrow a modern term) mechanisms of the body are designed to maintain all parts and organs within the range of a satisfactory *krasis* in terms of their functions/actions.

Next, it is important to recognize that the animal body is divided into three major functional systems:

1. The brain, spinal cord, and nerves, both cranial and spinal; these are responsible for motor and sensory functions.
2. The heart and arteries; these are responsible for the

vital force and preservation of the innate heat (*vide infra*).

3. The liver and veins; these are responsible for the nutrition of all the bodily parts.

Other structures are subsidiary to and dependent on these main systems and their components. Further, the working of such a system is dependent on its *dunamis* (capacity, faculty, power), and there may be more than one *dunamis* per system. Galen recognizes the imprecision of his fundamental concept of *dunamis*, writing in his *On the Natural Faculties* (*Physical Capacities*):[78]

> The so-called *haematopoietic* faculty in the veins, then, as well as all the other faculties, fall within the category of relative concepts; primarily because the faculty is the cause of the activity, but also, accidentally, because it is the cause of the effect. But if the cause is relative to something—for it is the cause of what results from it, and of nothing else—it is obvious that the faculty also falls into the category of the relative; and so long as we are ignorant of the true essence of the cause which is operating, we call it a faculty.

Nonetheless, the concept of *dunamis* is critical to Galen's physiology. Initiated by their capacities, the various structures carry out their functions (*energeiai*), which become manifest in their actions (*erga*). For example, the stom-

---

[78] *De naturalibus facultatibus*, Book 1, chapter 4 (II.9–10K); translation after A. J. Brock, *Galen on the Natural Faculties*, LCL (with minor modifications).

ach, which Galen often uses to exemplify a mechanism or concept and which is a component in the third (vegetative, nutritive) system, "attracts" the ingested food through its attractive capacity, retains it while it is being processed through its retentive capacity, alters it in this process through its alterative capacity, and then passes it on through its expulsive capacity. The nutriment, so processed in the stomach, then moves on to the liver (the headquarters, as it were, of the nutritive system), and the process of transformation into blood is set in motion. This allows the food to provide nutrition for the other structures of the body. This triad of *dunamis* (capacity), *energeia* (function), and *ergon* (action) is, then, one critical component of Galen's physiology.

Two other factors that are also of major importance are *pneuma* (or really *pneumas*) and innate heat. In the *MM* Galen states that there are three *pneumas*, one associated with each of the three major systems identified above. There is a psychic *pneuma*, a vital *pneuma*, and a physical *pneuma*. Ultimately these *pneumas* are derived from the inspired air and are distributed by the arterial system but may undergo modification before being distributed within their respective systems. Thus the *pneuma* is "processed" in the *rete mirabile* at the base of the brain (a structure which Galen did not realize was absent in the human) before becoming the psychic *pneuma* and entering the brain to be distributed by the nerves. For health, the system of *pneumas* needs to be functioning in a normal way.

"Innate heat" is another key concept which Galen inherited from his ancient authorities, in this instance Hippocrates and particularly Aristotle. He considered this innate heat to have its seat in the heart and arteries and to be supplied in the formation of the fetus, as the following statement indicates:

> We do not posit masses and pores as elements in the body, nor do we declare that heat comes from motion or friction or some other cause. Rather, we suppose the whole body breathes and flows together, the heat not acquired or subsequent to the generation of the animal, but itself first, original and innate. This is nothing other than the nature and soul of life so that you would not be wrong in thinking heat to be a self-moving and constantly moving substance.[79]

Thus, the innate heat is located centrally in the heart, its maintenance is aided by respiration, and it is distributed to the rest of the body through the arteries. However, unlike the other aspects of Galenic physiology previously mentioned, it does not play a large role in his treatment methods as described in the *MM*.

Galen details his views on pathology in three works referred to in the *MM* as required reading for students of that treatise. In the first two works he sets out his pathophysiology, which is based on the concept of *dyskrasia*. In general terms, a *dyskrasia* may arise from a change in the balance of the elemental qualities occurring within the substance of the involved part itself from either internal or external causes or from an inflow of material (flux) which alters the balance, or from a combination of both. He divides the *dyskrasias* into those that are "regular" and those that are "irregular." In the regular *dyskrasias* there is uni-

---

[79] *De tremor, palpitatione, convulsion et rigore*, VII.616K.

formity in the imbalance of the four elemental qualities that involves the part or the whole. There are eight possible *dyskrasias* of this sort: four "simple" *dyskrasias*, in which there is a preponderance of one elemental quality (hot, cold, moist, or dry) only, and four "compound" *dyskrasias*, in which there is a preponderance of one of the four possible combinations (hot and moist, hot and dry, cold and moist, cold and dry). These regular *dyskrasias* are described in the work on *krasis* itself (*De temperamentis*), which also describes the normal physiology, in the work *On the Causes of Diseases*, and in the final book (Book 6) of *On the Preservation of Health*. The irregular *dyskrasias*, which are the subject of a short treatise entitled *On Irregular Dyskrasias*, are those in which more than one form of *dyskrasia* exists in different parts of the patient at the same time. He notes in this work that there is an unspecified number of such *dyskrasias*. Importantly, also, in Galen's scheme, *dyskrasias* are the agents of disturbances of the soul, i.e., mental symptoms and diseases. In the third work, which is his major treatise on anatomical pathology, *On the Affected Parts*, Galen begins with two books on issues of diagnosis considered particularly from a topographical viewpoint. The remaining four books then deal with diseases according to an anatomical division.

A further group of treatises of particular importance for the foundation of his method are the four works on the classification and causation of diseases and symptoms. They are important for the following four reasons.

1. They set out definitions of the essential terms for the *MM*: health (*hygieia*), disease (*nosos*), affection (*pathos*), symptom (*symptoma*), condition (*diathesis*),

function (*energeia*), and according to/contrary to nature (*kata phusin/para phusin*).

2. The two works on differentiae of diseases and symptoms establish a comprehensive classification of the conditions that require treatment.

3. The two works on causation of diseases and symptoms analyze the mode of causation of these abnormalities on the premise that every change from accord with nature to contrary to nature has one or more causes, recognizable (at least potentially) by either reason or observation.

4. There are descriptions of a wide variety of diseases and symptoms which help the doctor's understanding of the mechanisms of the diseases he must treat.

Next, and penultimately, there are the three substantial treatises on pharmacology—one on the *krasis* and potency of a large number of simple medications and two on compound medications, one of which is organized according to the classes of materials and the other according to the affected places for which they are to be used.[80] Apart from the obvious need for knowledge of the basic makeup and availability of the medications, the methodical doctor must have a knowledge of their various potencies, means of application, ease of penetration into tissues, and side effects.

The final book that Galen refers to repeatedly in the

---

[80] These are, respectively, *De simplicium medicamentorum temperamentis et facultatibus* (XI.379–892K and XII.1–377K), *De compositione medicamentorum secundum locos* (XII.378–1007K and XIII.1–361K), and *De compositione medicamentorum per genera* (XIII.362–1058K).

MM is his work *On the Preservation of Health*. In the opening paragraph of the present introduction, the division of the doctor's function into prophylactic and therapeutic components is noted as a point of emphasis for Galen. Obviously this work is primarily concerned with the prophylactic, but both prophylaxis and treatment depend on the same theoretical foundation, so it can be seen as a necessary complement to his *MM* in the comprehensive functioning of the doctor. Moreover, in his *On the Preservation of Health*, there is no small amount of pathological and therapeutic information.

In summary, then, in working by method (that is, Galen's method), the doctor comes to the patient with a firm commitment to a continuum theory of matter in his understanding of the structure of the human body. He is equipped also with a thorough grounding in anatomy and physiology. The sick patient is going to be suffering from one (or perhaps more) of the diseases from among the three classes of Galen's basic classification: a disturbance of *krasis* of a part or the whole; an organic disease involving size, number, conformation, or position; or a dissolution of continuity affecting either an *homoiomerous* or an organic part. A diagnosis needs to be made which includes the nature of the disease and the part or parts affected. Possible causal factors need to be identified and evaluated. Other factors must be taken into account—factors such as the patient's age, habitus, and customs and the place and climatic conditions. As far as possible an assessment should be made of the individual characteristics of the patient when healthy, although Galen recognizes the inevitable inexactitude in such an assessment.

Having made this comprehensive evaluation, the doctor must arrive at the sum total of therapeutic indications. If there is only one indication—for example, cooling for a hot *dyskrasia*—the matter may be relatively simple. If there are multiple indications, an order of priority needs to be established. Treatment measures can then be initiated. When medications are to be used, their compositions and potencies must be known. The overriding objectives in each of the three classes of diseases are, respectively, as follows:

1. Restoration of a normal *krasis* in the simple or compound *dyskrasias*, usually through the exhibition of opposites.
2. Restoration of an accord with nature in organic parts that are contrary to nature in terms of size, number, conformation, or position—at least if the change is sufficient to interfere with function. This may involve surgery or other measures, depending on circumstances.
3. Restoration of continuity or union where there is dissolution of continuity or union. This may involve surgical measures directly with appropriate postoperative care (e.g., immobilization in a fracture) or treatment by medications and other measures in cases such as infected wounds or chronic ulcers.

In addition, symptoms consequent to the primary disease can be treated with symptomatic measures. Examples are the symptoms that may accompany fevers, which Galen covers in Book 12 of his *MM*. If the treatment measures are proving ineffectual, or even harmful, the situation can be reevaluated theoretically (i.e, the concept of the disease mechanism and its causation) and on the basis of prior experience. Then new approaches to therapy can be devised until the desired outcome is achieved. It is also of importance for the doctor to make an accurate assessment of prognosis as far as possible, both to inform the patient and to guide the treatment. This, in its briefest essence, is Galen's method of medicine as articulated in the work of that name.

5. THE *METHOD OF MEDICINE* (MM)

This is the work that sets out Galen's method of medical practice most completely. Buried in the middle of Book 9 of this treatise, Galen makes the following statement about his composition of the *MM*:

> You shouldn't be surprised, then, that although I bear witness to Hippocrates' discovery of the therapeutic method, I myself turned my hand to writing this particular treatise. I came to this book, as I said a little earlier, not because the method itself was entirely undiscovered but because it was lacking in some respects, since I found that none of my predecessors had completed the method. Indeed, some did not know it at all while those who did know it were unable to add what was lacking. (633K)

Of course, much ancient writing has been lost, and medical treatises are no exception. But certainly in what we have remaining there is no comparable systematic exposition of a complete method of medical practice. The *MM* is complete not in the sense of considering all diseases in a "head to heel" arrangement but insofar as the underlying theory is established and the method formulated on the basis of this theory in relation to all classes of disease in Galen's own classification. Paradigmatic conditions are considered and principles are illustrated by case reports. The underlying message is that if the student is able to gain a thorough grasp of these principles, clarified by the examples of their application, he will then be able to confront any disease which comes before him in a reasoned and effective manner. The *MM* reads like a handbook for an experienced practicing doctor—a postgraduate text rather than a text for medical students, which would fit with its variable and somewhat restricted use in later teaching establishments.

The work itself has a somewhat curious initial history, having been written in two parts whose composition was separated by an interval of approximately twenty years. The first part, comprising Books 1–6 and dedicated to Hiero, was probably completed in the first half of the 170s, a decade of great literary production for Galen. We know essentially nothing about Hiero, the dedicatee, although Nutton speculates that he "must be assumed to have been an extremely competent practitioner, and we are told by Galen that he had a detailed knowledge of anatomy and a long-standing and intimate acquaintance with Galen and other doctors."[81] One may assume also that Hiero studied with Galen and accompanied him on his rounds, at least in some instances. The second part, comprising Books 7–14, was dedicated to Eugenianus, also a doctor and friend who, like Hiero, seems to have witnessed Galen at work. The reason given by Galen at the beginning of Book 7 for

[81] V. Nutton in Kudlien and Durling, *Galen's Method of Healing*, p. 5.

his initial abandonment of the project—that Hiero had died while abroad—is hardly likely to have been the whole story. The date of composition of the second part is uncertain but is quite probably in the 190s (even the late 190s) and after the writing of the three major works on pharmacology, which are frequently referred to throughout these last eight books.

So the two parts were separated in time of composition by approximately two decades. Nevertheless, the transition between them is relatively seamless,[82] and the overall structure of the work is such that the later part takes up where the first part left off in terms of Galen's scheme of classification, with only a minor preamble to the new dedicatee. The earlier part finishes with the completion of the books on the treatment of diseases of dissolution of continuity which affect both *homoiomerous* and organic parts. The later part starts with disorders of *krasis* which essentially affect *homoiomerous* structures and concludes with disorders of organic parts involving particularly abnormalities of magnitude, number, position, and conformation. Three points of note are: (a) the overall sequence of theory, dissolution of continuity, *dyskrasias,* and diseases of organic parts; (b) the particular attention given to fevers in the section on *dyskrasias*; (c) the impression of poor organization and haste of composition of the final two books, which may simply indicate the author's wish to bring the massive work to completion as he advanced through his seventh decade or, perhaps, that he was in-

---

82 One noticeable difference is the more practical and less polemical tone of the later-written part, and perhaps a higher proportion of case reports.

tending to deal with these matters at greater length in a planned work on surgical treatment, this being a major component of treatment of many (although by no means all) of these problems. The contents of the subdivisions are summarized below, while the subject matter of each chapter of each book is outlined in the synopses of content preceding each volume.

Section 1: Theory (Books 1 and 2): The first two books establish the theoretical foundation of Galen's system of medicine generally and his method of treatment more specifically. This involves stating the definitions of the basic concepts and entities: health, disease, affection, condition, symptom, function, and action. Galen considers the important aspects of causation, touches on the basic division between *homoiomeres* and organic parts, and gives some account of the theory of the four elemental qualities and the role of their imbalance (*dyskrasia*) in the creation of disease. He also refers to his classifications of diseases and symptoms. A particular feature of these two books is their polemical nature, incorporating vicious and at times *ad hominem* attacks on individuals and sects whose theories run counter to Galen's own. Such attacks are especially directed at Thessalus and the Methodic sect, but the followers of Erasistratus and the Empirics are by no means immune. The polemic is adorned with bravura literary flourishes and is accompanied by lamentation about the overall decline of the standards of medical practice in general.

Section 2: Diseases Due to Disorder of Continuity (Books 3–6): Book 3 begins with a consideration of "indication" (*endeixis*), a factor which is fundamental to treatment decisions. There is also some consideration of how knowledge is acquired—it must either be through reason or through experience. Galen deals in order with the management of simple wounds, wounds or ulcers with a cavity, tissue loss (in particular skin loss), overgrowth of flesh (exuberant granulation tissue), and the ichors (serous fluids) that may flow from a wound. Book 4 is primarily concerned with the management of chronic wounds and ulcers in both superficial and deep structures. The concepts of *kakoethia* (chronicity, "malignancy") and *kakochymia* (a bad state of the humors) are introduced. Also stressed is the need to insure that the tissue underlying or surrounding a wound or ulcer is in good condition if healing is to be achieved. Several specific components of treatment—particularly purging and phlebotomy—are discussed in detail. In the opening section of Book 5 Galen focuses on the essential processes of the healing of wounds and ulcers (dissolution of continuity): bringing about union (conglutination), creating new flesh (enfleshing), reduction of excess flesh, and scar formation (cicatrization). The management of hemorrhage from various sites is considered in the later chapters. Finally, there is detailed discussion of the treatment of wounds and ulcers in the respiratory structures— the upper and lower airways and the lungs themselves. In Book 6 there is consideration of inflammation in wounds and ulcers, its effects, and its management. Then, sequentially, Galen deals with the treatment of wounds of nerves/ sinews, ligaments, the abdomen, fractures of long bones, and skull fractures.

Section 3: Diseases Due to *Dyskrasia*, Including Fevers (Books 7–12): *Dyskrasias* are diseases of *homoiomeres*. The concept of *dyskrasia* depends on the theory of the four qualities (hot, cold, moist, and dry) as the elemental components of structure. In theory, there is *eukrasia* and there are eight possible *dyskrasias*—four "simple" *dyskrasias*, involving a preponderance of one only of the four qualities, and four "compound" *dyskrasias*, involving a preponderance of one of the nonexclusive pair of qualities—that is, hot and moist, hot and dry, cold and moist, and cold and dry. In Book 7 the treatment of *dyskrasias* in general is considered, with particular focus on the *homoiomerous* components of the stomach as an example. In general terms, *dyskrasia* can be due to a change occurring primarily within the affected structure itself or to inflowing material adversely affecting the proper balance (*krasis*) of the qualities. Book 8 begins with a detailed consideration of fever, which is identified as a particular form of hot *dyskrasia*. Stoppage of the skin pores is seen as a key factor in the causation of fever. The last sections of Book 8 are devoted to the first kind (*differentia*) of fever—the ephemeral fever. The essential features of this are that it has only a single paroxysm and the total duration of the fever is one day. In Book 9, Galen turns to continuous (synochial, nonintermittent) fevers, which may also be termed polyhemeral. These fevers have a single continuous paroxysm extending over a number of days. A crucial factor in their causation is putrefaction of humors. Important in the management of such fevers are the patient's strength or capacity (*dunamis*), the use of phlebotomy, and the taking of cold water. Book 10 returns to a general consideration of the treatment of fevers. There is particular focus on the role of fasting in causing and prolonging such fevers. Several case reports are provided to illustrate and support Galen's arguments. In the concluding chapters of Book 10 attention is given to hectic fevers. Book 11 is primarily concerned with the treatment of continuous fevers caused by putrefaction of humors. The essential component of their treatment is opposition—for example, the opposition of cold to heat. The differences in the three kinds of fever—ephemeral, polyhemeral due to putrefaction of humors, and continuous—are outlined and their implications for treatment discussed. Specific and detailed consideration is given to the treatment of putrefaction. Book 12 is devoted to the symptoms which may accompany fevers and their management. The two main symptoms considered are syncope and pain.

Section 4: Diseases Due to Abnormal Swellings/ Diseases of Organic Parts (Books 13–14): Book 13 is almost entirely about inflammation—how it is caused and, in particular, how it is to be treated. Which part is inflamed has an important bearing on treatment. Several different parts are considered: liver, spleen, head (brain and eye). Book 14 begins with the treatment of erysipelas, starting with the features that distinguish it from inflammation. Scirrhous and edematous swellings are then considered, followed by the treatment of the specific swellings involving the penis (priapism) and tongue. Other swellings discussed include "malignant" pustules (*anthrakes*), glandular (scrofulous) swellings, and abscesses. There is then consideration of diseases due to either excess or deficiency. The main example of the former is obesity. Examples of the latter include congenital absence of tissue (missing digits, hypospadias) and focal or general atrophy. The final three chapters concern, respectively, the treatment of various kinds of warts, hair problems (alopecia, baldness, *ptilosis*), and the eyes (pterygium, chalazion, cataract). At the very end there is a brief mention of the treatment of gastrointestinal worm infestations. Nutton's comment on Book 14—that it "resembles a very hasty combination of stray thoughts and lacks any strong central core, either thematic or paradigmatic"[83]—is entirely apt.

Galen's *MM* is, then, a systematic account of medical treatment and its underlying theory and methodology. By no means every disease is considered, nor is every remedy or form of treatment. The assumption is that if the student has grasped the principles and their method of application, if he knows how to further his own knowledge and expertise by a judicious mix of theoretical formulation and practical experience, and if he has access to Galen's pharmacological texts and the other specific treatises mentioned above, and if he studies them assiduously, he is equipped to practice medicine in a rational and successful fashion.

What subsequently happened to this great tome on the practice of medicine? Certainly many of Galen's methods were preserved in the writings of the medical encyclopedists during the several centuries immediately following his death. The fate of the work as a whole from then on may be briefly recounted in relation to the sequence given below. The *MM* was included in the Syriac and Arabic translations listed as the first two stages of the translation/preservation process. Specifically, it was included in Sergius' translations in the sixth century and in those of Hunain ibn Ishâq in the ninth century. It was then translated into Latin by all three of the eleventh- and twelfth- century translators, as follows: (a) by Constantine the African from the Greek as the *Megategni*, which was a paraphrastic trans-

---

[83] See Nutton. in Kudlien and Durling, *Galen's Method of Healing*, p. 8.

lation of the whole work; (b) by Gerard of Cremona as the *De ingenio sanitate*, which was a translation from the Arabic of the whole work; (c) by Burgundio of Pisa as the *Terapeutika*, which was a translation from the Greek of Part 2 (i.e., Books 7–14) minus the last part of Book 14.

Subsequent translations have been few in number and mostly partial. They are listed below in chronological order.

1. The important translation of the whole work from Greek into Latin by Thomas Linacre. This went through fifteen printings between 1519 and 1609 and was, with minor modifications, used for the Latin versions in the collected works edited by Chartier and Kühn.

2. The translation of Books 3–6 into English by the surgeon Thomas Gale, printed in London in 1586.

3. The translation of the whole work into English (albeit with parts of each chapter omitted—essentially the polemical passages and other digressions) by Peter English, printed in Edinburgh in 1656.

4. Four translations of parts of Books 1 and 2 into German as dissertations presented between 1898 and 1900 (three in Berlin and one in Kiel).[84]

5. The translation of Books 1 and 2 into English with detailed commentary by R. J. Hankinson, published in 1991.

6. The translation of Books 1 and 2 into French by J. Boulogne, published in 1992.

[84] For bibliographical details of these three short dissertations, see J. Boulogne (2009), p. 35.

7. The translation of the whole work into French by J. Boulogne, published in Paris in 2009.

6. TERMINOLOGY

Despite Galen's repeated protestations that names are not important and that it is only matters that matter, he devotes considerable attention to the definition of a group of key terms in the opening two books of his *MM* and particularly in his four treatises on the classification and causation of diseases and symptoms and his work on nomenclature specifically, all of which are referred to on a number of occasions in his *MM*.[85] It is essential for the doctor to have a clear concept of what actually constitutes health and disease and their concomitants if he is to perform his prophylactic and therapeutic tasks adequately. What follows is a series of definitions of and comments on the important terms in Galen's method, divided into three sections: basic definitions, transliterated terms, and other, translated terms of significance.

Basic Definitions

Health (ὑγίεια)**:** First, for Galen, health is something that positively exists; it is not just the absence of disease. He attacks the Methodic Olympicus in Book 2 of the *MM* (X.137K) because he takes the latter position. Two definitions of health are offered by Galen in his *On the Dif-*

---

[85] The last is *De nominibus medicis*; see M. Meyerhof and J. Schacht, *Galen über die medizinischen Namen* (Arabic text, German translation, Berlin, 1931).

ferentiae of Diseases; one is functional and the other structural, as follows:[86]

1. Health exists when the functions (*energeiai*) of the body are in accord with nature (*kata phusin*).
2. Health exists when the constitution (*kataskeue*) of the organs by which the body functions is in accord with nature (*kata phusin*).

However, understanding of these definitions depends on the definitions of the constituent terms: function, constitution, and accord with nature. In terms of Galen's own concepts of structure and function, the definition of health in the pseudo-Galenic *Definitiones medicae* is perhaps more enlightening: "Health is a *eukrasia* in accord with nature of the primary humors in us or the unhindered functioning of the natural capacities (*dunameis*). Health is a *eukrasia* of the four primary elemental qualities from which the body is composed (i.e., hot, cold, moist, and dry)."[87] Whether there is also a third, intermediate condition between health and disease is an issue not addressed in either the *MM* or the four treatises on diseases and symptoms. It is, however, considered at some length in Galen's *Art of Medicine* (I.307–313K).

Disease (νόσος, νόσημα): Like health, disease for Galen is a specific entity. Again, both structural and functional definitions are offered in the treatise *On the Differentiae of Diseases*—disease is "either some constitution contrary to nature or a cause of damaged function" (VI.837–8K). Disease, then, occurs when the balance of

---

[86] *De differentiis morborum*, VI.836–37K.
[87] *Definitiones medicae*, XIX.382K.

the primary constituents of the body, whether these be the four elemental qualities or humors, or something else (e.g., particles and pores on the Methodic scheme), are disturbed to such an extent as to harm function. However, function can also be harmed by structural changes at a macroscopic level, as in organic diseases where there are abnormalities of size, number, position, or conformation, or where there is dissolution of continuity.

Affection (πάθος, πάθημα): In Urmson's modern definition relating particularly to Aristotle's *Metaphysics*, V.21 (1022b15–21), an affection is "what happens to anything that undergoes, suffers or experiences anything."[88] In this sense an affection is not necessarily pathological. Indeed, the distinction between health, disease, and affection is not altogether clear despite Galen's statement to the contrary.[89] Nor is the distinction between affection (*pathos*) and condition (*diathesis; vide infra*) clear, although it might be said that the former is a change in progress while the latter is an established change.

Symptom (σύμπτωμα): Galen provides a detailed definition of "symptom" in Book 1 of his *MM*, which prompts Hankinson to write: "This (i.e. symptom) is a type of [condition/*diathesis*], that is of a body or part of a body constituted in a certain way, but one which has no causal bearing on any of the *energeiai* (i.e. functions). It will be apparent from this that a *sumptoma* differs from its contemporary homophone, either in its general or its medically exact use (although in many cases it reasonably ap-

---

[88] J. O. Urmson, *The Greek Philosophical Vocabulary* (London, 1990), p. 126.

[89] *De symptomatum differentiis*, VII.44K.

proximates to the former, as Galen's examples suggest)."[90] However, in his *On the Differentiae of Symptoms* Galen states unequivocally that "the specific characteristic of a symptom is this: it is contrary to nature."[91] This suggests a closer correspondence with modern usage than Hankinson claims, and is in fact how the term is used in the *MM*. In effect, a definition might be that a symptom is a condition contrary to nature that does not adversely affect function. Two other, related terms are ἐπιγέννημα (epiphenomenon) and συνδρομή (syndrome). As neither is used to any extent in the *MM*, they are not considered here.

Condition (διάθεσις): A modern English dictionary definition of the term "diathesis," very definitely in current medical use, is as follows: "A particular condition or habit of the body, esp. one predisposing to certain diseases."[92] This would serve for Galen's use and might favor simply transliterating the term which, for him, is a key element of several of the other definitions. We have, however, opted for "condition" as the translation. Three statements by Galen on the term follow:[93]

1. "For each thing that exists is in some sense in a condition, whether it is healthy, diseased, or neither."
2. "Sometimes an affection arises from a certain cause

---

[90] See R. J. Hankinson, *Galen on the Therapeutic Method: Books 1 and 2* (Oxford, 1990), p. 152.

[91] *De symptomatum differentiis*, VII.51–52K.

[92] *The Chambers Dictionary*, 11th ed. (2008).

[93] The three sources are, respectively, *De symptomatum differentiis*, VII.43K, *Methodus medendi*, X.63K, and *De locis affectis*, VIII.25K.

but in some way is not yet a stable condition if the
cause is separated. Sometimes it has already come
about or is still coming about. Often, when the cause
has gone, the coming about ceases and it is already a
stable condition."

3. "There is nothing else to be cured by doctors apart
from the condition of bodies."

Constitution (κατασκευή): Although translated by us
as "constitution," *kataskeue* is more or less equivalent to
diathesis. Thus, in the *MM* Galen writes: "If health is some
condition or constitution in accord with nature, so disease
will be some condition or constitution contrary to nature."[94]

State (ἕξις): The distinction between "state" and "condition" is clearly expressed by Aristotle as follows:[95] "A
state differs from a condition by the latter being easily
changed whereas the former is longer lasting and more difficult to change. States are also conditions but conditions
are not necessarily states. For those who are in states are
also in a certain condition in some way on account of these,
but those who are in a certain condition are not always also
in a state."

Capacity (δύναμις): This is a particularly important
term in the *MM*. Not only is it used frequently, but it is also
found in three distinct contexts. First, it is found in the
strictly "physiological" sense, as in Galen's important and
fundamental (to the *MM*) work, *On the Natural Faculties
(Physical Capacities)*. Second, it is used in relation to a pa-

[94] *Methodus medendi*, X.52K.
[95] Aristotle, *Categories* VIII.9a8–13.

tient's ability to tolerate a particular treatment, and third, it is used in relation to the strength, power, or potency of medications. The term is given detailed consideration by Aristotle in *Metaphysics* V.12, where he writes:[96] "Capacity, then, is the source, in general, of a change or movement in another thing or in the same thing *qua* other, and also the source of a thing's being moved by another thing or by itself *qua* other." Phillips says of Galen's use of *dunamis* in his *On the Natural Faculties* (*Physical Capacities*):[97] "The notion of *dunamis* in this book is very pervasive and mostly verbal, being a development in medicine, not of *dunamis* as known in *Ancient Medicine*, but of the Aristotelian *dunamis* as potentiality contrasted with *energeia*, activity or actuality, also Aristotelian." Galen himself recognizes the difficulty, writing in his work *The Faculties of the Soul Follow the Mixtures of the Body*:[98]

> Many of the wise are openly in confusion on this matter, having an incorrect understanding of "capacity." They seem to me to wrongly conceive of "capacity" as something which dwells in substances, as we do in houses, not being aware that the effective cause of each thing that comes about is conceived of in relation to something else, and that there is some name for this cause as of such a thing that is separate and per se. But in it, in relation to what is brought

96 *Metaphysics* 1019a18–21. Translation after W. D. Ross, in J. Barnes, *The Complete Works of Aristotle: The Revised Oxford Translation* (Princeton, 1984), vol. 2, p. 1609.

97 E. D. Phillips, *Aspects of Greek Medicine* (Philadelphia, 1987), p. 176.

98 *Quod animi mores*, IV.769K.

about from it, the "capacity" is of what is brought about, and because of this we say that substance has as many capacities as it has functions (*energeiai*).

Function (ἐνέργεια): This term is taken to represent the functional expression of the capacity (*dunamis*). LSJ lists one meaning as "physiological function," with reference to a passage in Galen's *On the Preservation of Health*. This is taken to be the sense intended in Galen's series of definitions foundational to his method in the *MM*. The relevant passage reads as follows:[99]

> Certainly one must not, therefore, determine those who are healthy and those who are diseased simply by strength or weakness of functions, but one must attribute "in accord with nature" (*kata phusin*) to those who are healthy in contrast to "contrary to nature" (*para phusin*) to those who are diseased; that is, for the former to be a healthy condition (*diathesis*) in accord with nature effecting functions, and for the latter to be a diseased condition (*diathesis*) contrary to nature harming function.

Debru has argued that "the concept of function (from the Latin *functio*) does not occur in antiquity in the sense with which it has been used since the seventeenth century."[100] It is, however, clearly the modern concept of the term "function" that applies to what Galen is describing. Linacre, for example, in his translation of the *MM* and of

[99] *De sanitate tuenda*, VI.21K.
[100] A. Debru, "Physiology," in Hankinson, *Cambridge Companion to Galen*, p. 265.

the four treatises on the classification and causation of diseases and symptoms, uses *actio* and *functio* interchangeably for *energeia*.

Action (ἔργον): We have taken *ergon* to be the action carried out by the performance of the function. On function expressed in action, Galen writes in Book 1 of the *MM*: "For it is agreed, then, in this case, by all men and not only doctors but also by those they meet, that it is [the eye's] action (*ergon*) to see. And whether I say 'action' (*ergon*) or 'function' (*energeia*) certainly makes no difference now in this case."

On the interrelation of these three terms, Galen writes:[101] "I shall call the action (*ergon*) what has already been brought about and 'filled up' by the function (*energeia*) of these, for example the blood, flesh, and nerve. I term the active movement the function and the capacity (*dunamis*) the cause of this." Brock, in the introduction to his translation of Galen's *On the Natural Faculties* (*Physical Capacities*), summarizes the use of the three terms as follows:[102] "Any of the operations of the living part may be looked on in three ways, either (a) as a *dunamis*, faculty, potentiality; (b) as an *energeia*, which is the *dunamis* in operation; or (c) as an *ergon*, the product or effect of the *energeia*."

Use (χρεία): This is not a term used to any significant extent in the *MM*. Nevertheless, it is important for an understanding of Galen's anatomical views, forming as it does part of the title of one of his major works on the subject, *On the Use of the Parts*. May's clear definition, which in-

101 *De facultatibus naturalibus*, I.2.
102 Brock, *Galen: On the Natural Faculties*, pp. xxx–xxxi.

cludes the distinction between "use" (χρεία) and "function" (ἐνέργεια), is as follows: "The Greek χρεία of the title . . . does not mean function as one might naturally suppose. Function is more nearly ἐνέργεια or 'action' in Galen's terms. Χρεία means for him rather the suitability of a part for performing its action, the special characteristics of its structure that enable it to function as it does."[103]

Accord with nature, nonaccord with nature, contrary to nature (κατὰ φύσιν, οὐ κατὰ φύσιν, παρὰ φύσιν): The first and third of these terms are of particular importance in Galen's basic definitions. The slightly cumbersome translations are used to identify and emphasize the technical nature of these terms and are preferred over such possible alternatives as "normal/abnormal" and "natural/unnatural," although in certain nondefinitional contexts one or other of these pairs may be used. The middle term above—"nonaccord with nature"—is not used in either the *MM* or the four treatises on diseases and symptoms. It is, however, prominent in Galen's *Art of Medicine*. The following passage from the pseudo-Galenic *Medical Definitions* clarifies the meanings of these terms and the relationship between them, and also further clarifies Galen's concepts of health and disease.

> Health is that which is in accord with nature. Disease is that which is contrary to nature. What is "natural" (φύσει) but neither "in accord with nature," nor already "contrary to nature," is like someone being very thin, or dry, or thick-set, or fat, or sharp-

[103] See May, *Galen on the Usefulness of the Parts of the Body*, vol. 1, p. 9.

nosed, or grey, or snub-nosed, or grey-eyed. Those who are thus are not in a condition "in accord with nature" for they have gone beyond "balance" but neither are they "contrary to nature" for they are not hindered in function. Something that is "non-natural" (οὐ φύσει) is neither "contrary to nature," nor "in accord with nature," nor "natural." Examples are those who have *leuke*, leprous warts, warts and the like. Such people are not "in accord with nature" as they are outside what accords with nature, but they are not "contrary to nature" as they are not impeded in the functions that accord with nature. These things are not, however, "natural" in that they are not present *ab initio*, i.e. from the initial genesis. They remain, therefore, "non-natural." What is "non-natural" by definition is close to what accords with nature and what is contrary to nature.[104]

Transliterated Terms (* indicates terms still in use)

Adiapneusis (ἀδιαπνευστία): Failure of transpiration/perspiration.

Diapedesis*(διαπήδησις): Transudation from blood vessels to tissues. The modern definition is "the passage of blood or any of its formed elements through the intact walls of blood vessels" (S).

Hegemonikon (ἡγεμονικόν): This refers to the authoritative or commanding faculty or capacity of the soul as the center of consciousness and neurological function generally. There was prolonged uncertainty as to whether

---

[104] *Definitiones medicae*, XIX.384–85K.

it was located in the brain or the heart—although Galen had no doubt it was in the former, *contra* Aristotle, among others.

Homoiomere/homoiomerous (ὁμοιομέρεια/ὁμοιο-μερής): Essentially the term means "having parts like each other"—that is, of consistently uniform structure. It is a term of Aristotelian origin (*Parts of Animals*, II, 648a6–655b27). Galen's definition in *MM* is that "a part is *homoiomerous*, as the name itself also clearly shows, which is divisible into similar parts throughout, like the vitreous and the crystalloid and the specific substance of the eye" (X.48K). In his *On the Differentiae of Diseases*, he lists arteries, veins, nerves, bone, cartilage, ligaments, membranes, and flesh as *homoiomerous* structures and makes it clear that these are components of organic bodies and are themselves formed from the primary elements (VI.841K).

Ichor* (ἰχώρ): Used in the sense of "serum" or "serous or sero-purulent discharge." It closely corresponds to the modern definition as "a thin watery discharge from an ulcer or unhealthy wound" (S). The same term has therefore been retained without italicization in our translation.

Kachexia* (καχεξία): This is taken as a general term indicating a "bad state of the body" (see Hippocrates, *Aphorisms* III.21). In this sense it differs from the more specific modern usage to describe "a general weight loss and wasting occurring in the course of a chronic disease or emotional disturbance" (S).

Kakochymia/euchymia (κακοχυμία/εὐχυμία): This is taken to be a pair of terms used nonspecifically to indicate respectively any unhealthy or healthy state of the four humors.

Kakoethical (κακοήθης): This term is retained in the

sense of "chronic," "intractable," or "incurable." LSJ's gloss for medical purposes is "malignant" and is used, for example, by both Jones and Lloyd in Hippocrates, *Aphorisms* VI.4. We have avoided this rendering, given the modern connotation of the epithet when applied to an ulcer.

Krasis/eukrasia/dyskrasia* (κρᾶσις/εὐκρασία/ δυσκρασία): The basic meaning of *krasis* is "blending" or "mixing." In Galen's physiology and pathophysiology this has a specific application to the four elemental qualities. *Eukrasia* exists when the krasis or mixing of these qualities lies within the normal range; *dyskrasia* refers to an abnormality of the mixing and is a major cause of disease.

Paremptosis (παρέμπτωσις): The basic meaning of "influx" or "entrance" is applied, in the pathophysiological theory of Erasistratus, to the spillover of excess blood in the veins into the arteries through minute "anastomoses." This interferes with the passage of *pneuma* and has an important role in the causation of disease, particularly inflammation.

Pikrocholic/melancholic* (πικρόχολος/μελαγχολικός): *Picrocholic* means full of yellow bile or "bilious"— i.e., adversely affected by yellow bile, the presumed consequences of which are nausea and irritability. *Melancholic* means full of black bile or "melancholic"—i.e., adversely affected by black bile, the consequences of which are depression of the spirits and sadness.

Plethora* (πληθώρα): Basically an excess of blood in the veins. Galen devotes a monograph to the topic (*De plenitudine*, VII.513–583K). For Erasistratus this term (and therefore the process it refers to) has a particular significance as the forerunner to *paremptosis* (*vide supra*).

Pneuma (πνεῦμα): In ancient physiology (e.g., Hippocrates) this term had a number of meanings. Particularly with Erasistratus it was used to describe an air- or spirit-like material, derived from the inspired air, which traveled in the arteries either alone (Erasistratus) or with blood (Galen) and was distributed throughout the body. In Galen's system there were three forms of *pneuma*, one associated with each of the three "systems" described in section 4 above (see also *MM* XII.839–40K). *Pneuma* became particularly important in the physiological and pathophysiological theories of the Pneumatist school. For a succinct summary of the concept, see the introduction to May's (1968) translation of Galen's *On the Use of the Parts*, vol. 1, pp. 46–49.

Proegoumenic/prokatarktic (προηγούμενος/προκαταρκτικός): The following two brief definitions are taken from the commentary on the four books on the classification and causation of diseases and symptoms prepared by J. du Bois and published in Paris in 1539.[105] (a) προηγούμενος—that is, preceding or internal—is an affection or movement outside nature occurring in the animal itself. (b) προκαταρκτικός—that is, evident and external, which, approaching externally, forcefully alters and changes bodies.

Translated Terms

Community (κοινότης): The literal meaning is "shar-

---

[105] J. du Bois, *Methodus sex librorum Galeni in differentiis et causis morborum et symptomatum in tabellas sex* (Paris, 1539), p. 4.

ing in common" or "community." In Methodic theory the term is specifically applied to the three "communities" or "generalities" of diseases: (a) constriction of the pores with obstruction; (b) dilatation of the pores with flux; (c) a combination of constriction and obstruction.

Constriction/dilatation ($\sigma\tau\acute{\epsilon}\gamma\nu\omega\sigma\iota\varsigma/\epsilon\mathring{\upsilon}\rho\acute{\upsilon}\tau\eta\varsigma$): Particularly applied to the postulated states of the "theoretical" pores of Methodic theory but also used in their general sense.

Contingent/accidental ($\kappa\alpha\tau\grave{\alpha}$ $\sigma\upsilon\mu\beta\epsilon\beta\eta\kappa\acute{o}\varsigma$): A term used with $\kappa\alpha\tau'$ $\acute{\epsilon}\alpha\upsilon\tau\acute{o}$. We have translated this as "contingent" or "accidental" in the senses 2–4 listed under "accidental" in the *OED*—this despite Urmson's objection.[106]

Differentia ($\delta\iota\alpha\phi\rho\acute{\alpha}$): Frequently used in the *MM*, and particularly in the four treatises on diseases and symptoms with the specific meaning the term carries in logic and taxonomy. When used thus it is rendered "differentia." In other contexts the standard (i.e., nontechnical) meaning of "difference" is used.

Dissolution of continuity ($\lambda\acute{\upsilon}\sigma\iota\varsigma$ $\sigma\upsilon\nu\epsilon\chi\epsilon\acute{\iota}\alpha\varsigma$): A fundamental term in Galen's classification of diseases describing one of the three classes. Throughout Galen's works there is some variation in the components of the term— e.g., $\delta\iota\alpha\acute{\iota}\rho\epsilon\sigma\iota\varsigma$ or $\delta\iota\alpha\phi\theta\rho\acute{\alpha}$ instead of $\lambda\acute{\upsilon}\sigma\iota\varsigma$, and $\acute{\epsilon}\nu\omega\sigma\iota\varsigma$ instead of $\sigma\upsilon\nu\acute{\epsilon}\chi\epsilon\iota\alpha$.

Element ($\sigma\tau\omega\chi\epsilon\hat{\iota}o\nu$): Galen uses this term both in the specific sense of a primary structural component of matter (the sense broadly that has endured in modern science) and in the more general sense of a fundamental com-

---

[106] See Urmson, *Greek Philosophical Vocabulary*, pp. 85–86.

ponent of any system (compare *On the Differentiae of Diseases*, VI.840K and VI.836K, for the respective uses). Galen was in no doubt what the primary elements (or elemental qualities) of matter were, and also how important it was for the doctor to know this. The pseudo-Galenic *Definitiones medicae* offers the following definition, which summarizes Galen's position: "An element is that from which, as primary and most simple, all things arise and to which, as most simple and least, all things are resolved. So Athenaeus the Athenian says in his third book. The elements of medicine are, as certain of the ancients understood, hot, cold, moist and dry, from which, appearing primary, simplest and least, man is put together, and to which, as appearing last, simplest and least, man is resolved into" (XIX.356K).

Humor (χυμός): The following definition, from the *Definitiones medicae* (XIX.457–8K), is applicable to Galen's most common use of the term: "Humor in Hippocrates is invariably applied to the humors in the body which make up our structure—that is, blood, phlegm and the two biles, yellow and black. In Plato and Aristotle the gustatory quality which each of these has in us is also termed humor. These are the qualities of sharpness, dryness, harshness, acridness, saltiness, sweetness and bitterness."

Indication/indicator (ἔνδειξις, σκοπός): *Endeixis* is an important term in Galen's method and has been a particular point of discussion in recent times. Galen himself describes it in the *MM* as "a reflection of the consequence" and gives detailed consideration to the term in the opening section of Book 3. In essence, his use of "indication" appears to be close to the present usage as defined in

Stedman (S): "The basis for initiation of a treatment for a disease . . . may be furnished by a knowledge of the cause (causal indication), by the symptoms present (symptomatic indication), or by the nature of the disease (specific indication)." It is the last that Galen is particularly concerned with. The term "indicator," which is sometimes used to translate σκοπός rather than the more usual "aim" or "objective," is taken to apply to what furnishes the basis for the indication and/or is the target of the indicated treatment.

Innate heat (ἔμφυτον θερμόν): This is a feature of all animal bodies while they are living. In sanguineous animals its source is in the heart, from which it is distributed to the other parts of the body. Galen's views on innate heat were derived from Hippocrates and Aristotle. For those men, it was formed at the time of the organism's initial development but was maintained and cooled as required by respiration. Others (notably Erasistratus and Asclepiades) considered that body heat was not innate but acquired from outside sources.

Pore (πόρος): In Galen's usage this term generally applies to channels that are macroscopic and visible, such as the bile ducts or urethra, as distinct from the "theoretical" pores postulated by Asclepiades. To quote Vallance: "Galen uses the word in a variety of ways, some of which look remarkably close to those he attributes to Asclepiades. But most often Galen's pores are visible passages: the urethra (or ureter), for instance, the 'bile-ducts', the windpipe, the 'spermatic ducts', the ethmoid passages, the 'optic passage' and the 'acoustic passage'. Galen is always keen to set himself up as someone who does not believe what he cannot see by experiment and observation, and he frequently qualifies πόρος with αἰσθητός."[107]

Putrefaction (σῆψις): The process of decay or fermentation. In the *MM* the term is generally found in one of two contexts: in reference to abnormal change in a humor and in reference to presumed inflammatory change in a wound or ulcer. "Putrefaction" is used in both contexts, although "sepsis" would serve in the second case and even "digestion" perhaps in the first.

Superfluity (περίττωμα): What is over and above, particularly after the digestion of food. We have almost invariably rendered περίττωμα as "superfluity"; other possibilities include "residue," "surplus," and even "excretion" or "excrement."

7. LANGUAGE AND STYLE

Fachprosa (Technical Prose) as an Expression of Literate Greek within Atticism

The term "Atticism" refers to the concerted and influential attempt by men of high education, beginning in the first century BC but predominantly from late in the first century AD onward, to prescribe what was acceptable Greek (and Latin) style. By this they meant that Attic grammatical norms (syntax, orthography, morphology, phonology, lexicon) in use in the fourth and fifth centuries BC were to be the yardstick of true cultural attainment in Greek in the Roman imperial period. Despite the dismissive comment

---

[107] Vallance, *Lost Theory of Asclepiades of Bithynia*, pp. 50–51.

by Galen's contemporary the *rhetor* and Atticizing ideologue Phrynichus of Byzantium, not all doctors were uneducated (ἀμαθής) when it came to writing. Galen is one of
several men of the imperial period who fell into that group
of highly educated, Atticizing writers of technical treatises
in Greek whose work could be described stylistically as
prose that belongs to a layer in between popular speech
and highly literary Greek.[108] It is not that he was not capable of producing the latter—indeed, in one of the styles he
employs in *MM* he does just that. Rather, his chosen task,
medical treatises produced for doctors (not for laymen),
determined the style to be adopted: *Fachprosa*. This involved a certain linguistic pragmatism.[109] As with so much
else, Galen was in no doubt about his capabilities in Greek;
but he saw that his goal was to provide clear instruction for
the next generation of doctors, not to be an ideologue for
Atticism.

In seeking to determine the consistency of Galen's
achievement as a "pragmatic Atticizer," we must recognize
the problem of accepting Kühn's text as authoritative in
matters of orthography, morphology, and even syntax. It
may also have to be allowed that some of the MSS for the
text of Galen have "tidied up" what later copyists perceived to be Atticizing or non-Atticizing inconsistencies.
Even allowing for this, however, it emerges that Galen is

---

108 For "Zwischenschichtsprosa," see L. Rydbeck, *Fachprosa,
vermeintliche Volkssprache und Neues Testament,* Studia Graeca
Upsaliensia 5 (Uppsala, 1967), pp. 188–92.

109 See W. Herbst, "Galeni Pergamani de Atticissantium
studiis testimonia collecta atone examinaten." Dissertation, Leipzig, 1911.

not a "hard-line" Atticistic ideologue in his writing. Yet some features of his language use may not be able to be settled definitively; one of these may be his concern for aspect.

Several factors may account for variation and inconsistency, including haste in dictation reflecting an inadvertent slipping into more current, colloquial (i.e., "normal"-register) language. It is also possible that the amanuensis copying at Galen's dictation is responsible for some of the orthographic inconsistencies. Galen will have pronounced his Greek as a man of his period, for significant vowel shifts in Greek had occurred some centuries earlier. The amanuensis may not have made consistent allowance for this in transcribing at Galen's dictation, and these features then failed to be picked up at a checking of the text once copied out.

Stylistic Variatio *as a Mark of* Galen's Erudite Control of Greek

It is not merely in his use of technical terminology and syntax that Galen provides variety for his reader; at a broader level, he alters his style quite distinctively. The highly technical vocabulary is largely confined to the dominant stylistic mode: no-nonsense instruction in medical treatment. Some of this specialist terminology is of course retained in his second style, the numerous case histories he includes to illustrate the treatment he has given to patients. These passages are frequently invested with human interest, but always serve a greater purpose: to illustrate how successful Galen was in his treatment of patients, and often in explicit contrast to other doctors. Extended polemical sec-

tions (largely in Books 1 and 2) have their own highly
wrought stylistic features, but not the technical language
which would largely be the preserve of doctors. The polemical portions of the work constitute Galen's third style
in *MM* and are replete with rhetorical characteristics such
as would be found in any writer of the Second Sophistic
who wished to display his cleverness to the coterie of intellectual peers and those who aspired to that: orators like
Dio Chrysostom (fl. AD II), biographers like Philostratus
(fl. AD III), essayists like Lucian (fl. AD II), and some of the
Church fathers like Basil and his brother Gregory (fl. AD
IV). Galen is highly literate, highly erudite, but what he is
composing does not require him to be highly literary. The
polemical sections merely display that he can achieve this
where appropriate.

The dominant mode of medical instruction is what
qualifies Galen to be thought of as a writer of *Fachprosa*.
The other two styles he employs provide a change of pace
and variety. His indubitable interest in style and in the use
of rhetorical features in the period is put into service to his
goal: achieving his didactic purpose in a forthright and
clear manner. However, it would be quite wrong to imagine that those other styles were irrelevant to his overarch-
ing didactic aim. These other styles, and particularly the
case histories, are a means to an end: they engage the
reader in a different manner and maintain interest in the
topic being presented. The intent of the polemic is to confirm for the reader (if there were any serious doubt!) that
Galen is in a direct line of descent from Hippocrates as *the*
medical authority par excellence: he has no peer in his own
time or in the recent past. This authoritativeness is reinforced throughout the *MM* (but perhaps more frequently

in Books 7–14, which resume and complete the treatise after a twenty-year hiatus) by his multitude of cross-references to his other works. The intent of the polemic is to sweep away the approaches taken by his rivals from different philosophical schools within medicine; above all this means the Methodics. Once the ground is largely cleared in the first two books, he can then proceed to his course of instruction, dealing in succession with ulcers/wounds, fractures, fevers, etc. The case histories illustrate the application of his instruction to real-life situations—though, unsurprisingly for a man of Galen's powerful ego, apart from a single exception at 7.8 (504.4–506.9K), we only hear about his successful treatments.

Variatio is a crucial feature of the *MM*: to maintain the reader's engagement throughout such a long treatise, Galen includes variety at a macro as well as a micro level. Macro is the stylistic changes already mentioned. Micro-level *variatio* includes such features as word choice (at least eight different words are used to refer to "book" or "treatise," for example), word order, ringing the changes on syntactic constructions, literary quotations and allusions, the occasional inclusion of asides, and short digressions.

Instruction in medical procedure is the style which dominates *MM* after the polemical and more explicitly philosophical first two books. Galen gives some relief from it by inserting case histories and occasional (but rarer in the later books) passing polemic. After Book 2 the default style is the instructional one. In view of the advice being provided about treatment of medical conditions, two features may be highlighted.

1. Deliberate impersonalization: Galen refers to himself in the first-person singular comparatively rarely, and more frequently uses plural for singular, except to say "I undertook this particular treatment." When he is cross-referring, or referring to what doctors should do, he frequently uses the perfect or aorist passive third person: "this has been discussed" = "I have discussed this." Impersonal verbs are visible everywhere. χρή is much more common than δεῖ or ἀναγκαῖον (ἐστίν), which both nevertheless still occur in instructional contexts.
2. Direct instruction: This is often couched less directly. Imperatives occur, but third-person imperatives, imperatival infinitives, hortatory subjunctives, and potential optatives are all quite common as different stylistic ways in which Galen imparts his advice about medical and related procedures.

Case histories in the work bring life to the theory and give substance to the instructional sections. It would be an exaggeration to say that Galen does this for light relief from the theory. However, it is undeniable that there is an element of self-promotion about it. The spread of the case histories across the books is uneven: none in Books 1–4 (none would be expected in Books 1 and 2, given their subject matter), only one in each of Books 11 and 13, but several in each of Books 5–10, 12, and 14. This suggests that at a certain point Galen began to include them; i.e., they were an afterthought, not part of the original conception of the work. But they tail off somewhat as he comes toward the concluding books of the treatise: most of those in books 12 and 14 are relatively brief. Perhaps this may be understandable when we recall that Galen was now an old man, intent on completing a major treatise covering many diverse topics, a treatise which had been subject to a hiatus of many years. The total number of case histories is fifty-two. The length varies considerably, from a line or two to several pages in Kühn. The brevity or allusiveness of some may mean that they should scarcely qualify as case histories, but simply as instances which he has witnessed or attended to and chooses to mention in passing. Sometimes more than one is provided to illustrate the particular medical treatment he is discussing; but by no means every topic is allocated one. Only occasionally does one follow straight on from another. A few case histories are included to show how Galen's medical opponents failed to treat patients properly, leading to their death: e.g., 6.2 (390.4–12K), 13.15 (909.10–916.3K). The case histories are, incidentally, one of the main sources for the extrapolation of social history in the *MM*. Not that this was the intent; their pedagogical contribution to the treatise was the rationale for their inclusion.

Philosophical polemic is a third style encountered in the *MM* and is mainly directed at Thessalus, but also includes Olympicus and other Methodics in general. Galen does criticize the Empirics and the Dogmatics as well, though not as harshly as the Methodics. His criticism of Thessalus and the Methodic School is especially trenchant in Book 1, and its vapor trail is to be found throughout the *MM*.

The continuing appeal of Methodic medicine to doctors, from its rise probably in the first century BC and over the next two centuries into Galen's time, clearly irked Galen very considerably, and it may be more than their

wrongheadedness which offended him. He claims to be
defending the great ones of the past (Hippocrates above
all) who are derided by the Methodics, but it may just as
much be the very continuing popularity of the Methodic
hairesis in medical circles—there were still known Methodic doctors in the sixth century AD—that got under his
skin. To call a group after its founder often amounted to
casting aspersions on it, and Galen's invention (apparently)
of the epithet *Thessaleios*[110] as a way of referring to the
Methodics is a typical instance. Θεσσάλειος occurs thirty-
three times in *MM*, but not evenly spread across the fourteen books. Galen employs the adjective in five other
places outside *MM*; apart from this, it occurs nowhere else
in Greek literature. The device of the posthumous attack
on his philosophical and medical opponents is an indication of how strong their influence remained in Galen's
time—so alive to Galen were those long dead! The Methodics were more disparate than Galen's broad-brush polemic suggests, and his attack on Thessalus is a device to
demonize all his contemporaries who identified with that
school.

Features of particular note in polemical sections include the use of the sarcastic superlative to mock Galen's
opponents. Particularly visible is ἀμεθοδώτατος (most
amethodical), e.g., 1.3 (27.5K), 5.10 (346.11–16K), 6.4
(421.5K). Galen uses this pun on numerous occasions—
overmuch, indeed, almost to the point of cliché—against
the Methodics in general and Thessalus in particular.
Other superlatives employed sarcastically of Thessalus in-

---

110 Not to be confused with *Thessalios*, the adjective connected with Thessaly.

clude ἀναισχυντότατος (most shameless), γενναιότατος (most noble), θαυμασιώτατος (most wondrous), σοφώτατος (most sapient). Ridicule of Thessalus' books is another distinctive motif, e.g., 1.2 (18.11K).

Thessalus ὁ δεύτερος Ἀσκληπιός (the second Asclepius) at Book 3.7 (208.13K) is an especially telling piece of mock adulation. The claim to have written his treatise at Asclepius' dictation in Egyptian Thebes, coupled with the point that Asclepius had a son called Thessalus, goes only some way toward making the point. The complex development of Book 1.2 is the main reason for proposing that, while most of the work was produced by dictation, some of it may have been written out by Galen himself. The close interlocking of the various kinds of rhetorical features, the conceits, word choice, etc., point to this as a very carefully conceived showpiece, perhaps an actually written-out section once delivered as a display piece at a public lecture. This is Galen showing off his literary credentials as he begins.

Why does Galen bother to attack someone long dead whose work he regards as so flawed? He may be seeking to undermine what he regards as Thessalus' continuing pernicious influence among contemporary doctors in the second half of the second century, for the Methodic school was undoubtedly still very active, as Soranus' profile demonstrates. Alternatively, Galen uses the attack on another doctor as a device by which he can draw attention to his own achievement. This becomes clear during the course of Book 1.2, when we see how many of his own works Galen refers to: ten of them. This has a twofold effect for the reader/listener. First, Galen lauds and refers to the medical and philosophical great men of the past and implicitly places himself in their company by referring to his own treatises. Second, this feature is an apologetic device at the very outset of the work to emphasize to his readers that he is the absolutely right—indeed, the only possible—person equipped by his practical experience and theoretical knowledge to write such an all-encompassing work on medicine.

Book Divisions, Quotations, Cross-References

MM is no haphazard jumble put together on the run, even though there are portions which suggest a lack of coherence, e.g. Book 14. It is clear that Galen invested considerable thought in the arrangement of his material. The very fact that Galen returned to the treatise late in the second century after a two-decade hiatus indicates that he had conceived the entire work as a coherent treatment of the subject, as a unity. Furthermore, the book divisions are his. The addresses to his two successive patrons are an indication of this. He addresses Hiero in Books 1, 2, and 3; then, in Book 7, we find his first address to Eugenianus by name as dedicatee of the second half of the work. Galen addresses him by name again in Books 8 and 10, all mentions occurring in the initial chapter of a book and, with one exception, in the opening couple of sentences of that book. Despite the long break in the execution of the work as a whole, it does not appear that he revised the first six books when he resumed the task of completing the treatise: some intentions foreshadowed there were not fulfilled in the last eight books.[111]

---

[111] Nutton, in Kudlien and Durling, *Galen's Method of Healing*, pp. 4, 7–8.

A further indication of the separation into discrete books by Galen himself is provided at 6.5 (425.15K). Galen refers here to his third and fourth books of the present treatise, which have already been criticized by others for longwindedness (μακρολογία). Although it cannot be ruled out that this comment was added by Galen when writing a later book and acknowledging a reaction to his prolixity in earlier ones, it is more likely that it shows the books were initially distributed piecemeal, not the whole treatise (or not even Books 1–6) at one time. Why Books 3 and 4? These are the "beginnings of treatment" by Galen following the introductory two books, whose focus was mainly polemic and philosophy.

The numerous cross-references to his other treatises are not primarily for show, except in Book 1, when they are used as part of establishing his authority to expose Thessalus and the Methodics. Galen clearly expects the reader to have read his theoretical works before the *MM*, which is the culmination (but not a summary) of his earlier treatises.

Quotations and allusions are of several kinds. He cross-refers to other parts of the present treatise, e.g., 5.7 (335.13–16K), an instance of foreshadowing a matter to be dealt with later. He also refers to other works by himself, e.g., 1.2 (14.11–15.11K). In this section he refers to ten of his other treatises, giving titles. Third, Galen refers to numerous works by others. Some are general, passing mentions; others are quotations, sometimes brief but occasionally quite extended, especially in the case of Hippocrates. Positive quotations include particularly the numerous references to Hippocrates but also to Plato and Aristotle.

Negative quotations and references mainly concern Methodic works, especially those of Thessalus.

Figurative Language

Similes occur in some quantity, but several are rather stereotyped. Examples include 1.4 (35.3K, "but like the Euripus they ebb and flow [in their arguments]"); 1.9 (71.6K, "It would be terrible that it were permissible for them to speak incorrectly like tyrants while we are not allowed to use [correct] Greek"). The ὡς τύραννος (like a tyrant) simile occurs several times of doctors. Extended figures may begin with a simile; for example, 5.15 provides a lengthy simile of walking along a road on two legs or limping on one: likewise, in 9.6, a person who wishes to achieve the goal of the medical craft must use both "legs": method in the theories in general and practice in them individually.

Metaphors are not very frequent, though a few are memorable. Several are quite extended. Examples include 1.1 (6.4, 6K, three Italian doctors and their pupils make an admirable *khoros*), 1.2 (10.15–11.9K, extended agonistic figure in the polemic against Thessalus), 2.3 (88.3K, the language of fighting is employed a good deal here, and elsewhere), 7.2 (459.1–5K, Hippocrates' works need good farmers who will sow, achieve increase, and bring his work to completion). Most previous doctors destroyed his seed. Galen sees himself as a farmer cultivating what Hippocrates had sown.

Rhetorical features of all kinds abound. Very frequent are alliteration, anaphora, crasis as well as elision, ellipse, litotes, parataxis. Reasonably common are hendiadys, hy-

perbole (especially in polemical sections). Not common
are chiasmus, hiatus, hyperbaton. Rare are euphemism,
homoioteleuton, kyklos, rhetorical questions (but especially in polemical sections). Galen quite frequently uses
"triples" (three infinitives, three nouns, etc.) as a stylistic
feature to clarify or reinforce his point; perhaps this is a
kind of hyperbolic hendiadys, though to give three examples of anything is a long-standing rhetorical device.

It has been claimed that Galen's rhetorical skills "do not
enhance his stature as a doctor or as a man."[112] Yet it is un-
thinkable that any person from Greco-Roman antiquity
who was well educated and highly trained in any branch
of learned study would not employ unquestioningly all
the armory that was available to him. This is exactly what
Galen does whenever he deems it appropriate. While the
display pieces are rhetorically memorable, we should not
get them out of proportion in *MM*, for their function is to
serve a much larger and more serious goal: by exposing in
such damning fashion the weaknesses of other schools
(above all the Methodics), he can then maintain his readers' focus firmly on the explication of his own method of
medical treatment.

8. TEXT AND TRANSLATION

In preparing a translation of a work such as Galen's *MM*, it
is worthwhile to consider the nature of the likely reader-
ship. In our view, now and for the foreseeable future, the
main group of readers will be those with a serious focus on
the history of ancient Western science and medicine. Doc-

[112] Ibid., p. 14.

tors with a more general interest in early medicine may also find this a work of interest, although the number of doctors well trained in classical languages must now be very small compared with even the quite recent past. For classicists without a long suit in ancient philosophy, Galen is likely to be of relatively little interest. His oeuvre is not high literature, nor does it offer the linguistic stimulus of documentary texts. Of course, he comes into his own as an exponent of *Fachprosa*, as outlined in the previous section.

On the matter of the text, the present work does not have the ambition to be a true edition of *MM*. Our base text is Kühn, but this has been altered in a number of ways.

First, we have tacitly updated the text from the early nineteenth-century German orthographic conventions in use in Kühn's day. The vast majority of these will not even be noticed by the reader but include certain aspects of accentuation, the iota subscript, and the breathing mark (especially over double medial *rho* (-ῥῥ-). In this class, too, is our tacit correction of obvious typographical errors in Kühn[113] and similar errors transmitted through the TLG #5 electronic copy of Kühn. There is not a multitude of these, and they have not been introduced without due consideration of whether the different spelling may reflect a different MS reading. So, for example, we have rarely attempted to "tidy up" the text for consistency, since there is considerable variety in the use of Atticistic features.

---

[113] E.g., 2.5 (104.16K) εὐλόγως, 3.4 (196.3K) ἐπιπάττειν, 3.9 (217.12K) τὸ νῦν ἡκωμένον, 4.2 (240.2K) ὑπερκειμένων, 4.7 (304.4K) ἀπεπτήσαντες, 4.7 (304.13–14K) τὸν . . . λόγον. All references in the present volume are to Kühn vol. 10, comprising the *MM*, unless a particular volume is specified.

Changes applied to our text in this category total somewhere between 2,500 and 3,000, and can vary considerably between different books (280-plus for Book 5, about 150 for Book 6).

In a separate category are changes we have applied in capitalization and punctuation. Thus, we mark the start of direct speech, the first letter of a book title, or a technical term (e.g., Ἐμπειρικός) with a capital letter. Alterations to punctuation are more conservative of Kühn's practice, but where sense appears to be held back by his punctuation, then we have intervened. The reader will see, too, that we have inserted paragraph breaks into the Greek text; these align as closely as possible with where we judge new paragraphs are appropriate in the English translation. In this regard, readers should take it as a sign of our general reluctance to alter too much of the Kühn punctuation when they encounter something other than a period (usually a semicolon) at the end of one of our paragraphs in the Greek.

Our third category of changes is much smaller: textual emendations. At the suggestion of Vivian Nutton, we have looked at the readings of the British Library MS (twelfth century) of *MM*. This is a MS full of interest for a variety of reasons, but we have limited ourselves to noting readings which in our view are clearly superior to those in the MSS on which Kühn's printed text is based. This MS, which we have abbreviated as B in the textual notes, exhibits many other differences, e.g., in word order and in orthography; but we have very rarely noted these unless they are of consequence for another reason. So the reader should understand that we are not attempting to provide here a full collation of B against K(ühn). This is a MS which will undoubtedly repay fuller study in another context. We have also given consideration to the alterations to the text of Books 1 and 2 proposed by R. J. Hankinson in his 1991 translation and philosophical commentary. He made use of two Paris MSS, and a number of his emendations to Kühn's text based on those MSS (or his own conjectures) have been attractive to us and accepted. In some of these cases, these two MSS (P1 and P2) align with B against K. The reader who has access to Kühn may notice that there are a fair number of places where the Latin text (abbreviated KLat in this volume) is not a translation of K but is clearly drawing on other MSS reflecting different readings.

The sheer number of these changes taken together means that it is inevitable that we have overlooked some features which should have been altered. In the first category the alterations are nearly all of a mechanical kind; the second involves a blend of the mechanical with some judgment; the third requires judgment virtually alone. The decisions we have made about how to present the text reflect our view of who our primary reader is, as outlined above. Our aim, then, is an improved and serviceable text, but a finally authoritative Greek text has not been our goal here.

On the matter of the translation, we have made use of the previous translations listed on pp. lxxvii–lxxviii, apart from nos. 4 and 6. Linacre's complete Latin translation went through fifteen versions/printings between the time of its first appearance in 1519 and its last printing in 1609. Brock, in the introduction to his 1916 translation of Galen's *On the Natural Faculties*, has described Linacre's translation of that work as "marked by minute accuracy and elegant Latinity." There is no need to alter this description when referring to Linacre's translation of the *MM*.[114] We have made use of the 1542 printing and the 1562 version of the *MM* in the *Galeni Omnium Operum Sexta Classis* published in Venice. The former has useful original marginal notes which include comments on the text. Thomas Gale's early English version has been of help, particularly with the surgical descriptions in Book 6. Peter English's seventeenth-century English translation has been frequently consulted. His opening note to the "gentle reader" is of some interest in relation to the recognition of the continuing importance of the work to the middle of the seventeenth century:

> I have but a few words to say to thee now. Only I desire thee to entertain this book as thy darling, as being matchlesse in its kind. It is not only absolutely necessary for directing thee in any practice of Physick, but also without the knowledge of it, it is impossible to administer any Cure safely, unlesse it be at randome, like a blind man throwing his staffe at a Dog.

Given this work's focus on the practical aspects of Galen's *MM* (Peter English omits much of the polemical material), we have found it helpful for clarification of procedures and methods and for the English translation of practices and medications. Hankinson's recent translation of Books 1 and 2 has, with its detailed commentary, helped to clarify

---

[114] As mentioned earlier, it is basically Linacre's translation which appears along with the Greek text for the *MM* in the two collections of Galen's works due respectively to René Chartier (1679) and Carl-Gottlob Kühn (1821–1833).

some of the more general philosophical issues addressed in these opening books. Boulogne's 2009 French translation appeared only after completion of our own translation, but we have been able to look through it, particularly to examine points of difficulty.

On the translation itself, the general objective is that characteristically claimed by translators: to provide a smoothly readable version in the language of the translation while remaining faithful to the language of the original—an objective much easier to state than to achieve! Moreover, in our even approaching such an aim, Galen's Greek presents certain specific and substantial problems quite apart from the problems of the text itself. In our view there are two particularly intrusive problems. The first is how to deal with Galen's complex sentence construction— what Hankinson has called his "syntactically and paratactically involved style." The second problem is how to deal with what are, in effect, technical terms of critical importance in Galen's own system of medicine, especially when these reflect structural and functional concepts now outmoded. To make matters worse, some of these terms remain in use today, albeit with a somewhat different meaning in some cases. A subsidiary and related problem is how to deal with the names of diseases, symptoms, medications, and other treatment methods—that is, whether to retain the original Greek term transliterated, use the Latin version, or attempt to find the correct English equivalent.

In brief, in our attempt to render Galen's elaborate Greek *Fachprosa* into modern English that may be read with relative ease (bear in mind that this is a medical textbook), we have adopted several specific strategies. First, we have been prepared to split up Galen's long and involved sentences and to change the order of the clauses where this seemed to improve clarity without unduly sacrificing fidelity to the original. Second, we have not attempted to translate every Greek particle, particularly as they can often be functionally replaced by punctuation in creating a modern English version. Third, we have given ourselves some license in dealing with the voices, moods, and tenses of the Greek verbs where not to do so would result in an English sentence that reads awkwardly. Nevertheless, despite these three "liberties," we have attempted to provide an English translation that can be matched with the Greek without undue difficulty.

Finally, a word on the title. There have to date been several English renderings, beginning with Peter English's *Method of Physick*. We have opted for *Method of Medicine* over the two other recent renderings, *Method of Healing* and *On the Therapeutic Method*, because in the former the term "healing" strikes rather an odd note and in the latter the work is much wider in scope than a text on therapeutics, covering, as it does, the whole range of medical practice. It is, in effect, the equivalent of a combination of a modern textbook on medicine with one on surgery. In his recent translation, referred to above, Boulogne has titled the work *Méthode de traitment,* which is, perhaps, the most literal translation and would have been our first alternative after *Method of Medicine*.

9. DISEASES AND SYMPTOMS

Abscess (ἀπόστημα): This includes the modern pyogenic abscess but is not confined to this. Galen classifies it as a disease of "excess." See also *MM*, 984K ff., where treatment by incision is mentioned.

Alopecia (ἀλωπεκία): Described as being like mange in foxes (LSJ). It is similar in description to the modern disease of the same name. In the *MM* (Book 14, Chapter 18) it is linked with other varieties of hair loss (baldness, ophiasis). Galen distinguishes between these on causal grounds (1014K ff.).

Alphos (ἀλφός): Listed in LSJ as "dull-white leprosy, esp. on the face." It is not leprosy in the modern sense but a form of skin depigmentation, possibly psoriatic. Galen classifies it as a *dyskrasia* of *homoiomerous* bodies due to inflow of a substance. See also Ce, 5.28.19.

Anesthesia, dysesthesia (ἀναισθησία, δυσαισθησία): Loss of sensation and disordered sensation—probably quite close to modern usage. Galen lists the former as a symptom due to a cold *dyskrasia*.

Aneurysm (ἀνεύρυσμα): In the *MM* Galen describes the false aneurysm that may form after an arterial wound.

Anthrax (ἄνθραξ): Listed in LSJ as "carbuncle or malignant pustule"; the possibility of smallpox is raised. Other sources (e.g., *EANS*) describe it as an infected wound. Whether there is any connection with anthrax in the present sense is unknown.

Apepsia, bradypepsia, dyspepsia (ἀπεψία, βραδυπεψία, δυσπεψία): Absence or failure of digestion, slowed digestion and disordered or impaired digestion.

Apnea, dyspnea, orthopnea (ἄπνοια, δύσπνοια, ὀρθόπνοια): Failure of respiration, disordered or difficult respiration, and difficulty breathing when lying flat—all as in modern usage.

Apoplexy (ἀποπληξία): Sudden collapse with paralysis; presumably close to modern usage as a descriptive term. Ascribed to a cold *dyskrasia* by Galen. See M, p. 510 for Aretaeus' description and her comment on this.

Arthritis (ἀρθρῖτις): A nonspecific term for diseases of the joints, possibly inflammatory and possibly including gout.

Ascarides (ἀσκαρίδες): A form of intestinal worm infestation—see G, *MM* 1004, 1014, and 1021K.

Ascites (ἀσκίτες): A form of dropsy as a collection of abnormal fluid. For a definition see XIX.424K.

Atheroma (ἀθέρωμα): A tumor full of gruel-like matter—see G, *MM*, 985K and XIX.440K for a definition.

Atonia (ἀτονία): Weakness or debility of a generalized or focal type—see G, VI.853–54K.

Atrophy (ἀτροφία): A nonspecific loss of substance; similar to modern usage—see G, VI.89K.

Avulsion (ἀπόσπασμα): This is taken as being similar to modern usage—a tearing away with separation, as with a tendon from a bone.

Boil (δοθιήν): A boil or small abscess.

Bubo (βουβών): Glandular swelling in the groin; the equivalent to modern inflammatory lymphadenopathy or lymphadenitis.

Cancer (καρκίνος): An eroding sore or ulcer. Used by Galen as a term to describe a superficial abnormality attributed to black bile—see G, VI.874–75K.

Cardialgia (καρδιαλγία): Heartburn—described by Galen as "a sensory symptom of the opening of the stomach distressed by mordant humors." (G, VII.135–36K).

Catalepsy (κατάληψις): A term with several meanings, including collapse, rigidity, and mental disturbance. For a definition and varieties, see G, XIX.414K (as κάτοχος).

Cataract (ὑπόχυμα): Taken to be closely equivalent to modern usage—see G, *MM*, 119, 990, 1019K, and VII.89 and 95K.

Catarrh (κάταρρος): A nasal discharge or flux from the head—see G, VII.107K and XIV.742K.

Cephalalgia (κεφαλαλγία): A nonspecific term for headache or pain in the head—see G, VII.58K.

Ceria (κηρία): Tapeworm—listed in the *MM* with helminthes and ascarides (1004K).

Chalazion (χαλάζιον): A small cyst growing on the eyelid. The term is now used for a tarsal cyst—see G, VI.862–63K.

Cholera (χόλερα): A disease marked by simulataneous diarrhea and vomiting. See G, XIV.730K and XIX.421K and also M, p. 340, who includes Celsus' description.

Coloboma (κολόβωμα): Refers to a part lost by mutilation. The term has now come to mean any defect, whether congenital, pathological, or artificial (S).

Coma (κῶμα): A reversible loss of consciousness. Possibly equivalent to κάρος and λήθαργος.

Consumption (φθίσις): Wasting—usually due to pulmonary tuberculosis. See Gr, pp. 177–97.

Convulsion (σπασμός): Listed by Galen along with apoplexy, epilepsy, and tremor as a primary *dyskrasia* of cold (VI.850K). Si writes: "The Greek term *spasmos* meant both a continued contraction by a tetanic stimulus and an alternating violent contraction and relaxation of skeletal muscle. Both types of movement are also symptoms of epilepsy" (p. 245).

Coryza (κόρυζα): Like catarrh, a flux from the head. The two terms are frequently found together.

Cynanche (κυνάγχη): A nonspecific term for an acute infection involving the structures of the throat—i.e., tonsils, uvula, pharynx, larynx, and epiglottis.

Delirium (παρακοπή, παραφροσύνη): Probably similar to the modern sense; i.e., confused, agitated, and excited behavior. Described by Galen at VII.60K.

Dislocation (ἐξάρθρησις): Grouped by Galen with παράρθρησις as a disease involving change of position—see G, VI.870K and VII.36K.

Dropsy (ὕδερος): Edema, presumably of various kinds. Related by Galen to maldistribution of nutritive materials—see G, VII.62K.

Dysentery (δυσεντερία): Probably a nonspecific term to indicate frequent watery stools, possibly containing blood and mucus (similar to present usage). For Galen's classification, see VII.246–47K.

Ecchymosis (ἐκχύμωσις): An extravasation of blood into the skin or superficial tissues, as in current usage—see G, *MM*, 232K.

Edema (οἴδημα): This appears to be a general term for a type of swelling defined by its characteristics on palpation and not limited to local or generalized fluid collections. Galen lists it as a disease of *homoiomerous* bodies due to inflowing material (VI.849K).

Elephas (ἐλέφας): Taken to be the same as ἐλεφαντίασις. This is not elephantiasis in the modern sense. It may refer to true leprosy—see Gr, pp. 168–76.

Empyema (ἐμπύημα): An internal collection of pus, as in present usage.

Encanthis (ἐγκανθίς): A fleshy tumor at the inner angle of the eye. See Galen, *On the Use of the Parts*, Book 10, Chapter 11, and Ce, 7.7.5.

Epilepsy (ἐπιληψία): Similar to present usage. See
G, VIII.193K ff. for Galen's identification of three types of
epilepsy.

Epinoctis (ἐπινυκτίς): A form of pustule that is painful at night—see Ce, 5.28.15.

Eruption (ἐξάνθημα): A general term for skin eruptions, as in present usage.

Erysipelas (ἐρυσίπελας): A disease characterized
by skin discoloration (redness, yellowness). The modern
erysipelas is defined as "a specific, acute, superficial cutaneous cellulitis caused by β-haemolytic streptococci and
characterized by hot, red, oedematous, brawny and
sharply defined eruptions usually accompanied by constitutional symptoms" (S). Galen considers erysipelas in
Book 13 of the *MM* (946K ff.). Gr writes: "The term erysipelas in Greek medical parlance designates various diseases
that 'redden the skin' and also diffuse, purulent inflammations of internal organs, but in its commonest sense it designates a group of skin diseases with hot, painful reddish
swelling, now thought to be streptococcal dermatitis" (p.
129). See also G, VI.849K.

Eschar (ἐσχάρα): A scab on a wound, as in modern
usage.

Fatigue (κόπος): In Galen this is a wide-ranging
concept. In *On the Preservation of Health* he writes:
"There are seven opinions on the concept of fatigue"; he
lists three simple forms and four compound forms—see G,
VI.189K ff.

Fever (πυρετός): As in modern usage but without the
actual measurement of temperature. The various types of
fever are the subject of Books 8–12 of the *MM*.

Fracture (κάταγμα): As in modern usage, and considered in Book 6 of the *MM* as an example of dissolution of continuity.

Gangrene (γάγγραινα): Taken as approximately equivalent to the modern use—"extensive necrosis from any cause" (S). See G, XI.135K (definition), VII.22 and 75K, and VII.720 and 726K.

Gout (ποδάγρα): Presumably the same disease as that to which the term is presently applied. See Gr, pp. 72–73.

Headache: See Cephalalgia.

Heatstroke (ἔγκαυσις): Presumably the same meaning as now. Interpreted by Galen as a hot *dyskrasia*.

Hemiplegia (παρχπληγίχ, παραπληξία): For a definition, see G, XVI.826K and XVIIA.332K; see also *MM* (638K). According to LSJ the term is also used for "madness, derangement."

Herpes (ἕρπης): A skin affliction of uncertain nature. For Galen's definition, see XI.74K and XIX.440K. For the relationship to erysipelas, see *MM*, Book 14 (1004–5K). For herpetic ulceration, see *MM*, 83K.

Hydrops: See Dropsy.

Hypopyon (ὑπόπυος): In general this means tending to suppurate or be mixed with pus—see G, XII.804K and XIV.774K. In the *MM* it is mentioned specifically in relation to the eye (1019K).

Hysteralgia (ὑστεραλγία): Pain of uterine origin—see G, *MM*, 83K.

Ileus (εἰλεός): Used as a general term for dysfunction of the retentive capacity in relation to the gastrointestinal tract—see G, VII.69 and 220K. Listed in LSJ as "intestinal obstruction" but may also include the paralytic ileus of modern usage.

Induration (σκίρρωσις): Ancient usage is probably

not far removed from the current sense—"the process of becoming extremely firm and hard, or having such physical features" (S). See G, XI.718, 720 and 726K and XIII.933 and 950K (in relation to inflammation).

Inflammation: See Phlegmone and Phlogosis. Inflammation is discussed by Galen in detail in Book 13 of the *MM* and is there characterized by firmness, tension, redness, and a throbbing sensation as well as a tendency to go on to suppuration. All are key features of inflammation as understood today. What is different is the concept of mechanism, which Galen identifies as an influx of blood primarily.

Inguinal hernia (ἐντεροπλοκήλη [containing bowel] and ἐπιπλοκήλη [containing omentum]): See G, VI.870K.

Insomnia (ἀγρυπνία): Linked with coma by Galen as a symptom of the sensory component of the soul (VII.58K). Both, he says, are "due to involvement of the 'primary sense' itself which is . . . common to all sensations."

Lepra (λέπρα): Not leprosy but an unidentified skin disease associated with scaling and depigmentation—see Gr, pp. 162–63. Attributed to black bile and linked with *alphos* and *leuke*—see G, XIV.757K ff. and XIX.427K.

Lethargy (λήθαργος): As in present usage but may include drowsiness and forgetfulness. See G, *MM*, 929–31K and M, pp. 502–3.

Leuke (λεύκη): A skin disease named for its color (or lack thereof)—see G, VII.75 and 226–28K and Gr, pp. 165–67.

Leukophlegmatic dropsy (λευκοφλεγμασία): A form of dropsy. See G, XIV.746K. Galen describes it as being caused by a distribution of phlegm through the whole body (G, VII.224K).

Lithiasis (λιθίασις): Listed in LSJ as "the disease of the stone." It is clearly identified by Galen in the *MM* (917K) as being linked with the genitourinary system.

Marasmus (μαρασμός): Wasting or withering—see G, VII.315 and 317K. Also applied to a type of fever—see G, VII.326K.

Melancholia (μελαγχολία): A melancholy state attributed to an excess of black bile. A cold, dry *dyskrasia*—see G, I.522K; as a symptom, see G, VII.203K.

Meliceris (μελικηρίς): A cyst or wen resembling a honeycomb—see G, VI.863K, VII.35K and *MM*, 985K.

Narke (ναρκή): A symptom rather than a disease, which is defined as "a combination of disturbed sensation and disturbed movement involving the whole body or the limbs and due to cooling or compression" (G, VII.108–9K). Classified as a cold *dyskrasia*—see also *MM*, 917K and XIX.424K.

Nephritis (νεφρῖτις): Taken as a nonspecific term for kidney disease.

Noma (νομή): A form of spreading ulcer—*MM* 326K. The term is now confined to a gangrenous stomatitis (cancrum oris) and a similar process involving the labia majora (S).

Odontalgia (ὀδονταλγία): Toothache.

Ophiasis (ὀφίασις): A bald patch on the head of serpentine or winding form; attributed by Galen to nutritional failure and linked to leuke and alopecia—see VII.63K.

Ophthalmia (ὀφθαλμία): An inflammatory disease of

the eye with discharge, possibly severe conjunctivitis—see M, pp. 1006–19 but particularly p. 1016.

Otalgia (ὠταλγία): Earache—see G, XVIIB.261K for a definition and also VII.58K and *MM*, 83K.

Palpitation (παλμός): Classified by Galen as a form of disordered movement—see VII.159K ff.

Paralysis (παράλυσις): Similar to the modern sense but includes sensory as well as motor functions—see Si, pp. 227–28.

Peripneumonia (περιπνευμομία): See Pneumonia.

Phagadaena (φαγέδαινα): A form of eroding ulcer—see G, *MM*, 83K.

Phlegmone (φλεγμονή): The standard term for inflammation and inflammatory swellings. It is the major topic in Book 13 of the *MM*. The term *phlegmon* remained in medical use until recently to denote a localized inflammation.

Phlogosis (φλόγωσις): A descriptive term for the fiery red heat of inflammation. Galen suggests it was also used as a term for inflammation itself—see *MM*, Book 13.

Phlyktaina (φλύκταινα): A term for a blister or pustule that has burst and is ulcerated—see Ce, 5.28.15 (he calls it "the worst kind of pustule").

Phrenitis (φρενῖτις): Inflammation of the brain. Termed by Si "delirium with fever"—see his discussion on pp. 270–72. M (p. 508) states that "Aretaeus' treatment of phrenitis indicates that this was essentially symptomatic febrile delirium but may have included meningitis and cerebritis."

Phthoe (φθόη): Taken as equivalent to phthisis—see G, VII.29 and 279K.

Phyma (φῦμα): Tumor or tubercle; Gr (p. 188) writes: "The word *phuma* corresponds primarily to our terms 'abscess' and 'tubercle', but also functions as the name for certain forms of cancer and hydatid cyst." See G, VI.849K.

Plague (λοιμός): Essentially the same meaning as currently—"any disease of wide prevalence and/or excessive mortality" (S). The Great Plague of Athens (430–427 BC) described by Thucydides (2.47–54) may have been, as M suggests (p. 325), a mixed epidemic. More recent evidence suggests it was typhoid fever. The plague in Rome referred to by Galen may have been true bubonic plague (due to *Pastuerella pestis*—see M, p. 363).

Pleuritis (πλευρῖτις): Pleurisy, although Gr (p. 131) suggests the description may apply to lobar pneumonia. See G, VIII.326K and XIX.420K (definition).

Pneumonia (περιπνευμομία): A term for inflammation of the lungs, which may equate with the modern lobar pneumonia—see G, VII.174K and Gr, p. 131.

Polyp (πολύπους): Similar to the modern meaning referring to a nasal polyp—see G, VII.106K.

Priapism (πριαπισμός): Persistent enlargement/erection of the penis without sexual desire, as in current usage—see G, VI.869K.

Psora (ψώρα): A skin disease of uncertain nature associated with itching—see G, VII.849–50K.

Pterygium (πτερύγιον): Similar to modern usage in describing hypertrophied bulbar conjunctival tissue growing from the medial canthus of the eye to the edge of the cornea or beyond—see G, VI.862K.

Ptilosis (πτίλωσις): A disease of the eyelids in which

the edges become inflamed and swollen and the eyelashes fall out—see G, *MM*, 1004 and 1014K.

Rhyas (ῥυάς): An eye disease associated with continuous watery discharge—see G, VI.870 and *MM*, 1002K.

Rigor (ῥῖγος): May be equivalent to rigor in the modern sense; described by Galen as an "irregular shaking and agitation of the whole body"—see G, VII.145K and *MM*, 1002K.

Rupture (ῥῆγμα): A rupture, tearing, or laceration of tissue—see G, *MM*, 160 and 232K.

Sarcocele (σαρκοκήλη): A form of scirrhus involving the testes—see G, VII.729 and *MM*, 1004K.

Satyriasis (σατυρίασις): Priapism with sexual desire —perhaps due to an inflammatory disease involving the genitalia. See M, p. 518 and pp. 610–11, who includes ancient descriptions.

Sciatica (ἰσχιάς): A term for a symptom probably similar to modern usage; i.e., pain in the back and hip radiating into the leg. In ancient times likely to have been mainly due to hip disease—see G, VI.849K and M, p. 493.

Scirrhus (σκίρρος): Listed in LSJ as a "hardened swelling or tumour, induration." This is similar to modern usage; i.e., "obsolete term for any fibrous indurated area, especially an indurated carcinoma" (S).

Scrofula (χοιράς): Cervical lymphadenopathy, probably of tuberculous origin—see Gr, pp. 178, 196.

Shivering (φρίκη): Corresponds to the modern usage. Grouped by Galen with the disordered movements—see VII.147K.

Sicus (σύκωσις): An ulcer resembling a fig ripe to the point of bursting, particularly on the eyelids—see *MM*, 82K.

Spasm (σπάσμα): A complex term; listed by LSJ in one sense as "sprain or rupture of muscle."

Sphacelus (σφάκελος): A form of gangrenous necrosis particularly involving bone.

Staphyle (σραφυλή): Refers, as a disease, to inflammation of the uvula with swelling—see G, VII.263K and *MM*, 82K.

Staphyloma (σταφύλωμα): Listed by LSJ as a "defect in the eye inside the cornea"—see G. VII.734K, XIX.435K, XIX.439K, and Ce, 7.7.11.

Steatoma (στεάτωμα): A sebaceous tumor, perhaps equivalent to the modern sebaceous cyst in some instances—see G, VII.22K (cause), *MM*, 985K (treatment) and XIX.440K (definition).

Swooning (λιποψυχία): Probably identical in meaning to λιποθυμία and meaning fainting in the modern sense—see G, VII.136 and 194K (causes) and M, p. 510, who includes Aretaeus' description and mentions that the term remained in use through the eighteenth century.

Syncope (συγκοπή): A sudden, generalized collapse —much like the present use of the term but with broader connotations, See G, VII.127K and *MM*, 805K for causes, and Si, pp. 251–53 for detailed consideration.

Tenesmus (τεινεσμός): A vain attempt to evacuate *per rectum*. The meaning seems very similar to the modern definition: "painful and ineffectual straining to empty the bowels" (S).

Tetanus (τέτανος): A term that currently applies to the acute neurotoxicity due to infection with *Clostridium tetani* which is marked by intense muscle spasm, including severe involvement of the masseter muscles ("lockjaw"). Tetanic spasms more generally refer to prolonged muscle spasm due to repeated rapid stimuli. It seems probable that the ancient descriptions of tetanus do refer to the effects of *C. tetani* infection.

Torpor (κάρος): Like coma, a reversible loss of consciousness which may include deep sleep.

Tremor (τρόμος): As in the present usage. It was classified by Galen as a symptom due to a disturbance of the motor component of the psyche.

Ulcer (ἕλκος): This is a problematic term. It was used by Galen to refer in a general way to dissolution of continuity involving a surface, whether external or internal. It ranges in application from a fresh wound through a chronic and possibly infected wound to what would now be referred to as an ulcer, which may arise in various places due to various causes. The term may also refer to ruptured vesicles or pustules (i.e., "sores"). Where the context allows, the appropriate specific term is used in our translation. Where the statement is general, it is translated as "wound and ulcer" or "wound or ulcer."

Warts: Three varieties, as follows; (a) thin-necked or pedunculated (ἀκροχορδών); (b) sessile (μυρμηκία); and (c) a large warty excrescence (θύμος).

Wound (ἕλκος): See Ulcer.

10. MEDICATIONS

Absinth (Absinthium): See Wormwood.

Acacia (ἀκακία): *Acacia arabica*; also *A. nilotica, A. pontica,* and *A. maritima*; drying agent; D, I.133; G, XI.814K; Ce, pp. xv–xvi.

Agrimony (εὐπατόριον): *Agrimony eupatorium*; used for wounds and ulcers; D, IV.41; G, XI.79K; Cu, pp. 12–15.

Alexanders (ἱπποσέλινον): *Smyrnium olustratum*; Cretan alexanders; D, III.78; G, XII.128K.

All-heal (πάνακες): *Ferulago galbanifera*; several varieties, e.g., of Hercules, of Aesculapius; many uses; D, III.55–57; G, XII.95K; Cu, pp. 10–11; T, 9.7.2.

Aloe (ἀλόη): *Aloe vera*, *A. vulgaris*; bitter aloes; hemostatic, for wound conglutination, purgative, component of eye salves and ear lotions; D, III.25; G, XI.822K; Ce, p. xviii.

Alum (στυπτερία): Also alumen; a term for a group of alum or ferrous sulfate-containing substances; strong drying agent; D, V.123; G, XII.236K; for a detailed list of varieties, see Ce, pp. xviii–xix.

Ambrosia: Term for a compound antidote (among other things); for the potion, see G, XI.824K, XIII.64K, and XIV.149K; D, III.129 lists *Artemisia compestris* under Ambrosia.

Andron, troche of: A multi-component troche or pastille compounded by Andron from pomegranate flowers, oak gall, myrrh, birthwort, vitriol, fissile alum, and Cyprian misu marinated in sweet wine—see *EANS*, p. 80.

Aphrogala (ἀφρόγαλα): Frothed milk; G, X.468K.

Aphronitron (ἀφρόνιτρον): Listed by LSJ as a "form of native sodium carbonate" but in L&S as an "efflorescence of saltpeter (potassium nitrate)"; various uses; D, V.131; G, XI.695–96K and XII.210–13K.

Apomel (ἀπόμελι): Listed in LSJ as a mixture of water and honey—a kind of "inferior mead" but elsewhere as a vinegar/honey mixture, e.g., "a kind of decoction prepared of honey or an honeycomb mixed with vinegar, and boiled a short time" (Chambers, *Cycl. Supp.* 1753 in *OED*); possibly equivalent to oinomeli (D, V.16) or oxymeli (D, V.22).

Galen's description in *De sanitate tuenda* VI.274K is in keeping with the LSJ description.

Aristolochia (ἀριστολοχία): Plants from the genus *Aristolochia* (birthwort); the root yields an irritant glucoside used in poultices; D, III.4–6; G, XI.683K and 835–36K; Ce, p. xxi.

Aromatic reed (κάλαμος ἀρωματικός): *Acorus calamis*; sweet flag; rhizome dried and eaten or oil pressed from it; D, I.17; G, XI.405–6K and XII.6K ff.; Ce, p. xvi.

Artomel (ἀρτόμελι): Plaster or poultice of bread and honey; G, X.692 and 781K.

Asparagus (ἀσφάραγος): *Asparagus officianalis* or *acutifolius*; the stem may be eaten directly; a decoction is prepared from the root; D, II.152; G, XI.841K; Cu, pp. 28–30.

Asphalt (ἄσφαλτος): Asphaltos, bitumen, pitch; different sources; D, I.99; G, XII.375K.

Ass's milk (ὄνου γάλα): G. VI.682K ff. and XII.265K.

Athanasia (ἀθανασία): a compound antidote—for details of various recipes, see *EANS*, pp. 57–58; G, XIII.203K and XIV.148K.

Balsam (βάλσαμον): *Balsamodendron opobalsamum*; Balsam tree; D, I.18; G, XI.846K and XII.554K; used as aromatic herb—*Chrysanthemum balsamita*, costmary; Ce, p. xxvii: Cu, p. 94.

Barley (κριθή): *Hordeum sativum*; various forms—groats, meal, cake, water; D, II.108, 109; G, VI.501K and XII.44K.

Bdellium (βδέλλιον): Aromatic gum from *Balsamodendrum africanum* (LSJ); also seed from the Palmyra

INTRODUCTION

palm and the Doum palm; D, I.80; G, XI.849K ff; Ce, p. xxii.

Bean (κύαμος): *Vicia faba, Kuamos hellenikos*; also *Nelumbium speciosum* (the Egyptian bean); D, II.127, 128; G, XII.49K and, for powers of the Egyptian bean, VI.532K.

Beeswax (κηρός): Cera; used as a discutient, emollient, and enfleshing agent; D, II.105; G, XIII.411K; Ce, p. xxvi.

Bread and honey cataplasm/poultice: See Artomel.

Brimstone (θεῖον): Sulfur, used either burned or unburned; D, V.124; G, XII.903K.

Cadmia (καδμεία): Calamine; for preparation and uses, see D, V.84 and G, XII.219–20K; Ce, p. xxiii.

Cankerwort (ἐλατίνη): *Linaria spuria*; D, IV.40; G, XII.873K.

Caper (κάππαρις): *Capparis spinosa*; D, II.204; G, XII.9K ff.

Cardamom/cardamomum (κάρδαμον): *Lepidarum sativum*, cress; *Eletarria cardamomum*; seeds from Malabar and Sri Lanka produce aromatic oil; D, II.185; G, XII.11–12K; for various external uses, see Ce, p. xxv.

Castor (κίκι): *Ricinus communis*; castor oil (*cicinium oleum*); D. IV.164 and for oil I.38; G. XI.649K; Ce, p. xxvi.

Castoreum (καστόρειον): Material derived from testes of beavers; used in eye and ear salves; D, II.26; G, XII.337–41K; Ce, p. xxv.

Catmint (καλάμινθος): *Nepeta cataria*; various uses, including as diuretic; D, III.43; Ce, p. xliv; Cu, p. 201.

Celery (σέλινον): *Selinon agrion* (*Ranunculus repens*), Selinon keraion (*Apium graveolens*); D, III.74 and 75; G, XI.834K and XII.158K.

Celtic spikenard: See Nard; D, V.67; for powers, G, XII.85K; for use on liver, G, XIII.209K.

Centaury (κενταύριον): *Centaurea salonitata*; for the different forms, see D, III.240–42; G, XII.19–20K; Ce, p. xxv–xxvi; Cu, pp. 76–77, 167.

Cephalicum (κεφαλικόν): A compound remedy for the head; G, XIII.541K ff. and XIV.765K.

Cerussa: See Lead (a).

Chalcanthum (χάλκανθος): Copperas water; used for flatworm infestation; D, V.114; for source, powers, and uses, see G, XII.238K ff.

Chalcitis (χαλκίτης): copper ore; used for erysipelas and herpes; used in eye medications; D, V.115; G, XI.688K and XII.241K; Ce, p. xvi.

Chalk, washed (τίτανος): Used as a drying and cicatrizing agent; D, V.150.

Chamomile (χαμαιμήλον): *Matricaria chamomilla*; earth apple; G, XI.562 and 833K; for preparation and uses, see Cu, pp. 67–68.

Chaste tree seed (ἄγνος): *Vitex agnus-castus*; used as purgative, for headache, and in poultices; D, I.135; G, XI.807–9K.

Chian mastich: See Mastich.

Cinnamon (κίνναμωμον): *Cinnamomum cassia/verum*; D, I.13; G, XII.26K; Ce, xxvi–xxvii.

Colocynth (κολοκύνθη/ος): *Lagenaria vulgaris*; D, IV.178; G, XII.34K.

Copper, burned (χαλκὸς κεκαυμένος): Possibly cuprous oxide; D, V.87; G, XII.242K; Ce, p. xvii, for various preparations of copper.

Copper, flake (λεπὶς χαλκοῦ): Flakes of cuprous oxide prepared by hammering; D, V.89; Ce, p. xxvii.

Copper, flower (ἄνθος χαλκοῦ): Grains of cuprous oxide prepared by quenching heated copper; D, V.88.

Coriander (κορίαννον): *Coriandrum sativum*; used as diuretic and externally; D, III.71; G, XII.36K ff; Ce, p. xxvii.

Cretan alexanders: See Alexanders.

Crocus: See Saffron.

Cucumber (σίκυος): *Cucumis sativus*; D, II.162; G, XII.121–22K; Cu, p. 102.

Cumin (κύμινον): *Cuminum cyminum*; D, IV.178; G, XII.52K and XIII.119K.

Cyperus (κύπειρον, κύπερος): *Cyperus rotundus*; D, I.4; G, XII.54, 472, 961K; T, 4.10.5.

Date palm (βάλανος φοίνικος): Fruit of *Phoenix dactylifera*; from Egypt; D, I.148; G, XII.151K.

Diaspermaton: Medication made from seeds; analgesic and hypnotic; G, *MM*, 372K and XIII.978K.

Dill (ἄνηθον): *Anethum graveolens*; D, III.67; G, XI.832K and XIII.316K; Cu, pp. 105–6.

Diphryges (διφρυγής): Baked clay from copper mines (LSJ); sulfide and oxide of copper mixed with iron and zinc ores; used for cleansing and treatment of abscesses; D, V.120; G, XII.214K ff.

Dropwort (οἰνάνθη): *Spiraea filipendula*; oenanthe; D, III.135 (oinanthe as *Pedicularis tuberose*).

Egyptian thorn (ἄκανθα Αἰγυπτία): Egyptian acanthus; D, I.133; T, 9.1.2.

Endive (ἴντυβος): *Chicorium endivia* (chicory), *C. intybus*; used for eye inflammations, erysipelas; D, II.160; G, VI.628K and XII.119K; Cu, p. 115.

Epithymum (ἐπίθυμον): *Cuscula epithymum*; dodder of thyme; D, IV.179; G, XI.875K; Cu, p. 108–9.

Euphorbium (εὐφόρβιον): *Euphorbia resinifera*; spurge; D, IV.165 (for several varieties); G, XI.879K and XIII.270K ff.

Fenugreek (τῆλις): *Trigonella foenum-graecum*; used in various mixtures; D, II.124; G, VI.537K and XII.141K; Ce, pp. xxxiii–xxxiv.

Fleawort (ψύλλιον): *Plantago psyllinum*; D, II.151; G, XI.740K; Ce, p. xlviii; Cu, pp. 128–29.

Frankincense (λιβανωτός, λίβανος): Gum of *Boswellia carteri, B. sacri*; D, I.81; G, XII.60K; Ce, p. xxxix.

Galena (μολύβδαινα): See Lead (b).

Goatwort (τράγιον): *Tragium columnae* or *Hypericum hircinum*; D, IV.5.

Grapevine (ἄμπελος): *Vitis vinifera*; Ampelos oinophoros; D, V.1.

Hazelwort (ἄσαρον): *Asarum europeieum*; European wild ginger; D, I.9; G, XI.840K.

Hellebore (ἐλλέβορος): *Veratrum album, Helleboras niger, H. officianalis*; white and black hellebore; purgative and emetic; D, IV.150–52; G, XI.874K; Ce, pp. lviii–lix.

Hematite (αἱματίτης): D, V.144 and 145 for sources and preparation.

Hemlock (κωνειόν): *Conium maculatum*; D, IV.79.

Henbane (ὑοσκύαμος): *Hyoscyamus albus, H. niger*; D, IV.69; Cu, pp. 150, 152.

Higry-pigry (πίκρα): *Hiera picra*; made from aloes and canella bark; G, XIII.129, 131K.

Honey (μέλι): Widely used alone or in mixtures; D, II.101; G, XI.671K ff. and XII.70K.

Horehound (πράσιον): *Marrubium vulgare*; D, III.119; G, XII.107K; Ce, p. xliii; Cu, p. 158.

Houseleek (ἀείζωον): *Sempervivum arboretum*; D, IV.89–90; G, XI.740, 813K; Cu, pp. 160–61.

Hyssop (ὕσσωπος): *Hyssopus officianalis*; G, XII.149K; Cu, pp. 156–57.

Illyrian iris (ἶρις Ἰλλυρική): D, I.1; G, XI.135K; Ce, p. xxxvii.

Iris (ἶρις): *Iris pallida*; wide range of uses; D, IV.22; Ce, p. xxxvii.

Isis (ἶσις): May refer to different things, including types of plasters—see *EANS*, p. 446.

Ladanum (λήδανον): *Cistus creticus;* D. I.128; G. XII.28; Ce, p. xxxviii.

Lead (μόλυβδος): Five forms listed in Ce, p. xlviii, as follows (a–c referred to by Galen in *MM*): (a) *Cerussa* (ψιμύθιον), white lead (lead acetate), used for recent wounds, D, V.103; G, XII.243K (powers and uses), XIII.416K (preparation). (b) *Galena* (μολύβδαινα), lead sulfate, hemostatic, D, V.100. (c) *Litharge* (λιθάργυρος), *spuma argenti*, treated lead oxide, D, V.102. (d) *Plumbum album*, possibly tinstone. (e) *Plumbi stercus*, lead slag, lead dross, D, V.97.

Linseed (λινόσπερμον): *Linum usitatissimum*; Flax; D, II.125; G, VI.549K and XII.62K.

Litharge (λιθάργυρος): See Lead (c).

Mandrake (μανδραγόρας): *Mandragora officianalis*; used as soporific and anodyne; D, IV.76; G, XI.751K and XII.67K; Ce, pp. xli–xlii; also listed in LSJ as belladonna (*Atropa belladonna*), T, 6.2.9.

Manna (μάννα): Manna of frankincense; same powers as frankincense but weaker; D, I.83; G, *MM*, 887–88K and XII.845K.

Mastich (σχῖνος): *Pistacia lentiscus*; also termed lentiscum; used for ulceration, dysentery, hemorrhage; D, I.89; G, XII.135K, XIII.35K and for Chian mastich, XII.68 and 180K; Ce, p. xxxix; T. 9.1.2.

Melikraton (μελίκρατον): Mulse; mixture of honey with milk, water, and wine, or honey and water (hydromel); Hippocrates, *Aphorisms* V.41; G, VI.741K.

Mercury (λινοζῶστις): Possibly *Mercurialis annua*; D, IV.191; G, XII.63K and XIV.760K.

Misu (μίσυ): Misy, copperas; a copper ore found in Cyprus; D, V.117; G, XI.688K and XII.241K.

Mustard (σίναπι): Used in plasters; D, II.142; G, I.682K and XI.870K; Ce, p. liv.

Myrobalanos (μυροβάλανος): *Balanos myrepsica*; Ce, p. xxii.

Myrrh (σμύρνα): *Commiphora myrrha*; different sources, various uses; D, I.77; G, XII.81 and 127K; Ce, p. xliii.

Myrtle (μυρσίνη): *Myrtus communis*; used as a cooling agent and in plasters; D, I.155; G, *MM*, 330K and XII.81K ff; Ce, p. xliii.

Nard (νάρδος): *Nardostachys jatamansi* and other varieties; also called spikenard; D, I.6–8; G, XII.84–85K and XIII.209K; Ce, p. xliv.

Navelwort (κοτυληδών): *Cotyledon umbilicus*, *C. sterilis*: G, XII.41K and XIII.386K.

Nightshade (στρύχνος): Several species (four listed in LSJ); according to Spencer (Ce, p. lv), all yield scopolamine; D, IV.72–74 (*Physalis alkengi*, *Withania somnifera*, *Datura stramomium*).

Oak gall (κηκίς): *Galla*; used externally as astringent, erodent, and excedent; produced in some species of oak by the gall fly; D, I.146; G, XII.24K ff.

Oil of balsam: See Balsam.

Olive oil (ἔλαιον): D, I.30 and 31.

Omphacium (ὀμφάκιον): Juice of unripe olives and grapes; cleaning agent for wounds and ulcers; G, VI.426K and XI.788K.

Opium (ὄπιον): Poppy juice, opium; D, IV.65; G, XIII.269K.

Opoponax (ὀποπάναξ): Gum of *Opoponax hispidus*; Hercules' woundwort; used in various mixtures; D, III.55; G, XII.94K ff.; XIII.62; Ce, p. xlv.

Oregano (ὀρίγανον): An acrid herb; several varieties; D, III.32–34; G, XIV.140K; Ce, p. xlv; Cu, pp. 182–83.

Oxymel (ὀξύμελι): A vinegar/honey mixture; D, V.22 (for preparation); G, VI.271ff.

Oxyrhodinum (ὀξυρρόδινον): Vinegar and oil of roses mixture; D, I.29; G, XI.559K.

Panax (πανάκεια): *Panaces*, all-heal; an emollient mucilage; G, XI.863K; Ce, p. xlv.

Papyrus (πάπυρος): *Cyperus papyrus*; used for fistulae, wounds, and ulcers; D, I.115; G, XII.94K; Ce, p. xlvi.

Pasion, troche of: Prepared from copper flake, burned copper, sal ammoniac, alum, and verdigris heated in the sun with frankincense then added—see *EANS*, p. 627.

Pennyroyal (βλήχων): *Mentha pulegium*; D, III.36; G, XI.882K; Ce, p. xlii.

Pepper (πέπερι): *Piper nigrum, P. album,* and *P. longum*; D, II.189; G, XII.97K (uses of all three forms); Ce, p. xlvii.

Pine (πεύκη): *Pinus pinea* and other varieties; various products (cones, resin) and uses; D, I.86–88; Ce, p. xlvii.

Pitch (πίσσα): Used as emollient and in preparation of plasters; D, I.94 and 95; G, XI.734K and XIII.709K.

Plantain (ἀρνόγλωσσον): *Plantago major*; D, II.153; G, XIII.320K; Ce, p. xlvii–xlviii; Cu, pp. 224–25.

Polyeides, troche of: Prepared from aloes, alum, calcanthum, myrrh, pomegranate flowers, and bull gall ground in dry wine—see *EANS*, p. 682.

Pomegranate (ῥόα/ῥοιά): *Punica granatum*; for various forms (including the rind), see D, I.151–54; G, VI.603K and XI.847K.

Pompholyx (πομφόλυξ): Impure zinc oxide; D, V.85; G, XII.234–35K; for use as an emplastic, G, XII.634K; for use in the eyes, G, XII.699K.

Poppy (μήκων): *Papaver somniferum, P. rhoeas* (wild poppy), *P. argemone* (prickly poppy); D, IV.64–66; G, VI.548K and XII.74K; Ce, p. xlv–xlvi.

Propolis (πρόπολις): Bee glue; a resinous substance gathered by bees for use in hive-building; used for nerve wounds and other things; D, II.106; G, XII.108K.

Ptisan (πτισάνη): A medicinal drink made from barley; see Galen's *De ptisana*, VI.816–31K, and for powers and uses, G, XV.452K.

Purpura (πορφύρα): Dye from the purple fish (genus of Murex gastropods); D, II.4; G, XII.344 and 348K.

Purslane (ἀνδράχνη): *Portulaca oluracea*; D, II.151; G, VI.634K, XI.740, 751K; Cu, pp. 231–32.

Quince juice (μῆλον κυδώνιον): *Cydonia vulgaris*; multiple uses; D, I.160; G, VI.602K and XII.76K.

Radish (ῥαφανίς): *Raphanus sativus*; D, II.137; G, XII.111K (powers and uses).

Rosaceum (ῥόδινος): Rhodinum; for preparation, see D, I.53: also G, XI.538K.

Rue (πήγανον): *Ruta graveolens*; D, III.52, 53; G, XI.809K; Ce, p. li.

Rupos (ῥύπος): Grime from different sources—baths, wrestling halls, gymnasia; D, I.34–36.

Safflower (κνῆκος): *Cnicus* sp. or *Carthamus tincturius*; D, IV.190; G, XI.610–12K.

Saffron (κρόκος): *Crocus sativus*; D, I.25; G, XII.48K; Ce, pp. xxviii–xxix.

Sagapine (σαγάπηνον): Probably *Ferula persica*; also its gum; D, III.95; G, XII.117K; Ce, p. li.

Scammony (σκαμμωνία): *Convolvulus scammonia*, *C. farinosus*; used in purging mixtures and with barley in poultices; D, IV.171; G, IV.760K; Ce, p. liii.

Scolopendrium (σκολόπενδριον): *Scolopendrium officinale*; hart's tongue; D, III.121; G, XI.746K; Cu, pp. 145, 147.

Sinopian earth (Σινωπικὴ μίλτος): A red earth found in Cappadocia; D, V.111.

Sorrel (ὀξαλίς): *Rumex acetosa*, *R. patienta*, *R. crispis*; curled dock (ὀξυλάπαθον); D, II.140; G, VI.794K and XV.405K.

Spikenard: See Nard.

Stinging nettle (ἀκαλήφη): *Urtica pilulifera*; D, IV.94; G, VI.639K, XI.817K; Ce, p. lviii; Cu, pp. 202–3.

Storax (στύραξ): *Storax officianalis*; used for promoting suppuration and for treating wounds; D, I.79; G, XI.767K and XII.131K; Ce, p. lvi.

Sycamore (συκόμορον): Fruit of the sycamore fig (*Ficus sycomorus*); D, I.181.

Tamarisk (μυρίκη): *Tamarix tetranda* (Greece); *Tamarix articulata* (Egypt); used as a repressive and cooling agent; D, I.118; G, XI.746K (use of root); G, XII.80K ff.; Ce, p. lvii: Cu, pp. 281–82.

Terebinth (τερέβινθος/τέρμινθος): *Pistachia terebinthus*; terebinthus; resin from turpentine tree; D, I.91; G, XII.113–14 and 137K; Ce, p. lvii.

Thapsia (θαψία): *Thapsia garganica*; a strong counterirritant; D, IV.157; G, XI.885K.

Thyme (θύμον): *Thymbra capitata*; Cretan thyme; D, III.44; G, XI.887K ff.

Tragacanth (τραγάκανθα): *Astragalus gummifer*, also *A. aristatus*, *A. parnasei*, *A. creticus*; D, III.23; G, XII.143K and XIII.10K.

Turpentine: See Terebinth.

Verdigris (ἰός): Basic cupric acetate; D, V.91; G, XII.218K.

Vetch (ὄροβος): *Vicia ervilia*; meal of bitter vetch; D, II.131.

Vinegar (ὄξος): Used alone or in mixtures (e.g., oxymel); D, V.21–25; G, XII.90K (medicinal powers).

Wax: See Beeswax.

White lead (cerussa): See Lead (a).

Wild lettuce (θριδακίνη): *Lactuca scariola*; D, II.166; G, XI.887K; Cu, pp. 170–71.

Wine (οἶνος): For the variety of wines, see D, V.7–82 and G, VI.334–39K.

Wormwood (ἀψίνθιον): *Artemisia absintheum*, also *A. pontica* and *A. maritima*; absinthium; carminative and diuretic; D, III.26; Ce, p. xv; Cu, pp. 307–13.

BIBLIOGRAPHY

TEXTS AND TRANSLATIONS OF THE
METHODUS MEDENDI

Boulogne, J. *Galien. Méthode thérapeutique, livres I et II.* 2 vols. Villeneuve-d'Ascq: Université Charles-de-Gaulle-Lille 3, 1992.

———. *Méthode de traitment.* Paris: Gallimard, 2009.

English, Peter. *Galen's Method of Physick.* Edinburgh: 1656.

Gale, Thomas. *Certaine Works of Galen's called Methodus Medendi.* London: Thomas East, 1586.

Hankinson, R. J. *Galen on the Therapeutic Method: Books 1 and 2.* Oxford: Oxford University Press, 1991.

Kühn, C-G. *Claudii Galeni Opera Omnia.* 20 vols. Leipzig, 1821–1833 (reprint Hildesheim: Georg Olms Verlag, 1997), volume 10, pp. 1–1021.

Linacre, Thomas. *Cl. Galeni Methodi Medendi, vel De Morbis Curandi.* Lyon: G. Rovire, 1546.

———. *Galeni Methodi Medendi.* In *Galeni Omnium Operum Sexta Classis.* Venice: Vincentium Valgrisium, 1562.

TRANSLATIONS OF OTHER
GALENIC WORKS

Boudon, V. *Galien: Exhortation á l'étude de la medicine, Art medical*. Paris: Les Belles Lettres, 2002.

Boudon-Millot, V. *Galien: Introduction general, Sur l'ordre de ses propres livres, Sur ses propres livres, Que l'excellent médicin est aussi philosophe*. Paris: Les Belles Lettres, 2007.

Brain, P. *Galen: On Bloodletting*. Cambridge: Cambridge University Press, 1986.

Brock, A. J. *Galen: On the Natural Faculties*. Loeb Classical Library. Cambridge, MA: Harvard University Press, 1963 [1916].

Daremberg, C. *Oeuvres anatomiques, physiologiques et médicales de Galien*. Paris: J-P. Baillière, 1854–1856.

De Lacy, P. H. *Galen: On the Doctrines of Hippocrates and Plato*. 2 vols. CMG, V.4.1.2. Berlin: Akademie-Verlag, 1978.

———. *Galen: On the Elements according to Hippocrates*. CMG, V.1.2. Berlin: Akademie-Verlag, 1996.

Duckworth, W. H. L., M. C. Lyons, and B. Towers. *Galen: On Anatomical Procedures. The Later Books: IX.6–XV*. Cambridge: Cambridge University Press , 1962.

Edlow, R. B. *Galen: On Language and Ambiguity*. Leiden: E. J. Brill, 1977.

Grant, M. *Galen on Food and Diet*. London: Routledge, 2000.

Green, R. M. *A Translation of Galen's Hygiene*. Springfield, IL: C. C. Thomas, 1951.

Hankinson, R. J. *Galen: On Antecedent Causes*. Cambridge: Cambridge University Press, 1998.

Johnston, I. *Galen: On Diseases and Symptoms*. Cambridge: Cambridge University Press, 2006.

May, M. T. *Galen: On the Usefulness of the Parts of the Body*. 2 vols. Ithaca, NY: Cornell University Press, 1968.

Meyerhof, M., and J. Schacht. *Galen über die medizinischen Namen*. Berlin: Abh. Akad. Wiss., 1931.

Nutton, V. *Galen: On My Own Opinions*. CMG, V.3.2. Berlin: Akademie-Verlag, 1999.

———. *Galen: On Prognosis*. CMG, V.8.1. Berlin: Akademie-Verlag, 1979.

Powell, O. *Galen on the Properties of Foodstuffs*. Cambridge: Cambridge University Press, 2003.

Siegel, R. E. *Galen: On the Affected Parts*. Basel: S. Karger, 1976.

Singer, C. *Galen: On Anatomical Procedures*. Oxford: Clarendon, 1956.

Singer, P. N. *Galen: Selected Works*. Oxford: Oxford University Press, 1997.

Walzer, R., and M. Frede. *Three Treatises on the Nature of Science*. Indianapolis: Hackett, 1985.

GENERAL WORKS

Celsus. *De Medicina*. Translated by W. G. Spencer. 3 vols. Loeb Classical Library. Cambridge, MA: Harvard University Press, 1935–1938.

Conrad, L. I., M. Neve, V. Nutton, R. Porter, and A. Wear. *The Western Medical Tradition (800 BC to AD 1800)*. Cambridge: Cambridge University Press, 1995.

Culpepper, Nicholas. *The English Physician Enlarged (Culpepper's Herbal)*. London: Folio Society, 2007 [1653].

BIBLIOGRAPHY

Dioscorides. *The Greek Herbal of Dioscorides.* Translated by John Goodyer, edited by R. T. Gunther. New York: Hafner, 1968 [1934].

Garofalo, I. *Erasistrati Fragmenta.* Pisa: Giardini Editori e Stampatori, 1988.

Grmek, M. D. *Diseases in the Ancient Greek World.* Baltimore: Johns Hopkins University Press, 1991.

Hankinson, R. J., ed. *The Cambridge Companion to Galen.* Cambridge: Cambridge University Press, 2008.

Keyser, P. T., and G. L. Irby-Massie, eds. *The Encyclopedia of Ancient Natural Scientists.* Oxford: Routledge, 2008.

Kudlien, F., and R. J. Durling, eds. *Galen's Method of Healing.* Leiden: E. J. Brill, 1991.

Longrigg, J. *Greek Rational Medicine.* London: Routledge, 1993.

Mettler, C. C. *The History of Medicine.* Philadelphia: Blakiston, 1947.

Nutton, V. *Ancient Medicine.* London: Routledge, 2004.

———, ed. "The Unknown Galen." *Bulletin of the Institute of Classical Studies*, suppl. 77 (2002).

Steckerl, F. *The Fragments of Praxagoras and His School.* Leiden: E. J. Brill, 1958.

Urmson, J. O. *The Greek Philosophical Vocabulary.* London: Duckworth, 1990.

Vallance, J. *The Lost Theory of Asclepiades of Bithynia.* Oxford: Clarendon, 1990.

Van der Eijk, P. J. *Diocles of Carystus: A Collection of Fragments with Translation and Commentary.* 2 vols. Leiden: E. J. Brill, 2000–2001.

Von Staden, H. *Herophilus: The Art of Medicine in Early Alexandria.* Cambridge: Cambridge University Press, 1989.

BIBLIOGRAPHY

MANUSCRIPTS

Kühn (= K) vol. X has provided the base text for ours printed here.

The Latin text printed in K (abbreviated by us as KLat in this volume) was produced three hundred years before K was printed, and so is not a translation or a correction of K's Greek text. It clearly draws on other MSS than those used by K, reflecting different readings in the Greek. This may sometimes alert us to a problem in K; but generally we have not privileged the Latin translation over K's Greek text.

For a list of MSS of the *MM*, see Diels.[115] The following manuscripts are referred to in our textual notes with the abbreviation listed.

 B—British Library MS Add. 6898 (London; 12th cent.)[116]
 P1—Parisinus Gr. 2160 (Paris; 14th cent.)
 P2—Parisinus Gr. 2171 (Paris; 15th cent.)[117]

---

[115] Hermann Diels, *Die Handschriften der Antiken Ärtze* (Leipzig, Zentralantiquariat der Deutschen Demokratischen Republik, 1970 reprint), pp. 91–93.

[116] We are not attempting to provide here a full collation of B against K. B exhibits many other differences, e.g., in word order and in orthography, and it is interesting for other reasons as well. But we have very rarely noted these.

[117] We have not directly consulted the two Paris MSS. We have made use of some of their readings for Books 1 and 2 as they are reported by Hankinson, *Galen on the Therapeutic Method*, App. 1, pp. 235–37.

Boulogne (2009) 11, 31, draws upon these three MSS for his translation and also upon three others as well as two fragmentary MSS. We have included no references to these other five in our textual notes.

ABBREVIATIONS

Ce   Celsus. *De Medicina*. Translated by W. G. Spencer. Loeb Classical Library. 3 vols. Cambridge, MA: Harvard University Press, 1935–1938.

CMG   Corpus Medicorum Graecorum

Cu   Nicholas Culpepper. *The English Physician Enlarged (Culpepper's Herbal)*. London: Folio Society, 2007 [1653].

D   Dioscorides. *The Greek Herbal of Dioscorides*, translated by John Goodyer [1653]. Edited by R. T. Gunther. New York: Hafner, 1968 [1933].

EANS *The Encyclopedia of Ancient Natural Scientists*. Edited by P. T. Keyser and G. L. Irby-Massie. London: Routledge, 2008.

G   Galen. References to the *MM* are indicated by the Kühn page number; references to other Galenic works are indicated by the Kühn volume and page numbers. His three major pharmacological treatises are *De simplicium medicamentorum temperamentis et facultatibus*, XI.379–892K and XII.1–377K; *De compositione medicamentorum secundum locos*, XII.378–1007K and XIII.1–361K; *De compositione medicamentorum per genera*, XIII.362–1058K.

Gr   M. D. Grmek. *Diseases in the Ancient Greek World*. Baltimore, MD: Johns Hopkins University Press, 1991.

L&S   C. T. Lewis and C. Short. *A Latin Dictionary*. Oxford: Clarendon, 1993 [1879].

LCL   Loeb Classical Library.

LSJ   H. G. Liddell, R. Scott, and H. Stuart Jones. *A Greek-English Lexicon*. 9th ed. (1940), with revised suppl. by P. G. W. Glare. Oxford: Clarendon, 1996.

M   C. C. Mettler. *The History of Medicine*. Philadelphia: Blakiston, 1947.

OCD   *Oxford Classical Dictionary*. Edited by S. Hornblower and A. Spawforth. 3rd ed. Oxford: Clarendon, 1996.

OED   *Oxford English Dictionary*. 12 vols. Oxford: Oxford University Press, 1978 [1933].

S   *Stedman's Medical Dictionary*. 27th ed. Baltimore: Lippincott, Williams and Wilkins, 2000.

Si   R. E. Siegel. *Galen on the Affected Parts*. Basel: S. Karger, 1976.

T   Theophrastus. *Enquiry into Plants*. Translated by A. Hort. Loeb Classical Library. 2 vols. Cambridge, MA: Harvard University Press, 1916, 1926.

SYNOPSIS OF CHAPTERS

BOOK I

1. Following the dedicatory remarks to Hiero, which include Galen's explanation for his delay in providing the requested *Method of Medicine*, he laments the decline in standards among doctors in general and the lack of discrimination among patients in their selection of a doctor. He singles out Thessalus and the Methodics as the extreme example of this decline in standards, particularly when compared to the era of the great schools of Cos and Cnidus.

2. Galen begins his virulent attack on Thessalus, mixing ad hominem arguments with derisory remarks on his teaching, which compares so unfavorably with that of the ancients. The sustained polemic is peppered with literary allusions and references to previous luminaries in medicine and the natural sciences, as well as to other philosophers and logicians.

3. The attack on Thessalus now focuses on the issue of classification, particularly the gross oversimplification of dividing diseases into two major classes only (fluxion and obstruction), with a nebulous third class combining the two. Galen broadens the discussion to classification generally and again brings in, as his allies, his two most admired

philosophers, Plato and Aristotle, and others to aid him in his contemptuous dismissal of Thessalus.

4. This chapter completes the first salvo of the attack on Thessalus by examining the two ways of acquiring knowledge, reason and experience. In identifying the fundamental element in his system as the "communities," Thessalus (according to Galen) has used neither and is quite unable to demonstrate the existence or nature of his supposed "communities" in any satisfactory way.

5. Having dispatched the upstart Methodics, Galen now begins to establish the foundation of his own method of treatment. First, he defines the starting point, and second, he examines the key concepts on which the method is based, beginning with health and disease. A digression ensues on the issue of naming generally.

6. Consideration is given to some of the distinctions important in the theoretical basis of Galen's method: between functioning actively and being affected passively, between the different applications of the term "part" in relationship to the whole, and between *homoiomeres* and organs. The eye is used here, as elsewhere, as an example.

7. Starting from the axiom that nothing happens without a cause, Galen examines the nature of causation in diseases. In considering this, it needs to be clearly recognized that health and disease must fall within the same class. Thus, if health lies in functions that are in accord with nature, then disease must lie in functions that are contrary to nature. The same applies if health is defined as a condition that is in accord with nature. Galen embarks on a further attack on the Methodics, particularly Julianus, for their failure to define disease and to distinguish disease

from affection. The key point for Galen himself is that the conditions of bodies are the causes of diseases acting by impairing functions and so are the proper objects of treatment.

8. There is, however, a third class apart from conditions and functions, which is that of causes affecting conditions. When a disease is present because of damaged function consequent upon an altered condition, the cause responsible for the altered condition may be either still operative or no longer so. Galen makes the distinction between diseases and symptoms. The latter are due to changed conditions that are neutral in terms of function. A distinction is also made between internal and external antecedent causes.

9. After a further digression directed at Olympicus, Galen identifies the four things that exist in relation to the body which may or may not be in accord with nature: functions, constitutions/conditions, the things which precede the first two, and the things which are consequent upon them. Most of the chapter is, however, about the confusion of the Methodics regarding terms and definitions.

BOOK II

1. Galen lists those things that are contrary to nature (abnormal) in his conceptual scheme: damaged functions, conditions responsible for the damage, causes of the conditions, and the symptoms that follow them. Although there may be some doubt where "disease" is located in this scheme, this is not critical. What is critical is to apply treatment to eradicate the condition in the particular case.

Time should not be wasted on sterile terminological dispute. Nevertheless, agreement on terminology is necessary for effective communication of ideas and specifically for teaching.

2. Galen gives examples of the different ways in which diseases are named. This provides insight into apparent anomalies in nomenclature. He refers to his treatises on the differentiae of diseases and symptoms. These, he says, must be studied before the present treatise on treatment can be effectively utilized.

3. First Galen stresses the need to know the elemental composition of the body. Then he gives further description of those things that are contrary to nature (causes, diseases, and symptoms, in this case), providing examples of each and giving thought as to how they are to be distinguished.

4. To understand, categorize, and classify diseases, it is necessary to know what causes normal function and what disturbs it. Two examples are given—taste and touch. Arguments, even ridicule, are directed against the Methodics and Erasistrateans, as well as the Empirics to a lesser extent. Galen concludes by considering abnormalities in the balance of the four elemental qualities (*dyskrasias*), either singly or in combination, as causes of abnormal function, and the principles of restoration of normality by reestablishing the correct balance.

5. The bedrock of the Dogmatic or Rationalist tradition in medicine is the knowledge of its theoretical basis—the physical components of the body, functions, conditions, causes, etc. Of course, experience plays a role, but not to the exclusion of theory, as the Empirics claim. In addition,

demonstration and reasoned argument are essential. It is this theoretical foundation that is the starting point for devising and evaluating the various forms of treatment. The other schools are ridiculed for their failure to recognize this. The chapter ends with a further lamentation about present-day doctors, whom Galen thinks, in the majority of cases, are more concerned with wealth and reputation than the pursuit of truth.

6. Galen asserts that the first and essential step in establishing a rational method of medicine is to determine the total number of diseases and to classify them appropriately. This requirement is ignored by the other schools, particularly the Methodics. Galen refers especially to his four treatises on diseases and symptoms and the division therein of diseases into the *dyskrasias* of the *homoiomeres*, disorders of conformation, number, magnitude, and position of the organic parts, and dissolution of continuity—that is, six classes of diseases in all.

7. The method of medicine, and specifically of treatment, to be set out by Galen is based on indication (*endeixis*). This is a theoretical construct independent of experience. To discover cures for each of the diseases, it is necessary to know precisely what "disease" is. Before getting to the point, Galen embarks on a long digression about the distinction between what is one in form and what is one in number and how names are devised and applied in different circumstances. The argument is particularly directed against Themison. The purpose of the argument for Galen is to establish that the key concepts in his scheme, such as disease, condition, symptom, and affection, actually exist in bodies and can be related to indication.

BOOK III

1. Galen states that indication (*endeixis*) is the starting point for the discovery of cures for all diseases. However, it is only the starting point, and in many instances is known to laymen. What the doctor adds is knowledge of how to carry out what the indication indicates. According to Galen, this knowledge is acquired either by experience, which takes time, or by theory—there is no third path. In whatever way it is acquired, it also involves knowing what can and cannot be achieved by the measures available.

2. Galen considers first a wound in a fleshy part. A simple wound requires union; a wound with a cavity requires filling of the cavity plus union. How to achieve these objectives can only be known by either experience or reason; there is no other way, as Thessalus and his followers claim. Galen emphasizes this point in relation to enfleshing medications, particularly the compound medication cephalicum. Harmful treatments, especially oil in a wound with a cavity, are also considered, as are the different responses of different patients to the same medication. Some principles of the preparation of multicomponent medications are outlined. Both the Methodics and the Empirics come in for further criticism when their methods are compared to Galen's method of treatment.

3. The cure of hollow wounds (i.e., those with a cavity) is discussed. The two primary requirements for filling of the cavity are healthy (i.e., *eukratic*) underlying flesh and the inflow of blood in the right quantity and of the right quality. Problems arise if there are superfluities making the wound moist or filthy. Drying medications are needed to deal with thin superfluities and purifying medications to

deal with thick superfluities. Specific medications are considered.

4. The basic treatment of the uncomplicated wound without a cavity or skin loss is conglutination. Fleshy structures will maintain the union of their own accord; hard and dry structures need something to keep them together —e.g., encircling bandages, sutures, or fibulae. Drying medications may also be used. Wounds need to be dried, cleansed, and drawn together where possible. If there is a cavity, it needs to be filled with flesh. Some consideration is given to the nature of medications used in wound healing

5. Galen states that treatment of the wound with tissue loss needs regeneration of flesh, which in turn needs blood. The problem of regenerating skin is considered. Galen takes it to be impossible to regenerate skin as such, so the need arises to make the regenerated tissue sufficiently like skin to be able to perform the functions of skin. For this, there are medications that are drying and contracting. Some specific examples are considered.

6. The overgrowth of flesh in a wound or ulcer is considered. The therapeutic aim is removal of excess flesh, and the means are medications that are strongly drying. These are similar to the medications that are cleansing and scarinducing. Examples are given. Only those working by Galen's method are able to make the appropriate changes in treatment to meet different circumstances.

7. In contrast, the so-called method of the Methodics is lacking when it comes to deciding on the treatment for wounds, in particular because it doesn't take into account the nature of the affected part. According to Galen, treatment must also be tailored to the individual patient, espe-

cially their *krasis*. The Empiric has some awareness of this, albeit nontheoretical, whereas the Methodic has none.

8. The need to ensure that the underlying flesh is in good condition (i.e., *eukratic*) when attempting to heal a wound is stressed. Cleansing and removal of excess flesh can be achieved by medications alone. Other important factors are considered, such as the multiple potencies of some medications which can, in fact, be conflicting, the *krasis* of the surroundings, and the season. In addition, more moist natures require more moist medications, and so on.

9. In deciding on the treatment of a wound, the key factors are the *krasis* of the whole body, of the affected part, and of the ambient air, and the nature of the affected part. These may be in opposition to one another. Galen discusses how to deal with this and how to decide on the order of treatment if several factors are involved—e.g., an inflamed and contaminated wound with a cavity. The matter of treating the most dangerous condition first is considered.

10. A summary is given of the differentiae of wounds, with particular attention to differences of form, magnitude, and chronicity. Galen makes a plea for accurate terminology in describing a wound. He emphasizes that the chronicity of a wound per se indicates nothing specific. The need to establish an outflow for ichors from a wound is considered.

BOOK IV

1. Galen continues the discussion of dissolution of continuity as a class of diseases variously named according to

the part involved. He begins with some general remarks about simple and compound conditions. The causation of wounds and ulcers (*helkos*) and the basic requirements for their cure are considered. The importance of the underlying flesh being in a good state (*eukratic*) is emphasized.

2. How to treat abnormalities in the underlying flesh that will prejudice the treatment of the overlying wound or ulcer is outlined. The treatment of swellings associated with wounds or ulcers is described, as is the place of excision in facilitating healing. The need to prevent the flow of bad humors into the affected part and the need to reestablish balance in terms of the four qualities for healing to take place are both discussed.

3. According to Galen, the primary indication for treatment doesn't come from the *prokatarktic* (external antecedent) cause; it comes from the condition. Also, causes can't be treated if they are no longer operating. The distinction between therapy and prophylaxis is made. Empirics may take the *prokatarktic* cause as part of the syndrome and include it in considerations of treatment—an example is a scorpion sting. *Prokatarktic* causes do contribute to diagnosis. Galen criticizes the Empirics and stresses that *prokatarktic* causes have nothing to do with indications. The case of an ulcer arising from an abscess is considered. Further consideration is given to the distinction between therapy and prophylaxis.

4. Two long quotations from Thessalus on the treatment of *kakoethical* (chronic and intractable) ulcers are given. Thessalus' method of treatment comes under heavy criticism from Galen, not surprisingly. He berates Thessalus for taking chronicity as an indication. He then presents a very detailed criticism of Thessalus' approach to the di-

agnosis and management of wounds and ulcers. According to Galen, Thessalus is deeply ignorant of the use of medications in the treatment of ulcers. A hypothetical case of a *kakoethical* ulcer is considered. Galen returns to his own basic contention: the primary indication is taken from the condition. A criticism of Methodic terminology is offered.

5. Ulcers described as *kakoethical* are considered. The key features are chronicity and difficulty of cure. Chronicity is not, however, an indicator of treatment. It is a sign of the bad condition of the affected part and/or a generalized *kakochymia*. Chronicity is a sign, *kakochymia* is a condition, and evacuation is the treatment. He gives a series of quotations from Hippocrates on chronicity in wounds and ulcers. The possible role of varices is considered. The importance of purging the whole body is stressed. Measures are described for producing suppuration when this is desirable. The significance of associated bruising in regard to treatment is discussed, as is the place of incision. In summary, there is one general cure for wounds and ulcers, and there is no therapeutic indication to be taken from chronicity. According to Hippocrates, drying is the fundamental component of treatment for all wounds and ulcers. Further criticism is directed at Thessalus regarding the treatment of ulcers.

6. There is additional discussion of the Hippocratic teaching on the treatment of wounds and ulcers. In identifying the therapeutic indications, a key factor is the severity of the disease or condition. Galen considers the differing roles of phlebotomy and purging, as well as the specifics of purging in the treatment of wounds and ulcers. The distinction is made between the upper and lower body cavities (chest and abdomen) in relation to purging. The

Hippocratic position on phlebotomy in the treatment of chronic wounds and ulcers is defined—in particular, his recommendation to create a flow of blood from a recent wound as a way of preventing inflammation. A general statement on medications to draw away other humors is provided.

7. There is further discussion of the origins of the indications for treatment. The importance of the position and conformation of the affected part as indicative factors is stressed. Differences in the nature and timing of treatment for ulcers in the stomach and esophagus are considered. Some differences between internally and externally administered medications are identified. Various medications are described. The method of application of medications for ulcers of the mouth and pharynx is described, as are the particular features of medications for the trachea. The treatment of ruptures and ecchymoses is detailed.

ΓΑΛΗΝΟΥ ΘΕΡΑΠΕΥΤΙΚΗΣ
ΜΕΘΟΔΟΥ

METHOD OF MEDICINE

ΒΙΒΛΙΟΝ Α[1]

1Κ 1. Ἐπειδὴ καὶ σύ με πολλάκις, ὦ Ἱέρων[2] φίλτατε, καὶ
ἄλλοι τινὲς νῦν ἑταῖροι παρακαλοῦσι θεραπευτικὴν
μέθοδον αὐτοῖς γράψαι, ἐγὼ δὲ μάλιστα μὲν καὶ ὑμῖν
χαρίζεσθαι βουλόμενος, οὐχ ἥκιστα δὲ καὶ τοὺς μεθ᾽
ἡμᾶς ἀνθρώπους ὠφελῆσαι καθ᾽ ὅσον οἷός τέ εἰμι
προαιρούμενος, ὅμως ὤκνουν τε καὶ ἀνεβαλλόμην
ἑκάστοτε διὰ πολλὰς αἰτίας, ἄμεινον εἶναί μοι δοκεῖ
καὶ νῦν αὐτὰς διελθεῖν, πρὶν ἄρξασθαι τῆς πραγματείας, ἔχουσι γάρ τι χρήσιμον εἰς τὰ μέλλοντα ῥηθήσεσθαι.

2Κ   κεφάλαιον μὲν οὖν ἁπασῶν αὐτῶν ἐστι τὸ κιν-
δυνεῦσαι | μάτην γράψαι, μηδενὸς τῶν νῦν ἀνθρώπων
ὡς ἔπος εἰπεῖν ἀλήθειαν σπουδάζοντος, ἀλλὰ χρή-
ματά τε καὶ δυνάμεις πολιτικὰς καὶ ἀπλήστους ἡδο-
νῶν ἀπολαύσεις ἐζηλωκότων ἐς τοσοῦτον ὡς μαίνε-
σθαι νομίζειν εἴ τις ἄρα καὶ γένοιτο σοφίαν ἀσκῶν
ἡντιναοῦν. αὐτὴν μὲν γὰρ τὴν πρώτην καὶ ὄντως
σοφίαν, ἐπιστήμην οὖσαν θείων τε καὶ ἀνθρωπίνων
πραγμάτων, οὐδ᾽ εἶναι νομίζουσι τὸ παράπαν· ἰατρι-

---

[1] Κ; ΠΡΩΤΟΝ (om. ΒΙΒΛΙΟΝ) Β
[2] Ἱέρον Β

BOOK I

1. Since you, my dearest Hiero,[1] [have called upon me] 1K
many times, and now also certain other colleagues are calling upon me to write a method of medicine for them, and
since I especially wished to oblige you [all], and no less also
made a choice to help those who will come after us, as far
as I am able, but have, however, been hesitating and delaying each time for many reasons, it seems to me better to go
over these reasons now, before I begin the treatise, as they
do have some relevance to what is going to be said.

The chief reason of all is the risk of writing in vain, as al- 2K
most nobody nowadays is, one might say, eager for truth.
Instead, people strive after money, political power, and
an insatiable enjoyment of pleasures to such an extent
that they would consider someone mad if he were to gain
expertise in any area whatsoever. They think the truly primary form of wisdom, which is knowledge of matters
divine and human, doesn't exist at all. However, they do

[1] On Hiero, to whom the first six books are dedicated, V.
Nutton, in F. Kudlien and R. J. Durling (1991), p. 5, writes: "[He]
must then be assumed to have been an extremely competent medical practitioner, and we are told by Galen that he had a detailed
knowledge of anatomy and a long-standing and intimate acquaintance with Galen and other doctors."

3

κὴν δὲ καὶ γεωμετρίαν καὶ ῥητορικὴν ἀριθμητικήν τε
καὶ μουσικὴν ἁπάσας τε τὰς τοιαύτας τέχνας εἶναι
μὲν ὑπολαμβάνουσιν, οὐ μὴν ἐπί γε³ τὸ τέλος αὐτῶν
ἰέναι δικαιοῦσιν. ἀλλ' ἔμοιγε καὶ τῶν πάνυ δοκούντων
με φιλεῖν ἔνιοι πολλάκις ἐπετίμησαν ὡς πέρα τοῦ
μετρίου τὴν ἀλήθειαν σπουδάζοντι καὶ ὡς οὔτ' ἐμαυ-
τῷ⁴ μέλλοντι χρησίμῳ γενήσεσθαι παρ' ὅλον τὸν
βίον οὔτε ἐκείνοις, εἰ μὴ σχολάσαιμι μέν τι τῆς
τοσαύτης περὶ τὴν ἀλήθειαν σπουδῆς, προσαγορεύ-
οιμι δὲ περιερχόμενος ἔωθεν, εἰς ἑσπέραν τε συνδει-
πνοῖμι τοῖς δυναμένοις· ἐκ τούτων γὰρ καὶ φιλεῖσθαι
καὶ προσάγεσθαι καὶ τοὺς τεχνίτας πιστεύεσθαι,⁵ οὐκ
ἐκ τῆς οἰκείας παρασκευῆς· οὐδὲ γὰρ εἶναι τοὺς κρί-
3K νοντας | ἐκείνην, ἁπάντων δι' ὅλης ἡμέρας ἀσχολουμέ-
νων, ἔωθεν μὲν ἐν προσαγορεύσεσι κοινῇ, μετὰ ταῦτα
δ' ἤδη σχιζομένων, ἐπὶ μὲν τὴν ἀγορὰν καὶ τὰς δίκας
οὐ σμικροῦ τινος ἔθνους, ἐπὶ δ' αὖ τοὺς ὀρχηστάς τε
καὶ τοὺς ἡνιόχους ἑτέρου πλείονος, οὐκ ὀλίγου δέ
τινος ἄλλου τοῖς κύβοις, ἤ τισιν ἔρωσιν, ἢ λουτροῖς, ἢ
μέθαις, ἢ κώμοις σχολάζοντος, ἤ τισιν ἄλλαις ἡδο-
ναῖς τοῦ σώματος, ἐς ἑσπέραν δὲ κοινῇ πάντων αὖθις
συναθροιζομένων εἰς τὰ συμπόσια, κἀπειδὰν ἐμπλη-
σθῶσιν οἴνου, οὐ λύρας ἐν κύκλῳ περιφερομένης, ἢ
κιθάρας, ἤ τινος ἄλλου τῶν μουσικῶν ὀργάνων ὧν
ἅπτεσθαι πάλαι κατὰ τὰς τοιαύτας συνόδους καλὸν
ἐνενόμιστο καὶ δεινῶς αἰσχρὸν τοὐναντίον ἦν, ἀλλ'
οὐδὲ λόγων τινῶν ἀνακοινουμένων, οἵους ἐν τοῖς συμ-

4

accept that medicine, geometry, rhetoric, arithmetic, music, and all such arts do exist, but they don't think it worthwhile to pursue them, at least not to their fulfillment. But also, even some who seem particularly well-disposed toward me have often reproached me for having an excessive zeal for truth. [They say] that, throughout my whole life, I shall never be of use, either to myself or to them, unless I take some time off from such a pursuit for truth and go around greeting people in the early morning and dining with those who are powerful in the evening. It is [they say] from these activities that craftsmen are approved of, accepted and trusted. It is not from their particular attainment, for there are no judges of that because they are occupied for the whole day, spending the early mornings in salutations in public, and, after that, when they have already split up, a not inconsiderable crowd goes off to the forum and the law courts, another crowd, larger again, goes off to dances and chariot races, while another crowd, by no means small, spends its time in dicing, amorous adventures, bathing, drinking, carousing, or indulging in certain other pleasures of the body. However, when evening falls, they all come together again for symposia. There, when they have drunk their fill of wine, neither the lyre nor cithara, nor any of the other musical instruments is passed around in a circle—instruments which, in ancient times, were thought of as good to make use of at such gatherings (the opposite being taken as particularly shameful), nor do they put forward arguments such as occurred at the sym-

3K

---

3 γε om. B   4 οὔτ᾽ ἐμαυτῷ B; οὔθ᾽ ἑαυτῷ K

5 καὶ φιλεῖσθαι τοὺς τεχνίτας B (om. καὶ προσάγεσθαι καὶ πιστεύεσθαι)

ποσίοις συνέγραψαν ἡμῖν οἱ παλαιοὶ γινομένους, ἀλλ᾽
οὐδ᾽ ἄλλου τῶν καλῶν οὐδενός, ἀλλὰ προπινόντων μὲν
ἀλλήλοις, ἀμιλλωμένων δὲ περὶ μεγέθους ἐκπωμάτων.
ἄριστος γὰρ ἐν τούτοις οὐχ ὁ πλείστων ἁψάμενος
ὀργάνων μουσικῶν ἢ λόγων φιλοσόφων, ἀλλ᾽ ὁ παμ-
πόλλας καὶ μεγίστας ἐκπιὼν κύλικας·

4K   ὥστ᾽ ἔμοιγε καὶ περὶ τὴν ἕω | δοκοῦσιν ἔτι μεθύειν
οἱ πολλοὶ τῶν τοιούτων, καί τινες αὐτῶν ὄζουσιν οἴνου
σαφῶς οὕτως ὡς ἄρτι προσενηνεγμένοι. ὥστ᾽ εἰκότως,
ἐπειδὰν νοσεῖν ὑπάρξωνται, μετακαλοῦνται τῶν ἰατρῶν[6] οὐ τοὺς ἀρίστους, οὕς γε μηδὲ πώποτε κρῖναι
προὐθυμήθησαν ὑγιαίνοντες, ἀλλὰ τοὺς συνηθεστά-
τους τε ἅμα καὶ κολακευτικωτάτους, οἳ καὶ ψυχρὸν
δώσουσιν, ἢν αἰτηθῶσι, καὶ λούσουσιν, ἢν κελευ-
σθῶσι, καὶ χιόνα καὶ οἶνον ὀρέξουσι καὶ πᾶν ὑπ-
ηρετήσουσι τὸ προσταττόμενον ὥσπερ ἀνδράποδα,
ἔμπαλιν ἐκείνοις τῶν ἰατρῶν τοῖς παλαιοῖς Ἀσκληπιάδαις, οἳ τῶν νοσούντων ἠξίουν ἄρχειν ὡς στρατηγοὶ
στρατηγουμένων καὶ βασιλεῖς ὑπηκόων, οὐκ ἄρχεσθαι καὶ δεσπόζεσθαι, καθάπερ Γέται καὶ[7] Τίβιοι καὶ
Φρύγες καὶ Θρᾷκες ἀργυρώνητοι. οὔκουν οὐχ ὁ κρείτ-
των τὴν τέχνην, ἀλλ᾽ ὁ κολακεύειν δεινότερος ἐντι-
μότερος αὐτοῖς ἐστι, καὶ τούτῳ ἅπαντα βάσιμα καὶ
πόριμα, καὶ τῶν οἰκιῶν ἀνεῴγασιν αἱ θύραι τῷ τοιούτῳ, καὶ πλουτεῖ τε ταχέως οὗτος καὶ πολὺ δύναται,
καὶ μαθητὰς ἔχει τοὺς ἐκ κοιτῶνος καλοὺς[8] ὅταν
ἔξωροι γένωνται.

posia which the ancients recorded for us, nor do they do anything else noble. Instead, they drink toasts to one another, competing over the size of their drafts. For the best among them is not the one who plays most musical instruments or engages in most philosophical arguments, but the one who quaffs the most and the biggest bowls of wine.

So to me, at least, the majority of such men still seem drunk around dawn, and some of them smell so clearly of wine it is as if they had just now been plying themselves with it. As a result, when they become sick, naturally they do not call in the best doctors, whom they never showed themselves eager to pick out when they were healthy. Instead they choose those doctors to whom they are most accustomed and who are, at the same time, those most inclined to flattery. These doctors will give them cold water if they ask for it, and will bathe them if they demand it, and set out snow and wine, and will comply with every order, like slaves—quite the opposite to those Aclepiadian doctors of ancient times who thought it right to rule the sick, like generals rule armies and kings rule subjects rather than be ruled and dominated like Getae, Tibians, Phrygians, or Thracians who are bought with silver. Thus it is not the man who is better at the craft [of medicine] but the man who is cleverer at flattery who is more honored among them. For him, everything is accessible and provided; the doors of houses stand open to such a man. He quickly becomes rich and very powerful, and has pretty boys from the bedchamber as his students when they become too old.

4K

---

6 τῶν ἰατρῶν om. B, recte fort.

7 Γέται καί om. B

8 B, Pl; πολλούς, K

5K   καὶ τοῦτο κατανοήσας ὁ Θεσσαλὸς | ἐκεῖνος οὐ τὰ
ἄλλα μόνον ἐκολάκευε τοὺς ἐπὶ τῆς Ῥώμης πλου-
σίους, ἀλλὰ καὶ τῷ μησὶν ἐξ ἐπαγγείλασθαι διδάξειν
τὴν τέχνην ἑτοίμως ἐλάμβανε μαθητὰς παμπόλλους.
εἰ γὰρ οὔτε γεωμετρίας οὔτε ἀστρονομίας οὔτε διαλεκτικῆς οὔτε μουσικῆς οὔτε⁹ ἄλλου τινὸς μαθήματος
τῶν καλῶν οἱ μέλλοντες ἰατροὶ γενήσεσθαι δέονται,
καθάπερ ὁ γενναιότατος ἐπηγγείλατο Θεσσαλός, ἀλλ᾽
οὐδὲ μακρᾶς ἐμπειρίας χρήζουσι καὶ συνηθείας τῶν
ἔργων τῆς τέχνης, ἕτοιμον ἤδη προσιέναι παντὶ τῷ¹⁰
γενησομένῳ ῥᾳδίως ἰατρῷ. διὰ τοῦτο καὶ σκυτοτόμοι
καὶ τέκτονες καὶ βαφεῖς καὶ χαλκεῖς ἐπιπηδῶσιν ἤδη
τοῖς ἔργοις τῆς ἰατρικῆς, τὰς ἀρχαίας αὐτῶν ἀπο-
λιπόντες τέχνας. οἱ μὲν γὰρ τὸν ῥῶπον διατιθέμενοι
καὶ περὶ πρωτείων ἐρίζουσι. καὶ διὰ τοῦτο κἀγὼ γρά-
φειν ὤκνουν θεραπευτικὴν μέθοδον, ἣν εἰσηγήσαντο
μὲν ἄνδρες παλαιοί, τελειῶσαι δ᾽ ἐπεχείρησαν οἱ μετ᾽
αὐτούς.

    καὶ πρόσθεν μὲν ἔρις ἦν οὐ σμικρά, νικῆσαι τῷ
πλήθει τῶν εὑρημάτων ἀλλήλους ὀριγνωμένων τῶν ἐν
Κῷ καὶ Κνίδῳ· διττὸν γὰρ ἔτι τοῦτο τὸ γένος ἦν τῶν
6K ἐπὶ | τῆς Ἀσίας Ἀσκληπιαδῶν, ἐπιλιπόντος τοῦ κατὰ
Ῥόδον· ἤριζον δ᾽ αὐτοῖς τὴν ἀγαθὴν ἔριν ἐκείνην, ἣν
Ἡσίοδος ἐπήνει καὶ οἱ ἐκ τῆς Ἰταλίας ἰατροί, Φιλι-

---

⁹ μουσικῆς οὔτε *om.* B
¹⁰ τῷ B; *om.* K

Because that man Thessalus[2] recognized this, he not 5K
only used to flatter the rich in Rome in various ways but
also, by promising to teach the craft in six months, readily
attracted a great number of students. For if those who
would become doctors have no need of geometry, astronomy, dialectic, music, or any of the other noble disciplines,
as the most high-minded Thessalus proclaimed, and further, if they have no need of extensive experience in, or familiarity with, the practices of the craft, there is now a
ready way forward for anyone who wants to become a doctor easily. Because of this, cobblers, carpenters, dyers, and
blacksmiths may now leap into the practices of medicine,
forsaking their own original crafts. And these men, when
they have displayed their meagre talents, also contend for
preeminence. This is why I myself have been hesitant to
write about a method of medical treatment—a method
which the ancients introduced, and which those who came
after them have tried to bring to completion.

In past times, too, there was no little contention as
those in Cos and Cnidus strove to prevail over each other
in the number of their discoveries. There were still two
groups of Asclepiads in Asia, even when the one on Rhodes 6K
had failed.[3] And the Italian doctors, Philistion, Empedo-

---

2 Thessalus, fl. first century AD, is the main target of Galen's
vituperation throughout the work but particularly in this first
book. He may be taken as having established the Methodic sect.

3 Galen accepts the orthodox view of two founding schools of
medicine in the Aegean in the fifth century BC. There is no real
information on a further, distinct school at Rhodes.

στίων τε καὶ Ἐμπεδοκλῆς καὶ Παυσανίας καὶ οἱ τούτων ἑταῖροι· καὶ τρεῖς οὗτοι χοροὶ θαυμαστοὶ πρὸς
ἀλλήλους ἁμιλλωμένων ἐγένοντο ἰατρῶν· πλείστους
μὲν οὖν καὶ ἀρίστους χορευτὰς ὁ Κῷος εὐτυχήσας
εἶχεν, ἐγγὺς δ' ἔτι τούτου¹¹ καὶ ὁ ἀπὸ τῆς Κνίδου,
λόγου δ' ἦν ἄξιος οὐ σμικροῦ καὶ ὁ ἀπὸ τῆς Ἰταλίας.
ἀλλ' οὐδεὶς τούτων οὔτε ἔωθεν ἐπὶ τὰς τῶν πλουσίων
ἐφοίτα θύρας προσαγορεύσων αὐτοὺς οὔτ' εἰς ἑσπέραν δειπνησόμενος, ἀλλ' ὥσπερ Ἡσίοδος φησιν,¹²

Εἰς ἕτερον γάρ τίς τε ἰδὼν ἔργοιο χατίζει¹³
πλούσιον, ὃς σπεύδει μὲν ἀρόμμεναι ἠδὲ
    φυτεύειν,

οὕτω κἀκεῖνοι διὰ παντὸς ἤριζον ἀλλήλοις οὐκ
ἀροῦν ἢ φυτεύειν γῆν, σμικρότερα γὰρ ταῦτα τοῦ τῶν
Ἀσκληπιαδῶν γένους καὶ Ἀσκραίῳ πρέποντα ποιη-
τῇ, ἀλλ' ἀσκεῖν καὶ αὔξειν ἀεὶ¹⁴ καὶ τελειοῦν πει-
7K ρᾶσθαι τὴν Ἀπόλλωνός τε καὶ Ἀσκληπιοῦ | τέχνην.
νυνὶ δ' ἀπόλωλε μὲν ἡ ἀγαθὴ ἔρις, ἢ σμικρὸν ἔτι καὶ
ἀμυδρὸν αὐτῆς ἐν ἀνθρώποις ἐστίν· ἐπικρατεῖ δ' ἡ
πονηρὰ καὶ ὁ ἀποτρέψων οὐδεὶς οὐδ' ὁ ἰασόμενος,
ὥσπερ Ἡσίοδος,

Μηδέ σ' Ἔρις κακόχαρτος ἀπ' ἔργου θυμὸν
    ἐρύκοι.

¹¹ B; τούτῳ K   ¹² K; ἐποίησεν B, P1, P2
¹³ B; χατίζων K   ¹⁴ ἀεί om. B

10

cles, Pausanias and their colleagues[4] contended with them also in that noble kind of rivalry which Hesiod praised. So there were these three admirable troupes of doctors vying with each other. The Coan [school] achieved success by having the greatest number of pupils and the most able, but the [school] from Cnidus was not far behind it, while that from Italy was worthy of no little regard. But none of these frequented the doors of the rich, either to greet them in the early morning, or to dine with them in the evening. Rather, as Hesiod says,

> For someone who is in need of work looks to another, a rich man, who is eager to plow and plant.[5]

And so those men were continually contending with each other, not to plow or sow the earth, for these things are too trivial for Asclepiads although suitable for the Ascraean poet, but to practice, constantly strengthen, and try to bring to perfection the craft of Apollo and Asclepius. Nowadays, however, noble rivalry has perished, or rather 7K only a small and faint part of it still exists among men. Worthless contention is dominant and there is nobody who will avert or remedy it. As Hesiod [says]:

> Do not let Strife, rejoicing in evil, curb your will to work.[6]

---

[4] Philiston: a contemporary of Plato and teacher of Eudoxus. None of his original writings survive. Empedocles (ca. 492–432 BC) was from Acragas in Sicily. He is renowned primarily as a philosopher, although he is also regarded by some as the founder of the Sicilian school of medicine. Pausanias was a pupil of Empedocles.   [5] *Works and Days* 21–22.   [6] *Works and Days* 28.

11

GALEN

αὕτη γὰρ ἡ Ἔρις, ὡς ὁ θειότερος αὖ πάλιν Ἡσιόδου
ποιητής φησιν·[15]

Ἡ δ᾽ ὀλίγη μὲν πρῶτα κορύσσεται, αὐτὰρ ἔπειτα
οὐρανῷ ἐστήριξε κάρη, καὶ ἐπὶ χθονὶ βαίνει.

2. Ὑπὸ ταύτης τῆς ἔριδος ἐκμανεὶς ὁ Θεσσαλὸς
ἐκεῖνος Ἱπποκράτει τε καὶ τοῖς ἄλλοις Ἀσκληπιάδαις
ἐπιτιμᾷ, καὶ κοινὸν τῆς οἰκουμένης θέατρον ἐν ταῖς
ἑαυτοῦ βίβλοις πληρῶν, ἐπ᾽ ἐκείνου κρίνεται καὶ νικᾷ
καὶ στεφανοῦται κατὰ τῶν παλαιῶν ἁπάντων, ἀνακη-
ρυττόμενος αὐτὸς ὑφ᾽ ἑαυτοῦ. ταυτὶ μὲν οὖν ἔν τε τῷ
Περὶ τῶν κοινοτήτων ἐποίησε κἂν Τοῖς συγκριτικοῖς,
ἐν ἅπασι δὲ τοῖς ἄλλοις ὑβρίζων οὐ παύεται, καθάπερ,
8K   οἶμαι, καὶ δι᾽ ὧν ἐπιστέλλει Νέρωνι, | κατ᾽ ἀρχὰς μὲν
εὐθέως γράφων αὐτοῖς ὀνόμασιν οὕτως·

Παραδεδωκὼς νέαν αἵρεσιν καὶ ὡς μόνην ἀληθῆ
διὰ τὸ τοὺς προγενεστέρους πάντας ἰατροὺς
μηδὲν παραδοῦναι συμφέρον πρός τε ὑγείας
συντήρησιν καὶ νόσων ἀπαλλαγήν.

ἐπὶ προήκοντι δὲ τῷ γράμματι προϊών φησιν ὡς
Ἱπποκράτης μὲν ἐπιβλαβῆ τὴν παράδοσιν πεποίηται,
ἐτόλμησε δὲ καὶ τοῖς Ἀφορισμοῖς ἀντιλέγειν, ἀσχη-
μοσύνην ἀσχημονήσας μεγίστην, καὶ δείξας ὅτι μηδ᾽
εἰσήχθη πρός τινος εἰς τὴν Ἱπποκράτειον θεωρίαν
μηδ᾽ ἀνέγνω παρὰ διδασκάλου[16] τὰ συγγράμματα

15 φησιν om. B
16 διδασκάλων B

12

For on this Strife, as the poet even more divine than Hesiod says:

> At first she armed herself only slightly, but then,
> raising her head to the heavens, trampled the earth.[7]

2. Driven mad by this contention, that Thessalus criticizes Hippocrates and the other Asclepiads and, filling the general stage of the inhabited world with his books, he is judged against that man, and conquers. He is crowned over all the ancients, and proclaims himself champion. He did this very thing, then, in the works *On Communities* and *On Comparisons*.[8] Nor does he stop committing outrages in all the other works, like, I suggest, through those [writings] he sent to Nero when he starts right away with these very words:

8K

> I have established a new sect and, as all doctors who came before passed on nothing useful regarding either the preservation of health or the relief of disease, it is the only true sect.[9]

As he proceeds in the letter, he says that Hippocrates had created a tradition that was harmful. He even dared to criticize the *Aphorisms*, and so brought the greatest disgrace on himself, and showed that he had neither been introduced by anyone to the Hippocratic theory, nor had he read his writings with a teacher. Nevertheless, such a man

---

7 *Iliad* 4.442–43.

8 None of Thessalus' writings are extant. We are mainly reliant on the notably antagonistic Galen for information about him.

9 This is taken to be a direct quotation following Linacre, although no reference is given and no source is extant.

αὐτοῦ· καὶ ὅμως ὁ τοιοῦτος ἑαυτὸν οὐκ αἰδεῖται στεφανῶν. διό μοι δοκῶ κἀγώ, καίτοι γε οὐκ εἰθισμένος ἐξελέγχειν πικρῶς τοὺς σκαιούς, ἐρεῖν τι πρὸς αὐτὸν ὑπὲρ τῆς τῶν παλαιῶν ὕβρεως.

τί πειρᾷ διαβάλλειν ὦ οὗτος τὰ χρηστὰ διὰ τὸ παρὰ τοῖς πολλοῖς εὐδοκιμεῖν, ἐνὸν ὑπερβάλλεσθαι τοῖς ἀληθέσιν, εἰ φιλόπονός τέ τις εἴης καὶ ἀληθείας ἐραστής; τί δὲ τῇ τῶν ἀκροατῶν ἀμαθίᾳ συμμάχῳ κέχρησαι κατὰ τῆς τῶν παλαιῶν βλασφημίας; μὴ τοὺς ὁμοτέχνους τῷ πατρί σου κριτὰς καθίσῃς ἰα-
9K τρῶν, τολμηρότατε Θεσσαλέ· νικήσεις | γὰρ ἐπ᾽ αὐτοῖς[17] καὶ καθ᾽ Ἱπποκράτους λέγων καὶ κατὰ Διοκλέους καὶ κατὰ Πραξαγόρου καὶ κατὰ πάντων τῶν ἄλλων παλαιῶν, ἀλλ᾽ ἄνδρας παλαιούς,[18] διαλεκτικούς, ἐπιστημονικούς, ἀληθὲς καὶ ψευδὲς διακρίνειν ἠσκηκότας, ἀκόλουθον καὶ μαχόμενον ὡς χρὴ διορίζειν[19] ἐπισταμένους, ἀποδεικτικὴν μέθοδον ἐκ παίδων μεμελετηκότας, τούτους εἰς τὸ συνέδριον εἰσάγαγε δικαστάς, ἐπὶ τούτων τόλμησον Ἱπποκράτει τι μέμψασθαι, τούτων κρινόντων ἐπιχείρησόν τι τῇ μιαρᾷ καὶ βαρβάρῳ σου[20] φωνῇ πρὸς Ἱπποκράτην διελθεῖν, πρῶτον μὲν ὡς οὐ χρὴ φύσιν ἀνθρώπου πολυπραγμονεῖν· ἔπειτα δὲ ὡς εἰ καὶ τοῦτο συγχωρήσειέ τις, ἀλλ᾽ ὅτι γε κακῶς αὐτὴν ἐζήτησεν ἐκεῖνος καὶ ψευδῶς ἀπεφήνατο σύμπαντα.

[17] νικήσεις γὰρ ἐπ᾽ αὐτοῖς K (ἐν pro ἐπ᾽ B); καὶ γὰρ αὐτοὺς κρίτας χρώμενος νικήσας γὰρ ἐν αὐτοῖς P1, P2; καὶ γὰρ

feels no shame when he awards himself the crown. Accordingly, I think it falls to me to say something to him regarding his insolence toward the ancients, although it is certainly not my custom to refute harshly those who are foolish.

Why, my man, do you try to discredit those things that are good in order to be thought well of by the multitude, when it is possible to excel in those things that are true, if you are diligent and love the truth? Why do you make use of the ignorance of your listeners as an ally in the slander of the ancients? Do not, most brazen Thessalus, appoint your father's fellow craftsmen as judges of doctors. With these 9K men you will, indeed, triumph when you speak against Hippocrates, Diocles, Praxagoras, and all the other ancients. Bring, rather, to the seat of judgment the men of old—men who were skilled in dialectic and capable of knowledge, who were practiced in distinguishing truth and falsehood, who knew how to differentiate consequence and contradiction as they ought, and men who had given careful attention to the demonstrative method from childhood. Dare to find some fault with Hippocrates in front of them. Attempt, with your uncouth and barbaric voice, to proceed against Hippocrates when those men are in judgment, first, on the grounds that man should not busy himself about the nature of man, and next, on the grounds that, even if he were to concede that he should, Hippocrates had sought it in the wrong way and had, in fact, spoken altogether falsely.

---

aëtoêv ὄv krÉtav xrómenov nikÔsav Ᾱp‰ aëtoÍv *conj.* Hankinson

18 ἄνδρας ἰατροὺς παλαιούς B

19 γνωρίζειν B   20 σου *om.* B

τίς οὖν ἔσται κριτής; εἰ βούλει, Πλάτων, ἐπειδὴ
τοῦτον γοῦν οὐκ ἐτόλμησας λοιδορεῖν. ἐγὼ μὲν γὰρ
οὐδὲ τοὺς μαθητὰς αὐτοῦ φύγοιμ᾽ ἄν, οὔτε τὸν Σπεύ-
σιππον οὔτε τὸν Ξενοκράτην· τὸν Ἀριστοτέλην δὲ κἂν
παρακαλέσαιμί σε κριτὴν ὑπομεῖναι καὶ σὺν αὐτῷ
Θεόφραστον· εὐξαίμην δ᾽ ἄν σε καὶ Ζήνωνα καὶ Χρύ-
σιππον ἅπαντάς τε τοὺς ἀπ᾽ αὐτῶν ἑλέσθαι κριτάς. |
10K   οὐδεὶς τούτων, ὦ τολμηρότατε Θεσσαλέ, τῶν Ἱπποκράτους κατέγνω περὶ φύσεως ἀνθρώπου δογμάτων, ἃ
τὴν ἀρχὴν οὔτ᾽ ἀνεγνωκέναι μοι δοκεῖς οὔτ᾽, εἴπερ
ἀνέγνως, συνιέναι· καὶ εἰ συνῆκας δέ, κρῖναι γοῦν
ἀδύνατον ἦν σοι, τραφέντι μὲν ἐν γυναικωνίτιδι παρὰ
πατρὶ μοχθηρῶς ἔρια ξαίνοντι. μὴ γὰρ ἀγνοεῖσθαί
μοι δόκει τὸ θαυμαστόν σου γένος καὶ τὴν ἀοίδιμόν
σου παιδείαν, μηδ᾽ ὡς ἐν κωφῷ θεάτρῳ λοιδορεῖν
Ἱπποκράτην τε καὶ τοὺς ἄλλους παλαιούς· ἀλλὰ τίς
ὢν καὶ πόθεν, ἐκ ποίου γένους, ἐκ ποίας ἀνατροφῆς, ἐκ
ποίας παιδεύσεως, ἐπίδειξον πρότερον, εἶθ᾽ οὕτως
λέγε, τοῦτ᾽ αὐτὸ πρῶτον μαθών, ὦ θρασύτατε, ὅτι
λέγειν οὐκ ἐφεῖται πᾶσι δημοσίᾳ ἐν οὐδεμιᾷ τῶν
εὐνομουμένων πόλεων, ἀλλ᾽ εἴ τις ἐπίσημός ἐστι καὶ
γένος ἔχει καὶ ἀνατροφὴν δεῖξαι καὶ παιδείαν ἀξίαν
τοῦ δημηγορεῖν, τούτῳ συγχωροῦσιν ἀγορεύειν οἱ
νόμοι· σὺ δ᾽ οὐδὲν τούτων ἔχων ἐπιδεῖξαι τολμᾷς ὦ
γενναιότατε κατηγορεῖν Ἱπποκράτους, καὶ καθίζεις
μὲν ἐν ταῖς ληρώδεσί σου βίβλοις δικαστὰς τοὺς
Ἕλληνας, ἀποφαίνῃ δ᾽ αὐτὸς οὐκ ἀναμείνας ἐκείνους
11K   καὶ στεφανοῖς σεαυτόν, ἐνίοτε μὲν κατὰ πάντων | τῶν

Who, then, will be a judge? Plato, if you wish, since at least you have not dared to revile him. Nor would I shun those who were his pupils, Speusippus and Xenocrates. And I would call upon you to submit to Aristotle as judge, and Theophrastus with him. I would pray for you to choose both Zeno and Chrysippus as judges, and all those who were their followers. None of these men, most audacious 10K Thessalus, condemned the teachings of Hippocrates on the nature of man which, to begin with, you do not seem to me either to have read or, if you have read them, to have understood. And if you did understand them it would, at the very least, be impossible for you to judge them since you are someone brought up in women's quarters with a father who, in his sorry plight, carded wool. Don't, I tell you, make it seem that your wondrous family or your famous education are unknown, or that you revile Hippocrates and the other ancients, as in a theater of the deaf, but first reveal who you are and where you are from; that is, from what kind of family, with what kind of upbringing, and with what kind of education, and then speak like this, having realized first, my overweening friend, that it is not permitted to everyone to speak publicly in any of the well-ordered cities. Only to the man who is outstanding and shows he has a family, upbringing, and education worthy of speaking in the assembly do the laws grant the right to speak in public. But you, my most noble fellow, who can show none of these things, dare to accuse Hippocrates and in your ridiculous books you place the Greeks as judges, yet you obviously do not wait for them but award yourself the crown, sometimes over all doctors and sometimes simply 11K

17

ἰατρῶν, ἐνίοτε δὲ κατὰ πάντων ἁπλῶς Ἑλλήνων. τοῦτο
γάρτοι τὸ θαυμαστόν ἐστι τόλμημα τοῦ σοφωτάτου
Θεσσαλοῦ, νικῆσαι μὲν ἅπαντας ἰατρούς, αὐτὸν ἀγω-
νιστήν, αὐτὸν ἀγωνοθέτην, αὐτὸν κριτὴν γενόμενον·
ἐφεξῆς δὲ καὶ τοὺς ἄλλους Ἕλληνας εἰς ἀγῶνα
προσκαλέσασθαι, ῥήτορας, γεωμέτρας, γραμματι-
κούς, ἀστρονόμους, φιλοσόφους, εἶτ᾽ ἐν αὐτοῖς κατα-
στάντα, καὶ τῇ τῶν ἐριουργῶν ἑρμηνείᾳ χρησάμενον,
ἀξιοῦν ἁπάντων εἶναι πρῶτον· ἰατρικὴν μὲν γὰρ ἁπασῶν τῶν τεχνῶν πρωτεύειν, ἑαυτὸν δὲ τοὺς ἰατροὺς
ἅπαντας νενικηκέναι. τοῦτο μόνον ἐκ τύχης ἀληθῶς
συνελογίσατο Θεσσαλός· εἰ γὰρ ἰατρικὴ μὲν ἀπασῶν
ἐστι τῶν τεχνῶν ἀρίστη, πρῶτος δ᾽ ἐν αὐτῇ Θεσσαλός, εἴη ἂν οὕτω γε πάντων ἀνθρώπων πρῶτος καὶ
Σωκράτους δηλονότι καὶ Λυκούργου καὶ τῶν ἄλλων,
οὓς ὁ Πύθιος ἐπήνεσεν ἢ ὡς ἀγαθούς, ἢ ὡς σοφούς, ἢ
ὡς Μουσῶν θεράποντας, ἢ ὡς Διὸς ὑπηρέτας, ἢ ὡς
ἄλλο τι θεοφιλὲς ἔχοντας.

ἄγε δὴ λοιπὸν ὕμνους ᾀδόντων ἅπαντες Θεσσαλοῦ,
καὶ γραφόντων ἐπινίκια μέλη, καὶ κοινὸν τῆς οἰκουμένης τὸ θέατρον γενέσθω, καὶ παρελθὼν ᾀδέτω τις
ὡς παρὰ τοῖς | ἱστοῖς τραφεὶς ἐνίκησε μὲν Δημοσθέ-
νην καὶ Λυσίαν καὶ τοὺς ἄλλους ῥήτορας, ἐνίκησε δὲ
Πλάτωνα καὶ Σωκράτην καὶ τοὺς ἄλλους φιλοσόφους,
ἐνίκησε δὲ καὶ Λυκοῦργον καὶ Σόλωνα καὶ τοὺς ἄλλους νομοθέτας, ἐστεφάνωται δὲ κοινῇ κατὰ πάντων
ἀνθρώπων, ῥητόρων, φιλοσόφων, νομοθετῶν. εἰ γὰρ
δὴ γεωμετρῶν ἔτι καὶ γραμματικῶν καὶ μουσικῶν

12K

18

over all Greeks. For surely it is amazing effrontery on the part of the surpassingly sapient Thessalus, to overcome all doctors by making himself competitor, organizer and judge. And then, too, he calls other Greeks to the contest—rhetoricians, geometricians, grammarians, astronomers and philosophers—and standing among them and speaking in the style of wool workers, he deems himself worthy of being first among all of them since he places medicine first of all the arts, and he judges himself to have vanquished all doctors. On the first point only does Thessalus reason correctly, but quite by chance. For if medicine is the most noble of all the arts and Thessalus is the most noble of its practitioners, he would, in this way, be first of all men and obviously greater than Socrates, Lycurgus and the others, or those whom the Pythian praised as noble, or wise, or attendants of the Muses, or servants of Zeus, or possessing in any other way favor from the gods.

Well then, let everyone sing victory songs about Thessalus. Let them write epinician lyrics, and let the theater of the civilized world be his public. Let someone come forward to sing of how he, Thessalus, reared beside the 12K looms, overcame Demosthenes, Lysias and the other orators, overcame Plato, Socrates and the other philosophers, overcame Lycurgus, Solon and the other lawmakers, and has been crowned publicly over all men—orators, philosophers and lawmakers. If I were to mention by name geometricians, as well as grammarians and musicians after

ὀνομαστὶ μνημονεύοιμι μετὰ τὰς τηλικαύτας νίκας,
ὑβρίζειν δόξω τὸν ἄνθρωπον· ὅπου γὰρ Λυκοῦργος
καὶ Σόλων καὶ Πλάτων καὶ Σωκράτης καὶ Πυθαγόρας
ἐνικήθησαν, ἦπου ἄρα καλὸν ἔτι μνημονεύειν Ἱππάρ-
χου καὶ Ἀρχιμήδους καὶ Ἀριστοξένου καὶ Ἀριστάρ-
χου καί τινων ἑτέρων τοιούτων οὐδενὸς ἀξίων, ὡς ἂν
εἴποι Θεσσαλός; ἀλλὰ τίς ἡμῖν οὕτω μεγαλόφωνος
ποιητὴς ὃς ᾄσεται ταῦτα; τίνος Ὁμήρου νῦν εὐπορή-
σομεν ἐν ἑξαμέτρῳ τόνῳ τὴν Θεσσάλειον ὑμνήσοντος
νίκην; ἢ τίνος μελοποιοῦ κατὰ Πίνδαρον ᾄσοντος
ὑψηλῶς ἐν διθυράμβοις ὡς πάλαι τὸν Διόνυσον, οὕτως
νῦν τὸν Θεσσαλόν; ἢ τούτων μὲν οὐδενὸς χρῄζομεν,
13K   Ἀρχιλόχου δέ | τινος ἢ Ἱππώνακτος ἰάμβους γραφόν-
των, ἤ τινος τῶν ἀπὸ τῆς τραγικῆς σκηνῆς, ὃς ἐρεῖ
πρὸς αὐτόν·

Μέν᾽ ὦ ταλαίπωρ᾽ ἀτρέμα σοῖς ἐν δεμνίοις,
ὁρᾷς γὰρ οὐδὲν ὧν δοκεῖς σάφ᾽ εἰδέναι.

ὄνειρον Ὀρέστειον διηγῇ Θεσσαλέ. ὅποι[21] τοῦτο τὸ
θέατρον, ἐν ᾧ νικᾷς Ἱπποκράτην; τίνες οἱ κριταὶ
καθεδοῦνται; τίνες οἱ ἀγωνοθετοῦντες; ἆρα βούλει
πρῶτον Πλάτωνος ἀναγνῶμεν τὴν ψῆφον; ἴσως γὰρ
οὐκ ἀναίνῃ τοιοῦτον ἑλέσθαι κριτήν· ἀλλά τοί φησιν
οὗτος αὐτοῖς ὀνόμασι·

[21] B; οἷον K

such victories, I shall seem to insult the man. For where Lycurgus, Solon, Plato, Socrates, and Pythagoras have been conquered, is it then still a good thing to mention Hipparchus, Archimedes, Aristoxenus, and Aristarchus and certain other such men who are entirely worthless, according to Thessalus? But which of us is so grandiloquent a poet that he might sing to us of these things? What Homer shall we find available now to hymn the victory of Thessalus in hexameters? Or what lyric poet, who will sing now of Thessalus in this way as, in ancient times, Pindar sang sublimely of Dionysus in dithyrambs? Or is it none of these men we need, but rather an Archilochus or Hipponax writing iambics, or one of those from the tragic stage who will say to him:

13K

> Rest quiet in your bed, miserable one,
> for you see none of the things you think you know
>   clearly.[10]

You describe an Orestian dream, Thessalus. Where is this theater in which you vanquish Hippocrates? Who are the judges who will be sitting? Who are those presiding at the contest? Do you wish us to recognize the vote of Plato first? Perhaps you do not refuse to select such a man as judge. But surely he says in these very words:[11]

---

10 Euripides, *Orestes* 258–59.

11 See *Phaedrus* 270C–D. There are some minor textual variations between the text as it appears in Plato and that given by Galen.

Ψυχῆς οὖν φύσιν ἀξίως λόγου κατανοῆσαι οἴει
δυνατὸν εἶναι ἄνευ τῆς τοῦ ὅλου φύσεως;
Εἰ μὲν Ἱπποκράτει τῷ τῶν Ἀσκληπιαδῶν δεῖ τι
πείθεσθαι, οὐδὲ περὶ σώματος, ἄνευ τῆς
μεθόδου ταύτης.

Καλῶς γὰρ, ὦ ἑταῖρε, λέγεις· χρὴ μὲν πρὸς τῷ
Ἱπποκράτει τὸν λόγον ἐξετάζοντας σκοπεῖν εἰ
συμφωνεῖ.

Φημί.

Τῷ τοίνυν περὶ φύσεως σκοπεῖν τί ποτε λέγει
Ἱπποκράτης τε καὶ ὁ ἀληθὴς λόγος; ἆρ᾽ οὐχ
ὧδε; δεῖ διανοεῖσθαι περὶ τῆς ὁτουοῦν φύσεως,
πρῶτον μὲν εἰ ἁπλοῦν ἢ καὶ πολυειδές ἐστιν
14K   οὗ πέρι βουλησόμεθα,[22] | αὐτοί τε εἶναι
τεχνικοὶ καὶ ἄλλους δυνατοὶ ποιεῖν. ἔπειτα δὲ
ἂν μὲν ἁπλοῦν ᾖ, σκοπεῖν τὴν δύναμιν αὐτοῦ,
τίνα πρὸς τί πέφυκεν εἰς τὸ δρᾶν ἔχον, ἢ τίνα
εἰς τὸ παθεῖν ὑπό του· ἐὰν δὲ πλείω εἴδη ἔχῃ,
ταῦτα ἀριθμησάμενον, ὅπερ ἐφ᾽ ἑνός, τοῦτο
ἰδεῖν ἐφ᾽ ἑκάστου, τὸ τί ποιεῖν αὐτὸ πέφυκεν,
ἢ τὸ τί παθεῖν ὑπό του.

ἤκουσας, ὦ γενναιότατε, Πλάτωνος ὁμοίᾳ μεθόδῳ
τὰ κατὰ τὴν ψυχὴν ἀξιοῦντος εὑρίσκειν, οἵᾳ περ
Ἱπποκράτης τὰ κατὰ τὸ σῶμα· πότερον ἔτι βούλει
πολλὰς πολλαχόθι αὐτοῦ τῶν συγγραμμάτων ἐκλέξω
σοι ῥήσεις, ἐν αἷς ζηλοῖ τὸν Ἱπποκράτην πάντων

---

[22] B; βουλευσόμεθα K

[Socrates:] Do you think, then, it is possible to understand the nature of the soul in a way that is worth discussing without understanding the nature of the whole?

[Phaedrus:] If, in fact, we must put our trust in Hippocrates, one of the Aesclepiads, we have no understanding of the body without this method.

[Socrates:] You are right, my friend. We ought to examine closely the argument in addition to Hippocrates to see if it is consistent.

[Phaedrus:] I agree.

[Socrates:] Moreover, in the considerations about its nature, what do Hippocrates and the true argument state? Is it not this? Regarding the nature of anything whatsoever we must think first whether that thing about which we wish to be 14K expert ourselves, and to be able to make others so, is simple or multiform. Then, if it is simple, we must consider its capacity, whether it is by nature able to act, and on what, or whether it is acted upon, and by what. If, on the other hand, it is multiform, we must enumerate the forms and consider with reference to each of them, whether it has the nature to act, and on what, or to be acted upon, and by what.

You have heard, my very high-minded friend, that Plato thought it worthwhile to discover what pertains to the soul by a similar method to that which Hippocrates used for what pertains to the body. Do you still want me to pick out for you the numerous passages in many places of his treatises in which he commends Hippocrates particularly,

23

μάλιστα τῶν ἔμπροσθεν αὐτοῦ γεγονότων; ἢ τοῦτο
μὲν ἐν ἑτέρᾳ πραγματείᾳ πεποιηκώς, ἐν ᾗ περὶ τῶν
Ἱπποκράτους καὶ Πλάτωνος δογμάτων ἐπισκέπτομαι,
εἰς ἐκείνην ἀναπέμψω τὸν βουλόμενον; ἀποδέδεικται
γάρ, ὡς ἐγὼ νομίζω, πάνυ σαφῶς ἡ περὶ πλεῖστά τε
καὶ μέγιστα δόγματα συμφωνία τῶν ἀνδρῶν· μετα-
βὰς δὲ τὸν ἕτερον ἤδη σοι καλέσω χορὸν μάρτυρα,
τὸν ἐκ τοῦ περιπάτου, τὰς Ἱπποκράτους ἀρχὰς τῆς
15K φυσιολογίας τιθέμενον; | ἀλλά τοι καὶ περὶ τούτου
δέδεικταί μοι δι' ἑτέρων ὑπομνημάτων, ὧν ἓν μέν ἐστι
τὸ Περὶ τῶν καθ' Ἱπποκράτην στοιχείων, ἐφεξῆς δ'
ἕτερα τρία τὰ Περὶ κράσεων, εἶθ' ἑξῆς ἕτερα δύο, τὸ
μὲν Περὶ τῆς ἀνωμάλου δυσκρασίας, ἐκ τῆς Περὶ
κράσεων ἔτι πραγματείας ὑπάρχον, ἄλλο δὲ Περὶ τῆς
ἀρίστης κατασκευῆς τοῦ σώματος, εἶτ' ἐπὶ τούτοις τὰ
Περὶ φυσικῶν δυνάμεων τρία· ταῦτ' οὖν εἴπερ ἀνα-
γνοίη τις, ἐπιγνώσεται σαφῶς ἐξηγητὴν ὄντα τῶν
περὶ φύσεως λογισμῶν Ἱπποκράτους Ἀριστοτέλη.
καὶ μὲν δὴ καὶ περὶ τῆς τῶν νοσημάτων διαφορᾶς,
ὁπόσα τέ ἐστι καὶ ὁποῖα, καὶ περὶ συμπτωμάτων
ὡσαύτως, ἔτι τε καὶ τῶν καθ' ἑκάτερον αἰτιῶν, Ἱπποκράτης μὲν πρῶτος ἁπάντων ὧν ἴσμεν ὀρθῶς ὑπάρ-
ξασθαι φαίνεται, μετ' αὐτὸν δ' Ἀριστοτέλης ἐπὶ

---

¹² *De placitis Hippocratis et Platonis libri ix*, V.181–805K.
There is a translation by P. H. de Lacy in CMG V.4.1.2 (Berlin,
1978).

¹³ The works are as follows: *De elementis secundum Hippocratem libri iii*, I.413–508K (translation by P. H. de Lacy, CMG

among all those who came before him? I have done this in another work in which I undertake a review of the teachings of Hippocrates and Plato, and to which I refer anyone who wishes [to learn more].[12] For the accord between the two men has, I think, been very clearly demonstrated in most, and the most important, of their doctrines. Shall I now go on and call for you another troupe as witness, that from the Peripatos, to confirm the Hippocratic principles of natural science? But I have, in fact, provided demonstration about this in other treatises, of which one is *On the Elements according to Hippocrates*; and next, the three books of *On Krasias*; and next, two others, the one *On Anomalous Dyskrasia*, which takes its point of origin from the work *On Krasias*, and the other *On the Best Constitution of the Body*, and, in addition to these, the three books of *On the Physical Capacities*.[13] If, indeed, someone were to read these, he would clearly realize that Aristotle expounded the arguments of Hippocrates on nature. And in particular, concerning the differentiae of diseases, how many there are and of what kinds, and likewise concerning symptoms, as well as the causes of both diseases and symptoms, we are aware that Hippocrates seems to be the first of all those whom we know to have made a correct start while, after him, Aristotle set things out to the fullest ex-

15K

V.1.2, Berlin, 1996); *De temperamentis libri iii*, I.509–694K (translation by P. N. Singer, 1997); *De facultatibus naturalibus libri iii*, II.1–214K (translation by A. J. Brock, 1916, LCL); *De optima corporis nostri constitutione*, IV.737–49K (translation by R. J. Penella and T. S. Hall, *BHM* 47, 1973, pp. 282–95); *De inaequali intemperie*, VII.733–52K (translation by M. Grant, 2000).

πλεῖστον ἐξηγήσατο· εἴσεται δὲ καὶ περὶ τούτων ὁ
βουληθεὶς ἀναγνῶναι τὰ καθ' ἕκαστον αὐτῶν ὑπομνή-
ματά μοι γεγραμμένα.

ὥστ' εἴπερ οἱ ἐκ τοῦ Περιπάτου κριταὶ καθίσαιεν,
Ἱπποκράτης μέν, οἶμαι, νικήσει, Θεσσαλὸς δ' ὡς
ἀναίσχυντός τε καὶ ἰταμὸς ἐκβληθήσεται. εἰ δὲ τοὺς
ἀπὸ τῆς Στοᾶς φιλοσόφους εἰς τὸ συνέδριον εἰσ-
16K αγαγόντες ἐπιτρέψαιμεν καὶ τούτοις τὴν | ψῆφον, ἐξ
ὧν αὐτοὶ τίθενται δογμάτων, ἐκ τούτων Ἱπποκράτην
στεφανώσουσι. τὸ γὰρ θερμὸν καὶ τὸ ψυχρὸν καὶ τὸ
ξηρὸν καὶ τὸ ὑγρὸν Ἱπποκράτης μὲν πρῶτος εἰσ-
ηγήσατο, μετ' αὐτὸν δ' Ἀριστοτέλης ἀπέδειξεν·

ἕτοιμα δ' ἤδη παραλαβόντες οὐκ ἐφιλονείκησαν οἱ
περὶ τὸν Χρύσιππον, ἀλλ' ἐκ τούτων τὰ σύμπαντα
κεκρᾶσθαι λέγουσι, καὶ ταῦτ' εἰς ἄλληλα πάσχειν καὶ
δρᾶν καὶ τεχνικὴν εἶναι τὴν φύσιν, ἅπαντά τε τἄλλα
τὰ περὶ φύσεως Ἱπποκράτους δόγματα προσίενται,
πλὴν περὶ μικροῦ τινός ἐστιν αὐτοῖς ἡ διαφορὰ πρὸς
Ἀριστοτέλη. λέγοντος γὰρ Ἱπποκράτους ὀρθῶς ὡς
Σύμπνουν καὶ σύρρουν ἐστὶν ἅπαν τὸ σῶμα, καὶ
πάντα συμπαθέα τὰ τῶν ζῴων μόρια, προσίενται μὲν
ἀμφότεροι τουτί, διαφέρονται δὲ ἐν τῷ τὰς μὲν ποιότητας μόνας τὸν Ἀριστοτέλη δι' ἀλλήλων ἰέναι καὶ
κεράννυσθαι πάντη, τοὺς δ' ἀπὸ τῆς Στοᾶς οὐ ταύτας

tent.[14] And anyone who is willing to read the treatises I have written on each of these matters will also know about them.

The consequence is that, if those from the Peripatos were to sit in judgment, I believe Hippocrates would gain the victory, while Thessalus, so shameless and reckless, would be thrown out. If, on the other hand, we were to bring forward philosophers from the Stoa to the council chamber and entrust the vote to them, on the basis of 16K the doctrines they themselves have put forward, they will crown Hippocrates. For Hippocrates was the first to propose [the elemental qualities of] hot, cold, dry and moist and, after him, Aristotle proved them.

And the followers of Chrysippus, when they accepted these things already to hand, were not embroiled in contention. Rather, they say that all things are compounded from these [four elemental qualities], and that these things are affected by and act on each other, and that nature is proficient. And they approve all the other doctrines of Hippocrates regarding nature, apart from one minor point which is a difference between them and Aristotle. For when Hippocrates correctly says that "the whole body is animated by one spirit and flows together," and that "all the parts of living creatures have an affinity," both accept this very point. However, they differ in this: Aristotle held that the qualities alone interpenetrate each other and are mixed together completely, whereas those from the Stoa

[14] The four books referred to are *De differentiis morborum*, VI.836–80K, *De morborum causis*, VII.1–41K, *De symptomatum differentiis*, VII.42–84K, and *De symptomatum causis*, VII.85–272K. There is a translation of all four by I. Johnston, (2006).

μόνας, ἀλλὰ καὶ τὰς οὐσίας αὐτὰς ὑπολαμβάνειν. ὅτι
δὲ τοῦτο διορίζεσθαι περιττὸν ἰατρῷ, καὶ ὡς ἀρκεῖ
μόνον ὁμολογηθέντα εἰς τὰ τῆς ἰατρικῆς ἔργα τὰ πρὸς
ἀμφοτέρων ἀποδεικνύμενα, καὶ ὡς αἱ ποιότητές τε καὶ
17K αἱ δυνάμεις | ἐν τοῖς κεραννυμένοις ὅλαι δι' ὅλων ἀνα-
μίγνυνται, δέδεικταί μοι πρόσθεν ἤδη καὶ νῦν, εἴ τι
δεήσει, δειχθήσεται. ὥστε καὶ κατὰ Πλάτωνα καὶ
κατὰ τοὺς ἐκ τοῦ Περιπάτου καὶ κατὰ τοὺς ἐκ τῆς
Στοᾶς ἡ Ἱπποκράτους νικᾷ φυσιολογία· καὶ πολὺ δὴ
μᾶλλον ἐκ τῆς φυσιολογίας ἅπαντες ἐπιδεικνύουσιν οἱ
προειρημένοι φιλόσοφοι μὴ δύνασθαί τινα καλῶς
ἰάσασθαι τὰ νοσήματα, πρὶν ὅλου τοῦ σώματος ἐπισκέψασθαι τὴν φύσιν.

ἆρ' οὖν ἐνίκησεν ἂν ἐν τούτοις τοῖς φιλοσόφοις ὁ
Θεσσαλὸς ἀγωνιζόμενος ὑπὲρ τῶν πρωτείων, οἳ τῆς
ἑαυτῶν ἁπάσης φυσιολογίας Ἱπποκράτην προὑστή-
σαντο; τί δέ, εἰ τοῖς γεωμέτραις, ἢ τοῖς ἀστρονόμοις,
ἢ τοῖς μουσικοῖς, ἢ τοῖς ῥήτορσιν ἐπιτρέψειε τὴν
κρίσιν; ἆρ' οἰόμεθα καὶ τούτους Ἱπποκράτην παρ-
ελθόντας ἕτερόν τινα στεφανώσειν; ἐγὼ μὲν οὔτ' ἄλλον τινὰ πέπεισμαι τὰ πρωτεῖα λήψεσθαι, καὶ πάντων
ἥκιστα τὸν ἰταμώτατον Θεσσαλόν· οὐδεὶς γὰρ οὕτως ἠτίμησεν οὐ γεωμετρίαν, οὐκ ἀστρονομίαν, οὐ
μουσικήν, οὐ ῥητορικήν, ὡς ἐκεῖνος, ὥστε ταύτῃ γ' ἐν
ἐχθρῶν θεάτρῳ γένοιτ' ἂν ὁ ἀγὼν αὐτῷ. ἀλλ' ἴσως
18K τούτους μὲν οὐκ ἂν εἰς | τὸ θέατρον ἐκάθισεν, οὕς γε
αὐτὸς φθάνων ἐχθροὺς ἐποιήσατο, μόνοις δὲ τοῖς ἐν
διαλεκτικῇ γυμνασθεῖσι φιλοσόφοις, ὡς ἂν ἀληθῶν

suppose that not these qualities only but also the substances themselves [are mixed completely].[15] I have already shown previously that it is redundant for the doctor
to make this distinction, and that it is quite sufficient for
the practice of medicine to agree with what both [Hippoc-
rates and the Stoics] have demonstrated, which is that the
qualities and the capacities in those things that have been   17K
mixed are thoroughly blended together throughout. And I
will show this again now if need be. As a consequence, according to Plato, as well as to the Peripatetics and the
Stoics, the natural science of Hippocrates triumphs, and
much more, all the previously mentioned philosophers
have shown, on the grounds of natural science, that it is impossible for anyone to cure diseases properly without considering the nature of the body in its entirety.

So then, would Thessalus, when he is competing for
first prize, have triumphed among those philosophers
who made Hippocrates the champion of their whole natural science? What if he were to entrust the judgment to
geometers, astronomers, musicians, or orators? Do we
think that these men, too, would pass over Hippocrates
and crown someone else? I am not persuaded that anyone
else will take first place, least of all the absolutely reckless
Thessalus. Nobody has disdained geometry, astronomy,
music and rhetoric like this man, so the contest would take
place in a theater of those antagonistic to him. But perhaps
he would not have brought these people together in the
theater—people whom he had made his enemies in ad-   18K
vance—but would entrust the judgment only to philoso-

15 See Aristotle, *De generatione et corruptione* 1.10 (328a, 26–
28), and Alexander of Aphrodisias, *De mixtione* in *Supplementum
Aristotelicum*, 2.473.

τε καὶ ψευδῶν λόγων τὸ κριτήριον ἠσκηκόσιν, ἐπιτρέψειε τὴν κρίσιν. ἀλλ' ἐὰν τοὺς περὶ Πλάτωνα καὶ
Ἀριστοτέλη καὶ Χρύσιππον ὡς ἀγυμνάστους ἐν τῇδε
παρέλθωμεν, οὐχ εὑρήσομεν ἑτέρους. εἰ τοίνυν οὔτε
τοὺς ἀπὸ τῶν ἄλλων τεχνῶν ὑπομένει δικαστὰς ὁ
Θεσσαλὸς οὔθ' οἱ διαλεκτικώτατοι τῶν φιλοσόφων
οἴσουσιν αὐτῷ τὴν ψῆφον, ὑπὸ τίνων ἔτι κριθήσεται
νικᾶν; τίνες πληρώσουσιν αὐτῷ τὸ θέατρον; τίνες
ἀναγορεύσουσιν; τίνες στεφανώσουσιν; αὐτὸς ἑαυτὸν
δηλονότι, τοῦτο γὰρ ἐν ταῖς αὐτοῦ²³ βίβλοις ταῖς
θαυμασταῖς ἐποίησεν, αὐτὸς ἑαυτὸν καὶ κρίνας καὶ
στεφανώσας καὶ ἀναγορεύσας.

3. Ἀλλ' ἴσως ὑπενόησε τοῦτο αὐτὸ τιμὴν αὐτῷ
γενήσεσθαι²⁴ καὶ μνήμης ἀφορμήν, εἰ λοιδορησάμε-
νος τοῖς ἀρίστοις ἀνδράσιν ἀναγκάσειεν ἡμᾶς ἀντιλέγειν αὐτῷ. ἀλλ' οὕτω γε καὶ Ζωΐλος ἔνδοξος τὴν
Ὁμήρου μαστίζων εἰκόνα καὶ Σαλμωνεὺς τὸν Δία
19K   μιμούμενος καὶ ἄλλο πλῆθος οὐκ | ὀλίγον ἐπιτρίπτων
ἀνθρώπων, ἢ τοὺς βελτίονας οὐκ αἰδουμένων, ἢ καὶ
τοῖς θεοῖς αὐτοῖς λοιδορουμένων. ἀλλ' οὐκ ἀγαθὴν
οὗτοί γε δόξαν ὑπελίποντο σφῶν αὐτῶν, οὐδὲ ζηλοῖ
νοῦν ἔχων ἀνὴρ οὐδεὶς οὔτε τὸν Ὁμηρομάστιγα Ζω-
ΐλον οὔτε τὸν παραπλῆγα Σαλμωνέα, καίτοι τοῖς μὲν
φιλολοιδόροις ζηλωτὸς ὁ Ζωΐλος, τοῖς δ' ἱεροσύλοις ὁ
Σαλμωνεύς. ἀλλὰ τί τοῦτο; καὶ γὰρ οἱ βαλαντιοτόμοι

²³ B; ἑαυτοῦ K
²⁴ B; τοῦτ' αὐτῷ τιμὴν γενήσεσθαι K

phers trained in dialectics since they are practiced in the way of judging between true and false arguments. But if we are to pass over the followers of Plato, Aristotle, and Chrysippus as being unpracticed in this matter, we shall not find others. If Thessalus does not submit to judges from other disciplines, and those philosophers most skilled in dialectics will not cast their vote in his favor, by whom will he be judged the victor? Who will fill the theater for him? Who will proclaim him in public? Who will crown him? Clearly he will have to do these things himself. And this is what he did in those marvelous books of his in which he judges, crowns and proclaims himself [victor].

3. But perhaps he supposed this very thing would bring him honor and provide the starting point of his being remembered—that having abused the best men, he would compel me to speak against him. In fact, it was just in this way that Zoilus found fame for whipping the image of Homer, Salmoneus for imitating Zeus, and that by no means small crowd of cunning men who either did not respect their betters, or who even reviled the gods themselves. But, in truth, these men left behind no good opinion of themselves. Indeed, no sensible man envies either the Homer-whipping Zoilus or the mad Salmoneus. And yet, Zoilus is admired by abusers and Salmoneus by the sacriligeous.[16] But what of this? For cutpurses also admire

19K

---

[16] Zoilus of Amphipolis was a fourth-century Cynic philosopher who wrote several critical works, none of which is extant. Most notable was the work "Against Homer's poetry." Salmoneus, the son of Aeolus, is said to have imitated Zeus by driving around in a chariot making a noise like thunder and flinging torches as lightning. Tradition has it that Zeus hit him with a real thunderbolt for his troubles.

τὰ τῶν βαλαντιοτόμων ζηλοῦσι καὶ οἱ προδόται τὰ
τῶν προδοτῶν καὶ οὐδείς ἐστιν ἁπλῶς ἄνθρωπος ὃς
οὐκ ἂν σχοίη χορὸν οἰκεῖον ἐν ᾧ στεφθήσεται. καὶ
εἴπερ ἔγραψε Θεσσαλὸς ὡς ἐν μαγείροις καὶ βαφεῦσι
καὶ ἐριουργοῖς καὶ σκυτοτόμοις καὶ ὑφάνταις τε καὶ
κναφεῦσιν ἀγωνιζόμενος, ἀποίσεται τὴν νίκην καὶ
καθ᾽ Ἱπποκράτους καὶ οὐδεὶς ἂν ἡμῶν ἀντεῖπεν· ἐπεὶ
δὲ πάντας ἀνθρώπους καθίζει δικαστάς, ἐκ τῶν πάντων δ᾽ ἐστὶ δήπου καὶ Πλάτων καὶ Ἀριστοτέλης καὶ
Θεόφραστος καὶ Χρύσιππος, οὐκ ἂν ἔτι πάσας μόνος
ἀποστρέφοιτο τὰς ψήφους, ἀλλ᾽ ἴσως ἔνεσται δίκην
ἐφέσιμον ἀγωνίσασθαί τινι. κἂν γὰρ Ἱπποκράτης
καταφρονήσῃ, μικρότερον ἑαυτοῦ νομίσας ἀγωνίσασθαι πρὸς Θεσσαλόν, ἀλλ᾽ ἴσως Ἐρασίστρατος οὐ
20K καταφρονήσει, | καὶ πολύ γε μᾶλλον Ἡρόφιλος, καὶ
τούτων ἔτι μᾶλλον Ἀσκληπιάδης ἄλλοι τε πολλοὶ
τῶν νεωτέρων ἰατρῶν ἔχοντές τι φύσει φιλόνεικον οὐ
καταφρονήσουσι τῆς ὕβρεως, ἣν εἰς ἅπαντας ἅμα
τοὺς Ἕλληνας ὑβρίζει Θεσσαλός, ἀλλ᾽ εἰς τὸ μέσον
τε προάξουσιν, ἐπιδείξουσί τε τοῖς Ἕλλησιν ἁπάσας
αὐτοῦ τὰς βίβλους ἀμαθίας ἐσχάτης μεστάς, ὃς τοσαῦτά τε καὶ τηλικαῦτα γράψας βιβλία καὶ τοσαύτας
ληρήσας ἐπῶν χιλιάδας, ἀπόδειξιν οὐδεμίαν οὐδαμόθι
τῶν ἑαυτοῦ συγγραμμάτων ἐπεχείρησεν εἰπεῖν, ἀλλ᾽
ὡς τύραννος κελεύει δύο μόνα εἶναι τὰ πάντα κατὰ
δίαιταν νοσήματα, ῥοῶδες καὶ στεγνόν, οὐκ εἰδὼς ὅτι
διαφοράν τινα νοσημάτων εἴρηκεν, ἐγνωσμένην μὲν
καὶ τοῖς ἔμπροσθεν ἰατροῖς, ὡς ἐπιδείξομεν, ἀλλ᾽

the deeds of cutpurses and traitors admire the deeds of traitors, and, quite simply, there is no man who does not have his own troupe among whom he will be crowned. In fact, if Thessalus wrote as though competing among cooks, dyers, wool workers, shoemakers, weavers, and fullers, he would carry off the victory against Hippocrates as well, and none of us would have spoken against this. However, since he makes all men sit as judges, and presumably Plato, Aristotle, Theophrastus and Chrysippus are among them, he alone would no longer garner all the votes, although perhaps he would be able to take one of them on in a court of appeal. But even if Hippocrates were to feel scorn, considering it beneath his dignity to compete with Thessalus, well perhaps Erasistratus will not be disdainful, much less   20K
Herophilus, and even less than these men, Asclepiades and many other of the more modern doctors who are by nature somewhat fond of contention and will not be contemptuous of the insolence which Thessalus directs simultaneously at all the Greeks. Rather, they will advance him to a central position and will make a display to the Greeks of all his books, full as they are of the utmost ignorance—a man who wrote so many books and of such length, and who said so many foolish things. But no demonstration did he attempt to articulate anywhere at all in his own writings. Instead, like a tyrant, he decrees that all diseases are of two kinds only, in terms of regimen—fluxion and obstruction.[17] He did not realize that he had spoken of one differentia of diseases, and one known to previous doctors, as I shall

[17] See the Introduction, section 2, for a summary of Methodic theory.

οὐδεὶς ἦν οὕτως ἀπαίδευτος ὡς τὰς διαφορὰς τῶν
νοσημάτων αὐτὰ νομίζειν εἶναι τὰ νοσήματα καὶ τῆς
θεραπείας τὴν ἔνδειξιν ἐξ ἐκείνων λαμβάνειν ὑπερβὰς
τὴν οὐσίαν. ἀλλὰ τοῦτο τὸ σφάλμα τοῦ Θεσσαλοῦ
σμικρὸν μὲν ὦ Ζεῦ καὶ θεοί, σμικρότατον, ὃ καὶ
παιδάριον ἐν ἐλευθέροις μαθήμασι τεθραμμένον εὐ-
θέως γνωρίσειεν· ὅμως δ' οὖν τοῦτο τὸ σφάλμα τὸ |
21K   σμικρὸν εἰς τοσοῦτον ἐπῆρεν αὐθαδείας αὐτὸν ὥστε
νομίζειν εὑρηκέναι τι μέγα καὶ σεμνόν.

ὁμοίως[25] εἰ καί τις εἰπὼν πᾶν ζῷον ἢ λογικὸν
ὑπάρχειν ἢ ἄλογον, ἄλλο τι νομίζει καὶ μὴ διαφορὰς
εἰρηκέναι ζῴων, ὡσαύτως οὖν τούτῳ κἀκείνου ῥηθέν-
τος, ἅπαν ζῷον ἢ θνητόν ἐστιν ἢ ἀθάνατον· ἡ γὰρ ἐν
ἑκάστῃ τῶν διαφορῶν ἀντίθεσις ὅλη κατὰ πάντων
λέγεται τῶν εἰδῶν· ἅπαν οὖν ζῷον ἢ ἄγριόν ἐστιν ἢ
ἥμερον· ἅπαν οὖν ζῷον ἢ ὑπόπουν ἐστὶν ἢ ἄπουν·
ἅπαν οὖν ζῷον ἢ κερασφόρον ἐστὶν ἢ ἄκερον· καὶ
οὐδέν γε τιμιωτέραν ἑτέρας ἑτέραν ἀντίθεσιν ἐν ταῖς
διαφοραῖς ἔστιν εὑρεῖν, οὐδὲ μᾶλλον ὑπάρχουσαν
ἅπασι τοῖς κατὰ μέρος. ἀλλ' οὐ χρὴ περὶ ζῴων ἐρωτη-
θέντας ὁπόσα τὰ πάντα ἐστὶ ἀποκρίνασθαι μίαν ἀντίθεσιν διαφορῶν· οὕτω μὲν γὰρ ἔσται δύο τὰ πάντα,
καὶ οὐδὲν μᾶλλον ἢ λογικὸν καὶ ἄλογον, ἢ θνητὸν καὶ
ἀθάνατον, ἢ ἄγριον καὶ ἥμερον, ἢ τῶν ἄλλων τις
ἀντιθέσεων. εἰ δὲ τὰς διαφορὰς ἐάσας τις, ὡσπερούν[26]
ἐστι δίκαιον, ἵππον ἀποκρίναιτο καὶ βοῦν καὶ κύνα
22K   καὶ ἄνθρωπον, ἀετόν τε καὶ μέλιτταν καὶ | μύρμηκα καὶ

show. But none of these doctors was so uneducated as to think that the differentiae of diseases are the diseases themselves, or to take from them the indication for treatment, passing over the substance itself. But, O Zeus and you gods, this error by Thessalus is simplistic, absolutely simplistic, such that even a young child, educated in liberal studies would immediately recognize it. Nevertheless, it was this simplistic error that raised him to such a degree of insolence that he thought he had discovered something important and significant. 21K

It is just as if someone were to say that every animal is either rational or irrational, thinking he had stated something other than the differentiae of animals. Similar to this is the statement that every animal is either mortal or immortal. For in each case a complete antithesis of differentiae can be posited concerning all the kinds; for example, that every animal is either wild or tame; that every animal either has feet or is without feet; that every animal is either horned or hornless. And, in fact, among the differentiae, it is not at all possible to find one antithesis that is more important than another, or that inheres in all these individually. But one should not, when asked how many kinds of animals there are in all, respond with one antithesis of differentiae for in this way everything will be two [in kind] in all, but no longer rational or irrational, or mortal or immortal, or wild or tame, or any one of the other antitheses. If, however, someone were to leave aside the differentiae, as is, in fact, right, and were to reply "horse," or "cow," or "dog," or "man," or "eagle," or "bee," or "ant," or 22K

---

25 *conj.* nos; ὁμοίς ὡς εἰ; ὅ μοι ὡς εἰ B
26 B, Pl, P2; ὡς οὖν K

λέοντα καὶ πρόβατον, ἅπαντά τε τἆλλα κατ' εἶδος
ἐπέλθοι ζῷα, δῆλον ὡς οὗτος ὀρθῶς ἀποκεκριμένος
ἐστὶ τῷ πυθομένῳ ὁπόσα τὰ πάντ' ἐστὶ ζῷα· κἂν εἰ
πολλὰ μὲν διέλθοι τῷ λόγῳ ζῷα, πάντα δ' ἐξαριθμήσασθαι μὴ δυνατὸν εἶναι λέγοι, καὶ οὕτως ἂν εἴη
δεόντως ἀποκεκριμένος.

ὁμοίας οὖν οὔσης τῆς ζητήσεως ἐπὶ τοῦ τῶν νοσημάτων ἀριθμοῦ παρὰ πᾶσι τοῖς παλαιοῖς ἰατροῖς, καὶ
τῶν μὲν εἰπόντων ἑπτὰ τὰ πάνθ' ὑπάρχειν αὐτά, τῶν δ'
ἐλάττω τούτων ἢ πλείω, πάντων δ' οὖν εἰς τὰ κατὰ τὴν
οὐσίαν εἴδη βλεπόντων, οὐκ εἰς τὰ κατὰ τὴν δια-
φοράν· οὐδεὶς γὰρ ἦν οὕτως ἀπαίδευτος οὐδ' ἀμαθὴς
λογικῆς θεωρίας ὡς διαφορὰν εἰδῶν εἰπεῖν ἀντ' οὐ-
σίας· ὁ δ' ἐκ τῆς γυναικωνίτιδος ἐκπηδήσας Θεσσαλὸς ἐπιτιμᾷ τηλικούτοις ἀνδράσιν, οὐ γένος ἔχων
εἰπεῖν, οὐκ ἀνατροφήν, οὐ παιδείαν οἵαν ἐκείνων ἕκαστος, ὁ μὲν Ἀριστοτέλους, ὁ δὲ Πλάτωνος, ὁ δὲ Θεοφράστου γενόμενος ὁμιλητής, ἤ τινος ἄλλου τῶν ἐν τῇ
λογικῇ θεωρίᾳ γεγυμνασμένων ἀνδρῶν. ὡς οὖν εἴ τις
23K ἐρωτηθεὶς ὁπόσα τῆς | φωνῆς τὰ πάντ' ἐστὶ στοιχεῖα,
δύο φήσειεν ὑπάρχειν, ἤτοι γὰρ φωνῆεν εἶναι φήσει
πάντως ἢ σύμφωνον ὅπερ ἂν εἴη στοχεῖον φωνῆς,
ἀληθὲς μὲν εἴρηκεν, οὐ μὴν πρός γε τὴν ἐρώτησιν
ἀπεκρίνατο, κατὰ τὸν αὐτόν, οἶμαι, τρόπον ὅστις ἂν
ὁπόσα τὰ πάντ' ἐστὶ νοσήματα διελέσθαι βουληθεὶς
ὑπερβῇ μὲν εἶδός τι λέγειν νοσήματος, οἶον ἤτοι
φλεγμονήν, ἢ σκίρρον, ἢ οἴδημα, διαφορὰς δ' εἴπῃ
μόνας, εἴτ' οὖν στεγνὸν καὶ ῥοῶδες, εἴτ' ἀραιὸν καὶ

"lion," or "sheep," and went on to all the other animals according to species, clearly he would have answered correctly someone who asked how many kinds of animals there are in all. And even if he were to cover many animals in the discussion but were to say that it is not possible to enumerate all of them, he has still answered as he should.

Similar, then, was the inquiry into the number of diseases carried out by all the doctors of old, some of them saying there were seven in all, and others saying there were fewer or more than these, but all of them looking toward the kinds in terms of substance and not in terms of differentiae. For none of them was so poorly educated or so ignorant of logical theory as to speak of the differentiae of kinds as opposed to substance. Thessalus, however, springing forth from the women's quarters, censures such men, although he himself has neither the breeding worth speaking of, nor the education, nor the learning that each of them [possessed], one a pupil of Aristotle, another of Plato, another of Theophrastus, or any other of those men trained in logical theory. It is as if someone who was asked how many elements of speech there are in all were to say there are two because, he will claim, whatever is an element of speech is, in all cases, either a vowel or a consonant. He has said something true but he has not, in fact, answered the question. In the same way, I think, if someone who wished to distinguish of what sort all the kinds of diseases are, were to pass over what is spoken of as the kind of disease, like inflammation, induration, or edema, and were to speak of differentiae alone, like obstruction and fluxion,

23K

πυκνόν, εἴτε σκληρὸν καὶ μαλακόν, εἴτε συντεταμένον καὶ κεχαλασμένον, ἀληθὲς μὲν εἴρηκεν, οὐ μὴν πρός γε τὴν ἐρώτησιν ἀπεκρίνατο. πρῶτον μὲν γὰρ οὐδὲ πᾶσα διαφορὰ προστιθεμένη τῷ γένει συντελεῖ τι πρὸς τὴν τοῦ εἴδους γένεσιν, ἀλλ' ἥτις ἂν ἐκ τῆς τοῦ γένους οἰκείας ᾖ διαιρέσεως· αὗται γάρ εἰσιν εἰδο-ποιοὶ μόναι τῶν διαφορῶν, αἱ δ' ἄλλαι πᾶσαι περιτ-ταί. ζώου μὲν γὰρ οἰκεῖαι διαφοραὶ τὸ θνητὸν καὶ ἀθάνατον, ἄλογόν τε καὶ λογικόν, ἥμερόν τε καὶ ἄγριον, ὅσα τ' ἄλλα τοιαῦτα· μαλακὸν δὲ καὶ σκλη-ρόν, καὶ βαρὺ καὶ κοῦφον, καὶ ἀραιὸν καὶ πυκνόν, καὶ μέγα καὶ μικρόν, οὐ ζώου, ἀλλ' οὐσίας εἰσὶ διαφοραί.

24K | καὶ τοίνυν εἰ μὲν προστεθείη τῷ ζώῳ τὸ μαλακὸν καὶ τὸ σκληρόν, ἢ τὸ πυκνὸν ἢ τὸ ἀραιόν, ἢ τὸ μικρὸν ἢ τὸ μέγα, πλεῖον οὐδὲν εἰς εἴδους γένεσιν συντελέσει· εἰ δ' ἤτοι λογικὸν καὶ ἀθάνατον, ἢ λογικὸν καὶ θνητόν, εἴη ἂν τὸ μὲν εἴδει θεός, τὸ δὲ ἄνθρωπος· οὕτω δὲ κἂν εἰ προσθείης τῷ λογικῷ ζώῳ διττὰς οἰκείας διαφοράς, τὸ πεζὸν καὶ τὸ δίπουν, εἶδος ἐργάσῃ τι καὶ οὕτως, τὸν ἄνθρωπον·

ὅθεν ἀδύνατόν ἐστιν οὐδενὸς τῶν ὄντων εἰδοποιοὺς εὑρεῖν διαφορὰς ἄνευ τοῦ τὸν ὁρισμόν, ἢ τὸν λόγον τῆς οὐσίας ἀκριβῶς αὐτοῦ περιγράψασθαι. δεύτερον δ' ἐπὶ τούτου σφάλμα τοῖς ἀγυμνάστοις περὶ λόγον, ἐπειδὰν ἐξευρήσουσι μίαν τινὰ διαφορᾶς ἀντίθεσιν, εἶδός τι τοῦ προβεβλημένου γένους ὑπολαμβάνειν εὑρηκέναι, ὥσπερ ὀλίγον ἔμπροσθεν ὑπὲρ τῶν τῆς φωνῆς στοιχείων ἐλέγετο. φωνῆεν γάρ τις εἰπὼν καὶ

or like rarefaction and condensation, or like hardness and softness, or like tension and relaxation, he has said something true but has not, in fact, answered the question. For first, not every differentia that is added to the genus contributes something to the creation of the species, but only whatever differentia is derived from the appropriate division of the genus. These alone are species-forming among the differentiae, while all the others are superfluous. For the appropriate differentiae of [the genus] "animal" are mortal and immortal, irrational and rational, tame and wild, and other such things. Soft and hard, heavy and light, rarefied and dense, and large and small are not differentiae of "animal" but of "substance." Therefore, if softness or hardness, or denseness or looseness of texture, or smallness or largeness is added to "animal," this will contribute nothing more to the creation of the species. If, however, rational and immortal, or rational and mortal [are added], this would be, on the one hand, the species "god" and, on the other hand, the species "man." In like manner, if you were to add to "rational animal" two appropriate differentiae, footed and bipedal, you will also, in this way, make a species, [namely] "man."

    On these grounds, it is impossible to discover species-forming differentiae of any being without defining precisely its boundary or the basis of its actual substance. Second, in regard to this, an error is made by those untrained in reasoning who, whenever they discover some one antithesis of differentia, suppose they have discovered some species of the proposed genus, as was said a little earlier with regard to the elements of speech. For someone who

24K

σύμφωνον οὔπω τὰ πάντα στοιχεῖα τῆς ἀνθρώπου
φωνῆς εἴρηκεν, ἀλλὰ δύο τὰς πρώτας γενικὰς δια-
φοράς· εἰ δὲ τὰ μὲν φωνήεντα τέμνων αὖθις εἰς μακρὰ
25K καὶ βραχέα καὶ δίχρονα, τὰ σύμφωνα | δ᾽ εἰς ἡμίφωνά
τε καὶ ἄφωνα, καὶ αὖθις τὰ μὲν μακρὰ διχῇ, καθάπερ
οὖν καὶ τὰ βραχέα, τὰ δ᾽ αὖ δίχρονα τριχῇ· καὶ δὴ καὶ
τὰ ἄφωνα πρῶτον μὲν εἰς δασέα καὶ ψιλὰ καὶ μέσα,
καὶ τούτων ἕκαστον αὖθις τριχῇ, τὰ δ᾽ ἡμίφωνα
πάλιν, εἰ καὶ ταῦτα κατὰ τὴν οἰκείαν τέμοι τομήν, ἵνα
μὴ μακρολογῶ περιττῶς, οὕτως ἂν ἐξεύροι²⁷ τὰ τέτταρα καὶ εἴκοσι στοιχεῖα τῆς φωνῆς ᾗ χρώμεθα. τὸ
μὲν γὰρ εἰπεῖν αὐτὸ τοῦτο μόνον, ὡς ἔστι τῶν στοιχείων τῆς φωνῆς τὰ μὲν φωνήεντα, τὰ δὲ σύμφωνα,
τεχνικὸν οὔπω ποιεῖ τὸν ἀκροατὴν οὐδ᾽ ἀκριβῶς ἐπι-
στήμονα συμπάντων τῶν στοιχείων· ἀλλ᾽ ἐὰν διελό-
μενος εἰς βραχέα καὶ μακρὰ καὶ δίχρονα, βραχέα μὲν
εἶναι φῇ δύο, τό τε ε καὶ τὸ ο, μακρὰ δ᾽ ὁμοίως δύο, τό
τε η καὶ τὸ ω, δίχρονα δὲ τρία, τό τε ἄλφα καὶ τὸ ι καὶ
τὸ υ, τεχνικὸν οὕτω ποιήσει τὸν ἀκούσαντα περὶ τῶν
φωνηέντων ἁπάντων· ὡσαύτως δὲ καὶ περὶ τῶν συμ-
φώνων κατὰ τὸν αὐτὸν τρόπον.

οὕτως οὖν καὶ ὅστις ἐπιχειρεῖ λέγειν ὑπὲρ τοῦ τῶν
νοσημάτων ἀριθμοῦ, πόσα τὰ σύμπαντ᾽ ἐστίν, οὐ χρὴ
τοῦτον ἐν τῇ πρώτῃ καταμεῖναι διαφορᾷ, τέμνοντα δ᾽
αὐτὴν ἐπεξιέναι, μέχρι περ ἂν ἐπί τι τῶν ἐσχάτων
26K εἰδῶν ἀφίκηται | τῶν μηκέτι τμηθῆναι δυναμένων εἰς

says "vowel" and "consonant" has not yet mentioned all the elements of human speech but only the two primary, generic differentiae. If, however, he were to divide vowels further into long, short, and dichronous, and to divide consonants into semivowels and mutes, and then further divide the long and short [vowels] into two and the dichronous [vowels] into three, and moreover, if he were to divide first the mute consonants into aspirated, unaspirated and intermediate, and divide each of these again into three, and the semivowels again, and if he were also to divide these according to their proper division, so that I do not go on at unnecessary length, in this way he would discover the twenty-four elements of speech we use. Just to say this alone—that some elements of speech are vowels and some are consonants—does not yet make the listener proficient or accurately knowledgeable about all the elements. But if, having divided [the vowels] into short, long and dichronous, he were to say that there are two that are short (*epsilon* and *omikron*), and likewise that there are two that are long (*eta* and *omega*), and three that are dichronous (*alpha*, *iota* and *upsilon*), he will in this way make the listener proficient regarding all the vowels. And similarly too, he will make the listener proficient regarding the consonants in the same way.

In this way, therefore, whoever attempts to make a statement about the number of diseases, how many there are in all, should not stop at the first differentia but go on dividing differentiae until he comes to one of the lowest species (*infimae species*), one of those which cannot be fur-

25K

26K

---

27 τέμοι . . . ἐξεύροι B (τέμνοι *ex* KLat *secet et* ἐξεύροι *ex* inveniat *conj.* Hankinson); τέμνοις . . . ἐξεύροις K, P1, P2

ἕτερον εἶδος. ὅτι δ' οὐ τοῦ τυχόντος ἐστὶ τοῦτο ποιεῖν,
ἀλλ' ἀνθρώπου γεγυμνασμένου μεγάλως ἐν τῇ διαιρε-
τικῇ μεθόδῳ, μαθεῖν ἔνεστι τῷ βουλομένῳ πρῶτον μὲν
ἅπαντα ἀναγνόντι κατὰ τὴν ἀρχὴν τοῦ Φιλήβου Πλάτωνι γεγραμμένα περὶ τῆς τοιαύτης μεθόδου, μετὰ
ταῦτα δὲ τόν τε Σοφιστὴν ἀναλεξαμένῳ καὶ τὸν Πολι-
τικόν· ἔτι δὲ μᾶλλον αὐτῷ χαλεπώτερον φανεῖται τὸ
πρᾶγμα²⁸ τὸ πρῶτον Περὶ μορίων ζῴων Ἀριστοτέλους
ἀναγνόντι· πειρᾶται μὲν γὰρ ἐν ἐκείνῳ τὰς διαφορὰς
ἁπάσας ἐξαριθμήσασθαι τῶν ζῴων, ἀπορίας τε παμ-
πόλλας κινήσας, μόγις ὑπόπτως τε καὶ δεδιὼς²⁹ ἀπο-
φαίνεσθαί τι τολμᾷ.

εἶτ' Ἀριστοτέλους τε καὶ Πλάτωνος οὕτω μέγα καὶ
χαλεπὸν εἶναι νομιζόντων εἰς τὰς οἰκείας διαφορὰς
ἀκριβῶς τὰ γένη τέμνειν καὶ μετ' αὐτοὺς Θεοφράστου
τε καὶ τῶν ἄλλων φιλοσόφων ἐξεργάζεσθαι πειρωμένων τὸν τρόπον, ὡς οὔπω κατορθωμένον οὐδὲ παρ'
ἐκείνοις, ὁ τολμηρότατος Θεσσαλὸς ἁπλῶς ἀποφηνάμενος ἀξιοῖ πιστεύεσθαι δύο τὰ πάντ' εἶναι κατὰ
δίαιταν νοσήματα τὰ γοῦν ἁπλᾶ καὶ πρῶτα καὶ οἷον
στοιχεῖα, | τρίτον γὰρ ἐξ αὐτῶν ἄλλο γεννᾶται τῷ
λόγῳ σύνθετον, ἐπιπεπλεγμένον ἐξ ἀμφοῖν. ἀλλ' εἴπερ
μεθόδῳ τινὶ ταῦτ' ἐξεῦρες, ὥσπερ οὖν ἀλαζονεύῃ, τί
οὐχὶ καὶ ἡμῖν ἔφρασας αὐτήν, ἀλλὰ πᾶν τοὐναντίον, ἢ

27K

----

²⁸ K, B; γράμμα P1, P2;   ²⁹ B; δειλῶς K

----

¹⁸ The relevant passages are *Philebus* 12 (LCL, Plato VIII, p.

42

ther subdivided into another species. It is possible for someone who so wishes to read first something written by Plato about such a method at the beginning of the *Philebus*, and, after that, to read through the *Sophist* and the *Politicus*,[18] to learn that doing this is not a matter of chance but [can only be done] when a man has been thoroughly trained in the method of division. The matter will seem rather more complex to someone who has read the first book of Aristotle's *On the Parts of Animals* for he tries, in that [work], to enumerate all the differentiae of animals and, when he is disturbed by the very many difficulties, he barely ventures to give an opinion, [and does so] provisionally and with trepidation.[19]

Aristotle and Plato thought it was such a major and difficult task to divide the genera accurately into the appropriate differentiae, just as Theophrastus did after them, and the other philosophers who tried to bring the method to completion, that it hasn't yet been successfully accomplished by those men. Nevertheless, the extraordinarily overbold Thessalus thinks he is worthy of credence when he pronounces baldly that all diseases are of two kinds according to regimen—at any rate, those that are simple and primary, and elements, as it were, for another third kind 27K arises compounded from these according to the theory, having been made up from both of them. But if, by some method, you have discovered these things, as in fact you boast, why have you not also told us about it, but instead, in

242ff), *Sophist* 218C–232B (LCL, Plato VII, pp. 270–318), and *Politicus* throughout.

[19] See Aristotle, *De partibus animalium* 642b5ff and notes c and d in the LCL Aristotle XII, pp. 78–79.

κατὰ τοὔνομα τὸ σεμνόν, ᾧ προσαγορεύεις σαυτόν,
ἀμεθοδώτατε καὶ προπετέστατε, τὴν ἀπόφασιν ἐποι-
ήσω, μηδ᾽ οὖν μηδὲ τῆς ἀρχῆς αὐτῆς ἐφαψάμενος, ἀφ᾽
ἧς ἀναγκαῖόν ἐστιν ἄρξασθαι τὸν μέλλοντα καλῶς
οὑτινοσοῦν πράγματος ἐξευρήσειν εἴδη τε καὶ διαφορὰς οἰκείας; Περὶ παντὸς γάρ, ὦ παῖ, μία ἀρχὴ
ἀρίστη, εἰδέναι περὶ ὅτου ἡ ζήτησις, ἢ πάντα ἁμαρ-
τάνειν ἀνάγκη, Πλάτων πού φησιν, οὐκ εἰς τὸ διαιρεῖν
μόνον ὁτιοῦν ἀξιῶν ἡμᾶς ἀπ᾽ αὐτῆς ἄρχεσθαι τοῦ
ζητουμένου τῆς οὐσίας, ἀλλ᾽ εἰς ἅπαν ἀεὶ χρῆσθαι
σκέμμα τῷ τοιούτῳ τρόπῳ τῆς ἀρχῆς.

ἐχρῆν μὲν οὖν κἀνταῦθα τί ποτέ ἐστιν νόσημα καὶ
τί σύμπτωμα καὶ τί πάθος ἀκριβῶς εἰπόντα, καὶ
διορισάμενον ὅπῃ ταὐτόν ἐστιν ἕκαστον τῶν εἰρημένων καὶ ὅπῃ μὴ ταὐτόν, οὕτως ἤδη πειρᾶσθαι τέμνειν
εἰς τὰς οἰκείας διαφορὰς αὐτά, καθ᾽ ἣν ἐδίδαξαν ἡμᾶς
οἱ φιλόσοφοι μέθοδον· ἢ εἴπερ ἑτέραν τινὰ βελτίω |
τῆς παρ᾽ ἐκείνων γεγραμμένης ἐξεῦρες, αὐτὸ τοῦτο
πρότερον ἀγωνίσασθαι, καὶ δεῖξαι καὶ διδάξαι τοὺς
Ἕλληνας ὡς ὁ παρὰ τοῖς ἱστοῖς τραφεὶς ὑπερεβάλετο
μὲν Ἀριστοτέλη καὶ Πλάτωνα μεθόδοις λογικαῖς, κατ-
επάτησε δὲ Θεόφραστόν τε καὶ τοὺς Στωϊκοὺς ἐν
διαλεκτικῇ, φανερῶς δ᾽ ἐξήλεγξε τοὺς ἑταίρους αὐτῶν
ἅπαντας, οὐδὲ τίνα ποτ᾽ ἐστὶ τὰ πρῶτα νοσήματα
γινώσκοντας, τὸν Ἡρόφιλον ἐκεῖνον τὸν διαλεκτικόν,
καὶ τὸν συμφοιτητὴν αὐτοῦ Φιλότιμον, καὶ τὸν δι-
δάσκαλον αὐτοῦ Πραξαγόραν τὸν ἀπὸ Ἀσκληπιοῦ,
καὶ σὺν τούτοις τε καὶ πρὸ τούτων Ἐρασίστρατον,
Διοκλέα, Μνησίθεον, Διευχῆ, Φιλιστίωνα, Πλειστό-

28K

complete opposition to that revered name with which you name yourself, you, a man most unmethodical and rash, made an assertion without having grasped even the very origin itself from which it is essential for anyone who intends to discover the species of anything at all and their proper differentiae to begin? For, as Plato says somewhere, "in everything, my boy, there is one best starting point, which is to know what the search is about, otherwise everything inevitably goes wrong."[20] And he (Plato) thinks it right for us to take our starting point from the actual substance of what is being sought, not only in relation to dividing anything whatsoever, but also always to use this kind of starting point in relation to everything.

Here too it is necessary to say precisely what a disease is, and a symptom, and an affection, and to distinguish in what way each of the things spoken of is the same and in what way not the same, and only then endeavor to divide them in this way into the proper differentiae according to the method which the philosophers taught us. Or, if you have discovered some other, better method than that which they have written about, you should first resolve the issue, and then show and teach the Greeks how someone raised among the looms has surpassed Aristotle and Plato in logical methods, and has trampled underfoot both Theophrastus and the Stoics in dialectics, and has clearly refuted all their students who do not even know what the primary diseases are—men like Herophilus the dialectician, his fellow pupil Philotimus, his teacher Praxagoras, the follower of Aesclepius, and their contemporaries and predecessors Erasistratus, Diocles, Mnesitheus, Dieuches, Phil-

28K

---

[20] See both *Sophist* 242B and *Phaedrus* 237B–C. This is not an exact quotation.

νικον, αὐτὸν Ἱπποκράτην. τὸ δ᾽ ἁπλῶς ἀποφήνασθαι
δύο εἶναι τὰ πάντα πάθη κατὰ δίαιταν, οὐ μέθοδον,
οὐκ ἀπόδειξιν, οὐ πιθανὴν πίστιν, οὐ παραμυθίαν,
οὐδ᾽ ὅλως οὐδὲν ἄλλο προσθέντα, πλὴν εἰς τοὺς παλαιοὺς βλασφημήσαντα, προστάττοντός ἐστιν ἔργον,
οὐ διδάσκοντος.

ἔστω, σιωπᾷς, ἐκ ποίας εὗρες αὐτὰ μεθόδου λογι-
κῆς· ἀλλά τοι κἂν κριτήριόν γέ τι τῶν λόγων τῆς
ἀληθείας ἐχρῆν σε παρασχέσθαι. τοῦ μὲν γὰρ εὑρεῖν
29K τὸ ζητούμενον | αἱ λογικαὶ μέθοδοι τὴν δύναμιν ἔχου-
σι, τοῦ δὲ πιστώσασθαι τὰ καλῶς εὑρημένα δύο ἐστὶν
ἅπασιν ἀνθρώποις κριτήρια, λόγος καὶ πεῖρα. πρὸς
γοῦν τὸν ἐρωτήσαντα διὰ τί τῷδέ τινι τῷ πυρέττοντι
συνεχώρησας ὕδατος πιεῖν ψυχροῦ, δύο εἰσὶν ἀποκρί-
σεις, ἡ μὲν ἑτέρα γένεσίν τε καὶ φύσιν ἐκδιδάσκουσα
πυρετοῦ, καὶ περὶ τοῦ τῶν νόσων καιροῦ διεξιοῦσα,
καὶ κατὰ τὸν αὐτὸν τρόπον ὕδατος ψυχροῦ φύσιν
ἐξηγουμένη, κἀπειδὰν ταῦτα διεξέλθῃ, πειρωμένη διδάσκειν, ὡς τῷ τοιῷδε νοσήματι κατὰ τὸν τοιόνδε
καιρὸν εὔλογόν ἐστι ἴαμα γενέσθαι τὸ ὕδωρ τὸ ψυ-
χρόν· ἡ δ᾽ ἑτέρα τῶν ἀποκρίσεων οὐδενὸς τούτων τῆς
φύσεως ἐφαψαμένη καταφεύγει πρὸς τὴν πεῖραν, ἐν
τοιῷδε νοσήματι καὶ καιρῷ τὸ ψυχρὸν ὕδωρ ἑωρᾶσθαι
φάσκουσα πολλάκις ὠφελεῖν. ἐχρῆν οὖν, οἶμαι, καὶ
τὸν Θεσσαλὸν ἤτοι πεῖραν ἢ λόγον ἐφ᾽ οἷς ἀποφαίνε-
ται κριτήριον ἐπάγειν, οὐχ ὡς τύραννον ἡμῖν ἐπιτάτ-
τειν, ἀξιοῦντα πιστεύεσθαι χωρὶς ἀποδείξεως. Καὶ
τίνα, φασίν, ἀκούειν ἀπόδειξιν ἀξιοῖς; οὕτω γὰρ ἀντε-

istion, Pleistonicus and Hippocrates himself. The bald pronouncement that all affections are two in terms of regimen, setting out neither method, nor demonstration, nor persuasive argument, nor solution, nor anything else at all apart from slander of the ancients, is the work of one who gives orders and not of one who teaches.

So be it. You are silent as to the kind of logical method by which you discovered these things. At least you should have supplied some basis for judging the truth of your arguments. For, on the one hand, logical methods have the power to discover what is sought while, on the other hand, there are, for all men, two criteria for believing in things that have been correctly discovered—reason and experience. Indeed, to someone who asks why you agreed to a drink of cold water for a person with a fever, there are two replies. The one teaches about the genesis and nature of fever, about the appropriate times in diseases, and, in the same way, explains the nature of cold water and, whenever it goes over these things, attempts to teach how, in this particular disease in relation to this particular time, it happens that cold water is the reasonable treatment. The other response touches on nothing about the nature of these things, but has recourse to experience, asserting that, in this particular disease at this particular time, cold water has often been seen to be of help. So then, in my view, Thessalus must focus on either experience or reason as the criterion in giving his account of these things and not, like a dictator, order us around, thinking it right that we should trust him without demonstration. "But," they say, "what kind of demonstration do you think it right to hear?"—for

29K

47

ρωτῶσιν ἡμᾶς οἱ ἀπ' αὐτοῦ· καὶ δικαίως γε τοῦτο
30K ποιοῦσιν, οὐδ' εἰς ἔννοιάν | ποτε παρελθόντες ἀποδεί-
ξεως, ὡς ἂν οὔτε γεωμετρίας οὔτ' ἀριθμητικῆς οὔτε
διαλεκτικῆς οὔτε ἀναλυτικῆς οὔθ' ὅλως λογικῆς τινος
ἁψάμενοι θεωρίας. ἀποκριτέον οὖν αὐτοῖς, ὡς Ὀψὲ
πάνυ μανθάνειν ἐφίεσθε τί ποτ' ἐστὶν ἀπόδειξις, καὶ
ὡς οὐκ ἐνδέχεται χρόνῳ βραχεῖ λεπτῆς γνώμης δεομένη παρακολουθῆσαι θεωρίᾳ μήτ' ἠσκημένους ἀκούειν ἀκριβῶν λόγων ἐν διαστροφῇ τε πολυχρονίῳ γε-
γονότας. ἐκείνους μὲν οὖν ἀποπέμψωμεν, ὡς μηδὲ
συνιέναι δυναμένους ἀληθῶν μαθημάτων, μήτιγε δὴ
μαθεῖν ἢ κρῖναι καλῶς.

4. Ἡμεῖς δὲ μετὰ τῶν ἠσκημένων τε ἅμα παρακολουθεῖν ἀποδείξει καὶ φύσει συνετῶν, οὐ γὰρ δὴ ὄνους
Θεσσαλείους ἐπαγγελλόμεθα διδάσκειν, ἐπὶ τὸ προκείμενον ἐξ ἀρχῆς ἴωμεν, εὐθὺς ἅμα τῇ διδασκαλίᾳ
τῆς θεραπευτικῆς μεθόδου καὶ ὧν ἐσφάλησαν οἱ
πλεῖστοι τῶν ἰατρῶν ἐπιχειρησάντων ἐξευρεῖν αὐτὴν
ἐξηγούμενοι τὰς αἰτίας· εἰς γάρ τοι τὴν βεβαιοτέραν
πίστιν τῶν ἀληθῶν οὐδὲ τοῦτο σμικρὸν φαίνεται συν-
31K τελεῖν. πρῶτον μὲν οὖν εὐλαβηθῶμεν ἀμφοῖν | ἅμα
μεμνῆσθαι, μεθόδου τε λογικῆς καὶ πείρας ἀλόγου·
πρόκειται γὰρ οὐ περὶ πάσης εὑρέσεως ἰαμάτων εἰπεῖν νῦν, ἀλλὰ μόνης τῆς κατὰ μέθοδον· ὥσπερ καὶ
περί γε τῆς ἐμπειρικῆς ἡμῖν τε δι' ἑτέρου γράμματος
εἴρηται καὶ αὐτοῖς τοῖς[30] Ἐμπειρικοῖς καλουμένοις
ἰατροῖς ἐπὶ πλεῖστον ἐξείργασται. καὶ οὕτως ἂν εὐξαί-

---

[30] τοῖς B, P1, P2; om. K

so his followers question us in turn. And, indeed, they do this with reason, never having arrived at any notion of demonstration, since they would not have come to grips with geometry, arithmetic, dialectics, analysis, or logical theory of any kind. I must reply to them, then, [by saying]: "You are aiming to learn very late in the day what demonstration is, and it is not possible to follow in a moment a theory which requires a fine intelligence, nor for those who are practiced in long-term distortion to listen to precise logic." Let us, then, dismiss these people as not having the capacity to understand true studies, much less to learn and judge properly. 30K

4. Let us proceed instead in the company of those who are both trained to follow exposition and are naturally intelligent (for we certainly do not profess to give instruction to those asinine Thessaleians) to what was proposed at the outset, and immediately, along with the teaching of the therapeutic method, expound the reasons why the majority of doctors, when they attempt to discover this method, slipped into error, because this seems to bring about, to no small extent, a stronger confidence in the truth. First, let us take care not to pay attention to both things simultaneously, i.e. logical method and irrational experience, for it is not proposed to speak now about the whole discovery of cures, but only that which relates to method just as I have also spoken about the empirical [discovery of cures] in another work,[21] and this has been dealt with more fully by the so-called Empiric doctors themselves. And so I would pray 31K

---

21 As R. J. Hankinson (1991) has pointed out, this is more likely to be *De empirica subfiguratione* than *De experientia medica*. Both works are translated in R. Walzer and M. Frede (1985).

μὴν καὶ τοὺς Λογικοὺς ἅπαντας ἰατροὺς ἔχεσθαι τοῦ
προκειμένου, καὶ μὴ συγχεῖν, μηδὲ ταράττειν, μηδὲ
συνάγειν εἰς ταὐτὸν ἀναλογισμόν τε καὶ πεῖραν, ἀλλ᾽
ἑκάτερον ἰδίᾳ μεταχειρίζεσθαι καὶ σκοπεῖσθαι τίνα
δύναμιν ἔχει καὶ πόσον εἰς τὸ τέλος τῆς τέχνης
συνεργεῖ.

τὸ τοίνυν μεθόδῳ τι ζητεῖν ἐξευρεῖν ἀντίκειται μὲν
τῷ κατὰ τύχην τε καὶ αὐτομάτως· ἔστι δὲ τὸ τοιοῦτον
μετά τινος ὁδοῦ καὶ τάξεως, ὡς εἶναί τι πρῶτον ἐν τῇ
ζητήσει καὶ δεύτερον καὶ τρίτον καὶ τέταρτον καὶ
οὕτως ἐφεξῆς τἆλλα σύμπαντα, μέχρι περ ἂν ἀφίκη-
ταί τις ἐπ᾽ αὐτὸ τὸ προκείμενον ἐξ ἀρχῆς. οἱ μὲν οὖν
ἀπὸ τῆς ἐμπειρίας καλῶς ποιοῦντες ὁμολογοῦσιν ὡς
οὔτε τῆς εὑρέσεως οὔτε τῆς διδασκαλίας ἀναγκαία
32K τάξις ἐστὶ παρ᾽ | αὐτοῖς· ἄτεχνον γάρ τι καὶ ἄλογον ἡ
πεῖρα καὶ τύχης ἀγαθῆς δεόμενον εἰς τὴν τῶν ζητουμένων εὕρεσιν. ὅσοι δὲ λόγον ἡγεμόνα τῆς εὑρέσεως
ἐποιήσαντο καὶ τάξιν, ὁδόν τε μίαν τὴν ἐπὶ τὸ τέλος
ἄγουσαν ὑπέθεντο, τούτοις ἀναγκαῖον μὲν ἦν ἀπὸ
πρώτου τινὸς ἀρξαμένοις ὁμολογουμένου πᾶσιν ἀνθρώποις, οὕτως ἤδη μετιέναι πρὸς τὰ λοιπά· ποιοῦσί
γε μὴν οὐχ οὕτως, ἀλλὰ καὶ τὰς ἀρχὰς οἱ πλεῖστοι
διαφωνουμένας λαμβάνουσιν, οὐκ ἀποδείξαντες δὲ
ἐπὶ τὰ λοιπὰ κατὰ τὸν αὐτὸν τρόπον μετέρχονται,
νομοθετοῦντες μᾶλλον ἢ ἀποδεικνύντες. ἅπαντα δ᾽
αὐτοῖς τὰ τοιαῦτα συμβαίνει διὰ τὸ μηδὲν ὑπὲρ ἀποδείξεως ἐπεσκέφθαι πρότερον, ἀλλ᾽ ἅμα τε τοῖς ζητου-
μένοις ἐφίστασθαι καὶ τολμᾶν χρῆσθαι πρὸς τὴν

that all the Rationalist doctors too will hold themselves to the proposition, and not confound or confuse or bring together as one, analogy and experience, but try out each individually, and consider what power each has, and how much it contributes to the goal of the craft.

Thus, to seek to discover something by method stands in opposition to doing so by chance and spontaneously, for such an approach requires a certain path and order so that there is something first in the search, and then something second, and third, and fourth and so on with respect to all the other [steps] in sequence until one arrives at the very thing that was proposed at the outset. Those who employ the empirical approach are doing the right thing when they agree that, for them, there is no necessary order either of discovery or teaching. Experience is something 32K that is unsystematic and irrational, and requires good fortune for the discovery of those things being sought. However, those who made reason and order their guides to discovery, and took as foundational that there is a single path leading to the objective are constrained by a necessity to start from some first point agreed upon by all men, and only then progress toward the rest. However, the majority do not do this but rather take disputed starting points and, without having provided demonstration, go on in like manner to the rest, laying down the law instead of providing demonstration. All such things happen to them because they have not given prior consideration to demonstration. And yet, at the same time, they apply themselves to what is being sought and dare to use demonstrations to support

πίστιν αὐτῶν ἀποδείξεσιν, ὅμοιόν τι ποιοῦσιν ἀνθρώπῳ μετρεῖν ἐπιχειροῦντι σφαῖραν, ἢ κύβον, ἢ
κῶνον, ἢ κύλινδρον, ἤ τι τοιοῦτον ἕτερον, οὔτε γεωμετρίας οὔτε λογιστικῆς ἐπιστήμονι θεωρίας, ἀλλὰ
μηδὲ πῆχυν, ἢ παλαιστήν, ἢ πόδα παρεσκευασμένῳ,
κἄπειτα ἀγανακτοῦντι πρὸς τοὺς ἀπόδειξιν ζητοῦντας, |

33K ἢ καὶ σιωπᾶν ἀξιοῦντας. ὡς γὰρ κἀκεῖ γελοῖος ὁ
φάσκων ὀρθογωνίου τριγώνου, τῆς μὲν ἑτέρας τῶν
περὶ τὴν ὀρθὴν γωνίαν πεντάποδος, εἰ οὕτως ἔτυχεν,
ὑπαρχούσης, τῆς δ' ἑτέρας δωδεκάποδος, οὐ τριάκοντα ποδῶν γίγνεσθαι τὸ ἐμβαδόν, ἀλλὰ τετταράκοντα,
καὶ τούτων μηδεμίαν ἀπόδειξιν ἔχων εἰπεῖν, οὕτω
κἀνταῦθα γελοῖος ὁ ἀποφηνάμενος μὲν ὁτιοῦν, ἀποδεῖξαι δ' οὐ δυνάμενος.

ὡς οὖν ἐπὶ[31] τῆς κατὰ τὸ τρίγωνον ἀποδείξεως, οὐ
γὰρ ἀφεκτέον ἡμῖν ἐστι τοῦ παραδείγματος, ἀπεληλα-
κόσιν ἤδη τοῦ λόγου τοὺς ἀπαιδεύτους Μεθοδικούς,
αὐτὸ μὲν τὸ προκείμενον ἐκ δυοῖν τούτων ἐπεραίνετο
προτάσεων, μιᾶς μὲν τῆς τὸ περιεχόμενον χωρίον ὑπό
τε τῆς πεντάποδος καὶ δωδεκάποδος, ἑξηκοντάπουν
γίγνεσθαι, δευτέρας δὲ τῆς ἥμισυ τὸ[32] τρίγωνον ἐκείνου τοῦ χωρίου λεγούσης καὶ δεικνυούσης ὑπάρχειν,
ἑκατέρα δὲ πάλιν τούτων ἑτέρων τινῶν εἰς ἀπόδειξιν
ἐδεῖτο προτάσεων, εἶτ' ἐκεῖναι πάλιν ἑτέρων, ἄχρι περ
ἂν ἐπὶ τὰς πρώτας ἀνέλθωμεν, αἳ οὐκέτ' ἐξ ἀλλήλων,[33]
οὐδὲ δι' ἀποδείξεως, ἀλλ' ἐξ ἑαυτῶν ἔχουσι τὴν
πίστιν, οὕτως, οἶμαι, κἀπὶ τῶν τὴν ἰατρικὴν τέχνην

34K ἀποδεικνυμένων | ἁπάντων εἰς πρώτας τινὰς ἀναποδεί-

52

their belief. They act like someone who tries to measure a sphere, cube, cone, or cylinder, or some other such thing, but has no knowledge of either geometry or logical theory, and provides himself with neither cubit, span, nor foot rule, and then becomes vexed with those who seek a demonstration, or think he should be silent. For just as some- 33K one would be ludicrous who asserts that, in the case of a right-angle triangle, if one of the sides enclosing the right angle is five feet, as it might happen to be, and the other is twelve feet, the area is not thirty feet but forty feet, and to say this is so without giving any demonstration, so here too, someone who declares anything whatsoever without being able to provide a demonstration would be laughable.

So in the demonstration regarding the triangle—for there is no need for us to resile from the example since we have already expelled the uneducated Methodics from the discussion—the proposition itself was reached from these two premises: the first is that the area enclosed by the five feet and the twelve feet is sixty feet, and the second is the claim that the triangle is half that area, and showing that it is. However, each of these again requires certain other premises for demonstration, then those others again, until we come to those premises that are primary, which no longer have their proof from one another or from demonstration, but from themselves. The same applies too, I think, in the case of demonstrations in the medical craft. In 34K all instances, there must be reduction to certain primary

---

31 ἐπί B; om. K
32 τό B; om. K
33 αἵ οὐκέτ' ἐξ ἀλλήλων B; αἱδὲ οὐκ ἐξ ἄλλων K

κτους προτάσεις καὶ ἐξ ἑαυτῶν πιστὰς ἀνάγεσθαι
χρῆναι πάντα. καὶ εἴπερ οὕτως ἅπαντες ἐπεχείρησαν
εἰπεῖν τι περὶ τῆς θεραπευτικῆς μεθόδου, πάντως ἄν
που καὶ συνεφώνησαν ἀλλήλοις, ὥσπερ οἱ ἀριθμητι-
κοί τε καὶ γεωμέτραι καὶ οἱ λογιστικοί· μαθεῖν γοῦν
ἔστι παρ' ἐκείνων εὐθὺς κατ' ἀρχὰς ὁποῖον μέν τι
δηλοῦται πρὸς ἑκάστου τῶν ὀνομάτων οἷς μέλλουσι
χρῆσθαι, τίνας δὲ προτάσεις ἀναποδείκτους παραλή-
ψονται πρὸς τὸν λόγον, ἅσπερ δὴ καὶ ἀξιώματα καλοῦσιν, οἷον ὅτι γραμμὴν μὲν ὀνομάζω μῆκος ἀπλα-
τές, ἐπιφάνειαν δὲ τὸ μῆκος καὶ πλάτος μόνον ἔχον,
καὶ τρίγωνον μὲν τόδέ τι, τετράγωνον δὲ τόδέ τι, καὶ
τῶν ἄλλων ὁμοίως ἕκαστον· εἶθ' ὅτι καὶ τοῖς τοιούτοις
ἀξιώμασι χρήσοιτο, προειπὼν ὡς τὰ τῷ αὐτῷ ἴσα καὶ
ἀλλήλοις ἐστὶν ἴσα, καὶ ἐὰν ἴσοις ἴσα προστεθῇ, τὰ
ὅλα ἴσα ἔσται· μετὰ ταῦτ' ἤδη πειρᾶται δεικνύναι τὰ
θεωρήματα, μηδὲν τούτων ἔξωθεν ὧν ἐξ ἀρχῆς ὑπέθετο προλαμβάνων. οἱ πολλοὶ δὲ τῶν ἰατρῶν, ὡς
οἶσθα καὶ αὐτός, Ἱέρων κράτιστε, πόθεν ἤρξαντο τῆς
35K εὑρέσεως ἣν εὑρηκέναι φασὶν ἐρωτώμενοι | τοσοῦτον
ἀποδέουσι τοῦ λέγειν ἀναποδείκτους τε καὶ ἅπασιν
ὁμολογουμένας ἀρχάς, ὥστ' οὐδ' ἀποκρίνεσθαι σύμφωνον ἑαυτοῖς οὐδὲν ἐξευρίσκουσιν, ἀλλ' Εὐρίπου
δίκην ἄνω τε καὶ κάτω μεταβάλλονται, τἀναντία τιθέ-
μενος ἕκαστος ἑαυτῷ τοῦ λόγου προϊόντος ὧν ἐξ
ἀρχῆς ὑπέθετο.

φαινομένας γοῦν εἰπὼν εἶναι τὰς κοινότητας ὁ σοφώτατος Θεσσαλός, ὀλίγον ὕστερον οὐ μόνον οὐδένα

54

and undemonstrable premises, and from these all things must draw their proof. Indeed, if everyone attempted to say something about the therapeutic method in this way, they would be in harmony with each other in every respect, just like the arithmeticians, geometers, and logicians. At any rate, it is possible to learn from such men right from the outset what is signified by each of the terms they are going to use, and what undemonstrable premises they will assume with respect to the argument, which in actual fact they call axioms. For example, I call a length with no breadth a "line," while what has length and breadth only, I call a "surface," and this a "triangle," and that a "quadrilateral," and each of the other things likewise. Then one might also use such axioms, putting forward the proposition that those things equal to the same thing are also equal to each other, and that, if equals are added to equals, the totals [so created] will be equal and, after this, attempt to demonstrate the theorems, assuming beforehand nothing outside those things which were proposed at the outset. Most doctors, as you yourself also know, my dearest Hiero, when asked to say where they began the discovery of what they have discovered, are to such an 35K extent deficient in stating indemonstrables and starting points agreed by all that they can make no reply that is consistent among themselves but, as the argument proceeds, they ebb and flow like the Euripus, each one postulating things that are the opposite of those things he postulated at the beginning.

At all events, that most sapient Thessalus says the "communities" are apparent, yet a little later says not only

τῶν ἔμπροσθεν ἰατρῶν ἰδεῖν αὐτάς φησιν, ἀλλ᾽ οὐδὲ
τὸν πρῶτον γεννήσαντα Θεμίσωνα· τούτῳ γὰρ οὖν δὴ
μόνῳ παραχωρεῖ καθάπερ πατρὶ τέκνα γνήσια τὰς
τερατώδεις ἐκείνας κοινότητας. εἶθ᾽ οἱ μετ᾽ αὐτοὺς
ἅπαντες ἀλλήλοις τε καὶ τῷ Θεσσαλῷ διηνέχθησαν,
οὔτε τὰς αὐτὰς εἰσηγούμενοι κοινότητας οὔθ᾽ ὅλως
ἀλλήλοις ὁμολογοῦντες οὐδὲ καθ᾽ ἕν, ὥσπέρ σοι καὶ
τοῦτο πολλάκις ἀπέδειξα παρόντων αὐτῶν τῶν Μεθο-
δικῶν·

ἴσως δ᾽ ἄν που καὶ γράψαιμι κατὰ πολλὴν σχολὴν
ὑπὲρ τῆς διαφωνίας αὐτῶν, ἀλλὰ νῦν γε τοσοῦτον εἰς
τὰ προκείμενα προσήκει λαβεῖν, ὡς ἐχρῆν ἀρχηγοὺς
αἱρέσεως καθισταμένους αὐτοὺς ἐξηγήσασθαι πρό-
36K τερον ἐφ᾽ ὅτου πράγματος ἕκαστον | τῶν ὀνομάτων
ἐπιφέρουσιν, ὥσπερ οὖν καὶ οἱ Ἐμπειρικοὶ ποιοῦσι,
φαίνεσθαι μὲν λέγοντες τὰ ταῖς αἰσθήσεσιν ὑπο-
πίπτοντα, γινώσκεσθαι δὲ τὰ μνημονευόμενα, φαίνεσθαι δ᾽ ἅμα καὶ γινώσκεσθαι τὰ καὶ πρότερόν ποτε
ταῖς αἰσθήσεσιν ὑποπεσόντα καὶ νῦν ὁμοίως ὑπο-
πίπτοντα. πότερον οὖν οὕτω καὶ αὐτοὶ φαίνεσθαι λέγουσι τὰς κοινότητας ὡς αἰσθήσει γνωριζομένας, ἢ
καὶ τὰ διὰ λόγου λαμβανόμενα φαινόμενα καλοῦσιν;
οἱ μὲν γὰρ ἀπὸ τῆς Ἐμπειρίας οὐ πάνυ τι συγχωροῦσιν οὐδὲν τῶν τῷ λόγῳ μόνῳ δοκούντων ἐγνῶσθαι
φαινόμενον ὀνομάζειν· οἱ δ᾽ αὖ παλαιοὶ φιλόσοφοι
διττὸν γένος εἶναί φασι τῶν φαινομένων, ἓν μέν, ὅπερ

---

22 Themison of Laodicea (ca. 90–40 BC) is regarded, on some-

that no previous doctors have seen them, not even their originator Themison;[22] but that, in fact, to him alone did those monstrous "communities" yield, like legitimate off-spring to their father. Then all those who followed differed from each other, and from Thessalus, neither proposing "communities" that were the same, nor agreeing in any way with each other in relation to any one single point, and this is exactly what I have frequently demonstrated to you when the Methodics themselves were present.

But perhaps, when I have plenty of time, I could, I suppose, write about their disagreements, but now, at least, it is appropriate just to deal with what pertains to the matter lying before us, which is that it is necessary for those who set themselves up as the founders of a sect to show first to what matter they relate each of the terms. This is what the 36K Empirics do when they say that those things which fall under the senses are apparent, whereas those things that are remembered are known, and that those things that at some time previously fell under the senses and now like-wise fall under the senses are, at one and the same time, apparent and known. So, then, do [the Methodics] them-selves say that the "communities" are apparent as being known by perception or do they also call apparent those things accepted through reason? For the Empirics abso-lutely do not accept that any of those things which seem to be known by reason alone are to be called apparent. The philosophers of old, in turn, say there is a twofold class of things that are apparent (phenomena): one component

what inconclusive evidence, as the "founder" of Methodism and is said to have written four books, one of which was titled *The Method*.

καὶ τοῖς Ἐμπειρικοῖς ὁμολογεῖται, τῶν αἰσθήσει τινὶ
διαγινωσκομένων, οἷον λευκοῦ καὶ μέλανος καὶ σκλη-
ροῦ καὶ μαλακοῦ καὶ θερμοῦ καὶ ψυχροῦ καὶ τῶν
ὁμοίων, ἕτερον δὲ τῶν ὑποπιπτόντων νοήσει κατὰ
πρώτην ἐπιβολὴν ἀναπόδεικτον, ὡς τὰ τῷ αὐτῷ ἴσα
καὶ ἀλλήλοις ὑπάρχειν ἴσα, καὶ ἐὰν ἴσοις ἴσα προστεθῇ, καὶ τὰ ὅλα ἴσα γίγνεσθαι, καὶ ἐὰν ἀπὸ ἴσων ἴσα
ἀφαιρεθῇ, καὶ τὰ λοιπὰ ἴσα εἶναι. τοῦ τοιούτου γένους
εἶναί φασι καὶ τὸ μηδὲν ἀναιτίως γίγνεσθαι· καὶ πάντ᾽
37K ἐξ ὄντος τινός, ἐκ δὲ | τοῦ μηδόλως ὄντος οὐδέν· οὕτω
δὲ καὶ τὸ φθείρεσθαι μηδὲν εἰς τὸ τελέως[34] οὐκ ὄν, καὶ
τὸ περὶ παντὸς ἀναγκαῖον ἢ καταφάσκειν ἢ ἀπο-
φάσκειν, ἕτερά τε τοιαῦτα πολλά, περὶ ὧν ἐν ταῖς
λογικαῖς πραγματείαις ἐπισκέπτονται, καὶ ἡμῖν δὲ εἰς
ὅσον οἷόν τε σαφέστατα διὰ τῶν Περὶ[35] ἀποδείξεως
ὑπομνημάτων εἴρηται.

περὶ τούτων ἐν ταῖς τοιαύταις ἀρχαῖς, ἃς δὴ καὶ
λογικὰς ὀνομάζομεν, ἀμφισβητοῦσιν ἔνιοι τῶν φιλοσόφων ἐρίζοντες· ἀλλ᾽ ἐκεῖνοι μὲν ἄχρι γοῦν τοσούτου
σωφρονοῦσιν, ὡς ἀπιστεῖν ἀποδείξει πάσῃ, γινώ-
σκοντες, οἶμαι, κἂν μὴ λέγωσιν, ὡς αὐτὸ γοῦν τοῦτο
βεβαίως ἐπίστανται, τὸ μηδὲν ἀποδειχθῆναι δύνασθαι, τῶν λογικῶν ἀρχῶν ἀπιστουμένων· ὅσοι δ᾽ ἄχρι
τοσούτου σκαιοὶ καὶ ἀνόητοι τυγχάνουσιν ὄντες, ὡς
μηδὲ αὐτῷ τούτῳ παρακολουθεῖν, ἀποδεικνύναι μὲν
πειρῶνται, τίνες δέ εἰσι καὶ ποῖαι καὶ πόσαι τῶν

---

[34] τελέως B, P1, P2; τέως K   [35] B; ὑπέρ K

58

(and here there is agreement with the Empirics) comprises those things discerned by a sense, such as whiteness or blackness, hardness or softness, hot or cold, and suchlike, while the other comprises those things which fall under the intellect at their first apprehension and are indemonstrable—for example, things that are equal to the same thing are equal to each other, and that if equals are added to equals the wholes are equal, and that if equals are subtracted from equals the remainders are equal. They also claim that the nonexistence of anything without a cause is part of such a class, and that everything comes from some existing thing, while nothing comes from something that does not exist at all. So too, [they say that] nothing is destroyed to what is completely nonexistent, and that it is necessary for everything to be either confirmed or denied, and many other such propositions which they consider in their treatises on logic, and which I have also spoken of with the greatest possible clarity through the treatise *On Demonstration*.[23]

37K

Some philosophers, since they are contentious, dispute about these things subsumed under such principles which, indeed, we call logical as well. But they are, at least, sufficiently sensible to distrust all demonstration, knowing, I think, even if they do not say so, enough to be assured of this very point—that nothing can be demonstrated when the logical principles are not to be trusted. However, those who are actually so foolish and unintelligent as not to follow this very position, do attempt to provide demonstrations. There are, however, certain kinds and numbers of

[23] Galen's major work on logic, *De demonstratione*, is no longer extant.

ἀποδείξεων ἀρχαὶ μήτε γινώσκειν μήτε ζητεῖν ἐθέλειν
μήτ᾽ ἄλλου διδάσκοντος ἀκούειν ὑπομένειν, ἀλλ᾽
ἁπλῶς ἀποφαίνεσθαι καὶ φθέγγεσθαι ῥήματα μηδ᾽ ὅ
τι σημαίνει σαφῶς εἰπεῖν δυνάμενοι. εὐλόγως οὖν
38K ἑκατοντάβιβλοι πραγματεῖαι γράφονται | τοῖς ἀπ᾽ αὐ-
τῶν, ἅμα μὲν ζητοῦσι καθ᾽ ὅτου πράγματος ἕκαστον
τῶν ὀνομάτων ὁ Θεσσαλὸς ἐπέφερεν, ἅμα δ᾽ οὐχ
εὑρίσκουσιν οὐδὲν τοιοῦτον ᾧ συμφωνήσει πάντα τὰ
κατὰ μέρος ὑπ᾽ αὐτοῦ λεγόμενα. τίνες γὰρ οὖν αἱ
φαινόμεναι κοινότητές εἰσιν, ἢ πῶς φαινόμεναι, λέγειν οὐκ ἔχουσιν, οὐδ᾽ ἂν πολλαπλασίους ἄλλας γρά-
ψωσι βίβλους. ἤτοι γὰρ αἰσθήσει πάντως ὑποπίπτειν
χρὴ τὸ φαινόμενον, ἢ νοήσει κατὰ μίαν ἐπιβολὴν
ἀθρόως, ἑκάτερα χωρὶς ἀποδείξεως· εἴ τι δ᾽ ἐκπέπτωκεν ἐκ τοῦ κατὰ μίαν προσβολὴν εἰς γνῶσιν ἥκειν,
εὐθὺς μὲν τοῦτο καὶ διαπεφώνηται πάντως καὶ ἀποδείξεως δεῖται καὶ τέχνην οὐδεμίαν ἀπὸ τοιούτου
πράγματος ἄρχεσθαι προσήκει.

  ταῦτ᾽ οὖν εἰ μὲν ἐγυμνάσαντο κατὰ τὰς λογικὰς
μεθόδους, αὐτοί τ᾽ ἂν ᾔδεσαν ἡμῶν τε οὐκ ἂν μάτην
κατέτριβον τὸν χρόνον· ἐπεὶ δ᾽ ἀγύμναστοι καὶ ἀμα-
θεῖς ὄντες, ἐξ ἀπονοίας ἐτόλμησαν ἀποδείξει χρῆσα-
σθαι, πρὶν ὅ τί ποτέ ἐστιν ἀπόδειξις μαθεῖν, ἀναγκαῖον ἤδη τοὺς τοιούτους ἅπαντας σφάλλεσθαι καὶ
ληρεῖν μακρά, καὶ μηδὲ τοῖς ὀρθῶς ἀποδεικνύουσιν
ἀκολουθεῖν, ἀλλ᾽ ἀναλίσκειν μάτην τὸν χρόνον. μὴ
39K τοίνυν αὐτοῖς | μηδ᾽ ὡς ζῴοις λογικοῖς ἔτι διαλεγώ-
μεθα, μηδ᾽ ἀντιλέγωμεν μακρά, πρὶν ἂν ἐθελήσωσι

principles of demonstration that they are unwilling either
to know or to seek [to know], or to allow themselves to
learn from some other teacher. Rather, they simply make
assertions and utter words without being able to say clearly
what they signify. With good reason, then, do their acolytes
write hundred-volume treatises as, at one and the same
time, they seek to discover to what matter Thessalus applies each of his terms, but fail to discover any such thing
with which all the particular terms stated by him are consistent. They are not able to say what the apparent "communities" are, or how they are apparent, [and could] not,
even if they were to write many times as many other books.
For something that is apparent must either fall completely
under perception or completely under reason at its first apprehension, in each case apart from demonstration. And if
something has failed to come to the intellect in one apprehension, it is immediately both questionable in every way
and in need of demonstration. In no art is it appropriate to
start from such a thing.

Now in regard to this, if these men had undertaken
training in logical methods, they would have known this
themselves and would not have wasted our time in vain.
But because they are untrained and ignorant, and due to
their laziness dared to make use of demonstration before
they even learned what demonstration is, it is inevitable
that all such men actually err and talk a lot of nonsense,
and do not even follow those who provide correct demonstrations, but fruitlessly squander their time. Let us not,
therefore, discourse any more with them as though with
rational creatures, nor speak against them at great length

38K

39K

μαθεῖν οἷόν τι πρᾶγμά ἐστιν ἀπόδειξις, ὅπως τε δεῖ
τὸν μέλλοντα καλῶς αὐτῇ χρήσασθαι γεγυμνάσθαι.

5. Καί σοι τὸν ἑξῆς λόγον ἤδη ἅπαντα ποιήσομαι,
χρώμενος ταῖς μεθόδοις ἃς ἐν τοῖς Περὶ τῆς ἀποδείξεως ὑπομνήμασι κατεστησάμην. ὅτι τε γὰρ ἀρχαὶ
πάσης ἀποδείξεώς εἰσι τὰ πρὸς αἴσθησίν τε καὶ
νόησιν ἐναργῶς φαινόμενα καὶ ὡς ἐπὶ πάντων τῶν
ζητουμένων εἰς λόγον χρὴ μεταλαμβάνεσθαι τοὔνομα, δι᾿ ἐκείνων ἀποδέδεικται· νυνὶ δ᾿ ὅπως μὲν ᾖ
εὑρίσκειν, ἢ ἀποδεικνύναι προσήκει, λέγειν οὐ πρόκειται, τοῖς δ᾿ ἤδη μεμαθηκόσι τε καὶ ἠσκηκόσιν ἅμα
μὲν ἀποδοῦναί τινα καρπὸν τῶν πόνων εὐκαιρότατον,
ἐξευρόντας οὐ σμικρὸν πρᾶγμα τὸ νῦν ἡμῖν προ-
κείμενον· ἅμα δ᾿ εἴ τινες ἐπιθυμηταὶ τῆς μεγίστης
τέχνης εἰσίν, ἣ περὶ τὴν ψυχὴν τοῦ ἀνθρώπου κατα-
γίνεται, προγυμνάσαι καὶ τούτους εὔλογον ἐν τοῖς
σμικροτέροις· τούτου γὰρ χρὴ μάλιστα κατὰ πάσας
τὰς μεθόδους ἀντέχεσθαι, τοῦ γυμνάζεσθαι κατ᾿ αὐ-
40K τὰς | ἐπὶ πολλῶν πολλάκις προβλημάτων μικροτέρων,
πρὶν ἐπιχειρεῖν τοῖς μείζοσιν.

ἤδ᾿ οὖν ἡμῖν ἀρχὴ τῆς ἀληθοῦς ἔστω διδασκαλίας,
ἣν ἂν εὐθὺς ἀπ᾿ ἀρχῆς ἐποιησάμεθα, ζητοῦντές τε τὴν
τέχνην αὐτοὶ καὶ ποδηγοῦντες ἑτέρους μηδέπω δι-
εστραμμένους οὕτως ὥστ᾿ ἐπεὶ πρόκειται θεραπείας
εὑρεῖν ἁπάντων τῶν νοσημάτων, ἀναγκαῖον ἐπίστασθαι πρότερον ὁπόσα τὰ σύμπαντά ἐστιν· ἀλλ᾿ ἐπεὶ
μήτε διαφορὰς μήτε εἴδη δυνατὸν ἐξευρεῖν γένους
μηδενὸς ἄνευ τοῦ βεβαίως αὐτὸ τὸ τεμνόμενον ἐπί-

before they are willing to learn what sort of thing demonstration is, and how someone intending to use it properly must be trained.

5. I shall now set out in order for you the whole argument using the methods which I established in my work *On Demonstration*. It was shown in those writings that the origins of every demonstration are the things clearly apparent to sensation and reason, and that, in the case of all things being inquired into, it is necessary to assign a name to the argument. At the moment, I don't propose to say how it is appropriate either to discover or to demonstrate. Rather, I propose in part to give some of the fruits of my labors that are most seasonable for those who have already learned and practiced [these things], because I have discovered that what lies before us now is no insignificant matter. In part, also, I propose that, if some are to set their hearts on the greatest art, which is that relating to the soul of man, it is reasonable for them to train first in the lesser arts. One must hold fast to this [rule] particularly in all the methods: to exercise oneself in these methods frequently 40K in the many minor problems before attempting those that are major.

Let us make this, then, the starting point of the true teaching, which we ought to have done right from the beginning if we are seeking the art ourselves and guiding others, who have not yet been perverted, in such a way. Since what is proposed is to discover treatments for all diseases, it is essential to know beforehand how many [diseases] there are in all. But because it is impossible to discover either the differentiae or the kinds of any genus without certain knowledge of the actual thing being divided, we must

στασθαι, χρὴ δήπου καὶ νῦν ὅ τί ποτέ ἐστι νόσημα τῷ
λόγῳ διελθεῖν, ἵν᾽ οὕτως ἐπιχειρήσωμεν ὀρθῶς αὐτοῦ
τῇ διαιρέσει.

πῶς οὖν ἐξεύρωμεν αὐτὸ ὀρθῶς μεθόδῳ; πῶς δ᾽
ἄλλως ἢ ὡς ἐν τοῖς Περὶ ἀποδείξεως ἐλέγετο; τῆς
ἐννοίας πρότερον ὁμολογηθείσης, ἧς χωρὶς οὐχ οἷόν
τέ ἐστιν εὑρεθῆναι τὴν οὐσίαν τοῦ προκειμένου πρά-
γματος· αὐτὴν δὲ τὴν ἔννοιαν ὁμολογουμένην ἅπασιν
ἐλέγομεν χρῆναι λαμβάνειν, ἢ οὐδ᾽ ἂν ἀρχὴν δεόντως
ὀνομάζεσθαι. τίς οὖν ὑπὸ πάντων ἐστὶν ἀνθρώπων
ὁμολογουμένη περὶ τοῦ νοσεῖν ἔννοια; καὶ κατὰ τίνος
41K μάλιστα φέρουσιν ὑποκειμένου πράγματος | τουτὶ τὸ
ῥῆμα τὸ νοσεῖν; ἆρ᾽ οὐκ ἐπειδὰν μὲν ἀνεμπόδιστοι
ταῖς ἐνεργείαις ἁπάντων ὦσι τῶν τοῦ σώματος μορίων, ὑγιαίνειν τε σφᾶς αὐτοὺς τηνικαῦτά φασι καὶ
οὐδὲν οἴονται δεῖσθαι τῶν ἰατρῶν, ἐπειδὰν δὲ τῶν
κατὰ φύσιν ἔργων τοῦ σώματος ὁτιοῦν αἰσθάνωνται
σφισιν ἢ κακῶς ἢ μηδόλως ἔτι γινόμενον, ἡγοῦνταί γε
νοσεῖν ἐν ἐκείνῳ τῷ μέρει τοῦ σώματος, οὗ τὴν ἐνέργειαν ὁρῶσι βεβλαμμένην, ἰατρῷ τε συμβούλῳ χρῶνται περὶ τῆς ἰάσεως; ἐγὼ μὲν οὕτως ὁρῶ πάντας
ἀνθρώπους τῷ τε τῆς ὑγείας καὶ τῷ τῆς νόσου χρωμένους ὀνόματι, καὶ τὴν ἔννοιαν ἣν εἶπον ἅπαντας
διασῴζοντας ἐπί τε τούτων αὐτῶν καὶ ἔτι πρὸς τούτοις
οὐδὲν ἧττον ἐπὶ τῶν παρακειμένων αὐτοῖς ὀνομάτων τε
καὶ ῥημάτων ἁπάντων. καὶ γὰρ ὑγιαίνειν ἐκεῖνον ὑπ-
ειλήφασιν ᾧ μηδεμία βέβλαπται μηδενὸς ἐνέργεια
μορίου, καὶ νοσεῖν ᾧ βέβλαπται· καὶ ὑγιαίνων οὗτος

also now, of course, go over what "disease" is by way of a concept, so that in this way we might attempt a correct division of it.

How, then, are we to find this out correctly by method? How else than by what was said in [my work] *On Demonstration*? First, the concept must be agreed upon: without this it is not possible for the substance of the matter being proposed to be discovered. As for the concept itself, it has been my practice to say that we must accept the one agreed upon by all, otherwise it would not be possible to name a suitable starting point. What concept concerning disease is agreed upon by all men? And to what underlying thing especially do they apply this particular term "disease"? Is it not the case that, whenever there are no impediments to the functions of all the parts of the body, under these circumstances people say they are healthy and think they have no need of doctors whereas, whenever they become aware that any one whatsoever of the natural actions of the body is occurring either badly or not at all, they consider themselves to be diseased, at least in that particular part of the body whose function they see to be damaged, and they do have recourse to medical consultation regarding the treatment? I see all men using the terms "health" and "disease" in this way, and this is the concept which I stated all men maintain in the case of these very names and, as well as these, no less in the case of all the names and terms which are etymologically related to them. For they also consider that person to be healthy in whom no function of any part [of the body] is damaged, and someone to be diseased in whom there is damage. And this person, in whom

41K

ὀνομάζεται παρ' αὐτοῖς ᾧ πάντα τοῦ σώματος τὰ
μόρια κατὰ φύσιν ἐνεργεῖ, καὶ νοσῶν ᾧ βέβλαπταί τι·
καὶ οὐδεὶς ὅλως Ἑλλήνων οὔτ' ὠνόμασεν ἄλλως οὔτ'
ἐπ' ἄλλό τι πρᾶγμα φέρει τῶν εἰρημένων ὀνομάτων |
42K ἕκαστον, ὡς ἐπὶ πλεῖστον ἐδείξαμεν ἐν τῇ τῶν ἰατρικῶν ὀνομάτων ἐξηγήσει, καὶ αὐτοῦ γε τούτου μέμνησό
μοι διὰ παντὸς τοῦ λόγου μάλιστα, διότι τὰς μὲν τῶν
ὀνομάτων ἐξηγήσεις ἐκ τῆς τῶν Ἑλλήνων συνηθείας
ποιησόμεθα, καθότι κἀν τοῖς περὶ τῆς ἀποδείξεως
ὑπομνήμασιν ἐλέγετο· τὰς δὲ τῆς οὐσίας αὐτῆς τοῦ
πράγματος εὑρέσεις τε καὶ ζητήσεις καὶ ἀποδείξεις
οὐκέτ' ἐκ τῶν τοῖς πολλοῖς δοκούντων, ἀλλ' ἐκ τῶν
ἐπιστημονικῶν λημμάτων, ὑπὲρ ὧν τοῦ τρόπου τῆς
εὑρέσεως ἐν ἐκείνοις εἴρηται.

λαβόντες οὖν ἀρχὴν ὁμολογουμένην ἅπασιν, ὡς ἐν
Τῇ θεραπευτικῇ μεθόδῳ τοῦτ' εἴη τὸ προκείμενον,
ὑγείαν ἐκπορίζεσθαι τοῖς νενοσηκόσι σώμασι, τουτέστι τὰς κατὰ φύσιν ἐνεργείας τῶν μορίων, εἴ που³⁶
βεβλαμμέναι τύχοιεν, ἐπανορθοῦσθαι· τὸ μετὰ τοῦτ'
ἤδη ζητήσομεν ὁπόσα τὰ σύμπαντά ἐστι κατὰ τὸν
τόπον ἀλλήλοις παρακείμενα πράγματα, μή που τύ-
χωμέν τινα τοῦ λόγου προϊόντος ἢ νοσήματα νομί-
σαντες, ὅταν ᾖ παραπλήσια τούτοις, ἢ ὑγείαν, ὅταν
καὶ τῇ ταύτης φύσει πλησιάζῃ. προκεχειρίσθω δέ
τινα μόρια σαφηνείας ἕνεκεν, ἐφ' ὧν ὁ λόγος ἡμῖν
περανθήσεται· |

43K πρῶτον μὲν ἁπάντων ὀφθαλμός· ὁμολογεῖται γὰρ

³⁶ εἴ που P1, P2; εἴπερ K

all the parts of the body function in accord with nature, is called healthy compared to them, and someone in whom there is damage, diseased; and on the whole, none of the Greeks either name differently, or apply each of the terms mentioned to some other matter, as I showed in great detail in the explanation of medical terms.[24] I urge you to bear this point particularly in mind throughout the entire discussion because I shall make the interpretation of names on the basis of the customary usage of the Greeks, as I said in the work *On Demonstration*. But bear in mind too that the discoveries, investigations, and demonstrations of the actual substance of the matter no longer come from the opinions of the many. Rather, they come from premises based on knowledge, the manner of discovery of which was spoken of in those [writings].

42K

Therefore, having taken as a starting point that which is agreed by all, what is proposed in *The Method of Medicine* is that health is to be provided for bodies that have become diseased; that is to say, to restore the functions of the parts to normal wherever they should happen to have been damaged. After this, I shall examine how many other things there are in all that are closely related in terms of "position," lest we should somehow happen, as the argument progresses, to think that some of them are diseases whenever they resemble them, or health whenever they approximate to the nature of this. Let us, however, pick out certain parts [of the body] for the sake of clarity, through which our argument will be developed to a conclusion.

First of all [let us select] the eye, for there is agreement

43K

24 Presumably *De nominibus medicis,* translated into German from the Arabic by M. Meyerhof and J. Schacht (1931).

οὖν ἐπὶ τούτου πᾶσιν ἀνθρώποις, οὐκ ἰατροῖς μόνον,
ἀλλὰ καὶ τοῖς τυχοῦσιν, ὡς ἔστιν ἔργον αὐτῷ τὸ
βλέπειν. εἴτε δ' ἔργον εἴποιμι κατὰ τὸν λόγον, εἴτ'
ἐνέργειαν, οὐδὲν ἔν γε τῷ νῦν διαφέρει· κατὰ δὲ τὸν
αὐτὸν τρόπον οὐδ' εἰ τὸ βλέπειν εἴποι τις ἔργον εἶναι
τῶν ὀφθαλμῶν, οὐδ' εἰ τὴν βλέψιν, οὐδ' εἰ τὴν ὄψιν ἢ
τὴν ὅρασιν, ἢ ὅπως ἂν ἄλλως ὀνομάσῃ, διαφέρει· καὶ
γὰρ εἰ σολοικίζων ὀνομάσοι, πρός γε τὴν αὐτὴν τοῦ
πράγματος ἐπιστήμην οὐδὲν τοῦτο βλάπτει, μόνον εἰ
καθ' ὅτου πράγματος φέρει τοὔνομα, διηγήσοιτο
σαφῶς, ἐν τούτῳ γάρ ἐστι τὸ κῦρος τῆς διδασκαλίας.
ὀνομαζέσθω τοίνυν ὀφθαλμὸς μὲν τὸ μόριον τοῦ
σώματος, οὐδὲν οὐδ' ἐνταῦθα διαφέρον εἴτε μέρος εἴτε
μόριον εἴποι τις· ὅ τι γὰρ ἂν ᾖ τοῦ παντὸς συμπλη-
ρωτικόν, ἐκεῖνο μόριόν τε καὶ μέρος ὀνομάζεται, τοῦ
ὅλου δηλονότι σώματος, οὗ συμπληρωτικὸν ὑπάρχει.
ἐν γὰρ τῷ πρός τι τὸ μέρος· ὅλου γὰρ καὶ παντός ἐστι
τὸ μέρος, ὥσπερ, οἶμαι, καὶ τὸ πᾶν καὶ τὸ ὅλον πρὸς
τὴν τῶν οἰκείων μερῶν τε καὶ μορίων ἀναφορὰν ὀνο-
44K   μάζεται, | καὶ ἔστιν ὥσπερ τὸ δεξιὸν πρὸς τὸ ἀριστε-
ρὸν καὶ τὸ ἀριστερὸν πρὸς τὸ δεξιόν, οὕτω καὶ τὸ πᾶν
πρὸς τὸ μέρος καὶ τὸ μέρος πρὸς τὸ πᾶν. εἴ τις οὖν
ταύτην φυλάττων τὴν ἔννοιαν αἱρεῖται μέρος λέγειν,
οὐ μόριον, ἢ εἴ τις ἔμπαλιν οὐ μόριον, ἀλλὰ μέρος,
ἐμοὶ μὲν οὐδὲν εἰς τὴν εὕρεσιν τῶν πραγμάτων ἐμποδίζει, δείκνυσι δ' αὐτὸν ὀψιμαθῆ τῆς τῶν Ἑλλήνων
φωνῆς· ὥς πέρ γε καὶ εἴ τις ὅλον καὶ τὸ πᾶν διορίζει,
καὶ οὗτος ἀγνοεῖ τὴν τῶν Ἑλλήνων διάλεκτον.

in this case by all men, not only doctors but also anyone at all, that its action is to see. Whether I say action or function in the course of the argument makes no difference, at least for the moment. In the same way, if someone should say that "looking" is the action of the eyes, or the "act of sight," or "vision," or the "act of seeing," or whatever else one might wish to call it, it makes no difference. Even if someone were to apply names incorrectly, it causes no harm to the actual knowledge of the matter, as long as the name being applied to a particular matter is set out explicitly, for in this lies the validity of the teaching. Let the eye, then, be called a part of the body, insofar as it makes no difference here if one says some component (*meros*) or part (*morion*). For whatever constitutes an essential part of the whole is called a part or a component, the whole, clearly, being the body of which it is an essential part. In this [body] the part is in relation to something because it is also the part of a totality and of a whole so that, in my view, the whole and the totality are so named with reference to its own parts or components. And just as the right is named with reference 44K to the left, or the left to the right, so also the whole is named with reference to the part, or the part to the whole. If someone, while adhering to this concept, chooses to say "component" (*meros*) and not "part" (*morion*), or conversely "part" (*morion*) and not "component" (*meros*), as far as I'm concerned this presents no hindrance to the discovery of the matter but shows him to be laggard in learning the language of the Greeks. Similarly, if someone makes a distinction between the whole (*holos*) and the totality (*pan*), he, too, is ignorant of the Greek language.

εἴρηται δ᾽, ὡς οἶσθα, περὶ τῆς τῶν ὀνομάτων χρήσεως ἐπὶ πλέον ἑτέρωθι, καὶ νῦν ὅσον ἀναγκαῖον εἰς
τὸ προκείμενον δίειμι, τοῦτ᾽ ἐνδεικνύμενος μόνον, ὡς
οὐ χρὴ περιέλκεσθαι τοῖς ὀνόμασιν, οὐδὲ τοὺς ἐν
τούτοις διαφερομένους ἤδη κἂν τοῖς πράγμασιν αὐτοῖς ἡγεῖσθαι διαφέρεσθαι. καὶ τούτου δ᾽ αὐτοῦ πάντας ὡς ἔπος εἰπεῖν ὁρᾷς ἀγυμνάστους, οὐ τοὺς ἰατροὺς
μόνον τοὺς νῦν ὄντας, ἀλλὰ καὶ τῶν φιλοσόφων τοὺς
πλείστους· ὀλίγοι γὰρ αὐτῶν ἴσασι διακρίνειν τὰς ἐν
τοῖς ὀνόμασι διαφωνίας τῶν ἐν τοῖς πράγμασιν· ἀλλ᾽
ἐδείχθη καὶ ἡ τούτου μέθοδος ἐν τῇ λογικῇ θεωρίᾳ,
45K καὶ νῦν ἥκει καιρὸς αὐτῆς, | εἴ πέρ ποτε καὶ ἄλλοτε.
τίς δ᾽ ἦν ἡ μέθοδος; ἀπὸ[37] τῆς τῶν πραγμάτων ἄρξασθαι διαφορᾶς, οὐκ ἀπὸ τῆς τῶν ὀνομάτων, καὶ δεῖξαι
λόγου χάριν ἀλλήλοις παρακείμενα τέτταρα πράγματα, κἄπειθ᾽ ἑξῆς ἀποδείξει βεβαιώσασθαι τὸ μήτε
πλείω τούτων εἶναι μήτ᾽ ἐλάττω τὰ κατὰ τὸ προκείμενον σκέμμα περιεχόμενα· μετὰ τοῦτο δ᾽ ἤδη καὶ
καθ᾽ ἕκαστον τῶν πραγμάτων ἴδιον ὄνομα θέμενον,
οὕτω περαίνειν ἅπαντα τὸν ἑξῆς λόγον, οὐκέτ᾽ οὐδα-
μόσε μετατιθέντα καὶ μεταφέροντα τῶν ὀνομάτων οὐδέν, ἀλλ᾽ ἀκριβῶς διαφυλάττοντα καθ᾽ οὗπερ ἂν αὐτὸς
ἐξ ἀρχῆς ἐπιτίθηται πράγματος. καὶ γὰρ σαφὴς οὕτως ἡ διδασκαλία γίνεται καὶ τῶν παρὰ τὰς ὁμωνυ-
μίας σοφισμάτων ἐκτός, καὶ ῥᾳδίως ἐξελέγχεται τὰ
μάτην προσκείμενα καὶ διὰ ταχέων εὑρίσκεται τὰ

[37] ἀπό B; ἢ ἀπό P1, P2, K; ἢ ἀπό conj. Hankinson

More has been said elsewhere, as you know, on the use of terms,[25] so now I shall go over the matter just as far as is necessary, showing only this—that we must not be distracted by names, nor should those who differ in these names be thought to differ also in the matters themselves. And, as one might say, you see that everyone is unpracticed in this very matter, and not only the doctors of our own day, but also most of the philosophers. Few of these men know to distinguish the disagreements on names from those on the matters. But the method for this was shown by logical theory and now is the proper time to apply it, if, indeed, 45K any one time is better than another. What, in fact, is the method? It is to start from the differentiae of the matters and not from the differentiae of names, and to show, for the sake of argument, that there are four matters closely connected to each other, and then, in sequence, to confirm by demonstration that there are neither more nor fewer than these comprising the subject lying before us. Only then, when a specific name is assigned to each of the matters, do we in this way draw the whole argument to a conclusion point by point without changing or transferring any of the names in any way, but strictly preserving them for the particular matter to which they were assigned from the beginning. And so, in this way, the instruction becomes clear and free of captious arguments over similar names. Things proposed unnecessarily are readily refuted and

25 See R. B. Edlow (1977).

λείποντα, καὶ τά τε διαφωνούμενα καὶ τὰ συμφωνού-
μενα μάλιστα ἐν ταῖς τοιαύταις ἑρμηνείαις ἀκριβῶς
γνωρίζεται.

6. Λεγέσθω δὴ πάλιν ἡμῖν ἀναλαβοῦσιν. ὄψις μὲν
ὀφθαλμῶν ἐνέργεια, διάλεξις δὲ γλώττης, βάδισις δὲ
σκελῶν· ἡ δὲ ἐνέργεια πάλιν αὕτη κίνησις δραστική·
46K τούτων δ᾽ | αὐτῶν ἡ μὲν κίνησις ἐξάλλαξις τοῦ προϋ-
πάρχοντος, ἡ δραστικὴ δὲ ἡ ἐξ ἑαυτοῦ, ὥσπέρ γε καὶ
παθητικὴ κίνησις ἡ ὑπό[38] τινος τῶν ἔξω· οἷον ἡ μὲν
πτῆσις ἐνέργεια τοῦ ζῴου τοῦ πτηνοῦ[39] καὶ ἡ βάδισις
τοῦ βαδιστικοῦ· τὸ δ᾽ ὑφ᾽ ἑτέρου φερόμενον, ὡς ἀμεί-
βειν τόπους, οὐκ ἐνεργεῖν, ἀλλὰ πάσχειν ἐστίν. ἐνήρ-
γησε μὲν γὰρ ὁ βαδίσας ἐκ Πειραιέως ἐπὶ Σούνιον,
ἐκινήθη γὰρ δραστικῶς, τουτέστιν ἐξ ἑαυτοῦ τε καὶ
κατὰ τὴν οἰκείαν φύσιν· ἔπαθε δὲ ὁ πλεύσας ἐπὶ τὸ
Σούνιον ἐκ τοῦ Πειραιέως, ἠνέχθη γὰρ ὑπὸ τῆς νεώς.

ἐπεὶ δ᾽ ἐξάλλαξιν εἶπον εἶναι τοῦ προϋπάρχοντος
τὴν κίνησιν, ἐξαλλάττεται δὲ διχῶς τὸ προϋπάρχον, ἢ
κατὰ ποιότητα, ἢ κατὰ τόπον, ἡ μὲν οὖν κατὰ τόπον
ἐξαλλαγὴ αὐτοῦ φορὰ ὀνομάζεται, ἡ δὲ κατὰ ποιότητα
μεταβολή, ἀλλοίωσις.[40] ὥστε εἶναι φορὰν μὲν ἐξάλλαξιν,[41] ἢ ἀλλαγήν, ἢ μεταβολὴν τοῦ προϋπάρχοντος,[42] ἐξεπίτηδες γὰρ ἐχρησάμην πολλοῖς ὀνόμασιν,
αὐτὸ τοῦτ᾽ ἐνδείκνυσθαι βουλόμενος, ὡς ἔνεστι παμπόλλους ὁρισμοὺς ποιεῖν ἑνὸς πράγματος, ἐν ταῖς

---

[38] B; ἀπό K   [39] B; τοῦ πτηνοῦ (om τοῦ ζῴου) K
[40] ἡ μὲν οὖν κατὰ τόπον ἐξαλλαγὴ αὐτοῦ φορὰ ὀνομάζεται, ἡ δὲ κατὰ ποιότητα μεταβολή, ἀλλοίωσις K; τὴν μὲν

omissions rapidly discovered. Also, particularly, inconsistencies and consistencies in such explanations are accurately recognized.

6. So then, let me say this as I resume the argument. Sight is the function of the eyes, speech of the tongue, and walking of the legs. Again, the function itself is active movement, and the movement of these very things is a change of the previously existing thing. Active movement arises from the thing itself, just as passive movement arises from something else external. For example, flying is the function of what flies and walking of what walks, but to be carried by something else, e.g. to change place, is not to function but to be affected. Thus, someone who walks from Peiraeus to Sunium functions because he goes forward actively—that is to say, both from himself and by virtue of his own nature—whereas someone who sails from Peiraeus to Sunium is affected because he is carried by the ship.

When I said that movement is a change of the previously existing thing, what previously existed can change in two ways—either in qualities or in position. Change in position is called motion, while change with respect to qualities is called alteration. So motion can be change, or interchange, or exchange, or transfer in relation to a preexisting position. I have deliberately used many terms since I want this particular point to be clear: that it is possible to create many definitions for the one thing, which differ only in the

46K

οὖν κατὰ τόπον ἐξαλλαγὴν αὐτοῦ, φορὰν ὀνομάζω, τὴν δὲ κατὰ ποιότητα, μεταβολήν, καὶ ἀλλοίωσιν B

41 B; ἢ ὑπάλλαξιν post ἐξάλλαξιν add. K
42 B; τόπου post προϋπάρχοντος add. K

φωναῖς μόνον, οὐκ ἐν τοῖς νοήμασι διαφέροντας, ἀλ-
47K λοίωσιν δὲ ἢ μεταβολὴν κατὰ | τὸ ποιόν, ἢ ἀλλαγὴν
τῆς προϋπαρχούσης ποιότητος, ἢ ὑπαλλαγὴν κατὰ τὸ
ποιόν, ἢ ὑπάλλαξιν ποιότητος, ἢ ὅπως ἂν ἄλλως
ἐλπίσῃς μάλιστα συνήσειν τοῦ λεγομένου τὸν ἀκού-
οντα· τὸ γὰρ πολυειδὲς τῆς ἑρμηνείας εἰς τοῦτο ἔστω
σοι χρήσιμον. ἡ μὲν οὖν ὄψις, αὖθις γὰρ ἐπὶ τὸν
ὀφθαλμὸν ἰτέον, ἐνέργεια τοῦ μέρους ἐστίν· ὁ δ᾿
ὀφθαλμὸς αὐτὸς τὸ τοῦ ζῴου μόριον, οὐδὲν γὰρ, ὡς
εἴρηται, διαφέρει μόριον εἰπεῖν, ἢ μέρος. ὄργανον δὲ
ὀνομάζω μέρος ζῴου τελείας ἐνεργείας ἀπεργαστικόν,
οἷον ὀφθαλμὸν ὄψεως καὶ γλῶτταν διαλέκτου καὶ
σκέλη βαδίσεως· οὕτω δὲ καὶ ἀρτηρία καὶ φλὲψ καὶ
νεῦρον, ὄργανά τε καὶ μόρια ζῴων ἐστί. κατὰ ταύτην
γοῦν τὴν χρῆσιν τῶν ὀνομάτων οὐ πρὸς ἡμῶν μόνον,
ἀλλὰ καὶ πρὸς τῶν παλαιῶν Ἑλλήνων ὁρισθεῖσαν, ὁ
μὲν οὖν ὀφθαλμὸς ὀνομασθήσεται καὶ μόριον ζῴου
καὶ μέρος καὶ ὄργανον· ὁ δὲ κερατοειδὴς χιτὼν μόριον
μὲν καὶ μέρος, ὄργανον δ᾿ οὔ· κατὰ ταὐτὰ δὲ καὶ ὁ
ῥαγοειδὴς καὶ ὁ ἀραχνοειδὴς καὶ ὁ ἀμφιβληστρο-
ειδής· ἕκαστος γὰρ τούτων πρῶτον μὲν καὶ μάλιστα
μόριόν ἐστιν ὀφθαλμοῦ, διότι δ᾿ οὗτος προσώπου, |
48K διὰ τοῦτο κἀκεῖνοι κατὰ δεύτερον ἤδη λόγον· οὕτω δὲ
καὶ τοῦ σώματος ὅλου, διότι καὶ τὸ πρόσωπον ὅλου
τοῦ σώματός ἐστι μόριον.

---

26 On the anatomical terminology relating to the eye, see
Celsus VII.7.13B–C (LCL Celsus, *On Medicine III*, pp. 346–48)

words and not in the concepts. Alteration, on the other hand, is a change with respect to quality, or a change of a 47K previously existing quality, or an exchange in respect to quality, or a variation of quality, or however else you might particularly hope the listener to understand what was said, for let the diversity of the referring be useful to you for this purpose. Sight then—for one must go back to the eyes once more—is a function of the component (*meros*), while the eye itself is a part (*morion*) of the animal for, as has been said, it makes no difference to say part (*morion*) or component (*meros*). I call an organ a component (*meros*) of an animal which performs a complete function: for example, the eye [effects] sight, the tongue speech, the legs walking, and in like manner, an artery, a vein and a nerve are both organs and also parts of animals. At all events, in accordance with this use of terms defined not only by us alone but also by the Greeks of old, the eye will be called a part (*morion*) of an animal, and a component (*meros*), and an organ, whereas the external "tunic" (cornea, sclera) is a part (*morion*) and a component (*meros*) but not an organ, and it is the same for the choroid membrane, the arachnoid membrane and the retina, for each of these is primarily and particularly a part (*morion*) of the eye. But because the eye is part of the face, these are also parts of the face in 48K a secondary sense, in the same way as they are also parts of the whole body because the face is a part of the whole body.[26]

and Galen, *De usu partium*, Book 10 (translation by M. T. May, 1968, vol. 2, p. 463ff). For Aristotle on the part-whole relationship, see *De caelo* 302a31–32, 302b25, *De generatione animalium* 715a10–11, 722a18–21, and *Meteorologica* 388a13–20.

ὁμοιομερὲς δέ ἐστι μόριον, ὡς καὶ τοὔνομα αὐτὸ
σαφῶς ἐνδείκνυται, τὸ διαιρούμενον εἰς ὅμοια πάντη
μόρια, καθάπερ ἐν ὀφθαλμῷ τό θ' ὑαλοειδὲς καὶ
τὸ κρυσταλλοειδὲς καὶ τῶν χιτώνων ἡ ἴδιος οὐσία.
δείκνυται δὲ καὶ ταῦτα ἐπὶ πλέον ἐν τοῖς Τῶν ἀνατο-
μικῶν ἐγχειρήσεων ὑπομνήμασιν, ἐνταῦθα δὲ ἀρκεῖ
μόνων ἡμῖν ὧν[43] εἰς τὰ παρόντα δεόμεθα μνημονεῦ-
σαι· δεόμεθα δὲ καθ' ἕκαστον μόριον ἐπιδεῖξαι πλείω
πράγματα, διαφέροντα μὲν ἀλλήλων, οὐχ ὁρώμενα δὲ
ἐνίοις τῶν ἰατρῶν· ἔφαμεν δὲ τοῦτο χρήσιμον ὑπάρχειν εἴς τε τὸ χρῆσθαι τοῖς ὀνόμασιν ὀρθῶς, οὗπερ
ἕνεκα καὶ νῦν αὐτὸ μετεχειρισάμεθα, καὶ μέντοι καὶ
πρὸς αὐτὴν τὴν προκειμένην μέθοδον ἀναγκαιότατον
ἐπιδειχθήσεται. τὸ μὲν γὰρ ὄργανον ὀφθαλμός, ἐνέργεια δ' ἡ ὄψις· ἐν δ' αὐτοῦ τῶν μορίων ὁμοιομερές τε
καὶ πρῶτον ὄργανον ὄψεως, τὸ κρυσταλλοειδὲς ὑγρόν,
ὡς ἐν τοῖς περὶ αὐτῶν λόγοις ἀποδέδεικται· τοῦτο γάρ
49K   ἐστι τὸ δεόμενον ἀλλοιωθῆναι πρός τινος τῶν | ἔξωθεν
χρωμάτων, ἵν' ἴδῃ τὸ ζῷον. ἀλλοιοῦσθαι δ' οὐκ ἠδύνατο, μὴ καθαρὸν ἀκριβῶς καὶ διαφανὲς γινόμενον·
οὕτω δ' εἶναι καὶ καθαρὸν καὶ διαφανὲς οὐκ ἠδύνατο
χωρὶς τῆς νῦν ὑπαρχούσης αὐτῷ[44] κράσεως· ἐδείχθη
γὰρ ἕκαστον τῶν ὄντων τοιοῦτον ὂν οἷόν πέρ ἐστι διὰ
τὴν τοῦ θερμοῦ καὶ ψυχροῦ καὶ ὑγροῦ καὶ ξηροῦ
κρᾶσιν· ὥστ' εἴ τι τούτων ἐξαλλαχθείη μεγάλως, ἢ
οὐκ ὄψεται τὸ ζῷον, ἢ κακῶς ὄψεται.

[43] μόνων ἡμῖν ὧν B; μόνον εἰπεῖν ὧν K   [44] B; αὐτῆς K

A part (*morion*) is a *homoiomere* if it is divisible in its entirety into like parts, as the name itself clearly indicates, just as, in the eye, the transparent vitreous and crystalline, and the specific substance of the tunics are. These are things that were shown in greater detail in my treatise *On Anatomical Procedures*[27] although here it is enough just to speak of those things which we need to recall for our present purpose. We need to show that the things pertaining to each part are many, and they differ from each other, and are not observed by some doctors. I said that this is useful in the correct employment of names, which is why I also dealt with it now; and of course, it will also be shown that it is absolutely essential to the very method being proposed. The organ is the eye while sight is the function. One of its parts is *homoiomerous* and is the primary organ of sight, which is the crystalline humor (lens), as has been demonstrated in my works on these, since this is what needs to be altered by one of the colors externally for the animal to see.   49K However, it cannot be altered unless it is perfectly clear and transparent, and it cannot be clear and transparent like this apart from the mixture that now constitutes it. For it was shown that each existing thing is as it is because of the mixture of hot, cold, moist, and dry, so that, if any of these [qualities] is altered greatly, the animal will either not see, or will see badly.

[27] There is, in fact, very little on the eye in *De anatomicis administrationibus*, the work referred to here; see II.443–44K. The eye and the mechanism of sight is dealt with in considerable detail in Book 10 of *De usu partium,* as mentioned in the previous note.

ἀλλὰ τοῦτο μὲν οὔπω γινώσκομεν, ἀρχόμενοι ζητεῖν τὴν τέχνην, οὐδὲ χρὴ τῶν ἔπειτά τι μελλόντων
ζητεῖσθαι προλαμβάνειν ὡς ἐπισταμένους, οὐδ᾽ ἐγὼ
τούτου χάριν ἐμνημόνευσα τῶν ὑπὲρ τοῦ κρυσταλλοειδοῦς μοι δεδειγμένων ἐν ἑτέροις, ἀλλ᾽ ἕνεκα τῆς
τῶν νῦν μελλόντων ῥηθήσεσθαι σαφηνείας. ὁρῶντες
γὰρ ὀφθαλμὸν ἀκριβῶς ἐνεργοῦντα, καὶ αὖθις μὴ
βλέποντα, καὶ τὸ μὲν ὑγείαν αὐτοῦ, τὸ δὲ νόσον ἢ
πάθος ἢ ὅ τι βούλει καλοῦντες, οὐδὲν γὰρ τοῦτο
διαφέρει πρός γε τὰ παρόντα, ζητοῦμεν ἑξῆς τίς ποτ᾽
ἐστὶν ἡ τῆς βλάβης αἰτία.

50K   7. Πόθεν, φήσεις, ἐπὶ τοῦτ᾽ ἐλθόντες; ἐξ | ἀναπο-
δείκτου μὲν ἀξιώματος, ὁμολογουμένου δὲ πᾶσιν, ὅτι
πρὸς τὴν νόησιν ἐναργὲς ὑπάρχει. τί δὲ τοῦτ᾽ ἔστι; τὸ
μηδὲν χωρὶς αἰτίας γίνεσθαι· τούτου γὰρ μὴ συγχωρηθέντος, οὐδὲ ζητεῖν δυνάμεθα τὴν αἰτίαν τοῦ βεβλάφθαι τὴν ὄψιν, ἢ ἀπολωλέναι παντελῶς· ἀλλ᾽ ἐπεὶ
τῶν πρὸς νόησιν ἐναργῶν ἐστιν, ὑποθέμενοί τινα
τῆς βλάβης ὑπάρχειν αἰτίαν, ἐπὶ τὸ ζητεῖν αὐτὴν
ἀφικνούμεθα. ταύτην οὖν τὴν αἰτίαν, εἴ τε διάθεσίν
τινα σώματος, εἴ τέ πως διακείμενον σῶμα προσαγορεύειν ἐθέλοις, οὐδὲν μὲν εἴς γε τὰ παρόντα διαφέρει·
πάντως δ᾽ οὖν ἤτοι τὸ νόσημα αὐτὸ φήσεις ὑπάρχειν
αὐτήν, ἢ εἴπερ τὸ νόσημά ἐστιν ἡ βλάβη τῆς ἐνεργείας, ἡ βλάπτουσα διάθεσις αὐτὴν αἰτία τοῦ νοσήματος ὑπάρξει. καὶ γίνεται κἀνταῦθα πάλιν ὑπὲρ ὀνόματος ἡ ἀμφισβήτησις, ἤτοι τὴν ἐν τοῖς ὀφθαλμοῖς
διάθεσιν, ὑφ᾽ ἧς ἡ ὄψις βλάπτεται, νόσον ἡμῶν ὀνο-

But we do not yet know this, as we are at the beginning of our investigation of the art. Nor should we presuppose as knowledge any of the next things we intend to investigate. It isn't for this purpose that I have made mention of things about the crystalloid that I demonstrated in other [works], but for the clarity of those things that will be said. For when we see, the eye is functioning correctly, and when we fail to see, it is the converse. We call the former health and the latter disease, or affection, or whatever you wish, for this makes no difference, at least in the present context. What we seek next is the cause of the damage.

7. From where, you will ask, do we proceed with this? From an indemonstrable axiom, but one which is agreed 50K by all, in that it is clear to the understanding. And what is this? That nothing happens without a cause. Unless this is agreed upon, we are unable to investigate the cause of the damage to vision, or of its complete destruction. But since this is one of the things clear to the understanding, when we have postulated there to be some cause of the damage, we proceed to the search for it. With respect to this cause, whether you wish to call it a certain condition of the body, or the body being in some kind of state, makes no difference, at least to the matter before us. At all events, you will either say that the disease itself is it (the cause) or, if the disease is the damage of function, then the condition damaging it will be the cause of the disease. And here, too, the dispute is again about a name in that we name either the condition in the eyes by which vision is damaged, or the ac-

μαζόντων, ἢ αὐτὴν τὴν βλάβην τῆς ἐνεργείας· ἀλλ᾽
εἴτε τὴν βεβλαμμένην ἐνέργειαν ἐθέλοι τις ὀνομάζειν
νόσον, ἀνάγκη δήπου τοῦτον πολὺ πρότερον ὑγείαν
ὑποθέσθαι τὴν κατὰ φύσιν ἔχουσαν ἐνέργειαν· εἴτε
51K τὴν διάθεσιν, ὑφ᾽ ἧς ἡ | ἐνέργεια βλάπτεται, καὶ
τοῦτον πολὺ πρότερον ἐπὶ τῆς κατὰ φύσιν εἴτ᾽ οὖν
διαθέσεως εἴτε καὶ κατασκευῆς ἐθέλει καλεῖν, ἐπιφέρειν τὸ τῆς ὑγείας ὄνομα. τὸ δ᾽ ἐν ταῖς ἐνεργείαις
ὑποθέμενον εἶναι τὴν ὑγίειαν, ἐν ταῖς διαθέσεσιν
ὑπολαμβάνειν συνίστασθαι τὴν νόσον, ἢ ἔμπαλιν ἐν
μὲν τῇ κατασκευῇ τῶν μορίων τὴν ὑγείαν, ἐν δὲ τῇ
βλάβῃ τῶν ἐνεργειῶν τὴν νόσον, ἄξιον τῶν τε ἄλλων
μεθοδικῶν ἐστι καὶ δὴ καὶ τοῦ τῆς ἐμπληξίας αὐτῶν
ἀρχηγοῦ Θεσσαλοῦ. πάντες γοῦν σχεδὸν οἱ ἀπὸ τῆς
ἀμεθόδου τε καὶ μανιώδους ταύτης αἱρέσεως τὴν μὲν
ὑγείαν εὐστάθειαν τῶν κατὰ φύσιν ἐνεργειῶν εἶναί
φασι καὶ ἰσχύν, τὴν δὲ νόσον οὐκ ἔτι βλάβην ἐνεργείας καὶ ἀσθένειαν, ἀλλ᾽ οἱ μὲν διάθεσίν τινα σώματος, οἱ δὲ σῶμά πως διακείμενον· ἧς τίς ἂν εὑρεθείη
μείζων ἐμπληξία; τοῦτο μέντοι κἂν ὁ τυχὼν ἐξεύροι,
τὸ μὴ δεῖν ἐν ἑτέρῳ μὲν γένει τὴν ὑγείαν, ἐν ἑτέρῳ δὲ
τὴν νόσον, ἀλλ᾽ ἐν ταὐτῷ πάντως ἄμφω τίθεσθαι· τὰ
γὰρ ἐναντία κατὰ πλεῖστόν ἐστιν ἀλλήλων διεστηκότα ἐν τῷ αὐτῷ γένει, καθάπερ λευκὸν καὶ μέλαν, ἐν
γὰρ ἀμφοῖν γένος τὸ χρῶμα.

καὶ τοίνυν εἴπερ ἐναντία ἐστὶν ὑγεία καὶ νόσος, ἐν
52K ᾧπερ ἂν ᾖ τῷ | γένει τῶν κατὰ φύσιν ἡ ὑγεία, τούτου
τοῦ γένους ἐν τῷ παρὰ φύσιν ἡ νόσος ὑπάρξει· ὥστε

tual damage of the function, a disease. But if someone should wish to name the damaged function a disease, it is, I presume, necessary for him to postulate much earlier that health is to have the function which accords with nature. And if he wishes to call [disease] the condition by which the function is damaged, this man must also apply the term "health" much earlier to either the condition or constitution, whichever he wishes to call it, that accords with nature. It is [a claim] worthy of the other Methodics, and in particular of Thessalus, the founder of their stupidity, to postulate that health subsists in the functions and to take disease to subsist in the conditions, or conversely, to postulate that health subsists in the constitution of the parts and disease in the damage of functions. At any rate, nearly all of those from this methodless and mad sect say that health is stability of the natural functions, and strength, whereas disease is not damage of functions, and weakness, but, according to some, a certain condition of the body and, according to others, the body being in a certain condition. Is there any greater stupidity to be found? However, anyone could find this out—that one must not place health in one genus and disease in another; both should be absolutely in the same [genus]. For opposites are those things separate from each other to the greatest degree in the same genus, like white and black, there being one genus for both—that of color. 51K

In fact, if health and disease are opposites, in whatever class of things which are in accord with nature health may be, disease will be of that same class of things when they 52K

εἰ μὲν ἐνέργεια κατὰ φύσιν ἡ ὑγεία, πάντως δή που
παρὰ φύσιν ἐνέργειά τις ἡ νόσος ἐστίν· εἰ δ᾽ ἤτοι
διάθεσίς τις ἢ κατασκευὴ κατὰ φύσιν ἡ ὑγεία ἐστί,
καὶ ἡ νόσος ἐξ ἀνάγκης ἔσται διάθεσίς τις ἢ κατασκευὴ παρὰ φύσιν. ὁ μὲν οὖν Θεσσαλὸς οὐδ᾽ ἐπεχείρησεν ὅλως ἀφορίσασθαι νόσον, ἀλλὰ χρὴ μαντεύ-
εσθαι κατὰ τίνος ἐπιφέρει τοὔνομα πράγματος. ὅτι
μὲν γὰρ οὐδὲν διαφέρειν ἡγεῖται νόσημα πάθους ἐπ-
εδείξαμέν σοι δι᾽ αὐτῶν τῶν συγγραμμάτων αὐτοῦ,
παράλληλα τιθέντος ἄμφω καὶ μεταλαμβάνοντος ἑκάτερον εἰς θάτερον, ὡς οὐδὲν διαφέρον ἢ οὕτως ἢ
ἐκείνως εἰπεῖν· οἱ δ᾽ ἀπ᾽ αὐτοῦ πάντες ἄνω καὶ κάτω
στρέφονται, λυγιζόμενοί τε καὶ παρακαλυπτόμενοι,
καὶ πάντα ποιοῦντες ὡς ἤτοι παντάπασιν ἀσαφῶς
εἰπεῖν ἢ μηδ᾽ ὅλως, ὥσπερ αὐτὸς ὁ Θεσσαλὸς καὶ πρὸ
τούτου Θεμίσων ὁ τὴν ῥίζαν αὐτοῖς τῆς ἐμπληξίας
ταύτης ὑποθέμενος.

εἰ δή σοι τὰ Πρόκλου καὶ Ῥηγίνου καὶ Ἀντιπάτρου
53K λέγοιμι, καὶ πρὸς | τούτοις Εὐδήμου καὶ Μνασέου καὶ
Φίλωνος καὶ Διονυσίου, λάθοιμ᾽ ἂν ἐμαυτὸν ἐκπεσὼν
τῆς προκειμένης νῦν πραγματείας, ἐπιστημονικῆς τε
οὔσης καὶ τὸ χρήσιμον αὐτὸ πειρωμένης ἐκδιδάσκειν.
ἀλλὰ τῆς μὲν ἐκείνων διαφωνίας ἴσως ἄν ποτε καὶ
ὕστερον εἴη μνημονεῦσαι, καὶ σὺν αὐτοῖς γε τοῖς νῦν
εἰρημένοις τοῦ πάντα σοφώτερον ἐπιταράξαντός τε
καὶ συγχέαντος αὐτῶν τὰ πράγματα Μενεμάχου, καὶ
τοῦ ληρώδους Ὀλυμπικοῦ, καὶ μετ᾽ αὐτὸν[45] Ἀπολλω-

45 αὐτὸν B, P1; αὐτοῦ K

are contrary to nature, so that if health is normal function, it follows that disease is, in all respects, some function which is somehow abnormal. If, however, health is either some condition or constitution that is normal, disease will also necessarily be some condition or constitution that is abnormal. Thessalus did not actually attempt to define disease. Rather, we must rely on divination as regards the matter to which he applies the name. I have shown you by way of his writings that he thinks there is no difference between a disease and an affection since he applies both [terms] indifferently, and changes from one to the other as if there were no difference in speaking of it like this or like that. And all those who follow him turn themselves upside down, contorting themselves and hiding their tracks and doing everything they can to speak as obscurely as possible, or to say nothing at all, just as Thessalus himself did, and before him Themison, who laid down the root of this stupidity for them.

Certainly, if I were to state for you the [doctrines] of Proclus, Rheginus, Antipater, and besides these, of Eude- 53K mus, Mnaseas, Philo, or Dionysius, I would be digressing, not realizing that I had wandered away from the matter currently before us, namely the matter of knowledge, and the attempt to give thorough instruction in what is actually useful.[28] But perhaps at some later time it may be possible to mention the discord of those men and, in addition to those who have now been mentioned, the works of Mene-machus who caused even more trouble and created confusion more cleverly than they did, and of the frivolous Olympicus, and his successors Apollonides and Soranus,

[28] Little is known about any of the members of this initial group of Methodics; see R. J. Hankinson (1991), pp. 144–45.

νίδου καὶ Σωρανοῦ καὶ τοῦ νῦν ἔτι ζῶντος Ἰουλιανοῦ·
τούτῳ μέν γε καὶ ἡμεῖς ἐνετύχομεν, ἵνα καὶ παρὰ
ζῶντος ἀνθρώπου φωνῆς ἐκμάθωμεν λήρους μακρούς,
εἶχε δ᾽ οὖν οὐδ᾽ οὗτος λέγειν ὅ τί ποτ᾽ ἐστὶ πάθος καὶ
νόσημα. καὶ τεκμήριόν γε τούτου μέγιστον· ἐτῶν γὰρ
ἤδη πλειόνων ἢ εἴκοσι γεγονότων ἐξ οὗπερ ἡμεῖς ἐπὶ
τῆς Ἀλεξανδρείας αὐτῷ τούτῳ συνεγενόμεθα, γεγρα-
φὼς εἰσαγωγὰς ἄλλας ἐπ᾽ ἄλλαις, ἀεὶ γὰρ αὐτὰς
μετατίθησί τε καὶ μεταρρυθμίζει τῷ μηδέποτ᾽ ἀρκεῖσθαι ταῖς γραφείσαις, κατ᾽ οὐδεμίαν αὐτῶν ἐτόλμη-
σεν εἰπεῖν ὅ τί ποτ᾽ ἐστὶ νόσος, καίτοι γε μηδὲν πρὸς
54K ἔπος ἐν αὐταῖς διεξέρχεται | μέχρι τοῦ καὶ τὰ τοιαῦτα
ζητεῖν, εἰ ζωγραφία χρήσιμος ἰατροῖς ἐστιν· ἀλλ᾽
ὅμως τοσαῦτά τε καὶ τοιαῦτα γράφων, καὶ δῆλος ὤν,
ὥσπερ καὶ Μενέμαχος, ὅτι σαφῶς ἔγνωκε τῆς Μεθοδικῆς αἱρέσεως τὴν ἀτοπίαν, οὐδέπω καὶ τήμερον
ἔγραψεν ἐν ταῖς εἰσαγωγαῖς ὅ τί ποτε νόσον ἢ πάθος
ὀνομάζει.

ἐμοὶ δ᾽ οὖν ἐρομένῳ ποτ᾽ αὐτὸν οὕτω μακρῶς τε
ἅμα καὶ ἀσαφῶς διῆλθεν, ὡς ὧν μὲν ἔλεγε συνιέναι
μηδενός, ἀναγκασθῆναι δὲ τό γε τοσοῦτον εἰπεῖν πρὸς
αὐτόν, ὡς διαφέρεσθαί μοι δοκοίη πρὸς Ὀλυμπικόν,
καίτοι πάππον αὐτοῦ τῆς διδασκαλίας ὄντα· μαθητὴς
γάρ ἐστιν οὗτος ὁ Ἰουλιανὸς Ἀπολλωνίδου τοῦ Κυ-
πρίου, ἐκεῖνος δ᾽ ἦν Ὀλυμπικοῦ φοιτητής. ὁ τοίνυν
Ὀλυμπικός, ὡς ἔφην, ὁρίσασθαι τολμήσας ὑγείαν τε

---

[29] More is known about the members of this second grouping.

and of Julianus who is still alive today (in fact, I have met him),[29] so that, from the voice of a living person, we might examine thoroughly these great absurdities. However, even he cannot say what an affection or a disease is. And there is, in fact, very substantial evidence of this, for already, during the more than twenty years that have elapsed since I met with the man himself in Alexandria, he has written one elementary treatise after another, constantly rearranging and emending them, never satisfied with what he has written. In none of them, however, has he ventured to say what a disease is. Indeed, he details nothing to the purpose in them, even going so far as to look into such things as whether painting is useful to doctors. But for all that, since he wrote so many and such a variety of things, it was clear, as was the case with Menemachus also, that he was aware of the absurdity of the Methodic sect, and yet never to this day has he written in his elementary treatises what it is he calls "disease" and what "affection."   54K

Once, when I questioned him, he went over things at such length and so obscurely that I understood nothing of what he said, and was compelled to say to him this much at least—that he seemed to me to differ from Olympicus, although the latter was the grandfather of his teaching. For this Julianus was a pupil of Apollonides of Cyprus, while the latter was a disciple of Olympicus. Moreover, as I said, Olympicus had the courage to define health and affection.

All were Methodics. For the first four, see *EANS*, pp. 546–47, 588, 109, and 749–51 respectively. Julianus, against whom the rest of the paragraph is directed, is dealt with more fully by Galen in his *Adversus ea quae Iuliano in Hippocratis aphorismos enuntiata sunt. Contra Juliano*, XVIIIA.246–99K.

καὶ πάθος, τὴν μὲν ὑγείαν διάθεσιν ἔφησε κατὰ ἐκτότητα νόσου· τὸ δ' αὖ πάθος τροπὴν τοῦ κατὰ φύσιν εἰς
τὸ παρὰ φύσιν, ἐπίμονον. ἔστι μὲν δὴ καὶ τούτων
ἑκάτερον ἀλογίας παμπόλλης ἀνάπλεων, ἣν καὶ τότε
διῆλθον τῷ Ἰουλιανῷ καὶ νῦν ἐπὶ κεφαλαίων ἐρῶ.

55K   τὸ γοῦν συγχέον, ἔφην, ἐστὶν ἐκεῖνο, τὸ μὴ μόνον
ἁπλῶς οὕτως εἰπεῖν τὸν | Ὀλυμπικὸν ὑγείαν εἶναι διά-
θεσιν κατὰ ἐκτότητα νόσου, ἀλλὰ προσθεῖναι τῷ
λόγῳ ἣν διάθεσιν ὁριζόμεθα εὐστάθειαν τῶν κατὰ
φύσιν ἐνεργημάτων καὶ ἰσχύν· οὐ γὰρ ἔχω συμβαλεῖν
εἴτε ἐν τῇ τῶν ἐνεργειῶν εὐσταθείᾳ μόνῃ τὴν ὑγείαν,
εἴτε ἐν τῇ τοῦ σώματος διαθέσει, εἴτ' ἐν ἀμφοῖν
ὑποτίθεται· τάχα δ' ὥσπερ εἴωθε χρῆσθαι τοῖς τῶν
Ἑλλήνων ὀνόμασιν ἀλλοκότως τε καὶ τεταραγμένως
ἅμα τοῖς ἄλλοις ἅπασι Μεθοδικοῖς, οὕτω καὶ νῦν οὐκ
ἐπὶ τὸ σῶμα τὴν διάθεσιν, ἀλλ' ἐπὶ τὰς ἐνεργείας
ἀναφέρει, ὥστε ἡμᾶς ἀκοῦσαι τοῦ λόγου κατὰ τοῦτον
τὸν τρόπον· ὑγεία ἐστὶ διάθεσις ἐνεργειῶν κατὰ ἐκτότητα νόσου. δίκαιον δ' ἦν, οἶμαι, προσθεῖναι τῷ
λόγῳ δυοῖν θάτερον αὐτόν, ἢ ἐνεργειῶν, ἢ σώματος,
ἵν' ἤτοι γένηται τοιοῦτος ὁ λόγος, ὑγεία ἐστὶ διάθεσις
ἐνεργειῶν κατὰ ἐκτότητα νόσου· ἢ νὴ Δία τοιοῦτος,
ὑγεία ἐστὶ διάθεσις σώματος κατὰ ἐκτότητα νόσου·
καὶ μέν γε καὶ εἰ ἄμφω συνθεῖναι προήρετο, καὶ οὕτως
ἐνεχώρει σαφῶς τε ἅμα καὶ διὰ βραχέων εἰπεῖν, ὑγεία
ἐστὶ διάθεσις ἐνεργειῶν τε καὶ σώματος κατὰ ἐκτότητα νόσου.[46]

56K   τί δ', ὅταν ἐπιφέρων εἴπῃ, ἣν διάθεσιν | ὁριζόμεθα

86

He said that health was a condition in relation to the absence of disease whereas an affection was a change from what was in accord with nature to what was contrary to nature that persists. But each of these [definitions] is full of the utmost nonsense, which is what I said to Julianus at the time, and shall now say in summary.

At the very least, I said, the confusion is this: not only did Olympicus simply say that health was a condition related to the absence of disease, but added to the definition that "we define this condition as stability of the natural functions, and strength." I cannot make out if health is postulated to depend solely on the stability of the functions, or on the condition of the body, or on both. Perhaps, as he was accustomed to using the terms of the Greeks both unusually and in a confusing manner along with all the other Methodics, now also in this way he does not apply "condition" to the body but to the functions, so that we are to understand the argument in the following way: "health is a condition of the functions in the absence of disease." It would be right, I think, to add to the definition one or other of these two things—either "of the functions" or "of the body," so that such a statement becomes either: "health is a condition of the functions in relation to the absence of disease," or like this, by Zeus, that: "health is a condition of the body in the absence of disease." But if he had made the choice to combine both together, it would have allowed him to say clearly and, at the same time, concisely that health is a condition of the functions and of the body in relation to the absence of disease.

But what about when he says as a rider that "we define

55K

56K

---

46 ἢ νὴ Δία . . . ἐκτότητα νόσου K; *om.* B (= 55.15–18K)

εὐστάθειαν τῶν κατὰ φύσιν ἐνεργημάτων καὶ ἰσχύν;
πότερον μέρος ὑποληπτέον εἶναι τοῦτο τοῦ προειρη-
μένου καὶ χρὴ συνάπτειν ἡμᾶς ὅλον τὸν λόγον ὡδί
πως· ὑγεία ἐστὶ διάθεσις σώματος κατὰ ἐκτότητα
νόσου καὶ εὐστάθεια τῶν κατὰ φύσιν ἐνεργημάτων
καὶ ἰσχύς· ἢ τέλειός ἐστιν ὁ λόγος οὗτος αὐτὸς καθ᾽
ἑαυτόν, ὅ τί ποτ᾽ ἐστὶν ὑγεία διδάσκων, ὥσπέρ γε καὶ
ἤρεσεν ἐνίοις τῶν Μεθοδικῶν, εὐστάθειαν ἀποφηνα-
μένοις εἶναι τῶν κατὰ φύσιν ἐνεργειῶν τὴν ὑγείαν;
ἀλλ᾽ εἴπερ οὗτος τέλειος, ὁ προειρημένος οὐκ οἶδ᾽ ὅ τι
διδάσκει, διάθεσιν εἶναι λέγων τὴν ὑγείαν. ἐκεῖνο μὲν
γὰρ ὃ ἔφη, τὸ κατὰ ἐκτότητα νόσου, τοιοῦτόν ἐστιν
οἷον καὶ παῖδα γελάσαι. εἰ γὰρ δὴ συγχωρήσομεν
οὕτως ὁρίζεσθαι, δηλονότι καὶ ἡ νόσος ἔσται διάθεσις
σώματος κατὰ ἐκτότητα ὑγείας, ἵνα ἕκαστος τῶν ὅρων
ἡμῖν οὐ τοῦ τί ποτ᾽ ἐστὶ τὸ ὑποκείμενον, ἀλλὰ τοῦ τί
ποτ᾽ οὐκ ἔστι, γένηται διδάσκαλος.

Ἐάσθω δ᾽, ἔφην, εἰ βούλει καὶ ταῦτα, καὶ γὰρ
πάρεργά πώς ἐστιν· ἀλλ᾽ ἐκεῖνό γε παρελθεῖν τε καὶ
παριδεῖν οὐκ ἐγχωρεῖ, τὸ κατὰ μὲν τὴν τῆς ὑγείας
διδασκαλίαν ἅπαντα προσέρχεσθαι ταῖς ἐνεργείαις |
57K ἤτοι μόναις ἢ μετὰ τοῦ συγχέαι καὶ περιπλέξαι καὶ
ἀναμῖξαί πως ἀσαφῶς τὸ τῆς διαθέσεως ὄνομα,
καθάπερ ὁ Ὀλυμπικός· ἐν δὲ τῷ τοῦ πάθους οὐκέτι
μεμνῆσθαι τῶν ἐνεργειῶν· ἀπέχρησε γὰρ εἰπεῖν αὐτῷ,
πάθος ἐστὶ τροπὴ τοῦ σώματος ἐκ τοῦ κατὰ φύσιν εἰς
τὸ παρὰ φύσιν ἐπίμονος. Ἐχρῆν δ᾽, ἔφην, ἐν ταῖς
ἐνεργείαις, ἢ ἐν ταῖς διαθέσεσιν, ἄμφω τάττειν αὐτόν.

the condition as a stability of the natural functions, and strength"? Must we understand this to be part of what was previously said and so, particularly, must we join together the whole definition as follows: "health is a condition of the body in the absence of disease and stability of the natural functions, and strength"; or is the definition itself complete on its own, since it teaches what health is, at least to the satisfaction of some of the Methodics, who assert that health is a stability of the natural functions? But if this [definition] is complete, I don't know what the previously articulated one teaches, when it says that health is a condition. For what that phrase—"in the absence of disease"—says is such that even a child would laugh. Certainly, if we agree to it being defined in this way, clearly also disease will be a condition of the body in the absence of health, so that each of the definitions becomes for us a teaching, not of what the matter is that is being proposed, but of what it is not.

"Let us allow this," I said, "if these things are what you wish, for they are somehow subordinate matters." But what cannot be passed over and overlooked is the association of all things related to the teaching of health to the functions alone, or to somehow confound, complicate, and mix it obscurely with the term "condition," just as Olympicus [does]. However, in the [definition] of affection, nothing is mentioned anymore about functions. It is enough for him to say that an affection is a deviation of the body from what accords with nature to what is contrary to nature that is persistent. "He ought," I said, "to have assigned both either to the functions or to the conditions."

57K

89

ὃ δέ μοι πρὸς ταῦτ᾽ ἀπεκρίνατο, καὶ ἤδη μέν σοι
πολλάκις εἶπον, Ἱέρων κράτιστε, καὶ νῦν τ᾽ ἀνα-
μνῆσαι προσήκει, τὸ μηδὲν εἶναι θαυμαστόν, ἐν μὲν
τῇ τῶν ἐνεργειῶν εὐσταθείᾳ σὺν ἰσχύι τετάχθαι τὴν
ὑγείαν, ἐν δὲ τῇ παρὰ φύσιν τοῦ σώματος διαθέσει
τὴν νόσον· Οὐ γάρ ἐστιν ἐναντία, καθάπερ σὺ νομίζεις, ἔφησεν, ἔστι γάρ τι μέσον αὐτῶν, ὃ μήθ᾽ ὑγεία
μήτε νόσος ἐστίν. ἀκούσας οὖν ἐγὼ τὸν λόγον τοῦτον
ἐχωρίσθην ἐκπεπληγμένος τε καὶ λυπούμενος ἅμα,
χρὴ γὰρ ὁμολογεῖν τὸ συμβάν· ἔμπροσθεν μὲν γὰρ
οὐδενὶ τῶν ἐν τοιαύτῃ δόξῃ τελέως ἐνετετυχήκειν ἐμ-
πλήκτῳ, τότε δ᾽ ἐντυχὼν πρῶτον εἰκότως ἐξεπλάγην,
οὐχ ὅτι μόνος ἐκεῖνος οὕτως ἦν ἀναίσθητος, ἀλλ᾽ ὅτι
58K   πολλῷ σκαιοτέρους | ἑαυτοῦ τοσούτους εἶχε μαθητάς,
οἳ κατὰ τὴν ἀρχὴν αὐτήν[47] τῆς διδασκαλίας ὁρῶντες
οὕτως ἐσφαλμένους τοὺς Μεθοδικούς, οὐκ ἀφίστανται
τῆς αἱρέσεως, ἢ εἴπερ οὐδ᾽ ὅλως ὁρῶσι, τελέως εἰσὶν
ἀπόπληκτοι.

τί γὰρ δὴ καὶ πρὸς ἔπος οὐκ εἶναι τὴν νόσον
ἐναντίον ὑγείᾳ, διότι μέσον αὐτῶν ἐστί τι; δῆλον γὰρ
ὡς οὐδὲ τὸ λευκὸν ἐναντίον ἔσται τῷ μέλανι, διότι
μέσον αὐτῶν ἐστι τὸ ξανθόν τε καὶ τὸ φαιόν, ἐρυθρόν
τε καὶ ὠχρὸν ἕκαστόν τε τῶν ἄλλων χρωμάτων· οὐδὲ
τὸ θερμὸν τῷ ψυχρῷ, καὶ γὰρ καὶ τούτων ἐστὶ μέσα
χλιαρόν τε καὶ εὔκρατον. οἱ μὲν δὴ σοφώτατοι Μεθοδικοὶ κατὰ τὴν ἀρχὴν εὐθέως πεπτωκότες οὐ σμικρὸν
οὐδὲ τὸ τυχὸν πτῶμα τί ἂν ἔτι τῶν ἐφεξῆς ἀληθῶν
καταμάθοιεν; οὐδὲ ἓν δήπου, δειχθήσεται γὰρ ἅπαντα
τὰ κατὰ τὴν ἰατρικὴν τέχνην ἐκ τούτων ἠρτημένα καὶ

What he replied to me on this matter, and what I have often said to you before now, most excellent Hiero, and what it is now appropriate to recall, is that it is no surprise that health, on the one hand, is placed in the stability and strength of the functions while disease, on the other hand, is placed in the condition of the body that is contrary to nature. "For they are not opposites as you think," he said, "since there is something intermediate between them which is neither health nor disease." When I heard this, I retired from this argument, being at once astounded and distressed—I must confess what happened—for I had never previously encountered anyone so completely stupefied by such a doctrine. But then, when I met one for the first time, I was naturally amazed, not because that man alone was so stupid but that he had so many pupils far 58K
more unfortunate than himself. Those men either saw the Methodics falling into error in such a way at the very foundation of their teaching or, if they failed to see this, were totally stupefied.

For what, I ask, can be said about disease not being the opposite of health because there is something intermediate between them? It is clear on these grounds that white will not be the opposite of black because yellow, gray, red, pale and each of the other colors are intermediate between them. Nor would heat be the opposite of cold because tepid and temperate are between them. What, then, might those most sapient Methodics understand of truths that follow in a connected manner when they have fallen into a calamity neither small nor inconsequential right from the start? Not one thing, it would seem, for it will be shown that all things pertaining to the art of medicine depend

---

47 B; τὴν αὐτὴν ἀρχὴν K

δεόντως, εἴ γ᾽ ἐν ταῖς μεθόδῳ τινὶ συνισταμέναις
τέχναις ἀρχὴ τῆς συστάσεως ἡ τοῦ τέλους ἐστὶν
ἔννοια. πεπλημμέληται μὲν οὖν καὶ ἄλλοις πολλοῖς
εἰς τὴν τοῦ τέλους ἔννοιαν οὐκ ὀλίγα, τῶν μὲν τὸ
ὑγιάζειν ὡς τὸ πολὺ τέλος εἶναι λεγόντων τῆς ἰατρι-
κῆς, τῶν δὲ τὰ σύμφορα πράττειν ὡς πρὸς τὴν ὑγείαν, |
59K τῶν δ᾽ ἐκκόπτειν τὰς νοσώδεις αἰτίας, τῶν δὲ τὰ παρ᾽
ἑαυτῶν ἅπαντα ποιεῖσθαι, τῶν δ᾽ ὡς ἂν ἑκάστῳ παρα-
στῇ καὶ δεήσῃ, καὶ περὶ τούτων ἰδίᾳ διορίσασθαι·
ἀλλ᾽ οὐδεὶς οὕτως ἔμπληκτος ὡς ἐν ἄλλῳ μὲν γένει
τὴν ὑγείαν, ἐν ἄλλῳ δὲ ὑποθέσθαι τὴν νόσον, ἀλλ᾽
ἤτοι ταῖς κατὰ φύσιν ἐνεργείαις προσέχων ἢ ταῖς
κατασκευαῖς τῶν μορίων, ἃς ἔνιοι διαθέσεις ὀνομά-
ζουσιν· εἴτε δ᾽ ἐν ταῖς κατὰ φύσιν ἐνεργείαις ἐστὶ τὸ
ὑγιαίνειν, ἐν ταῖς παρὰ φύσιν ἔσται τὸ νοσεῖν· εἴτε ἐν
ταῖς κατασκευαῖς ταῖς κατὰ φύσιν, ἐν ταῖς παρὰ
φύσιν ἔσται κατασκευαῖς ἡ νόσος· εἴτ᾽ ἐν ταῖς διαθέσεσιν, ἐν ταύταις καὶ τὸ νοσεῖν. οὐδὲ γὰρ οὐδὲ
βαθείας τινὸς εἰς τοῦτο θεωρίας ἐστὶ χρεία, μόνον δ᾽
ἀπόχρη τὸ μὴ διεστράφθαι.

τίς γὰρ οὐκ οἶδεν ὡς εἰ τὸ βλέπειν ὑγιαίνειν ἐστίν,
ὅτι τὸ νοσεῖν ἔσται τὸ ἀμβλυώττειν, ἢ ὅλως τὸ μὴ
βλέπειν; τίς δ᾽ οὐ συνίησιν ὡς εἰ τὸ ἀκούειν ὑγιαίνειν
ἐστίν, ὅτι νοσεῖν ἔσται τό τε μόγις ἀκούειν καὶ τὸ μηδ᾽
ὅλως ἀκούειν; οὕτω δὲ καὶ εἰ τὸ πέττειν ὑγιαίνειν ἐστί,
τὸ ἀπεπτεῖν τε καὶ δυσπεπτεῖν ἔσται νοσεῖν; καὶ εἰ τὸ
60K κινεῖσθαι | καθ᾽ ὁρμὴν ἔστιν ὑγεία, νόσος ἂν εἴη
δήπου σπασμὸς καὶ παλμὸς καὶ παράλυσις καὶ τρό-

on these [truths], and necessarily so, if the basis of their composition, at least in the arts put together by a certain method, is the concept of an objective. And thus, to no small extent has error beset many others when it comes to the concept of the objective, since some say that health is the objective of medicine for the most part, and others that it is to create the circumstances conducive to health, others that it is to eradicate the causes of diseases, others that it is to do everything they can, others that one should provide for each person what he may require, and to make distinctions in these things individually. But no one is so stupid as to propose that health is in one class and disease in another, rather than putting them either in functions that accord with nature or in the constitutions of the parts which some call conditions. If health is in the functions in accord with nature, disease will be in the functions contrary to nature, and if it is in the constitutions in accord with nature, disease will be in constitutions contrary to nature, and if it is in conditions, disease will be in these too. Nor is there any need for some weighty theory for this. It is quite enough not to be perverse.

For who does not know that, if to see is to be healthy, then to be diseased will be to see dimly or not at all? And who does not understand that, if to hear is to be healthy, then to be diseased will be to hear with difficulty or not at all. Or, in like manner also, if to digest is to be healthy, will not to digest at all or to do so abnormally be to be diseased? And if to move voluntarily is health, disease would be, I presume, spasm, or palpitation, paralysis, or tremor, or,

59K

60K

93

μος καὶ συλλήβδην εἰπεῖν ἅπαν ὅ τί περ ἂν ἤτοι
τελέως ἀναιρεῖ τὴν καθ᾽ ὁρμὴν κίνησιν ἢ ἐμποδίζει γέ
πως αὐτήν. ὡσαύτως δὲ εἰ τὸ κατὰ φύσιν αἰσθάνεσθαι
τῆς ὑγείας ἐστίν, ἡ ἀναισθησία καὶ δυσαισθησία καὶ
νάρκη καὶ ὀδύνη νόσοι γενήσονται· καὶ εἰ τὸ τεταγμέ-
νως ἀναπνεῖν ὑγεία, ἄπνοια καὶ δύσπνοια νόσος. ἀλλ᾽
εἴπερ ταῦτα νόσοι, πρόδηλον ὡς αἱ διαθέσεις τῶν
μορίων ὑφ᾽ ὧν ἀποτελοῦνται νόσων εἰσὶν αἰτίαι, καὶ
οὐ χρὴ λέγειν οὔτε φλεγμονὴν οὔτε σκίρρον οὔτ᾽
ἐρυσίπελας οὔτε ἀπόστασιν οὔθ᾽ ἕλκος οὔτε οἴδημα
νοσήματα· καὶ εἴπερ ταῦτα νοσήματα, πρόδηλον ὡς
οὐδὲν ἐκείνων νόσημα. δύο γάρ ἐστι γένη πραγμάτων
οὐδὲν ὁμοίων ἀλλήλοις,[48] ἀλλὰ πάντῃ τε διαλλαττόν-
των καὶ ὅλῃ τῇ φύσει διαφερόντων· ὀνομάζουσι δὲ τὸ
μὲν ἕτερον τῶν γενῶν σῶμα, τὸ δ᾽ ἕτερον ἐνέργειαν.

ὀφθαλμὸς μὲν οὖν καὶ γλῶττα καὶ οὖς καὶ σκέλος
ἕκαστόν τε τῶν τοιούτων σῶμά πως ἔχον ἐστίν· ὄψις
δὲ καὶ ἀκοὴ καὶ διάλεξις καὶ βάδισις ἐνέργειαι τῶν
61K εἰρημένων σωμάτων. εἴπερ οὖν ἐν | τῷ πως ἔχειν τὰ
σώματα τὸ νοσεῖν ἐστιν, ἐν τῷ πως ἔχειν τὰς ἐνεργείας τὸ νοσεῖν οὐκ ἔσται· εἰ δέ γ᾽ ἐν τούτῳ τὸ νοσεῖν
εἴη, πρόδηλον αὖ πάλιν ὡς οὐκ ἔστιν ἐν τῇ τῶν
σωμάτων διαθέσει. τὸ μέντοι τὴν μὲν διάθεσιν αἰτίαν
εἶναι, τὴν δὲ ἐνέργειαν τὸ γιγνόμενον ὑπὸ τῆς τοῦ
σώματος διαθέσεως, ὁμολογεῖσθαι χρὴ καὶ φυλάττεσθαι παντὸς μᾶλλον, ὥστε καὶ ὅστις ἀγνοεῖ τοῦτο,
περί τι τῶν ἀναγκαίων ἔσφαλται πραγμάτων· ὁ δ᾽
ἤτοι τὴν βλάβην τῆς ἐνεργείας ἢ τὴν διάθεσιν τοῦ

in short anything that entirely does away with voluntary movement, or at least hinders it somehow. Similarly, if natural sensation is health, then loss of sensation (anesthesia) or disordered sensation (dysesthesia) as well as numbness and pain will be diseases. And if to breathe regularly is health, apnea and dyspnea are diseases. But if, in fact, these things are diseases, it is clear that the conditions of the parts through which they are brought about are causes of diseases, and we ought not to say that inflammation, induration, erysipelas, abscess, wound/ulcer and edema are diseases. But if these latter are diseases, it is clear that none of the former are diseases. For the two classes of things are not the same but are in every way distinct, and differ in their whole nature. They name one of the classes with respect to a body and the other with respect to a function.

Thus eye, tongue, ear, and limb, and each one of such things are, in some way, bodies, whereas sight, hearing, speech, and walking are functions of the aforementioned bodies. If disease is bodies being in a certain state, then disease will not be the functions being in a certain way. If, however, disease were to lie in this, then it is also clear, conversely, that it is not in the condition of the bodies. The fact is, and this must be agreed upon and maintained above all, that the condition is the cause while the function is what occurs due to the condition of the body, so that someone who is ignorant of this is in error with regard to one of the essential matters. However, if someone calls the damage of function or the condition of the body a disease,

61K

---

48 P1; ἀλλήλων B; *om.* K

σώματος ὀνομάζων νόσημα, κἂν εἰ μὴ δεόντως ὀνο-
μάζοι, δύναται γοῦν ὀρθὴν ἔχειν τὴν δόξαν ὑπὲρ
αὐτῶν τῶν πραγμάτων· ἔστι δ᾽ οὐκ ἐκ τῶν ὀνομάτων
τὸ καλῶς ἰάσασθαι τὰς νόσους, ἀλλ᾽ ἐκ τῆς τῶν
πραγμάτων ὀρθῆς ὑπολήψεως. εὐθὺς δὲ καὶ τοῦτ᾽ αὐτὸ
πολλοὺς τῶν ἰατρῶν ἔστιν εὑρεῖν ἀγνοοῦντας, καὶ
νομίζοντας ἐν πράγμασί τι διαφέρεσθαι τοὺς τὰς
διαθέσεις τῶν σωμάτων ἡγουμένους εἶναι νοσήματα
πρὸς τοὺς ἐν ταῖς βλάβαις τῶν ἐνεργειῶν ὑπολαμ-
βάνοντας αὐτὰ συνίστασθαι· καὶ τούτων πάντων τῶν
ἁμαρτημάτων, ὅπερ εἴρηταί τε πολλάκις ἤδη καὶ αὖ-
62K θις εἰρήσεται, ἓν αἴτιον ὑπάρχει τὸ | μὴ γεγυμνάσθαι
κατὰ τὴν λογικὴν μέθοδον τοὺς ἐπιχειροῦντας ὁτιοῦν
ἐξευρίσκειν λογικῶς, ἀλλ᾽ ἅμα μὲν ἀποχωρεῖν τῆς
ἐμπειρίας, ὡς γεγυμνασμένους τὸν λογισμόν, ἅμα δ᾽
ἀγυμνάστους ὄντας ἐν αὐτῷ σφάλλεσθαι μέγιστα.
μυριάκις γοῦν ὑπὲρ ὀνομάτων αὐτοὺς εὑρίσκω διαφερομένους ὡς ὑπὲρ πραγμάτων· αὖθις δ᾽ ἄν, εἰ τύχοι,
πρᾶγμά τι μέγιστον ἀγνοοῦντες, ὄνομα νομίζουσιν
ἀγνοεῖν, ὥς πέρ γε κἀπὶ τοῦ προκειμένου νῦν ἡμῖν οὐκ
ἴσασι διακρίνειν, ὡς ἡ μὲν κατασκευὴ τῶν σωμάτων
αἰτίας ἔχει λόγον, ἡ δ᾽ ἐνέργεια τὸ πρὸς ἐκείνης ἐστὶν
ἀποτελούμενον, οὐδ᾽ ὡς τὸ θεραπευόμενον ἡ τοῦ σώματός ἐστι διάθεσις· ἕπεται γὰρ ἐξ ἀνάγκης ταύτῃ
κατὰ φύσιν μὲν ἐχούσῃ κατὰ φύσιν ἐνεργεῖν, ἐξιστα-
μένῃ δὲ τοῦ κατὰ φύσιν εὐθὺς καὶ τὴν ἐνέργειαν εἰς τὸ
παρὰ φύσιν ἐκτρέπειν.

ἐν τούτῳ δὲ τὸ πᾶν ἐστι, καὶ τοῦτο ἀρχὴ καὶ οἷον

even if he is not using names as he should, he can, nonetheless, hold the correct opinion about the matters themselves. For curing diseases properly does not come from the names but from the correct conception of the matters. And it is immediately possible to find many doctors who are ignorant of this very thing too, since they think there is some difference in terms of the matters between those who suppose diseases are conditions of bodies and those who assume they subsist in damage of the functions. But as I have already said, and often, and will say again, there is one cause of all these errors. This is that those who attempt   62K
to investigate logically in any way whatsoever without having been trained in the logical method, but at the same time shun experience as if they had been trained in logic, although they are in fact untrained in it, err very greatly. Times without number I find them disputing about names as though about facts. Moreover, as may happen, when they are ignorant of some very important matter, they think they are ignorant of the name, which is the case in the matter presently before us, where they do not know to distinguish that it is the constitution of bodies which has the ground of cause whereas the function is what is brought about by that, nor that what is to be treated is the condition of the body. For it follows, of necessity, from the condition being in accord with nature, that function is in accord with nature whereas, when the condition departs from an accord with nature, function also immediately changes to being contrary to nature.

The whole matter lies in this; this is the beginning and,

στοιχεῖόν τι πρῶτον ἁπάσης τῆς θεραπευτικῆς ὑπάρχει μεθόδου· τὸ δὲ εἴτ᾽ αὐτὸ τοῦτο χρὴ προσαγορεύειν
νόσον, εἴτε τὴν βλάβην τῆς ἐνεργείας, ὑπὲρ ὀνόματός
ἐστιν ἀμφισβητούντων. εἰρήσεται μὲν οὖν τί μοι καὶ
περὶ τῆς τῶν ὀνομάτων χρήσεως, ὥσπερ εἴρηται καὶ
63K πρόσθεν ἤδη δι᾽ ἑτέρων. | ἀλλὰ νῦν οὔπω διαστέλλο-
μαι περὶ αὐτῶν, ἵν᾽ ἔργῳ τοῦτ᾽ αὐτὸ μᾶλλον βεβαιώ-
σωμαι, καὶ δείξω τίς ἀρχὴ καὶ ῥίζα τῆς θεραπευτικῆς
ἐστι μεθόδου, περὶ ἣν εὐθὺς ἄλλοι τε πολλοὶ τῶν
Λογικούς τε καὶ Δογματικοὺς ἑαυτοὺς ὀνομασάντων
καὶ οἱ βέλτιστοι σφάλλονται Μεθοδικοί. τοῦτο μὲν
οὖν καὶ ἤδη πως φαίνεται τοῖς συνετοῖς, ὡς οὐδὲν
ἄλλο ἐστὶ τὸ θεραπευόμενον ὑπὸ τῶν ἰατρῶν πλὴν ἡ
τῶν σωμάτων διάθεσις, ὡς ἐν τῷ μετὰ ταῦτα λόγῳ
δειχθήσεται.

8. Τὸ δὲ τὴν ἄγνοιαν ἐπανορθώσασθαι τῶν μὴ
γινωσκόντων ὅσα τὰ σύμπαντά ἐστι πράγματα κατὰ
τὸν ἐνεστῶτα λόγον ἀλλήλοις παρακείμενα, νῦν ἡμῖν
προὔκειτο. φαίνεται γὰρ ἓν μέν τι γένος εἶναι τῶν
σωμάτων αὐτῶν, ἕτερον δὲ τὸ τῶν ἐνεργειῶν· καὶ τὸ
μὲν τῶν σωμάτων ἡγεῖσθαί τε καὶ ποιεῖν τὰς ἐνεργείας, ἕπεσθαι δ᾽ ἐκείνας κατὰ φύσιν μὲν ἔχουσι τοῖς
σώμασιν ἀμέμπτως τε καὶ κατὰ φύσιν αὐτὰς δια-
κειμένας, παρὰ φύσιν δ᾽ ἐχόντων ἢ μὴ γιγνομένας
παντάπασιν, ἢ παρεμποδιζομένας γε πάντως. τρίτον
δ᾽ ἐπὶ τούτοις ἐστὶ γένος τὸ τῶν ἐργαζομένων τὰς

as it were, a primary element of the whole method of medicine. But whether one should term this itself the disease, or the damage of function is a matter for people who dispute over names. I shall, then, say something about the use of names, as I have already done before in other works.[30] However, for the moment, I shall make no further distinctions about these things so that I might establish this very thing particularly in action, and I shall show what the origin and root of the method of medicine is—[a subject] about which many others who call themselves Logicians and Rationalists, as well as the very fine Methodics, are at once in error. What is also already apparent to those who are to some degree wise is that the object of treatment for doctors is nothing else apart from the condition of bodies, as will be shown in the argument that follows.

63K

8. The task now lying before us is to correct the ignorance of those who do not know how many things there are in all that are grouped with each other in the present argument. For there seems to be one class of the bodies themselves and another of the functions, and that of the bodies seems to precede and create the functions while those functions which follow in bodies that are normal are themselves in a faultless and natural state. If, however, the bodies are contrary to nature, [the functions] either do not occur at all or are, at least, altogether hampered. There is a third class in addition to these, which is that of the causes

30 See specifically *De captionibus penes dictionem*, XIV.582–98K (translation, R. B. Edlow [1977]) and *De nominibus medicis* (Arabic text and German translation by M. Meyerhof and J. Schacht [1931]). Galen, however, mentions the issue of naming frequently in a variety of his works.

64K διαθέσεις αἰτίων· ὃν γὰρ ἡ διάθεσις ἔχει πρὸς | τὴν
ἐνέργειαν λόγον, τοῦτον ἕτερόν τι χρὴ πάντως ἔχειν
πρὸς τὴν διάθεσιν, ἑνὶ μόνῳ διαλλάττον τῷ τὴν μὲν
διάθεσιν ἅμα ταῖς ἐνεργείαις ὑπάρχειν καὶ μὴ δύνασθαί ποτε μήτε τὴν κατωρθωμένην ἐνέργειαν εἶναι
χωρὶς τῆς τῶν σωμάτων κατὰ φύσιν διαθέσεως μήτε
τὴν βεβλαμμένην ἄνευ τοῦ καὶ τὰ σώματα βεβλάφθαι. τὰ δ' αἴτια τῆς διαθέσεως ταύτης τῆς ἐμποδιζούσης τὴν ἐνέργειαν δύναται μὲν καὶ μηκέτ' εἶναι,
δύναται δὲ καὶ νῦν ἔτι παραμένειν· ἕτερα δ' οὖν πάντως ἐστὶ τῶν διαθέσεων αὐτῶν σοι, καὶ τοῦτο τρίτον
εὕρηται γένος ἕτερον ἐνεργείας τε καὶ τῆς ἐργαζομένης αὐτὴν διαθέσεως.

ἐπ' αὐτῷ δ' ἄλλο τέταρτον γένος διαθέσεως, ὅσα
τοῖς σώμασιν ὑπάρχει κατὰ φύσιν τε καὶ παρὰ φύσιν
ἔχουσι, μηδὲν μήτ' ὠφελοῦντα μήτε βλάπτοντα τὰς
ἐνεργείας· οἷον εἰ τύχοι τὸ χρῶμα τοῦ σώματος παντὸς ἢ μέλαν ἐκ λευκοῦ γιγνόμενον, ἐν ἡλίῳ διατρι-
ψάντων ἐπὶ πλέον, ἢ λευκὸν ἐκ μέλανος, ἐν σκιᾷ
διαιτηθέντων, ἢ ἐρυθρὸν λουσαμένων, ἢ ὠχρὸν φοβηθέντων.[49] οὔτε γὰρ ἐνέργεια τοῦτ' ἔστιν οὔτε διάθεσις
σώματος ἐνεργείας αἰτία, καὶ πολὺ δὴ μᾶλλον οὐδ' ἡ
65K τὰς παρὰ | φύσιν ἐργαζομένη διαθέσεις αἰτία, σύμ-
πτωμα δ' ἐστὶ συμβαῖνον ἐξ ἀνάγκης ἐπὶ ταῖς δια-
φόροις τῶν σωμάτων ἀλλοιώσεσιν, εἴτ' οὖν κατὰ φύσιν, εἴτε καὶ παρὰ φύσιν ἔχοιεν.

ἐπειδὴ τοίνυν ἤδη τέτταρα γένη διώρισται, κἂν τῷ
ταῦτα γινώσκειν ἢ μὴ τὸ καλῶς ἄρχεσθαι τῆς θερα-

100

bringing about the conditions. For the ground which the condition has in relation to function, something else must 64K have in relation to the condition, differing in one respect only, which is that the condition exists at the same time as the functions and there can never be a successful function apart from the condition of bodies being normal, nor a damaged function without the bodies also having been damaged. It is, however, possible for the causes of this condition which hinders function either to be no longer in existence or to be still remaining. [The causes], let me insist to you, are altogether different from conditions themselves; and this third class is found which is different from function and from the condition bringing the function about.

In addition to this, there is another, fourth class of conditions comprising those that exist in bodies that are either in accord with nature or contrary to nature (normal or abnormal), but which neither benefit or damage the functions. For example, it might happen that the color of the whole body either becomes dark having been pale, as in those who spend too much time in the sun, or pale having been dark, as in those who live their lives in the shade, or red as a result of washing, or pale as a result of fear. But this is neither a function nor a condition of the body causing functions, much less the cause which brings about abnormal conditions. It is a symptom that is a necessary accompaniment due to different alterations of bodies whether they are normal or abnormal.

Therefore, since four classes have by now been distinguished, and I shall show that whether you know these or

49 ἢ ἐρυθρὸν . . . φοβηθέντων K; om. B

πευτικῆς μεθόδου δείξομεν ὑπάρχον, ἐξέστω λοιπὸν
τῷ βουλομένῳ κατ᾽ αὐτῶν ἃς ἂν ἐθέλῃ τίθεσθαι προσ-
ηγορίας· οἷον, εἰ βούλοιτο, τὴν μὲν παρὰ φύσιν τῶν
σωμάτων διάθεσιν, ὅταν ἐνέργειάν τινα βλάπτῃ,
νόσημα προσαγορευέτω, αὐτὴν δὲ τὴν βλάβην τῆς
ἐνεργείας ἐξαίρετόν τι σύμπτωμα νοσήματος· ὅσα δ᾽
ἄλλως συμβέβηκεν, ὥσπερ τὰ χρώματα, καὶ ταῦτ᾽, εἰ
βούλοιτο, καλείτω συμπτώματα, διοριζέτω μέντοι τῆς
βλάβης τῶν ἐνεργειῶν αὐτά, καὶ εἴπερ ἐκεῖνα ἐξαί-
ρετα συμπτώματα νοσημάτων ὀνομάζει, ταῦτ᾽ οἰκεῖά
τε καὶ ἴδια καλείτω, καί τινα πρὸς τούτοις, εἰ βούλοιτο, μήτ᾽ οἰκεῖα μήτ᾽ ἴδια, συμπίπτοντα δὲ κατά τινα
τύχην· τέταρτον δ᾽ ἐπὶ τοῖσδε γένος τιθέσθω τὸ τῶν
νοσωδῶν αἰτίων, καὶ τούτων τὰ μὲν ἐν αὐτῷ τοῦ ζῴου |
66K τῷ σώματι συνιστάμενα προηγούμενα καλείτω, τὰ
δ᾽ ἔξωθεν προσπίπτοντα προκατάρχοντα. θέμενος δ᾽
οὕτως ἢ ἄλλως ὅπως ἂν ἐθέλῃ σαφῶς καὶ χρησίμως
τοῖς ἀκούουσι, μηκέτι μετατιθέσθω, μηδ᾽ ἐξαλλαττέτω
τὴν χρῆσιν, ἀλλ᾽ ἀεὶ φυλαττέτω παρ᾽ ὅλον τὸν λόγον,
ἵνα καὶ μανθάνωμεν ἃ λέγει ῥᾳδίως, καὶ τὰς ἀντιλογίας καὶ τοὺς ἐλέγχους πρός τι σαφὲς καὶ δι-
ωρισμένον ποιώμεθα.

πῶς καὶ τίνα τρόπον; ἐνδείξασθαι γὰρ ἔτι τοῦτ᾽
αὐτὸ χρὴ διὰ τοὺς ἀναισθήτους Μεθοδικούς. ἔστω
τινὰ λέγειν ὡς ἡ μὲν φλεγμονὴ διάθεσίς ἐστι παρὰ
φύσιν, τὸ δ᾽ ἔργον τοῦ φλεγμαίνοντος μέρους τὸ
βεβλαμμένον οἰκεῖον ἐξαίρετον τοῦ πάθους σύμπτω-

not, this is the proper beginning of the method of medicine, let it be left to someone to apply whatever terms he might wish to these classes. For example, let him, if he wants to, call the condition of bodies contrary to nature, whenever it damages a certain function, a disease, and the actual damage of function, some specific symptom of disease. Those things that have come about otherwise, such as colors, let him also call symptoms if he wishes. Nevertheless, let him distinguish these from what damages functions and, if he names those specific symptoms of diseases, let him call them proper and peculiar, and any in addition to these, if he wishes, neither proper nor peculiar, but symptoms occurring by chance. Apart from these, let him put forward a fourth class, that of causes of disease. Of these, let him call those which exist in the actual body of the animal *proegoumenic* causes and those which befall 66K [the animal] from without, *prokatarchontic* causes.[31] Having set [the matter] out like this, or in any other way he might wish that is clear and useful to his audience, let him make no more changes, nor alter the usage, but always preserve the argument in its entirety so that we too might easily understand what he says, and might make our opposing arguments and refutations to any part of it clear and distinct.

How and in what way? For it is still necessary to demonstrate this very point on account of the senseless Methodics. Let someone say that inflammation is a condition contrary to nature whereas the damaged action of the inflamed part is a proper and specific symptom of the af-

31 On Galen's use of causal terminology, see the Introduction, section 6, and I. Johnston (2006), pp. 31–37.

μα, ποδῶν μὲν βάδισις, ὀφθαλμῶν δὲ ὄψις, ὤτων δ᾽
ἀκοή· τὸ δ᾽ ἔρευθος, εἰ τύχοι, καὶ ἡ τάσις, ἥ τ᾽
ἀντιτυπία καὶ ὁ παρὰ φύσιν ὄγκος ὁ ταῖς φλεγμοναῖς
ἑπόμενος, ἕτερόν τι γένος εἴτε συμπτωμάτων, εἴτε
συμβεβηκότων, εἴθ᾽ ὅπως ἂν ἄλλως ἐθέλῃ τις ὀνομάζειν, ἀλλ᾽ οὖν ὅτι γε μὴ ταὐτὸ γένος ἐστὶ τῇ βλάβῃ
τῶν ἐνεργειῶν, ἴστω τε καὶ διοριζέσθω σαφῶς· ἡ πλη-
θώρα δ᾽, εἰ τύχοι, τῆς φλεγμονῆς αἰτία προηγουμένη, |
67K καὶ ταύτης προκατάρχουσα τὸ πλῆθος τῶν ἐδεσμά-
των. ὡς οὖν ἐγὼ καὶ παραδείγματα πεποίημαι σαφῆ
τοῦ λόγου καὶ τέτταρα γένη διώρισμαι καὶ τὰς αἰτίας
καὶ ἐννοίας αὐτῶν εἴρηκα, κατὰ τὸν αὐτόν, οἶμαι,
τρόπον ἐχρῆν ποιῆσαι τὸν Θεσσαλὸν ἐπὶ τοσούτοις τε
καὶ τηλικούτοις ἀνδράσι καθ᾽ ὧν ἑαυτὸν ἀνεκήρυττε,
μέλλοντα νεωτέραν αἵρεσιν συνίστασθαι· νυνὶ δ᾽ οὔτε
αὐτὸς οὐδὲν εἶπε σαφὲς οὔτέ τις τῶν ἀπ᾽ αὐτοῦ.

9. Τολμήσας γοῦν ὁ Ὀλυμπικὸς ἀφορίσασθαι τί
ποτ᾽ ἐστὶ πάθος, οὐ πάθους, ἀλλὰ συμπτωμάτων εἴρηκεν ἔννοιαν. ὅλως μὲν οὖν οὐδ᾽ ὅ τί ποτ᾽ ἐστὶ τὸ πάθος,
οὐδ᾽ ὅπῃ τοῦ νοσήματος διαφέρει, γινώσκουσιν· ἀλλὰ
τοῦτο μὲν ἐν τοῖς ἑξῆς διοριῶ, πάντα γὰρ ἅμα λέγειν
οὐκ ἐγχωρεῖ. συγχωρηθέντος δ᾽ αὐτοῖς τοῦ ταὐτὸν
εἶναι νόσημά τε καὶ πάθος, ἴδωμεν ὅ τί ποτέ φασι.
Πάθος ἐστὶ τροπὴ τοῦ σώματος ἐκ τοῦ κατὰ φύσιν
εἰς τὸ παρὰ φύσιν ἐπίμονος. εἶτα μικρὸν προελθὼν
φησιν· Ἰστέον δ᾽ ὅτι διαφέρει πάθος συμπτώματος·
πάθος μὲν γάρ ἐστιν, ὡς ὀλίγον ἔμπροσθεν ἔφην, διά-
68K θεσις | παρὰ φύσιν τοῦ σώματος ἐπίμονος· σύμπτωμα

fection—walking of the feet, sight of the eyes, hearing of the ears. On the other hand, the redness (if it occurs), or the tension, or the hardness, or the swelling contrary to nature, are what follow inflammations and are some other class, either of symptoms or of accidentals, or however else someone might wish to name them. But the same class is not one of damage of functions—let him recognize this and clearly distinguish it. *Plethora*, if it occurs, is a *pro-egoumenic* cause of inflammation and the *prokatarktic* 67K cause of this is an abundance of foods. So, then, I have not only created clear examples of the argument, but I have also differentiated the four classes, and have spoken of the causes and concepts of these. It behooved Thessalus, I think, to do the same thing, if he intended to establish a new sect and proclaim himself superior to so many men of such standing. But, as it is, he says nothing that is clear, nor does any one of those who follow him.

9. Olympicus, at least when he makes so bold as to define what an affection is, articulates a concept of symptoms, not of affections. On the whole, then, they (the Methodics) know neither what an affection is nor how it differs from a disease. But I shall make this distinction in due course—it is not possible to say everything all at once. If, however, we concede to them that disease and affection are the same thing, let us see what it is they say: "An affection is a change of the body [which goes] from being in accord with nature to being contrary to nature, and is persisting." Having gone on a little further, he says: "One must know that an affection differs from a symptom. For an affection is, as I said a little earlier, a condition of the 68K body which is contrary to nature and persisting, whereas a

δὲ ὃ τῷ πάθει συμβαίνει, εἰδικὴν ὥς πέρ τινα καὶ
μερικωτέραν ἐν τοῖς παρὰ φύσιν ἔχον τύπωσιν. αὕτη
μὲν ἡ θαυμαστὴ ῥῆσις Ὀλυμπικοῦ τοῦ σοφοῦ, τολμή-
σαντος ἀφορίσασθαι πάθος τε καὶ σύμπτωμα· τοσ-
ούτων δ' ἐστὶν ἁμαρτημάτων μεστὴ ὥστέ μοι παρ-
ίσταται τὸ τοῦ μωροῦ τοῦ πρὸς κόσκινον εἰπόντος οὐχ
εὑρίσκειν ὅ τι βύσειεν ἢ μὴ βύσειεν αὐτοῦ. τί γὰρ δὴ
καὶ πρῶτον ἐξ αὐτῶν εἴποι τις, ἢ τί παραλίποι; πάντα
μὲν γὰρ ἐξελέγχειν ὅσα κακῶς ἀποφαίνονται μακρὸν
ἂν εἴη.

ἢ ἐκ τοῦ κατὰ φύσιν εἰς τὸ παρὰ φύσιν τροπὴ
πᾶσα νόσος ἐστίν, εἰ μόνον αὐτῇ προσείη τὸ ἐπίμονον; ἀλλὰ τὴν ἄχροιαν ὑμεῖς αὐτοὶ καὶ τὴν ἀτρο-
φίαν ἐν τοῖς συμπτώμασιν, οὐκ ἐν τοῖς πάθεσιν
ἀριθμεῖτε· τί δ' ἡ κακοχυμία; τί δὲ ἡ ἔνδεια; τί δὲ ἡ
καχεξία; τί δὲ τὸ πλῆθος; οὐ παρὰ φύσιν; εἰ τοίνυν
αὐτοῖς προσείη τὸ ἐπίμονον, ἐν τοῖς νοσήμασιν
ἀριθμηθήσονται.[50] καὶ μὴν οὐδ' αὐτοὶ βούλεσθε, καὶ
καλῶς γε τοῦτο ποιεῖτε· προσεῖναι γὰρ χρὴ τῷ παρὰ
69K φύσιν εἶναι τὴν διάθεσιν ἐνέργειάν | τινα πρὸς αὐτῆς
βλάπτεσθαι· μέχρι δ' ἂν ἀβλαβεῖς αἱ πᾶσαι φυλάτ-
τωνται, κἂν μυριάκις ἐξαλλάττηται καὶ τρέπηται καὶ
μεταβάλληται τὸ σῶμα, νόσος οὔπω τῶν διαθέσεων
ἐκείνων ἐστὶν οὐδεμία.

[50] B; ἀριθμηθήσεται K

---

[32] The source of this allusion, perhaps from a comic writer or
possibly simply proverbial, is unknown.

[33] Plethora, kakochymia, and kachexia are among a small

symptom is what happens contingent upon the affection, although it has a delineation that is specific and, as it were, more particular among the things contrary to nature." This is the remarkable statement of Olympicus the wise when he was bold enough to distinguish affection from symptom. It is a statement filled with so many errors that for me it stands comparison with the dullard when he said to the sieve that he could not discover what would plug it up and what would not.[32] For what, really, might someone say first out of these things, or what leave aside? It would be a lengthy matter to refute all the things they have pronounced on wrongly.

Is every kind of change from what accords with nature to what is contrary to nature a disease providing only that duration is associated with it? But you yourselves number pallor and atrophy among the symptoms, and not among the affections. What of *kakochymia*? What of deficiency? What of *kachexia*? What of *plethora*?[33] Are these not contrary to nature? If duration is associated with them, they will be numbered among the diseases. However, you yourself do not want this, and you do well in this regard. For due to the condition being contrary to nature we should allow that some function is harmed by it. Whilever all the functions are preserved undamaged, even if the body is changed, turned, or altered in ten thousand ways, none of those conditions is, as yet, a disease. 69K

number of terms transliterated, as discussed in the Introduction. The first means a fullness of the veins, the second a bad state of the humors, and the third, still in use today in the Latinized form, has the meaning here of "a bad state of the body" (Hippocrates, *Aphorisms* 31). Galen makes the distinction between the second two in Book 4 (263K).

τό γέ τοι τῆς θεραπείας δεόμενον οὐδὲν ἄλλο ἐστὶ
πλὴν τῆς βλαπτούσης τὴν ἐνέργειαν διαθέσεως. οὐ
μὲν γὰρ δεόμεθα πρώτου καὶ μάλιστα πάντων, ἡ κατὰ
φύσιν ἐστὶν ἐνέργεια· δι᾿ ἐκείνην δὲ καὶ τῆς κατὰ
φύσιν εἴτε διαθέσεως εἴτε κατασκευῆς ὀνομάζειν
ἐθέλοις. ὁρᾶν γὰρ δεόμεθα καὶ ἀκούειν καὶ
διαλέγεσθαι καὶ βαδίζειν, οὐκ ὀφθαλμῶν, οὐδ᾿ ὤτων,
οὐδὲ γλώττης, οὐδὲ σκελῶν· εἰ γοῦν ἦν ὁρᾶν δι᾿ ἑτέρου
μορίου, τίς ἂν ἦν ὀφθαλμῶν ἡ χρεία; καὶ εἴπερ ἦν
ἀκούειν δι᾿ ἄλλου τινὸς ὀργάνου, τί τῶν ὤτων
ἐδεήθημεν ἄν; οὕτω δὲ καὶ τῆς γλώττης καὶ τῶν
σκελῶν οὐκ ἂν δήπουθεν οὐδὲν ὄφελος ἦν ἡμῖν, εἰ
διαλέγεσθαι καὶ βαδίζειν οἷόν τ᾿ ἦν ἄνευ τούτων. τοῦ
μὲν οὖν ὁρᾶν δι᾿ ἑαυτὸ⁵¹ χρῄζομεν· ὀφθαλμῶν δὲ οὐ δι᾿
ἑαυτούς,⁵² ἀλλὰ διὰ τοῦτο. καὶ γλώττης δὲ καὶ ὤτων
καὶ σκελῶν, οὐχ ἵνα ἔχωμεν ὄργανα καὶ πολλὰ μόρια,
70K χρῄζομεν, ἀλλὰ διαλέξεως ἕνεκα καὶ ἀκοῆς καὶ | βαδί-
σεως. ὅταν γοῦν νεκρωθῇ τι μόριον ἀποτμηθῆναι
δυνάμενον, οἷον δάκτυλος, ἢ πούς, ἢ ἄκρα χείρ, οὐκ
ἀνεχόμεθα βαστάζειν ἀργὸν αὐτό, καὶ περιφέρειν
οἷον ἄχθος ἀλλότριον, ἐναργῶς δηλοῦντες ἐν τούτῳ
ὅτι μὴ τῶν μορίων αὐτῶν, ἀλλὰ τῶν ἐνεργειῶν χρῄζομεν. ὥσπερ οὖν ὅλον τὸ μόριον τῆς ἐνεργείας ἕνεκα
ἔχειν δεόμεθα, κατὰ τὸν αὐτόν, οἶμαι, τρόπον καὶ
τῆς κατὰ φύσιν αὐτοῦ κατασκευῆς διὰ τὴν ἐνέργειαν
ὀρεγόμεθα. ὡς γὰρ καὶ πρόσθεν ἐλέγετο, λόγον αἰτίας
ἡ κατασκευὴ πρὸς τὴν ἐνέργειαν ἔχει· τὰ δὲ ἐξ ἀνάγκης ἑπόμενα ταῖς κατασκευαῖς ἀφ᾿ ὧν ἐνεργοῦμεν

108

Surely that which requires treatment is nothing other than the condition which damages function. Function to be in accord with nature is what we need first, and most of all. And it is on account of that we need the condition or, if you prefer, the constitution to be in accord with nature. For what we need is to see, hear, talk and walk, not eyes, ears, tongue and limbs. If, in fact, there was sight through another part, what need would there be for eyes? And if there was hearing through some other organ, what need would we have of ears? Likewise, I presume, there would be no benefit for us from tongue or limbs, if it were possible to talk and walk without them. We need vision for its own features; we do not need eyes for themselves but for vision. And we need a tongue, ears and limbs not so that we might have organs and many parts but for the sake of speech, hearing, and walking. At all events, whenever some part is made gangrenous and it can be amputated, like a finger, or a foot, or the extremity of an arm, we do not put up with bearing this uselessly and carrying it around like an unnatural burden. This shows clearly that it is not the parts we need but the functions. Therefore, just as we need to have the whole part for the sake of the function, in the same way, I think, we also desire the constitution itself to be in accord with nature because of the function. For as was also said before, the constitution has the ground of cause in relation to function. Those things that necessarily follow the constitutions from which we function are called

70K

---

51 *conj.* Hankinson; αὐτόν B; ἑαυτῶν P1, P2, K
52 αὐτούς B

ὑγιαινόντων μὲν ἡμῶν συμβεβηκότα, νοσούντων δὲ συμπτώματα καλεῖται.

καὶ τέτταρα ταῦτ᾽ ἐστὶ γένη πάντων τῶν περὶ τὸ σῶμα κατὰ φύσιν τε καὶ παρὰ φύσιν ἐχόντων ἡμῶν, ἐνέργειαι, κατασκευαί, τὰ προηγούμενα τούτων, τὰ ἑπόμενα· τιθέσθω λοιπὸν ὁ βουλόμενος ὀνόματα καθ᾽ ἕκαστον αὐτῶν ἰδίᾳ, κἂν εἰ Δίωνα, κἂν εἰ Θέωνα βούλοιτο καλεῖν ὁτιοῦν ἐξ αὐτῶν, οὔ μοι διαφέρει, μόνον ἴστω τοῦτο καὶ φυλαττέτω διαπαντός, ὡς τέτ-
71K ταρα τὰ | πάντ᾽ ἐστὶν ἀλλήλοις παρακείμενα πρά-γματα. ἐπεὶ δὲ κατὰ τοῦτο τοῦ λόγου γέγονα, δοκῶ μοι δικαίαν ἀξίωσιν ἐνεγκεῖν, ἵν᾽ ὡς ἡμεῖς ἐκείνοις συγ-χωροῦμεν ἄττα ἂν γ᾽ ἐθέλωσιν ὀνόματα τίθεσθαι, κατὰ τὸν αὐτὸν τρόπον κἀκείνους ἡμῖν συγχωρεῖν Ἑλληνικοῖς τε χρῆσθαι καὶ παλαιοῖς· ἢ δεινὸν ἂν εἴη σολοικίζειν μὲν ἐκείνοις ἐξεῖναι καθάπερ τυράννοις, Ἑλληνίζειν δ᾽ ἡμῖν οὐκ ἐξεῖναι. καλείτωσαν, εἰ βού-λοιντο, τὴν ὑγείαν εὐστάθειαν τῶν[53] ἐνεργειῶν, καίτοι δέδεικται πρὸς ἡμῶν ὡς ἡ διάθεσίς τε καὶ ἡ κατα-σκευὴ τῶν μορίων, ἀφ᾽ ἧς κατὰ φύσιν ἐνεργοῦμεν, ὑγεία πρὸς ἁπάντων Ἑλλήνων ὀνομάζεται· καὶ τοῦτο θέμενοι τὴν ὑγείαν, ὅμως τὴν νόσον οὐκ ἐνεργείας βλάβην, ἀλλὰ παρὰ φύσιν ἡγείσθωσαν εἶναι διάθε-σιν.

ὡς οὖν ἡμεῖς ἐκείνους μήθ᾽ Ἑλληνιστὶ μήτε δια-λεκτικῶς ὀνομάζοντας οὐ κωλύομεν, οὕτω κἀκεῖνοι συγχωρείτωσαν ἡμῖν Ἑλληνιστί τε ἅμα καὶ δια-λεκτικῶς οὐχ ἅπασαν τὴν παρὰ φύσιν διάθεσιν, ἀλλ᾽

"contingent attributes" when we are healthy and symptoms when we are diseased.

And so there are these four classes of all the things that exist in the body when we are in accord with nature (normal) and when we are contrary to nature (abnormal): functions, constitutions, the things which precede them, and the things which are consequent upon them. Let it be the case, further, that anyone who wishes to give names to each of these things separately, even if he should wish to call them Dion or Theon or something else of the sort—it makes no difference to me—let him know this alone and preserve it throughout, as all four things are closely related 71K to each other. Since I have reached this point in the argument, it seems to me a fair demand to make of them that just as I allow them to apply whatever names they might wish, in the same way they should allow me to use [the names] that are Greek and ancient. It would be a terrible thing if it were permissible for them to speak incorrectly like dictators, whereas it was not permitted to me to use correct Greek. Let them, if they wish, call health stability of the functions, despite my having shown that it is the condition or constitution of the parts from which we function in accord with nature that is called health by all Greeks. And if they do posit health to be this, nevertheless they should not posit injury of function to be disease, but should consider it to be a condition contrary to nature.

So then, as I do not prevent them from applying names that are neither Greek nor logical, let them in the same way allow me to apply the name "disease," according to Greek and logical use, not to every condition that is con-

---

53 B; αὐτῶν K

ἥτις ἂν ἐνέργειαν βλάπτῃ νόσημα προσαγορεύειν·
ἥτις δ' ἂν παρὰ φύσιν μὲν ᾖ, μὴ μέντοι βλάπτῃ γ'
ἐνέργειαν, οὐ νόσον, ἀλλὰ σύμπτωμα νοσήματος. |
72K αὖθις δ' ὥσπερ ἐκεῖνοι τὸ ἐπίμονον προστιθέασιν, οὐ
δηλοῦντες ἄχρι πόσων ὡρῶν ἡ παρὰ φύσιν αὕτη
διάθεσις παραμείνασα νόσος ἐστίν, οὕτως ἡμῖν συγχωρείτωσαν ἀφαιρεῖν τὸ ἐπίμονον· εἴτε γὰρ τρισὶν
ὥραις, εἴτε τέτρασιν, εἴτε καὶ ἡμίσει μόνον ὥρας ὅλῳ
τις τῷ σώματι καταληφθείη σφοδρῶς, ὡς μήτ' αἰσθάνεσθαι μήτε κινεῖσθαι, τοῦτον ἡμεῖς ἀπόπληκτον ὀνο-
μάζομεν· ὥσπερ εἰ καὶ σπασθείη σύμπαντι τῷ σώματι, καὶ τοῦτον ἐπίληπτον, οὔθ' ὡρῶν ἀριθμὸν οὔθ'
ἡμερῶν ἔτι προσλογιζόμενοι. μόνης γὰρ τῆς τοῦ πράγματος φύσεως, οὐ τῆς τοῦ χρόνου ποσότητος ὑπάρχει δηλωτικὰ τὰ τοιαῦτα τῶν ὀνομάτων, ὥσπερ οἶμαι
καὶ λευκὸν καὶ μέλαν καὶ θερμὸν καὶ ψυχρόν· ἢ
θαυμαστὸν ἂν εἴη τὸ ὕδωρ τὸ θερμὸν οὐκ εἶναι θερμόν, ἂν μὴ δι' ὅλης ἡμέρας ὑπάρχοι τοιοῦτον, ἢ τὸν ἐξ
ὥραις πυρέξαντα μὴ πεπυρεχέναι, χρῆναι γὰρ καὶ
τοῦτον, εἴπερ ἐπύρεξεν, ἐπίμονον ἔχειν τὸ πάθος·

καίτοι τίς ὁ χρόνος οὗτός ἐστιν· ὁ κρίνων τὸ ἐπίμονον καὶ τὸ μὴ τοιοῦτον οὐδεὶς αὐτῶν ὥρισεν, ἆρά γε
73K ἡμερῶν τις ἀριθμός, ἢ μηνῶν, ἢ ὡρῶν, | ἢ διὰ τί
λέγουσιν ἐπίμονον, ἐνὸν εἰπεῖν πολυχρόνιον, ἢ τοῦτο
μὲν καὶ μετατιθέντες ἔνιοι ἐξ αὐτῶν δύσλυτον ὀνομάζουσιν. ἀλλὰ τοῦτό γε τὸ δύσλυτον οὐ νοσήματος
ἁπλῶς, ἀλλὰ χρονίου νοσήματός ἐστιν ἴδιον, ὥσπερ
γε, οἶμαι, καὶ τὸ ῥᾳδίως λυόμενον ὀξέος. τὸ δ' οἴεσθαι

trary to nature, but only to whatever might harm function. Whatever might be contrary to nature and yet does not, in fact, harm function is not a disease but a symptom of disease. Again, just as those men add "persisting" but do not make clear how many hours this condition contrary to nature must last until it is a disease, so let them allow me to do away with the term "persisting." For if someone were to suffer a severe collapse of the whole body such that he had neither feeling nor movement, whether this lasts for three hours, or four, or only half an hour, we call it "apoplexy." Similarly, if someone were to suffer a convulsion in the whole body, we call this "epilepsy" without making an additional reckoning of the hours or days. For such terms are indicative of the nature of the matter alone and not of its duration, just as, I think, are white and black, or hot and cold. It would be surprising for hot water not to be hot if it was not hot through the whole day, or for someone who was febrile for six hours not to have a fever on the basis that the affection would need to be persisting for him to have a fever. 72K

And further, not one of them has defined what this time is that determines whether something is persisting or not —whether it is a number of days, months, or hours, or why they say "persisting" when it is possible to say "long-lasting," or also why some of them change this term and call it "difficult of resolution." But, in fact, this "difficult of resolution" is not simply characteristic of a disease but is specific of chronic disease, just as, I think, "easy of resolution" is of acute [disease]. Is it not the height of ignorance to 73K

διαφέρειν ἢ δύσλυτον, ἢ ἐπίμονον, ἢ χρόνιον εἰπεῖν,
ἆρ' οὐκ ἐσχάτης ἀμαθίας ἐστίν; ἔτι δὲ θαυμαστότερον, ὅταν οὗτοι μὲν ὥσπερ ἐξ ὕπνου βαθέος ἐγερ-
θέντες ἐπιχειρῶσι διορίζεσθαι πάθος συμπτώματος, ὁ
δὲ τῆς ἐμπληξίας αὐτῶν ἡγεμὼν ἐν τῷ δευτέρῳ περὶ
μεθόδου γράφει· Τὰ γὰρ αὐτὰ προηγησάμενα μὲν
πάθη λέγεται, ἐπιγενόμενα δὲ συμπτώματα· καίτοι
τοῦτό γε πολὺ θαυμαστότερον ὧν ἐκεῖνοι λέγουσι, τὴν
τοῦ ἥπατος φλεγμονήν, εἰ μὲν εὐθὺς εἰσβάλοι κατὰ
τὴν πρώτην ἡμέραν, πάθος εἶναι συγχωρεῖν, εἰ δ' ἐφ'
ἑτέρῳ τινὶ γένοιτο, κατὰ τὴν δευτέραν ἢ τρίτην, εἰς τὰ
συμπτώματα μετατιθέναι. καίτοι τί λέγω δευτέραν
ἡμέραν; ἄμεινον γὰρ εἰπεῖν ὥραν δευτέραν ἀπὸ τῆς
εἰσβολῆς τοῦ νοσήματος. οὐ γὰρ δή που κατὰ μὲν τὴν
74K δευτέραν ἡμέραν ἡ τοῦ ἥπατος φλεγμονὴ | σύμπτωμα
γενήσεται, κατὰ δὲ τὴν δευτέραν ὥραν ἀπὸ τῆς ἀρχῆς
ἄλλο τι καὶ οὐ σύμπτωμα· τὸ γὰρ ἐπιγίγνεσθαί τινι
προηγουμένῳ πάντως που καὶ τοῦθ' ἕξει. ἀλλὰ τὸ
οὕτω, φασί, ταχέως ἐπιγιγνόμενον οὐδὲν διαφέρει τοῦ
συνεισβάλλοντος.

πάλιν οὖν αὐτὸν ἐχρῆν εἰρηκέναι σαφῶς ὁπόσαις
ὥραις ὁρίζεται καὶ διακρίνει τοῦ συνεισβάλλοντος τὸ
ἐπιγιγνόμενον. ὁ Θεσσαλὸς μὲν δὴ τοιοῦτος. οἱ δὲ
περὶ τὸν Ὀλυμπικόν, ὡς ἂν εἰς ἄκρον ἥκοντες σοφίας,
οὐχ οὕτω διορίζουσι πάθος συμπτώματος, ἀλλὰ τὸ
μὲν πάθος ὡς προείρηται, τὸ σύμπτωμα δὲ τὸ τῷ

---

34 Presumably Thessalus is being referred to here. He is cred-

think it makes a difference to say "persisting," "difficult of resolution," or "chronic"? It is still more remarkable whenever these people, as if stirred from a deep sleep, attempt to differentiate affection from symptom, which is what the leader of their stupidity writes in the second [book] of his *On Method*:[34] "For when these same things come first they are called affections, but when they occur afterward they are called symptoms." And indeed, this is far more remarkable than those people who say that inflammation of the liver, if it comes on immediately on the first day, is accepted as being an affection whereas, if it occurs at another time, the second or third day, it is placed among the symptoms. And indeed, why do I say second day? For it would be better to say the second hour from the onset of the disease. For surely it cannot be that inflammation of the liver during the second day will become a symptom whereas, during the second hour from the onset, it was something else and not a symptom. It will be a symptom simply by supervening on what preceded it in some way. But what is like this, they say, when it supervenes quickly, does not differ from what appears together with it.

74K

Again, therefore, it behooves him to say clearly by how many hours he defines it, and how he distinguishes the epiphenomenon from what appears together with it. Thessalus, at least, does such a thing. On the other hand, those who follow Olympicus, as if they had reached the pinnacle of wisdom, do not distinguish affection from symptom in this way but say the affection is as previously stated, whereas the symptom is what occurs along with an affec-

ited with a work *On Method*. See *EANS*, p. 805 for a list of works ascribed to him.

πάθει συμβαῖνον ὑπάρχειν φασί, θαυμαστῶς πάνυ
καὶ σαφῶς ἐξηγησάμενοι τὴν οὐσίαν αὐτοῦ. τί γὰρ δὴ
καὶ ὂν τὸ σύμπτωμα, ὃ τῷ πάθει συμβέβηκεν, ἐχρῆν,
οἶμαι, προσθεῖναί τε καὶ διορίσασθαι, ἆρά γε διάθεσίς τίς ἐστι σώματος, ἢ βλάβη τινὸς ἐνεργείας, ἢ
συναμφότερον. ἐκεῖνοι μὲν οὖν οὐ λέγουσιν, ἡμᾶς δὲ
δηλονότι μαντεύσασθαι χρή.

   τὸ δὲ καὶ προσθεῖναι τῷ λόγῳ τοῦτ᾽ αὐτόν, εἰδικήν,
ὥσπερ καὶ μερικωτέραν ἔχον ἐν τοῖς παρὰ φύσιν
ἐντυπώσιν, ὑπερβολὴν οὐκ ἀπολέλοιπε σαφηνείας,
75K ἅμα τῷ | καὶ τοῖς ὀνόμασιν Ἑλληνιστὶ καὶ παγκάλως
ἑρμηνεύεσθαι, εἰδικώτερόν τινα τύπον ἐν τοῖς παρὰ
φύσιν ἔχειν τὸ σύμπτωμα. τί ποτ᾽ οὖν ἐστι τὸ γενι-
κώτερον ἔχον τὸν τύπον; οὐ γὰρ εἴρηκας εἰ χωρὶς τῆς
πρὸς ἐκεῖνο παραβολῆς ἐγχωρεῖ τὸ εἰδικώτερον ἐξευρεῖν. εἰ δ᾽ ὅλως πρὸς οὐδὲν παραβάλλοντες εἰδικώτερον ὀνομάζουσιν, ἀκριβῶς τε πάνυ καὶ σαφῶς ἑρμη-
νεύουσι, καίτοι διὰ συντόμων τε ἅμα καὶ σαφῶν οἷόν
τ᾽ ἦν εἰπεῖν ὡς τὰ παρὰ φύσιν ἅπαντα τὰ κατὰ τὸ
σῶμα τῶν ζῴων ἤτοι νοσήματ᾽ ἐστίν, ἢ αἴτια, ἢ
συμπτώματα· κοινοῦ δ᾽ αὐτοῖς ὄντος τοῦ παρὰ φύσιν,
ἡ νόσος μὲν ἐνέργειαν βλάπτει, τὸ δ᾽ αἴτιον ταύτης
προηγεῖται, τὸ σύμπτωμα δ᾽ ἕπεται ταύτῃ, διττὸν ὂν
τὴν φύσιν, ἐνεργείας μὲν βλάβη τὸ ἕτερον, διάθεσις
δέ τις ἀκολουθοῦσα τῷ νοσήματι τὸ λοιπόν. ἀλλὰ
γάρ, ὥσπερ ἔφην, εἰ πάντα τις ἐπέρχοιτο τὰ σφάλ-
ματ᾽ αὐτῶν, οὐκ ἂν ἐπιθείη τέλος τῷ λόγῳ, καὶ γινώσκεις τοῦτο ἀκριβῶς καὶ σύ, φίλτατε Ἱέρων, ὅτι μηδὲ
τὸ χιλιοστὸν αὐτῶν μέρος ἐξελέγχειν ἐπεχείρησα.

tion, thus explicating its substance quite wonderfully and clearly. But, in my view, they ought to have added and defined what kind of thing a symptom is which appears together with an affection; whether it is some condition of the body, or damage of some function, or both together. As those men do not say, quite clearly we must resort to divination.

And to add "specific" to the definition, as it also gives the impression of those things contrary to nature being more subdivisible, does not forsake extreme clarity. At the same time, interpreting with names that are Greek, if it is 75K altogether done properly, means that symptom has a certain more specific form of expression among those things contrary to nature. What is it that has the more generic type? For you have not said whether it is possible to discover what is more specific apart from comparison with that (i.e., the generic). If they use the more specific term without comparing it to anything, they interpret it very precisely and clearly. Nevertheless, it was possible to state succinctly and, at the same time, clearly that all things contrary to nature in the bodies of animals are either diseases, causes, or symptoms. What is common to them is being contrary to nature. The disease damages function, the cause precedes the disease, and the symptom follows it, its nature being twofold—the one being damage of function, and the other being some condition which follows the disease. But, as I said, if someone were to go through all their errors, they would never put an end to the discussion. And you will realize this precisely, my dearest Hiero, in that I have not attempted to refute a thousandth part of them.

τοσοῦτον οὖν ἔτι προσθεὶς ἐνταυθοῖ που κατα-
76K παύσω τὸ πρῶτον γράμμα, διότι κατὰ τὴν | ἀρχὴν τῆς
μεθόδου σφάλλονται πολλοὶ τῶν ἰατρῶν, οἱ μὲν ἀπὸ
Θεσσαλοῦ καὶ Θεμίσωνος, οἵπερ δὴ καὶ Μεθοδικοὺς
ἑαυτοὺς ὀνομάζουσιν, ἔσχατά τε καὶ μέγιστα σφάλ-
ματα, σὺν αὐτοῖς δ' οὐκ ὀλίγοι τῶν Ἀναλογιστικῶν τε
καὶ Δογματικῶν καὶ Λογικῶν ὀνομαζομένων. εἰ μὴ
γὰρ ἐξεύροι τις ἁπάσας τὰς διαθέσεις ὑφ' ὧν ἐνέργεια
βλάπτεται, τὸ πλῆθος αὐτῶν τῶν νοσημάτων ὁπόσον
τ' ἐστὶ καὶ ὁποῖον ἀδύνατον ἀκριβῶς ὁρισθῆναι· τοῦτο
δ' οὐδ' ἐπιχειρήσαντες ἔνιοι ποιῆσαι τυράννων δίκην
ἀποφαίνονται τὰ δόξαντά σφισι χωρὶς ἀποδείξεως.
ἔνιοι δ' οὐ μόνον οὐκ ἀπέδειξαν, ἀλλ' οὐδὲ παρὰ τῶν
ἀποδεικνύντων μανθάνουσι· καὶ τό γε πλεῖστον γένος,
ὡς οἶσθα, τῶν νῦν ἐπιπολαζόντων ἰατρῶν, ἔστι τοι-
οῦτον· καὶ θαυμαστὸν ἴσως οὐδέν· ὅπου γὰρ καὶ
τῶν φιλοσόφων οἱ πολλοὶ χωρὶς ἀποδείξεως ἀξιοῦσι
πιστεύεσθαι, τί χρὴ θαυμάζειν τινὰ τῶν ἰατρῶν; οὐδὲ
γὰρ σχολή γε αὐτοῖς ἔστιν ἀλήθειαν ζητεῖν, ἕωθεν
μὲν ἐν ἀσπασμοῖς διατρίβουσιν, οὓς αὐτοὶ καλοῦσιν
ἀσπασμούς, εἰς ἑσπέραν δ' ἐμπιπλαμένοις τε καὶ
μεθυσκομένοις.

77K   ἀλλὰ κατὰ τὸν παλαιὸν | αὐλητήν, ὦ Ἱέρων, ἁμιλ-
λαίμην ἂν καὶ ταῖς Μούσαις· αἰσχρὸν γὰρ αὐλητὴν
μὲν οὕτως εὑρεθῆναι φιλόκαλον, οὐ μέγα τὸ πρᾶγμα
κατορθοῦντα, μέθοδον δὲ θεραπευτικὴν ἐκ παλαιοῦ
μὲν ζητουμένην, ἀκριβῶς δ' οὔπω γεγραμμένην, ἐξευρεῖν τε καὶ τελειῶσαι δυναμένους ἡμᾶς ὀκνεῖν καὶ

If, then, I add just this much, I shall put an end to the first book here, because many doctors get frustrated by the method at the start. On the one hand, there are those who follow Thessalus and Themison, who actually call themselves Methodics, and who make the most extreme and significant errors and, along with them, not a small number of those who call themselves Analogists, Dogmatics, or Rationalists. Unless someone were to discover all the conditions by which function is damaged, the great number of actual diseases, how many there are, and of what sort, could not be determined precisely. Since some don't even attempt to do this, like dictators they declare their opinions without demonstration. Some, on the other hand, not only do not provide a demonstration but do not even learn from those who do provide demonstrations. And, as you know, the largest class of doctors who are fashionable now is of this kind. Perhaps this is no surprise. Where the majority of philosophers also think themselves worthy of credence without demonstration, why should you be surprised if some doctors [do so too]? There is not, in fact, the free time for them to seek truth when, in the early morning, they busy themselves with greetings, which they call "salutations," while in the evening they eat to excess and get drunk.

76K

But like the ancient flute player, Hiero, I too would contend with the Muses. For it would be shameful for a flute player to be found so enthusiastic in this way when he successfully accomplishes nothing of significance, while I, who am able to discover and complete the method of medicine, which has been sought from ancient times but not yet written about accurately, hesitate, delay and defer [do-

77K

μέλλειν καὶ ἀναβάλλεσθαι διὰ τὴν ἐπιπολάζουσαν ἐν
τῷ νῦν χρόνῳ ῥᾳθυμίαν. ὥστ᾽ ἔμπαλιν ἤδη μοι δοκῶ
διακεῖσθαι νῦν ἢ πρόσθεν· οὐδὲ γὰρ ὑμῖν χάριν οἰκείαν δίδωμι, προτρεψαμένοις με τὴν θεραπευτικὴν
μέθοδον ἅπασαν ἐφεξῆς διελθεῖν. ὁ μὲν δὴ πρῶτός μοι
λόγος ἐνταυθοῖ τελευτάτω, τοῦ δ᾽ ἑξῆς παντὸς ὁ δεύτερος ἀρχέσθω τοῦτον τὸν τρόπον.

ing this] due to the prevailing idleness of the present time. As a consequence, I now seem to be in the opposite position to before. I am not giving you the proper reward—you who entreated me to go over the whole therapeutic method step by step. So let me bring the first book to completion here and begin the second in sequence of the whole [work] in the following way.

ΒΙΒΛΙΟΝ Β

1. Τῶν συμβαινόντων τοῖς σώμασιν ἐν τῷ παρὰ φύσιν ἔχειν, Ἱέρων κράτιστε, τέτταρες ἐδείχθησαν αἱ πᾶσαι διαφοραί, μία μὲν αὐτῆς τῆς βεβλαμμένης ἐνεργείας, ἑτέρα δὲ τῆς ἐργαζομένης αὐτὴν διαθέσεως, ἄλλη τε τρίτη τῶν ταύτης αἰτιῶν, καὶ τετάρτη τῶν ἐξ ἀνάγκης ἑπομένων αὐτῇ συμπτωμάτων. ὅτι μὲν οὖν ἤτοι πάντα ταῦτ' εἶναι χρὴ τὴν νόσον, ἢ τινα τούτων, ἢ πάντως γ' ἓν ἐξ αὐτῶν, ἕτοιμον συλλογίσασθαι· μηδενὸς γὰρ παρὰ τὰ προειρημένα τοῖς νοσοῦσιν ὑπάρχοντος, οὐδὲ
ἔξω τούτων ἔσται τὸ νόσημα. λείπεται | τοίνυν ἢ τὸ πάντων ἄθροισμα λέγειν τὴν νόσον εἶναι, ἢ τινα τούτων, ἢ ἕν γέ τι πάντως. ἀλλὰ τὸ μὲν ἐξ ἁπάντων ἄθροισμα πρὸς τῷ μηδ' εἰρῆσθαι πρός τινος οὐδ' ἐγχωρεῖ λεχθῆναι· τί γὰρ ἔσται νόσου αἴτιον, ἢ τί σύμπτωμα νοσήματος, εἰ τὸ πάντων ἄθροισμα νόσημα νομισθήσεται; οὐδὲν[1] δήπουθεν. ἀναγκαῖον οὖν ἀπολιπεῖν δύο ἄλλα γένη παρὰ τὰς νόσους, ἕτερον μὲν τῶν ἐργαζομένων αὐτὰς αἰτιῶν, ἕτερον δὲ τῶν ἑπομένων μὲν ἐξ ἀνάγκης, λυπούντων δ' οὐδὲν τὸν ἄνθρωπον, ἀλλ' εἰ ταῦτ' ἀφέλοιμεν, ἐν δυοῖν ἐστι τούτοιν ἡ νόσος, ἢ ταῖς βεβλαμμέναις ἐνεργείαις, ἢ ταῖς ἐργαζομέναις αὐτὰς διαθέσεσι. καὶ δὴ καὶ δι-

BOOK II

1. Most excellent Hiero, all the four differentiae of things
contrary to nature which befall bodies were shown to be
the following: One is the actual function that has been
damaged, another is the condition that brings this damage
about, another and third, consists of the causes of this condition, and the fourth comprises the symptoms which necessarily follow it. That all of these, or some of them, or at
least one of them, must then be the disease is readily de-
duced for, as nothing exists in those who are diseased apart
from the aforementioned things, disease will not fall outside them. It remains, then, to say whether disease is the
aggregate of all them, or some of them, or is one of them at
least. But not only has nobody ever claimed that disease is
the aggregate of all these [differentiae]; it is not even possible to make this claim. For what will be a cause of disease,
or a symptom of disease, if the aggregate of all of these is
thought to be the disease? Nothing, clearly! Therefore, it is
necessary to set aside two other classes apart from the diseases, one comprising the causes that bring them about,
and the other the things that follow of necessity but do not
distress the person at all. But if we do set these [two
classes] aside, disease must lie in the remaining two; that
is, the damaged functions or the conditions that bring

---

1 οὐδέν B, P1, P2; οὐδὲ ἕν K

ἠνέχθησαν εὐθὺς ἐκ παλαιοῦ καὶ περὶ τοῦδε καὶ νῦν
ἔτι διαφέρονται πάντες οὐκ ἰατροὶ μόνον, ἀλλὰ καὶ
φιλόσοφοι, τῶν ἐνεργειῶν μὲν τὰς βλάβας ἕτεροι, τῶν
δ᾽ ἐργαζομένων αὐτὰς διαθέσεων ἕτεροι προσαγο-
ρεύσαντες νοσήματα.

τὸ μὲν οὖν διαφέρεσθαι τοὺς ἄνδρας ἐν οὕτως
ἀσαφέσι πράγμασιν οὐδὲν θαυμαστόν· τὸ δὲ μὴ δια-
γιγνώσκειν ὡς ὑπὲρ ὀνόματος ἐρίζουσιν ἐπιτιμήσεως
80K ἄξιον. εἴπερ γὰρ ὡμολόγηται πρὸς ἁπάντων Ι ἡ θεραπεία τῆς ἐμποδιζούσης τὴν ἐνέργειαν εἶναι διαθέσεως,
οὐδὲν ἔτι χρήσιμον εἰς τὰ τῆς τέχνης ἔργα τὸ διελέσθαι πότερα τὴν διάθεσιν, ἢ τὴν βεβλαμμένην
ἐνέργειαν ὀνομαστέον ἐστὶ νόσημα. ἑκατέρως γὰρ
ὀνομαζόντων, ὁ κάμνων ὑγιαίνων ἀποδειχθήσεται
μόνον εἰ τὰ δέοντά τις ἰάματα προσφέροι ταῖς δια-
θέσεσιν· αὗται γάρ εἰσιν ἃς ἀλλοιοῦν χρὴ καὶ μετα-
βάλλειν καὶ τελέως ἐκκόπτειν, οὐχ αἱ βλάβαι τῶν
ἐνεργειῶν. οὐδεὶς γοῦν ἰᾶται τὸ χωλεύειν βαδίζοντα,
καὶ γὰρ γελοῖον, ἀλλὰ τὴν ἐργαζομένην αὐτὸ διάθεσιν, οἷον τὴν φλεγμονήν, εἰ διὰ ταύτην χωλεύει· καὶ
ταύτην καὶ καταντλεῖ καὶ καταπλάττει καὶ σχάζει καὶ
διαφορεῖ καὶ παντὶ τρόπῳ λύειν ἐπιχειρεῖ·

τὸ γὰρ ὀρθῶς βαδίζειν ἕπεται ταύτῃ λυθείσῃ, καὶ
οὐδὲν ἔτι δεόμεθα τὴν χωλείαν ἐπανορθοῦσθαι τῆς
φλεγμονῆς οἰχομένης· οὐδὲ γὰρ ὑπομένει τι τῆς βεβλαμμένης ἐνεργείας, ἐὰν ἐκκόψῃ τις ἀκριβῶς τὴν
ἐργαζομένην αὐτὴν διάθεσιν, ἔστ᾽ ἂν δ᾽ ὑπολείπηταί
τι τῆς διαθέσεως, ἀνάγκη καὶ τὴν ἐνέργειαν ἀνάλογον

124

them about. However, right from ancient times there has been dispute about precisely this, and even now everyone, not only doctors but also philosophers, enters the dispute, some identifying diseases with damage of function and others with the condition bringing the damage about.

Little wonder, then, that people disagree on such uncertain matters. What does, however, warrant criticism is the failure to recognize that they are wrangling about names. For if it is agreed by all that treatment is directed at 80K the condition hindering function, it is of no use to the practice of the craft to distinguish whether you must name the condition or the damaged function the disease. Whichever definition is used, patients will be made healthy only if someone applies the required cures for the conditions insofar as it is these conditions which you must change, transform and eradicate completely, and not the damages of functions. At all events, nobody cures the lameness in walking—the very idea is ridiculous. But [you cure] the condition that brings this about; for example, the inflammation, if someone is lame because of this. It is this that you bathe, poultice, incise and disperse, and try to resolve in every way.

Walking properly depends on this being resolved. We have no further need to correct the lameness once the inflammation has gone. Nothing remains of the damaged function if you comprehensively eradicate the condition bringing it about. If, however, something of the condition still remains, the function, too, is necessarily damaged in

ἐκείνη βεβλάφθαι. ταύτην οὖν τὴν διάθεσιν εἴτε νόση-
μα καλεῖν, εἴτε πάθος, εἴτ᾽ αἰτίαν νοσήματος, εἴτε |
81K πάθους ἐθέλοι τις, οὐδὲν εἰς τὴν θεραπείαν οὔτ᾽ ὄφελος
οὔτε βλάβος ἐντεῦθεν· ἀλλ᾽ οὐδ᾽ εἰ Θεωνά τις ἢ Δίωνα
προσαγορεύσας αὐτήν, ἔπειτ᾽ ὀρθῶς ἰῷτο, βλάψειεν
ἂν οὐδ᾽ οὗτος οὐδὲν τὸν νοσοῦντα· κἂν εἰ τελέως δέ
τις ἀνώνυμον ἀπολιπὼν αὐτὴν ἃ χρὴ προσφέροι τῷ
κάμνοντι βοηθήματα, πρὸς τῷ μὴ βλάπτειν μηδέν,
οὗτος ἔτι κάλλιστα θεραπεύσει. διδάσκειν μέν τοι
βουλόμενος ἕτερον ἃ γινώσκει, δεήσεταί τε πάντως
ὀνομάτων ἐπὶ τοῖς πράγμασιν, ὅρον τε τῆς χρήσεως
αὐτῶν ἕξει τὴν σαφήνειαν· ὁ γὰρ ὡς ἂν ὁ μανθάνων
ἐκμάθοι σαφέστατα μάλιστα σπουδάζων ὀνομάζειν,
ἄριστος διδάσκαλος. ἐπεὶ τοίνυν καὶ ἡμεῖς ἐν τούτῳ
νῦν καθεστήκαμεν, ἀνάγκη μέν που θέσθαι τοῖς πράγμασιν ὀνόματα· τὸ δ᾽ εἰ καὶ σαφῶς, ἡμῖν σκοπεῖσθαι
πάρεστιν. ἡ μὲν δὴ τὴν ἐνέργειαν ἐμποδίζουσα διάθεσις ὀνομαζέσθω νόσος· εἴ τι δ᾽ ἕπεται τῇδε, σύμ-
πτωμα· τὸ δ᾽ ἐργαζόμενον αὐτήν, αἴτιον.

2. Οὕτω δὲ τούτων διωρισμένων ἐπιβλέπειν ἀκριβῶς χρὴ τὴν ἀνωμαλίαν τῶν ὀνομάτων, ἃ κατὰ τῶν
82K νοσημάτων | ἐπήνεγκαν οἱ πρῶτοι θέμενοι· πολλαχόθι
μὲν γὰρ ἀπὸ τοῦ βεβλαμμένου μορίου τὰ ὀνόματα,
πλευρῖτις καὶ περιπνευμονία καὶ ἰσχίας καὶ ποδάγρα
καὶ νεφρῖτις καὶ ἀρθρῖτις, ὀφθαλμία τε καὶ κεφαλαλγία καὶ δυσεντερία· πολλαχόθι δ᾽ ἀπὸ τοῦ συμπτώματος, εἰλεὸς καὶ τεινεσμὸς καὶ σπασμὸς καὶ
παλμὸς καὶ τρόμος καὶ παράλυσις, ἀπεψία τε καὶ

proportion to that. Therefore, whether you wish to call this condition a disease, or affection, or cause of a disease, or cause of an affection, there is neither benefit nor harm for the treatment as a result. Indeed, even if someone were to call it Theon or Dion, as long as he treats it correctly he would do no harm to the diseased person. And if someone leaves it completely nameless, but applies the remedies that are necessary to the patient, in addition to doing no harm, he will still be treating it in the best possible way. But surely, if someone wishes to teach another the things he knows, he will require names for the matters, and will have clarity as his criterion in the use of these. The best teacher is the man who zealously pursues this issue of nomenclature so that the student may learn with the utmost clarity. Accordingly, since I, too, am now engaged in this [teaching], it is presumably necessary to apply names to the matters. To do this clearly is my present objective. So let disease be called the condition hindering function while, if something follows this, let it be called a symptom, and what brings it about, a cause.

2. So, having established these definitions, it is necessary to look closely and precisely at the inconsistency of the names which those who first applied them assigned to diseases. Very often, they derived the names from the damaged part (pleuritis, peripneumonia, sciatica, gout, nephritis, arthritis, ophthalmia, headache, and dysentery), very often from the symptom (ileus, tenesmus, spasm, palpitation, tremor, paralysis, apepsia, dyspnea, apnea, insomnia,

81K

82K

δύσπνοια καὶ ἄπνοια καὶ ἀγρυπνία καὶ παραφροσύνη
καὶ κῶμα· πολλαχόθι δ᾽ ἀπ᾽ ἀμφοῖν ἅμα, ὡς κεφαλαλγία καὶ ὠταλγία καὶ καρδιαλγία καὶ ὀδονταλγία
καὶ ὑστεραλγία· πολλαχόθι δ᾽ ἀπὸ τῆς δοξαζομένης
αἰτίας, ὡς ἡ μελαγχολία μὲν ὑπὸ πάντων, αἱ χολέραι
δὲ ὑπὸ τῶν Κνιδίων ἰατρῶν, ἴσως δὲ καὶ ὁ λευκο-
φλεγματίας ὕδερος ἐντεῦθεν· ἐνίοτε δὲ ἀπὸ τῆς πρός τι
τῶν ἐκτὸς ὁμοιότητος, ἐλέφας καὶ καρκίνος καὶ πολύπους καὶ σταφυλὴ καὶ λεύκη καὶ μυρμηκία καὶ ἀθέρωμα καὶ στεάτωμα καὶ σταφύλωμα καὶ μελικηρὶς καὶ
ἄνθραξ, ἀλωπεκία τε καὶ ὀφίασις καὶ σύκωσις καὶ
σατυριασμὸς καὶ πριαπισμός·

τῶν νοσημάτων δ᾽ αὐτῶν ὀνόματα μήτε τόπου ἐφα-
πτόμενα πεπονθότος μήτε τῆς ποιούσης αἰτίας ὀλίγα,
φλεγμονὴ καὶ γάγγραινα καὶ σκίρρος, ἐρυσίπελάς τε
83K καὶ | ἀπόστημα καὶ οἴδημα καὶ ἐμπύημα καὶ ἕλκος
ἐξάρθρημά τε καὶ κάταγμα καὶ σπάσμα καὶ ῥῆγμα
καὶ κολόβωμα καὶ δοθιὴν καὶ ἴονθος καὶ φῦμα· καίτοι
καὶ τούτων αὐτῶν ἔνια τὰ μὲν καὶ τὸν τόπον τοῦ
σώματος, ἤτοι τὸ πεπονθὸς μέρος ἐμφαίνειν ἔοικεν,
ἔνια δὲ ἀπὸ τοῦ πλεονεκτοῦντος ὀνομάζεσθαι[2] συμ-
πτώματος· εἰ δ᾽ ἄρα τι καὶ χωρὶς παρεμφάσεως ὀνομάζεται, τάς γ᾽ ἐν αὐτῷ διαφορὰς καὶ τοῦτο πολυειδεῖς
ἔσχηκεν, οἷον ἕλκος, εἰ καὶ μὴ συνεχείας ἦν ἡ λύσις
ἐν σαρκώδει μορίῳ, καὶ ταύτῃ παραδηλοῦν ἐδόκει τὸν

[2] Β; ὀνομάζεται Κ

delirium and coma), very often from both simultaneously (cephalalgia, otalgia, cardialgia, odontalgia and hysteralgia) and very often from what was thought to be the cause, such as what was called melancholia generally but cholerae by the Cnidan doctors and perhaps leucophlegmatic dropsy as well.[1] Sometimes they were named from their similarity to external things in some respect, like elephas, cancer, polyp, staphyle, leuke, warts, atheroma, steatoma, staphyloma, meliceris, anthrax, alopecia, ophiasis, sicus, satyriasis, and priapism.

Names of the diseases themselves which have no connection to the affected place or to the effecting cause are few: phlegmone (inflammation), gangrene, scirrhus (induration), erysipelas, apostema (abscess), edema, empyema, wounds and ulcers, dislocation, fracture, spasm, rupture, coloboma, boil, eruption, and phuma. And indeed, some of these very terms do seem to indicate the place in the body or the affected part, while others seem to be named from the predominant symptom. And if something is named apart from signification, it has differentiae in it and these are diverse. For example, in the case of *helkos*,[2] even if there is no dissolution of continuity in a fleshy part (and

83K

---

[1] This reads as if this is one disease given three different names according to ideas on its causation. If so, it is not clear what the disease is.

[2] *Helkos* is a particularly problematic term as far as translation is concerned. For Galen, it is essentially dissolution of continuity involving a surface, whether external or internal. Sometimes it is best rendered as "wound," sometimes as "infected wound," sometimes as "ulcer," and sometimes as "sore." It is often used to cover all four possibilities. In what follows, one of the four possibilities is used if it is clearly indicated. When *helkos* is used in a more general sense (as above), it is translated as "wound or ulcer."

πεπονθότα τόπον, ἀλλ' αἵ γε κατὰ μέρος αὐτοῦ διαφοραὶ ποικίλαι τοῖς ὀνόμασι, χειρώνειον καὶ τηλέφιον
καὶ καρκίνος, ἕρπης τε καὶ φαγέδαινα, καὶ πάνθ' ὅσα
τοιαῦτα, τὰ μὲν ἀπὸ τῶν πρώτως ἰασαμένων, ὡς τὸ
χειρώνειον· ἔνια δ' ἀπὸ τῶν πεπονθότων, ὡς τὸ τηλέ-
φιον· ἀπὸ δὲ τῆς πρὸς τὸ ζῷον ὁμοιότητος ὁ καρκίνος·
ἢ φαγέδαινα δ' ἀπὸ τοῦ συμπτώματος, ὥσπέρ γε καὶ
οἱ ἕρπητες. ἀλλ' ἡ μὲν φαγέδαινα πάντως ἐστὶν ἕλκος
ἐσθιόμενον, ἢ ἀναβιβρῶσκον, ἢ ὅπως ἂν ἐθέλῃ τις
ὀνομάζειν· ὁ δ' ἕρπης οὔθ' ἕλκος ἀεί, καὶ ὁπότε μεθ'
84K   ἑλκώσεως, οὐ κατέχων | τὴν ἀρχαίαν ἕδραν, ἐπινέμε-
ται τὰ πλησίον, ἀλλ' ὥσπερ τοὔνομα δηλοῖ, δίκην
ἕρποντος θηρίου, καταλείπει μὲν τὰ πρότερα, μετέρχε-
ται δ' ἐφ' ἕτερα. κοῖλον δ' ἕλκος καὶ ῥυπαρὸν καὶ
καθαρόν, ὁμαλές τε καὶ ὑπερσαρκοῦν, οἰκειοτέρας μὲν
ἔσχηκε τὰς προσηγορίας, οὐ μὴν ὡσαύτως γε πάσας,
ἀλλὰ τὸ μὲν ὁμαλὲς ἀπὸ τῆς οἰκείας διαφορᾶς, ὡσαύτως δὲ καὶ τὸ κοῖλον ἢ ὑπερσαρκοῦν· ἔναιμον δὲ καὶ
καθαρὸν καὶ ῥυπαρὸν οὐ κατὰ τὰς οἰκείας διαφοράς,
ἀλλ' ἀπὸ τῶν ἔξωθεν ὀνομάζεται συμπτωμάτων.

οὕτως οὖν ἀνωμάλου τῶν ὀνομάτων τῆς θέσεως
τοῖς ἀρχαίοις γεγενημένης, καὶ πολὺ μᾶλλον, ὅταν
ἐπινυκτίδα καὶ ἀκροχορδόνα καὶ νυκτάλωπα προσ-
αγορεύσωσι, τὸ μὲν ὅτι νύκτωρ ἐγένετο, τὸ δ' ὅτι κατ'

---

3 Chiron, one of the three centaurs, was traditionally regarded
as the teacher of Asclepius. Telephus was the son of Hercules and
Auge. He was wounded while fleeing from Achilles when his foot
was caught in vine placed by Dionysus. He was healed by Achilles'
spear. The animal referred to is, of course, the crab.

by this it seems to suggest the affected place), its individual differentiae are varied in names—chironium, teleph-
ium, cancer, herpes, phagedaena, and all other such terms.
Some [are named] from those who first cured them, like
chironium, some from those who were affected, like te-
lephium, while cancer gets its name from the similarity to
the animal.[3] Phagedaena, however, [takes its name] from
the symptom, just as herpetic [ulcers] also do. But phagedaena is, in general, an ulcer that eats away or erodes, or
whatever someone might wish to term it. Herpes is not always an ulceration, although whenever it is accompanied
by ulceration, it does not occupy its original position, but   84K
feeds on the neighboring area like a crawling beast, as the
name makes clear, leaving its former position to spread to
other [places]. Hollow wounds or ulcers that are putrid
and clean, level and raised, have more fitting names, although not all in the same way. The level [wound or ulcer]
is named from the specific differentia, as are those that are
hollow and those with an excess of flesh (i.e. are raised).
The hemorrhagic, clean, and putrid wounds or ulcers are
not named in relation to the specific differentiae, but from
the external symptoms.

In such a way, then, did anomalies arise in the application of names by the ancients, and much more so when
they designated something epinoctis, thin-necked wart or
nyctalopia;[4] the first because it occurs at night, the second

4 There are some questions about these terms. We have taken
ἐπινυκτίδα to be what is now termed eponychia, given that it is
very painful at night. ἀκροχορδόνα is listed in a modern medical
dictionary as an old term for a skin tag while νυκτάλωπα
(nyctalopia) remains in use as a term for "decreased ability to see
in reduced light" (S).

ἄκρας ὀχεῖται τῆς ἐπιφανείας τοῦ δέρματος, τὸ δ᾽ ὅτι
τῆς νυκτὸς ἀποφαίνει μὴ βλέποντας, ἕτερά τε πολλὰ
τοιαῦτα ποιῶσιν, εἰ γὰρ ἐπεξίοιμι πάντα, κινδυνεύσω
ἴσως³ σπουδάζειν δοκεῖν τὸ πάρεργον⁴ ὃ φεύγειν
ἐκέλευσα, πειρᾶσθαι οὖν χρὴ παντὶ τρόπῳ τὸν τῆς
ἀληθείας αὐτῆς ὀρεγόμενον ἀποχωρεῖν μὲν τοῦ προσ-
δοξαζομένου τοῖς ὀνόμασιν, ἐπὶ δὲ τὴν οὐσίαν τῶν
πραγμάτων αὐτὴν ἰέναι καὶ ταύτην ἐπισκέπτεσθαι καὶ
85K   ζητεῖν, ὁπόσα τὰ σύμπαντ᾽ ἐστὶ | νοσήματά τε καὶ
συμπτώματα, καὶ προσέτι τὰ προηγούμενα τούτων
αἴτια.

τοῦτ᾽ οὖν ἡμεῖς ἐποιήσαμεν ἐν ἑτέροις ὑπομνήμασιν, ὧν ἐστι περὶ μὲν τοῦ πλήθους τῶν νοσημάτων
ἕν, ἐπιγέγραπται δὲ Περὶ τῆς τῶν νοσημάτων διαφορᾶς, ἕτερον δὲ Περὶ τῆς τῶν συμπτωμάτων ἐστὶ
διαφορᾶς· οὕτω δὲ καὶ τὰς αἰτίας αὐτῶν ἐπειράθημεν
ἐξευρεῖν ἑκατέρας ἰδίᾳ, τάς τε τῶν νοσημάτων καὶ τὰς
τῶν συμπτωμάτων ἁπάντων, ὡς μηδὲν ἔτι λείπειν,
ἀλλ᾽ ἑτοίμην εἶναι τὴν παρασκευὴν ἅπασιν εἰς τὴν
νῦν ἡμῖν προκειμένην πραγματείαν. ὅθεν οὐδ᾽ ἀνα-
γινώσκειν ἔτι τὰ μετὰ ταῦτα ῥηθησόμενα συμβουλεύω, πρὶν ἐν ἐκείνοις γυμνάσασθαι· παρακούσας γάρ
τις οὕτω πολλῶν θεωρημάτων οὔτ᾽ αὐτὸς ὠφεληθήσεται καὶ μάτην ἐγκαλέσει τοῖς ὀρθῶς λεγομένοις.

---

³ ἴσως B; om. K   ⁴ τὸ πάρεργον B; om. K

---

⁵ On the two recurring causal terms "proegoumenic" and

because it is borne on the outermost surface of the skin, and the third because it signifies failure of vision at night. And they make many other such terms. But if I were to go over them all, perhaps I would be in danger of seeming to be serious about something of secondary importance—something I gave instructions to avoid. Anyone who yearns for the truth should attempt to rid himself in every way of what is believed in regard to names, go to the very substance of the matters, reflect on this, and seek out how many diseases and symptoms there are in all and, over and above this, their *proegoumenic* causes.[5]   85K

I have done this in other treatises, of which there is one about the number of diseases entitled *On the Differentiae of Diseases*, and another *On the Differentiae of Symptoms*. In this way, too, I have attempted to discover the causes of all diseases and symptoms, each one specifically, so that nothing is lacking and everything is prepared and ready for us in respect to the matter now lying before us.[6] For this reason, I would advise people not to read further what will be said in what follows before becoming practiced in those [treatises]. Otherwise, failing to understand the many theories in this manner, they will not benefit themselves and will quarrel to no purpose with what is said correctly.

"prokatarktic," which may be understood as "internal antecedent" and "external antecedent," see the Introduction, section 6.

[6] Four treatises that are foundational to Galen's theory of medicine detail the classification and causation of diseases and symptoms. They are as follows: *De differentiis morborum*, VI.836–80K; *De morborum causis*, VII.1–41K; *De symptomatum differentiis*, VII.42–84K; and *De symptomatum causis*, VII.85–272K.

3. Ἐν ἐκείνοις μὲν οὖν ἅπαντα κατὰ μέρος ἐπεξέρ-
χομαι, τά τε νοσήματα καὶ τὰ συμπτώματα καὶ τὰς
αἰτίας· ἐνταυθοῖ δὲ δύο ἔτι προσθεὶς ταῦτα, ἀναγκαῖα
γινώσκεσθαι τοῖς ἀσκήσουσι τὴν θεραπευτικὴν μέθοδον, ἐπὶ τὸ χρῆσθαι τοῖς εὑρισκομένοις τηνικαῦτα
86K   μεταβήσομαι. τίνα δὲ | τὰ δύο ταῦτ᾽ ἐστὶν ἃ μέλλω
λέξειν; ἓν μὲν ὅπῃ διαφέρει νόσημα πάθους· ἕτερον δὲ
ὅτι χωρὶς τοῦ γνῶναι τὰ στοιχεῖα τοῦ σώματος, ἐξ ὧν
πρῶτον γέγονεν, ἀμήχανον ἐξευρεῖν τὰ νοσήματα.
ταῦτ᾽ οὖν ἐγὼ μὲν πειράσομαι διελθεῖν ἐπιμελέστατα,
τοὺς δ᾽ ἀναλεξομένους αὐτὰ παρακαλῶ μὴ πρότερον
ἐπ᾽ αὐτὴν μετιέναι τὴν θεραπευτικὴν μέθοδον, πρὶν
ὁπόσα τὰ πάντα ἐστὶ νοσήματα καὶ αὐτοὺς ζητῆσαι
κατὰ μόνας, καὶ τοῖς ὑφ᾽ ἡμῶν γεγραμμένοις ἐπιμελῶς ἐντυχεῖν. ὡς οὖν ταῦτα ποιησάντων, ἄρξομαι
τοῦ λόγου.

τρεῖς ἐδείχθησαν οὖσαι διαθέσεις ἐν τῷ σώματι
παρὰ φύσιν· αἰτίων τε καὶ νοσημάτων καὶ συμπτωμάτων. αἰτίων μὲν οἷον τοῦ πλήθους, ἢ τῆς διαφθορᾶς·
νοσημάτων δὲ οἷον τῆς φλεγμονῆς, ἢ τοῦ ἕλκους·
συμπτωμάτων δὲ οἷον τῆς ἀχροίας, ἢ τῆς ἰσχνότητος.
ἔξωθεν δὲ τούτων ἐστὶ τὰ ἀμέτρως ἐκκρινόμενα τοῦ
σώματος, ἢ παρὰ φύσιν ἐπεχόμενα, καὶ τῶν ἐνεργειῶν
αἱ βλάβαι, κοινῇ μὲν ἅπαντα προσαγορευόμενα συμπτώματα, γένος δ᾽ οὐχ ἓν ὄντα.⁵ διάθεσις μὲν γάρ τίς
ἐστι σώματος ἡ ἀχροία· τὸ δὲ ἐκκρινόμενον ἢ ἐπεχό-
μενον ἕπεται μὲν διαθέσει· διάθεσις⁶ δ᾽ οὐκ ἔστιν· |
87K   οὕτω δὲ καὶ ἡ ἐνέργεια βεβλαμμένη τε καὶ ἀβλαβὴς

134

3. In those treatises I go through all [these] things individually—diseases, symptoms and causes. But here two further things are added which those who will practice the therapeutic method must know. I shall then turn to the use of the things discovered. What are these two things I am about to speak of? One is in what way a disease differs from an affection, and the other is that it is impossible to discover the diseases without a knowledge of the elements of the body; that is, those from which it is made in the first place. I shall therefore attempt to go over these things very carefully, and I exhort those who will read about them not to advance to the therapeutic method itself before they search out, one by one, how many diseases there are in all, and then carefully read the things I have written. Now, assuming they have done this, I shall begin my exposition.

86K

The conditions in the body that are contrary to nature (abnormal) were shown to be three in number: causes, diseases, and symptoms. Examples of causes are excess or destruction; examples of diseases are inflammation or ulceration; and examples of symptoms are pallor or thinness. Apart from these, there are immoderate excretions from the body, or abnormal retentions, or damages of functions. All are commonly called symptoms, but they are not one class. Pallor is a condition of the body, whereas excretion or retention is consequent upon, but is not, a condition. Also the function, whether damaged or undamaged, is not

87K

---

5 ὄντα B; ἔχοντα K
6 B, P1, P2; διαθέσει om. K

οὖσα διάθεσις μὲν οὐκ ἔστιν, ἕπεται δὲ ἐξ ἀνάγκης τῇ
τοῦ μορίου διαθέσει.

τὸ μὲν οὖν οἴδημα καὶ ἡ φλεγμονὴ τῶν ἁπλῶς
ὄντων ἐστί, κατὰ ταῦτα δὲ καὶ τὸ πλῆθος, εἰ τύχοι, τοῦ
αἵματος, ἢ τοῦ σώματος ἡ ὠχρότης· ἡ δ' ἐνέργεια τῶν
μὲν ἁπλῶς ὄντων οὐκ ἔστιν, ἢ οὐχ ὁμοίως γε τούτοις
ὄντων· οὐδένα γὰρ αὐτῆς χρόνον ὑπομένει τὰ μόρια,
καθάπερ οὐδὲ τὰ τῆς λέξεως, οὐδ' ὅλως κινήσεως
οὐδεμιᾶς, ἀλλ' ἕκαστον τούτων ἐν τῷ γίνεσθαι τὸ
εἶναι λαμβάνει. διττοῦ δ' ὄντος γένους κινήσεως, τοῦ
μὲν κατὰ τόπον, τοῦ δὲ κατὰ ποιότητα, φορὰ μὲν
τὸ πρότερον, ἀλλοίωσις δὲ τὸ δεύτερον ὀνομάζεται.
πᾶσα μὲν οὖν ἐνέργεια κίνησίς ἐστι δραστική· πᾶσα
δ' ἀλλοίωσις κίνησις παθητικὴ τοῦ ἀλλοιουμένου,
πάσχει γάρ τι τὸ ἀλλοιούμενον. αἱ τοίνυν διαθέσεις,
ἐπειδὰν ἀλλοιοῦνται, κινοῦνται· παυσάμεναι δὲ τοῦ
κινεῖσθαι, ἠλλοίωνται μέν, ἀλλοιοῦνται δ' οὐκ ἔτι. πᾶν
γὰρ τὸ ὁπωσοῦν ἔχον ἔν τινι πάντως ἐστὶ διαθέσει· τὸ
88K δ' ἐν δυσλύτῳ διαθέσει καθ' ἕξιν | ἤδη διάκειται·
ἀλλοιοῦται μὲν ὁ μελαινόμενος, ἠλλοίωται δὲ ὁ μελαν-
θείς· ὥστ' εἶναι τὴν ἀλλοίωσιν γένεσιν ποιότητος, ἢ
διαθέσεως, ἢ ὅπως ἂν ἐθέλῃς ὀνομάζειν. οὐ μάχεται δὲ
τὸ λέγειν ἀλλαγὴν εἶναι τοῦ προϋπάρχοντος τὴν ἀλλοίωσιν τῷ λέγειν γένεσιν αὐτὴν εἶναι ποιότητος· ἅμα
γὰρ ἄμφω συμπίπτει, καὶ ἡ πρόσθεν ὑπάρχουσα τῷ

---

[7] In what follows, "change" rather than "movement" is used to

a condition but a necessary consequence of the condition of the part.

Edema and inflammation are simple entities as, in the same way, are excess of blood or pallor of the body, should they occur. A function, on the other hand, is not a simple entity, or at least it is not like these entities, for the parts of it do not endure for any period of time, just as the parts of speech don't, or any change at all does not. On the contrary, each of these acquires its existence by coming into being. Since there are two classes of change, that in relation to place and that in relation to quality, the former is called "movement" and the latter "alteration."[7] Every function is an active change, while every alteration is a passive change of what is altered insofar as what is altered has something happen to it. Accordingly, conditions, whenever they are altered, undergo change. When they cease being changed, they have been altered, but are no longer still being altered. Now anything that exists in any way whatsoever is always in a certain condition while what is in a condition that is difficult to break down is already fixed   88K in a permanent state. What is *being* made black is being changed, but what has *been* made black has been changed, so that alteration is the creation of a quality, or of a condition, or of whatever else you might wish to call it. To say that alteration is a transformation of what previously existed is not at odds with saying it is the creation of a quality, for both happen at the same time. That is, there is a change

render κίνησις. For a succinct discussion of this issue, see J. O. Urmson (1990), pp. 90–91. For the relevant Aristotle references, see *Physics* 200b26ff., and particularly in relation to health and disease, *Metaphysics* 1042a32ff.

σώματι μεταβάλλει,[7] καὶ νῦν ἄλλη γίγνεται. τοῦ γοῦν ἐν ἡλίῳ διατρίψαντος ἀλλοιοῦται μὲν ἡ λευκότης, γεννᾶται δὲ ἡ μελανότης· καὶ τοῦ παρὰ πυρὶ θαλπομένου μεταβάλλει μὲν ἡ ψυχρότης, γίγνεται δὲ ἡ θερμότης.

ὅταν δὲ τοῦδέ τινος, ὃ οὐκ ἔστιν οὐσία, γένεσιν εἶναι λέγωμεν, οὐ ταὐτὸν δηλοῦμεν ἐν τῇ λέξει τῇδε κἀπειδὰν ἁπλῶς ὀνομάσωμεν γένεσιν· ἡ μὲν γὰρ ἁπλῶς ὀνομαζομένη γένεσις ὁδός ἐστιν εἰς οὐσίαν, ἡ δὲ τοῦδέ τινος γένεσις, εἰς τὴν ὡς ἂν εἴποι τις ὕπαρξιν ἐκείνου. ἀλλὰ τοῦτο μὲν ἐν παρέργῳ λελέχθω, ὃ δὲ ἐν τῷ λόγῳ μάλιστα προὔκειτο, σχεδὸν ἤδη διώρισται, τὸ τὰ μὲν ἐν γενέσει τε καὶ μεταβολῇ καὶ ἀλλοιώσει καὶ ἁπλῶς εἰπεῖν ἐν κινήσει τοῦ εἶναι μεταλαμβάνειν, 89K τῶν δ' ὑπομένειν τὴν οὐσίαν· ὑγεία μὲν οὖν | καὶ νόσος, ὅσαι τε συμπτωμάτων ἢ αἰτίων εἰσὶ διαθέσεις, ἢ ἕξεις, ὑπομενόντων εἰσίν· αἱ δ' ἐνέργειαι πᾶσαι καὶ αἱ καθ' ὁτιοῦν ἀλλοιώσεις ἐν τῷ γίνεσθαι τὸ εἶναι κέκτηνται, καὶ τὸ καθ' ὁτιοῦν κινούμενον σῶμα κατ' ἐκεῖνο πάσχει, καὶ ἡ κίνησις αὐτοῦ πάθος ἐστίν.

οἱ μὲν οὖν παλαιοὶ καὶ τὰς ἐν τῷ κατὰ φύσιν ἔχειν ἁπάσας κινήσεις, ὅσαι γε μὴ δραστικαί, πάθη προσαγορεύουσιν, ὥσπερ οὖν ἐνεργείας τὰς δραστικάς, οὕτω καὶ αὐτὰς τῶν αἰσθήσεων τὰς ἀλλοιώσεις ὁ Πλάτων ὀνομάζει πάθη· τοῖς νεωτέροις δ' οὐκ οἶδ'

---

[7] B (cf. mutatur KLat), recte conj. Hankinson; μεταβολή K, P1, P2

in what previously existed in the body and now it becomes different. Thus, the whiteness of someone who spends time in the sun alters and blackness is generated. In like manner, the coldness of someone who is warmed by a fire changes and warmth occurs.

Whenever we speak of the generation of this something that is not a substance, we do not signify the same thing with this locution as when we simply use the term "generation." For what is called generation simply is a path to substance whereas the generation of something is, you might say, [the path] to the existence of that thing. But I speak of this by way of an aside. What is particularly proposed in my argument, and is already all but defined, is that some things partake of existence in generation, mutation, and alteration and, to speak generally, in change, but there are others whose substance remains. Health and disease, and those symptoms and causes that are conditions or states, are among those things that persist. However, all functions and alterations of any kind whatsoever have acquired their existence in generation, and the body that is changed in any respect whatsoever is affected in relation to that, and the change is an affection of it. 89K

The ancients called all changes that were in the category of "according to nature" affections, at least those that were not active, just as they called the active ones functions. In this way too, Plato called the actual changes of the sense perceptions affections.[8] For the moderns it seems

8 Plato, *Timaeus* 61d–66c.

ὅπως δόξαν, ἐπὶ τῆς παρὰ φύσιν μόνης κινήσεως
κεῖται τοὔνομα. ἰδίως μὲν οὖν τὸ πάθος ἐπὶ πάσης τῆς
ἔξωθεν κινήσεως ἐλέγετο παρὰ τῶν παλαιῶν, ἤδη δὲ
καταχρώμενοι καὶ τὰς ἐκ πάθους μὲν γεγενημένας τῶν
διαθέσεων, οὐκέτι δ᾽ ἐν κινήσει, πάθη προσαγορεύ-
ουσιν· οὐ μὴν χρονιώτερόν γε οὐδὲ δυσλυτώτερον ἡ
διάθεσις τῆς ἕξεως, ὥσπερ οὐδὲ ἡ ἀρρωστία· ἀλλ᾽ αἱ
τοιαῦται νομοθεσίαι τῶν ὀνομάτων ὑπὸ τῶν νεωτέρων
ἐπεισήχθησαν.

    εἴρηται δὲ ἐπιπλέον ὑπὲρ τῶν ἰατρικῶν ὀνομάτων
90K ἑτέρωθι, | καὶ νῦν οὐ τοῦτο πρόκειται σκοπεῖν, ἀλλ᾽
ὅπως ἡμεῖς χρησόμεθα, διελέσθαι μόνον ἀναγκαῖον
ἔδοξε σαφηνείας ἕνεκα. τὴν γὰρ ἐναντίαν ὑγείᾳ διάθεσιν, ὑφ᾽ ἧς ἐνέργειαν λέγομεν βλάπτεσθαι, νόσημα
μόνον προσαγορεύομεν, εἴτε πολυχρόνιος, εἴτε ὀλιγο-
χρόνιος, εἴτ᾽ ἐν ἀκαρεῖ χρόνῳ γίγνοιτο· τὰς δ᾽ ἄλλας
ἁπάσας τὰς προηγουμένας τούτων ἐν αἰτίας λόγῳ
διαθέσεις παρὰ φύσιν, αὐτὸ τοῦτο μόνον, αἰτίας, οὐ
πάθη· τὰ δ᾽ ἑπόμενα ταύταις, ὅσα μὲν ἐνεργειῶν εἰσι
βλάβαι, συμπτώματά τε καὶ πάθη, κατὰ ταὐτὰ δὲ καὶ
τὰς ἀμέτρους ἐκκρίσεις ἢ ἐπισχέσεις· ὅσαι δὲ διαθέσεις, ὥσπερ καὶ ἡ ἄχροια, πρὸς τῷ τοῦ πάθους τε
καὶ τοῦ συμπτώματος ὀνόματι διαθέσεις ὀνομάζομεν,
ὥσπερ οὖν καί εἰσι. κοινὸν μὲν δὴ τούτων ἁπάντων τὸ
παρὰ φύσιν καὶ τῶν αἰτίων καὶ τῶν νοσημάτων καὶ
τῶν συμπτωμάτων· ἴδιον δὲ τῶν μὲν νοσημάτων τὸ

(and I don't know how) the term is to be found in the case of change contrary to nature only. "Affection" was used specifically by the ancients in respect of every change from without, but now [the moderns] misuse [the term] and call those conditions that arise from an affection but are no longer in a state of change, affections, whereas, in fact, the condition is neither more enduring nor more difficult of resolution than the state, just as weakness is not. But such rules of terminology have been introduced by the moderns.

More has been said about medical terminology elsewhere.[9] It is not proposed to consider this now, but rather how I shall use it, distinguishing only what seems necessary for the sake of clarity. I apply [the term] "disease" only to the condition that is opposite to health, by which I mean the function is damaged, whether it (i.e. the disease) is of long or short duration, or momentary. All other conditions contrary to nature that precede this and have the ground of cause, I term causes alone and not affections. I call those things that follow these causes, when they are damages of functions, symptoms and affections in the same way as I do disproportionate excretions and retentions. Some conditions, like pallor, I do call conditions but, in addition, I give them the name of affection or symptom because that is what they are. What is common to all of these, and this includes causes, diseases, and symptoms, is that they are contrary to nature. What is specific to diseases is the dam-

90K

---

[9] The recurring reference to Galen's work on medical terminology is the *De nominibus medicis*, translated from the Arabic text by M. Meyerhof and J. Schacht (1931). There is also the pseudo-Galenic *Definitones medicae*, XIX.346–462K.

βλάπτειν ἐνέργειαν, τῶν δὲ συμπτωμάτων τὸ τούτοις
ἕπεσθαι, τῶν δὲ αἰτίων τὸ προηγεῖσθαι. οὔτ' οὖν ὅστις
κίνησιν εἶπε παρὰ φύσιν εἶναι τὴν νόσον οἶδεν ὃ
λέγει, καθάπερ ἐν τῷ πρὸ τούτου λόγῳ διήλθομεν
91K ἐνίους τῶν | Μεθοδικῶν οὕτως ἀφορίσασθαι προσ-
θέντας ἐκ περιττοῦ τὸ ἐπίμονον· οὐδ' ὅστις τροπὴν ἐκ
τοῦ κατὰ φύσιν εἰς τὸ παρὰ φύσιν, οὐδὲν γὰρ μᾶλλον
αἰτίας, ἢ νοσήματος, ἢ συμπτώματος ὁ λόγος· ἅπαντα
γὰρ ταῦτα διαθέσεις εἰσὶ παρὰ φύσιν, ἀλλ' εἰ μὲν
ὀλιγοχρόνια, δῆλον ὡς ὀξέα, εἰ δ' αὖ[8] δύσλυτα, χρόνια. διοίσει δ' οὐδὲν ἢ νόσον, ἢ νόσημα λέγειν, ὥσπερ
οὐδὲ πάθος, ἢ πάθημα.

καὶ μὲν δὴ καὶ ὅτι τὸ πάθους ὄνομα καὶ κατὰ τοῦ
νοσήματος ἐπιφέρουσιν οἱ παλαιοί, καθάπερ καὶ τὴν
ἀρρωστίαν καὶ τὴν ἀσθένειαν, ἐπιδέδεικται καὶ τοῦτ'
ἐν τοῖς Περὶ τῶν ἰατρικῶν ὀνομάτων, καὶ ὡς οὐδὲν
διαφέρει λέγειν ἀρρωστίαν ἢ ἀρρώστημα· καὶ μέν γε
καὶ ὡς τοὺς νοσοῦντας αὐτοὺς οὐ νοσοῦντας μόνον,
ἀλλὰ καὶ ἀρρωστοῦντας καὶ ἀσθενοῦντας καὶ κάμνον-
τας ὀνομάζουσιν, ἐπιδέδεικται δὲ καὶ τοῦτο δι' ἐκείνων
τῶν ὑπομνημάτων. λοιπὸν δ' ἂν εἴη νῦν, οὗπερ ἕνεκα
ταῦτ' εἴρηται πάντα, προσθέντας ἐπί τι τῶν ἑξῆς ἤδη
92K μετιέναι. τί δὲ τοῦτ' ἔστιν; οὐκ | ἄλλο τοῦ πολλάκις
ἤδη καὶ πρόσθεν εἰρημένου, τοῦ πρῶτόν τε καὶ μάλιστα τοῦτο σπουδάζειν τοὺς ἰατρούς, καὶ τοῦτο σχεδὸν
αὐτῶν ἔργον ὑπάρχειν ἴδιον, ἐκκόπτειν τὰς νόσους·

---

[8] B; δέ (αὖ om.) K

age to function; what is specific to symptoms is that they follow diseases; what is specific to causes is that they precede diseases. Anyone who says that disease is change contrary to nature doesn't know what he is talking about, just like some of the Methodics I considered in the previous   91K
book, i.e. those who make the definition by the superfluous addition of "persisting." The same applies to someone [who says disease is] "a change from what accords with nature to what is contrary to nature," for that statement is no more a definition of a disease than it is of a cause or a symptom, for all these are conditions contrary to nature. If they are of short duration, clearly they are acute, and if in turn they are difficult of resolution, they are chronic. It will make no difference whether you say disease (*nosos*) or disease (*nosema*), just as it does not if you say affection (*pathos*) or affection (*pathema*).

Furthermore, it has been shown in my treatise *On Medical Terms* that the ancients applied the term "affection" (*pathos*) to disease, just as they did to debility and weakness, and that it makes no difference to say debility (*arrōstia*) or debility (*arrōstema*). Moreover, that these men not only called those who were diseased, "diseased," but also "debilitated," "weak," and "suffering" was pointed out in those treatises. What remains [for me] to add now is the purpose for which I have said all these things. Then I shall proceed, in order, to what follows. What is this? It is nothing other than what has often already been said previously—that the primary and most important endeavor for   92K
doctors, and this is to all intents and purposes their specific function, is to eradicate diseases. As soon as this is done,

εὐθὺς γὰρ ἅμα τούτῳ καὶ ἡ βλάβη τῆς ἐνεργείας
οἴχεται, καὶ τἆλλα συμπτώματα πάντα συναναιρεῖται.
χρῄζουσι μὲν γὰρ πάντες οἱ ἄνθρωποι πρώτης καὶ
μάλιστα τῆς κατὰ φύσιν ἐνεργείας, δι' ἐκείνην δὲ καὶ
τῆς ὑγείας· καὶ ἀποθέσθαι γε βούλονται τὴν βλάβην
τῆς ἐνεργείας, καὶ διὰ τοῦτο καὶ τὴν νόσον·

οὐ μὴν τῇ γε βλάβῃ τῆς ἐνεργείας, ἀλλὰ τῇ νόσῳ
προσφέρουσι τὰ βοηθήματα, τουτέστι τῇ παρὰ φύσιν
διαθέσει τῇ βλαπτούσῃ τὴν ἐνέργειαν. ὅστις οὖν οὐκ
οἶδεν αὐτῶν τῶν κατὰ φύσιν ὑπαρχόντων τοῖς μορίοις
τά τ' ἄλλως συμβεβηκότα καὶ τὰ τῆς ἐνεργείας αἴτια
διορίσαι, πῶς τοῦτον εἰκὸς ἐξευρεῖν τὴν διάθεσιν ὑφ'
ἧς πρώτως ἡ ἐνέργεια βλάπτεται; τὰ μὲν γὰρ ἄλλως
συμβεβηκότα τοῖς σώμασι, κἂν μυριάκις ἀλλοιωθείη,
βλάπτειν τὴν ἐνέργειαν οὐ δύναται,[9] ἕως ἂν ὑφ' ὧν
ἐγίγνετο κατὰ φύσιν ἔχῃ πάντα· τούτων δ' εἴπέρ τι
κἂν ἐν ἀλλοιωθῇ, βλαβῆναι τὴν ἐνέργειαν εὐθὺς |
93K   ἀναγκαῖον εἰς τοσοῦτον εἰς ὅσον περ καὶ ὠφελεῖται
κατὰ φύσιν ἔχοντος.

4. Ἐμοὶ μὲν οὖν εἴρηται τὸ πᾶν, καὶ δέδεικται
σαφῶς ἤδη τοῖς γε δυναμένοις ἕπεσθαι λόγοις ἀληθέσιν, ὡς οὐκ ἐγχωρεῖ ὁπόσα τὰ πάντ' ἐστὶ νοσήματα,
μεθόδῳ περιλαβεῖν, εἰ μή τις εἰδείη ὁπόσα τὰ πάντ'
ἐστὶν ὑπάρχοντα κατὰ φύσιν ἔχοντι τῷ σώματι τῆς
ἐνεργείας αἴτια· μανθάνειν δ' οὔπω δυνατόν ἐστι τῶν
εἰρημένων οὐδέν, ὅσοι σκαιότεροί τέ εἰσι καὶ ἀργοὶ
τὴν διάνοιαν, ἢ τοῖς τῆς Μεθοδικῆς αἱρέσεως λήροις
ἐνετράφησαν. αὖθις οὖν κἀκείνοις, ὃ καθόλου νῦν

144

with it the damage to function is gone, and all the other symptoms are completely eradicated. For what all people need first and foremost is function that is in accord with nature, and through that, health. What they wish for is removal of damage to function, and through that, disease.

It isn't to the damage of function but to the disease that they apply remedies, which is to say, to the abnormal condition damaging function. Therefore, if someone does not know to make a distinction, among those things that are normal for the parts, between those that are random and contingent and that are causes of function, how is this person likely to discover the condition due to which function is primarily damaged? For those things that are random and contingent in bodies, even if they are altered ten thousand times, are not able to damage function whilever all those things from which they arise are in accord with nature. But if even one of these is altered, the function is, of necessity, immediately damaged to the same degree as it is 93K benefited when it is in accord with nature.

4. I have, then, said everything, and have already clearly shown, at least to those who are capable of following true arguments, that it is impossible for someone to comprehend by method how many diseases there are altogether if he does not know how many causes of function there are in all in a body that is in accord with nature. It is not at all possible for those who are rather stupid and lazy, or those reared on the nonsenses of the Methodic sect, to understand any of those things spoken of. Therefore, let me now go over once more, point by point, for the sake of

---

9 B, P1, P2; δύνανται K

εἴρηται τοῖς συνετοῖς, ἐπέλθωμεν κατὰ μέρος, ἕν τι
καὶ δεύτερον οἷον παραδείγματα τῷ λόγῳ προχει-
ρισάμενοι.

διὰ τί γὰρ ἡ γλῶττα τῶν χυμῶν αἰσθάνεται, τῶν δ'
ἄλλων μορίων οὐδέν; ἆρά γε διὰ χρόαν, ἢ διὰ τὴν
θέσιν, ἢ διὰ τὸ μέγεθος, ἢ διὰ τὸ σχῆμα; πασχούσης
γὰρ αὐτῆς, οἶμαι, καὶ μηκέτ' αἰσθανομένης τῶν χυμῶν ἤτοι τὴν χρόαν ἐπανάξομεν εἰς τὸ κατὰ φύσιν, εἰ
κατὰ ταύτην εἶχε τὴν ἐνέργειαν, ἢ τῶν ἄλλων ἕκαστον
94K   τῶν εἰρημένων, εἰ κατ' ἐκεῖνο· | κἂν εἰ κατ' ἄλλο δέ τι
παρὰ ταῦτα, δῆλον ὡς κατ' ἐκεῖνο μόνον, εἴπερ ἂν
αὐτὴν ἐπανάγοιμεν εἰς τὸ κατὰ φύσιν, οὐδὲν τῶν
ἄλλων ἔτι δεησόμεθα. φέρε γὰρ ὅτι πυκνὴ τοῖς πόροις
ἐστὶν εἰς τοσόνδε, διὰ ταῦτ' αὐτὴν αἰσθάνεσθαι τῶν
χυμῶν· ἆρ' οὐ τὴν ἐκείνων συμμετρίαν μέν, ὁπόθ'
ὑγιαίνουσι, φυλάξομεν, τὴν ἀμετρίαν δ' αὖθις ὁπότε
νοσοῦσιν, ἐπανορθωσόμεθα; φέρε δ' εἰ οὕτως ἔτυχε,
διότι συμμέτρως ἔχει θερμότητα,[10] αἰσθητικὴν εἶναι
τὴν γλῶτταν τῶν χυμῶν· ἆρ' οὐ κἀνταῦθα πρόδηλον
ὡς τῶν ἄλλων ἁπάντων ἀμελήσαντες, ἐκεῖνο φυλάξομεν αὐτῆς μόνον, ἀφ' οὗ τὴν ἐνέργειαν ἐκέκτητο; φέρε
δ' εἰ ξηρότητός τε καὶ ὑγρότητος ὧδέ πως ἔχουσα, διὰ
τοῦτ' αἰσθάνοιτο, τίς οὐκ ἂν ἁπάντων τῶν ἄλλων
ἀμελῶν εἰς τοῦτ' ἀποβλέψει μόνον αὐτῆς, ὅπως μήθ'
ὑγροτέρα τοῦ δέοντος ἔσται μήτε ξηροτέρα, τίς δ' οὐκ
ἂν εἴπερ τοῦτ' ἐστὶν ἀληθές, ἐξ ἑτοίμου συνελογίσατο
δύο εἶναι τὰ πάντα τῆς γλώσσης νοσήματα, τὸ μὲν
ὑγρόν, τὸ δὲ ξηρόν; ὥσπερ αὖ καὶ εἰ θερμότητι καὶ

those people who are intelligent what has been said in general, and provide one or two examples for the argument.

Why does the tongue perceive flavors while other parts do not? Is it because of its color, position, size or form? In my view, when it is affected and no longer perceives the flavors, we shall either restore the color to normal, if the function is dependent on this, or each one of the other things mentioned, if it is dependent on them. If, however, it is something else apart from these, it is clear that, in that one thing alone, if we were to restore it to normal, we would no longer have need of the others. Suppose the reason that it perceives flavors is because its pores have a certain density. Shall we not preserve the due proportion of these when they are healthy, and, on the other hand, rectify the disproportion when they are sick? Or suppose, if it should happen so, that the tongue perceives flavors because it has the right proportion of heat. Is it not quite clear here that, neglecting all the other [factors], we shall preserve only that feature of it from which it had acquired the function? Or suppose, somehow, there is [a balance] of dryness and moisture and that the tongue perceives because of this. Should someone not pay attention to this alone, that is, how it will be neither moister nor drier than it should be, neglecting all other things? And who will not, if this is true, readily deduce that all the diseases of the tongue are two in number, one moist and one dry? Likewise, too, if the tongue should have perception due to a

94K

---

10 B, P1, P2; θερμότητος K

ψυχρότητι συμμέτρῳ τὴν αἴσθησιν ἔχοι, τίς οὐκ ἂν
κἀνταῦθα δύο εἶναι τὰ νοσήματα αὐτῆς ἐνόησεν, ἀμε-
95K   τρίαν θερμότητός τε καὶ ψύξεως; | ὥσπερ εἰ καὶ τῇ τῶν
πόρων συμμετρίᾳ τὴν αἴσθησιν ἐκέκτητο, πρόχειρον
ἦν δήπου κἀνταῦθα λογίσασθαι πάντως ὑπὸ τῆς ἀμετρίας αὐτὴν βλαβήσεσθαι, διττὴν δὲ ταύτην ἔσεσθαι,
πύκνωσίν τε καὶ μάνωσιν τῶν πόρων. ἆρ᾽ οὖν ἔτι λέγω
πολλὰ τοὺς ἀναισθήτους ἐπάγων, εἰ καὶ μηδ᾽ ἄλλο,
τοῦτο γοῦν ἐννοῆσαι, τὸ μὴ δύνασθαί τι μήθ᾽ εὑρεῖν
μήτ᾽ ἀποδεῖξαι τὸ πλῆθος τῶν νοσημάτων, ἄνευ τοῦ
γνῶναι, τίνα μὲν τῶν ὑπαρχόντων τοῖς μορίοις αἴτια
τῆς ἐνεργείας ἐστί, τίνα δ᾽ ἄλλως τούτοις συμβέβηκεν; ἢ καὶ δεύτερόν τι καὶ τρίτον ἔτι παράδειγμα
προχειρίσομαι; πολλάκις γὰρ ὑπὸ τοῦ πλήθους αὐτῶν
τιτρώσκονται τῶν ἀνοήτων αἱ ψυχαί.

φέρε τοίνυν αὖθις ὡδί πως αὐτοὺς ἐρωτήσωμεν. ἆρ᾽
αἰσθάνεται τὸ σῶμα θερμῶν καὶ ψυχρῶν, καὶ σκλη-
ρῶν καὶ μαλακῶν, καὶ λείων καὶ τραχέων, καὶ ἁπλῶς
ἁπάντων τῶν ἁπτῶν, ὅτι λευκὸν τὴν χρόαν ἐστίν, ἢ ὅτι
μέλαν, ἢ ὅτι πυρρόν, ἢ ἁπλῶς εἰπεῖν ὅτι τοιόνδε τὴν
χρόαν· ἢ κατ᾽ οὐδὲν μὲν τούτων, δι᾽ ἄλλο δέ τι;
96K   πρόδηλον γὰρ οἶμαι παντί, τὸ φυλάττειν αὐτῷ | χρῆ-
ναι μόνον ἐκεῖνο τῷ μέλλοντί[11] γε αἰσθήσεσθαι καλῶς, ἐξ οὗπερ ἐκέκτητο μόνου τὸ καλῶς αἰσθάνεσθαι.
εἰ μὲν γὰρ ἐκ τοῦ λευκὸν εἶναι τοῦτ᾽ ἐκέκτητο, περὶ
παντὸς ἐχρῆν ποιεῖσθαι καὶ φυλάττειν τοῦτο καὶ φεύγειν τὸ μέλαν· εἰ δ᾽ ἔμπαλιν ἐκ τοῦ μέλαν ὑπάρχειν ἦν
αἰσθητικόν, ἀποδιδράσκειν ἐχρῆν, οἶμαι, καὶ δεδιέναι

148

balance of hot and cold, who would not, in this case, think
there are here also two diseases of the tongue, a disproportion of heat and a disproportion of cold? Similarly, if it had   95K
acquired perception through a balance of pores, it is presumably easy to reason here that it will be especially damaged by an imbalance, and that there will be two forms of
this—a constriction and a dilatation of the pores. Must I
say much more to persuade the foolish, so that, even if
nothing else, they at least understand that it is not possible
either to discover or to demonstrate the number of diseases without knowing which of the things existing in the
parts are causes of function and which are otherwise contingent? Shall I provide a second, and even a third example, for often the minds of the foolish are harmed by the
sheer number of them?

Well then, let me put the question to them again in this
way. Does the body perceive hot and cold, hard and soft,
smooth and rough, and, in general, all things touched, because it is white in color, or black, or red, or to speak generally, some sort of color, or is it none of these things but
something else? It is clear to everyone, I think, that it is   96K
necessary to preserve in that person who is going to perceive properly only that from which proper perception is
acquired because, if this had been acquired from being
white, one ought to make it of the utmost importance to
preserve this and to get rid of black. But if, on the other
hand again, perception is from black, it is necessary, I

---

11 B; τῷ *om.* K

τὰς ἄλλας ἁπάσας χρόας· οὕτω δὲ καὶ εἰ διότι ξανθὸν
ἢ πυρρόν ἐστι, διὰ τοῦτ' αἰσθάνοιτο, φευκτέον ἐστίν,
οἶμαι, τὰς ἄλλας ἁπάσας χρόας, ὡς ἀναισθησίας ἢ
δυσαισθησίας ἀπεργαστικάς.

κατὰ μὲν δὴ καὶ εἰ τῷ σκληρὸν εἶναι τὴν αἴσθησιν
εἶχε, τῷ μαλακὸν γενέσθαι βλαβήσεται· καὶ εἰ τῷ
πυκνὸν εἶναι, τῷ μανὸν ἀπεργασθῆναι· καὶ εἰ συμμετρίᾳ πόρων ᾐσθάνετο, πρὸς τῆς ἀμετρίας δήπου
βλαβήσεται· καὶ καθόλου τοῦτ' αὐτὸ μόνον ὑπάρχειν
χρὴ πρὸς τὴν αἴσθησιν, ἀφ' οὗ τὴν αἴσθησιν εἶχε,
καὶ τοῦτ' ἐπανορθοῦσθαι μόνον, ἐπειδὰν ἐξίσταται τῆς
φύσεως, ὑφ' οὗ τὴν αἴσθησιν βλάπτεται. ἆρ' οὖν
δεήσει τρίτου παραδείγματος, ἢ καὶ ταῦθ' ἱκανά; τοῖς
μὲν συνετοῖς, οἶμαι, καὶ ταῦτ' ἐστὶ περιττά, τὸ καθ-
όλου συνιέναι δυναμένοις ἄνευ τῶν παραδειγμάτων, |

ἀμαθέσι δὲ καὶ σκαιοῖς καὶ φιλονείκοις, ἴσως οὐδ' εἰ
τρίτον προστεθείη παράδειγμα, πλέον οὐδέν. ἀλλ'
ὅμως ἐπειδή περ εἴρηται δύο, καὶ κατατρίβουσιν ἀεὶ
μάτην ἡμῶν τὸν χρόνον, εἴη ἂν καὶ νῦν οὐκ ἀπεικὸς ἐν
αὐτοῖς ἔτι προσθεῖναι παράδειγμα. καὶ δὴ καὶ προ-
βεβλήσθω μὲν ὅπως ἀπεπτοῦσαν ἐπανορθωσόμεθα
γαστέρα· τὸν δὲ λόγον οὐ πρὸς τοὺς Μεθοδικοὺς ἔτι
μόνους, ἀλλ' ἤδη καὶ πρὸς ἐκείνους ποιησόμεθα τῶν
Λογικῶν οἳ νομίζουσι μεθόδῳ τινὶ δύνασθαι καὶ λόγῳ
τὴν τέχνην συστήσασθαι χωρὶς τοῦ γνῶναι τὴν πρώτην αἰτίαν τῆς ἐνεργείας, ἣν δὴ καὶ προσεχῆ καλεῖν
εἰώθασιν.

ἔστω δή τινα λέγειν, ἀπὸ γὰρ τῶν πρόχειρον ἐχόν-

think, to shun and fear all the other colors. In a similar manner also, if it is because of yellow or red that there is perception, all these other colors must be avoided, I think, as being what create anesthesia or dysesthesia.

And further, if it is through being hard that [a body] has perception, by it becoming soft perception will be damaged, and if it is through being constricted, perception [will be damaged] by its being dilated. And if it perceives through a balance of pores, it will presumably be harmed by an imbalance of pores. In general, there is that which alone is necessary for perception and from which there is perception, and it is only this that must be restored whenever it departs from nature, due to which perception is harmed. Will there be need for a third example, or is this enough? To those who are intelligent, I think, even these [examples] are superfluous as they are able to understand the whole matter without examples. But for those who are ignorant, foolish, and argumentative, perhaps they would be no better off even if a third example were to be added. But all the same, since in fact two examples have been mentioned, and they constantly waste my time in vain, it would not be unreasonable now to add one more example for them. Let me raise [the question] of how we shall restore a stomach that is not digesting. I advance the argument not for the Methodics alone, but also for those of the Rationalists who think they are able, by some method and theory, to bring together the art without a knowledge of the primary cause of the function which they are, in fact, accustomed to call [the] proximate [cause].

And indeed, let one of them speak, for it is better to be-

97K

τῶν τὴν ἀτοπίαν ἄρξασθαι βέλτιον, ἵν᾽ ἐπαγάγωμεν
αὐτούς, εἰ οἷόν τε, κατὰ βραχὺ πρὸς τὸ καὶ τῶν
ἀμυδροτέρων αἰσθάνεσθαι· λέγειν οὖν ὑποκείσθω τινὰ
διότι πολλαῖς ἐφεξῆς ἡμέραις ὅδε τις ἄνθρωπος ὁ νῦν
ἀπεπτῶν, ἐπὶ γάλακτος μόνου διαιτηθείς, ἠλλοίωσε
τὸ τῆς γαστρὸς χρῶμα, καὶ λευκὸν ἐποίησεν ἀντ᾽
ἐρυθροῦ, διὰ τοῦτ᾽ αὐτῷ βεβλάφθαι τὴν ἐνέργειαν·
οἶμαί σε γελᾶν ἤδη, καὶ δικαίως γελᾶν· ἀλλ᾽ εἴπερ |
98K εἰδείης, ὡς ἴσον ἐστὶ καὶ τούτῳ περὶ χρωμάτων εἰπεῖν
ὁτιοῦν ἄνευ τοῦ προσθεῖναι τὴν ἀπόδειξιν καὶ σοὶ περὶ
τῆς τῶν πόρων, εἰ οὕτως ἔτυχε, συμμετρίας, ἢ ἄλλης
ἡστινοσοῦν διαθέσεως, οὐκ οἶμαί σε γελάσειν εὐ-
λόγως· ἢ γὰρ κἀπὶ σαυτῷ τὸν γέλωτα κίνησον, ἢ
μηδ᾽ ἐφ᾽ ἑτέρῳ. ἔστω γὰρ ἰταμὸν εἶναι τὸν τὸ χρῶμα
τῆς γαστρὸς αἰτιώμενον τοῦ μὴ πέττειν καλῶς καὶ
φάσκειν ὡς ἐπειδὴ κατὰ φύσιν ἔχουσα, τὴν χρόαν
ἐνερευθής ἐστι, νῦν δ᾽ ἀπειργάσθη λευκὴ ἀκριβῶς, διὰ
τοῦτ᾽ ἀπεπτήσειν ἐξ ἀνάγκης αὐτήν, ἡδέως ἂν ἀκούσαιμί σου τὴν πρὸς τοῦτον ἀντιλογίαν· ἐγὼ μὲν γὰρ
οὐδ᾽ ἐπινοῆσαι δύναμαι τρόπον ἕτερον αὐτῆς, ἄνευ τοῦ
κελεῦσαι τῷ ταῦτ᾽ εἰπόντι δεῖξαι πρότερον, εἰ διὰ τὴν
χρόαν ὅλως ἐνεργεῖ κατὰ φύσιν ἡ γαστήρ· σὺ δὲ
εἴπερ ἔχεις, ἡδέως ἂν ἀκούσαιμί σου. ἀλλ᾽ οὔτε ἔχεις
οὔθ᾽ ἕξεις εἰπεῖν ἕτερόν τινα τρόπον ἀντιλογίας πρὸς
τὸν τὴν χροιὰν αἰτιώμενον τῆς ἀπεψίας ἀλλ᾽ ἢ τὴν
πρόκλησιν τοῦ δεῖξαι πῶς ἐκ τοῦ κατὰ φύσιν χρώ-
ματος ἡ γαστὴρ εἶχε τὸ πέττειν.

εἶτ᾽ ἐκεῖνος μὲν οὐ πιστευθήσεται τὴν χρόαν αἰτιώ-

gin from those who have absurdity ready to hand so that we might lead them, if at all possible, little by little to an awareness of more obscure matters. Assume, then, he says that this particular person, who has been fed for many days in succession with milk alone, is now unable to digest because the color of the stomach is changed and made white instead of red, and that is why the function is damaged in it. I think you would immediately laugh—and you would laugh rightly. But if you realize that there is an equivalence 98K between this man saying anything whatsoever about colors without adding the [required] demonstration and you saying something about the balance of the pores, if it happened to be so, or about any other condition whatsoever, I don't think it would be reasonable for you to laugh. Either direct the laughter at yourself, or at least not at another. Suppose the person who imputes the failure of proper digestion to the color of the stomach is headstrong, and says that when it is normal its color is somewhat red whereas now that it has been made completely white, because of this it will, of necessity, be unable to digest, I would be happy to hear you refuting him. For I cannot think of any other way of refutation apart from bidding the one who says this to show first that it is entirely because of color that the stomach functions normally. If you really could do this, I would gladly listen to you. But you do not and will not have any other method of refutation to offer to someone who attributes the failure of digestion to its color, apart from challenging him to show how the stomach does digest because its color is normal.

If that man will not be believed when he imputes the

μενος τῆς ἀπεψίας, πρὶν δεῖξαι κατὰ τοῦτ᾽ ἐνεργοῦσαν |
99K αὐτήν, σὺ δ᾽ ἤτοι τὴν ἀμετρίαν λέγων τῶν πόρων ἢ
ὁτιοῦν ἄλλο πιστευθήσῃ πρὸ τοῦ δεῖξαι πῶς ἐνεργεῖ
κατὰ τὴν ἐν ἐκείνῳ τῷ γένει συμμετρίαν; Ἀλλ᾽ οὐδὲ
τοῦτο λέγω, φησίν, οὐδ᾽ ἄλλο τι τὸ προσεχὲς τῆς
πέψεως αἴτιον, ἀλλ᾽ ὅλως ἀγνοεῖν ὁμολογῶ. καὶ μὴν εἰ
τῷ μὲν τὴν χρόαν αἰτιωμένῳ τῆς ἐνεργείας ἀναγκαῖόν
ἐστι καὶ τῆς βλάβης αἰτιᾶσθαι, τῷ δὲ τὴν συμμετρίαν
τῶν πόρων, καὶ τούτῳ τὴν ἀμετρίαν τῶν αὐτῶν τούτων
πόρων· καὶ τῷ τὴν εὐκρασίαν τῶν τεττάρων ποιοτήτων, θερμότητος καὶ ψυχρότητος καὶ ὑγρότητος καὶ
ξηρότητος, καὶ τούτῳ τὴν δυσκρασίαν τῶν αὐτῶν·
ἀναγκαῖον ἔσται καὶ σοὶ τὸ κατὰ φύσιν ὑποθεμένῳ
πρότερον, οὕτως ἐξευρεῖν τὸ παρὰ φύσιν, εἰ δὲ μὴ
γινώσκεις τὸ κατὰ φύσιν, οὐδὲ τὸ παρὰ φύσιν οἶσθα·
καὶ γὰρ δὴ καὶ ὑμῶν αὐτῶν ἀκούω λεγόντων πρὸς
τοὺς Ἐμπειρικοὺς ἰατροὺς ὡς οὐκ ἐνδέχεται γνῶναι τὸ
παρὰ φύσιν, εἰ μὴ πρότερον εἰδείη τις τὸ κατὰ φύσιν.
Ἀλλὰ γιγνώσκω, φησί, τὸ κατὰ φύσιν· ἆρά γε σύμ-
100K παν, ἢ μέρος αὐτοῦ | τι; καὶ τουτὶ τὸ μέρος ὃ γινώσκεις
ἆρά γε τὸ τῆς ἐνεργείας ἐστὶν αἴτιον, ἢ ἄλλως ὑπάρχει τῇ γαστρί; τί γὰρ δὴ καὶ γινώσκεις; αὐτῆς
θέσιν δηλαδὴ καὶ μέγεθος καὶ πλοκὴν καὶ διάπλασιν·
ἀλλ᾽ οὐδὲν τούτων ἐστὶ τῆς ἐνεργείας αἴτιον.

ἀλλ᾽ οὐδὲ ἀγνοεῖταί τι τούτων τοῖς Ἐμπειρικοῖς,
ὁμολογοῦσί τε γὰρ χρῆσθαι τῇ κατὰ περίπτωσιν
ἀνατομῇ καὶ ταῦτ᾽ ἐξ ἐκείνης μανθάνειν, οὐ μὴν ἐνεργείας τε καὶ χρείας μορίων. Ἀλλ᾽ οἶδά, φησι, καὶ τὴν

154

failure of digestion (apepsia) to the color until he shows
that digestion functions due to color, will you really be be-   99K
lieved when you say it is the imbalance of the pores, or
whatever else, before you show how it functions due to balance in that class? "But I don't assert this," he says, "or that
anything else is the proximate cause of digestion; I confess
that I am completely ignorant." And further, if it is necessary for the one who imputes the function to the color to
also impute the damage [to color], it is also necessary for
the one who [imputes function] to the balance of the pores
to do the same with regard to imbalance of these same
pores, and for someone [who imputes function] to an
eukrasia of the four qualities—hot, cold, moist and dry—
to do the same with respect to a *dyskrasia* of these. It will
be necessary also for you to propose what is normal first,
and in this way discover what is abnormal. For if you don't
know what is normal then neither do you know what is abnormal. Furthermore, I hear you yourself saying to the
Empiric doctors that it is impossible to know what is abnormal without first knowing what is normal. "But I do
know," he says, "what is normal." Do you in fact know it all
or just some part of it? And is the part you do know in fact   100K
the cause of function, or is it something else in the stomach? For what, indeed, do you know? You know, of course,
its position, size, structure and conformation. But none of
these things is a cause of function.

However, none of these things is unknown to the Empirics, for they acknowledge that they use the anatomy that
pertains to experience and they learn these things from
that, but not the functions and the uses of the parts. "But,"
he says, "I know the function too. It is a wrapping around

155

ἐνέργειαν· ἔστι γὰρ περιστολὴ καὶ τρίψις. ἀλλ᾽ εἰ μὴ
τὴν αἰτίαν εἰδείης αὐτῆς, οὐκ εἴσῃ τὴν νόσον· εἰ γὰρ ἡ
εὐκρασία τῶν τεττάρων ποιοτήτων αἰτία τῆς ἐνεργείας
ἐστίν, ἡ δυκρασία πάντως τῆς βλάβης αἰτία ἔσται·
σὺ δ᾽ οἴει φλεγμονὴν καὶ σκίρρον, οἴδημά τε καὶ
ἀπόστημα, καὶ τἄλλα ὅσα τοῖς ὀφθαλμοῖς ἰδεῖν ἔστι,
μόνα τῆς γαστρὸς εἶναι παθήματα· καίτοι γ᾽ οὐδὲ
ταῦτα τοῖς Ἐμπειρικοῖς ὁμοίως ὀφθαλμοῖς μόνοις καὶ
χερσὶ καὶ ταῖς ἄλλαις αἰσθήσεσι καταμανθάνεις,
ἀλλ᾽ ἐπὶ τὴν οὐσίαν αὐτῶν ἀνέρχεσθαι πειρᾷ, καὶ
ταύτην ἐξευρίσκειν ἀκριβῶς, οὐκ ἀρκούμενος τοῖς
φαινομένοις αἰσθήσει συμπτώμασιν, ἃ τοῖς Ἐμπει-
101K ρικοῖς ὁρίζει τε καὶ | περιγράφει τὴν συνδρομήν· οὕτω
γὰρ ἀξιοῦσιν ὀνομάζειν αὐτοὶ τὸ τῶν συμπτωμάτων
ἄθροισμα τῶν ὑπαρχόντων τῷ πεπονθότι τόπῳ. καὶ
τὴν ἔνδειξίν γε τῆς θεραπείας οὐκ ἐκ τῶν φαινομένων
λαμβάνεις συμπτωμάτων· οὐδὲ γὰρ εἰ παρὰ φύσιν
ὄγκος, οὐδ᾽ εἰ ἀντίτυπος, οὐδ᾽ εἰ ὀδυνηρός, οὐδ᾽ εἰ
ἐρυθρός, ἀλλ᾽ εἰ σφήνωσις ἐν τοῖς πέρασι τῶν ἀρτηριῶν ἐπὶ παρεμπτώσει σκοπεῖς καὶ τὴν θεραπείαν, ὡς
αὐτὸς ἔφης, πρὸς τοῦτ᾽ ἀναφέρων ἐξευρίσκεις. ἢ γὰρ
οὐχ οὗτος ὁ Ἐρασιστράτου τρόπος τῆς διδασκαλίας
ἐν τοῖς Περὶ πυρετῶν, ὥσπερ αὖ Διοκλέους μὲν ἕτερος,
Πραξαγόρου δ᾽ ἄλλος, Ἀσκληπιάδου δ᾽ ἄλλος; ὥστ᾽
οὐκ ἀπὸ τῶν περὶ τὸ φλεγμαῖνον μέρος φαινομένων

---

10 This is a term with several different (but related) meanings,
one of which has a particular theoretical significance for Erasis-

and a rubbing." Well, if you don't know the cause of this
function, you don't know the disease. For if the *eukrasia* of
the four qualities is a cause of function, the *dyskrasia* will
undoubtedly be a cause of damage. You, however, think
that inflammation, induration, edema, abscess and other
such things that are visible to the eyes are the only affections of the stomach. Nevertheless, you don't only observe
closely those things with the eyes, hands, and other senses,
like the Empirics, but you try also to get to their substance
and discover it precisely. Nor are you satisfied with the
symptoms apparent to perception which, for the Empirics,
define and determine the "syndrome," for so they see fit to   101K
name the collection of symptoms existing in the affected
place. And you don't take the indication for treatment
from the apparent symptoms. You don't consider whether
the swelling is unnatural, hard, painful or red, but whether
there is obstruction at the ends of the arteries due to
paremptosis,[10] and you discover the therapy, as you yourself say, by referring to this. Is this not the way of teaching
of Erasistratus in [his work] *On Fevers*, just as Diocles had
another again, Praxagoras another, and Asclepiades yet
another?[11] Thus, the indication for remedies was not, for

tratus; see the Introduction, Section 6, on terminology. See also
the pseudo-Galenic *Introductio sive medicus*, XIV.777K, where
the meaning is probably similar to that intended here—in effect,
arterial embolism.

[11] None of the works of these writers is extant, although each
has a relatively recent study or collection of fragments: for Erasistratus, I. Garofalo (1988); for Diocles of Carystus, P. J. van der
Eijk (2000); for Praxagoras, F. Steckerl (1958); and for Asclepiades, J. Vallance (1990).

συμπτωμάτων ἡ ἔνδειξις αὐτοῖς γίγνεται τῶν βοηθημάτων, ἀλλ' ἀπὸ τῆς οὐσίας αὐτῆς· οὐ γὰρ εἰ παρὰ
φύσιν ὄγκος, οὐδ' εἰ ἀντίτυπος, οὐδ' εἰ πόνος σφυγμώ-
δης, ἀλλ' εἰ παρέμπτωσίς τε καὶ σφήνωσις ἐν τοῖς
ἐσχάτοις τῶν ἀρτηριῶν, ἢ ἔμφραξις ἐν τοῖς πέρασι
τῶν φλεβῶν, ἢ σῆψίς τις τῶν χυμῶν, ἢ λόγῳ θεω-
ρητῶν ὄγκων ἔντασις, ἐν λόγῳ θεωρητοῖς ἀραιώμασιν
ἐπισκοποῦνται.

102K   ὥστε ἕκαστος | τούτων ἀπὸ τῶν τῆς διαθέσεως τοῦ
φλεγμαίνοντος μέρους, οὐκ ἀπὸ τῶν ἑπομένων αὐτῇ
συμπτωμάτων ἔνδειξιν τῶν βοηθημάτων λαμβάνει.
κατὰ τὸν αὐτόν, οἶμαι, τρόπον καὶ ὅστις αἰτιᾶται τὸ
θερμὸν καὶ ψυχρὸν καὶ τὸ ξηρὸν καὶ τὸ ὑγρόν· ἀλλ'
οὗτος μὲν εἰ καὶ χωρὶς φλεγμονῆς, ἢ ἕλκους, ἢ ἀπο-
στήματος, ἤ τινος ἑτέρου τοιούτου, μόνῳ τῷ ψυχροτέρα[12] γεγονέναι μὴ πέπτοι καλῶς ἡ γαστήρ, εὐπορεῖ
τῶν βοηθημάτων· οἱ δὲ τὰς φλεγμονὰς καὶ τοὺς σκίρ-
ρους καὶ τἆλλα ὅσα τοῖς ὀφθαλμοῖς ἔστι θεάσασθαι
μόνα νομίζοντες εἶναι νοσήματα, γελοίως πάνυ τὰς
χωρὶς τούτων ἀπεψίας ἀτονίᾳ τῆς κοιλίας γίγνεσθαί
φασιν, ὥσπερ διάθεσίν τινα λέγοντες τὴν ἀτονίαν
ἰδίαν ἐξαίρετον, ἀλλ' οὐχ ὥσπερ καὶ τοῖς ἐκπυϊσκο-
μένοις τε καὶ σκιρρουμένοις καὶ φλεγμαίνουσι καὶ
ἄλλως ὁπωσοῦν πεπονθόσιν ὑπάρχειν. πάντα γὰρ
ταῦτα τὰ πάθη, κἂν ἐν γαστρὶ κἂν ἐν ἥπατι κἂν ἐν
θώρακι κἂν ἐν ὁτῳδήποτε γένηται, παραχρῆμα τὸ
μέρος ἀτονώτερον ἐργάζεται περὶ τὴν ἰδίαν ἐνέργειαν·

these men, on the basis of the apparent symptoms relating to the inflamed part, but on the basis of the substance itself. For they did not consider whether a swelling was unnatural, or hard, or pulsating painfully, but whether there was paremptosis or obstruction in the ends of the arteries, or a blockage at the limits of the veins, or putrefaction of the humors, or stasis of the theoretical particles in the theoretical pores, both identified by reason.

So each of these men takes the indication for remedies from the aspects of the condition of the inflamed part, and not from the symptoms that follow the condition. I think anyone who attributes the cause to heat, cold, moisture, or dryness does so in the very same way. For if the stomach does not digest properly in the absence of inflammation, ulcer, abscess, or any other such thing, but only because it has become colder, he will have plenty of remedies. Those who think that only such things as inflammations, indurations, and the other similar things that are visible to the eyes are diseases, say quite absurdly that, apart from these, failure of digestion (apepsia) occurs due to weakness (atonia) of the stomach,[12] as if saying that atonia is some specific and removable condition, and not what exists in things that are suppurating, indurated, inflamed or otherwise affected in some way. For all these affections that occur in the stomach, liver, thorax, or wherever else, immediately make the part weaker in terms of its specific

12 There is variation in the terminology for the stomach. Galen here uses *gaster* in the first instance and *koilia* in the second. Sometimes the latter is clearly used to refer to the abdomen generally.

---

12 B; ψυχρά K

ἀλλ' οὐ τοῦτ' ἄρ' ἦν αὔταρκες αὐτοῖς εἰς τὴν τῶν
βοηθημάτων ἔνδειξιν, ἢ μάτην ζητοῦσι τὰς διαθέσεις, |
103K   ἀλλ' ἐπ' αὐτὴν ἀνέρχονται τὴν οὐσίαν τοῦ νοσήματος,
ὡς οὐκ ἐνὸν ἄλλως εὐπορῆσαι τῆς προσηκούσης
ἰάσεως.

οὔκουν ἔτι τὸν ἔλεγχον ἐξ ἡμῶν ἀναμένουσιν, ἀλλ'
αὐτοὶ σφᾶς αὐτοὺς ἐξελέγχουσιν οἱ τὴν ἀτονίαν εἶναι
λέγοντες τὸ πάθος, ἐν οἷς οὐδὲν ὧν ἐκεῖνοι παθῶν
ὡρίσαντο πεπονθυίας τῆς γαστρὸς ἀπεπτεῖ τὸ ζῷον.
οὔτε γὰρ ἴδιον, ἀλλὰ κοινὸν ἁπάντων λέγουσι, καὶ τὴν
θεραπείαν οὐδὲ κατ' αὐτοὺς ἐκείνους δυνάμενον ἐνδείξασθαι εὐλόγως. ὄνομα γάρ ἐστι ψιλὸν τὸ ῥωννύναι
τὴν ἀτονίαν, καὶ οἷον σκοπὸς μᾶλλον, οὐ θεραπεία. τί
γὰρ χρὴ ποιοῦντας ῥώμην ἐντιθέναι τοῖς ἀρρωστοῦσι
περὶ τὴν ἐνέργειαν οὐ λέγουσιν. ἐν τούτῳ δ' ἦν ἡ
θεραπεία. καὶ χωρὶς τοῦ τὴν διάθεσιν εὑρεθῆναι τῆς
γαστρὸς εὐπορῆσαι βοηθημάτων ἀδύνατον· εἰ μὲν
γὰρ ἔψυκται, θερμαντέον, εἰ δ' ὕγρανται, ξηραντέον·
ὡσαύτως δὲ καὶ εἰ μὲν ἀμέτρως τεθέρμανται, ψυκτέον,
εἰ δ' ἐξήρανται, ὑγραντέον. οὗτοι μὲν ἁπλοῖ τρόποι
τῆς ἰάσεως τέτταρες. ἕτεροι δὲ τέτταρες σύνθετοι, εἰ
μὲν ψυχροτέρα καὶ ξηροτέρα τὴν κρᾶσιν ἡ γαστὴρ
104K   ἐγένετο, θερμαντέον τ' ἐστὶ | καὶ ὑγραντέον αὐτήν· εἰ
δὲ ὑγροτέρα καὶ θερμοτέρα, ξηραντέον τέ ἐστι καὶ
ψυκτέον· οὕτω δὲ καὶ εἰ μὲν θερμοτέρα τε καὶ ξηροτέρα, ψυκτέον τε καὶ ὑγραντέον, εἰ δ' ὑγροτέρα τε καὶ
ψυχροτέρα, ξηραντέον τε καὶ θερμαντέον· ὥστε καὶ αἱ

function. But this is not enough for them as an indication for remedies, nor do they seek in vain the conditions, but 103K return to the actual substance of the disease, as if it were not possible to find the appropriate means of cure otherwise.

So these men do not await refutation by me. Rather, they refute themselves when they say that weakness (atonia) is an affection in those cases in which the organism fails to digest although the stomach is suffering none of the affections which they defined. But what they speak of is not something specific but something common to all things and, by their own say-so, it is not possible for treatment to be indicated rationally. For the term "strengthening the weakness" is an empty phrase, and is rather more like an objective than a treatment. For they don't say what it is they must do to strengthen those who are weak in terms of function, and yet treatment depends on this. Without discovering the condition of the stomach, it is impossible to find the remedies. For if it is cold, it must be heated; if it is moist, it must be dried. In like manner, too, if it has been disproportionately heated, it must be cooled and if disproportionately dried, it must be moistened. These are the four simple methods of cure. There are, however, four compound [ways]: if the stomach has become too cold and too dry in terms of *krasis*, it must be 104K heated and moistened; if it is too moist and too hot, it must be dried and cooled. Likewise, if it is too hot and too dry, it must be cooled and moistened; and if it is too moist and too cold, it must be dried and heated. Thus, there are eight

διαθέσεις ὀκτὼ τῆς γαστρὸς αὐτῆς, ὡς ἐκεῖνοι λέγουσιν, ἀτονίας αἰτίαι, καὶ οἱ τρόποι τῆς ἰάσεως ὀκτώ.

5. Καὶ οὐκ ἐγχωρεῖ λέγειν οὐδενὶ τῶν Δογματιζόντων ὁμοίως τοῖς Ἐμπειρικοῖς ὡς οὐδὲν δέοιντο
γιγνώσκειν, εἴθ᾽ ὑπάρχουσιν, εἴτε μή· τελέως γὰρ
ἀνατρέψουσι τὴν Λογικὴν αἵρεσιν, ὁμολογήσαντες
εὐπορεῖν μὲν τῆς θεραπείας, ἀγνοεῖν δὲ τὴν διάθεσιν·
ἐκ πείρας γὰρ δήπου πάντες εὐπορήσουσι τῆς ἰάσεως,
εἴπερ μὴ ἐκ τῆς τοῦ πράγματος αὐτοῦ φύσεως ἔνδειξιν
ἔλαβον. οἱ μὲν οὖν Ἐμπειρικοὶ καὶ τῷ μὴ δύνασθαι
νομίζειν εὑρεθῆναί τι τῶν ἀδήλων, καὶ τῷ μὴ δεῖσθαι,
κἂν εὑρεθῇ, τετηρῆσθαι γὰρ αὐτοῖς τὰς θεραπείας ἐπὶ
ταῖς φαινομέναις συνδρομαῖς, εὐλόγως οὔτε γιγνώσκειν φασὶν εἰ ὀκτὼ διαθέσεις εἰσὶ καθ᾽ ἃς ἡ γαστὴρ
105K ἀτονεῖ, καὶ | χωρὶς τῆς τοιαύτης περιεργίας εὐπορεῖν
τῶν ἰαμάτων· οἱ δὲ καὶ τὸν λόγον ὁμολογοῦντες ἔχειν,
ᾧ καὶ περὶ τῶν ἀδήλων διασκέπτονται, καὶ τὴν εὕρεσιν αὐτῶν ἔνδειξιν ἰαμάτων παρέχεσθαι φάσκοντες,
οὐκ οἶδ᾽ ὅπως οὐκ αἰδοῦνται λέγοντες ἢ μὴ γινώσκειν
εἰ ὑπάρχουσιν αἱ ὀκτὼ διαθέσεις, ἢ μὴ δεῖσθαι πρὸς
τὰς ἰάσεις αὐτῶν. οὐ γὰρ τοῦτ᾽ ἀπόχρη μόνον εἰπεῖν,
ὡς οὐκ ἴσασιν, ἀλλ᾽ ἐξελέγξαι προσήκει τοὺς εἰδέναι
φάσκοντας, ὡς οὐκ ἀληθεύουσιν· ἄχρι δ᾽ ἂν μήτ᾽
αὐτοὶ τοῦτο ποιῶσιν, ἕτεροί τε πολλὰς ἀποδείξεις
λέγωσι τοῦ πᾶν σῶμα διὰ τὴν ἐκ τῶν τεττάρων ποιὰν
κρᾶσιν ἐνεργεῖν, εὐλογώτερον ἐκείνοις πιστεύειν, εἰ
μή τι ἄρα προφάσεις ψιλὰς λέγοντες ἀξιώσουσι
πιστότεροι τῶν τὰς ἀποδείξεις λεγόντων εἶναι. καὶ

conditions of the stomach itself which are causes of weakness (as those men say), and eight ways of cure.

5. It is not permissible for any of the Dogmatics, as it is for the Empirics, to say that they need to know nothing about whether these things exist or not. For they will completely overturn the Rationalist sect if they admit that they have found a way of treatment but are ignorant of the condition. Of course, they will all find a way of cure from experience, if they don't take an indication from the nature of the matter itself. The Empirics, who do not think it is possible for anything hidden to be discovered, and who think it is not needed even if it is discovered, for the treatments have been observed by them on the basis of the apparent syndromes, quite reasonably say they do not know if there are eight conditions in relation to which the stomach becomes weak; and so they find remedies without such over-elaboration. However, I do not know how those who profess that they do have a theory with which they examine those things that are hidden, and say that the discovery of these things provides an indication for remedies, are not embarrassed when they say that either they don't know if there are eight conditions, or that they have no need of them for cures. It is not enough [for them] simply to say that they don't know; they also need to refute those who claim they do know, as not speaking the truth. So long as these men do not do this, and others speak of many demonstrations of the whole body functioning because of a certain *krasis* of the four [qualities], it is more reasonable to believe the latter, at least if those who make unsupported claims do not think they are more worthy of credence than

105K

μὴν ἐκεῖνοι μὲν εἰ καὶ μηδὲν ἄλλο, πείθειν γοῦν καὶ
διδάσκειν τοὺς ἀκροατάς, οὐ βιάζεσθαι καὶ προστάττειν ἐπιχειροῦσιν· οὗτοι δ' αὐτοὶ[13] τοὐναντίον ὡς
τύραννοι κελεύουσι μὴ ζητεῖν τῆς ἐνεργείας τὴν αἰτίαν. ἀλλ' ἡμεῖς μὲν καὶ Διονύσιον καὶ Φάλαριν καὶ
τοὺς ἄλλους τυράννους διὰ τοῦτο μισοῦμεν, ὅτι κελεύουσι καὶ προστάττουσιν, οὐ πείθουσι καὶ διδάσκου-
106K   σιν, | ὡς Σόλων καὶ Δράκων καὶ Λυκοῦργος.

Ἀλλ' ἐγώ, φησι, ἐν τοῖς ὅροις μένω τῆς τέχνης,
ὑμεῖς δὲ ἀποχωρεῖτε, καὶ πρὸς τὰς ἄλλας ἀρχὰς ἡμᾶς
ἀνάγειν ἐπιχειρεῖτε τῆς φυσικῆς θεωρίας. εἶτα οὐκ
ἀποδείξεις, ὦ γενναιότατε, κἂν αὐτὸ τοῦτο, τίνες εἰσὶν
οἱ ὅροι τῆς ἰατρικῆς θεωρίας καὶ τίνα χρὴ γινώσκειν
τὸν μέλλοντα λόγῳ ποιήσασθαι τὴν εὕρεσιν τῶν βοηθημάτων, ἀλλὰ μορμολυξάμενος οἴει καταπλήξειν
ἡμᾶς; ἀκούω καὶ σοῦ λέγοντος ὡς οὐ χρὴ σκοπεῖσθαι
τῆς ἐνεργείας τὴν αἰτίαν· ἀκούω δὲ καὶ τῶν Ἐμπειρικῶν ὡς οὐδὲ τὰς ἐνεργείας αὐτὰς ἐπισκέπτεσθαι
προσῆκεν· ἀκούω δὲ καὶ τοῦ λέγοντος ὡς οὐ μόνον
ἐπισκεπτέον εἶναι δεῖ αὐτάς, ἀλλὰ καὶ τὰς αἰτίας ὑφ'
ὧν γίγνονται ζητητέον. ἆρ' οὖν κελεύεις με γίνεσθαι
τῶν ἀδίκων κριτῶν, οἳ μὴ περιμείναντες ἁπάντων
ἀκοῦσαι τῶν ἀμφισβητούντων ἀλλήλοις, ἑνὶ φέροντες

13 Β; αὖ Κ

13 Unlike the earlier passage referring to tyrants, Galen now
gives two specific examples: Dionysius, the tyrant of Syracuse who

those offering demonstrations. Furthermore, even if those men do nothing else, they at least attempt to persuade and teach their pupils rather than compel and command them. But these very men, in complete contrast, issue orders like tyrants not to search for the cause of the function. But we hate Dionysius, Phalaris, and the other tyrants because of this—that they order and command, and do not persuade and teach, like Solon, Draco and Lycurgus.[13]

106K

"But I remain within the boundaries of the art," he says, "whereas you depart [from them] and try to lead us toward the other principles of physical theory." So then, my most noble friend, will you not even demonstrate this very thing; that is, what the boundaries of medical theory are, and what someone who intends to make the discovery of remedies according to reason must know? Do you think, rather, that by assuming a fearsome expression, you will terrify us? And I hear you say it is not necessary to examine the cause of function. But I also hear the Empirics say it is not their concern to give consideration to the functions themselves. And yet I hear as well the man who says that it is not only necessary for these to be looked into, but it is necessary also to seek the causes from which they arise. Are you, then, demanding that I become one of those unjust judges who do not wait to hear all the parties contend-

ruled from 367 to 357 BC, and Phalaris of Acragas (ca. 570–549 BC), who was the first major Sicilian tyrant. In comparison, Solon (sixth century BC) was an early Athenian lawmaker and poet, highly regarded by Herodotus, Draco (seventh century BC) was Solon's notable predecessor at Athens, famed for the severity of his laws, and Lycurgus here probably refers to the traditional founder of Sparta's *eunomia*.

ἔδοσαν τὴν ψῆφον; ἢ πρῶτον μὲν ἀκοῦσαι τοὺς λό-
γους ὑμῶν ἑκάστου καταμόνας, εἶτ' ἀλλήλοις παρα-
βαλεῖν καὶ διασκέψασθαι τίς ἑαυτῷ τε καὶ τοῖς φαινομένοις ὁμολογεῖ καὶ τίς οὔτε τοῖς φαινομένοις οὔθ'
107K ἑαυτῷ; καὶ μὴν εἰ τοῦτο | ποιήσαιμι, τῶν μὲν Ἐμπειρι-
κῶν ἀκούσαιμι κἂν παραμυθεῖσθαι γοῦν πειρωμένων
ἃ λέγουσιν, εἰ καὶ μὴ βεβαίως ἀποδεικνύουσιν· ὑμῶν
δ' οὐδὲ τοῦτο. τίς γὰρ ἢ παραμυθίαν ὑμῶν, ἢ ἀπόδειξιν εἰπεῖν ἐπεχείρησεν ἡδέως ἂν ἀκούσαιμι, δι' ἣν οὐ
χρὴ ζητεῖν τῆς ἐνεργείας τὴν αἰτίαν; ἡ μὲν γὰρ
ἔμπροσθεν ὑπ' ἐμοῦ ῥηθεῖσα μέθοδος ἀπέδειξεν ὡς
δεῖ ζητεῖν· ὑμεῖς δ' οὔτ' ἀπόδειξιν οὐδεμίαν[14] οὔτε
λόγον οὐδένα πιθανὸν ἐπεχειρήσατε εἰπεῖν, ἀλλ' ἀνα-
τείναντες τὰς ὀφρῦς ἐπιτιμᾶτε μόνον ἡμῖν σεμνῶς,
ἀποχωρεῖν τῆς ἄκρας φυσιολογίας κελεύοντες καὶ μὴ
ζητεῖν οὕτω φύσιν ἀνθρώπου καταμαθεῖν ὡς οἱ φιλόσοφοι καταμανθάνουσιν, ἄχρι τῶν πρώτων στοιχείων
ἀνιόντες τῷ λόγῳ καὶ τοῦτο ὑμῖν ἀπόχρη μόνον εἰπεῖν,
ὡς ἀρτηρίαν καὶ φλέβα καὶ νεῦρον ἀρχὰς προσεχεῖς
καὶ οἷον στοιχεῖα χρὴ τίθεσθαι τῆς περὶ τὸν ἄνθρωπον φυσιολογίας.

καί τις ἐπήνεσεν ἐν τούτῳ τὸν Ἡρόφιλον εἰπόντα
κατὰ λέξιν οὕτως· Ἔστω ταῦτα εἶναι πρῶτα, εἰ καὶ μή
ἐστι πρῶτα. τὸν δ' εἰς ἀπόδειξιν προκαλούμενον ἐξ-

---

[14] ἀπόδειξιν ὡς οὐ χρὴ ζητεῖν οὐδεμίαν B

---

[14] This reference is undoubtedly to Hippocrates' *On the Na-*

ing with each other, but give their vote to one, or that I first listen to each of your arguments one at a time, and examine and consider among them which is consistent with itself and with the phenomena, and which is consistent neither with itself nor with the phenomena? And if I were to do this, I would at least listen to the Empirics when they at- 107K tempt to justify what they say, even if they don't offer a certain demonstration. But you do not even do this. I would gladly give a hearing to whichever one of you attempted to provide an explanation or demonstration as to why it is not necessary to seek the cause of the function. For the method I stated previously showed that it is necessary to seek this. But you don't attempt any demonstration nor do you articulate any credible argument. Instead, you just raise your eyebrows and rebuke us haughtily, telling us to abandon the high peaks of natural science and not to seek to understand the nature of man in the way the philosophers understand it—that is, advancing by reason as far as the primary elements.[14] It should be enough for you to say this alone: that we should posit artery, vein and nerve as proximate principles[15] and we should lay down elements, as it were, of the natural science that pertains to man.

Someone praised Herophilus when he spoke these exact words: "Let these things be primary even if they are not primary."[16] But when someone challenges you to provide

---

ture of Man and Galen's own De elementis secundum Hippocratem (I.413–508K). Galen also wrote a commentary on Hippocrates' work (XV.1–173K).

15 The reference is to Erasistratus' "triplokia"—i.e., nerves, veins, and arteries.

16 See H. von Staden (1989), pp. 117–19.

ἐλέγχοντά τε τὰς ὑποθέσεις τῶν ταῦτα δοξαζόντων
108K ἑαυταῖς μαχομένας ἀπωθεῖσθε καὶ φεύγετε | καὶ τὴν
ἀρχὴν οὐδὲ παρέχετε τὰ ὦτα καὶ καταφρονεῖν προσ-
ποιεῖσθε καὶ μισόλογοι γίγνεσθε νῦν, οἱ τὸν λόγον
καὶ τὴν ἀπόδειξιν ἐπανατείνομενοι τοῖς Ἐμπειρικοῖς.
ὅτι γὰρ ἑαυτοῖς οἱ λόγοι διαφέρονται ἁπάντων τῶν ἐξ
ἡμίσεος Δογματιζόντων, εὐφωρότατόν ἐστι τοῦτο τῷ
κἂν βραχὺ γεγυμνασμένῳ κατὰ τὰς ἀποδεικτικὰς
μεθόδους. ἐπειδὰν μὲν γὰρ φλεγμαίνῃ γαστὴρ καὶ διὰ
τοῦτο πέττειν ἀρρωστῇ, τίς ἡ τῆς φλεγμονῆς ἐστιν
αἰτία ζητεῖν δικαιοῦσι, κἀντεῦθεν εὐποροῦσι τῶν ἰαμάτων, ἀποχωροῦντες τῆς ἐμπειρικῆς εὑρέσεως· ἐπειδὰν δὲ χωρὶς φλεγμονῆς, ἢ τοιούτου τινὸς ἄλλου
παθήματος, ὑπὸ δυσκρασίας μόνης ἀρρωστῇ πέττειν,
ἐνταῦθα πάλιν ἐκ τῆς ἐμπειρίας αὐτῆς[15] ἡ τῶν βοηθημάτων εὐπορία. καὶ μὴν ἀλλήλοις μὲν ταῦτα μάχεται, τὰ δὲ τῶν Ἐμπειρικῶν ὁμολογεῖ, καὶ ἀποδείκνυσί
τε καὶ περαίνει τὸ σφέτερον ἐξ ὧν αὐτοὶ ὑμεῖς συγ-
χωρεῖτε λημμάτων.

εἰ γὰρ ὅλως δυνατόν ἐστιν ἐπὶ φαινομένοις συμ-
πτώμασι τετηρῆσθαι θεραπείαν, ἀγνοουμένης τῆς
διαθέσεως, οὐκ ἐπὶ μὲν τῆσδε δυνατόν, ἐφ' ἑτέρας δ'
ἀδύνατον, ἀλλ' ἐπὶ πασῶν ὁμοίως ἔσται δυνατόν.
109K τοιγαροῦν | οὐδ' ἐνταῦθα λόγον οὐδένα λέγειν ἕξετε
τοῦ μὴ τὴν ἐμπειρίαν αὐτάρκη γίγνεσθαι πρὸς τὴν
τῶν βοηθημάτων εὐπορίαν, ἐφ' οἷς τὴν διάθεσιν εὑρεῖν ἀδυνατεῖτε. πάντα οὖν ὡς τύραννοι προστάττετε,
χρῆσθαι δ' ἀποδείξεσιν οὔτ' αὐτοὶ βούλεσθε, βέλτιον

demonstration and refute the hypotheses of those holding
a belief in these things by showing they are mutually exclusive, you reject and run away from him, and do not even   108K
lend your ears to begin with. You pretend to despise him,
and now you become haters of argument, you who held up
both argument and demonstration against the Empirics. It
is very easy to see, even for someone only slightly practiced
in the demonstrative methods, that the arguments of all
the "semi-Dogmatics" conflict with each other. So, whenever the stomach is inflamed, and because of this digestion is weak, they think it right to seek out the cause of
the inflammation and, on that basis, find ways of treatment, eschewing empirical discovery. But whenever, in
the absence of inflammation or some other such affection,
digestion is weak due to a *dyskrasia* alone, the provision of
remedies is, on the contrary, from experience itself. Furthermore, these actions are inconsistent with each other,
whereas those of the Empirics are consistent, and they
demonstrate and conclude their own business from the
premises that you yourselves agree on.

If it is possible, in general, to make trial of a treatment
on the basis of the apparent symptoms even though the
condition is not known, it would not be possible in some
cases and impossible in others, but will be equally possible
in all cases. For that very reason you will not be able to   109K
state here any argument that experience is not sufficient in
itself for the provision of remedies in those instances in
which you are unable to discover the condition. Therefore,
as tyrants do, you order all these things, although you yourselves are unwilling to use demonstrations—for it is better,

15 αὐτοῖς B, P1, P2

γὰρ ἴσως εἰπεῖν τοῦτο τοῦ μὴ δύνασθαι, καὶ τοῖς
βουλομένοις τε ἅμα καὶ δυναμένοις οὐχ ἕπεσθε. τί
ποτ᾽ οὖν ἄλλο εἰσὶν ὑμῶν οἱ λόγοι πλὴν ἔρις καὶ
φιλονεικία καὶ πρόκλησις εἰς λοιδορίας καὶ μάχας,
οἵας καὶ τῶν ὑμετέρων διδασκάλων τις ἐποιεῖτο διὰ
παντός, ἢ καταγελῶν εἴ τις ἐφθέγξατο θερμὸν καὶ
ψυχρόν, ὡς βαλανεῦσι μᾶλλον, οὐκ ἰατροῖς προσ-
ηκόντων ὀνομάτων, ἢ σφοδρῶς ἐπιτιμῶν, ὡς ἀποχω-
ροῦντι πόρρω τῆς ἰατρικῆς, ἢ τὴν Ἐρασιστράτου
προχειριζόμενος ἀξιοπιστίαν. ἀλλὰ ταύτην μὲν πρῶτον ἀκούσας ἥσθην, δεύτερον δὲ καὶ τρίτον ἀκούων
ἐμίσησα, βωμολοχίᾳ μᾶλλον, οὐκ ἰατρικῇ πρέπειν
ἡγησάμενος. εἰ γὰρ ἅπαξ ἡ τῶν κελευσάντων μὴ
προσωτέρω χωρεῖν ἀξιοπιστία μάρτυς ἱκανὴ πρὸς
110K ἀπόδειξιν εἶναι νομισθήσεται, λῆρος ἤδη | μακρὸς
ἔσται πάντα, καὶ πέρας οὐδὲν ἐν τοῖς διαλόγοις ἀλλ᾽ ἢ
τοῦθ᾽ ὅπερ νῦν ὁρᾶτε γιγνόμενον, ἔχθρα καὶ μάχη καὶ
λοιδορία. τοῖς γὰρ ἀποχωρήσασι μὲν τῶν λογικῶν
ἀποδείξεων, ὅτι δ᾽ Ἡρόφιλος οὕτως ἐκέλευσεν ἢ Ἐρασίστρατος, ἀξιοῦσι πιστεύειν, ἀνάγκη πᾶσαν λοιδο-
ρίαν καὶ μάχην ἀκολουθῆσαι, τὰ θαυμαστὰ τῶν νῦν
διαλόγων ἆθλα.

φέρε γὰρ ἑτέρου μέν τινος λέγοντος ὡς τῷδέ τινι
τῷ μὴ πέπτοντι καλῶς ἡ γαστὴρ δύσκρατος ἐπὶ τὸ
ξηρότερόν τε καὶ ψυχρότερον ἐγένετο, καὶ διὰ τοῦτ᾽
αὐτὴν ὑγραντέον τ᾽ ἐστὶ καὶ θερμαντέον, ἑτέρου δέ
τινος, ἐκτροπῆς τοῦ κατὰ φύσιν ἐπὶ τὸ ψυχρότερόν τε
καὶ ὑγρότερον ἀπεργασθείσης, θερμὰ καὶ ξηρὰ τὰ

perhaps, to say this than to say you are unable to—and you do not follow those who both are willing to and, at the same time, are able to. For what else are these arguments of yours but strife and contentiousness, and a challenge to abuse and dispute, such as one of your teachers also used to engage in continually, either mocking if someone spoke about hot and cold, as being terms more suitable for bath-house attendants than doctors, or vehemently censuring them for straying far from the medical art, or putting forward Erasistratus as an authority. Although, when I first heard this, I was pleased, on the second and third hearing I hated it, thinking it more suitable for buffoonery than for the medical art. For if just once the credibility of those who forbid us to advance any further will be thought to be sufficient evidence for demonstration, everything will now   110K be great nonsense, and there will be no end to the debates but that which you now see occurring—enmity, conflict and abuse. For those who depart from logical demonstrations and see fit to believe because Herophilus and Erasistratus urged them to, it is inevitable that every abuse and contention will follow. These are the wonderful prizes for the debates of our own day.

Well then, let us suppose there is someone who says that, in a person who does not digest properly, the stomach is *dyskratic* in terms of being too dry and too cold and, because of this, we must moisten and warm it, whereas someone else claims that the departure from normal is brought about by [the stomach] being too cold and too moist, and

διαιτήματα προσφέρεσθαι συμβουλεύοντος· καὶ ἄλλος τις τρίτος παρελθών, ὡς μὲν οὐκ ὀρθῶς εἴρηται τῶν εἰρημένων ὁτιοῦν μηδ' ἐπιχειρήσειεν ⟨ἂν⟩[16] ἀντειπεῖν, μόνον δ' ἐπιτιμῶν ὡς περιττὰ ζητοῦσι, καὶ μάρτυρα τὸν Ἐρασίστρατον ἢ τὸν Ἡρόφιλον ἐπάγοιτο· πῶς οὐχ, ὅπερ ἔφην, ἀρχὴ διαφορᾶς ἐντεῦθεν ἔσται καὶ λοιδορίας τῆς πρὸς ἀλλήλοις; ἀνάγκη γὰρ δήπου κἀκείνους, Ἀθήναιον καὶ Μνησίθεον καὶ Διοκλέα καὶ
111K Πλειστόνικον, | Ἱπποκράτην τε καὶ Φιλιστίωνα καὶ μυρίους ἑτέρους τοιούτους ἐπικαλέσασθαι μάρτυρας. εἰ γὰρ δὴ κατὰ μάρτυρας χρὴ διαιρεῖσθαι τὸν λόγον, οὐ σμικρῷ τινι κρατήσουσιν· ὅτι τε γὰρ τῆς νοσώδους δυσκρασίας εἴδη πολλὰ καὶ ὅτι καθ' ἕκαστον ἡ θεραπεία διάφορος οὐχ Ἱπποκράτην μόνον, ἢ ἄλλους παμπόλλους ἰατρούς, ἀλλὰ καὶ Πλάτωνα καὶ Ἀριστοτέλην καὶ Θεόφραστον καὶ Ζήνωνα καὶ Χρύσιππον, ἅπαντάς τε τοὺς ἐλλογίμους φιλοσόφους παρεχόμενοι μάρτυρας· ὅτι τε χωρὶς τοῦ τὴν φύσιν εὑρεθῆναι τοῦ σώματος ἀκριβῶς οὐχ οἷόν τ' ἐστὶν οὔτε περὶ νοσημάτων διαφορᾶς ἐξευρεῖν οὐδὲν οὔτε ἰαμάτων εὐπορῆσαι προσηκόντως, ἅπαντας πάλιν τοὺς νῦν εἰρημένους μοι φιλοσόφους τε καὶ ἰατρούς, οὐ προστάττοντας μὰ Δί' ὡς οὗτοι δίκην τυράννων, ἀλλ' ἀποδεικνύντας παρέξονται.

πρὸς ταῦτ' οὖν οἱ τὸ θερμὸν καὶ ψυχρὸν βαλανέων, οὐκ ἰατρῶν ὀνόματα φάσκοντες εἶναι βωμολοχεύσονται δηλονότι καὶ γελωτοποιήσουσιν, ἢ μωρούς, ἢ Φρύγας, ἢ σχολαστικοὺς διηγούμενοι· συνίσασι γὰρ

advises the application of a regimen directed at heat and dryness. Then some other third person could come along and, without even attempting to gainsay anything that has been said, simply censure those who seek superfluous things, calling upon Erasistratus and Herophilus as witnesses. How will this not be a starting point for dispute and abuse among them, as I said? For it is necessary, I presume, for those men also to call upon witnesses— Athenaeus, Mnesitheus, Diocles, Pleistonicus, Hippocrates, Philistion and other such men in countless numbers— and if the argument should really be determined on the basis of witnesses, they will prevail by no small margin. That there are many kinds of pathological *dyskrasia* and that the treatment is different for each, they provide as witnesses not only Hippocrates and a great many other doctors, but also Plato, Aristotle, Theophrastus, Zeno, and Chrysippus, as well as all the noted philosphers. That without the nature of the body being discovered precisely it is impossible either to find out about the differentiae of diseases, or to find suitable means of remedies, they will again provide all these philosophers and doctors now spoken of by me—men who do not, by Zeus, command like these people in the manner of tyrants, but will provide demonstrations.

111K

In these matters, then, those who claim that hot and cold are the terms of bathhouse attendants and not of doctors will clearly be indulging in ribaldry and making mockery, describing them as fools, or Phrygians, or pedants, for

---

16 ἂν conj. nos

ἑαυτοῖς οὐ μόνον ἀποδεικτικὸν ἐπισταμένοις οὐδέν,
112K ἀλλ᾽ οὐδ᾽ ὅ τι | ποτέ ἐστιν ἀπόδειξις ἐπαΐουσιν. ἐκ
τούτων οὖν τῶν σκωμμάτων ἀνάγκη γενήσεσθαι διαφορᾶς ἀρχήν· ἵνα γὰρ τοῦ πρώτου πάντων ὧν οἱ
χωρὶς ἀποδείξεως φλυαροῦντες οὐκ ὀκνοῦσι λέγειν
ἐπιμνησθῶ, σκέψαι πῶς ἀναγκαῖόν ἐστιν ἀκολουθῆσαι μάχην αὐτῷ. πρὸς γὰρ τὰς ἀναποδείκτους φάσεις
αὐτῶν καὶ τοὺς ἀξιοπίστους μάρτυρας, ὅταν ἕτεροί
τινες ἐνδοξοτέρους τε καὶ πολὺ πλείονας ἀντιπροτεί-
νωνται μάρτυρας, ἀναγκαῖον ἢ συγχωρεῖν καὶ ἡτ-
τᾶσθαι κατ᾽ ἄμφω νενικημένους, ἔν τε τῷ μὴ συνακο-
λουθῆσαι πρὸς τὴν ἀπόδειξιν κἂν τῷ κεκρατῆσθαι
πρὸς τοῦ πλήθους τῶν μαρτύρων, ἢ ἀναισχυντήσαν-
τας Ἐρασίστρατον ἁπάντων ἐκείνων τῶν μαρτύρων
ἀποφαίνεσθαι πιστότερον. ἀνάγκη γὰρ ἐνταῦθα τὸν
μὲν εἰπεῖν ὡς οὐκ ἦν πιστότερος οὔτε τῶν περὶ τὸν
Ἱπποκράτην καὶ Μνησίθεον ἰατρῶν οὔτε τῶν περὶ τὸν
Ἀριστοτέλη τε καὶ Πλάτωνα φιλοσόφων, τὸν δ᾽ ὡς
ἀντειπεῖν· εἶτ᾽ ἄνω καὶ κάτω τῆς τοιαύτης ἀντιλογίας
φερομένης οὕτως ἀπαίδευτά τε καὶ φιλόνεικα[17] προ-
αχθῆναι τὸν ἕτερον αὐτῶν εἰπεῖν ὡς Οὐκ ἔσται οὕτω
σοι καλῶς, ἢν Ἐρασίστρατον ἀτιμάζῃς. ταυτὶ γὰρ
113K ὁρᾷς ἑκάστης ἡμέρας, ὦ Ἱέρων, γιγνόμενα κατὰ | τοὺς
τῶν ἰατρῶν διαλόγους·

τοιαύτης δ᾽ ἅπαξ ἀνοιχθείσης ὁδοῦ, πάντ᾽ ἐπιρρεῖ
τὰ τῶν γυναικῶν ἤδη ῥήματα καὶ κακῶς εἰπόντες
ἀλλήλους, οὐ διδάξαντές τι χρηστὸν ἢ μαθόντες
ἀπαλλάττονται. καὶ τῆς τοιαύτης ἀσχημοσύνης οὐκ

174

they realize that they themselves not only know nothing about demonstration, but they have no understanding at all of what it is. From these jokes there will inevitably arise a source of difference. So let me mention the first of all the things they do not hesitate to say when they talk nonsense without [providing] demonstration, and consider how, inevitably, conflict follows this. Whenever others bring forward a far greater number of more highly regarded witnesses against the undemonstrated statements of these men and their plausible witnesses, it is necessary for them either to concede that they have been defeated and are worsted in both respects—that they do not attend to demonstration, and that they have been overcome by the quantity of witnesses—or else to declare quite shamelessly that Erasistratus is more credible than all those witnesses. For it is necessary to say here that he was not more credible than the doctors who follow Hippocrates and Mnesitheus, or the philosophers in the circle of Plato and Aristotle, and for the other to argue against this. When this sort of argument has gone back and forth in this ignorant and contentious way, the latter is led to say, "It will not go well for you if you dishonour Erasistratus." You see this sort of thing happening every day, Hiero, in the debates among doctors.

112K

113K

Once this sort of path has been opened up, all the words of women now flow along it, and they abuse one another and then go away, neither learning nor teaching anything useful. And it cannot be said that those who shun demon-

---

17 B, K; ἀπαιδεύτου τε καὶ φιλονείκου P1, P2, *recte fort.*

ἔστιν εἰπεῖν ὡς οὐχ οἱ τὰς ἀποδείξεις ἀποδιδράσκον-
τες ἄρχουσιν· ἀποδιδράσκουσι δ᾽, ὡς οἶσθα, πολυειδῶς, οἱ μὲν σεμνῶς ἐπιτιμήσαντες μόνον, οἱ δὲ κομ-
ψευσάμενοί τι βωμολοχικόν, οἱ δ᾽ εἰς γέλωτα καὶ
χλεύην ἐξάγοντες τὸν διάλογον· εἰ δέ τις καὶ τολ-
μήσειε παραμεῖναί τε τῷ λόγῳ καὶ τῶν ἀποδείξεων
ἐπακοῦσαι, μάλιστα μὲν οὐδ᾽ ἕπεται τὴν ἀρχήν, οὐ
γὰρ ἐνδέχεται τὸν ἀγύμναστον ἀποδεικτικῆς μεθόδου
τοῖς χρωμένοις αὐτῇ παρακολουθεῖν·

εἰ δ᾽ ἄρα καὶ μέχρι τινὸς παρακολουθήσειεν, ἀλλὰ
τῷ πάντως ἐπαμύνειν ἐθέλειν οἷς ἐνετράφη δόγμασιν,
ἐπιχειρῶν ἀντιλέγειν, εἶτ᾽ ἐξελεγχόμενος, ἀπέραντα
καὶ ἀσυλλόγιστα καὶ περιττὰ καὶ ληρώδη φλυαρῶν,
ἀγανακτεῖ καὶ καταρᾶται τοῖς διαλεκτικοῖς, ὡς κακῶν
αἰτίοις, ὅτι δηλαδὴ τὴν κόρυζαν ἀπομύττουσιν αὐτῶν
καὶ θεραπεύειν πειρῶνται προσφέροντες οὐ μέλι καὶ
114K πλακοῦντας, ἀλλὰ | σκόροδά τε καὶ κρόμμυα, τὰ καὶ
τοὺς κορυζῶντας ἀλεκτρυόνας ἰώμενα. παραγέγονας
γὰρ δὴ μυριάκις αὐτοῖς ὡς ὑπὸ σκορόδων ὄντως καὶ
κρομμύων τῶν ἐλέγχων ἀναγκαζομένοις δακρύειν·
οἶσθα δὲ δήπουθεν ὡς καὶ πολλοὶ πολλάκις ἡμῖν
ἐξωμολογήσαντο καταμόνας αἰσθάνεσθαι μὲν ἤδη
τῶν κατὰ τὴν σφετέραν αἵρεσιν ἀτόπων, οὐ δύνασθαι
δ᾽ ἔν γε τῷ φανερῷ μεταθέσθαι διὰ τὸ μήτ᾽ ἄλλα
γινώσκειν ἀφ᾽ ὧν τιμηθήσονται καὶ τοῖς πολλοῖς τῶν
ἀνθρώπων ἐφθακέναι ἀπὸ τούτων γιγνώσκεσθαί τε
καὶ τιμᾶσθαι. διὰ ταῦτα τοίνυν κἀγὼ πολλάκις ἀνεβαλλόμην ὑπομνήματα γράψαι μεθόδου θεραπευ-

strations are not the source of such disgraceful conduct. They shun [demonstration], as you know, in various ways. There are those who just haughtily censure it; there are those who invent something ludicrous; and there are those who lead the debate toward mockery and jest. If, however, one of them does dare to remain for the argument, and listens to the demonstrations, in the first place and above all he does not follow them, since it is impossible for someone unpracticed in the method of demonstration to follow those who use it.

If, however, one of them were to follow closely up to a certain point but, because he wishes to defend at all costs the doctrines he was brought up on, he attempts a counterargument, he is then refuted as talking inconclusive, invalid, superfluous and silly nonsense. Then he becomes irritated and brings curses down on those skilled in dialectics as agents of evil because quite clearly they wipe the snot from people's noses and attempt to treat them, not by providing honey and flat cakes, but by giving them garlic 114K and onions, which are also the cures for cocks with nasal discharge. For you have been present on countless occasions when they have been driven to tears by the refutations, just as they would really be by garlic and onions. You know, of course, that many of them have often confessed to me privately that they now perceive the absurdities of their own sect, but are unable to change their view, at least openly, because they know nothing else for which they will be held in regard, and they are already recognized and honored by the majority as a result of these things. Accordingly, because of this, I have often put off writing treatises

τικῆς, ὡς ἂν ἀκριβῶς εἰδὼς ὀλιγοστοὺς τῶν νῦν
ἀνθρώπων ὑπ' αὐτῶν ὠφεληθησομένους. εἰ μὴ γὰρ
μεγάλη τις γένοιτο καὶ δαιμονία μεταβολὴ τῶν ἀν-
θρωπείων πραγμάτων, οἴχεται πάντα τὰ καλὰ καὶ
συγκέχυται καὶ διέφθαρται, μηδενὸς ἀλήθειαν σπουδάζοντος, ἀλλὰ τὸ δόξαι μόνον. οἶσθα γὰρ δήπου καὶ
σὺ σαφῶς ὡς οὐδὲ πέντε τοῖς πᾶσιν ἀνθρώποις ἐνετύχομεν εἶναι μᾶλλον ἢ φαίνεσθαι σοφοῖς ὀρεγομένοις.
καὶ μὴν εἰ μή τις ὀρεχθείη σοφίας αὐτῆς δι' ἑαυτήν, |
115K οὐδὲ καιρὸν ἕξει τοῦ γυμνάσασθαι κατὰ τὰς λογικὰς
μεθόδους, ἀλλὰ περὶ πλοῦτον καὶ δόξαν καὶ δύναμιν
πολιτικὴν ἐσπουδακώς, περὶ τὴν ἐν ἐκείνοις ἀσχολίαν
ἅπαντα κατατρίψει τὸν βίον.

6. Ἐάσαντες οὖν αὐτούς, πάλιν ἐπὶ τὸ προκείμενον
ἴωμεν. ἔστι τὸ προκείμενον ἐξ ἀρχῆς, ὡς εἰ μή τις
ἅπαντα τὸν ἀριθμὸν τῶν νοσημάτων ἐξεύροι μεθόδῳ,
πταίσει μέγιστον πταῖσμα κατὰ τὴν ἀρχὴν εὐθὺς
αὐτῆς τῆς θεραπευτικῆς μεθόδου· πρόδηλον γὰρ ὡς
τοσούτους χρὴ τρόπους εἶναι τῆς ἰάσεως ὅσαιπερ καὶ
αἱ τῶν νοσημάτων ἰδέαι. τὸ τοίνυν μήτ' ἄπειρα ποιῆσαι τὰ νοσήματα ταῖς κατὰ μέρος ἰδιότησι προσ-
έχοντας μήτ' εὐθὺς ἐν τοῖς πρώτοις καταμεῖναι γε-
νέσιν οὐ τοῦ τυχόντος ἐστίν, ἀλλ' ἀνδρός, ὡς καὶ
πρόσθεν ἐδείκνυτο, πάνυ γεγυμνασμένου κατὰ τὰς
διαιρετικὰς μεθόδους. ἀρχὴ δὲ τῆς διαιρέσεως αὐτῶν,
ὥς που καὶ τοῦτ' ἐλέγετο, τὸν λόγον τῆς οὐσίας τοῦ
διαιρουμένου πράγματος ἀφορίσασθαι. καὶ τοίνυν
ἐδείκνυτο πάντως μὲν ἔν τι τῶν παρὰ φύσιν ὑπαρ-

on the method of medicine because I know very well that few people nowadays would be benefited by them. For unless some great and miraculous change were to occur in human affairs, all good things get lost, confused and destroyed, and nobody is eager for truth, but only for reputation. You know also, I presume, and clearly, that I have not encountered five in all who desire to be wise rather than to appear to be [wise]. And furthermore, if someone does not desire wisdom for its own sake, he will not take any opportunity to gain practice in the logical methods but, having an established desire for wealth, reputation and political power, he will waste his whole life in the pursuit of those things. 115K

6. Therefore, having done with these people, let me return again to the matter in hand. This is what was proposed at the outset: unless someone discovers the total number of diseases by method, he will take a giant false step right at the start of the therapeutic method itself. It is quite clear that there must be the same number of forms of treatment as there are kinds of diseases. Accordingly, the man who avoids creating an infinite number of diseases by attending to the specific instances individually, and who does not stop immediately at the first classes is no ordinary man. He is a man who is particularly practiced in the methods of division, as was shown earlier. A first principle of their division is to mark off the definition of the substance of the matter being divided, as I also said somewhere else. So it was shown that disease is, assuredly, one of the things that

χόντων νόσημα. τεττάρων δ' ὄντων τῶν παρὰ φύσιν,
116K ἤτοι τῆς βεβλαμμένης ἐνεργείας, | ἢ τῆς ἐργαζομένης
αὐτὴν διαθέσεως, ἢ τῆς¹⁸ ταύτην ποιούσης αἰτίας, ἢ
τῶν ἑπομένων αὐτῇ συμπτωμάτων, εἴτε τὴν βλάβην
τῆς ἐνεργείας εἴτε καὶ τὴν ἐργαζομένην αὐτὴν διάθεσιν ἐθέλοι τις ὀνομάζειν νόσον, οὐδὲν τοῦτο τὴν θεραπευτικὴν μέθοδον ὑπαλλάττειν ἐδείκνυμεν, εἰ τοῦθ' ἓν
μόνον γιγνώσκοι, τὸ τὴν πρώτην θεραπείαν, ἣν δήπου
καὶ προσεχῆ καλοῦσιν ἔνιοι, τῆς τὴν ἐνέργειαν ἐμποδιζούσης εἶναι διαθέσεως. ἐπιδεδεῖχθαι δ' ἡμῖν ἐλέγομεν ὡς ταύτην εὐλογώτερον εἴη προσαγορεύειν νόσημα, μὴ μέντοι κωλύειν ἡμᾶς εἴ τις ἐθέλοι τὴν μὲν τῆς
ἐνεργείας βλάβην ὀνομάζειν νόσημα, τὴν δ' ἐργαζομένην αὐτὴν διάθεσιν αἰτίαν τοῦ νοσήματος.

ὑποθέμενοι δὲ καλεῖσθαι νόσημα διάθεσιν παρὰ
φύσιν ἐνέργειαν βλάπτουσαν ἐζητήσαμεν ἐφεξῆς
ὁπόσα τὰ σύμπαντ' ἐστὶ νοσήματα. πρόδηλον δ' ἦν ἐν
τούτῳ τὸ δεῖν ἐξευρεῖν πρῶτον, εἴ τις ὁδῷ καὶ τάξει
μέλλει προϊέναι καὶ μὴ καθάπερ οἱ πολλοὶ τῶν ἰατρῶν
ὡς τύραννοι προστάττειν, ἥτις ποτὲ διάθεσίς ἐστιν ἡ
τῆς ἐνεργείας αἰτία δραστική. ταύτην οὖν ἡμεῖς μὲν
εὐκρασίαν ἐλέγομεν εἶναι θερμοῦ καὶ ψυχροῦ, ὑγροῦ
117K καὶ ξηροῦ· καὶ διὰ τοῦθ' ἡ πρώτη νόσος ἡ | ἐν τοῖς
ὁμοιομερέσι, τῇ δυσκρασίᾳ τούτων ἐδείκνυτο γίγνεσθαι.

ἕτερος δέ τις ἐν ὄγκοις καὶ πόροις θήσεται τὴν
τούτων συμμετρίαν, καὶ διὰ τοῦτ' ἀμετρίᾳ τῶν πόρων

180

is contrary to nature. However, there are four things contrary to nature: function that has been damaged, the condition bringing this about, the cause creating the condition, and the symptoms which follow it. I demonstrated that if someone wishes to term "disease" either the damage of function or the condition bringing this about, this does not change the method of treatment in any way, provided he knows this one thing alone—that the primary treatment (which is, I presume, what some call proximate) is of the condition hindering function. I have shown, as I said, that it is more reasonable to call this a disease. I shall not, however, stand in the way of someone who might wish to call the damage of function "disease," and the condition bringing this about the "cause" of the disease.

Having established that a condition contrary to nature which damages function is to be called a disease, I sought out, as a next step, how many diseases there are in all. And it was absolutely clear in this that if someone intends to proceed in an orderly way, and not by giving orders like a tyrant as many doctors do, what must be discovered first is whatever the condition is that is the effective cause of function. I said that this is a *eukrasia* of hot and cold, moist and dry. And because of this the primary disease, which is in the *homoiomeres*, was shown to come about through a *dyskrasia* of these [qualities].

Someone else will, however, place [the effective cause of function] in the balance of corpuscles and pores and, because of this, will place disease in organisms in an imbal-

116K

117K

---

18 B, P1, P2; τήν K

αὐτῶν νοσήσειν τὰ ζῷα. τὸ δὲ μήτ' αὐτὸν ἀποφήνασθαι τολμῆσαι τῆς ἐνεργείας τὴν αἰτίαν ἐν ὁτῳδήποτε
γένει τῶν ὄντων ἐστί, μήτε τοῖς λέγουσιν ἀντειπόντα
νομίζειν ἔτι λόγῳ καὶ μεθόδῳ προϊέναι, δεινῶς ἐλέγομεν εἶναι μοχθηρόν, ἅμα μὲν ἄφυκτον ἐργαζόμενον
τὴν ἐκ τῶν Ἐμπειρικῶν κατηγορίαν, ἅμα δὲ αὑτῷ
μαχόμενον· ἐξ ἡμίσεος γὰρ δὴ τοὺς τοιούτους εἶναι
Λογικούς· ὅπως μὲν δὴ γίγνεται φλεγμονὴ καὶ σκίρρος καὶ οἴδημα καὶ πάνθ' ὅσα τοιαῦτα, πολυπραγμο-
νοῦνται, ὅτι δὲ καὶ χωρὶς τούτων ἁπάντων κατὰ δυσκρασίαν μόνην ἐνέργεια βλάπτεται μὴ γινώσκονται,
ἀλλ' ἐμπειρικῶς τὰ τοιαῦτα θεραπεύονται.

ὅστις οὖν βούλεται γνῶναι πόσον ἁμαρτάνουσιν οἱ
τοιοῦτοι καὶ πόσον τι πλῆθος ὑπερβαίνουσι νοσημάτων καὶ ὡς πολὺ πλέον ἀγνοοῦσιν ἢ γιγνώσκουσι,
τὸ Περὶ διαφορᾶς νοσημάτων ἀναλεξάσθω γράμμα·
μαθήσεται γὰρ ὡς ὀρθῇ μὲν ὁδῷ πρῶτος ἁπάντων
118K Ἱπποκράτης ἐχρήσατο, δέον δ' αὐτὴν τελειῶσαι | τοὺς
μετ' αὐτόν, οὐχ ὅπως οὐδεὶς ἐτελείωσεν, ἀλλὰ καὶ τὰ
καλῶς εὑρημένα διέφθειραν οἱ πλεῖστοι. πλησίον δὲ
τοῦ τελειῶσαί τε καὶ συμπληρῶσαι τὴν ὑφ' Ἱπποκράτους παραδοθεῖσαν ὁδὸν οἱ περὶ τὸν Ἀριστοτέλην
τε καὶ Θεόφραστον ἀφίκοντο, καὶ εἰ χρὴ τἀληθὲς
εἰπεῖν, ἐτελείωσαν δυνάμει διορισάμενοι τὸ μὴ ταὐτὸν
εἶναι γένος τῶν νοσημάτων ἔν τε τοῖς ὁμοιομερέσι
σώμασιν ἔν τε τοῖς ὀργανικοῖς ὀνομαζομένοις. ὑπὸ

---

[17] This is, of course, the Methodic position. For a summary of

ance of these same pores.[17] I said that someone who neither dares to declare whatever class of existents the cause
of function is in, nor refutes those who do, and still thinks
he proceeds by logic and method, is terribly mistaken
since, at one and the same time, he makes the charge of the
Empirics inescapable and he contradicts himself. In fact,
such people are "semi-Dogmatics." They busy themselves
with how inflammation, induration, edema, and all other
such things come about, yet they don't know that, apart
from all these things, function is damaged in *dyskrasia*
alone, so they treat such things in the manner of the Empirics.

Therefore, let anyone who wishes to know the degree
to which such people are mistaken, how great a number of
diseases they overlook, and how many more things they are
ignorant of than they know, read the book *On the Differentiae of Diseases*.[18] For he will learn how Hippocrates was
the first of all to use the right path, and how, although   118K
his successors needed to complete this path, nobody did
bring it to completion. Instead, the majority destroyed the
things that had been discovered properly. Aristotle, Theophrastus and their followers came close to completing and
filling out the path handed down by Hippocrates and, truth
to tell, by distinguishing that the classes of diseases in *homoiomerous* bodies and in the so-called organic structures
were not the same, they did virtually bring it to comple-

their theory, see the Introduction, section 2. For a more detailed
account, see J. Vallance (1990).

[18] *De morborum differentiis*, translated by I. Johnston (2006),
pp. 131–57. In fact, Hippocrates is not mentioned by name in this
work.

μὲν γὰρ τῶν ὁμοιομερῶν τὰς ἐνεργείας γίγνεσθαι καὶ
διὰ τοῦτ' εἶναι καθ' ἕκαστον τῶν ὀργάνων ἕν ἴδιον
ὁμοιομερές. ὅσα δ' ἄλλα μετὰ τούτου συμπληροῖτο
πᾶν ὄργανον, ἕνεκα χρείας τινὸς ἐκείνου τοῦ πρώτου
τῆς ἐνεργείας αἰτίου γεγονέναι. καὶ τούτων μέντοι
πάλιν αὐτῶν ἑκάστου κατὰ μόνας ὑπάρχειν ἐνέργειαν,
οἷον ἐπὶ τῶν ὀφθαλμῶν. ἄμεινον γὰρ ἴσως, ὡς ἐν
ἑτέροις ἐπὶ πλέον ἐδείξαμεν, ἐνταυθοῖ διὰ βραχέων
ὑπομνήσεις ποιήσασθαι.

τὸ μὲν τῆς ὄψεως ὄργανόν ἐστι τὸ κρυσταλλοειδὲς
ὑγρόν, ἕκαστον δὲ τῶν ἄλλων μορίων ἐκείνου χάριν
ἐγένετο. καὶ πάντων εἰρήκαμεν αὐτῶν τὰς χρείας ἐν τῷ
119K δεκάτῳ τῆς Περὶ χρείας μορίων πραγματείας. | ἀλλ' εἰ
καὶ ὅτι μάλιστα τοῦ κρυσταλλοειδοῦς ἕνεκεν ἐγένετο
σύμπαντα, κατὰ μέρος γοῦν ἕκαστον αὐτῶν ἐνεργείας
τινὸς μετέχει, κοινῆς μὲν ὅλῳ τῷ ζῴῳ φλὲψ καὶ ἀρτηρία καὶ νεῦρον· οἱ δ' ὑμένες οἱ κατὰ τὸν ὀφθαλμόν, ὡς
ἂν τρεφόμενοι δηλονότι καὶ τῶν φυσικῶν ἐξ ἀνάγκης
μετέχουσι δυνάμεων, ὥστε καὶ τῶν κατ' αὐτὰς ἐνεργειῶν. ὅταν μὲν οὖν τὸ κρυσταλλοειδὲς ὑπὸ δυσκρασίας νοσήσῃ, βλάπτεται μὲν ἡ τῶν ὀφθαλμῶν ἐνέργεια πάντως, ἀλλ' οὐκ ἔστιν ὡς ὀργάνων αὐτῶν τὸ
νόσημα. τὸ δ' ὑπόχυμα καλούμενον οὐδενὸς μὲν ὁμοι-
ομεροῦς ἐστι πάθους, ὅλων δὲ τῶν ὀφθαλμῶν ὡς
ὀργάνων.

οὕτω δὲ κἂν εἰ γλίσχρων τινῶν ἢ παχέων χυμῶν
ἔμφραξις ἐν τοῖς πέρασι τῶν κατὰ τὰ σιμὰ τοῦ ἥπατος εἴη φλεβῶν, ἐμποδισθήσεται μὲν ἡ ἀνάδοσις,

tion. For it is through the *homoiomeres* that functions occur, and because of this, there is one specific *homoiomere*
for each of the organs. However many other things there
are that complete the whole organ along with this exist for
the sake of some use of that primary cause of its function.
And, of course, there is again a function of each of these
things individually, like in the case of the eyes. It is better,
perhaps, since I have set this out at greater length in other
places, to provide a brief reminder at this point.[19]

The organ of sight is the crystalline humor while each
of the other parts exists for the sake of that. I have stated
the uses of all of them in the tenth book of my treatise *On
the Use of the Parts*. But if it is the case that they too all ex-   119K
ist especially for the sake of the crystalline [humor], each
of them individually partakes of some function, one which
vein, artery, and nerve partake of in common with them in
the whole organism whereas the membranes in the eye, as
they are clearly nourished and, of necessity, partake of the
natural capacities, consequently also partake of the functions relating to these capacities. So whenever the crystalline [humor] is diseased due to a *dyskrasia*, the function of
the eyes is comprehensively damaged, but this is not as a
disease of organs themselves. On the other hand, what is
termed "cataract" is not an affection of anything *homoiomerous*, but of the whole eye as an organ.

Similarly, if there is an obstruction of certain viscid and
thick humors at the ends of the veins in the concavity of the
liver, distribution will be impeded, and the affection will

---

[19] See *De usu partium*, Book 10, III.760–89K, where Galen
gives a very detailed account of the structure and function of the
eyes. See also M. T. May (1968) for a translation.

ὅλου δ' ἔσται τοῦ ἥπατος ὡς ὀργάνου τὸ πάθος,
οὐδενὸς τῶν ὁμοιομερῶν αὐτοῦ μορίων νοσήσαντος. εἰ
δὲ δυσκρασία καταλάβοι τὰς φλέβας, αὐτῶν μὲν
ἐκείνων ἔσται τὸ νόσημα πρῶτον, κατὰ συμβεβηκὸς
δὲ καὶ τοῦ ἥπατος. Ἐρασίστρατος μὲν οὖν ἔσφαλται
περὶ τὴν οὐσίαν αὐτῆς τῆς[19] φλεγμονῆς. οὔτε γὰρ ἐν
120K τοῖς πέρασι | τῶν ἀρτηριῶν γίγνεται σφήνωσις ἐξ
ἀνάγκης ἐν τοῖς φλεγμαίνουσι μορίοις οὔτε πνεῦμα
μόνον ἐν τῷ κατὰ φύσιν αἱ ἀρτηρίαι περιέχουσιν, ὡς
ἐν τοῖς περὶ τούτων λογισμοῖς ἀπεδείξαμεν.

εἰ δ' οὖν ἐστί τι τοιοῦτον πάθος οἷον ἐκεῖνος οἴεται
φλεγμονή, καὶ σκίρρος τοιοῦτον οἷον ἐκεῖνος νομίζει,
καὶ τῶν ἄλλων ἕκαστον, ὡς αὐτὸς μὲν ἀσαφῶς ἐπὶ
πολλῶν, οἱ δ' ἀπ' αὐτοῦ πειρῶνται διέρχεσθαι σαφέστερον, ὀλίγου δεῖν ἀπαθῆ καταλείπει τὰ στερεά,
μόνον ἑλκωθῆναι δυνάμενα καὶ διατμηθῆναι καὶ θλι-
βῆναι καί τι τοιοῦτον ἕτερον ὑπομεῖναι πάθημα.
νοσεῖν δ' αὐτὰ δι' ὅλων ἑαυτῶν οὐδαμόθι φησὶ νόσους
τοιαύτας οἵας ἡμεῖς ἀπεδείξαμεν εἶναι τὰς ὀκτὼ δυσκρασίας. καὶ μὴν ὁρᾶταί γε σύμπαντα τὰ σώματα,
μέχρι καὶ τῶν δυσπαθεστάτων, οἷον χαλκοῦ καὶ λίθου
καὶ σιδήρου, θερμαινόμενά τε καὶ ψυχόμενα καὶ ξη-
ραινόμενα καὶ ὑγραινόμενα, καὶ θαυμαστὸν εἰ ἀρτηρία μόνη καὶ φλὲψ καὶ νεῦρον οὐδὲν τοιοῦτον πείσεται, καὶ τούτου θαυμαστότερον, εἰ πείσεται μέν,
ἐνεργήσει δὲ ἀμέμπτως, οἷον ἐπὶ τῆς καρδίας, εἰ |

19 αὐτῆς τῆς P1 P2; αὐτὴν τῆς B; αὐτῆς καὶ K

be of the whole liver as an organ since none of its *homoi-omerous* parts will be diseased. If, however, a *dyskrasia* involves the veins, the disease will primarily be of those [veins] themselves and only incidentally of the liver. Therefore, Erasistratus was wrong about the essential nature of inflammation itself. It is not that blockage necessarily occurs in the ends of the arteries in inflamed parts, nor that the arteries contain *pneuma* alone in what is in accord with nature, as I showed in my considerations on these things.[20]

120K

If inflammation is the sort of affection which that man thinks it is, and induration such as he thinks, and each of the others, as he obscurely [considered] in his many [writings][21] and as his successors attempted to go over more clearly, he leaves aside the solid parts as all but impassible, in that they would only be able to be wounded, severed, or compressed, or suffer some other such affection. He says that these are in no place diseased throughout their entirety with the kinds of diseases I showed the eight *dyskrasias* to be. And yet we do in fact see all substances, right up to the most resistant, like bronze, stone, and iron, heated, cooled, dried and moistened. It would be remarkable if only arteries, veins, and nerves were not affected in this way. And it would be more remarkable still, if they are affected but function faultlessly, as for example in the case of the heart, should this happen [to be affected], whose ca-

20 See, for example, *De causis procatarcticis*, XIV.714–15.

21 None of his writings is extant. For fragments, see I. Garofalo (1988).

121K τύχοι, δύναμις μέν τίς ἐστι καὶ κατ' αὐτὸν τὸν Ἐρασίστρατον, ᾗ διαστέλλεται καὶ συστέλλεται. καὶ
βλάπτεσθαι δὲ δήπου ταύτην χρή, τῆς καρδίας ἐξαι-
ρεθείσης ζῶντος τοῦ ζῴου, καθάπερ πολλάκις ὁρῶμεν
ἐν ταῖς ἱερουργίαις γιγνόμενον· εἰ γὰρ μηδὲν βλάπτεται, κινηθήσεται διαπαντός, οὐχ ἕως χρόνου τινός, ὡς
νῦν φαίνεται. δῆλον οὖν ὅτι βλάπτεται καὶ διὰ τοῦτο
παύεται κινουμένη. τίς οὖν ἡ βλάβη, καλῶς εἶχεν
ἐπισκέψασθαι, δυναμένης γε δηλονότι τὴν βλάβην
ἀναδέξασθαι τῆς καρδίας καὶ πρὶν ἐξαιρεθῆναι τοῦ
ζῴου. τίς οὖν ἄλλη πλὴν δυσκρασίας ἐστίν; οὔτε γὰρ
τὸ σχῆμα φαίνεται μεταλλαττόμενον αὐτῆς, οὔτε κοιλότης τις, οὔτε σύνδεσμος οὔτε στόμιον, ἀλλ' οὐδ'
ἄλλο μόριον οὐδὲν ἀπολλύμενον, ἀλλὰ μόνον ἡ φυσικὴ κρᾶσις ἐξαλλαττομένη. ταῦτ' οὖν ἅπαντα τῶν
ὁμοιομερῶν, ὡς εἴρηται, νοσήματα τυγχάνοντα, τελείως αὐτῷ παραλέλειπται. τὸ γὰρ δὴ τοῦ αἵματος ἐν
τοῖς πέρασι τῶν ἀρτηριῶν σφηνωθέντος ἐνέργειάν
τινα βλαβῆναι τῶν ἀρτηριῶν ὡς ὀργάνων ἐστὶ τὸ
πάθος· ὡς δ' ὁμοιομερῶν σωμάτων, ὀκτὼ μὲν αἱ κατὰ
122K ψιλὰς τὰς ποιότητας δυσκρασίαι, | μετὰ ῥευμάτων δ'
ὀκτώ.

χρὴ τοίνυν, ὅστις τὰς τούτων ἀποδείξεις ἐπιστήμῃ
βούλεται περιλαβεῖν, ἀπὸ τοῦ Περὶ τῶν στοιχείων
ἄρξασθαι λόγου, κἄπειθ' ἑξῆς ἕκαστον ἀναλέξασθαι
τῶν ἄλλων, ὡς εἴρηται καὶ πρόσθεν. ἔστι δ' ἐφεξῆς
μὲν ἐκείνῳ τὰ Περὶ κράσεων ὑπομνήματα. καὶ τούτων

pacity, even according to Erasistratus himself, is to expand 121K
and contract. And this must certainly be damaged if the
heart is taken out of the living animal, as we frequently see
happening at sacrifices. For if it is not damaged, it will continue to move constantly, and not just for a time, as now appears to be the case. It is clear, then, that it is injured, and
because of this, it ceases to move. It is right to consider
what the damage is, since clearly the heart is also able to
suffer the damage before it is removed from the animal.
What else is it apart from *dyskrasia*? For its conformation
is obviously not undergoing change, nor is its hollowness,
ligaments or orifice. Indeed, no other part is being destroyed at all—only the natural *krasis* is changing. Thus, all
these diseases that occur in *homoiomeres*, as I said, are
completely left aside by him. For the damage to a certain
function when the blood is blocked at the ends of the arteries is the affection of the arteries as organs, whereas [the
affections of arteries] as *homoiomerous* bodies, the *dys-*
krasias in terms of bare qualities, are eight in number and 122K
those with fluxions are [also] eight in number.[22]

Anyone who wishes to grasp the demonstrations of
these things through scientific knowledge ought to start
from my work *On the Elements [according to Hippocra-*
tes], and then read through each of the others in turn, as
was said earlier. Following that, there is the treatise *On*
Krasias (On Mixtures), and after these the one *On Irregu-*

---

[22] The fluxions are yellow and black bile, blood, and phlegm.
See *De morborum causis*, VII.22–23K.

GALEN

ἐφεξῆς τὸ Περὶ τῆς ἀνωμάλου δυσκρασίας. εἶτα τὰ
Περὶ τῶν φυσικῶν δυνάμεων, ὅσα τ᾽ ἄλλα περὶ τῶν
ψυχικῶν εἴρηται παθῶν ἐφεξῆς ἑκάστης ἰδίᾳ. τούτοις
δ᾽ ἕπεται τὰ Περὶ χρείας μορίων, οἷς τὰ Περὶ τῶν
νοσημάτων τε καὶ συμπτωμάτων διαφορᾶς.

οἱ πολλοὶ δὲ τῶν ἰατρῶν, οὔτε τῇ πείρᾳ μόνῃ
προσέχοντες τὸν νοῦν, ἐνὸν αὐτοῖς ἀγαθοὺς ἰατροὺς
γίγνεσθαι καὶ κατὰ τὴν τῶν Ἐμπειρικῶν ἀγωγήν,
ὀριγνώμενοί τε τοῦ τελείου, κἄπειτα χωρὶς ἀποδείξεως
ἀποφάσεσι πιστεύοντες, ἢ μοχθηραῖς ἀποδείξεσι
παραλογισθέντες, οὐ μόνον οὐδὲν ἐξευρίσκουσι χρηστόν, ἀλλὰ καὶ τὰ διὰ τῆς ἐμπειρίας ἐγνωσμένα
διαφθείρουσιν. οὐ γὰρ δήπου σμικρὰν ἔχει δύναμιν ὁ
λόγος ὡς πρὸς τὸ κοσμῆσαι τὴν ἐμπειρίαν ἢ δια-
φθεῖραι, ἀλλ᾽ ὅσον ὁ χρηστὸς ἐπικοσμῶν προστίθη-
σιν, τοσοῦτον | ἢ καὶ πλέον ὁ μοχθηρὸς ἀφαιρεῖ. καὶ
ταῦτ᾽ ἀκούεις ἐμοῦ[20] λέγοντος ἑκάστοτε τοῖς πολλοῖς
τῶν ἰατρῶν, ὅσοι πρὶν γυμνάσασθαι κατὰ τὰς λογικὰς μεθόδους ἢ ἀποδεικνύναι τι πειρώμενοι παρα-
λογίζονται σφᾶς αὐτούς, ἢ διαιρεῖν ὁτιοῦν εἰς εἴδη τε
καὶ διαφοράς, εἶτα κἀνταῦθα κακῶν μαγείρων δίκην

123K

[20] ἐμοῦ B, P1, P2; om. K

[23] De elementis secundum Hippocratem, I.413–508K; De temperamentis, I.509–694K; De inaequali intemperie, VII.733–52K;
and De naturalibus facultatibus, II.1–214K. The first has been
translated by P. H. de Lacy (1996), the second by P. N. Singer
(1997), the third by M. Grant (2000), and the fourth by A. J. Brock
(1916).

190

lar Dyskrasia and then *On the Natural Capacities*,[23] and those treatises in which each of the affections of the *psyche* is spoken of specifically and in order.[24] Following these, there is [the work] *On the Uses of the Parts*, and following these again, the works *On the Differentiae of Diseases* and *On the Differentiae of Symptoms*.[25]

But the majority of doctors do not direct their attention to experience alone, although it would be possible for them to become good doctors too in terms of the system of the Empirics. Instead, they desire perfection, either believing claims without [supporting] demonstrations or misleading themselves by unsound demonstrations, so they not only discover nothing useful, but they also destroy those things that have become known through experience. For reason, certainly, has no small capacity for bringing order to experience or for destroying it, but whatever the man of integrity adds to it by way of adornment, so much and even more the unsound man destroys. You have heard 123K me saying these things time and again to many of the doctors who, before they become practiced in the Rationalist methods, either attempt to demonstrate something and mislead themselves by fallacious reasoning, or divide anything at all into kinds and differentiae, and then, like bad

---

24 *Quod animi mores corporis temperamenta sequuntur*, IV.767–822K; *De proprium animi cuiuslibet affectuum dignotione et curatione*, V.1–57K; and *De animi cuiuslibet peccatorum dignotione et curatione*, V.58–103K. All three are translated by P. N. Singer (1997). 25 *De usu partium*, III.1–939K and IV.1–366K; translated by M. T. May (1968). *De differentiis morborum*, VI.836–80K and *De symptomatum differentiis*, VII.42–84K, both translated by I. Johnston (2006).

οὐ κατ' ἄρθρα τέμνουσιν, ἀλλὰ συντρίβουσί τε καὶ
θλῶσι καὶ διασπῶσιν, ὥσπερ κἀπὶ τοῦ νῦν ἡμῖν
προκειμένου. συμβουλεύω δὴ πᾶσιν, ὡς οἶσθα, τοῖς
τοιούτοις τῇ πείρᾳ προσέχειν τὸν νοῦν. οὐ σμικρὸς
γὰρ ὁ κίνδυνος ἅπαντι τῷ μειζόνων ἢ καθ' ἑαυτὸν
ὀρεγομένῳ πραγμάτων μήτ' ἐκείνων ἐφικέσθαι καὶ
τῶν ἐνδεχομένων γνωσθῆναι παντάπασιν ἀτυχῆσαι.

τοῖς οὖν καὶ πεφυκόσιν εἶναι ἄριστα καὶ τοῖς
μανθάνειν ἄγουσι σχολήν, αὖθις ἡμεῖς διαλεγώμεθα,
τοσοῦτον ἀναμνήσαντες αὐτοὺς ὧν εὐθὺς κατ' ἀρχὰς
εἴπομεν, ὡς οὐ προσήκει συγχεῖν ἅμα καὶ φύρειν
ἀμφότερα, τά τ' ἐκ τῆς πείρας εὑρισκόμενα καὶ τὰ
διὰ μόνου τοῦ λόγου, ἀλλ' ὑπὲρ ἑκατέρων ἰδίᾳ δια-
λεχθέντας, αὖθις ἄμφω συναγαγεῖν. εἰρηκότες οὖν
124K   ἡμεῖς ὑπὲρ τῆς ἐμπειρικῆς | εὑρέσεως ἑτέρωθι, περὶ
τῆς λογικῆς ἐν τοῖσδε τοῖς ὑπομνήμασι προὐθέμεθα
διελθεῖν. καί μοι δοκῶ σαφῶς ἤδη δεδειχέναι, τοῖς γε
τὰ περὶ τῆς τῶν νοσημάτων τε καὶ συμπτωμάτων
διαφορᾶς ἀνεγνωκόσι, πρὸς οὓς ὁ μετὰ ταῦτα πᾶς
ἔσται μοι λόγος, ὡς εὐθὺς ἐν ἀρχῇ μέγιστον πτῶμα
πεπτώκασιν οἱ περὶ τὸν Θεσσαλόν. ἦν μὲν γὰρ οὐ
σμικρὸν οὐδὲ τὸ Ἀσκληπιάδειον πτῶμα, διὰ τὸ κατ'
ἀρχὰς ἐσφάλθαι τὸν ἄνδρα περὶ τὰ τοῦ σώματος
στοιχεῖα, πολὺ δ' ἔτι μεῖζον αὐτοῦ καὶ ἀνιατότερον
ἐποίησαν οἱ περὶ τὸν Θεσσαλόν, εἰς δύο μὲν ἅπαντα
τὰ κατὰ δίαιταν νοσήματα διαθέσεις ἀναγαγόντες
ὁμοίως ἐκείνῳ, πολλοὺς δὲ τῶν θεραπευτικῶν σκοπῶν

butchers, do not cut at the joints,[26] but beat, crush, and tear apart just as [they do] in the matter now before us. Certainly I advise everyone, as you know, to pay attention to such things on the basis of experience. For the danger is not trifling to anyone who desires to attain something beyond his capability in that he fails to achieve those things he takes upon himself and altogether fails in the things that can be understood.

Therefore, let me again take up the discussion with those who are, by nature, the best and who have the time to learn, reminding them of those things I said right at the start—that it is not appropriate to confuse and mix up both things, i.e. those discovered through experience and those discovered by reason alone. Rather, it is proper to discuss each of them individually and then bring both together. I have spoken about the empirical conception elsewhere; I propose to go over in detail the Rationalist [conception] in these treatises. And it seems to me I have already shown clearly, at least to those who have read the treatises on the differentiae of diseases and symptoms (for it is to them my whole argument to follow will be directed), that right at the start the followers of Thessalus took a great tumble.

124K

Now the Asclepiadian tumble was by no means small because the man erred right at the beginning regarding the elements of the body.[27] But what the Thessaleians did was far worse than this and more incorrigible. Like Asclepiades, they reduced all the diseases connected with regimen to two conditions, but they also did away with many of

26 This is Plato's image in *Philebus* 265e.

27 This is the fundamental difference between atomic theories of structure and theories involving the four elemental qualities.

ἀφελόντες, οἷς ἐκεῖνος ἐχρήσατο. χείριστον δὲ καὶ
ἀνιατότερον ἁμαρτάνοντες, ὅτι μήτε τὰς τῶν ἐνεργειῶν βλάβας, ἀλλὰ μηδὲ τὰς αἰτίας αὐτῶν τὰς διαθέσεις ὑπολαμβάνουσιν εἶναι νοσήματα, μόναις δὲ
ταῖς κενώσεσιν ἐπεχομέναις τε καὶ πλεοναζούσαις
ἀξιοῦσι προσέχειν τὸν νοῦν, οὐδ' οὖν οὐδὲ τί ποτ' ἐστὶ
τὸ πέρα τοῦ δέοντος ἢ κενοῦσθαι τὰ ἐκ τοῦ σώματος, ἢ
ἐπέχεσθαι διδάξαντες ἡμᾶς σαφῶς. ἢ γὰρ ὡς πρὸς
τὴν δύναμιν, ἢ ὡς πρὸς τὴν αἰτίαν, ἢ ὡς πρὸς τὴν |
125K διάθεσιν, ἢ ὡς πρὸς τὸ κατὰ τὴν ὑγείαν ἑκάστῳ
τετηρημένον ἀναφέρεσθαι χρὴ τὴν τήρησιν. ὅθεν,
οἶμαι, καὶ πόλεμος οὐ σμικρὸς τοῖς ἀπ' αὐτῶν ἐγένετο
κατά τε ἄλλα πάντα διενεχθεῖσι καὶ περὶ τῆς τῶν
παθῶν ἐννοίας τε καὶ ὑπάρξεως. ἀλλ' εἰ νῦν κινήσαιμι
τὴν περὶ τῆς διαφωνίας αὐτῶν διέξοδον, ἀπάξω τοῦ
χρησίμου τὸν λόγον.

ὡς οὖν ἀνεγνωκόσιν ἤδη τὰ περὶ τῆς τῶν νοσημάτων τε καὶ συμπτωμάτων διαφορᾶς ὑπομνήματα
καὶ πρὸς τούτοις ἔτι τὰ τῶν αἰτίων αὐτῶν, ἔτι τε πρὸς
τούτοις ἐκεῖνα σύμπαντα διεληλυθόσιν ὧν ὀλίγον ἔμπροσθεν ἐμνημόνευσα, τὸν ἑξῆς ἅπαντα ποιήσομαι
λόγον, ἀρξάμενος ἐνθάδε. ἐπειδὴ τὰς ἐνεργείας ἁπάσας ἐδείξαμεν ὑπὸ τῶν ὁμοιομερῶν γιγνομένας σωμάτων, τὰ δ' ἄλλα πάντα τὰ καθ' ἕκαστον ὄργανον
μόρια χρείαν τινὰ τούτοις παρέχοντα, διττὸν δήπου
γένος ἔσται νοσημάτων, ἕτερον μὲν ἐν τοῖς ὁμοιο-
μέρεσι σώμασιν, ἕτερον δὲ ἐν τοῖς ὅλοις ὀργάνοις· ἐν
μὲν τοῖς ὁμοιομερέσιν αἱ δυσκρασίαι· τῶν δ' ὅλων

the therapeutic objectives which that man made use of. Worse, and more difficult to correct, they were mistaken in that they took neither the damages of functions nor even the conditions that were the causes of these to be diseases, thinking it worthwhile to direct their attention to the evacuations alone, either retentions or excesses, but not teaching us clearly what constitutes more than is required, either of an evacuation of things from the body, or of a retention. We ought to direct attention either to the capacity, or to the cause, or to the condition, or to what has been 125K observed in each of these during health. Whence, I think, no small battle arose among those of their number who disagreed about everything else, as well as about the concept and existence of the affections. But if I were now to apply myself to the issue of the discord among them, I would be diverting the discussion away from what is useful.

I shall, therefore, fashion the whole discussion that follows for those who have already read the treatises on the differentiae of diseases and symptoms, and, in addition to these, those on their causes, and over and above these, all those I made mention of a little earlier; and I shall make a start here. Since I showed that all functions arise by the agency of *homoiomerous* bodies whereas all the other parts relating to each organ provide a certain use for them, there will be, of course, a twofold class of diseases: one in *homoiomerous* bodies and the other in whole organs. In the *homoiomeres* there are the *dyskrasias*. Of the whole

ὀργάνων ἓν μὲν τὸ παρὰ τὴν διάπλασιν, ἓν δὲ τὸ παρὰ
τὸν ἀριθμὸν τῶν μορίων, ἄλλο δὲ τὸ παρὰ τὸ ποσὸν
ἑκάστου, καὶ τέταρτον τὸ παρὰ τὴν θέσιν, κοινὸν δὲ
126K   τῶν ὁμοιομερῶν καὶ τῶν ὀργανικῶν | μορίων νόσημά
ἐστιν ἡ τῆς συνεχείας λύσις. ἐξ οὖν ἐστι τὰ πάντα τῶν
νοσημάτων γένη· ἓν μὲν ἴδιον τῶν ὁμοιομερῶν, ἡ
δυσκρασία, τέτταρα δὲ ἑκάστου τῶν ὀργάνων, ὡς
εἴρηται νῦν ἤδη, καὶ πρὸς τούτοις ἔστι κοινὸν ὀργανικῶν τε καὶ ὁμοιομερῶν ἡ τῆς συνεχείας λύσις. αἱ δὲ
καθ' ἕκαστον αὐτῶν διαφοραὶ μέχρι τῶν ἐσχάτων
εἰδῶν ἐν τῷ Περὶ τῆς τῶν νοσημάτων διαφορᾶς εἴ-
ρηνται.

7. Τούτων οὕτως ἐχόντων ἤδη λεκτέον ὑπὲρ τῶν
θεραπευτικῶν ἐνδείξεων, αὐτὸ τοῦτο πρότερον ἐξηγη-
σαμένους τὸ τῆς ἐνδείξεως ὄνομα. τὴν γὰρ οἷον ἔμφα-
σιν τῆς ἀκολουθίας ἔνδειξιν λέγομεν. εὑρίσκεται μὲν
κἀκ τῆς πείρας τὸ ἀκόλουθον, ἀλλ' οὐχ ὡς ἐμφαινό-
μενον τῷ ἡγουμένῳ. καὶ διὰ τοῦτο τῶν Ἐμπειρικῶν
οὐδεὶς ἐμφαίνεσθαί φησι τῷδέ τινι, τόδε τι. καίτοι γε
ἀκολουθεῖν λέγουσι τόδε τῷδε καὶ προηγεῖσθαι τόδε
τοῦδε καὶ συνυπάρχειν τόδε τῷδε, καὶ ὅλως ἅπασαν
τὴν τέχνην τήρησίν τε καὶ μνήμην φασὶν εἶναι τοῦ
τί σὺν τίνι καὶ τί πρὸ τίνος[21] καὶ τί μετὰ τίνος[22]
127K   πολλάκις | ἑώραται. τὸν τοίνυν ἐξ αὐτῆς τῆς τοῦ πρά-
γματος φύσεως ὁρμώμενον ἐξευρίσκειν τὸ ἀκόλουθον

[21] πρὸ τίνος B (conj. quoque Hankinson); πρὸς τίνος P1,
P2, K   [22] τί μετὰ τί P1; τί μετὰ τίνος B, P2, K

organs, one [kind of disease] is because of the conformation, one because of the number of parts, another because of the magnitude of each, and a fourth because of the position. Common to both the *homoiomeres* and the organic parts is the disease that is the dissolution of continuity.[28] 126K There are, then, six classes of diseases in all. One, *dyskrasia*, is specific to *homoiomeres*, four are specific to each of the organs, as I said just now, and, in addition to these, and common to organs and *homoiomeres*, there is dissolution of continuity. The differentiae in relation to each of these, right up to the ultimate kinds, have been considered in my work *On the Differentiae of Diseases*.

7. These things being thus, we must now speak about the therapeutic indications after first explaining this very thing—the term "indication." We say that an indication is a reflection, as it were, of what is consequent. The consequent is discovered from experience, but not as something that is apparent in the antecedent. And for this reason none of the Empirics speaks of anything being reflected by anything else. Yet they say that this is consequent upon that, or that this is antecedent to that, or that this and that coexist, and they say that in general the whole art [of medicine] is the observation and recollection of what has been observed in conjunction with what, and what prior to what, and what in association with what on many occasions. Therefore, the person who sets out to discover what 127K is consequent from the actual nature of the matter without

---

[28] A disease class first specifically identified by Galen—see *De differentiis morborum*, VI.871–72K. Diseases of this class are the subject of Books 3–6 of the present treatise.

ἄνευ τῆς πείρας ἐνδείξει τὴν[23] εὕρεσιν ἔστι πεποιῆ-
σθαι.

διωρισμένου δὲ καὶ τοῦδε πάλιν ἀναμνήσαντες
ὅπερ ἤδη καὶ πρόσθεν εἴπομεν, ὡς ἡ θεραπευτικὴ
πᾶσα μέθοδος ἄνευ τῆς ἐμπειρίας προέρχεται καὶ ὡς
οὐκ ὀρθῶς ποιοῦσιν οἱ συνάγοντες εἰς ταὐτὸν καὶ
συγχέοντες ἀμφοτέρας τὰς διδασκαλίας, ἐμπειρικήν
τε καὶ λογικήν, ἐχώμεθα τῶν ἑξῆς. εἴη δ᾽ ἂν πρῶτον
ἁπάντων τῶν ἐφεξῆς, ὅπερ καὶ πρῶτον ἁπάντων ἕπεται τοῖς ὑποκειμένοις. ἕπεται δὲ πρῶτον καὶ μάλιστα
τὸ δι᾽ ἐνδείξεως ἅπασαν γίγνεσθαι τὴν θεραπευτικὴν
μέθοδον. ὅσον γὰρ ἀποκεχώρηκε τῆς ἐμπειρίας, ἔνδειξις ὀνομάζεται σύμπαν. ὥστε καὶ ὅστις ἀκριβῶς
βούλεται συστήσασθαι τὴν θεραπευτικὴν μέθοδον,
ἄρξασθαι μὲν αὐτὸν ἀπὸ τῶν πρώτων ἐνδείξεων χρή,
μεταβῆναι δὲ ἐντεῦθεν ἐπὶ τὰς ἐφεξῆς, εἶτ᾽ αὖθις ἐπὶ
τὰς ἐκείνων ἐχομένας, καὶ τοῦτο ποιοῦντα μὴ παύσασθαι πρὶν ἐφικέσθαι τοῦ τέλους αὐτοῦ.[24]

τέλος δ᾽ ἐστὶ τῆς νῦν ἡμῖν προκειμένης πραγματείας ἐξευρεῖν ἑκάστου τῶν νοσημάτων ἰάματα. τίς
128K οὖν | ἀρχὴ τῆς ἐπὶ τοῦτο φερούσης ὁδοῦ; τοῦ νοσή-
ματος ἡ γνῶσις, ὁποῖόν τι τὴν φύσιν ἐστίν, ὡς ἀπεδείχθη καὶ πρόσθεν. εἰ γὰρ δὴ τὸ θεραπευόμενον
αὐτὸ τοῦτ᾽ ἔστιν, εὔλογον δήπου καὶ τῶν ἐνδείξεων
ἐντεῦθεν ἄρξασθαι. τίς οὖν ἡ γενικὴ καὶ κοινὴ πάντων
τῶν νοσημάτων ἔνδειξις εὑρεῖν χρὴ πρῶτον, εἶτα
ἐντεῦθεν ἐπὶ τὰς κατ᾽ εἴδη προελθεῖν. ἀνάγκη γὰρ δὴ
τὰς νόσους ἁπάσας ἑνὸς καὶ ταὐτοῦ μεθέξει νόσους

[drawing on] experience is making the discovery by indication.

Having established this distinction, let me call to mind again what I already spoke about earlier—that the whole therapeutic method proceeds independent of experience and that those who combine both teachings, empirical and rational, into one thing, and compound them together are wrong—and let me deal with what comes next. First of all things in order is also that which is first of all things that follow those things laid down. What follows first and foremost is that the whole therapeutic method is based on indication. For whatever is distinct from experience is all called indication, so that anyone who wishes to formulate the therapeutic method accurately should begin from the primary indications and move on from there to those things that follow, and then again, in turn, to those things associated with these, and not stop doing this until he reaches its completion.

The goal of the matter now lying before us is to discover cures for each of the diseases. What, then, is the beginning 128K of the path leading to this? The knowledge of disease— what kind of thing it is by nature—as was also shown before. For surely, if this is the actual thing to be treated, it is reasonable here, I presume, to start from the indications. First, it is necessary to discover the generic and common indication of all diseases, and then proceed from here to those indications based on kinds. Now it is necessary that all diseases are called diseases by virtue of their sharing in

---

23 ἐνδείξει τήν B, P1, P2; ἐνδείξεις καί K
24 αὐτοῦ B, P1; αὐτῶν K

ὀνομάζεσθαι καθάπερ, οἶμαι, καὶ ἄνθρωπον καὶ βοῦν
καὶ κύνα καὶ τῶν ἄλλων ἕκαστον. ἓν γὰρ καὶ ταὐτὸν ἐν
ἅπασι τοῖς ἀνθρώποις ἐστί. διὸ καὶ τῆς αὐτῆς προσηγορίας ἅπαντες ἐτύχομεν ἄνθρωποι καλεῖσθαι. παραπλησίως δὲ κἀν τοῖς κυσὶν ἅπασιν ἕν τι καὶ ταὐτόν
ἐστιν, ἐφ' ὃ δὴ καὶ τὴν διάνοιαν ἐπερειδόμεθα νοῆσαι
βουληθέντες τὸν κύνα. καὶ μὲν δὴ καὶ τοῖς ἵπποις
ὁμοίως ἕν τι καὶ ταὐτὸν ἅπασιν ἐστὶν ᾗ πάντες ἵπποι
καλοῦνται. μάθοις δ' ἂν ἐναργέστερον ἐπὶ τῶν ὁμωνύ-
μων αὐτό. τοῖς μὲν γὰρ τετράποσι ζῴοις ἅπασι τοῖς
ὑλακτικοῖς ἓν καὶ ταὐτὸν ὑπάρχει, τὸ τετράποσί τ'
εἶναι σύμπασι καὶ ὑλακτικοῖς. τοῖς δ' ἐναλίοις θηρίοις
129K τοῖς ἁρπακτικοῖς, ἃ | δὴ καὶ αὐτὰ κύνας ὀνομάζομεν,
ἓν αὖ κἀκείνοις ὑπάρχει ταὐτόν, οὐχ ὑπάρχον τοῖς
ἐπιγείοις. ὥστε μηδενὸς ἐκεῖνα τούτοις κοινωνεῖν ἄλλου κατὰ τὴν τῶν κυνῶν φύσιν πλὴν ὀνόματος. ἀνθρώπῳ μέντοι πρὸς ἄνθρωπον, οἷον Σωκράτει πρὸς
Ἀλκιβιάδην, οὐκ ὀνόματος μόνον, ἀλλὰ καὶ τῶν ὑπαρχόντων ἐστὶν ἡ κοινωνία· καὶ γὰρ καὶ ζῷα καὶ δίποδα
καὶ πεζὰ καὶ λογικὰ καὶ θνητὰ καὶ ὅλως οὐδὲν ἂν
εὕροις ὑπάρχον οὐδενὶ τῶν κατὰ μέρος ἀνθρώπων ᾗ
ἄνθρωπος, ὃ μὴ καὶ τοῖς ἄλλοις ἅπασιν[25] ὑπάρχει.
τοῖς μέντοι χερσαίοις κυσὶ πρὸς τοὺς ἄλλους θαλατ-
τίους ὑπάρχει πολλὰ διαφέροντα καὶ κατὰ τὴν τοῦ
σώματος ἰδέαν καὶ κατὰ τὸ τῆς ψυχῆς ἦθος. ἥμερον
γὰρ τοῦτο καὶ φιλάνθρωπον, ἐπίβουλον δ' ἐκεῖνο καὶ
ἄγριον, καὶ χερσαῖον μὲν τοῦτο, θαλάττιον δ' ἐκεῖνο,
καὶ τὸ μὲν τετράπουν, τὸ δὲ οὔ, καὶ τὸ μὲν ὑλακτικόν,

one and the same thing, just as, I think, man, dog, cow and each of the other [animals] do, for there is one same thing in all men. It is because of this that all men happen to be called by the same name. Similarly too, in all dogs there is some one same thing which we direct our attention to if we wish to conceive of "dog." Further, in all horses also, there is likewise one same thing on the basis of which all are called "horse." You would understand this more distinctly in the case of homonyms, for there is this one and the same thing in all four-footed animals that bark, which is that they are all four-footed and barking. In those wild and preda- 129K
tory sea creatures, which we actually also call dogs, there is again one and the same thing belonging to them which does not belong to those on dry land. Thus they have noth-ing else in common with terrestrial dogs apart from the name. However, in one man in relation to another man, for example, in Socrates in relation to Alcibiades, the com-monality is not only one of name but also of what pertains to them. For, in fact, they are both animals, terrestrial bi-peds, rational and mortal, and, in general, you would find nothing belonging to man *qua* man that does not also be-long to all others. However, in terrestrial dogs compared to the others that are sea-dwelling, there are many differ-ences, both in the form of the body and in the disposition of the soul. For the one is tame and gets on well with hu-mans, whereas the other is treacherous and wild; one is terrestrial whereas the other is marine; one is a quadruped but the other is not; one barks but the other does not. But

---

25 ἅπασιν B (ἅπασι P1); ἀνθρώποις K

τὸ δὲ οὐχ ὑλακτικόν. οὐ μὴν τῶν ἐπιγείων κυνῶν ὁ μὲν
ὑλακτικός ἐστιν, ὁ δὲ οὐχ ὑλακτικός, καὶ τετράπους
μὲν ὅδε τις, ἕτερος δὲ μὴ τοιοῦτος, ἀλλὰ πᾶσι μὲν
αὐτοῖς ἓν εἶδός ἐστιν ᾗ κύνες ὀνομάζονται καὶ οὐ
130K μόνον ταῖς οὐσίαις ἔοικεν ὑπάρχειν | τὸ τοιοῦτον,
ἀλλὰ καὶ τοῖς συμβεβηκόσιν αὐτοῖς ἢ ὡς διαθέσεσιν,
ἢ ὡς ἐνεργήμασιν, ἢ ὡς παθήμασιν.

οἷον ἄνθρωπος περιπατῶν ἀνθρώπου περιπατοῦν-
τος οὐδὲν διαφέρει κατ' αὐτὸ τὸ περιπατεῖν, καὶ και-
όμενος δὴ καιομένου καὶ τεμνόμενος τεμνομένου καὶ
λευκὸς λευκοῦ καὶ μέλας μέλανος· ἐν μέντοι τῷ μᾶλλόν τε καὶ ἧττον ἕκαστον τούτων οὐ σμικρὰν ἔχει
διαφοράν· οἷον λευκὸς μᾶλλον ἢ ἧττον· ἀλλ' ᾗ λευκός,
ἕν τι καὶ ταὐτὸν ἑτέρῳ λευκῷ κέκτηται· καθάπερ καὶ ᾗ
ἄνθρωπος, ἕν τι ταὐτὸν ἀνθρώπῳ τῷ τυχόντι. καὶ καθ'
ἕκαστον δὴ τῶν σημαινομένων ἐν ἅπασιν ὑπάρχει
ταὐτόν· οὕτω δὴ καὶ τὸ νοσεῖν καὶ τὸ ὑγιαίνειν· τὸ μὲν
τοῖς νοσοῦσιν ἅπασιν ὑπάρχει, τὸ δὲ τοῖς ὑγιαί-
νουσιν, ἓν καὶ ταὐτὸν ἑκάτερον· καὶ ὥσπερ ἐκ τῆς
ἄνθρωπος φωνῆς ἕν, οὕτω κἀκ τῆς ὑγείας ἓν σημαίνεται. δηλοῖ δὲ καὶ ἡ καθ' ἑκάστην ἡμέραν ἡμῖν
γιγνομένη πρὸς ἀλλήλους διάλεκτος, ὡς ἐν οἷς οὐκ
ἔστιν ὁμωνυμία, τὸ σημαινόμενον ἓν ὑπάρχει. λέγοντος γάρ τινος ὑπὸ ἀνθρώπου πληγῆναι λίθῳ τὴν
κεφαλήν, οὐδενὶ τῶν ἀκουόντων ἀσαφὴς ὁ λόγος, οὐδ'
131K ἀμφίβολος, ὥσπερ εἰ καταβρωθῆναί τις, εἰ | οὕτως
ἔτυχε, Κορίσκον ὑπὸ κυνὸς διηγεῖτο· Τίνος γὰρ κυνός;

among terrestrial dogs, it is not that one is barking and another is not, or that one is four-footed and another is not like this—in all of them there is one form on the basis of which they are called dogs, and it seems that they are not only like this in their substances at least, but also in those things that are contingent to them, such as conditions, functions, or affections.

130K

For example, one man who walks does not differ from another man who walks in respect to the walking itself; nor, certainly, does one man being cauterized differ from another being cauterized, nor does one being cut differ from another being cut, nor does one who is white differ from another who is white, nor does one who is black differ from another who is black. Nevertheless, there is no small difference in terms of more or less with respect to each of these qualities. For example, whiteness is more or less, but insofar as there is the possession of whiteness, it is the same in one as it is in another; just as also, in being a man there is one thing that is the same for whoever happens to be a man. And in respect to each of the things signified, one thing is the same for all. It is like this, too, with being diseased and being healthy. What is in all those who are diseased and what is in all those who are healthy is one and the same in either case. And just as by the term "man" one thing is signified, so too is it the case for "health." This is clear from the conversation that occurs between each of us every day when, in those things for which there is no homonym, one thing is signified. For when someone says he has been hit on the head with a stone by a man, the statement is not obscure or ambiguous to anyone who hears it, as it would be if someone were to report, should it happen to be the case, that Coriscus was devoured by a dog. "By

131K

203

ὁ ἀκούσας ἐρήσεται διότι, οἶμαι, δύο ἐστὶν εἴδη
κυνῶν, τὸ μὲν ἐπίγειον, τὸ δὲ ἐνάλιον. οὐ μὴν ὑπὸ
τίνος γε λίθου καὶ τίνα τὴν κεφαλὴν ἐρωτήσει· καὶ
γὰρ λίθου παντὸς ἓν εἶδος ᾗ λίθος ἐστὶ καὶ κεφαλῆς
ἁπάσης ᾗ κεφαλή, κυνὸς δ' οὐχ ἓν ᾗ κύων, ὥσπερ οὐδὲ
γλώττης ᾗ γλῶττα. καὶ γὰρ καὶ αὐλοῦ καὶ ὑποδή-
ματος καὶ ζῴου μόριον ἡ γλῶττα. καὶ εἴ τινος ἀκού-
σαις οἰκέτῃ προστάσσοντος ὠνήσασθαι γλῶτταν,
ἄδηλόν ἐστιν ἥντινα λέγει γλῶτταν· οὐ μὴν εἰ γαστέρα τις, ἢ κύστιν ἢ ἧπαρ ὠνήσασθαι κελεύοι. καθ'
ἕκαστον οὖν τῶν σημαινομένων ἕν τι πρᾶγμά ἐστιν
ὑποκείμενον, οὐ μὴν καθ' ἑκάστην γε τῶν φωνῶν ἕν·
ἐνίοτε μέντοι σημαίνεται μόνον πρὸς τῆς φωνῆς, ὑπόκειται δὲ οὐδέν. ἀλλὰ περὶ μὲν τῶν οὕτω λεγομένων οὐ
πρόκειται νῦν διελθεῖν. ἐν οἷς δὲ οὐ σημαίνεταί τι
μόνον ἐκ τῆς φωνῆς, ἀλλὰ καὶ πρᾶγμά τί ἐστιν
ὑποκείμενον, ὅσαπερ ἂν ᾖ τὰ σημαινόμενα, τοσαῦται
καὶ αἱ τῶν πραγμάτων ὑπάρχουσιν ἰδέαι· τῆς μὲν
φωνῆς ἓν σημαινούσης ἓν ἐξ ἀνάγκης ἐστὶ καὶ τὸ τοῦ
πράγματος εἶδος. |

132K   ἀριθμῷ μέντοι πολλὰ ταῦτα ἐγχωρεῖ γενέσθαι,
καθάπερ τὸ α. καὶ διὰ τοῦτο ἑπτὰ μὲν τὰ φωνήεντά
φαμεν ὑπάρχειν, στοιχεῖα δὲ τέτταρα καὶ εἴκοσι τὰ
σύμπαντα, κατὰ τὴν ἡμετέραν δηλονότι διάλεκτον,
ἐπὶ τὸ κοινὸν ἁπάντων εἶδος ἀποβλέποντες ἓν ὑπάρχον, οὐκ ἐπὶ τὰ κατὰ μέρος, ἐπὶ τὰ ἐν χάρταις καὶ
ξύλοις καὶ διφθέραις καὶ λίθοις γεγραμμένα, πάμ-
πολύ τι πλῆθος ὄντα καὶ μηδ' ἀριθμηθῆναι δυνάμενα

204

what dog," the listener will ask, because I think, there are
two kinds of dogs: one terrestrial and the other marine.
But he will certainly not ask by what stone, or what head.
For there is one form for every stone by which it is a stone,
and for every head by which it is a head, but there is not
one form of dog by which it is a dog, just as there is not one
of tongue by which it is a tongue, for a tongue is part of a
pipe, and of a shoe, and of an animal. And if you heard
someone giving an order to a slave to buy a tongue, it
would not be clear which tongue he is referring to. But if
someone were to direct him to buy a stomach, bladder or
liver, it would be clear. In relation to each of the things signified, there is, then, some one thing underlying it, but not
one in relation to each of the terms. Sometimes, however,
something is only signified by the term, and nothing underlies it. But it is not our present task to expatiate about
things spoken of in this way. In those instances where
something is not only signified by the term, but there is
also some matter underlying, there are as many forms
of matters existing as there are things signified. When the
term signifies one thing there is, of necessity, one form of
the matter.

In number, however, it is possible for many of these   132K
things to occur, as with the letter *alpha*. And because of
this, when we say there are seven vowels, and twenty-four
elements altogether, this clearly relates to our language,
since we are looking at what is the one common form of everything and not at the individual [letters] as having been
written on papyrus, wood, parchment, or stone, which are
very many and cannot be counted, and which extend al-

καὶ σχεδὸν εἰς ἄπειρον ἐκτεινόμενα· δύναται γοῦν
ἄχρι τοῦ παντὸς αἰῶνος α καὶ β καὶ γ γράφεσθαι
μυρία, κατὰ ταὐτὰ δὲ καὶ τῶν ἄλλων ἕκαστον γραμ-
μάτων. ἀλλὰ τά γε σύμπαντα τέτταρα καὶ εἴκοσι τὸν
ἀριθμὸν εἶναί φαμεν, οὐ τὰ κατὰ μέρος προχειρι-
ζόμενοι, τὰ δ' εἴδη μόνον, καθ' ὧνπερ, οἶμαι, καὶ τὰ
ὀνόματα φέρομεν. ἄλφα γὰρ οὐ τουτὶ μέν τι λέγεται
τὸ γεγραμμένον ἐν χάρτῃ, τουτὶ δ' οὐ λέγεται τὸ
γεγραμμένον ἐν ξύλῳ, ἀλλὰ καὶ τοῦτο κἀκεῖνο, κἂν εἰ
κατὰ τῆς γῆς γράψαις, κἂν εἰ κατὰ λίθου, κἂν εἰ
καταξύσαις, κἂν εἰ διὰ χρωμάτων. καὶ οὐδὲ πολλὰ
τοὺς παῖδάς τις διδάσκει α καὶ β καὶ γ καὶ τῶν ἄλλων
ἕκαστον, ἀλλ' ἓν μὲν ἕκαστον, ὁμοῦ δὲ σύμπαντα
133K τέσσαρα καὶ εἴκοσι. οὕτως δὲ κἂν ἵππον ἕνα | δείξεις,
ἢ κάμηλον παιδί, θεασάμενος αὖθις ἕτερον ἵππον, ἢ
κάμηλον ἑτέραν, οὐκ ἐρωτᾷ τί ποτ' ἐστὶ τὸ ζῷον, ἀλλὰ
τὸ μὲν ἵππον ὀνομάζει, τὸ δὲ κάμηλον. καὶ ταὐτόν γε
εἶναι ἐκεῖνό φησι τοῦτο τὸ πρόσθεν ὁραθὲν τῷ νῦν
ὁρωμένῳ. καίτοι τὸ μέν, εἰ οὕτως ἔτυχεν, ἀπέθανεν,
ἕτερον δ' ἐστὶ τὸ νῦν ὁρώμενον. οἶνον δὴ λέγουσιν οἱ
ἄνθρωποι τὸν αὐτὸν χθὲς καὶ τήμερον πεπωκέναι, τῷ
εἴδει δηλονότι τὸν αὐτόν· ἐνίοτε δέ φασι τρεῖς οἴνους
πεπωκέναι τήμερον, ἢ νὴ Δία ἕνα, πανταχοῦ πρὸς τὸ
εἶδος ἀποβλέποντες, ἐπικεῖσθαί τε μίαν, εἰ τύχοι,
σφραγῖδα πεντεκαίδεκα θύραις, ἐν ἅπασι τούτοις ἐπὶ
τὸ εἶδος ἀναφέροντες τὸν λόγον. οὕτω δὲ ἐναργές ἐστι
καὶ φύσει πᾶσιν ὑπάρχει καὶ ἀνθρώποις καὶ βοσκή-
μασιν ἕτερον μέν τι ὡς ὑποκείμενον κατ' οὐσίαν,

most to infinity. One would be able, in the space of a whole lifetime, to write *alpha* and *beta* and *gamma* innumerable times, and the same with each of the other letters. But when we say these are altogether twenty-four in number, we do not choose those individually but the forms alone, in respect of which, I believe, we apply the names here. For *alpha* is not said of this particular something that is written on papyrus, or this particular thing that is written on wood, but it is this and that, even if you write it on earth, or on stone, or if you inscribe it, or if [you write it] with colors. And nobody teaches children many *alphas* and *betas* and *gammas* and each of the other [letters], but each single one, and altogether for the whole twenty-four. Likewise, if you show one horse or camel to a child, when the child later sees another horse or camel, he won't ask what the animal is, but names one a horse and the other a camel. And he says that what he saw before is the same as what he sees now, and the same, even though, as may happen, the first one dies and the one now seen is another. Men say that the wine they have drunk was the same yesterday as it is today since it is clearly the same in kind. Sometimes they say they have drunk three wines today, or, by Zeus, one, but in all cases they are looking at the kind, and if they say one seal is placed, should it so happen, on fifteen doors, in all these [instances] they are applying the term to the form. In this way it is clear, and is innate in everyone, both humans and beasts, to recognize one thing as underlying in terms of

133K

ἕτερον δὲ ὡς εἶδος ἓν ἐπινοεῖν, ὥστε καὶ τοῖς ὄνοις,
οἵπερ ἁπάντων τῶν θρεμμάτων ἀνοητότατοί γε δοκοῦ-
σιν ὑπάρχειν, ἄλλο μὲν τὸ κατ᾽ εἶδος ἕν, ἄλλο δὲ τὸ
κατ᾽ ἀριθμόν, εἰς διάγνωσιν ἥκει. θεασάμενος γοῦν
κάμηλον ὁ ὄνος ἐξίσταταί τε καὶ φεύγει καὶ δέδιεν, εἰ
μηδέποτε τύχοι θεασάμενος· εἰ μέν τοι συνεθισθείη |
134K τῷ θεάματι, κἂν ἄλλην αὐτῷ καὶ ἄλλην ἐπιδείξῃς
κάμηλον, οὐκέτι δέδιεν ὑπὸ συνηθείας, ἀλλ᾽ ὡς ἓν
εἶδος ὁρᾷ κἀκείνην ᾗ συνειθίσθη καὶ ταύτην ᾗ πρώτως ἐντυγχάνει. οὕτω δὲ καὶ τοὺς ἀνθρώπους οὐ δέδιεν
ὑπὸ συνηθείας, ἀλλ᾽ ὡς ἓν εἶδος ὁρᾷ καὶ τούτους· εἰ
μέντοι θεάσαιτο τὸν ὀνηλάτην, οὐχ ὡς ἄνθρωπον
μόνον, ἀλλὰ καὶ ὡς τόν δέ τινα γνωρίζει καὶ σείει γε
τὰ ὦτα πολλάκις καὶ τὴν κέρκον κινεῖ καὶ ὀγκᾶται καὶ
σκιρτᾷ θεασάμενος, ἐμφαίνων ὅτι γνωρίζει τὸν οἰκεῖον. τοῦτον μὲν δὴ καὶ ὡς ἄνθρωπον καὶ ὡς συνήθη
γνωρίζει· τὸν δὲ νῦν αὐτῷ πρῶτον ὀφθέντα, καθ᾽ ὅσον
μὲν ἄνθρωπον ὡσαύτως, ὡς συνήθη δ᾽ οὐχ ὡσαύτως.

ὥστ᾽ οὐ μόνον ἡμεῖς, ἀλλ᾽ ἤδη καὶ οἱ ὄνοι τὸ μὲν ὡς
ἀριθμῷ ταὐτὸν ὁρῶσί τε καὶ διαγινώσκουσι καὶ
μέμνηνται, τὸ δὲ ὡς εἴδει. καὶ τὸν Δίωνα τὸν ὀνηλάτην, ἔστω γάρ, εἰ τύχοι οὕτως λεγόμενος, ἄλλως
μὲν ὡς ἄνθρωπον, ἄλλως δὲ ὡς Δίωνα γνωρίζουσιν οἱ
συνήθεις ὄνοι, τὸ μέντοι κοινὸν εἶδος αὐτοῦ καὶ πρὸς
τοὺς ἄλλους ἀνθρώπους ὡς ἀνθρώπου λαμβάνοντες,
τὸ δὲ ἴδιον ἐξαίρετον ὡς Δίωνος μόνου.

135K καὶ τοσοῦτον τοίνυν δέον τοὺς παλαιοὺς | φιλοσό-
φους ἐπαινεῖν, ὡς μέγα τι καὶ σοφὸν ἐξευρόντας, ὅτι

208

substance, and another one thing as the form, so that even donkeys, which seem to be the most unintelligent of all domesticated animals, also come to the distinction between what is different in respect to form, and what is different in respect to number. At any rate, when a donkey sees a camel, it becomes frantic and flees, and is fearful, if it should happen never to have seen one. If, however, it has become accustomed to the sight, and you had shown it one camel after another, it would no longer be afraid due to habituation, since it sees the one form in that to which it has become accustomed, and this which it encounters for the first time. In the same way too it is not afraid of men due to habituation, since it also sees the one form in them. If, however, it sees the donkey driver, [it recognizes him] not only as a man but also as someone it knows, and shakes its ears often, and moves its tail, and brays, and leaps up when it sees him, revealing that it knows the familiar. It recognizes this person both as a man and as someone it is accustomed to. On the other hand, the man now seen by it for the first time, [it recognizes] in the same way as a man, but not like one it is accustomed to.

So it is not only us but now donkeys too who see one thing as being the same in number, and distinguish and remember it, and another thing as being the same in form. Donkeys that are used to Dion the donkey driver—for let him be so named—recognize him in one way as a man and in another way as Dion, taking his common form and the relation to other men as being of a man, and what is specific and distinctive about him as being of Dion alone.

To such a degree, then, our praise for the ancient philosophers as having discovered something important and

134K

135K

τὸ ταὐτὸν καὶ τὸ ἕτερον καὶ τὸ ἓν καὶ τὸ οὐχ ἓν οὐ
μόνον κατ᾽ ἀριθμόν, ἀλλὰ καὶ κατ᾽ εἶδος χρὴ νοεῖν,
ὥστε καὶ τοῖς ὄνοις φημὶ τοῦτο ὑπάρχειν φύσει.
πρόσκειται μὲν οὖν ὑπὸ τῶν παλαιῶν φιλοσόφων, ὡς
οὐ μόνον ἀριθμῷ καὶ εἴδει λέγεταί τι ταὐτόν, ἀλλὰ καὶ
τῷ γένει. οὐ μὴν ἤδη γέ πω τοῦδε χρῄζω πρὸς τὰ
παρόντα· μόνον γὰρ ἀρκεῖ μοι τὸ δεῖξαι τῶν ὄνων
ὑπάρχοντας ἀναισθητοτέρους ὅσοι μὴ συγχωροῦσιν
ἕτερον μέν τι τῷ εἴδει τὸ ἕν, ἕτερον δ᾽ ἀριθμῷ λέγεσθαι, καὶ μᾶλλον ἔτι τοὺς ἕνα μὲν τὸν φρενιτικὸν
εἶναι λέγοντας καὶ ἕνα τὸν Ἐμπειρικόν, ἕνα δὲ τὸν
ἄνθρωπον εἶναι μὴ συγχωροῦντας, ἢ μὴ γινώσκοντας
ὡς εἴδει μὲν ἓν ὁ ἄνθρωπος, ἀριθμῷ δ᾽ οὐχ ἕν. οὐδ᾽ ὁ
Σωκράτης μὲν ἓν καὶ τὸ εἶδος καὶ τὸν ἀριθμόν, ὁ
φρενιτικὸς δὲ τὸ μὲν εἶδος εἷς, οὐχ εἷς δέ ἐστι τὸ
πλῆθος. οὐ γὰρ ἐνδέχεται Δίωνα καὶ Σωκράτην καὶ
Θέωνα καὶ Κορίσκον ἅμα πάντας, εἰ τύχοι, φρενιτί-
ζοντας ἕνα τῷ πλήθει τοὺς τέσσαρας ὑπάρχειν, ἀλλὰ
τὸ μὲν εἶδος ἕνα, τὸ πλῆθος δ᾽ οὐχ ἕνα.

136K   παραλογώτερον δέ τι τῶν | Ἐμπειρικῶν ἰατρῶν
ἐστιν, ὅτι καὶ τὸν Ἐμπειρικὸν ἕνα λέγουσιν, εἶτ᾽
ἐρωτηθέντες πῶς ἕνα φασὶ τὸν ζῶντα τῷ τεθνεῶτι, καὶ
τὸν ἐπὶ τῆς Ἑλλάδος τῷ κατ᾽ Αἴγυπτον, ἀποκρίνονται
πρὸς τοῦτο θαυμαστὴν ἀπόκρισιν. ᾗ γάρ φασιν Ἐμπειρικός ἐστι, ταύτῃ καὶ εἷς. τοῦτο γὰρ δὴ τῆς ἐσχάτης ἀναισθησίας ἐστίν, εἰ προστιθέντες τὸ ᾗ καὶ τὸ
ταύτῃ, μηδ᾽ ὧν αὐτοὶ φθέγγονται συνίασιν. εἰ γὰρ δὴ
ταύτῃ γε Σεραπίων καὶ Μηνόδοτος εἷς ἐστὸν ᾗ Ἐμπει-

wise—that we ought to perceive the same and the different, and the one and not one, not only in relation to number, but also in relation to form—must be tempered by the fact that this is, as I say, also innate in donkeys. What is added by the ancient philosophers is that something is said to be the same not only in number and form, but also in class. I do not, at least for now, have need of this for my present purpose. For it is enough for me just to show that those who do not agree that it is one thing to say that something is one in form and another to say it is one in number are more stupid than donkeys. More stupid still are those who say it is one thing to be phrenitic and one to be an Empiric, but do not agree that it is one thing to be a man, or do not know that man is one in form but not in number. Nor is Socrates one in form and number, whereas someone who is phrenitic is one in form but not one in number. It is not possible that Dion, Socrates, Theon and Coriscus, if it should happen that they were all phrenitic at the same time, were one in number, since there are four of them. But they are one in form although not in number.

More contrary to reason is something the Empiric doctors say: that "Empiric" is one thing. But when they are asked how they say that someone living is the same as someone dead, or someone in Greece is the same as someone in Egypt, they give a remarkable answer to this [question]. For, they say, "by virtue of" being an Empiric, he is also one in this way. Truly it is a mark of the utmost stupidity if they add "by virtue of" and "in this way" without being cognizant of what they are saying. For if, in fact, Serapion and Menodotus are one "in this way" "by virtue of" being

136K

ρικοί, κατ' ἄλλα δήπουθεν οὐχ εἷς ἔσονται. ὥστ' εἴ γε
παντοίως εἷς ἦν, ἐκ περιττοῦ καὶ μάτην ἄν, οἶμαι,
προσέκειτο τὸ ᾗ καὶ τὸ ταύτῃ, παρὸν ἁπλῶς εἰπεῖν ὡς
εἷς ἐστι Σεραπίων καὶ Μηνόδοτος.

οὕτως οὖν ὡς ὑπὲρ αὑτοῦ μόνου Μηνοδότου τὸν
λόγον ποιούμενος, οὐκ ἂν προσθήκης δεηθείης, ἀλλ'
ἁπλῶς ἂν εἴποις, εἷς ἐστι Μηνόδοτος. εἰ τοίνυν Μηνόδοτος μὲν εἷς ἁπλῶς, Μηνόδοτος δὲ καὶ Σεραπίων
οὐχ ἁπλῶς εἷς, ἀλλ' ᾗ Ἐμπειρικοί, πάντως δήπουθεν
αὐτοῖς ἐστιν ἕτερ' ἄττα καθ' ἃ δύο εἰσὶ καὶ οὐχ εἷς
ἀμφότεροι, καὶ γίνεται τοῦτο ἐκεῖνο τὸ πρὸς τῶν |
137K παλαιῶν φιλοσόφων εἰρημένον, ἕτερον μὲν ἀριθμῷ
καὶ ταὐτὸν καὶ ἕν, ἕτερον δὲ τῷ εἴδει, καὶ μηδὲν εἶναι
θαυμαστόν, εἰ Μηνόδοτος Σεραπίωνι κατά τι μὲν ὁ
αὐτός ἐστι καὶ εἷς, κατά τι δὲ οὐχ ὁ αὐτὸς οὐδ' εἷς. ᾗ
μὲν γὰρ Ἐμπειρικὸς ὁ αὐτός, ᾗ δ' ὁ μὲν σιμός, ὁ δὲ
γρυπός, ᾗ μέλας, ᾗ λευκός, ᾗ μέγας, ᾗ μικρός, οὐχ ὁ
αὐτός. ἆρ' οὖν οὕτως ἐστὶν ἑκάτερος αὐτῶν ἄνθρωπος,
ὡσεὶ ᾗ γρυπὸς ᾗ σιμός, ᾗ οὕτως ὡς Ἐμπειρικός; ᾗ κἂν
παῖς τοῦτό γε νοήσειεν, ὡς ᾗ μὲν ἄνθρωπος εἷς ἐστιν,
ᾗ δ' ὁ μὲν σιμός, ὁ δὲ γρυπός, οὐχ εἷς.

ἆρ' οὖν οὐκ ἐσχάτης ἀναισθησίας, ἢ φιλονεικίας, ἢ
οὐκ οἶδ' ὅ τί ποτε καὶ προσειπεῖν ἄξιον, ἕνα μὲν
ὁμολογεῖν εἶναι τὸν φρενιτικὸν ᾗ φρενιτικός, ὡσαύτως
δὲ καὶ τὸν ληθαργικόν τε καὶ πλευριτικόν, οὐδένα δὲ
τὸν ἄνθρωπον ᾗ ἄνθρωπος· καὶ τὸν μὲν Ἐμπειρικὸν
ἕνα λέγειν ᾗ Ἐμπειρικός, οὐχ ἕνα δὲ τὸν ἵππον ᾗ
ἵππος, ἐνὸν ἀκοῦσαι λέγοντος Ἀριστοτέλους τε καὶ

Empirics, in other respects, presumably, they will not be one. So if, in fact, they are one in all kinds of ways, it would be superfluous and pointless, I think, to add "by virtue of" and "in this way," when it is possible simply to say that Serapion and Menodotus are one.

It would be similar if you were to make the argument about Menodotus himself alone, since you would not need any addition, but could simply say "Menodotus is one thing." If, therefore, Menodotus is simply one thing whereas Menodotus and Serapion are not simply one thing, but only "by virtue of" being Empirics, then assuredly there are, for them, other things in relation to which they are two and not one, and this is what has been stated by the philosophers of old—that it is one thing to be one and the same in number, but another thing to be one and the same in form, and there is nothing remarkable about Menodotus being the same as, and one with Serapion in respect to one thing, but not one and the same in some respect. Is it in this way, then, that each of them is a man, like being hook-nosed or snub-nosed, or is it, in this way, like being Empirics? Even a child would know this at least—that "by virtue of" being a man they are one, but "by virtue of" being snub-nosed or hook-nosed, they are not one.

Is it not the utmost stupidity or contentiousness— I don't know what the best term for it is—to grant that the man with phrenitis is one thing "by virtue of" being phrenitic and the same in the case of the man with lethargy and the man with pleurisy, but not to grant that a man is one thing "by virtue of" being a man, and also to say that the man who is an Empiric is one thing "by virtue of" being an Empiric whereas a horse is not one thing "by virtue of" being a horse? It is possible to listen to Aristotle and Theo-

137K

Θεοφράστου δύνασθαί τι τῷ μὲν εἴδει ταὐτὸν ὑπάρχειν ἕτερον ἑτέρῳ, τῷ δ' ἀριθμῷ μὴ ταὐτόν, ἔτι δὲ
τούτων ἔμπροσθεν αὐτοῦ τοῦ κἀκείνοις ὑφηγησα-
138K μένου τὴν τοιαύτην | διαστολὴν τῶν σημαινομένων
ἐπακοῦσαι λέγοντος, ὡς οὐδὲν θαυμαστόν ἐστιν ἓν
εἶναι τὰ πολλὰ καὶ τὰ πολλὰ ἕν. οὕτω γὰρ σαφῶς
ἅπαντα τοῦτον τὸν λόγον ὁ Πλάτων διῆλθεν ἐν ἀρχῇ
τοῦ Φιλήβου, ὥστ' ἐγὼ μὲν καὶ τοῖς ἀναισθήτοις
αὐτὸν εἶναι νομίζω σαφῆ.

γνωρίζουσι γοῦν οἱ ὄνοι καὶ ἄνθρωπον καὶ κάμηλον καὶ βοῦν, καὶ τόνδέ τινα τὸν ἄνθρωπον καὶ τήνδέ
τινα τὴν κάμηλον, καὶ τόνδέ τινα τὸν βοῦν. οὕτω δὲ
καὶ ὁδὸν οὐ μόνον ἁπλῶς ὡς ὁδόν, ἀλλὰ καὶ ὡς τήνδέ
τινα γνωρίζουσιν. ἐπίστησον γοῦν ὄνον ἐπ' ἀρχὴν
ὁδοῦ μὴ γνωρίμου καὶ θέασαι πῶς αὐτὴν βαδίζει τε
καὶ διέρχεται πᾶσαν, οὐκ ἐκτρεπόμενος ἑκατέρωσε,
πλὴν εἰ μὴ τύχοι που σχιζομένη, δῆλον ποιῶν ὡς αὐτὸ
τὸ εἶδος ὅ τί ποτ' ἐστὶν ὁδοῦ μέμνηται καὶ γιγνώσκει
σαφῶς. βαδίζει γοῦν τὴν τετριμμένην· καθ' ὅσον δὲ
ἀγνοεῖ σφάλλεται· οὐ γὰρ δὴ τήν γε ἄτομον καὶ μίαν
τῷ ἀριθμῷ μεμνημένος ἀπ' ἐκείνης ἣν οὐκ οἶδε βαδίζειν δύναται. δῆλον δ' ὅτι τὴν ὁδὸν ταύτην, ἣν νῦν
βαδίζει πρῶτον, ᾗ μὲν ὁδὸς ὡς εἴδει γινώσκων βαδίζει, καθ' ὅσον δὲ ἀριθμῷ μία, κατὰ τοσοῦτον ἀγνοεῖ
139K τῷ τε μηδαμῶς | πρὸς τὰς ἀτρίπτους ἐκτρέπεσθαι καὶ

---

29 See, for example, Aristotle, *Metaphysics* 1015b–1017a and

phrastus when they say that there is a capability for some
one thing to be the same as another in form but not the
same in number, and even before these men, to the one
who showed the way to such a distinction between things   138K
signified, and to pay heed to him when he says there is
nothing remarkable in one thing being many, or in many
things being one.[29] For Plato went over this whole argument lucidly at the beginning of the *Philebus*, so I think it is
clear even to idiots.

Anyway, donkeys recognize man, camel and ox, and this
particular man, this particular camel, and this particular
ox. So too do they recognize a road, not only simply as a
road, but also as this particular [road]. At any rate, make a
donkey stand at the start of a road it doesn't recognize and
see how it walks and goes along the whole [road], not turning to either side unless the road should happen to divide
somewhere, making it apparent that it is the actual form,
whatever is characteristic of a road, that it remembers and
knows clearly. At any rate, it walks [the road] that has been
well trodden. To the extent that it does not know [the
road], it makes mistakes, for certainly it is not able to walk
along the road that is undivided and single in number because it has a memory [of it] from that road which it does
not know. It is clear that, in respect to this road which it
now walks for the first time, it walks because it recognizes
it as being a road in form. However, as for it being one in
number, it is ignorant because nowhere does it turn aside   139K
toward untrodden [roads], and because, in the case of what
is divided into two, it will not know which road it must go

Theophrastus, *Metaphysica* 4b7ff. Their predecessor is, of
course, Plato.

τῷ καθ᾽ ὃ σχίζεται μὴ γινώσκειν ὁποίαν ἰτέον· ὅπερ
ἠπίστατο ἂν ἀκριβῶς, εἰ δεύτερον αὐτὴν ἢ τρίτον
ἔτυχε νῦν βαδίζων. ἐπειδὴ γὰρ ἕτερον μὲν οἶδεν,
ἕτερον δ᾽ ἀγνοεῖ, καθ᾽ ὅσον τὸ μὲν κοινὸν εἶδος ὁδοῦ
γινώσκει, τὸ δ᾽ ἴδιον ταύτης ἤ τινος ἀγνοεῖ, καθ᾽ ὅσον
μὲν οἶδεν οὐ σφάλλεται, βαδίζει γοῦν τὴν τετριμ-
μένην, καθ᾽ ὅσον δ᾽ ἀγνοεῖ σφάλλεται πολλάκις ἐν
ταῖς τριόδοις, οὐκ εἰδὼς ὁποίαν ἕληται. διττὰς οὖν
ἔχουσι γνώσεις καὶ οἱ ὄνοι· τῶν μὲν κοινῶν εἰδῶν
ἑτέρας, τῶν δ᾽ ἰδίων ἄλλας. λοιπὸν εἴτε ἓν εἶδος ἐκεῖνο
ἐθέλοις καλέσαι τὸ κοινόν, εἴτε γένος, εἴτε κοινότητα,
φυλάττων αὐτοῦ τὴν ἔννοιαν, ἣν ἐγὼ νῦν ἐξηγοῦμαι,
περὶ μὲν ὀνομάτων ἀμφισβητήσεις, οὐ μὴν μεταθεῖ-
ναί γε δυνήσῃ τὸ πρᾶγμα.

καίτοι πρὸς μὲν τὴν τῶν ὀνομάτων θέσιν ἴσως
ἕτερος ἀμφισβητήσει παραπλησίως σοι, τῆς περὶ τὰ
πράγματα θεωρίας ἀγύμναστος. οὐ μὴν ἡμεῖς γε
ἀμφισβητήσομεν, ἀλλ᾽ ἐκείνου μόνον ἀξιώσομέν σε
μεμνῆσθαι τοῦ παρὰ Πλάτωνος λεγομένου· ἐν γὰρ δὴ
140K τὰ πολλὰ εἶναι | καὶ τὸ ἓν πολλά, θαυμαστῶς λεχθέν,
καὶ οὐ²⁶ ῥᾴδιον ἀμφισβητῆσαι τῷ τούτων ὁποτερο-
νοῦν τιθεμένῳ· εἰ γὰρ δὴ τοῦτο διασῴζοις, οὐκέθ᾽ ἕξεις
ἐρίζειν, ὥσπερ νῦν ἐρίζεις τὰ μὲν ὑπὸ τῆς ἀμαθίας, τὰ
δ᾽ ὑπὸ τῆς φιλονεικίας ἀγόμενος. ἀλλ᾽ εἴτέ τις ἕνα
λέγοι τὸν φρενιτικόν, ἕνα συγχωρήσεις ὑπάρχειν· εἴτε
πολλούς, καὶ οὕτω συγχωρήσεις· ὡσαύτως δὲ καὶ τὸν
Ἐμπειρικόν τε καὶ Δογματικὸν καὶ τὸν Μεθοδικόν·
οὕτω δὲ τὸν ἰατρὸν ἕνα τε καὶ πολλοὺς φήσεις· ἕνα μὲν

down—which is something it would have known accurately if it had happened now to be walking it for the second or third time. Since it knows the one thing but does not know the other —that is, to the extent that it knows the common form of a road but not the specifics of this particular road—it does not err and walks the well-trodden road whereas, to the extent that it doesn't know, it errs often at crossroads, not knowing which one it should choose. So donkeys also have two kinds of knowledge: one of the common forms and one of the specifics. Finally, if you wish to call that one common thing a form, or class, or community, preserving the concept of it I am now expounding, you will be disputing over names, but you will not be able to change the facts.

And yet, perhaps, someone else similarly unpracticed in the theory about [these] matters will dispute the assigning of names with you. I will not enter the dispute. Rather, I think it right for you to remember only what was said by Plato: that the many are one and the one is many. A remarkable statement! Nor is it easy to take issue with someone who assumes either of these two [positions].[30] For if you keep this in mind, you will no longer be able to contend as you now contend, since you are led on partly by ignorance and partly by contentiousness. But if someone should say the "phrenitic" is one, you will concede that he is one; if [he should say it is] many, also in the same way you will agree, and in like manner also with respect to the Empiric, the Dogmatic, and the Methodic. In this way you will say the doctor is one and also many: one "by virtue of" be-

140K

30 See Plato's *Philebus* 14c.

---

26 K; οὐ *om.* P1, B (τὸ λεχθέν)

ᾗ ἰατρόν, οὐχ ἕνα δὲ τῷ κατὰ μέρος πλήθει. οὐ γὰρ δὴ
ἐπὶ μὲν τοῦ Ἐμπειρικοῦ τὸ ᾗ προσθήσεις, ἀφαιρήσεις
δὲ ἐπὶ τοῦ ἰατροῦ, οὐδὲ ἐπὶ μὲν τοῦ ἰατροῦ προσθήσεις, ἀφαιρήσεις δὲ ἐπ' ἀνθρώπου, οὐδὲ τὸν φρενιτικὸν μὲν ἕνα φήσεις ᾗ φρενιτικός, τὸν νοσοῦντα δ'
οὐχ ἕνα. καὶ γὰρ καὶ οὗτος ᾗ νοσῶν εἷς ἐστιν.

ἐπιλαθοῦ τοίνυν ἤδη ποτὲ τῶν λήρων ἐκείνων, οὓς
ἐν ἄλλοις βιβλίοις ἐρίζων λέγεις, ἀξιῶν δειχθῆναί σοι
τὸν ἄνθρωπον αὐτὸν καθ' ἑαυτὸν μόνον ἄνευ τῶν κατὰ
μέρος, ὥσπερ αὐτὸς δεῖξαι δυνάμενος τὸν Ἐμπειρικὸν
ἄνευ Μηνοδότου καὶ Σεραπίωνος καὶ τῶν ἄλλων τῶν
141K   κατὰ μέρος, ἢ νὴ Δία τὸν φρενιτικὸν | ἄνευ τῶν κατὰ
μέρος φρενιτικῶν. ἐν τίνι τοίνυν τὸ σφάλμα καὶ πόθεν
ἡ ἐκτροπὴ τοῦ καὶ τῶν ὄνων αὐτοὺς γίγνεσθαι μωρο-
τέρους; ἐξ ὧνπερ καὶ ἄλλα μυρία σφάλλονται. μεταβῆναι γὰρ ἐπὶ τὰς οὐσίας τῶν πραγμάτων ἀπὸ τῶν
ἐννοιῶν ἐπιχειροῦντες, εἶθ' ὡς ἀγύμναστοι τῆς λογικῆς θεωρίας σφάλλονται, συνανατρέποντες τῇ περὶ
τούτων ἀπορίᾳ καὶ τὰς ἐννοίας. ἐκδέχεται γὰρ αὐτοὺς
ἐνταῦθα τὸ περὶ γενῶν καὶ εἰδῶν ζήτημα σφῆλαι
δυνάμενον, οὐ μόνον ἀγυμνάστους ἀνθρώπους ἐν ταῖς
λογικαῖς μεθόδοις, ἀλλὰ καὶ τῶν γεγυμνασμένων τι-
νάς, ἐὰν μὴ προσέχωσιν ἀκριβῶς τὸν νοῦν. ἀλλ' οὐ
χρὴ διότι περὶ τῆς οὐσίας ἀποροῦσι τῶν πραγμάτων,
ἀφίστασθαι τῶν ἐναργῶν ἐννοιῶν· οὐδ' ἡγεῖσθαι σοφὸν ἐξευρηκέναι τι τοὺς μὲν Ἐμπειρικούς, ἐὰν ἐν
εἴπωσιν, ἄνευ τοῦ προσθεῖναι κατὰ ποῖον σημαινόμενον ἕν ἐστι, τοὺς δὲ Μεθοδικούς, ἐὰν ἀντὶ γένους, ἢ

ing a doctor but not one "by virtue of" the number considered individually. For you will not, on the one hand, add the phrase "by virtue of" to "the Empiric" and, on the other hand, take it away in the case of "the doctor"; nor will you add it in the case of "the doctor" but take it away in the case of "man"; nor will you say the "phrenitic" is one "by virtue of" being phrenitic but the person diseased is not one, for this person, too, by virtue of being diseased, is one.

Therefore, finally forget now those absurdities that, in a contentious spirit, you state in other books, demanding that man in himself and alone be shown to you without the individual examples, as if the Empiric [man] can be shown without Menodotus, or Serapion, or the others individually or, by Zeus, the phrenitic man without the phrenitics individually. In what, then, is the error, and from what source comes the change that makes them more foolish than donkeys? It is on the basis of these things that they make countless other mistakes. In attempting to make the transition from the concepts of the matters to their substances, as if unpracticed in logical theory, they make mistakes and, because of their perplexity in these matters, they overturn the concepts as well. For the inquiry regarding classes and forms awaits them here, which has the capacity to baffle not only men unpracticed in logical methods, but also some who have had extensive practice, if they don't focus their minds with precision. But it is unnecessary for them to depart from clear concepts just because they are at a loss concerning the substance of the matters. Nor should they suppose the Empirics have discovered something profound, if they say a thing is one without adding what kind of thing is signified, or the Methodics, if they

141K

219

εἴδους, ἢ κοινοῦ κοινότητα λέγωσιν. ἐμοὶ μὲν γὰρ
ἄμεινον ἐδόκει σαφῶς τῆς ἐννοίας ἤδη διωρισμένης,
ὡς ᾗ μὲν φρενιτικοί, ταύτῃ πάντες εἷς· ᾗ δ' ὁ μὲν νέος,
ὁ δὲ γέρων, ἢ ἰσχνός, ἢ παχύς, ἢ ἀνήρ, ἢ γυνή, |
142K   ταύτῃ πολλοί, χρήσασθαι λοιπὸν ἑρμηνείᾳ παλαιᾷ
καὶ συγκινδυνεῦσαι κατὰ τὴν λέξιν Ἀριστοτέλει καὶ
Θεοφράστῳ καὶ Πλάτωνι. πάντα τὰ τοιαῦτα τῷ μὲν
εἴδει λέγουσιν ἓν ὑπάρχειν, τῷ πλήθει δ' οὐχ ἕν· οὐ
φρενιτικὸν μόνον, ἢ ληθαργικόν, ἢ Ἐμπειρικόν, ἀλλὰ
καὶ Δογματικὸν καὶ Μεθοδικὸν καὶ ἄνθρωπον καὶ
ἵππον καὶ ἄνδρα καὶ γυναῖκα καὶ τῶν ἄλλων ἕκαστον.
εἰ δ' ἐπὶ τὰ κατὰ μέρος ἔλθοις, οἷον τήνδε τὴν γυναῖκα
τὴν δειχθῆναι δυναμένην, ταύτην οὐκ ἐγχωρεῖ τῷ μὲν
εἴδει λέγειν ἕν, τῷ πλήθει δὲ πολλά, κατ' ἄμφω γὰρ ἕν
ἐστιν ἡ δειχθῆναι δυναμένη γυνή, καὶ τῷ εἴδει καὶ τῷ
πλήθει, ὅπερ δὴ καὶ τῷ ἀριθμῷ καλοῦμεν.

οἱ δέ γε οὐχ οὕτως ποιοῦσιν, ἀλλ' οἱ μὲν κοινότητας ὀνομάζουσιν, ὥσπερ οὐ μᾶλλον ἀπορηθῆναι δυνα-
μένας εἰδῶν καὶ γενῶν, οἱ δ' ᾗ μὲν τόδε τι λέγουσιν
ὑπάρχειν ἕν· ᾗ δ' οὐχ ἕν, οὐκέτι λέγουσιν ἓν ὑπάρ-
χειν.27 ἐχρῆν γὰρ δήπου καὶ τούτους ὥσπερ δή ποτε ὅ
τε Μηνόδοτος καὶ Σεραπίων καὶ Θεοδᾶς καὶ Γλαυκίας,
Ἀπολλώνιός τε καὶ Καλλικλῆς καὶ Διόδωρος καὶ
143K   Ἡρακλείδης | καὶ Λύκος, εἷς ἅπαντες ὑπάρχουσιν ᾗ
Ἐμπειρικοί, οὕτω πάλιν ᾗ οὐχ εἷς ἅπαντες, ἀλλὰ
πάμπολλοί τινές εἰσιν, ἐξηγήσασθαι· ἐν αὐτῷ γὰρ τῷ

27 οἱ δ' ᾗ μὲν . . . ὑπάρχειν K, quem pro tem. accipe quod

say "community" instead of class, kind, or common aspect. For it seems to me better, when the concept has already been clearly defined, that "by virtue of" being phrenitics all are one, whereas "by virtue of" being young, or old, or thin, or fat, or a man, or a woman, they are many, to use 142K thereafter an ancient expression, running the risk in respect of language in company with Aristotle, Theophrastus, and Plato. They say that all such things are one in kind but not one in quantity, and not only phrenitic, or lethargic, or Empiric, but also Dogmatic, Methodic, human being, horse, man, woman and each of the others. If, however, you were to come to these individually—for example, the particular woman that can be pointed out—it is not possible to say she is one in form but many in quantity for, in relation to both, the woman who can be pointed out is one in form and in quantity, which we also call number.

In fact, they do not act in this way. Rather, some name "communities" as if these can be less problematic than kinds and classes, while others say something is one "by virtue of" being this particular thing—although, "by virtue of" not being one, they no longer say it is one. It also behooves them, of course, to explain how Menodotus, Serapion, Theodas, Glaucias, Apollonius, Callicles, Diodorus, Heraclides, and Lycus are all one "by virtue of" being Em- 143K pirics, but, on the contrary, how they are not all one but many particular people.[31] For in the very act of explaining

[31] All the men named are presumably Empirics, although details are scanty in several cases; for further brief details, see the Introduction, section 2 for some and *EANS* for the remainder.

---

non constat inter mss. B et P1 similiores, sim. autem P2 et K. Plur. mss inspectanda.

ταῦτ' ἐξηγεῖσθαι πάντως ἄν που κατενόησαν ὡς ἓν καὶ
πολλὰ ταὐτὸν εἶναί τε καὶ λέγεσθαι²⁸ δυνατόν ἐστι.
Μηνόδοτος οὖν καὶ Σεραπίων ᾗ μὲν Ἐμπειρικοὶ εἷς,
καὶ νὴ Δία γε ᾗ ἰατροὶ καὶ ᾗ ἄνθρωποι.

τί δὲ ᾗ ζῷα, καλὸν ἐρέσθαι τοὺς Ἐμπειρικούς, ἆρά
γε καὶ ταύτῃ²⁹ Μηνόδοτος καὶ Σεραπίων εἷς ἐστι; εἰ
μὲν γὰρ μὴ φαῖεν, οὐδ' ἡμεῖς συγχωρήσομεν ᾗ Ἐμπειρικοί, ταύτῃ γίγνεσθαι τοὺς δύο ἀνθρώπους ἕνα.
συγχωρούντων δὲ καὶ ταύτῃ τοὺς δύο γίνεσθαι ἕνα,
καθ' ὅσον ἄμφω ζῷα, εὐθὺς μὲν ὑπομνήσομεν, ὡς
ὀρθῶς ἄρα πρὸς τῶν παλαιῶν φιλοσόφων ἐλέγετο τὸ
μὲν ἀριθμῷ, τὸ δὲ εἴδει, τὸ δὲ γένει ταὐτόν τε καὶ ἓν
ὑπάρχειν. ἑξῆς δὲ πάλιν ἐρησόμεθα, φρενιτικὸς Μηνόδοτος, φρενιτικὸς Σεραπίων, πότερον ὁ αὐτός ἐστιν
ἢ ἕτερος; ἀποκρινομένων δὲ ταύτῃ φρενιτικὸν εἶναι
καὶ ἕνα καὶ τὸν αὐτὸν ἀμφοτέρους ᾗ φρενιτικοί, πάλιν
144K ἐρησόμεθα, τί δὲ καθὸ νοσοῦντες | οὐ καὶ ταύτῃ εἷς
ἄμφω ἐστόν; εἰ μὲν οὖν μὴ φαῖεν, οὐδ' ἡμεῖς συγχωρήσομεν ᾗ φρενιτικοί. συγχωρησάντων δὲ ἐρησόμεθα
τί δηλονότι πρᾶγμα μίαν ἰδέαν ἔχον, ἐφ' οὗ τοῦτο τὸ
ὄνομα φέρουσιν ἅπαντες ἄνθρωποι, νόσον. οὐ γὰρ δὴ
φρενῖτις μέν τι γενήσεται πρᾶγμα μίαν ἰδέαν ἔχον
καὶ ταύτῃ ποιοῦν ἅπαντας ἕνα τοὺς δεξαμένους αὐτό,
νόσος δ' οὐχ ὡσαύτως ἕνα ποιήσει πάντας οἷς ἂν
ἐγγένηται. Ἀλλ' οὐκ ἔστι, φησίν, οὐδὲν οὕτως ἀφω-
ρισμένον εἶδος ἢ ζῴου ἢ νοσήματος ὡς ἀνθρώπου καὶ

these things, they would understand somehow or other how it is possible to say that the same thing is both one and many. Thus, Menodotus and Serapion are one "by virtue of" being Empirics, but also, by Zeus, "by virtue of" being doctors and men.

What of "by virtue of" being animals—is it right to ask the Empirics whether, at least also in this, Menodotus and Serapion are one? For if they say no, neither will we concede that the two men are one "by virtue of" being Empirics. If, however, they do concede that in this way the two men are one, to the extent that both are animals, we will immediately remind [them] how it used to be stated correctly by the ancient philosphers that things can be one and the same in number, form or class. Further again, we will ask them: are phrenitic Menodotus and phrenitic Serapion, the same or different? If they reply that both are phrenitic in this way, and are one and the same insofar as they are phrenitic, we will ask again: in terms of having a disease, are not both also one in this way? If they say no, neither will we concede that "by virtue of" being phrenitics [they are one]. If they do agree, we will ask what this matter is which has a single form to which all men apply this term, "disease." For phrenitis will certainly not be some matter having a single form "by virtue of" which it makes everyone that receives it one, but disease will not, in like manner, make everyone in whom it might occur, one. "But this is not so," he says, "for there is no distinct kind either of 'animal' or of 'disease,' as there is of 'man' or 'phrenitis.'"

144K

---

28 πολλὰ ταὐτὸν εἶναί τε καὶ λέγεσθαι B; πολλὰ καὶ ταὐτὸν εἶναί τε λέγεσθαι P1, P2, K

29 καὶ ταύτῃ B P1; κατὰ ταῦτα K

φρενίτιδος. τί φὴς ὦ οὗτος; ἆρά γε οὐδὲν αἱ φωναὶ
δοκοῦσί σοι σημαίνειν, ἥ τε ζῷον καὶ ἡ νόσος, ἀλλ᾽
ὁμοίως ἐκφωνεῖσθαι τῷ βλίτυρι καὶ σκινδαψός; ἢ
σημαίνουσι μέν, οὐδὲν δ᾽ ὑπόκειται πρᾶγμα ταῖς φωναῖς, ὡς ἐν τῷ Σκύλλα καὶ Κένταυρος, ἢ καὶ σημαίνουσι καὶ τὸ σημαινόμενον ἐν ὑπάρχει; εἰ μὲν γὰρ
οὐδέν ἐστι πρᾶγμα τὸ δηλούμενον ὑπὸ τῆς ζῷον ἢ τῆς
νόσημα φωνῆς, οὐκ ὀρθῶς λέγεις τὸν ἄνθρωπον εἶναι
ζῷον ἢ τὴν φρενῖτιν νόσον. εἰ δ᾽ ἔστι καὶ λέγεις
ἀληθῶς, τουτὶ μὲν τὸ προσερχόμενον ζῷον εἶναι, ἢ
τὴν φρενῖτιν νόσον,[30] τοῦτον δ᾽ εἰ τύχοι τὸν κατα-
145K κείμενον | ‹φρενίτιδι›[31] ἄνθρωπον νοσεῖν, ἔστι τι πάν-
τως τῶν ὑπαρχόντων αὐτοῖς, ἐφ᾽ οὗ φέρεις ἕκαστον
τῶν ὀνομάτων.

ἀλλ᾽ οὐ γεγύμνασαι νοεῖν αὐτά, καίτοι γε ἐκ τῶν
πρώτων εἰσαγωγῶν ὄντα τῆς λογικῆς θεωρίας. τί οὖν
τοῦτο πρὸς τὸ ἀληθές; οὐ δήπου γὰρ ἐξ ὧν ἂν σὺ μὴ
συνίεις, ἐκ τούτων χρὴ κρίνεσθαι τὴν ἀλήθειαν, ἀλλ᾽
ἐξ ὧν ἂν καὶ συνετός τις ὢν φύσει καὶ μαθὼν καὶ
ἀσκήσας καὶ μὴ φιλονεικῶν καὶ τιμῶν τἀληθές, ὧν
οὐδὲν ὑπάρχει σοι· καίτοι μὰ τοὺς θεοὺς οὐκ οἶδ᾽ εἴ τι
προσδεῖταί τινος φύσει συνετοῦ τά γε τοιαῦτα. τίς
γὰρ οὐκ οἶδεν ὡς οὐ ταὐτὸν σημαίνει Σωκράτης καὶ
σιμός, ἀλλὰ τὸ μὲν Σωκράτης ὅλης τῆς ὑποκειμένης
οὐσίας ἐστὶν ὄνομα, τῶν δ᾽ ἄλλων ὀνομάτων οὐδὲν

---

[30] ἢ τὴν φρενῖτιν νόσον K; om. B, P1, P2 (cf. KLat)
[31] conj. Hankinson ex phrenitide KLat

What are you saying, you wretch? Don't even the words "animal" and "disease" have any significance to you, but are pronouncements similar to *blituri* and *scindapsus*?[32] Or do they signify [something], but no matter underlies the words, as in the cases of "Scylla" and "centaur," or do they both signify, and the thing signified is one? For if there is no clear matter indicated by the terms "animal" and "disease," you are not correct in saying that man is an animal or phrenitis is a disease. If there is, and what you say is true, that this one approaching is an animal or that phrenitis is a disease, and if it should happen that this man lying down is sick with phrenitis, there is, at all events,   145K something that exists in both on the basis of which you apply each of the terms.

But you are not practiced enough to understand these things even though they are among the first things introduced in logical theory. What, then, has this to do with truth? It is necessary to judge the truth, not from the things which, I presume, you do not understand, but from those things that someone who is naturally intelligent and is taught, someone who is practiced and not contentious, and who respects truth (none of which you are) would [know]. And yet, by the gods, I do not know whether such matters need someone who is naturally intelligent. For who does not know that Socrates and snub-nosed do not signify the same thing, but that "Socrates" is the name of the whole underlying substance whereas none of the other

32 Although these words are both used as standard nonsense words in Greek, they do have a meaning as musical terms; see R. J. Hankinson's (1991) discussion, pp. 220–21.

κατὰ τῆς τοῦ σώματος οὐσίας ἁπάσης λέγεται; οὔτε
γὰρ ὁ σιμὸς οὔθ᾽ ὁ προγάστωρ οὔθ᾽ ὁ φαλακρός, ἀλλὰ
τὸ μὲν τοῦ σχήματος τῆς ῥινός ἐστιν ὄνομα, τὸ δὲ τῆς
ἐνδείας τῶν ἐν τῇ κεφαλῇ τριχῶν, τὸ δὲ τοῦ μεγέθους
τῆς γαστρός. καὶ ταῦτα μέν ἐστι τὰ κατὰ μόρια.
λευκὸν δ᾽ εἰ φήσαιμεν ἢ μέλανα Σωκράτην, κατὰ
πάντων, οἶμαι, τῶν μορίων τοῦ σώματος ἐπιφέρομεν
146K τὰς προσηγορίας, | οὐ μὴν τὴν οὐσίαν γε ἅπασαν,
ἀλλ᾽ ἕν τι τῶν συμβεβηκότων αὐτῇ δηλοῦμεν, τὸ
χρῶμα, καὶ μέντοι κἂν εἰ παχύν, ἢ λεπτὸν εἴποιμεν, ἢ
σκληρόν, ἢ μαλακόν, ἢ δασύν, ἢ ψιλόν, ἤ τι τῶν
ἄλλων ἕκαστον ἃ τῷ Σωκράτει συμβέβηκεν, οὐ κατὰ
πάσης οὐδ᾽ οὕτω δηλονότι τῆς οὐσίας ἐπιφέρομεν τὴν
προσηγορίαν, ἀλλ᾽ ἕν τι τῶν συμβεβηκότων αὐτῇ
δηλοῦμεν. οὕτω δὲ καὶ τὸ καθῆσθαι καὶ τὸ περιπατεῖν
καὶ τὸ κινεῖσθαι καὶ τὸ κοιμᾶσθαι καὶ τὸ ἐγρηγορέναι
καὶ τῶν ἄλλων ἕκαστον τῶν τοιούτων ὀνομάτων οὐ
κατ᾽ οὐδενὸς δήπου τῶν ὄντων ἐπιφέρομεν, ἀλλά τι
τῶν ὑπαρχόντων Σωκράτει δηλοῦμεν· ἃ κατὰ τὸν ἔμπροσθεν λόγον ἢ ἐνεργείας ἐλέγομεν ὑπάρχειν, ἢ
παθήματα τούτων, ἤ τινας διαθέσεις. ἄμεινον οὖν σε
καὶ νῦν ἔτι τούτῳ τῷ τρόπῳ χρησάμενον γυμνάσασθαι, καθ᾽ ὅ τι κἂν τοῖς ἔμπροσθεν ἐδείκνυμεν, οὐκ
ἀπὸ τῶν ὀνομάτων, ἀλλ᾽ ἀπὸ τῶν πραγμάτων ἀρξάμενον. ἄρξαι δ᾽ ἀπὸ σαυτοῦ πρῶτον καὶ σκέψαι, πότερον
ἁπλοῦν τι πρᾶγμα ὑπάρχεις, ἢ σύνθετον, ἆρά γε ποὺς
ὑπάρχεις ἢ ὀφθαλμὸς ἢ ῥὶς ἢ κεφαλή; δῆλον γὰρ ὅτι
τούτων οὐδὲν οὔτε χωρὶς τούτων, ἀλλὰ κἀκ τούτων τε

terms is used in relation to the whole substance of the
body—that is, neither snub-nosed, potbellied nor bald,
which are terms for the shape of the nose, the lack of hair
on the head, and the size of the belly [respectively]? These
are terms applied to the parts. If, however, we were to say
Socrates is pale or dark, we are, I think, applying the terms
to all parts of the body but not in fact to the whole sub-   146K
stance. Rather, we are indicating one of the things incidental to it—the color. And further, if we say fat or thin, hard
or soft, hairy or bare, or any one of the other things which
happen incidentally to Socrates, even in this way we are
quite clearly not applying the name to the whole substance, but are indicating one of the things incidental to it.
In like manner also, sitting down, walking around, moving,
sleeping and being awake, and each of the other such
terms, we presumably do not apply to any existing things,
but use them to indicate one of the things existing in Socrates which, in relation to the earlier discussion, we said were
functions, or affections of functions, or certain conditions.
It would be better still, even now, for you to practice using them in this way, as I demonstrated in the earlier discussion, beginning not from names but from real things.
Begin from yourself first, and consider whether you are a
simple or compound thing: are you, that is, a foot, or an
eye, or a nose, or a head? It is clear that you are none of
these things, nor are you separate from them, but are com-

147K κἀκ τῶν ἄλλων ἀπάντων μορίων, ἑκάστου | τὴν οἰ-
κείαν ἔχοντος θέσιν, ὅλως ὑπάρχεις συγκείμενος.

ὑποκείσθω δή σοι τοὔνομα Θεμίσων. ἀλλ' ὅταν γε
φῶ Θεμίσωνα χωλὸν εἶναι, τὸ μὲν χωλὸν ἐπὶ τῆς τῶν
ποδῶν φέρω διαθέσεως, τὸ δὲ Θεμίσων τοῦ παντὸς ἦν
ὄνομα. καὶ μὲν δὴ καὶ σιμὸς καὶ τυφλὸς ἀπὸ μέρους ὁ
Θεμίσων ὀνομάζεται· πυρρὸς δὲ καὶ παχὺς οὐκ ἀπὸ
μέρους, ἀλλ' ἀπὸ διαθέσεων ἐνυπαρχουσῶν τῷ παντὶ
παραπλησίως τῷ περιπατῶν καὶ καθήμενος καὶ δια-
λεγόμενος καὶ ζῶν. ἆρ' οὖν ταῦτα μὲν γνωρίζεις ὡς
οὐκ ἔστι δηλωτικὰ τῆς ὅλης οὐσίας τῆς σῆς, ἀλλὰ τὰ
μὲν ἀπὸ μορίου τινὸς ὠνόμασται, τὰ δ' ἀπὸ διαθέσεως
μιᾶς· ὅταν δὲ ἀγαθὸν εἴπῃ τίς σε καὶ δίκαιον, οὐκέτι
γνωρίζεις ὡς καὶ ταῦτα διαθέσεών ἐστιν ὀνόματα τῶν
ἐπιγιγνομένων τῇ σῇ ψυχῇ; καὶ μὴν εἴ γε γνωρίσαις
ὡς ἀνάλογον ἔχει ταῦτα τῷ λευκὸς καὶ τῷ μέλας, ὡς
γὰρ ἐκεῖνα τῶν τοῦ σώματος, οὕτω ταῦτα τῶν τῆς
ψυχῆς ἐστι διαθέσεων ὀνόματα, γνωριεῖς, οἶμαι, καὶ
ὡς ὁ τεχνίτης καὶ ὡς ὁ ἄτεχνος ἀπὸ τῶν τῆς ψυχῆς
διαθέσεων ὀνομάζονται· καὶ τεχνίτην δ' εἰ νοήσαις
ὅθεν ὀνομάζεται, νοήσεις, οἶμαι, καὶ τὸν ἰατρὸν ὅθεν
ὠνόμασται. τοῦτον δ' εἰ νοήσαις ὅθεν ὀνομάζεται, οὐκ |
148K ἂν ἔτι σοι δεήσει πολλῆς πραγματείας ἐξευρεῖν ἐφ'
ὅτου ποτὲ τὸ ἐμπειρικὸς ὄνομα τέτακται.

τοῦτο δ' αὐτὸ τί ποτέ ἐστιν ὃ κελεύω σε ποιεῖν;
οὐδὲν σεμνὸν οὐδὲ μέγα. τὸ γὰρ διαιρεῖν τὰς κατηγο-

---

33 Themison of Laodicea was a pupil of Asclepiades and prob-

228

pounded from these things and also from all other parts, each having its proper position.   147K

So then, let us suppose your name is Themison.[33] But whenever, in fact, I say that Themison is lame, I apply the term "lame" to the condition of the feet, whereas Themison is the name of the whole. And furthermore, Themison is called snub-nosed and blind from a part [of his body], whereas he is called ruddy and fat not from parts but from conditions inherent in the whole in a closely similar manner to "walking," "sitting," "speaking," and "living." Do you not realize, then, that these [terms] are not signifiers of your whole substance, but that there are those named from a certain part and those named from a single condition? And whenever someone says you are good and just, do you not now realize that these are names of conditions supervening on your soul? And further, if you were to realize that these are analogous to "pale" and "dark," for those are names of conditions of the body in the same way as the former are names of conditions of the soul, you will realize, I think, how skilled and unskilled [people] are named from conditions of the soul. If you know from what source the skilled person is named, you will also know, I think, from what source the doctor is named. And if you were to know this, you would not need much work to discover what the   148K term "Empiric" has been assigned to at some time.

What is this that I am asking you to do? It is nothing grave and important. For the division of categories is the

ably lived and worked in Rome toward the end of the first century BC. He has some claim to be the founder of the Methodic sect. Here, however, the name is just used as an example in Galen's argument.

ρίας ἀρχὴ τῆς λογικῆς ἐστι θεωρίας· ἧς ὅτι παντελῶς
ἀμαθῶς ἔχετε δηλοῦται δι᾽ ὧν εἰκῆ φλυαρεῖτε. καὶ νῦν
οὖν σωφρονήσαντες αὖθις ἄρξασθε τὰ τῷ σώματι
συμβεβηκότα κατονομάζειν· οἷον ὅτι λευκός ἐστιν ὅδε
καὶ μέλας, ἢ νὴ Δία θερμὸς ἱκανῶς, ὡς μὴ φέρειν
ἀλύπως τὴν θέρμην· εἶτα τὴν οὕτω πολλὴν θερμασίαν
ὡς κάμνειν τὸ σῶμα δι᾽ αὐτὴν καὶ καλῶς ἐνεργεῖν μὴ
δύνασθαι, τῷ προσαγορεύοντι πυρετὸν ἐπιτρέψατε·
πάντες γὰρ ἄνθρωποι τὸν οὕτω θερμὸν πυρέττειν
φασί. καὶ οὐδὲν μέγα ποιήσετε μεταλλάττοντες τὸ
ὄνομα, πλὴν κατατρίψετε ὑμῶν τὸν χρόνον. ἀλλ᾽ ἐκεῖνο μᾶλλον, ὦ οὗτος, εἰ βούλει, ποίησον, ὅταν εἴπῃς
Θεμίσων πυρέττει καὶ Δίων πυρέττει καὶ πολλοὺς ἐφεξῆς οὕτως ὀνομάσῃς πυρέττοντας, ἐπίσκεψαι προσέχων τὸν νοῦν, ἆρα ἐν ἅπασιν αὐτοῖς ἓν καὶ ταὐτόν
149K ἐστι τὸ πυρέττειν ἢ ἕτερον. εὑρήσεις | γὰρ ἓν μὲν καὶ
ταὐτὸν τῷ εἴδει, τῷ πλήθει δέ, ὅπερ καὶ ἀριθμῷ καλοῦμεν, οὐχ ἕν. ἄλλως γὰρ οὔτ᾽ ἀποκρίνασθαί σοι δυνατὸν οὔτε νοῆσαι. εἷς οὖν ὁ πυρέττων ᾗ πυρέττει νὴ
Δία· καὶ γὰρ ὁ παραφρονῶν εἷς ᾗ παραφρονεῖ. τί δ᾽ ὁ
πυρέττων τε ἅμα καὶ παραφρονῶν, ἆρ᾽ οὐχὶ καὶ οὗτος
εἷς ᾗ πυρέττει τε ἅμα καὶ παραφρονεῖ; πρόδηλον καὶ
τοῦτ᾽, οἶμαι, παντί.

κείσθω τοίνυν κατ᾽ ἀμφοῖν τούτοιν ἓν ὄνομα, τὸ
πυρέττειν λέγω καὶ παραφρονεῖν, καὶ καλείσθω φρενιτικὸς ὁ τοιοῦτος· εἰ δ᾽ οὐ νοεῖς ὅπως κατ᾽ ἀμφοῖν ἓν
ὄνομα τίθεται, τάχ᾽ ἂν ἀναμνήσαιμί σε τῶν ὑπ᾽ αὐτοῦ
σου λεγομένων ὀνομάτων. ἵππον γὰρ δήπου καλεῖς τι,

first principle of logical theory. That you are completely ignorant of this is shown by the nonsense you heedlessly utter. Therefore, having now come to your senses, begin again to name those things that are incidental to the body. For example, that this person is pale, or dark, or, by Zeus, so hot that he cannot bear the heat without pain. Then, in this way, permit someone to give the name "fever" to heat so great that the body suffers because of it and cannot function properly, for all men say that someone heated in this way is febrile. But you will do nothing substantial by changing the name, apart from wasting your time. However, you would do better, you wretch, should you so wish, whenever you say Themison is febrile, or Dion is febrile, or you name many, one after another in the same way, if you direct your attention to considering whether it is one and the same thing to be febrile for all of them, or different. For you will find that it is one and the same in form, but in magnitude, which we also call number, it is not one. It is impossible for you to answer or to understand otherwise. So the person who is febrile "by virtue of" having a fever is one, by Zeus, and the person who is delirious is one "by virtue of" being delirious. And what about the person who is febrile and, at the same time, delirious? Is he not also one "by virtue of" being febrile and delirious? This, I believe, is clear to everyone.

149K

Accordingly, let there be one name for both of these—I refer to being febrile and being delirious—and let such a person be called "phrenitic." If you do not understand how one name is applied to both, perhaps I should remind you of names mentioned by you yourself. For something that is

τὸ ζῷον δηλονότι τὸ χρεμετιστικόν; ἆρ' οὖν ἡγῇ σὺ
διαφέρειν ἢ ἵππον εἰπεῖν ἢ ζῷον χρεμετιστικόν; ἐγὼ
μὲν γὰρ οὐχ ἡγοῦμαι. καὶ μὴν εἰ τοῦθ' οὕτως ἔχει κατ'
ἀμφοῖν ἐκείνων τῶν ὀνομάτων, ἵνα συντομώτερον εἴπῃς, ἵππον ἐπέθου. οὕτω δὲ κἂν εἴ τι πεζὸν καὶ δίπουν
ζῷον, ἀντὶ τοῦ διὰ τριῶν ὀνομάτων ἐνδείξασθαι, δι'
ἑνὸς ἐθελήσῃς δηλῶσαι, καλέσεις ἄνθρωπον. καὶ τό
150K γε διαλύειν | ἕκαστον τῶν ὀνομάτων εἰς λόγον οὕτω
γίνεται. καὶ μὴν καὶ τὸ συντιθέναι τὸν λόγον εἰς ἓν
ὄνομα κατὰ τὸν εἰρημένον ἀποτελεῖται τρόπον, ὅταν
τῶν θ' ἁπλῶν ἑκάστου τὴν ἔννοιαν ἔχῃς κατὰ τοὔνομα
καὶ δυνατὸς ᾖς ἐκ δυοῖν ἁπλοῖν ἔννοιαν αὖθις ἑτέραν
ἐργάσασθαι σύνθετον, εἶτ' ἐπ' αὐτῆς ὄνομα θέσθαι·
κἄπειτα πάλιν αὖθις ἐκείνῃ τῇ συνθέτῳ προσθεὶς
ἕτερον ἁπλοῦν, ἐκ τριῶν ἁπλῶν ἔννοιαν αὖθις ἀπεργα-
σάμενον μίαν, ἐπενεγκεῖν τι καὶ κατὰ ταύτης ὄνομα.
πῶς καὶ τίνα τρόπον; οὐ γὰρ ἀποκνήσω γυμνάζων
τοὺς σωθῆναι βουλομένους ἐκ τῆς πολυχρονίου ταύτης ἀπαιδευσίας ἐπὶ πλέον ἐπεκτεῖναι τὸν λόγον.

ἡ μὲν θερμότης ἁπλοῦ πράγματος ὄνομα. καὶ μὲν
δὴ καὶ ἡ βλάβη τῆς ἐνεργείας ἁπλοῦν τι πρᾶγμα.
τοσαύτη δὲ θερμότης ὡς ἤδη βλάπτειν ἐνέργειαν
οὐκέθ' ὁμοίως ἁπλοῦν. εἰ τοίνυν καὶ περὶ σύμπαν
γένοιτο τὸ σῶμα, πολὺ δὴ μᾶλλον οὐκέθ' ἁπλοῦν.
ἵν' οὖν μὴ πολλὰ λέγωσιν οἱ ἄνθρωποι, συντομίαν
ἀσκοῦντες φύσει τὴν τοιαύτην θερμότητα πυρετὸν
151K ὀνομάζουσιν. | ἑτοιμότερον γάρ ἐστιν εἰπεῖν πυρέττειν
Δίωνα τοῦ τοσαύτην θερμότητα ἔχειν ἐν ἅπαντι τῷ

an animal and neighs, you call, I presume, a horse. Do you think, then, that saying "horse" is different from saying "an animal that neighs"? I do not think so. For if this is the case, you apply the term "horse" in relation to both of those names, so that you might speak more briefly. Similarly too, if some animal is footed and bipedal, and instead of indicating this by three names, you wish to signify it by one name, you will call it a "man." The resolution of each name   150K into a definition occurs in this way. Further, the putting together of the definition into a single name is accomplished in the way that was stated; whenever you have the concept of each of the single things according to its name, you can, from the two simple concepts, create another concept again, which is composite, and then attach a name to this. And thereafter, when you apply another simple [term] to that composite [concept], making again one [composite] concept from three simple ones, you attach some name to this. How and in what way? For I shall not hesitate to extend the argument still further, exercising those who wish to be saved from their entrenched ignorance.

"Heat" is the name of a simple thing. And further, damage of function is a simple thing. But heat which is now such as to damage function is no longer, in a similar way, simple. Moreover, if it should also happen to involve the whole body, much more is it no longer simple. Therefore, so that men should not say many things, being inclined by nature to the practice of brevity, they call such heat "fever." For it is more expedient to say that Dion has a fever   151K than to say he has an amount of heat in his whole body such

σώματι ὡς βεβλάφθαι πολλὰς ἐνεργείας. ὅταν μὲν
οὖν αὐτὴν τὴν διάθεσιν δηλῶσαι βουληθῶσι, πυρετὸν
ὀνομάζουσιν, ὅταν δὲ τὸν ἔχοντα τὴν διάθεσιν, ἀπ'
ἐκείνης παρονομάζουσι καὶ καλοῦσι πυρέττοντα· καθάπερ ἀπὸ τῆς λευκότητος τὸν λευκὸν καὶ ἀπὸ τῆς
μελανότητος τὸν μέλανα. συνθέτου δὴ πράγματός
ἐστιν ὄνομα πυρετὸς καὶ πολὺ μᾶλλον ὁ πυρέττων·
ἁπλοῦν δέ γε παραφροσύνη. ἀλλ' εἰ προστεθείη τὸ
ἁπλοῦν τοῦτο τῷ συνθέτῳ, φρενιτικὸς μὲν ὁ ἄνθρωπος, ἡ διάθεσις δ' αὐτοῦ φρενῖτις ὀνομάζεται· καθάπερ, οἶμαι, καὶ ὁ ἄνθρωπος αὐτός, ἵνα μὴ λέγηται
ζῷον λογικὸν θνητόν, ἕνεκα συντομίας ἄνθρωπος ὠνο-
μάσθη, λόγου τινὰ δύναμιν ἐχούσης τῆς ἄνθρωπος
προσηγορίας· καὶ τοῦτ' ἔστιν ὃ καλοῦσιν οἱ παλαιοὶ
φιλόσοφοι τὸν λόγον εἰπεῖν τοῦ ὀνόματος. οὐ μὴν εἰς
ἄπειρόν γε προσάγουσιν, ἀλλ' ἄχρι τῶν ἁπλῶν ἀνέρχονται. τὸν γὰρ ἄνθρωπον, ἐπειδὰν διαλύσῃς εἰς ζῷον
καὶ λογικὸν καὶ θνητόν, καὶ αὖθις λύσεις τὸ ζῷον εἰς
οὐσίαν αἰσθητικήν· οὐ μὴν τήν γ' οὐσίαν ἔτι λῦσαι
152K   δυνήσῃ, καθάπερ οὐδὲ τὴν αἴσθησιν. ἁπλοῦν | γὰρ
ἤδη καὶ πρῶτόν ἐστιν ἑκάτερον τούτων. ᾗ καὶ θαυμάζειν ἐπέρχεταί μοι τῶν φρενιτικὸν μέν τινα καὶ
ἄνθρωπον εἶναι συγχωρούντων, νόσημα δὲ καὶ ζῷον
οὐ συγχωρούντων. ὅμοιον γάρ ἐστι τοῦτο τῷ τὰ μὲν
σύνθετα συγχωρεῖν, ἀμφισβητεῖν δὲ περὶ τῶν ἁπλῶν·
ὥσπερ οὐ προτέρων τῇ φύσει τῶν ἁπλῶν ὑπαρχόντων.

Οὐκ εἶδον, φησίν, αὐτὸ καθ' ἑαυτὸ τὸ ζῷον· ἀλλ'
οὐδὲ ἄνθρωπον, ὦ μωρέ, καίτοι λέγεις εἶναι σαυτὸν

that many functions have suffered damage. Thus, whenever they wish to indicate the condition itself, they use the term "fever," and whenever there is a person who has the condition, they derive the name from that condition, and call him "febrile." Similarly, "pale" [is derived from] pallor and "swarthy" from swarthiness. Actually, fever is the name of a composite thing as, to a much greater degree, "being febrile" is. Delirium, though, is a simple thing, but if this simple thing is added to the composite, the man is termed "phrenitic," and his condition "phrenitis." Similarly also, I think, man himself—so that one does not speak of him as an animal that is rational and mortal— is called "man" for the sake of brevity, the term "man" having a certain power of definition. And this is what the ancient philosophers called, "to articulate the definition of the term." Nor do they proceed to infinity, but only go as far as the simple things. When you resolve "man" into "animal," "rational" and "mortal," you will also further resolve "animal" into "sentient substance." But you cannot resolve "substance" any further, just as you cannot resolve "sentient." Each of these is already simple and primary. For this reason also, it strikes me as amazing that some accept there can be "phrenitic" and "man," but do not accept there can be "disease" and "animal." For this is tantamount 152K to agreeing on the matter of composite things, but disputing about simple ones, as if simple things were not prior by nature.

"But," he says, "I haven't seen animal in itself." Nor [have you seen] man in himself, you fool, although you say

ἄνθρωπον. ἢ τοῦτο μὲν ὁμολογήσεις, τὸ δὲ καὶ ζῷον
ὑπάρχειν οὐχ ὁμολογήσεις;

Οὐκ ἐθεασάμην, φησίν, καθ᾽ ἑαυτὴν οὐδαμόθι νό-
σον· οὐδὲ γὰρ φρενῖτιν ἐθεάσω ποτὲ μόνην, ἀλλ᾽ ἐπὶ
Θέωνος, ἢ ἐπὶ Δίωνος, ἢ ἐπ᾽ ἄλλου τινὸς ἀνθρώπου.
ὥστε τοῦτό γε τελέως ἠλίθιον, εἰ διότι μηδαμόθι
τεθέασαι νόσημα μόνον αὐτὸ καθ᾽ ἑαυτό, διὰ τοῦτο
νομίζεις μηδ᾽ εἶναι νόσημα· οὕτω γὰρ οὐδὲ πυρετόν,
οὐδὲ φρενῖτιν, οὐδ᾽ ἄλλο τῶν τοιούτων οὐδὲν εἶναι
συγχωρήσεις, ὡς οὐδὲ τούτων γε τεθέασαί τι μόνον
αὐτὸ καθ᾽ ἑαυτό. βέλτιον δ᾽ ἦν οὐχ οὕτως, ἀλλ᾽ ὥσπερ
εἴρηται πρόσθεν, ἀπὸ τῶν πραγμάτων αὐτῶν ἄρξα-
153K σθαι καὶ θεάσασθαι | τῇ διανοίᾳ πόσα τὰ σύμπαντά
ἐστιν ἁπλᾶ· κἄπειθ᾽ ἑκάστῳ θέμενον ἴδιον ὄνομα,
συμπλέκειν ἐξ αὐτῶν ἤδη τὰ σύνθετα.

ἐγγιγνέσθω δὴ τῷ ὑποκειμένῳ σώματι τουθ᾽ ἓν
πρῶτον, τὸ αἰσθάνεσθαι. πότερον οὐ καλέσεις ζῷον ᾧ
τουθ᾽ ὑπάρχει; καὶ μὴν ὑπὲρ ὀνόματος οὕτως ἀμφισβητήσεις. ἀλλ᾽ οὐδὲ εἶναι φήσεις αἰσθανόμενον
σῶμα; καὶ μὴν οὕτω γε τῶν πραγμάτων αὐτῶν κατα-
ψεύσῃ. ἀλλὰ καὶ σῶμα συγχωρῶν αἰσθανόμενον εἶναί
τι καὶ κατὰ τοῦ τοιούτου σώματος τοὔνομα τοῦτο τὸ
ζῷον λέγεσθαι, τολμήσεις φάναι μηδὲν εἶναι τὸ ζῷον;
οὐκοῦν οὐδὲ τὸ λευκὸν οὐδέν ἐστιν, οὐδὲ τὸ βαδίζον
οὐδὲ τὸ τρέχον; ἀπὸ γὰρ τῶν συμβεβηκότων ἑαυτῷ τὸ
σῶμα προσαγορεύεται λευκόν, βαδίζον καὶ τρέχον.
αὐτὰ δὲ τὰ συμβεβηκότα τὸ μὲν λευκότης ὀνομάζεται,
τὸ δὲ βάδισις, τὸ δὲ δρόμος. κατὰ δὲ τὸν αὐτὸν τρόπον
αἴσθησις μὲν ἕν τι τῶν ὑπαρχόντων τοῖς σώμασιν,

you are a man yourself. Will you agree on this but not agree that "animal" also exists?

"I have never seen," he says, "disease in itself anywhere." Neither have you ever seen phrenitis alone but only in Theon or Dion, or some other person. So it is absolutely stupid if, because you have never seen disease alone and of itself, you think that disease does not exist. For on this basis, you will not concede that there is fever, phrenitis, or any other such thing, because you have not seen any one of these things alone and of itself. It is better not to do this but, as I said before, to start from the matters themselves and determine by thought how many simple things there are in all, and then to confer on each of them its own specific name, and then to put together the compound from these. 153K

Suppose there is this one primary thing inherent in the underlying body—to have sensation. Will you not call that in which this exists an animal? But even so, you will be arguing over terminology. Or will you say a body is not capable of sensation? Really, in doing this you will be in error about the matters themselves. But if you concede that a body is something that is capable of sensation, and that referring to such a body this term "animal" is used, will you dare to deny that the animal exists? Is there, accordingly, no "pallor," or no "walking," or no "running"? For a body is said to be "pale," or to "walk," or to "run" from those things accidental to itself, and the accidentals themselves called "pallor," "walking," and "running." In the same way, sensation is one of the things existing in bodies, the body it-

αἰσθανόμενον δὲ αὐτὸ τὸ σῶμα· τοῦτ' οὖν καὶ ζῷον
ὀνομάζεται. τίς οὖν θεασάμενος αἰσθανόμενον σῶμα,
παρεὶς τὸ ζῷον ὄνομα ζητήσει τι κατ' αὐτοῦ λέγειν
ἕτερον; ἆρ' οὖν νοεῖται μόνον τὸ σῶμα καθάπερ Κέν-
154K   ταυρος, ἢ καὶ τυγχάνει τι τῆς προσηγορίας | ταύτης
ὑποκείμενον πρᾶγμα; δῆλον ὡς καὶ τυγχάνει. τί δέ,
νοεῖται μόνον ἡ αἴσθησις, ἢ καί τι τῶν τοῖς σώμασιν
ὑπαρχόντων ἐστίν; ἐμοὶ μὲν δοκεῖ καὶ τοῦτ' εἶναι
πρόδηλον ὡς ἕν τι τῶν ἐν τοῖς σώμασιν ὑπαρχόντων
ἐστὶ καὶ ἡ αἴσθησις.

κἂν μὴν εἰ μήτε τὸ σῶμα νοεῖται μόνον, ἀλλὰ καὶ
ἔστι, μήθ' ἡ αἴσθησις, ἔστι γὰρ καὶ ἥδε, πῶς ἄμφω
συντιθέντα τὸ σύνθετον οὐκ ὂν ποιήσει; γελοῖον γὰρ
ἤδη τοῦτό γε, σῶμα μὲν εἶναί τι καὶ αἴσθησιν, αἰσθανόμενον δὲ οὐδὲν εἶναι σῶμα· καὶ τούτου γελοιότερον,
αἰσθανόμενον μὲν εἶναι σῶμα, ζῷον δ' εἶναι μηδέν,
ὥσπερ ἄλλο τι καὶ οὐ τοῦθ' ὑπάρχον ζῷον, ἢ διαφέρον
τι τῷ λόγῳ δηλοῦν ἐπιχειρεῖν ὁτιοῦν ἢ ὀνόματι, τῆς δ'
αὐτῆς ἀτοπίας ἔχεται καὶ τὸ μὴ συγχωρεῖν εἶναί τι
νόσον· εἰ γὰρ οὐδέν ἐστι διάθεσις, οὐδὲ νόσος ἔσται
τι. δοθείσης δ' εἶναι διαθέσεως, ἔσται τι καὶ νόσος·
ἥτις γὰρ ἂν ἐνέργειαν βλάπτῃ διάθεσις, ἐκείνη νόσος
ἐστίν.

Ἀλλ' οὐκ ἔχεις μοι δεῖξαί, φασι,[32] νόσον αὐτὴν
καθ' ἑαυτήν. οὐδὲ γὰρ φρενῖτιν, ὦ οὗτος, οὐδὲ πυρετόν.
155K   ἀλλ' ὅμως καὶ ταῦτα συγχωρεῖς | ὑπάρχειν καὶ ἄλλα
πολλά. τὴν γὰρ μικρολογίαν τῶν ὀνομάτων, ἣν ἐκομ-
ψεύσαντό τινες τῶν φιλοσόφων, ἀνατρέπουσαν ἅπα-

self being capable of sensation. And this, then, is called an animal. Who, then, seeing a body capable of sensation, will pass over the name "animal" and seek to say something else in relation to it? Is the body only a concept then, as in the case of the centaur, or does there also happen to be some underlying matter for this term? It is clear that this 154K does happen. And is sensation something in concept only, or is it also something which exists in bodies? It seems clear to me that sensation is also one of the things existing in bodies.

Further, if the body is not only conceived of, but actually exists, and sensation is not [only conceived of] but exists too, how will the combination of both not make a composite entity? Now this is absurd—that a body is something which exists, as is sensation, but a sensing body does not exist. And even more absurd than this is that there is a perceiving body but not an animal, as if something else and not this was an animal, or that there was a difference between trying to indicate anything whatsoever by a definition and by a name. Not to concede that disease exists is of a piece with this very same absurdity. For if no condition exists, there will be no disease. However, if it is granted that condition exists, then disease will exist too. For whatever condition damages function is a disease.

"But," he says, "you cannot show me a disease in itself." Nor, you wretch, can I show you phrenitis or fever. Nevertheless, you do concede that these things exist, and many 155K others. I refrain for the present from speaking about the logic-chopping of terminology which some philosphers

---

32 φησι conj. nos; φασι omnes

σαν τὴν ἐν τῷ βίῳ συνήθειαν, ὡς μὴ δ᾽ ἐκείνους[33] αὐτῇ
χρῆσθαι δύνασθαι κατὰ τὰ σφῶν αὐτῶν συγγράμματα, παραιτοῦμαι λέγειν τὰ νῦν, ἑτέρωθι διειλεγμέ-
νος ὑπὲρ αὐτῶν ἐπὶ πλέον. εἰρηκὼς οὖν οὐδὲν ἧττον
ὅσα χρὴ κἂν τοῖς Περὶ τῶν στοιχείων λογισμοῖς,
λέγω δὲ μικρολογίαν, ἐν ᾗ διαιροῦνται κατὰ γένη τό
τε ὂν καὶ τὸ ὑφεστός. ἀδιαφόρως γὰρ ἡμῖν κἀνταῦθα
καὶ κατὰ τὸν ἑξῆς λόγον εἰρήσεται ταῦτα.

πάντας δ᾽ ἐν πᾶσιν ἐξελέγχειν ἀδύνατον. ἀλλὰ γὰρ
περὶ τοῦ μὴ μόνον ἔννοιαν εἶναι νοσήματος ἰδίαν,
ἀλλὰ καὶ πρᾶγμά τι τῆς προσηγορίας ταύτης τυγ-
χάνον ὑποκεῖσθαι, κατά γε τὸ παρὸν ἀρκεῖ λελέχθαι
ταῦτα. σαφέστερον δ᾽ ἔτι τοῦτ᾽ αὐτὸ νοηθήσεται τοῦ
λόγου προϊόντος, ἐπειδὰν ὁ περὶ πρώτων ἐνδείξεων
περαίνηται λόγος. ὅσα δὲ περὶ νοσήματος εἴρηται
νῦν, ἡγοῦμαι καὶ περὶ συμπτώματος εἰρῆσθαι καὶ
πάθους, ὑγείας τε καὶ ἀρτιότητος, ἰσχύος τε καὶ δυνά-
156K μεως ἁπάντων τε τῶν | ἄλλων ὧν ὀνόματά τε καὶ
νοήσεις εἰσὶ κατά τινων ὑποκειμένων λεγόμενα. πάντα
γὰρ ταῦτα τοῖς σώμασιν ὑπάρχει, τὰ μὲν ὡς διαθέσεις, τὰ δ᾽ ὡς ἐνέργειαι, τὰ δ᾽ ὡς πάθη· καὶ τὰ μὲν
ὡς κατὰ φύσιν ὄντα, τὰ δ᾽ ὡς παρὰ φύσιν, ἔνδειξίς τε
καθ᾽ ἕκαστον αὐτῶν ἰδία γίνεται, παρεωραμένη τοῖς
πλείστοις τῶν ἰατρῶν.

[33] μὴ δ᾽ ἐκείνους B (conj. simil. Hankinson); μὴ δι᾽ ἐκείνους
K, P1, P2

quibble about, and which overturns all that is customary in life. Not even those men can use it according to their own writings.[34] I have argued about these things at length elsewhere, since I have said as much as is necessary in my work *On the Elements [according to Hippocrates]*—I speak of the logic-chopping in which what exists and what subsists are distinguished according to their class. I shall speak of these things making no distinction, both here and in the discussion that follows.

It is impossible to refute all people in all matters. But concerning this, at least for the present it will be enough that I have said this: not only is there a specific concept of disease, but also there is a real thing that happens to underlie this term. This will be understood even more clearly as the argument proceeds, after the discussion of the primary indications reaches its conclusion. And all that has now been said about disease, I consider has also been said about symptom and affection, health and soundness, strength, and capacity and all the other things of which names and concepts are used in relation to underlying things. For all these things exist in bodies, some as conditions, some as functions, and some as affections. Some of them are as entities in accord with nature, whereas others are as entities contrary to nature. A specific indication occurs in relation to each of these, one that is disregarded by the majority of doctors.

156K

34 Presumably a reference to the Stoics.

ΒΙΒΛΙΟΝ Γ

157K 1. Εἴπερ οὖν, ὦ Ἱέρων, ἡ ἔνδειξις ἐκ τῆς τοῦ πράγματος φύσεως ὁρμωμένη τὸ δέον ἐξευρίσκει, τὴν ἀρχὴν
τῆς τῶν ἰαμάτων εὑρέσεως ἐκ τῆς τῶν νοσημάτων
αὐτῶν ἀνάγκη γίγνεσθαι· καὶ γὰρ καὶ ἄτοπον ἕτερον
μὲν εἶναι τὸ ἐνδεικνύμενον τὴν θεραπείαν, ἕτερον δὲ τὸ
θεραπευόμενον· ἕκαστον γὰρ ὑπὲρ ἑαυτοῦ τι δύναται
δηλῶσαι μᾶλλον ἢ ὑπὲρ ἄλλου. τοῦτο μὲν δὴ κἀν τοῖς
ἐφεξῆς ἔσται σαφέστερον. ἐπεὶ δὲ πάντες ὁμολογοῦσιν ἐκ τῶν διαθέσεων τὰς πρώτας ἐνδείξεις λαμ-
158K βάνειν, οὐ χρὴ μηκύνειν ἔτι περιττῶς τὸν λόγον | ἀπο-
δεικνύντας ὡς ἐντεῦθεν ἄρχεσθαι προσήκει, μᾶλλον δ'
ὅτι μήτε τὸ ξύμπαν τοῦτ' ἐστὶ μήθ' ὅλως μέγα τι
μέρος, ὡς οἱ Μεθοδικοὶ νομίζουσιν, ἀλλὰ σμικρότα-
τόν τε καὶ ἀρχὴν μόνον ἐπιδεῖξαι πειραθῶμεν. αὐτοὶ
δή φασιν ἐκεῖνοι τὸν μὲν ἐν τῇ κύστει λίθον, ὅτι τῷ
γένει παρὰ φύσιν, ἐνδείκνυσθαι τὴν ἄρσιν. οὕτω δὲ
καὶ τὰς ἀκροχορδόνας καὶ τὰς μυρμηκίας ἀθερώματά
τε καὶ στεατώματα καὶ μελικηρίδας, ὅσα τ' ἄλλα
τοιαῦτα. τὸ δ' εἰς τὸν ὄσχεον ἐμπεπτωκὸς ἔντερον, ὅτι
τῷ τόπῳ παρὰ φύσιν, ἅπαντά τε τὰ ἐξηρθηκότα τὴν
εἰς τὴν οἰκείαν χώραν ἐπάνοδον ἐνδείκνυται. καὶ μὴν

242

BOOK III

1. Therefore, Hiero, if the indication, which takes its origin   157K
from the nature of the matter, reveals what is needed, the
starting point for the discovery of the cures necessarily
arises from the nature of the diseases themselves. Moreover, it would be paradoxical if what indicates the treatment is different from what is being treated, because each
thing is able to reveal something about itself more than it is
able to reveal something about another thing. This will
certainly be clearer in what follows. Since everyone agrees
to take the primary indications from the conditions, it is
not necessary to prolong the argument unduly once I have   158K
shown that it is appropriate to begin here. Instead, I shall
attempt to show that this is neither the whole argument
nor actually a large part of it, as the Methodics think, but a
very small part and only the beginning. Those very men say
that a stone in the bladder, by being in the class "contrary
to nature" indicates its removal. And the same applies in
the case of thin-necked warts, sessile warts, atheromata,
steatomata, melicerides and other such things. Bowel that
has herniated into the scrotum, by being in an unnatural
place, indicates the return to its proper place, as do all
those things that are displaced. Indeed, no craft as yet ex-

οὐδὲν τούτων οὐδέπω τεχνικόν, ἀλλ᾽ ὅπερ, οἶμαι, καὶ
τοῖς ἰδιώταις ἅπασιν ὑπάρχει γινώσκειν· ἐμβληθῆναι
γοῦν ἑαυτῶν κελεύουσι τὸ κῶλον, ὅταν ἐξηρθρηκότος
αἰσθάνωνται καὶ ἀφαιρεθῆναι τὴν ἀκροχορδόνα καὶ
τὸ ἕλκος εἰς οὐλὴν ἀχθῆναι καὶ τὸ ῥεῦμα τῆς κοιλίας
ἐπισχεθῆναι.

τὸ δὲ δι᾽ ὧν χρὴ ταῦτα ποιεῖν οὐκ ἴσασι. καὶ τοῦτ᾽
ἔστιν ὃ χρὴ προστιθέναι τὸν ἰατρόν. ὥστε ἡ ἀπὸ τῶν
νοσημάτων ἔνδειξις ἀρχὴ μέν ἐστι καὶ οἱονεὶ ὁρμη-
τήριόν τι τῆς θεραπευτικῆς μεθόδου, τῆς τέχνης δ᾽
159K οὔπω | τῆς ἰατρικῆς μόριον οὐδέν, ἢ οὐκ ἀξιόλογόν γε
μόριον, οὐδὲ ἴδιον, ἀλλ᾽ ὅπερ καὶ τοῖς ἰδιώταις ὑπάρχει κοινόν. ὁ τοίνυν ἐξευρεῖν δυνάμενος ὑφ᾽ ὧντινων
ἔσται τὸ δηλούμενον ἐκ τῆς πρώτης ἐνδείξεως, οὗτός
ἐστιν ὁ τῶν νοσημάτων θεραπευτής· καὶ εἰ μὲν διὰ τῆς
ἐμπειρίας εὕροι, τηρητικός τέ τις καὶ Ἐμπειρικὸς ὀνο-
μασθησόμενος, εἰ δὲ διὰ λόγου τινός, ἢ μεθόδου,
Λογικός τε καὶ Μεθοδικὸς καὶ Δογματικός. οὐκοῦν ὁ
μὲν ἰδιώτης, ἄνωθεν γὰρ ταὐτὸ ῥητέον, ἥκει παρὰ τὸν
ἰατρόν, ἐμβαλεῖν κελεύων τὸ κῶλον, ἢ διαπλάσαι τὸ
συντετριμμένον ὀστοῦν, ἢ ἐξελεῖν τὴν μελικηρίδα. τὸ
δ᾽ ὅπως χρὴ τούτων ἕκαστον ποιῆσαι τῆς ἰατρικῆς
ἐστι τέχνης εὕρημα. οἱ μὲν οὖν Ἐμπειρικοὶ δι᾽ ἐμπειρίας εὑρίσκεσθαι πάντα φασίν· ἡμεῖς δὲ τὰ μὲν ἐμ-
πειρίᾳ, τὰ δὲ λόγῳ. μήτε γὰρ ἐκείνην ἱκανὴν εἶναι
πάντα μήτε μόνον εὑρίσκειν τὸν λόγον.

οὐ μὴν ἀξιοῦμέν γε συγκεχυμένην ποιεῖσθαι τὴν
διδασκαλίαν, ἀλλ᾽ ἰδίᾳ μὲν τὴν ἐμπειρικήν, ἰδίᾳ δὲ

ists for these matters other than that which is, in my view, also known by all laymen. At all events, they direct that their own limb be put back into place whenever they realize it is dislocated, that a thin-necked wart be removed, that a wound be brought to a scar, and that a flux of the stomach be stopped.

But what they don't know is how they ought to do these things. This is what the doctor must add. As a result, the indication from the diseases is a beginning and starting point, as it were, for the therapeutic method, and is not as yet any part of the medical art, or at least not a noteworthy 159K or specific part, but something also common to laymen. Therefore, the person who is able to discover by whatever means what will be revealed from the primary indication is the one who treats the disease. And if he finds out through experience, he will be called an "observer" or an "Empiric" whereas, if he finds out through some theory or method, [he will be called] a "Rationalist," or "Methodic," or "Dogmatic." Therefore the layman, for we must be consistent, comes to the doctor directing him to put the limb back into place, or to set the broken bone, or to remove the meliceris. However, the means necessary for doing each of these things is the invention of the medical art. The Empirics say all these things are discovered through experience. I say that some are discovered through experience; but some through reason, because experience alone is not enough to discover everything, nor is reason.

However, I think it is important not to make the teaching confused, but to identify separately the empirical and

τὴν λογικήν, ἵν' ὅσην ἑκατέρα δύναμιν ἔχῃ σαφῶς
εὑρεθῇ. καὶ νῦν ἡμῖν πρόκειται περὶ τῆς λογικῆς
εὑρέσεως εἰπεῖν.

160K   ἆρ' οὖν ἔχομέν | τινα μέθοδον ᾗ χρώμενοι τῶν εἰρη-
μένων ἕκαστον εὑρήσομεν; ἀνελεῖν λέγω τὸ περιττὸν
τῷ γένει καὶ μεταθεῖναι τὸ τὴν οἰκείαν χώραν ὑπηλ-
λαχός, ἑνῶσαί τε τῆς συνεχείας λελυμένον. ἢ τὴν
ἐμπειρικὴν ὑπ' αὐτὰ παρακαλέσομεν; ἐγὼ μὲν καὶ
πάνυ πέπεισμαι μέθοδον ὑπάρχειν τινὰ τῆς τῶν
ζητουμένων εὑρέσεως, ἧς ἀρχὴν εἶναι τὴν ἐκ τῶν
νοσημάτων ἑκάστου προσπίπτοντα σκοπόν. ἡ γὰρ
τῆς συνεχείας λύσις τὴν ἕνωσιν ἐπιζητεῖ· κατὰ μὲν
ὀστοῦν κάταγμα λεγομένη, κατὰ δὲ τὸ σαρκῶδες μέρος ἕλκος, ὥσπερ γε καὶ τὸ τραῦμα καὶ τὸ ῥῆγμα καὶ
τὸ σπάσμα, τὸ μὲν ἐν σαρκώδει μορίῳ διὰ τοῦ τρωθῆναι γεγονός, τὸ δὲ ῥῆγμα καὶ τὸ σπάσμα χωρὶς τοῦ
τρωθῆναι, σαρκώδους μὲν ἐν τῷ ῥήγματι μορίου τῆς
συνεχείας λυθέντος, νευρώδους δὲ ἐν τῷ σπάσματι.
τούτων ἁπάντων ὁ μὲν σκοπὸς ἕνωσις. εἴτε δ' οἷόν τε
τυχεῖν αὐτοῦ καθ' ἅπαν, εἴτ' οὐκ ἐγχωρεῖ πολλαχόθι,
τοῦτ' αὐτὸ πρῶτον ἤδη τεχνίτου γινώσκειν. ἰδιώτης
γὰρ οὐδεὶς οἶδεν οὔθ' ὅτι τῶν φρενῶν τὸ νευρῶδες οὔθ'

---

1 The term σκοπός is sometimes rendered "indicator" rather
than the more usual "aim" or "objective," depending on context.
Linacre was aware of the difficulty, translating σκοπός as *indi-
catio* here with a marginal note to the effect that it is different
from ἔνδειξις, which is clearly a technical term for Galen.

2 Another somewhat problematical term is ἕλκος, which is

the rational, so that whatever power each one has may be clearly revealed. And the task before us now is to speak about rational discovery.

Do we, then, have some method, using which we will discover each of the aforementioned things? I say it is to take away what is in excess in the class, change the place of what is altered in respect to its proper place, and unite what has suffered dissolution of continuity. Or shall we invoke the empirical [method] for these? I, too, am very much persuaded that there is a certain method for the discovery of the things sought, the beginning of which is the indicator[1] that comes from each of the diseases. For the dissolution of continuity requires union. In a bone [this dissolution] is called a fracture, while in a fleshy part it is called a wound (*helkos*),[2] just as in fact it is also called a wound (*trauma*), rupture or tear. It is a wound when the wounding occurs in a fleshy part, whereas rupture or tearing occurs apart from wounding, the former when there is dissolution of continuity in the rending of a fleshy part, and the latter when it arises in rupture of a sinewy part.[3] What is indicated (the goal) for all these things is union. Whether it is possible for this to happen everywhere, or is not possible in many places, is now primarily a matter for the expert to know. No layman knows that neither the sinewy part of the diaphragm, nor the small intestines

considered at some length in the Introduction, section 6. In this book it clearly corresponds to "wound" in modern terms. Context determines the choice between "wound" and "ulcer."

[3] A third term with variable meaning is *neuron* and its cognates (as above). The options are "nerve" and "sinew," the choice again depending on context.

161K ὅτι τὰ λεπτὰ τῶν ἐντέρων | οὐκ ἐγχωρεῖ δέξασθαι τὸν
σκοπόν, οὐ μὴν οὐδὲ περὶ πόσθης, οὐδὲ περὶ τοῦ
λεπτοῦ τῶν γνάθων οἶδεν· ἀλλ' οὐδ' εἰ τερηδὼν ὀστοῦ
δύναται θεραπευθῆναι, καθάπερ ἐν σαρκὶ διάβρωσις·
οὐδ' εἰ τὸ κάταγμα συμφῦναι, καθάπερ τὸ τραῦμα,
κατὰ ταὐτὰ δὲ οὐδ' εἰ πωρωθῆναι δύναται γιγνώσκει·
ὡσαύτως δὲ καὶ περὶ τῶν ἐν τῇ κεφαλῇ καταγμάτων ὁ
ἰδιώτης οὐδὲν οἶδεν, εἴτε χρὴ τὴν πώρωσιν ἀναμένειν,
εἴτ' ἄλλως ἰᾶσθαι. πολὺ δὲ μᾶλλον οὐδὲ εἰ καρδίας
τρωθείσης ἢ πνεύμονος ἢ γαστρὸς ἢ ἥπατος ἐλπίζειν
χρὴ τὴν ἴασιν· οὐδ' ὅλως οὐδὲν οὐκέτι περαιτέρω τοῦ
πρώτου σκοποῦ γιγνώσκει τῶν ἰδιωτῶν οὐδείς.

τοῦτ' οὖν αὐτὸ πρῶτον ἤδη τῆς τέχνης ἔργον, ἤτοι
τυχεῖν ἐλπίζειν τοῦ τέλους ἢ ἀπογινώσκειν τοῦ τυχεῖν·
διττὴ δ' ἡ γνῶσις αὐτοῦ καὶ τρίτην οὐκ ἐγχωρεῖ
γενέσθαι· διὰ μὲν τῆς ἐμπειρίας ἡ ἑτέρα, μακροῦ
δηλονότι χρόνου δεομένη· διὰ δὲ τῆς αὐτοῦ τοῦ πράγματος φύσεως ἡ ἑτέρα· καὶ γὰρ τὴν οὐσίαν ἑκάστου
τῶν μορίων ἐπισκέψεται καὶ τὴν ἐνέργειαν καὶ τὴν
χρείαν καὶ τὴν θέσιν, ἐξ ὧν ὁρμωμένη τό τ' ἀδύνατον
162K ἰαθῆναι προγνώσεται καὶ τοῦ | δυνατοῦ δέξασθαι τὴν
ἴασιν ὑπὲρ τῆς τῶν βοηθημάτων εὑρέσεως ἐπισκέψεται.

2. Πρόδηλον δ' ὡς ἀπὸ τῶν ἁπλουστάτων ἄρξεται.
τί δ' ἁπλούστερον ἕλκους ἐπιπολῆς ἐν σαρκώδει
μορίῳ; τοῦτ' οὖν εἰ μὲν ἁπλῶς ἕλκος εἴη, σκοπὸς
αὐτοῦ τῆς ἰάσεως ἕνωσις· εἰ δὲ σὺν κοιλότητι, διττὸς
μὲν ὁ σκοπός, ὅτι καὶ ἡ διάθεσις διττή· συνεχείας μὲν

can "accept" what is indicated, and he certainly does not   161K
know about either the prepuce or the thin part of the
cheeks. Besides, he does not know if caries of the bone
can be treated, and the same with an erosion in flesh, or
whether a fracture knits, or a wound heals. Similarly, he
does not know if a callus can be made hard. In like manner,
too, the layman does not know, concerning fractures in the
head, whether it is necessary to await callus formation or to
effect a cure in another way. Much more, however, does he
not know if he should hope for a cure when the heart has
been wounded, or the lung, stomach or liver; nor, in general, does any layman know anything beyond the primary
objective.

This, then, is now the very first task of the craft—to
know whether there is hope of achieving the desired outcome or not. This knowledge has two components; it is not
possible for there to be a third. One is knowledge from experience, which clearly requires a long time. The other is
knowledge from the nature of the matter itself, which
takes into account the substance of each of the parts, and
their function, use, and position. Proceeding from these
factors, not only will there be prior knowledge of what can-   162K
not be cured and of what can respond to the cure, but also
there will be consideration of the discovery of remedies.

2. It is clear that [we should] begin from the most simple [diseases]. What is simpler than a superficial wound in
a fleshy part? If this wound is simple, the objective of its
cure is union. If it has a cavity, the objective is twofold in
that the condition is also twofold—the wound is a dissolu-

λύσις τὸ ἕλκος, ἀπώλεια δὲ οὐσίας τινὸς οἰκείας τῷ
ζώῳ ἡ κοιλότης. εὑρίσκεται δὲ κἀνταῦθα πολλάκις ὁ
ἕτερος τῶν σκοπῶν ἀδύνατος· οἷον εἰ μὴ μόνον ἡ
σάρξ, ἀλλὰ καὶ τὸ ὑποκείμενον ὀστοῦν ἀπολωλὸς
εἴη· πληρωθῆναι γὰρ ἀκριβῶς ἡ τοιαύτη κοιλότης οὐ
δύναται, ἀλλ᾽ ἐπουλωθῆναι μέν, ὅπερ ἦν ἕλκους ἴασις,
ἀνίατος δὲ ἡ κοιλότης καταλειφθήσεται. τοῦτ᾽ οὖν
αὖθις αὐτὸ πάντως μὲν ἤτοι διὰ τῆς ἐμπειρίας ἢ διὰ
τοῦ λόγου χρὴ γνῶναι· ὁ Θεσσαλὸς δὲ οὔτε τούτοις
χρῆται καὶ τρίτον οὐδὲν προστίθησιν, εἶτ᾽ οὐκ αἰδεῖται ληρῶν, ἀλλ᾽ ἐᾷ τοῦτο· τὸ κοῖλον δ᾽ ἕλκος ἐν
σαρκώδει μορίῳ χωρὶς τοῦ πεπονθέναι τι τῶν ὑποκειμένων ὅπως ἰασώμεθα λεγέτω παρελθὼν ὁ Θεσσά-
163K   λειος | ἰατρός. Ἐμβαλόντες, φησί, τὸ σαρκωτικὸν
φάρμακον· εὖ γε τῆς εὐχερείας, ἴσως δ᾽ ἀναισθησίας
εἰπεῖν ἦν ἄμεινον, εἰ σαρκωτικὸν εἰπὼν ἀπηλλάχθαι
δοκεῖ τοῦ ζητουμένου· εἰ γὰρ ἤδη τὸ σαρκωτικὸν
ἐπιστάμεθα, τί ζητοῦμεν ἔτι; λέγε μοι τὸ σαρκωτικὸν
ὅ τί ποτ᾽ ἐστίν, ᾧ μέλλεις χρῆσθαι; λιβανωτόν, οἶμαι,
φήσεις, ἴριν ἢ ἀριστολοχίαν ἢ ὀρόβινον ἄλευρον ἢ
πάνακα· τῶν γὰρ ξηρῶν φαρμάκων πρῶτον μνημο-
νεύσω. ταῦτ᾽ οὖν εἰπέ μοι πόθεν εὗρες; Ἐκ τῆς πείρας,
φησί. τί δὴ οὖν ἔτι προσέθηκας σύ; τὸ μὲν γὰρ ὅτι
χρὴ πληροῦν τὸ κοῖλον οἶδε δήπου καὶ ὁ ἰδιώτης. τὸ δ᾽
ἐξ ὧν καὶ δι᾽ ὧν φαρμάκων, ἐδίδαξεν ἡ πεῖρα.

Θεσσαλὸς δ᾽ οὔθ᾽ ὡς Ἐμπειρικὸς οἶδε τὸ φάρμακον
οὔθ᾽ ὡς Λογικός. ὡς Ἐμπειρικὸς μέν, ὅτι μὴ βούλεται·
ὡς Λογικὸς δέ, ὅτι μὴ δύναται· ἐπεὶ ὅτι γε ὡς Ἐμ-

tion of continuity, while the cavity is a destruction of some substance proper to the organism. In this situation, it is often found that one of the objectives is impossible; for example, if not only the flesh is destroyed but also the underlying bone. A cavity of this kind cannot be filled up perfectly but it can be scarred over, which is a cure of the wound, although the cavity will be left behind incurable. This itself is something which, in general, we must know either through experience or through reason. Thessalus, however, does not use [either of] these means, nor does he add a third. And he is not embarrassed by his humbug, but allows it. Let the Thessaleian doctor come forward and say how we will cure a hollow wound in a fleshy part when there is no involvement of anything underlying. "By apply- ing an enfleshing (sarcotic) medication," he says. Well, it would be better to speak of his recklessness, or perhaps of his stupidity if, having mentioned "enfleshing," he thinks he is absolved from the search. If we already know what is enfleshing, why would we look any further? Tell me, at some point, what this "sarcotic" is that you intend to use? Frankincense, I think you will say, or iris, or aristo- lochia, or meal from bitter vetch, or panax—for I shall mention first the dry medications. Tell me, from what source did you discover these? "From experience," he says. What more is there for you to still add? Even the lay- man, presumably, also knows that we must fill the cavity. However, experience teaches us from what and by which medications.

163K

Thessalus does not, however, know the medication as the Empiric knows it or as the Dogmatic knows it. He does not know it as the Empiric knows it because he does not wish to, and he does not know it as the Dogmatic knows it

251

πειρικὸς οἶδεν, ἀκριβῶς ἐγὼ τοῦτο γινώσκω. δυοῖν γὰρ ὄντοιν ἁπάσης εὑρέσεως ὀργάνων, ἐμπειρίας καὶ λόγου, ὁ τὸ μὲν εὑρημένον ἐπιστάμενος, εἰπεῖν δ' οὐκ ἔχων αὐτοῦ τὸν λόγον, εὔδηλός ἐστιν ἐκ τῆς ἐμπειρίας

164K εὑρηκώς. ἵνα | τοίνυν εἰδῇ πόσον ἁμαρτάνει, μικρὸν ἡσυχάσας ἀκροατὴς ἡμῶν γενέσθω· βούλομαι γάρ τινα διαλεχθῆναι τῷ μονὴν τὴν ἐμπειρίαν πρεσβεύοντι·

δίκαιον γὰρ οἶμαι κἀκεῖνον εἰπεῖν ὅπως εὗρε τουτὶ τὸ σαρκωτικὸν φάρμακον τὸ ξηρόν, ὃ δὴ κεφαλικὸν ὀνομάζουσι· σύγκειται δὲ ἐξ ἴρεως καὶ ἀριστολοχίας ὀρόβου τε καὶ λιβανωτοῦ καὶ μάννης. ἔστι καὶ ἕτερόν τι ᾧ πρὸς τοῖς εἰρημένοις καὶ φλοιὸς πάνακος ἐπεμβάλλεται· καὶ μὲν δὴ καὶ ἕτερόν ἐστιν ᾧ καὶ καδμεία πεπλυμένη προσεπεμβάλλεται. λεγέτω τοίνυν ὑπὲρ τούτων ὅπως εὑρέθη. Καὶ τί μοί, φησι, ζητεῖν ὑπὲρ τῆς εὑρέσεως αὐτῶν, ἀλλ' οὐ τοῖς εὑρημένοις ὀρθῶς χρῆσθαι; ταυτὶ μὲν οὖν εὐθὺς κατ' ἀρχὰς ἀποφαίνονται, κατὰ σύμβασιν δέ, καλοῦσι γὰρ οὕτως αὐτοὶ καὶ τῷ ῥήματι τούτῳ, ποτὲ μὲν ἐξ ὀνειράτων ἐνδέχεσθαι τὰ τοιαῦτα εὑρῆσθαί φασιν, ἔστι δ' ὅτε κατὰ δή τινα τύχην ἐκχυθῆναι τὸ ἕτερον εἰς τὸ ἕτερον, εἶτά τινα τῷ μικτῷ τολμῆσαι χρήσασθαι, τῆς τόλμης δ' οὐ λέγειν τὴν ἐλπίδα. ταυτὶ μὲν οὖν πρόδηλος λῆρος.

ὁ δὲ τρίτος αὐτοῖς τρόπος τῆς εὑρέσεώς ἐστιν

---

4 On this medication, see Galen, *De compositione medicamentorum per genera* 2.3, XIII.541K ff.

because he is unable to, since what the Empiric knows is precisely what I know. There are two "instruments" for every discovery—experience and reason. Someone who knows what has been discovered but is not able to state the reason for it has clearly made his discovery from experience. Accordingly, that he might know how much he errs, let him be my silent listener for a short while, as I wish certain matters to be discussed with someone who privileges experience alone.

164K

In my view it is only right for that person also to say how he discovered that this particular enfleshing medication, which is dry and which they actually call cephalicum,[4] is compounded from iris, aristolochia, bitter vetch, frankincense, and manna. And there is also another thing, in addition to those mentioned, which is put in—the bark of panax. And furthermore, there is yet another thing added to it which is washed cadmia. Accordingly, let him say how they were discovered. "But why," he will say, "is it necessary for me to speak about the search for the discovery of these constituents, but not about how to use correctly those that have been discovered?" These particular things, therefore, are apparent straightaway at the outset, but they appear "by coincidence," for these men speak of them like this and with this term. They say it is sometimes possible for such things to be discovered from dreams, and sometimes again that by some chance one thing merges into another. So then [they say] that someone has the courage to make use of the mixture, but they don't speak of the expectation of that courage. These particular claims are transparent humbug.

The third way of discovery for them is really inferential.

165K ὄντως ἐπιλογιστικός· ἑκάστου | γὰρ ἐκείνων ἁπλῶν
ἰδίᾳ τις πεπειραμένος ὡς σαρκωτικῶν, κἄπειθ᾽ εὑ-
ρίσκων ἐνίοτε μὴ σαρκοῦντα, προσεπελογίσατο μὴ
πάσῃ φύσει πᾶν ἁρμόττειν. εἰ γὰρ ὃν οὐκ ἐσάρκωσεν
ἡ ἀριστολοχία, τοῦτον ὁ λιβανωτὸς ἐσάρκωσεν, ᾧ δ᾽ ὁ
λιβανωτὸς οὐχ ἥρμοττε, τούτῳ τῆς ἴρεως προσαχθεί-
σης ἀπήντησε τὸ δέον, εὔλογον, οἶμαι, μὴ πάντας ὑπὸ
πάντων ὁμοίως διατίθεσθαι· τούτου δ᾽ ἅπαξ εἰς ἐπι-
λογισμὸν ἐλθόντος ἄμεινον ἔδοξεν ὡς οἷόν τε πλεῖστα
τῶν ὁμοειδῶν εἰς ταὐτὸν ἀναμίξαι, ἵν᾽ ἑκάστη φύσις
σώματος εὐπορῇ τοῦ προσήκοντος. καὶ μήν, ὦ ἑταῖρε,
ἐν τῇ συμπλοκῇ τῶν εἰδῶν οὐ φυλάττονται τῶν οἰκείων οὐσιῶν αἱ ἐνέργειαι, ὡς ἐπὶ ἑνὸς ἑκάστου εἴδους
τῷ ὠφελεῖν εἰς νόσον ἥνπερ χρὴ θεραπεύειν εὐπορεῖν
τοῦ προσήκοντος. εἰ μὲν γὰρ ἤτοι τὴν φύσιν ἠδύναντο
τοῦ σώματος ἐξευρεῖν ἢ τοῦ προσφερομένου φαρμάκου τὴν δύναμιν, οὐδὲν ἂν ἴσως ἐδέησεν αὐτοῖς τῆς
τοιαύτης ποικιλίας, ἐν ἑκάστοτε φάρμακον ἐφ᾽ ἑνὶ
σώματι τὸ συμφέρον εὑρίσκειν δυναμένοις. ἐπεὶ δ᾽
ἀγνοοῦσιν ἑκάτερον, κακῶς ἀναμιγνύουσιν ἅπαντα,
166K πολλαῖς φύσεσιν ἁρμόττον ἐπιτεχνήσασθαι | βουλό-
μενοι ἓν φάρμακον.

τοῦτον τὸν τρόπον τῆς συνθέσεως τῶν φαρμάκων
ἐγὼ πείθομαι τοῖς πρώτοις τῶν ἰατρῶν ἐπινενοῆσθαι

For if someone has tried out each of those simple medica- 165K
tions individually as sarcotics, then, when he discovers that
sometimes one is not enfleshing, he has provided further
proof that not everything is suitable for every nature. For if
frankincense created flesh in a particular person when
aristolochia did not, or if in someone for whom frankincense was not suitable what was needed followed when iris
was applied, it would be a reasonable inference, I think,
that not all people are affected in the same way by all
things. Once [the doctor] has come to this inference, it
would seem better, as far as possible, to mix most of the like
forms in the same medication so that each bodily nature
has an abundance of what is appropriate. And yet, my
friend, in the combination of the forms, the actions of the
specific substances are not preserved such that, in the case
of each single kind of body, there is an abundance of what
is beneficial for the disease we must treat.[5] For if they
were able to discover either the nature of the body or the
potency of the medication being applied, perhaps there
would be nothing lacking for them among such diversity,
as they would be able to discover one medication which is
useful when applied in one body on each occasion. But
since they don't know either thing (i.e. the nature of the
body or the potency of the medication), they mix everything badly when they wish to devise a single medication 166K
suitable to many natures.

I believe this manner of synthesis of medications was
invented by the first doctors and I accept it as an ancient

[5] Linacre has a marginal note on this sentence that part is
missing from some manuscripts. His Latin version has been translated; see Linacre (1546), p. 122.

καὶ ὡς ἀρχαῖον εὕρεμα προσίεμαι. τοσοῦτόν γε μὴν
ἀποδεῖν ἡγοῦμαι τῆς ὄντως μεθόδου θεραπευτικῆς,
ὅσον εὐλογώτερός ἐστι τῶν ἐγχεομένων εἰς ἄλληλα
κοσκίνων. εἰ γὰρ μὴ λογίζεται πρῶτον μὲν ὡς μόνης
τῆς ἐξ ὁμοειδῶν φαρμάκων συνθέσεως, οὐ μὴν τῆς γ᾽
ἐξ ἐναντίων εἴρηκε τὴν μέθοδον. ἔπειθ᾽ ὡς ἐν τῷ
πλήθει τῆς μίξεως ἓν μέν, εἰ τύχοι, τὸ τῷ πάσχοντι
προσῆκόν ἐστι φάρμακον, ἐγχωρεῖ δὲ καὶ μηδέν, ἑπτὰ
δ᾽ ἢ ὀκτὼ τῶν οὐκ οἰκείων· ὥστε πλείοσιν ἀριθμοῖς
βλάψαι τὸ τοιοῦτον ἢ ὠφελῆσαι· ταῦτ᾽ εἰ μὴ λογίζεται, πλέον αὐτὸν ἀγνοεῖν ἢ γιγνώσκειν τοῦ πράγματος εἴποιμ᾽ ἄν.

ἔλαιον γοῦν ἐγχεόμενον ἕλκει κοίλῳ πάντων ἐναν-
τιώτατον φάρμακον· εἰ γὰρ ἐθελήσεις οὕτω θεραπεύειν, αὐτῇ γνώσεις τῇ πείρᾳ ῥυπαρὸν καὶ βρυῶδες
ἀποτελούμενον τὸ ἕλκος. εἰ δὲ καὶ ἡ ὥρα τοῦ ἔτους
θερμὴ τύχοι καὶ ὁ ἄνθρωπος εἴη κακοχυμώτερος, ἢ
167K   φύσει | ῥευματικώτερος ἢ καὶ περὶ τὴν δίαιτάν τι
πλημμελοίη, κίνδυνος τούτῳ σαπῆναι τὸ μόριον ἐν ᾧ
τὸ ἕλκος ἐγένετο. κίνδυνος δὲ κἂν εἰ κηρῷ μόνῳ χρῷο,
κἂν εἰ τήκων ἐλαίῳ· ταυτὶ μὲν οὖν διασήψει σοι τὸ
ἕλκος· εἰ δὲ ἰὸν λειώσας ἐμπλάττῃς, οὐ διασήψει μὲν
οὗτός γε οὐδαμῶς, ὀδύνην δ᾽ ἐργάσεται καὶ δῆξιν οὐ
σμικράν, ἀνάβρωσίν τε καὶ φλεγμονήν· εἰ δὲ ἐπιπλέον
χρήσαιο, καὶ σπασμόν. ἐπεὶ τοίνυν οὔτε τὸ ἔλαιον
οὔτε ὁ ἰὸς οὔτε ὁ κηρὸς ἕλκος κοῖλον σαρκῶσαι
δύνανται, δῆλον ὡς οὐδὲ μίξει ποτ᾽ αὐτὰ τῶν ἀπὸ τῆς
ἐμπειρίας οὐδείς·

discovery. Yet in fact I think it is deficient as a true method of treatment to the extent that it is more applicable to the situation when sieves pour their contents into one another. For if he does not take into account first that which is only from the synthesis of like medications, he has not, in fact, spoken of the method of synthesis from opposites. So, in the many components of the mixture, it may happen that there is one medication appropriate to the patient, although it is also possible there is none, or that there are seven or eight that are not appropriate. So such a medication with a greater number [of components] will harm rather than help and, if he does not take these things into account, I would say he is more ignorant than knowledgeable about the matter.

At any rate, oil, when it is poured on a hollow wound, is the most inimical medication of all [to healing] for, if you do wish to treat in this way, you will know from experience itself that the wound is made filthy and foul-smelling. And if it happens to be a hot time of the year, or if the person is rather *kakochymous*, or more subject to flux by nature, or also if there is something wrong with the regimen, there is for this man a danger of putrefaction involving the part in which the wound exists. There is also a danger if you use either wax alone, or wax dissolved in oil; these particular things will putrefy the wound for you. If, however, you apply triturated verdigris, this will in no way putrefy, although it will bring about pain and no little biting, erosion and inflammation. If you use still more, it will bring about convulsions as well. Since, therefore, neither oil, verdigris nor wax is able to enflesh a hollow wound, it is clear that none of those [men] who work on the basis of experience will ever mix them.

167K

ἀλλ᾽ ἐγὼ μίξω γε τῷ δέοντι μέτρῳ καὶ ταῦτα καὶ
ἄλλα μυρία φάρμακα τῶν βλαπτόντων ἰδίως ἕλκος
κοῖλον. εἰ γὰρ μὴ ταῖς αὐταῖς δυνάμεσι βλάπτοιεν,
ἀλλ᾽ ὑπεναντίαις, ἄμετρα δήπουθέν ἐστιν ὡς πρὸς
ἕλκους κοίλου πλήρωσιν. ἀλλ᾽ ὅπως ἐκ δυοῖν ἀμέτροιν
κράσεων ἓν ἀποτελεῖται σύμμετρον, ἐν τοῖς περὶ φαρμάκων συνθέσεως ἐμάθομεν λογισμοῖς. οὔκουν ἔτι
χαλεπὸν ἐξ ἐλαίου καὶ κηροῦ καὶ ἰοῦ συνθεῖναι φάρ-
168K μακον σαρκωτικόν· εἰ γὰρ εἰδείης ὡς | ξηραίνεσθαι
μετρίως δεῖται τὸ τοιοῦτον ἕλκος, οὐ ξηραίνει δ᾽ οὔτε ὁ
κηρὸς οὔτ᾽ ἔλαιον, εἰδείης ἂν ὡς οὔτε ἑκάτερον οὔτ᾽
ἄμφω πληρώσουσιν ἕλκος κοῖλον· οὐ μὴν οὐδ᾽ ὁ ἰὸς
μόνος, ἀμέτρως γὰρ ξηραίνει. μίξας οὖν ἅπαντα συμμέτρως ξηρὸν ἐργάσασθαι δυνήσῃ φάρμακον· ὁπόσον
δ᾽ ἑκάστου χρὴ τὸ μέτρον εἶναι δέδεικται μὲν ἤδη
μοι κἀν τοῖς περὶ φαρμάκων συνθέσεως ὑπομνήμασιν, δειχθήσεται δὲ καὶ νῦν, εἰ δεηθείη, τοῦ λόγου
προϊόντος. ἀποπέμψαι γάρ με χρὴ πρῶτον ἀπὸ τῶν
ἐφεξῆς λόγων τὸν ἀμέθοδον ἐκεῖνον Θεσσαλόν, ἐνδει-
ξάμενον αὐτῷ πόσον ἁμαρτάνει τοῦ δέοντος. φρονίμῳ
γὰρ ἀνθρώπῳ καὶ τὰ νῦν εἰρημένα σαφῶς ἐνδείκνυται
τὴν θεραπευτικὴν μέθοδον ὁποίαν τινα εἶναι χρή.
ἀλλὰ γὰρ οὐ πρὸς τοὺς τοιούτους ὁ λόγος· ὥστε
ἀναγκαῖον ἔτι διαλεχθῆναι πρὸς αὐτοὺς ἐνθένδε ποθὲν
ἀρξάμενον.

But I will mix, in the required amount, both these and countless other medications that are individually harmful to a hollow wound. If [the medications] are harmful not by the same potencies but by those that are opposite, presumably they are disproportionate for the filling of a hollow wound. But we did learn in the discussions about the composition of medications how a mixture from two immoderate medications makes one moderate medication. So there is no longer any problem about compounding a sarcotic medication from oil, wax and verdigris. If you know that such a wound or ulcer needs to be moderately dried, and that neither wax nor oil dries, you would know that neither each one singly nor both together would fill up a hollow wound or ulcer. And neither would verdigris alone, for it dries excessively. But then, when you mix all these, you are able to make a moderately drying medication. What the amount of each must be, I have already shown in the treatises on the synthesis of medications,[6] and will show again now if needs be as the argument proceeds. For it is first necessary for me to dismiss that "methodless" Thessalus from the discussions to follow, once I have shown him how far he strays from what is right. And to the sensible man those things now spoken of demonstrate clearly what sort of thing the therapeutic method must be. But the argument is not directed to such people, so it is still necessary here for the origin to be discussed with them.

168K

[6] We have been unable to locate the recipe for the preparation of this compound medication in either *De compositione medicamentorum secundum locos* (XII.378–1007K and XIII.1–361K) or *per genera* (XIII.362–1058K). For the preparation of verdigris, see Dioscorides, V.91.

ἅπασα κοιλότης παρὰ φύσιν ἐνδείκνυται τὴν πλή-
ρωσιν· ὥστε καὶ ἡ ἐν τῷ σαρκώδει μορίῳ· αὕτη δὲ ἡ
πλήρωσις σκοπὸς τῆς τῶν ἰαμάτων εὑρέσεως γίγνε-
169K ται. ἵνα δ᾽ εὑρεθῇ τὰ πληρώσαντα καὶ | λόγου δεόμεθα
συχνοῦ καὶ πολλῶν τῶν κατὰ μέρος ἐνδείξεων, καὶ
μεθόδου λογικῆς ἀκριβοῦς· ἐθεάσω γοῦν πολλάκις
ἕλκη δυσίατα μὴ δυναμένους θεραπεῦσαι μήτε τοὺς
τὴν ἐμπειρίαν πρεσβεύοντας ἰατροὺς τούτους δὴ τοὺς
πολυφαρμάκους, ἀλλὰ μηδὲ τοὺς τὸν ἀναλογισμὸν
ἐπαγγελλομένους ἅπαντας.

οἱ γὰρ Θεσσάλειοι Μεθοδικοὶ μὲν τοὔνομα, ταῖς δ᾽
ἀληθείαις Ἀμέθοδοι, καθάπερ τινὲς ὄνοι λύρας οὐδ᾽
ἐπαΐειν ἱκανοὶ τῆς τοιαύτης θεωρίας εἰσί, μή τοί γε δὴ
λογισμῷ τὸ δέον ἐξευρίσκειν. ἐθεάσω δὲ πολλάκις
ἐπὶ τῶν τοιούτων ἑλκῶν τοὺς μὲν ἀπὸ τῆς ἐμπειρίας
ἄλλοτ᾽ ἐπ᾽ ἄλλο μεταβαίνοντας φάρμακον, οὐ μὰ Δία
λογισμοῦ τινος ἐξηγουμένου τῆς μεταβάσεως, ἀλλ᾽
ἐπειδὴ πολλῶν μὲν ἐπειράθησαν πληρούντων ἕλκη
κοῖλα, τὴν δ᾽ ὡς αὐτοὶ καλοῦσιν ἰδιοσυγκρασίαν, ἐφ᾽
οἷς ἕκαστον αὐτῶν εὐδοκίμησεν οὔτε διαγινώσκειν
οὔτε μεμνῆσθαι δύνανται, διὰ τοῦτο καὶ νῦν οὐκ ἐπι-
στάμενοι μὲν ἐφ᾽ ὅ τι χρὴ μεταβαίνειν, ἐλπίζοντες δ᾽
ἐν πολλῇ τῇ κατὰ μέρος διεξόδῳ πάντως εὑρεθή-
σεσθαί ποτε τὸ προσῆκον, ἄλλοτ᾽ ἐπ᾽ ἄλλο μεταπη-
δῶσι, τύχῃ μᾶλλον ἢ λογισμῷ τὴν τοῦ συμφέροντος |
170K εὕρεσιν ἐπιτρέποντες. ὅμοιοι δ᾽ αὐτοῖς εἰσι, κἂν μὴ
θέλωσιν, ὅσοι τῶν Δογματιζόντων ἐπὶ τὰς φυσικὰς
ἀρχὰς τῶν σωμάτων οὐκ ἐδυνήθησαν ἀναβῆναι τῷ

Every cavity contrary to nature indicates [the need] for filling, so this also applies in a fleshy part, and this filling is itself the indicator of the discovery of the cures. In order that the things which are filling are discovered, we need considerable discussion, many indications individually, and a method that is logical and precise. At all events, you often see intractable wounds or ulcers, which neither these doctors who give primacy to experience and so rely on polypharmacy, nor all those who profess to follow the course of reason are able to treat. 169K

Now the Thessaleians, while Methodics by name, are, however, "Amethodics" when it comes to matters of truth, just as some asses are toward the lyre, nor are they capable of understanding such a theory, and certainly not of discovering by reasoning what is needed. On the other hand, you have often seen, in such wounds or ulcers, those who rely on experience change sometimes from one medication to another without, by Zeus, providing any rationale for the change. But since they make trial of many agents for filling hollow wounds or ulcers, as they call the particular characteristic, they are unable to either recognize or remember for what aspects each of the agents was held in high regard and, because of this, they now do not know which one they ought to change to. Hoping, no doubt, that what is appropriate will, at some time, be discovered by many individual trials, they jump from one to another, entrusting the discovery of what is useful more to chance than to reason. Some of the Dogmatics are like them, even if they don't wish [to be]; [that is,] those who are not able to advance in the argument as far as the natural origins of 170K

λόγῳ. καὶ γὰρ αὐτοί, καθότι πρόσθεν ἐδείξαμεν, ἐξ
ἡμίσεώς εἰσιν Ἐμπειρικοί, οἳ οὐκ ἠδυνήθησαν δια-
λαβεῖν περὶ τῶν πρώτων στοιχείων. περὶ δὲ τῶν ἀμεθόδων τούτων Θεσσαλείων τί ἄν τις καὶ λέγοι; μόνοι
τοίνυν οἱ ὄντως μεθόδῳ θεραπεύοντες ἐξευρίσκουσί τε
τὸ δέον ἢ φάρμακον ἢ διαίτημα καθ' ἕκαστον τῶν
τοιούτων ἑλκῶν ἐπιδεικνύουσι τε τὰ σαφέστατα διὰ
τῶν ἔργων αὐτῶν ὁπηλίκον ἀγαθόν ἐστι καὶ ὅσον φῶς
παρέχει πρὸς τὰς ἰάσεις ἡ περὶ φύσεως πραγματεία.

καὶ γὰρ δὴ καὶ ὡς τοῖς συνεχῶς ἀφ' ἑτέρου φαρμάκου μεταβαίνουσιν ἐφ' ἕτερον ἐνίοτε παρορᾶται καὶ
καταφρονεῖται τὸ χρήσιμον, ἐπέδειξά σοι πολλάκις
ἑνὶ φαρμάκῳ τὰ τοιαῦτα τῶν ἑλκῶν θεραπεύσας ὧν
ἔφθανον ἐκεῖνοι κεχρῆσθαι. κατεφρονήθη δ' εἰκότως ἡ
δύναμις τοῦ τοιούτου φαρμάκου διά τε τὴν ἀκαιρίαν
τῆς χρήσεως, οὐ μόνον οὐδὲν ὠφελῆσαι δόξαντος,
ἀλλὰ καὶ προσβλάψαι, καὶ διὰ τὸ μηδὲν ἐνίοτε σαφὲς
171K ἐργάζεσθαι | τὴν πρώτην χρῆσιν. ἐθεάσω δὲ καὶ
ὀφθαλμῶν ὀδύνας σφοδροτάτας ἰασαμένους ἡμᾶς ἢ
λουτροῖς ἢ οἴνου πόσεσιν ἢ πυρίαις ἢ φλεβοτομίαις ἢ
καθάρσεσιν, ἐφ' ὧν οὐδὲν ἄλλο ἔχουσιν οἱ πολλοὶ τῶν
ἰατρῶν ἢ ταυτὶ τὰ δι' ὀπίου καὶ μανδραγόρου καὶ
ὑοσκυάμου συντιθέμενα φάρμακα, μεγίστην λώβην
ὀφθαλμῶν· οὐδὲ γὰρ οὐδ' ἄλλῳ τινὶ τὴν ἐν τῷ παραχρῆμα δόκησιν τῆς ἀνωδυνίας ἀλλ' ἢ τῷ νεκροῦν τὴν
αἴσθησιν ἐργάζονται. καὶ πολλοὺς οἶσθα μετὰ τὰς
τοιαύτας χρήσεις τῶν φαρμάκων, ἐπειδὰν ἀμετρότερον προσαχθῇ, μηκέτ' ἐπανελθόντας εἰς τὸ κατὰ

bodies. For they, too, just as I showed before, are "semi-Empirics"—those who have not been able to understand about the primary elements. And what might someone say about these "amethodical" Thessaleians? Only those who truly treat by method both discover the required medication or regimen for each of such wounds or ulcers and display with the utmost clarity by their actions how great a good the treatise on nature is and how much light it provides regarding cures.[7]

Certainly, I too have often shown you that I have treated such wounds with a single medication from among the medications which those men have mixed beforehand —a medication whose usefulness is sometimes overlooked and neglected by those who change continually from one medication to another. In all likelihood, the potency of such a medication was disregarded because it was used at an inopportune time—a time when the medication not only seemed to be of no benefit but even to be harmful, and because sometimes it had no apparent effect during the first use. You have also seen me cure very severe pains of the eyes with either baths, drinks of wine, vapor baths, phlebotomy or purging, in cases where the majority of doctors have nothing else to offer apart from those medications compounded from opium, mandrake and henbane, to the very great detriment of the eyes. For they bring about the impression of pain relief in the short term by no other means than the destruction of the sensation [of the eyes]. And you know that many people, after the use of these kinds of medications whenever they are applied to

171K

---

[7] It is not entirely clear which treatise is referred to here. It is probably *De elementis secundum Hippocratem*.

φύσιν, ἀλλ' ἀρξαμένους μὲν ἐντεῦθεν ἀμυδρῶς καὶ
μόγις ὁρᾶν, ἐν τῷ χρόνῳ δ' ὑποχύσεσιν ἢ μυδρι-
άσεσιν ἢ φθίσεσιν ἢ ῥυτιδώσεσιν ἁλόντας.

οἶσθα δὲ δήπου συνδιατρίψας ἡμῖν εὐθὺς ἐκ μει-
ρακίου, μηδὲ παρ' ἑνὶ τῶν διδασκάλων θεασαμένους
ἡμᾶς ἔργον τοιοῦτον, ἀλλ' ἐξευρόντας αὐτοὺς τῷ
λογισμῷ· καὶ ὅτι γε πολλῷ χρόνῳ τὸν ἀφορισμὸν
ἀνεσκεψάμην ἐκεῖνον, Ὀδύνας ὀφθαλμῶν ἀκρητοπο-
σίη ἢ λουτρὸν ἢ πυρίη ἢ φλεβοτομίη ἢ φαρμακείη
λύει, καὶ ὡς ἐκ τῆς ἄλλης ἀκριβείας Ἱπποκράτους
172K   ἤλπιζον μηδ' ἐνταῦθα | μήτε ψεῦδός τι μήτ' ἀδύνατον
λέγεσθαι· καὶ ὡς τοῦτ' ἦν με τὸ προτρέψαν ἐπὶ τὴν
ζήτησιν, ἕως οὗ καὶ ταύτην τὴν Ἱπποκράτους ὁδὸν
ἐξεῦρον διορίσασθαι, πότε καὶ πῶς ἐφ' ἑκάστου τῶν
εἰρημένων χρηστέον. ὃ καὶ δῆλον ἐποίησα πολλοῖς
τῶν θεασαμένων τὰ τοιαῦτα, πηλίκη μέν ἐστιν ἡ τῆς
θεραπευτικῆς μεθόδου δύναμις, ἡλίκον δὲ κακὸν εἰρ-
γάσαντο μὴ φυλάξαντες τὴν παλαιὰν ἰατρικὴν οἱ τὰς
νεωτέρας αἱρέσεις συστησάμενοι. ταῦτά τοι καὶ ὑμεῖς
καίτοί γε ἄκοντά με κατ' ἀρχὰς ἠναγκάσατε, λιπα-
ροῦντες διεξελθεῖν ἅπασαν τήνδε τὴν πραγματείαν ἣν
εὔχομαι μὲν τοῖς θεοῖς ὄνησίν τινα καὶ τοῖς ἄλλοις
ἀνθρώποις γενέσθαι, βραχυτάτην δ' ἔχω τὴν ἐλπίδα
διὰ τὴν κατέχουσαν νῦν ὀλιγωρίαν μὲν τῶν καλῶν,
ἐπίδοσιν δὲ εἰς τιμὴν πλούτου καὶ δόξης καὶ πολι-
τικῶν δυνάμεων· ἐφ' ἃ τοῖς ἐκτραπεῖσιν οὐκ ἐνδέχεται

---

[8] On this last, see Rufus, fr. 78.

excess, never return to normal, but from that point on begin to see indistinctly or with difficulty, and over time suffer from cataracts, mydriasis, miosis or contractions of the eyes.[8]

You know, of course, having spent time with me right from your youth, that I have not seen such an action in the presence of one of my teachers, but have myself made the discovery by the process of reason, and that over a long period, I have examined closely that aphorism: "Drinking neat wine, or bathing, or a vapor bath, or phlebotomy, or a medication resolve pains of the eyes."[9] And on the basis of the accuracy elsewhere in Hippocrates, I expected that here nothing false or impossible was being said. So this was what gave direction to my search until, following the Hippocratic path, I discovered the way to determine when and how I must use each of the things mentioned. Clearly I also did this for the many who observed such things—that is, how great the power of the therapeutic method is and what great harm those men cause who do not preserve the ancient medical art but adhere to the newer sects. Mind you, on these things, in actual fact you brought pressure to bear on me, although I was hesitant at the beginning when you entreated me to go through the whole treatise, which I pray to the gods is of some benefit to other men also. However, I have very little hope because of the overpowering contempt nowadays for good things and the addiction to the respect for wealth, reputation and political power, due to which it is impossible for those who are devoted to these things to discover the truth in any of its existing forms. But

172K

[9] See *Aphorisms*, VII.46. Neither of the two different versions given exactly corresponds to Galen's text.

τἀληθὲς ἐν οὐδενὶ τῶν ὄντων ἐξευρεῖν. ἀλλὰ ταῦτα μὲν
ὅπῃ τῷ θεῷ φίλον, οὕτω τελευτήσει.

τὴν δ' οὖν θεραπευτικὴν μέθοδον, ἀσκηθεῖσαν μὲν
τοῖς παλαιοῖς ἰατροῖς, ὀλιγωρουμένην δὲ νῦν ἀνακτη-
σώμεθα καθ' ὅσον οἷοί τ' ἐσμέν, αὖθις ἀναλαβόντες |
173K τὸν λόγον ἐπὶ τοῦ προκειμένου παθήματος ἕλκους
κοίλου. περὶ μὲν δὴ τῆς πρώτης εὑρέσεως τῶν σαρ-
κωσόντων τὸ τοιοῦτον ἕλκος φαρμάκων ἀρκείτω τὰ
μικρῷ πρόσθεν εἰρημένα,[1] καὶ συγχωρείσθω δ', εἰ
βούλει, τοῖς Ἐμπειρικοῖς ἃ λέγουσιν ἅπαντα. περὶ δὲ
τῆς τῶν εὑρημένων χρήσεως ἐπὶ μὲν τῶν ἔργων αὐτῶν
ἐπέδειξά σοι πολλάκις· οὐδὲν δ' ἧττον καὶ νῦν ἐπιδεῖξαι τῷ λόγῳ πειράσομαι πῶς ἐν οἷς ἂν μηδὲν
δράσῃ τὸ σύνηθες ἑκάστῳ φάρμακον, ἐπ' ἄλλο μεταβαίνειν εὐμηχάνως τε καὶ τεχνικῶς ἀποροῦσιν οἱ
Ἐμπειρικοί. καὶ τοῦτ' εὐλόγως γίνεται· τοῦ γὰρ πρώτου φαρμάκου τῆς ἀποτυχίας τὴν αἰτίαν ἀγνοοῦντες,
οὐδὲ φυλάξασθαι δήπουθεν αὐτὴν ἐπὶ τοῦ δευτέρου
δύνανται. ἀγνοουμένης γὰρ ἔτι τῆς αἰτίας δι' ἣν
ἐνεργεῖ τὸ φάρμακον, οὐδὲ δι' ἣν ἀποτυγχάνει γνῶναι
δυνήσονται. ταύτης δ' ἀγνοουμένης οὐδ' ἐφ' ἕτερον ἔτι
μεταβαίνειν εὐλόγως ἐγχωρεῖ, φυλάξασθαι γὰρ οὐδ'
ἐπ' ἐκείνου δυνήσονται τὴν αὐτὴν αἰτίαν.

3. Εἴπωμεν οὖν ἡμεῖς ἤδη τὴν Ἱπποκράτειόν τε ἅμα
καὶ ἀληθῆ μέθοδον ἑλκῶν κοίλων ἰάσεως· ἄρχεσθαι |
174K δὲ δήπουθεν αὐτὴν ἐκ τῆς οὐσίας χρὴ τοῦ πράγματος.
ἐπεὶ τοίνυν ἐν τοῖς κοίλοις ἕλκεσι πρόκειται γεννῆσαι

to the extent that these things are pleasing to the god, so they will be accomplished.

Let me, then, revive the method of medicine practiced by the doctors of the past but nowadays held in contempt, insofar as I can, taking up again the argument in the case of the affection before us—the hollow wound or ulcer. Regarding the first discovery of the "sarcotic" medications for such a lesion, let what has been said a little earlier be sufficient and concede, if you will, to the Empirics everything they say. About the use of the discoveries, I demonstrated to you their actions on many occasions. No less shall I now attempt to demonstrate by theory how, among these, a medication that is in common use does not act in each [disease], and how the Empirics don't have the wherewithal to change over to another medication skillfully and according to the rules of the craft. And this is to be expected because, if they are ignorant of the cause of the failure of the first medication, they won't be able to look out for this in the case of the second medication. When the cause by which the medication acts remains unknown, they won't be able to recognize the reason for its failure. And since the cause is not known, it is no longer possible to change to another medication in any rational manner, for they will not be able to look out for the actual cause in that case.

3. So let me now speak of the Hippocratic and, at the same time, true method of cure of hollow wounds and ulcers, and it is clearly necessary to begin this from the substance of the matter. Accordingly, since in hollow wounds and ulcers our task is to recreate the flesh that has

173K

174K

τὴν ἀπολωλυῖαν σάρκα, δεῖ γινώσκειν περὶ² σαρκὸς
γενέσεως, ὡς ὕλη μὲν αὐτῆς αἷμα χρηστόν, ὁ δ᾽ οἷον
δημιουργός τε καὶ τεχνίτης ἡ φύσις. ἀλλ᾽ οὐχ ἁπλῶς
εἰπεῖν χρὴ φύσιν, ἀλλὰ προσθεῖναι τὴν τίνων καὶ ποῦ.
δῆλον δὲ ὅτι τῶν ὑποκειμένων σωμάτων οἷς σὰρξ
ἐπιτρέφεσθαι μέλλει, τούτων ἡ φύσις ἔσται δημι-
ουργὸς τῆς γενηθησομένης σαρκός. ἀλλ᾽ ἡ φύσις
ἑκάστου τῶν σωμάτων ἐδείχθη κατά τινα θερμοῦ καὶ
ψυχροῦ καὶ ξηροῦ καὶ ὑγροῦ κρᾶσιν ἀποτελεῖσθαι.
δῆλον οὖν ὡς ἡ τούτων εὐκρασία κατὰ τὸ ὑποκείμενον
μόριον ᾧ μέλλομεν ἐπιθρέψειν τὴν λείπουσαν σάρκα
τὸν λόγον ἕξει τοῦ δημιουργοῦ. πρῶτον μὲν οὖν ἡμῖν
σκεπτέον ἐπὶ παντὸς ἕλκους κοίλου δύο ταῦτα, τό θ᾽
ὑποκείμενον εἰ εὐκράτως ἔχει, τουτέστιν εἰ κατὰ
φύσιν. ἐδείχθη γὰρ ἡ ἐν τοῖς ὁμοιομερέσι σώμασιν
ὑγεία τῶν τεττάρων οὖσα ποιοτήτων εὐκρασία καὶ
προσέτι τὸ αἷμα τὸ ἐπιρρέον, εἰ χρηστόν τε καὶ σύμ-
175K   μετρον· | εἰ μὲν δὴ καὶ τούτων τι μοχθηρῶς ἔχοι,
πολλαὶ διαθέσεις γίγνονται παρὰ φύσιν·

ἡμῖν δ᾽ ὑπόκειται μία κοιλότης ἐν σαρκώδει μορίῳ.
ὑποκείσθω τοίνυν ὑγιεινόν τε τὸ χωρίον ἥ τ᾽ ἐπιρροὴ
τοῦ αἵματος ἄμεμπτος ἐν ποσότητι καὶ ποιότητι. καὶ
τούτων οὕτως ἐχόντων οὐδὲν ἂν ἔτι κωλύοι τὴν πρώτην γένεσιν τῆς σαρκὸς ἄμεμπτον γενέσθαι, μηδενὸς
δεηθεῖσαν ἔξωθεν φαρμάκου· τῶν γὰρ αἰτίων ἀμφοτέρων ὑφ᾽ ὧν γίγνεται παρόντων καὶ μηδενὸς τῶν
ἔξωθεν ἐμποδὼν ὄντος, οὐκ ἐνδέχεται κωλυθῆναι τὴν
τῆς σαρκὸς γένεσιν. ἀλλ᾽ ἐν αὐτῷ δὴ τῷ γεννᾶσθαι

been destroyed, it is necessary to know about the generation of flesh, and that its material is useful blood, and that the "demiurge" or "craftsman," as it were, is Nature. But we must not simply say "Nature" but add the nature of what things and how. It is clear that the flesh of the bodies underlying those wounds will be what causes growth, and the nature of these will be the "demiurge" of the flesh that will be regenerated. But the nature of each of the bodies was shown to consist of a certain *krasis* of heat, cold, dryness and moisture. It is clear that the *eukrasia* of these [qualities] in the underlying part will have the ground of the "demiurge" by which we will cause the growth of the flesh that is lacking. First, then, we must consider in every hollow wound and ulcer these two things: whether what is underlying is *eukratic*—that is to say, if it is in accord with nature, for it was shown that health in *homoiomerous* bodies lies in a *eukrasia* of the four qualities—and, in addition, if the flow of blood is of the right quality and quantity. If, however, one of these things is in a bad state, many abnormal conditions arise.

175K

One, I suggest, is hollowness in a fleshy part. Assume that the place is healthy and the flow of blood without fault in terms of quantity and quality. If things are thus, nothing should still prevent the primary genesis of flesh from occurring faultlessly without the need of any medication externally because, as both causes from which this genesis occurs are present and there are no external hindrances, it is impossible for the genesis of flesh to be prevented. But in the actual generation of the primary flesh, two super-

----

2 B; τὶ περί om. K

τὴν πρώτην σάρκα περίττωμα διττὸν ἀνάγκη γίγνεσθαι, καθότι καὶ τοῦτ᾽ ἐν τοῖς περὶ φύσεως εἴρηται
λογισμοῖς, ὡς ἁπάσῃ τῇ κατὰ ποιότητα μετακοσμή-
σει τῆς τροφῆς ἕτερον μὲν παχύτερον, ἕτερον δὲ
λεπτότερον ἕπεται περίττωμα. τούτων τῶν περιττω-
μάτων καὶ καθ᾽ ὅλον τὸ σῶμα γιγνομένων, ἀεὶ τὸ μὲν
λεπτότερον ἢ ἄδηλός ἐστι διαπνοῇ· γίγνεται δὲ καὶ
δήλη πολλάκις, ὅταν ἤτοι τὸ ἔμφυτον ἀρρωστήσῃ
θερμὸν ἢ τροφῇ χρήσηται πλείονι τοῦ δέοντος, ἤ τις
176K ἐπαχθῇ τῷ ζῴῳ κίνησις σφοδροτέρα. τὸ δ᾽ ἕτερον | ὁ
ἐπιτρεφόμενός ἐστι τοῖς σώμασιν ἡμῶν ῥύπος· καὶ δὴ
κἂν τοῖς ἕλκεσιν ἰχὼρ μὲν καλεῖται τὸ λεπτὸν περίττωμα, ῥύπος δ᾽ ἕλκους τὸ παχύ. καὶ διὰ μὲν τὸ λεπτὸν
περίττωμα ὑγρὸν τὸ ἕλκος γίγνεται, διὰ δὲ τὸ παχὺ
ῥυπαρόν· καὶ δεῖται διὰ τοῦτο διττῶν φαρμάκων, ὡς
μὲν ὑγρὸν τῶν ξηραινόντων, ὡς δὲ ῥυπαρὸν τῶν καθαιρόντων αὐτό. κατ᾽ οὐδένα τοίνυν χρόνον τῆς φύσεως
ἀργούσης οὐδεὶς ἔσται καιρὸς ἐν ᾧ μὴ ταῦτ᾽ ἄμφω
κατὰ τὸ κοῖλον ἕλκος ἀθροισθήσεται· ὥστε οὐδὲ χρόνος ἔσται καθ᾽ ὃν οὐ δεήσεται τῶν φαρμάκων ἀμφοτέρων, τοῦ τε ξηραίνοντος καὶ τοῦ καθαίροντος. ὁποῖον
μὲν οὖν εἶναι χρὴ τῷ γένει τὸ φάρμακον εὕρηται.

ἀλλ᾽ οὐκ ἀρκεῖ τοῦτο, χρὴ γάρ τι τῶν κατ᾽ εἶδος
ἐξευρεῖν ὃ προσαχθήσεται. πόθεν οὖν ἐκεῖνο κἀκ τίνος
εὑρεθήσεται μεθόδου, ἢ τῆς ἐν τοῖς Περὶ φαρμάκων
ἁπλῶν δυνάμεως εἰρημένης; ἐδείκνυμεν γὰρ ἐν ἐκείνοις τὰ μὲν ξηραίνοντα, τὰ δ᾽ ὑγραίνοντα, τὰ δὲ
ψύχοντα, τὰ δὲ θερμαίνοντα τῶν φαρμάκων· ἔνια δὲ

fluities necessarily arise, in that it has been stated in the accounts of nature that in every change in the qualities of nutriment, whether they are thicker or thinner, a superfluity follows. And when these superfluities arise in the whole body, in respect to the thinner, transpiration is always imperceptible; whereas it often becomes perceptible whenever either the innate heat becomes weak, or it uses greater nourishment than is necessary, or some overly strong movement burdens the organism. The other is the filth caused to grow in our bodies. And in wounds and ulcers the thin superfluity is called an "ichor" and the thick superfluity is called the "filth of a wound." Furthermore, due to the thin superfluity a wound becomes moist, while due to the thick superfluity it becomes filthy. Because of this there is need of a twofold [approach to] medications; that is, there is need of those that dry what is moist, and those that purify the actual filth. Accordingly, since at no period of time does nature remain idle, there will be no moment at which both these (i.e. moisture and filth) will not be collected together in a hollow wound or ulcer; so there will be no time at which there will not be need of both medications, the drying and the purifying. It has been shown what kind the medication must be in terms of class.

176K

But this is not enough; it is necessary to discover which particular medications in terms of kind will be applied. How and by what method will that be discovered? Surely it will be from what is stated about potency in my treatise *On the [Mixtures and] Potencies of Simple Medications*? For I showed in that work which medications cause drying, moistening, cooling and heating and which, by virtue of

κατὰ συζυγίαν ἢ θερμαίνοντα καὶ ξηραίνοντα, ἢ ψύ-
177K χοντα | καὶ ὑγραίνοντα, ἢ θερμαίνοντα καὶ ὑγραίνον-
τα, ἢ ψύχοντα καὶ ξηραίνοντα· εἶναί τε καθ' ἕκαστον
αὐτῶν ἄπειρον μέν τι τῷ πλήθει τὸ μᾶλλόν τε καὶ
ἧττον· εἰς δὲ τὴν χρείαν τὴν ἰατρικὴν ὅροις εὐσήμοις
περιγραφόμενον, πρώτης τινὸς ἐν αὐτοῖς γινομένης
τάξεως καὶ δευτέρας καὶ τρίτης καὶ τετάρτης. ἐκ ποίας
οὖν τάξεως ἔσται τὸ σαρκωτικὸν φάρμακον, ὃ δὴ
μετρίως ἔφαμεν χρῆναι ξηραίνειν τε καὶ ῥύπτειν; ἐκ
τῆς πρώτης δηλονότι· μᾶλλον γὰρ ἐπιταθὲν ὡς μὴ
μόνον ἐκδαπανᾶν τὸ περιττὸν τῆς ἀπορρεούσης ὑγρότητος, ἀλλὰ καὶ αὐτοῦ τοῦ ἐπιρρέοντος αἵματος ἅπτεσθαι, κωλύσει τὴν σάρκωσιν ἀναλίσκον αὐτῆς τὴν
ὕλην. ἐδείχθη δὲ τοιαῦτα, λιβανωτός τε καὶ κρίθινον
ἄλευρον καὶ κυάμινον ὀρόβινόν τε καὶ ἶρις ἀριστολοχία τε καὶ καδμεία καὶ πάναξ καὶ πομφόλυξ· ἅπαντα δὲ ταῦτα ἀλλήλων ἐδείκνυτο διαφέροντα τῷ τε
μᾶλλον καὶ ἧττον. καὶ τῷ μὲν ἁπλᾶς ἔχειν τὰς ἐπικρα-
τούσας δυνάμεις, τὰ δὲ συνθέτους. ἀριστολοχία μὲν
γὰρ καὶ πάναξ μᾶλλον ξηραίνει τῶν ἄλλων καὶ θερ-
178K μότερα τὴν φύσιν ἐστί· | τὸ δὲ κρίθινον καὶ τὸ κυάμι-
νον ἄλευρον ἧττον πολὺ ἐκείνων ξηραίνει καὶ ἥκιστα
θερμότητος μετέχει· λιβανωτὸς δὲ θερμὸς μέν ἐστι
μετρίως, ἧττον δὲ τούτων ξηραίνει, ὥστε τινὰς φύσεις
σωμάτων οὐδὲ ξηραίνει τὴν ἀρχήν· ὀρόβινον δὲ καὶ
ἶρις ἐν τῷ μεταξὺ τούτων τε καὶ ἀριστολοχίας καὶ
πάνακός ἐστιν.

ὅπερ δ' ὁ λόγος ἐκίνησε χρησίμως αὖθις ἀναλάβω-
μεν. ὁ γάρ τοι λιβανωτὸς ὑγρὰν μὲν φύσιν σώματος

conjunction, are both heating and drying, or cooling and 177K
moistening, or heating and moistening, or cooling and drying. And, in relation to each of these, there is infinite variation in terms of more and less in amount whereas, for medical use, this is circumscribed by distinct boundaries, there
being a certain order in them of first, second, third, and
fourth. From what kind of order will the enfleshing medication be that I said was necessary to dry and clean moderately? Obviously it is from the first order, and it is raised to
a higher level as it doesn't only consume the excess of
outflowing moisture but also, since it destroys the inflowing blood itself, it will prevent the growth of flesh, consuming the material of this. Such things were shown—frankincense, barley meal, meal of bitter vetch, iris, aristolochia,
cadmia, panax and pompholyx. All these things were demonstrated to differ from each other in terms of more or
less. It was also demonstrated that some have simple prevailing potencies while others have compound ones. For
aristolochia and panax dry more than the others and are
hotter in nature. Barley meal and the barley bran dry much 178K
less than they do and partake least of heat. Frankincense,
however, is moderately hot but dries less than these, so
that it does not dry certain bodily natures at the start. Bitter vetch and iris are in between these and aristolochia and
panax.

Let me reiterate what the discussion has usefully produced. Frankincense can certainly produce flesh in a body

σαρκῶσαι δύναται, ξηρὰν δ' οὐ δύναται· χρὴ γὰρ
ἐπίστασθαι περὶ τῶν πρώτων ἐνδείξεων ὡς δύο ἐστὸν
αὐτῶν αἱ διαφοραί, τοῦ μὲν κατὰ φύσιν τὴν φυλακὴν
ἐνδεικνυμένου καὶ διὰ τοῦτο ὁμοίων ἑαυτοῦ δεομένου,
τοῦ δὲ παρὰ φύσιν τὴν ἀναίρεσιν τὴν ἑαυτοῦ καὶ διὰ
τοῦτο τῶν ἐναντίων· φθείρεται γὰρ πᾶν εἰς ἐναντία τε
καὶ δι' ἐναντίων. τὸ μὲν οὖν ἕλκος ὅσῳπερ ἂν ὑγρότερον ᾖ, τοσούτῳ δεῖται φαρμάκου ξηραίνοντος μᾶλ-
λον· ἡ φύσις δ' αὐτοῦ τοῦ σώματος ὅσῳπερ ἂν ὑγροτέρα τύχῃ, τοσούτῳ δεῖται φαρμάκου ξηραίνοντος
ἧττον· ὥστε τῶν ἴσην ὑγρότητα ἐχόντων ἑλκῶν τὸ
μὲν ἐν ξηροτέρᾳ τῇ τοῦ κάμνοντος κράσει μᾶλλον
179K   ξηραίνεσθαι δεῖται, τὸ δ' ἐν ὑγροτέρᾳ | τοσούτῳ κατα-
δεέστερον, ὅσῳπερ ἂν καὶ ἡ φύσις τῆς φύσεως ἀπο-
λείπηται· τὴν γὰρ ἐπιτρεφομένην σάρκα παραπλησίαν εἶναι χρὴ τῇ προϋπαρχούσῃ. ξηροτέρας οὖν
οὔσης τῆς ἀρχαίας ξηροτέραν χρὴ γενέσθαι καὶ τὴν
νέαν, ὥστε ἐπὶ πλεῖον αὐτὴν δεῖ ξηραίνεσθαι, καὶ
ὅσῳπερ ἂν ᾖ ἐπὶ πλέον ξηρά, ἐπὶ τοσούτῳ καὶ τὸ
προσαγόμενον φάρμακον εἶναι ξηραντικώτερον. ἐπὶ
δέ γε τῆς ὑγροτέρας φύσεως εἰς τοσοῦτον αὖ πάλιν
ἧττον ξηραινόντων χρεία ἐστὶ φαρμάκων, εἰς ὅσον καὶ
ἡ σὰρξ ἧττόν ἐστι ξηρά.

τοιαύτην οὖν ἔχει κρᾶσιν λιβανωτός, ὡς πρὸς ἀν-
θρωπίνην φύσιν σώματος. πρὸς μὲν γὰρ τὰς εὐκρά-
τους καὶ μέσας ὁμολογεῖ, τῶν δ' ὑγρατέρων ἀτρέμα
ξηραντικώτερος ὑπάρχει, ὥσπερ οὖν αὖ καὶ τῶν
ἄκρως ξηρῶν ὑγρότερος ἀτρέμα. δεόντως οὖν ἐπὶ μὲν

of a moist nature but not in one of a dry nature. What you must know about the primary indications is that there are two differentiae of these: what is in accord with nature indicates preservation and, for this reason, has need of things like itself, while what is contrary to nature indicates removal, and for this reason has need of those things opposite to itself, for all destruction is to opposites and through opposites. Therefore, the wound or ulcer stands more in need of a drying medication to the extent that it is more moist. [Conversely] to the extent that the nature of the body itself happens to be more moist, it is less in need of a drying medication. So, of wounds or ulcers that are equally moist, that in a patient with a drier *krasis* needs to be dried more, whereas that in a patient with a more moist *krasis* is less in need to the extent that the one nature departs from the other nature. For the flesh that is being created ought to be closely similar to that which existed before. Therefore, when the original flesh was drier, the new flesh must become drier, so that this needs to be dried still more; and to the extent to which it is still more dry, the medication being applied also [needs to be] more drying to the same extent. But, on the contrary, in a more moist nature, the extent to which the flesh itself is less dry determines the extent to which there is need of those medications that dry less.

179K

Thus, frankincense has the sort of *krasis* that is consonant with the human bodily nature: to the *eukratic* and middling [natures], it is agreeable; for the more moist [natures], it is slightly more drying; and again, to those that are extremely dry, it is slightly more moistening. Neces-

ἐνίων ἑλκῶν τε καὶ φύσεων ὁ λιβανωτὸς ἐκπυΐσκει
μέν, οὐ μὴν καὶ σαρκοῖ· κατὰ δέ τινας ἤδη καὶ σαρκοῖ.
παραφυλάξας οὖν εὑρήσεις ὁμολογοῦν τῷ λόγῳ τὸ
φαινόμενον. ἐν μὲν γὰρ ταῖς ὑγροτέραις φύσεσι σαρ-
κωτικός ἐστιν, ἐν δὲ ταῖς ξηροτέραις οὐκέτι· καὶ κατὰ
μὲν τὰ μετρίως ὑγρὰ τῶν ἑλκῶν οἷός τε σαρκοῦν |
180K ἐστι, κατὰ δὲ τὰ λίαν ὑγρὰ παντάπασιν ἀδύνατος.

ὁρᾷς οὖν ἤδη σαφῶς ὅσων δεῖ θεωρημάτων ἀνδρὶ
μέλλοντι κατὰ μέθοδον ὀρθὴν ἕλκος ἰᾶσθαι; ἐπειδὴ
γὰρ εὑρέθη πάντως ὑγρότης ἐνυπάρχουσα τῷ πάθει,
τὸ ξηραῖνον ἐνεδείξατο φάρμακον. ἀλλ᾽ ἐπεὶ τὰ μὲν
αὐτῶν μᾶλλον ξηραίνει, τὰ δ᾽ ἧττον, ἔκ τε τῆς τῶν
ἑλκῶν διαφορᾶς τὸ χρήσιμον ἐλήφθη κἀκ τῆς τοῦ
κάμνοντος φύσεως. ὥστ᾽ οὐ μόνον ἀνάγκη περὶ φύσεως σώματος ἐπεσκέφθαι τῷ μέλλοντι κατὰ τρόπον
ἰατρεύσειν ἕλκος, ἀλλὰ καὶ τὴν περὶ φαρμάκων θεωρίαν ἀκριβῶς ἐκμεμαθηκέναι καὶ κράσεως σώματος
ὑγρᾶς καὶ ξηρᾶς ἐπίστασθαι γνωρίσματα.

θέασαι τοίνυν ὅση τῶν Μεθοδικῶν ἐστιν ἡ περὶ τὰς
ἀποφάσεις τόλμα, τοῦθ᾽ ἓν μόνον ἀρκεῖν αὐτοῖς ἡγουμένοις εἰς ἕλκους ἴασιν κοίλου, τὸ γινώσκειν ὅτι
πληρωτέον τέ ἐστιν αὐτὸ καὶ σαρκωτέον· οὐ γὰρ ἐν
τούτῳ γε τὸ θεραπεύειν ἐστίν, ἀλλ᾽ ἐν τῷ τὸ σαρκῶσον
ἐξευρεῖν. Ἀλλ᾽ εὕρηταί, φησι, τὸ σαρκῶσον τῇ πείρᾳ.
λέγε τοίνυν καὶ τὸ θεραπεῦσον ἐκ τῆς πείρας εὑρῆ-
181K σθαι· καὶ μὴ μάτην φρυάττου | μηδ᾽ ἀνατείνου τὴν
μέθοδον. καίτοι καὶ παρ᾽ αὐτοῖς τοῖς Ἐμπειρικοῖς ἡ
χωρὶς διορισμοῦ πεῖρα κατέγνωσται· γράφουσι γοῦν

276

sarily then, in some wounds and ulcers and in some natures, frankincense causes suppuration but does not, however, also produce flesh. In some [natures] it does actually also produce flesh. If you consider this, you will find that what is observed agrees with the theory. In more moist natures frankincense is flesh-producing, while in more dry natures it is no longer so; and in regard to moderately moist wounds and ulcers it can produce flesh, while in those that are exceedingly moist it is altogether unable [to do so].   180K

So do you now see clearly the need of such principles for a man who intends to cure a wound or ulcer by the right method? For when it is found, in general, that moisture is present in the affection, it indicates a drying medication. But since some of these medications dry more and some less, the use is taken from the difference between the wounds or ulcers and from the nature of the patient. So not only is it essential for someone who intends to cure a wound or ulcer properly to give consideration to the nature of the body; it is also essential for him to have learned thoroughly the theory of medications and to know the signs of a moist and dry *krasis* of the body.

Look, then, at how great the rashness of the Methodics is in their assertions when they claim that this one thing is sufficient on its own for the cure of a hollow wound or ulcer—namely, the knowledge that you must fill it and enflesh it. For treatment does not, in fact, lie in this but in the discovery of what is enfleshing. "But what is enfleshing is discovered by experience," says [the Methodic]. Just say, then, that what is curative is found from experience and do not pointlessly crow about and exalt your method. Indeed,   181K
among the Empirics themselves, experience without discrimination is condemned. At all events, in the treatises

277

ἐν τοῖς περὶ φαρμάκων ὑπομνήμασιν· ἔμπλαστρος
πρὸς ἁπαλόχρωτας καὶ παῖδας καὶ γυναῖκας· ἴσασί τε
τὸν λιβανωτὸν ἐπὶ τῶν τοιούτων φύσεων ἕλκη κοῖλα
μηδὲν ἔχοντα σύμπτωμ' ἕτερον, ἀνατρέφοντα καὶ
πληροῦντα. πότερον δ' ὑγρὰ τὰ τοιαῦτα σώματ' ἐστὶ
καὶ διὰ τοῦτο δεῖται μετρίως ξηραινόντων φαρμάκων,
ἢ ἄλλη τις αἰτία τοῦ συμβαίνοντός ἐστιν, οὐκ ἐπίστανται. καὶ γὰρ αὖ καὶ πρὸς τὰ γεροντικὰ σώματα
γεγραμμένον εὑρήσεις ἕτερον φάρμακον, ἄλλο δέ τι
πρὸς τὰ δυσεπούλωτα καὶ ὀχθώδη τῶν ἑλκῶν, καὶ
πολλοὺς ἄλλους διορισμοὺς ἐν ἅπασι τοῖς θεραπευ-
τικοῖς ὑπομνήμασι γράφουσιν, ἐξ ὧν ὡς οἷόν τε πρὸς
τὴν ἰδιότητα τῆς θεραπευομένης φύσεως ἐξευρίσκουσι
τὸ συνοῖσον φάρμακον. ἅπαντες γὰρ οἱ διορισμοὶ
κατὰ τὰς τέχνας ἀπὸ τοῦ κοινοῦ πειρῶνται τὸ ἴδιον
χωρίζειν· καὶ ὅσῳπερ ἄν τις πλείω διορίσηται, πλησι-
έστερον ἀφικνεῖται τοῦ ἰδίου, τοῦτο δ' αὐτὸ τὸ³ |
182K   ἀκριβῶς ἴδιον, οὔτε γραφῆναι δυνατόν ἐστιν οὔτε
λεχθῆναι· διὸ καὶ τῶν Ἐμπειρικῶν τοῖς μάλιστα τῶν
ἔργων τῆς τέχνης φροντίσασι καὶ σχεδὸν ἅπασι τοῖς
Δογματικοῖς ὡμολόγηται τὸ μηδεμίαν οἷόν τ' εἶναι
γραφῆναι θεραπείαν ἀκριβῶς, ἀλλὰ τὸ λεῖπον εἰς τὸν
στοχασμὸν τῆς τοῦ κάμνοντος φύσεως οἱ μὲν ἐκ τῆς
ἑκάστου τῶν θεραπευόντων οἰκείας τριβῆς, οἱ δ' ἐκ τοῦ
λογικῶς τετεχνᾶσθαι φασὶ χρῆναι προστιθέναι· οὐδεὶς δ' αὐτῶν οὕτως ἦν εὐχερής, ὡς ἅπαντος ἕλκους
κοίλου φάρμακον ἓν ἔχειν ἐπαγγέλλεσθαι σαρκω-
τικόν· οὐ γὰρ εὑρήσεις ἐν οὐδενὶ τοιοῦτον φάρμακον,

about medications they write to apply plasters to those who are soft-skinned, children and women, and they know that in such natures frankincense causes growth and fills up hollow wounds and ulcers that have no other symptom. Whether such bodies are moist and, because of this, need moderately drying medications, or whether there is some other cause of what happens, they do not know. For once more, also, in respect to aged bodies, you will find another medication is written about, and another in respect to wounds and ulcers that are hard to cicatrize and are swollen; and they write of many other distinctions in all their therapeutic treatises. From these it is possible for them to discover the medication suitable for the particular character of the nature being treated, for all the distinctions in crafts attempt to separate the specific from the general and, to the extent that someone might make a further distinction, the nearer he comes to the specific, although this very thing is precisely specific, and cannot either be written or stated. On which account, also, among both those Empirics who particularly give thought to the tasks of the art, and almost all the Dogmatics, there is agreement that it is impossible for any treatment to be written down precisely. They say there is something remaining which comes down to conjecture about the nature of the patient. Some say this must be added from the specific practice of each [doctor] providing treatment and some say from being devised skillfully on a logical basis. None of them are so tolerant of imprecision as to assert that there is one enfleshing medication for every hollow wound or ulcer, for you will not find a medication of such a kind to cure every

182K

3 B; τὸ *om.* K

οἷον πᾶν ἕλκος κοῖλον ἰᾶσθαι, ἀλλὰ παρὰ τὸ πλῆθος
τῆς ὑγρότητός τε καὶ τοῦ ῥύπου καὶ αὐτὴν τοῦ κάμνοντος τὴν κρᾶσιν ὑπαλλάττεσθαι χρὴ τὸ φάρμακον.
ἐάσαντες οὖν ἐνταῦθα τὴν ἀναισχυντίαν τῶν Μεθοδικῶν ἴδωμεν ὅ τι ποτὲ λέγουσιν οἱ ἀπὸ τῆς ἐμπειρίας,
ἐκ τῆς ἰδίας ἑκάστου τριβῆς καὶ γυμνασίας εἰσφέ-
ρεσθαί τι χρῆναι πρὸς τὴν τῶν οἰκείων τῷ κάμνοντι
φαρμάκων εὕρεσιν ἀξιοῦντες.

183K ὡς γὰρ καὶ πολλάκις εἰρήκαμεν, οὐδὲν μὲν τῶν
κατὰ τὴν ἰατρικὴν πραγμάτων καὶ φαρμάκων[4] ἄρρητον ὑπάρχει κατ' εἶδος, ἀλλ' ὃ μήτε ῥηθῆναι μήτε
γραφῆναι μήθ' ὅλως διδαχθῆναι δύναται τὸ ποσόν
ἐστιν ἐν ἑκάστῳ· καὶ δὴ κἀπὶ τῶν ἑλκῶν ἡ μὲν ὑγρότης καὶ ὁ ῥύπος οὐκ ἄρρητα, τὸ ποσὸν δ' ἄρρητον ἐν
ἑκατέρῳ· καίτοι κἀνταῦθα προσέρχεσθαί πως βουλόμεθα τῇ δηλώσει πλησίον, ὀλίγον καὶ πολὺν λέγοντες
ῥύπον καὶ λεπτὸν καὶ παχὺν καὶ παντελῶς ὀλίγον καὶ
λίαν πολὺν καὶ μέτριον καὶ σύμμετρον καί πως ἄλλως
οὕτως ὀνομάζοντες πολυειδῶς, ἵν' ὡς οἷόν τε πλησίον
ἀφικώμεθα τῆς δηλώσεως τοῦ ποσοῦ. πρόσχες οὖν
ἤδη μοι τὸν νοῦν ἀκριβῶς, ἵν' εἰδῇς ὅσον πλεονεκτεῖ
τὸ μεθόδῳ ποιεῖν ὁτιοῦν τοῦ δι' ἐμπειρίας μόνης. ἔστω
γὰρ ἐγνῶσθαι τόδε τι τὸ φάρμακον ἕλκους κοίλου
σαρκωτικὸν ἐπὶ τῶν ὡς ἂν μὲν ἡμεῖς εἴποιμεν ὑγροτέρων τὴν κρᾶσιν, ὡς δ' ὁ τηρητικός τε καὶ Ἐμπειρικός, ἁπαλοχρώτων τε καὶ παίδων καὶ γυναικῶν, εἶτα
νῦν τῷ τοιούτῳ προσαγόμενον ὀνῆσαι μηδέν. ἡμεῖς
μὲν οὖν ζητήσωμεν κατὰ τί μηδὲν ὠφέλησεν, εἰς δύο

hollow wound or ulcer in everyone. Rather, besides the abundance of moisture and filth, the medication must alter the actual *krasis* of the patient. Therefore, if we accept here the impudence of the Methodics, let us see what they say—those who, on the basis of experience, think it right that something ought to contribute to the discovery of the medications that are appropriate to the patient from the specific practice and exercise of each person.

For as I too have often said, none of the matters and medications pertaining to the craft of medicine is inexpressible in terms of kind, but the quantity cannot in each case be stated, or written, or in a word, taught. Further, in the case of wounds and ulcers, the moistness and filth are not inexpressible whereas the quantity in each is inexpressible. And indeed, we wish somehow to come near to expressing this, saying slightly or greatly filthy, thin, thick, extremely slight, very great, average or in due proportion, or however else, naming so diversely that as far as possible we come near to the expression of quantity. Pay strict attention to me now so that you may know how doing anything whatsoever by method gains an advantage over doing it by experience alone. For suppose it is the case that this medication for a hollow wound or ulcer is known to be enfleshing in those whom we might say are more moist in terms of *krasis* or, as the observer and the Empiric might say, in soft-skinned women and children, and now there is no benefit when it is applied to such a person. Let us, then, investigate why it brings no benefit, referring to these two

183K

---

4 καὶ φαρμάκων om. B, *recte fort.*

τούτους ἀναγαγόντες σκοπούς· ἢ γὰρ ἐνδεέστερον ἢ |
184K ἀμετρότερον ἐξήρανε· καὶ σημεῖά γε τούτων τόν τε
ῥύπον ἕξομεν καὶ τὸν ἰχῶρα. εἰ μὲν γὰρ πλείων ὁ
ῥύπος, ὑγρότερόν τε ὅλον εἴη τὸ ἕλκος, ἐνδεέστερον
ἐξήρανεν· εἰ δὲ καθαρόν τε καὶ ἄνικμον εὑρεθείη,
περαιτέρω τοῦ προσήκοντος. εὐθὺς δὲ καὶ τὸ ποσὸν
τοῦ συμμέτρου μᾶλλον ἢ ἧττον ἐκ τοῦ ποσοῦ τῶν
γνωρισμάτων εἰσόμεθα· καὶ τοσούτῳ δυνησόμεθα τὸ
ἐφεξῆς φάρμακον ἢ ξηρότερον ἢ οὐ τοιοῦτον προσ-
ενεγκεῖν.

ὁ δ᾽ Ἐμπειρικὸς ὅτι μὲν οὐκ ἐσάρκωσε τόνδέ τινα,
τὸ προσαχθὲν φάρμακον ὁρᾷ· μὴ γινώσκων μέντοι
πότερον τῷ μᾶλλον ἢ τῷ ἧττον ξηρᾶναι, μεταβαίνειν
ἐφ᾽ ἕτερον ἀδυνατεῖ. κατὰ δὲ τὸν αὐτὸν τρόπον καὶ οἱ
περὶ τὸν Ἐρασίστρατόν τε καὶ Ἡρόφιλον ἐξ ἡμισείας
ὥσπερ καὶ πρόσθεν ἐδείξαμεν ὄντες Δογματικοὶ κακῶς ἰατρεύουσιν ἕλκος· μόνα γὰρ ἐπιχειροῦσι λογικῶς θεραπεύειν ὅσα τῶν ὀργανικῶν ἐστι μορίων ἴδια
νοσήματα· τὸ δ᾽ ἕλκος, ὥσπερ καὶ πρόσθεν εἴρηται,
κοινόν ἐστιν ὁμοιομερῶν τε καὶ ὀργανικῶν, ὥστε καὶ
τοῦτο κατὰ τοσοῦτον ἐμπειρικῶς θεραπεύουσι, καθ᾽
ὅσον ἐν τοῖς ὁμοιομερέσι πέφυκε γίνεσθαι. καὶ μὲν δὴ
κἂν τῷ τὰς ἀπολωλυίας τελέως οὐσίας ἢ κεκολο-
185K βωμένας ἐπιχειρεῖν | θεραπεύειν, κἀνταῦθα ἀναγκαῖον
αὐτοῖς ἐστιν ἀποπίπτειν πολλαχῇ τοῦ λογικῶς. εἰ γὰρ
αὐτὸ τὸ ἀπολωλὸς οὐσία τίς ἐστιν ὁμοιομερής, ἀναγκαῖόν ἐστι τὸν προνοούμενον αὐτοῦ τῆς γενέσεως ὑπὲρ
ἁπάσης τῆς φύσεως ἐπίστασθαι. περὶ μὲν δὴ τούτων

indicators; whether it dried too little or too much, and in   184K
fact we have the signs of these things in respect to filth and
the ichor. For if the filth is greater, the wound or ulcer as a
whole is too moist and is dried too little whereas, if it is
found to be clean and without moisture, it is dried beyond
what is appropriate. We will know immediately the quantity
of the balance in terms of more or less from the number of
signs, so we will be able in such a way to apply as the next
medication one which is either more drying or not.

The Empiric, however, sees that the applied medication did not create flesh in this instance, but nevertheless
does not know whether to dry more or less, and is unable to
change to another medication. In the same way, too, the
followers of Erasistratus and Herophilus, being "semi-
Dogmatics," as we also showed before, treat a wound or
ulcer badly, for they only attempt to treat logically such
diseases as are specific to the organic parts, whereas the
wound or ulcer, as I also said before, is common to both
homoiomeres and organic [parts]. But, to the extent that it
arises in the *homoiomeres* by nature, they treat it empirically. Indeed, even in this, if they attempt to treat completely destroyed or badly damaged substances, here too   185K
it is inevitable that, in many instances, they fall short of
what is logical. If what is actually destroyed is some *homoiomerous* substance, it is essential for the person who gives
forethought to the genesis of this to know about its whole
nature. I shall certainly speak again about these matters. I

καὶ αὖθις εἰρήσεται. τὸ δὲ μὴ τυχὸν εἶναι πρᾶγμα,
καλῶς ἕλκους προνοήσασθαι καὶ ὡς ἡ πρώτη πασῶν
ἔνδειξις, ἡ καὶ τοῖς ἰδιώταις γινωσκομένη πολλοστόν
ἐστι μόριον τῆς θεραπείας, ἐναργῶς ἀποδεδεῖχθαι
νομίζω· καὶ γὰρ ὅτι δραστικαὶ ποιότητές εἰσι θερμότης τε καὶ ψυχρότης καὶ ὑγρότης καὶ ξηρότης ἀναγκαῖον ἀποδεδεῖχθαι καὶ τούτοις ἐφεξῆς ἅπαντα τὰ
περὶ κράσεων ἐγνῶσθαι κατά τε τὸ ἡμέτερον σύγ-
γραμμα καὶ τἆλλα πάντα τὰ τούτῳ πλησιάζοντα.

νῦν μὲν οὖν ὁ λόγος ἐφ᾽ ἕλκους εἴρηται κοίλου,
μόνην αὐτὴν τὴν κοιλότητα θεραπευόντων ἡμῶν· ἡ
γὰρ ὡς ἕλκους θεραπεία κατὰ τὸ παρὸν οὔπω λέλεκται. συνίσταται δὲ καὶ ἥδε κατὰ τὴν αὐτὴν μέθ-
οδον· ἀπό τε γὰρ τῆς τοῦ θεραπευομένου⁵ κράσεως
λαμβάνεται καὶ προσέτι τῆς τῶν φαρμάκων δυνά-
186K   μεως· εἴρηται δ᾽ ἄμφω ταῦτα τοῦ περὶ τῶν | στοιχείων
λόγου, μὴ συγχωρηθέντος γὰρ ἐν τῇ μεθόδῳ γενέσεως καὶ φθορᾶς αἰτίας εἶναι τὰς τέτταρας ποιότητας,
οὔτ᾽ ἄρξασθαι τῆς μεθόδου δυνατὸν οὔτε προελθεῖν
οὔτε τελειῶσαι· τὸ δ᾽ ἐκείνας ἐπιδεῖξαι δρώσας τε καὶ
πασχούσας εἰς ἀλλήλας τῆς περὶ τῶν στοιχείων ἐστὶ
θεωρίας. ὅπερ οὖν ἐν τοῖς ἔμπροσθεν ἐπεδείξαμεν, ὑπὸ
τοῦ νῦν ἐνεστῶτος λόγου μαρτυρεῖται, τὸ μηδὲν δύνασθαι πραγματεύσασθαι περὶ μηδενὸς τῶν ὁμοιομερῶν
τὸν ἰατρὸν ἄνευ τῆς φυσικῆς ὀνομαζομένης θεωρίας.
ἀλλ᾽ ἐκεῖ μὲν ἐπὶ τῶν ὁμοιομερῶν ἀπεδείχθη μόνον,
ἐνταῦθα δ᾽ ἤδη πως ὁ λόγος ἐμφανίζει μηδὲ ἐπὶ τῶν
ὀργανικῶν ὁλόκληρον ἐξευρεῖν δύνασθαι τὴν θερα-

think, however, it has been clearly shown that it is not a matter of chance to give proper forethought to a wound or ulcer, nor that the primary indication of all, which is known even to laymen, is just a small part of the treatment. For it is also essential to have established that the active qualities are heat, cold, moisture and dryness, and after this, everything else about *krasias* (mixtures) is known from my book, as are all other things pertaining to this.[10]

Therefore, at this point in the discussion of a hollow wound, what has been spoken of is our treatment of the cavity only; the treatment of the wound as a wound hasn't yet been stated for the present. However, this too takes place according to the same method, for it arises from the *krasis* of the person being treated and, as well as this, from the potency of the medications. Both these factors were covered in the discussion about elements. On the question of method, unless it is agreed that the causes of genesis and destruction are the four qualities, it is not possible to start the method, nor to advance it, nor to bring it to completion. To show how those qualities act on and are acted on by each other pertains to the theory about elements. Thus, what I demonstrated in the previous discussion is that no doctor is able to treat systematically any of the *homoiomeres* without what may be termed a "physical theory." But there it was shown only in the case of *homoiomeres*, whereas here the discussion already makes it clear in a certain way that it is not possible to discover any complete

186K

---

[10] This is taken to be a reference to *De temperamentis libri III*, I.509–694K as a whole.

---

5 B; θεραπεύοντος K

πείαν μηδένα χωρὶς τοῦ κἀκείνης προσάψασθαι· δειχθήσεται δ' ἐναργέστερον ἔτι ταὐτὸ τοῦτο παρ' ὅλην
τὴν πραγματείαν.

4. Ἐπὶ δὲ τὴν τοῦ ἕλκους θεραπείαν μόνου μετέρ-
χεσθαι καιρός· εἴη δ' ἂν μόνον ἐπειδὰν μήτε διάθεσις
αὐτῷ συμπαρῇ μηδεμία μήτε σύμπτωμα. μὴ τοίνυν
ἔστω μήτε ῥευματικὸν τὸ ἡλκωμένον μόριον μήτε
κακόχυμον μήθ' | ὅλως δύσκρατον· ἀλλὰ μηδὲ κοιλό-
της αὐτῷ συνέστω, μηδὲ τοῦ δέρματος ἀπώλεια μηδεμία. καὶ γὰρ αὖ τοῦτο παρορῶσιν οἱ πολλοὶ τῶν
ἰατρῶν, οὐ συνιέντες ὡς ἐπειδὰν ἕλκος κοῖλον πλη-
ρωθὲν ὁμαλὲς μὲν ὑπάρχῃ, πλατὺ δέ, διττὴ καὶ νῦν
ἐστιν ἐν τῷ μορίῳ διάθεσις, ἑτέρα μὲν οὐσίας δέρματος ἀπώλεια, δευτέρα δὲ συνεχείας λύσις. ἐπειδὰν μὲν
οὖν αὐτὸ τοῦτο μόνον ᾖ συνεχείας λύσις, ἤτοι τῆς
ἐπιδερμίδος ἢ καὶ τοῦ δέρματος ἅπαντος ἢ καὶ τῆς
ὑποκειμένης ἅμ' αὐτῷ σαρκός, ἕλκος ἐστὶν οὕτω τὸ
πάθημα καὶ δεῖται κολλήσεως μόνης. εἰ γὰρ συν-
αχθείη πρὸς ἄλληλα τὰ χείλη τοῦ δέρματος, οὐδέν
ἐστι μεταξὺ τοῦ δέρματος ἑτερογενές, ὥσπερ ἐπὶ τοῦ
πεπληρωμένου τε καὶ ὁμαλοῦ ἕλκους· ἐπ' ἐκείνου γὰρ
οὐχ ἅπτεται τὰ πέρατα τοῦ ἕλκους ἀλλήλων, ἀλλ' ἐκ
τῆς ἡλκωμένης ἁπάσης χώρας ἀπόλωλε τὸ δέρμα καὶ
χρὴ γεννῆσαι δήπουθεν αὐτό· κατὰ μέντοι τὸ διῃρη-
μένον ὑπό τινος ὀξέος κολλήσεως δεῖ μόνης, οὐ μὴν
καὶ γενέσεως δέρματος. ὅταν οὖν ἕλκους ἁπλοῦ προκείμενον ᾖ θεραπείαν εὑρεῖν, ὑποτίθεσθαι χρὴ τῷ
λόγῳ διαίρεσιν σαρκώδους μέλους χωρὶς ἀπωλείας |

treatment in the case of the organic bodies apart from the application of theory. This will be made even more apparent throughout the entire treatise.

4. It is time now to pass on to the treatment of the wound per se whenever it exists in isolation with neither a condition nor a symptom accompanying it. Let us assume that the wounded part is not subject to flux, is not *kakochymous*, and is not on the whole *dyskratic*. But let there be no hollowness present with it, nor any destruction of the skin. For again, the majority of doctors also overlook this, not realizing that whenever a hollow wound is filled and is level but flat, there is now a twofold condition in the part, the one being loss of the substance of the skin, and the other, dissolution of continuity. Whenever there is this dissolution of continuity alone, either of the epidermis or of the whole skin, or also of the underlying flesh along with it, a wound is in this way the affection, and needs conglutination alone. If the margins of the skin are drawn together with each other, there is nothing in between of a different class to skin, just as in the case of the wound that has been filled and is level. In the latter case, the opposite sides of the wound do not contact each other but the skin of the whole wounded region is lost and there is need, obviously, to regenerate this. However, in relation to what has been divided by something sharp, there is need of conglutination alone and not of the generation of skin as well. Therefore, whenever what lies before us is to discover the treatment of a simple wound, what must be taken as foundational in the discussion is the division of the fleshy part

187K

188K μορίου. τὸ δέ γε πλατὺ τὸ ἐπουλώσεως δεόμενον ἕλκος
ἀπολώλεκε τελέως τὴν καλουμένην ἐπιδερμίδα. ταύτην οὖν γεννῆσαι χρὴ καὶ πρὸς ἑαυτὴν ἑνῶσαι· καὶ δύ'
ἐνταῦθα πρόκεινται σκοποί, καθάπερ ἐπὶ τοῦ κοίλου·
διότι καὶ ἡ διάθεσις ἐπ' ἀμφοῖν ἐστι διττή. τίνι τοίνυν,
φήσει τις αὐτῶν ἴσως, Ὁμαλὲς ἕλκος τοῦ κοίλου
διενήνοχεν, εἰ καὶ διάθεσις ἐπ' ἀμφοῖν ἐστι διττὴ καὶ
διττὸς ὁ σκοπὸς τῆς θεραπείας; πλήθει τῶν ἀπολωλότων, ὦ βέλτιστε, μορίων. ἐπὶ μὲν γὰρ τοῦ κοίλου καὶ ἡ
ἐπιδερμὶς μὲν ἀπόλωλε καὶ ἡ τοῦ δέρματος δὲ φύσις ἡ
λοιπὴ πᾶσα καὶ τῆς ὑποκειμένης σαρκὸς οὐκ ὀλίγον
ἐνίοτε μέρος· ἐπὶ δὲ τοῦ πεπληρωμένου σὰρξ μὲν
οὐκέτι λείπει, τὸ δ' ἔξωθεν σκέπασμα λείπει. τίς μὲν
οὖν ἡ τῶν τοιούτων ἑλκῶν ἐστιν ἴασις ἐφεξῆς ἐροῦμεν·
ἐν δὲ τῷ παρόντι τοῦ μόνον ἕλκους ὄντος, ἑτέραν δὲ
μηδεμίαν ἔχοντος διάθεσιν, ὁποίαν τινὰ χρὴ τὴν θεραπείαν ποιεῖσθαι λέγωμεν.

ἐπεὶ τοίνυν διαίρεσις μόνον ἐστίν, ἅμα χρὴ τὰ
πέρατα γενέσθαι τῶν διῃρημένων· ἢ οὐ τοῦτο μόνον,
189K ἀλλὰ καὶ μεῖναι | συνελθόντα; διττὴ δ' ἡ τῶν συν-
ελθόντων μονή· τὰ μὲν γὰρ δι' ἑαυτῶν, τὰ δὲ δι' ἄλλων
μένει· δι' ἑαυτῶν μὲν ὅσα συμφύεται, δι' ἄλλων δὲ τά
τε συνδούμενα καὶ τὰ κολλώμενα. τὰ μὲν δὴ συμ-
φυόμενα πάντως χρὴ μαλακὰ τὴν φύσιν εἶναι. τοιοῦτον δὲ ἥ τε σὰρξ ἐστιν αὐτὴ καὶ ὅσα σαρκώδη
μόρια κατὰ τὴν σύστασιν. ὅσα δ' ἐστὶ σκληρὰ καὶ
ξηρά, συμφῦναι μὲν οὐ δύναται, κόλλης δέ τινος ἢ

without its destruction. The flat wound that is in need of 188K
scarring over has completely destroyed the so-called epidermis. It is therefore necessary to regenerate this and
reunite it with itself, so here two objectives lie together,
just as in the case of the hollow [wound], because the condition in both cases is also twofold. To which, perhaps, one
of them[11] will say: "In what way is a level wound differentiated from a hollow wound, if in both cases the condition
and the aim of treatment is twofold?" By the magnitude of
the destroyed parts, my good man! For in the case of the
hollow [wound], not only is the epidermis destroyed, but
also the whole remaining nature of the skin and the underlying flesh is sometimes [affected] to no small extent. In
the case of a wound that has been filled, the flesh is no
longer lacking but the external covering is lacking. Next, I
shall say what the cure of such wounds is. For the present,
let me speak about the kind of treatment we must carry out
when there is a wound alone without any other condition.

Accordingly, when there is division alone, the margins
of what has been divided should be brought together; and
not only this but, having come together, they should also
remain so. Things brought together remain so in two ways: 189K
of their own accord and by means of other things. Those
that do so of their own accord grow together, whereas
those that do so through other means are bound together
or conglutinated. Now those things that grow together
must be entirely soft in nature. Flesh itself is such a thing,
as are those parts that are fleshy in consistency. Those that
are hard and dry cannot grow together and require some

---

[11] Presumably "they" are the Methodics.

δεσμοῦ δεῖται πρὸς τὸ μεῖναι συναχθέντα. τῶν μὲν δὴ
τοιούτων σωμάτων ἡ ἴασις ἐν τοῖς ἑξῆς εἰρήσεται.

περὶ δὲ τῶν ἑνωθῆναι δυναμένων ὁ λόγος περαι-
νέσθω, ζητούντων ἡμῶν κἀνταῦθα τὸ τῆς συμφύσεως
αἴτιον. ἔστι δ' ὥσπερ ἐπὶ τῶν κοίλων ἑλκῶν ἡ φύσις
αἰτία τῆς σαρκώσεως, οὕτω κἀπὶ τῶν ἁπλῶν ἑλκῶν
τῆς συμφύσεως· ὅθεν ἐὰν συναγάγῃς εἰς ταὐτὸν ἀκριβῶς τὰ διεστηκότα, χωρὶς τῆς ἄλλης ἁπάσης τῆς
ἔξωθεν ἐπιτεχνήσεως συμφύεται. καί σοι γέγονεν
αὖθις ἕτερος σκοπὸς ὁ τῆς συναγωγῆς, ἵν' ἐντεῦθεν
ὁρμώμενος ζητήσῃς ἐξ ὧν τοῦτο ποιήσεις. ἢ γὰρ
190K δεσμὸν ἐν κύκλῳ περιλαβὼν ἐκ δυοῖν ἀρχῶν, | ἢ
ῥαφάς, ἢ ἀγκτῆρας ἐπιθείς, ἢ τινὰ τούτων, ἢ πάντα
συνάξεις εἰς ταὐτὸ τὰ διῃρημένα. χρὴ δὲ μήτε μαλακὸν εἶναι πάνυ καὶ οἷον βρυῶδες τὸ περιβαλλόμενον,
ἵν' ἀσφαλῶς συνέχῃ, μήθ' οὕτω σκληρὸν ὡς θλίβειν·
ἀλλὰ μηδὲ τὴν ἐπιβολὴν ἢ οὕτω χαλαρὰν ὡς μηδὲν
ἀνύειν, ἢ οὕτω σφοδρὰν ὡς θλίβουσαν ὀδύνην ἐργάζεσθαι. ταῦτ' εἰ ποιήσαις καὶ εἴη τὸ ἕλκος μόνον ἄνευ
κακοχυμίας, ἢ ῥεύματος, ἢ δυσκρασίας, ἢ φλεγμονῆς,
ἤ τινος ἄλλης κακώσεως, ἑνωθήσεται πάντως. εἰ δ'
ἤτοι διὰ τὸ μέγεθος ἀδύνατον εἴη μέχρι τοῦ βάθους
ἀκριβῶς ἀλλήλοις παρατεθῆναι τὰ κεχωρισμένα σώματα, μήτε τῶν ῥαμμάτων μήτε τῶν ἀγκτήρων μήτε
τῆς ἐπιδέσεως ἀφικνεῖσθαι δυναμένης αὐτῶν, ἢ φθά-
νοι τις ἰχὼρ αὐτόθι συνειλεγμένος, ἢ καί τις ὀδύνη
συνοῦσα, κολληθῆναι τὸ τοιοῦτον ἕλκος ἀδύνατον ἐπὶ
μόνῃ τῇ συναγωγῇ·

glue or binding for what has been brought together to remain so. The cure of such bodies will be spoken about in what follows.

But let me complete the discussion about those things that can be united, since what we are seeking here is the cause of the coalescence. As in the case of the hollow wounds, where Nature is the cause of flesh production, so too, in the case of simple wounds, Nature is the cause of coalescence. As a consequence, if you bring together accurately the [tissues] that have been set apart, they grow together without any other artificial contrivance externally. And let me tell you, the indicator of the bringing together becomes different again, so that having started out from here, you will seek out those things through which you will achieve this. For when you encompass the wound in an encircling bandage with two points of origin, or place sutures or a fibula, or one of these things, or all of them, you will bring what has been divided to the same point. And it is necessary that what is used to encompass [the wound] is neither unduly soft, nor as it were flabby, so that it holds it together safely but is not so hard as to cause compression. But the application should not be so loose as to achieve nothing nor so strong as to cause pain by compression. If you do these things, and if it is a wound alone without *kakochymia*, flux, *dyskrasia*, inflammation, or some other abnormality, it will unite completely. If, on the other hand, because of the magnitude, it is impossible for the separated bodies to be apposed accurately right to the depths, or it is impossible for sutures, fibulae or binding to come near to them, or some ichor has collected in the spot beforehand, or pain is present as well, primary closure (conglutination) of such a wound is out of the question.

190K

291

τό τε γὰρ ὀδυνώμενον ἐρεθίζει τι πλέον ἐπιρρεῖν· εἰ
δὲ καὶ τὸ ἴσον ἐπιρρεῖ τὸ κατὰ φύσιν, ἀλλ' ἤ γε
δύναμις ἀρρωστοῦσα τῶν ὀδυνωμένων τε ἅμα καὶ
191K τετρωμένων | μορίων οὐκ οἴσει τὸ ἴσον, ἀλλ' ὡς ὑπὸ
πλείονος βαρυνθήσεται, κἀκ τούτου πάντως μὲν ἰχῶ-
ρες περιττοί, θαυμαστὸν δ' εἰ μὴ καὶ φλεγμονὴ γενήσεται. καὶ μὲν δὴ καὶ εἰ χωρὶς ὀδύνης ὁ ἰχὼρ ἐν τῷ
μεταξὺ τῶν συναχθέντων χειλῶν τοῦ ἕλκους εἴη
παρακείμενος, ἢ καί τις χώρα γίγνοιτο μεταξὺ κενὴ
μὲν ἰχῶρος, ἀέρος δὲ πλήρης, οὐκ ἐνδέχεται κολληθῆναι τὸ τοιοῦτον ἕλκος ἐκ μόνης τῆς συναγωγῆς· ὅ τε
γὰρ ἰχὼρ ἤδη διακόπτει τὴν ἕνωσιν αἵ τε μεταξὺ τῶν
ἑνωθησομένων χῶραι κεναὶ κωλύουσιν ἅψασθαι τὰς
ἐπιφανείας ἀλλήλων· ὥστ' ἐκεῖνά γε τὰ μέρη τοῦ
ἕλκους ἡ φύσις δεῖται προσαρκῶσαι πρότερον, ἵνα
συμφύσῃ· μικρὰ δὲ δήπουθέν ἐστιν οὕτως, εἰ καλῶς
συναχθῇ τὸ ἕλκος, ὡς μιᾶς ἡμέρας ἢ τὸ πλεῖστόν γε
δεῖσθαι δυοῖν. ἐν οὖν τούτῳ τῷ χρόνῳ φαρμάκου
χρεία ξηραίνοντος τὸ μόριον, ἵν' εἴτέ τις ἤδη παρακείμενος ἰχὼρ εἴη, τοῦτον ἐκδαπανήσῃ καὶ τὸν μέλλοντα συρρεῖν εἰς τὰς κενὰς χώρας κωλύσῃ. νῦν οὖν
πάλιν ἀναμνήσθητί μου τοῦ σαρκωτικοῦ φαρμάκου
τοῦ μετρίως ξηραίνοντος, ἵν' εἰδῶμεν εἴτε ξηραντικώ-
192K τερον | αὐτοῦ χρὴ τὸ κολλητικὸν ὑπάρχειν εἴτε μή. τὸ
μὲν δὴ σαρκωτικὸν εἰ σύμπαν ἐξεδαπάνα τὸ ἐπιρρέον
αἷμα, τὴν ὕλην ἂν οὕτως ἀφῃρεῖτο τῆς σαρκώσεως. τὸ
δέ γε κολλητικὸν ἢ οὐδ' ὅλως δεῖται γενέσεως σαρκός,
ἢ σμικρᾶς παντάπασιν· ὥστε μᾶλλον αὐτὸ χρὴ ξη-

If there is a wound that is painful, provoking excessive inflow, or if the inflow is normal, but the capacity of the parts both wounded and weakened by pain will not toler- 191K ate the normal inflow but will be weighed down by it as if by a greater flux, and from this the ichors are especially excessive, it would be surprising if inflammation didn't arise. Moreover, if ichor without pain is present between the apposed margins of the wound, or also if some space empty of ichor but filled with air occurs in between, it is impossible for such a wound to be conglutinated with a single apposition because the ichor now breaks down the union and the empty spaces between the [margins] that are to be united prevent the parts contacting one another, so that in those parts of the wound Nature requires prior assistance for them to coalesce. Obviously these factors are so minor that, if the wound is coapted well, it needs one or two days at the most [to heal]. Within this time there is need of a medication which dries the part in that, if some ichor is already present, it will consume this and prevent future flow into the empty spaces. Now recall once again my enfleshing medication that is moderately drying, in order that we may know whether what is conglutinat- 192K ing needs to be more drying than this or not. Certainly, if what is enfleshing entirely consumes the flowing blood, it would in this way take away the material of flesh production. In fact, what is conglutinating either does not need generation of flesh at all or only very little. As a result, there is a greater necessity for this to dry than to produce

ῥαίνειν τοῦ σαρκωτικοῦ. ταύτῃ τε οὖν ἀλλήλων διοίσει
μικράν τινα διαφοράν, ἑτέραν τε μεγάλην, ᾗ τὸ μὲν
σαρκωτικὸν εὐθὺς χρὴ καὶ ῥυπτικὸν ὑπάρχειν, ἵνα μὴ
μόνον ξηραίνῃ τὸ περιττὸν τῆς ὑγρότητος, ἀλλὰ καὶ
τὸν ῥύπον ἀφαιρῇ· τὸ δὲ κολλητικὸν οὐ ῥύπτειν οὐδὲ
ἀποσμᾶν, ἀλλὰ τοὐναντίον ἅπαν εἰς ταὐτὸν συνάγειν
ἅπασαν τὴν οὐσίαν· ὅπερ, οἶμαι, πέφυκε δρᾶν ὅσα
τῶν φαρμάκων αὐστηρὰ καὶ στύφοντα καλεῖται· ταῦτα γὰρ εἰς ταὐτὸ συνάγειν καὶ πιλεῖν, οὐκ ἀπορρύ-
πτειν, οὐδὲ καθαίρειν πέφυκεν. ὥστε μάλιστα πάντων
φυλαξώμεθα τὸ στῦφον φάρμακον, ἔνθα σαρκῶσαι
πρόκειται δυσαπολύτως ἐμπλάσσον τοῖς ἕλκεσι τὸν
ῥύπον·

193K   οἶνος οὖν ἄριστον φάρμακον ἑλκῶν ἁπάντων ᾗ
ἕλκη. εἰ δὲ καὶ μὴ προσθείημεν τῷ | λόγῳ ᾗ ἕλκη,
ταὐτόν, οἶμαι, νοήσεις· ὑπὲρ γὰρ τοῦ μὴ παρακοῦσαί
τινα πρόσκειται χάριν ἀναμνήσεως, οὐχ ὡς ἀναγκαῖόν τι διοριζόμενον. ὡς εἴ γέ μοι μεμνημένος εἴης
τῶν ἐν τῷ πρὸ τούτου βιβλίῳ λόγων ἁπάντων, τῶν
περὶ τῶν καθ' ἕκαστον ὄνομα σημαινομένων τε καὶ
ὑποκειμένων πραγμάτων, οὐδὲν ἔτι σοι δεήσομαι τὰ
τοιαῦτα διορίζεσθαι, μόνον δὲ ἀρκέσει μοι καθ' ἕκαστον αὐτῶν διελέσθαι τὰς ἁπλᾶς διαθέσεις τῶν συνθέτων, ὑπὲρ ὧν ἤδη μέν πού τι πρόσθεν εἴρηται,
ῥηθῆναι δ' ἀναγκαῖον ἔσται καὶ νῦν, οὐ τοσοῦτον
αὐτοῦ τοῦ πράγματος ἕνεκεν, ἀλλ' ὅτι νομίζουσιν οἱ
πολλοὶ τῶν ἰατρῶν ὑπὸ τῆς λέξεως ἐξαπατώμενοι
διαφορὰς ἑλκῶν εἶναι τὸ κοῖλον καὶ ὁμαλές, ἔναιμον

flesh. And in this way, materials will differ from each other in terms of both a minor and a major difference, since what is enfleshing must also be immediately cleansing, so that it not only dries the excess of moisture but also takes away the filth. What conglutinates does not cleanse nor does it wipe away. On the contrary, it brings the whole substance together as one, which is, I think, what those medications that are called harsh and astringent in nature do. For these medications are by their nature able to join into one and to press close but not to cleanse thoroughly or purify. As a result, let us above all guard against the astringent medications in that here, where what confronts us is to create flesh, they cause the filth to adhere to wounds in such a way that it is difficult to remove.

Wine is the best medication for all wounds insofar as they are wounds. And even if I do not add to the discussion 193K what wounds are, you will, I think, understand this [as I do], for to prevent misunderstanding, something is added as a reminder, not as something it is necessary to define. So if, in fact, you are reminded by me of all the discussions in the book prior to this one—those concerning the matters that are signified and underlying in relation to each term— I shall no longer need to distinguish such things for you. It will be enough for me just to divide off the simple conditions from the compound in relation to each of these. Something has already been said previously somewhere about these, but now it will need to be said again, not so much for the sake of the matter itself, but because the majority of doctors, being deceived by the term, think that the differentiae of wounds are hollow and flat, bleeding and

τε καὶ παλαιόν, ῥυπαρόν τε καὶ καθαρόν, ἀφλέγμαν-
τόν τε καὶ φλεγμαῖνον. ἀναγκαῖον οὖν ἔσται διελέσθαι τίνες μὲν αἱ οἰκεῖαι διαφοραὶ τῶν ἑλκῶν εἰσι,
τίνες δ᾽ ἐπιπλοκαὶ διαθέσεων ἑτέρων. ἀλλὰ τοῦτο μὲν
ὀλίγον ὕστερον·

ἡ δὲ συνήθης διδασκαλία τοῖς παλαιοῖς, ἥνπερ δὴ
καὶ νῦν ηὐξάμην ἀσκηθῆναι, κατὰ φύσιν ὑπάρχει, |
194K μάλιστα τῶν ἁπλῶν ἑκάστης διαθέσεως ἴδιον ἴαμα
λεγόντων αὐτῶν καὶ μάλιστα πάντων Ἱπποκράτους. ἡ
γάρ τοι μέθοδος ἡ θεραπευτικὴ κατὰ τοῦτον ἂν μάλιστα προΐοι τὸν τρόπον, ὑπὲρ ἑκάστου τῶν ἁπλῶν ἰδίᾳ
διελθόντων ἡμῶν· ἔπειτ᾽ αὖθις ἐπὶ τοῖς συνθέτοις
ἅπασιν ἑτέραν μίαν ἐπιδειξάντων μέθοδον· ὥσπερ καὶ
εἰ δύο ἦν ὄντως κατὰ δίαιταν νοσήματα, τό τε στεγνὸν
καὶ τὸ ῥοῶδες, ἰδίαν ἑκατέρου θεραπείαν εἰπόντας,
οὕτως ἐχρῆν ἐπιπεπλεγμένου μνημονεύειν, ὡς οἱ περὶ
τὸν Θεσσαλὸν ἀξιοῦσι, τὸν αὐτόν, οἶμαι, τρόπον,
ἐπειδὰν τῶν μὲν ἑλκῶν ᾗ ἕλκη πάντων ἓν εἶδος ὑπάρχει, τῶν φλεγμονῶν δ᾽ ᾗ φλεγμοναί, καὶ τούτων ἕτερον εἶδος ἕν, ἰδίᾳ μὲν χρὴ τῶν ἑλκῶν, ἰδίᾳ δὲ τῶν
φλεγμονῶν εἰπόντας θεραπείας, οὕτως ἤδη συνάπτειν
εἰς ταὐτὸν ἀμφοτέρας. τοῦτ᾽ οὖν εἰ ποιήσαιμεν, ἕλκη
μὲν ἅπαντα ξηραίνεσθαί τε ἅμα καὶ στύφεσθαι δεό-
μενα, κατὰ τὴν εἰρημένην μέθοδον εὑρήσομεν, οὐ μὴν
καὶ ῥύπτεσθαί γε· κοιλότητα δ᾽ ἐν σαρκὶ ξηραίνεσθαι
μὲν καὶ ῥύπτεσθαι, στύφεσθαι δ᾽ οὐκέτι.

καὶ δὴ κατὰ τὸν αὐτὸν τρόπον ὃν ἔμπροσθεν εἴπο-
195K μεν ἐπὶ τῶν κοίλων ἑλκῶν, | ἀνάλογον καὶ νῦν ἐπι-

chronic, filthy and clean, and noninflamed and inflamed. It will be necessary, then, to distinguish what the proper differentiae of wounds and the combinations of other conditions are. But [more on] this a little later.

The customary teaching by the ancients, which is actually what I also wish to be practiced now, is in accord with nature. They particularly say that there is a specific 194K cure for the simples of each condition, and most of all Hippocrates [says this]. For truly the therapeutic method would go forward especially in this manner, if we were to go over each of the simple conditions individually. On the other hand, if we demonstrated another, single method for all the compound conditions, just as if there were really two diseases in relation to regimen—obstruction and fluxion—when we spoke of a specific treatment of each, in the same way it would be necessary to make mention of what has been combined, as the followers of Thessalus think is right. Similarly, I believe, whenever there exists one form of all wounds as a wound, and of inflammations as an inflammation another single form, it would be necessary to speak of the treatment of wounds specifically and of inflammations specifically, and in this way now to join both into the same. If we do this, we will discover that all wounds need to be simultaneously dried out and drawn together in accord with the stated method, but not in fact to be cleansed also. On the other hand, we will find that a cavity in flesh [needs to] be dried out and cleansed, but no longer to be drawn together.

And further, just as I said before in the case of hollow wounds, we shall now also analogously consider the nature 195K

σκεψόμεθα τοῦ σώματος τὴν φύσιν, εἰ μαλακὴ καὶ
βρυώδης, ἢ σκληρὰ καὶ ξηρὰ καὶ σύντονος. ἡ μὲν γὰρ
προτέρα καθ' ὅσον ὑγροτέρα, κατὰ τοσοῦτον καὶ τῶν
φαρμάκων ἧττον ξηραινόντων δεήσεται· ἡ δευτέρα δὲ
καθ' ὅσον ξηροτέρα, κατὰ τοσοῦτον αὖ καὶ ἥδε καὶ
σφοδρότερον ξηραινόντων δεήσεται καὶ μᾶλλον στυφόντων. ὁ γοῦν Ἐμπειρικός, οἶμαι, κἀνταῦθα παίδων
μὲν καὶ γυναικῶν καὶ ἀπαλοσάρκων μνημονεύσει,
νεανίσκους καὶ γεωργοὺς καὶ θαλαττουργοὺς ἀντι-
τάττων αὐτοῖς· οὐ μὴν ὅτι γε διὰ μὲν τὴν ὑγρότητα
τῆς κράσεως ἐπὶ παίδων καὶ γυναικῶν ἑώραται τὰ
τοιαῦτα τῶν φαρμάκων εὐδοκιμοῦντα· διὰ δὲ τὴν
ξηρότητα πάλιν ἕτερα, θερισταῖς καὶ ναύταις ἁρμότ-
τοντα συνιέναι δυνάμενος, οὔτε τῆς καθ' ἕκαστον
σῶμα θεραπείας ἀκριβῶς στοχάσεται καὶ τῆς ἀποτυχίας οὐχ εὑρήσει τὴν αἰτίαν. ὥστε οὐδὲ τῆς ἐπὶ τὸ
βέλτιον εὐπορήσει μεταβολῆς, ὁπόταν ἀποτυγχάνῃ
τὰ διὰ τῆς ἐμπειρίας αὐτῷ προεγνωσμένα. τοῦτο μὲν
δὴ καθόλου περὶ τῶν φαρμάκων εἴρηταί μοι τῶν
κολλητικῶν· ἑξῆς δ' ἄλλη τις μέθοδος εἰς τὴν σκευ-
196K   ασίαν τε καὶ | τὴν σύνθεσιν αὐτῶν διαφέρουσα προσ-
έρχεται· τοῖς μὲν γὰρ κοίλοις ἕλκεσιν ὃ βουλόμεθα
προσφέρομεν εὐθύς, εἴτ' οὖν ξηρὸν εἴθ' ὑγρὸν φάρ-
μακον· ἐγχωρεῖ γὰρ ἐπιπάττειν ἢ ἐμπλάττειν αὐτὰ
παντὶ μορίῳ τοῦ ἕλκους· ἐπὶ δὲ τῶν ἄχρι βάθους
ἱκανοῦ γεγενημένων τραυμάτων, ἐπειδὰν ἅπαξ συν-
αγάγωμεν τὰ χείλη, ψαῦσαι τῶν ἐν τῷ βάθει διῃρη-
μένων οὐκ ἐγχωρεῖ. χρὴ τοίνυν οὐχ ἁπλῶς εἰ ξηραν-

of the body—if it is soft and flabby, or hard, dry and contracted. First, to the degree that it is moister, so also it will require the drying medications less. Second, to the degree that it is drier, so it will again now require stronger drying medications and astringent medications more. At all events, the Empiric, I think, will here also call to mind children and women, and those with soft flesh, contrasting these with young men, farmers and people who earn their living from the sea. It is not because of the moistness of the *krasis* in children and women that he has seen such medications as highly regarded, nor again is it because of the dryness that he is able to recognize others suitable for reapers and sailors. Nor will he make an accurate estimation of the treatment in relation to each body, or discover the cause of failure, so that he will not procure change for the better whenever he fails with those things previously known by him through experience. I stated this in general terms regarding the conglutinating medications. Next, some other method comes to the fore, which pertains to the preparation and composition of these medications. For we immediately apply what we wish to hollow wounds, whether this is a dry or moist medication. It is possible to sprinkle or smear these on every part of the wound. In the case of wounds that have reached a considerable depth, as soon as we first bring the margins together, it is not possible to contact those things that are separated in the depths. Accordingly, we must not simply consider whether the

196K

τικόν ἐστι καὶ αὐστηρὸν μετρίως τὸ φάρμακον, ἀλλ᾽ εἰ
καὶ μέχρι τοῦ βάθους ἐξικνεῖσθαι δυνατὸν ἐπισκοπεῖ-
σθαι. ψιμμύθιον γοῦν καὶ λιθάργυρος στύφει καὶ
ξηραίνει μετρίως· ἀλλ᾽ ἐὰν ἐπιπάσσῃς αὐτὰ δίκην
τέφρας ἐν κύκλῳ τοῦ τετρωμένου, πλέον οὐδὲν ἀνύ-
σεις· οὐ γὰρ διϊκνεῖται τῶν οὕτω ξηρῶν φαρμάκων εἰς
τὸ βάθος ἡ δύναμις. ὑγρότητος οὖν αὐτοῖς δεήσει
τινός, ἵν᾽ ὁποῖόν τι τῶν ἐμπλαστικῶν φαρμάκων, ἢ καὶ
τῶν ὑγροτέρων τι γένηται. τοῦτο μὲν οὖν τῆς περὶ
συνθέσεως φαρμάκων πραγματείας ἐστὶν ἴδιον, οὐκ
αὐτῆς τῆς θεραπευτικῆς μεθόδου· καὶ εἰ δόξαιμεν
αὐτοῦ δεῖσθαί τε πρὸς τὰ παρόντα, κἂν ἐπὶ προήκοντι
τῷ λόγῳ μνημονεύσαιμεν. |

5. Ἐπὶ δὲ τὸ τῆς οὐλῆς δεόμενον ἕλκος ἐπάνειμι,
περὶ οὗ μικρὸν ἔμπροσθεν ἔλεγον ὡς ὁ πρῶτος μὲν
εἴη καὶ τούτου σκοπὸς ἐκ τούτου γένους τοῦ κοίλου.
γεννῆσαι γὰρ χρή τι τῶν ἀπολωλότων, οὐχ ἁπλῶς
ἑνῶσαι τὰ διεστηκότα· τρόπον δ᾽ ἕτερον ἐπὶ τούτου
γεννᾶται τὸ λεῖπον ἢ ὂν ἐπὶ τοῦ κοίλου. ἐν ἐκείνῳ μὲν
γὰρ τὸ αἷμα, τούτῳ δ᾽ ἡ σὰρξ ὕλη. πληροῦται μὲν οὖν
τὸ κοῖλον ὑπὸ τῆς γεννωμένης σαρκός, τὴν γένεσιν ἐκ
τοῦ αἵματος ἐχούσης· εἰς οὐλὴν δὲ ἀφικνεῖται τὸ ἤδη
πεπληρωμένον ὑπὸ τοῦ γεννωμένου δέρματος, ἐκ τῆς
ὑποβεβλημένης σαρκὸς τὴν γένεσιν ἔχοντος· ἀλλὰ
σὰρξ μὲν ἡ αὐτὴ τῷ εἴδει τῇ διεφθαρμένῃ δύναται
γεννηθῆναι κατὰ τὸ κοῖλον ἕλκος· δέρμα δ᾽ οὐκ ἐνδέχεται γεννηθῆναι τοιοῦτον ἀκριβῶς οἷον ἦν τὸ

medication is moderately drying and constricting, but also whether it is able to reach to the depths. At any rate, white lead and litharge[12] constrict and dry moderately but, if you sprinkle these like ashes around the part that has been wounded, you will accomplish nothing more, for the potency of the medications that dry like this does not reach to the depths. They will need some moisture so that it may be one of the emplastic medications of the moister kind. This, however, is proper to the matter of the synthesis of medications and not to the matter of the therapeutic method itself. And if we should decide that we need this for our present purposes, we may call it to mind as the discussion proceeds.

5. I shall return to the wound that stands in need of a   197K
scar, which I spoke of a little earlier as having its first indicator from this class of hollowness. For it is necessary to generate something of what has perished and not simply unite what has separated. However, what is lacking is in this instance regenerated in another way than in the case of a hollow wound, because the material in that is blood whereas in this it is flesh. The cavity, then, is filled by the regenerated flesh which has its origin from the blood. What has already been filled comes to a scar through the generated skin which has its origin from the underlying flesh. But flesh that is the same in kind to that which has been destroyed can be regenerated in the hollow ulcer, whereas it is not possible for generated skin to be exactly of

12 See Dioscorides, V.103 and V.102 respectively, for the preparation and use of these medications. Also see Galen, *De compositione medicamentorum per genera*, XIII.407K ff. on cerussa (white lead) and XIII.394K ff. on litharge.

διεφθαρμένον, ἀλλ' ὅμοιον μέν τι δέρματι καὶ τὴν
χρείαν αὐτοῦ δυνάμενον ἀποπληροῦν, οὐ μὴν ἀκριβὲς
δέρμα. διὰ τί μὲν οὖν οὐχ οἷόν τ' ἐστὶν ἡμῖν γεννῆσαι
δέρμα τὸ ἅπαξ ἀπολλύμενον, ὥσπερ σάρκα καὶ πι-
μελὴν γεννῶμεν, ἐκ τῶν φυσικῶν ἐστι προβλημάτων·

ὅπως δ' ἄν τις μιμήσαιτο καὶ φύσιν καὶ χρείαν δέρ-
198K ματος, | ἐκ τῆς νῦν ἐνεστώσης πραγματείας, ἧς τὴν
μέθοδον ἤδη λέγομεν. ἐπειδὴ πρόκειται σκεπάσαι τὴν
σάρκα συμφύτῳ τινὶ σκεπάσματι, τοῦτο γάρ ἐστι τὸ
εἰς οὐλὴν ἀγαγεῖν τὸ ἕλκος, ἤτοι δέρμα γεννητέον
ἡμῖν ἐστιν, ἢ τῆς σαρκὸς τὸ ἐπιπολῆς δέρματι παρα-
πλήσιον ἐργαστέον· ἀλλ' οὐκ ἐγχωρεῖ γεννῆσαι δέρμα, τὸ λοιπὸν ἄρα πειρατέον ἐργάζεσθαι. τίς οὖν ὁ
τρόπος τῆς ἐργασίας; ἡ ἀλλοίωσις δηλονότι· σαρκὸς
γάρ τι μόριον οὐκέτι σάρκα μένειν, ἀλλ' οἷον δέρμα
γενέσθαι βουλόμεθα· πῶς οὖν ἀλλοιωθήσεται; κατά
τινα τῶν ἀλλοιουσῶν δηλονότι ποιοτήτων· ἥκει γὰρ
αὖθις ἐνταῦθα, κἂν μὴ θέλωμεν, ὁ περὶ τῶν στοιχείων
λόγος, οὗ χωρὶς οὐδὲ ἐπουλωτικὸν ἔστιν εὑρεῖν
φάρμακον, οὐ μόνον σαρκωτικὸν ἢ κολλητικόν. ἐπεὶ
τοίνυν τὸ δέρμα τῆς σαρκὸς ξηρότερόν ἐστι καὶ
πυκνότερον, εἰ ξηραίνοιμεν καὶ στύφοιμεν τὴν σάρκα,
δέρματι παραπλησίαν ἐργασόμεθα. τὸ μὲν κεφάλαιον
ἔχεις ἤδη τῶν ἐπουλωτικῶν φαρμάκων, ἀλλ' οὐκ ἀρκεῖ
τοῦτο· καὶ γὰρ τὰ κολλητικὰ ξηραίνοντά τε ἦν καὶ
199K στύφοντα. ὅπῃ | ποτ' οὖν διοίσει ταῦτ' ἐκείνων, εἰς
αὐτὴν ἀποβλέπων τὴν οὐσίαν τῶν πραγμάτων ἐξευρήσεις. ἐπειδὴ γὰρ ἐν μὲν ταῖς κολλήσεσι τῶν ἡλκω-

the kind that was destroyed, although it is somewhat like
skin and is able to fulfill the use of skin despite not exactly
being skin. And this is why it is not possible for us to regenerate the skin that has been completely lost in the way we
regenerate flesh and fat, since it is derived from the [class
of] natural barriers.

How someone might imitate the nature and use of skin
is now the matter in question. I speak now about the   198K
method of this. Since what lies before us is to cover the
flesh with some united covering membrane, for this is to
bring the wound to a scar, we must either regenerate skin
or create a surface on top of the flesh resembling skin. But
as it is not possible to regenerate skin, what remains is that
we must attempt to make [such a surface]. What, then, is
the way of doing this? It is change, obviously. For we wish
some part of the flesh to remain flesh no longer but to become skin, as it were. How will it be changed? Clearly it
will be in relation to some of its changing qualities. For
here again there arises, even if we do not wish it to, the discussion about the elements, without which there is no discovery of a cicatrizing medication, much less one which is
enfleshing or conglutinating. Since skin is drier and thicker
than flesh, if we dry and contract the flesh, we will make it
like skin. You already have the chief point of the cicatrizing
medications, but this is not enough. The conglutinating
medications are also drying and contracting. You will dis-   199K
cover the way in which these medications will somehow
differ from those by directing your attention to the actual
substance of the matter. For since, in the conglutination of

μένων ξηραίνεσθαι χρὴ τὸ ἐπιρρέον, ὡς ἀπέριττον
μένειν τὸ πεπονθὸς μέρος, ἐν δὲ ταῖς ἐπουλώσεσιν οὐ
μόνον τὸ ἐπιρρέον, ἀλλὰ καὶ τὸ περιεχόμενον ἐν ταῖς
σαρξὶν ὑγρὸν ἐκδαπανᾶσθαι προσήκει, πολὺ δήπου
ξηρότερον εἶναι χρὴ τὸ συνουλωτικὸν φάρμακον τοῦ
κολλητικοῦ· τῷ μὲν γὰρ κολλήσοντι, σκοπὸς εἷς οὗτος
μόνος ἐκδαπανῆσαι τὸ περιττὸν τοῦ κατὰ φύσιν, τῷ δὲ
οὐ τοῦτο μόνον, ἀλλὰ καὶ αὐτοῦ τοῦ κατὰ φύσιν
ἅψασθαι· κηκὶς οὖν ὀμφακῖτις ἐνταῦθα καὶ τὰ τῆς
ῥοιᾶς λέμματα καὶ τῆς Αἰγυπτίας ἀκάνθας ὁ καρπός,
μετρίως ξηραίνοντα φάρμακα· χαλκῖτις δὲ καὶ χαλκὸς
κεκαυμένος καὶ λεπὶς χαλκοῦ καὶ μίσυ καὶ στυπτηρία
σχιστὴ πολὺ τούτων σφοδρότερα· μίσυ μὲν καὶ χαλκῖτις μάλιστα, μετριώτερον δ' ἡ λεπὶς τοῦ χαλκοῦ· καὶ
τούτου μετριώτερον ὁ κεκαυμένος χαλκός, εἰ δὲ καὶ
πλύναις αὐτόν, τὸ ἀδηκτότατον ἕξεις φάρμακον. ἔστι
δὲ καὶ τοῦτο ἤδη τῆς περὶ φαρμάκων συνθέσεως πρα-
200K γματείας, | ἑπομένης τῇ θεραπευτικῇ μεθόδῳ. τὸ μὲν
γὰρ τὰς δυνάμεις τῶν φαρμάκων γνῶναι προηγεῖται
τῆς θεραπευτικῆς μεθόδου· καὶ λέλεκται περὶ αὐτῶν
ἑτέρωθι· τὸ δὲ συνθεῖναι τὰ φάρμακα μετὰ τὴν θερα-
πευτικήν ἐστι μέθοδον. ὅταν γὰρ αὕτη μὲν διδάξῃ τὰ

13 Peter English lists the agents as follows: unripe Oake-
apples, Rinde-pile, fruit of Egyptian thorn, Red Vitriol, burnt
Brasse, Offall of Brasse and Vitriol. References to Dioscorides are
as follows: oak gall, I.146; rind of pomegranate, I.153; various
kinds of Akantha, III.14–20; chalcitis, V.115; burned copper, V.87;
scales of copper, V.89; *misu*, V.117; alum, V.123.

wounds, it is necessary to dry up the inward flow, so it is necessary for the affected part to remain without superfluity. In those wounds being cicatrized, it is appropriate to consume not only the flow but also the surrounding moisture in the flesh, so the cicatrizing medication must of course be very much more drying than the conglutinating medication, because in what will conglutinate there is this one objective alone, which is to consume what is in excess of normal, whereas in the other case (i.e. cicatrizing) there is not only this objective, but also that of binding what is normal. Thus here, unripe oak gall, the rind of pomegranate and the fruit of the Egyptian thorn are moderately drying medications. Chalcitis, burned copper, scales of copper, *misu* and divided alum are very much stronger than these, especially *misu* and chalcitis, whereas scales of copper are more moderate and burned copper more moderate than this, and if you wash it, you will have the least mordant medication.[13] This now pertains to the matter of the compounding of medications that is subsequent to the therapeutic method. Knowledge of the potencies of the medications precedes the therapeutic method and I have written about these elsewhere.[14] The compounding of medications, however, comes after the therapeutic method. For whenever this instructs generally—I speak of

200K

[14] The treatises on medications are repeatedly referred to throughout this work. The main ones are *De simplicium medicamentorum temperamentis et facultatibus*, XI.379–892K and XII.1–377K; *De compositione medicamentorum secundum locus*, XII.378–1007K and XIII.1–361K; and *De compositione medicamentorum per genera*, XIII.362–1058K. It is presumably the order of study of these works that is being spoken of here.

καθόλου, λέγω δὲ τὸ ξηραίνειν ἢ ὑγραίνειν, ἢ ψύχειν ἢ
θερμαίνειν, καὶ ἤτοι μετρίως τοῦτο δρᾶν, ἢ σφοδρῶς,
ἢ ἀμυδρῶς, εἰδῶμεν δὲ καὶ τὴν τῶν ἁπλῶν φαρμάκων
ἑκάστου δύναμιν ἰδίᾳ καθ᾽ ἑαυτὴν ἐπεσκεμμένοι, τηνικαῦτα πῶς ἄν τις ταῦτα μίξειεν ἐπιτηδείως τῇ χρείᾳ
προσήκει σκέπτεσθαι· γίνεται γοῦν οὕτως διττή τις ἡ
περὶ τῶν φαρμάκων μέθοδος· ἑτέρα μὲν ἡ τῆς δυνάμεως αὐτῶν, ἑτέρα δὲ ἡ τῆς συνθέσεώς τε καὶ σκευ-
ασίας. ἀλλὰ γὰρ ἐπὶ τὸ λεῖπον ἔτι τῆς περὶ τῶν ἑλκῶν
ἀπιέναι χρὴ μεθόδου.

6. Λείπει δ᾽, ὡς οἶμαι, τὸ περὶ τῶν ὑπεραυξανο-
μένων σαρκῶν εἰπεῖν, ὃ δὴ καὶ ὑπερσάρκωσιν ὀνομάζουσιν οἱ πλείους τῶν ἰατρῶν. ἔστι δὲ καὶ τοῦτο
νόσημα τοῦ γένους τοῦ παρὰ τὸ ποσόν, ἢ τὸ πηλίκον
201K τῶν μορίων· | ἐξέστω γὰρ ὡς ἂν ἐθέλοις ὀνομάζειν· ἐκ
ταὐτοῦ δὲ γένους καὶ ἡ κοιλότης ἦν, ὑπὲρ ἧς προ-
ειρήκαμεν. ὡς οὖν ὃ καλοῦσιν ἕλκος κοῖλον οὐχ ἕν
ἐστι πάθος, ἀλλὰ κοιλότης τε ἅμα καὶ ἕλκος, οὕτως
ἕλκος ὑπερσαρκοῦν οὐχ ἕν ἐστι πάθος, ἀλλ᾽ ὑπερ-
σάρκωσίς τε ἅμα καὶ ἕλκος, ἐνδείκνυται δὲ τὸ τῷ
μεγέθει παρὰ φύσιν τὴν πρώτην ἔνδειξιν, ἣν δὴ καὶ
σκοπὸν τῆς τῶν ἰαμάτων εὑρέσεως ἐλέγομεν εἶναι, τοῦ
πλεονάζοντος τὴν ἀφαίρεσιν· ὑπὸ φαρμάκων δ᾽ αὕτη
γίνεται μόνον, οὐκέθ᾽ ὑπὸ φύσεως, ἀνάπαλιν ἢ ὡς ἐπὶ
σαρκώσεως καὶ κολλήσεως εἶχεν· ἐκεῖνα μὲν γὰρ τῆς
φύσεως αὐτῆς ἐστιν ἔργα, τῶν φαρμάκων τὰ διακω-
λύοντα τὰς ἐνεργείας αὐτῆς ἐκκοπτόντων· ἡ δὲ τῶν
ὑπεραυξηθεισῶν σαρκῶν καθαίρεσις οὐδὲν μὲν τῆς

drying, moistening, cooling, or heating and doing this either moderately, strongly, or weakly—we also know the potency of each of the simple medications since we have given consideration to this specifically. And then we consider in what circumstances it is appropriate for someone to mix these so they are suitable for use. At any rate, in this way there is a twofold method regarding medications. One pertains to their potency and the other to their synthesis and preparation. But we must return to what still remains of the method regarding wounds and ulcers.

6. What does remain, I think, is to speak about the increased growth of flesh which the majority of doctors also call overgrowth of flesh (exuberant flesh). This too is a disease from the class that relates to the size or magnitude of the parts, for let it be permissible to name it as you might wish. And a cavity (hollowness), about which I have spoken previously, is also from this same class. Therefore, as what people call a hollow wound is not one single affection but hollowness and a wound simultaneously, in the same way, a wound with excess flesh is not one single affection but an overgrowth of flesh and a wound simultaneously. And the wound, by its unnatural size, displays its primary indication, which I also said is the indicator of the discovery of cures; that is, the removal of what is excessive. This only occurs through medications and no longer through the agency of Nature, contrary to what obtains in the growth of flesh and the conglutination of wounds, for those are actions of Nature itself, medications eradicating those things that impede its (i.e. Nature's) functions. The reduction of the overgrowth of flesh is not an action of Nature; it occurs

201K

φύσεώς ἐστιν ἔργον, ὑπὸ δὲ τῶν ἰσχυρῶς ξηραινόντων
γίνεται φαρμάκων. παράκειται δὲ ταῦτα τὰ φάρμακα
τοῖς τε ῥύπτουσιν ἰσχυρῶς καὶ τοῖς ἐπουλοῦσιν, ὡς
πολλοὺς διαμαρτάνοντας ἐνίοτε τὸ καθαιρετικὸν φάρ-
202K μακον ἢ ὡς ῥύπου καθαρτικόν, ἢ ὡς | εἰς οὐλὴν ἄγον
παραλαμβάνειν· οἷον αὐτίκα τὸ μίσυ καὶ ἡ χαλκῖτις εἰ
ὑγρᾷ φύσει προσάγοιτο, τῶν καθαιρόντων μᾶλλον ἢ
τῶν ἐπουλούντων ἐστίν· ὅθεν εἴ ποτε τοιούτοις ἀναγ-
κασθείημεν χρῆσθαι πρὸς ἐπούλωσιν, ἑτέρων δηλονότι μὴ παρόντων, ὡς ἐλαχίστοις αὐτοῖς χρησόμεθα,
μόνον τὸν πυρῆνα τῆς μήλης καθιέντες εἰς ἄκρον
λελειωμένα τὰ φάρμακα· κἄπειθ᾽ οὕτως οἷον χνοῦν
τινα τοῖς τῆς ἐπουλώσεως δεομένοις ἐπιβάλλομεν
μορίοις. εἰ δὲ καὶ καθαιρεῖν βουλοίμεθα τὰ ὑπερ-
έχοντα, δαψιλέστερον ἐπιθήσομεν. ἰὸς δὲ τούτων ἐστὶ
καθαιρετικώτερος, ὡς ὅλως ἐκπεπτωκέναι τοῦ γένους
τῶν ἐπουλούντων· εἰ δὲ καὶ καύσειας αὐτά, δριμύτερα
μὲν ἧττον, ἐπουλωτικώτερα δὲ ποιήσεις. εἰ δὲ καὶ
πλύναις, ἠπιώτερα.

μέμνησαι δὲ δήπου καὶ σὺ τὸν ἄνευ λογισμοῦ
θεραπεύοντά ποτε τὸ ῥυπαρὸν ἕλκος, τῷ συνήθει φαρμάκῳ τῷ χλωρῷ, μιγνύντα μὲν αὐτῷ τὸ μέλι, πολλαῖς
δὲ ἐφεξῆς ἡμέραις εὑρίσκοντα ῥυπαρὸν ὁμοίως· εἶτ᾽
ἀπορούμενόν τε καὶ ὅπη μεταβῇ μὴ γινώσκοντα· συν-
203K έβαινε | γὰρ οὐ καθαίρεσθαι μόνον τὸν ῥύπον, ἀλλὰ
καὶ συγκαθαιρεῖσθαί τι καὶ συντήκεσθαι τῆς ὑποκειμένης σαρκός, ἰσχυροτέρου τοῦ φαρμάκου τῆς τοῦ
κάμνοντος ὑπάρχοντος φύσεως. εἶθ᾽ ὁ μὲν ἰατρὸς ἀεὶ

through medications that are strongly drying. These medications are closely connected with those that cleanse vigorously and cause cicatrization, so that many err at times with respect to the reducing medication, taking it to be one that cleanses the filth or leads to a scar. For example, *misu* and chalcitis, if you apply them to a moist nature, are more of the reducing than the scar-inducing sort. Whence, if at some time we are compelled to use such things for the purpose of scar production (other things presumably not being to hand), we use them very sparingly, sending down the head of the probe only, after triturating the medications to an extreme degree. And then, in like manner, we apply a powder alone to the parts that are in need of cicatrization. If, however, we also wish to remove excess [flesh], we will apply it more abundantly. Verdigris is more reducing than these so that it altogether stands out among the class of cicatrizing agents.[15] And if you burn those so they are less sharp, you will make them more cicatrizing. If you also wash them, you will make them more soothing.

202K

Presumably you remember, too, the person who was once, without any reasoning, treating a filthy wound with the customary green medication, having mixed honey with it, and who discovered after many days in succession that it was just as filthy. Then he was bereft of ideas and did not know which way to turn, for what happens is that not only is the filth removed, but also something of the underlying flesh is removed with it, and is dissolved when the medication is stronger than the nature of the patient. Then the doctor is always in the habit of mixing more of the honey

203K

---

[15] Dioscorides describes the preparation and use of two types of verdigris; see V.91 and V.92.

πλέον ἀνεμίγνυε τῷ φαρμάκῳ τοῦ μέλιτος, ἵνα δὴ
σφοδρότερον καθήρειεν, ὡς ἐλλιπῶς τοῦ προτέρου
τοῦτο δράσαντος. ἐγίγνετο δὲ πᾶν τοὐναντίον· εἰς
ὅσον γὰρ ἐπετείνετο τῇ δριμύτητι τὸ προσφερόμενον,
εἰς τοσοῦτον συνετήκετο μὲν ἡ ὑποκειμένη σάρξ, ὁ δὲ
τῆς συντήξεως ῥύπος εὑρισκόμενος ἐπὶ τοῦ ἕλκους
ἐξηπάτα τὸν ἰατρόν, ὡς οὐδὲν ἀνύοντος τοῦ φαρμάκου.
τούτου μὲν δὴ περὶ τὴν διάγνωσιν, οὐ μόνον περὶ τὴν
θεραπευτικὴν μέθοδον ἡ ἄγνοια· καὶ γὰρ μάλιστα καὶ
ῥυπαρὸν καὶ ὑγρὸν ὁμοίως φαίνεται τὸ ἕλκος ἐπ᾽
ἀμφοτέρων τῶν φαρμάκων, ἀλλά τοι κοιλότερον μὲν
ἐπὶ τῶν ἰσχυρῶν τε καὶ συντηκόντων γίγνεται· καὶ
προσέτι τοῖς χείλεσιν ὀχθῶδες, ἐρυθρόν τε καὶ ὑπο-
φλεγμαῖνον, ἔστιν ὅτε δὲ καὶ δάκνεται σαφῶς ὁ ἄνθρωπος ὑπὸ τοῦ τοιούτου φαρμάκου·

204K   τὸ δ᾽ ἧττον ἢ | προσήκει ξηραῖνον οὔτε δῆξιν οὔτε
τῶν ἄλλων οὐδὲν ὧν εἶπον ἐργάζεται. δῆλον δ᾽, οἶμαι,
κἀπὶ τούτων ἐστὶν ὡς ὁ μὲν Ἐμπειρικός, εἰ καὶ ὅτι
μάλιστα διωρισμένῃ χρήσαιτο τῇ πείρᾳ, τό γε μεταβαίνειν ἐπὶ τὸ προσῆκον εὐμηχάνως οὐκ ἔχει. μόνῳ δ᾽
ὑπάρχει τοῦτο τῷ κατὰ μέθοδον ἰατρεύοντι, τὴν ὄντως
δηλονότι μέθοδον, ἣν ἐγὼ νῦν διέρχομαι.

7. Τὴν γὰρ τῶν ἀμεθόδων Θεσσαλείων μέθοδον
ὄνομα μόνον οἶσθα δήπου κενόν, ἔρημον ἔργου παν-
τός· οἵ γε τοσαύτης τε καὶ τηλικαύτης οὔσης μεθόδου
περὶ τὴν τῶν ἑλκῶν ἴασιν οὔτε τοῖς τῶν Ἐμπειρικῶν
ἐχρήσαντο διορισμοῖς εἰς τὴν τῶν φαρμάκων εὕρεσιν
οὔτ᾽ ἀπὸ τῆς φύσεως αὐτῆς τῶν πραγμάτων ἔλαβον

with the medication, so that it actually purifies more strongly, just as it purified deficiently when he did this previously. Everything that is contrary occurs because, to the extent that the application was increased in its sharpness, so to this degree the underlying flesh was dissolved, the revealed filth of the colliquescence in the wound deceiving the doctor [into thinking] that the medication accomplished nothing. The ignorance of this relates to the diagnosis and not only to the therapeutic method. And especially also, the wound or ulcer appears to an equal degree filthy and moist in the case of both medications, but becomes more hollow in the case of those that are strong and liquefying. And it is raised at the margins as well, and red, and somewhat inflamed, and sometimes also the person clearly feels the bite of such a medication.

It is appropriate that the medication dries less and does not cause biting nor any of the other things I spoke of. It is, I think, clear in relation to these things that the Empiric, even if he uses experience that reflects particular discrimination, is not in fact skillful in changing to what is appropriate. This is [still] reserved only for the man who heals by the method that is obviously the true method, and the one I am now going over. 204K

7. You know, I presume, that the method of the amethodical Thessaleians is just an empty name devoid of all function. In fact, although there was such a great and substantial method for the cure of wounds, those people did not use the distinctions of the Empirics for the discovery of medications, nor did they take up the indication from

τὴν ἔνδειξιν, ὡς οἱ Δογματικοί· μόνον δ᾽ εἰπόντες ὃ καὶ
τοῖς ἰδιώταις γνωρίζεται, τὸ δεῖσθαι τὸ μὲν κοῖλον
ἕλκος πληρώσεως, τὸ δὲ πλῆρες ἐπουλώσεως, τὸ δ᾽
ὑπερσαρκοῦν καθαιρέσεως, καὶ τὸ μὲν ῥυπαρὸν καθάρσεως, τὸ δὲ καθαρὸν ἐπουλώσεως, τὸ δὲ ἔναιμον καὶ
κολλήσεως, ἑλκῶν θεραπείας οἴονταί τινα μέθοδον
εἰρηκέναι· τοσοῦτον ἀποδέουσι γιγνώσκειν ὡς ταῖς
205K μὲν ὑγροτέραις | φύσεσι τῶν ἧττον ξηραινόντων φαρ-
μάκων ἐστὶ χρεία, ταῖς δὲ ξηροτέραις τῶν μᾶλλον. ὃ
τοίνυν παρ᾽ ὅλον τὸν λόγον ἐφάνη σαφῶς αὖθις ἀνα-
ληπτέον· ἵν᾽ ἡμεῖς τε μάλιστα προσέχωμεν αὐτῷ τὸν
νοῦν, οἵ τ᾽ ἄλλοι πάντες οἱ τὴν παλαιὰν μέθοδον δια-
φθείροντες ἐναργέστερον γνῶσιν ὅσον ἁμαρτάνουσιν.

ἄρξομαι δ᾽ ἀπὸ τῶν σαρκώσεως δεομένων ἑλκῶν,
ἕν τι τοῦτο παράδειγμα προχειρισάμενος, ἐπειδὴ καὶ
φθάνω τὸν λόγον ὑπὲρ αὐτοῦ πεποιημένος. εἶθ᾽ ἑξῆς
περὶ πάσης ὁμοῦ τῆς ἰάσεως ἐν τῷ καθόλου ποιήσομαι τὸν λόγον. ἐφάνη τοίνυν οὐ τῷ λόγῳ μόνον,
ἀλλὰ καὶ τῇ πείρᾳ σκοπουμένοις, οὐ τῶν αὐτῶν
ἅπασα φύσις δεομένη φαρμάκων, ἀλλ᾽ αἱ μὲν ἀσθε-
νέστεραι καὶ μαλακώτεραι τῶν μαλακωτέρων, αἱ δ᾽
ἰσχυρότεραι καὶ ξηρότεραι τῶν ἰσχυροτέρων. οὕτω δὲ
κἀπὶ τῶν εἰς οὐλὴν ἀγομένων ἑλκῶν εἶχε καὶ προσέτι
τῶν κολλήσεως δεομένων. ἁπλῶς γὰρ οὐδὲν τῶν ἰσχυρῶν φαρμάκων αἱ μαλακαὶ φέρουσι φύσεις. ἐν δὲ τῇ
διεξόδῳ ταύτῃ τοῦ λόγου κατάφορον γίγνεται σαφῶς
ὅτι τε τὴν φύσιν ἐπισκεπτέον ἐστὶ τοῦ κάμνοντος, ὅτι
206K τε καθ᾽ ἕκαστον ἄνθρωπον | ἰδίᾳ τίς ἐστι θεραπεία·

312

the actual nature of the matters as the Dogmatics did. After simply stating what was known even by laymen— namely, that a hollow wound or ulcer needs to be filled, one that is filled needs to be scarred over, one that has an excess of flesh needs to be reduced, one that is filthy needs to be cleaned, one that is clean needs to be scarred over and one that is blood-filled (recent) needs to be conglutinated—they think they have stated a method of treatment for wounds: that's how far they fall short of knowing that the need for drying medications is less in more moist natures but more in those that are drier. Accordingly, we must again take up what was clearly apparent throughout the whole discussion so that we direct our attention particularly to this, and so that all those others who corrupt the age-old method may know more clearly how much they are mistaken.

205K

I shall begin with the wounds that require enfleshing, choosing this as one example, since I have also previously made the discussion about this. Then next, I shall make the discussion about every common cure in general. Thus, it seemed to those considering [the matter] not by reason alone, but also by experience, that not every nature requires the same medications; those that are weaker and softer need softer medications and those that are stronger and drier need stronger medications. Along the same lines, in wounds being brought to cicatrization, there is in addition a need for conglutination. For soft natures simply tolerate none of the strong medications. In the course of the same discussion it becomes clearly apparent that it is the nature of the patient we must consider because the treat-

206K

καὶ τρίτον ἐπὶ τούτοις ὡς ἐπειδὴ τὸ τῆς ἑκάστου
φύσεως ἴδιον ἄρρητόν ἐστι καὶ πρὸς τὴν ἀκριβεστά-
την ἐπιστήμην ἄληπτον, οὗτος ἂν ἄριστος ἰατρὸς εἴη
τῶν κατὰ μέρος ἁπάντων νοσημάτων, ὁ μέθοδόν τινα
πορισάμενος ἐξ ἧς διαγνωστικὸς μὲν τῶν φύσεων
ἔσοιτο, στοχαστικὸς δὲ τῶν ἑκάστης ἰδίων ἰαμάτων.

τὸ δ᾽ οἴεσθαι κοινήν τινα ἁπάντων ἀνθρώπων εἶναι
θεραπείαν ἐσχάτως ἠλιθιόν ἐστιν· ὅπερ οἱ ἀναισθη-
τότατοι νομίζουσι Μεθοδικοί. καὶ διὰ ταῦθ᾽ ἑστάναι
τὰ τῆς ἰατρικῆς ἔφασαν ἅπαντα θεωρήματα, τουτέστιν ἐπιστημονικὰ καὶ βέβαια ταῖς γνώσεσιν ὑπάρχειν. εἶναί τε τὴν γνῶσιν αὐτῶν τέχνην τινὰ κοινοτήτων, οὐκ ἰδιοτήτων, ὡσπερεὶ τὸν κοινὸν καὶ γενικὸν
ἄνθρωπον θεραπεύοντες, οὐ τοὺς κατὰ μέρος. ὡς οὖν
ἐν τοῖς ἄλλοις ἅπασιν εὐθέως κατὰ τὰς ἀρχὰς ἐσφάλησαν, οὕτω κἀν τῷδε· θεραπεύεται μὲν γὰρ οὐχ ὁ
κοινὸς καὶ γενικὸς ἄνθρωπος, ἀλλ᾽ ἡμῶν ἕκαστος,
ἄλλος ἄλλην ἔχων δηλονότι κρᾶσίν τε καὶ φύσιν. οἱ δ᾽
207K   οἴονται μίαν θεραπείαν ἁπάντων ἀνθρώπων | εἶναι·
ἐγὼ δ᾽ εἰ καὶ τὴν ἑκάστου φύσιν ἀκριβῶς ἠπιστάμην
ἐξευρίσκειν, οἷον ἐπινοῶ τὸν Ἀσκληπιόν, αὐτὸς ἂν ἦν
τοιοῦτος· ἐπεὶ δ᾽ ἀδύνατον τοῦτο, τὸ γοῦν ἐγγυτάτω
προσιέναι καθόσον ἀνθρώπῳ δυνατὸν αὐτός τε ἀσκεῖν
ἔγνωκα καὶ τοῖς ἄλλοις παρακελεύομαι. πειρῶνται μὲν
οὖν εἰς ὅσον οἷόν τε καὶ οἱ ἀπὸ τῆς ἐμπειρίας, ἀποχωρεῖν μὲν τῶν κοινῶν, προσέρχεσθαι δὲ τοῖς ἰδίοις·
ἀλλ᾽ ὅσον καὶ τούτοις ἐνδεῖ πρὸς τὸ τέλειον εἴρηται
πρόσθεν. οὐ γὰρ ἐπὶ παίδων, ἢ γυναικῶν, ἢ γερόντων,

ment is specific to each person. And third, in addition to these factors, since what is specific to each nature is inexpressible and incomprehensible in terms of very precise knowledge, the person who provides a method on the basis of which he would be a diagnostician of natures and an estimator of the specific cures for each [nature] will be the best doctor for all the individual diseases.

To think there is some common treatment for all people is foolish in the extreme. But this is what the Methodics, men who are absolutely lacking in perception, think. And because of this, they are in the habit of saying that all their theories of medicine stand, that is to say, are scientific and secure in their means of knowing. And they are in the habit of saying that their knowledge is a craft of "communities" and not of specifics, just as if they were treating a "common" and generic person and not a series of individuals. Thus, as they tripped up in all other things right at the beginning, so too did they trip up in this, for it is not the "common" and generic person that is treated but each one of us, having clearly a different *krasis* (temperament) and *physis* (nature). They think, however, there is one treatment for all people, and if I had also known how to discover precisely the nature of each person, like I think Aesculapius did, I would myself be like him. But since this is impossible, I have decided to approach as closely as is possible for a man, and myself, to practice this, and to exhort others [to do so]. The Empirics try as far they can to go away from the common and approach the specific, but I said before how much they fall short of perfection. For it is not that you must separately distinguish children, women,

207K

ἢ μαλακὴν ἐχόντων καὶ λευκὴν τὴν σάρκα καὶ ὅσα
τοιαῦτα, ὡς ἐκεῖνοι ποιοῦσι, προσδιοριστέον ἐστίν,
ἀλλ᾽ ὅπως ὑγρότητος ἢ ξηρότητος ἔχει τὸ σῶμα. τοὺς
μὲν οὖν Ἐμπειρικοὺς ἰατροὺς ἄλλων τε πολλῶν ἕνεκεν
ἀποδέχεσθαι χρὴ καὶ μάλισθ᾽ ὅταν προσέρχεσθαι
πειρῶνται καθόσον ἐγχωρεῖ τῇ τοῦ κάμνοντος
ἰδιότητι. μετὰ γὰρ τοὺς διορισμοὺς ἅπαντας οὓς
διορίζονται, καὶ τὸν ἀπὸ τῶν ἐθῶν ἐπάγουσιν, ὡς
κἀντεῦθεν εὐπορήσαντες οἰκειοτέρων τῷ κάμνοντι
βοηθημάτων. εἰρήσεται δ᾽ ἡμῖν ἐν τοῖς ἑξῆς ἐπὶ |
208K πλέον ὑπὲρ τῶν ἐθῶν, κἀκεῖ ἀποδείξομεν ὑπὲρ τοῦ
γνῶναι τὴν ἰδιότητα τῆς τοῦ κάμνοντος φύσεως, ἐξευ-
ρῆσθαι τοῖς παλαιοῖς καὶ τὸν ἀπὸ τοῦ ἔθους διο-
ρισμόν.

τοῦτον οὖν ἐπὶ τοῖς ἄλλοις οἱ Ἐμπειρικοὶ παρα-
λαμβάνουσι καὶ πρὸς τούτῳ καὶ αὐτὸν τὸν ἰατρόν, εἰ
πολλάκις εἴη παραγεγονὼς τῷ νοσοῦντι, βέλτιον ἂν
ἰᾶσθαί φασι τοῦ μὴ παραγεγονότος· εἶθ᾽ ὅταν ταῦτα
πάντα προσθῶσιν, οὔπω βεβαίαν οὐδ᾽ ἐπιστημονικὴν
ἔχειν φασὶ τῆς ἰδίας τοῦ κάμνοντος ἰάσεως τὴν γνῶσιν. ὁ δ᾽ ἀναισχυντότατος Θεσσαλὸς ἓν μόνον εἰδώς,
ὅτι τὸ κοῖλον ἕλκος πληρωτέον, ἑστῶτά τε καὶ βεβαιά
φησι τὰ τῆς ἰατρικῆς εἶναι θεωρήματα. καίτοι τοῦτό
γε πάντες, ὡς εἴρηται καὶ πρόσθεν, ἄνθρωποι γινώ-
σκουσιν, οὐχ οἱ νῦν μόνον, ἀφ᾽ οὗ Θεσσαλός, ὁ
δεύτερος Ἀσκληπιός, εἰς ἀνθρώπους ἧκεν, ἀλλὰ καὶ οἱ
πρὸ Δευκαλίωνος, οἶμαι, καὶ Φορωνέως, εἴπερ γε
κἀκεῖνοι Λογικοί τε ἦσαν. ἀλλὰ πρὸς τῷ γινώσκειν ὡς

the aged and those having soft, pale flesh and other such things as they do; what you must separately define is how the body is in terms of moistness and dryness. It is necessary for the Empiric doctors to accept [this] because of many other factors, and particularly whenever they attempt to come as far as is possible to what is specific for the patient. After all, in the distinctions they do make, they also bring forward that based on customs, as here too they have recourse to more specific remedies for the patient. In what follows I shall say even more about customs; here I 208K shall offer clarification about knowing what is specific in the nature of the patient, and I shall show that the distinction based on custom was known to the ancients.

The Empirics, then, accept this [distinction] in addition to other matters, and besides this, they also say that the doctor himself, if he is often in attendance on the sick person, would be better able to effect a cure than if he were not in attendance. Then, when they add all these things, they say they still do not have a secure and scientific knowledge of the specific cure of the patient. But the most shameless Thessalus, who knows one thing alone—that you must fill the hollow wound—says his theories of medicine are established and firmly based. And yet all men know this, as I said before, and not only those of the present day, from the time when Thessalus, the second Aesculapius, came among men, but also, I believe, those before Deucalion and Phoroneus, at least if those men were also Dogmatics.[16] But in addition to knowing that the hollow

16 Deucalion and Phoroneus were ancient, semimythical figures; *OCD*, pp. 460 and 1175 respectively. Galen's point is about the ancient awareness of method in medicine.

σαρκωτέον ἐστὶ τὸ κοῖλον ἕλκος, ἔτι κἀκεῖνο συν-
ίεσαν, ὡς ὁ γινώσκων τὰ φάρμακα τὰ σαρκώσοντα
τοιοῦτον ἕλκος, ἐκεῖνος ἰατρός ἐστιν.

209K   εἰ μὲν οὖν ἐξ ἐμπειρίας εὕρηται ταῦτα, | δῆλον ὡς
ἐμπειρικῶς ἡμῖν ἰατρευτέον ἐστίν· εἰ δὲ ἐκ λόγου,
λογικῶς· οὐ γὰρ δὴ ἄλλο μὲν εὕρηκεν, ἄλλῳ δέ τινι
νῦν ἐπιδεξίως χρήσεται. ἀλλὰ περὶ μὲν τούτου πρὸς
τοὺς Ἐμπειρικούς ἐστιν ἡ ἀμφισβήτησίς τις ἡμῖν·
ὅπερ δὲ λέγων ἀπέλιπον, ἡ ὄντως ἰατρικὴ τῆς τοῦ
κάμνοντος ἐστόχασται φύσεως· ὀνομάζουσι δέ, οἶμαι,
τοῦτο πολλοὶ τῶν ἰατρῶν ἰδιοσυγκρασίαν, καὶ πάντες
ἀκατάληπτον ὁμολογοῦσιν ὑπάρχειν· καὶ διὰ τοῦτο
καὶ αὐτὴν τὴν ὄντως ἰατρικὴν Ἀσκληπιῷ καὶ Ἀπόλ-
λωνι παραχωροῦσιν. ἤρτηται δὲ ὁ λόγος οὗτος σύμπας ἀπὸ διττῶν ἀρχῶν· ἀπὸ μὲν τῶν ἐναργῶς φαινομένων τοῖς Ἐμπειρικοῖς τε καὶ Τηρητικοῖς, ἀπὸ δὲ τῶν
στοιχείων τοῖς Λογικοῖς. ὅτι τε γὰρ ἄλλον ἄλλο
φάρμακον ὠφελεῖ σχεδὸν ἤδη καὶ οἱ παῖδες ἐπίσταν-
ται· συμφωνεῖ δὲ τούτῳ καὶ ὁ ἀπὸ τῶν στοιχείων
λογισμός. εἰ γὰρ ὑπόθοιο πεντεκαίδεκα διαφορὰς
εἶναι κατὰ τὸ μᾶλλόν τε καὶ ἧττον ἐν ταῖς κράσεσι
τῶν ἀνθρώπων ἐπὶ μόνης τῆς ὑγρᾶς φύσεως, ἀνάγκη
δήπου σε καὶ τῶν φαρμάκων οἷς μέλλεις χρήσασθαι
πεντεκαίδεκα διαφορὰς ἐπίστασθαι, καὶ τὰς μὲν
210K   μᾶλλον, τὰς δὲ ἧττον ξηραινούσας, ἵν᾽ | ἑκάστῃ φύσει
τὸ προσῆκον ἐξευρίσκῃς. εἰ δὲ καὶ τῆς ξηροτέρας
φύσεως ἄλλας πεντεκαίδεκα διαφορὰς ὑποθέμενος
ὡσαύτως κἀπ᾽ ἐκείνης ἄλλων πεντεκαίδεκα δέοιο φαρ-

wound or ulcer is something you must enflesh—they do still understand that—they realize that the one who knows the medications that are enfleshing in such a wound is the doctor.

Therefore, if these things are discovered through experience, it is clear that he must cure the wound empirically. If, on the other hand, they are discovered by reason, he must cure it rationally. For certainly, if he discovers nothing different, he will now use something else appropriately. But we have some dispute about this with the Empirics. What I omitted to say is that what is truly the art of medicine is to make an estimation of the nature of the patient. I believe many doctors call this "idiosyncrasy" and all agree that it is incomprehensible. Because of this, they leave the true art of medicine to Aesculapius and Apollo. This argument in its entirety has a dependence on two "principles"—that from the things which are clearly apparent to Empirics and "Observers," and that from the elements to the Rationalists. Even children almost know already that different medications are of benefit to different people, while reasoning derived from the elements also agrees with this. For if you were to postulate that there are fifteen differentiae in terms of more or less in the *krasias* (temperaments) of people, in the case of the moist nature alone, it is I presume necessary that you also know fifteen differences of medications which you intend to use, and that some are more drying and some less, so that for each nature you may discover what is appropriate. And if you also postulate fifteen other differentiae of the drier nature, in that nature you will similarly need fifteen other medica-

209K

210K

319

μάκων, ἔσται σοι τὰ πάντα τριάκοντα φάρμακα πρὸς
τριάκοντα φύσεις ἡρμοσμένα, καὶ τούτοις προσηκόντως χρῆσθαι δυνήσεται μόνος ὁ περὶ κράσεως σωμάτων ἀκριβῶς ἐπεσκεμμένος.

ἆρ᾽ οὖν εἰ μὲν ὅλον τὸ σῶμα εἴη ξηρότερον τὴν
κρᾶσιν, ὑπὸ τῶν ξηραντικωτέρων ὠφεληθήσεται φαρμάκων; εἰ δὲ μόριον αὐτοῦ τι τῶν ἄλλων φύσει ξηρότερον ὑπάρχοι, τῶν ἧττον ξηραινόντων δεήσεται; ἢ
πρόδηλον κἀνταῦθα τὸ μὲν ξηρότερον τῇ κράσει μόριον τῶν ξηραντικωτέρων, τὸ δ᾽ ὑγρότερον τῶν ἧττον
ξηραινόντων προσδεῖσθαι; καὶ τοῦτ᾽ οὖν ὅλον παραλέλειπται τοῖς ἀμεθόδοις Θεσσαλείοις, ἓν ἐπὶ παντὸς
μορίου φάρμακον ἡγουμένοις ἁρμόττειν. οἱ δ᾽ ἀπὸ τῆς
Ἐμπειρίας ὅσον πλεονεκτοῦσι κἂν τῷδε τῶν Θεσσαλείων Μεθοδικῶν, τοσοῦτον ἀπολείπονται τῶν ὄντως
μεθοδικῶν τε καὶ λογικῶν. ἔχουσι γὰρ δὴ κἀκεῖνοι
πρὸς τῆς πείρας διδαχθέντες | ἄλλο μὲν τῶν ἐν ὀφθαλ-
μοῖς ἑλκῶν, ἄλλο δὲ τῶν ἐν ὠσίν, ἢ ἄρθροις, ἢ σαρξίν,
ἢ δέρματι μόνῳ φάρμακον. ἀλλ᾽ ὅτι γε κἀνταῦθα
μεταβαίνειν ἐφ᾽ ἕτερον ἀδυνατήσωσιν, ἐκ τῶν ἔμπροσθεν εἰρημένων εὔδηλον.

8. Ἐπεὶ δὲ καὶ περὶ τούτων αὐτάρκως διώρισται,
πάλιν ἐπὶ τὴν ἀρχὴν ἀνέλθωμεν τοῦ λόγου, μιγνύντες
ἁπάσας τὰς συμπιπτούσας ἕλκει διαθέσεις, ἀπὸ πρώτης ἀρξάμενοι τῆς δυσκρασίας. εἰ γὰρ ἤτοι πρόσθεν
εἴη κατὰ δή τινα συντυχίαν, ἢ καὶ παρ᾽ αὐτὸν τῆς
ἑλκώσεως τὸν χρόνον ἡ ἡλκωμένη σὰρξ γένοιτο θερμοτέρα τοῦ δέοντος, ἢ ψυχροτέρα, δεήσει τὸ φάρμακον οὐ μόνον ξηραίνειν μετρίως, ἀλλὰ καὶ θερμαίνειν

211K

tions, so you will have thirty medications in all suitable for thirty natures. Only the person who has made accurate observations of the *krasis* in bodies will be able to use these medications appropriately.

Thus, if the whole body is too dry in terms of *krasis*, will it be benefited by the more drying medications whereas, if some one part of it is more dry in nature than the others, will it need less of those [medications] that are drying? Or is it clear that the part which is more dry in *krasis* needs in addition more of those medications that are drying, whereas the part that is moist needs less of those medications that are drying? All of this has been left aside by the amethodical Thessaleians, who think that one medication is suitable for every part. The Empirics have as much of an advantage over the Thessaleian Methodics in this as they are inferior to those who are truly methodical and rational. Those men, taught as they are by experience, certainly have one medication for wounds in the eyes, another for wounds in the ears, another for wounds in the joints, another for wounds in the flesh, and another for wounds in the skin alone. But the fact that here too they are unable to change to another medication is clear from what has been said previously.

211K

8. However, since I have also established a sufficient distinction regarding these matters, let me return again to the beginning of the argument and bring together all the conditions that befall a wound, beginning from the primary *dyskrasia*. For if it is either before its occurrence or at the actual time of the wounding that the wounded flesh becomes warmer or colder than it should be, it will require a medication that is not only moderately drying, but also

ἢ ψύχειν εἰς τοσοῦτον, εἰς ὅσον ἡ ὑποκειμένη σὰρξ
ἐξέστη τοῦ κατὰ φύσιν· οὐ γὰρ ἐγχωρεῖ σάρκωσιν, ἢ
πλήρωσιν, ἢ κόλλησιν, ἢ ἐπούλωσιν ἕλκους ὀρθῶς
ποτε γενέσθαι τῆς ὑποκειμένης σαρκὸς ἐχούσης κακῶς, οὐδὲ εἰκῆ πρόσθεν ἐλέγομεν ἔργα φύσεως εἶναι
σύμπαντα ταῦτα. κάθαρσιν μέντοι τῶν ῥυπαρῶν καὶ
καθαίρεσιν τῶν ὑπεραυξηθέντων ἐγχωρεῖ γενέσθαι

212K καὶ χωρὶς τοῦ κατὰ φύσιν ἔχειν | τὴν σάρκα· μόνον
γὰρ τῶν φαρμάκων ἦν ἔργα. διὸ καὶ μείζων ἡ πρόνοια
γιγνέσθω σοι τῆς εὐκρασίας τῶν ἡλκωμένων μορίων,
ὁπότε σαρκοῦν ἢ κολλᾶν ἢ ἐπουλοῦν ἐθέλεις αὐτά.
σῴζεσθαι γὰρ δεῖ τὰς κινήσεις τῆς φύσεως αἷς εἵπετο
τῶν εἰρημένων ἕκαστον· οὐ σωθήσονται δ' ἄλλως εἰ
μὴ πάντη κατὰ φύσιν ἔχοι τὸ μόριον. ὥσπερ οὖν εἰ
φλεγμονή τις ἅμα τῷ ἕλκει τύχοι, πρὶν ταύτην λῦσαι,
σαρκοῦν, ἢ κολλᾶν, ἢ ἐπουλοῦν οὐκ ἂν οὐδεὶς ἐπεχείρησεν αὐτό, κατὰ τὸν αὐτόν, οἶμαι, τρόπον εἰ καὶ
χωρὶς φλεγμονῆς εἴη μόνη δυσκρασία τῶν εἰρημένων,
οὐδὲν ἐλπίσομεν γενέσθαι πρὶν ἐκείνην ἰᾶσθαι. πάλιν
οὖν ἐντεῦθεν ἔνδειξίς τις εἰς τὴν τῶν ἔμπροσθεν εἰρημένων φαρμάκων εὕρεσιν γίνεται· ξηραίνοντα μὲν
γὰρ ἦν ἅπαντα, διέφερε δ' ἀλλήλων ἐν τῷ μᾶλλόν τε
καὶ ἧττον. οὐ μὴν ὅπως γε τοῦ θερμαίνειν ἢ ψύχειν
εἶχεν εἴρηταί που πρόσθεν, ἀλλ' ἡ μέθοδός πως ἀναγ-
κάζει καὶ τοῦτ' ἐρευνᾶσθαι. οὐ γὰρ ἁπλῶς εἰ ξηραῖνον,
ἀλλ' εἰ μὴ καὶ σφόδρα θερμαῖνον, ἢ ψῦχον ἐπισκέπτεσθαι χρή.

213K φεύξῃ | τοιγαροῦν ὑοσκύαμον καὶ μανδραγόραν

heating or cooling to the degree that the underlying flesh departs from normal. It is not possible for enfleshing, filling, conglutination or cicatrization of a wound to occur properly at any time when the underlying flesh is bad. Nor was I without purpose when I said before that these are all actions of Nature. Nevertheless, it is also possible for cleansing of what is filthy and removal of what is overgrown to occur apart from there being normal flesh because these are simply actions of the medications. On which account, too, let your prior consideration about the *eukrasia* of the wounded parts be greater when you wish to enflesh, conglutinate, or cicatrize them. It is necessary that the actions of Nature, which each of the things mentioned follow, be preserved. They will not otherwise be preserved unless the part is entirely in accord with nature. Therefore, just as when some inflammation happens together with the wound, nobody would attempt to enflesh, conglutinate or cicatrize before resolving the inflammation, in the same way, I think, if even apart from the inflammation, there should be a mono-*dyskrasia* of those things spoken of, we shall not expect anything to occur before that is cured. Again here a certain indication arises toward the discovery of the previously mentioned medications, because all those that are drying are different from one another in terms of more or less. In fact, not only was how they are heating or cooling spoken of before to some degree, but the method also compels us to search this out in some way. It is not simply necessary to consider whether a medication is drying, but also whether it is strongly heating or cooling as well.

Accordingly, you will avoid henbane, mandrake and

212K

213K

323

καὶ κώνειον, ὡς πέρα τοῦ μετρίου ψύχοντα, καίτοι
ξηραίνει γε εἰς τοσοῦτον, εἰς ὅσον ἕλκος ξηραίνεσθαι
ὀφείλει. καὶ ῥητίνη καὶ πίττα καὶ ἄσφαλτος, εἰ καὶ
ξηραίνει συμμέτρως, ἀλλὰ πέρα γε τοῦ προσήκοντός
ἐστι θερμά· καὶ διὰ τοῦτο οὐκ ἄν τις αὐτοῖς χρήσαιτο
μόνοις ἄνευ τοῦ τοῖς ἀτρέμα ψύχουσιν ἐπιμίξας, ἐν ἐξ
ἁπάντων εὔκρατον ἀπεργάσασθαι φάρμακον. εἰ δὴ
ταῦθ᾿ οὕτως ἔχει, καθάπερ οὖν ἔχει προσεπιβλέπειν
δεήσει καὶ τὴν τοῦ περιέχοντος ἡμᾶς ἀέρος κρᾶσιν·
οἷον γὰρ φάρμακόν τι καὶ οὗτος ἔξωθεν προσπίπτων
τοῖς σώμασιν, ἐπειδὰν ἀμέτρως ἔχῃ θερμότητος ἢ
ψύξεως, ἐμποδὼν ἵσταται τῇ θεραπείᾳ. χρὴ τοίνυν
ἀντιπεπονθέναι τὰ φάρμακα ταῖς ἀμετρίαις αὐτοῦ.
καὶ διὰ τοῦτο καὶ Ἱπποκράτης ψυχροτέροις μὲν τῇ
δυνάμει χρῆται κατὰ τὰς θερμὰς ὥρας, θερμοτέροις δὲ
κατὰ τὰς ψυχράς. οἶσθα δὲ δήπου κἀνταῦθα τῶν
ἀναισθήτων τινὰ Μεθοδικῶν ὁμολογήσαντα μὲν ἐπιβλέπειν ὅπως ἔχει θερμότητος ἢ ψύξεως ὁ περιέχων
ἀὴρ τὸν κάμνοντα, μὴ μέντοι τὰς ὥρας τοῦ ἔτους
214K ἐπισκέπτεσθαι συγχωροῦντα, ὥσπερ | τῶν ὀνομάτων
τῶν κατὰ τὰς ὥρας βλαπτόντων ἢ ὠφελούντων, ἀλλ᾿
οὐ τῆς κράσεως αὐτῶν, ἢ οὐ διὰ ταύτην ἀποβλε-
πόντων εἰς αὐτὰς τῶν παλαιῶν ἰατρῶν.

ἀλλὰ γὰρ ὅτι μὲν ἀναγκαῖόν ἐστι τῷ μέλλοντι
μεθόδῳ τινὶ θεραπεύσειν ἕλκος, ἐπί τε τὰ στοιχεῖα
πρῶτα καὶ μάλιστα παραγίνεσθαι καὶ τὰς ὥρας τοῦ
ἔτους καὶ τὰς κράσεις τῶν σωμάτων ὅλων τε καὶ κατὰ
τὰ μόρια ἐπιβλέπειν ἱκανῶς οἶμαι δεδεῖχθαι. πάλιν δ᾿

324

hemlock as more than moderately cooling, although they are in fact drying to the degree that the wound needs to be dried. And there are also pine resin, pitch and asphalt, although they do also dry moderately; nevertheless, they are hot to a greater degree than is appropriate, and because of this, nobody would use them on their own without mixing [them] with things that are gently cooling to make a single *eukratic* medication from all [the components]. If this is actually the situation, to the extent that it is, there will be the need to look in addition at the *krasis* of the ambient air for, just as with a medication, this too impacts on bodies externally, and whenever it is disproportionately hot or cold, stands in the way of treatment. Accordingly, it is necessary that the medications [given] act in a contrary way to its imbalances. And because of this, Hippocrates also used medications that were colder in potency in the hot seasons of the year and hotter in the cold seasons. You know, of course, that here too one of the stupid Methodics, having agreed to observe whether the air surrounding the patient was hot or cold, nevertheless did not agree to consider the seasons of the year, as if the names of the seasons were 214K harmful or helpful, but not their *krasis*, or that it was not because of this *krasis* that the doctors of old considered them.

But it has, I think, been demonstrated sufficiently that it is essential for anyone intending to treat a wound by a certain method to pay particular attention to the primary elements, the seasons of year and the *krasis* of bodies as a whole, and also to look at the parts. On the other hand, we

ἀναμνηστέον κἀνταῦθα τὸ καὶ πρόσθεν εἰρημένον ἐπὶ
τῆς κατὰ τὸ ξηρόν τε καὶ ὑγρὸν ἐνδείξεως· ὡς γὰρ ἐπ᾽
ἐκείνων ἡ μὲν ὑγροτέρα φύσις ὑγροτέρων ἐδεῖτο τῶν
φαρμάκων, ἡ δὲ ξηροτέρα ξηροτέρων, οὕτως καὶ νῦν ἡ
μὲν θερμοτέρα θερμοτέρων, ἡ δὲ ψυχροτέρα ψυχρο-
τέρων δεήσεται, ἔμπαλιν δὴ τῆς ἐνδείξεως γιγνομένης
ἀπὸ τῶν παρὰ φύσιν τε καὶ κατὰ φύσιν· τὰ μὲν γὰρ
κατὰ φύσιν ὁμοίων ἑαυτοῖς ἐστιν ἐνδεικτικά, τὰ δὲ
παρὰ φύσιν ἐναντίων, εἴ γε τὰ μὲν φυλάττεσθαι, τὰ δὲ
διαφθείρεσθαι χρή.

9. Τὸ μὲν οὖν καὶ τὰς κράσεις τῶν σωμάτων καὶ τὰς
ὥρας τοῦ ἔτους καὶ τὰς φύσεις τῶν μορίων ἐπιβλέ-
215K πειν | χρῆναι τὸν μέλλοντα καλῶς ἕλκος ἰάσασθαι
δεδεῖχθαί μοι νομίζω σαφῶς· καὶ ὡς μὲν πρῶτος
σκοπὸς τῆς ἰάσεως ἐκ τῆς διαθέσεως λαμβάνεται
μόνης, ἐξευρεῖν δὲ οὐκ ἔτι ἐντεῦθεν ἐγχωρεῖ τὰ βοηθήματα, πρὶν ἐπί τε τὰ στοιχεῖα τῶν σωμάτων ἀναβῆναι καὶ τοῦ κάμνοντος ἐπισκέψασθαι τὴν κρᾶσιν,
ὅλου τε τοῦ σώματος καὶ τοῦ πεπονθότος μέρους,
εὐθὺς αὐτῷ καὶ τὴν τοῦ περιέχοντος κρᾶσιν συνεπι-
σκεπτομένους· ἥτις ἐκτείνεται κἀπὶ τὰς ἐπιδήμους
καταστάσεις καὶ προσέτι τὰς χώρας. ὅτι δὲ πολλάκις
ἐναντίαι ἐνδείξεις γίγνονται κατὰ μίαν θεραπείαν,
ὅπως τε χρὴ μεταχειρίζεσθαι τὰς τοιαύτας, εἰρήσεται
μὲν ἐπιπλέον ἐν τοῖς ἐφεξῆς, εἴη δ᾽ ἂν οὐκ ἄπο τρόπου
καὶ νῦν ἐπὶ βραχὺ διελθεῖν ὑπὲρ αὐτῶν. οὐδὲν γὰρ
οἶμαι θαυμαστὸν ὑγροτέραν μὲν ὑπάρχειν τὴν κρᾶσιν
τοῦ κάμνοντος, αὐτὸ δὲ τὸ πεπονθὸς μόριον ξηρό-

must also remember here what was previously said in the case of the indication that relates to dry and moist; for as in those, the moister nature always needs moister medications, and the drier nature, drier medications. So now also the hotter nature will need hotter medications and the colder nature, colder medications, there being a contrary situation, surely, when the indication is from these things contrary to nature than when it is from those things in accord with nature. The things that are indicated by an accord with nature are those things like themselves, and by a contrariety to nature, those things opposite to themselves, if it is necessary to preserve the former and destroy the latter.

9. What I have shown clearly, I think, is that the person who is going to cure a wound properly ought to pay close attention to the *krasias* of the bodies, the seasons of the year and the natures of the parts, and that the primary indicator of the cure is taken from the condition alone. However, it is not yet possible to discover the remedies here before proceeding to the elements of the body and considering the *krasis* of the patient, both of the whole body and of the affected part, and to jointly consider with this right away the *krasis* of the surroundings, which extends to local conditions and regions as well. I shall state at greater length in what follows that contrary indications frequently arise in relation to a single treatment, and how we must handle such [indications], although it would not be out of place to go over them briefly now also. For it is, I think, not surprising for the *krasis* of the patient to be

215K

τερον, ἢ τοῦτο μὲν ὑγρότερον, ἅπασαν δὲ τὴν κρᾶσιν
ξηροτέραν· ὡσαύτως δὲ καὶ κατὰ θερμότητα καὶ ψῦξιν
ὑπεναντίως ἔχειν τῇ κράσει τὸ μόριον πρὸς τὸ ὅλον.
ὥσπερ οὖν εἰ τὸ πᾶν σῶμα τῆς μέσης ὑπῆρχε κρά-
216K σεως, ἣν ἀρίστην ἐδείκνυμεν, οὐδὲν ἂν ἕνεκά | γε τῆς
τοῦ κάμνοντος φύσεως ἐνεωτερίζομεν ἐν τοῖς φαρμάκοις, οὕτως ἐπειδὰν ἤτοι ξηρότερον ἢ ὑγρότερον, ἢ
ψυχρότερον ἢ θερμότερον ᾖ τοῦ δέοντος, ἐπιτείνειν εἰς
τοσοῦτον χρὴ τὰς δυνάμεις τῶν φαρμάκων, εἰς ὅσον
καὶ τὸ σῶμα φυσικῆς ἐπείληπται δυσκρασίας. οὐ γὰρ
δὴ ἐπιλελήσμεθά γε, τίς μὲν ἡ φυσικὴ δυσκρασία, τίς
δ' ἡ παρὰ φύσιν. εἴρηται γὰρ ὑπὲρ αὐτῶν ἐν ἄλλοις
καὶ μάλιστ' ἐν τῷ Περὶ τῆς ἀνωμάλου δυσκρασίας
γράμματι.

φέρε τοίνυν ὅλην τὴν κρᾶσιν τοῦ κάμνοντος σώματος ὑγροτέραν εἶναι καὶ διὰ τοῦτο δεῖσθαι τῶν ἧττον
ξηραινόντων φαρμάκων, αὐτὸ δὲ τὸ πεπονθὸς μόριον
τῶν φύσει ξηροτέρων ὑπάρχειν, οἷά περ ἐλέγομεν
εἶναι τὰ ἧττον σαρκώδη. τοιαῦτα δ' ἐστὶ τά τε κατὰ
τοὺς δακτύλους καὶ τὰ ἄρθρα καὶ τὰ ὦτα καὶ τὴν ῥῖνα
καὶ τοὺς ὀφθαλμοὺς καὶ τοὺς ὀδόντας, ἁπλῶς δ' εἰπεῖν
ἵνα χόνδροι πολλοὶ καὶ ὑμένες καὶ σύνδεσμοι καὶ
ὀστᾶ καὶ νεῦρα, πιμελὴ δὲ καὶ σὰρξ ἢ οὐδ' ὅλως, ἢ
ἐλαχίστη, διάφορος δ' ἐν τούτοις ἡ ἔνδειξις ἀπό τε τοῦ
πεπονθότος μέρους ἐστὶ καὶ τῆς φύσεως τοῦ κάμνον-
217K τος. ὥστε εἰ μὲν ὅσῳ τοῦ κάμνοντος | ἡ κρᾶσις ὑγρο-
τέρα πέφυκε τοῦ συμμέτρου, τοσούτῳ καὶ τὸ μόριον
εἴη ξηρότερον τοῦ συμμέτρου, μήτε προστιθέναι τι

328

more moist, while the affected part itself is more dry, or this to be more moist and the whole *krasis* more dry. In like manner too, in relation to heat and cold, there may be an opposition in *krasis* between the part and the whole. Thus, just as when the whole body is of moderate *krasis*, which we showed was best, we would change nothing in the medications for the sake of the nature of the patient, so whenever the body is more dry, more moist, more cold, or more hot than it should be, it is necessary to increase the potencies of the medications to the degree that the body has been taken over by a natural *dyskrasia*. Nor, certainly, will we lose sight of what is a natural *dyskrasia* and what is an unnatural *dyskrasia*. I spoke about these *dyskrasias* in other [works] and particularly in the treatise *On Irregular Dyskrasia*.[17]

Suppose, therefore, the whole *krasis* of the patient's body is more moist, and because of this, needs less of the drying medications, whereas the affected part itself is among those things that are more dry in nature, of the sort which I said were less fleshy. Examples are found in the fingers, joints, ears, nose, eyes and teeth, and in summary, in a place where there is much cartilage, membrane, ligament, bone and nerve but very little fat and flesh, or none at all. In these places, the indication from the affected part is different to that from the nature of the patient. As a result, if the part is drier than normal to the same extent that the *krasis* of the patient is more moist in nature than is normal, I undertake neither to add nor take away

216K

217K

---

[17] *De inaequali intemperie*, VII.733–52K (translated by M. Grant, 2000).

μήτ' ἀφαιρεῖν τοῦ φαρμάκου, τοιοῦτον δὲ προσφέρειν,
οἷον ἂν ἐπὶ τοῦ συμμέτρου τῇ κράσει σώματος ἐν
συμμέτρῳ τῇ κράσει μορίῳ γεγονότος ἕλκους παρ-
ελάβομεν. εἰ δὲ πλέον εἴη τὸ μόριον τοῦ μετρίου
ξηρότερον, ἢ ὅσῳ τοῦ σώματος ἡ κρᾶσις ὑγροτέρα,
τοσοῦτον ἐπιτείνεσθαι χρὴ ξηρότητι τὸ φάρμακον,
ὅσον ὑπερβάλλει τὸ μόριον τῆς ὅλης κράσεως. οἷον εἰ
τέσσαρσι μὲν ἀριθμοῖς εἴη τὸ ἡλκωμένον μέρος ξηρότερον τοῦ συμμέτρου, τρισὶ δ' ἀριθμοῖς ἡ φύσις τοῦ
νοσοῦντος ὑγροτέρα τῆς εὐκράτου, πρόδηλον ὡς ἑνὶ
τοῦ συμμέτρου μορίου τὸ νῦν ἡλκωμένον ἔσται ξηρο-
τέρου δεόμενον φαρμάκου. ὅτι δὲ ἅπαντα ταῦτα στο-
χασμῷ λαμβάνεται καὶ ὅτι κάλλιστα δυνατός ἐστι
στοχάζεσθαι ὁ γεγυμνασμένος ἐν τοῖς περὶ τούτων
λογισμοῖς ἄντικρυς δῆλον.

ἐπὶ μὲν δὴ τῶν τοιούτων ἁπάντων ἐναντίαι πολλάκις ἐνδείξεις καθ' ἕνα γίνονται χρόνον· οὐδὲν γὰρ ἔτι
218K δέομαι λέγειν ὑπὲρ τῶν κατὰ θερμόν | τε καὶ ψυχρὸν
ἐνδείξεων ἀνάλογον τοῖς εἰρημένοις νοεῖσθαι δυνα-
μένων· ἐφ' ἑτέρων δὲ καὶ τοῖς χρόνοις ἐφ' οἷς εὐθὺς αἱ
ἐνδείξεις τέμνονται, καὶ χρὴ τὴν μὲν ἡσυχάσαι κατά
γε τὴν ἀρχὴν τῆς θεραπείας, ἐνεργῆσαι δὲ ἑτέραν·
οἷον ὅταν ἕλκος ᾖ κοῖλόν τε ἅμα καὶ ἱκανῶς ῥυπαρόν·
αἱ μὲν γὰρ διαθέσεις αἱ παρὰ φύσιν ἐν τούτοις τρεῖς
εἰσιν, ἕλκος καὶ κοιλότης καὶ ῥύπος. ἡ δὲ τῆς ἰάσεως
τάξις ἀπὸ τῆς ἀναιρέσεως τοῦ ῥύπου τὴν ἀρχὴν ἔχει,
τῷ μήτε κολληθῆναί τι, μήτε σαρκωθῆναι δύνασθαι,
πρὶν καθαρὸν γενέσθαι. δευτέραν δὲ χώραν ἡ τῆς

anything by way of the medication, whereas I would undertake to apply such a medication in the case of a body balanced in *krasis*, when a wound has occurred in a part that is balanced in *krasis*. If the part is drier than normal by as much as the *krasis* of the body is moister, it is necessary to increase the medication to the extent that the dryness of the part exceeds the whole *krasis*. If, for example, the wounded part is four magnitudes more dry than normal, and the nature of the diseased person three magnitudes more moist than the *eukratic*, it is clear that the part which is now wounded will be in need of a medication drier by one magnitude than a balanced part. It is, however, patently obvious that all these things are arrived at by guesswork, and that someone practiced in calculations about these matters is best able to carry out the estimation.

So then, in the case of all such things, opposite indications often arise at one time. I need say nothing further about the indications in relation to heat and cold since they can be understood analogously to what has been said. In other cases also, there are times when the indications are immediately divided and it is necessary to set aside one at the beginning of treatment and to activate another—for example, whenever a wound is hollow and at the same time excessively filthy. For the conditions that are contrary to nature in these cases are three: a wound, a cavity and filth. However, the order of the cure starts with the removal of the filth, in that it is not possible for the wound to be conglutinated or enfleshed before it becomes clean. The cure of the cavity will take second place, for if we were either to

218K

κοιλότητος ἴασις ἕξει· εἰ γὰρ ἤτοι κολλήσαιμεν, ἢ
ἐπουλώσαιμεν, ἢ καθόλου φάναι θεραπεύσαιμεν τὸ
ἕλκος, οὐκέτι ἐγχωρεῖ πληρῶσαι τὴν κοιλότητα. φέρε
τοίνυν μὴ μόνον ταῦτ' εἶναι τὰ τρία περὶ τὸ μέρος,
ἀλλὰ καὶ φλεγμονήν, ἢ ἐρυσίπελας, ἢ γάγγραναν, ἤ
τινα δυσκρασίαν ἁπλῆν ἢ σύνθετον, ἆρ' οὐκ ἐνταῦθα
πρόδηλον ὡς εἰ μή τις πρότερον ἐκείνην ἰάσαιτο,
πληρῶσαι σαρκὶ τὸ κοῖλον ἕλκος οὐκ ἐγχωρεῖ;
λέλεκται γὰρ καὶ πρόσθεν ὡς ἡ τῆς σαρκὸς γένεσις ἐκ
τῆς   ὑποκειμένης   ἄρχεται   τῆς   ὑγιοῦς·   ἐκ
219K φλεγμαινούσης δὲ καὶ | δυσκράτου καὶ ἁπλῶς εἰπεῖν
νοσούσης, οὐκ ἐγχωρεῖ γεννηθῆναι νέαν σάρκα.

σκοπὸς οὖν ἐν ἁπάσαις ταῖς τοιαύταις ἐπιπλοκαῖς
ἔστω σοι τριττός. εἷς μὲν ὡς ὁ ἐξ αἰτίων τοῦ μέλ-
λοντος ἔσεσθαι λαμβανόμενος· ὁ δὲ ἕτερος ὡς ὁ τὸν
ὧν οὐκ ἄνευ λόγον ἔχων· ὁ δὲ τρίτος ὡς ὁ τῶν
ἐπειγόντων τε καὶ κατεπειγόντων ὀνομαζόμενος. ἡ μὲν
γὰρ εὐκρασία τῆς ὑποκειμένης σαρκὸς αἰτίας λόγον
ἔχει, συμφύουσά τε τὸ ἡλκωμένον αὐτῇ καὶ ἀναπλη-
ροῦσα τὸ κοῖλον. ἡ δὲ καθαρότης τοῦ ἕλκους τὸν ὧν
οὐκ ἄνευ λόγον· καὶ ταύτην ὁ ῥύπος διακόπτων κωλύει
τὴν θεραπείαν. ἔχει δὲ καὶ αὐτὸ τὸ ἕλκος ὡς πρὸς τὴν
κοιλότητα τὸν ὧν οὐκ ἄνευ λόγον. εἰ γὰρ εἰς οὐλὴν
ἀχθείη τὸ ἕλκος, οὐκέθ' οἷόν τε σαρκῶσαι τὴν κοιλότητα. πρὸς ταῦτ' οὖν ἀποβλέπων ἐξευρήσεις τὴν
τάξιν τῆς ἰάσεως· οἷον ἡ φλεγμονὴ καὶ κοιλότης καὶ
ἕλκος καὶ ῥύπος ἅμα κατὰ ταὐτὸν ὑπάρχει μόριον· ὅτι
χρὴ πρῶτον μὲν τὴν φλεγμονήν, δεύτερον δὲ τὸν

332

conglutinate or cicatrize, or to speak generally, if we were to treat the wound beforehand, it would no longer be possible to fill the cavity. Suppose, therefore, that it is not only these three things that involve this part, but also inflammation, erysipelas, gangrene, or some simple or compound *dyskrasia*. Is it not clear here that, unless someone were to cure that beforehand, it would not be possible to fill the hollow wound with flesh? For I have also said before that the genesis of flesh begins from healthy underlying flesh, whereas from flesh that is inflamed or *dyskratic*, or in a word diseased, it is not possible for new flesh to be regenerated.

219K

In all such combinations, let your indicator be threefold. One indicator will be that taken from the causes of what is about to exist. The second indicator is like that which has the ground of *sine qua non*, and the third indicator is what may be termed pressing or urgently requiring attention. The *eukrasia* of the underlying flesh has the ground of cause, what is wounded being united by this and the cavity filled. The cleanliness of the wound has the ground of those things *sine qua non*, and the filthiness, since it interrupts this, hinders the treatment. And the wound itself, by virtue of the cavity, has the ground of those things *sine qua non*. If the wound is brought to a scar, it is no longer possible to fill the cavity with flesh. If you pay attention to these things, you will discover the order of the cure. For example, if inflammation, hollowness, wound, and filthiness are present at the same time in the same place, it is necessary to cure the inflammation first, the

ρύπον, τρίτον δὲ ἰάσασθαι τὴν κοιλότητα, καὶ τέταρτον τὸ ἕλκος. ἐν μὲν δὴ τοῖς εἰρημένοις ἥ τε τάξις καὶ
ἡ τῶν σκοπῶν εὕρεσις ἐντεῦθεν. ὁ δὲ τοῦ | κατεπεί-
γοντος σκοπὸς ἐν τούτοις μὲν οὐκ ἔστιν, ἐν ἄλλοις δ'
ἐστίν· ἀφ' ἧς γὰρ κινδυνεύει πρώτης καὶ μάλιστα
διαθέσεως ὁ ἄνθρωπος, ἐκείνην πρῶτον ἰατέον. ἐνίοτε
δὲ οὐ πρώτην μόνον, ἀλλὰ καὶ μόνην αὐτήν· οἷον εἰ
νυγείσης κεφαλῆς μυὸς ἀκολουθήσειε σπασμός, εἶτα
πρὸς μηδενὸς τῶν οἰκείων ἰαμάτων καθίσταιτο· διατεμὼν γὰρ ὅλον τὸν μῦν ἐγκάρσιον, ἰάσῃ μὲν τὸν
σπασμόν, ἀλλὰ πηρώσεις τινὰ τῶν τοῦ μορίου κινή-
σεων. οὕτω δὲ καὶ φλεβὸς ἢ ἀρτηρίας αἱμορραγούσης
ἀμέτρως ὁ διατεμὼν ὅλον ἐγκάρσιον τὸ ἀγγεῖον οὐκέτι μὲν ἰάσασθαι δύναται τὸ ἕλκος αὐτοῦ· τὸν δ' ἐκ τῆς
αἱμορραγίας κίνδυνον ἐπέσχεν. ἀλλὰ καὶ νεῦρον νυ-
γὲν ἀναγκαζόμεθα πολλάκις ἐγκάρσιον διακόπτειν,
ὅταν ἤτοι σπασμούς, ἢ παραφροσύνας, ἢ ἀμφότερα
μεγάλα καὶ δυσίατα βλέπωμεν ἑπόμενα τῇ τρώσει.
κατὰ δὲ τὸν αὐτὸν τρόπον ἐξάρθρημα μεθ' ἕλκους
ἐπειδὰν γένηται κατά τι τῶν μειζόνων ἄρθρων, τὸ μὲν
ἕλκος ἰώμεθα, τὸ δὲ ἐξάρθρημα καταλείπομεν ἀνία-
τον· ὅτι καὶ τοῦτ' ἐγχειρούντων ἰάσασθαι, σπασμοὶ
τοὐπίπαν | ἕπονται. τρίτος οὖν οὗτος σκοπός ἐστιν ὁ
πρὸς τὸ κατεπεῖγον γιγνόμενος, ἕτερος ἐκείνων τῶν
δύο τῶν ὀλίγον ἔμπροσθεν εἰρημένων. οὐ γὰρ ταὐτόν
ἐστιν ἢ ὡς αἴτιόν τι σκοπεῖν, ἢ ὡς τὸν ὧν οὐκ ἄνευ
λόγον ἔχον, ἢ ὡς κατεπεῖγον. ἀλλὰ καὶ ὡς τὸ κατεπεῖγον ἐνίοτε τοιοῦτόν ἐστιν, ὡς ἀνίατον ἀναγκάζειν

filthiness second, the hollowness third, and the wound fourth. So then, the order and discovery of the indicators are here in what has been said. However, the indicator of what is urgent is not in these things but in others. You must first treat that condition from which the person is primarily and particularly in danger. Sometimes the condition is not only the primary one, but also the only one. For example, if, when the head of a muscle is pierced, a spasm follows which is settled by none of the specific cures, you will cure the spasm by cutting the whole muscle across, but you will incapacitate some of the movements of the part. So too, when a vein or artery is hemorrhaging excessively, someone who cuts the whole vessel across transversely is no longer still able to cure the wound, although he has put an end to the danger from the hemorrhage. But also, we are often compelled to cut transversely across a pierced nerve, whenever we see either spasms or derangements which are significant and difficult to treat following the wounding. And in the same way, whenever a dislocation arises with a wound in one of the major joints, we must cure the wound but leave the dislocation as incurable in that, if we also attempt to cure this, spasms generally follow. This third indicator, then, is what is directed toward what is most urgent; it is different from the other two that were spoken about a little earlier in that it is not the same to consider something as a cause, or as having the ground of *sine qua non*, or as being urgent. But also, what is urgent is sometimes such as to compel another condition to be left

220K

221K

ἑτέραν ἀπολιπέσθαι διάθεσιν, εἴρηται, καὶ ὡς ἡ διάθεσις αὕτη πολλάκις ὑφ' ἡμῶν αὐτῶν γίνεται, τοῦτο μὲν
ἐπὶ τῶν νενυγμένων νεύρων, ἢ τενόντων, ἢ αἱμορρα-
γούντων ἀγγείων, τοῦτο δὲ ἐπὶ τῶν κατὰ τὰς κεφαλὰς
τετρωμένων μυῶν· ἐπὶ μὲν γὰρ ἐξαρθρήματος ἅμα καὶ
ἕλκους οὐκ αὐτὸ ποιοῦμεν, ἀλλὰ μόνον οὐκ ἰώμεθα τὸ
γενόμενον. εἰρήσεται δὲ κἂν τοῖς ἑξῆς ἔτι περὶ τούτων
ἐπιμελέστερον.

10. Ἐν γὰρ τῷ παρόντι συγκεφαλαιώσασθαι βούλομαι τὸν ἐνεστῶτα λόγον ἐπὶ τὰς οἰκείας διαφορὰς
τῶν ἑλκῶν ἐπανελθὼν, ἵν', εἴ τις κἀντεῦθεν ἔνδειξις
ἰαμάτων ἐστί, μηδὲ ταύτην παραλίπωμεν. τὸ μὲν οὖν
φλεγμαῖνον ἕλκος καὶ τὸ σηπόμενον ἀναβιβρωσκό-
222K μενόν τε καὶ γαγγραινούμενον | ἐρυσιπελατῶδές τε
καὶ καρκινῶδες ἀνώδυνόν τε καὶ ὀδυνῶδες, τά τ' ἄλλα
τοιαῦτα λέγουσιν ὡς διαφορὰς ἑλκῶν, εἰ μὲν ἄλλως
τις διέρχοιτο θεραπείαν ἐμπειρικὴν ἀναγράφων, οὐκ
ἀμφισβητητέον αὐτῷ διαφορὰς ἑλκῶν ὀνομάζοντι·
μυριάκις γὰρ εἴρηται τὸ μὴ δεῖν ὑπὲρ τῶν ὀνομάτων
ἐρίζειν· εἰ δ' ὡς ἐντεῦθεν μέλλων ἐρεῖν τι τεχνικὸν
ὑπὲρ ἐνδείξεων, ἐπιδεικτέον αὐτῷ τὰς μὲν εἰρημένας
ἁπάσας διαθέσεις ὑπάρχειν συνθέτους, ἄλλας δ' εἶναι
διαφορὰς ἕλκους ἁπλοῦ καὶ μόνου, χωρὶς ἑτέρας τινὸς
ἐπιπεπλεγμένης αὐτῷ διαθέσεως. εἰ γὰρ ἁπλῶς διαιρέσεως γενομένης ὑπό τινος ὀξέος τὸ σχῆμα τοῦ
τρώσαντος ἐναπομαχθείη τῷ διῃρημένῳ, γένοιντ' ἂν
οὕτως ἑλκῶν διαφοραὶ πάμπολλαι, λοξῶν, εὐθειῶν,
ἑλικοειδῶν, ἀγκιστροειδῶν, ἄλλως ὁπωσοῦν ἐχόντων.
αὗται μὲν οὖν αἱ διαφοραὶ πᾶσαι παρὰ τὸ σχῆμα.

as incurable, as was said, and this condition itself often occurs iatrogenically, as in the case of pierced nerves or sinews, or hemorrhaging vessels, or in the case of muscles that have been wounded in their heads. In the case of dislocation coincident with a wound, we do not do this; rather we simply do not cure what has happened. Still more will be said about these matters in what follows.

10. For the present, I wish to summarize the established argument by returning to the specific differentiae of wounds, so that, if there is also here some indication of cures, we do not leave this out. Therefore, in respect of the inflamed wound, the putrefying erosion, gangrene, erysipelas, cancers (both painless and painful), and other such things which [doctors] speak of as differentiae of wounds and ulcers, if someone, when describing them, were to go over the empirical treatment differently, we must not dispute with him if he names these differentiae of wounds. I have said countless times that there is no need to contend about names. If, however, we are about to say something practical about indications, as here, we must point out to him that all the conditions spoken of are compound, whereas other differentiae of a wound are simple and single, not having any other condition combined with them. If, when a division occurs simply due to something sharp, the form of what is wounded takes an impression from what has divided it, in this way very many differentiae of wounds will arise, [such as] oblique, straight, spiral or uncinate, or whatever else there is. All these are differentiae pertaining to form.

222K

παρὰ δ᾽ αὖ τὸ μέγεθος ἐν τῷ μᾶλλόν τε καὶ ἧττον
ἕτεραι μυρίαι· καὶ γὰρ μικρὸν καὶ μέγα καὶ μεῖζον καὶ
μικρότερον ἕλκος ἕλκους λέγεταί τι καὶ γίνεται· καὶ
223K   μὲν δὴ καὶ βραχὺ καὶ μακρὸν ἐπιπολῆς τε καὶ | βαθύ,
καὶ καθ᾽ ἕκαστον αὐτῶν τὸ μᾶλλόν τε καὶ ἧττον ἐν τῇ
κατὰ τὸ μέγεθος, ἢ τὸ πηλίκον, ἢ τὸ ποσόν, ἢ ὅπως ἂν
ἐθέλοι τις ὀνομάζειν διαφορᾷ. καὶ εἴπερ ταῦτα οὕτως
ἔχει, πάντως δήπου καὶ ὁμαλὲς καὶ ἀνώμαλον ἕλκος
ἐν τῷ βάθει τῆς διαιρέσεως ἔσται. κατὰ μῆκος γάρ, εἰ
οὕτως ἔτυχεν, ἀνεσχισμένου τοῦ μηροῦ τὸ μὲν ἄνω
μέρος τῆς διαιρέσεως ἐνδέχεται βαθύ, τὸ κάτω δὲ
ἐπιπόλαιον ὑπάρχειν, ἢ ἔμπαλιν ἐπιπολῆς μὲν τὸ ἄνω,
βαθὺ δ᾽ εἶναι τὸ κάτω. καὶ μὲν δὴ καὶ τὸ διεσπάσθαι
κατά τι, ἢ τοὐπίπαν καὶ διατετμῆσθαι καὶ τοῦ τρώσαντος ὑποδύντος ὑπὸ τὸ δέρμα λοξόν, μέρος μέν τι
τοῦ ἕλκους φαίνεσθαι, μέρος δ᾽ ἕτερον ὑπὸ τῷ δέρματι
κατακεκρύφθαι, καὶ τοῦτο ἢ ἐκ τῶν ἄνωθεν εἶναι
μερῶν, ἢ ἐκ τῶν κάτωθεν, ἢ ἐκ τῶν πλαγίων, ἅπαντα
καὶ ταῦθ᾽ ἑλκῶν εἰσι διαφοραί. παρὰ δ᾽ αὖ τὸν χρόνον
ἕτεραι διαφοραὶ τῶν ἑλκῶν, παλαιὸν καὶ ἔναιμον ἢ
πρόσφατον ὀλιγοχρόνιόν τε, καὶ πολυχρόνιον, ἐν
ἅπασι δ᾽ αὐτοῖς τὸ μᾶλλόν τε καὶ ἧττον πάμπολυ.
224K   κατὰ μὲν αὐτὴν τοῦ ἕλκους τὴν φύσιν | αὗται δια-
φοραί, κυριώταται μὲν αἱ κατὰ τὴν οὐσίαν τοῦ πράγματος ἥ τε παρὰ τὸ σχῆμα καὶ ἡ παρὰ τὸ ποσὸν τῆς
διαιρέσεως, ἤτοι κατὰ τὸ μῆκος, ἢ βάθος, ἢ κατ᾽
ἀμφοτέρας τὰς διαστάσεις, ὁμαλότητά τε καὶ ἀνωμαλίαν τὴν ἐν τούτοις. ἔξωθεν δὲ προσιοῦσαι τὸν ὦν

338

Pertaining to size in terms of more or less, there is also a myriad of others for small and large; larger and smaller are terms used of a wound and do occur. Moreover, there is also short or long of the surface, and in the depths, and in relation to each of these, more or less in the differentiae, in relation to magnitude, size, amount or whatever someone might wish to call it. And if these things are so, then of course there will in general be a regular and an irregular wound in the depth of the division. If it should happen that the thigh is torn open longitudinally, it is possible for the division of the part above to be deep and of the part below to be superficial, or conversely, for the division of the part above to be superficial and of the part below deep. Furthermore, when there is tearing away of something, or in general something has been cut through, and the wound goes under the skin obliquely, one part of the wound is apparent whereas another part is concealed under the skin, and this is either from the parts above, or from the parts below, or from those [torn] obliquely. All these are differentiae of wounds too. In terms of time also, there are other differentiae of wounds—long-standing and bleeding, recent and acute, chronic—while in all these there are very many degrees in respect to more and less.

In relation to the actual nature of the wound, these are the differentiae. The most characteristic are those pertaining to the substance of the matter, which relate to the form and amount of the division, or pertain to the length or depth, or to both dimensions, and to the regularity and irregularity in these. Those things that come into play exter-

223K

224K

339

οὐκ ἄνευ λόγον ἔχουσαι· παρά τε τὸν χρόνον ἐν ᾧ τὸ
ἕλκος, οὕτω γὰρ τὸ μὲν πρόσφατον καλεῖται, τὸ δὲ
παλαιόν, καὶ παρὰ τὸ φαίνεσθαί τε καὶ μὴ φαίνεσθαι
πᾶν ἢ μέρος. ἤδη δὲ καὶ παρὰ τὸν τῆς γενέσεως
τρόπον ἐν τῷ τμηθῆναι πᾶν ἢ διασπασθῆναι πᾶν· ἤ τι
μὲν τετμῆσθαι μέρος αὐτοῦ, διεσπάσθαι δ᾽ ἕτερον. εἰ
δὲ καὶ τὰς παρὰ τὸν τόπον ἐν ᾧ γέγονε τὸ ἕλκος
ἐκλογίζοιο διαφοράς, οἷον εἰ πέρας μυός, εἰ ἀρχὴ
μυός, εἰ τὸ μέσον τοῦ μυός, εἰ δέρμα ἐστὶ τὸ ἡλκωμένον, εἰ ἧπαρ ἢ γαστήρ, εἶεν ἂν δήπου καὶ αὗται
διαφοραὶ τῶν ἑλκῶν. ταῦτα μὲν οὖν οὕτως ἔχει, οὐκ
ἀπὸ τῆς οἰκείας αὐτῶν φύσεως, ἀλλ᾽ ἀπὸ τῶν χωρίων
ἐν οἷς συνίστανται τὴν γένεσιν ἔχουσα. ὅταν δ᾽ εἴποι
τις ἤτοι φλεγμαῖνον ἕλκος, ἢ ὑπερσαρκοῦν, ἢ κοῖλον, |

225K εἴ τ᾽ οἴηται[6] παραπλησίας εἰρηκέναι διαφορὰς ἑλκῶν,
ἃς νῦν ἤδη πέπαυμαι λέγων, οὗτος ἐξ ἀνάγκης ἐν τῇ
θεραπευτικῇ μεθόδῳ σφαλήσεται.

τὸ γὰρ φλεγμαῖνον ἕλκος οὑτωσὶ λεγόμενον ὅμοιον
μὲν ἔχει τὸ τῆς ἑρμηνείας σχῆμα τῷ μικρὸν ἕλκος, οὐ
μὴν τό γε δηλούμενον ὅμοιον ὑπάρχει. τὸ μὲν γὰρ
ἐπιπολῆς ἢ βαθὺ κατηγορήσαντες τοῦ ἕλκους, οἰκείαν
αὐτοῦ διαφορὰν ἐμηνύσαμεν· τὸ φλεγμαῖνον δ᾽ οὐδ᾽
ὅλως ἐστὶν ἕλκους διαφορά· δύναται γὰρ φλεγμῆναι
μόριον καὶ χωρὶς ἕλκους. ὅθεν οἶμαι καὶ τὴν λέξιν
ἐνταυθοῖ μὲν ὑπαλλάξαι δυνατόν· εἰ γὰρ εἴποις ἕλκος
τῷδέ τινι γεγονέναι μετὰ φλεγμονῆς, οἰκειότερόν γε
τῷ πράγματι καὶ σαφέστερον ἑρμηνεύσεις· οὐ μὴν εἰ

nally have the ground of *sine qua non* and depend on the time for which the wound exists, so it is called recent or old; and depending on whether it is visible or not, it is called whole or part. Now there is also the manner of its creation, whether the whole is cut through or torn asunder, or one part of it has been cut through but another part torn asunder. And if you reckon the differentiae on the basis of the place in which the wound has occurred—for example, if it is at the end of the muscle, or the beginning of the muscle, or the middle of the muscle, or if the skin has been wounded, or the liver or stomach—these would be, of course, differentiae of wounds. If these things are so, they have their genesis not from their own specific nature but from the places in which they exist. But whenever someone speaks of an inflamed wound, or an exuberant ulcer, or a hollow [wound or ulcer], if he thinks that he has articulated differentiae of wounds that are similar, which differentiae I have now already stopped speaking about, he will inevitably be mistaken in the method of treatment.

For the inflamed wound, when spoken of in this way, has a similar form of interpretation to that in respect to a small wound, but what in fact is signified is not similar. This is because, when we speak about the superficiality or depth of the wound, we disclose a specific differentia of it. And being inflamed is not entirely a differentia of a wound. For it is possible for a part to be inflamed without a wound, from which, I think, it is also possible to change the terminology here. For if you were to say a wound has occurred in such and such a part along with inflammation, you will be describing it more specifically and more clearly, but this is

225K

---

6 B; ἢ κοῖλον, οἴεται K

φαίης μετὰ μεγέθους μὲν τῷδε, μετὰ σμικρότητος δὲ
ἄλλῳ γεγονέναι. καὶ γὰρ οἰκειότερόν τε τῷ πράγματι
καὶ σαφέστερον ἑρμηνεύσεις, εἰ τῷδε μέν τινι φαίης
ἕλκος μέγα γεγονέναι, τῷ δὲ αὖ μικρόν. ὅθεν εἰ οἷόν τ᾽
ἦν καὶ τὴν λέξιν ὑπαλλάττειν ὡς καὶ τῷ λεγομένῳ
πράγματι πρεπωδεστέραν ἐργάζεσθαι καὶ τοῖς ἀκού-
σουσι σαφεστέραν, οὐ χρὴ κατοκνεῖν οὕτω ποιεῖν·
ἀρχὴ γὰρ τοῦ μὴ σοφίζεσθαι περὶ τὰ πράγματα τὸ
226K   καὶ τῇ | λέξει χρῆσθαι διωρισμένῃ.

τίς οὖν ἐν τοῖς τοιούτοις ἡ μέθοδος; εἰπεῖν γὰρ χρὴ
παράγγελμά τι καὶ οἷον σκοπὸν ᾧ προσέχοντες τὸν
νοῦν ἀεὶ δυνησόμεθα διορίζεσθαι ταχέως εἴτε διαφορὰν εἴρηκέ τις ἡστινοσοῦν διαθέσεως, εἴτ᾽ ἐπιπλο-
κὴν ἑτέρας. ἔστω δή σοι διορισμὸς ὅδε· τὸ δυνάμενον
ἰδίᾳ ποτὲ καὶ καθ᾽ ἑαυτὸ συστῆναι, τοῦτ᾽ οὐκ ἄν ποτε
γένοιτο τῶν ἄλλων οὐδενὸς διαφορά. μέγεθος μὲν οὖν
καὶ σμικρότης, ὁμαλότης τε καὶ ἀνωμαλία καὶ χρόνος
καὶ σχῆμα τῶν ἑτέροις συμβεβηκότων ἐστίν. ἕλκος δὲ
καὶ φλεγμονὴ καὶ γάγγραινα καὶ σηπεδὼν ἕκαστον
ἰδίᾳ τε καὶ καθ᾽ αὑτὸ δύναται συστῆναι, διαθέσεις
γάρ τινές εἰσι τοῦ σώματος ἡμῶν παρὰ φύσιν, οὐ τὰ
ταῖς διαθέσεσιν ἐξ ἀνάγκης συμβεβηκότα. πᾶσι μὲν
γὰρ τοῖς εἰρημένοις ἐξ ἀνάγκης συμβέβηκεν ἤτοι
μικροῖς ἢ μεγάλοις ὑπάρχειν, ἢ ὁμαλέσιν, ἢ ἀνω-
μάλοις, ἢ προσφάτοις, ἢ παλαιοῖς, ἢ φαίνεσθαι προ-
χείρως, ἢ κεκρύφθαι καὶ μὴ βλέπεσθαι· τὸ φλεγμαί-
νειν δ᾽ οὐκ ἔστι τῶν συμβεβηκότων ἕλκει, καθάπερ
οὐδὲ τὸ σήπεσθαι καὶ γαγγραινοῦσθαι. πάντα γὰρ

not the case if you were to say it has occurred along with largeness in this part, or with smallness in another part. And you will be describing the matter more specifically and more clearly, if you were to say that a large wound occurs in this part, or again, a small wound. From which, if it were possible by changing the terminology to bring about something more appropriate in the matter being spoken of and clearer to those listening, you must not shrink from doing this. The starting point of not being sophistical about matters is to use terminology that is defined.   226K

What, then, is the method in such things? For it is necessary to articulate some instruction or objective, as it were, with which, when we focus our attention [on it], we are always able to distinguish quickly if someone has stated a differentia of any condition whatsoever, or if another condition is involved. So then, let this be your definition: what can exist separately in some way and of itself would not at any time be a differentia of anything else. Therefore, largeness and smallness, regularity and irregularity, and time and form are among the contingent attributes in other things. A wound, inflammation, gangrene and putrefaction are each separate and able to exist independently in that they are conditions of our bodies contrary to nature, and not things contingent to the conditions of necessity, for they are necessarily contingent to all the things spoken of, whether they are small or large, regular or irregular, recent or long-standing, readily apparent or concealed and not visible. But inflammation is not one of those things occurring contingently to a wound just as putrefaction and gan-

ταῦτ᾽ ἐστὶν ἐκ τοῦ τῶν νοσημάτων γένους, εἴ γε παρὰ |
227K   φύσιν εἰσὶ διαθέσεις καὶ βλάπτουσιν ἐνέργειαν.

ἑτέρῳ δ᾽ αὖ πάλιν τρόπῳ ἕλκος ὀδυνώμενον ἢ ἕλκος
ῥυπαρὸν λέγεται μὲν ὥς τις ἕλκους διαφορά, σύνθετον
δέ τι δηλοῦται κἀνταῦθα, πλὴν ἕτερον τρόπον ἢ ὡς
φλεγμαῖνον ἕλκος ἐλέγετο καὶ σηπόμενον. ἐκεῖ μὲν
γὰρ διάθεσις ἡ φλεγμονὴ καὶ ἡ σηπεδών· ἐνταυθοῖ δὲ
ὅ τε πόνος καὶ ὁ ῥύπος ἐκ τοῦ τῶν συμπτωμάτων
γένους. οὕτω δὲ κἀπειδὰν εἴπῃ τις ἕλκος, ἢ κακόχυμον, ἢ ῥευματικόν, ἢ ἀναβιβρωσκόμενον, αἰτίαν
συνεμφαίνει τῇ διαθέσει. καὶ δῆλον ἐκ τῶν τοιούτων
ὡς οἷον στοχεῖά τινα τῆς θεραπευτικῆς ἐστι μεθόδου
τὰ πρῶτά τε καὶ ἁπλᾶ καὶ ἀσύνθετα νοσήματα, καὶ
διὰ τοῦτ᾽ ἐν τῷ περὶ τῆς διαφορᾶς τῶν νοσημάτων
ὑπομνήματι πάντ᾽ ἐξηριθμησάμεθα ταῦτα. διοίσει δ᾽
οὐδὲν ἢ πρῶτα λέγειν, ἢ ἁπλᾶ· καὶ γὰρ εἰ πρῶτον,
ἁπλοῦν, καὶ εἰ ἁπλοῦν, πρῶτον· ὥστε καὶ στοιχειῶδες.
ἔνδειξις δὲ ἰάσεως ἀπὸ τῶν διαφορῶν οὐχ ἁπασῶν
γίνεται. τὸ γὰρ πρόσφατον ἢ παλαιὸν ἕλκος οὐδὲν
ἐνδείκνυται, καίτοι δοκεῖ τισιν, ἀλλὰ παραλογίζονται |
228K   σφᾶς αὐτούς, ὡς κἂν τοῖς κατὰ δίαιταν ἑτέραν μὲν
ἀρχῆς, ἑτέραν δ᾽ ἐπιδόσεως, ἄλλην δ᾽ ἀκμῆς τε καὶ
παρακμῆς ἔνδειξιν εἶναι λέγοντες· ὑπὲρ ὧν ἐπὶ πλέον
ἐν τοῖς ἑξῆς ἐρεῖν μέλλοντες, οὐ δεόμεθα νῦν μηκύνειν
τὸν λόγον· ἀλλ᾽ ὅσον εἰς τὰ παρόντα μόνον αὔταρκες
ἐροῦμεν.

τὸ ἕλκος τὸ πρόσφατον, ἐπειδὴ τοὐπίπαν ἄνευ τε

grene are not. For all these are from the class of diseases, if they are conditions contrary to nature and harm function.   227K

In another way again, a wound is said to be painful or filthy, as a differentia of a wound. However, here something compound is signified, but in another way than by saying it is inflamed or putrefying, whereas in the former case, the pain and filth are from the class of symptoms. In such a way also, whenever someone mentions *kakochymia*, or subject to flux, or eroding, in respect to a wound or ulcer, he is indicating a cause at the same time as the condition. And clearly, among those things that are, as it were, elements of the method of treatment, there are the primary, simple and uncombined diseases, and because of this, we enumerated all these in the treatise *On the Differentiae of Diseases*.[18] It will make no difference whether we say primary or simple, for if something is primary it is simple, and if it is simple it is primary, so that it is also elementary. An indication of a cure arises from the differentiae but not from all of them. A recent or long-standing wound indicates nothing and yet to some it seems to do so. But they mislead themselves if they say that in   228K wounds there is an indication according to regimen that is different at the beginning, during the progression, during the peak, and during the abatement. As I intend to say still more about these things in what follows next, I do not need to prolong the discussion now, but will say only what is sufficient for the present purposes.

They think that a recent wound, because it generally

---

[18] *De differentiis morborum*, VI.836–80K. For an analysis of Galen's classification, see I. Johnston (2006), pp. 65–80.

διαθέσεως ἑτέρας ἐστὶ καὶ σύμπτωμα μηδὲν μηδέπω
ἔχει συνόν, ἑτέραν οἴονται⁷ ποιεῖσθαι τὴν ἔνδειξιν τοῦ
παλαιοῦ· τὸ δ᾽ οὐχ οὕτως ἔχει. τὸ γὰρ αὐτὸ τοῦτο
μόνον ἕλκος· ἔστι δὲ τοιοῦτον ᾧ μήτε κοιλότης τις
σύνεστι μήτ᾽ ὀδύνη μήτε ῥύπος, ἁπασῶν τε τῶν ἄλλων ἀπήλλακται διαθέσεων, αὐτῆς δὲ μόνης δεῖται
τῆς ἰδίας ἰάσεως, ἧς ὁ σκοπὸς ἔνωσις, ἢ κόλλησις,
ἢ σύμφυσις, ἢ συνέχεια. μυριάκις γὰρ εἴρηται τὸ
καλεῖν ὡς ἂν ἐθέλῃ τις, ἔνθα μηδὲν βλάπτεται τὸ
πρᾶγμα. εἴτ᾽ οὖν πρόσφατον εἴη τὸ τοιοῦτον ἕλκος
εἴτε παλαιόν, ἀεὶ τῆς αὐτῆς δεῖται θεραπείας, οὐδὲν
τῆς ἀπὸ τοῦ χρόνου διαφορᾶς ἴδιον ἐνδεικνυμένης. εἰ
μέντοι κοιλότητα βαθεῖαν ἔχει κατακεκρυμμένην ὑπὸ
229K τῷ δέρματι, | σκέπτεσθαι⁸ πότερον ἐκ τῶν ἄνωθεν
μερῶν εἴη, ὡς ὑπορρεῖν ἐξ αὐτῆς τοὺς ἰχῶρας κατάν-
τεις, ἢ κάτωθεν, ὡς αὐτόθι συνίστασθαι.

τῶν μὲν οὖν ὑπορρύσεις ἐχόντων ἡ αὐτὴ θεραπεία
τοῖς ἄλλοις, τῶν δ᾽ οὐκ ἐχόντων ἡμᾶς χρὴ μηχανᾶ-
σθαί τινας ἐκροάς· διττὴ δ᾽ ἡ μηχανή· ποτὲ μὲν ἀνα-
τέμνοντί σοι τὴν κοιλότητα σύμπασαν, ἐνίοτε δὲ ἀντι-
διαιροῦντι μόνον ἐν τῷ πυθμένι. τὸ δ᾽ ὅτε χρὴ τούτων
ἑκάτερον δρᾶν ἥ τε τῶν χωρίων ἐνδείξεται φύσις καὶ
τὸ τοῦ ἕλκους μέγεθος. εἰ μὲν γὰρ καὶ τὰ χωρία
σφαλερὰν ἔχει τὴν διαίρεσιν καὶ τὸ ἕλκος εἴη μέγα,
βέλτιον ἀντιδιαιρεῖν, εἰ δὲ τἀναντία, τὸ ἀνατέμνειν
ἄμεινον. ἡ δ᾽ ἐπίδεσις ἀρχέσθω μὲν ἐκ τῶν ἄνωθεν,

---

⁷ B (cf. putant KLat); οἷόν τε K

exists without another condition and doesn't yet have any symptom combined with it, produces an indication that is different from a wound that is long-standing. But this is not the case. It is itself a wound pure and simple. It is such that there is no hollowness present with it, nor pain, nor filthiness, and it is free from all other conditions and requires the specific cure of itself alone, of which the aim is union, conglutination, growing together, and [restoration of] continuity. For I have said countless times that you may call something whatever you wish when it causes no harm to the matter. Whether such a wound is recent or long-standing, it always needs the same treatment; the differentia based on time indicates nothing specific. If, however, it has a deep cavity that has been hidden under the skin, consider whether it involves superficial parts, in which case the ichors flow out in a downward direction from it, or involves deep parts, in which case they remain on the spot.

229K

For those [wounds], then, which have flow downward, the treatment is the same as for the others, whereas for those that do not, we need to contrive some outflow. The contriving is of two kinds: sometimes it is [achieved] by cutting open the cavity in its entirety, and sometimes simply by making a counter-incision in the base. The nature of the places and the size of the wound indicate when you should do each of these things. If the places also make division dangerous and the wound is large, it is better to make a counter-incision. If the opposite applies, laying open is better. However, the bandaging must begin in the parts

---

8 BK; ⟨χρή⟩ *fort.* nos (*cf.* oportet KLat)

τελευτάτω δὲ κάτω ἵνα περ ἡ ἐκροή. ὅτι δὲ καὶ ἡ παρὰ
τὰ τετρωμένα μόρια σύμπαντα διαφορὰ τῶν ἑλκῶν
ἐπικαιροτάτη πρὸς ἔνδειξιν τῆς ἰάσεως ἔμπροσθεν
εἴρηται. ἀλλ' ἐκείνη μὲν ὡς ὁμοιομερῶν, ἧς δὲ νῦν
ἐμνημονεύσαμεν, ὡς ὀργανικῶν ἐστιν ἔνδειξις. εἰρήσεται μὲν δὴ καὶ περὶ τῆς ἢ ὡς ὁμοιομερῶν, ἢ ὡς
ὀργανικῶν σωμάτων ἐνδείξεως ἐπὶ πλέον ἐν τοῖς ἑξῆς·

230K   ἐν δὲ τῷ παρόντι πάλιν ἐπὶ τὰς | οἰκείας διαφορὰς
τῶν ἑλκῶν ἰτέον· εἶτ' ἐγκάρσιον ἢ εὐθύ, καὶ μέχρι
βάθους ἢ ἐπιπολῆς, καὶ μικρὸν ἢ μέγα διοριστέον. τὰ
μὲν γὰρ ἐγκάρσια διὰ τὸ τὰ χείλη μᾶλλον αὐτῶν
διεστηκέναι τε καὶ ἀφεστηκέναι τῆς συναγωγῆς ἀκρι-
βεστέρας δεῖται· ὥστε καὶ ῥαφαῖς καὶ ἀγκτῆρσιν ἐπὶ
τούτων χρηστέον. ὅσα δὲ κατὰ τὰ μῆκος τῶν μυῶν
ἐγένετο, ταῦτ' ἐκ δυοῖν ἀρχῶν ἐπιδῶν οὔτε ῥαφῶν οὔτε
ἀγκτήρων δεήσῃ. εἰ δ' ἄλλως ἐπιδεῖν ἐθελήσαις ἢ
ἀγκτῆρσιν καὶ ῥαφαῖς, ἀρκέσουσιν ἢ ἐλάχισται παντελῶς αἱ ῥαφαί. καὶ τὰ μὲν μεγάλα τῶν ἑλκῶν ἐπὶ
μᾶλλον ξηραίνουσι θεραπεύσεις φαρμάκοις, εἴ τι τῶν
ἔμπροσθεν εἰρημένων μέμνησαι· τὰ δὲ σμικρὰ καὶ τὸ
μετρίως ξηραῖνον αὐτάρκως ἰάσεται. τὰ δ' εἰς βάθος
διήκοντα πάντως μὲν ἤδη καὶ μεγάλα δεῖται δὲ τῆς ἐκ
δυοῖν ἀρχῶν ἐπιδέσεως καὶ τοῦ μὴ προπετῶς κολληθῆναι τὰ χείλη· τὰ δ' εἰς βάθος τε καὶ μῆκος ἐπὶ πολὺ
προήκοντα διχῇ τ' ἂν εἴη μεγάλα καὶ διττὴν ἔχει τὴν
ἔνδειξιν, ὡς καὶ τῶν πάνυ ξηραινόντων δεῖσθαι φαρ-
231K μάκων, καὶ μὴ συνάγεσθαι προπετῶς τὰ χείλη | καὶ ἐκ
δυοῖν ἀρχῶν ἐπιδεῖσθαι καὶ ῥάπτεσθαι διὰ βάθους.

348

above and finish at those below where the outflow is. It has been stated previously that the differentia which pertains to all the wounded parts is most advantageous as an indication of the cure. But in the case of *homoiomerous* [parts], that [differentia] which I just now called to mind is an indication, as in the case of organic [parts]. Still more will also be said, of course, in what follows about the indication as pertaining to either *homoiomeres* or to organic bodies.

For the present, we must again go to the specific differentiae of wounds. We must distinguish whether [the wound] is oblique or straight, and whether it extends deeply or is superficial, and whether it is small or large. For oblique [wounds], because their margins are more separated and apart, require greater precision in being apposed, so that we should use both sutures and fibulae in these cases. However, for those wounds that occur in the long axis of the muscles, when you bind these from the two ends, you will need neither sutures nor fibulae. If you do wish to bind otherwise, either with fibulae or sutures, the least number of sutures in total will suffice. Larger wounds you will treat with medications that dry out more, if you recall something of what was previously said. Those that are small, moderate drying will cure sufficiently. Those that penetrate completely to the depths and have already become noticeably large need to be bound from the two ends and not to have the margins prematurely conglutinated. On the other hand, those that are both deep and very long, as they are big in two directions, have also a twofold indication; that is, they require strong drying medications and not to have the margins brought together prematurely, and they require to be bound from the two ends and sutured

230K

231K

οὕτω δὲ κἂν εἰ πολλὰς ἐπιπεπλεγμένας ἴδοις διαφοράς, ἑκάστην ἰδίαν ἔνδειξιν ἔχουσαν, εἰ μὲν μὴ
μάχοιντο, πάσαις χρῆσθαι κράτιστον· εἰ δέ πῃ καὶ
διαφέροιντο, πῶς χρὴ διορίζεσθαι περὶ τῶν τοιούτων
εἴρηται μέν που κἀν τοῖς ἔμπροσθεν, εἰρήσεται δὲ κἀν
τοῖς ἐφεξῆς ἐπιπλέον. ἤδη γάρ μοι καιρὸς εἶναι δοκεῖ
καταπαύειν ἐνταυθοῖ τὸ τρίτον τῶνδε τῶν ὑπομνημάτων. ἐν δὲ τῷ μετ᾽ αὐτὸ τετάρτῳ περὶ τῶν ἅμα τοῖς
ἕλκεσιν ὡς τὸ πολὺ γινομένων διαθέσεων ὁ λόγος
ἡμῖν ἔσται. συναναγράψωμεν δ᾽ αὐταῖς καὶ τὰς τῶν
προηγουμένων αἰτίων θεραπείας.

deeply. Thus, even if you see many differentiae intermingled, each having a specific indication, if they are not conflicting, it is best to use all of them. If, however, they also differ in some way, how we must distinguish among them was spoken of to some extent in what has gone before and will be expanded on in what follows. For already it seems to me timely to bring the third of these books to an end here. In the fourth, after this one, my discussion will deal with conditions arising frequently in conjunction with wounds. Along with these, I shall write about the treatments of the *proegoumenic* (internal antecedent) causes.

ΒΙΒΛΙΟΝ Δ

1. Ἕν τι γένος ἦν νόσου καὶ ἡ τῆς συνεχείας λύσις, ἐν ἅπασι μὲν τοῦ ζῴου τοῖς μέρεσι γινομένη, προσαγορευομένη δ' οὐχ ὡσαύτως ἐν ἅπασιν. ἕλκος μὲν γὰρ ἐν σαρκώδει μορίῳ, κάταγμα δ' ἐν ὀστῷ, σπάσμα δ' ἐν νεύρῳ καλεῖται. τούτου δὲ τοῦ γένους ἐστὶ καὶ τὸ ἀπόσπασμα καὶ τὸ ῥῆγμα καὶ τὸ θλάσμα, τὸ μὲν ἐν συνδέσμῳ γινόμενον, τὰ δ' ἐν ἀγγείοις τε καὶ μυσὶν ἐκ βιαίας πληγῆς ἢ καταπτώσεως ἤ τινος ἑτέρας ἰσχυρᾶς κινήσεως. ἡ δ' ἐκχύμωσις ὡς τὰ πολλὰ μὲν ἅμα τῷ θλασθῆναί τε καὶ ῥαγῆναι γίνεται, συμπίπτει δέ |

ποτε καὶ κατὰ ἀναστόμωσιν ἀγγείων καὶ τὴν καλουμένην ὑπό τινων διαπήδησιν, ἕτερόν τι γένος συνεχείας λύσεως ὑπάρχουσαν τηνικαῦτα. καὶ μὴν καὶ κατὰ ἀνάβρωσιν ἐνίοτε διαφθείρεται τὸ συνεχὲς ἐν τοῖς τοῦ ζῴου μέρεσιν· ἀλλ' ἤδη μικτὴ διάθεσις τοῦτο· συνεφάπτεται γὰρ ἑτέρου γένους νοσήματος, ὑπὸ τὸ ποσὸν τῶν μορίων πεπτωκότος· ὥσπερ ἐπὶ τῶν κοίλων

---

[1] The Greek terms are given primacy in this opening statement. Subsequently, the English terms in brackets are used and where there is more than one possibility, context determines

BOOK IV

1. There is one particular class of diseases, dissolution of continuity, which, although it occurs in all parts of the organism, is not similarly named in them all. Thus, it is called *helkos* (wound, ulcer, sore) in a fleshy part, *katagma* (fracture) in a bone and rupture in a *neuron* (nerve, sinew, tendon). *Apospasma* (avulsion), *rhēgma* (laceration) and *thlasma* (bruising)[1] are also of this class, the former occurring in tendons and the latter two in vessels and muscles from a violent blow, or a falling down, or some other strong movement. Ecchymosis occurs along with bruising and rupture in many instances. However this happens, whether from anastomosis of vessels or from what is called *diapedesis* by some, it is another class of dissolution of continuity under these circumstances.[2] And further, sometimes the continuity in the parts of the organism is destroyed by erosion, but this is already a mixed condition, being connected with another class of disease since it falls under the quantity of the parts, as I showed previously in

232K

233K

which is used. See also section 6, on terminology, and section 9, on diseases and symptoms in the Introduction.

[2] These two terms, *anastomosis* and *diapedesis*, are both still in use. *Anastomosis* has, however, a quite different meaning now. Linacre has "by an opening of the mouths of vessels"; see his p. 172.

ἑλκῶν ἔμπροσθεν ἐδείκνυμεν. ἔστι γὰρ οὖν καὶ αὐτῶν
τούτων ἡ γένεσις διττή, ποτὲ μὲν ἐκ περιαιρέσεως
ἀποτελουμένη, ποτὲ δὲ ἐξ ἀναβρώσεως· ἀλλ᾽ ἡ μὲν
περιαίρεσις ὅπως γίνεται πρόδηλον· ἡ δὲ ἀνάβρωσις
εἰ μὲν ἔνδοθεν ἐξ αὐτοῦ τοῦ ζῴου τὴν γένεσιν ἔχει,
χυμῶν ἐστι μοχθηρῶν ἔγγονος· εἰ δὲ ἔξωθεν, ἐπὶ
φαρμάκοις ἢ πυρὶ συνίσταται. καὶ δὴ καὶ προσέχειν
χρὴ τὸν νοῦν, ὥσπερ καὶ πρόσθεν ἐλέγετο, καὶ διορίζεσθαι τὰς ἁπλᾶς διαθέσεις τῶν ἐπιπεπλεγμένων·
ἁπλῆν μὲν γὰρ ἐφ᾽ ἁπλῷ νοσήματι καὶ τὴν θεραπείαν,
οὐχ ἁπλῆν δὲ ἐπὶ συνθέτῳ ποιεῖσθαι προσῆκον. ἥτις
μὲν οὖν ἐστι μέθοδος ἐπὶ ταῖς τῶν συνθέτων ἰάσεσιν
ἔμπροσθεν εἴρηται. χρὴ δ᾽ οὐ τὸ καθόλου μόνον αὐτῆς
234K   ἐκμαθεῖν, ἀλλὰ κἂν τοῖς | κατὰ μέρος γεγυμνάσθαι.

καὶ γὰρ οὖν κἂν τούτοις ἑτέρων ἐστὶ χρεία μεθόδων
πολλῶν ὡς ἂν εἴποι τις μερικῶν· ἐφ᾽ ἑκάστου γὰρ
εἴδους νοσήματος ἴδιον εἶδός ἐστι μεθόδου. πάλιν οὖν
ὅσον ὑπόλοιπόν ἐστι τῆς τῶν ἑλκῶν ἰάσεως, ἐν τῷδε
τῷ γράμματι λεγέσθω τὴν ἀρχὴν ἡμῖν ἐνθένδε ποιη-
σαμένοις. ἕλκος ἅπαν ἤτοι μόνον ἐστὶν αὐτὸ καθ᾽
ἑαυτό, μήτε συνεισβαλούσης αὐτῷ διαθέσεως ἑτέρας
μήτε προηγησαμένης μήτε ἀκολουθησάσης, ἢ μετά
τινος ἑτέρας ἤτοι μιᾶς ἢ καὶ πλειόνων συνίσταται. καὶ
τούτων τῶν διαθέσεων ἔνιαι μὲν οὐ μόνον εὐθὺς ἐξ
ἀρχῆς ἐποιήσαντο ἕλκος, ἀλλὰ καὶ νῦν ἔτι καὶ μεῖζον
ἐργάζονται· τινὲς δὲ τὸν ὦν οὐκ ἄνευ λόγον ἔχουσιν
ὡς πρὸς τὴν ἴασιν· ἀλλὰ περὶ μὲν τούτων εἴρηται
πρόσθεν, ὑπὲρ δὲ τῶν μεῖζον ἐργαζομένων τὸ ἕλκος ἐν

the case of hollow wounds and ulcers.[3] The genesis of these is twofold, brought about in part by a stripping away, and in part by erosion. How the stripping away occurs is clear. However, the erosion, if it has its genesis from within the organism itself, is a by-product of bad humors whereas, if its genesis is external, it arises from medications or fire. Furthermore, as I also said before, it is necessary to direct attention to distinguishing the simple conditions from those that are compound for, in a simple disease, it is appropriate to also make the treatment simple, while in a compound disease it is not appropriate to make the treatment simple. What the method is in regard to the cures of compound diseases was spoken of earlier. Not only is it necessary to learn this thoroughly in general terms, but also to become practiced in it in individual cases.

234K

Even in these cases there is the need for many other methods which are, one might say, particular, in that there is a specific kind of method for each kind of disease. Therefore, let me again say whatever remains to be said about the cure of a wound, making a start from here, in this book. Every wound either exists by itself alone, there being no other condition appearing together with it, or preceding or following it, or it coexists with some other condition, either one or more. And some of these conditions not only produce a wound right from the start but also make it still larger, while some have the ground of *sine qua non* in respect of the cure. But I spoke about these earlier. In this [book] I shall speak about those things that make the

3 Book 3 above.

τῷδε λεχθήσεται. διττὸς μὲν οὖν ὁ ἐπ' αὐτῶν σκοπός,
ἢ ἐκκόψαι τελείως ἐκ τοῦ σώματος τὰς τοιαύτας διαθέσεις, ἢ νικῆσαι τὴν ἀπ' αὐτῶν βλάβην. ἀλλὰ τοῦτο
μὲν ἐπειδὰν σμικρὰ παντελῶς ἡ διάθεσις ὑπάρχῃ,
δυνατὸν ἐργάσασθαι· μεγάλης δ' οὔσης τὸ ἕλκος εἰς
οὐλὴν ἀγαγεῖν οὐκ ἐνδέχεται, πρὶν ἐκείνην ἰάσασθαι. |

235K τίνες οὖν αἱ τοιαῦται διαθέσεις καὶ πόσαι σκεπτέον
ἡμῖν ἀκριβῶς ἐνθένδε ποθὲν ἀρξαμένοις ὅθεν κἀν τοῖς
ἔμπροσθεν ἠρξάμεθα. πᾶν ἕλκος, εἴτε μετὰ κοιλότητος εἴτε καὶ μόνον ὑπάρχει, τῆς θ' ὑποκειμένης
σαρκὸς δεῖται κατὰ φύσιν ἐχούσης καὶ μηδενὸς
μεταξὺ παρεμπίπτοντος εἰς τὰ κολληθησόμενα χείλη,
καθάπερ πολλάκις γίνεται, τρίχα καὶ ψάμμον καὶ
ῥύπον, ἔλαιόν τε καί τι τοιοῦτον ἕτερον ἐμποδίσαι τὴν
κόλλησιν, ἀλλὰ ταῦτα μὲν οἷον συμπτώματά τινα τῶν
ἑλκῶν ἐστι, κωλῦσαι μὲν ὁπότε παρείη τὴν ἴασιν
δυνάμενα, ποιῆσαι δ', εἰ μὴ παρείη, μὴ δυνάμενα.

τῆς δ' ὑποκειμένης σαρκὸς ἡ διάθεσις αἰτίας λόγον
ἔχει πρὸς τὸ γινόμενον· ἐξ αὐτῆς γὰρ καὶ δι' αὐτὴν ἥ
τε κόλλησις τῶν διεστώτων καὶ ἡ σάρκωσις τῶν
κοίλων γίνεται. χρὴ τοίνυν ταύτην ἀκριβῶς κατὰ
φύσιν ἔχειν, ἵν' ἑκάτερον ἐκείνων ἀμέμπτως ἐπιτελῆ-
ται· τὸ καλῶς δ' ἔχειν αὐτὴν κατὰ τὴν οἰκείαν ὑπάρχει
κρᾶσιν, ὥσπερ καὶ τοῖς ἄλλοις ἅπασιν. εὔκρατον μὲν
οὖν ἀκριβῶς εἶναι προσήκει τὴν ὑποκειμένην σάρκα
πρὸς κόλλησίν τε καὶ σάρκωσιν ἑλκῶν. ἆρ' οὖν ἀρκεῖ

236K τοῦτο μόνον, | ἢ καὶ τὸ ἐπιρρέον αἷμα χρηστὸν καὶ
σύμμετρον εἶναι χρή; ἐμοὶ μὲν καὶ τοῦτο παντὸς

wound larger. There is a twofold aim regarding these: either to completely eradicate such conditions from the body or to overcome the harm arising from them. At least whenever the condition is in all respects small, this can be achieved. However, when it is large, it is not possible to bring the wound to a scar before that condition is cured. Therefore, we must carefully consider what such condi- 235K tions are, and how many there are, starting with those we started with before. Every wound, whether it exists with a cavity or alone, needs the underlying flesh to be in accord with nature, and for there to be nothing lying between the margins to be conglutinated, as often happens when hair, sand, dirt, oil, or some other such thing hinders the conglutination. But these things are, as it were, symptoms of the wounds which, when present, are able to prevent the cure —something they can't do if they are not present.

The condition of the underlying flesh has the ground of cause in relation to what happens, for it is both from this and due to this that either the conglutination of separated [margins] or the enfleshing of cavities occurs. Therefore, it is necessary for this [underlying] flesh to be exactly in accord with nature so that each of those things is faultlessly accomplished. But to be right is for it to have its proper *krasis* just as it also is for all other things. Therefore, it is appropriate for the underlying flesh to be precisely *eukratic* in respect of the conglutination and enfleshing of wounds. Is this alone enough or must the blood which 236K flows in be good for its purpose and in due proportion? What seems to me to be true above all is that blood which

μᾶλλον ἀληθὲς εἶναι δοκεῖ· τό τε γὰρ διεφθαρμένον
αἷμα τοσοῦτον ἀποδεῖ πρὸς κόλλησιν ἢ γένεσιν σαρκὸς ἐπιτήδειον ὑπάρχειν, ὥστ' αὐτὸ πολλάκις ἀναβι-
βρώσκειν καὶ ἑλκοῦν τὸ σῶμα· τό τε πολὺ πλάδον ἐν
τοῖς ἡλκωμένοις περιττὸν ἐργαζόμενον ἐμποδὼν ἵσταται ταῖς ἰάσεσιν, ὥς που καὶ πρόσθεν ἐδείκνυτο. καὶ
τρεῖς οὗτοι τρόποι τῶν δυσιάτων ἑλκῶν ἐοίκασιν ὑπ-
άρχειν· ὅ τ' ἐκ τῆς δυσκρασίας τῆς ὑποκειμένης σαρκὸς καὶ ὁ ἐκ τῆς μοχθηρίας τοῦ τ' ἐπιρρέοντος αἵματος, καὶ τρίτος ὁ ἐκ τῆς ποσότητος. ἢ οὐχ ὧδε χρὴ τὴν
διαίρεσιν, ἀλλ' ὡδὶ ποιήσασθαι μᾶλλον; ὡς τῶν δυσιάτων ἑλκῶν τὰ μὲν διὰ τὴν δυσκρασίαν τῆς ἡλκωμένης σαρκός, τὰ δὲ διὰ τὸν ἐπιρρέοντα χυμὸν γίνεται
τοιαῦτα· καὶ ὡς τῆς μὲν δυσκρασίας δύο ἔστωσαν
διαφοραί, ποτὲ μὲν ταῖς ποιότησι μόναις οὐ κατὰ
φύσιν ἐχούσης τῆς ὑποκειμένης σαρκός, ἐνίοτε δὲ καὶ
μετ' ὄγκου τινὸς ἐπικτήτου. τῆς δ' ἐπιρροῆς ἕτεραι
δύο, τό τε ποσὸν καὶ τὸ ποιὸν τῶν ἐπιρρεόντων χυμῶν·
237K ἐνίοτε δὲ καὶ μίγνυσθαι συμβέβηκέ | τινας τῶν εἰρη-
μένων διαθέσεων, ἢ καὶ πάσας ἅμα. χρὴ δ' οὐ πασῶν
δήπουθεν ἅμα λέγεσθαι τὴν μέθοδον τῆς ἰάσεως, ἀλλ'
ἑκάστης ἰδίᾳ.

2. Τῆς μὲν οὖν σαρκὸς αὐτῆς ἰάσῃ τὴν δυσκρασίαν, εἰ μὲν αὐχμώδης καὶ ξηρὰ φαίνοιτο, τέγγων
εὐκράτῳ πολλάκις ὕδατι. καθ' ἑκάστην δὲ χρῆσιν ὁ
σκοπὸς ἔστω σοι τῆς καταντλήσεως, ὅταν πρῶτον εἰς
ἔρευθός τε καὶ ὄγκον αἴρηται τὸ μόριον, ἀφίστασθαι
τηνικαῦτα· διαφορήσεις γὰρ ὁ εἵλκυσας καταιονῶν

is corrupted is so lacking in terms of being useful for conglutination and the generation of flesh that it itself often erodes and ulcerates the body. Also, the abundant humor existing in the wounded parts acts as a hindrance to the cures by creating a superfluity, as was also shown somewhere before.[4] And these appear to be the three kinds of wounds that are difficult to cure: one because of a *dyskrasia* of the underlying flesh, one because of a bad quality of the inflowing blood, and a third because of the quantity [of the inflow]. Or should we not make such a division, but rather the following? That among wounds that are difficult to heal, there are those that are due to the *dyskrasia* of the wounded flesh and those that are due to the inflowing humor, and that there must be two differentiae of the *dyskrasia*: at one time when the underlying flesh is not in accord with nature by the qualities alone, and at another time with some added swelling. And there are two other differentiae of the flow in respect of the quantity and quality of the inflowing humors. Sometimes it happens that 237K some of the aforementioned conditions are mixed, or all of them at the same time. It is presumably not necessary to state the method of cure of all of these conditions at once, but of each individually.

2. You may cure the *dyskrasia* of the flesh itself, if it appears parched and dry, by moistening it frequently with *eukratic* water. In each such use let your indicator to stop perfusion be the time when the part is first raised to redness and swelling because, if you perfuse further, you will disperse what you have attracted. As a result, you will

4 See Book 2, 117–18K.

ἐπιπλέον· ὥστ᾽ οὐδὲν ἔσται σοι πλέον. ἀλλὰ καὶ τῶν
φαρμάκων ἡ δύναμις ὑγροτέρα τις ἔστω τῆς ἔμπροσθεν ἐπὶ τῆς ὑγιοῦς σαρκὸς παρηνημένης· εἰ δ᾽
ὑγροτέρα τοῦ κατὰ φύσιν ἡ σὰρξ φαίνοιτο, τὰ ἐναντία
ποιητέον, ἐπιτείνοντα μὲν τῶν φαρμάκων τὴν δύναμιν
ἐπὶ τὸ ξηρότερον, ὕδατι δὲ μηδ᾽ ὅλως χρώμενον· ἀλλ᾽
εἰ καὶ ἀποπλῦναι δέοι τὸ ἕλκος, οἶνος, ἢ ὀξύκρατον,
ἢ ἀφέψημα πόας αὐστηρᾶς παρασκευαζέσθω. κατὰ
ταῦτα δὲ τὴν μὲν θερμοτέραν τοῦ δέοντος σάρκα
ψυκτέον, τὴν δὲ ψυχροτέραν θερμαντέον. ἔσται δὲ
ἑκατέρα δήλη καὶ χροιᾷ καὶ ἁφῇ καὶ τῇ τοῦ κάμνοντος
238K   αἰσθήσει· | ποτὲ μὲν γὰρ πυρώσεως ὁμολογοῦσιν
αἰσθάνεσθαι, ποτὲ δ᾽ ἐπιδήλου τινὸς ψύξεως κατὰ τὸ
μόριον· καὶ χαίρουσιν ἢ τοῖς ψυχροῖς φαρμάκοις ἢ
τοῖς θερμοῖς· καὶ τοῖς μὲν ἐρύθημα λεπτὸν ἐπανθεῖ,
τοῖς δὲ ἐπὶ τὸ λευκότερον ἡ χροιά. ταυτὶ μὲν οὖν οὐ
τῆς παρούσης ἐστὶ πραγματείας διορίζειν· οὐ γὰρ
διαγνωστικὴν μέθοδον, ἀλλὰ θεραπευτικὴν ἐνεστη-
σάμεθα· τῇ δὲ ἀκολουθίᾳ πως τοῦ λόγου συνεξέδρα-
μεν· αὖθις οὖν ἐπανέλθωμεν ἐφ᾽ ἅπερ ἐξ ἀρχῆς προὐθέμεθα.

τῶν σὺν ὄγκῳ τινὶ παρὰ φύσιν ἡλκωμένων μορίων
ἰᾶσθαι χρὴ πρότερον τὸν ὄγκον· ἥτις δὲ τῶν παρὰ
φύσιν ἐστὶν ὄγκων ἁπάντων ἴασις ἐν τοῖς ἑξῆς εἰρή-
σεται· νυνὶ δ᾽ ὅσον ἐξ αὐτῶν συνῆπται τῇ τῶν ἑλκῶν
θεραπείᾳ ῥητέον. ἐπειδὰν τὰ χείλη μόνα τῶν ἑλκῶν
ἐπὶ πλέον ἀχροίας ἢ σκληρότητος ἥκοι, περιτέμνειν

achieve nothing more. But also, let the potency of the medications be somewhat more moist than previously advised in the case of healthy flesh. If, however, the flesh seems more moist than normal, you must do the opposite, increasing the potency of the medications to a greater dryness, using no water at all. But if the wound or ulcer does need to be washed, prepare wine, oxykraton,[5] or a decoction of an astringent herb. On the same basis, you must cool flesh that is hotter than it should be and heat flesh that is colder. Each will be clear from the color and feel [of the flesh] and from the perception of the patient, for sometimes patients admit to a feeling of burning, and sometimes of unusual coldness in the part, and they will welcome either cold or hot medications respectively. In some a slight redness appears on the surface, while in others the skin color is whiter. These are not, however, distinctions to be made in the present treatise, for I am not establishing a diagnostic method but a therapeutic one. I have, to some extent, gone off at a tangent in the discussion. Therefore, let me return once more to the matters I raised at the beginning.

238K

When parts are ulcerated in association with some abnormal swelling, it is necessary to cure the swelling first. What the cure of all unnatural swellings is, I shall speak about in what follows. In this discussion now I must speak about as much of these as is connected to the treatment of ulcers.[6] Only when the margins of the ulcer reach a greater degree of decoloration and hardness is it necessary to ex-

---

5 Described in L&S (under posca) as "an acidulous drink of vinegar and water"; see Pliny *HN*, 27.4.12 #29 and the *OED*, where there is reference to this passage.

6 "Ulcer" is now used instead of "wound" for *helkos* as the discussion has moved on to obviously chronic lesions.

αὐτὰ χρὴ μέχρι τῆς ὑγιοῦς σαρκός· ἐπειδὰν δὲ καὶ
μέχρι πλέονος ἡ διάθεσις ἐκτείνηται, σκέψις ἐνταῦθα
γίνεται πότερα περικοπτέον ἅπαν τὸ παρὰ φύσιν
ἐστίν, ἢ θεραπευτέον ἐν χρόνῳ. καὶ δῆλον ὡς καὶ τῇ
239K τοῦ κάμνοντος εἰς τοῦτο προσχρῆσθαι | δεῖ προθυμίᾳ·
τινὲς μὲν γὰρ ἐν χρόνῳ πλέονι θεραπεύεσθαι βούλονται χωρὶς τομῆς· ἔνιοι δὲ πᾶν ὁτιοῦν ὑπομένειν
εἰσὶν ἕτοιμοι τοῦ θᾶττον ὑγιᾶναι χάριν. οὕτω δὲ κἀπὶ
τῶν ἐπιρρεόντων τοῖς ἡλκωμένοις μέρεσι μοχθηρῶν
χυμῶν ἡ μὲν ὡς ἡλκωμένων ἴασις ἐν τῷδε λελέξεται, ἡ
δ᾽ ὡς κακοχυμίας ἢ πλήθους ἐν τοῖς ἰδίοις ἐκείνων
λογισμοῖς. ὅταν οὖν ὀλίγῳ τε πλείω καὶ μὴ πολλῷ
φαυλότερος ᾖ τοῦ κατὰ φύσιν ὁ ἐπιρρέων τοῖς ἡλκωμένοις χυμός, ἀποτρέπειν αὐτὸν καὶ ἀναστέλλειν
προσήκει, στύφοντά τε καὶ ψύχοντα τὰ πρὸ τῶν ἡλκωμένων χωρία. χρὴ δὲ καὶ τὴν ἐπίδεσιν ἄρχεσθαι μὲν
ἀπὸ τοῦ πεπονθότος, ἐπινέμεσθαι δὲ ἐπὶ τὸ ὑγιές, ὡς
ἐν Τοῖς κατάγμασιν ἐκέλευσεν ὁ Ἱπποκράτης. ἀλλὰ
καὶ τὰ τοῖς ἕλκεσιν αὐτοῖς προσαγόμενα φάρμακα
ξηραντικώτερα τῶν τοῖς ἁπλοῖς ἕλκεσι προσαγομένων ὑπαρχέτω.

μὴ δυναμένης δὲ ὑπὸ φαρμάκων κρατηθῆναι τῆς
ἐπιρροῆς τὴν αἰτίαν αὐτῆς ἐπισκεψάμενον, ἐκείνην
ἐκκόπτειν πρότερον. εἰ μὲν οὖν δι᾽ ἀτονίαν τινὰ τοῦ
δεχομένου τὸ ῥεῦμα μορίου τοῦτο συμβαίνει, ταύτην
240K ἰατέον· εἴη δ᾽ ἂν ἔτι τοῦτο τῶν ἡλκωμένων | μορίων

cise them as far as healthy flesh. When the condition extends further, the issue arises as to whether you must excise everything that is contrary to nature, or treat over a period of time. On this point it is clear that you also need to 239K take into account the wishes of the patient, in that some want to be treated over a longer time without excision, while some are prepared to submit to anything at all for the sake of a more rapid return to health. The cure of bad humors flowing into the ulcerated parts as ulcerating agents has been addressed in this work; the cure of *kakochymia* and abundance as ulcerating agents has been addressed in the specific considerations of those [conditions].[7] Whenever the humor flowing into the ulcerated parts is not very much more in amount and not much worse than normal, it is appropriate to divert and repel it by contracting and cooling the places lying before those that are ulcerated. And it is necessary to start the binding from what has been affected and extend it to what is healthy, as Hippocrates directed in *Fractures*.[8] But also, the medications applied to ulcers themselves must be more drying than those applied to simple wounds.

If the flow cannot be controlled by medications, after looking into its cause, eradicate that first. If the flow occurs due to some weakness of the part receiving the flux, you must cure this weakness. Besides, this may be a specific cure for ulcerated parts. If, however, it is due to abundance 240K

[7] See, respectively, *De temperamentis*, I.664K, and *De plenitudine*, VII.547K.   [8] Galen makes several references in this work to the Hippocratic technique of binding or bandaging; see Hippocrates, *Fractures IV* in particular, although bandaging is discussesd throughout that treatise.

οἰκεία τις ἴασις· εἰ δὲ διὰ πλῆθος ἢ κακοχυμίαν ἤτοι
παντὸς τοῦ σώματος ἢ τινος τῶν ὑπερκειμένων μορίων, ἐκεῖνα πρότερον ἐπανορθωτέον. ἡ μὲν οὖν ἀτονία
τοῦ μέρους, δι᾽ ἣν ἐπ᾽ αὐτὸ πλείους τοῦ δέοντος
ἀφικνοῦται χυμοί, πάντως μὲν ἐπὶ δυσκρασίᾳ γίνεται,
οὐ μὴν ἁπάσῃ γε ἕπεται ἀτονία δυσκρασίᾳ· καὶ διὰ
τοῦτο πολλάκις μὲν αὐτὸ τοῦτο μόνον ἡ ἡλκωμένη
σὰρξ δύσκρατός ἐστιν, οὐ μὴν καὶ ἄτονος· ἐνίοτε δ᾽
ἄμφω, δύσκρατός τε ἅμα καὶ ἄρρωστος· αἱ γὰρ ἐπὶ
πλέον[1] ἐκτροπαὶ τῆς δυσκρασίας ἀτονίας εἰσὶν αἰτίαι
τοῖς πεπονθόσιν. ἰατέον δὲ ταύτας, ὡς καὶ πρόσθεν
εἴρηται, τὰς μὲν θερμὰς ψύχοντα, τὰς δὲ ξηρὰς ὑγραίνοντα, καὶ τὰς μὲν ψυχρὰς θερμαίνοντα, τὰς δὲ ὑγρὰς
ξηραίνοντα· καὶ δὴ καὶ κατὰ συζυγίαν εἰ ψυχρότερός
τε ἅμα καὶ ὑγρότερος ὁ τόπος εἴη, θερμαίνοντά τε καὶ
ξηραίνοντα· κἀπὶ τῶν ἄλλων ὡσαύτως, ἀεὶ ταῖς κρα-
τούσαις ποιότησι τὰς ἐναντίας προσάγοντα.

λογισμὸς δὲ τούτου τοιόσδε· τὸ κατωρθωμένον
ἅπαν οὐκ ἐν ζῴοις μόνον ἢ φυτοῖς, ἀλλὰ καὶ τοῖς
ἄλλοις ἅπασι σύμμετρόν τί ἐστι καὶ μέσον ἁπάντων
241K τῶν διημαρτημένων· ὅτου | γὰρ ἂν μήτ᾽ ἀφελεῖν ἔστιν
μήτε προσθεῖναι μηδὲν ἢ μόριον ἢ ποιότητα πάντῃ
τοῦτ᾽ ἀμέμπτως ἔχει· τὸ δ᾽ ἀφαιρέσεως τινος ἢ προσθήκης χρῇζον ἐκπέπτωκε μὲν ἤδη τῆς ἀρίστης κατασκευῆς, ἐπανελθεῖν δ᾽ αὐτὴν ἑτέρως ἀμήχανον αὐτῷ
χωρὶς τοῦ τὸ μὲν περιττὸν ἀφελεῖν, τὸ δὲ ἐλλεῖπον
προσθεῖναι. περὶ μὲν δὴ τῶν μορίοις τισὶν ἐλλειπόν-
των ἢ πλεοναζόντων ἕτερος λόγος·

364

or *kakochymia*, either of the whole body or of one of the overlying parts, you must correct those things first. Weakness of the part, due to which humors come to it in excess of requirements, always arises due to a *dyskrasia*, although weakness does not in fact follow every *dyskrasia*. And because of this, the ulcerated flesh is itself only *dyskratic*, but not also weak. Sometimes, however, it is both; that is, *dyskratic* and weak at the same time. What is more, the deviations are causes of the *dyskratic* weakness in the affected parts. You must cure these, as I said before, by cooling those that are hot, moistening those that are dry, heating those that are cold, and drying those that are moist. Furthermore, in a conjunction, if the place is colder and more moist at the same time, [treat it] by heating and drying, and the same with the other conjunctions, always applying the opposites to the prevailing qualities.

The rationale of this is as follows: every correction of all these qualities that have gone wrong, not only in animals and plants so affected but also in everything else, lies in an equilibrium and balance, for whatever it is impossible to 241K either remove anything from or add anything to, whether it be a part or a quality, is entirely without fault. If, however, it requires some removal or addition, it has already departed from the best constitution, and it is impossible to restore this in one way or another without removing what is in excess or adding what is deficient. In fact, there is another discussion about the deficiencies and excesses in certain parts.[9]

9 See *De morborum causis*, chapter 8, VII.34-35K.

---

1 B; ἐπιπλέον K

ἐν οἷς δὲ ἐπικρατεῖ τις ποιότης, εὐθὺς μὲν ἐνταῦθα
νενικῆσθαι τὴν ἐναντίαν ἀναγκαῖον, εὐθὺς δὲ καὶ τὴν
ἐπανόρθωσιν ἐκ τῆς τέως κεκρατημένης, αὖθις ἀντεισ-
αγομένης ἀνάγκη γίνεσθαι. ψύχων γὰρ τὸ τεθερ-
μασμένον ἅμα μὲν ἀντεισάξεις τὸ λοιπόν, ἅμα δὲ καὶ
καθαρεῖς τὸ πλεονάζον. ὥστε ἀνάγκη πᾶσα τῶν κατὰ
δυσκρασίαν τινὰ τοῦ κατὰ φύσιν ἐξεστηκότων τὴν
ἴασιν γίνεσθαι διὰ τῶν ἐναντίων τῇ δυνάμει· οὕτω μὲν
ἡ δι᾽ ἀτονίαν ὑπὸ ῥεύματος ἐνοχλουμένη σάρξ, ἤ τι
μόριον ἕτερον σαρκῶδες· ἐπειδὰν τὴν τῆς δυσκρασίας
πρότερον ἰαθῇ διάθεσιν, ἐφεξῆς δηλονότι καὶ τὴν τῆς
ἑλκώσεως ἰαθήσεται, οὐκ ἄλλως μὲν νῦν θεραπευ-
242K θεῖσαν² | τὴν δυσκρασίαν, ἄλλως δ᾽ εἰ χωρὶς ἕλκους
ἐπεπόνθει. ᾧ καὶ δῆλον ὡς οὐχ ἕλκους ἐστίν, ἀλλὰ
δυσκρασίας ἴδιος ἡ τοιαύτη πᾶσα θεραπεία. κατὰ δὲ
τὸν αὐτὸν τρόπον, εἰ δι᾽ ἕτερόν τι μόριον ἢ καὶ τὸ
σύμπαν σῶμα πληθωρικὸν ἢ κακόχυμον ὑπάρχον
ἐπιρρέον τι τοῖς ἡλκωμένοις μέρεσι μοχθηρὸν ἰάσασθαι χρὴ πρότερον ἢ τὸ τοῦ ῥεύματος αἴτιον ἢ καὶ τὸ
σύμπαν σῶμα. κατὰ τοῦτ᾽ οὖν καὶ κιρσοὺς πολλάκις
ὑπερκειμένους τῶν ἡλκωμένων μορίων ἰασώμεθα πρότερον, ἵν᾽ ἐφεξῆς ἰασώμεθα τὸ ἕλκος, καὶ τῶν σπλη-
νωδῶν τὸν σπλῆνα καὶ τῶν ἄλλο τι μόριον ἐπίσημον
πεπονθότων ἐκεῖνο πρότερον ἐκθεραπεύσαντες, οὕτως
ἐπὶ τὴν τῶν ἑλκῶν ἴασιν ἀφικόμεθα. ἀλλ᾽ οὐδεμία τῶν
ἰάσεων τούτων αὐτοῦ τοῦ ἕλκους ἐστίν, ἀλλά τινος
ἑτέρας διαθέσεως ἤτοι γεννώσης ἢ αὐξανούσης τὸ
ἕλκος.

366

In those in which some quality prevails, it is here immediately necessary for the opposite to be overcome and, in respect of the restoration of what has been overcome up to that time, it is necessary that this be reintroduced. By cooling what has been heated, you will at one and the same time restore the deficiency and reduce the excess. Consequently, it is absolutely necessary for the cure of those things that have departed from an accord with nature by virtue of a *dyskrasia* to occur through those things that are opposite in capacity. This applies when flesh, or some other fleshy part is afflicted by weakness due to a flux. Whenever you cure the condition of the *dyskrasia* first, what follows, clearly, is that the condition of the ulceration will be cured, although you have treated the *dyskrasia* no differently than if it had occurred apart from ulceration. From this it is also clear that every such treatment is specific, not to the wound or ulcer, but to the *dyskrasia*. In the same way, if something bad is flowing to the ulcerated parts because either some one part or the whole body is *plethoric* or *kakochymous*, it is first necessary to cure the cause of the flux or also the whole body. Therefore, in the same way too, I often cured tortuous veins (varices) overlying the ulcerated parts so that I could next cure the ulcer. And, in the case of people suffering splenic disease, or people in whom some other important part has been affected, when I have first thoroughly treated the spleen, or the part in question, I shall come to the cure of the ulcer. But none of these cures is of the ulcer itself, but of some other condition which either gives rise to, or exacerbates, the ulcer.

242K

---

2 B; θεραπευθεῖσα K

3. Καὶ γὰρ αὖ καὶ τοῦτο καιρὸς διορίσασθαι ἤδη,
τὸ μηδὲν τῶν προκαταρξάντων τῆς διαθέσεως αἰτίων
ἐνδείκνυσθαι τὴν θεραπείαν, ἀλλὰ τὴν μὲν ταύτης
ἔνδειξιν ἀπ᾽ αὐτῆς ἄρχεσθαι τῆς διαθέσεως, ἐξευ-
243K ρίσκεσθαι δὲ | τὰς κατὰ μέρος ἐνεργείας ἀπό τε τοῦ
πρώτου σκοποῦ καὶ τῆς τοῦ πεπονθότος μορίου φύσεως καὶ τῆς τοῦ περιέχοντος κράσεως, ὅσα τε ἄλλα
τούτοις ἐστὶν ὁμογενῆ. συνελόντι γὰρ εἰπεῖν ἀπ᾽
οὐδενὸς τῶν μηκέτι ὄντων ἔνδειξιν τοῦ συμφέροντος
ἔνεστι λαβεῖν. ἀλλ᾽ ἐπεὶ πολλάκις εἰς διάγνωσιν τῆς
διαθέσεως, ἀδήλου παντάπασιν ὑπαρχούσης καὶ τῷ
λόγῳ καὶ ταῖς αἰσθήσεσιν, ἀναγκαζόμεθα πυνθάνε-
σθαι περὶ τοῦ προκατάρξαντος αἰτίου, δόκησις τοῖς
πολλοῖς γίνεται κἀκεῖνο συνενδείκνυσθαι τὴν ἴασιν·
τὸ δ᾽ οὐχ οὕτως ἔχει. μαθήσῃ δ᾽ ἐναργῶς ἐφ᾽ ὧν
ἐγχωρεῖ ἀκριβῶς γνῶναι τὴν διάθεσιν. εἴτε γὰρ ἐκχύμωσις, εἴθ᾽ ἕλκος, εἴτε ἐρυσίπελας, εἴτε σηπεδών, εἴτε
φλεγμονὴ κατά τι μέρος ὑπάρχει, περιττὸν ζητεῖν τὸ
αἴτιον ποιῆσαν, εἰ μὴ καὶ νῦν ἔτι ποιεῖ· οὕτως γὰρ ἅμα
τε τὸ γεγονὸς θεραπεύσομεν ἤδη ἅμα τε τὸ ποιοῦν ἔτι
ποιεῖν διακωλύσομεν. εἰ δ᾽ ἐποίησε μέν, ἀπηλλάγη δέ,
τὸ μὲν γεγονὸς ἰασόμεθα, τὸ δὲ οὐκέτι ὂν οὐδ᾽ ἂν
ἐκκόπτειν προαιρώμεθα, δυνησόμεθα· τῶν μὲν γὰρ
ὄντων αἱ θεραπεῖαι, τῶν δὲ ἔσεσθαι μελλόντων αἱ
244K προφυλακαί· τὰ δὲ μήτ᾽ ὄντα μήτε βλάψαι | προσ-
δοκώμενα καὶ τοῦ θεραπευτικοῦ καὶ τοῦ προφυλακτικοῦ μέρους τῆς τέχνης ἐκπέπτωκεν.

3. It is time now to make this distinction again—that none of the *prokatarktic* causes of the condition indicates the treatment. The indication of treatment starts from the condition itself, while it is discovered in respect of the functions individually from the primary indicator, the nature of the affected part, the *krasis* of the ambient air, and such other things as are cognate with these. In short, it is not possible to take an indication of any value from something that does not still exist. But because, when it comes to a diagnosis of the condition, it is often completely obscure to both reason and the senses, we are compelled to inquire about the *prokatarktic* cause, it being an opinion held by many that this contributes to the indication of the cure. However, this is not so. You will learn clearly from which things it is possible to recognize the condition accurately. If ecchymosis, ulcer, erysipelas, putrefaction, or inflammation exists in some part, it is superfluous to seek the effecting cause, if this is not now still acting. So we shall treat, at one and the same time, what has already occurred, and we shall prevent what is producing it from still acting. If, however, the latter has acted and gone, we shall cure what has occurred, but we shall be unable to eradicate what no longer exists, even if we should wish to do so. Treatments pertain to those things that exist; prophylactic measures pertain to those things that will exist in the future. Those things that neither exist, nor are expected to cause harm, fall outside the scope of both the therapeutic and the prophylactic parts of the craft.

243K

244K

ὥστε οὔτε ἔνδειξις ἀπ᾽ αὐτῶν ἐστιν εἰς θεραπείαν
οὔτε προφυλακή τις, ἀλλ᾽ ἢ μόνον, ὡς εἴρηται, πρὸς
τὰς ἐκπιπτούσας τὴν ἡμετέραν ἐπίγνωσιν διαθέσεις ἡ
γνῶσις τοῦ προκατάρξαντος αἰτίου χρησίμη, τοῖς δ᾽
ἀπὸ τῆς Ἐμπειρίας ἰατροῖς ὡς μέρος τῆς ὅλης συνδρομῆς, ἐφ᾽ ᾗ τετηρήκασι τὴν θεραπείαν καὶ τὸ προκατάρξαν αἴτιον ἐνίοτε προλαμβάνεται, καθάπερ ἐπί
τε τῶν λυττώντων κυνῶν καὶ τῶν ἰοβόλων ἁπάντων
θηρίων, ἤδη δὲ καὶ τῶν Δογματικῶν ἐκείνων, ὅσοι
χωρὶς ἐνδείξεως λογικῆς ἀπὸ τῆς ἐμπειρίας μόνης
ὁμολογοῦσι θεραπεύειν τὰ τοιαῦτα. καὶ γὰρ καὶ τούτοις ὡς ἓν μέρος τῆς ὅλης συνδρομῆς τὸ προκατάρξαν
αἴτιον ζητεῖται, τοῖς δ᾽ ἐκ μὲν τῆς ἔμπροσθεν πείρας
ἐγνωκόσι τῶν ἰοβόλων θηρίων τὰς δυνάμεις, ἔνδειξιν
δὲ θεραπείας ἀπ᾽ αὐτῶν λαμβάνουσιν, οὐκ εἰς ἔνδειξιν
ἰάσεως τὸ προκατάρξαν αἴτιον γνωσθέν, ἀλλ᾽ εἰς τὴν
τῆς παρούσης διαθέσεως ἐπίγνωσιν συντελεῖ.

φέρε γὰρ ἐπίστασθαι μὲν τὸν ἰὸν τοῦ σκορπίου
ψυχρὸν εἶναι τῇ δυνάμει καὶ λαμβάνειν ὡς ἀπὸ ψυ-
245K χροῦ | τὴν τῆς ἰάσεως ἔνδειξιν, ἔχειν δὲ μηδὲν μή πω
σημεῖον ὅτι τοιαύτη τις ἐν τῷδε τῷ σώματι διάθεσις
ὑπάρχει, δῆλον γὰρ ὡς εἰ πυθοίμην ὅτι σκορπίος ὁ
πλήξας, ἐκθερμαίνειν πειράσομαι τό τε σύμπαν σῶμα
καὶ τὸ νενυγμένον ὑπ᾽ αὐτοῦ μόριον, οὐκ ἀναμείνας ἔτι
τὴν πεῖραν, ἀλλ᾽ ἀπ᾽ αὐτῆς τοῦ πράγματος τῆς
φύσεως λαβὼν τὴν ἔνδειξιν. ἐδείχθη γὰρ ἐν τοῖς περὶ
φαρμάκων ὑπομνήμασιν, ἐν οἷς ἠξίωσα γεγυμνάσθαι
πρότερον, ὅτῳ μέλλει τι καὶ τῶν νῦν λεγομένων ὄφε-

Consequently, there is no indication from these things with regard to treatment or prophylaxis. As I said, the knowledge of the *prokatarktic* cause is useful only in respect of the conditions which fall outside our recognition. Yet for Empiric doctors the *prokatarktic* cause is sometimes taken as part of the whole syndrome, on the basis of which they make trial of the treatment, as in the case of rabid dogs and all venomous creatures. Now there are those Dogmatics who admit that they treat such things from experience alone quite apart from the logical indication. And indeed, the *prokatartktic* cause is sought by them as one part of the whole syndrome, although for those who know the potencies of venomous creatures from prior experience and take an indication of treatment from these potencies, knowledge of the *prokatarktic* cause does not contribute to the indication of cure, but to the recognition of the present condition.

Suppose I know the poison of the scorpion is cold in terms of potency, and take the indication of cure as being 245K from the coldness, without as yet having any sign that such a condition exists in this particular body. Clearly, if I believe that a scorpion was what stung [the person], I shall attempt to heat the whole body thoroughly as well as the part that has been pierced by it. I won't wait for further experience, but will take the indication from the very nature of the matter. For it was shown in the treatises on medications, with which I think it worthwhile for anyone who intends to benefit from what is now being discussed to be-

λος ἔσεσθαι, μηδεμίαν ἄνευ πείρας εὑρίσκεσθαι δύνα-
μιν· ἦν γὰρ ἂν δήπου μακάριον εἴ τις ἐκ τοῦ θεάσασθαι λιθάργυρον, ἢ καστόριον, ἢ κανθαρίδας εὐθέως
ἐγίνωσκεν αὐτῶν τὰς δυνάμεις. ἀλλ᾽ ὥσπερ ἐν ἅπασιν
αἱ διαμαρτίαι τοῖς ὑπερβάλλουσι τοῦ μέτρου καὶ τοῖς
ἐλλείπουσιν, οὕτω κἀνταῦθα γίνονται· καὶ δὶς διὰ
πασῶν, οὐχ ἅπαξ, ὡς ἔοικεν ἀντᾴδουσιν ἀλλήλοις οἵ
τε μηδέπω καὶ τήμερον ὁμολογοῦντες ἐπίστασθαί γε
τὰς δυνάμεις τῶν φαρμάκων ἐπὶ τοσαύτῃ πείρᾳ, οἵ τε
καὶ πρὸς τῆς μιᾶς πείρας ἀξιοῦντες ἐπίστασθαι· καὶ
γὰρ καὶ τοῦτο προπετές, εἰ χρὴ προπετὲς εἰπεῖν τὸ
246K   ἀδύνατον, | καὶ θάτερον ἢ τελέως ἀναισθήτων ἐστὶν ἢ
φανερῶς ἐριζόντων.

ἀλλὰ γάρ, ὡς ἔφην, οὐ χρὴ νῦν περὶ τούτων ἀκούειν ποθεῖν, εἰρημένων ἐπὶ πλέον ἔν τε τῷ τρίτῳ τῶν
περὶ κράσεων κἂν τοῖς περὶ φαρμάκων ὑπομνήμασιν·
ἀλλ᾽ εἰς διάγνωσιν τῶν διαθέσεων ἔνια τῶν προκαταρξάντων αἰτίων συντελεῖ· ἔνθα δ᾽ οὐδὲν λανθάνει τῆς
παρούσης διαθέσεως, οἴχεται καὶ τοῦ προκατάρξαντος
τος ἡ χρεία· εἴρηται μὲν οὖν μοι κἂν τοῖς ἔμπροσθεν
ὡς οὐ δεῖ συνάπτειν ἐς ταὐτὸν ἀμφοτέρας τὰς διδασκαλίας, ἀλλ᾽ ἰδίᾳ μὲν τὴν Ἐμπειρικήν, ἰδίᾳ δὲ
ποιεῖσθαι τὴν Λογικήν. ἀναμεμνήσθω δὲ κἂν νῦν ὡς

---

10 There is the general statement that nothing of the medical
craft is discovered apart from experience in the pseudo-Galenic
Introductio sive medicus (XIV.676K). No statement of the sort referred to (i.e., on potencies) was located in the three treatises on

come familiar, that no potency is discovered apart from experience.[10] Of course, it would be a blessing if someone, by looking at litharge, castoreum or the cantharides, immediately knew their potencies. But, as in all things, errors arise due to those who exceed the mean or fall short, and so too do they arise here. And not only once but twice, it seems, they are thoroughly out of tune with each other, there being those who even today don't acknowledge that they know the potencies of the medications from such experience, and those who think they know them from a single experience. Truly this is rash, if we must say that rash refers to what is impossible; otherwise they are either absolutely stupid or obviously contentious.

246K

But, as I said, we must not now be desirous of hearing about these things, since they were spoken of at greater length in the third of the treatises on *krasis* and in those on medications.[11] But some of the *prokatarktic* causes do contribute to a diagnosis of the conditions. However, where nothing of the existing condition eludes us, the usefulness of the *prokatarktic* [cause] also vanishes. Therefore, I said in what has gone before that there is no need to bring both teachings together as one. Rather, we should make the Empirical and Rational distinct. Bear this in mind, as I propose now to go over the Rationalist teaching

medications listed in Book 3, n. 14. Galen's descriptions of the three medications mentioned may be found in his *De simplicium medicamentorum temperamentis et facultatibus* at XII.224K ff., XII.337-41K, and XII.363K ff.

[11] Book 3 of *De temperamentis*, I.646-94K (translated by P. N. Singer, 1997, pp. 266–89), and the treatises on medications referred to in the previous note.

ἐπειδὴ πρόκειται μόνην τὴν Λογικὴν ἐν τοῖσδε τοῖς
ὑπομνήμασι διελθεῖν, εἰ δὲ καὶ μὴ προσκέοιτό που
περί τινος τῶν λεγομένων, ὡς οὐχ ἁπλῶς ἐστιν ἀληθές, ἀλλὰ μόνοις τοῖς κατὰ μέθοδον ἰατρεύουσιν,
ἀκόλουθον αὐτῶν λογίζεσθαί τινα τοῦτο καὶ προστιθέναι παρ' ἑαυτοῦ. νυνὶ μὲν γὰρ ἡμεῖς προσεθή-
καμεν ὡς οὐδὲν τῶν προκαταρξάντων αἰτίων εἰς ἔνδειξιν θεραπείας ἐστὶ χρήσιμον, ἀλλὰ εἰς διάγνωσιν
247K   ἐνίοτε | διαθέσεως, ὁμολογοῦντες ὡς ἐν τοῖς ἐμπειρι-
κῶς ἰωμένοις ὁτιοῦν, ἔν τι τῶν τῆς ὅλης συνδρομῆς
μορίων ἐστὶ καὶ τὸ προκατάρχον αἴτιον, εἴτ' οὖν
λογικῶς τἆλλα θεραπεύοιεν εἴτε δι' ἐμπειρίας ἅπαντα·
κατὰ δὲ τὸν ἐφεξῆς λόγον οὐκ ἀναγκαῖον ἂν εἴη
προσγράφειν τοῦτο.

πάλιν οὖν ἐπὶ τὸ προκείμενον ἐπανέλθωμεν, ἀρχὴν
ὁμολογουμένην λαβόντες ᾗ κἂν τοῖς ἔμπροσθεν ἤδη
κεχρήμεθα φάσκοντες, τὴν τῆς θεραπείας δεομένην
διάθεσιν αὐτὴν εἶναι τὴν τὸν πρῶτον σκοπὸν ἐν-
δεικνυμένην· ἐκ δὲ τούτου τἆλλα πάντα λαμβάνεσθαι.
τούτῳ δ' ὅτι τῷ σκοπῷ κοινωνίαν οὐδεμίαν ἔχει τῶν
προκαταρχόντων αἰτίων οὐδὲν ἐξ αὐτῶν μάλιστα τῶν
ἑλκῶν, ὅθεν περ ὁ λόγος ὡρμήθη, μαθήσῃ. γεγενήσθω
γοῦν ἕλκος ἐξ ἀποστήματος· ἀλλ' εἰ τοῦτο, δῆλον ὡς
ἐκ μοχθηρῶν χυμῶν· οὕτω γὰρ εἴωθεν ἡ φύσις ἐν
νόσοις ἐκκαθαίρουσα τὸ σῶμα τὸ περιττὸν ἅπαν
ὠθεῖν ἐπὶ τὸ δέρμα· καὶ τούτῳ μὲν οὖν ἑλκωθῆναι
συμβαίνει, τῷ δ' ὅλῳ σώματι ἐκκεκαθάρθαι. τίς οὖν ἡ
τῶν τοιούτων ἑλκῶν ἴασις; οἷά περ καὶ ἡ τῶν ἄλλων

alone in these treatises. If it is something not related in some way to one of the things being discussed, inasmuch as it is not absolutely true but only true for those who treat by method, calculate what one of their followers would add from his own experience. What I now propose is that no *prokatarktic* cause is useful as an indication for therapy, but that it is sometimes useful for the diagnosis of a condition, since I concede that, for those who cure in any way empirically, the *prokatarktic* cause is also one of the parts of the whole syndrome, whether they treat some things rationally or everything empirically. It should not be necessary to write this again in the discussion that follows.

247K

Therefore, let me return once more to what was proposed, taking as an agreed principle what I have already used previously when I said that the actual condition that requires treatment is what reveals the primary indicator, and that it is from this that everything else is taken. From this you will learn that none of the *prokatarktic* causes has anything in common with the indicator, and especially in ulcers, from which the discussion took its origin. Let us assume, at any rate, that an ulcer arises from an abscess.[12] But if this is the case, it is clear that it is from bad humors, for this is how, in diseases, Nature customarily clears out the body, forcing all superfluity towards the skin. Therefore, it is by the whole body being cleared out that ulceration occurs. What, then, is the cure of such ulcers? It is

[12] Here *helkos* clearly refers to what in modern terminology is an ulcer.

ἁπάντων οἷς οὐκ ἐπιπλέκεται διάθεσις οὐδεμία κακο-

248K ήθης. | ἀλλ᾽ εἴ περ τοῦθ᾽ οὕτως ἔχει, δῆλον ὡς οὐδεμία
παρὰ τῆς ποιησάσης τὸ ἕλκος αἰτίας ἔνδειξις εἰς τὴν
θεραπείαν ἐγένετο. καὶ μὴν εἴ περ ἔμενεν ἡ κακοχυμία, πάντως ἄν που καὶ παρ᾽ αὐτῆς τὴν ἔνδειξιν
ἐλάβομεν. ἀλλὰ καὶ ἄλλως ἄτοπον ἦν δεῖσθαι θεραπείας τὸ μηκέτ᾽ ὄν, ἢ ἐνδείκνυσθαι θεραπείαν τὸ μὴ
δεόμενον αὐτῆς· ὥστε παντοίως ἄτοπον ἐκ τοῦ προκατάρξαντος αἰτίου ἔνδειξιν λέγειν γίνεσθαι θεραπείας. ἐπεὶ τοίνυν οὐ τοῦτο, δῆλον ὡς τὸ παρὸν αἴτιον
ἔνδειξιν ποιήσεται.

τίς οὖν ἡ ἔνδειξις; ἀκριβολογουμένῳ μὲν ἡ προφυ-
λακτικὴ προσαγορευομένη, καταχρωμένῳ δ᾽ ἡ θερα-
πευτική· καὶ γὰρ καὶ αὐτῶν τῶν ἑλκῶν τῆς ἰάσεως, εἴθ᾽
ἁπλῶς ἕλκη μόνον εἴτε καὶ μετὰ κοιλότητος ὑπάρχει
κατὰ τὸν ἀκριβῆ λόγον ἡ ἴασις ἐκ τοῦ φεύγειν τε καὶ
προφυλάττεσθαι τὰ λυπήσοντα τὴν φύσιν ἀποτελεῖται. καὶ ὅλως ἐφ᾽ ὧν τὸ γινόμενον αὐτῆς τῆς φύσεως
ἔργον ἐστίν· ὡς κόλλησις ἕλκους καὶ σάρκωσις, ἐκ
τοῦ προφυλακτικοῦ γένους ἐστὶν ἡ τῶν τοιούτων ἐπι-
μέλεια· ἀλλ᾽ ὅμως ἴασις λέγεται πρὸς ἁπάντων ἀν-
θρώπων. καὶ τούτῳ διώρισται τοῦ προφυλακτικοῦ |

249K μέρους τῆς τέχνης, τῷ διάθεσιν μὲν ὑπάρχουσαν ἤδη
τινὰ νοσερὰν ἐκκόπτεσθαι, κατὰ τὸ ἕτερον εἶδος τῆς
προφυλακτικῆς, κωλύεσθαι δὲ γίνεσθαι τὴν μηδέπω
γεγενημένην κατὰ τὸ ἕτερον.

ὥστε κἀνταῦθα περὶ ὀνομάτων ἐρίζοντες ἀγνοοῦσιν
οἱ νεώτεροι τῶν ἰατρῶν. ἐχρῆν δ᾽ αὐτούς, εἰ περὶ

like that of all the other ulcers in which no *kakoethical* condition is implicated. But if this is the case, it is clear that no 248K
indication regarding treatment arises from the cause
which produces the ulcer. If, however, the *kakochymia*
were still present, we would somehow have taken the indication entirely from this. And apart from anything else, it
would be strange for something that no longer exists to require treatment, or for something to indicate treatment
that does not need it. So in every way it would be strange to
say that the indication of treatment arises from the *prokatarktic* cause. Therefore, although this is not so, it is
clear that a cause which is present will provide an indication.

What indication, then? In precise terms, it is what is
called prophylactic; in terms of use, it is what is called therapeutic, inasmuch as in the case of the ulcer itself, whether
it is simply an ulcer alone or is one of those with a cavity,
strictly speaking the cure is accomplished by avoiding and
guarding against things which will distress Nature. And in
general, in the case of these things, what has occurred is
an action of Nature itself. Thus, the conglutination and
enfleshing of an ulcer is the responsibility of those things
from the prophylactic class, although "cure" is the term
used by everybody. And for this reason, there is a distinction to be made in the prophylactic part of the craft be- 249K
tween the eradication of some already existing disease
condition, which is one kind of prophylaxis, and preventing the occurrence of what has not yet happened, which is
another kind of prophylaxis.

Consequently, here too, younger doctors who argue
about names are ignorant. What they ought to do, if they

πραγμάτων ἐσπούδαζον, ἐξευρεῖν ὡς δύο εἰσὶν αἱ
πρῶται διαφοραὶ τῶν ἐνεργειῶν τοῖς ἰατροῖς. ἢ γὰρ
τὰς οὔσας ἤδη διαθέσεις ἐξ ὧν πράττουσι θεραπεύουσιν, ἢ τὰς οὐκ οὔσας γενέσθαι κωλύουσι. τὸ μὲν
δὴ τὰς οὔσας ἐκκόπτειν, εἴτε τὰ διακόπτοντα τὰς
ἐνεργείας τῆς φύσεως ἐκποδὼν ποιουμένους εἴτε καὶ
αὐτούς τι διὰ τῶν φαρμάκων ἐργαζομένους, ἅπαντες
ἄνθρωποι θεραπεύειν ὀνομάζουσι, τὸ δὲ κωλύειν γενέσθαι προφυλάττεσθαι. καὶ δὴ καὶ τὰ μετὰ κακοχυμίας
ἡλκωμένα θεραπεύουσιν οἱ λόγῳ τε καὶ μεθόδῳ τῇ
τέχνῃ προσιόντες, ἅμα μὲν ἐκείνην ἐκκαθαίροντες,
ἅμα δὲ τὰ διακόπτοντα τὰς κινήσεις τῆς φύσεως
ἀναιροῦντες. ἄμφω δ᾽ ἐστὶν ἀκριβολογουμένῳ ταῦτα
προφυλακτικά. κωλύει γάρ, ὡς κἂν τῷ πρὸ τούτου
δέδεικται λόγῳ, πάντα τὰ τοιαῦτα ῥύπον ἐπιτρέφε-
σθαι τοῖς ἕλκεσιν, ἢ ὑγρότητα πολλήν, ἢ μοχθηράν. |

250K   4. Οὐκ οὖν ἐν ὀνόμασι μικρολογεῖσθαι καλόν, ἀλλ᾽
ἄμεινον εἰπεῖν τινα μέθοδον ἰάσεως ἑλκῶν, οἵαν ἡμεῖς
ἔν τε τῷ πρὸ τούτου λόγῳ κἂν τῷδε διεξῆμεν. ἐγὼ μὲν
γὰρ καὶ θαυμάζω τὴν ἀναισθησίαν τοῦ Θεσσαλοῦ,
γράφοντος ὡδί πως ὑπὲρ τῆς τῶν κακοηθῶν ἑλκῶν
ἰάσεως·

Εἰσὶ δὲ σφόδρα ἀναγκαῖαι καὶ αἱ κοινότητες αἱ
τῶν χρονίων ἑλκῶν καὶ μὴ ὑγιαζομένων, ἢ
κατουλουμένων καὶ πάλιν ἀναλυομένων· πρὸς
τῷ ἐπὶ μὲν τῶν μὴ συμφυομένων σκέπτεσθαι τί
ἐστι τὸ ἐμποδίζον καὶ τοῦτ᾽ αἴρειν, τὸ δ᾽ ἐπου-
λούμενον καὶ ἀναξαινόμενον ἀναγκάζειν κρα-

are serious about these matters, is to discover that there are two primary differences in the functions of doctors. They either treat already existing conditions by the things they do, or they prevent conditions that have not occurred. To eradicate conditions that now exist, either by removing those things that interrupt the functions of Nature, or by acting on them through medications, is what all men call "treatment"; to prevent them occurring is "prophylaxis." Furthermore, those who treat what has been ulcerated in association with *kakochymia,* proceeding by reason and method, simultaneously purge the *kakochymia* and remove those things interrupting the actions of Nature. Both these things are, in a strict sense, prophylactic. As has been demonstrated in the discussion prior to this one, this prevents all those things which maintain the filth in an ulcer; that is, either excessive or bad moisture.

4. No good [will come] from a hair-splitting examina-   250K
tion of names; better to speak about a method of cure for wounds and ulcers such as I went through in the discussion prior to this one, and in this one itself. For I marvel at the stupidity of Thessalus when he writes about the cure of *kakoethical* ulcers as follows:

> The "communities" of ulcers that are chronic and unhealed, or that have scarred over and broken open again, are extremely pressing. On this point, in the ulcers that have not united, consider what the hindrance is and remove this. When there is scarring that has broken open again, it is necessary to re-

379

τεῖν τῆς οὐλῆς, μετασυγκρίνοντας τὸ πάσχον
μέρος, ἢ καὶ κοινῶς ὅλον τὸ σῶμα καὶ δυσπαθὲς
τοῦτο ποιεῖν διὰ τῶν τοῦτο δρώντων βοηθημάτων.

ταυτὶ μὲν οὖν ὁ Θεσσαλὸς ἐν τῷ περὶ χειρουργίας
βιβλίῳ κατ᾽ ἀρχὰς εὐθὺς προειπὼν ἐν τοῖς ἐφεξῆς ἐπὶ
πλέον ὧδέ πως ὑπὲρ αὐτῶν τούτων γράφει·

Τὰ δὲ χρόνια τῶν ἑλκῶν καὶ μὴ ὑγιαζόμενα, ἢ
κατουλούμενα καὶ ἀναξαινόμενα ἐμφαίνει· τὰ
μὲν εἰς οὐλὴν μὴ συνερχόμενα ἐκκόπτειν τὰ
251K κωλύοντα τὴν σύμφυσιν | γίνεσθαι καὶ νεωτερο-
ποιεῖν τοὺς πεπονθότας τόπους καὶ παραπλήσια
ποιήσαντας τοῖς νεοτρώτοις πάλιν ἐναίμως
ἰᾶσθαι, κἂν μὴ κρατηθῇ, παρηγορεῖν τὴν φλεγμονὴν καὶ τὴν λοιπὴν προσάγειν ἐπιμέλειαν·
τὰ δ᾽ εἰς οὐλὴν ἐρχόμενα καὶ ἀναλυόμενα, κατὰ
μὲν τοὺς παροξυσμοὺς καὶ τὰς ἑλκώσεις ὁμοίως θεραπεύειν τοῖς προσφάτως φλεγμαίνουσι,
καταπλάσμασι τοῖς παρηγοροῦσιν, ἕως ἂν παύ-
σηται ἡ ἀγανάκτησις· ἐνδούσης δὲ συνεργεῖν
εἰς ἐπούλωσιν· μετὰ δὲ ταῦτα φοινίσσειν τὰ
κύκλῳ μέρη, πλατὺν περιλαμβάνοντας τόπον τῷ
διὰ τοῦ νάπυος μαλάγματι, ἤ τινι ἑτέρῳ μετα-
βάλλειν δυναμένῳ, καὶ τὴν εὐπάθειαν ἀναιρεῖν.
μὴ ληγόντων δὲ καὶ κοινῶς ὅλου τοῦ σώματος
ἐπιμέλειαν ποιεῖσθαι, μετασυγκρίνοντας αὐτὸ
διὰ γυμνασίων ποικίλων καὶ αἰώρας καὶ ἀνα-
φωνήσεως παρόντων ἐμπείρων, καὶ διαίτης κατὰ

---

13 Here and in the two subsequent instances we have followed

pair the scar by altering the state of the pores of the affected part, or also of the whole body jointly, and this is not easy to do with the remedies which [normally] do this.[13]

This, then, is what Thessalus proclaims in his book about surgery, right at the start, and what he enlarges on in what follows, when he writes on these same matters thus:

Those wounds and ulcers that are chronic and unhealed, or have scarred over and broken open again indicate [the following]. In those that do not unite in a scar, eradicate those things that are preventing the union and "refresh" the affected places, making them like recent wounds again, to cure when bleeding. And even if it is not overcome, mitigate the inflammation and apply the rest of the treatment. In those [wounds and ulcers] that have come to scarring and broken down, treat the things that are irritating and ulcerating, as you would in recent inflammations, soothing them with poultices until the pain and irritation has ceased. Then encourage [the wound or ulcer] to close over into a scar. After this, redden the parts in a circle, surrounding the flat place with the emollient made from mustard, or from something else able to bring about change and achieve comfort. If there is still no abatement, attend to the care of the whole body generally, altering the state of the pores using various exercises, passive and vocal, with experienced people present.

251K

Linacre (pp. 185–86) in taking the statement attributed to Thessalus by Galen as a direct quotation from a work no longer extant.

πρόσθεσιν αὐξανομένης τε καὶ μειουμένης, ἀρχῆς ἐντιθεμένης διὰ τὸν ἀπὸ ῥαφανίδων ἔμετον.
χρῆσθαι δὲ καὶ τῇ τοῦ λευκοῦ ἐλλεβόρου δόσει
καὶ τοῖς ἄλλοις ἅπασιν οἷς χρώμεθα ἐπὶ τῶν |
252K ὑπαγομένων διαίτῃ χρονίων καὶ δυσαποτρίπτων
παθῶν.

αὕτη μὲν ἡ τοῦ Θεσσαλοῦ ῥῆσις. ἄξιον δὲ θαυ-
μάσαι τἀνθρώπου τὴν ἀναισθησίαν ἢ τὴν τόλμαν· εἰ
μὲν αὐτὸς ἑαυτὸν ἀνέπεισεν ὡς ὀρθῶς λέγει, τὴν
ἀναισθησίαν· εἰ δ' ἐπιστάμενος ὡς οὐδὲν λέγει παρα-
κρούεσθαι τοὺς ἀναγινώσκοντας ἅπαντας ἤλπικε, τὴν
τόλμαν.

ἐκ τῶν χρονίων ἑλκῶν, ὦ γενναιότατε, τίς ἔνδειξις
γίνεται θεραπείας; ἐγὼ μὲν γὰρ οὔτ' ἐκ τῶν προσφάτων οὔθ' ὅλως ἐκ χρόνου κατ' οὐδὲν τῶν νοσημάτων
ἐξεῦρον οὐδεπώποτε τὴν θεραπείαν, ἀλλ' ἐξ αὐτῆς τῆς
διαθέσεως, ἣν ἰᾶσθαί μοι πρόκειται. καθόλου γὰρ ἐὰν
εἰς τὸν χρόνον ἀποβλέπῃ τις, ὡς ἔνδειξιν παρ' αὐτοῦ
λαμβάνειν, ἑτέραν μὲν πάντως ἡ δευτέρα τῶν ἡμερῶν,
ἑτέραν δ' ἡ τρίτη παρέξει τὴν ἔνδειξιν· οὕτως δὲ καὶ ἡ
τετάρτη τῆς πέμπτης ἑτέραν· καὶ τούτων ἁπασῶν ἡ
ἕκτη καὶ τῶν ἄλλων ἑκάστη τῶν μετὰ ταύτας. ὥστ'
οὐκέτι τὰς διαθέσεις ἃς θεραπεύομεν ἐπισκεψόμεθα
καὶ παρ' αὐτῶν ἔνδειξιν ληψόμεθα; καί τοί γε τούτου
ἀλογώτερον οὐδ' ἐπινοῆσαι δυνατόν ἐστι. πῶς οὖν
ἀναγκαῖαι αἱ κοινότητες αἱ τῶν χρονίων ἑλκῶν εἰσιν,
253K οὐδέν | γε ἐνδείκνυσθαι δυναμένου τοῦ χρόνου καθ'
ἑαυτόν; οὐ δήπου γὰρ ἐπειδὰν ὑπὸ κακοχυμίας ἕλκος

If the food intake has been increased, decrease this too, making a start with vomiting induced by radishes. Also use the administration of white hellebore and all the other things that we use in those affections subject to regimen that are chronic and hard to get rid of.

252K

This is Thessalus' statement. Either the foolishness or the audacity of the man is worthy of wonder. If he convinced himself that he spoke correctly, it is foolishness. If he knew he was talking nonsense, but had hoped to deceive all his readers, it is audacity.

What indication of treatment arises, my most noble friend, from chronic wounds and ulcers? Neither from these, nor from those that are acute, nor from the time in general, have I ever discovered the treatment in any disease. Rather, it is from the condition itself, which lies before me to cure. In general, if someone pays attention to the time, so as to take an indication from this, no doubt the second day will provide another indication, the third day another, and in the same way also, the fourth day another and different from the fifth day, and different from all these, the sixth, and each of the others after these. Consequently, will we no longer consider the conditions which we are treating and take an indication from these [days]? Indeed, it is impossible to think of anything more illogical than this. How, then, are the "communities" of the chronic ulcers necessary when the time of itself is in fact unable to indicate anything? For we will not, I presume, take a dif-

253K

ἀναβιβρώσκηται, διάφορον ἔνδειξιν ἀπ᾽ αὐτοῦ ληψόμεθα μετὰ τέτταρας μῆνας ἧς εὐθὺς ἐξ ἀρχῆς ἐλάβομεν. ἐγὼ μὲν οὐδ᾽ ἂν ἐάσαιμι χρονίσαι τὸ τοιοῦτον
ἕλκος, ἀλλ᾽ εὐθέως ἀπὸ τῆς ἀρχῆς ἐκκόψαιμι τὴν
αἰτίαν αὐτοῦ. καὶ γὰρ καὶ γνωρίζειν δυνατόν ἐστι τὴν
διάθεσιν ἀπὸ τῆς ἀρχῆς ὡς τὰ πολλά, καὶ τὴν ἔνδειξιν
ἀπὸ τῆς διαθέσεως λαμβάνειν ἀναγκαῖον. ὁ χρόνος δὲ
τί πλέον ἡμᾶς διδάξει τοῦ τῶν ἡμερῶν ἀριθμοῦ, μὰ
τοὺς θεούς, οὐκ ἔχω συμβαλεῖν, πλὴν εἰ τοῦτο λέγειν
ἠβουλήθη ὁ Θεσσαλός, ὡς εἰς διάγνωσιν τῶν τοιούτων ἑλκῶν ἀναγκαῖον ἀναμεῖναι τὸν χρόνον. ἀλλ᾽
οὕτω γε πρῶτον μὲν ἂν ἰδιώτης εἴη παντάπασιν, εἰ
μηδέποτε πρὸ τοῦ χρονίσαι τὸ ἕλκος ὁμολογεῖ δια-
γνῶναι δύνασθαι τὴν διάθεσιν. ἔπειτα δὲ σαφῶς ἂν
ἔτι καὶ τοῦθ᾽ ὁμολογήσειεν, ὡς ἐξ ἄλλου μὲν ἡ τῆς
ἰάσεως ἔνδειξις, ἐξ ἄλλων δὲ ἡ διάγνωσις γίνεται τῆς
διαθέσεως.

ἔστω γάρ τι συμβάλλεσθαι τὸν χρόνον εἰς τὴν
διάγνωσιν· ἀλλ᾽ ἥ γε ἔνδειξις τῆς ἰάσεως οὐκ ἐκ τοῦ
254K χρόνου. τί γὰρ | ἂν εἴη πρὸς ἔπος, εἴ τι χρονίζει τῶν
ἑλκῶν, ἐκκόπτειν τὰ κωλύοντα τὴν σύμφυσιν γίνεσθαι
καὶ νεωτεροποιεῖν τοὺς πεπονθότας τόπους; εἰ γὰρ διὰ
ῥεῦμα κακόηθες, ὦ γενναιότατε, τὰ χείλη τοῦ ἕλκους
ἐν διαθέσει τινὶ γέγονε, τί πλέον ἕξομεν, ἂν περι-
κόψωμεν αὐτὰ πρὶν ἰάσασθαι τὸ ῥεῦμα; μεῖζον ἐργασόμεθα δηλονότι τὸ ἕλκος, ὥσπερ καὶ ποιοῦσιν ἔνιοι
τῶν ὁμοίως ἐκείνῳ θεραπευόντων ἕλκη. τῆς γὰρ αἰτίας
μενούσης τῆς καὶ πρότερον αὐτὰ σκληρὰ καὶ τυλώδη

ferent indication from this, when an ulcer is eroded by *kakochymia*, after four months than we took right at the start. I would not allow such an ulcer to become chronic, but would eradicate its cause right at the start. Furthermore, it is possible to recognize the condition from the start in many cases, and it is necessary to take the indication from the condition. What more the time will teach us other than the sum of the days, I am, by the gods, unable to guess, unless Thessalus wanted to say this: that for the diagnosis of such ulcers it is necessary to wait a certain time. But if this were so, he would first be altogether a layman, if he admits that he is never able to diagnose the condition before the ulcer becomes chronic. And then, clearly, he would also be admitting that the indication of the cure arises from one thing, while the diagnosis of the condition arises from others.

For suppose that time contributes something to the diagnosis, but in fact the indication of the cure is not from the time. What would be the point, if any, in the ulcers that are chronic, of eradicating those things that are preventing union occurring and "refreshing" the affected places? For if, my most noble fellow, due to a *kakoethical* flux, the margins of the ulcer are in a certain condition, what more would we gain should we cut all around these before curing the flux? Quite clearly we shall make the ulcer bigger, just as some do when they treat ulcers like him. If the cause, which previously made the margins hard and cal- 254K

GALEN

ποιησάσης οὐδὲν ἔσται πλέον ἐκ τοῦ περιτέμνειν
ἄλλο γε ἢ μέγεθος ἕλκους· πάλιν γὰρ ἐκεῖνα τὰ
περιτμηθέντα τοῖς πρότερον ὁμοίως ἔσται τυλώδη καὶ
σκληρά. καί τοί γ' οὐδ' αὐτὸ τοῦτο προσέθηκεν ὁ
σοφώτατος Θεσσαλός, ὡς ἐκκοπτέον ἐστὶ τὰ τυλώδη
καὶ σκληρὰ καὶ κακόχροα τῶν ἡλκωμένων μορίων,
ἀλλ' ἁπλῶς ἐκκόπτειν κελεύει τὰ κωλύοντα τὴν σύμφυσιν καὶ νεωτεροποιεῖν. εἰ μὲν οὖν ἐκκόπτειν τὰ
κωλύοντα τὴν σύμφυσιν αἴτια συνεβούλευε, παλαιός
τ' ἂν ἦν ὁ τοιοῦτος λόγος, ἐγώ τε οὐδὲν ἂν ἐμεμφόμην
αὐτῷ, παρήνηται γὰρ ὑπὸ πάντων σχεδὸν τῶν πα-
λαιῶν ἰατρῶν, ὅσοι γε λόγῳ | τινὶ καὶ μεθόδῳ περὶ
θεραπείας ἑλκῶν ἔγραψαν, ὡς ἐκκοπτέον ἐστὶ τὰς
ἐργαζομένας αἰτίας αὐτά, καθάπερ, οἶμαι, καὶ τῶν
ἄλλων ἀπάντων νοσημάτων. οὐ γὰρ δὴ ἐπὶ μὲν τῶν
ἑλκῶν ἔτι μενούσης τῆς ποιούσης αὐτὰ αἰτίας κάλλιον
ἐκείνην πρότερον ἐκκόπτειν, ἐπὶ δὲ τῶν ἄλλων νοσημάτων οὐ κάλλιον, ἀλλ' ἐπὶ πάντων ἁπλῶς ὧν τὸ
ποιοῦν ἔτι πάρεστιν ἀπ' ἐκείνου τῆς θεραπείας ἀρ-
κτέον.

εἰ δὲ τὰ κωλύοντα τὴν σύμφυσιν οὐκ ἐπὶ τῶν αἰτίων
ἁπάντων ὅσα τοῦτο πέφυκε δρᾶν, ἀλλ' ἐπὶ τῶν χειλῶν
εἴρηκε μόνον, ὡς ἐξ ὧν ἐπιφέρει δῆλός ἐστιν, πλέον
ἀγνοεῖν ἔοικεν ἢ γινώσκειν εἰς ἑλκῶν ἴασιν. εἴη μὲν
γὰρ ἂν ποτε καὶ τοῦτο μόνον αἴτιον τοῦ μὴ θεραπεύεσθαι τὸ ἕλκος· εἴη δ' ἂν οὐδὲν ἧττον, ὡς εἴρηται,
καὶ ἡ χωρὶς ὄγκου παρὰ φύσιν ἐν τοῖς ἡλκωμένοις
μέρεσι δυσκρασία καὶ ἡ μετ' ὄγκου μέν τινος, ἀλλ' οὐ

386

lous, remains operative, nothing will be gained from the excision other than making the ulcer bigger, for those margins that are cut around will become hard and callous like they were previously. And indeed, the most sapient Thessalus did not add this: that we must cut around those ulcerated parts that are callous, hard and of a bad color. Rather, he simply directs us to eradicate those things preventing union and to "refresh." If he did advise the eradication of the causes preventing union, and such was the reasoning of the ancients, I would have no quarrel with him, for this was what was recommended by almost all the doctors of old, or at least those who wrote about the treatment of ulcers based on some theory and method: that is, that you must eradicate the causes which bring them about, just as, I believe, is also the case with all other diseases. It is certainly not the case with ulcers that, when the cause creating them still remains, it is better to eradicate that first, whereas with other diseases, it is not better. Rather, in all cases (i.e. ulcers and other diseases), when what caused them is plainly still present, we must begin the treatment from that.

255K

If, however, he is saying that those things which prevent union are not among all the causes which by nature do this, but only in the case of the margins, as he clearly does from the things he brings up, he seems to me more ignorant than knowledgeable when it comes to the cure of ulcers. For sometimes this might be the sole cause of the ulcer not being treatable. However, no less might it be a *dyskrasia,* either without an abnormal swelling in the ulcerated parts, or with one, but one which absolutely does not need to be

πάντως τοῦ γε περιτομῆς δεομένου· καὶ πρὸς τούτοις
ἔτι σκιρρὸς ὑπερκείμενος, ἢ σπλὴν μέγας, ἤ τις ἐν
ἥπατι κακοπραγία καὶ χωρὶς τούτων ἁπάντων ἀτονία
256K τοῦ μέρους αὐτοῦ τοῦ πεπονθότος, | ἐπίτασις οὖσα
δυσκρασίας καὶ ἥδε· καὶ μὲν δὴ καὶ ἡ καθ᾽ ὅλον τὸ
σῶμα κακοχυμία μέγιστον τῶν αἰτίων ὅσα λυμαίνε-
σθαι τοῖς ἕλκεσι πέφυκεν. ἐνοχλεῖ δ᾽ οὐδὲν ἧττον
αὐτοῖς καὶ ἡ καλουμένη πληθώρα.

τούτων ἕκαστον εἰ κελεύοι ἐκκόπτειν Θεσσαλός,
ἐπαινῶ τὸν ἄνθρωπον, ὡς ἑπόμενον τοῖς παλαιοῖς· εἰ
δὲ τὰ χείλη μόνον, ἓν ἐκ πολλῶν ἔγνωκε, ὃ μηδὲ τοὺς
αἰπόλους λανθάνει. εἰ γὰρ σκληρὰ καὶ τετυλωμένα
καὶ πελιδνὰ καὶ μέλανα καί τινα ἄλλην ἐπίσημον
ἄχροιαν ἔχοντα θεάσαιτό τις αἰπόλος ἕλκους χείλη,
πάντως τολμήσει περικόπτειν αὐτά. καὶ γὰρ τοι³ καὶ
προχειρότατόν ἐστι τὸ περικόψαι· μεῖζον δέ γε καὶ
τεχνικώτερον ἰᾶσθαι φαρμάκοις. Θεσσαλὸς δὲ οὔτε
τῶν ὑπὸ φαρμάκων δυναμένων μαλαχθῆναι χειλῶν εἰς
γνῶσιν ἧκέ ποτε, καὶ γὰρ καὶ λέγουσιν αὐτὸν ἀπο-
στῆναι τελέως τοῦ τοιούτου μέρους τῆς τέχνης, ὥσπερ
οὖν ἐμφαίνει καὶ αὐτός, οὔθ᾽ ὅλως ἐμπειρίαν ἢ λογικὴν ἐπιστήμην ἔοικεν ἔχειν οὐδενὸς φαρμάκου· καθότι
καὶ τοῦτο διὰ τοῦ περὶ φαρμάκων ἐνδείκνυται βιβλίου.
ἀλλὰ περὶ μὲν τῶν ἐν ἐκείνοις οὐκ ὀρθῶς εἰρημένων
257K ἐπὶ προήκοντι τῷ λόγῳ | διαλέξομαι· περὶ δὲ τῆς τῶν
χρονίων ἑλκῶν ἰάσεως, ἣν ἐν τῇ προγεγραμμένῃ
ῥήσει Θεσσαλὸς ἐποιήσατο, πρόκειταί μοι τό γε νῦν
εἶναι διελθεῖν.

cut out. And in addition to these factors, there may be an overlying scirrhosity, or an enlarged spleen, or a bad condition of the liver, or apart from all these, a weakness of the affected part itself, this being an intensification of the *dyskrasia*. Furthermore, a *kakochymia* of the whole body is the most significant of the causes that are by nature harmful to ulcers. But no less disturbing to them is so-called *plethora*.

256K

If Thessalus were to give instruction to eradicate each of these things, I would commend the man as following the ancients. If, however, it is the margins only, he knows one thing among many, and a thing which does not even elude goatherds. For if a goatherd were to see the margins of an ulcer hard, callous, livid and black, or having some other notable discoloration, he would certainly have the courage to excise them. And in fact, the excision is very easily done. It is, however, better and more skillful to cure with medications. Thessalus, on the other hand, has never come to the realization that the margins [of an ulcer] can be softened by potent medications, for they say he distanced himself completely from this part of the craft, just as he himself also reveals, and he seems to have no empirical or theoretical knowledge of any medication. This is also revealed by his book on medications. But I shall speak about what was incorrectly stated in those [works] as the discussion proceeds. The matter that I now propose to go over is that concerning the cure of chronic ulcers, which Thessalus related in the previously quoted passage.

257K

---

³ τι B

ἄμεινον μὲν ἦν δήπου μὴ χρόνια καλεῖν, ἀλλὰ
κακοήθη ταῦτα, καὶ τὴν φύσιν αὐτῶν ἐκδιηγήσασθαι
καὶ τὰς αἰτίας τῆς γενέσεως εἰπεῖν καὶ τὴν θεραπείαν
ἑκάστου, τὴν μὲν ὡς ἐφ᾽ ἕλκει κοινὴν ἁπάντων αὐτῶν
οἵαν ἐν τῷ τρίτῳ γράμματι διῆλθον· ἰδίαν δ᾽ ἐφ᾽
ἑκάστου, κατὰ τὸ τῆς ἐργαζομένης αἰτίας εἶδος, ὡς ἐν
τούτῳ τῷ λόγῳ διωρισάμην. ὁ δὲ οὐδὲν τούτων ποι-
ήσας καὶ νεωτεροποιεῖν τοὺς ἡλκωμένους τόπους ἀξιοῖ
καὶ παραπλήσια τοῖς νεοτρώτοις ἀπεργασάμενος
ἐναίμους ἰᾶσθαι. τοῦτο μέν γε ναί, μὰ τὸν Ἀσκληπιόν,
ἐναργῶς ἄν τις γνωρίσειε τοῖς ἔργοις τῆς τέχνης
ἐγγεγυμνασμένος, ὡς ὑπ᾽ ἀνθρώπου γέγραπται ταῦτα
μηδέποτε προνοήσαντος ἕλκους. ἐναίμως ἰᾶσθαι
δύναταί τις, ἕλκος χρόνιον ὅμοιον τοῖς νεοτρώτοις
ἐργασάμενος, ἀγκτῆρσι συναγαγὼν ἢ ῥάψας αὐτοῦ
τὰ χείλη· ἢ τούτων μὲν οὐδενί, ἐναίμῳ δέ τινι φαρμάκῳ καὶ μόνῃ σὺν αὐτῷ θαρρήσας ἐπιδέσει; τίς οὐκ
258K   οἶδεν ὡς πᾶν ἕλκος κακόηθες εὐθὺς καὶ | κοῖλόν ἐστιν,
ὡς ἂν ἐξ ἀναβρώσεως γενόμενον; ἆρ᾽ οὖν, ὦ σοφώτατε
Θεσσαλέ, πρὶν σαρκωθῆναι τὸ κοῖλον ἕλκος, εἰς σύμφυσιν ἀχθῆναι δύναται; ἢ οὐ τοῦτ᾽ ἔστι τὸ ἐναίμως
ἰᾶσθαι; μάτην τοίνυν αὐτὸς σὺ τῶν κοίλων ἑλκῶν τὸν
σκοπὸν οὐ κόλλησιν, ἀλλὰ πλήρωσιν ἔγραψας. εἰ δὲ
καὶ μὴ δι᾽ ἑαυτὸ κοῖλον ἦν ἅπαν ἕλκος κακόηθες, ἀλλά
τοί γ᾽ ἐν τῷ νεωτεροποιεῖν, αὐτοῦ τὰ χείλη περι-

Presumably it is better not to call these chronic but *kakoethical* (chronic and intractable), and to set out in detail their nature, and to speak of the causes of their genesis and the treatment of each, as I did go over the treatment that is common to all [wounds and] ulcers, insofar as they are [wounds and] ulcers, in the third book. What is specific to each, in terms of the kind of effecting cause, is as I have distinguished in this discussion. He, however, does none of these things, but considers it right to "refresh" the ulcerated places, and having made them like recent wounds, to cure them while they are bleeding. By Asclepius, anyone practiced in the actions of our craft would clearly know that these things have been written by a man who has never given any thought to a wound or ulcer. Is anyone able to cure what is bleeding, [say] a chronic wound or ulcer, having made it like a recent wound, by bringing its margins together with fibulae[14] or suturing them, or with none of these things, but with some blood-stanching medication, placing his confidence in binding alone together with this medication? Who does not know that every *kakoethical* wound or ulcer is at once also hollow, as it would be   258K if it occurred due to erosion? Is it possible then, most sapient Thessalus, for a hollow wound or ulcer to be brought to union before it is filled with flesh? Or is this not to cure what is filled with blood? Accordingly, you yourself wrote incorrectly that the objective in hollow ulcers is not conglutination but filling. If any *kakoethical* ulcer is not hollow in and of itself, certainly in the "refreshing," when we cut

---

[14] "Fibula" is the Latin term for the Greek ἀγκτήρ, a type of pin used for bringing wounds together; see Celsus, V.26(23) and the Introduction to LCL, *Celsus*, vol. II, p. lxi.

κόπτοντας ὡς σὺ κελεύεις, ἐξ ἀνάγκης οἶμαι καὶ
κοῖλον γίνεται καὶ πλείστην ἴσχει τῶν χειλῶν τὴν
διάστασιν· ὥστ᾽ οὐκ οἶδα πῶς ἔτι κολλήσεις αὐτὸ καὶ
συμφύσεις ἐναίμως. εἰ γὰρ προσάγειν ἐπιχειρήσεις
βιαίως τὰ διεστῶτα πάμπολυ χείλη, φλεγμανεῖ μὲν ἐξ
ἀνάγκης, οὐ συμφύσεται δέ. τούτου καὶ μόνου συνιέναι μοι δοκεῖ καὶ Θεσσαλός· ἐπιφέρει γοῦν, κἂν μὴ
κρατηθῇ, παρηγορεῖν τὴν φλεγμονήν. ἄμεινον δὲ ἦν
γράψαι καὶ μὴ κρατηθέντων παρηγορεῖν τὴν φλεγμονήν, ἐξ ἀνάγκης γὰρ οὐ κρατηθήσεται. ἀλλ᾽ εἰ καὶ
τοῦτο συγχωρηθείη τῷ Θεσσαλῷ καὶ παρέλθοιμεν
αὐτὸ καὶ μὴ λίαν ἀκριβῶς ἐξετάζοιμεν, ὅτι γε τελέως
259K ἀποκεχώρηκε | τῆς κοινότητος ἧς αὐτὸς ὑπέθετο πρό-
δηλον παντί. εἰ γὰρ τὸ ἐμποδίζον ἐξαιρήσομεν, οὐδὲν
ἔτι περὶ τῆς τῶν χρονίων ἑλκῶν ὡς χρονίων κοινότητος ληψόμεθα.

ἀλλ᾽ ἔστω καὶ τοῦτο. θεασώμεθα δὲ τὰ ἐφεξῆς,
γράφει γοῦν ὧδε·

Τὰ δ᾽ εἰς οὐλὴν ἐρχόμενα καὶ ἀναλυόμενα κατὰ
μὲν τοὺς παροξυσμοὺς καὶ τὰς ἑλκώσεις ὁμοίως
θεραπεύειν τοῖς προσφάτως φλεγμαίνουσι.

μετὰ δὲ ταῦτα φησί· Φοινίσσειν τὰ κύκλῳ μέρη τῷ διὰ
τοῦ νάπυος μαλάγματι. τί φῄς, ἄνθρωπε, κἂν δριμύ,
κἂν θερμὸν ῥεῦμα τὸ φερόμενον ᾖ, φοινίσσειν χρὴ
νάπυϊ τὸ μόριον; ἵν᾽ ὅπερ ἐν πολλῷ χρόνῳ πάσχειν
ὑπὸ τοῦ ῥεύματος ἔμελλεν, ὑπὸ τοῦ Θεσσαλείου ταχέως πάθοι φαρμάκου, πᾶν ἑλκωθέν τε καὶ ἀναβρω-

away its margins as you direct, it necessarily becomes hollow, I believe, and maintains a very considerable separation of the margins. As a consequence, I do not know how you will still conglutinate and unite it when it is bleeding because, if you attempt to bring the widely separated margins together forcibly, there is inevitably inflammation, and there will be no union. And Thessalus seems to me to focus on this alone. At any rate, he adds that, even if the inflammation is not overcome, you will mitigate it. It would be better to write *when* the inflammation is not overcome, for inevitably it will not be overcome. But even if this too were to be conceded by Thessalus, we would pass over it without very precise examination, so it is clear to everyone 259K that he has totally abandoned the "community" which he himself postulated. If we take away what is causing the hindrance, we will get nothing else anymore about the "community" of chronic ulcers as being chronicity.

But enough of this. Let us see what follows. Anyway, he writes thus:

> Those [ulcers] that have come to scarring and are breaking down are, in their exacerbations and ulcerations, to be treated in like manner to those that have recently become inflamed.

After this, he says: "Redden the parts all around with the rubifacient made from mustard." Why do you say, my good man, that it is necessary to redden the part with mustard, even if a sharp or hot flux was what is carried in? Is it so that what was going to be affected by the flux over a long time might be affected quickly due to the Thessaleian medication, everything being ulcerated and eroded? The

θέν; τὰς γὰρ διὰ ψύξιν ἢ ὑγρότητα πολλὴν ἄνευ
θερμασίας ἐπιφανοῦς ἀτονίας τῶν μερῶν φοινιγμοῖς
ἐθεράπευον οἱ παλαιοί. σὺ δ' ἐξῆς ἐπὶ πάντων χρᾷ,
πρῶτον μὲν αὐτὸ τοῦτο μὴ διορισάμενος, εἴτε δι'
ἀτονίαν τοῦ μέρους, εἴτε διὰ κακοήθειαν τοῦ ῥεύματος,
οὐ θεραπεύεται τὸ ἕλκος. ἔπειτα δ' ὑπαλλάττων τὴν
260K   τάξιν, ὅταν γὰρ κατακαύσας τῷ | νάπυϊ τὸ μέρος ἀνύ-
σῃς μηδέν, ἐπὶ τὴν τοῦ παντὸς σώματος ἔρχῃ θερα-
πείαν· ἔμπαλιν δ', οἶμαι, καὶ τῷ λόγῳ καὶ τῇ πείρᾳ
περὶ τούτων ἔγνωσται, τὸ σύμπαν σῶμα πρότερον
ἀπέριττον ἐργασαμένους τολμᾶν ἐπιφέρειν τι τῷ μορίῳ θερμαῖνον καὶ δριμὺ φάρμακον. ἕλκειν γὰρ ἐφ'
ἑαυτὰ πέφυκεν ἐξ ὅλου τοῦ σώματος ἅπαντα τὰ τοιαῦτα δίκην σικύας. ἐὰν μὴ φθάσῃς κενώσας αὐτό,
χορηγίαν ῥεύματος ἐγκαταλείψεις τῷ δριμεῖ φαρμάκῳ. τοῦτο καὶ τοῖς Ἐμπειρικοῖς ἰατροῖς ὡμολόγηται καὶ τοῖς Δογματικοῖς· τοῦτο καὶ τοῖς ἀρίστοις
ἐδόκει τῶν φιλοσόφων· ἐπειδὴ γὰρ κἀκείνων μέμνηται
Θεσσαλός, οὐ χεῖρον αὐτοὺς ἐπικαλέσασθαι μάρτυρας, ὡς ὀφθαλμὸν οὐκ ἐγχωρεῖ καλῶς ἰάσασθαι πρὸ
τῆς ὅλης κεφαλῆς, οὐδὲ ταύτην ἄνευ τοῦ παντὸς
σώματος. οὕτως Ἀριστοτέλης καὶ Πλάτων ἐγίνωσκεν
ὑπὲρ νοσημάτων ἰάσεως· οὕτω δὲ καὶ Ἱπποκράτης καὶ
Διοκλῆς καὶ Πραξαγόρας καὶ Πλειστόνικος καὶ πάντες οἱ παλαιοί.

Θεσσαλὸς δὲ μόνος ἔμπαλιν ἐπὶ τὸ διὰ τοῦ νάπυος
ἥκει φάρμακον πρῶτον· εἶθ' ὕστερον ἐπιμελεῖται τοῦ
261K   παντὸς σώματος· οὔκουν οὐδ' ἐνταῦθα | φρονίμως

ancients treated the weaknesses of the parts, due to marked cold and moisture without conspicuous heat, with rubefacients. You, however, use them regularly in all cases without first distinguishing whether it is because of the weakness of the part or the *kakoethical* nature of the flux that the ulcer is not [effectively] treated. And then you change the order. For when you accomplish nothing after burning the part with the mustard, you come to the treatment of the whole body. Conversely, I think, those who know about these things from both theory and experience, having previously rendered the whole body free of superfluity, venture to apply some medication that is hot and pungent to the part. For all such [medications] naturally draw from the whole body toward themselves like a cupping glass. If you do not evacuate the whole body beforehand, you will leave behind an abundance of the flux with the pungent medication. This was a matter of agreement among both the Empiric and the Dogmatic doctors, and also seemed right to the best philosophers. Seeing that Thessalus remembered those men too, it is no bad thing to call them as witnesses [to the fact] that it is not possible to cure an eye properly before curing the whole head, or to cure the head without curing the whole body. This is how Aristotle and Plato understood the cure of diseases, as also did Hippocrates, Diocles, Praxagoras, Pleistonicus and all the ancients.

Thessalus alone, contrariwise, comes first to the medication made from mustard, and then later takes care of the whole body, so he does not here propose anything at all in a

260K

261K

οὐδὲν ὑποτιθέμενος. ἐνὸν γὰρ ἅπαξ ἐκκενώσαντα τὸ
σῶμα καθαίροντι φαρμάκῳ, μετὰ τοῦτο χρηστῶς ἀνα-
τρέφειν, ἀναφωνήσεώς τε μέμνηται καὶ γυμνασίων
αἰωρήσεών τε καὶ διαίτης ἐκ περιόδου μεταβαλλομέ-
νης ᾳμι τινος ἀπὸ ῥαφανίδων ἐμέτου· κἄπειτα τὸν
κολοφῶνα τούτοις ἐπάγει, τὸν ἐλλέβορον αὐτόν, ὁ
χωρὶς περιεργίας ἐπαγγειλάμενος ἅπαντα θεραπεύειν.
ἐγὼ δ᾽ οὐδ᾽ ἐπινοῆσαι δύναμαι πῶς ἄν τις χεῖρον, ἢ
μακρότερον, ἢ περιεργότερον ἕλκος ἰάσαιτο.

φέρε γάρ, ἵν᾽ ὥσπερ ἔργῳ πολλάκις ἑωράκαμεν,
οὕτω καὶ τῷ λόγῳ πλάσωμεν ἄνθρωπον ἰάσεως ἕλκους
κακοήθους δεόμενον. ἔστω τις ὑγιαίνων μὲν τἄλλα,
κνησάμενος δ᾽ ἐξαίφνης ὁτιοῦν μόριον, εἰ βούλει πῆχυν, ἐγειράτω παραχρῆμα φλύκταιναν· εἶτ᾽ αὖθις καὶ
αὖθις κνησμῶδες γιγνέσθω ταὐτὸ τοῦτο μόριον· ἐκρα-
γείσης δὲ τῆς φλυκταίνης ἕλκος κακόχρουν, ἀνω-
μάλως ἀναβιβρωσκόμενον γενέσθω· καὶ ταῦτ᾽ ἐν τρισὶν ἢ τέτταρσιν ἡμέραις ἀπὸ τῆς ἀρχῆς συμπιπτέτω.
λεγέτω δή τις ἐνταῦθά μοι τῶν Θεσσαλείων ἰατρῶν
ὅντινα χρὴ τρόπον ἰᾶσθαι τὸ τοιοῦτον ἕλκος. ἐγὼ μὲν
262K   γάρ φημι | κακόηθές τε πάντως ὑπάρχειν αὐτό, καὶ
διὰ τοῦτο συνεπισκέψομαι παραχρῆμα τὴν τοῦ παντὸς σώματος διάθεσιν, ὁποία τίς ἐστιν. εὑρήσω γὰρ
ἔκ τε τῶν περὶ τὸ ἕλκος συμπτωμάτων κἀκ τῶν περὶ
σύμπαν τὸ σῶμα φαινομένων σημείων, ὁποῖος μάλιστα τὴν ἰδέαν ἐστὶν ὁ πλεονάζων χυμός· καὶ τοῦτον
ἐκκενώσω φαρμάκῳ παραχρῆμα· καὶ οὐκ ἀναμενῶ

396

sensible way. For having evacuated the body once only with a purging medication, after this he nurtures it beneficially, and mentions vocal and passive exercises, a periodically changing regimen, and vomiting induced by radishes. And then, as the culmination of these measures, he introduces hellebore itself, and claims, without further elaboration, to treat everything. I cannot imagine how anyone could cure a wound or ulcer in a worse, or more time-consuming and ineffectual way.

Suppose we paint a picture in words of a man requiring cure of a *kakoethical* ulcer such as we have often seen in practice. Suppose it is someone who is healthy in other respects and suddenly becomes itchy in any part whatsoever—the forearm, if you wish—and that it immediately becomes raised into a pustule. Then, suppose this same part is repeatedly affected by itching and, when the pustule bursts open, the ulcer is of a bad color and irregularly eroded. And suppose this happens within three or four days from the onset. Then let one of the Thessaleian doctors here tell me in what way I ought to cure such an ulcer. I say this is, in every respect, a *kakoethical* ulcer, and because of this, I shall immediately consider what the condition of the whole body is as well. I shall discover from the symptoms pertaining to the ulcer and from the visible signs pertaining to the whole body, what kind of humor is most in excess, and I shall immediately evacuate this with a medication. I shall not wait for some condition that is

262K

τὸν πῆχυν ὅλον τἀνθρώπου διάθεσίν τινα κακοήθη
καὶ δυσίατον σχεῖν.

οἱ δ' ἀπὸ τοῦ Θεσσαλοῦ, τὰς ἐκείνων δηλονότι
φυλάττοντες ὑποθήκας, πρῶτον ἀναμενοῦσι χρόνιον
γενέσθαι τὸ ἕλκος, ἵν' εἰς τὴν θαυμαστὴν ἐμπέσῃ
κοινότητα τῶν χρονίων ἑλκῶν, ὥσπερ οὐκ ὂν ἄμεινον
μακρῷ κακοηθῶν ἑλκῶν, ἀλλὰ μὴ χρονίων ἐνδεικτικὴν
θεραπείας ὑποθέσθαι κοινότητα. εἶτα δυοῖν θάτερον, ἢ
ἐκκόψουσι καὶ νεωτεροποιήσουσι καὶ συνάξουσιν ὡς
εἰς κόλλησιν, ἢ πρῶτον μὲν τῷ διὰ τοῦ νάπυος
χρήσονται φαρμάκῳ, τούτου δ' ἀνύσαντος μηδὲν ἐπὶ
τὰς ἀναφωνήσεις τε καὶ τὰς αἰωρήσεις καὶ τὰ ἄλλα
γυμνάσια καὶ τὰς τῆς διαίτης κατὰ περιόδους μετα-
βολὰς ἀφίξονται· κἄπειτα καὶ τοῖς ἀπὸ ῥαφανίδων
263K ἐμέτοις | χρήσονται, καὶ μηδὲ τούτων ἰασαμένων τὸ
ἕλκος ἐλλέβορον δώσουσιν· ἂν δὲ μηδ' οὗτος ἀνύσῃ
μηδέν, ἀποπέμψουσιν εἰς Λιβύην τὸν ἄνθρωπον· ἔτι
γὰρ τοῦτ' ἔδει προσγεγραφέναι τὸν Θεσσαλὸν ἐπὶ τῇ
θαυμαστῇ τῶν ἑλκῶν τῶν κακοηθῶν ἰάσει. κατατρίβει
γοῦν ἐν ἀναφωνήσεσιν, αἰώραις τε καὶ τοῖς τοιούτοις
ὥσπερ καχεξίαν, ἀλλ' οὐ κακοχυμίαν θεραπεύων. καὶ
τί θαυμαστόν, εἰ μήτε γνωρίζειν ὁμολογοῦσιν ἄρτι
συνιστάμενον ἕλκος κακόηθες, ἀναμένουσί τε χρόνιον
αὐτὸ γενέσθαι καὶ πολλάκις μὲν ἐπουλωθῆναι, πολλάκις δ' ἀναλυθῆναι πρὸ τοῦ γνῶναι τί ποιητέον
ἐστίν; ὅπου καὶ τοὺς ὁπωσοῦν πυρέξαντας ὑπερβάλ-

---

15 The distinction between these terms is considered in the

kakoethical and difficult to cure to involve the man's whole forearm.

Thessaleians, however, if they clearly adhere to their own precepts, will first wait for the ulcer to become chronic so that it may fall into the wondrous "community" of chronic ulcers, as though this were not much better than the *kakoethical* ulcers, but without the "community" of chronicity to suggest an indication of treatment. Then there are two alternatives: either they will excise, "refresh," and bring together [the margins] as for conglutination, or they will first use the medication made from mustard, and when this accomplishes nothing, they will proceed to vocal, passive, and other exercises, and the periodically changing regimen. Then they will use vomiting induced by radishes, and when these measures fail to cure the ulcer, they will give hellebore. Should this achieve nothing, they will send the person off to Libya, for Thessalus ought to have written this as well, in addition to his wondrous cure of *kakoethical* ulcers. At all events, he wastes time on vocal and passive exercises and such things just as if he is treating *kachexia* rather than *kakochymia*.[15] And what is there to wonder at, if at one time they do not admit to recognizing a *kakoethical* ulcer existing acutely, and they wait for it to become chronic and often scarred over, and frequently broken down, before knowing what must be done? And they think it right for those who are fe-

263K

Introduction, section 6, on terminology. In summary, *kakochymia* is a disorder of the humors defined in *De probis pravisque alimentorum sucis*, VI.749K and Book 13 of the *MM* (891K), while *kachexia* is similar in meaning to the Latinized form still in use—a bad general state of the body with wasting.

λειν ἀξιοῦσι τὸν διὰ τρίτης ἡμέρας ἤτοι γενησόμενον
ἢ μὴ γενησόμενον παροξυσμόν· οὕτως ἀκριβῶς ἄρα
τὴν περὶ κρίσεων ἐκμεμαθήκασι θεωρίαν, ἢ τῆς μελ-
λούσης ἀκμῆς τοῦ νοσήματος ὑπάρχουσι προγνωστι-
κοί. τί δὴ συμβαίνει πολλάκις; ἐπὶ τῆς κλίνης κατα-
σήπεσθαι τοὺς ἀνθρώπους ὑπ᾽ αὐτῶν, ἀπηλλάχθαι
δυναμένους εὐθὺς ἐν τῇ δευτέρᾳ τῶν ἡμερῶν.

οὐχ ἅπαξ γὰρ ἡμεῖς, ἢ δίς, ἢ τρίς, ἀλλὰ μυριάκις
264K   αὐτοί τε πολλοὺς τῶν | πυρεξάντων ἐλουσάμεθα, ἅμα
τῷ παύσασθαι τὸν πρῶτον παροξυσμόν· τούς τε δι-
δασκάλους ἡμῶν ἐθεασάμεθα ταὐτὸ τοῦτο ποιοῦντας·
ἀδεῶς τε τοῦ λοιποῦ διαιτᾶσθαι συνεχωρήσαμεν, ὡς
οὐκ ἂν ἔτι πυρέξοντας, οὓς ὁ σοφώτατος Θεσσαλός, ὁ
τὴν πρώτην διάτριτον ἐξευρών, ἐταρίχευσεν ἂν ὅλαις,
οἶμαι, τρισὶ λιμοκτονήσας ἡμέραις· εἶθ᾽ οὕτως ἔθρε-
ψεν ἄν, οἶμαι, δηλαδὴ μετρίως τεταρταίους. εἶτα κατ᾽
ὀλίγον ἀνακομίζων μόλις ἑκταίους ἢ ἑβδομαίους ἀπέ-
λυσεν ἂν ἐπὶ τὰ συνήθη τοὺς ἅπαξ πυρέξαντας. οὕτως
ἀεὶ κατασήπουσι τοὺς ἀνθρώπους ἐν τοῖς πάθεσι, κἂν
ἀπαλλαγῆναι ῥᾳδίως αὐτῶν ἦν δυνατόν.

ὀλιγίσταις οὖν ἡμέραις οἷόν τε θεραπευθῆναι
κακόηθες ἕλκος ἀρχόμενον ὁ Θεσσαλὸς εἰς ἐνιαυτὸν ἢ
καὶ πλείονα χρόνον ἐκπίπτειν ἐᾷ. τὸ γὰρ ἀναμένειν
πολλάκις μὲν αὐτὸ συνουλωθῆναι, πολλάκις δ᾽ ἀναλυθῆναι, ἵν᾽ εἰδῇ εἰ κακόηθες, κἄπειτα τῆς θεραπείας
ἀρξάμενον οὐδ᾽ οὖν οὐδὲ τότε καθαίρειν εὐθύς, ἀλλὰ

brile in any way whatsoever to go beyond the third day, whether a paroxysm will occur or not. In this way, they are either completely conversant with the theory about crises, or they are prescient regarding the impending peak of the disease. So what does in fact often happen? Patients who could be up and about straightaway on the second day, in their hands rot away in their beds.[16]

Not once only, or two or three times, but on countless occasions, I myself bathed many of those who were febrile at the time of cessation of the first paroxysm. And I saw my teachers doing this same thing, and was untroubled in allowing the regimen to continue so they would not still be febrile—these patients whom the most sagacious Thessalus, discovering the first three-day period, would have caused to waste away, starving them, I imagine, for three whole days. Then, I believe, he would nourish them for four days, moderately of course. Next, having gradually and with difficulty carried them through six or seven days, he would bring back those who were once febrile to their customary situation. So he always allowed those people to waste away like this in their affections—even those who could easily have been relieved.

Therefore, Thessalus allows an incipient *kakoethical* ulcer that can be treated in a very few days to degenerate for a year or an even longer time. For the delay frequently allows it to become scarred over, and often to break down again, so that he may know if it is *kakoethical*, and then, neither having begun the treatment nor at that time

264K

[16] To give added force to his criticism of the Methodics, Galen foreshadows his attack on them for their management of fevers in later books.

τῷ διὰ τοῦ νάπυος μὲν πρῶτον, εἶτ᾽ αἰώραις ἀναφωνή-
σεσί τε καὶ διαίταις χρῆσθαι, κἄπειτα ῥαφανῖσιν, εἶθ᾽
265K   οὕτως ἐλλεβόρῳ, τί ἄλλο ἢ ἐνιαυτὸν | ἀναμένοντός
ἐστιν; εἶτ᾽, ὦ πρὸς θεῶν, ἐξ ἡμερῶν, ἢ τὸ πλεῖστον
ἑπτά, δυναμένου τἀνθρώπου τεθεραπεῦσθαι, μῆνας
ἀναμενοῦμεν πολλούς, ἵνα δηλαδὴ πρῶτον μὲν γνῶ-
μεν εἰ χρόνιόν ἐστιν, ἔπειτα δ᾽ ἀρξώμεθα τῆς θεραπείας; καὶ τίς ἦν ἀνάγκη χρονίων ἑλκῶν ἰδίαν ὑποθέσθαι
κοινότητα, μηδὲν εἰς τὰς ἰάσεις ἡμᾶς ὠφελοῦσαν; ἐνὸν
μὴ χρονίων, ἀλλὰ κακοηθῶν, οὐ κοινότητα μὰ Δία
οὐδὲ τούτων ἐνδεικτικήν, ἀλλὰ θεραπείαν γράψαι.
συμβέβηκε μὲν γάρ τισιν ἕλκεσί τε καὶ νόσοις κακοή-
θεσιν ὑπάρχειν, οὐ μὴν ἀπὸ τούτου γε ἡ τῆς θεραπείας ἔνδειξις, ἀλλ᾽ ἡ μὲν διάθεσις αὐτὴ τὸν πρῶτον
τῆς ἰάσεως ὑπαγορεύει σκοπόν· ἐξ ἐκείνου δ᾽ εὑρίσκεται τὰ ποιητέα καθ᾽ ὃν ἐγὼ διελήλυθα τρόπον. ὥστε
τοῦτ᾽ ἔστι τὸ μεθόδῳ θεραπεύειν, ὃ ποιοῦμεν ἡμεῖς
ἑπόμενοι τοῖς παλαιοῖς· εἴ γε χρὴ τὴν μέθοδον ὁδόν
τινα εἶναι καθόλου μίαν ἁπάντων κοινὴν τῶν κατὰ
μέρος. ὁ δέ γε κἂν τούτῳ σφάλλεται καὶ τὸ πάντως
ὑπάρχον τοῖς ὁτιοῦν μεθόδῳ ποιοῦσι, τοῦτο τὴν μέθ-
οδον αὐτὴν εἶναι νομίζει. γνῶσιν μὲν γὰρ ἔχειν |
266K   ἀναγκαῖόν ἐστι τὸν μεθόδῳ πᾶν ὁτιοῦν ἐργαζόμενον
ὁμοιότητός τε καὶ ἀνομοιότητος, οὐ μὴν αὐτό γε τοῦτ᾽
ἔστιν ἡ μέθοδος, ὁμοίου τε καὶ ἀνομοίου γνῶσις. οὐδὲ
τοῦτο λέγει Πλάτων ἢ Ἀριστοτέλης, ὧν τολμᾷ κατα-
ψεύδεσθαι Θεσσαλός.

    ἀλλὰ γὰρ οὐ τοῦ παρόντος καιροῦ ταῦτ᾽ ἐξελέγ-

purged immediately, he first uses the medication prepared
from mustard, and then passive and vocal exercises, and
regimen, and next radishes, and then, in the same way, hellebore. What is this if not delaying for a year? By the gods,   265K
in a person who could have been treated in six or, at the
most, seven days, must we wait many months, so that we
might first know clearly if it is chronic, and then begin the
treatment? And why is it necessary to postulate a "community" specific to chronic ulcers, if it gives us no help with
our treatments? Although it is possible [to do so], do not
write of chronic [ulcers] but of *kakoethical* ones, and not of
a "community" indicative of these, by Zeus, but of their
treatment. With some ulcers and diseases, it does happen
that they are *kakoethical*, but the indication of treatment is
not in fact taken from this. Rather, it is the condition itself
that suggests the primary indicator of the cure. We discover what is to be done from that in the manner which I
recounted in detail. This is to treat by method, which is
what we who follow the ancients do. If there should be
some methodical path it will, in general, be one common
to all [conditions] in turn. In fact, even in this he is mistaken and thinks it is true that for those who do anything
whatsoever by method, this is the actual (i.e. the right)
method. It is necessary for someone who does anything at
all by method to have knowledge of similarity and differ-   266K
ence, but not [to believe] that similarity and dissimilarity is
itself the method. Neither Plato nor Aristotle says this
which Thessalus dares to falsely claim about them.

But now is not the time to refute this claim. I shall re-

χειν. αὖθις οὖν ἐπὶ τὴν θεραπευτικὴν μέθοδον ἐπάνειμι καὶ δείξειν ἐπαγγέλλομαι τήν τε ἀρχὴν αὐτῆς μίαν
ἐν ἁπάσαις ταῖς ἰάσεσι, τήν τε ἀπὸ τῆς ἀρχῆς ὁδὸν
ἕως τοῦ τέλους ὁμοίαν ἐν ἅπασι τοῖς κατὰ μέρος. ὥστ᾽
εἰ καὶ καθ᾽ ἕκαστον πάθος ἰδίᾳ τις φαίνοιτο μέθοδος
ἰάσεως, ἀλλὰ τό γε κοινὸν ἐφ᾽ ἁπάσαις γένος ἓν
ὑπάρχει. ἄρχεσθαι μὲν γὰρ ἀεὶ χρὴ τῆς ἐνδείξεως ἀπὸ
τῆς διαθέσεως, ἣν θεραπεύειν ἐπιχειροῦμεν· ἐπισκέπτεσθαι δὲ καὶ διορίζεσθαι πότερον ἤδη πέπαυται τὸ
ποιῆσαν αἴτιον τὴν διάθεσιν, ἢ καὶ νῦν ἔτι συνεπαύξει
τε καὶ ποιεῖ· κἄπειτα πεπαυμένου μὲν ἐπὶ τὴν ἐν τῷ
τρίτῳ τῶνδε τῶν ὑπομνημάτων εἰρημένην μέθοδον
ἰτέον· ἔτι δὲ ποιοῦντος ἐπὶ τὴν ἐν τῷδε. τῇ γὰρ αὐτῇ
267K   μεθόδῳ τῇδε καὶ φλεγμονῆς | καὶ πυρετοῦ καὶ πάντων
ἁπλῶς τῶν νοσημάτων τὰς ἰάσεις ἐξευρήσομεν, εἰ μὲν
μηκέτι γίγνοιτο μηδέν, μὴ προσχρώμενοι τοῖς προ-
ηγησαμένοις αἰτίοις, ἀλλ᾽ ἐξ αὐτῆς μόνης τῆς διαθέσεως ὁρμώμενοι· εἰ δέ τι καὶ νῦν γίγνοιτο, καὶ
διττὸν σκοπὸν τῆς θεραπείας ὑποτιθέμενοι καὶ τἄλλ᾽
ἐξῆς ὡς εἴρηται ποιοῦντες.

ἀλλὰ γὰρ καὶ τῆς ἀναισθησίας τῶν ἑπομένων τῷ
Θεσσαλῷ θαυμάζειν ἄξιον· οὐκ ἐπειδὰν ἐν τοῖς τοιούτοις ἁμαρτάνωσιν, ἀλλ᾽ ὅτι δυσπαθείας τε καὶ μετα-
συγκρίσεις, ἀτονίας τε καὶ ῥώσεις καὶ πολλὰ τοιαῦθ᾽
ἕτερα λέγοντες ὀνόματα σημαινόμενα πρὸς αὐτῶν,

17 Presumably Galen is referring to the distinction between
the treatment of an as yet uncomplicated wound and that of a

turn once more to the therapeutic method, and will undertake to show that it has the one point of origin in all cures, and that the path from beginning to end is the same in all particulars. Consequently, if a specific method of cure is apparent for each affection, there is a single class in common for all cures. For it is always necessary to begin the indication from the condition we are trying to treat, although it is also necessary to consider and determine whether the cause which produced the condition has already ceased, or is currently still helping to increase [the condition] and acting. If it has ceased, we must go to the method described in the third book of this treatise; if it is still acting, we must go to the method in this book.[17] For by this same method, we shall discover the cures of inflammation, fever, and in short, of all diseases. If there is nothing still occurring, we would not be making use of the *proegoumenic* causes but would make a start from the condition itself alone. If, however, there is at the time something else also occurring, we would postulate a second indicator of treatment and do the other things in order, as was said.

267K

But I also think it right to be amazed at the stupidity of those who follow Thessalus. It is not that they are mistaken in such things, but that they speak of *dyspathia* and *metasyncrisis*,[18] of weakness and strength, and many other such things, using terms that signify something to them, but

chronic inflamed wound, which might properly be termed an ulcer, and lesions like this—for example, an abscess or pustule that has burst and is chronically discharging.   [18] In this further rant against the Methodics, we have simply transliterated the technical terms, which Galen thinks are meaningless anyway. For a detailed discussion of the theory, see J. Vallance (1990).

οὐδέπω καὶ νῦν ἐρωτηθέντες, ἀποκρίνασθαι δύνανται.
τί γάρ ἐστι τὸ μετασυγκρίνειν τὴν ἕξιν ἐπὶ τῶν χρονι-
ζόντων ἁπάντων οὔθ᾽ ὡσαύτως ἀλλήλοις οὔτε σαφῶς
οὔτε νουνεχῶς ἀποκρίνονται. εἰ μὲν οὖν ἢ παλαιὸν ἢ
παρά τινι τῶν Ἑλλήνων ἦν γεγραμμένον τοὔνομα,
τάχ᾽ ἂν ἴσως ἐξ ὧν ἐκεῖνοι γράφουσιν ἐνοήσαμεν ἐφ᾽
ὅτου πράγματος ἐπιφέρουσιν αὐτό· νυνὶ δέ, τῆς γὰρ
τούτων ἐμπληξίας ἐστὶν οἰκεῖον, ἀπὸ τῆς Ἀσκληπιάδου γεγενημένον ὑποθέσεως, ὥσπερ καὶ τἆλλα
268K   αὐτῶν | δόγματα δίκαιοι δήπουθέν εἰσι τοὺς ἰδίους
ὀνείρους ἐξηγεῖσθαι· ὅθεν συγκρίνεσθαι τὰ σώματα
καὶ διακρίνεσθαι τοῖς ὄγκους καὶ πόρους ὑποθεμένοις,
ἢ ἄτομα καὶ κενόν, ἢ ὅλως ἀπαθῆ καὶ ἀναλλοίωτα τὰ
πρῶτα στοιχεῖα, μόνοις ἐγχωρεῖ λέγειν, ὥσπερ οὖν
καὶ λέγουσι καὶ συνεχῶς αὐτοῖς χρῶνται τοῖς ὀνόμασι. καὶ δῆτα καὶ ὁ Θεσσαλὸς ἐν τῷ κανόνι ταύτας
κατασκευάζων τὰς ἀρχὰς νεωτεροποιεῖ μέν τι κἀκεῖ
παρὰ τὰ Θεμίσωνί τε καὶ Ἀσκληπιάδῃ δοκοῦντα·
διδάσκει δ᾽ οὖν ὅμως τὴν ἑαυτοῦ γνώμην οὐκ ἀσαφῶς.
οὐ γὰρ ἁπλῶς ὡς Ἀσκληπιάδης ἐν συμμετρίᾳ μέν τινι
πόρων τὸ ὑγιαίνειν ἡμᾶς ὑποθέμενος, ἐν ἀμετρίᾳ δὲ τὸ
νοσεῖν, ἐπάνοδον εἶναι τὴν θεραπείαν εἰς τὴν ἀρχαίαν
συμμετρίαν τῶν πόρων ὑπέλαβεν, οὕτω καὶ ὁ Θεσσαλός, ἀλλὰ τὸν τρόπον τῆς ποροποιΐας ὅλον ὑπαλλάττεσθαι νομίζει, κἀκ ταύτης τῆς ὑπολήψεως ἥκει τὸ
μετασυγκρίσεως ὄνομα, ταὐτὸν δηλοῦν δυνάμει τῷ
τῆς μεταπoροποιήσεως.

[19] We have followed Linacre in assuming that the unstated

[what this is] they cannot even today answer when asked. For they do not distinguish either clearly or sensibly what the state of *metasyncrisis* is in the case of all chronic [ulcers],[19] even to one another in the same way. If it is a term, either an ancient one or one written by one of the Greeks, perhaps from what those men write we would know to what matter they are applying it. Now however, since it is a characteristic of their stupidity arising from the hypothesis of Asclepiades,[20] as do the rest of their theories also, they are right, I suppose, to interpret their peculiar dreams, with their postulations of bodies coming together and separating, and of *onkoi* (corpuscles) and *poroi* (pores), or atoms and void, and it is possible for them alone to speak of altogether impassible and immutable first elements, as they do when they speak of and continually use these terms. And to be sure, Thessalus too, in his canon, when he formulated these principles, created something novel there besides the suppositions of Themison and Asclepiades. Indeed, he teaches this conceptual scheme of his not without clarity. He does not simply postulate, as Asclepiades does, that our being healthy depends on a certain balance of *poroi*, whereas our being sick depends on an imbalance, and he does not simply take treatment to be a return to the original balance of the *poroi*. Thessalus does think along these lines, but he thinks that the whole manner of the state of the pores is changed, and from this assumption comes to the term *metasyncrisis* which signifies the same as the term *metaporopoiesis* in terms of force.

268K

noun is "ulcer," although Galen could be making a more general claim—for example, about conditions or diseases.

[20] Asclepiades was, in a sense, the founder of Methodic theory.

οὐκ ἐχρῆν δ᾽ αὐτὸν ἐν οἷς ἀποχωρεῖν τῶν ἀδήλων
κελεύει καὶ μόναις προσέχειν τὸν νοῦν ταῖς ἐναργῶς
269K φαινομέναις κοινότησιν, ἐν τούτοις | ἔτι Δογματικοῖς
χρῆσθαι τοῖς ὀνόμασιν. Ἀλλὰ μὴ δογματικῶς ἄκουε
λέγοντος αὐτοῦ, φασιν, ἀλλ᾽ ἀφελῶς· εἰώθασι γὰρ
οὕτως ἀντιλαμβάνεσθαί τινες τῶν ἀπ᾽ αὐτοῦ, πάλιν
ἐφ᾽ ἕτερον ἡμᾶς ἄγοντες ὄνομα τὴν ἀφέλειαν, ἣν οὐδ᾽
αὐτὴν ἐγὼ γοῦν ἔχω νοῆσαι τί δηλοῖ. εἰ μὲν γὰρ ὡς
αὐτοὶ καὶ τοῦτ᾽ ἐξηγοῦνται, πάλιν εἰς ἕτερον ὄνομα
μεταλαμβάνοντες ληρωδέστερον τὸ βιωτικῶς, εἶτ᾽
αὖθις καὶ τοῦτ᾽ ἐξηγούμενοί φασι δηλοῦσθαι πρὸς
αὐτοῦ τὸ τοῖς πολλοῖς τῶν ἀνθρώπων ὡσαύτως, ἴσον
ἂν εἴη δήπου τὸ ἀφελῶς τῷ μὴ διηρθρωμένως μηδ᾽
ἀκριβῶς, ἀλλ᾽ ἀτέχνως τε καὶ χωρὶς ἐπιστήμης ἁπά-
σης· φθέγγονται μὲν γὰρ οἱ προπετέστεροι τῶν ἀνθρώπων ὀνόματα τεχνικὰ μετά τινων ὑπονοιῶν οὐδὲν
ἐχουσῶν ἔρεισμα, τοῖς δ᾽ ἐρωτήσασιν ὅ τί ποτε δη-
λοῦσιν οὐκ ἔχουσιν ἀποκρίνασθαι σαφῶς. εἰ δὲ τοῦθ᾽
ὁμολογοῦσι καὶ οἱ Θεσσάλειοι πεπονθέναι, φθέγγεσθαι μέν τινα, μὴ γινώσκειν δ᾽ ἀκριβῶς ἃ λέγουσιν,
αὐτὸ δήπου προσίενται τὸ πρὸς ἡμῶν αὐτοῖς ὀνειδι-
ζόμενον. ἡ γοῦν μετασύγκρισις εἰ μὲν ἐπὶ τοῦ τὴν |
270K ποροποιίαν ἐναλλάττεσθαι λέγοιτο, νοῦν μὲν ἕξει τινὰ
καὶ δηλώσει τι πρᾶγμα, ληρώδης δ᾽ ἔσται πολυειδῶς.
οὔτε γὰρ ἐξ ὄγκων καὶ πόρων τὰ σώματα ἡμῶν συν-
έστηκεν οὔτ᾽ εἰ καὶ τοῦτ᾽ ἀληθὲς ἦν, ἔχει τις δεῖξαι
πῶς ἐξαλλάττει τὸ νᾶπυ τὴν ποροποιίαν, οὔτ᾽ εἰ καὶ
τοῦτ᾽ εἶχέ τις δεῖξαι, κατὰ τὴν ἀκολουθίαν ἣν τῆς

But in these matters he ought not to have gone away from the unseen things and exhorted us to turn our attention to the manifestly apparent "communities" alone, still using the Dogmatic terms in these. "But," they say, "do not listen when he speaks 'dogmatically' but only when he speaks simply." For some of his followers are accustomed to apprehend it in this way, directing us back again to another term in respect of simplicity—a simplicity which is such that I, at any rate, do not grasp what it signifies. But if, as they themselves explain it, they change from a term in common use to another, quite silly term, and when they come to explain this in turn, they say what is signified by him is like what is signified by the majority of people, this is the equivalent presumably of explaining what is simple in a way that is neither clearly articulated nor precise, but is naive and devoid of all science. For these overreckless men spout technical terms with deep meanings devoid of foundation, and when asked at some time what they signify, they have no clear answer. If even the Thessaleians admit that they are affected in this way, and that they say certain things without knowing precisely what they are saying, then they are accepting the very thing we reproach them for. Anyway, *metasyncrisis*, if it is said in the case of a change in the state of the pores, will have a certain sense and will signify something, but it will be in a foolish and complicated way. Our bodies are not composed of *onkoi* and *poroi*.[21] Nor, even if this were true, is anyone able to show how mustard changes the state of the *poroi*. And even if somone were able to show this, he would not be in

269K

270K

[21] On the nature of *onkoi* (corpuscles) and *poroi* (pores), see J. Vallance (1990), chapter 1, pp. 7–43.

αἱρέσεως αὐτῶν, ἀρκεῖσθαι φασκόντων ταῖς φαινομέναις κοινότησι. μὴ τοίνυν μηδὲ χρήσθωσαν τῷ
ὀνόματι, μηδὲ πρᾶγμαθ᾽ ἡμῖν παρεχέτωσαν· ἔνεστι
γὰρ δήπου καὶ χωρὶς τοῦ χρήσασθαι τῷ τῆς μετασυγκρίσεως ὀνόματι τὴν θεραπείαν εἰπεῖν τῶν χρονι-
ζόντων ἑλκῶν ἑτέροις ὀνόμασιν, ὥσπερ καὶ οἱ Ἐμπειρικοὶ ποιοῦσιν.

ὅτι δὲ καὶ ἡ τῆς ἀτονίας προσηγορία κατὰ τὸν
αὐτὸν τρόπον αὐτοῖς φλυαρεῖται δέδεικται πρόσθεν ἐν
τῷ δευτέρῳ λόγῳ. εἰ μὲν γὰρ ὡς Ἐμπειρικοὶ προσ-
φέρονται τοὔνομα, πλέον οὐδὲν δηλοῦσι τοῦ μὴ σῴζεσθαι τὴν ἐνέργειαν· εἰ δέ τινας ὑποτίθενται δυνάμεις
τὸ ζῷον διοικεῖν, οἵας ἡμεῖς τε λέγομεν ἅπαντές
τε σχεδὸν οἱ παλαιοί, πρὸς τῷ τοῖς Ἀσκληπιάδου
δόγμασιν ἐναντία τίθεσθαι καὶ τῶν ἀδήλων τε καὶ
271K   διαπεφωνημένων | ἐφάψονται, καίτοι φεύγειν ταῦτα
παρακελευόμενοι. τί λέγεις ὦ ἄνθρωπε; τὸ μετασυγκρίνειν ἀποσαφήνισον ἡμῖν. εἰ μὲν γὰρ τὸ τοὺς πόρους ὑπαλλάττειν, καὶ ψευδῆ καὶ τῶν ἀδήλων ἐφάπτῃ·
εἰ δ᾽ αὐτὸ τοῦτο τὸ ῥώννυσθαί τε καὶ ὑγιάζεσθαι τὸ
μόριον τοῦ σώματος, ἢ τὸν ἄνθρωπον ὅλον, οὐδὲν ἂν
πλέον ἐνταῦθα τῶν Ἐμπειρικῶν ἀποφαίνῃ, πλὴν ὀνόματος. γιγνώσκουσι γὰρ δήπου κἀκεῖνοι τῶνδέ τινων
προσαγομένων τῶν βοηθημάτων ὑγιάζεσθαι τὸν ἄνθρωπον, ἀλλὰ τί ποιούντων αὐτῶν οὐκ ἴσασιν. οὔτε
γὰρ εἰ τοὺς πόρους ὑπαλλάττουσιν αἱ δυνάμεις τῶν
βοηθημάτων, οὔτ᾽ εἰ συμμετρίαν αὐτοῖς ἐκπορίζουσιν,
οὔτ᾽ εἰ σύμπαν ἀλλοιοῦσι κατὰ ποιότητα τὸ θεραπευ-

agreement with their sect, since they say they are satisfied with the apparent "communities." And so let them not use this term or present the matter to us. For it is possible, I presume, to speak of the treatment of chronic ulcers with other terms apart from using the term *metasyncrisis*, just as the Empirics do.

It has also been shown before (in the second book) that the term "weakness" (*atonia*) is used nonsensically by them in the same way. For if they apply the term as the Empirics do, they signify nothing more than the nonpreservation of function. If, however, they propose that certain capacities, of the kind we and almost all the ancients speak of, govern the organism and, in addition to this, they postulate things contrary to the opinions of Asclepiades, they touch on things that are obscure and are points of disagreement. And yet they exhort us to avoid these things. What, 271K my dear chap, are you talking about? Make clear to us what the meaning of *metasyncrisis* is. If it is that the *poroi* undergo change, you are being deceptive and are touching on obscurities. If, on the other hand, it is that this particular part of the body, or the whole person, is strong and healthy, you would be making clear here nothing more than the Empirics do without the term. For even those men, I presume, know that when some of these remedies are applied, the person becomes healthy. What they do not know, when they do these things, is why. For it is possible for one of the Empirics to say that the potencies of the remedies do not change the pores, or produce balance in them, or change

ὅμενον μόριον, ἔχει τις εἰπεῖν τῶν Ἐμπειρικῶν. ἐκεῖνοι
μὲν οὖν σωφρονοῦσιν, ἓν μόνον ἐπίστασθαι λέγοντες,
ὡς τῷ τοιῷδε νοσήματι κατὰ τόνδε τὸν καιρὸν προσφερομένου τοῦ διὰ νάπυος φαρμάκου, πολλάκις ἐτή-
ρησαν ὠφέλειαν ἀκολουθοῦσαν. οὐ μὴν μεθόδους γε
φθέγγονται καὶ τὰς ὀφρῦς ἀνατείνουσι καὶ σεμνύνον-
ται τῇ τοιαύτῃ γνώσει καὶ τοῖς παλαιοῖς λοιδοροῦνται
272K καὶ τὸν Ἱπποκράτην τὸ | μηδὲν ὑπειλήφασιν, ἀλλ᾽
αὐτὸν τοὐναντίον ἐπαινοῦσί τε καὶ σχεδὸν ἅπαντά
φασιν ἀληθεύειν αὐτόν.

ὁ δὲ καὶ τούτου καὶ τῶν ἄλλων ἰατρῶν ἁπάντων
καταφρονήσας Θεσσαλὸς ἕλκους κακοήθους Ἐμπειρικὴν ἀναγράφων διδασκαλίαν οὐκ αἰσθάνεται· καίτοι γ᾽ εἰ καὶ τοῦτο δεόντως ἐποίησεν, ἦν ἄν τι πλέον
ἐξειργασμένος· ἀλλὰ γὰρ οὐδὲ τοῦτο ποιεῖν ἔοικεν,
ὑπαλλάττων τὴν τάξιν τῶν βοηθημάτων καὶ πρότερον
χρώμενος τῷ τοῦ πεπονθότος μέρους, πρὶν ἂν τὸ
σύμπαν σῶμα παρασκευάσαι. τοῦτο γὰρ ὑπερβολὴν
ἀμαθίας ἔχει· μόνον γοῦν σχεδόν τι τοῖς ἰατροῖς
ἅπασιν ὡμολόγηται καίτοί γε τῶν πλείστων διαπεφω-
νημένων, τὸ πᾶν σῶμα κενὸν καὶ ἀπέριττον ἐργάζεσθαι, πρὶν ὁτιοῦν μόριον ἰσχυροῖς ὑποβάλλειν βοη-
θήμασιν. εἴτε γὰρ τῇ πείρᾳ κρίνειν ἐθέλει τις ἄν, εἴτε
καὶ τῷ λογισμῷ, τρίτον γὰρ οὐδὲν ἕτερον κριτήριον
οὔτε κατ᾽ ἄλλην τέχνην οὔτε καθ᾽ ὅλον τὸν βίον
ἔχομεν, εὑρήσει μέγιστον κακὸν ὑπάρχον, ὅταν τοῦ
παντὸς σώματος ἐπικουρίας δεομένου, πρὶν ἐκείνου
προνοήσασθαι, τῷ πεπονθότι μορίῳ προσφέρει τις

the whole part being treated in terms of quality. Those men, then, are of sound mind when they claim to know one thing alone; that in this particular disease, and at this particular time, when they apply the medication made from mustard, they often observe a benefit that follows. At least they don't talk about methods, or raise their eyebrows, or exalt themselves with such knowledge, or revile the ancients and accept nothing Hippocratic but, on the contrary, they praise him and say that he speaks the truth in almost every instance.

272K

Thessalus, however, since he despises both Hippocrates and all other doctors, does not understand the Empiric teaching on *kakoethical* ulcers when he describes it. Indeed, if he had done this as he ought, he would have achieved rather more. But he does not seem to do even this, changing the order of the remedies and using them first on the affected part before providing for the whole body. This betokens an excess of ignorance. Although they disagree on most things, the one thing that almost all doctors do agree on is to make the whole body empty and without superfluity before subjecting any part of it whatsoever to strong remedies. If anyone wishes to judge, either by experience or by reasoning—and we have no other, third criterion, whether in relation to another craft or to life as a whole—he will discover that it is very harmful, whenever the whole body requires succor, if he gives thought to the affected part before the whole body, and applies any sort of

273K ὁτιοῦν δριμὺ καὶ θερμὸν φάρμακον· | ἕλκει γὰρ ἐφ᾽
ἑαυτὸ δίκην σικύας ἐξ ὅλου τοῦ σώματος τὰ περιτ-
τώματα καὶ στηρίζει δυσλύτως κατὰ τὸ πεπονθὸς
μέρος.

ἄξιον οὖν ἐρέσθαι τοὺς Θεσσαλείους, πόθεν ἐπῆλθε
τῷ Θεσσαλῷ τοιαῦτα φλυαρεῖν ὑπὲρ ἑλκῶν κακοηθῶν
ἰάσεως· οὔτε γὰρ Ἐμπειρικὸς οὐδεὶς τῶν πρόσθεν οὔτε
Λογικὸς ἀνὴρ οὕτως ἔγραψεν· ἀλλὰ μὴν οὐδ᾽ αὐτὸς ὁ
Θεσσαλός, οὐδὲ τῶν ἀπ᾽ αὐτοῦ τις τολμήσειεν εἰπεῖν ἢ
τῇ πείρᾳ συμφωνεῖν ἢ τῷ λογισμῷ τὴν τοιαύτην τάξιν
τῶν βοηθημάτων. οὐ μὴν οὐδὲ δεῖξαι δύνανται, πῶς ὁ
χρόνος, οὐχ ἡ διάθεσις ἐνδείκνυται· καὶ τὸ τούτου
μεῖζόν ἐστι, πῶς αὐτὸς ὁ Θεσσαλός, ἀξιῶν σκέπτεσθαι τί τὸ ἐμποδίζον ἐστὶ τὴν συνούλωσιν τῶν ἑλκῶν,
καὶ τοῦτ᾽ ἐκκόπτειν, οὐχὶ τελέως ἐστὶν ἀναίσθητος;
ἅμα μὲν οὐκ εἰδὼς ὡς τοῦτ᾽ ἀρκεῖ μόνον, ἡ χρονιότης
δὲ τῶν ἑλκῶν οὐδέν ἐστι πρὸς ἔπος, ἅμα δὲ ὡς οὐκ ἐφ᾽
ἑλκῶν μόνον, ἀλλὰ κἀπὶ τῶν ἄλλων ἁπάντων νοσημάτων τοῦτο ποιητέον ἐστίν, ὡς οἱ παλαιοὶ παραινοῦσιν.
ἀλλὰ πρὸς ταῦτα μὲν ἡμῖν οὐδὲν ἀποκρίνονται· παρ-
ακοὰς δὲ ἑκάστοτε λέγοντες ὡς δῆθεν ἀκριβῶς μεμα-
274K θηκότες ἢ τὴν Ἱπποκράτους, | ἢ τὴν ἄλλου τινὸς τῶν
παλαιῶν γνώμην, ὀρθῶς φασι τὸν Θεσσαλὸν ἀποφήνασθαι χρονίων ἑλκῶν εἶναί τινα κοινότητα μίαν.
οὕτω γοῦν καὶ Ἱπποκράτην γινώσκειν ἐν τῷ Περὶ
ἑλκῶν ὧδέ πως γράψαντα· Καὶ ἀπὸ τῶν πεπαλαιωμένων ἑλκέων ξυμφέρει αἷμα ποιέειν ἀπορρέειν πυκινά, ὅπως ἂν δοκέῃ καιρὸς εἶναι.

414

sharp and hot medication. This draws to itself the super-   273K
fluities of the whole body, like a cupping glass, and fixes
them indissolubly in the affected part.

It is, then, worth asking the Thessaleians how it came to
Thessalus to talk such nonsense about the cure of *kakoethical* ulcers. For no Empiric of those who came before,
nor any Dogmatic, wrote in this way. But not even Thessalus himself, nor any of those who follow him, will dare to
say they agree with such an order of remedies on the basis
of either experience or reasoning. Nor are they able to
show how the time rather than the condition provides the
indication. And much more than this, how is this Thessalus, who thinks it worthwhile to consider what is hindering the cicatrization of the ulcer and excise it, not absolutely stupid? At one and the same time, he does not know
that this is sufficient alone, and that the chronicity of
wounds and ulcers is of no relevance, and that this does not
apply to wounds and ulcers alone, but also must be done to
all other diseases, as the ancients recommend. But they
have no answer for us on these matters, saying on each occasion that there has been a misunderstanding and that
they have, would you believe, learned accurately the Hip-   274K
pocratic concept or that of another of the ancients, and
they say Thessalus is right to declare that there is one
"community" of chronic wounds and ulcers. At least they
do know that Hippocrates, in the [work] *On Wounds* (*Ulcers*), wrote as follows: "It is beneficial to make blood flow
away from long-standing wounds and ulcers repeatedly in
whatever way seems opportune."[22]

22 Hippocrates, *Peri helkōn* 2, LCL, *Hippocrates*, vol. VIII,
pp. 344-45.

τάχα οὖν ἄμεινον ἂν εἴη, καίτοι μὴ προηρημένον
με περὶ τῆς Ἱπποκράτους γνώμης ἐνταυθοῖ διέρχεσθαι, δηλῶσαί τι κἂν διὰ κεφαλαίων ὑπὲρ αὐτῆς· εἴη
δ᾽ ἂν οὐδὲν ἧττον καὶ τῆς τῶν παλαιῶν διανοίας
ἐξήγησις ὅδε ὁ λόγος. ἐκεῖνοι γὰρ οἱ ἄνδρες, ἅτε
μήπω δουλεύοντες αἱρέσει δογμάτων, ἀλλὰ καθαρᾷ
καὶ ἁπλῇ τῇ διανοίᾳ σπουδάζοντες ἐξευρίσκειν τι
χρηστὸν εἰς τὰς ἰάσεις, ἔμελλον δήπου τὰ μὲν ἐκ τῆς
πείρας εὑρήσειν, τὰ δὲ ἐκ τοῦ λόγου· καὶ γράψειν γε
τὰ εὑρημένα πολλαχόθι μὲν χωρὶς τοῦ προσθεῖναι τὸν
τρόπον τῆς εὑρέσεως, ἐνίοτε δὲ καὶ σὺν τούτῳ· καὶ
τοῦτό γε ποιήσειν αὐτὸ τῆς ὠφελείας ἕνεκα τῶν ἀνα-
γινωσκόντων· εἰ μὲν γὰρ εἰς τὴν ἐπιδέξιον χρῆσιν τῶν
εὑρημένων ἤλπιζόν τι συντελέσειν τοῖς ἔπειτα τὸν
275K   τρόπον τῆς εὑρέσεως γνωσθέντα, | τηνικαῦτα μὲν
ἀκριβῶς ἔγραφον· εἰ δὲ μή, περιττόν τε λέγειν ἡγοῦν-
το καὶ παρέλειπον. ὅτι γὰρ εἴ πέρ τι καὶ ἄλλο, καὶ
ἡ βραχυλογία τοῖς παλαιοῖς ἐτετίμητο, πάντες ἤδη
τοῦτο γινώσκουσι κἂν ἐγὼ μὴ λέγω· καὶ διά γε ταύτην
τὴν αἰτίαν οὐχ Ἱπποκράτης μόνον, ἀλλὰ καὶ οἱ ἄλλοι
παλαιοὶ τὸ μέσον ὑπερβαίνοντες ἐνίοτε τῷ πρώτῳ τὸ
τρίτον συνάπτουσιν. εἰ γὰρ σημεῖον μὲν εἴη τὸ πρῶτον τοῦ δευτέρου, τούτῳ δ᾽ ἐξ ἀνάγκης ἕποιτο τὸ
τρίτον, οὕτως ἐπιφέρουσι τῷ πρώτῳ τὸ τρίτον ὑπερβαίνοντες τὸ δεύτερον. ἔδειξα δὲ πολλάκις τοιαῦτα
τούς τ᾽ ἄλλους παλαιοὺς καὶ μάλιστα πάντων τὸν
Ἱπποκράτην γράψαντα, καὶ χρὴ τὸν βουλόμενον
ἐθάδα γενέσθαι παλαιᾶς ἑρμηνείας ἐν ἐκείνοις γυμνά-

Although I have not previously chosen to discourse on the opinion of Hippocrates here, perhaps it would be better to make known something about this, even if only in summary. This same discussion would also be no less a statement of the thought of the ancients. For those men, inasmuch as they were not yet slaves to any school of opinions, were eager to discover, by understanding pure and simple, what was useful for cures. They intended, I presume, to discover some through experience and some through reason, and to write about those discoveries in many places without adding the manner of discovery, although sometimes with this as well, at least if it would be of benefit for the readers. Since they anticipated to some extent that knowing the manner of discovery would contribute something to the skillful use of the discoveries by those who followed, then under those circumstances they   275K
wrote precisely. If not, they believed that to speak was superfluous and omitted [to do so]. Apart from anything else, this was because brevity had been prized by the ancients—everyone already knows this, even if I do not say [it]. For this very reason, not only Hippocrates but also the other ancients, if they passed over the middle, sometimes connected the third to the first. For if the first was a sign of the second, and the third followed this of necessity, in this way they impute the third to the first, passing over the second. I have shown often that the other ancients, and most of all Hippocrates, wrote such things, and it behooves someone who wishes to become familiar with the ancient

σασθαι. νυνὶ δ᾽ αὐτὸ τὸ προβεβλημένον ἐξηγήσομαι μόνον.

5. Ὅσα γὰρ τῶν ἑλκῶν, ἁπάντων ὀρθῶς καὶ δεόντως γιγνομένων ὅμως οὐ θεραπεύεται, καλεῖται μὲν ὑπὸ τῶν ἰατρῶν κακοήθη, χρονίζει δὲ πάντως ὅταν τὴν ὡς ἑλκῶν μόνην αὐτοῖς τις ἐπάγει θεραπείαν. ἥτις δ᾽ ἐστὶ τῶν ἑλκῶν ὡς ἑλκῶν ἴασις ἐν τῷ πρὸ τούτου λόγῳ διώρισται. ταῦτα | γοῦν τὰ ἕλκη καὶ κακοήθη καὶ πεπαλαιωμένα καὶ χρονίζοντα καλοῦσιν, ἀδιαφόρως χρώμενοι τοῖς ὀνόμασιν ἐπ᾽ αὐτῶν. καὶ δὴ καὶ πρὸς τὸ διαγνῶναι τὴν διάθεσιν, ὅτι κακοήθης, ἅμα τοῖς ἄλλοις γνωρίσμασι καὶ τὸ χρονίζειν αὐτὰ πάντων τῶν δεόντων γιγνομένων ἔχει τινὰ μοῖραν. οὐ μὴν τοῦτό γε αὐτὸ χρονίζειν ἢ χρόνια καλεῖσθαί τε καὶ εἶναι, τὴν προσήκουσαν ἐνδείκνυται θεραπείαν· ἀλλ᾽ ἐκ μὲν τούτου τὸ μοχθηρῶς διακεῖσθαι τὸ ἡλκωμένον μόριον ἔνεστι συλλογίσασθαι· τούτου δ᾽ εὑρεθέντος εὐπορῆσαι τῆς θεραπείας. πῶς καὶ τίνα τρόπον; εἰ μὲν μόνα τὰ περιέχοντα μόρια τὴν ἕλκωσιν οὕτως εἴη διακείμενα, ταῦτ᾽ ἐξιασάμενον· εἰ δὲ σύμπαν τὸ σῶμα κακοχυμίας τινὸς εὑρίσκοιτο μεστόν, ἐκείνην ἐκκενώσαντα. σημεῖον μὲν οὖν τῆς κακοχυμίας τὸ χρονίζειν τὰ ἕλκη· τοῦ συμφέροντος δ᾽ ἡ εὕρεσις, οὐκ ἐκ τοῦ χρονίζειν, ἀλλ᾽ ἐκ τῆς κακοχυμίας.

ὥστ᾽ εἶναι τρία ταῦτ᾽ ἐφεξῆς ἀλλήλων, τὸ σημεῖον, τὴν διάθεσιν, τὴν θεραπείαν· σημεῖον μὲν τὸ χρονίζειν· διάθεσιν δὲ τὴν κακοχυμίαν· θεραπείαν δὲ τὴν ταύτης κένωσιν. καὶ κατὰ τοῦτο πολλάκις τοὺς παλαι-

interpretations to be practiced in those things. Now I shall explain the actual proposition alone.

5. Doctors call *kakoethical* those ulcers which, despite everything being done correctly and properly, are nevertheless not cured, and to all intents and purposes become chronic whenever someone applies to them the treatment that is solely for ulcers. What the cure is of ulcers as ulcers has been defined in the book prior to this one. Anyway, they call these ulcers *kakoethical*, long-standing and chronic, using the terms for them without distinction. And indeed, when it comes to diagnosing the condition—that it is *kakoethical*, along with the other notable features—the chronicity is one part of all the essential aspects. It is not actually this chronicity itself, or being called and being chronic, which indicates the appropriate treatment, but from this [chronicity] it is possible to infer the bad state of the ulcerated part. Once this is discovered, you will find the means of treatment. How and in what manner? If only those parts containing the ulcerated area are affected in this way, you will cure these completely. If, however, the whole body is found to be full of *kakochymia*, you evacuate that. Chronicity in ulcers is, then, a sign of *kakochymia*. The discovery of what is useful is not, however, from the chronicity but from the *kakochymia*.

276K

Therefore, there are these three things that follow each other: the sign, the condition, and the treatment. Chronicity is the sign, *kakochymia* is the condition, and the evacuation of the *kakochymia* is the treatment. In regard

419

277K οὓς | ὑπερβαίνοντας τὸ μέσον ἐπὶ τὸ τρίτον εὐθέως
ἀπὸ τοῦ πρώτου παραγίνεσθαι, ὥσπερ καὶ Ἱπποκράτης ἐποίησεν εἰπών· Καὶ ἀπὸ τῶν πεπαλαιωμένων
ἑλκῶν ξυμφέρει αἷμα ποιέειν πυκινά, ὅπως ἂν δοκέῃ
καιρὸς εἶναι· οὐ τῆς παλαιότητος δήπουθεν ἐνδειξαμένης τὴν θεραπείαν, ἀλλὰ τῆς μοχθηρίας τοῦ αἵματος. ἐπιφέρων γοῦν αὐτὸς ἐρεῖ· Κωλύει γὰρ μάλιστα
μὲν τὰ τοιαῦτα ἕλκεα ὑγιαίνεσθαι, ἔπειτα δὲ καὶ
τἆλλα σύμπαντα αἵματος σηπεδών, καὶ ὅ τι ἐξ αἵματος μεταστάσιος γεγένηται. καὶ δὴ καὶ μετ᾽ ὀλίγον
αὖθις ὑπὲρ τῶν μὴ συνιόντων εἰς οὐλὴν ἑλκῶν διεξιών,
Οὐδ᾽ ἤν, φησι, τὰ περιέχοντα τοῦ ἕλκεος μελανθῇ
αἵματος σηπεδόνι, ἢ καὶ κιρσοῦ παρέχοντος τὴν ἐπιρ-
ροήν, οὐδὲ ταῦτα ἐθέλει συνιέναι, ἢν μὴ τὰ περιέχοντα
τοῦ ἕλκεος ὑγιέα ποιήσῃς. εἶτα καὶ περὶ τῶν κιρσῶν
τῆς ἰάσεως γράφει. καὶ πρὸς τούτοις ἔτι καθάρσεως
μέμνηται τοῦ σύμπαντος σώματος ἐπί τε ἄλλοις τισὶ
τρώμασι καὶ οἷς σφακελίσαι κίνδυνος, ἕρπησί τε καὶ
πᾶσι τοῖς ἐσθιομένοισιν· οὕτω δ᾽ ὀνομάζειν εἴωθε τὰ
ἀναβιβρωσκόμενα. καὶ μὲν δὴ κἂν τοῖς ἐφεξῆς πάλιν
278K ὧδέ πώς φησιν· Ἐπὶ παντὶ | ἕλκει, ἐρυσιπέλατος ἐπι-
γενομένου, κάθαρσιν ποιέεσθαι παντὸς τοῦ σώματος.

κ καὶ ὅλως εἰ θελήσαις ἐπιμελῶς διελθεῖν τὸ Περὶ
τῶν ἑλκῶν βιβλίον, εὑρήσεις αὐτὸν ἀεὶ μὲν ἀπὸ τῶν
διαθέσεων τὴν ἔνδειξιν λαμβάνοντα· προσχρώμενον
δέ ποτε τῷ χρόνῳ πρὸς τὴν τῆς διαθέσεως διάγνωσιν.
ὅτι δ᾽ οὕτω ταῦτ᾽ ἔχει μάθοις ἂν ἐκ πρώτης μὲν ἀρχῆς

to this, the ancients often passed over the middle to come   277K
straight to the third from the first, just as Hippocrates
also did when he said: "And it is useful to make the blood
flow repeatedly from long-standing ulcers in whatever way
seems opportune."[23] It is not, of course, the chronicity
which indicates the treatment but the bad condition of the
blood. At any rate, he himself goes on to say: "For it particularly prevents such ulcers being restored to health, as also
does every other putrefaction of blood, and whatever has
arisen from a transformation of the blood."[24] And indeed,
shortly after, when he again goes over ulcers not coming
together to form a scar, he says: "If the parts surrounding
the ulcer become black due to putrefaction of blood, or
also due to a varix providing the flow, they are not able to
unite unless you make those parts healthy."[25] Then he
writes about the cure of varices. In addition to these [ob-
servations], he mentions as well purging of the whole body
for certain other wounds in which there is also a danger of
gangrene, for the herpetic ulcers, and for all those that are
"eaten away" (for this is how he is accustomed to name erosions). And furthermore, in what follows, he again speaks
thus: "For every ulcer, when erysipelas supervenes, carry   278K
out purging of the whole body."[26]

In general, if you wish to go over his book *On Wounds*
(*Ulcers*) carefully, you will find he always takes the indication from the conditions, although he sometimes makes
use of the time in regard to the diagnosis of the condition.
That this is the case, you may learn from the very begin-

23 See n. 22 above.
24 Hippocrates, *Peri helkōn*, pp. 346-47.
25 Op. cit., pp. 368–69.   26 Loc. cit.

τοῦ συγγράμματος, ἐχούσης ὧδε· Ἕλκεα ξύμπαντα οὐ
χρὴ τέγγειν πλὴν οἴνῳ· ὅτι πολλάκις ἑτέρα διάθεσις
ἐπιπλακεῖσα τῷ ἕλκει κωλύει τὴν ὡς ἕλκους προσφέρεσθαι θεραπείαν. καὶ τὴν αἰτίαν διδάσκων φησί·
Τὸ γὰρ ξηρὸν τοῦ ὑγιέος ἐγγυτέρω ἐστί, τὸ δ' ὑγρὸν
τοῦ μὴ ὑγιέος. εἶθ' ἑξῆς· Τὸ γὰρ ἕλκος ὑγρόν ἐστι· τὸ
δὲ ὑγιὲς ξηρόν ἐστι. καὶ διὰ τοῦτο καθ' ὅλον τὸ σύγ-
γραμμα τῆς θεραπείας τῶν ἑλκῶν ἁπάσης σκοπὸν
ποιησάμενος τὸ ξηραίνειν, οὕτως ἤδη τὰ κατὰ μέρος
ἐξευρίσκει, σὺν τῷ καὶ πολλάκις ἀναμιμνήσκειν ἡμᾶς
τοῦ σκοποῦ. ἔν τε γὰρ τῷ γράψαι, Τῶν δὲ ἑλκέων ὅ τι
μὲν ἂν ὀξεῖ βέλει ἢ[4] διατμηθῇ ἢ διακοπῇ, ἐνδέχεται
καὶ ἔναιμον φάρμακον τὸ κωλῦον διαπύειν καὶ ἀναξη-
ραῖνον· γίνεται γὰρ ἀπορρέοντος τοῦ αἵματος ξηρότε-
ρον. | καὶ πάλιν· Ὁκοῖα δ' ἂν καθαρθέντα καλῶς καὶ
ἐς τὸ δέον ἀεὶ ἐπὶ τὸ ξηρότερον θεραπεύεται, πλὴν εἰ
θλασθῇ. καὶ πάλιν, Ὅ τι δ' ἂν μὴ δύνηται προσθεῖναι, ἡ σὰρξ ὑγρὴ ἐοῦσα αἰτίη ἐστίν· ἐν τοῖς τοιούτοις
ἅπασιν ἀναμιμνήσκει τοῦ πρώτου σκοποῦ τῶν ἑλκῶν
τῆς ἰάσεως.

Ἕλκους γὰρ ᾗ ἕλκος ἐστὶν ἴαμα τὸ ξηραίνεσθαι
μετρίως· εἴρηται δ' ἡ ἀπόδειξις ἐν τῷ πρὸ τούτου
βιβλίῳ. τοῦ μέντοι μεθ' ἑτέρας διαθέσεως ἧς πρώτης
χρὴ ποιήσασθαι τὴν ἐπιμέλειαν, οὐκ ἔθ' ὡς ἕλκους
ἐστὶν ἡ θεραπεία μόνου, ἀλλὰ πρώτα μὲν ἐκείνης τῆς
διαθέσεως, ἐφεξῆς δὲ τοῦ ἕλκους· εἴτε γὰρ φλεγμονὴ

279K

---

4 ἢ om. videtur B, recte fort.

ning of the book, which has the following: "All ulcers should not be moistened other than with wine."[27] This is because often another condition interwoven with the ulcer prevents the application of the treatment for ulcers. And when he teaches the cause, he says: "For dryness is nearer to health, whereas moistness is nearer to not being healthy."[28] Then next [he says]: "For the ulcer is moist, while what is healthy is dry."[29] Because of this, since he made drying the objective of every treatment of ulcers throughout the whole treatise, he already reveals in this way particular instances by which he reminds us often of this objective. Thus, in this [work] he wrote: "In those wounds which are cut through or gashed by a sharp arrow, it is possible for a blood-stanching medication to prevent suppuration and drying out. For when blood flows, drying occurs." And again: "Those wounds that are purged properly and to the extent that is necessary are always treated toward the more dry unless there is bruising." And again: "If union cannot come about, the cause is the moist flesh." In all such instances he reminds us of the primary objective of the cure of ulcers.

279K

The cure of an ulcer *qua* ulcer is to dry moderately. The demonstration was set out in the book prior to this one. Of course, when the ulcer occurs with another condition which demands primary care, the treatment is no longer that of an ulcer alone, but first of that condition and next after that of the ulcer. For if there is some inflammation,

---

27 This is the opening sentence of Hippocrates' *Peri helkōn*, pp. 342-43. 28 These two statements immediately follow the opening sentence. 29 For this and the several immediately following references, see Hippocrates, *Peri helkōn*, p. 343ff.

τις, εἴτε μελανότης, εἴτ᾽ ἐκχύμωσις, εἴτ᾽ ἐρυσίπελας,
εἴτ᾽ οἴδημα περὶ τὴν ἡλκωμένην συσταίη σάρκα,
πρώτης ἐκείνης χρὴ ποιεῖσθαι τὴν θεραπείαν. ἀλλ᾽ ὅτι
γε τὸ ἕλκος ἐν τούτῳ τῷ χρόνῳ μὴ ὅτι θεραπεύεται
προσηκόντως, ἀλλὰ καὶ πολὺ μεῖζον ἑαυτοῦ γίνεται,
παντί που δῆλον· εἴτε γὰρ θλασθείη τὰ πέριξ χωρία
τοῦ ἕλκους, εἴτε φλεγμονή τις, εἴτ᾽ ὄγκος ἕτερος ἐν
αὐτοῖς συσταίη, τὴν οἰκείαν ἐκείνης τῆς διαθέσεως
ἴασιν ἐξευρήσομεν, εὖ εἰδότες ὡς οὐχ οἷόν τ᾽ ἐστὶν |
280K   ἰαθῆναι τὸ ἕλκος πρὶν ὑγιᾶναι τὸ χωρίον ἐν ᾧ
συνέστη. διὰ τοῦτ᾽ οὖν καὶ αὐτὸς ὁ Ἱπποκράτης ἀνα-
μιμνήσκων ἡμᾶς ὧν εὐθὺς ἐν ἀρχῇ τοῦ συγγράμματος ἀπεφήνατο, τά τ᾽ ἄλλα τὰ μικρῷ πρόσθεν
εἰρημένα προσέγραψε καὶ μέντοι καὶ τάδε·

> Τῶν δ᾽ ἑλκέων ὅ τι μὲν ἂν ὀξεῖ βέλει ἢ διατμηθῇ,
> ἢ διακοπῇ, ἐνδέχεται καὶ ἔναιμον φάρμακον τὸ
> κωλῦον διαπύειν καὶ ἀναξηραῖνον. εἴ τις δ᾽ ὑπὸ
> τοῦ βέλους ἐθλάσθη τε καὶ διεκόπη σάρξ, ταύ-
> την ἰατρεύειν, ὅπως διάπυος ὡς τάχιστα γένη-
> ται· ἧττόν τε γὰρ φλεγμαίνει καὶ ἀνάγκη τὰς
> σάρκας τὰς θλασθείσας καὶ κοπείσας καὶ σα-
> πείσας καὶ πῦον γεννωμένας ἐκτακῆναι, ἔπειτα
> βλαστάνειν νέας σάρκας.

δηλοῖ γὰρ ἐν τούτῳ τῷ λόγῳ σαφῶς ὡς μόνας
ἐκείνας τῶν ἐν τοῖς ἡλκωμένοις μέρεσι γινομένων
διαθέσεων οὐ χρὴ ξηραίνειν ἐφ᾽ ὧν ὅ τι τάχιστα
γεννῆσαι βουλόμεθα πῦον, εὐθὺς συνεμφαίνων ὅτι
μετὰ σήψεώς τινος γεννᾶται τὸ πῦον. ἅπαντα δὲ τὰ
σηπόμενα θερμῷ καὶ ὑγρῷ τοῦτο πάσχει. καὶ τοίνυν

blackness, ecchymosis, erysipelas or edema existing in the flesh around what is ulcerated, we must make the treatment of that primary. Anyway, it is clear to everyone that, unless the ulcer is being treated properly during this time, it becomes much larger than it was. If the areas around the ulcer are bruised, or there is some inflammation, or some other swelling exists in them, we will find the specific cure of that condition, knowing full well that it is not possible for the ulcer to be cured before the place in which it exists is made healthy. Because of this, Hippocrates himself also reminded us of those things he had stated right at the start of the book when he wrote, in addition to the other things mentioned a little earlier, as follows: 280K

> In the case of wounds that are cut through or gashed by a sharp arrow, it is possible for a blood-stanching medication to prevent suppuration and drying out. However, if some flesh is bruised and gashed by the arrow, treat this in such a way that suppuration is produced as quickly as possible because then it will be less inflamed. Of necessity, the flesh which has been bruised, beaten and putrefied, and has generated pus, dissolves away and then produces new flesh.

He clearly makes known in this work that, among the conditions occurring in the wounded or ulcerated parts, it is not necessary to dry only those in which we wish pus to be generated as quickly as possible. He directly indicates at the same time that pus is generated with some putrefaction. However, all things that putrefy suffer this due to heat and moisture. Therefore, we also apply plasters made

καὶ τὰ διὰ τῆς ὠμηλύσεως καταπλάσματα θερμαίνοντά τε καὶ ὑγραίνοντα προσφέρομεν ἐπὶ πασῶν τῶν
281K ἐκπυῆσαι δεομένων | διαθέσεων. ὠμήλυσις γὰρ δι'
ὑδρελαίου καὶ ἄρτος δι' ὑδρελαίου καὶ καταιόνησις δι'
ὕδατος θερμοῦ πολλοῦ καὶ ἡ τετραφάρμακος δύναμις,
ἅπαντά τε τὰ θερμαίνοντα καὶ ὑγραίνοντα διαπυΐσκει
τάχιστα. διὰ τοῦτο καὶ τοῖς φλεγμαίνουσι μορίοις,
ἐπειδὰν ἤδη σφύζῃ σφοδρότερον, ὡς ἀπελπισθῆναι
τὴν χωρὶς διαπυήσεως ἴασιν, ἐπ' αὐτῶν ἅπαντες οἱ
παλαιοὶ τὰ τοιαῦτα προσφέρουσι φάρμακα, πρότερον
δ' οὔ. καὶ τοῦτο καὶ αὐτὸς ὁ Ἱπποκράτης ἐναργῶς
ἡμᾶς διδάσκει κατά τε τὴν προγεγραμμένην ῥῆσιν, ἐν
ᾗ κελεύει τὰ μὲν χωρὶς τοῦ τεθλάσθαι τετρωμένα μόρια ξηραίνειν ὡς μάλιστα, τὰ δ' ἅμα θλάσει τινὶ γε-
γενημένα διαπυΐσκειν ὡς τάχιστα. καὶ μέντοι κἀπειδὰν εἴπῃ,

> Τὰ δὲ ἕλκεα ὅσα μὴ καλῶς καθαρθέντα ἐς τὸ
> δέον, ἀεὶ πρότερον ἄρξεται βλαστάνειν, ταῦτα
> ὑπερσαρκέει μάλιστα· ὁκοῖα δ' ἂν καθαρθέντα
> καλῶς καὶ ἐς τὸ δέον ἀεὶ ἐπὶ τὸ ξηρότερον
> θεραπεύεται, πλὴν εἰ θλασθῇ, ταῦτα οὐχ ὑπερ-
> σαρκέει ὡς ἐπιπολύ·

καὶ γὰρ καὶ ἐνταῦθα τὸ πλὴν εἰ θλασθῇ προσκείμενον
282K ἀναμιμνήσκει τοῦ κατὰ τὴν | προγεγραμμένην λέξιν
εἰρημένου, τοῦ χρῆναι πάντα ξηραίνεσθαι πλὴν τῶν
θλασθέντων.

---

30 Compounded from wax, resin, pitch, and fat; see *De sim-*

426

from barley meal that are both heating and moistening in all conditions requiring suppuration. For barley meal 281K made with a water-oil mixture, bread made with a water-oil mixture, irrigation with copious hot water, the "tetrapharmaceutical potency,"[30] and all those things that are heating and moistening, very quickly cause thoroughgoing suppuration. Because of this too, all the ancients applied such medications to parts that are inflamed, whenever they are already throbbing quite severely such that a cure is despaired of without suppuration, but not before this. This is something Hippocrates himself also clearly teaches us in the previously quoted statement in which he recommends that parts that have been wounded without bruising be dried to the maximum extent, while those parts [in which wounding] has occurred along with some bruising be brought to thoroughgoing suppuration as quickly as possible. Indeed, he says,

> Those wounds that are not purified properly and to the necessary extent before new growth begins always have the greatest excess of flesh, while wounds that are purified properly and to the extent that is necessary are always treated by what is more drying unless they are bruised, as they do not have an excess of flesh to any great extent.[31]

The addition here "unless they are bruised" reminds us of 282K what was said in the previously written statement—that all wounds and ulcers need to be dried except those that are bruised.

---

plicium medicamentorum temperamentis et facultatibus, Book 2, XII.328K.   [31] This is not an exact quotation; see Hippocrates, *Peri helkōn*, pp. 348–49.

οὐδὲ γὰρ ὁπότε τὰ φλεγμαίνοντα καταπλάσσεται
θερμαίνοντι καὶ ὑγραίνοντι καταπλάσματι, κατὰ πρῶτον λόγον γίνεται τοῦτο· τοῦτ᾽ ἔστιν οὐχ ὡς ἴαμα τῆς
διαθέσεως, ἀλλ᾽ ὡς παρηγορία τοῦ συμπτώματος·
ἐπεί τοι τὰ τῶν φλεγμονῶν αὐτῶν ἰάματα τῆς ξηροτέρας ἐστὶ δυνάμεως. ἄκουσον γοῦν λέγοντος τοῦ
Ἱπποκράτους, Καταπλάσματα οἰδημάτων καὶ φλε-
γμασίης τῆς ἐν τοῖς περιέχουσιν, εἰ ἑφθῇ φλόμος, καὶ
τῆς τριφύλλου τὰ φύλλα ὠμὰ καὶ τοῦ ἐπιπέτρου τὰ
φύλλα ἑφθὰ καὶ τὸ πόλιον· ἅπαντα γὰρ ταῦτα ξηραίνειν πέφυκε, καθότι κἀν τοῖς περὶ φαρμάκων ὑπομνήμασιν ἐλέγετο. καὶ ἡ σύντομος θεραπεία τῶν φλε-
γμαινόντων μορίων, διὰ τῶν τοιούτων ἐπιτελεῖται
φαρμάκων, ἃ ἤτοι τελέως ἐξιᾶται τὴν διάθεσιν· ἢ εἰ
καὶ καταλείπει τι βραχὺ διαπύϊσκον, ἑτέρου χρήζει
φαρμάκου δριμέος ἐκκενοῦν δυναμένου τὸ πῦον· ἢ
εἴπερ λεπτὸν εἴη τὸ περιέχον δέρμα καὶ θᾶττον ἀπαλ-
λάξαι τὸν κάμνοντα βουλόμεθα, τομῆς ἐστι χρεία. ἡ
283K δὲ διὰ τῆς ὠμηλύσεως ἀγωγὴ τῶν φλεγμαινόντων | ἐκ
τοῦ παρηγορικοῦ τρόπου τῆς τέχνης ἐστίν, οὐ τοῦ
θεραπευτικοῦ τε καὶ ἀγωνιστικοῦ· ἀλλὰ περὶ μὲν τῆς
τῶν τοιούτων διαφορᾶς ἐν τοῖς ἑξῆς πλέον ἐροῦμεν.

ὅτι δὲ τὰ ἕλκη πάντα ξηραίνειν ὁ Ἱπποκράτης
κελεύει καὶ ὅτι τὸν σκοπὸν εἶναι τῆς ἰάσεως ἀπεφήνατο τῆς διαθέσεως ἐνδειξαμένης, οὐ τοῦ χρόνου,
σαφῶς ἤδη μοι δεδεῖχθαι νομίζω. εἰ δέ τις ἐπὶ μᾶλλον
πεισθῆναι βούλεται, τῷ περὶ τῶν ἑλκῶν βιβλίῳ τἀν-
δρὸς ἐπιπλέον ὁμιλησάτω πάντα, γνώσεται γὰρ ἐναρ-

According to the first statement, this does not occur when those wounds that are inflamed are poulticed with a heating and moistening cataplasm. This is not applied as a cure of the condition but as a paregoric of the symptom, since surely the cures of inflammations themselves are of a more drying potency. At any rate, listen when Hippocrates says: "Cataplasms for swelling and inflammation involving the surrounding parts [are to be of] boiled mullein, the uncooked leaves of the trefoil (clover), the boiled leaves of sedum and hulwort."[32] All these are drying by nature in the manner spoken of in the treatises on medications. A shortened treatment of the inflamed parts is accomplished by such medications, which either completely get rid of the condition or, if anything suppurating remains even to a slight degree, there is need of another sharp medication which is able to clear out the pus. If, however, the surrounding skin is thin and we wish to release the patient more quickly, there is need of an incision. The carrying away of the inflammation through barley meal is from the paregoric part of the craft and not from the therapeutic or "aggressive" part. But I shall speak more about the difference between such things in what follows.

283K

I have, I think, already clearly shown that Hippocrates recommends drying of all wounds and ulcers, and that he declared the indicator of the cure to be from the indicating condition and not from the time. If, however, anyone wishes to be persuaded further, let him attend all the more to Hippocrates' book on wounds and ulcers and he will clearly know this very thing: that there is one cure of all

32 Hippocrates, *Peri helkōn* 11, pp. 352–53.

γῶς αὐτό τε τοῦτο τὸ μίαν εἶναι πάντων ἑλκῶν ἴασιν
καθόλου τὴν ὑφ᾽ ἡμῶν ἐν τῷ πρὸ τούτου λόγῳ δε-
δειγμένην, ἔτι τε πρὸς τούτῳ κἀκεῖνο μαθήσεται, τὸ
μηδεμίαν ὑπάρχειν ἔνδειξιν ἀπὸ τοῦ χρόνου μήτ᾽ ἐπὶ
τῶν ἑλκῶν μήτ᾽ ἐπὶ τῶν φλεγμονῶν μήθ᾽ ἁπλῶς ἐπ᾽
ἄλλης ἡστινοσοῦν διαθέσεως.

ἐπεὶ δὲ κατὰ τοῦτο τοῦ λόγου γεγόναμεν, ἐπιδεῖξαι
δίκαιον ὡς οὐ μόνον ὧν ἄρτι διεληλύθαμεν εὑρετὴς ὁ
Ἱπποκράτης ἐστίν, ἀλλὰ καὶ τῶν ἄλλων ἁπάντων ὅσα
χρὴ γινώσκειν τὸν μέλλοντα καλῶς ἕλκος ἰάσασθαι.
φαίνεται γὰρ οὐ μόνον τῶν ἄνευ τινὸς ἑτέρας δια-
284K θέσεως ἑλκῶν ἐξευρὼν τὴν ἴασιν, | ὡς ἐν τῷ ξηραίνειν
ἐστίν, ἀλλὰ καὶ τῶν διαθέσεων ἁπασῶν, ἑκάστης ἰδίᾳ
κατ᾽ εἶδος. ἤτοι γὰρ οὐκέτ᾽ ἐπιρρεῖ τῷ δεδεγμένῳ τὴν
ἕλκωσιν μορίῳ μοχθηρὸς χυμός, ἢ ἐπιρρεῖ· μηκέτι
μὲν οὖν ἐπιρρέοντος, αὐτὸ μόνον ἰᾶσθαι χρὴ τὸ
πεπονθός· εἰ μὲν ἤτοι πελιδνόν, ἢ μέλαν, ἢ ἐρυθρὸν
εἴη, σχάζοντάς τε καὶ τοῦ αἵματος ἀφαιροῦντας· εἶθ᾽
οὕτως παραχρῆμα μὲν ἐπιθέντας, ὡς αὐτὸς ἔλεγε,
σπόγγον ξηρότερον μᾶλλον ἢ ὑγρότερον· οὐ γὰρ
ἀγνοήσειν οἶμαί τινα τὸ ἢ μόριον ἀποφάσεως ἔχον
ἐνταῦθα δύναμιν, ὡς εἰ καὶ οὕτως εἶπε, ξηρότερον,
οὐχ ὑγρότερον· ἔπειτα δὲ τοῖς ξηραίνουσι φαρμάκοις
χρωμένους, εἶτ᾽ εἰ πάλιν δεήσειεν, αὖθις αἵματος
ἀφαιροῦντας· εἶτ᾽ αὖθις τὰ τοιαῦτα ποιοῦντας ἄχρις
ἂν ἐξυγιασθῇ τελέως· εἰ δὲ τὰ χείλη σκληρὰ καὶ
τυλώδη φαίνοιντο, περιτέμνοντας αὐτά. καὶ γὰρ δὴ
καὶ περὶ τούτων φησί· Τῶν δ᾽ ἑλκέων τὰ κυκλοτερῆ ἢν

wounds and ulcers in general, [and it is] the one I have
shown in the book prior to this one. In addition to this, he
will learn that there is no indication from the time—not in
the case of wounds and ulcers, not in the case of inflammations, and not, in short, in the case of any other condition
whatsoever.

Since I have come to this point in the discussion, it is
fitting to show that Hippocrates is not only the discoverer
of those things I went over just now, but also of all the other
things someone who intends to cure a wound or ulcer
properly must know. Not only did he quite clearly discover
the cure of wounds and ulcers not associated with some
other condition, which lies in drying, but also of all other   284K
conditions, each one individually in terms of kind. For the
bad humor either no longer flows to the part receiving the
ulceration, or it does flow. If it is no longer flowing, it is
necessary to cure only what is actually affected. If this is
livid, black or red, it is necessary to cure by scarifying
and releasing the blood, and then immediately applying a
sponge that is more dry rather than more moist, as he said.
I do not believe anyone will be ignorant about the part
which the force of negation has here, as he stated it in this
way—"drier not more moist." Thereafter, use the drying
medications, and if needed again, a further removal of
blood, and next in turn do the same things again until such
times as health is restored completely. If, however, the
margins [of the ulcer] appear hard and callous, excise
them. Indeed, he speaks further about these matters as
follows: "If ulcers that are circular are somewhat concave,

ὑπόκοιλα ᾖ, ἐν κύκλῳ περιτέμνειν χρὴ τὰ ἀφεστῶτα, ἢ
πάντα, ἢ τὰ ἡμίσεα τοῦ κύκλου, κατὰ μῆκος τοῦ
ἀνθρώπου.

γέγραφε δὲ καὶ περὶ τῶν ἅμα τοῖς ἕλκεσιν ὄγκων |
285K ἁπάντων, ὡς χρὴ θεραπεύειν ἕκαστον· ὡσαύτως δὲ καὶ
περὶ τῶν κιρσῶν· ὅταν καὶ διὰ τούτους ἕλκη δυσίατα
γίγνηται, δῆλον ὡς ἐπιρρέοντός τινος ἐξ αὐτῶν τοῖς
ἡλκωμένοις μορίοις. οὕτως δὲ κἀπειδὰν ἐξ ὅλου τοῦ
σώματος ἡ ἐπιρροὴ γίγνηται, καθαίρειν κελεύει τὸ
πᾶν ἐν οὐδενὶ τούτων ἀπὸ τοῦ χρόνου τὴν ἔνδειξιν
λαμβάνων· ἐπεί τοι καὶ γελοῖον ἀπὸ μιᾶς κοινότητος
ἐνδείξεις οὕτω πολλὰς καὶ διαφερούσας καὶ πολλάκις
ἐναντίας γίγνεσθαι. εἰ γὰρ καὶ συγχωρήσαιμεν ἔνδειξίν τινα περὶ τοῦ χρόνου λαμβάνεσθαι, τίς ποτέ
ἐστιν αὐτὴ δίκαιον εἰπεῖν, αὐτὴν ἑνὶ κεφαλαίῳ περι-
λαβόντα, καθάπερ ἐπὶ τῶν ἄλλων ἁπάντων ποιοῦμεν
οὐχ ἡμεῖς μόνον, ἀλλὰ καὶ αὐτὸς ὁ Θεσσαλός. ἐν γοῦν
ἐνδείκνυται καθόλου τὸ στεγνὸν πάθος αὐτῷ τὸ χα-
λᾶν· ὥσπερ γε καὶ τὸ ῥοῶδες ἐν ἕτερον τὸ στέλλειν.
ἀλλὰ καὶ κατ' αὐτὰ τὰ ἕλκη τὸ μὲν ῥυπαρὸν καθαί-
ρεσθαι δεῖται, τὸ δὲ κοῖλον πληροῦσθαι· καὶ τὸ μὲν
ὁμαλὲς ἐπουλοῦσθαι, τὸ δὲ ὑπερσαρκοῦν καθαιρεῖ-
σθαι, καὶ κατ' αὐτὸν ἐκεῖνον· λεξάτω τοίνυν ἡμῖν οὕτω |
286K κἀπὶ τοῦ κεχρονισμένου τι τοιοῦτον ἕτερον ἕν, ὡς ἐπ'
ἐκείνων ἑκάστου· ἀλλ' οὐκ ἔχει· καὶ γὰρ καὶ περιτέμνειν αὐτά φησι χρῆναι. καίτοι τίς ἂν ἔνδειξις αὕτη
νοῦν ἔχουσα περὶ τοῦ χρόνου γίγνοιτο; καὶ τῷ διὰ τοῦ

it is necessary to cut around in a circle those things being removed, either the whole of the circle or half, along the length of the person (i.e. vertically)."[33]

He has also written about all the swellings [that occur] together with ulcers, that we must treat each one, and in like manner also about the varices.[34] Whenever, due to these [varices], ulcers become hard to heal, it is clear that there is some flow from them to the ulcerated parts. In the same way too, whenever the flow occurs from the whole body, he recommends purging the whole [body], in no instance of these taking the indication from the time. For surely it is ludicrous that from one "community" there arise indications which are numerous, different and often conflicting. And if we were to agree to take some indication from the time, whatever that indication is, we would be right to speak of it as encompassed under one heading, just as we do in the case of all the others—and not only us but even Thessalus himself. The affection of constriction indicates one thing to him, at least in general terms, and that is relaxation. In the same way too, flux indicates one other thing, and that is repression. But also in ulcers themselves, there is need to purify the filth, fill the cavity, and cicatrize the flat [ulcer] but reduce the exuberant [flesh], according to the author himself. Therefore, let him tell us if chronicity in the case of a wound or ulcer is another one thing like those are. But he cannot. For in fact, he says you should also cut around them. And indeed, what actual indication that makes sense would arise from the time?

285K

286K

33 See Hippocrates, *Peri helkōn*, pp. 348–49.

34 Swellings are considered in *Peri helkōn*, 10 and 11, and varices in 25.

νάπυος χρῆσθαι φαρμάκῳ, καθ' οὗ τὸ κενὸν ὄνομα
φθέγγεται, τὴν μετασύγκρισιν; ἔτι τε πρὸς τούτοις,
τοῖς ἀπὸ ῥαφανίδων ἐμέτοις; καὶ τελευτῶν ἐπειδὰν
μηκέθ' εὑρίσκῃ μηδέν, ἐλλεβόρῳ· ἀλλὰ ταῦτα μέν, ὡς
ἔφην, κἂν τοῖς ἑξῆς ἐπὶ πλέον εἰρήσεται, δεικνύντων
ἡμῶν ὡς οὐδὲν ἐπ' οὐδενὸς νοσήματος ὁ χρόνος ἐνδείκνυται, σημεῖον μέντοι πολλάκις γίγνεται τῆς διαθέσεως.

6. Ἐπάνειμι δὲ πάλιν ἐπὶ τὸν Ἱπποκράτην· θαυμάζω γὰρ τῆς ἀκριβείας τὸν ἄνδρα κἂν τοῖς ἄλλοις
ἅπασιν, οὐχ ἥκιστα δὲ κἂν τῷ μὴ παραλιπεῖν εἰς
ἔνδειξιν διαφέροντα σκοπὸν οὐκ ἐφ' ἑνὸς μόνον ἢ
δυοῖν, ἀλλ' ἐπὶ πάντων ἁπλῶς τῶν νοσημάτων. ἔστι δ'
οὗτος ὁ ἀπὸ τῆς ἰσχύος τῆς διαθέσεως λαμβανόμενος·
οὐ μόνον οἱ Μεθοδικοὶ παρεῖδον, οὐδὲν γὰρ τοῦτό γε
287K   θαυμαστόν, ἀλλὰ καὶ τῶν Λογικῶν οἱ | πλεῖστοι· καὶ
καθ' ἕτερον τρόπον ἅπαντες οἱ Ἐμπειρικοί. ἐπειδὰν
γὰρ ἐπὶ τῇ πληθωρικῇ καλουμένῃ συνδρομῇ κένωσιν
ἑαυτοῖς τετηρῆσθαι λέγωσιν, ἄντικρυς ὁμολογοῦσιν,
ὡς εἰς οὐδὲν ἄλλο τῶν περὶ τὸν κάμνοντα γιγνομένων
ἀποβλέποντες, ἐπὶ τὸ κενοῦν παραγίγνονται. καὶ οὐ
τοῦτό φημι διότι καὶ αἱ καθάρσεις κενώσεις εἰσίν, οὐδ'
αὗται πρὸς τῆς πληθωρικῆς διδασκόμεναι συνδρομῆς,
ἀλλ' ὅτι καὶ τὴν φλεβοτομίαν αὐτὴν ἐνίοτε, καίτοι μὴ
παρούσης τῆς πληθωρικῆς συνδρομῆς, δίκαιόν ἐστι
παραλαμβάνειν. εἰ γὰρ ἰσχυρὸν εἴη τὸ νόσημα καὶ
ῥώμη δυνάμεως, οὐκ ἔστιν ὅστις οὐκ ἂν φλεβοτομή-
σειε τῶν ὡμιληκότων τοῖς ἔργοις τῆς τέχνης.

Does he use a medication made from mustard for that on which he bestows the empty name, *metasyncrisis*? Further, on top of this, does he use vomiting induced by radishes? And as his final step, does he use hellebore when he finds nothing [else works]? But these things, as I said, will be spoken of further in what follows when we show that the time indicates nothing in the case of any disease. It is, however, often a sign of the condition.

6. I shall return again to Hippocrates, for I am amazed at the precision of the man, not only in all other things, but also by no means least in his not neglecting to distinguish the indicator when it comes to an indication, and not just in one or two diseases, but in absolutely all diseases. He is the one who takes [the indication] from the severity of the condition—something which not only the Methodics overlooked (this at least is not surprising), but also the majority of the Rationalists, as in another way did all the Empirics. For whenever, in the so-called "plethoric syndrome," they say evacuation has been observed by them, they admit outright that they disregard all the other occurrences involving the patient and undertake evacuation. I do not say this because purgings are also evacuations, or because it is these that are taught in relation to the "plethoric syndrome," but that sometimes, with respect to phlebotomy itself, even when the plethoric syndrome is not present, it is appropriate to have recourse to this. For if the disease and the strength of capacity are both strong, there is nobody familiar with the actions of the craft who would not carry out phlebotomy.

287K

αὐτοὺς γοῦν ὁρῶμεν τοὺς Ἐμπειρικούς, ἐπειδὰν ἐκ
καταπτώσεώς τινος ἢ ἄλλης πληγῆς θλασθῇ μέρη
τινὰ τοῦ σώματος ἰσχυρῶς, ἐπὶ τὴν φλεβοτομίαν
ἐρχομένους· καίτοι μικρὸν ἔμπροσθεν ὑγίαινεν ἐκεῖνος, μηδεμίαν ἔχων πληθωρικὴν συνδρομήν. ᾧ δῆλον
ὡς οὐχ οὗτός ἐστιν ὁ σκοπὸς τῆς φλεβοτομίας, ἀλλ' ἥ
τε τοῦ νοσήματος ἰσχὺς καὶ ἡ ῥώμη τῆς δυνάμεως,
ἀφωρισμένων τοῦ λόγου τῶν παιδίων. καὶ γὰρ αὖ καὶ
288K   καθ' ἕτερον τρόπον, εἴ τις ὑγιαίνων | ἔτι καὶ μηδὲν
μηδέπω βεβλαμμένος ἐν τῇ πληθωρικῇ γένοιτο συνδρομῇ, τοῦτον οὐκ ἀνάγκη φλεβοτομεῖν· ἀλλ' ἀρκεῖ
τῷ μὲν ἀσιτία, τῷ δὲ ὀλιγοσιτία, τῷ δ' ὑπαγωγὴ
γαστρός, ἢ κάθαρσις, ἢ πλείω λουτρά· τῷ δέ τινι καὶ
γυμνάσιον ἤρκεσε μόνον ἢ τρίψις πολλή· φλεβοτομία
δ' οὐκ ἐξ ἀνάγκης, οὐδ' ὑπ' αὐτῶν τῶν Ἐμπειρικῶν
τοῖς οὕτως ἔχουσι προσάγεται. κατὰ δὲ τὸν αὐτὸν
τρόπον οὐδὲ ἡ κάθαρσις ἐπὶ μόνῳ πλήθει χυμῶν
μοχθηρῶν δεόντως παραλαμβάνεται· ἀλλ' ὥσπερ ἡ
φλεβοτομία διά τε πλῆθος αἵματος καὶ ἰσχυρὰν νόσον, οὕτω καὶ ἡ κάθαρσις διά τε πλῆθος ἑτέρου τινὸς
χυμοῦ καὶ ἰσχὺν νοσήματος.

περὶ μὲν τῆς φλεβοτομίας ἐν ἑτέρῳ τέ μοι διῄρηται
λόγῳ κἂν τοῖς ἑξῆς εἰρήσεται· περὶ δὲ τῆς καθάρσεως
ἐν τῷδε τῷ λόγῳ δίειμι· χρῄζουσι γὰρ αὐτῆς οἱ
κάμνοντες οὐχ ὡς τὸ λυποῦν περίττωμα καθαιρούσης
μόνον, ἀλλὰ καὶ ὡς ἀντισπώσης τε καὶ κενούσης· καὶ

Anyway, we see Empirics themselves, whenever certain parts of the body are bruised severely by a fall or some other blow, proceeding to phlebotomy. And indeed, this is when the person in question was healthy a little while before, and had no plethoric syndrome. It is clear from this that [the plethoric syndrome] is not the indicator for phlebotomy. Rather, it is the severity of the disease and the strength of the capacity, although this argument does not apply to children. Also, in another way, if someone is healthy and has not yet been harmed by the plethoric syndrome, it is not necessary to carry out phlebotomy on this person. In some cases, fasting, moderation of diet, purging of the stomach downward, purification, or more frequent baths are sufficient. In one particular case, exercise alone and much rubbing were enough. Phlebotomy is not necessarily introduced by the Empirics themselves to those who are like this. In the same way, neither is purification necessarily undertaken on the basis of a large amount of bad humors alone, but just as phlebotomy is undertaken due to a large amount of blood and a severe disease, so purging is undertaken because of a large amount of some other humor and the severity of the disease.

288K

I have gone over [the topic of] phlebotomy in another discussion.[35] I shall speak [more about it again] in what follows. In this discussion I shall go over purging, for patients have need of this, not only to purge the distressing superfluity, but also to draw it in the opposite direction and evac-

[35] Presumably the three treatises on the subject: XI.147–86K, XI.187–249K, and XI.250–316K. All have been translated by P. Brain (1984).

διὰ τοῦθ᾽ Ἱπποκράτης ἔν τε τοῖς ἄλλοις ἅπασι συγγράμμασι κἂν τῷ Περὶ τῶν ἑλκῶν ἐπισκοπεῖται καὶ
289K   τὴν ἰσχὺν τοῦ νοσήματος εἰς ἔνδειξιν | καθάρσεως.
Ὑποκάθαρσις γάρ, φησι, τῆς κάτω κοιλίης ξυμφέρει
τοῖς πλείστοισι τῶν ἑλκέων καὶ ἐν τρώμασιν ἐν κεφαλῇ ἐοῦσι καὶ ἐν κοιλίῃ καὶ ἐν ἄρθροισι καὶ ὅσα
σφακελίσαι κίνδυνος καὶ ὅσα ῥάπτεται καὶ τοῖς ἐσθι-
ομένοισι καὶ ἕρπησι καὶ τοῖσιν ἄλλοισι τοῖσι πε-
παλαιωμένοισι τὰ ἕλκεα καὶ ὁκοῖα δ᾽ ἂν μέλλῃ τις
ἐπιδέειν, ὑποκαθαίρειν τὴν κάτω κοιλίην. ἐν τούτῳ τῷ
λόγῳ σαφῶς ἡμᾶς ἐδίδαξεν ὅτι καὶ[5] τοῖς ἕλκεσιν
ἅπασι καὶ τοῖς τρώμασιν,[6] ὅταν ἰσχυρὰ γένηται
κάθαρσις, συμφέρει. τριχῶς γὰρ οὐ μόνον τούτων,
ἀλλὰ καὶ τῶν ἄλλων παθῶν ἁπάντων ἰσχυρῶν γιγνομένων, ἢ διὰ τὸ κύριον τοῦ πεπονθότος μέρους, ἢ διὰ
τὸ μέγεθος τῆς διαθέσεως, ἢ διὰ τὴν κακοήθειαν,
ἑκάστου τούτων ἰδίᾳ φαίνεται μεμνημένος ὁ Ἱπποκράτης, ἐπὶ μὲν τῶν ἐν τῇ κεφαλῇ καὶ κοίλια τρωμάτων τὸ κύριον ἐμφαίνων τοῦ τετρωμένου μορίου.

κοιλίαν δ᾽ ὅτι μὴ τὴν κάτω μόνην ἀκούειν νῦν χρή,
ἀλλὰ καὶ τὴν ἄνω, πρόδηλον οἶμαι παντί· διαιρουμένου γὰρ τοῦ μεταξὺ τραχήλου καὶ σκελῶν κύτους
290K   εἰς δύο μεγίστας κοιλότητας, | ἡ πρώτη μὲν ὑπὸ τοῦ

---

[5] B; καί om. K   [6] Galen uses the Ionic form of this word
several times in the following lines, perhaps unconsciously so after having just included it in the immediately preceding quotation
from Hippocrates.

uate it. Because of this, Hippocrates in all the other treatises, and even in the one *On Wounds (Ulcers)*, also considered the severity of the disease as an indication for 289K purging. "For," he says, "to purge the lower cavity[36] downward is beneficial in the majority of ulcers, and in wounds in the head, abdomen, and joints. Also purge the belly downward in those ulcers where there is a danger of gangrene, and those that are sutured, and in the erosions, herpetic ulcers, and other ulcers that have become long-standing. In the case of whatever anyone is intending to bind, purge the lower cavity downward." In this discussion, he clearly taught us that in all wounds and ulcers, whenever the purification is strong, it is beneficial, for there are three aspects, not only of these affections, but also of all other affections that are strong—the importance of the affected part, the magnitude of the condition and the *kakoethia*—and Hippocrates clearly made mention of each of these individually in the case of wounds in the head and abdomen, thus indicating the importance of the wounded part.[37]

I believe it is clear to everyone that it is not only necessary to hear now about the cavity below, but also about the cavity above. For the trunk between the neck and the legs is divided into two very large cavities; the first is enclosed 290K

36 In this context *koilia* is a body cavity, the upper one being the thorax and the lower one the abdomen; see Hippocrates, *Art.* 46, and Galen, *In Hippocratis librum de acutorum victu commentarii*, XV.896K.

37 See Hippocrates, *Peri helkōn* 5, pp. 348–49.

θώρακος, ἡ δευτέρα δ' ὑπὸ τοῦ περιτοναίου περι-
έχεται. καὶ δὴ τῶν τρωμάτων ὅ τι ἂν εἴη εἴσω τοῦ
θώρακος, ἢ εἴσω τοῦ περιτοναίου διασχῇ, κίνδυνον οὐ
σμικρὸν ἐπιφέρει, καὶ μάλισθ' ὅταν συντρώσῃ τι τῶν
ἔνδον· ἀλλὰ καὶ ὅτι ταχέως κακοήθη γίνεται πάντα τὰ
ἐν τοῖς ἄρθροις τρώματα, καὶ τοῦτο σχεδὸν ἅπαντες
ἴσασιν, ἐκ μὲν τῆς πείρας μόνης μεμαθηκότες οἱ
ταύτῃ μόνῃ προσέχοντες τὸν νοῦν, ἐκ δὲ τῆς φύσεως
αὐτῶν τῶν τετρωμένων ὀργάνων οἷς ἐσπουδάσθη
φύσεως σώματος ἐπιστήμην ἔχειν. ὅπου γὰρ τένοντες
καὶ νεῦρα καὶ ἄσαρκα καὶ ὀστώδη χωρία, κίνδυνος
ἐνταῦθα καὶ ὀδυνηθῆναι καὶ ἀγρυπνῆσαι καὶ σπασθῆ-
ναι καὶ παραφρονῆσαι. ταῦτά τε οὖν τὰ τρώματα καὶ
πρὸς τούτοις ὅσα ράπτεται, τουτέστιν ὅσα οὕτως ἐστὶ
μεγάλα ὡς ραφῆς χρῄζειν, ἢ εἰ μὴ ταύτης, ἀλλ'
ἐπιδέσεως γοῦν, ὑποκαθαίρεσθαι δεῖται. λέλεκται δ'
ἐν τῷ πρόσθεν λόγῳ διότι χρὴ τὰ μεγάλα τῶν ἑλκῶν ἢ
ραφαῖς, ἢ ἐπιδέσεσι συνάγεσθαι.

καὶ μὲν δὴ καὶ ὅσα σφακελίσαι κίνδυνος, ἐν μεγέθει δηλονότι φλεγμονῆς ἐστι. καὶ τοίνυν καὶ τὰ ἐσθι-
291K όμενα, | τουτέστι τὰ ἀναβιβρωσκόμενα, κακοήθη τε
ἅμα καὶ κακοχυμίας ἐστὶν ἔκγονα. καὶ οἱ ἕρπητες δ'
ἐπὶ χολώδει περιττώματι συνίστανται· καὶ τὰ ἄλλα
σύμπαντα τὰ παλαιούμενα κατά τινα τοιαύτην γίνεται
πρόφασιν· ὥστ' εὐλόγως ἐπὶ πάντων τούτων ὑποκαθαίρειν συμβουλεύει. καὶ μὲν δὴ καὶ προελθὼν ἔτι
τάδε φησίν· Ἐπὶ παντὶ ἕλκει ἐρυσιπέλατος ἐπιγενο-
μένου κάθαρσιν ποιέεσθαι τοῦ σώματος ἐφ' ὁπότερα

by the chest wall and the second by the peritoneum. Further, should a wound penetrate the chest wall or peritoneum, it carries no little danger, particularly when it wounds one of the [structures] within at the same time. But also, that all wounds in the joints quickly become *kakoethical* is something almost everyone knows, both those who have learned from experience alone, directing their attention solely to this, and those who have learned from the nature of the wounded organs themselves—that is, those by whom a knowledge of the nature of the body is diligently pursued. For wherever there are tendons and nerves, and fleshless and bony places, there is the danger of suffering pain, sleeplessness, spasms and delirium. These wounds and, in addition to these, those that are sutured, that is to say, those that are large enough to need suturing, or if not suturing, at least binding, require a downward purging. This is why it has been said in the earlier discussion that large wounds and ulcers need to be brought together with sutures or bindings.

Furthermore, in ulcers where there is a danger of mortification, this obviously lies in the magnitude of the inflammation. Moreover, those that are eaten away, that is to say, those that are eroded, are *kakoethical,* and at the same time, are born of *kakochymia.* The herpetic ulcers arise from a bilious superfluity, as do all the other long-standing [ulcers] from some such causes, so it is reasonable in all these cases that he (i.e. Hippocrates) recommends downward purging. Proceeding further, he says this: "In every ulcer, if erysipelas supervenes, carry out a purging of the body in whichever direction is beneficial for the ulcer, ei- 291K

ξυμφέρει τῷ ἕλκει, εἴτε ἄνω εἴτε κάτω· τούτου δ᾽ αὐτοῦ
πάλιν ἡμᾶς τὸν διορισμὸν ἐν τῷ περὶ χυμῶν ἐδίδαξεν,
ἀντισπᾶν μὲν κελεύων εἰς τἀναντία, παροχετεύειν δ᾽
εἰς τὰ πλάγια· καὶ μὲν δὴ καὶ ὡς ἐπειδὰν μάλιστα
ῥέπῃ, τότε ἀντισπαστέον· εἴρηται καὶ περὶ τούτου κατ᾽
ἐκεῖνο τὸ βιβλίον. ὥστε καὶ νῦν, εἰ μὲν ἔτι φέροιτο
σφοδρῶς τὸ ῥεῦμα, διὰ τῶν ἐναντίων ἀντισπάσομεν·
ἄνω μὲν γενομένου τοῦ ἕλκους κάτω καθαίροντες, εἰ δ᾽
ἐν τοῖς κάτω μέρεσι συσταίη, τὴν ἄνω κοιλίαν κε-
νοῦντες· ἤδη δὲ καὶ πεπαυμένου καὶ κατὰ τὸ μόριον
ἐστηριγμένου παροχετεύειν ἄμεινον· ἐγγυτέρω γὰρ ἡ
μετάληψις καὶ ἡ ὁρμὴ καὶ ἡ ὁλκὴ τᾶ καθαίροντι φαρ-
292K μάκῳ | ῥάων ἐκ τοῦ πλησίον.

ὅτι δ᾽ ὁ λόγος οὗτος ἤδη καὶ ἄλλου τινὸς ἅπτεται
τῶν τῆς τέχνης μερῶν, τοῦ περὶ τὴν τῶν χυμῶν ἴασιν,
οὐκ οἶμαί τινα λανθάνειν· ὅθεν κἂν τοῖς ἑξῆς αὐτὸν
ἀναγκαῖον ἔσται πάλιν ἐπαναλαβεῖν καὶ τελειῶσαι
σύμπαντα. νυνὶ δ᾽ ὅτι τὴν ἰσχὺν τοῦ νοσήματος, ἢν εἰ
καὶ μέγεθός τις ὀνομάζειν ἐθέλει, σκοπόν ἐστι ποιητέον ἡμῖν ἀφαιρέσεως αἵματος, ἢ καθάρσεως, καὶ ὡς
Ἱπποκράτης ἁπάντων πρῶτος ὧν ἴσμεν ἐξεῦρε τοῦτον
τὸν σκοπὸν ἐπιδεῖξαι βούλομαι. περὶ μὲν οὖν τῶν
ἄλλων νοσημάτων ἐν τοῖς ἑξῆς λόγοις ἐπιδείξω, περὶ
δὲ τῶν ἑλκῶν ἐν τῷδε. τὰ μὲν οὖν τῶν καθάρσεων ἤδη
μοι λέλεκται. τριχῶς γὰρ ἑκάστου νοσήματος ἰσχυ-
ροῦ γενομένου, διὰ τὸ κύριον τοῦ πεπονθότος μορίου,
διὰ τὸ μέγεθος τῆς διαθέσεως καὶ τρίτην τὴν κακοήθειαν αὐτοῦ, ἁπάντων τούτων ἐμνημόνευσεν Ἱπποκράτης ἐν τῷ περὶ[7] καθάρσεως λόγῳ.

442

ther upward or downward."[38] The determination of this itself, he taught us in the work on humors, directing us to draw away to the opposite [parts] or to divert to the sides. In fact, whenever it particularly inclines one way or another, you must at that time draw it away. There is discussion about this in that book. As a result, if the flux is still flowing strongly at the time, we will draw it off through the opposites. When the ulcer occurs above, we purge downward; if it exists in the parts below, we purge the upper cavity upward. If, however, the flux has already stopped flowing and has become fixed to the part, it is better to divert it because nearer transfer, movement and attraction by the purging medication is easier from that which is near.

292K

It does not, I think, escape anyone's notice that this discussion already also touches upon another of the parts of our craft—that about the cure of humors. Accordingly, it will be necessary to take this up again and bring it fully to completion. For now, we must make the strength of the disease—or magnitude, if someone wants to term it thus—our indicator for the removal of blood or purging, and I wish to show that Hippocrates was the first of all those we know to discover this indicator. I shall deal with the other diseases in the discussions that follow; I shall deal with wounds and ulcers in this one. I have already spoken of the matters pertaining to purging. For the severity of each disease hinges on three factors: the importance of the affected part, the magnitude of the condition, and third, the *kakoethicity* of it; and Hippocrates made mention of all of these in the discussion on purging.

---

[38] See Hippocrates, *Peri helkōn* 9, pp. 348–49.

---

7 B; τῆς K

τί δὴ οὖν, ἴσως φησί τις, οὐχὶ καὶ φλεβοτομεῖν
ἐνίοτε συμβουλεύει διὰ τὰς αὐτὰς προφάσεις; ἐμοὶ
γοῦν δοκεῖ καὶ τοῦτο κελεύειν, ἀλλὰ διὰ ταχέων τε καὶ
293K   μετ' ἀποδείξεως, ὡς αὐτῷ τε τούτῳ καὶ τοῖς | ἄλλοις
παλαιοῖς ἦν ἔθος. εἴσῃ δὲ πρῶτον μὲν ἀναγνοὺς τήνδε
τὴν ῥῆσιν αὐτοῦ· Ἕλκει νεοτρώτῳ παντί, πλὴν ἐν
κοιλίῃ, συμφέρει ἐκ τοῦ τρώματος αἷμα ῥυῆναι αὐτίκα
πλέον ἢ ἔλασσον· φλεγμαίνει γὰρ ἧσσον αὐτὸ τὸ
ἕλκος καὶ τὰ περιέχοντα.

μετὰ δὲ ταύτην ἐν τῷ Περὶ ἑλκῶν γεγραμμένην
ἀναμνησθεὶς ὧν ἐν τοῖς ἄλλοις ἅπασι συγγράμμασι
πολλάκις ὑπέθετο, μιμητὴν ἀξιῶν εἶναι τὸν ἰατρὸν οὐ
τῆς φύσεως μόνον, ἀλλὰ κἀκείνων ὅσα αὐτόματα
ὠφελεῖ, σαφῶς ἂν ἤδη τὴν γνώμην εἰδείης τοῦ παλαιοῦ περὶ τῆς τοῦ αἵματος ἀφαιρέσεως ἐπὶ τῶν ἰσχυρῶν
τραυμάτων· εἰ γὰρ δὴ συμφέρει μὲν αἷμα ῥυῆναι τοῖς
τοιούτοις, οὐκ ἐρρύη δέ, τὸ λεῖπον αὐτὸν χρὴ προσ-
τιθέναι· δηλοῖ δὲ τοῦτο κἀξ αὐτῶν ὧν ἐπιφέρει, συν-
άπτων γοῦν τῇ προειρημένῃ ῥήσει τήνδε φησί· Καὶ
ἀπὸ τῶν πεπαλαιωμένων ἑλκέων ξυμφέρει αἷμα ποιέειν ἀπορρέειν πυκινά, ὅκως ἂν δοκέῃ καιρὸς εἶναι,
καὶ ἀπ' αὐτῶν τῶν ἑλκέων καὶ ἀπὸ τῶν περιεχόντων τὸ
ἕλκος.

ἐπειδὴ γὰρ προειρήκει, Ἕλκει νεοτρώτῳ παντὶ ξυμ-
294K   φέρει αἷμα ῥυῆναι, γιγνώσκων | ὡς εἰ μὴ καὶ τῶν
κεχρονισμένων μνημονεύσειεν, οἰήσεταί τις ἐπὶ τῶν
προσφάτων μόνον οὕτως αὐτὸν ἀποφήνασθαι, διὰ
τοῦτο δεόντως προσέθηκε τὸ καὶ ἀπὸ τῶν πεπαλαιω-

Why, then, someone might perhaps ask, does he not sometimes recommend phlebotomy for the same reasons? Well, in fact, he does seem to me to order this, but briefly and with supporting proof, as was the custom for the man himself and for the other ancients. You will realize this first 293K if you read again this statement of his: "In every recent wound, other than in a body cavity, it is of benefit for blood to flow immediately from the wound more rather than less, for the wound itself and the surrounding parts become less inflamed."[39]

After this statement, written in his work *On Wounds (Ulcers)*, if you were to recall those things he often proposed in all the other treatises—it is a worthy aim for the doctor not only to be an imitator of Nature, but also of those things that are spontaneously beneficial—you would already have a clear idea of the knowledge of the ancient [doctor] about the removal of blood in severe wounds. Surely, if it is useful for blood to flow in such wounds but it does not flow, it behooves the doctor to add what is lacking. This is clear from those things he adds in conjunction with the previously quoted statement when he says this: "It is beneficial in long-standing wounds (ulcers) to make blood flow often in whatever way should seem to be opportune, both from the wound itself and from those parts surrounding the wound (ulcer)."[40]

He had previously said: "In every recent wound it is beneficial for blood to flow," knowing that if he were not to 294K mention wounds that have become chronic as well, someone would think him to have demonstrated this in the case of recent wounds only. Because of this, he was right to

[39] See Hippocrates, *Peri helkōn*, pp. 344–45.
[40] Loc. cit.

μένων ἑλκέων ἀφαιρεῖν τοῦ αἵματος. ἀλλ᾽ εἴπερ ἐκεῖνο
καθόλου παρ᾽ αὐτοῦ μεμαθήκαμεν, ὡς ἀρχομένων μὲν
τῶν ῥευμάτων ἀντισπᾶν προσῆκεν, ἐστηριγμένων δὲ
ἐν τῷ πεπονθότι μορίῳ τὴν κένωσιν ἢ ἀπ᾽ αὐτοῦ
ποιεῖσθαι τοῦ πεπονθότος μορίου, ἢ ὅτι μάλιστα πλη-
σιέστατα, πρόχειρον ἡμῖν καὶ νῦν συλλογίσασθαι
περὶ τῆς τοῦ αἵματος ἀφαιρέσεως, ὡς ἐν ἀρχῇ μὲν
πόρρωθεν, ἐξ ὑστέρου δ᾽ ἀπ᾽ αὐτῶν τῶν ἠλκωμένων
προσήκει ποιεῖσθαι.

καὶ μὲν δὴ καὶ τούτοις αὐτοῖς οἷς εἴρηκα προσθεὶς
ὡς τὸν πλεονάζοντα χυμὸν ἐκκενοῦν ὁ Ἱπποκράτης
συμβουλεύει, ποτὲ μὲν ἐπὶ τὴν τοῦ αἵματος ἀφαίρεσιν
ἄξεις, ὅταν τοῦτο κρατῇ, ποτὲ δ᾽ ἤτοι ξανθῆς, ἢ
μελαίνης χολῆς, ἢ φλέγματος ἀγωγὸν δώσεις φάρμακον, ἐκείνου μεμνημένος ἐν ἅπασι τούτοις, ὡς οὐκ
ἔστιν ἕλκους ἢ ἕλκος οὐδεμία τῶν τοιούτων ἰάσεων,
ἀλλ᾽ ἤτοι κακοχυμίας συμπαρούσης, ἢ πλήθους, ἢ
φλεγμονῆς, ἢ ἕρπητος, ἤ | τινος ἑτέρου τοιούτου· καὶ
μὲν δὴ καὶ ὡς ἐνίοτε τῶν συμβεβηκότων τι τοῖς
ἕλκεσιν ἔνδειξιν ἰδίαν ποιεῖται, καθάπερ καὶ τὸ μέγεθος. εἴρηται δὲ καὶ περὶ αὐτῶν ἐν τῷ πρὸ τούτου
γράμματι, τὰς διαφορὰς τῶν ἑλκῶν ἁπάσας, ὁπόσαι
τέ εἰσι καὶ ὁποῖαι καὶ τίς ἐφ᾽ ἑκάστου αὐτῶν ἔνδειξις,
ἐξηγησαμένου μου. τὸ δ᾽ ἀπὸ τῆς ἰσχύος τοῦ νοσήματος ἔνδειξιν γίγνεσθαι κενώσεως, ἐν ἐκείνῳ μὲν οὐκ
εἶπον τῷ λόγῳ, διότι τε μακροτέρας ἀποδείξεως ἐδεῖτο
καὶ τὴν τοῦ ὅλου σώματος ἐπιμέλειαν οὐ συνῆπτον ἐν
αὐτῷ τοῖς ἕλκεσιν, ἐνταῦθα δὲ διεξῆλθον ὅσον εἰς τὰ
παρόντα χρήσιμον.

also add [the recommendation] to withdraw blood from chronic wounds. But if we have learned that from him in general—that is, when fluxes are beginning it is appropriate to draw them in the opposite direction, whereas when they are fixed in the affected part, it is appropriate to make the evacuation from the affected part itself, or those parts particularly close to it—we are now ready to draw a conclusion about the removal of blood. [This is that], in the beginning, it is appropriate to make the removal from what is distant, but later from the wounded [parts] themselves.

Further, I would add to those things I have said, that Hippocrates recommends evacuation of the excess humor, and that sometimes you will do this by means of the removal of blood, whenever this predominates, and sometimes you will give a medication that draws away yellow or black bile, or phlegm, being mindful, however, of that man in all these things, in that none of these cures is of a wound (ulcer) *qua* wound (ulcer), but of the coincident *kakochymia*, or excess, or inflammation, or herpes, or some other 295K such thing. Moreover, sometimes one of those things occurring contingently in conjunction with wounds or ulcers produces a specific indication, just as the magnitude does. I spoke about these matters in the book prior to this one when I set out all the differentiae of wounds and ulcers, how many and of what sort they are, and what the indication is in each case. I did not say in that discussion that the indication for evacuation arises from the severity of the disease because it required a more lengthy demonstration, and because I did not link the care of the whole body with that of wounds and ulcers in that book. Here, however, I have covered as much as is useful for our present purpose.

GALEN

7. Ὁ γάρ τοι σύμπας λόγος ὑπὲρ τῆς τοιαύτης
ἐνδείξεως, ἣν ἀπὸ τῆς ἰσχύος φαμὲν τοῦ νοσήματος
λαμβάνεσθαι καὶ μετὰ ταῦθ᾽ ἡμᾶς ἀναμένει ῥηθῆναι,
καθάπερ καὶ ἡ ἀπὸ τῆς ἡλικίας, καὶ προσέτι καὶ ἡ ἀπὸ
τῆς τῶν χυμῶν ἰάσεως· οὕτω δὲ καὶ ἡ ἀπὸ τῶν πεπονθότων μορίων ἔνδειξις εἰς τὴν θεραπείαν γιγνομένη,
τελεώτερον ἐν τοῖς ἑξῆς ὑπομνήμασιν ἀποδοθήσεται.
νυνὶ μὲν γὰρ ὅσον ἀπὸ τῆς φύσεως αὐτῶν, τουτέστι
τῆς κράσεώς τε καὶ οὐσίας, οἷόν τ᾽ ἐστὶν | εἰς τὰς
ἰάσεις λαμβάνεσθαι λέλεκται μόνον· ἡ δ᾽ ἀπὸ τῆς
θέσεώς τε καὶ διαπλάσεως, ἔτι τε χρείας, ἀναισθησίας τε καὶ δυσαισθησίας ἔνδειξις οὐκ εἴρηται· λεγέσθω δὲ καὶ περὶ τούτων ὅσον εἰς τὴν τῶν ἑλκῶν ἴασιν
διαφέρει. τὸ μὲν οὖν αἰσθητικὸν μόριον ἀνωδύνως ὅτι
μάλιστα χρὴ πειρᾶσθαι θεραπεύειν· εἴρηται δ᾽ ἐν τοῖς
περὶ φαρμάκων ἡ τῶν ἀνωδύνων ὕλη. τὸ δὲ δυσαισθη-
τότερον ἐγχωρεῖ καὶ διὰ τῶν σφοδροτέρων, εἰ ἡ διάθεσις οὕτω κελεύει· καὶ μὲν δὴ καὶ τοῦ μὲν κυρίου μορίου
τὸν τόνον χρὴ φυλάττειν, ὡς ἐπὶ πλέον ἐν τοῖς περὶ
φλεγμονῆς λογισμοῖς ἀποδείξομεν· εἰ δέ τι μὴ τοιοῦτον, ἐγχωρεῖ τοῦτο καὶ τὴν χαλαστικὴν ἀγωγὴν τῆς
θεραπείας ἀλύπως δέχεσθαι. ταυτὶ μὲν οὖν ἐν τοῖς
ἐφεξῆς ἐπιπλέον ἐροῦμεν, ἐν δὲ τῷ παρόντι λόγῳ τὴν
ἀπὸ τῆς θέσεώς τε καὶ διαπλάσεως τῶν μορίων ἔνδειξιν ἔτι προσθέντες, οὕτω καταπαύσομεν καὶ τουτὶ
τὸ τέταρτον βιβλίον.

ἐντεῦθεν γοῦν ἐπενοήθη τὸν μὲν κατὰ τὴν κοιλίαν

7. The whole discussion is, then, about the sort of indication which I say to take from the severity of the disease. After this, what remains for me to state as well is the indication from age, and also that from the cure of the humors. In the same way, the indication pertaining to treatment that arises from the affected parts will be defined more completely in the books that follow. For now, I have said only as much as it is possible to take for the purpose of the cures from their nature, that is to say, from the *krasis* and the substance. The indication to be taken from the position 296K and conformation as well as from use, loss of sensation and disordered sensation, has not been discussed. Let me also say as much about these as pertains to the cure of wounds and ulcers. Thus, we must particularly attempt to treat painlessly a part that is sensitive. The material of those things that are anodyne was spoken of in the [writings] on medications.[41] It is also possible, however, [to treat] a part with quite disordered sensation by means of stronger medications, if the condition is such as to demand it. And we must also preserve the strength of the important part, as I will show at greater length in my deliberations on inflammation. If, on the other hand, it is not such a part, it is possible for this to receive the relaxing effect of the treatment painlessly. I shall say more about these particular things in what follows, but in the present discussion I shall just add the indication to be taken from the position and conformation of the parts, and in this way put an end to this, the fourth book.

Here, what is to be considered is that in ulceration in-

41 See, for example, *De simplicium medicamentorum secundum locos*, Book 11, XI.764K.

ἡλκωμένον πίνειν τὰ φάρμακα, τὸν δὲ κατὰ τὸν στό-
μαχον, οὐχ ἅπαξ οὐδ᾽ ἀθρόως ὅλα προσφέρειν, ἀλλὰ
297K κατὰ βραχύ τε καὶ συνεχῶς· ἐν γὰρ | τῷ παρέρχεσθαι
καὶ ψαύειν ἡ ὠφέλεια τούτοις ἐστίν, οὐκ ἐν τῷ περι-
έρχεσθαι καὶ πλησιάζειν ἐπὶ πλείονα χρόνον, ὥσπερ
τῇ γαστρί. καὶ μὲν δὴ καὶ ὡς χρὴ παχύτερα προσφέρειν ταῦτα καὶ γλίσχρα, παρὰ τῆς θέσεώς τε καὶ
διαπλάσεως ἡ ἔνδειξις. ἐπεὶ γὰρ δίοδός τις ὁ στόμα-
χός ἐστι τῶν ἐσθιομένων τε καὶ πινομένων, διὰ τοῦτο
πάντων τῶν ἔχεσθαί τε καὶ περιπήγνυσθαι καὶ προσ-
κολλᾶσθαι δυναμένων ἐστὶ χρεία φαρμάκων, οὐ τῶν
ἀποκλύζεσθαι καὶ διαρρεῖν ἑτοίμως πεφυκότων. περι-
πήγνυται μὲν οὖν παχέα, κολλᾶται δὲ τὰ γλίσχρα. τὰ
δ᾽ ἐν τοῖς παχέσιν ἐντέροις ἕλκη τῶν διὰ τῆς ἕδρας
ἐνιεμένων χρήζει μᾶλλον φαρμάκων· ἐγγυτέρω γὰρ
ταύτης ἐστί· τὰ δ᾽ ἐν τοῖς λεπτοῖς ἀμφοτέρων· πορ-
ρωτέρω γὰρ ἤδη ταῦτ᾽ ἐστὶ καὶ μέσα τῇ θέσει τῶν
ἄνωθέν τε λαμβανομένων καὶ κάτωθεν ἐνιεμένων φαρμάκων. κοινὴ δ᾽ ἐπὶ πάντων τῶν ἐντὸς μορίων ἔνδειξις
αἱρεῖσθαι μὲν τὰ συνηθέστατα τοῦ ζῴου τῇ φύσει καὶ
σιτία καὶ φάρμακα· φεύγειν δὲ καὶ ἀποτρέπεσθαι
298K τἀναντία· καίτοι γ᾽ ἐπὶ τῶν ἐκτὸς ἑλκῶν ἄλυπος | καὶ ἡ
τῶν τοιούτων χρῆσις, ἰοῦ καὶ χαλκοῦ κεκαυμένου καὶ
λεπίδος χαλκοῦ καὶ καδμείας καὶ πομφόλυγος καὶ
λιθαργύρου καὶ ψιμμυθίου. ταῦτ᾽ οὖν καὶ τὰ τοιαῦτα
μὴ προσφέρειν τοῖς ἐντός. εἴρηται δὲ περὶ τῆς φύσεως
αὐτῶν ἔν τε τῷ τρίτῳ Περὶ κράσεων κἂν τοῖς περὶ
φαρμάκων.

volving the stomach, [patients should] drink the medications, whereas in ulceration involving the esophagus, the whole dose should not be applied all at once and suddenly, but gradually and at frequent intervals because the benefit to be gained with these is in the passage and the contact, not in being surrounded and in contact over a longer time, as is the case for the stomach. Moreover, the indication from the position and conformation is that we should apply those medications that are thicker and viscid. Because the esophagus is the passageway of what is eaten and drunk, the need is for all medications that have the capacity to stick fast, that is, to congeal and adhere, and not for those of a nature to be washed off and flow through readily. The thick are those that congeal and the viscid are those that adhere. Ulcers in the large intestines have a greater need for medications inserted *per rectum* because this is nearer. Ulcers in the small intestines need both because this is further on and is in the middle in terms of position for medications taken from above (*per os*) and inserted from below (*per rectum*). The common indication for all the internal parts is to take both foods and medications that are most compatible with the nature of the organism, but on the other hand, to avoid and shun those things that are incompatible. And yet, the use of such things for ulcers that are external is harmless—[things such as] verdigris, burned copper, scales of copper, cadmia, pompholyx, litharge and white lead. But do not apply such things to internal parts. There was discussion about the nature of these in the third [book of the work] *On Krasias* (*Mixtures*) and in the books on medications.[42]

297K

298K

42 See Book 3, n. 14, for the three major works on medications. For the reference to *De temperamentis*, see I.649K.

αἱρεῖσθαι δὲ καὶ τὰς τροφάς, εἰ μὲν εἰς οὐλὴν
ἀγαγεῖν, ἢ κολλῆσαι βουλοίμεθα τὸ ἕλκος, αὐστηράς
τε καὶ γλίσχρας καὶ ἀδήκτους· εἰ δ᾽ ἀνακαθῆραι,
ῥυπτούσας μετρίως. εἰς μὲν δὴ τοῦτο πάντων ἄριστον
μέλι ἄπεφθον, τὰ δ᾽ αὐστηρὰ πόματα καὶ αἱ τοιαῦται
τροφαὶ πρόδηλοι παντί. καλῶ δ᾽ αὐστηρὸν ὅπερ καὶ
στῦφον ὀνομάζεται, τὸ στρυφνὸν δὲ ἐπιτεταμένον
ἐστὶν αὐστηρόν. ὅσα δὲ φάρμακα λαμβάνεται τοῖς
ἐντὸς ἄλυπα γέγραπται μὲν ἐν τοῖς περὶ φαρμάκων,
εἰρήσεται δὲ καὶ νῦν ὁ τύπος αὐτῶν. ὑποκυστὶς δὴ
βαλαύστιον καὶ κύτινοι ῥοιῶν καὶ κηκὶς καὶ ῥοιᾶς
λέμματα καὶ Σάμιος ἀστὴρ καὶ Λημνία σφραγὶς καὶ
χυλὸς ῥοῦ καὶ ῥόδων, ἀκακία τε καὶ τἄλλα ὅσα τοι-
αῦτα τοῖς ἐντὸς ἕλκεσιν ἀρήγοντα, βλάβην δ᾽ | οὐδε-
μίαν ἐργάζεται περὶ τὰ σπλάγχνα. διδόναι δ᾽ αὐτὰ διά
τινος τῶν στυφόντων ἀφεψήματος, ἢ μήλων κυδωνίων,
ἢ σχίνου, ἢ βάτου ἀκρεμόνων, ἢ ἀμπέλων, ἢ μύρτων,
ἢ καὶ δι᾽ οἴνου τινὸς τῶν αὐστηρῶν.

εὔδηλος δὲ ἡ τοῦ οἴνου χρῆσις, ὡς πεφυλάχθαι
χρὴ τὸν καιρὸν τῶν φλεγμονῶν· ἄλλως δ᾽ οὐδὲν κωλύει διδόναι. εὔδηλον δὲ ὡς καὶ ἀναλαμβάνειν χρὴ τὰ
τοιαῦτα φάρμακα, παρασκευάζοντα διά τε τῶν εἰρημένων ὑγρῶν καὶ προσέτι τραγακάνθης τε καὶ κόμμεως
ἐπιμιγνύντα καὶ μάλιστα τοῖς ἐν στομάχῳ προσάξειν
μέλλοντα. καὶ μὲν δὴ καὶ ἀνακογχυλίζεσθαι μὲν τοῖς
κατὰ τὴν φάρυγγα καὶ τὰ παρίσθμια προσφέροντα
κελεύειν χρή, κατέχειν δ᾽ ὕπτιον ἐπὶ πλεῖστον ἐν τῷ
στόματι χαλαροὺς ἐργασάμενον ἅπαντας τοὺς τῇδε

The nutriments of choice, if we wish to bring the wound or ulcer to scarring or conglutination, are those that are bitter, viscid and nonbiting. If, however, we wish it to be cleansed, the nutriments of choice are those that are moderately abstersive, and to this end, the best of all is unboiled honey, while bitter drinks and foods of this sort are known to everyone. I call bitter that which is also termed astringent and I call astringent that which is intensely bitter. I have written about those medications that are harmless when taken internally in the works on medications and an outline of these will now be given: hypocist, the flower of wild pomegranate, the flower of cultivated pomegranate, oak gall, the rind of pomegranate, Samian earth, Lemnian earth, the juice of pomegranates and roses, acacia arabica, and other such things that are beneficial to internal ulcers, while causing no harm to the internal organs. Give these things by way of one of the harsh concoctions: quince apples, mastich, blackberry branches, grapevines, myrtle, and by one of the bitter wines.

299K

It is clear, however, that the use of wine must be avoided at a time of inflammation; otherwise there is nothing to prevent us giving it. It is obvious, too, that these medications must be prepared by means of the previously mentioned liquids and with tragacanth and gum mixed in as well, particularly if you intend to apply them to ulcers in the esophagus. Furthermore, for ulcers of the pharynx and tonsils, we must direct that the things applied are gargled, whereas for ulcers involving the trachea, we must direct [the patient] to remain supine and hold [the medication] in the mouth for as long as possible while making all the

μῦς, ἐπὶ τῶν κατὰ τὴν ἀρτηρίαν ἑλκῶν· παραρρεῖ γὰρ
οὕτως ἀτρέμα καὶ κατὰ βραχύ, σαφῶς καὶ αἰσθητῶς
εἰς αὐτὴν τὴν ἀρτηρίαν τοῦ φαρμάκου· καὶ γὰρ κἂν τῷ
κατὰ φύσιν ἔχειν εὖ εἰδέναι χρὴ παρηθούμενον οὐκ
ὀλίγον ἐνταῦθα τοῦ πόματος. ἀλλ᾿ ὥσπερ ὑγιαινόν-
300K των, οὕτω | καὶ νοσούντων φυλάττεσθαι χρὴ τὸ πλέον,
ὡς βηχῶν κινητικόν. ἄχρι μὲν γὰρ ἂν ἐν κύκλῳ παρὰ
τὸν χιτῶνα τῆς ἀρτηρίας ὡσπερεὶ παρὰ τοῖχον ὕδωρ
φέρηται τὸ ὑγρόν, οὐκ ἐργάσεται βῆχα, τὸ δ᾿ εἰς τὰς
ὁδοὺς μέσας τοῦ πνεύματος ἐμπῖπτον εὐθὺς βηχώδεις
ἀποτελεῖ.

ταῦτά γε οὖν ἀπὸ τῆς θέσεως καὶ διαπλάσεως τῶν
μορίων εἴληπται πάντα· καὶ πρὸς τούτοις ἔτι τὸ συμ-
μιγῆναι μέλιτος ἅπασι τοῖς πρὸς τὰς ἑλκώσεις φαρμάκοις ἐπὶ τὸν κατὰ τὸν θώρακα καὶ τὸν πνεύμονα·
μόνα γὰρ εἴπερ ἐπὶ τούτων αὐστηρὰ προσφέροις φάρμακα, χρονίζει κατὰ τὴν γαστέρα. τῆς οὖν ἀναδόσεως
αὐτῶν ὄργανον ὑπάρχει τὸ μέλι καὶ ἔστιν οἷον ὄχημά
τι ταχείας φορᾶς, ἅμα τῷ μηδὲ βλάπτειν ἕλκη. κατὰ
δὲ τὸν αὐτὸν λόγον αὐτό τε τὸ μέλι καὶ τῶν οὔρησιν
κινούντων τινὰ μίγνυσθαι χρὴ τοῖς τῶν ἑλκῶν φαρμάκοις, ἐπειδὰν τὰ κατὰ τὴν κύστιν καὶ τοὺς νεφροὺς
ᾖ πεπονθότα. τὸ δὲ καὶ τὰς διαγνώσεις τῶν ἡλκωμένων μορίων ἀπό τε τῆς οὐσίας αὐτῶν καὶ τῆς
ἐνεργείας καὶ χρείας γίγνεσθαι καὶ τῆς θέσεώς τε καὶ
διαπλάσεως, εὔδηλον μὲν οἶμαι, κἂν ἐγὼ μὴ λέγω,
301K δείκνυται δ᾿ | αὐτάρκως κἂν ταῖς περὶ τῶν πεπονθότων
τόπων διαγνώσεσιν· ἀλλ᾿ οὐ πρόκειται νῦν περὶ ἐκεί-

454

muscles in it relaxed. In this way there is a gradual flow of the medication clearly and perceptibly to the trachea itself, for it is by this being in accord with nature that we must know well that a substantial amout of the beverage has filtered through. But just as with those who are healthy, so too with those who are sick, we must be more on our guard, since it provokes coughing. As long as the liquid is carried in a circle alongside the wall of the trachea, that is, if the liquid is carried against the side, it does not provoke coughing. If, however, it falls into the central channel of the inspired air, it immediately brings about coughing.

In fact, all these medications are taken on the basis of the position and conformation of the parts. In addition to these medications, there is the admixture of honey with all the medications for ulcers involving the chest wall and lung. For if you exhibit only bitter medications in these cases there is a delay in the stomach. Honey is an instrument of the distribution of these medications and is, as it were, something that facilitates their rapid passage as well as not harming ulcers. On the same basis, it is necessary to mix the honey itself and one of the diuretics with the medications for ulcers whenever the bladder and kidneys have been affected. It is, I think, clear, even if I do not say so, that the diagnoses of the ulcerated parts arise from their substance, function and use, and from their position and conformation. This is adequately demonstrated in the diagnoses concerning the affected places.[43] But I do not propose to say anything about those matters now. Therefore, I

300K

301K

---

[43] A general reference to the *De locis affectis libri III*, VIII.1-451K, translated by R. E. Siegel (1976).

νων λέγειν· αὖθις οὖν ἐπὶ τὴν θεραπευτικὴν μέθοδον
ἐπάνειμι. φημὶ δὴ καὶ ταῦτα καὶ ἄλλα πολλὰ τὴν τῶν
μορίων ἐνδείκνυσθαι θέσιν τε καὶ διάπλασιν· ἐπιδῆ-
σαι γὰρ τὸ ἡλκωμένον μόριον οὐκ ἐγχωρεῖ καλῶς
ἄνευ τοῦ λαβεῖν τὴν ἔνδειξιν ἢ ἐκ τῆς διαπλάσεως, ἢ
ἐκ τῆς θέσεως, ἢ ἐκ συναμφοτέρων· ἐνιέναι τε τὸν
αὐλίσκον τοῦ κλυστῆρος εἰς τὴν ἕδραν ἐπιτηδείως οὐχ
οἷόν τε χωρὶς τῆς τοιαύτης ἐνδείξεως. καὶ μὴν καὶ διὰ
τοῦ καυλοῦ φάρμακον ἐνιέναι πολλάκις εἰς τὴν κύστιν
ἀναγκαῖόν ἐστι. περὶ μὲν γὰρ τοῦ καθετῆρος οὐδὲν
δέομαι λέγειν, ὡς οὐχ οἷόν τέ ἐστι καλῶς χρήσασθαι
αὐτῷ χωρὶς τοῦ καὶ θέσιν ἀκριβῶς ἐπίστασθαι καὶ
διάπλασιν ὅλης τῆς κύστεως. ἐν μὲν δὴ τοῖς τοιούτοις
ἅπασι πρόδηλον ὡς οὐκ ὀλίγον εἰς τὴν ὅλην θεραπείαν ὁ πεπονθὼς τόπος συνενδείκνυται.

ἐπὶ δὲ τῶν καλουμένων ῥηγμάτων, πλέονες ἐνδείξεις φαίνονται συντρέχειν εἰς ταὐτό· καὶ γὰρ καὶ ἡ
ἀπὸ τῆς θέσεως ὀρθῶς ἂν ἐξετάζοιτο.[8] διότι γὰρ ἐν
302K βάθει τοῦ σώματός ἐστι καὶ κατακέκρυπται, | διὰ
τοῦτο καὶ τῆς θεραπείας ἐξηλλαγμένης παρὰ τὰ φαινόμενα δεήσεται. διότι δὲ σὺν ἐκχυμώσει μὲν πάντως,
ἐνίοτε δὲ καὶ σὺν περιθλάσει τῆς ἐρρωγυίας σαρκὸς
ἀποτελεῖται, διὰ τοῦτο πλείους ἰάσεις ἐνδείξεται· ἀεὶ
γὰρ τῷ πλήθει τῶν διαθέσεων οἱ πρῶτοι σκοποὶ τῶν
ἰάσεων ἰσάριθμοι. λεχθήσεται μὲν οὖν ἐπὶ πλέον ἐν
τοῖς περὶ τῆς φλεγμονῆς λογισμοῖς ὡς ἰσχυροτέρων
δεῖται φαρμάκων ἅπαντα τὰ διὰ βάθος πεπονηκότα
σώματα τῶν ἐπιπολῆς ἀρρωστούντων. δῆλον δ' οἶμαι

456

shall return again to the method of treatment. What I do say, certainly, is that the position and conformation of the parts indicate these and many other things, for it is not possible to bandage the ulcerated part properly without taking the indication from the conformation, or from the position, or from both together. And it is not possible to insert the tube of a clyster into the anus effectively apart from such an indication. Furthermore, it is often necessary to insert a medication through the urethra into the bladder. There is no need to say anything about the catheter other than it is not possible to use this properly without knowing precisely the position and conformation of the whole bladder. In all such instances it is surely quite clear that the affected place contributes in no small measure as an indication to the whole treatment.

In the case of the so-called ruptures, more indications appear to come together to the same point and, moreover, are properly evaluated on the basis of the position. For that reason, when [structures] are in the depths of the body and concealed, they will, because of this, need a completely 302K different treatment from those that are superficial. Since with ecchymosis above all, because it sometimes occurs with widespread bruising of the broken flesh, it will, for this reason, indicate more cures, for always the primary indicators of the cures are equal in number to the number of conditions. Therefore, I shall speak further [on this point], in the considerations on inflammation—that in those who are sick, all affected bodies that are deep require stronger medications than surface [structures]. And this much, I

---

8 B; ἐξετάζοντο K

καὶ νῦν ἤδη τό γε τοσοῦτον, ὡς ἐκλύεσθαι τὴν δύναμιν
ἀναγκαῖόν ἐστι τῶν ἐπιτιθεμένων ἔξωθεν φαρμάκων,
ὅταν ἐν τῷ βάθει κατακεκρυμμένον ᾖ τὸ δεόμενον τῆς
ἀπ᾽ αὐτῶν ὠφελείας· ἐπιτείνειν οὖν αὐτὴν εἰς τοσοῦτον
προσήκει εἰς ὅσον ἐκλύεσθαι μέλλει κατὰ τὴν εἰς τὸ
βάθος ὁδόν.

αἱ δ᾽ ἐκχυμώσεις ἅπασαι τὸν σκοπὸν τῆς ἰάσεως
κένωσιν ἕξουσιν· ὥστε θερμαινόντων αὐταῖς καὶ μετρίως ξηραινόντων ἐστὶ χρεία φαρμάκων. ὅσα γὰρ
ἰσχυρῶς ξηραίνει, διαφορεῖ μὲν εὐθὺς κατ᾽ ἀρχὰς
ἐπιδηλότερον τῶν ἀσθενεστέρων, ἀπολείπει δέ τι λεί-
303K ψανον τῆς διαθέσεως σκιρρῶδες καὶ δυσίατον. | εἰρή-
σεται μὲν οὖν κἀν τοῖς ἑξῆς περὶ τούτων ἀκριβέστε-
ρον, ἀλλὰ καὶ νῦν ὅσον εἰς τὰ παρόντα χρήσιμον
αὐτάρκως λέλεκται. τά τε γὰρ ὑγραίνοντα καὶ θερμαίνοντα φάρμακα καὶ ταῦτα δὴ τὰ συνήθως ἅπασιν
ὀνομαζόμενα χαλαστικὰ καὶ τούτων ὅσα βραχὺ μὲν
πρὸς τὸ ξηρότερον ἀποκεχώρηκεν, οὔπω δὲ σαφῶς
οὐδ᾽ ἐναργῶς ἐστι συντατικά, τῶν ἐκχυμωμάτων
ἁπάντων ἐστὶν ἰάματα. χρὴ δὲ δηλονότι καὶ ταῦτα
τοῖς τῷ ἐν βάθει τοῦ σώματος ῥήγμασι συνεπιτείνε-
σθαί τε τῇ δυνάμει καὶ δριμύτερα προσφέρεσθαι καὶ
τμητικώτερα καὶ τὸ σύμπαν εἰπεῖν ἐνεργέστερα τοσοῦτον εἰς ὅσον τοῦ δέρματος ἀποκεχώρηκε πρὸς τὸ
βάθος ἡ ἐκχύμωσις. ἐκ τῶν τοιούτων εἴη ἂν καὶ ἡ τῆς
σικύας χρῆσις ὠφέλιμος· ὄργανον δὲ καὶ αὕτη τοῖς
ἰατροῖς ἐξεύρηται βιαίας ὁλκῆς. ἐπειδὰν μέντοι δια-
φορηθῇ τὸ σύμπαν ἐκχύμωμα, ξηραίνειν ἤδη σφοδρό-

think, is already now clear—that of necessity there is some degree of loss of potency of medications applied externally, whenever what is hidden in the depths has the need of benefit from them. It is appropriate, then, to increase this [potency] to the extent that it is anticipated it will be released in its passage to the depths.

All the ecchymoses will have evacuation as the indicator of the cure, so that for them there is the need of heating and moderately drying medications. Those that dry strongly disperse immediately from the beginning more obviously than those that are weaker and leave behind a remnant of the condition that is scirrhous and difficult to cure. These matters will be spoken of more precisely in what follows, but for now enough to be useful has been said for our present purposes. The medications that are moistening and heating, and those that are customarily called "relaxing" by everyone, and those that incline a little toward the drier, but are not yet clearly and manifestly astringent, are cures of all the ecchymoses. Obviously we must also increase these things for the ruptures in the depths of the body and apply those that are sharper in potency and more cutting, and in summary, more active to the extent that the ecchymosis is further removed from the skin toward the depths. On the basis of such considerations, the use of the cupping glass would also be beneficial, this too being discovered by doctors to be an instrument of strong drawing [capacity]. Nevertheless, whenever the whole ecchymosis is dispersed, it is already

303K

τερον ἐγχωρεῖ τὸ ῥῆγμα καὶ συνάγειν ἐπιδέσει καὶ τὸ σύμπαν εἰπεῖν ἅπαντα πράττειν ὑπὲρ τοῦ συμφῦναι τὸ ἕλκος.

εἰ μὲν οὖν ἐν τάχει διαφορηθείη τὸ ἐκχύμωμα, προσίεται ῥᾳδίως τὴν σύμφυσιν ἡ ἐρρωγυῖα σάρξ· εἰ δ' ἐν χρόνῳ πλείονι διαφοροῖτο | ῥύπος ἀξιόλογον ὑποτρεφόμενον ἐν τῷ μεταξὺ τῶν χειλῶν ἵσταται τοῦ ἕλκους· ὥστ' οὐκέθ' οἷόν τε συμφῦναι τῷ ῥήγματι. καὶ διὰ τοῦτο πᾶν ὁτιοῦν αἴτιον ὑπομιμνήσκει ταῦτα· καὶ γὰρ ῥιγώσαντες καὶ ἀπεπτήσαντες καὶ πυρέξαντες καὶ σφοδρότερον ἐνεργήσαντες τοῖς τοιούτοις μορίοις εὐθέως ἀλγοῦσιν· οὐ γὰρ συνέφυ τὰ χείλη τοῦ ῥήγματος, ἀλλὰ παράκειται μόνον· ὥστε μικρὰ πρόφασις ἀφίστησί τε ῥᾳδίως ἀπ' ἀλλήλων αὐτὰ καὶ τὴν μεταξὺ χώραν ἐμπίπλησιν ὑγρότητος περιττῆς. καὶ τί γὰρ ἄλλο ἢ ἐκχύμωμα γίνεται συνεχῶς αὐτοῖς ὅμοιον τῷ κατ' ἀρχάς, ἡνίκα τὸ πρότερον ἡ σὰρξ ἐρράγη, πλὴν ὅτι νῦν ἰχωρός τινος μᾶλλον λεπτοῦ, κατ' ἀρχὰς δ' αἵματος ἦν τὸ ἐκχύμωμα; διὰ τοῦτο καὶ ῥᾷον νῦν ἡ κατ' ἀρχὰς διαφορεῖται. ταῦτα μὲν οὖν εἴρηταί μοι πρός γε[9] τὸν περὶ τῶν ἑλκῶν λόγον ἀποχρήσοντα, καὶ ἤδη τέλος ἐπιτίθημι καὶ τῷδε τετάρτῳ γράμματι.

9 B; τε K

possible to dry the rupture more strongly and to bring it together with a binding, and in summary, to do all those
things pertaining to union in the wound.

Therefore, if the ecchymosis is quickly dispersed, the
ruptured flesh is readily allowed to come to union. If, however, it is dispersed over a longer period, significant filth   304K
grows up in the space between the margins of the wound
or ulcer, so that it is no longer possible for the rupture to
unite. Because of this, any cause whatsoever suggests
these things because those who are cold, dyspeptic, feverish or functioning rather vigorously immediately feel pain
in such parts insofar as the margins of the rupture do not
grow together, but only lie beside each other, so that a
slight cause easily keeps them away from each other and
fills up the space between with moist superfluity. What
else other than an ecchymosis arises regularly from these
things like this at the beginning, when first the flesh is ruptured, except that now there is more of a thin ichor,
whereas the ecchymosis was blood in the beginning? Because of this also, it disperses more easily at the beginning.
This, then, will be enough for me to say in the discussion
on wounds and ulcers, and so I now put an end to this
fourth book.